NOT TO BE
TAKEN AWAY

KT-550-311

MEDICAL CENTRE
WATFORD GENERAL HOSPITAL
VICARAGE ROAD
WATFORD WD1 8HB

US 100
REF

CAMPBELL'S UROLOGY

Editor-in-Chief

Patrick C. Walsh, MD

David Hall McConnell Professor
Director, Department of Urology
The Johns Hopkins University School of Medicine
Urologist-in-Chief
The James Buchanan Brady Urological Institute
The Johns Hopkins Medical Institutions
Baltimore, Maryland

Editors

Alan B. Retik, MD

Professor of Surgery (Urology)
Harvard Medical School
Chief, Department of Urology
Children's Hospital
Boston, Massachusetts

E. Darracott Vaughan, Jr., MD

James J. Colt Professor of Urology
Weill Medical College of Cornell University
Chairman Emeritus
Department of Urology
The New York–Presbyterian Hospital
New York, New York

Alan J. Wein, MD

Professor and Chair, Division of Urology
University of Pennsylvania School of Medicine
Chief of Urology
University of Pennsylvania Health System
Philadelphia, Pennsylvania

Associate Editors

Louis R. Kavoussi, MD

Vice Chairman and Patrick C. Walsh Distinguished
    Professor of Urology
Director, Division of Endourology
The James Buchanan Brady Urological Institute
The Johns Hopkins Medical Institutions
Baltimore, Maryland

Andrew C. Novick, MD

Chairman, Urological Institute
The Cleveland Clinic Foundation
Professor of Surgery (Urology)
Ohio State University School of Medicine
Cleveland, Ohio

Alan W. Partin, MD, PhD

Bernard L. Schwartz Distinguished Professor of Urologic
    Oncology
The James Buchanan Brady Urological Institute
The Johns Hopkins Medical Institutions
Baltimore, Maryland

Craig A. Peters, MD

Associate Professor of Surgery (Urology)
Harvard Medical School
Associate Professor of Urology
Children's Hospital
Boston, Massachusetts

CAMPBELL'S UROLOGY

Eighth Edition

SAUNDERS

An Imprint of Elsevier Science

Philadelphia London New York St. Louis Sydney Toronto

SAUNDERS

An Imprint of Elsevier Science

The Curtis Center
Independence Square West
Philadelphia, Pennsylvania 19106

Volume 1: Part no. 9997618750
Volume 2: Part no. 9997618769
Volume 3: Part no. 9997618807
Volume 4: Part no. 9997618831
Set ISBN 0–7216–9058–0

CAMPBELL'S UROLOGY

Copyright © 2002, 1998, 1992, 1986, 1978, 1970, 1963, 1954, Elsevier Science (USA)

Copyright © renewed 1982 by Evelyn S. Campbell

All rights reserved. No part of this publication may be reproduced or transmitted in any form or by any means, electronic or mechanical, including photocopy, recording, or any information storage and retrieval system, without permission in writing from the publisher.

Notice

Medicine is an ever-changing field. Standard safety precautions must be followed, but as new research and clinical experience broaden our knowledge, changes in treatment and drug therapy may become necessary or appropriate. Readers are advised to check the most current product information provided by the manufacturer of each drug to be administered to verify the recommended dose, the method and duration of administration, and the contraindications. It is the responsibility of the treating physician, relying on experience and knowledge of the patient, to determine dosages and the best treatment for each individual patient. Neither the Publisher nor the editor assumes any liability for any injury and/or damage to persons or property arising from this publication.

THE PUBLISHER

Library of Congress Cataloging-in-Publication Data

Campbell's urology / editor-in-chief, Patrick C. Walsh; editors, Alan B. Retik . . . [et al.]—8th ed.
   p. cm.
Includes bibliographical references and index.
ISBN 0–7216–9058–0 (set)
1. Urology. I. Campbell, Meredith F. (Meredith Fairfax). II. Walsh, Patrick C.
III. Retik, Alan B. (Alan Burton).

RC871 .C33 2002
616.5—dc21

2001041122

Acquisitions Editor: Stephanie S. Donley
Developmental Editor: Hazel N. Hacker
Manuscript Editors: Tina Rebane, Jennifer Ehlers
Production Managers: Peter Faber, Norman Stellander, Mary Stermel

Printed in the United States of America

Last digit is the print number: 9   8   7   6   5   4   3   2   1

CONTRIBUTORS

Mark C. Adams, MD
Associate Professor of Urology and Pediatrics, Vanderbilt
    University School of Medicine, Nashville, Tennessee
    Urinary Tract Reconstruction in Children

Harold J. Alfert, MD
Department of Urology, The Johns Hopkins University
    School of Medicine; Assistant Professor, James
    Buchanan Brady Urological Institute, The Johns Hopkins
    Hospital, Baltimore, Maryland
    Retropubic and Suprapubic Open Prostatectomy

Rodney A. Appell, MD
Professor of Urology, Baylor College of Medicine;
    F. Brantley Scott Chair, Department of Urology, St.
    Luke's Episcopal Hospital, Houston, Texas
    Injection Therapy for Urinary Incontinence

Anthony Atala, MD
Associate Professor of Surgery, Harvard Medical School;
    Director, Genitourinary Reconstruction Program,
    Associate in Surgery (Urology), Children's Hospital,
    Boston, Massachusetts
    *Vesicoureteral Reflux and Megaureter; Tissue
        Engineering Perspectives for Reconstructive Surgery*

David M. Barrett, MD
Professor of Urology, Tufts University School of Medicine,
    Boston; CEO, Chairman, Board of Governors, and
    Senior Staff Consultant, Lahey Clinic, Burlington,
    Massachusetts
    Implantation of the Artificial Genitourinary Sphincter

Bruce J. Barron, MD
Professor, University of Texas Medical School, Houston,
    Texas
    Urinary Tract Imaging—Basic Principles

John M. Barry, MD
Head, Division of Urology and Division of Abdominal
    Organ Transplantation, Oregon Health and Science
    University; Staff Surgeon, University Hospital and
    Doernbecher Children's Hospital, Portland, Oregon
    Renal Transplantation

Stuart B. Bauer, MD
Professor of Surgery (Urology), Harvard Medical School;
    Senior Associate in Urology, Children's Hospital,
    Boston, Massachusetts
    *Anomalies of the Upper Urinary Tract; Voiding
        Dysfunction in Children: Neurogenic and Non-
        Neurogenic*

Clair J. Beard, MD
Assistant Professor of Radiation Oncology, Harvard
    Medical School; Co-Chair of Genitourinary Radiation
    Oncology, Brigham and Women's Hospital, Dana Farber
    Cancer Institute, Boston, Massachusetts
    Radiation Therapy for Prostate Cancer

Mark F. Bellinger, MD
Clinical Professor of Urology, University of Pittsburgh
    School of Medicine; Attending Physician, Children's
    Hospital of Pittsburgh, Pittsburgh, Pennsylvania
    *Abnormalities of the Testes and Scrotum and Their
        Surgical Management*

Mitchell C. Benson, MD
George F. Cahill Professor of Urology, Columbia
    University College of Physicians and Surgeons; Director
    of Urologic Oncology, New York–Presbyterian
    Hospital—Columbia Campus, New York, New York
    Cutaneous Continent Urinary Diversion

Richard E. Berger, MD
Professor of Urology, University of Washington Medical
    School, Seattle, Washington
    Sexually Transmitted Diseases: The Classic Diseases

Jay T. Bishoff, MD
Assistant Clinical Professor of Surgery, University of
    Texas Health Science, San Antonio; Director,
    Endourology Section, Wilford Hall Medical Center,
    Lackland AFB, Texas
    Laparoscopic Surgery of the Kidney

Jerry G. Blaivas, MD
Clinical Professor of Urology, Weill Medical College of
   Cornell University; Attending Surgeon, New York–
   Presbyterian Hospital and Lenox Hill Hospital, New
   York, New York
   *Urinary Incontinence: Pathophysiology, Evaluation, and
   Management Overview*

Jon D. Blumenfeld, MD
Associate Professor of Medicine, Weill Medical College of
   Cornell University; Associate Attending in Medicine,
   The Rogosin Institute, New York–Presbyterian Hospital,
   New York, New York
   Renal Physiology and Pathophysiology; The Adrenals

Joseph G. Borer, MD
Instructor in Surgery (Urology), Harvard Medical School;
   Assistant in Urology, Children's Hospital, Boston,
   Massachusetts
   Hypospadias

George J. Bosl, MD
Professor of Medicine, Weill Medical College of Cornell
   University; Chair, Department of Medicine, Memorial
   Sloan-Kettering Cancer Center, New York, New York
   Surgery of Testicular Tumors

Charles B. Brendler, MD
Professor and Chairman, Section of Urology, Department
   of Surgery, University of Chicago School of Medicine,
   Chicago, Illinois
   *Examination of the Urologic Patient: History, Physical
   Examination, and Urinalysis*

Gregory A. Broderick, MD
Professor of Urology, Mayo Medical School, Mayo Clinic,
   Jacksonville, Florida
   *Evaluation and Nonsurgical Management of Erectile
   Dysfunction and Priapism*

James D. Brooks, MD
Assistant Professor of Urology, Stanford University School
   of Medicine, Stanford, California
   Anatomy of the Lower Urinary Tract and Male Genitalia

Jeffrey A. Cadeddu, MD
Assistant Professor, Department of Urology, and Director,
   Clinical Center for Minimally Invasive Urologic Cancer
   Treatment, University of Texas Southwestern Medical
   Center, Dallas, Texas
   Other Applications of Laparoscopic Surgery

Steven C. Campbell, MD, PhD
Associate Professor of Urology; Codirector of Urologic
   Oncology, Loyola University Medical Center, Maywood,
   Illinois
   Renal Tumors

Douglas A. Canning, MD
Associate Professor in Surgery (Urology), The University
   of Pennsylvania School of Medicine; Director, Pediatric
   Urology, The Children's Hospital of Philadelphia,
   Philadelphia, Pennsylvania
   Evaluation of the Pediatric Urologic Patient

Michael A. Carducci, MD
Associate Professor of Oncology and Urology, Johns
   Hopkins University School of Medicine; Head, Drug
   Development Program—Oncology Center, Johns
   Hopkins Hospital, Baltimore, Maryland
   Chemotherapy for Hormone-Resistant Prostate Cancer

Lesley K. Carr, MD, FRCSC
Lecturer, Division of Urology, University of Toronto
   Medical School; Director of Women's Pelvic Health
   Centre, Sunnybrook and Women's College Health
   Sciences Centre, Toronto, Ontario, Canada
   *Vaginal Reconstructive Surgery for Sphincteric
   Incontinence and Prolapse*

Michael C. Carr, MD, PhD
Assistant Professor of Urology, Department of Surgery,
   University of Pennsylvania School of Medicine;
   Attending Surgeon, Pediatric Urology, Children's
   Hospital of Philadelphia, Philadelphia, Pennsylvania
   *Anomalies and Surgery of the Ureteropelvic Junction in
   Children*

Peter R. Carroll, MD
Professor and Chair, Department of Urology, University of
   California–San Francisco, San Francisco, California
   Cryotherapy for Prostate Cancer

H. Ballentine Carter, MD
Professor of Urology and Oncology, Johns Hopkins
   University School of Medicine, Baltimore, Maryland
   *Basic Instrumentation and Cytoscopy; Diagnosis and
   Staging of Prostate Cancer*

Michael B. Chancellor, MD
Professor of Urology; Director, Neuro-urology and Female
   Urology, University of Pittsburgh School of Medicine,
   Pittsburgh, Pennsylvania
   *Physiology and Pharmacology of the Bladder and
   Urethra*

Robert Chevalier, MD
Benjamin Armistead Shepherd Professor and Chair,
   Department of Pediatrics, University of Virginia;
   Attending Pediatrician, Children's Medical Center,
   University of Virginia Health System, Charlottesville,
   Virginia
   Renal Function in the Fetus, Neonate, and Child

Ralph V. Clayman, MD
Professor and Chairman, Department of Urology,
   University of California–Irvine, Irvine, California
   Basis of Laparoscopic Urologic Surgery

J. Quentin Clemens, BS, MD
Assistant Professor of Urology, Northwestern University
   College of Medicine, Chicago, Illinois
   Pubovaginal Slings

John M. Corman, MD
Assistant Clinical Professor, Department of Urology,
   University of Washington; Staff Urologist, Virginia
   Mason Medical Center, Seattle, Washington
   AIDS and Related Conditions

Paul J. Cozzi, MD
University of New South Wales Department of Surgery,
   Pitney Clinical Sciences Building, St. George Hospital,
   Sydney, Australia
   Surgery of Penile and Urethral Carcinoma

Juanita Crook, MD
Associate Professor of Radiation Oncology, University of
   Toronto; Radiation Oncologist, Princess Margaret
   Hospital, Toronto, Ontario
   Radiation Therapy for Prostate Cancer

Anthony V. D'Amico, MD, PhD
Associate Professor of Radiation Oncology, Harvard
   Medical School; Chief, Genitourinary Radiation
   Oncology, Brigham and Women's Hospital, Dana Farber
   Cancer Institute, Boston, Massachusetts
   Radiation Therapy for Prostate Cancer

Jean B. deKernion, MD
Professor and Chair, Department of Urology, University of
   California–Los Angeles, Los Angeles, California
   *Epidemiology, Etiology, and Prevention of Prostate
   Cancer*

Joseph Del Pizzo, MD
Assistant Professor of Urology, Section of Laparoscopic
   and Minimally Invasive Surgery, and Director of
   Laparoscopic Surgery, Department of Urology, Weill
   Medical College of Cornell University, The New York–
   Presbyterian Hospital, New York, New York
   The Adrenals

Theodore L. DeWeese, MD, PhD
Assistant Professor of Oncology, Johns Hopkins University
   School of Medicine, Baltimore, Maryland; Radiation
   Oncologist, Johns Hopkins Hospital, Baltimore,
   Maryland
   Radiation Therapy for Prostate Cancer

David A. Diamond, MD
Associate Professor of Surgery (Urology), Harvard Medical
   School; Associate in Urology, Children's Hospital,
   Boston, Massachusetts
   Sexual Differentiation: Normal and Abnormal

Caner Z. Dinlenc, MD
Assistant Professor of Urology, Albert Einstein College of
   Medicine; Physician-in-Charge of Endourology and
   Stone Disease, Beth Israel Medical Center, New York,
   New York
   Percutaneous Approaches to the Upper Urinary Tract

Roger Dmochowski, MD, FACS
Medical Director, North Texas Center for Urinary Control,
   Fort Worth, Texas
   *Surgery for Vesicovaginal Fistula, Urethrovaginal
   Fistula, and Urethral Diverticulum*

Steven G. Docimo, MD
Professor of Urology, University of Pittsburgh School of
   Medicine; Pittsburgh's Children's Hospital, Pittsburgh,
   Pennsylvania
   Pediatric Endourology and Laparoscopy

S. Machele Donat, MD
Assistant Attending Physician in Urology, Cornell
   University Medical College; Assistant Attending
   Surgeon, Memorial Sloan-Kettering Cancer Center, New
   York Hospital–Cornell Medical Center, New York, New
   York
   Surgery of Penile and Urethral Carcinoma

James A. Eastham, MD
Associate Professor, Memorial Sloan-Kettering Cancer
   Center, New York, New York
   Radical Prostatectomy

Mario A. Eisenberger, MD
Professor of Oncology and Urology, Johns Hopkins
   University; Active Full-Time Staff Physician, Johns
   Hopkins Hospital, Baltimore, Maryland
   Chemotherapy for Hormone-Resistant Prostate Cancer

Jack S. Elder, MD
Professor of Urology and Pediatrics, Case Western Reserve
   University School of Medicine, Cleveland, Ohio;
   Director of Pediatric Urology, Rainbow Babies and
   Children's Hospital, Cleveland, Ohio
   *Abnormalities of the Genitalia in Boys and Their
   Surgical Management*

Jonathan I. Epstein, MD
Professor of Pathology, Urology, and Oncology, The Johns
   Hopkins Medical Institutions, Baltimore, Maryland
   Pathology of Prostatic Neoplasia

Andrew P. Evan, PhD
Professor of Anatomy, Department of Anatomy and Cell
   Biology, Indiana University School of Medicine,
   Indianapolis, Indiana
   Surgical Management of Urinary Lithiasis

Robert L. Fairchild, PhD
Department of Immunology, Urological Institute, Cleveland
   Clinic Foundation, Cleveland, Ohio
   Basic Principles of Immunology in Urology

Diane Felsen, PhD
Associate Research Professor of Pharmacology in Urology,
Weill Medical College of Cornell University, New York,
New York
Pathophysiology of Urinary Tract Obstruction

Amr Fergany, MD
Fellow, Urological Institute, The Cleveland Clinic
Foundation, Cleveland, Ohio
Renovascular Hypertension and Ischemic Nephropathy

James H. Finke, PhD
Department of Immunology, Urological Institute, Cleveland
Clinic Foundation, Cleveland, Ohio
Basic Principles of Immunology in Urology

John M. Fitzpatrick, MCh, FRCSI, FRCS
Professor and Chairman, Academic Department of Surgery,
Mater Misericordiae Hospital and University College,
Dublin, Ireland
*Minimally Invasive and Endoscopic Management of
Benign Prostatic Hyperplasia*

Stuart M. Flechner, MD
Section of Renal Transplantation, Urological Institute, The
Cleveland Clinic Foundation, Cleveland, Ohio
Basic Principles of Immunology in Urology

Jenny J. Franke, MD
Assistant Professor, Department of Urology, Vanderbilt
University School of Medicine, Nashville, Tennessee
Management of Upper Urinary Tract Obstruction

John P. Gearhart, MD
Professor of Pediatric Urology and Professor of Pediatrics,
Johns Hopkins University School of Medicine; Chief and
Director of Pediatric Urology, Brady Urological Institute,
Johns Hopkins Hospital, Baltimore, Maryland
Exstrophy, Epispadias, and Other Bladder Anomalies

Glenn S. Gerber, MD
Associate Professor, Department of Surgery (Urology),
University of Chicago School of Medicine, Chicago,
Illinois
*Evaluation of the Urologic Patient: History, Physical
Examination, and Urinalysis*

Robert P. Gibbons, MD
Clinical Professor of Urology, University of Washington,
Seattle, Washington; Staff Urologist Emeritus, Section of
Urology and Transplantation, Virginia Mason Medical
Center, Seattle, Washington
Radical Perineal Prostatectomy

Inderbir S. Gill, MD, MCh
Head, Section of Laparoscopic and Minimally Invasive
Surgery, Urological Institute, and Director, The
Minimally Invasive Surgery Center, The Cleveland
Clinic Foundation, Cleveland, Ohio
Basis of Laparoscopic Urologic Surgery

Kenneth I. Glassberg, MD
Professor of Urology, Director of Division of Pediatric
Urology, State University of New York, Downstate
Medical Center, Brooklyn, New York
Renal Dysgenesis and Cystic Disease of the Kidney

David A. Goldfarb, MD
Head, Section of Renal Transplantation, Urological
Institute, Cleveland Clinic Foundation, Cleveland, Ohio
*Etiology, Pathogenesis, and Management of Renal
Failure*

Stanford M. Goldman, MD
Professor of Radiology and Urology, University of Texas–
Houston Medical School; Chief, Genitourinary
Radiology, Memorial Hermann Hospital, Houston, Texas
Urinary Tract Imaging—Basic Principles

Marc Goldstein, MD
Professor of Urology and Professor of Reproductive
Medicine, Weill Medical College of Cornell University;
Surgeon-in-Chief of Male Reproductive Medicine and
Surgery and Coexecutive Director, Cornell Institute for
Reproductive Medicine, New York Weill Cornell
Medical Center, New York, New York
*Surgical Management of Male Infertility and Other
Scrotal Disorders*

Edmond T. Gonzales, Jr., MD
Professor of Urology, Scott Department of Urology, Baylor
College of Medicine; Chief, Urology Service, Texas
Children's Hospital, Houston, Texas
Posterior Urethral Valves and Other Urethral Anomalies

Richard W. Grady, MD
Assistant Professor, The University of Washington Medical
School; Assistant Chief, Pediatric Urology, Children's
Hospital and Regional Medical Center, Seattle,
Washington
*Surgical Technique for One-Stage Reconstruction of the
Exstrophy-Epispadias Complex*

Asnat Groutz, MD
Lecturer, Sackler School of Medicine, Tel Aviv University;
Urogynecology Unit, Lis Maternity Hospital, Tel Aviv
Medical Center, Tel Aviv, Israel
*Urinary Incontinence: Pathophysiology, Evaluation, and
Management Overview*

Frederick A. Gulmi, MD
Assistant Professor of Urology, State University of New
York Health Sciences Center at Brooklyn; Attending
Urologist, Brookdale University Hospital and Medical
Center, Brooklyn, New York
Pathophysiology of Urinary Tract Obstruction

Michael L. Guralnick, MD, FRCSC
Assistant Professor of Surgery (Urology), Medical College
of Wisconsin, Milwaukee, Wisconsin
*The Neurourologic Evaluation; Retropubic Suspension
Surgery for Female Incontinence*

Misop Han, MD
Chief Urology Resident, Department of Urology, The
 Johns Hopkins University School of Medicine; Chief
 Resident, James Buchanan Brady Urological Institute,
 The Johns Hopkins Hospital, Baltimore, Maryland
Retropubic and Suprapubic Open Prostatectomy

Philip M. Hanno, MD
Attending Urologist, Hospital of the University of
 Pennsylvania; Medical Director, Clinical Effectiveness
 and Quality Improvement Department, University of
 Pennsylvania Health System, Philadelphia, Pennsylvania
Interstitial Cystitis and Related Disorders

Matthew Hardy, PhD
The Population Council, Rockefeller University, New
 York, New York
Male Reproductive Physiology

Harry W. Herr, MD
Professor of Urology, Cornell University Medical College;
 Attending Surgeon, Memorial Sloan-Kettering Cancer
 Center, New York Hospital–Cornell Medical Center,
 New York, New York
Surgery of Penile and Urethral Carcinoma

Sender Herschorn, BSc, MDCM, FRCSC
Professor and Chairman, Division of Urology, University
 of Toronto; Director, Urodynamics Unit, Sunnybrook
 and Women's College Health Sciences Centre, Toronto,
 Ontario, Canada
*Vaginal Reconstructive Surgery for Sphincteric
 Incontinence and Prolapse*

Stuart S. Howards, MD
Professor of Urology, University of Virginia Medical
 School; Chief, Pediatric Urology, Children's Medical
 Center, University of Virginia Health System,
 Charlottesville, Virginia
Renal Function in the Fetus, Neonate, and Child

Mark Hurwitz, MD
Assistant Professor of Radiation Oncology, Harvard
 Medical School; Vice Chief of Genitourinary Radiation
 Oncology, Brigham and Women's Hospital, Dana Farber
 Cancer Institute, Boston, Massachusetts
Radiation Therapy for Prostate Cancer

Jonathan P. Jarow, MD
Associate Professor of Urology, Johns Hopkins University
 School of Medicine, Baltimore, Maryland
Male Infertility

Thomas W. Jarrett, MD
Associate Professor and Chief, Division of Endourology,
 Johns Hopkins University School of Medicine; Chief of
 Endourology, Johns Hopkins Hospital, Baltimore,
 Maryland
*Management of Urothelial Tumors of the Renal Pelvis
 and Ureter*

Venkata R. Jayanthi, MD
Clinical Assistant Professor, Section of Pediatric Urology,
 Children's Hospital, Division of Urology, Department of
 Surgery, The Ohio State University Medical Center;
 Director, Resident Education, Section of Pediatric
 Urology, Children's Hospital, Columbus, Ohio
*Voiding Dysfunction in Children: Neurogenic and Non-
 Neurogenic*

V. Keith Jiminez, MD
Chief Resident, Department of Urology, Emory University
 School of Medicine, Atlanta, Georgia
Surgery of Bladder Cancer

Christopher W. Johnson, MD
Resident, Department of Urology, College of Physicians
 and Surgeons of Columbia University, and New York–
 Presbyterian Hospital—Columbia Campus, New York,
 New York
*Tuberculosis and Parasitic Diseases of the Genitourinary
 System*

Warren D. Johnson, Jr., MD
B. H. Kean Professor of Tropical Medicine and Chief,
 Division of International Medicine and Infectious
 Diseases, Weill Medical College of Cornell University;
 Attending Physician, New York–Presbyterian
 Hospital—Cornell Campus, New York, New York
*Tuberculosis and Parasitic Diseases of the Genitourinary
 System*

Gerald H. Jordan, MD
Professor and Chairman, Department of Urology, Eastern
 Virginia Medical School, Norfolk, Virginia
*Surgery for Erectile Dysfunction; Surgery of the Penis
 and Urethra*

David B. Joseph, MD
Professor of Surgery, University of Alabama at
 Birmingham, Birmingham, Alabama; Chief of Pediatric
 Urology, Children's Hospital, Birmingham, Alabama
Urinary Tract Reconstruction in Children

John N. Kabalin, MD
Adjunct Assistant Professor of Surgery, Section of
 Urologic Surgery, University of Nebraska College of
 Medicine, Omaha; Regional West Medical Center,
 Scottsbluff, Nebraska
*Surgical Anatomy of the Retroperitoneum, Kidneys, and
 Ureters*

Martin Kaefer, MD
Assistant Professor, Pediatric Urology, James Whitcomb
 Riley Hospital for Children, Indianapolis, Indiana
*Surgical Management of Intersexuality, Cloacal
 Malformations, and Other Abnormalities of the
 Genitalia in Girls*

Irving Kaplan, MD
Assistant Professor of Joint Center for Radiation Oncology,
 Harvard Medical School; Radiation Oncologist, Beth
 Israel Deaconess Medical Center, Boston, Massachusetts
Radiation Therapy for Prostate Cancer

Louis R. Kavoussi, MD
Patrick C. Walsh Distinguished Professor, Johns Hopkins
University School of Medicine; Vice Chairman, The
James Buchanan Brady Urological Institute, Johns
Hopkins Medical Institutions, Baltimore, Maryland
Laparoscopic Surgery of the Kidney

Akira Kawashima, MD, PhD
Associate Professor, Department of Radiology, Mayo
Medical School; Senior Consultant, Department of
Radiology, Mayo Clinic, Rochester, Minnesota
Urinary Tract Imaging—Basic Principles

Michael A. Keating, MD
Clinical Professor of Urology, University of South Florida,
Tampa, Florida; Chairman, Department of Children's
Surgery, Arnold Palmer Hospital for Children and
Women, Orlando, Florida
Vesicoureteral Reflux and Megaureter

Kurt Kerbl, MD
Associate Professor of Urology, Alle Kassen, Kirchdorf,
Austria
Basis of Laparoscopic Urologic Surgery

Adam S. Kibel, MD
Assistant Professor of Urologic Surgery, Washington
University School of Medicine; Attending Physician,
Barnes–Jewish Hospital, St. Louis, Missouri
Molecular Genetics and Cancer Biology

Stephen A. Koff, MD
Professor of Surgery, Ohio State University Medical
Center, Columbus, Ohio; Chief, Pediatric Urology,
Children's Hospital, Columbus, Ohio
*Voiding Dysfunction in Children: Neurogenic and Non-
Neurogenic*

John N. Krieger, MD
Professor, University of Washington; Staff Urologist, Puget
Sound VA Medical Center, Seattle, Washington
AIDS and Related Conditions

Lamk M. Lamki, MD
Professor of Radiology and Chief of Nuclear Medicine,
Department of Radiology, University of Texas Medical
School at Houston, Houston, Texas
Urinary Tract Imaging—Basic Principles

Jay C. Lee, MD
University of Washington, Seattle, Washington
Sexually Transmitted Diseases: The Classic Diseases

Herbert Lepor, MD
Professor and Martin Spatz Chairman, Department of
Urology, New York University School of Medicine;
Chief of Urological Surgery, New York University
Medical Center, New York, New York
*Evaluation and Nonsurgical Management of Benign
Prostatic Hyperplasia*

Ronald W. Lewis, MD
Witherington Chair in Urology, Professor of Surgery, Chief
of Urology, Medical College of Georgia, Augusta,
Georgia
Surgery for Erectile Dysfunction

Evangelos N. Liatsikos, MD
Instructor of Urology, University of Patras Medical School,
University Hospital, Rio-Patras, Greece
Percutaneous Approaches to the Upper Urinary Tract

David A. Lifshitz, MD
Lecturer, Sackler School of Medicine, Tel Aviv University,
Tel Aviv; Head, Endourology Service, Rabin Medical
Center, Petach Tikva, Israel
Surgical Management of Urinary Lithiasis

James E. Lingeman, MD
Clinical Professor, Department of Urology, Indiana
University School of Medicine; Director of Research,
Methodist Hospital Institute for Kidney Stone Disease,
Indianapolis, Indiana
Surgical Management of Urinary Lithiasis

Franklin C. Lowe, MD, MPH
Associate Professor of Clinical Urology, Columbia
University College of Physicians and Surgeons;
Associate Director, Urology, St. Luke's/Roosevelt
Hospital Center, New York, New York
*Tuberculosis and Parasitic Diseases of the Genitourinary
System; Evaluation and Nonsurgical Management of
Benign Prostatic Hyperplasia*

Tom F. Lue, MD
Professor and Vice Chairman, Department of Urology,
University of California, San Francisco, San Francisco,
California
*Physiology of Penile Erection and Pathophysiology of
Erectile Dysfunction and Priapism; Evaluation and
Nonsurgical Management of Erectile Dysfunction and
Priapism*

Donald F. Lynch, Jr., MD
Professor of Urology and Professor of Clinical Obstetrics
and Gynecology, Eastern Virginia School of Medicine;
Urologic Oncologist and Consultant Urologist, Sentara
Hospitals, Southside Virginia, Norfolk, Virginia, and
Virginia Beach, Virginia, and Howard and Georgianna
Jones Institute for Reproductive Medicine, Norfolk,
Virginia
Tumors of the Penis

Stanley Bruce Malkowicz, MD
Associate Professor of Urology, University of Pennsylvania
School of Medicine; Chief of Urology, Philadelphia VA
Medical Center, Philadelphia, Pennsylvania
Management of Superficial Bladder Cancer

David J. Margolis, MD, PhD
Associate Professor of Dermatology and Epidemiology,
University of Pennsylvania School of Medicine,
Philadelphia, Pennsylvania
*Cutaneous Diseases of the Male External Genitalia;
Color Atlas of Genital Dermatology*

Fray F. Marshall, MD
Professor of Urology, Emory University School of
  Medicine, Atlanta, Georgia
  Surgery of Bladder Cancer

Jack W. McAninch, MS, MD
Professor of Urology, University of California–San
  Francisco; Chief of Urology, San Francisco General
  Hospital, San Francisco, California
  Genitourinary Trauma

John D. McConnell, MD
Professor of Urology and Executive Vice President for
  Administration, The University of Texas Southwestern
  Medical Center, Dallas, Texas
  *Epidemiology, Etiology, and Pathophysiology of Benign
  Prostatic Hyperplasia*

W. Scott McDougal, MD
Walter S. Kerr, Jr., Professor of Urology, Harvard Medical
  School; Chief of Urology, Massachusetts General
  Hospital, Boston, Massachusetts
  Use of Intestinal Segments and Urinary Diversion

Elspeth M. McDougall, MD
Professor of Urologic Surgery, Vanderbilt University
  Medical Center, Nashville, Tennessee
  Percutaneous Approaches to the Upper Urinary Tract

Edward J. McGuire, MD
Professor of Urology, The University of Michigan, Ann
  Arbor, Michigan
  Pubovaginal Slings

James McKiernan, MD
Assistant Professor, Columbia University College of
  Physicians and Surgeons; Assistant Attending Physician,
  New York–Presbyterian Hospital, New York, New York
  Surgery of Testicular Tumors

Winston K. Mebust, MD
Emeritus Chair and Professor, Department of Urology,
  Kansas University Medical Center, Kansas City, Kansas
  *Minimally Invasive and Endoscopic Management of
  Benign Prostatic Hyperplasia*

Mani Menon, MD
Professor of Urology, Case Western Reserve University,
  Cleveland, Ohio; The Raj and Padma Vattikuti
  Distinguished Chair/Director, Vattikuti Urology Institute,
  Henry Ford Health System, Detroit, Michigan
  *Urinary Lithiasis: Etiology, Diagnosis, and Medical
  Management*

Anoop M. Meraney, MD
Fellow, Laparoscopic and Minimally Invasive Surgery,
  Cleveland Clinic Foundation Urological Institute,
  Cleveland, Ohio
  Basis of Laparoscopic Urologic Surgery

Edward M. Messing, MD
Chairman, Department of Urology, University of
  Rochester, Rochester, New York
  Urothelial Tumors of the Urinary Tract

Michael E. Mitchell, MD
Professor, The University of Washington Medical School;
  Chief, Division of Pediatric Urology, Children's Hospital
  and Regional Medical Center, Seattle, Washington
  *Surgical Technique for One-Stage Reconstruction of the
  Exstrophy-Epispadias Complex*

Joseph V. Nally, Jr., MD
Staff Nephrologist and Director of Fellowship Program,
  Department of Nephrology and Hypertension, Cleveland
  Clinic Foundation, Cleveland, Ohio
  *Etiology, Pathogenesis, and Management of Renal
  Failure*

Joel B. Nelson, MD
The Frederic N. Schwentker Professor and Chairman,
  Department of Urology, University of Pittsburgh School
  of Medicine; Attending Physician, UPMC Presbyterian
  Hospital, UPMC Shadyside Hospital, Pittsburgh,
  Pennsylvania
  Molecular Genetics and Cancer Biology

J. Curtis Nickel, MD
Professor of Urology, Queen's University; Staff Urologist,
  Kingston General Hospital, Kingston, Ontario, Canada
  Prostatitis and Related Conditions

Victor W. Nitti, MD
Associate Professor and Vice Chairman, Department of
  Urology, New York University School of Medicine,
  New York, New York
  Postprostatectomy Incontinence

H. Norman Noe, MD
Chief of Pediatric Urology, University of Tennessee Health
  Science Center; Chief of Pediatric Urology, LeBonheur
  Children's Medical Center, Memphis, Tennessee
  Renal Disease in Childhood

Andrew C. Novick, MD
Professor of Surgery (Urology), Ohio State University
  School of Medicine; Chairman, Urological Institute, The
  Cleveland Clinic Foundation, Cleveland, Ohio
  *Renovascular Hypertension and Ischemic Nephropathy;
  Renal Tumors; Surgery of the Kidney*

Carl A. Olsson, MD
Professor and Chairman, Department of Urology, College
  of Physicians and Surgeons, Columbia University;
  Director of Squier Urological Clinic and Chief of
  Urology, New York–Presbyterian Hospital, Columbia
  Presbyterian Campus, New York, New York
  Cutaneous Continent Urinary Diversion

John M. Park, MD
Assistant Professor of Urology and Director of Division of
Pediatric Urology, University of Michigan Medical
School, Ann Arbor, Michigan
*Normal and Anomalous Development of the Urogenital
System*

Alan W. Partin, MD, PhD
Professor of Urology, Oncology, and Pathology,
Department of Urology, The Johns Hopkins University
School of Medicine; Bernard L. Schwartz Distinguished
Professor of Urologic Oncology, The James Buchanan
Brady Urological Institute, The Johns Hopkins Medical
Institutions, Baltimore, Maryland
*The Molecular Biology, Endocrinology, and Physiology
of the Prostate and Seminal Vesicles; Retropubic and
Suprapubic Open Prostatectomy*

Christopher K. Payne, MD
Associate Professor of Urology, Stanford University
Medical School; Director, Female Urology and Neuro-
urology, Stanford Medical Center, Stanford, California
Urinary Incontinence: Nonsurgical Management

Craig A. Peters, MD
Associate Professor of Surgery (Urology), Harvard Medical
School; Associate Professor of Urology, Children's
Hospital, Boston, Massachusetts
*Perinatal Urology; Pediatric Endourology and
Laparoscopy*

Curtis A. Pettaway, MD
Associate Professor of Urology and Urologic Oncologist,
University of Texas, MD Anderson Cancer Center,
Houston, Texas
Tumors of the Penis

Robert E. Reiter, MD
Associate Professor, Department of Urology, University of
California, Los Angeles; Codirector, Prostate Cancer
Program, Jousson Comprehensive Cancer Center, Los
Angeles, California
*Epidemiology, Etiology, and Prevention of Prostate
Cancer*

Martin I. Resnick, MD
Lester Persky Professor and Chair, Department of Urology,
Case Western Reserve University School of Medicine;
Director, Department of Urology, University Hospitals of
Cleveland, Cleveland, Ohio
*Urinary Lithiasis: Etiology, Diagnosis, and Medical
Management*

Neil M. Resnick, MD
Professor and Chief, Division of Gerontology and Geriatric
Medicine, University of Pittsburgh Medical Center
Health System, Pittsburgh, Pennsylvania
Geriatric Incontinence and Voiding Dysfunction

Alan B. Retik, MD
Professor of Surgery (Urology), Harvard Medical School;
Chief, Department of Urology, Children's Hospital,
Boston, Massachusetts
*Ectopic Ureter, Ureterocele, and Other Anomalies of the
Ureter; Hypospadias*

Jerome P. Richie, MD
Elliott C. Cutler Professor of Surgery and Chairman of
Harvard Program in Urology (Longwood Area), Harvard
Medical School; Chief of Urology, Brigham and
Women's Hospital, Boston, Massachusetts
Neoplasms of the Testis

Richard C. Rink, MD
James Whitcomb Riley Hospital for Children, Indianapolis,
Indiana
*Surgical Management of Intersexuality, Cloacal
Malformations, and Other Abnormalities of the
Genitalia in Girls*

Michael Ritchey, MD
Professor of Surgery and Pediatrics, Director, Division of
Urology, University of Texas–Houston Medical School,
Houston, Texas
Pediatric Urologic Oncology

Ronald Rodriguez, MD, PhD
Assistant Professor of Urology, Medical Oncology, Cellular
and Molecular Medicine, Johns Hopkins University
School of Medicine, The James Buchanan Brady
Urological Institute, Baltimore, Maryland
*The Molecular Biology, Endocrinology, and Physiology
of the Prostate and Seminal Vesicles*

Claus G. Roehrborn, MD
Professor and Chairman, Department of Urology, The
University of Texas Southwestern Medical Center;
Attending Chief, Zale Lipshy University Medical Center,
Section of Urology, VA Medical Center, Dallas, Texas
*Epidemiology, Etiology, and Pathophysiology of Benign
Prostatic Hyperplasia*

Shane Roy, III, MD
Professor of Pediatrics, Section of Pediatric Nephrology,
University of Tennessee Health Science Center,
Memphis, Tennessee
Renal Disease in Childhood

Arthur I. Sagalowsky, MD
Professor of Urology, Chief of Urologic Oncology,
University of Texas Southwestern Medical School,
Dallas, Texas
*Management of Urothelial Tumors of the Renal Pelvis
and Ureter*

Carl M. Sandler, MD
Professor and Chairman of Surgery (Urology), The
University of Texas Medical School–Houston; Adjunct
Professor of Radiology, Baylor College of Medicine,
Houston, Texas
Urinary Tract Imaging—Basic Principles

Jay I. Sandlow, MD
Associate Professor, Director of Andrology and Male
  Infertility, University of Iowa Department of Urology,
  Iowa City, Iowa
Surgery of the Seminal Vesicles

Richard A. Santucci, MD
Assistant Professor, Wayne State University School of
  Medicine; Chief of Urology, Detroit Receiving Hospital,
  Detroit, Michigan
Genitourinary Trauma

Peter T. Scardino, MD
Chairman, Department of Urology, Memorial Sloan-
  Kettering Cancer Center, New York, New York
Radical Prostatectomy

Anthony J. Schaeffer, MD
Herman L. Kretschmer Professor and Chairman,
  Department of Urology, Northwestern University
  Medical School, Chicago, Illinois
Infections of the Urinary Tract

Steven J. Schichman, MD
Assistant Clinical Professor of Urology, Division of
  Urology, Department of Surgery, University of
  Connecticut, Farmington, Connecticut
The Adrenals

Peter N. Schlegel, MD
Acting Chairman and Associate Professor of Urology,
  Department of Urology, Weill Medical College of
  Cornell University; Acting Urologist-in-Chief, New
  York–Presbyterian Hospital–Weill Cornell Center, New
  York, New York
Male Reproductive Physiology

Steven M. Schlossberg, MD
Professor of Urology, Eastern Virginia Medical School,
  Norfolk, Virginia
Surgery of the Penis and Urethra

Richard N. Schlussel, MD
Department of Urology, Mount Sinai School of Medicine,
  New York, New York
*Ectopic Ureter, Ureterocele, and Other Anomalies of the
  Ureter*

Francis X. Schneck, MD
Clinical Assistant Professor of Urology, University of
  Pittsburgh School of Medicine; Attending Physician,
  Children's Hospital of Pittsburgh, Pittsburgh,
  Pennsylvania
*Abnormalities of the Testes and Scrotum and Their
  Surgical Management*

Mark Schoenberg, MD
Associate Professor, The James Buchanan Brady
  Urological Institute, Director, Urologic Oncology, Johns
  Hopkins University School of Medicine, Baltimore,
  Maryland
Management of Invasive and Metastatic Bladder Cancer

Martin J. Schreiber, Jr., MD
Staff Nephrologist, Department of Nephrology and
  Hypertension, Cleveland Clinic Foundation, Cleveland,
  Ohio
*Etiology, Pathogenesis, and Management of Renal
  Failure*

Fritz H. Schröder, MD, PhD
Professor of Urology, Erasmus University, Rotterdam, The
  Netherlands
Hormonal Therapy of Prostate Cancer

Peter G. Schulam, MD, PhD
Associate Professor and Chief, Division of Endourology
  and Laparoscopy, University of California–Los Angeles
  Medical Center, Los Angeles, California
Urinary Tract Imaging—Basic Principles

Ridwan Shabsigh, MD
Associate Professor of Urology, College of Physicians and
  Surgeons of Columbia University; Director, New York
  Center for Human Sexuality, New York–Presbyterian
  Hospital, New York, New York
Female Sexual Function and Dysfunction

Joel Sheinfeld, MD
Associate Professor, Weill Medical College of Cornell
  University; Vice Chairman, Department of Urology,
  Memorial Sloan-Kettering Cancer Center, New York,
  New York
Surgery of Testicular Tumors

Katsuto Shinohara, MD
Department of Urology, University of California–San
  Francisco, San Francisco, California
Cryotherapy for Prostate Cancer

Linda M. Dairiki Shortliffe, MD
Professor and Chair of the Department of Urology,
  Stanford University School of Medicine; Chief of
  Urology, Stanford University Medical Center; Chief of
  Pediatric Urology, Lucile Salter Packard Children's
  Hospital, Stanford, California
Urinary Tract Infections in Infants and Children

Mark Sigman, BS, MD
Associate Professor of Urology, Division of Urology,
  Department of Surgery, Brown University School of
  Medicine; Staff Urologist, Rhode Island Hospital and
  VA Hospital, Providence, Rhode Island
Male Infertility

Donald G. Skinner, MD
Professor of Urology, University of Southern California,
  Norris Comprehensive Cancer Center, Los Angeles,
  California
Orthotopic Urinary Diversion

Arthur D. Smith, MD
Professor of Urology, Albert Einstein College of Medicine, New York; Chairman, Long Island Jewish Medical Centre, New Hyde Park, New York
Percutaneous Approaches to the Upper Urinary Tract

Edwin A. Smith, MD
Assistant Clinical Professor of Urology and Director of Pediatric Urology, Emory University School of Medicine; Attending Pediatric Urologist, Children's Hospital of Atlanta, Atlanta, Georgia
Prune-Belly Syndrome

John J. Smith, III, MS, MD
Assistant Clinical Professor, Tufts University School of Medicine; Clinical Instructor of Surgery, Harvard Medical School, Boston; Senior Staff Consultant, Department of Urology, Lahey Clinic, Burlington, Massachusetts
Implantation of the Artificial Genitourinary Sphincter

Joseph A. Smith, Jr., MD
Professor and Chairman, Department of Urologic Oncology, Vanderbilt University, Nashville, Tennessee
Management of Upper Urinary Tract Obstruction

R. Ernest Sosa, MD
Associate Professor of Urology, New York–Presbyterian Hospital, Weill Medical College, Cornell University, New York, New York
Ureteroscopy and Retrograde Ureteral Access; The Adrenals

Graeme S. Steele, MD
Assistant Professor, Harvard Medical School; Associate Surgeon, Brigham and Women's Hospital, Boston, Massachusetts
Neoplasms of the Testis

John P. Stein, MD
Assistant Professor of Urology, University of Southern California, Norris Comprehensive Cancer Center, Los Angeles, California
Orthotopic Urinary Diversion

Stevan B. Streem, MD
Head, Section of Stone Disease and Endourology, Urological Institute, Cleveland Clinic Foundation, Cleveland, Ohio
Management of Upper Urinary Tract Obstruction

Li-Ming Su, MD
Assistant Professor of Urology and Director of Pelvic Laparoscopy and Stone Disease, Johns Hopkins Bayview Medical Center, The Brady Urological Institute, Johns Hopkins Medical Institutions, Baltimore, Maryland
Ureteroscopy and Retrograde Ureteral Access

Martha K. Terris, MD
Assistant Professor of Urology, Stanford University Medical Center, Stanford; Chief of Urology, Palo Alto Veterans Affairs Health Care System, Section of Urology, Palo Alto, California
Ultrasonography and Biopsy of the Prostate

E. Darracott Vaughan, Jr., MD
James J. Colt Professor of Urology, Weill Medical College of Cornell University; Chairman Emeritus, Department of Urology, New York–Presbyterian Hospital, New York, New York
Renal Physiology and Pathophysiology; Pathophysiology of Urinary Tract Obstruction; The Adrenals

Patrick C. Walsh, MD
David Hall McConnell Professor and Director of Department of Urology, The Johns Hopkins University School of Medicine; Urologist-in-Chief, The James Buchanan Brady Urological Institute, The Johns Hopkins Medical Institutions, Baltimore, Maryland
Anatomic Radical Retropubic Prostatectomy

George D. Webster, MB, FRCS
Professor of Surgery (Urology), Duke University, Durham, North Carolina
The Neurourologic Evaluation; Retropubic Suspension Surgery for Female Incontinence

Alan J. Wein, MD
Professor and Chair, Division of Urology, University of Pennsylvania School of Medicine; Chief of Urology, University of Pennsylvania Health System, Philadelphia, Pennsylvania
Color Atlas of Genital Dermatology; Pathophysiology and Categorization of Voiding Dysfunction; Neuromuscular Dysfunction of the Lower Urinary Tract and Its Management

Robert M. Weiss, MD
Donald Guthrie Professor of Surgery and Chief of Section of Urology, Yale University School of Medicine, New Haven, Connecticut
Physiology and Pharmacology of the Renal Pelvis and Ureter

Richard D. Williams, MD
Professor and Head, Rubin H. Flocks Chair, University of Iowa Department of Urology, Iowa City, Iowa
Surgery of the Seminal Vesicles

Howard N. Winfield, MD
Professor of Urology and Director of Laparoscopy and Minimally Invasive Surgery, Department of Urology, University of Iowa Hospitals and Clinics, Iowa City, Iowa
Other Applications of Laparoscopic Surgery

Gilbert J. Wise, AB, MD
Professor of Urology, State University of New York Health
  Science Center at Brooklyn; Director of Urology,
  Maimonides Medical Center, Brooklyn, New York
  *Fungal and Actinomycotic Infections of the
    Genitourinary System*

John R. Woodard, MD
Clinical Professor of Urology, Emory University School of
  Medicine, Atlanta, Georgia
  Prune-Belly Syndrome

Subbarao V. Yalla, MD
Professor of Surgery (Urology), Harvard Medical School;
  Chief, Urology Division, Boston Veterans Administration
  Medical Center, Boston, Massachusetts
  Geriatric Incontinence and Voiding Dysfunction

Naoki Yoshimura, MD, PhD
Associate Professor, Departments of Urology and
  Pharmacology, University of Pittsburgh School of
  Medicine, Pittsburgh, Pennsylvania
  *Physiology and Pharmacology of the Bladder and
    Urethra*

PREFACE

Eighth Edition of Campbell's Urology

The eighth edition of *Campbell's Urology* arrives at a momentous time—the dawn of a new millennium and the 100th anniversary of the American Urological Association. Appropriately, this new edition has been expanded from three to four volumes and completely revised to provide encyclopedic coverage of our expanding field. This revision has been accomplished with the aid of four outstanding new associate editors: Louis R. Kavoussi, MD, Patrick C. Walsh Distinguished Professor of Urology, Johns Hopkins University; Andrew C. Novick, MD, Chair, Institute of Urology, Cleveland Clinic; Alan W. Partin, MD, PhD, Bernard L. Schwartz Distinguished Professor of Urologic Oncology, Johns Hopkins University; and Craig A. Peters, MD, Associate Professor of Pediatric Urology, Harvard Medical School.

The content is organized into subject-oriented topics that are multi-authored and that, in effect, function like "mini" textbooks. Because this textbook is encyclopedic in scope, bold type is used to make it easier for readers to identify important topics and summaries of differing opinions. This edition is accompanied by a CD-Rom version that includes full text and references, with a web-based search engine that allows abstracts to be read via the Internet connected to Medline. The CD-Rom also includes an imaging atlas, a pathology atlas, and video clips of some of the most important operations. As in the past, the book is accompanied by a study guide that provides a structured approach to urologic education for residents, program directors, and certified urologists who must undergo the recertification process.

This new edition has 110 chapters, including 20 that are new and 46 with new authorship. Highlights of the new chapters include a self-standing chapter, "Basic Principles of Immunology in Urology," which includes information on both transplantation and cancer immunology. The subject of urinary incontinence has been divided into separate chapters that include "Postprostatectomy Incontinence" and "Urinary Incontinence: Nonsurgical Management." In the field of sexual dysfunction, there is a separate chapter entitled "Female Sexual Function and Dysfunction."

In the pediatric section, there are five new chapters: "Anomalies and Surgery of the Ureteropelvic Junction in Children," "Surgical Technique for One-Stage Reconstruction of the Exstrophy-Epispadias Complex," "Urinary Tract Reconstruction in Children," "Pediatric Endourology and Laparoscopy," and "Tissue Engineering Perspectives for Reconstructive Surgery."

The chapters on transitional cell carcinoma have also been subdivided to provide more complete coverage of "Management of Superficial Bladder Cancer," "Management of Invasive and Metastatic Bladder Cancer," and "Management of Urothelial Tumors of the Renal Pelvis and Ureter." In the area of prostate cancer, a chapter on cryotherapy has been added.

In the surgical section, new chapters include "Ureteroscopy and Retrograde Ureteral Access," "Surgical Management of Urinary Lithiasis," "Basics of Laparoscopic Urologic Surgery," "Laparoscopic Surgery of the Kidney," "Other Applications of Laparoscopic Surgery," and "Orthotopic Urinary Diversion." These new chapters and the other chapters, half of which have new authors, provide the most up-to-date knowledge in our field.

The editors are grateful for the support of the W.B. Saunders Company and especially to Richard Zorab and Stephanie Smith Donley, the editorial managers who have facilitated our interactions. We also wish to express our thanks to developmental editor Hazel Hacker; production managers Mary Stermel, Norman Stellander, and Peter Faber; copy editors Mimi McGinnis, Tina Rebane, and Jennifer Ehlers; and the staff of the W.B. Saunders Company for their patience and help in bringing this ambitious undertaking to publication.

On a personal note, I look back with great pride and pleasure to my association with this textbook since 1974 and to the privilege of being the senior editor for the past 20 years. Over this time, I have worked with an amazingly talented group of editors and authors in an effort to make certain that urologists around the world have had the latest and most authoritative knowledge at their fingertips. I am grateful for this opportunity.

PATRICK C. WALSH, MD
For the Editors

CONTENTS

Volume 2
V

97
Ureteroscopy and Retrograde Ureteral Access 3306
Li-Ming Su, MD, and R. Ernest Sosa, MD

98
Percutaneous Approaches to the Upper Urinary Tract 3320
Elspeth M. McDougall, MD, Evangelos N. Liatsikos, MD, Caner Z. Dinlenc, MD, and Arthur D. Smith, MD

99
Surgical Management of Urinary Lithiasis 3361
James E. Lingeman, MD, David A. Lifshitz, MD, and Andrew P. Evan, PhD

XIII
UROLOGIC SURGERY 3453

100
Basis of Laparoscopic Urologic Surgery 3455
Inderbir S. Gill, MD, MCh, Kurt Kerbl, MD, Anoop M. Meraney, MD, and Ralph V. Clayman, MD

101
The Adrenals 3507
E. Darracott Vaughan, Jr., MD, Jon D. Blumenfeld, MD, Joseph Del Pizzo, MD, Steven J. Schichman, MD, and R. Ernest Sosa, MD

IX

PEDIATRIC
UROLOGY

49
NORMAL AND ANOMALOUS DEVELOPMENT OF THE UROGENITAL SYSTEM

John M. Park, MD

The study of embryology provides a useful basis for the understanding of definitive human anatomy and various congenital disease processes. During the past two decades, a torrent of molecular information and novel experimental techniques has revolutionized the field of embryology. From the urologic surgeon's perspective, however, the classical, descriptive aspects of anatomic embryology continue to serve as an important reference point from which various congenital problems are solved. The aim of this chapter is to provide a concise, well-illustrated presentation of the essential facts in urogenital system development (Fig. 49–1), clarifying the important anatomic features and supplementing them with current molecular information. Deliberate efforts have been made to separate the molecular discussion from that of the descriptive embryology, in order to keep the main story of urogenital system development clear and understandable. To help with visualization of the key events, various drawings have been added, and these illustrations have been supplemented with adequate legends to help with easy review later on. It is not possible to cover every published information pertinent to the urogenital system development, and therefore only those with significant evidence are discussed. In particular, the experimental principles, such as in vitro organ culture techniques and molecular recombinant technology, are introduced, be-cause these novel methods of studying organ development will continue to change and enhance the current practice of urology.

KIDNEY DEVELOPMENT

Development of Three Embryonic Kidneys

Mammals develop three kidneys in the course of intrauterine life. **The embryonic kidneys are, in order of their appearance, the *pronephros*, the *mesonephros*, and the *metanephros*.** The first two kidneys regress in utero, and the third becomes the permanent kidney. Embryologically speaking, all three kidneys develop from the intermediate mesoderm. As the notochord and neural tube form, the mesoderm located on either side of the midline differentiates into three subdivisions: paraxial (somite), intermediate, and lateral mesoderm (Fig. 49–2). As the embryo undergoes transverse folding, the intermediate mesoderm separates away from the paraxial mesoderm and migrates toward the intraembryonic coelom (the future peritoneum). At this time, there is also progressive craniocaudal development of the bilateral longitudinal mesodermal masses,

1737

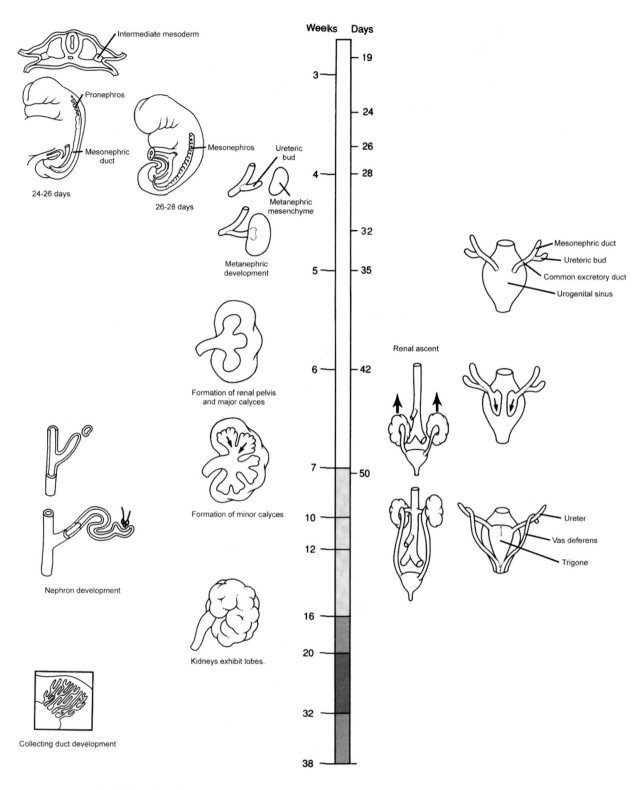

A. Kidney development
B. Ureter and bladder development

Figure 49–1. The timeline of urogenital system development. (Modified from Larsen WJ: Human Embryology. New York, Churchill Livingstone, 1997.)

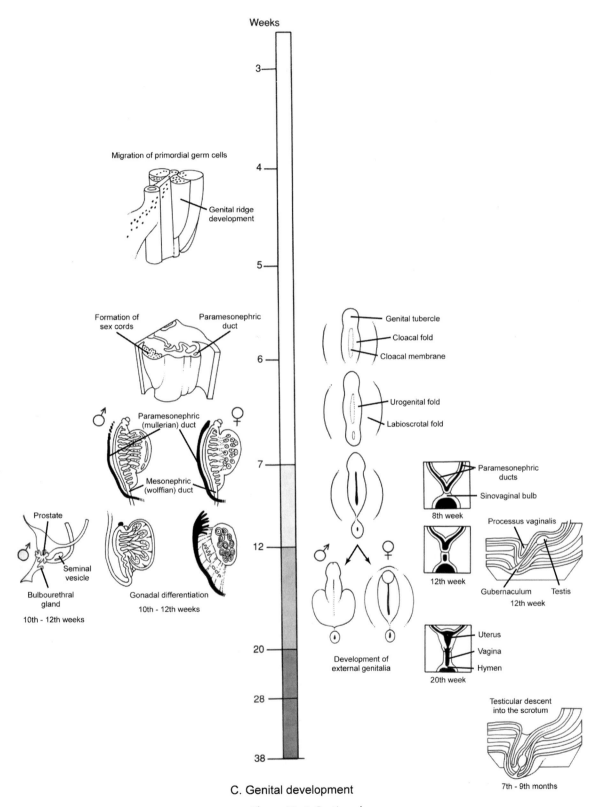

C. Genital development

Figure 49–1 *Continued*

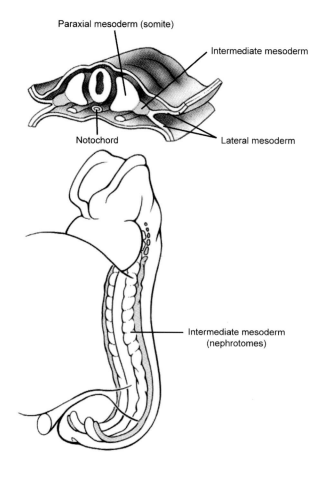

23 days

Figure 49–2. The intermediate mesoderm gives rise to paired, segmentally organized nephrotomes from the cervical to the sacral region. Cervical nephrotomes are formed early during the 4th week and are collectively referred to as the pronephros. (Modified from Larsen WJ: Human Embryology. New York, Churchill Livingstone, 1997.)

called *nephrogenic cords.* Each cord is seen bulging from the posterior wall of the coelomic cavity, producing the *urogenital ridge.*

Pronephros

The mammalian pronephros (plural, *pronephroi*) is a transitory, nonfunctional kidney, analogous to that of primitive fish. **In humans, the first evidence of pronephros is seen late in the 3rd week, and it completely degenerates by the start of the 5th week.** The pronephroi develop as five to seven paired segments in the region of the future neck and thorax (Fig. 49–3A). Development of the pronephric tubules starts at the cranial end of the nephrogenic cord and progresses caudally. As each tubule matures, it immediately begins to degenerate along with the segment of the nephric duct to which the tubules are attached.

Mesonephros

The second kidney, the mesonephros (plural, *mesonephroi*) is also transient, but in mammals it serves as an excretory organ for the embryo while the definitive kidney, the metanephros, begins its development (see Fig. 49–3B and C). There is a gradual transition from the pronephros to the mesonephros at about the 9th and 10th somite levels. Development of the *mesonephric ducts* (also called wolffian ducts) precedes the development of the mesonephric tubules. The mesonephric ducts can be seen at about the 24th day as a pair of solid longitudinal tissue condensations developing parallel to the nephrogenic cords in the dorsolateral aspect of the embryo. Their blind distal ends grow toward the primitive cloaca (see "Bladder and Ureter Development") and soon fuse with it at about the 28th day. This fused region later becomes a part of the posterior wall of the bladder. As the ducts fuse with the cloaca, they begin to form a lumen at the caudal end. This process of canalization then progresses cranially, transforming the solid condensations into the definitive mesonephric ducts.

Soon after the appearance of the mesonephric ducts during the 4th week, mesonephric vesicles begin to form. Initially, several spherical masses of cells are found along the medial side of the nephrogenic cords at the cranial end. This differentiation progresses caudally and results in the formation of 40 to 42 pairs of mesonephric tubules, but only about 30 pairs are seen at any one time, because the cranially located tubules start to degenerate beginning at about the 5th week. **By the 4th month, the human mesonephroi have almost completely disappeared, except for a few elements that persist into maturity. Certain elements of the mesonephroi are retained in the mature urogenital system as part of the reproductive tract.** In males, some of the cranially located mesonephric tubules become the efferent ductules of the testis. The epididymis and vas deferens are formed from the mesonephric (wolffian) ducts. In females, remnants of cranial and caudal mesonephric tubules form small, nonfunctional mesosalpingeal structures called the epoöphoron and the paroöphoron.

The mesonephric tubules differentiate into excretory units that resemble an abbreviated version of an adult nephron. Shortly after the cell clusters are formed, they develop lumens and take the shape of vesicles. As the vesicle elongates, each end curves in an opposite direction to form an S-shaped tubule. The lateral end forms a bud that connects with the mesonephric duct. The medial end lengthens and enlarges to form a cup-shaped sac, which eventually wraps around a knot of glomerular capillaries to form a renal corpuscle. The tuft of glomerular capillaries originating from a branch of the dorsal aorta invades the developing glomerulus, while an efferent arteriole empties into a subcardinal sinus.

Metanephros

The definitive kidney, or the metanephros (plural, *metanephroi*), forms in the sacral region as a pair of new structures, called the *ureteric buds*, sprouts from the distal portion of the mesonephric duct and comes in contact with the blastema of *metanephric mesenchyme* at about the 28th day (Fig. 49–4). The ureteric bud penetrates a condensing metanephric mesenchyme and begins to divide dichotomously. The tip of the dividing ureteric bud, called the *ampulla,* interacts with the metaneph-

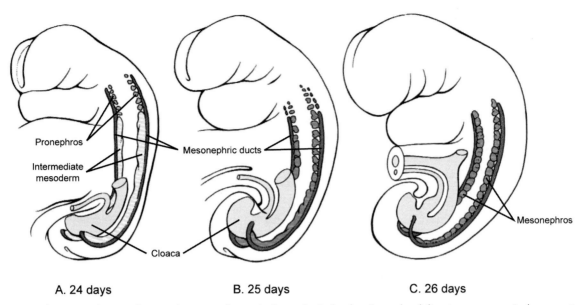

A. 24 days   B. 25 days   C. 26 days

Figure 49–3. Development of pronephros and mesonephros. *A,* Pronephroi develop in each of five to seven cervical segments, but these primitive renal structures degenerate quickly during the 4th week. The mesonephric ducts first appear on day 24. *B* and *C,* Mesonephric vesicles and tubules form in a craniocaudal direction throughout the thoracic and lumbar regions. The cranial pairs degenerate as caudal pairs develop, and the definitive mesonephroi contain about 20 pairs confined to the first three lumbar segments. (Modified from Larsen WJ: Human Embryology. New York, Churchill Livingstone, 1997.)

ric mesenchyme to induce formation of future nephrons (Fig. 49–5). As the ureteric bud divides and branches, each new ampulla acquires a cap-like condensation of metanephric mesenchyme, thereby giving the metanephros a lobulated appearance (Fig. 49–6).

The ureteric bud and metanephric mesenchyme exert reciprocal inductive effects toward each other, and the proper differentiation of these primordial structures de-

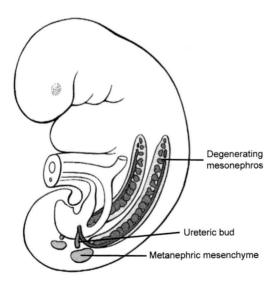

28 days

Figure 49–4. Metanephric mesenchyme condenses from the intermediate mesoderm during the early part of the 5th week and comes into contact with the ureteric bud, while the cranial mesonephroi continue to degenerate. (Modified from Larsen WJ: Human Embryology. New York, Churchill Livingstone, 1997.)

pends on these inductive signals (see "Molecular Mechanism of Kidney Development"). The metanephric mesenchyme induces the ureteric bud to branch, and, in turn, the ureteric bud induces the metanephric mesenchyme to condense and undergo mesenchymal-epithelial conversion. The nephron, which consists of the glomerulus, proximal tubule, loop of Henle, and distal tubule, is thought to derive from the metanephric mesenchyme, whereas the collecting system, consisting of collecting ducts, calyces, pelvis, and ureter, is formed from the ureteric bud (see Fig. 49–5).

In principle, all nephrons are formed in the same way and can be classified into fairly well-defined developmental stages (Larsson et al, 1983). The first identifiable precursors of the nephron are cells of metanephric mesenchyme that have formed a vesicle completely separated from the ureteric bud ampulla (stage I). Cells of the stage I renal vesicle are tall and columnar in shape, and they are stabilized by their attachments to the newly formed basement membrane (Fig. 49–7). The renal vesicle has not yet established a contact with the ampulla of the ureteric bud. The stage I renal vesicle then differentiates into an S-shaped stage II nephron that connects to the ureteric bud (Fig. 49–8). At this stage, the cup-shaped glomerular capsule is recognized in the lowest limb of the S-shaped tubule. The rest of the S-shaped tubule develops into the proximal tubule, the loop of Henle, and the distal tubule. When the cup-shaped glomerular capsule matures into an oval structure, the nephron has now passed into stage III of development (Fig. 49–9). Now the nephron can be divided into identifiable proximal and distal tubules. The stage IV nephron is characterized by a round glomerulus that closely resembles the mature renal corpuscle. The morphology of the proximal tubule resembles that of a mature nephron, whereas the distal segments are still primitive. In some species (e.g., the rodents), all stages of nephron develop-

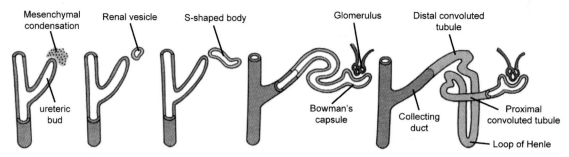

Figure 49–5. Development of the renal collecting ducts and nephrons. The tip of dividing ureteric bud induces the metanephric mesenchyme to condense; it then differentiates into a renal vesicle. This vesicle coils into an S-shaped tubule and ultimately forms Bowman's capsule as well as the proximal convoluted tubules, distal convoluted tubules, and loops of Henle. The ureteric bud contributes to the formation of collecting ducts. (Modified from Larsen WJ: Human Embryology. New York, Churchill Livingstone, 1997.)

ment are present at birth, whereas in others (e.g., the humans), all nephrons at birth are in varying steps of stage IV. Initially, vessels are seen in the cleft between the lower and middle portion of the S-shaped tubule, and they quickly branch into a portal system. Mesenchymal cells that do not become tubular epithelium either give rise to interstitial mesenchyme or undergo programmed cell death (apoptosis). **Overall, these events are reiterated throughout the growing kidney, so that older, more differentiated nephrons are located in the inner part of the kidney near the juxtamedullary region and newer, less differentiated nephrons are found at the periphery** (Fig. 49–10). **In humans, although renal maturation continues to take place postnatally, nephrogenesis is completed before birth.**

Development of the Collecting System

The bifurcation of the ureteric bud determines the eventual pelvicalyceal patterns and their corresponding renal lobules (Fig. 49–11). The first few divisions of the ureteric bud give rise to the renal pelvis, major and minor calyces, and collecting ducts. Thereafter, the first generations of collecting tubules are formed. When the ureteric bud first invades the metanephric mesenchyme, its tip ex-

pands to form an ampulla that will eventually give rise to the renal pelvis. By the 6th week, the ureteric bud has bifurcated at least four times, yielding 16 branches. These branches then coalesce to form two to four major calyces extending from the renal pelvis. By the 7th week, the next four generations of branches also fuse, forming the minor calyces. By the 32nd week, approximately 11 additional generations of bifurcation have resulted in approximately 1 to 3 million branches, which will become the collecting duct tubules.

Renal Ascent

Between the 6th and 9th weeks, the kidneys ascend to a lumbar site just below the adrenal glands (Fig. 49–12). The precise mechanism responsible for renal ascent is not known, but it is speculated that the differential growth of the lumbar and sacral regions of the embryo plays a role. As the kidneys migrate, they are vascularized by a succession of transient aortic sprouts that arise at progressively higher levels. These arteries do not elongate to follow the ascending kidneys, but instead degenerate and are replaced by successive new arteries. The final pair of arteries forms in the upper lumbar region and becomes the definitive renal arteries. Occasionally, a more inferior pair

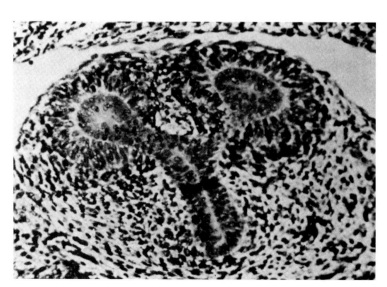

Figure 49–6. The ureteric bud divides to form enlarged tips, called ampullae, around which the metanephric mesenchyme condenses and begins nephron differentiation. (From Potter EL: Normal and Abnormal Development of the Kidney. Chicago, Yearbook Medical Publishers, 1972.)

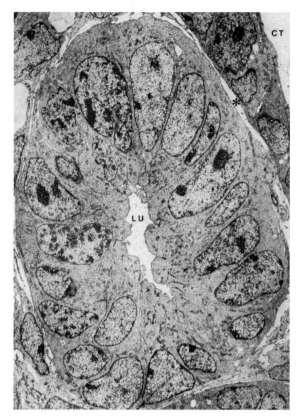

Figure 49–7. Stage I nephron development. The cells are tall with large nuclei, and the renal vesicle is separated from the developing collecting tubule (CT) by a narrow zone of low electron density (*). LU, lumen. (From Larsson L: J Ultrastruct Res 1975;51:119.)

of arteries persists as accessory lower pole arteries. **When the kidney fails to ascend properly, its location becomes ectopic.** If its ascent fails completely, it remains as a pelvic kidney. The inferior poles of the kidneys may also fuse, forming a horseshoe kidney that crosses over the ventral side of the aorta. During ascent, the fused lower pole becomes trapped under the inferior mesenteric artery and therefore does not reach its normal site. Rarely, the kidney fuses to the contralateral one and ascends to the opposite side, resulting in a cross-fused ectopy.

Molecular Mechanism of Kidney Development

In mammalian embryos, the permanent kidney is derived from the reciprocal inductive interactions between two primordial mesodermal structures, the ureteric bud and the metanephric mesenchyme. On induction by the ureteric bud, the metanephric mesenchyme undergoes a series of morphogenetic events that converts the mesenchyme to an epithelium and eventually generates most of the renal tubules. In turn, the metanephric mesenchyme provides a stimulus for continued growth and bifurcation of the ureteric bud, which eventually gives rise to the renal collecting ducts, calyces, renal pelvis, and ureter. Many of the early events in embryonic kidney development were first elucidated by manipulation of lower vertebrate embryos

and by use of a mammalian in vitro organ culture system. Clifford Grobstein's pioneering work in 1950s led to an organ culture technique whereby the metanephric mesenchyme is separated from the ureteric bud during the early part of kidney development and grown in vitro on a filter. An inducer tissue, such as ureter or spinal cord, cultured on the opposite side of the filter, then provides the inductive signal (Fig. 49–13). This ingenious experimental approach has established the kidney as a model system for studying the role of epithelial-mesenchymal interaction in organ development. The development of many other organs, including lung, salivary glands, gonads, prostate, and bladder, also requires epithelial-mesenchymal interaction for the controlled differentiation and proliferation of tissues.

Although much was known about the morphologic events of kidney development, the molecular mechanisms involved in these processes began to be identified only during the last few years (Fig. 49–14), largely by the identification of critical genes expressed during kidney development and the application of molecular recombinant techniques for single gene disruption (*gene knock-out*). **For a candidate gene to be unequivocally implicated in organ development, it must be expressed in a correct spatial and temporal manner relative to the developing organ, and when the gene is disrupted, normal organ**

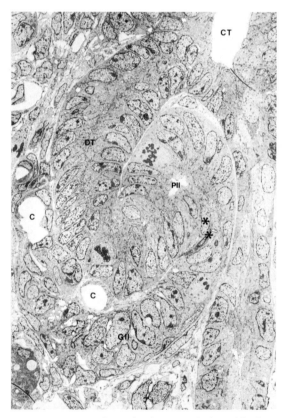

Figure 49–8. Stage II nephron development (S-shaped body). At this stage, the developing proximal tubule is recognizable (PII), and the future distal tubule (DT) is connected to the collecting tubule (CT). There are capillaries (C) in close proximity to the developing glomerulus (GII). The cells in the transition zone between the proximal tubule and glomerulus are marked with asterisks (*). (From Larsson L: J Ultrastruct Res 1975;51:119.)

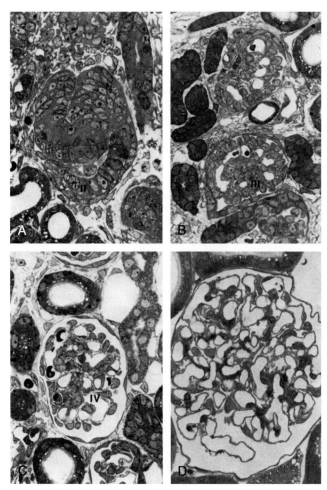

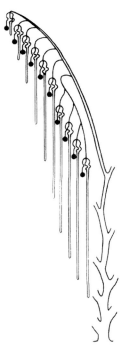

Figure 49–9. Stage III and IV nephron development as seen from a renal cortex of a 3-day-old rat. *A,* Stage II nephron with S-shaped body (II). *B,* Stage III nephron with oval-shaped glomeruli (III). *C,* Stage IV nephron resembles that of mature tubules and glomeruli (IV). *D,* Mature superficial glomerulus from adult rat kidney. (From Larsson L, Maunsbach AB: J Ultrastruct Res 1980;72:392.)

Figure 49–10. Schematic representation of progressive nephron differentiation. Older, more differentiated nephrons are located in the inner part of the kidney near the juxtamedullary region, and newer, less differentiated nephrons are found at the periphery. (From Potter EL: Normal and Abnormal Development of the Kidney. Chicago, Yearbook Medical Publishers, 1972.)

development must not occur. The advent of molecular biologic techniques has led to the identification of a large and growing number of genes expressed during kidney development. More than 200 genes and proteins are currently listed in the Kidney Development Database, and a detailed, up-to-date summary can now be accessed on a website (Davies and Brandli, 1991). However, to demonstrate that these genes are truly involved in kidney development, inactivation of the genes must lead to an abnormal kidney phenotype. A handful of genes are described here

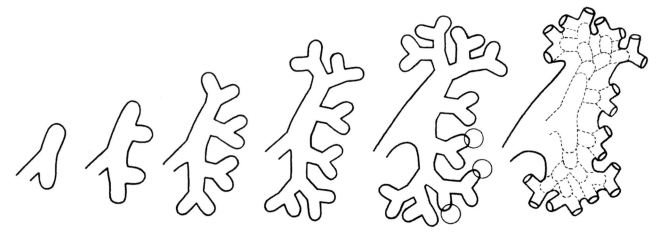

Figure 49–11. Dichotomous branching of the ureteric bud and subsequent fusion of the ampullae to form the renal pelvis and calyces. Circles indicate possible sites of infundibular development between the third, fourth, or fifth generations of branches and their subsequent expansions to give rise to the calyces. (From Potter EL: Normal and Abnormal Development of the Kidney. Chicago, Yearbook Medical Publishers, 1972.)

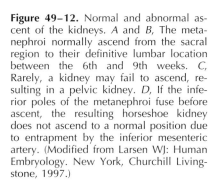

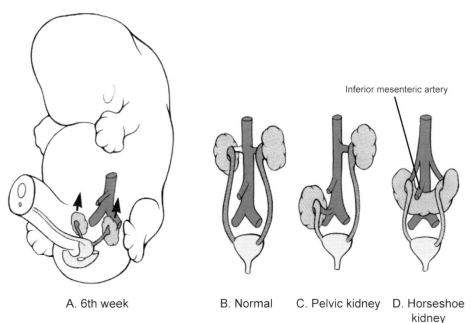

Figure 49–12. Normal and abnormal ascent of the kidneys. *A* and *B*, The metanephroi normally ascend from the sacral region to their definitive lumbar location between the 6th and 9th weeks. *C*, Rarely, a kidney may fail to ascend, resulting in a pelvic kidney. *D*, If the inferior poles of the metanephroi fuse before ascent, the resulting horseshoe kidney does not ascend to a normal position due to entrapment by the inferior mesenteric artery. (Modified from Larsen WJ: Human Embryology. New York, Churchill Livingstone, 1997.)

A. 6th week   B. Normal   C. Pelvic kidney   D. Horseshoe kidney

Inferior mesenteric artery

to illustrate some relevant points. There are now at least 11 genes that have been shown to play a critical role in kidney development via gene disruption studies (Lipschutz, 1998) (Table 49–1).

In creating a gene knock-out mouse, the totipotential embryonic stem cells are genetically altered and then microinjected into the cavity of an intact mouse blastocyst 2 to 3 days after fertilization. These stem cells can then populate any tissue of the developing mouse. If the altered stem cells contribute to the germ cells, the genomic information of the stem cells can be passed on to subsequent generations. **There are limitations, however, to the knowledge that can be gained from gene knock-out studies.** The first limitation involves *redundancy.* If a gene is crucial for development, it is logical to assume that whenever possible the organism will have a backup gene available that can replace the function of the crucial gene. When a gene is disrupted and no phenotypic abnormality is observed, redundancy is often invoked. Another limitation involves *embryonic lethality.* Many genes have multiple functions during development, and when the embryo dies very early, one does not get a chance to see whether the

Figure 49–13. Schematic representation of in vivo kidney development *(A)* and an in vitro transfilter organ culture system of Grobstein *(B)*. At an early stage of renal development, the metanephric mesenchyme is separated from the ureteric bud and cultured on a filter. If an inducer tissue, such as ureter or spinal cord, is grown on the opposite side of the filter, the metanephric mesenchyme will continue to differentiate into nephron structures. In the absence of inducer tissue, the metanephric mesenchyme will degenerate via apoptosis. (Modified from Vainio S, Muller U: Cell 1997;90:975.)

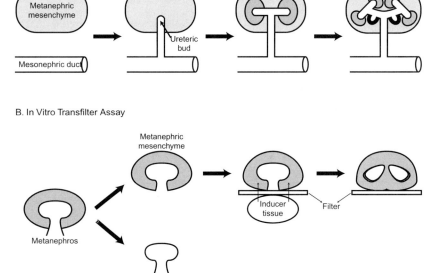

A. In Vivo Development

Metanephric mesenchyme

Mesenchymal condensations

Ureteric bud

Mesonephric duct

B. In Vitro Transfilter Assay

Metanephric mesenchyme

Metanephros

Inducer tissue

Filter

Ureteric bud

A. Ureter Induction

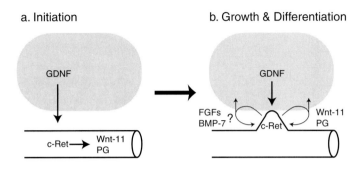

B. Tubule Induction

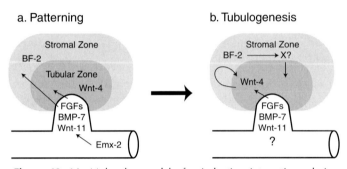

Figure 49–14. Molecular models for inductive interactions during early kidney development. *A,* Inductive signals that regulate the growth of the ureteric bud. (a) Initiation: Glial cell line–derived neurotrophic factor (GDNF) is secreted from the metanephric mesenchyme and activates the c-Ret receptor tyrosine kinase in the presumptive ureteric bud epithelium. This leads to induction of downstream factors such as Wnt-11 and proteoglycans (PG). (b) Growth and differentiation: Multiple molecules contribute to continued ureteric bud formation and branching, including mesenchymal proteins such as GDNF and ureteric bud factors such as Wnt-11, PG, BMP-7, and fibroblast growth factors (FGFs). Wnt-11 and PG might function as autocrine factors to maintain directional growth of the ureteric bud. Some of the ureteric bud signals may act on the mesenchyme as well. *B,* Signals involved in mesenchymal differentiation. (a) Patterning: The transcription factor Emx-2 regulates the ureteric bud epithelium expression of unidentified signaling molecules. Candidates are Wnt-11, BMP-7, and FGFs, and these factors may be involved in patterning the mesenchyme into two zones, a tubular one (Wnt-4 positive) and a stromal one (BF-2 positive). (b) Tubulogenesis: Cells from the ureteric bud and the stromal zone provide inductive signals for cells in the tubular zone to become nephrons. Here Wnt-4 is induced by ureteric bud signals and may then act as an autocrine factor in tubule development. (Modified from Vainio S, Muller U: Cell 1997;90:975.)

gene is involved in kidney development. One way to deal with this limitation is to use a tissue-specific method of gene disruption, which allows the gene knock-out to occur at a specific time and location during development. Currently, studies using combinations of gene expression analyses, gene knock-outs, and organ culture techniques are providing the most complete information. Several comprehensive reviews have been published on this topic (Saxen and Sariola, 1987; Bard et al, 1994; Patterson and Dressler, 1994; Lechner and Dressler, 1997; Vainio and Muller, 1997; Davies and Bard, 1998).

WT1 and PAX2

The classic transfilter assay of Grobstein is carried out with a mesenchyme isolated from rodent embryos at 11 to 12 days of gestation. By this time, kidney morphogenesis is well under way, and the ureteric bud has come into full contact with the condensing metanephric mesenchyme. This early phase of kidney development has now come into focus in molecular genetic experiments that address the functions of various transcription factors, signaling molecules, and receptors. The results of these experiments suggest that formation of the ureteric bud is initiated by inductive signals from the metanephric mesenchyme. The first evidence for this paradigm came from the analysis of mice lacking the transcription factor WT1, the product of the Wilms' tumor suppressor gene. During embryonic kidney development, WT1 is expressed in the metanephric mesenchyme but not in the ureteric bud. Mutant WT1 mice do not form ureteric buds, suggesting involvement of the transcription factor in the formation of ureteric bud. In organ culture, the WT1-deficient metanephric mesenchyme does not respond to inducer tissues, indicating that it may also confer mesenchymal competence for induction (Kreidberg et al, 1993). Other targeted mutations that cause defects in early kidney development include genes encoding the transcription factors PAX2 and LIM1 (Shawlot and Behringer, 1995; Torres et al, 1995). PAX2 is expressed in the mesonephric ducts and the ureteric buds from the murine embryonic day 12 onward. In *Pax2* gene knock-out mice, no mesonephric ducts, müllerian ducts, ureteric buds, or metanephric mesenchyme forms, and the animals die within 1 day after birth from renal failure (Torres et al, 1995). In humans, a *PAX2* gene mutation is related to a syndrome encompassing renal dysplasia, optic nerve colobomas, and vesicoureteral reflux (Sanyanusin et al, 1996). Further studies are required to establish their functions, but it seems likely that both *PAX2* and *LIM1* operate earlier than *WT1* does.

GDNF/c-RET

An important signaling molecule from the metanephric mesenchyme that regulates ureteric bud growth is glial cell line–derived neurotrophic factor (GDNF). In the mouse, targeted inactivation of c-RET, a member of the receptor tyrosine kinase superfamily, results in renal agenesis and dysplasia (Schuchardt et al, 1994). c-RET is expressed in the ureteric bud as it invades the metanephric mesenchyme. Later, its expression is confined to the bifurcating ampulla of the ureteric bud. The primary defect in the homozygous *c-Ret* gene knock-out mouse is a failure of the ureteric bud to emerge from the mesonephric duct and respond to signals from the metanephric mesenchyme (Schuchardt et al, 1996).

Although the importance of c-RET in kidney development had been clearly demonstrated, it was only recently that its ligand, GDNF, was identified. GDNF is a secreted glycoprotein that possesses a cystine-knot motif found in other growth factors such as platelet-derived growth factor (PDGF), nerve growth factor (NGF), and transforming growth factor–β (TGF-β). GDNF is expressed within the metanephric mesenchyme before ureteric bud invasion, and

Table 49–1. GENES CRUCIAL FOR THE DEVELOPMENT OF FUNCTIONAL KIDNEYS*

Gene	Type	MM	UB	Defect
WT1	Transcription factor	Yes	No	Renal agenesis
PAX2	Transcription factor	Yes	Yes	Renal agenesis
GDNF	TGF-β family member/ligand for c-RET	Yes	No	Renal agenesis or severe dysgenesis
c-RET	Receptor tyrosine kinase	No	Yes	Renal agenesis or severe dysgenesis
α8β1	Integrin	Yes	No	Renal agenesis or severe dysgenesis
WNT1	Secreted glycoprotein	Yes	No	Renal dysgenesis
BF2	Transcription factor	Yes	No	Abnormal stromal cells leading to renal dysgenesis
BMP7	TGF-β family member	Yes	Yes	Renal dysgenesis
PDGFB	PDGF and ligand for PDGFRβ	Yes	No	Absence of mesangial cells
PDGFRB	Receptor tyrosine kinase	Yes	No	Absence of mesangial cells
α3β1	Integrin	Yes	Yes	Abnormal glomerular podocytes and basement membrane

*Genes are listed in the order in which the developmental defects occur.

GDNF, glial cell line–derived neurotrophic factor; MM, metanephric mesenchyme expression; PDGF, platelet-derived growth factor; TGF, transforming growth factor; UB, ureteric bud expression.

Adapted from Lipschutz JH: Molecular development of the kidney: A review of the results of gene disruption studies. Am J Kidney Dis 1998;31:38–397.

later its expression is confined to the most peripheral mesenchyme of the developing kidney, where the induction of new nephrons occurs, complementing the expression pattern of c-RET at the ureteric bud ampulla. GDNF can promote ureteric bud growth in vitro, but more importantly, ureteric bud formation is impaired in *Gdnf* knock-out mice (Moore et al, 1996; Pichel et al, 1996; Sanchez et al, 1996), a phenotype strikingly similar to that of the c-*Ret* knock-out mice.

There is now compelling evidence that GDNF and c-RET are elements of the same signaling pathway that regulates ureteric bud development. High-affinity GDNF/c-RET interaction seems to require an adaptor molecule called GDNFR-α, which is attached to the cell surface (Jing et al, 1996). Continued bifurcation of the ureteric bud is probably generated by a refinement of the GDNF/GDNFR-α/c-RET signaling complex expression pattern. That is, expression is down-regulated in mature nephrons but continues at high levels in active areas of nephron formation. Candidate molecules that act downstream of GDNF/c-RET in the ureteric bud are proteoglycans (Vainio et al, 1989) and WNT11 (Kispert et al, 1996).

Signals Regulating Mesenchymal Differentiation

On induction by mesenchymal signals, the growing ureteric bud reciprocates by expressing signal molecules that regulate the differentiation of the metanephric mesenchyme. This process is not well understood, but some candidate molecules such as FGF2, BMP7, and WNT11 have emerged. There is also evidence that expression of these signaling molecules by the ureteric bud is regulated by the homeobox transcription factor EMX2. In *Emx2* gene knock-out mice, the ureteric bud forms and invades the metanephric mesenchyme, but its development is arrested and the mesenchyme does not differentiate (Miyamoto et al, 1997). It is not known whether the mesenchyme is a homogeneous cell population before interaction with the ureteric bud. It is clear, however, that the inductive signals from the ureteric bud patterns the mesenchyme into at least two different cell populations, a tubular one

and a stromal one. The tubular cell population is thought to derive from mesenchymal cells in direct contact with the ureteric bud ampulla, and they express PAX2, SDC1, and WNT4 (Vainio et al, 1989; Stark et al, 1994; Torres et al, 1995). The stromal cell population surrounds the tubular cells, and they express the transcription factor BF2 (Hatini et al, 1996).

Once the mesenchyme has been patterned, the cells in the tubular zone undergo morphogenesis to become renal tubular epithelial cells. There is evidence that this process depends not only on signals from the ureteric bud but also on signals from the mesenchyme itself. One of these autocrine signals may be WNT4, whose expression is induced in cells of the tubular zone on interaction with the ureteric bud. In *Wnt4* gene knock-out mice, the ureteric bud forms and invades the metanephric mesenchyme, but subsequent development of epithelial tubules is abolished (Stark et al, 1994). This suggests that two signals are essential for renal tubule formation—an initial ureteric bud derived signal (or signals) activating WNT4 expression in the metanephric mesenchyme, and WNT4 itself as a mesenchymal autocrine signal. Apparently, signals from the stromal cell population contribute to tubule formation as well, because tubulogenesis is perturbed in *Bf2* gene knock-out mice (Hatini et al, 1996).

The discovery that WNT4 acts as a downstream signal during the induction cascade leading to renal tubule formation leads to the question regarding the nature of the initial ureteric bud derived signal. In vitro data suggest a role for FGF2 and other uncharacterized factors secreted by the ureteric bud (Karavanova et al, 1996). Candidate molecules that may cooperate with FGF2 are WNT11 and BMP7 (Kispert et al, 1996; Vukicevic et al, 1996).

Cell Proliferation and Apoptosis

Although little is known regarding the mechanism by which cell proliferation and apoptosis are coordinated in the developing kidney, some clues are beginning to emerge. The product of the tumor suppressor gene *p53* is thought to regulate cell growth in two ways. It acts as a checkpoint in the cell cycle, and in a separate manner it controls apoptosis in response to stress (Polyak et al, 1996). In the developing kidney, p53 is normally expressed in comma- and S-shaped bodies (Schmid et al, 1991), but *p53* gene knock-out mice do not demonstrate any significant renal developmental anomaly (Donehower et al, 1995). In contrast, overexpression of wild-type p53 in the transgenic mice leads to small kidneys with fewer nephrons (Godley et al, 1996).

Widespread apoptosis occurs in the metanephric mesenchyme in the absence of inductive signals (Koseki et al, 1992). Therefore, it seems likely that induction of metanephric mesenchyme generates both survival and differentiation factors. Indeed, a number of growth factors, including epidermal growth factor (Weller et al, 1991) and basic fibroblast growth factor (Perantoni et al, 1995), can prevent cell death in cultured metanephric mesenchyme and may function as survival factors. During renal development, apoptotic cells are characteristically found between maturing nephrons in the metanephric mesenchyme (Koseki et al, 1992). Factors controlling apoptosis have been investigated, including BCL2, a form of cytoprotective protein. *Bcl2* gene knock-out mice develop cystic kidneys that are hypoplastic and have fewer nephrons (Nagata et al, 1996). In these mice, a dramatic increase in apoptosis within the metanephric mesenchyme was observed. These findings suggest that apoptotic regulation is required for normal renal development and that BCL2 may block apoptosis in many kidney cell types.

Renin-Angiotensin System

The renin-angiotensin system (RAS) is present and active during fetal life. It is generally thought that the major role of RAS in the fetus is to maintain the fetal glomerular filtration rate and ensure an adequate urine production (Lumbers, 1995). There is evidence that the RAS is also important for normal growth and development of the ureter and the metanephric kidney. The kidney is able to produce all components of the RAS, so the local (intrarenal) production of angiotensin II may play a critical role in this regard. Renin mRNA is detectable in the human mesonephros at about 30 days of gestation and in the metanephros at about 56 days (Schutz et al, 1996). A similar profile of expression is seen for angiotensinogen and angiotensin-converting enzyme (ACE). Both subtypes of angiotensin II receptors, AT_1 and AT_2, are expressed in the developing mesonephros and metanephros. AT_2 expression predominates in undifferentiated mesenchyme and declines with maturation, and this observation suggests the role of AT_2 in modulation of proliferation, apoptosis, and/or mesenchymal differentiation. AT_1 is expressed in more differentiated structures and may be involved in modulating later stages of renal vascular development and acquisition of classic angiotensin II–mediated effects of vasoconstriction and sodium reabsorption. The function of the AT_2 receptor is not defined completely, but it appears to play an important role in ureteral development (see "Role of the Renin-Angiotensin System in Ureteral Differentiation"). AT_2 is highly expressed in undifferentiated periureteral and peripapillary mesenchymal cells. AT_2 gene knock-out mice demonstrate a spectrum of congenital urinary tract abnormalities, in-

cluding ureteropelvic junction (UPJ) obstruction, multicystic dysplastic kidney, megaureter, vesicoureteral reflux, and renal hypoplasia (Nishimura et al, 1999).

Ten- to 12-month-old mutant mice lacking ACE are found to have abnormal renal vasculature and tubules as well as increased renin synthesis in interstitial and perivascular cells (Hilgers et al, 1997). Pharmacologic inhibition of ACE in the neonatal rat produces irreversible abnormalities in renal function and morphology (Guron et al, 1997), supporting the idea that an intact RAS is crucial for normal kidney development and maturation. In addition to the high rate of fetal loss, infants born to mothers treated with ACE inhibitors during pregnancy have increased rates of oligohydramnios, hypotension, and anuria (Shotan et al, 1994; Sedman et al, 1995). Babies with high umbilical cord renin concentrations have significantly smaller kidneys, and infants with intrauterine growth retardation have high angiotensin II levels in the blood (Konje et al, 1996).

Renal Vascular Development

The origin of the intrarenal vasculature is not completely understood. Until recently, it was thought that renal vasculature derived exclusively from branches off the aorta and other preexisting extrarenal vessels (angiogenic hypothesis). There is evidence, however, that the renal vessels may originate in situ, within the embryonic kidney from vascular precursor cells (vasculogenic hypothesis) (Loughna et al, 1996; Tufro et al, 1999). Using antibodies to FLK1, a vascular endothelial growth factor (VEGF) receptor present in angioblasts and mature endothelial cells, it was demonstrated that endothelial cell precursors are already present in the prevascular rodent kidneys before any vessels are discernible from a morphologic standpoint. When embryonic kidneys are cultured at the usual atmospheric oxygen concentration, vessels do not develop. However, if the explants are cultured in an atmosphere containing 5% oxygen, capillary sprouts develop within and outside the glomeruli, an effect that is inhibited by anti-VEGF antibodies (Tufro-McReddie et al, 1997). Depending on the developmental potential of the cells involved, both angiogenesis and vasculogenesis may play a role in the development of renal vasculature (Abrahamson et al, 1998).

BLADDER AND URETER DEVELOPMENT

Formation of the Urogenital Sinus

At the 3rd week of gestation, the cloacal membrane remains a bilaminar structure composed of endoderm and ectoderm. During the 4th week, the neural tube and the tail grow dorsally and caudally, projecting itself over the cloacal membrane, and this differential growth of the body results in embryo folding. The cloacal membrane is now turned to the ventral aspect of the embryo, and the terminal portion of the endoderm-lined yolk sac dilates and becomes the cloaca (Fig. 49–15). According to the embryonic theories of Rathke and Tourneux, the partition of cloaca into an

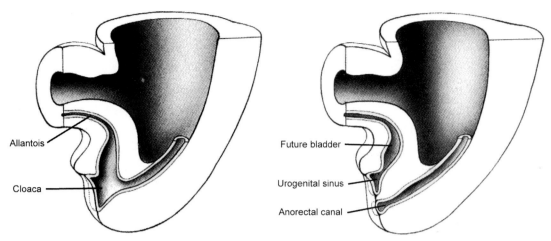

Figure 49–15. Development of the urogenital sinus. Between the 4th and 6th weeks, the cloaca is divided into an anterior urogenital sinus and a posterior anorectal canal. The superior part of the urogenital sinus, continuous with allantois, forms the bladder. The constricted narrowing at the base of the urogenital sinus forms the pelvic urethra. The distal expansion of the urogenital sinus forms the vestibule of the vagina in females and the penile urethra in males. (Modified from Larsen WJ: Human Embryology. New York, Churchill Livingstone, 1997.)

anterior urogenital sinus and a posterior anorectal canal occurs by the fusion of two lateral ridges of the cloacal wall and by a descending urorectal septum. This process is thought to occur during the 5th and 6th weeks, and it culminates in fusion of the urorectal septum with the cloacal membrane. **More recently, however, some investigators have challenged this classic view with evidence that there is neither a descending septum nor fusing lateral ridges of the cloacal wall** (van der Putte, 1986; Kluth et al, 1995). There is evidence that the urorectal septum never fuses with the cloacal membrane (Nievelstein et al, 1998). According to these new observations, the congenital cloacal and anorectal malformations, which were previously thought to occur as a result of a failure of septum formation and its fusion with the cloacal membrane, may in fact occur because of an abnormal development of the cloacal membrane itself (Nievelstein et al, 1998) (Fig. 49–16).

The mesonephric (wolffian) duct fuses with the cloaca by the 24th day and remains with the urogenital sinus during the cloacal separation. **The entrance of the mesonephric duct into the primitive urogenital sinus serves as a landmark distinguishing the cephalad vesicourethral canal from the caudal urogenital sinus. The vesicourethral canal gives rise to the bladder and pelvic urethra, whereas the caudal urogenital sinus forms the phallic urethra for males and the distal vaginal vestibule for females.**

Formation of the Trigone

By day 33 of gestation, the common excretory ducts (the portion of the mesonephric ducts distal to the origin of the ureteric buds) dilate and become absorbed into the urogenital sinus. The right and left common excretory ducts fuse in the midline as a triangular area, forming the primitive trigone. The ureteric orifice exstrophies and evaginates into the bladder by day 37 and begins

to migrate in a cranial and lateral direction within the floor of the bladder. During this process, the mesonephric (wolffian) duct orifice diverges away from the ureteric orifice and migrates caudally, flanking the paramesonephric (müllerian) duct at the level of the urogenital sinus. This is the site of the future verumontanum in males and vaginal canal in females (Fig. 49–17).

The mechanism of ureteric orifice incorporation into the developing bladder is inferred primarily from clinical observations of duplex kidneys. **The upper pole ureteric orifice rotates posteriorly relative to the lower pole orifice and assumes a more caudal and medial position. Weigert and Meyer recognized the regularity of this relationship between upper and lower pole ureteric orifices, which has come to be known as the Weigert-Meyer rule.** According to this concept, an abnormally lateral lower pole ureteric orifice may result from a ureteric bud's arising too low on the mesonephric duct, which causes premature incorporation and migration within the developing bladder. In such a ureteric orifice, vesicoureteral reflux is more likely to occur because of an inadequate intramural tunnel. In contrast, an abnormally caudal upper pole ureteric orifice may result from a ureteric bud's arising too high on the mesonephric duct. It may drain at the bladder neck and verumontanum, or it may remain connected to the mesonephric duct derivatives (e.g., vas deferens) (Mackie and Stephens, 1977; Schwarz and Stephens, 1978). In females, the ectopic upper pole ureter may insert into the remnants of the mesonephric (wolffian) ducts or into the vaginal vestibule (Fig. 49–18).

Anomalous development of the common excretory duct may lead to an ectopic vas deferens. In certain clinical situations, the vas deferens is connected to the ureter rather than the verumontanum, so that both ureter and vas drain into a common duct. This situation may occur when the ureteric bud arises too high on the mesonephric duct and the subsequent common excretory duct becomes too long, resulting in incomplete absorption into the developing bladder. **This anomaly, although rare,**

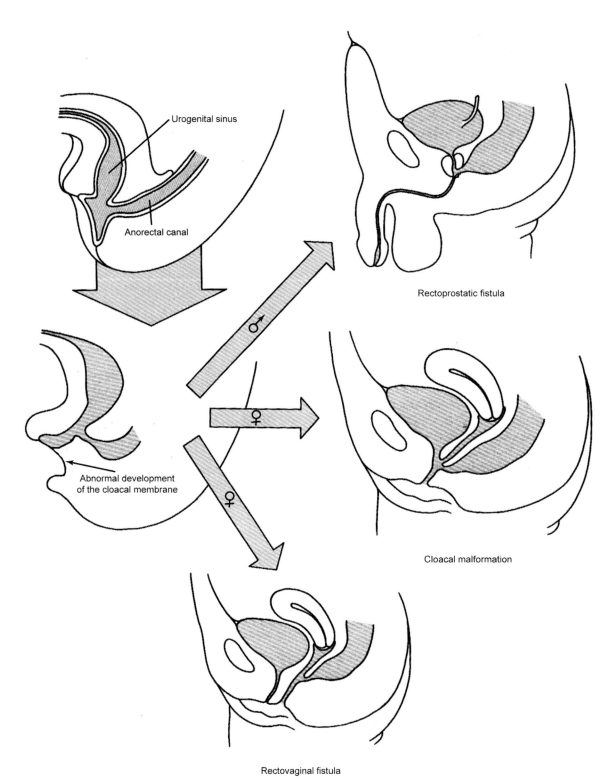

Figure 49–16. Abnormal development of cloacal membrane results in characteristic anomalies of the urogenital and lower gastrointestinal tract. (Modified from Larsen WJ: Human Embryology. New York, Churchill Livingstone, 1997.)

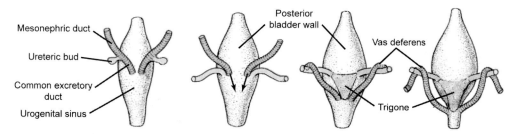

Figure 49–17. Incorporation of the mesonephric ducts and ureteric buds into the bladder wall. Between the 4th and 6th weeks, common excretory ducts, the terminal portion of the mesonephric ducts caudal to the ureteric bud formation, exstrophy into the posterior wall of the developing bladder. The triangular region of exstrophied mesonephric ducts forms the trigone of the bladder. This process brings the ureteric bud openings into the bladder wall, while the mesonephric duct openings are carried inferiorly to the level of pelvic urethra. (Modified from Sadler TW: Langman's Medical Embryology. Baltimore, Williams & Wilkins, 1985.)

should be kept in mind when evaluating male infants with epididymitis and ipsilateral hydronephrosis.

Development of the Ureter

In contrast to the previous discussion regarding the molecular aspects of ureteric bud–metanephric mesenchyme inductive interactions in forming the definitive kidney, very little is understood at the molecular level concerning the events of ureter development. There is only a small amount of descriptive information and speculative theories regarding the molecular mechanism of smooth muscle cell and urothelial differentiation. The ureter begins as a simple cuboidal epithelial tube, surrounded by loose mesenchymal cells, which acquires a complete lumen at 28 days of gestation in human. It was suggested that the developing ureter undergoes a transient luminal obstruction between 37 and 40 days and subsequently recanalizes (Alcaraz et al, 1991). It appears that this recanalization process begins in the midureter and extends in a bidirectional manner both cranially and caudally. In addition, another source of physiologic ureteral obstruction may exist as Chwalla's membrane, a two-cell-thick layer over the ureteric orifice that is seen between 37 and 39 days of gestation.

In humans, urine production is followed by proliferative changes in the ureteral epithelium (bilaminar by 10 weeks of gestation). The epithelium attains a transitional configuration by 14 weeks. The first signs of ureteral muscularization and development of elastic fibers are seen at 12 weeks of gestation. In both rats and humans, the ureteral smooth muscle phenotype appears later than that of the bladder. Smooth muscle differentiation is first detected in the subserosal region of the bladder dome and extends toward the bladder neck and urethra, whereas smooth muscle differentiation of the ureter occurs later within the subepithelial region in the ureterovesical junction, ascending toward the intrarenal collecting system (Baker and Gomez, 1998). **In the embryonic ureter and bladder it is likely that epithelial-mesenchymal interactions are important in the development of urothelium, lamina propria, and muscular compartments, but the exact nature of this induction process is unknown.** Before 10 weeks, elastic fibers are few in number, poorly developed and randomly arranged. After 12 weeks, these fibers become more numerous throughout the ureter and are seen with specific orientation (Escala et al, 1989).

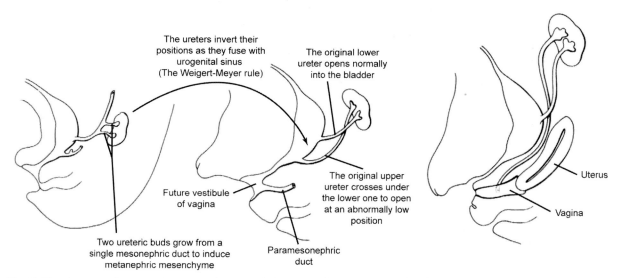

Figure 49–18. Development of an ectopic upper pole ureter draining into the vagina. (Modified from Larsen WJ: Human Embryology. New York, Churchill Livingstone, 1997.)

Role of the Renin-Angiotensin System in Ureteral Differentiation

One of the best-investigated mechanisms of ureteral development at this time involves the AT_2 gene. AT_1 was found to be expressed in mature glomeruli and in developing S-shaped bodies throughout the various stages of nephrogenesis. Both the temporal and spatial expression of AT_1 coincided with the differentiation and proliferation of glomerular mesangial and tubular cells. In contrast, AT_2 was expressed only in the mesenchymal cells adjacent to the stalk of the ureteric bud at early developmental stages and decreased markedly after birth (Kakuchi et al, 1995). The role of the AT_2 gene in ureteral development was further elucidated in AT_2 gene knock-out mice (Nishimura et al, 1999). These mice demonstrated a high incidence of congenital anomalies of the kidney and urinary tract (CAKUT), including UPJ obstruction, vesicoureteral reflux, ureterovesical junction obstruction, multicystic dysplastic kidney, hypoplastic kidney, and megaureter. It was speculated that CAKUT phenotypes may have been caused by delayed apoptosis in the undifferentiated mesenchymal cells surrounding the ureteric bud. These findings in AT_2 gene knock-out mice are especially fascinating in light of the fact that AT_2 gene mutations were also found in a selected cohort of patients with UPJ obstruction and megaureter (Hohenfellner et al, 1999).

Development of the Bladder and Continence Mechanisms

By the 10th week, the bladder is a cylindrical tube lined by a single layer of cuboidal cells surrounded by loose connective tissue. **The apex tapers as the urachus, which is contiguous with the allantois.** By the 12th week, the urachus involutes to become a fibrous cord, which becomes the *median umbilical ligament.* The bladder epithelium consists of bilayered cuboidal cells between the 7th and 12th weeks, and it begins to acquire mature urothelial characteristics between the 13th and 17th weeks. By the 21st week, it becomes four to five cell layers thick and demonstrates ultrastructural features similar to those of the fully differentiated urothelium. **Between the 7th and 12th weeks, the surrounding connective tissues condense and smooth muscle fibers begin to appear, first at the region of the bladder dome and later proceeding toward the bladder neck.** Collagen fibers first appear in the lamina propria and then later extend into the deeper wall between the muscle fibers (Newman and Antonakopoulos, 1989). **Embryologically speaking, the bladder comprises two regions: the trigone and the bladder body. The bladder body is derived from the endoderm-lined vesicourethral canal and the surrounding mesenchyme. The trigone has a different embryologic origin in that it develops from the incorporation of the common excretory ducts (the portion of mesonephric ducts caudal to the origin of the ureteric bud) into the base of the developing bladder.**

Bladder compliance is thought to change during gestation. **When studied in whole-organ preparations of fetal**

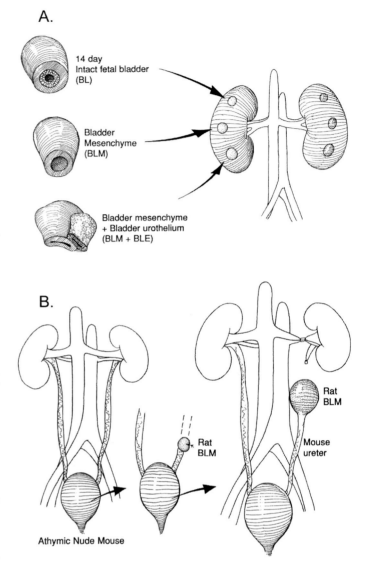

Figure 49–19. Tissue recombination experiments to study the role of epithelial-mesenchymal interaction in bladder smooth muscle development. *A,* Bladders were isolated from fetuses of 14-day pregnant rats. Intact bladder (BL), bladder mesenchyme alone (BLM), and bladder mesenchyme recombined with bladder epithelium (BLM+BLE) were grafted under the renal capsule of syngeneic hosts. BL and BLM+BLE grafts developed appropriately differentiated bladder smooth muscle, whereas BLM regressed with evidence of apoptosis. *B,* In situ induction of rat bladder smooth muscle by mouse ureteral epithelium. The left kidney was removed from an athymic nude mouse, and the BLM isolated from the fetus of a 14-day pregnant rat was grafted at the end of the ureteral stump. Rat BLM developed into a bladder-like structure with appropriate smooth muscle differentiation. (Reproduced from Baskin L, et al: J Urol 1996;156:1820.)

sheep bladders, bladder compliance is found to be very low during early gestation and to increase gradually thereafter (Coplen et al, 1994). The mechanism of these changes in bladder compliance is not known but may involve alterations in both smooth muscle tone and connective tissue composition. This phenomenon was also observed in developing human bladders (Kim et al, 1991). During gestation, the bladder wall muscle thickness increases and the relative collagen content decreases. The ratio of thick-to-thin collagen fibers also decreases, whereas the amount of elastic fibers increases. These changes in compliance seem to coincide with the time of fetal urine production, suggesting a possible role for mechanical distention (Baskin et al, 1994). In studies of organ culture explants of fetal mouse bladders, bladder distention promoted a more orderly development of collagen fiber bundles within the lamina propria, compared with decompressed bladder explants, suggesting that mechanical factors from accumulating urine may play a role during bladder development (Beauboeuf et al, 1998).

The epithelial-mesenchymal inductive interactions appear to be necessary for orderly differentiation and proper development of the bladder. A modified Grobstein technique was applied to study the mechanism of bladder smooth muscle cell differentiation (Baskin et al, 1996) (Fig. 49–19). Undifferentiated rat bladder epithelial and mesenchymal rudiments were separated before bladder smooth muscle cell differentiation and then recombined to grow within the immunologically compromised host (athymic nude mouse). In the presence of epithelial cells the mesenchymal cells differentiated into smooth muscle cells with sequential expression of appropriate muscle markers, whereas in the absence of epithelial cells they involuted with evidence of apoptosis. As in developing fetal bladders, histologically identifiable smooth muscle cells appeared in the outer bladder wall near the serosa rather than at the immediate epithelial-mesenchymal junction. The signaling mechanism for this inductive interaction is not known.

No functional study has been done to assess fetal continence mechanisms. Only a handful of ontogenic descriptions is available from human fetal specimens, providing a basis for speculative theories. A mesenchymal condensation forms around the caudal end of the urogenital sinus after the division of the cloaca and the rupture of the cloacal membrane. Striated muscle fibers can be seen clearly by the 15th week. At this time, the smooth muscle layer becomes thicker at the level of the bladder neck and forms the inner part of the urethral musculature. The urethral sphincter, composed of central smooth muscle fibers and peripheral striated muscle fibers, develops in the anterior wall of the urethra (Bourdelat et al, 1992). Beyond this point, sexual dimorphism develops in conjunction with the formation of the prostate in males and the vagina in females (Tichy, 1989). The urethral sphincter muscle fibers extend to the posterior wall of the urethra. In males, these fibers project to the lateral wall of the prostate; in females, the muscle fibers attach to the lateral wall of the vagina.

GENITAL DEVELOPMENT

Formation of Genital Ridges and Paramesonephric Ducts

During the 5th week, primordial germ cells migrate from the yolk sac along the dorsal mesentery to populate the mesenchyme of the posterior body wall near the 10th thoracic level (Fig. 49–20). **In both sexes, the arrival of primordial germ cells in the area of future gonads serves as the signal for the existing cells of the mesonephros and the adjacent coelomic epithelium to prolif-**

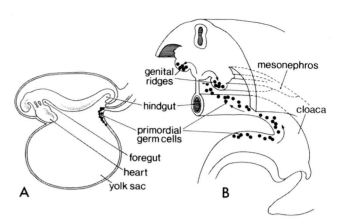

Figure 49–20. *A,* The site of primordial germ cell origin in the wall of the yolk sac in a 3-week-old embryo. *B,* Migratory path of the primordial germ cells along the wall of the yolk sac and dorsal mesentery into the developing genital ridges. (Modified from Sadler TW: Langman's Medical Embryology. Baltimore, Williams & Wilkins, 1985.)

erate and form a pair of *genital ridges* **just medial to the developing mesonephros** (Fig. 49–21). During the 6th week, the cells of the genital ridge invade the mesenchyme in the region of future gonads to form aggregates of supporting cells called *primitive sex cords.* The primitive sex cords subsequently invest the germ cells and support their development. The genital ridge mesenchyme containing the primitive sex cords is divided into cortical and medullary regions. Both regions develop in all embryos, but after the 6th week they pursue different fates in male and female embryos.

During this time, a new pair of ducts, called the *paramesonephric (müllerian) ducts,* begins to form just lateral to the mesonephric ducts in both male and female embryos (see Fig. 49–21). These ducts arise by craniocaudal invagination of thickened coelomic epithelium, extending all the way from the third thoracic segment to the posterior wall of the developing urogenital sinus. The caudal tips of the paramesonephric ducts are adherent to each other as they connect with the urogenital sinus between the openings of the right and left mesonephric ducts. The cranial ends of the paramesonephric ducts form funnel-shaped openings into the coelomic cavity (the future peritoneum).

Development of Male Genital Structures

Under the influence of *SRY* (the *s*ex-determining *r*egion of the *Y* chromosome; see "Molecular Mechanism of Sexual Differentiation"), cells in the medullary region of the primitive sex cords begin to differentiate into *Sertoli cells* while the cells of the cortical sex cords degenerate. **Sex cord cells differentiate into Sertoli cells only if they contain the SRY protein; otherwise, the sex cords differentiate into ovarian follicles.** During the 7th week, the differentiating Sertoli cells organize to form the *testis cords.* At puberty these testis cords associated with germ cells undergo canalization and differentiate into a system of seminiferous tubules. Direct cell-to-cell contact between de-

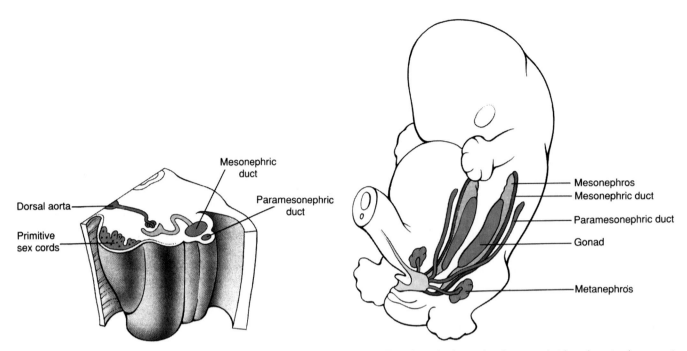

Figure 49–21. Formation of genital ridges and paramesonephric ducts. During the 5th and 6th weeks, the genital ridges form in the posterior abdominal wall just medial to the developing mesonephroi. The primordial germ cells induce the coelomic epithelial cells lining the peritoneal cavity and the cells of the mesonephros to proliferate and form the primitive sex cords. During the 6th week, the paramesonephric ducts develop lateral to the mesonephroi. The caudal tips of the paramesonephric ducts fuse with each other as they connect with the urogenital sinus. (Modified from Larsen WJ: Human Embryology. New York, Churchill Livingstone, 1997.)

veloping Sertoli cells and primordial germ cells is thought to play a key role in the proper development of male gametes. This interaction occurs shortly after the arrival of the primordial germ cells in the presumptive genital ridge. The testis cords distal to the presumptive seminiferous tubules also develop a lumen and differentiate into a set of thin-walled ducts called the *rete testis*. Just medial to the developing gonad, the tubules of rete testis connect with 5 to 12 residual tubules of mesonephric ducts, called *efferent ductules*. **The vas deferens develops from the mesonephric duct.** At this time, the testicle begins to round up, reducing its area of contact with the surrounding mesonephros. As the testicle continues to develop, the degenerating cortical sex cords become separated from the coelomic (peritoneal) epithelium by an intervening layer of connective tissue called the *tunica albuginea.*

As the developing Sertoli cells begin their differentiation in response to SRY, they begin to secrete a glycoprotein hormone called *müllerian-inhibiting substance* (**MIS**). **MIS causes the paramesonephric (müllerian) ducts to regress rapidly between the 8th and 10th weeks. Small müllerian duct remnants can be detected in the developed male as a small tissue protrusion at the superior pole of the testicle, called the *appendix testis*, and as a posterior expansion of the prostatic urethra, called the *prostatic utricle*** (Fig. 49–22). In female embryos, MIS is absent, so the müllerian ducts do not regress. The existence of MIS was first postulated in 1916 on the basis of evidence from freemartin calves (Behringer, 1994). Freemartin calves are female calves that share the womb with a male twin. These calves possess ovaries but, like their male twin, they lack müllerian derivatives and are therefore sterile. It was hypothesized that some substance

(now known as MIS) circulates from the bloodstream of the male calf to the bloodstream of the female calf and induces the müllerian ducts to regress. **Occasionally, genetic males have persistent müllerian duct structures (uterus and fallopian tubes), the condition known as *hernia uteri inguinale.*** In these individuals, either MIS production by Sertoli cells is deficient or the müllerian ducts do not respond to normal MIS levels.

During the 9th and 10th weeks, Leydig cells differentiate from mesenchymal cells of the genital ridge in response to the SRY protein. These endocrine cells produce testosterone. At an early stage of development, testosterone secretion is regulated by placental chorionic gonadotrophin, but eventually the pituitary gonadotrophins assume control of androgen production.

Between the 8th and 12th weeks, testosterone secretion by Leydig cells stimulates the mesonephric ducts to transform into the vas deferens. The cranial portions of the mesonephric ducts degenerate, leaving a small remnant of tissue protrusion called the *appendix epididymis*, and the region of mesonephric ducts adjacent to the presumptive testis differentiate into the epididymis. During the 9th week, 5 to 12 mesonephric ducts in the region of the epididymis make contact with the sex cords of the future rete testis. It is not until the 3rd month, however, that these mesonephric tubules actually establish communication with the rete testis as the efferent ductules. Meanwhile, the mesonephric tubules near the inferior pole of the developing testicle degenerate, sometimes leaving a remnant of tissue protrusion called the *paradidymis.*

The seminal vesicles sprout from the distal mesonephric ducts, whereas the prostate and bulbourethral glands develop from the urethra (Fig. 49–23). They

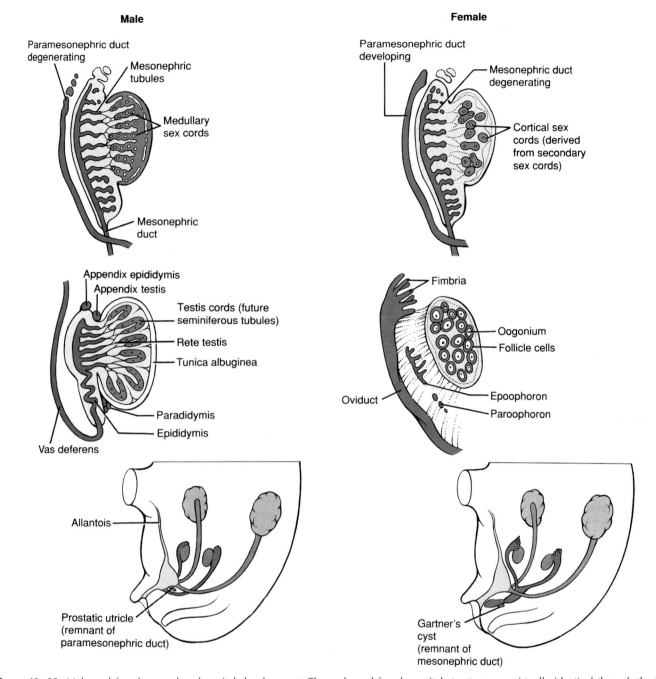

Male

Paramesonephric duct degenerating

Mesonephric tubules

Medullary sex cords

Mesonephric duct

Appendix epididymis
Appendix testis

Testis cords (future seminiferous tubules)

Rete testis

Tunica albuginea

Paradidymis

Epididymis

Vas deferens

Allantois

Prostatic utricle (remnant of paramesonephric duct)

Female

Paramesonephric duct developing

Mesonephric duct degenerating

Cortical sex cords (derived from secondary sex cords)

Fimbria

Oogonium

Follicle cells

Oviduct

Epoophoron

Paroophoron

Gartner's cyst (remnant of mesonephric duct)

Figure 49–22. Male and female gonad and genital development. The male and female genital structures are virtually identical through the 7th week. In males, SRY protein produced by the Sertoli cells causes the medullary sex cords to become presumptive seminiferous tubules and causes the cortical sex cords to regress. Müllerian-inhibiting substance (MIS) hormone produced by the Sertoli cells then causes the paramesonephric ducts to regress, leaving behind appendix testis and prostatic utricle as remnants. Appendix epididymis and paradidymis arise from the mesonephric ducts. In females, cortical sex cords invest the primordial germ cells and become the ovarian follicles. In the absence of MIS hormone, the mesonephric ducts degenerate and the paramesonephric ducts give rise to the fallopian tubes, uterus, and upper vagina. The remnants of the mesonephric ducts are found in the ovarian mesentery as the epoöphoron and paroöphoron, and in the anterolateral vaginal wall as the Gartner's duct cysts. (Modified from Larsen WJ: Human Embryology. New York, Churchill Livingstone, 1997.)

therefore have different embryologic origins. The glandular seminal vesicles sprout during the 10th week from the mesonephric ducts near their attachment to the pelvic urethra. The portion of the vas deferens distal to the developing seminal vesicle is thereafter called the *ejaculatory duct*. The prostate gland also begins to develop during the 10th week as a cluster of endodermal evaginations budding from the pelvic urethra. **These presumptive prostatic outgrowths are induced by the surrounding mesenchyme, and this process depends on the conversion of testosterone into dihydrotestosterone by 5α-reductase.** The prostatic outgrowths initially form approximately five independent groups of solid prostatic cords. By the 11th week, these cords develop lumens and glandular acini, and by the

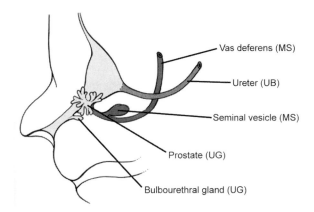

Vas deferens (MS)

Ureter (UB)

Seminal vesicle (MS)

Prostate (UG)

Bulbourethral gland (UG)

Figure 49–23. Development of male accessory sex glands. During the 10th week, the seminal vesicles sprout from the distal mesonephric ducts in response to testosterone, whereas the prostate and bulbourethral glands develop from the urethra in response to dihydrotestosterone. The vas deferens and seminal vesicle derive from the mesonephric ducts (MS), and the prostate and bulbourethral glands develop from the urogenital sinus (UG). UB, ureteric bud. (Modified from Larsen WJ: Human Embryology. New York, Churchill Livingstone, 1997.)

13th week, coincident with a rising testosterone level, the prostate begins its secretory activity. The mesenchyme surrounding the endoderm-derived prostatic acini differentiates into the smooth muscle and connective tissue of the prostate. As the prostate is developing, the paired bulbourethral glands sprout from the urethra just below the prostate.

Like renal and bladder development, prostatic development depends on mesenchymal-epithelial interactions, but under the influence of androgens (Cunha and Chung, 1981; Chung and Cunha, 1983). Studies using tissue recombination techniques have demonstrated that androgen receptor action in mesenchymal cells is essential for the induction of prostate and seminal vesicle development. This has led to the hypothesis that paracrine factors, which are produced by the mesenchyme under the influence of androgens, may control the development of the male reproductive tract. The identity of these androgen-regulated paracrine factors, however, has not been elucidated. It has been suggested that FGF10 may be a candidate mesenchymal regulator of epithelial growth in the prostate and seminal vesicle, but the FGF10 action does not appear to be regulated by androgen (Thomson and Cunha, 1999). It was demonstrated in mutant mice that the HOX family of homeobox genes may be involved in the proper differentiation of male accessory sex glands (Podlasek et al, 1997, 1999). In particular, HOXA13 and HOXD13 transcription factors are expressed in both urogenital sinus and mesonephric ducts, and the loss-of-function mutation of these genes (knock-out) results in agenesis of bulbourethral glands and defective morphogenesis of the prostate and seminal vesicles.

Development of Female Genital Structures

In female embryos, the primitive sex cords do not contain the Y chromosome, do not elaborate SRY pro- tein, and therefore do not differentiate into Sertoli cells. **In the absence of Sertoli cells and SRY protein, MIS synthesis, Leydig cell differentiation, and androgen production do not occur.** Consequently, male development of the genital ducts and accessory glands is not stimulated, and female development ensues. In females, the primitive sex cords degenerate and the mesothelium of the genital ridge forms the secondary cortical sex cords. These secondary sex cords invest the primordial germ cells to form the ovarian follicles. The germ cells differentiate into oogonia and enter the first meiotic division as primary oocytes. The follicle cells then arrest further germ cell development until puberty, at which point individual oocytes resume gametogenesis in response to a monthly surge of gonadotrophins.

In the absence of MIS, the mesonephric (wolffian) ducts degenerate and the paramesonephric (müllerian) ducts give rise to the fallopian tubes, the uterus, and the upper two thirds of the vagina. The remnants of mesonephric ducts are found in the mesentery of the ovary as the epoöphoron and paroöphoron, and near the vaginal introitus and anterolateral vaginal wall as Gartner's duct cysts (see Fig. 49–22). The distal tips of the paramesonephric ducts adhere to each other just before they contact the posterior wall of the urogenital sinus. The wall of the urogenital sinus at this point forms a small thickening called the *sinusal tubercle*. As soon as the fused tips of the paramesonephric ducts connect with the sinusal tubercle, the paramesonephric ducts begin to fuse in a caudal to cranial direction, forming a tube with a single lumen. This tube, called the *uterovaginal canal*, becomes the superior portion of the vagina and the uterus. The unfused, superior portions of the paramesonephric ducts become the fallopian tubes (oviducts), and the funnel-shaped superior openings of the paramesonephric ducts become the infundibula.

While the uterovaginal canal is forming during the 3rd month, the endodermal tissue of the sinusal tubercle in the posterior urogenital sinus continues to thicken, forming a pair of swellings called the *sinovaginal bulbs*. These structures give rise to the lower third of the vagina. The most inferior portion of the uterovaginal canal becomes occluded transiently by a block of tissue called the *vaginal plate*. The origin of the vaginal plate is not clear; it may arise from the sinovaginal bulbs, from the walls of the paramesonephric ducts, from the nearby mesonephric ducts, or from a combination of these tissues. The vaginal plate elongates between the 3rd to 5th month and subsequently becomes canalized to form the inferior vaginal lumen (Fig. 49–24).

As the vaginal plate forms, the lower end of the vagina lengthens, and its junction with the urogenital sinus migrates caudally until it comes to rest on the posterior wall of the definitive urogenital sinus (future vestibule of the vagina) during the 4th month. An endodermal membrane temporarily separates the vaginal lumen from the cavity of the definitive urogenital sinus. This barrier degenerates partially after the 5th month, but its remnant persists as the vaginal *hymen*. The mucous membrane that lines the vagina and cervix may also derive from the endodermal epithelium of the definitive urogenital sinus.

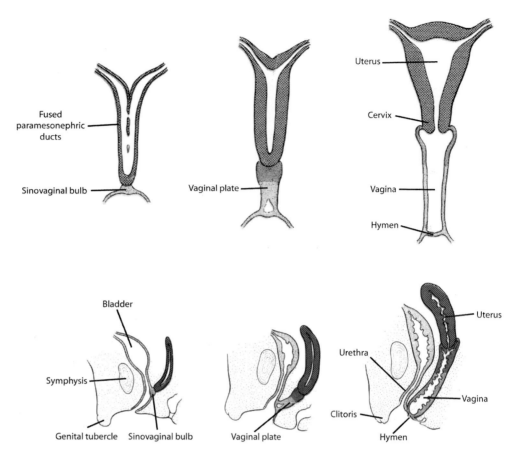

Figure 49–24. Development of uterus and vagina. During the 10th week, the paramesonephric ducts fuse at their caudal ends to establish a common channel and come into contact with a thickened portion of the posterior urogenital sinus called the sinovaginal bulb. This is followed by development of the vaginal plate, which elongates between the 3rd and the 5th month and becomes canalized to form the inferior vaginal lumen. (Modified from Sadler TW: Langman's Medical Embryology. Baltimore, Williams & Wilkins, 1985.)

Development of External Genitalia

The early development of the external genital is similar in both sexes. Early in the 5th week, a pair of swellings called *cloacal folds* develops on either side of the cloacal membrane. These folds meet just anterior to the cloacal membrane to form a midline swelling called the *genital tubercle* (Fig. 49–25). During the cloacal division into the anterior urogenital sinus and the posterior anorectal canal, the portion of the cloacal folds flanking the opening of the urogenital sinus becomes the *urogenital folds*, and the portion flanking the opening of the anorectal canal becomes the *anal folds*. A new pair of swellings, called the *labioscrotal folds*, then appears on either side of the urogenital folds (Fig. 49–26).

The most popular hypothesis of external genital development is based on work performed in the early part of the 20th century. Inherent to this type of analysis is that many of the conclusions are speculative and unproven in terms of mechanistic validity. Most embryology texts today quote the mechanism of urethral development proposed by Glenister (1954). The cavity of the urogenital sinus extends onto the surface of the enlarging genital tubercle in the form of an endoderm-lined *urethral groove* during the 6th week. This groove becomes temporarily filled by a solid endodermal structure called the *urethral plate*, but the urethral plate disintegrates and recanalizes to form an even deeper secondary groove. In males this groove is relatively long and broad, whereas in females it is shorter and more sharply tapered. In both sexes, an ectodermal *epithelial tag*

is at that time present at the tip of the genital tubercle (Fig. 49–27). The genital tubercle elongates to form the phallus, and a primordium of the glans clitoris and glans penis is demarcated from the phallic shaft by a coronary sulcus. The appearance of the external genital is similar in male and female embryos until the 12th week.

Starting in the 4th month, the effects of dihydrotestosterone on the male external genital become readily apparent. The perineal region separating the urogenital sinus from the anorectal canal begins to lengthen. The labioscrotal folds fuse in the midline to form the scrotum, and the urethral folds fuse to enclose the penile urethra. The penile urethra is completely enclosed by the 14th week. However, because the urethral groove does not extend onto the glans of the penis, the penile urethra may exist transiently as a blind-ending tube. **The formation of the distal glanular urethra may occur by a combination of two separate processes—the fusion of urethral folds proximally and the ingrowth of ectodermal cells distally.** It is generally thought that the stratified squamous lining of the fossa navicularis results from an ingrowth of surface ectoderm as far proximally as the valve of Guérin. The lacuna magna (also known as the sinus of Guérin), which can produce symptoms of hematuria and dysuria in some boys, may form as a result of dorsal extension of this ectodermal ingrowth. It has been suggested that the entire penile urethra might differentiate from the fusion of the urethral plate via the mechanism of epithelial-mesenchymal interactions (Kurzrock et al, 1999a, 1999b).

In the absence of dihydrotestosterone (in female em-

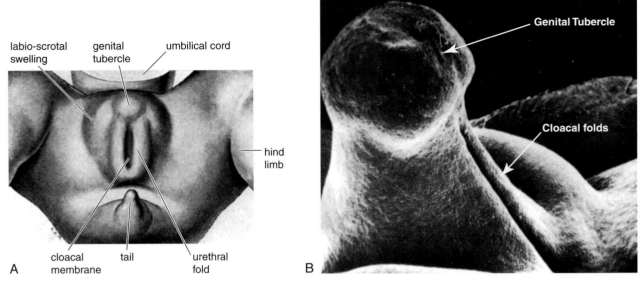

Figure 49–25. The early stages of cloacal fold development. (*A*, From Hamilton WJ, Mossman HW: Human Embryology Prenatal Development of Form and Function. New York, McMillan, 1976; *B*, from Waterman RE: Human embryo and fetus. In Hafez ESE, Kenemans P [eds]: Atlas of Human Reproduction. Hinghan, MA, Kluwer Boston, 1982.)

bryos), **the primitive perineum does not lengthen, and the labioscrotal and urethral folds do not fuse across the midline.** The phallus bends inferiorly, becoming the clitoris, and the definitive urogenital sinus becomes the vestibule of the vagina. The urethral folds become the labia minora, and the labioscrotal folds become the labia majora. **The external genitalia develop in a similar manner in genetic males who are deficient in 5α-reductase and therefore lack dihydrotestosterone.**

The information regarding the molecular mechanism of genital development is scant and incomplete. The transcription factor complex of *HOX4* genes, which has been shown to be important in the patterning and directional growth of various structures in the developing embryo, is expressed in a tissue-specific manner in the mouse genital tubercle (Dolle et al, 1991).

Gonadal Descent

During fetal development, the testes and the ovaries both descend from their original position near the 10th thoracic level. **In both sexes, the initial descent of the gonads depends on a ligamentous cord structure called the *gubernaculum*** (meaning "helm" or "rudder"). The testes complete their descent through the inguinal canal down to the scrotum, whereas the ovaries remain within the abdominal cavity. The mechanism of testicular descent is not known, but in the human fetus the most plausible theories are related to the development of the gubernaculum, processus vaginalis, inguinal canal, spermatic cord, and scrotum, because these structures differ substantially between male and female fetuses. Although it is not universally accepted that the gubernaculum holds the key to the mystery of gonadal descent, the development of this structure in the male is unique in that it offers the most obvious explanation of why the fetal testicle descends to the scrotum while the ovary does not.

During the 7th week, the gubernaculum forms within the longitudinal peritoneal folds on either side of the vertebral column. **The superior end of this cord is attached to the gonad, and its expanded inferior end, called the *gubernacular bulb*, is attached to the fascia between the developing external and internal oblique muscles in the region of the labioscrotal folds.** At the same time, a slight evagination of the peritoneum, called the *processus vaginalis*, develops adjacent to the gubernacular bulb. The inguinal canal is a caudal evagination of the abdominal wall that forms when the processus vaginalis expands inferiorly, pushing out a sock-like evagination through the abdominal wall layers. The first layer encountered by the processus vaginalis is the transversalis fascia, which lies just deep to the transversus abdominis muscle. Next, the processus picks up the muscle fibers of the internal oblique muscle, which go on to become the cremasteric muscle of the spermatic cord. Finally, the processus picks up a thin layer of the external oblique muscle, which becomes the external spermatic fascia. In males, the inguinal canal extends down to the scrotum and allows passage of the descending testicle. A complete inguinal canal also forms in females, but it appears to play no role in genital development. The processus vaginalis normally degenerates but occasionally remains patent, resulting in either a communicating hydrocele or an indirect inguinal hernia. During the 8th week, the processus vaginalis begins to elongate caudally, carrying along the gubernacular bulb.

The testicles descend to the level of internal inguinal ring by the 3rd month and complete their descent into the scrotum between the 7th and 9th month. During the early period, the relative growth of the lumbar vertebral column is probably responsible for the intra-abdominal descent of the testicles, whose position is relatively fixed by the gubernacular anchoring near the inguinal canal. The testicles remain near the internal inguinal ring between the 3rd and 7th month and later pass through the inguinal canal in response to the renewed shortening of the guber-

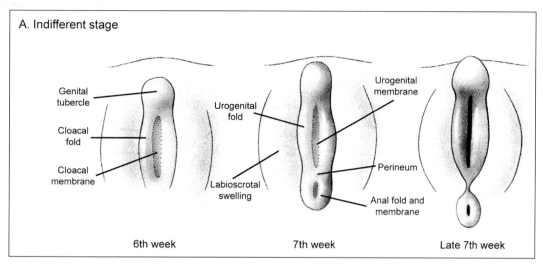

A. Indifferent stage

6th week · 7th week · Late 7th week

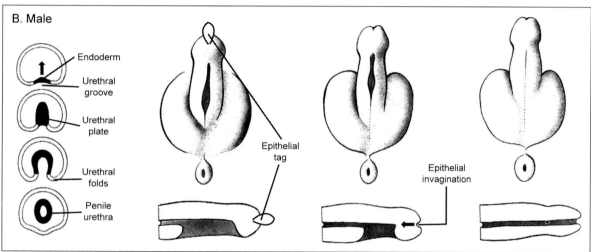

B. Male

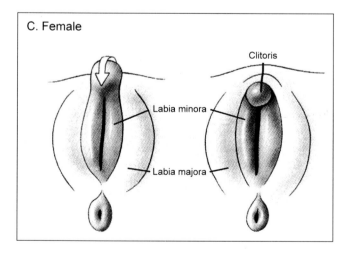

C. Female

Clitoris

Labia minora

Labia majora

Figure 49–26. Development of external genitalia in male and female fetuses. *A,* The external genitalia derive from a pair of labioscrotal swellings, a pair of urogenital folds, and an anterior genital tubercle. Male and female genitalia are morphologically indistinguishable until the 7th week. *B,* In males, the urogenital folds fuse and the genital tubercle elongates to form the penile shaft and glans. A small region of the distal urethra in the glans is formed by the invagination of surface epithelial tag. The fused labioscrotal folds give rise to the scrotum. *C,* In females, the genital tubercle bends inferiorly to form the clitoris and the urogenital folds remain separate to become the labia minora. The unfused labioscrotal folds form the labia majora. (Modified from Larsen WJ: Human Embryology. New York, Churchill Livingstone, 1997.)

naculum. This second phase of testicular descent appears to be a rapid process, probably occurring within a few days. The mechanism behind this latter event is not known, but there are several theories with varying degrees of evidence and speculation.

1. It has been suggested that active contraction by the gubernaculum and the surrounding cremasteric muscle fi-

bers provides the traction force necessary for this phase of testicular descent. Support for this theory was derived from studies of the genitofemoral nerve, which supplies the gubernaculum and the cremasteric muscle (Beasley and Hutson, 1987; Hutson et al, 1988). Division of the genitofemoral nerve in young rats resulted in the arrest of testicular descent.

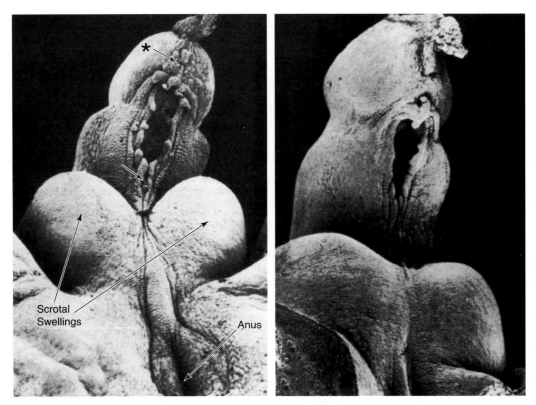

Figure 49–27. The epithelial tag and fusing urethral folds in the developing male external genital. The asterisk marks the urethral plate; age = 10 weeks; scanning electron micrograph. (From Waterman RE: Human embryo and fetus. In Hafez ESE, Kenemans P [eds]: Atlas of Human Reproduction. Hinghan MA, Kluwer Boston, 1982.)

2. Another plausible mechanism involves gubernacular shortening through the inguinal canal by means of rapid tissue swelling at its base. This morphologic change serves the secondary purpose of enlarging the inguinal canal, facilitating the passage of the testicles. In many large mammals, the gubernaculum swells in thickness until the diameter of the gubernaculum in the inguinal canal approaches that of the testicle. This process occurs primarily as the result of an increase in water and glycosaminoglycan contents as well as cellular hyperplasia and hypertrophy.

3. Increased abdominal pressure, created by the growth of the abdominal viscera and fetal respiratory efforts, may also aid the movement of the testicles through the canal. It should be noted, however, that this theory of increased intra-abdominal pressure as the force behind testicular descent does not explain the commonly observed asymmetric descent of the testes in humans. Furthermore, ovarian descent through the inguinal canal does not occur, although there is no apparent reason why the intra-abdominal pressure should be higher in males than in females.

Once they pass through the inguinal canal, the testicles remain within the subserosal fascia of the processus vaginalis, through which they descend toward the scrotum. Further descent from the external inguinal ring to the dependant portion of the scrotum may take more than 4 to 6 weeks. By the 9th month, just before normal term delivery, most testicles have completely entered the scrotal sac, and the gubernaculum is reduced to a small ligamentous band attaching the inferior pole of testis to the scrotal floor. The gonadotrophins and androgens appear to have a role as

well, although their target structures and mechanism of action remain undefined. It is generally accepted that the development of fetal spermatic vessels, vas deferens, and scrotum in regard to testicular descent is an androgen-dependent process, but this postulate has not been proven. Androgens may be responsible for the regulation of gubernacular changes leading to testicular descent. Clearly, both adequate lengthening of the spermatic vessels and vas deferens and development of the scrotum are important for full testicular descent.

The molecular mechanism of testicular descent is not known. It has been demonstrated that Leydig insulin-like hormone (Insl3) may be an important candidate molecule in the testicular descent (Nef and Parada, 1999). Insl3 is expressed in the developing testicles in rodents, and the Insl3 gene knock-out mice exhibited bilateral intra-abdominal testicles due to developmental abnormalities of the gubernaculum, with subsequent infertility.

The ovaries also descend and become suspended within the broad ligaments of the uterus. As in males, the female embryos develop a gubernaculum-like structure extending initially from the inferior pole of the gonad to the subcutaneous fascia of the presumptive labioscrotal folds. This female gubernaculum later penetrates the abdominal wall as part of a fully formed inguinal canal and becomes the *round ligament.* In females, although the gubernaculum does not shorten as it does in males, it still causes the ovaries to descend during the 3rd month (by anchoring the ovaries in the pelvis) and places them into a peritoneal fold (*the broad ligament of the uterus*). This translocation of ovaries appears to occur during the 7th week, when the gubernaculum becomes attached to the developing paramesonephric (müllerian) ducts. As the paramesonephric ducts fuse together in their caudal ends, they sweep out the broad ligaments and simultaneously pull the ovaries into these peritoneal folds. In the absence of androgens, the female gubernaculum remains intact and grows in step with the rest of the body. The inferior gubernaculum becomes the round ligament of the uterus and attaches the fascia of the labia majora to the uterus, while the superior gubernaculum becomes the ligament of the ovary, connecting the uterus to the ovary. As in males, the processus vaginalis of the inguinal canal is normally obliterated, but occasionally it remains patent to become an indirect inguinal hernia.

Molecular Mechanism of Sexual Differentiation

SRY

Mammalian embryos remain sexually undifferentiated until the time of sex determination. **When the Y-linked master regulatory gene, SRY, is expressed in the male, the epithelial cells of the primitive sex cords differentiate into Sertoli cells, and this critical morphogenetic event triggers subsequent testicular development.** Once the testicles are established, they produce androgens to give rise to the male phenotype. In the female gonads, no morphologic change is observable at the time of SRY expression. It follows from this general picture that in mammals sex determination is synonymous with testicle development, with the differentiation of Sertoli cells being the key event (McLaren, 1991). After three decades of search for the elusive mammalian testis-determining gene, the SRY gene was discovered in 1990 by Sinclair and colleagues

(Sinclair et al, 1990) (Fig. 49-28). Since then, research has focused on identifying the putative regulatory mechanism operating downstream of SRY and the genetic control of SRY expression. However, no new gene has been found thus far on the basis of analysis of the SRY protein or the SRY promoter. Subsequent studies of sex-reversed humans and the experimental induction of a variety of sex-reversing situations in rodents have identified a number of new genes involved in sex determination.

Although it has been known since 1921 that human males have an X and a Y chromosome, the role of these sex chromosomes in human sexual determination was not elucidated until 1959. This question was answered by the examination of two individuals with unique chromosome abnormalities: one female with Turner syndrome (45, X0 karyotype) and one male with Klinefelter syndrome (47, XXY karyotype). By 1966, analysis of many structurally aberrant Y chromosomes in humans led to the conclusion that **the information necessary to initiate male phenotypic development is present on the short arm of the Y chromosome.** The identity of the protein encoded by the testicle-determining region of the Y chromosome proved elusive.

In the mid-1980s, the DNA of sex-reversed males with 46,XX karyotype was examined. The genome in these individuals was found to contain small amounts of Y chromosome that had been translocated onto the X chromosome. Analysis of this DNA narrowed the location of the sex-determining region of the Y chromosome to a relatively small region within the short arm. This gene has since been designated as the SRY. The role of SRY in human sex determination was further supported by studies using mice (Greenfield and Koopman, 1996). The comparable genetic locus in mice (Sry) is activated and expressed in the genital ridge 11.5 days after coitus, just before the initiation of testicular development. Moreover, when the chromosomes

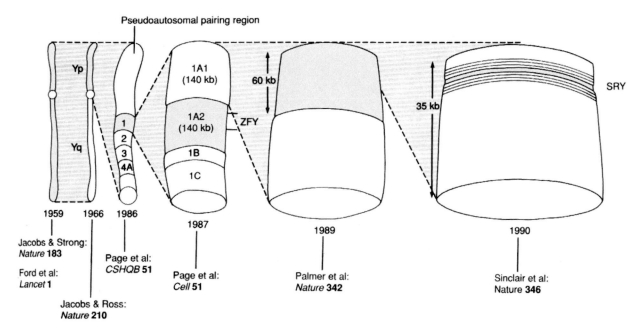

Figure 49–28. A 31-year history of the search for the sex-determining region of the Y chromosome, now designated as SRY. (Modified from McLaren A: Nature 1990;346:216.)

of a female XY mouse were analyzed with specific DNA probes for *Sry*, this locus was absent. Most importantly, it was demonstrated that insertion of *Sry* into one of the X chromosomes of genetically female mouse embryos converted the mice to phenotypic males. These transgenic female mice exhibited testicles, vas deferens, and an absence of the female reproductive tract.

It was thought that identification of the SRY protein would rapidly lead to the identity of downstream elements regulating male sexual development. So far, however, the binding of SRY protein to other genes or factors has not been demonstrated, and the molecular mechanism by which genes interact to determine sex remains speculative. It is now clear that only about 25% of sex reversals in humans can be attributed to disabling mutations of the *SRY*. Indeed, chromosomal deletions of 9p and 10q as well as duplications of Xp can also lead to a female phenotype in XY individuals despite an intact *SRY*.

WT1, SF1, SOX9, and DAX1

The activities of several new regulatory elements in male and female sexual differentiation have been described, including the Wilms' tumor gene (*WT1*), ste- roidogenic factor 1 (SF1), SOX9 (*SRY*-related transcription factor), and *DAX1* gene (Fig. 49–29).

Humans heterozygous for mutations in the *WT1* gene exhibit abnormalities of the genital system in addition to abnormalities in renal development (see "Molecular Mechanism of Kidney Development"). WT1 is expressed within the genital ridges during early gonad development in mouse and human embryos, before the expression of SRY. Therefore, it has been suggested that WT1 directly or indirectly induces the expression of SRY. In females with *WT1* mutations, the gonads may consist of undifferentiated streaks of mesenchyme. In *Wt1* knock-out mice, normal thickening of the genital ridge does not occur, even though primordial germ cells enter the presumptive gonadal tissue (Kreidberg et al, 1993).

Translocation mapping of sex-reversed patients with camptomelic dysplasia (CD) led to the identification of the *SRY*-related gene *SOX9*. 46,XY individuals with heterozygous mutations in *SOX9* show both CD and sex reversal, implying that *SOX9* is involved in both skeletal and sex determination (Foster et al, 1994). These individuals possess a normal *SRY* but may exhibit completely feminized genital structures. *SOX9* is related to *SRY* and may be structurally similar. Its gene product may, therefore, bind to

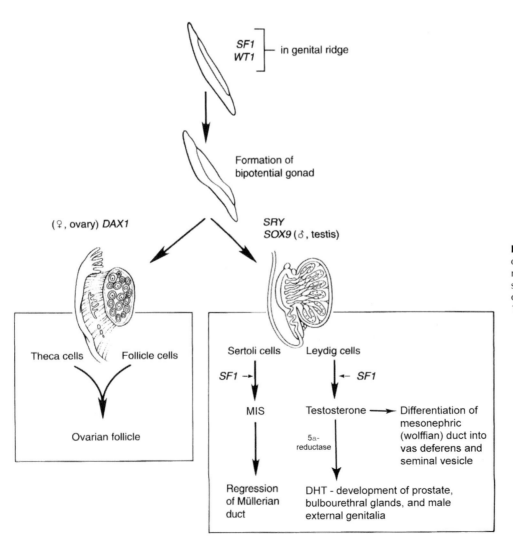

Figure 49–29. Molecular mechanism of male and female genital development. (MIS = müllerian inhibiting substance; DHT = dihydrotestosterone) (Modified from Marx J: Science 1995;270:901.)

DNA in a manner similar to the SRY protein. *SOX9* is expressed in differentiating Sertoli cells in male embryos of both mice and chickens (Morais da Silva et al, 1996).

SF1 is an orphan nuclear receptor; its best-known functions involve the regulation of steroid hydroxylase enzyme expression. This enzyme complex catalyzes multiple steps during the conversion of cholesterol to testosterone, and therefore SF1 may play an important role in the steroidogenic function of the Leydig cells. SF1 is expressed at an early stage of the genital ridge formation, and *Sf1* gene knock-out mice fail to develop gonads regardless of their genetic sex (Luo et al, 1994). These findings suggest that SF1, similar to WT1, shares a common pathway upstream of SRY, controlling the formation of the bipotential gonads. In addition, SF1 is expressed in developing Sertoli cells, implying a male-specific role (Ikeda et al, 1994), and it may be necessary in the activation of genes such as that for the MIS protein (Shen et al, 1994). As the bipotential gonad begins to differentiate, SF1 expression is maintained in the testicles but ceases in the ovaries.

The absence of a functional *DAX1* gene induces adrenal hypoplasia congenita and hypogonadotropic hypogonadism (Muscatelli et al, 1994). *DAX1* maps to the human Xp21 region, which contains *DSS* (dosage-sensitive sex reversal), a locus that causes male-to-female sex reversal when duplicated (Bardoni et al, 1994). This situation occurs despite an intact, normal *SRY*. *DAX1* gene expression persists in the developing ovaries but rapidly decreases in the testicles. This implies a key role for *DAX1* in sex determination. Because this gene is not required for testicular development, it has been suggested that *DAX1* may function as an ovarian inducer (Bardoni et al, 1994). In fact, *SRY* and *DAX1* may act antagonistically, and the precise degree and timing of their expression may be critical for the correct function of these genes during sex determination (Swain et al, 1998).

The molecular mechanisms by which *SRY* triggers testicular development are not known. Based on the available information, it seems likely that an antitestis factor produced by *DSS* (including the *DAX1* gene) functions to inhibit genes of the male pathway and that the role of *SRY* is to inhibit the action of *DSS,* permitting testis differentiation (Jimenez et al, 1996). According to this model, a single copy of *SRY* may be unable to counteract the effect of two active copies of *DSS*, so that male-to-female sex reversal would occur, as is observed in humans with a duplicate Xp21.

REFERENCES

Kidney Development

Abrahamson DR, Robert B, et al: Origins and formation of microvasculature in the developing kidney. Kidney Int Suppl 1998;67:S7–S11.

Bard JB, McConnell JE, et al: Towards a genetic basis for kidney development. Mech Dev 1994;48:3–11.

Davies JA, Bard JB: (1998). The development of the kidney. Curr Top Dev Biol 1998;39:245–301.

Davies JA, Brandli AW: The Kidney Development Database. Available at http://mbisg2.sbc.man.ac.uk/kidbase/kidhome.html and http://www.ana.ed.ac.uk/anatomy/kidbase/kidhome.html 1991

Donehower LA, Godley LA, et al: Deficiency of p53 accelerates mammary tumorigenesis in Wnt-1 transgenic mice and promotes chromosomal instability. Genes Dev 1995;9:882–895.

Godley LA, Kopp JB, et al: Wild-type p53 transgenic mice exhibit altered differentiation of the ureteric bud and possess small kidneys. Genes Dev 1996;10:836–850.

Guron G, Adams MA, et al: Neonatal angiotensin-converting enzyme inhibition in the rat induces persistent abnormalities in renal function and histology. Hypertension 1997;29(1 Pt 1):91–97.

Hatini V, Huh SO, et al: Essential role of stromal mesenchyme in kidney morphogenesis revealed by targeted disruption of Winged Helix transcription factor BF-2. Genes Dev 1996;10:1467–1478.

Hilgers KF, Reddi V, et al: Aberrant renal vascular morphology and renin expression in mutant mice lacking angiotensin-converting enzyme. Hypertension 1997;29:216–221.

Jing S, Wen D, et al: GDNF-induced activation of the ret protein tyrosine kinase is mediated by GDNFR-alpha, a novel receptor for GDNF. Cell 1996;85:1113–1124.

Karavanova ID, Dove LF, et al: Conditioned medium from a rat ureteric bud cell line in combination with bFGF induces complete differentiation of isolated metanephric mesenchyme. Development 1996;122:4159–4167.

Kispert A, Vainio S, et al: Proteoglycans are required for maintenance of Wnt-11 expression in the ureter tips. Development 1996;122:3627–3637.

Konje JC, Bell SC, et al: Human fetal kidney morphometry during gestation and the relationship between weight, kidney morphometry and plasma active renin concentration at birth. Clin Sci 1996;91:169–175.

Koseki C, Herzlinger D, et al: Apoptosis in metanephric development. J Cell Biol 1992;119:1327–1333.

Kreidberg JA, Sariola H, et al: WT-1 is required for early kidney development. Cell 1993;74:679–691.

Larsson L, Aperia A, et al: Structural and functional development of the nephron. Acta Paediatr Scand Suppl 1983;305:56–60.

Lechner MS, Dressler GR: The molecular basis of embryonic kidney development. Mech Dev 1997;62:105–120.

Lipschutz JH: Molecular development of the kidney: A review of the results of gene disruption studies. Am J Kidney Dis 1998;31:383–397.

Loughna S, Landels E, et al: Growth factor control of developing kidney endothelial cells. Exp Nephrol 1996;4:112–118.

Lumbers ER: Functions of the renin-angiotensin system during development. Clin Exp Pharmacol Physiol 1995;22:499–505.

Miyamoto N, Yoshida M, et al: Defects of urogenital development in mice lacking Emx2. Development 1997;124:1653–1664.

Moore MW, Klein RD, et al: Renal and neuronal abnormalities in mice lacking GDNF. Nature 1996;382:76–79.

Nagata M, Nakauchi H, et al: Apoptosis during an early stage of nephrogenesis induces renal hypoplasia in bcl-2-deficient mice. Am J Pathol 1996;148:1601–1611.

Nishimura H, Yerkes E, et al: Role of the angiotensin type 2 receptor gene in congenital anomalies of the kidney and urinary tract, CAKUT, of mice and men. Mol Cell 1999;3:1–10.

Patterson LT, Dressler GR: The regulation of kidney development: New insights from an old model. Curr Opin Genet Dev 1994;4:696–702.

Perantoni AO, Dove LF, et al: Basic fibroblast growth factor can mediate the early inductive events in renal development. Proc Natl Acad Sci U S A 1995;92:4696–4700.

Pichel JG, Shen L, et al: Defects in enteric innervation and kidney development in mice lacking GDNF. Nature 1996;382:73–76.

Polyak K, Waldman T, et al: Genetic determinants of p53-induced apoptosis and growth arrest. Genes Dev 1996;10:1945–1952.

Sanchez MP, Silos-Santiago I, et al: Renal agenesis and the absence of enteric neurons in mice lacking GDNF. Nature 1996;382:70–73.

Sanyanusin P, Schimmenti LA, et al: Mutation of the gene in a family with optic nerve colobomas, renal anomalies and vesicoureteral reflux. Nat Genet 1996;13:129.

Saxen L, Sariola H: Early organogenesis of the kidney. Pediatr Nephrol 1987;1:385–392.

Schmid P, Lorenz A, et al: Expression of p53 during mouse embryogenesis. Development 1991;113:857–865.

Schuchardt A, D'Agati V, et al: Defects in the kidney and enteric nervous system of mice lacking the tyrosine kinase receptor ret [see comments]. Nature 1994;367:380–383.

Schuchardt A, D'Agati V, et al: Renal agenesis and hypodysplasia in ret-k-mutant mice result from defects in ureteric bud development. Development 1996;122:1919–1929.

Schutz S, Le Moullec JM, et al: Early expression of all the components of the renin-angiotensin-system in human development [see comments]. Am J Pathol 1996;149:2067–2079.

Sedman AB, Kershaw DB, et al: Recognition and management of angiotensin converting enzyme inhibitor fetopathy. Pediatr Nephrol 1995;9: 382–385.

Shawlot W, Behringer RR: Requirement for Lim1 in head-organizer function [see comments]. Nature 1995;374:425–430.

Shotan A, Widerhorn J, et al: Risks of angiotensin-converting enzyme inhibition during pregnancy: Experimental and clinical evidence, potential mechanisms, and recommendations for use. Am J Med 1994;96: 451–456.

Stark K, Vainio S, et al: Epithelial transformation of metanephric mesenchyme in the developing kidney regulated by Wnt-4. Nature 1994;372: 679–683.

Torres M, Gomez-Pardo E, et al: Pax-2 controls multiple steps of urogenital development. Development 1995;121:4057–4065.

Tufro A, Norwood VF, et al: Vascular endothelial growth factor induces nephrogenesis and vasculogenesis. J Am Soc Nephrol 1999;10:2125–2134.

Tufro-McReddie A, Norwood VF, et al: Oxygen regulates vascular endothelial growth factor-mediated vasculogenesis and tubulogenesis. Dev Biol 1997;183:139–149.

Vainio S, Lehtonen E, et al: Epithelial-mesenchymal interactions regulate the stage-specific expression of a cell surface proteoglycan, syndecan, in the developing kidney. Dev Biol 1989;134:382–391.

Vainio S, Muller U: Inductive tissue interactions, cell signaling, and the control of kidney organogenesis. Cell 1997;90:975–978.

Vukicevic S, Kopp JB, et al: Induction of nephrogenic mesenchyme by osteogenic protein 1 (bone morphogenetic protein 7). Proc Natl Acad Sci U S A 1996;93:9021–9026.

Weller A, Sorokin L, et al: Development and growth of mouse embryonic kidney in organ culture and modulation of development by soluble growth factor. Dev Biol 1991;144:248–261.

Bladder and Ureter Development

Alcaraz A, Vinaixa F, et al: Obstruction and recanalization of the ureter during embryonic development. J Urol 1991;145:410–416.

Baker LA, Gomez RA: Embryonic development of the ureter and bladder: Acquisition of smooth muscle. J Urol 1998;160:545–550.

Baskin LS, Hayward SW, et al: Role of mesenchymal-epithelial interactions in normal bladder development. J Urol 1996;156:1820–1827.

Baskin L, Meaney D, et al: Bovine bladder compliance increases with normal fetal development. J Urol 1994;152:692–695; discussion 696–697.

Beauboeuf A, Ordille S, et al: In vitro ligation of ureters and urethra modulates fetal mouse bladder explants development. Tissue Cell 1998; 30:531–536.

Bourdelat D, Barbet JP, et al: Fetal development of the urethral sphincter. Eur J Pediatr Surg 1992;2:35–38.

Coplen DE, Macarak EJ, et al: Developmental changes in normal fetal bovine whole bladder physiology. J Urol 1994;151:1391–1395.

Escala JM, Keating MA, et al: Development of elastic fibres in the upper urinary tract. J Urol 1989;141:969–973.

Hohenfellner K, Hunley TE, et al: Angiotensin type 2 receptor is important in the normal development of the ureter. Pediatr Nephrol 1999;13: 187–191.

Kakuchi J, Ichiki T, et al: Developmental expression of renal angiotensin II receptor genes in the mouse. Kidney Int 1995;47:140–147.

Kim KM, Kogan BA, et al: Collagen and elastin in the normal fetal bladder. J Urol 1991;146:524–527.

Kluth D, Hillen M, et al: The principles of normal and abnormal hindgut development. J Pediatr Surg 1995;30:1143–1147.

Mackie GG, Stephens FD: Duplex kidneys: A correlation of renal dysplasia with position of the ureteric orifice. Birth Defects: Original Article Series 1977;13:313–321.

Newman J, Antonakopoulos GN: The fine structure of the human fetal urinary bladder: Development and maturation. A light, transmission and scanning electron microscopic study. J Anat 1989;166:135–150.

Nievelstein RA, van der Werff JF, et al: Normal and abnormal embryonic development of the anorectum in human embryos. Teratology 1998;57: 70–78.

Nishimura H, Yerkes E, et al: Role of the angiotensin type 2 receptor gene in congenital anomalies of the kidney and urinary tract, CAKUT, of mice and men. Mol Cell 1999;3:1–10.

Schwarz R, Stephens FD: The persisting mesonephric duct: High junction of vas deferens and ureter. J Urol 1978;120:592–596.

Tichy M: The morphogenesis of human sphincter urethrae muscle. Anat Embryol (Berl) 1989;180:577–582.

van der Putte SC: Normal and abnormal development of the anorectum. J Pediatr Surg 1986;21:434–440.

Genital Development

Bardoni B, Zanaria E, et al: A dosage sensitive locus at chromosome Xp21 is involved in male to female sex reversal. Nat Genet 1994;7: 497–501.

Beasley SW, Hutson JM: Effect of division of genitofemoral nerve on testicular descent in the rat. Aust N Z J Surg 1987;57:49–51.

Behringer RR: The in vivo roles of mullerian-inhibiting substance. Curr Top Dev Biol 1994;29:171–187.

Chung LW, Cunha GR: Stromal-epithelial interactions: II. Regulation of prostatic growth by embryonic urogenital sinus mesenchyme. Prostate 1983;4:503–511.

Cunha GR, Chung LW: Stromal-epithelial interactions: I. Induction of prostatic phenotype in urothelium of testicular feminized (Tfm/y) mice. J Steroid Biochem Mol Biol 1981;14:1317–1324.

Dolle P, Izpisua-Belmonte JC, et al: HOX-4 genes and the morphogenesis of mammalian genitalia. Genes Dev 1991;5:1767–1777.

Foster JW, Dominguez-Steglich MA, et al: Camptomelic dysplasia and autosomal sex reversal caused by mutations in an SRY-related gene. Nature 1994;372:525–530.

Glenister TW: The origin and fate of the urethral plate in man. J Anat 1954;88:413–424.

Greenfield A, Koopman P: SRY and mammalian sex determination. Curr Top Dev Biol 1996;34:1–23.

Hutson JM, Beasley SW, et al: Cryptorchidism in spina bifida and spinal cord transection: A clue to the mechanism of transinguinal descent of the testis. J Pediatr Surg 1988;23:275–277.

Ikeda Y, Shen WH, et al: Developmental expression of mouse steroidogenic factor-1, an essential regulator of the steroid hydroxylases. Mol Endocrinol 1994;8:654–662.

Jimenez R, Sanchez A, et al: Puzzling out the genetics of mammalian sex determination. Trends Genet 1996;12:164–166.

Kreidberg JA, Sariola H, et al: WT-1 is required for early kidney development. Cell 1993;74:679–691.

Kurzrock EA, Baskin LS, et al: Ontogeny of the male urethra: Theory of endodermal differentiation. Differentiation 1999a;64:115–122.

Kurzrock EA, Baskin LS, et al: Epithelial-mesenchymal interactions in development of the mouse fetal genital tubercle. Cells Tissues Organs 1999b;164:125–130.

Luo X, Ikeda Y, et al: A cell-specific nuclear receptor is essential for adrenal and gonadal development and sexual differentiation. Cell 1994; 77:481–490.

McLaren A: Development of the mammalian gonad: The fate of the supporting cell lineage. Bioessays 1991;13:151–156.

Morais da Silva S, Hacker A, et al: Sox9 expression during gonadal development implies a conserved role for the gene in testis differentiation in mammals and birds. Nat Genet 1996;14:62–68.

Muscatelli F, Strom TM, et al: Mutations in the DAX-1 gene give rise to both X-linked adrenal hypoplasia congenita and hypogonadotropic hypogonadism. Nature 1994;372:672–676.

Nef S, Parada LF: Cryptorchidism in mice mutant for Insl3. Nat Genet 1999;22:295–299.

Podlasek CA, Clemens JQ, et al: Hoxa-13 gene mutation results in abnormal seminal vesicle and prostate development. J Urol 1999;161:1655–1661.

Podlasek CA, Duboule D, et al: Male accessory sex organ morphogenesis is altered by loss of function of Hoxd-13. Dev Dyn 1997;208:454–465.

Shen WH, Moore CC, et al: Nuclear receptor steroidogenic factor 1 regulates the mullerian inhibiting substance gene: A link to the sex determination cascade. Cell 1994;77:651–661.

Sinclair AH, Berta P, et al: A gene from the human sex-determining region encodes a protein with homology to a conserved DNA-binding motif [see comments]. Nature 1990;346:240–244.

Swain A, Narvaez V, et al: Dax1 antagonizes Sry action in mammalian sex determination. Nature 1998;391:761–767.

Thomson AA, Cunha GR: Prostatic growth and development are regulated by FGF10. Development 1999;126:3693–3701.

50
RENAL FUNCTION IN THE FETUS, NEONATE, AND CHILD

Robert Chevalier, MD
Stuart S. Howards, MD

The development of renal function in the fetus and neonate can be viewed as a continuing evolution of interdependent morphologic and physiologic stages. During gestation, the functional changes are determined by increases in nephron number, growth, and maturation, while homeostasis of the fetus is maintained predominantly by the placenta. At birth, the kidney must suddenly assume this previously maternal role. The kidney's response to this demand is governed to a great extent by its anatomic development (gestational age at delivery), and important functional differences are seen in the premature and term neonate.

This chapter reviews the anatomic and functional aspects of fetal renal development, postnatal functional development, the evaluation of postnatal renal function, and the hormonal control of renal function during development through childhood.

ANATOMIC STAGES OF DEVELOPMENT

The major morphogenic stages of the human kidney appear quite early in development and, except for the last one, are transitory (Fig. 50–1) (Potter, 1972). **The pronephros appears at 3 weeks, never progresses beyond a rudimentary stage, and involutes by 5 weeks. The mesonephros is seen at 5 weeks of gestation, appears to have transitory function, and degenerates by 11 or 12 weeks. Its major role in renal development is related to the fact that its ductal system gives rise to the ureteric bud.** The latter is critical for development of the metanephric or definitive kidney. Studies have revealed that apoptosis is a primary mechanism responsible for the sequential development of the mammalian kidney. Apoptosis is a physiologic,

1765

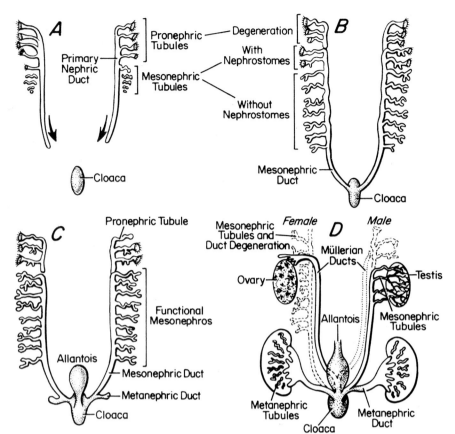

Figure 50–1. Relations of pronephros, mesonephros, and metanephros at various stages of development. To simplify, the tubules have been drawn as if they had been pulled out to the side of the ducts. The first rudimentary pronephros (A) is elaborated as a group of tubules emptying on either side into the primary nephric ducts, which extend caudad to discharge ultimately into the cloaca. A little later in development there arises a second group of tubules, more caudal in position than the pronephric tubules; these are the mesonephric tubules. In their growth they extend toward the primary nephric ducts and soon open into them (B). The plan (C) represents approximately the conditions attained by the human embryo toward the end of the 4th week. The diagram (D) depicts the conditions after sexual differentiation has taken place: female left side, male right side. The müllerian ducts arise in human embryos during the 8th week, in close association with the mesonephric ducts. The müllerian ducts are the primordial tubes from which the oviducts, uterus, and vagina of the female are formed. Note that although both mesonephric and müllerian ducts appear in all young embryos, the müllerian ducts become vestigial in the male and the mesonephric ducts become vestigial in the female. (From Patten BM: Human Embryology. New York, McGraw-Hill, 1968, p 450, with permission.)

programmed cell death that normally mediates the deletion of "unwanted" cells, such as the disappearance of uninduced metanephric mesenchyme (Koseki et al, 1992). **The metanephros begins its inductive phase after 5 weeks of gestation, and in the human nephrogenesis is completed by 34 to 36 weeks.** In the developing metanephric kidney, there is a centrifugal pattern of nephrogenesis and maturation, with the outer cortical nephrons being the last to complete development.

FUNCTIONAL DEVELOPMENT IN THE FETUS

Information regarding the functional development of the metanephric kidney is gained primarily through animal studies. One must be careful in extrapolating such data from species in which there is dissimilarity of structural maturation at comparable gestational ages. **Urine production in the human kidney is known to begin at about 10 to 12 weeks.** However, the placenta primarily handles salt and water homeostasis throughout gestation.

Fetal renal blood flow remains at a relatively low, stable rate in utero. The ratio of renal blood flow to cardiac output at 20 weeks is 0.03, whereas the postnatal ratio is between 0.2 and 0.3 (Rudolph and Heymann, 1976). This diminished renal blood flow is probably related to several different factors. The number of vascular channels is low early in gestation, and there is increased arteriolar resistance in these channels (Ichikawa et al, 1979; Robillard et al, 1987). Studies in animals have demonstrated a role for

renal innervation and for the renin-angiotensin system as chronic modulators of this effect (Robillard et al, 1987). These factors are discussed in greater detail later in this chapter.

The glomerular filtration rate (GFR) in the fetus is theoretically equal to the GFR of a single nephron times the number of functioning glomeruli. This is difficult to determine however, because the **GFR is much higher in juxtamedullary than in subcortical glomeruli** (Spitzer and Brandis, 1974). GFR parallels renal mass and correlates with gestational age as nephrogenesis continues from 10 to 12 weeks of gestation until 34 weeks (Smith and Robillard, 1989).

Fractional excretion of sodium (FENa) shows a negative correlation with gestational age. **The fetus produces hypotonic urine with high sodium content and in large volumes.** Potassium excretion similarly increases with gestation, which may be related to rises in fetal plasma aldosterone concentration. There is a maturational increase in glucose transport of the fetal kidneys. Other tubular functions, such as bicarbonate reabsorption and acid production, are low in the fetus. They are, however, each responsive to parathyroid excretion, intravascular volume, and acid infusion.

EVALUATION OF FETAL RENAL FUNCTION

Human fetal renal blood flow can be measured by color-pulsed Doppler ultrasound studies, which indicate that blood flow increases from approximately 20 ml/min at 25 weeks of gestation to more than 60 ml/min at 40 weeks (Veille et al, 1993). **Hourly human fetal urine production (determined by serial real-time bladder ultrasonography at 2- to 5-minute intervals) increases from 5 ml/hr at 20 weeks of gestation to 50 ml/hr at 40 weeks** (Rabinowitz et al, 1989). This extraordinary rate of diuresis would extrapolate to approximately 1 L/hr in the adult.

Because of urinary dilution, the human fetal urine sodium concentration is normally less than 100 mEq/L, chloride is less than 90 mEq/L, and osmolality is less than 200 mOsm/L (Crombleholme et al, 1990). Although urine values greater than these in fetuses with obstructive nephropathy have been correlated with a poor prognosis, reports indicate that sequential fetal urine samples must be obtained, both before and after intrauterine bladder shunting, to improve the predictive value (Evans et al, 1991; Johnson et al, 1994).

More recently, a urine total protein concentration of less than 20 mg/dl and β_2-microglobulin less than 4 mg/L have been shown to correlate with a favorable prognosis (Johnson et al, 1994). Other indices of tubular function include the measurement of amniotic fluid N-acetyl-D-glucosaminidase (NAG, an enzyme present in high concentration in proximal tubular cells) and of specific amino acids in fetal urine (Pachi et al, 1993; Eugene et al, 1994). Increased amniotic fluid NAG has been correlated with renal impairment of intrauterine growth retardation (Pachi et al, 1993), and fetal urine valine concentration is increased in fetuses with bilateral renal dysplasia and fetal or neonatal death (Eugene et al, 1994).

POSTNATAL FUNCTIONAL DEVELOPMENT

At birth, several dramatic events occur which alter renal function. The kidney's response to the changing milieu and its success at maintaining homeostasis are heavily influenced by the gestational age at delivery. Intrauterine factors can also significantly affect postnatal renal functional development: intrauterine growth retardation can permanently reduce the number of functioning nephrons (Merlet-Benichou et al, 1994). This may lead to renal failure manifesting at birth (Steele et al, 1988).

In a study of 500 normal neonates, Clark (1977) found that **every infant voided within the first 24 hours of life, regardless of gestational age.** After the first 2 days of life, oliguria is generally defined as a urine flow rate slower than 1 ml/kg/hr (Anand, 1982). However, infants receiving a restricted solute intake can remain in solute balance with urine flow rates as low as 0.5 ml/kg/hr.

The definition of polyuria is somewhat arbitrary, but any infant or child excreting more than 2000 ml/1.73 m² daily urine output should be evaluated further. It is important to distinguish pollakiuria (urinary frequency) from polyuria in the child, because the former can be a sign of emotional stress rather than a pathologic process (Asnes and Mones, 1973; Zoubek et al, 1990).

Renal blood flow increases sharply at birth, with a 5- to 18-fold rise having been demonstrated in different animal studies (Gruskin et al, 1970; Aperia and Herin, 1975). This reflects several factors. There is a redistribution of flow from the inner to the outer cortex (Aperia et al, 1977), and there is a drop in renal vascular resistance associated with increased intrarenal prostaglandins (Gruskin et al, 1970).

GFR doubles during the first week in term infants (Guignard et al, 1975). Because of the dependence of GFR on gestational age, GFR rises slowly for infants born before 34 weeks. After the neonate reaches a postconceptional age of 34 weeks, a rapid rise is then observed. **Factors responsible for this rapid rise include diminished renal vascular resistance** (Gruskin et al, 1970) **and increasing perfusion pressure, glomerular permeability, and filtration surface** (John et al, 1981). **In experimental animals, the increase in surface area for filtration accounts for most of the maturational increase in GFR** (Spitzer and Brandis, 1974). Serum creatinine, which reflects maternal levels at birth, also decreases by 50% in the first week of life in term or near-term infants. GFR continues to rise, reaching adult levels by 2 years of age (Rubin et al, 1949). Moreover, in very-low-birth-weight infants, GFR does not catch up to that of term infants of the same postconceptional age until more than 9 months after birth (Vanpee et al, 1992).

In the neonate, tubular function changes in association with the rise in GFR. There remains a blunted response to sodium loading, however, due to a lack of increase in FENa (Kim and Mandell, 1988). This appears to be related to the high circulating renin, angiotensin, and aldosterone levels and to a diminished renal response to atrial natriuretic peptide (see later discussion). Conversely, **premature infants of less than 35 weeks' gestation, subject to sodium deprivation may develop hyponatremia due to tubular immaturity and sodium wasting** (Roy et al, 1976; Engelke et al, 1978). Therefore, sodium supplementation is frequently required in premature infants.

In terms of concentrating ability, **the neonate can dilute fairly well (25 to 35 mOsm/L) but has limited concentrating capacity (600 to 700 mOsm/L)** (Hansen and Smith, 1953). The latter is even more restricted in the premature infant (500 mOsm/L). The factors responsible for this difference include anatomic immaturity of the renal medulla, decreased medullary concentration of sodium chloride and urea, and diminished responsiveness of the collecting ducts to antidiuretic hormone (Stanier, 1972; Schlondorff et al, 1978). By 8 years of age, the maximal concentrating ability of very-low-birth-weight infants is not different from that of term infants (Vanpee et al, 1992).

Acid-base regulation in the neonate is characterized by a reduced threshold for bicarbonate reabsorption (Svenningsen, 1974). Bicarbonate reabsorption is gradually increased with increasing GFR. There is also an inability to respond to an acid load. This improves by 4 to 6 weeks postnatally and is accentuated in the premature infant, who tends to be slightly acidotic in comparison with the adult.

Glucose transport matures with the rising GFR in the neonate. This is more readily observed in the premature infant because the fractional excretion of glucose is higher before 34 weeks of gestation (Arant, 1978).

Calcium/phosphate metabolism also changes shortly after birth. Parathyroid hormone (PTH) is suppressed at birth, and serum calcium falls. This secondarily causes an increase in PTH release. Initially tubular reabsorption of phosphate is high in the premature infant, and it remains so until regular feedings commence at term (Arant, 1978).

Although not generally identified as a significant renal compartment, the renal interstitium also undergoes developmental changes. After the differentiation of the interstitial mesenchyme and apoptotic destruction of unwanted undifferentiated interstitial cells, interstitial fibroblasts undergo changes, with decreasing expression of α smooth muscle actin and vimentin (Marxer-Meier et al, 1998). There is increasing evidence that the renal interstitium plays a crucial role in the maintenance of normal homeostasis, mediating cross-talk between tubular epithelial cells, extracellular matrix, fibroblasts, and endothelial cells (Fine et al, 1995; Zhuo et al, 1998). **Disruption of the interstitium by renal maldevelopment or injury would clearly be expected to impair ongoing development and tubular transport** (Wolf, 1999).

EVALUATION OF RENAL FUNCTION IN THE INFANT AND CHILD

Glomerular Function

Measurement of GFR in the infant is problematic for a number of reasons. The primary difficulty is obtaining an accurately timed urine collection in the incontinent patient without bladder catheterization. The second is the inherent inaccuracy in measurement of the most readily available index of GFR, plasma creatinine concentration: precision of the assay in most clinical laboratories is ±0.3 mg/dl.

CREATININE CLEARANCE
(ml/min/1.73 M²)

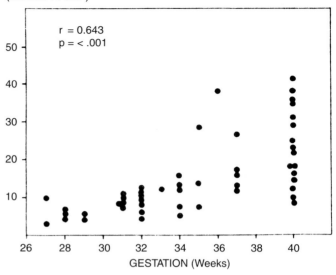

Figure 50–3. Creatinine clearance in relation to gestational age in clinically well infants studied from 24 to 40 hours after birth. (Reproduced from Siegel SR, Oh W: Renal function as a marker of human fetal maturation. Acta Paediatr Scand 1976;65:481–485.)

Therefore, the calculated GFR in the infant can be overestimated or underestimated by 100% under the best circumstances of sample collections. The third problem is the rapidly changing GFR with normal growth: GFR factored for adult surface area (1.73 m²) increases several-fold during the first 2 months of life (Fig. 50–2). Moreover, GFR increases with postconceptional age from 34 to 40 weeks' gestation (Fig. 50–3). Within the first 2 days of life, the plasma creatinine concentration reflects maternal levels and may not reflect the GFR of the infant. **By 7 days in the term infant, the plasma creatinine concentration is normally less than 1 mg/dl, whereas in preterm infants the level can remain as high as 1.5 mg/dl for the first month of life** (Trompeter et al, 1983). In view of these considerations, it is important to obtain serial values of serum creatinine. A progressive increase in serum creatinine during the neonatal period suggests renal insufficiency regardless of gestational age.

Long-term monitoring of GFR in children with urologic abnormalities should account for the increasing muscle mass that results in increasing serum creatinine concentration with age. A simple and reliable estimate of creatinine clearance (CCr) can be derived from the serum creatinine concentration and the patient's height using the empiric formula developed by Schwartz and colleagues (Schwartz et al, 1987):

$$CCr = k \times L/PCr$$

where CCr = creatinine concentration (ml/min/1.73 m²), k = a constant (0.33 for preterm infants, 0.45 for full-term infants, 0.55 for children), and L = body length (cm). **Although CCr is constant at 80 to 140 ml/min/1.73 m² after 2 years of age, the marked increase during the first 2 years of life should be taken into account when interpreting values for young infants.**

CREATININE CLEARANCE
(ml/min/1.73 M²)

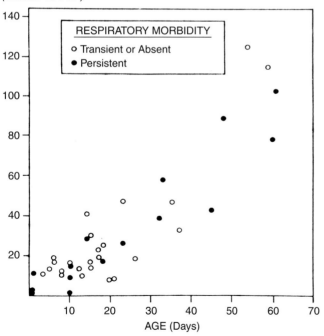

Figure 50–2. Creatinine clearance in relation to postnatal age during the first 60 days of life for preterm infants (mean birth weight, 1380 g; mean gestational age, 31 weeks). (From Ross B, Cowett RM, Oh W: Renal functions of low birth weight infants during the first two months of life. Pediatr Res 1977;11:1161–1164.)

A more accurate determination of GFR can be obtained by measuring CCr based on a 24-hour urine collection. As with the estimated CCr just described, the value should be corrected for adult surface area by multiplying by 1.73 and dividing by the patient's surface area (SA), derived from a nomogram (Cole, 1984):

$$\text{CCr (ml/min/1.73 m}^2\text{)} = \text{"uncorrected" CCr (ml/min)} \times 1.73/\text{SA}$$

Expression of all pediatric CCr measurements in this fashion should reduce confusion and ambiguity in comparing the results to expected normal ranges (see Figs. 50–2 and 50–3). It should be emphasized that the accuracy of the calculated CCr depends on the adequacy of the timed urine collection.

For more precise measurement of GFR, and to determine the relative contribution of each kidney to total GFR, a radiolabeled tracer that is cleared solely by glomerular filtration can be infused intravenously and plasma concentration of the isotope measured sequentially with concurrent scintigraphy. An agent frequently used for this purpose is technetium 99m-diethylenetriaminepentaacetic acid (Tc-DTPA). Although the precision of measurement of Tc-DTPA is greater than of creatinine and urine collection is not required, adequate venous access and patient cooperation during scintigraphy are necessary. The latter may limit the usefulness of the technique in infants and small children. As with CCr, measurement of GFR by Tc-DTPA clearance should be corrected for adult surface area, as described earlier.

Tubular Function

Sodium Excretion

In the fetus and neonate, external sodium balance is positive as a consequence of the sodium accretion necessary for rapid growth. In older infants and children, however, urinary sodium excretion is generally equivalent to sodium intake as long as the patient is in a steady state. **The 24-hour urine sodium excretion reflects the quantity of sodium ingested over the previous day and is normally 1 to 3 mEq/kg.** Patients with obligatory renal sodium losses ("salt wasting") must increase sodium intake to compensate for these ongoing losses. A diagnosis of salt-wasting nephropathy must be made while the patient is maintained on a restricted sodium intake (less than 1 mEq/kg/day) for 3 to 5 days. To prevent dangerous volume depletion or hyponatremia, the patient's blood pressure, weight, urine output, and serum sodium concentration should be closely monitored during the study. The 24-hour urine sodium excretion can also be helpful in monitoring compliance of patients on a restricted sodium intake, such as those with hypertension, nephrogenic diabetes insipidus, or nephrotic syndrome. Patients with sodium excretion greater than 3 mEq/kg/day may be counseled to improve their diets.

Of even greater clinical utility, the fraction of filtered sodium appearing in the urine (FENa) can be used to isolate the tubular from the glomerular contribution to so-dium excretion. This may be used to distinguish "prerenal" causes of oliguria from "renal parenchymal" or "postrenal" causes. A timed urine collection is not necessary, because sodium and creatinine concentration can be measured in a random urine sample (U_{Na} and U_{Cr}, respectively) obtained with a concurrent plasma sample (P_{Na} and P_{Cr}, respectively):

$$\text{FENa} = 100\%(U_{Na} \times P_{Cr})/(P_{Na} \times U_{Cr})$$

In the oliguric neonate (urine flow less than 1 ml/kg/hr), FENa less than 2.5% suggests a prerenal condition (Mathew et al, 1980)**; in the older infant or child, a value below 1% is consistent with prerenal oliguria.** Similar criteria can be used to differentiate causes of hyponatremia: FENa is increased in renal sodium wasting, adrenal insufficiency, and the syndrome of inappropriate antidiuretic hormone secretion (SIADH). In each case, the urine sample must be obtained (by bladder catheterization if necessary) before administration of any drugs that affect urine sodium excretion (e.g., diuretics).

Urinary Acidification

Although renal insufficiency can interfere with urinary acidification, retention of organic acids due to decreased GFR results in an increase in unmeasured anions. In renal tubular acidosis (RTA), this "anion gap" is in the normal range (5 to 15 mEq/L), and is defined as follows (values represent plasma concentration of respective electrolytes):

$$\text{Anion gap} = P_{Na} - [P_{Cl} + P_{HCO_3}]$$

The diagnosis of RTA should be considered in any infant or child with failure to thrive, because chronic systemic acidosis impairs growth. In addition, RTA can lead to nephrocalcinosis or nephrolithiasis (see later discussion).

A classification of RTA has been developed, based on the nephron segment affected and the transport defect involved. RTA can result from defective distal tubular acidification (type I), decreased threshold for proximal tubular bicarbonate reabsorption (type II), a combined proximal and distal abnormality (type III), or a distal defect involving impaired potassium secretion (type IV). **During the first 3 weeks of life, the threshold for bicarbonate reabsorption can be as low as 14.5 mEq/L in the normal infant** (Brown et al, 1978). This should not be regarded as RTA, because treatment with alkali has been shown not to alter growth and development in these infants (Brown et al, 1978). Congenital hydronephrosis can result in type I or type IV RTA in the infant or child (Hutcheon et al, 1976; Rodriguez-Soriano et al, 1983). **Appropriate evaluation and treatment are important to prevent the sequelae of RTA, which include growth retardation, osteodystrophy, nephrocalcinosis or nephrolithiasis, and polyuria.**

The approach to the infant or child with suspected RTA is shown in Figure 50–4. The presence of metabolic acidosis in the infant can be difficult to ascertain on the basis of serum total CO_2, because problems in obtaining the sample (e.g., venous access, small sample volume) can result in spuriously low values. It is therefore important to obtain the sample from a vein with good blood flow and to

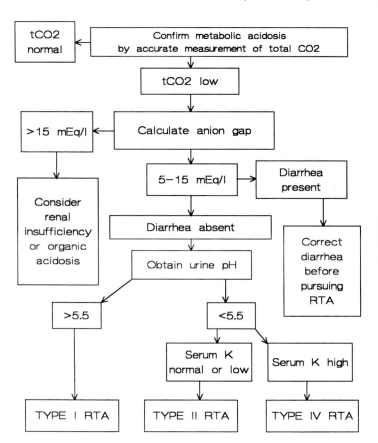

Figure 50–4. Evaluation of suspected renal tubular acidosis in the infant. See text for details.

transfer it expeditiously to the laboratory in a capped syringe on ice (as with arterial blood for blood gas analysis). Accurate measurement of urine pH is also crucial to making the diagnosis, and a urine sample should be obtained at the time of the blood sample from a freshly voided or bagged specimen. Urine should be withdrawn into a syringe, the air should be expressed, and the sample should be transferred immediately to the laboratory for measurement by pH meter (dipsticks are not sufficiently accurate). **A urine pH lower than 5.5 in the face of a total CO_2 concentration lower than normal for the patient's age suggests gastrointestinal bicarbonate loss or a defect in proximal tubular bicarbonate reabsorption with intact distal acidification (type II RTA), whereas an inappropriately high urine pH is consistent with distal or type I RTA. An elevated serum potassium concentration in the face of normal renal function suggests type IV RTA.**

Because of the difficulty in infants of pursuing bicarbonate infusion to rule out type II or acid infusion to rule out type I, alternate approaches have been developed to define the type of RTA. The simplest is to initiate alkali therapy with sodium bicarbonate or sodium citrate (Shohl's solution or Bicitra) at a dose of 3 mEq/kg/day divided in four doses. The aim is to increase serum total CO_2 to the normal range (generally greater than 20 mEq/L) and to raise urine pH above 7.8. Patients with type II RTA or infants with type I may require much greater doses of alkali (10 mEq/kg/day or more) to maintain a normal plasma total CO_2 concentration and to allow a normal growth rate. The fractional excretion of bicarbonate can then be calculated from random paired blood and urine samples, as for FENa (discussed earlier).

In contrast to types I and IV, in which the fractional bicarbonate excretion is less than 15%, the value in type II is greater than 15% owing to the reduced threshold for bicarbonate reabsorption (Chan, 1983). An alternate method to distinguish type II from other forms of RTA is to measure blood and urine partial pressure of carbon dioxide (PCO_2) after correction of acidosis with alkali therapy. In patients with type II the difference between urine and blood PCO_2 is greater than 20 mm Hg, and in those with type I it is less than 15 mm Hg (Donckerwolke et al, 1983).

A third option to identify patients with a distal tubular acidification defect (type I or IV) is to calculate the urinary anion gap (where values represent urinary concentration of respective electrolytes):

$$\text{Urinary anion gap (mEq/L)} = U_{Na} + U_K - U_{Cl}$$

Normal patients and those with intact distal urinary acidification have a negative urinary anion gap, whereas those with type I or IV RTA have a positive gap (Batlle et al, 1988).

Although the described studies should permit separation of type II from types I and IV RTA, the latter two forms are usually distinguishable (before treatment with alkali) by the presence of hyperkalemia in type IV but not type I. In addition, infusion of furosemide, 1 mg/kg, should result in acidification of urine in patients with type IV but not in those with type I (Stine and Linshaw, 1985).

Although there are a number of causes of RTA in children (Chan, 1983), **congenital obstructive nephropathy** (Hutcheon et al, 1976; Rodriguez-Soriano et al, 1983) and Fanconi syndrome should always be considered (see later discussion). **Serum electrolytes, calcium, phosphorus, PTH, and thyroid function tests should be obtained. A urinalysis should be performed, to screen for glucosuria. In addition, the urine amino acid pattern may reveal diffuse aminoaciduria. A 24-hour urine collection should be obtained for calculation of CCr, protein excretion, calcium excretion, and tubular reabsorption of phosphorus** (see later discussion). **Sonographic examination of the urinary tract should be performed not only to identify hydronephrosis but also to reveal nephrocalcinosis or nephrolithiasis that can develop in children with type I RTA.**

As described earlier, most infants and children with RTA respond well to alkali therapy (sodium bicarbonate or Shohl's solution). However, some patients with type IV RTA have persistent hyperkalemia despite correction of acidosis. This situation can be managed by administration of chlorothiazide, 10 to 20 mg/kg/day, or polystyrene sodium sulfonate (Kayexalate) 1 g/kg/day. Patients receiving diuretics need to be monitored closely for development of volume contraction, which can actually reduce potassium excretion. Infants receiving Kayexalate may undergo volume expansion from the exchange of sodium for potassium and may develop bowel obstruction from inspissated resin in the intestinal tract. As long as adequate GFR is maintained, treatment for most children with RTA caused by urologic abnormalities should continue indefinitely to ensure normal growth and to prevent complications such as nephrocalcinosis. **The dose of alkali may need to be adjusted every 3 to 6 months in the rapidly growing infant.**

Urinary Concentration

Most disorders of urinary concentration in infants and children are caused by renal maldevelopment (renal dysplasia or obstructive nephropathy), interstitial nephritis (pyelonephritis), or renal insufficiency. Additional causes include renal tubular acidosis, sickle-cell nephropathy, and medullary cystic disease. These generally result in a mild to moderate impairment in concentration, such that the urine specific gravity is greater than 1.005. Evaluation should include determinations of serum electrolytes, blood urea nitrogen (BUN), and creatinine; urinalysis and urine culture; renal ultrasonography; and possibly a voiding cystourethrogram. Infants with diabetes insipidus usually have a urine specific gravity consistently less than 1.005.

There is no physiologic definition of polyuria, and screening of urinary concentrating ability may be initiated based on parental concern regarding excessive voiding frequency. Measurement of urine output and interpretation of thirst in the infant is problematic. For these reasons, the infant with unexplained dehydration or hypernatremia should be screened for a urine concentrating defect.

A urine specific gravity greater than 1.020 generally rules out a serious abnormality of urinary concentration. In the young infant, overnight fluid restriction can result in dangerous volume depletion and hypernatremia. Such patients should undergo a formal water deprivation test in the hospital. This should begin with fluid restriction starting in the morning, with close monitoring of body weight and vital signs until loss of 3% body weight or

until the urine osmolality exceeds 600 mOsm in neonates or 800 mOsm in older infants and children. If tachycardia or hypotension develops at any time, the test should be terminated.

In patients who fail to produce a concentrated urine during water deprivation, fluid should be restricted on a separate day, and desmopressin (DDAVP, 10 μg for infants, or 20 μg for children) is instilled into the nostrils. Urine osmolality should be measured at 2-hour intervals for 4 to 6 hours. Renal response to DDAVP should be considered normal if the urine osmolality exceeds 600 mOsm for neonates or 800 mOsm for older infants and children. Such patients should be evaluated for central diabetes insipidus by a neurologist or endocrinologist.

Calcium Excretion

Urinary calcium excretion in the neonate is most easily assessed by determination of the calcium/creatinine ratio (mg/mg) in a random urine sample. In contrast to the older child, in whom a ratio exceeding 0.2 should be considered abnormal (Moore et al, 1978), **the ratio in the infant receiving breast milk can rise to 0.4 in the term infant and to 0.8 in the preterm neonate** (Karlen et al, 1985). **The most common cause of hypercalciuria in neonates is administration of calciuric drugs, such as furosemide and glucocorticoids, which are used in the management of bronchopulmonary dysplasia.** Such patients may be at risk for development of nephrocalcinosis or nephrolithiasis (Jacinto et al, 1988). This, in turn, may lead to renal dysfunction later in childhood (Downing et al, 1992). Although it may not be feasible to discontinue glucocorticoids, substitution of chlorothiazide for furosemide may reduce urinary calcium excretion.

Phosphorus, Glucose, and Amino Acid Excretion

Because the serum phosphorus concentration is higher in the neonate than in the older infant or child, **any neonate with a serum phosphorus concentration lower than 4 mg/dl should be evaluated for renal phosphorus wasting.** This can be accomplished in the neonate by measurement of phosphate and creatinine concentrations in urine (U_{PO_4} and U_{Cr}, respectively) and in a concurrent sample of plasma (P_{PO_4} and P_{Cr}, respectively) and calculation of the fractional tubular reabsorption of phosphorus (TRP):

$$TRP = 100\%[1 - (U_{PO_4} \times P_{Cr})/(P_{PO_4} \times U_{Cr})]$$

After the first week of life, the TRP should be greater than 95% in term infants and greater than 75% in preterm infants (Karlen et al, 1985). **After the neonatal period, the TRP should be greater than 85%.** Values below these ranges suggest a proximal tubular disorder, or hyperparathyroidism.

In preterm infants, the threshold for tubular glucose reabsorption is lower than in the term infant or in the older child. **The most common cause of glucosuria in hospitalized infants is intravenous infusion of dextrose at rates exceeding the tubular reabsorptive threshold.** Percent glucose reabsorption (micromoles per milliliter) is normally greater than 99% (Rossi et al, 1994).

As with glucose handling, the proximal tubule of the neonate is limited in its ability to reabsorb amino acids, compared with the older infant. This results in a generalized aminoaciduria that is normal during the neonatal period. Therefore, **in the evaluation of aminoaciduria, it is important to compare results with those of age-matched normal infants** (Brodehl, 1978). Normal values for fractional amino acid reabsorption have been determined for neonates, infants, and children (Rossi et al, 1994).

Fluid and Electrolyte Management in the Neonate

Fluid and electrolyte management in the neonate, particularly in the preterm infant, requires knowledge of functional renal maturation, as described earlier, and strict attention to detail. **There are significant hazards to overhydration of the neonate, including the opening of a symptomatic patent ductus arteriosus, cerebral intraventricular hemorrhage, and necrotizing enterocolitis. Severe underhydration, on the other hand, may lead to hypoglycemia, hyperbilirubinemia, and hyperosmolality. To replace the usual urinary losses, 50 to 80 ml per 100 kcal of formula is a reasonable starting point.** Insensible water losses can be large, particularly for the very-low-birth-weight infant in a radiant warmer (El-Dahr and Chevalier, 1990). As shown in Figure 50–5, **initial parenteral fluid requirements in preterm infants depend largely on the infant's environment in the neonatal care unit.** Moreover, the requirements (relative to body weight) decrease with increasing body weight.

In monitoring infants with urinary tract disorders, serial body weight measurements are extremely useful, as are repeated assessments of the cardiopulmonary status (El-Dahr and Chevalier, 1990). BUN and hematocrit values are not as useful in preterm infants as in older infants and children in view of their relatively low nitrogen intake and frequent blood sampling. **Once the physiologic postnatal diuresis has begun, 2 to 3 mEq/kg/day of sodium can be** prescribed. Neonates have higher plasma potassium concentration than older infants and children do (Chevalier, 1998). However, infants with high urine flow rates may have increased potassium losses. **Potassium chloride, 2 mEq/kg/day, can be added to the fluid prescription once urine output is established.** Hypernatremia in neonates is more often the result of insufficient water intake than excessive sodium intake. In general, hyponatremia is more common than hypernatremia, and it is often caused by excessive water intake, sometimes aggravated by increased antidiuretic hormone secretion (SIADH). The latter condition may result from perinatal asphyxia, intracranial hemorrhage, or pneumothorax. If SIADH is suspected, a trial of fluid restriction is appropriate.

HORMONAL CONTROL OF RENAL FUNCTION DURING DEVELOPMENT

Renin-Angiotensin System

Fetal and neonatal renal function is significantly modulated by a number of circulating hormones. The best studied is the renin-angiotensin system (RAS). Inasmuch as angiotensin II receptors have been identified in the fetal rat (term, 21 days) by the 10th day of gestation (Jones et al, 1989), and renin appears in the mesonephric and renal arteries by the 15th day (Richoux et al, 1987), a role for the RAS has been postulated in the process of angiogenesis. In the human fetus, renin is present in the transient mesonephros and can be identified as early as the 8th week of gestation in the metanephros (Celio et al, 1985). By the 19th day of gestation in the rat, both renin mRNA (demonstrated by in situ hybridization histochemistry) and the renin protein (demonstrated by immunocytochemistry) are distributed along arcuate and interlobular arteries (Gomez et al, 1986, 1989). However, **in the early postnatal period, renin becomes localized to the juxtaglomerular apparatus, which persists to adulthood** (Gomez et al,

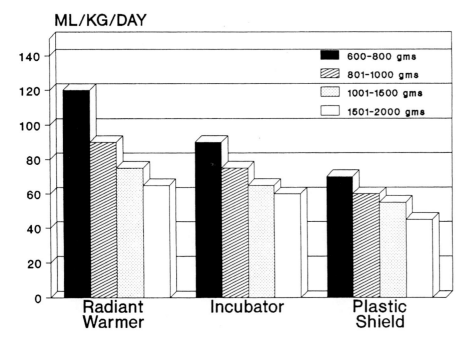

Figure 50–5. Initial (day 1 through day 3) parenteral fluid requirements in preterm infants according to body weight. (From El-Dahr SS, Chevalier RL: Special needs of the newborn infant in fluid therapy. Pediatr Clin North Am 1990;37:323–336.)

1986). In addition to these developmental changes in distribution of renin, there is an eight-fold decrease in the renal renin mRNA content during early development in the rat (Gomez et al, 1988a). These developmental changes are not irreversible: inhibition of angiotensin II formation by chronic intake of enalapril in the adult rat causes a redistribution of renin upstream along afferent arterioles and an increase in renal renin mRNA content reminiscent of the fetal pattern (Gomez et al, 1988b, 1990). In view of these findings, it is possible that, as a result of normal maturation, the sensitivity of the renal vasculature to angiotensin II increases, with secondary inhibition of renin gene expression.

Although plasma renin activity (PRA) remains low during fetal life (Pernollet et al, 1979), there is a marked increase during the perinatal period in most mammalian species, including humans (Wallace et al, 1980; Osborn et al, 1980; Siegel and Fisher, 1980; Fiselier et al, 1984). The mechanism underlying this increase in PRA, which is triggered by vaginal delivery (Jelinek et al, 1986), may relate to a rise in prostaglandin synthesis (Joppich and Houser, 1982) or increased sympathetic nervous activity (Vincent et al, 1980). However, studies in piglets failed to support the latter hypothesis (Osborn et al, 1980). It is likely that contraction of the extracellular space resulting from physiologic postnatal natriuresis contributes to the perinatal increase in PRA (Aperia et al, 1977).

In addition to developmental changes in renin synthesis, **the adrenal response to angiotensin increases during fetal and early postnatal life.** In the fetal lamb, furosemide infusion does not increase either PRA or plasma aldosterone concentration (Siegel et al, 1980). In late gestation, however, PRA increases without a mineralocorticoid response, and in the neonate both PRA and aldosterone concentration increase after furosemide infusion (Siegel et al, 1980). Maturation of the mineralocorticoid response can also be demonstrated by angiotensin II infusion, which results in greater plasma aldosterone concentrations in adult than in fetal sheep (Robillard et al, 1983). The physiologic significance of these events may rest in the response to hemorrhage, which causes a greater increase in PRA, plasma angiotensin II, and aldosterone in late than in early gestation in the ovine fetus (Robillard et al, 1982). Because blood pressure is maintained during moderate hemorrhage in late but not in earlier gestation (Robillard et al, 1982), the RAS may play a critical role in modulation of hemodynamics in the perinatal period. **Because of the critical dependence of the fetal and neonatal glomerular capillary pressure on angiotensin-mediated efferent arteriolar tone, fetal or neonatal GFR can fall precipitously after exposure to angiotensin-converting enzyme (ACE) inhibitors** (Martin et al, 1992). Both the potency and the duration of action of captopril are significantly greater in neonates than in older children (O'Dea et al, 1988). Moreover, in response to a reduction in renal mass, the remaining hyperfiltering immature nephrons are even more susceptible to the action of ACE inhibitors, which can induce renal failure and further nephron injury.

Atrial Natriuretic Peptide

Atrial natriuretic peptide (ANP), secreted by cardiac myocytes, has been shown to possess a number of sys-temic hemodynamic and renal effects, including an increase in GFR, natriuresis, diuresis, inhibition of renin and aldosterone release, vasorelaxation, and increase in vascular permeability (Goetz, 1988). Circulating ANP binds to specific receptors coupled to particulate guanylate cyclase, resulting in formation of cyclic guanosine monophosphate (cGMP), a second messenger responsible for the physiologic effects of ANP (Inagami, 1989). In addition, ANP binds to an even greater number of receptors not coupled to guanylate cyclase. Classified as "clearance" receptors, these are believed to contribute to the regulation of plasma ANP levels by removal of ANP from the circulation (Inagami, 1989). The precise role of ANP in the regulation of sodium and fluid homeostasis remains unclear, although evidence has accumulated to suggest that ANP plays a role in the physiologic adaptation of the fetus and neonate to its changing environment. ANP is present in the fetal rat heart shortly after completion of organogenesis (Dolan and Dobrozsi, 1987; Toshimori et al, 1987), and ANP mRNA first appears in the ventricles before becoming localized to the atria in the perinatal period (Wei et al, 1987). Compared with that of the mother, plasma ANP concentration in the fetus is significantly higher (Castro et al, 1988; Yamaji et al, 1988). Because metabolic clearance of ANP by the fetus exceeds that in the adult (Ervin et al, 1988), release of ANP from fetal cardiac myocytes must be far greater than in adults.

A number of stimuli have been shown to increase fetal plasma ANP levels. Acute volume expansion in the ovine fetus (Ross et al, 1987) and intrauterine blood transfusion in the human fetus (Robillard et al, 1988) raise plasma ANP concentration. Induction of atrial tachycardia in the fetal lamb results in hydrops and an increase in plasma ANP concentration (Nimrod et al, 1988). Fetal hypoxia has also been shown to result in contraction of circulating volume and an increase in the ANP level (Cheung and Brace, 1988). By increasing vascular permeability, ANP may contribute to regulation of blood volume in these pathologic states.

Atrial ANP content decreases in the perinatal period, with a subsequent increase during the first 15 days of postnatal life in the rat (Dolan et al, 1989). **This pattern is the opposite of that observed for plasma ANP concentration, which is elevated in the first several days of life and then decreases with maturation** (Weil et al, 1986; Kikuchi et al, 1988). It is likely that reduction in atrial ANP during the perinatal period results from increased release into the circulation. In preterm infants, plasma ANP levels are initially even higher than in full-term infants, and the ensuing postnatal decrease is correlated with decreasing atrial size and decreasing body weight (Bierd et al, 1990). It is therefore likely that ANP plays a role in physiologic postnatal natriuresis and diuresis. After the initial postnatal diuresis, however, the neonate enters a state of positive sodium balance necessary for rapid somatic growth.

The renal effects of infused ANP are reduced in the fetus compared with the adult (Brace et al, 1989; Hargrave et al, 1989). The natriuretic effect of ANP in the neonate is also reduced (Braunlich, 1987; Chevalier, 1988), and systemic clearance of ANP is increased (Chevalier, 1988). Moreover, compared with the adult, the neonatal renal natriuretic and diuretic response to acute volume expansion is attenuated (Schoeneman, 1980). However, chronic sodium loading of artificially reared preweaned rat pups increases the renal response to acute volume expansion, with an increase in the urinary excretion of cGMP (Muchant et al, 1995). It therefore appears that, rather than reflecting functional immaturity, the renal response to ANP in the neonate reflects an adaptation to the requirement for sodium conservation during this period.

Vasopressin

Similar to the adult, fetal and newborn sheep have been shown to respond to both osmolar and nonosmolar stimuli for release of arginine vasopressin (AVP) (Leake et al, 1979; Robillard et al, 1979). Despite circulating levels of AVP that can be significantly higher than in the adult (Pohjavuori and Fyhrquist, 1980), **the fetal collecting duct appears to be less sensitive than that of the adult to AVP** (Robillard and Weitzman, 1980). This may be a result of a reduced density of AVP receptors, which increase during early development (Rajerison et al, 1982). In addition, the tubular effects of vasopressin may be antagonized by increased prostanoid synthesis in early development (Melendez et al, 1990).

In the postnatal period, during which the collecting ducts develop full responsiveness to AVP, excessive or "inappropriate" AVP secretion due to birth asphyxia, intracerebral hemorrhage, or respiratory distress syndrome can result in severe hyponatremia (Kaplan and Feigin, 1978; Moylan et al, 1978; Stern et al, 1979). Conversely, infants born with nephrogenic diabetes insipidus do not respond to circulating AVP and may develop life-threatening hypernatremia.

Prostaglandins

Maternal serum prostaglandin concentration increases progressively during pregnancy (Reyes and Melendez, 1990). Because prostaglandins cross the placenta, blood levels are also elevated in the fetus and neonate (Reyes and Melendez, 1990). **Maternal administration of nonsteroidal anti-inflammatory drugs (NSAIDs), such as indomethacin, can result in prolonged renal insufficiency and oliguria in the neonate** (Buderus et al, 1993; Kaplan et al, 1994). Prolonged intrauterine exposure can also impair fetal renal development (Kaplan et al, 1994). Administration of indomethacin to neonates with patent ductus arteriosus also frequently results in decreased GFR and oliguria (Reyes and Melendez, 1990). Caution should be exercised in the administration of NSAIDs to any infant or child with a single functioning kidney or with renal impairment, because such patients are at increased risk for additional nephron injury and deterioration of GFR.

Nitric Oxide

Nitric oxide, a potent endothelium-derived relaxing factor, has multiple effects on renal function, including renal vasodilatation, regulation of tubuloglomerular feedback, and natriuresis (Bachmann and Mundel, 1994). Basal pro-

duction of nitric oxide in the third-trimester sheep fetus maintains baseline renal blood flow (Bogaert et al, 1993). In the neonatal pig, endogenous nitric oxide synthesis is also responsible for basal vasoconstrictor tone, and this effect is proportionately greater than in the adult (Solhaug et al, 1993). Renal endothelial nitric oxide production may be increased in early development as a response to increased vasoconstrictor influences described earlier. A counter-regulatory function of renal nitric oxide production was proposed, after studies of unilateral ureteral obstruction in the adult rat, in which endogenous renal nitric oxide activity parallels increased renal vascular resistance (Chevalier et al, 1992).

FUNCTIONAL RESPONSE OF THE DEVELOPING KIDNEYS TO MALFORMATION OR INJURY

Reduced Functioning Renal Mass

A reduction in the number of functioning nephrons in early development is most often the result of a congenital malformation or a perinatal vascular accident such as a renal embolus or renal vein thrombosis. Unilateral ureteral occlusion in the fetal lamb at midtrimester results in a 50% increase in contralateral kidney weight by 1 month (Peters et al, 1993). These findings are corroborated by two prenatal ultrasound studies of human fetuses with unilateral renal agenesis or multicystic kidney. In both reports, the single functioning kidneys were significantly longer than those in the control patients (Glazebrook et al, 1993; Mandell et al, 1993). **Such studies demonstrate unequivocally that compensatory renal growth can begin prenatally.** Because the placenta provides the excretory function for the fetus, an increased excretory burden on the kidney is not required to initiate compensatory growth. Rather, alterations in growth factors or inhibitors presumably modulate the prenatal changes.

Perhaps not surprisingly in view of the rapid growth of the normal kidney in the early postnatal period, **compensatory renal growth in the neonate greatly exceeds that in the adult** (Dicker and Shirley, 1973; Shirley, 1976; Hayslett, 1979). Whereas compensatory increase in renal mass in the adult is largely a result of cellular hypertrophy, hyperplasia is also stimulated in the uninephrectomized weanling rat (Phillips and Leong, 1969; Karp et al, 1971). Neonatal glomerular hypertrophy results also from increased glomerular basement membrane surface area and proliferation of mesangial matrix (Olivetti et al, 1980). As in the adult, the majority of the compensatory increase in renal mass in the neonate results from an increase in tubular volume (Hayslett et al, 1968; Horster et al, 1971).

Previously, compensatory renal growth in the uninephrectomized neonatal rat was thought to involve an increase in nephrogenesis of the remaining kidney (Bonvalet et al, 1972). **This was subsequently disproved by careful serial morphologic studies** (Kaufman et al, 1975; Larsson et al, 1980). In the guinea pig, approximately 20% of glomeruli are underperfused during the first several weeks of life and cannot be identified by uptake of colloidal carbon (India ink) injected in vivo (Chevalier, 1982a). After uninephrectomy at birth, however, these glomeruli are "recruited" within the first 3 weeks of life, resulting in an earlier increase in the number of perfused glomeruli per kidney (Chevalier, 1982b). The prior confusion regarding apparent compensatory nephrogenesis in animals subjected to uninephrectomy during early development was probably caused by incorrect descriptions of newly perfused glomeruli as newly formed glomeruli.

As with the enhanced increase in compensatory renal growth observed in the neonate with reduced renal mass, **the functional adaptation by remaining nephrons is greater in early development than in the adult**. In dogs subjected to 75% renal ablation at birth, GFR increased markedly and at 6 weeks of age was not different from that of sham-operated littermates (Aschinberg et al, 1978). However, dogs undergoing renal ablation at 8 weeks of age had a GFR 6 weeks later that was less than 50% that of sham-operated controls (Aschinberg et al, 1978). Reduced renal mass in the neonatal guinea pig or rat results in acceleration of the normal "centrifugal" functional nephron maturation, so that the compensatory increase in single-nephron GFR is greater in superficial than in deep nephrons (Chevalier, 1982a; Ikoma et al, 1990). These studies indicate that functional as well as morphologic correlates of compensatory renal growth are augmented in early postnatal development compared with the adult.

Sonography permits serial measurement of renal size in the fetus and after birth. Such "tracking" of renal size reflects the function of an abnormal contralateral kidney in infants with two functioning kidneys: an exaggerated rate of increase in renal size is correlated with contralateral renal function that contributes less than 15% of total function (O'Sullivan et al, 1992).

Congenital Urinary Tract Obstruction

The response of the developing kidney to ureteral obstruction differs from that of the adult kidney. **Complete unilateral ureteral obstruction (UUO) during midgestation in the fetal sheep results in dysplastic development of the ipsilateral kidney** (Beck, 1971). When UUO is imposed later in gestation, however, dysplastic changes do not develop (Glick et al, 1983). In the human infant, ureteral atresia in early gestation results in irreversible multicystic dysplasia of the ipsilateral kidney (Griscom et al, 1975). Ureteropelvic junction obstruction presumably develops later in gestation and causes less severe functional renal impairment, which may be minimized by early release of obstruction postnatally (King et al, 1984). These studies illustrate the critical importance of the timing of urinary tract obstruction with respect to renal development, and the greater susceptibility to injury of the fetal kidney.

Relief of temporary complete UUO in the neonatal rat allows recovery of normal GFR in the postobstructed kidney 1 month later, despite a 40% reduction in the number of nephrons (Chevalier et al, 1999a). However, the significant hyperfiltration of the remaining nephrons leads to progressive glomerular sclerosis, tubular atrophy, interstitial fibrosis, and deterioration of GFR (Chevalier et al, 1999b). These studies suggest that **after surgical relief of congeni-**

tal urinary tract obstruction, postoperative measurements of individual kidney GFR using radionuclide scans may be misleading, because functional adaptation by a population of nephrons may mask the deterioration of other nephrons. Follow-up studies extending well into adulthood are essential in defining the natural history of these patients.

Even in the early postnatal period, the maturing kidney appears to be more susceptible than the adult kidney to injury resulting from UUO. As in uninephrectomy (discussed earlier), partial UUO in the neonatal guinea pig results in a greater adaptive increase in GFR of the intact opposite kidney than does UUO in older animals (Taki et al, 1983). However, despite lower intraureteral hydrostatic pressure in neonatal than in adult guinea pigs (Chevalier, 1984), the decrement in GFR caused by ipsilateral UUO is more severe in younger than in older animals (Taki et al, 1983), and renal growth of kidneys with partial UUO since birth is arrested by 3 weeks of age (Chevalier, 1988). Morphologically, the neonatal guinea pig with ipsilateral partial UUO develops contraction of glomerular volume, glomerular sclerosis, and tubular atrophy (Chevalier et al, 1987). Most importantly, growth arrest cannot be prevented and function is not restored by release of obstruction after 10 days even though intraureteral pressure is normalized (Chevalier et al, 1988). In contrast, release of obstruction after a similar period in the adult animal does not cause renal atrophy but allows restoration of a normal glomerular perfusion pattern and renal blood flow (Chevalier et al, 1987).

As with UUO in the adult, chronic partial UUO in the neonatal guinea pig results in a marked increase in vascular resistance of the ipsilateral kidney. Whereas normal renal development in the guinea pig is characterized by a progressive increase in renal blood flow and recruitment of perfused glomeruli (Chevalier, 1982b; Chevalier 1983), these events are prevented by ipsilateral UUO at birth (Chevalier et al, 1987; Chevalier and Gomez, 1989). Normal renal growth and hemodynamic maturation can be restored, however, by removal of the intact opposite kidney at the time of ureteral obstruction (Chevalier and Kaiser, 1984). This suggests that growth factors regulated by total functional renal mass can modulate the response of the developing kidney to ipsilateral UUO.

The greater hemodynamic impairment of the neonatal kidney subjected to UUO may relate to the increased renal vascular resistance of the immature kidney and increased activity of the RAS (see earlier discussion). Renin content of the neonatal guinea pig kidney with ipsilateral UUO is increased compared with that of sham-operated controls, and release of obstruction returns the renin content to normal levels (Chevalier and Gomez, 1989). Inhibition of endogenous angiotensin II formation by chronic administration of enalapril to neonatal guinea pigs with UUO restores the normal maturational rise in renal blood flow, the number of perfused glomeruli, and the increase in glomerular volume of the ipsilateral kidney (Chevalier and Peach, 1985; Chevalier et al, 1987). Although administration of enalapril does not restore the renal blood flow of the neonatal guinea pig kidney after release of 5 or 10 days of ipsilateral UUO, enalapril reduces renal vascular resistance of the intact opposite kidney by 40% after release of contralateral UUO (Chevalier and Gomez, 1989). Moreover, the vasoconstrictor response of the intact kidney to exogenous angiotensin II is increased after release of contralateral UUO (Chevalier and Gomez, 1989). These studies indicate a dynamic functional balance between the two kidneys, which appears to be mediated or modulated by the intrarenal RAS.

As discussed earlier, the intrarenal distribution of renin changes dramatically during development. In the fetal and early postnatal periods, microvascular renin extends along interlobular and afferent arterioles, becoming localized to the juxtaglomerular region by the 20th postnatal day in the rat (Gomez et al, 1986). **In 4 week-old rats subjected to complete UUO during the first 2 days of life, renal renin content is increased in the obstructed kidney, and immunoreactive renin extends along the afferent arteriole** (El-Dahr et al, 1990a). Therefore, UUO from birth results in persistence of the fetal or early neonatal pattern even after the time of weaning (21 days). Furthermore, the proportion of juxtaglomerular apparatuses with renin gene expression (identified by in situ hybridization histochemistry) is increased in the obstructed kidney of 4-week-old rats (El-Dahr et al, 1990a). In addition to increased renin production and storage, neonatal UUO results in recruitment of renin-secreting cells by the renal cortex (Norwood et al, 1994). Four weeks of UUO in adult rats, however, does not alter the juxtaglomerular localization of renin (El-Dahr et al, 1990b). These studies indicate that the renal response to UUO is age dependent, with the neonate manifesting a greater activity of the RAS.

Perinatal Ischemia and Hypoxia

Renal dysfunction in the fetus and neonate is often the result of circulatory disturbances in the perinatal period. In response to hemorrhage or hypoxia, renal vascular resistance in the ovine fetus is increased while GFR is maintained, suggesting predominant efferent arteriolar vasoconstriction (Robillard et al, 1981; Gomez et al, 1984). This may be mediated, at least in part, by angiotensin (Robillard et al, 1982). Catecholamine release may be more important in mediating renal vascular resistance in early fetal life, whereas vasopressin appears to play a greater role in the more mature ovine fetus (Gomez et al, 1984). In the neonatal lamb, hypoxia increases plasma renin activity, aldosterone, and vasopressin (Weismann and Clarke, 1981). Although GFR is reduced during hypoxia, the effect does not change during the first month of life (Weismann and Clarke, 1981). The preterm infant, however, may have renal responses to ischemia and hypoxia that are more similar to the those of the fetus than those of the term neonate.

One of the homeostatic mechanisms for preservation of renal perfusion in the face of hypotension is autoregulation of renal blood flow. Compared with adult rats, **young rats manifest autoregulation of renal blood flow at lower perfusion pressures, commensurate with the lower mean arterial pressure during early development** (Chevalier and Kaiser, 1983). Whereas adult rats with prior uninephrectomy maintain autoregulation (albeit at higher levels of renal blood flow), **uninephrectomy at birth impairs autoregulation in young rats** (Chevalier and Kaiser, 1983). These observations raise the possibility that, after

reduction in functioning renal mass, the neonatal kidney may be at greater risk for renal ischemia in the face of superimposed hypotension. After temporary complete occlusion of the renal artery, however, mortality is greater in adult than in young rats (Kunes et al, 1978). Although this suggests that the neonatal kidney may be more resistant than the adult kidney to certain insults, **perinatal circulatory disorders can result in a variety of persistent glomerular and tubular functional abnormalities** (Dauber et al, 1976; Stark and Geiger, 1990).

Toxic Nephropathy

Neonates are increasingly exposed to a variety of potentially nephrotoxic agents. Fortunately, the developing kidney appears to be more resistant than the adult kidney to a number of toxic agents. Either sodium dichromate or uranyl nitrate, both experimental models of toxic acute renal failure, causes less renal injury in young than in adult animals (Pelayo et al, 1983; Appenroth and Braunlich, 1988). More relevant clinically, renal concentrations of aminoglycosides (Marre et al, 1980; Lelievre-Pegorier et al, 1985; Provoost et al, 1985) and cisplatin (Jongejan et al, 1986) are lower in young than in adult animals receiving high doses. This may be a result of the normally reduced perfusion of superficial cortical nephrons in the developing kidney, such that these nephrons receive a lower dose of toxin. Another possible cause is the proportionately greater renal mass compared to body weight in early development. Few studies have addressed the potential long-term impact of toxic renal injury, however. After uninephrectomy for Wilms' tumor, irradiation and chemotherapy cause greater impairment of compensatory renal growth in younger infants compared with older infants and children (Mitus et al, 1969; Luttenegger et al, 1975).

Recovery from Renal Injury: Relationship to Normal Development

Studies suggest that recovery from renal injury in the adult involves "recapitulation of phylogeny by ontogeny" (Hammerman, 2000). For instance, insulin-like growth factor 1 (IGF-1) plays a role in determining nephron number and nephron size and also can alter the course of recovery from ischemic acute renal failure or temporary ureteral obstruction (Chevalier et al, 2000; Hammerman, 2000). **Temporary ureteral obstruction in the neonatal rat delays maturation of the renal microvasculature, glomeruli, tubules, and interstitium** (Chevalier et al, 1999a). After relief of obstruction, some aspects of renal maturation proceed and others are permanently impaired (Chevalier et al, 1999b). Identification of the timing of expression of various genes involved in normal development may lead to insight into the reparative process and to new therapeutic interventions.

Implications of Congenital Renal Disease for Adult Function

Glomerular hyperfiltration and glomerular hypertrophy have been implicated in the progression of most forms of renal insufficiency (Brenner et al, 1982; Fogo and Ichikawa, 1989). **In view of the greater response by remaining nephrons, the neonate with reduced renal mass is theoretically at greater risk than the adult for long-term renal dysfunction.** In this regard, reduced renal mass causes greater proteinuria and glomerular sclerosis in the immature animal than in the adult (Celsi et al, 1987; Okuda et al, 1987; Ikoma et al, 1990). There is circumstantial evidence that intrauterine growth retardation is also accompanied by a nephron deficit, and that, in addition to renal insufficiency, it may lead to the development of hypertension in adulthood (Brenner and Chertow, 1994). Likewise, congenital unilateral renal agenesis in humans has been associated with focal glomerular sclerosis and progression to renal insufficiency in adulthood (Kiprov et al, 1982; Bhathena et al, 1985; Wikstad et al, 1988). More than 25% of children undergoing unilateral nephrectomy develop renal insufficiency and proteinuria in adulthood (Argueso et al, 1992). The critical question is what is the number of functioning nephrons below which progression is inevitable. In oligomeganephronia, a form of renal hypoplasia in which the number of nephrons is reduced to less than 50% of normal, glomeruli develop marked hypertrophy and sclerosis, leading to renal failure in later childhood (Elema, 1976; Bhathena et al, 1985). These considerations underscore the importance of attempting to maximize functional renal mass in the neonate or infant with renal impairment of any cause.

ACKNOWLEDGMENT

Original studies by Dr. Chevalier were supported by NIH grants AM25727, HL40209, and DK40558.

REFERENCES

Anatomic Development and Fetal Renal Function

Crombleholme TM, Harrison MR, Golbus MS, et al: Fetal intervention in obstructive uropathy: Prognostic indicators and efficacy of intervention. Am J Obstet Gynecol 1990;162:1239–1244.

Eugene M, Muller F, Dommergues M, et al: Evaluation of postnatal renal function in fetuses with bilateral obstructive uropathies by proton nuclear magnetic resonance spectroscopy. Am J Obstet Gynecol 1994; 170:595–602.

Evans MI, Sacks AJ, Johnson MP, et al: Sequential invasive assessment of fetal renal function and the intrauterine treatment of fetal obstructive uropathies. Obstet Gynecol 1991;77:545–550.

Ichikawa I, Maddox DA, Brenner BM: Maturational development of glomerular ultrafiltration in the rat. Am J Physiol 1979;236:F465–F471.

Johnson MP, Bukowski TP, Reitleman C, et al: In utero surgical treatment of fetal obstructive uropathy: A new comprehensive approach to identify appropriate candidates for vesicoamniotic shunt therapy. Am J Obstet Gynecol 1994;170:1770–1779.

Koseki C, Herzlinger D, Al-Awqati Q: Apoptosis in metanephric development. J Cell Biol 1992;119:1327–1333.

Pachi A, Lubrano R, Maggi E, et al: Renal tubular damage in fetuses with intrauterine growth retardation. Fetal Diagn Ther 1993;8:109–113.

Potter EL: Normal and Abnormal Development of the Kidney, vol 1. Chicago, Year Book, 1972.

Rabinowitz R, Peters MT, Vyas S, et al: Measurement of fetal urine production in normal pregnancy by real-time ultrasonography. Am J Obstet Gynecol 1989;161:1264–1266.

Robillard JE, Nakamura KT, Wilkin MK, et al: Ontogeny of renal hemodynamic response to renal nerve stimulation in sheep. Am J Physiol 1987;252:F605–F612.

Rudolph AM, Heymann MA: Circulatory changes during growth in the fetal lamb. Circ Res 1976;26:289–299.

Smith FG, Robillard JE: Pathophysiology of fetal renal disease. Semin Perinatol 1989;13:305.

Spitzer A, Brandis M: Functional and morphologic maturation of the superficial nephrons: Relationship to total kidney function. J Clin Invest 1974;53:279–287.

Veille JC, Hanson RA, Tatum K, et al: Quantitative assessment of human fetal renal blood flow. Am J Obstet Gynecol 1993;169:1399–1402.

Postnatal Functional Development

Anand SK: Acute renal failure in the neonate. Pediatr Clin North Am 1982;29:791–800.

Aperia A, Broberger O, Herin P: Renal hemodynamics in the perinatal period: A study in lambs. Acta Physiol Scand 1977;99:261–269.

Aperia A, Herin P: Development of glomerular perfusion rate and nephron filtration rate in rats 17–60 days old. Am J Physiol 1975;228:1319–1325.

Arant BS Jr: Developmental patterns of renal functional maturation compared in the human neonate. J Pediatr 1978;92:705–712.

Asnes RS, Mones RL: Pollakiuria. Pediatrics 1973;52:615–617.

Clark DA: Times of first void and first stool in 500 newborns. Pediatrics 1977;60:457–459.

Engelke SC, Shah RL, Vasan U, et al: Sodium balance in very low-birth-weight infants. J Pediatr 1978;93:837–841.

Fine LG, Norman JT, Ong A: Cell-cell cross-talk in the pathogenesis of renal interstitial fibrosis. Kidney Int 1995;49:S-48–S-50.

Gruskin AB, Edelmann CM Jr, Yuan S: Maturational changes in renal blood flow in piglets. Pediatr Res 1970;4:7–13.

Guignard JP, Torrado A, DaCunha O, et al: Glomerular filtration rate in the first three weeks of life. J Pediatr 1975;87:268–272.

Hansen JDL, Smith CA: Effects of withholding fluid in the immediate postnatal period. Pediatrics 1953;12:99.

John E, Goldsmith DI, Spitzer A: Quantitative changes in the canine glomerular vasculature during development: Physiologic implications. Kidney Int 1981;20:223–239.

Kim MS, Mandell J: Renal Function in the Fetus and Neonate. *In* King LR Jr (ed): Urologic Surgery in Neonates and Young Infants. Philadelphia, WB Saunders, 1988, pp 41–58.

Marxer-Meier A, Hegyi I, Loffing J, et al: Postnatal maturation of renal cortical peritubular fibroblasts in the rat. Anat Embryol (Berl) 1998; 197:143–153.

Merlet-Benichou C, Gilbert T, Muffat-Joly M, et al: Intrauterine growth retardation leads to a permanent nephron deficit in the rat. Pediatr Nephrol 1994;8:175–180.

Roy RN, Chance GW, Radde IC, et al: Late hyponatremia in very low birthweight infants (<1.3 kilograms). Pediatr Res 1976;10:526–531.

Rubin MI, Bruck E, Rapaport M: Maturation of renal function in childhood: Clearance studies. J Clin Invest 1949;28:1144.

Schlondorff D, Weber H, Trizna W, et al: Vasopressin responsiveness of renal adenylate cyclase in newborn rats and rabbits. Am J Physiol 1978;234:F16–F21.

Spitzer A, Brandis M: Functional and morphologic maturation of the superficial nephrons: Relationship to total kidney function. J Clin Invest 1974;53:279–287.

Stanier MW: Development of intra-renal solute gradients in foetal and postnatal life. Pfluegers Arch 1972;336:263–270.

Steele BT, Paes B, Towell ME, et al: Fetal renal failure associated with intrauterine growth retardation. Am J Obstet Gynecol 1988;159:1200–1202.

Svenningsen NW: Renal acid-base titration studies in infants with and without metabolic acidosis in the postnatal period. Pediatr Res 1974;8:659–672.

Vanpee M, Blennow M, Linne T, et al: Renal function in very low birth weight infants: Normal maturity reached during early childhood. J Pediatr 1992;121:784–788.

Wolf G: Vasoactive factors and tubulointerstitial injury. Kidney Blood Press Res 1999;22:62–70.

Zhuo JL, Dean R, Maric C, et al: Localization and interactions of vasoactive peptide receptors in renomedullary interstitial cells of the kidney. Kidney Int 1998;54(Suppl 67):S22–S28.

Zoubek J, Bloom DA, Sedman AB: Extraordinary urinary frequency. Pediatrics 1990;85:1112–1114.

Evaluation of Renal Function in the Infant and Child

Batlle DC, Hizon MH, Cohen E, et al: The use of the urinary anion gap in the diagnosis of hyperchloremic metabolic acidosis. N Engl J Med 1988;318:594–599.

Brodehl J: Renal Hyperaminoaciduria. *In* Edelmann CM Jr (ed): Pediatric Kidney Disease. Boston, Little, Brown, 1978, pp 1047–1079.

Brown ER, Stark A, Sosenko I: Bronchopulmonary dysplasia: Possible relationships to pulmonary edema. J Pediatr 1978;92:982–984.

Chan JCM: Renal tubular acidosis. J Pediatr 1983;102:327–340.

Chevalier RL: What are normal potassium concentrations in the neonate? What is a reasonable approach to hyperkalemia in the newborn with normal renal function? Semin Nephrol 1998;18:360–361.

Cole CH: The Harriet Lane Handbook, vol 10. Chicago, Year Book, 1984, p 331.

Donckerwolke RA, Valk C, van-Wijngaargen-Peterman MJ: The diagnostic value of the urine to blood carbon dioxide tension gradient for the assessment of distal tubular hydrogen secretion in pediatric patients with renal tubular disorders. Clin Nephrol 1983;19:254–258.

Downing GJ, Egelhoff JC, Daily DK, et al: Kidney function in very low birth weight infants with furosemide-related renal calcifications at ages 1 to 2 years. J Pediatr 1992;120:599–604.

El-Dahr SS, Chevalier RL: Special needs of the newborn infant in fluid therapy. Pediatr Clin North Am 1990;37:323–336.

Hutcheon RA, Shibuya M, Leumann E, et al: Distal renal tubular acidosis in children with chronic hydronephrosis. J Pediatr 1976;89:372–376.

Jacinto JS, Modanlou HD, Crade M: Renal calcification incidence in very low birth weight infants. Pediatrics 1988;81:31–35.

Karlen J, Aperia A, Zetterstrom R: Renal excretion of calcium and phosphate in preterm and term infants. J Pediatr 1985;106:814–819.

Mathew OP, Jones AS, James E, et al: Neonatal renal failure: Usefulness of diagnostic indices. Pediatrics 1980;65:57–60.

Moore ES, Coe FL, McMann BJ, et al: Idiopathic hypercalciuria in children: Prevalence and metabolic characteristics. J Pediatr 1978;92:906–910.

Rodriguez-Soriano J, Vallo A, Oliveros R: Transient pseudohypoaldosteronism secondary to obstructive uropathy in infancy. J Pediatr 1983;103:375–380.

Rossi R, Danzebrink S, Linnenburger K, et al: Assessment of tubular reabsorption of sodium, glucose, phosphate and amino acids based on spot urine samples. Acta Paediatr 1994;83:1282–1286.

Schwartz GJ, Brion LP, Spitzer A: The use of plasma creatinine concentration for estimating glomerular filtration rate in infants, children, and adolescents. Pediatr Clin North Am 1987;34:571–590.

Stine KC, Linshaw, MA: Use of furosemide in the evaluation of renal tubular acidosis. J Pediatr 1985;107:559–562.

Trompeter RA, Al-Dahhan J, Haycock GB, et al: Normal values for plasma creatinine concentration related to maturity in normal term and preterm infants. Int J Pediatr Nephrol 1983;4:145–148.

Hormonal Control of Renal Function During Development

Aperia A, Broberger O, Herin P, et al: Sodium excretion in relation to sodium intake and aldosterone excretion in newborn pre-term and full-term infants. Acta Paediatr Scand 1977;68:813–817.

Bachmann S, Mundel P: Nitric oxide in the kidney: Synthesis, localization, and function. Am J Kidney Dis 1994;24:112–129.

Bierd TM, Kattwinkel J, Chevalier RL, et al: The interrelationship of atrial natriuretic peptide, atrial volume, and renal function in premature infants. J Pediatr 1990;116:753–759.

Bogaert GA, Kogan BA, Mevorach RA: Effects of endothelium-derived nitric oxide on renal hemodynamics and function in the sheep fetus. Pediatr Res 1993;34:755–761.

Brace RA, Bayer LA, Cheung CY: Fetal cardiovascular, endocrine, and fluid responses to atrial natriuretic factor infusion. Am J Physiol 1989;257:R580–R587.

Braunlich HSS: Renal effects of atrial natriuretic factor in the rats of different ages. Physiologia Bohemslovaca 1987;36:119–124.

Buderus S, Thomas B, Fahnenstich H, et al: Renal failure in two preterm infants: Toxic effect of prenatal maternal indomethacin treatment? Br J Obstet Gynaecol 1993;100:97–98.

Castro LC, Law RW, Ross MG, et al: Atrial natriuretic peptide in the sheep. J Dev Physiol 1988;10:235–246.

Celio MR, Groscurth P, Imagami T: Onotogeny of renin immunoreactive cells in the human kidney. Anat Embryol (Berl) 1985;173:149–155.

Cheung CY, Brace RA: Fetal hypoxia elevates plasma atrial natriuretic factor concentration. Am J Obstet Gynecol 1988;159:1263–1268.

Chevalier RL: Renal effects of atrial natriuretic peptide infusion in young and adult rats. Pediatr Res 1988;24:333–337.

Chevalier RL, Thornhill BA, Gomez RA: EDRF modulates renal hemo-

dynamics during unilateral ureteral obstruction in the rat. Kidney Int 1992;42:400–406.

Dolan LM, Dobrozsi DJ: Atrial natriuretic polypeptide in the fetal rat: Ontogeny and characterization. Pediatr Res 1987;22:115–117.

Dolan LM, Young CA, Khoury JC, et al: Atrial natriuretic factor during the perinatal period: Equal depletion in both atria. Pediatr Res 1989;25:339–341.

Ervin MG, Ross MG, Castro R, et al: Ovine fetal and adult atrial natriuretic factor metabolism. Am J Physiol 1988;254:R40–R46.

Fiselier T, Monnens L, van Munster P, et al: The renin angiotensin aldosterone system in infancy and childhood in basal conditions and after stimulation. Eur J Pediatr 1984;143:18–24.

Goetz KL: Physiology and pathophysiology of atrial peptides. Am J Physiol 1988;254:E1–E15.

Gomez RA, Chevalier RL, Everett AD, et al: Recruitment of renin gene-expressing cells in adult rat kidneys. Am J Physiol 1990;259:F660–F665.

Gomez RA, Chevalier RL, Sturgill BC, et al: Maturation of the intrarenal renin distribution in Wistar-Kyoto rats. J Hypertension 1986;4(Suppl 5):S31–S33.

Gomez RA, Lynch KR, Chevalier RL, et al: Renin and angiotensinogen gene expression in the maturing rat kidney. Am J Physiol 1988a;254:F582–F587.

Gomez RA, Lynch KR, Chevalier RL, et al: Renin and angiotensinogen gene expression and intrarenal renin distribution during ACE inhibition. Am J Physiol 1988b;254:F900–F906.

Gomez RA, Lynch KR, Sturgill BC, et al: Distribution of renin mRNA and its protein in the developing kidney. Am J Physiol 1989;257:F850–F858.

Hargrave BY, Iwamoto HS, Rudolph AM: Renal and cardiovascular effects of atrial natriuretic peptide in fetal sheep. Pediatr Res 1989;26:1–5.

Inagami T: Atrial natriuretic factor. J Biol Chem 1989;264:3043–3046.

Jelinek J, Hackenthal R, Hilgenfeldt U, et al: The renin-angiotensin system in the perinatal period in rats. J Dev Physiol 1986;8:33–41.

Jones C, Millan MA, Naftolin F, et al: Characterization of angiotensin II receptors in the rat fetus. Peptides 1989;10:459–463.

Joppich R, Hauser I: Urinary prostacyclin and thromboxane A2 metabolites in preterm and full-term infants in relation to plasma renin activity and blood pressure. Biol Neonate 1982;42:179–184.

Kaplan SL, Feigin RD: Inappropriate secretion of antidiuretic hormone complicating neonatal hypoxic ischemic encephalopathy. J Pediatr 1978;92:431–433.

Kaplan BS, Restaino I, Raval DS, et al: Renal failure in the neonate associated with in utero exposure to non-steroidal anti-inflammatory agents. Pediatr Nephrol 1994;8:700–704.

Kikuchi K, Shiomi M, Horie K, et al: Plasma atrial natriuretic polypeptide concentration in healthy children from birth to adolescence. Acta Paediatr Scand 1988;77:380–384.

Leake RD, Weitzman RE, Weinberg JA, et al: Control of vasopressin secretion in the newborn lamb. Pediatr Res 1979;13:257–260.

Martin RA, Jones KL, Mendoza A, et al: Effect of ACE inhibition on the fetal kidney: Decreased renal blood flow. Teratology 1992;46:317–321.

Melendez E, Reyes JL, Escalante BA, et al: Development of the receptors to prostaglandin E2 in the rat kidney and neonatal renal functions. Dev Pharmacol Ther 1990;14:125–134.

Moylan F, Herin JT, Ktishnamoorthy K: Inappropriate antidiuretic hormone secretion in premature infants with cerebral injury. Am J Dis Child 1978;132:399–402.

Muchant DG, Thornhill BA, Belmonte DC, et al: Chronic sodium loading augments the natriuretic response to acute volume expansion in the preweaned rat. Am J Physiol 1995;269:R15–R22.

Nimrod C, Keane P, Harder J, et al: Atrial natriuretic peptide production in association with nonimmune fetal hydrops. Am J Obstet Gynecol 1988;159:625–628.

O'Dea RF, Mirkin BL, Alward CT, et al: Treatment of neonatal hypertension with captopril. J Pediatr 1988;113:403–406.

Osborn JL, Hook JB, Baile MD: Regulation of plasma renin in developing piglets. Dev Pharmacol Ther 1980;1:217–228.

Pernollet, MG, Devynck MA, Macdonald GJ, et al: Plasma renin activity and adrenal angiotensin II receptors in fetal newborn, adult and pregnant rabbits. Biol Neonate 1979;36:119–127.

Pohjavuori M, Fyhrquist F: Hemodynamic significance of vasopressin in the newborn infant. J Pediatr 1980;97:462–465.

Rajerison RM, Butten D, Jard S: Ontogenic Development of Kidney and

Liver Vasopressin Receptors. *In* Spitzer A (ed): The Kidney During Development: Morphology and Function. New York, Masson, 1982, pp 249–256.

Reyes JL, Melendez E: Effects of eicosanoids on the water and sodium balance of the neonate. Pediatr Nephrol 1990;4:630–634.

Richoux JP, Amsaguine S, Grignon G, et al: Earliest renin containing cell differentiation during ontogenesis in the rat. Histochemistry 1987;88: 41–46.

Robillard JE, Gomez RA, Meernik JG, et al: Role of angiotensin II on the adrenal and vascular responses to hemorrhage during development in the fetal lambs. Circ Res 1982;50:645–650.

Robillard JE, Weiner C: Atrial natriuretic factor in the human fetus: Effect of volume expansion. J Pediatr 1988;113:552–556.

Robillard JE, Weismann DN, Gomez RA, et al: Renal and adrenal responses to converting-enzyme inhibition in fetal and newborn life. Am J Physiol 1983;244:R249–R256.

Robillard JE, Weitzman RE: Developmental aspects of the fetal response to exogenous arginine vasopressin. Am J Physiol 1980;238:F407–F414.

Robillard JE, Weitzman RE, Fisher DA, et al: The dynamics of vasopressin release and blood volume regulation during fetal hemorrhage in the lamb fetus. Pediatr Res 1979;13:606–610.

Ross MG, Ervin MG, Lam RW, et al: Plasma atrial natriuretic peptide response to volume expansion in the ovine fetus. J Pediatr 1987;157: 1292–1297.

Schoeneman MJSA: The effect of intravascular volume expansion on proximal tubular reabsorption during development. Proc Soc Exp Biol Med 1980;165:319–322.

Siegel SR, Fisher DA: Ontogeny of the renin-angiotensin-aldosterone system in the fetal and newborn lamb. Pediatr Res 1980;14:99–102.

Solhaug MJ, Wallace MR, Granger JP: Endothelium-derived nitric oxide modulates renal hemodynamics in the developing piglet. Pediatr Res 1993;34:750–754.

Stern P, LaRochette F Jr, Little GA: Role of vasopressin in water imbalance in the sick newborn. Kidney Int 1979;16:956–959.

Toshimori H, Toshimori K, Oura C, et al: Immunohistochemical study of atrial natriuretic polypeptides in the embryonic, fetal and neonatal rat heart. Cell Tissue Res 1987;248:627–633.

Vincent M, Dessary Y, Annat G, et al: Plasma renin activity, aldosterone and dopamine-β-hydroxylase activity as a function of age in normal children. Pediatr Res 1980;14:894.

Wallace KB, Hook JB, Bailie MD: Postnatal development of the renin-angiotensin system in rats. Am J Physiol 1980;238:R432–R437.

Wei Y, Rodi CP, Day ML, et al: Developmental changes in the rat atriopeptin hormonal system. J Clin Invest 1987;79:1325–1329.

Weil J, Bidlingmaier F, Dohlemann C, et al: Comparison of plasma atrial natriuretic peptide levels in healthy children from birth to adolescence and in children with cardiac diseases. Pediatr Res 1986;20:1328–1331.

Yamaji T, Hirai N, Ishibashi M, et al: Atrial natriuretic peptide in umbilical cord blood: Evidence for a circulation hormone in human fetus. J Clin Endocrinol Metab 1988;63:1414–1417.

Functional Response of the Developing Kidneys to Malformation or Injury

Appenroth D, Braunlich H: Age dependent differences in sodium dichromate nephrotoxicity in rats. Exp Pathol 1988;33:179–185.

Argueso LR, Ritchey ML, Boyle ET Jr., et al: Prognosis of children with solitary kidney after unilateral nephrectomy. J Urol 1992;148:747–751.

Aschinberg LC, Koskimies O, Bernstein J, et al: The influence of age on the response to renal parenchymal loss. Yale J Biol Med 1978;51:341–345.

Beck AD: The effect of intra-uterine urinary obstruction upon the development of the fetal kidney. J Urol 1971;105:784–789.

Bhathena DB, Julian BA, McMorrow RG, et al: Focal sclerosis of hypertrophied glomeruli in solitary functioning kidneys of humans. Am J Kidney Dis 1985;5:226–232.

Bonvalet JP, Champion M, Wanstok F, et al: Compensatory renal hypertrophy in young rats: Increase in the number of nephrons. Kidney Int 1972;1:391–396.

Brenner BM, Chertow GM: Congenital oligonephropathy and the etiology of adult hypertension and progressive renal injury. Am J Kidney Dis 1994;23:171–175.

Brenner BM, Meyer TW, Hostetter TH: Dietary protein intake and the progressive nature of kidney disease: The role of hemodynamically mediated glomerular injury in the pathogenesis of progressive glomerular sclerosis in aging, renal ablation, and intrinsic renal disease. N Engl J Med 1982;307:652–659.

Celsi G, Bohman S-O, Aperia A: Development of focal glomerulosclerosis after unilateral nephrectomy in infant rats. Pediatr Nephrol 1987; 1:290–296.

Chevalier RL: Functional adaptation to reduced renal mass in early development. Am J Physiol 1982a;242:F190–F196.

Chevalier RL: Glomerular number and perfusion during normal and compensatory renal growth in the guinea pig. Pediatr Res 1982b;16:436–440.

Chevalier RL: Hemodynamic adaptation to reduced renal mass in early postnatal development. Pediatr Res 1983;17:620–624.

Chevalier RL: Chronic partial ureteral obstruction in the neonatal guinea pig II: Pressure gradients affecting glomerular filtration rate. Pediatr Res 1984;18:1271–1277.

Chevalier RL, Gomez RA: Response of the renin-angiotensin system to relief of neonatal ureteral obstruction. Am J Physiol 1989;255:F1070–F1077.

Chevalier RL, Gomez RA, Jones CA: Developmental determinants of recovery after relief of partial ureteral obstruction. Kidney Int 1988;33: 775–781.

Chevalier, RL, Goyal S, Kim A, et al: Renal tubulointerstitial injury from ureteral obstruction in the neonatal rat is attenuated by IGF-1. Kidney Int 2000;57:882–890.

Chevalier RL, Kaiser DL: Autoregulation of renal blood flow in the rat: Effects of growth and uninephrectomy. Am J Physiol 1983;244:F483–F487.

Chevalier RL, Kaiser DL: Chronic partial ureteral obstruction in the neonatal guinea pig I: Influence of uninephrectomy on growth and hemodynamics. Pediatr Res 1984;18:1266–1271.

Chevalier RL, Kim A, Thornhill BA, et al: Recovery following relief of unilateral ureteral obstruction in the neonatal rat. Kidney Int 1999a;55: 793–807.

Chevalier RL, Peach MJ: Hemodynamic effects of enalapril on neonatal chronic partial ureteral obstruction. Kidney Int 1985;28:891–898.

Chevalier RL, Sturgill BC, Jones CE, et al: Morphologic correlates of renal growth arrest in neonatal partial ureteral obstruction. Pediatr Res 1987;21:338–346.

Chevalier RL, Thornhill BA, Chang AY: Unilateral ureteral obstruction in neonatal rats leads to renal insufficiency in adulthood. Kidney Int 2000; 58:1987–1995.

Dauber IM, Krauss AN, Symchych PS, et al: Renal failure following perinatal anoxia. J Pediatr 1976;88:851–855.

Dicker SE, Shirley DG: Compensatory renal growth after unilateral nephrectomy in the newborn rat. J Physiol 1973;228:193–202.

El-Dahr SS, Gomez RA, Gray MS, et al: In situ localization of renin and its mRNA in neonatal ureteral obstruction. Am J Physiol 1990a;258: F854–F862.

El-Dahr S, Gomez RA, Khare G, et al: Expression of renin and its mRNA in the adult rat kidney with chronic ureteral obstruction. Am J Kidney Dis 1990b;15:575–582.

Elema JD: Is one kidney sufficient? Kidney Int 1976;9:308.

Fogo A, Ichikawa I: Evidence for the central role of glomerular growth promoters in the development of sclerosis. Semin Nephrol 1989;9:329–342.

Glazebrook KN, McGrath FP, Steele BT: Prenatal compensatory renal growth: Documentation with US. Radiology 1993;189:733–735.

Glick PL, Harrison MR, Noall RA, et al: Correction of congenital hydronephrosis in utero III: Early mid-trimester ureteral obstruction produces renal dysplasia. J Pediatr Surg 1983;18:681–687.

Gomez RA, Chevalier RL, Sturgill BC, et al: Maturation of the intrarenal renin distribution in Wistar-Kyoto rats. J Hypertension 1986;4(Suppl 5): S31–S33.

Gomez RA, Meernik JG, Kuehl WD, et al: Developmental aspects of the renal response to hemorrhage during fetal life. Pediatr Res 1984;18:40–46.

Griscom NT, Vawter GP, Fellers FX: Pelvoinfundibular atresia, the usual form of multicystic kidney: 44 unilateral and two bilateral cases. Semin Roentgenol 1975;10:125–131.

Hammerman MR: Recapitulation of phylogeny by ontogeny in nephrology. Kidney Int 2000;57:742–755.

Hayslett JP: Functional adaptation to reduction in renal mass. Physiol Rev 1979;59:137–164.

Hayslett JP, Kashgarian M, Epstein FH: Functional correlates of compensatory renal hypertrophy. J Clin Invest 1968;47:774–799.

Horster M, Kemler BJ, Valtin H: Intracortical distribution of number and volume of glomeruli during postnatal maturation in the dog. J Clin Invest 1971;50:796–800.

Ikoma M, Yoshioka T, Ichikawa I, et al: Mechanism of the unique susceptibility of deep cortical glomeruli of maturing kidneys to severe focal glomerular sclerosis. Pediatr Res 1990;28:270–276.

Jongejan HTM, Provoost AP, Wolff ED, et al: Nephrotoxicity of cisplatin comparing young and adult rats. Pediatr Res 1986;20:9–14.

Karp R, Brasel JA, Winick M: Compensatory kidney growth after uninephrectomy in adult and infant rats. Am J Dis Child 1971;121:186–188.

Kaufman JM, Hardy R, Hayslett JP: Age-dependent characteristics of compensatory renal growth. Kidney Int 1975;8:21–26.

King LR, Coughlin PWF, Bloch EC, et al: The case for immediate pyeloplasty in the neonate with ureteropelvic junction obstruction. J Urol 1984;132:725–728.

Kiprov DD, Colvin RB, McCluskey RT: Focal and segmental glomerulosclerosis and proteinuria associated with unilateral renal agenesis. Lab Invest 1982;46:275–281.

Kunes, J, Capek K, Stejskal J, et al: Age-dependent difference of kidney response to temporary ischaemia in the rat. Clin Sci Mol Med 1978;55: 365–368.

Larsson L, Aperia A, Wilton P: Effect of normal development on compensatory renal growth. Kidney Int 1980;18:29–35.

Lelievre-Pegorier M, Sakly R, Meulemans A, et al: Kinetics of gentamicin in plasma of nonpregnant, pregnant, and fetal guinea pigs and its distribution in fetal tissues. Antimicrob Agents Chemother 1985;28: 565–569.

Luttenegger TJ, Gooding CA, Fickenscher LG: Compensatory renal hypertrophy after treatment for Wilms' tumor. Am J Roentgenol Radium Ther Nucl Med 1975;125:348–351.

Mandell J, Peters CA, Estroff JA, et al: Human fetal compensatory renal growth. J Urol 1993;150:790–792.

Marre R, Tarara N, Louton T, et al: Age-dependent nephrotoxicity and the pharmacokinetics of gentamicin in rats. Eur J Pediatr 1980;133:25–29.

Mitus A, Tefft M, Fellers FX: Long-term follow-up of renal functions of 108 children who underwent nephrectomy for malignant disease. Pediatrics 1969;44:912–921.

Norwood VF, Carey RM, Geary KM, et al: Neonatal ureteral obstruction stimulates recruitment of renin-secreting renal cortical cells. Kidney Int 1994;45:1333–1339.

O'Sullivan DC, Dewan PA, Guiney EJ: Compensatory hypertrophy effectively assesses the degree of impaired renal function in unilateral renal disease. Br J Urol 1992;69:346–350.

Okuda S, Motomura K, Sanai T, et al: Influence of age on deterioration of the remnant kidney in uninephrectomized rats. Clin Sci 1987;72: 571–576.

Olivetti G, Anversa P, Melissari M, et al: Morphometry of the renal corpuscle during postnatal growth and compensatory hypertrophy. Kidney Int 1980;17:438–454.

Pelayo JC, Andrews PM, Coffey AK, et al: The influence of age on acute renal toxicity of uranylnitrate in the dog. Pediatr Res 1983;17: 985–992.

Peters CA, Gaertner RC, Carr MC, et al: Fetal compensatory renal growth due to unilateral ureteral obstruction. J Urol 1993;150:597–600.

Phillips TL, Leong GF: Kidney cell proliferation after unilateral nephrectomy as related to age. Cancer Res 1967;27:286–292.

Provoost AP, Adejuyigbe O, Wolff ED: Nephrotoxicity of aminoglycosides in young and adult rats. Pediatr Res 1985;19:1191–1196.

Robillard JE, Gomez RA, Meernik JG, et al: Role of angiotensin II on the adrenal and vascular responses to hemorrhage during development in the fetal lambs. Circ Res 1982;50:645–650.

Robillard JE, Weitzman RE, Burmeister L, et al: Developmental aspects of the renal response to hypoxemia in the lamb fetus. Circ Res 1981; 48:128–138.

Shirley DG: Developmental and compensatory renal growth in the guinea pig. Biol Neonate 1976;30:169–180.

Stark H, Geiger R: Renal tubular dysfunction following vascular accidents of the kidneys in the newborn period. J Pediatr 1990;83:933–940.

Taki M, Goldsmith DI, Spitzer A: Impact of age on effects of ureteral obstruction on renal function. Kidney Int 1983;24:602–609.

Weismann DN, Clarke WR: Postnatal age-related renal responses to hypoxemia in lambs. Circ Res 1981;49:1332–1338.

Wikstad I, Celsi G, Larsson L, et al: Kidney function in adults born with unilateral renal agenesis or nephrectomized in childhood. Pediatr Nephrol 1988;2:177–182.

51

PERINATAL UROLOGY

Craig A. Peters, M.D.

FETAL DIAGNOSIS

The impact of prenatal ultrasonographic (US) diagnosis on pediatric urology has been enormous, effectively creating a new class of disorders that require unique management approaches. Many of these patients are helped greatly with early diagnosis and prevention of secondary complications, particularly infection. Others, however, may be seen as being subjected to needless interventions because of prenatal findings of uncertain long-term clinical significance. The debate continues and will do so until a more practical understanding of the pathophysiology and an accurate assessment of these conditions' natural history is obtained. For now, we are obliged to deal with the information available and make clinical decisions based on the patient's condition and the parents' wishes. The chapter reviews the principles of prenatal urologic diagnosis and management and immediate care of the neonate with urologic problems.

Diagnostic Findings

Interpretation of any prenatal US image is based on a synthesis of specific findings to generate a differential diagnosis, exactly as is done postnatally. As with any single test, a definitive diagnosis may not always be made with certainty, and the ability to make a definitive diagnosis depends on the operator. The need for diagnostic accuracy, particularly when there is a spectrum of involvement, is also relative to the clinical situation. There are several essential elements to any prenatal US examination of the urinary tract that are used to define the possible diagnoses, and they are illustrated in Table 51–1. Recognizing these specific findings and their variations, and knowing the patterns of association that suggest specific diagnostic entities, will usually permit the perinatal urologist to make an accurate diagnosis that is adequate for the immediate perinatal period.

The **normal kidney** (Fig. 51–1) has an elliptical shape with distinctive internal echoes defined by the medullary pyramids and peripelvic echo complex. The renal cortex should be of uniform echogenicity, slightly less than that of the spleen or liver. **The echolucent pyramids, which should not be confused for dilated calyces, first become evident at about 20 weeks. Their absence later in gestation is abnormal.** The size of the normal kidney is important because it may reflect the condition of the contralateral kidney.

The renal parenchyma may be abnormally echogenic without having frank cysts. In some children this has been seen as an isolated finding without apparent negative sequelae, but it has also been associated with renal parenchymal disorders (Carr et al, 1995a). When associated with hydronephrosis, increased renal echogenicity suggests dysplastic changes, but this is not invariable unless there is profound hydronephrosis, often with decreasing amniotic fluid (AF) (Kaefer et al, 1997). The thickness of the parenchyma in the setting of hydronephrosis is important to note, but it does not predict decreased function. Often this thinning is caused simply by stretching of the parenchyma around a dilated collecting system. The label "cortical atrophy" should be discouraged.

Hydronephrosis is the most common abnormality found on prenatal US. It is seen in a wide spectrum, from pelvic

Table 51–1. ELEMENTS OF PRENATAL UROLOGIC ULTRASONOGRAPHIC DIAGNOSIS

Parameter	Comment	Possible Causes
Hydronephrosis	Variable severity; may include pelviectasis and/or caliectasis	Obstruction, reflux
Caliectasis	Intrarenal dilation; more indicative of significant pathologic process	Obstruction, reflux
Pelvic anterior-posterior diameter	Measured in the coronal plane, variable; in extremes may predict clinical outcome; caution should be exercised in over-reliance on these measurements	Increased in obstruction, reflux
Renal parenchyma	Echogenicity should be less than liver or spleen; lucent medullary pyramids should be seen	Increased echogenicity in dysplasia, obstruction, ARPKD
Urothelial thickening	Increased thickness of pelvic lining	Variable dilation as with reflux or occasionally obstruction
Duplication	Separation of renal pelvic sinus echoes when no hydronephrosis seen	Possible associated reflux or obstruction; look for dilated ureter and ureterocele
Cystic structures, renal	Simple cysts rare	MCDK, ADPKD
Cystic structures, intravesical	May be very large and fill bladder; thin walled	Ureterocele
Urinoma	Fluid collection around kidney; perinephric or subcapsular	Obstruction
Bladder filling	Fill and void cycles may be demonstrated over time	Urine production
Bladder wall thickness	Must be interpreted in context of bladder filling	Obstruction, neurogenic dysfunction
"Keyhole sign"	Dilated posterior urethral; difficult to image	Posterior urethral valves
Oligohydramnios	Markedly reduced amniotic fluid; usually considered as no pocket of fluid <2 cm	Poor urine output due to obstruction and/or renal failure

ARPKD, autosomal recessive polycystic kidney disease; MCDK, multicystic dysplastic kidney.

dilation that is barely noticeable to massive dilation taking up much of the fetal abdomen (Figs. 51–2 and 51–3). **Hydronephrosis is not a specific diagnosis, but a finding. The cause of the hydronephrosis is the diagnosis and will indicate the appropriate treatment.** The character of the hydronephrosis, however, is extremely important to permit a diagnosis and prognosis. A variety of grading systems have been used in the literature, all of which have similar strengths and limitations. Numerical grading systems convey a sense of quantification, as do renal pelvic anterior-posterior (AP) diameter measurements (Fernbach et al, 1993). The correlation between degree of hydronephro-

sis and postnatal outcome remains poor (see later discussion), which limits the value of an overprecise grading system. We have used the descriptive scale shown in Figure 51–4, with specific comment on the nature of calyceal dilation. AP diameter measurements are useful in a comparative sense, but there is variability in the reliability of these numbers. Practical thresholds have been developed from these measurements, but they should be used only as rough guidelines (Corteville et al, 1991). **When describing hydronephrosis, the pelvic and calyceal configuration must be included, as well as whether the condition is unilateral or bilateral.** It is best if the side of involvement is known, because this does not always correlate with post-

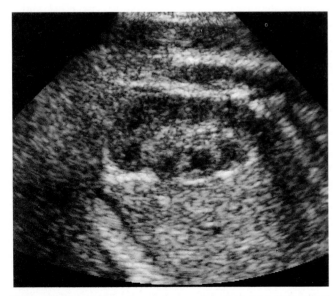

Figure 51–1. Ultrasound appearance of normal fetal kidney with echolucent medullary pyramids distinguishable from the more echogenic cortical parenchyma. The cortical parenchyma should be of lower echogenicity than adjacent liver or spleen.

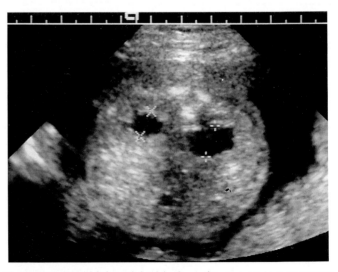

Figure 51–2. Mild bilateral fetal hydronephrosis seen in a transverse view. The bright area between the kidneys is the spine. The anterior-posterior (AP) pelvic diameter is measured in this view; however, calyceal configuration is not well seen.

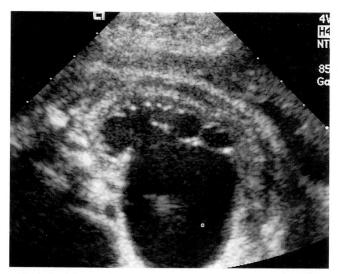

Figure 51–3. Severe fetal hydronephrosis with diffuse calyceal dilation arrayed around the markedly dilated renal pelvis. The renal parenchyma is stretched over the dilated collecting system, but this does not mean loss of functional potential. Corticomedullary differentiation is difficult to see in this configuration.

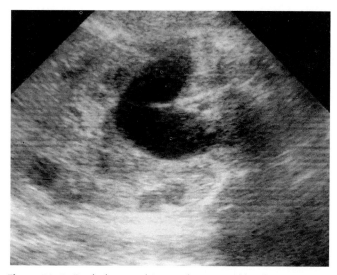

Figure 51–5. Fetal ultrasound image showing a dilated, tortuous ureter with the typical "folded sausage" shape. This may be associated with reflux, valves, ectopic ureters and ureteroceles, or ureterovesical junction obstruction.

natal findings and might suggest variability, perhaps because of reflux. Any variation in the degree of hydronephrosis during one examination is an important finding that is strongly suggestive of reflux.

Hydroureter may be more difficult to detect, but, if it is present, the appearance is characteristic. The markedly dilated ureter is seen in multiple adjacent cross sections, giving it a "folded sausage" look between the kidney and the bladder (Fig. 51–5). **In less severe cases, a dilated ureter is best detected behind a full bladder.** Ureteral peristalsis may be recognized as well. Confusion may occur if a duplex system has both ureters dilated, because resolution of these structures may not be possible.

Renal cysts may be seen in a variety of disorders and are usually multiple and heterogeneous in size. Multiple small cysts not resolved on US appear as a very bright, echogenic kidney, as is seen with autosomal recessive polycystic kidney disease (ARPKD), whereas the large macrocysts of a multicystic dysplastic kidney (MCDK) are readily apparent. **Cysts do not communicate visibly with**

each other, in contrast to dilated calyces. **A single upper pole cyst is probably not a cyst but a dilated upper pole.** A single cyst in the renal fossa may be an unusual MCDK, severe hydronephrosis without recognizable parenchyma, or a nonrenal structure, such as an intestinal duplication, a cystic tumor of the adrenal, or a loop of bowel.

The **bladder** is often neglected in fetal studies, because it is often difficult to image well. The bladder should be seen in a filled state on a fetal US, and occasionally voiding may be detected. If there is a question regarding renal function, bladder filling may be a useful sign of urine output. **The inability to identify a bladder on several studies should raise the question of bladder exstrophy.** The appearance of the bladder wall should be examined, because it may be a clue to bladder outlet obstruction, such as posterior urethral valves (PUV) or neurogenic dysfunction. This is a subjective observation, but, if it is present, is likely to be a real phenomenon. **Dilation of the posterior urethra, the "keyhole" sign, is strongly suggestive of PUV** (Fig. 51–6). Intravesical structures should be sought, particularly if a ureterocele may be present in association

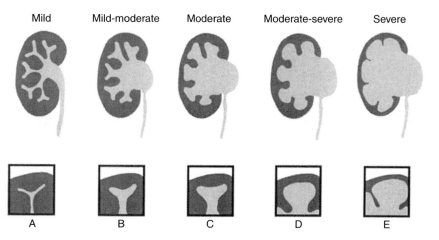

Figure 51–4. Diagram indicating appearance of progressive severity of hydronephrosis, including calyceal configuration. There is not always direct correlation between the degree of renal pelvic dilation and that of the calyces.

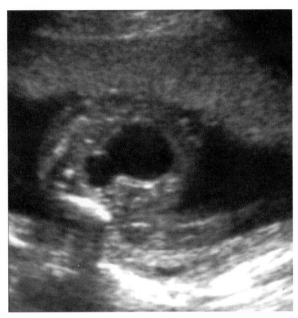

Figure 51–6. Fetal ultrasound at 22 weeks of a male fetus with posterior urethral valves. The bladder is thick walled and has a dilated posterior urethra (keyhole). Bilateral hydronephrosis, echogenic renal parenchyma, and a perinephric urinoma were also present.

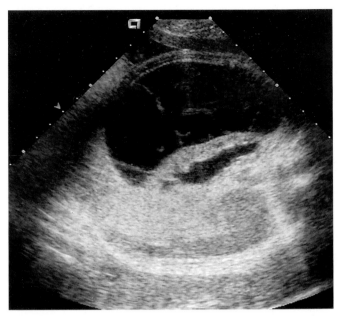

Figure 51–7. Appearance of a fetal perinephric urinoma associated with posterior urethral valves.

with a duplex system with upper pole hydronephrosis. An ectopic ureter, also associated with a dilated upper pole, may give the false appearance of an intravesical ureterocele, but the ureterovesical wall will be much thicker.

In some obstructive conditions, a **perirenal urinoma** may be present, indicating significant obstructive effect (Fig. 51–7). This usually appears as an anechoic structure around the kidney, at times with a thick outer rim that fuses with the kidney cortex, indicating a subcapsular urinoma. Urinary ascites may also be noted in the fetus with severe bladder outlet obstruction. The significance of a urinoma depends on the time of appearance and the anatomic basis. We have reported on perinephric urinomata associated with gradual involution of a previously hydronephrotic kidney, with no detectable function postnatally (Mandell et al, 1994). This probably indicates a high degree of obstruction, sufficient to induce a pop-off, but also permanent and severe injury to normal development. The pop-off effect may also serve to protect the kidney, but this is more often seen with PUV (Adzick, et al, 1985a).

A less commonly considered element of fetal US diagnosis is the characterization of the **external genitalia.** In cases where PUV is a diagnostic possibility, male gender is a required part of the diagnosis, but other conditions may depend on this determination. In situations where there is uncertainty as to the development of the external genitalia, careful examination may reveal particular aspects, such as phallic length, chordee, and the presence of scrotal testes. **Care must be exercised in this determination, because a virilized clitoris may appear as a small phallus, and without the presence of scrotal testes one cannot finalize a male assignment** (Benacerraf et al, 1989; Bromley et al, 1994). The appearance of a dilated, elongated penile urethra may be consistent with megalourethra, which is associated with the prune-belly syndrome, although isolated cases have been reported (Fig. 51–8).

Any assessment of the fetal urinary tract must include a comment on the AF volume. Although it is difficult to quantitate AF volume, and several systems exist to do so,

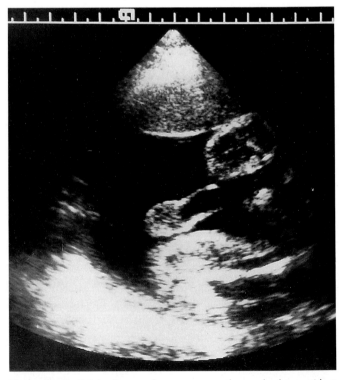

Figure 51–8. Fetal ultrasound appearance of a male fetus with a dilated and patulous urethra typical of a megalourethra. This may be seen in the prune-belly syndrome as well as in isolation. This child also had marked vesicoureteral reflux.

whether there is a noticeable reduction and what the time course of any change has been are important indicators of the health of the urinary tract (Queenan et al, 1972; Manning et al, 1981). **The time of onset of changes in the AF is critical and reflects a normal shift from being mostly a placental transudate to being predominantly a product of fetal urine** (Takeuchi et al, 1994). **This occurs after 16 weeks, and by 20 or 22 weeks most AF is fetal urine.** Therefore, oligohydramnios, the condition of reduced AF, may be caused by urinary tract obstruction and may become evident after only 18 or 20 weeks' gestation. It may also be the product of abnormal renal development without obstruction, such as bilateral MCDK or ARPKD (Stiller et al, 1988).

Concurrent with any fetal diagnosis of a urinary tract anomaly must be a thorough fetal survey, including all major systems, an estimate of fetal growth, and an evaluation of the AF and the placenta. If a major anomaly is identified, and particularly if any consideration for intervention is present, amniocentesis and karyotyping are considered essential elements of the evaluation. The incidence of concurrent chromosomal anomalies is relatively high in fetuses with urologic anomalies (Callan et al, 1990; Nicolaides et al, 1992).

Appearance of Major Diagnoses

A tentative fetal diagnosis may be made with US evaluation based on the association of the various elements already noted. Although a precise diagnosis may not always be made due to fetal imaging or overlap of some conditions, the differential diagnosis may be refined. Changes over time may also assist in making the ultimate diagnosis. The severity of certain conditions must be considered as well. It is difficult to make a firm prediction of outcome with postnatal imaging studies in many conditions, and in the fetus this possibility is even more restricted.

The usual appearance of a ureteropelvic junction (UPJ) obstruction is limited to some degree of pelvic and calyceal dilation, without any evidence of ureteral dilation. It is usually unilateral, and lesser degrees of dilation may at times be seen on the opposite side. Whether these dilations are all actually caused by a functional obstruction at the UPJ remains unclear, largely because of the huge spectrum of severity and the fact that surgery is rarely done for mild to moderate degrees of dilation. It is possible that some component of these cases is secondary to bladder hypertonicity, which is suggested by the extremely high proportion of male fetuses with these conditions. There is no postnatally validated degree of hydronephrosis that is truly "normal" or "physiologic." Mild degrees of dilation may reflect significant reflux, even without a dilated ureter.

Ureterovesical junction obstruction is characterized prenatally by dilation of the renal pelvis and ureter to the level of the bladder. The degree is also highly variable, and the amount of renal pelvic and calyceal dilation may be significant (Dorenbaum et al, 1986). The amount of dilation in the ureter may be greater distally than proximally. The ureters may be best seen at the level of the bladder, and some authors have used ureteral diameter measurements to attempt to prognosticate clinical outcome (Liu et al, 1994). The causes of the ureterovesical junction obstruction may be several, including primary obstruction of a normally positioned ureter or an ectopic ureter inserting into the bladder neck. Reflux may also produce a very similar pattern.

Vesicoureteral reflux (VUR) may be evident by a variable degree of collecting system dilation; however, there is no reliable way to predict the presence of reflux or its grade based on fetal US. Variable hydronephrosis during one examination or between examinations should always raise the suspicion of reflux and prompt postnatal evaluation. Reflux may occasionally be suspected on the basis of increased renal parenchymal echogenicity, which should prompt a postnatal voiding cystourethrogram (VCUG). Massive bilateral hydroureteronephrosis (HUN) may be present due to reflux in the megacystis-megaureter association yet appear similar to bladder outlet obstruction (Mandell et al, 1992a).

One of the most important, although at times challenging, fetal diagnoses is that of **posterior urethral valves.** The wide spectrum of severity seen in postnatal valves gives sufficient indication as to the range of possible fetal appearances of this condition. In some situations the diagnosis is obvious, but most such cases suggest a dismal prognosis. In other situations, the suspicion may be present but it remains unclear how aggressively to evaluate the patient in the postnatal period. The most severe manifestation of the condition may be seen early in gestation (even as early as 13 weeks), with bladder distention and bilateral hydronephrosis, associated with increased renal echogenicity (Bellinger et al, 1983; Reuter and Lebowitz, 1985; Barakat et al, 1991; Dinneen et al, 1993; Hutton et al, 1994; Gunn et al, 1995; Kaefer et al, 1997; Abbott et al, 1998). The latter may be indicative of renal dysplasia. On occasion, bladder dilation may be massive, taking up most of the fetal abdomen (Fig. 51–9). With gestational progression, the bladder may become thick walled and the posterior urethra may be recognized by its dilation (Fig. 51–10). By the middle of the second trimester (18 weeks), AF volume may begin to decrease owing to the decreasing contribution of the placenta to fluid volume and the increasing contribution of fetal urine, which is obstructed. **Second-trimester oligohydramnios (minimal AF) is usually associated with a lethal outcome in the immediate postnatal period due to pulmonary hypoplasia** (Barss et al, 1984). Oligohydramnios may develop later in gestation, and this may alter the prognosis. **Late-onset oligohydramnios (after 30 weeks) usually is not associated with pulmonary insufficiency, but it may pose obstetric risks** (Mandell et al, 1992c). PUV may also be manifest with a less obvious clinical picture, which may make it indistinguishable from other entities. In the setting of a distended bladder with dilated upper tracts, PUV, and also bilateral megaureters or bilateral reflux, are real possibilities (Abbott et al, 1998). On occasion, the dilated posterior urethra may be noted, and this is strongly suggestive of PUV. Other elements that might suggest the presence of PUV include perinephric urinomata, increased renal parenchymal echogenicity, and occasionally a thick-walled bladder. In the

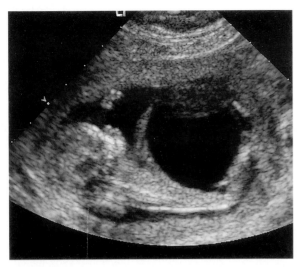

Figure 51–9. Massive bladder dilation is apparent in this early fetal ultrasound image showing megacystis, probably caused by posterior urethral valves. The bladder fills the entire abdomen and pushes the chest upward. Because of the early age of this fetus, oligohydramnios has not yet developed, but it can be expected to do so at 20 to 22 weeks.

setting of a dilated fetal bladder, bilateral HUN with increased parenchymal echogenicity is suggestive of PUV, and if oligohydramnios is seen at any time, the diagnosis becomes almost certain (Kaefer et al, 1997; Oliveira et al, 2000). However, significant reflux may have a very similar appearance in male fetuses, and only postnatal imaging can differentiate the two.

An unusual cause of fetal bladder outlet obstruction is apparent neurogenic dysfunction with bladder sphincter dyssynergy. This produces a dilated, thick-walled bladder with HUN. In the small group reported, a neurogenic cause

was hypothesized, but no clear neurologic lesion could be identified postnatally and the true underlying etiology was speculative (Bauer et al, 1989).

Ureterocele is one of the most definite diagnoses that may be made in the fetal period, although one of the more challenging (Schoenecker et al, 1985; Fitzsimons et al, 1986; Vergani et al, 1999). **The usual indication of the possibility of a ureterocele is the presence of upper pole hydronephrosis and a dilated ureter that may be traced to the bladder. Careful inspection of the bladder will then usually demonstrate an intravesical, thin-walled cystic structure associated with the base of the bladder** (Fig. 51–11). The communication with the dilated ureter may be seen as well. An alternative appearance is the association of an intravesical cystic structure with a cystic dysplastic upper pole without obvious hydronephrosis. This appearance may evolve such that the upper pole is no longer apparent and only the ureterocele is seen. This pattern is ureterocele disproportion, in which there is little ureteral dilation and a small dysplastic upper pole (Share and Lebowitz, 1989). **The absence of upper pole dilation should therefore not preclude the diagnosis of a ureterocele when the characteristic intravesical findings are noted.** Single-system ureteroceles, seen more frequently in boys, usually have associated hydronephrosis of the entire kidney, of variable degree.

In the setting of a ureterocele it is important to assess the contralateral renal unit, as well as the ipsilateral lower pole. Lower pole reflux may produce ipsilateral hydronephrosis, occasionally of massive degree. Contralateral reflux may be present as well, either in a single system or a duplex with lower pole reflux. **Bilateral hydronephrosis may imply bilateral reflux, but it may also indicate an element of bladder outlet obstruction caused by bladder neck prolapse of the ureterocele.** This has rarely caused oligohydramnios.

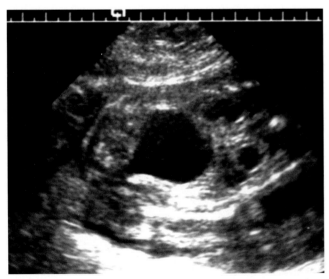

Figure 51–10. Ultrasound appearance of severe posterior urethral valves in a male fetus. The bladder is moderately distended and remains so. Both kidneys show moderately severe dilation with normal renal parenchyma. Amniotic fluid was normal. The child was delivered near full term without respiratory problems but with mild renal insufficiency and posterior urethral valves.

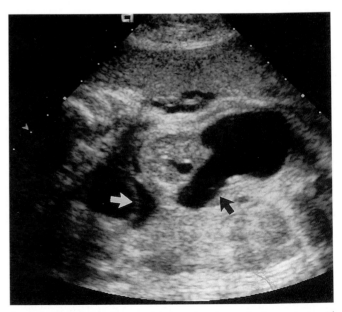

Figure 51–11. Fetal ultrasound image showing a duplex system with an intravesical ureterocele. There is marked upper pole hydronephrosis with a dilated ureter *(black arrow)* and a lower pole with mild pelvic dilation. The ureterocele *(white arrow)* is visible in the bladder.

Upper pole hydronephrosis in the fetus also suggests an ectopic ureter in the absence of an intravesical cystic structure; ureteral ectopia with obstruction is the presumed diagnosis. The dilated ureter may create a large impression on the back wall of the bladder, mimicking the appearance of a ureterocele. Although it is not always possible to accurately differentiate these entities, **the wall thickness of the ectopic ureter is much greater than that of the ureterocele, because the latter is made up only of attenuated ureteral wall, whereas the ectopic ureter impression includes the ureter and bladder walls.** The appearance of bilateral single-system ectopic ureters is quite distinct from that of the more common duplex ectopic ureters. Bilateral single ectopic ureters are usually associated with significant renal abnormality manifested by echogenic parenchyma and cysts, as well as minimal to no bladder filling. Reduced AF may be associated with severe renal impairment, as is frequently seen.

One of the most characteristic fetal US appearances is that of the MCDK. **The classic US appearance of an MCDK was initially defined by Sanders as being a non-reniform structure, with multiple noncommunicating fluid-filled cystic spaces, no central large cyst, and minimal to no recognizable renal parenchyma** (Bearman et al, 1976; Sanders and Hartman, 1984). The overall size of the cyst complex is quite variable, but its appearance is characteristic and immediately recognizable (Fig. 51–12). The absence of communication among the cystic structures, which is an essential part of the imaging diagnosis, is apparent on real-time imaging. In the severely hydronephrotic kidney, dilated calyces may appear to be noncommunicating on a static image, but the communications may be seen in dynamic views. The absence of US communication is in contrast to anatomic communication, usually through fine channels (Peters and Mandell, 1989; Borer et al, 1994). The amount of parenchyma is also variable, and there are examples of MCDKs that have a more substantial amount of parenchyma visible (Felson and Cussen, 1975).

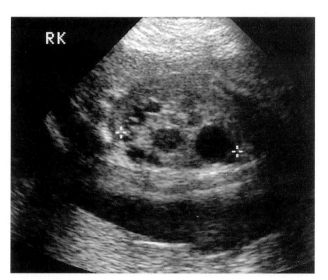

Figure 51–12. Multicystic dysplastic kidney with multiple, variable-sized cysts without a central large cystic area. There is a moderate amount of renal parenchyma that is echogenic. In some cases virtually no parenchyma is visible.

It is invariably echogenic and may be seen to contain small cysts. It is not oriented in any particular aspect of the cystic complex.

The **location of the MCDK** is typically in the usual renal position, but it may be seen in any position of an ectopic kidney, including the pelvis or as a crossed ectopic renal unit. In these cases, of course, the diagnosis may be more difficult in that other cystic anomalies may also be found in those positions.

Duplex systems may include a multicystic dysplastic moiety, usually the upper pole, but occasionally the lower. Associated ureteral pathology should then be sought, including ureteroceles or ureteral ectopia. This is best performed with a careful examination of the bladder.

The principal diagnostic confusion with MCDK is severe hydronephrosis. In such severe cases, the renal parenchyma is markedly attenuated, echogenic, and distorted by the dilated collecting system. The characteristic of most severely hydronephrotic kidneys is the presence of a central cystic structure that is medial and has multiple calyces arrayed about its lateral aspect. These are usually of similar size, and with real-time examination they may be seen to communicate with the central cystic structure. There are some cases in which this typical appearance is not evident, probably in the more severely affected kidneys, in which the dividing line between the hydronephrotic kidney and the MCDK becomes unclear (Felson and Cussen, 1975). When such ambiguity is present postnatally, it is best to assume that a salvageable kidney is present and plan the postnatal evaluation in that light.

The prenatal natural history of MCDK may be reflected in the varying appearance of the kidney with gradual involution (Avni et al, 1987). In some instances, the kidney becomes undetectable by US, either prenatally or in the postnatal period (Mandell et al, 1994). This observation raises the question of how many cases of absent kidneys are actually the end point of an MCDK that is nondetectable on US imaging. The functional consequences of this situation may not be relevant, but it is clear that some renal parenchyma, albeit dysplastic, is present.

Other diagnostic entities that may appear similar to an MCDK include any renal cystic disease with large cysts. This is in distinct contrast to the other common congenital cystic renal disease, ARPKD, which is characterized by large, uniformly echogenic kidneys without recognizable cysts (Smedley and Bailey, 1987; Townsend et al, 1988). The cysts in ARPKD are too small to be resolved by US. In contrast, congenital multilocular cystic nephroma has macrocysts detectable on US. This is a rare entity, characterized by segmental involvement of the kidney with variable-sized macrocysts (Eble and Bonsib, 1998). It is considered a neoplasm by many, but it is also viewed as a hamartomatous malformation. Other elements of this spectrum of congenital cystic malformations that includes cystic Wilms' tumor may also have a macrocystic appearance on US. These are rare and typically have larger amounts of parenchyma, and they will ultimately demonstrate function on postnatal imaging.

Nonrenal cystic lesions may also be confused for MCDK, although these are typically not in the renal fossa and may be confirmed to be nonrenal by the presence of two normal kidneys. These lesions include **mesen-**

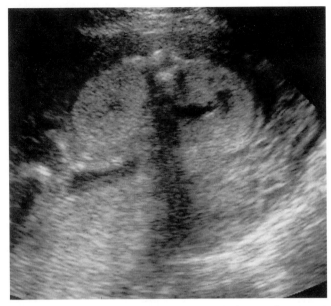

Figure 51–13. Bilaterally enlarged, echogenic kidneys without grossly apparent cysts are typical for autosomal recessive polycystic kidney disease (ARPKD). This appearance usually becomes apparent by 22 weeks of gestation, but not always. In early-onset cases, oligohydramnios is seen.

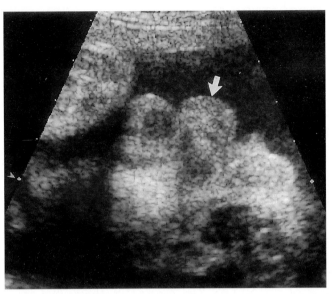

Figure 51–14. Fetal ultrasound image showing a low-set umbilical insertion, no evidence of bladder filling, normal kidneys, and a protuberance of tissue from the lower abdomen *(white arrow)*. The scrotum may be seen below the tissue protuberance. This pattern is typical of classic bladder exstrophy.

teric duplication cysts, neurenteric cysts, bronchogenic cysts (Bagolan et al, 2000), and the occasional cystic neuroblastoma (Kozakewich et al, 1998; Hamada et al, 1999). They are unlikely to be mistaken for an MCDK, but in the event of ambiguity, postnatal evaluation should permit resolution of any of these entities.

ARPKD, also called infantile polycystic kidney disease, does not appear cystic but is characterized by markedly enlarged, brightly echogenic kidneys (Lonergan et al, 2000) (Fig. 51–13). This appearance begins to develop before 20 weeks in most affected fetuses, but late development has been reported, making an early diagnosis difficult in affected families (Zerres et al, 1988; Edwards and Baldinger, 1989; Mandell et al, 1991). As yet, a specific chromosomal diagnosis is not available (Ceccherini et al, 1989). As the condition progresses, oligohydramnios develops and most of these infants die of pulmonary insufficiency with Potter's syndrome. Macrocystic disease associated with autosomal dominant polycystic kidney disease (ADPKD) has been reported in the fetus also, although with a very different prognosis (Reeders et al, 1986; McHugo et al, 1988; Ceccherini et al, 1989; Edwards and Baldinger, 1989; Novelli et al, 1989). The cysts are heterogeneous in size and location and may be few in number. It may be important to assess the family when this finding is noted, both to confirm the diagnosis and to identify affected members. The health insurance ramifications of this determination must be considered, however.

Renal agenesis is evidenced by the progressive absence of AF after 16 to 18 weeks, the time when fetal urine begins to constitute the bulk of the AF (Cardwell, 1988; Holmes, 1989; Sherer et al, 1990). The kidneys are not detectable, and no bladder filling is seen. The adrenal glands may be visible in their normal position, but with a linear appearance, the so-called "lying down adrenal" (Hoffman et al, 1992). A small thorax is evident later in gestation. The affected children represent the classic appearance of Potter's syndrome, with oligohydramnios, pulmonary hypoplasia, skeletal defects, low-set ears, and neonatal lethal pulmonary insufficiency.

An important and difficult diagnosis is that of the exstrophy conditions. Classic bladder exstrophy is characterized by the absence of bladder filling on repeated examinations, low-set umbilical cord, and abnormal-appearing external genitalia (Barth et al, 1990; Gearhart et al, 1995). The protrusion of the bladder plate may be apparent just below the umbilical cord (Fig. 51–14). The kidneys are normal, and there are rarely associated conditions. In sharp contrast, cloacal exstrophy is often associated with myelomeningocele, lower extremity abnormalities, and cardiac defects (Meglin et al, 1990; Kaya et al, 2000). Its lower abdominal appearance is often confused with an omphalocele, which is also present. Intestinal protrusion, as is seen postnatally, may or may not be evident on prenatal US (Austin et al, 1998). The diagnosis of either of these conditions requires careful counseling of the prospective parents as to the postnatal implications, and many families choose termination of the pregnancy. As a result, the diagnostic accuracy must be high and the diagnosis must be made at an early point in gestation.

Genital abnormalities are occasionally detected in utero, usually as penile anomalies such as hypospadias or severe chordee (Benacerraf et al, 1989; Mandell et al, 1995). Isolated epispadias is rarely detected in utero. The presence of a penile anomaly in utero should prompt a search for the testes to determine whether the fetus is male or female. Karyotyping may be appropriate as well. In the absence of testes in the inguinal canals or scrotum, the diagnosis of a male fetus should not be made. Severe virilization of females with congenital adrenal hyperplasia may produce a markedly enlarged clitoris. Inappropriate, prenatal sex assignment has been made in this context (Bromley et al, 1994).

Imperforate anus (Mandell et al, 1992b) and its extreme manifestation, cloacal malformation (Cilento et al, 1994), have been specifically detected prenatally, based on identification of various elements of these complex abnormalities.

Certain genitourinary abnormalities have been shown to be associated with other particular anomalies in other systems. **The finding of hydronephrosis has an association with Down's syndrome, with an incidence of 3.3% in fetuses with hydronephrosis** (Benacerraf et al, 1990). Although the incidence of Down's with isolated hydronephrosis is low, consideration of further evaluation in such cases may be appropriate, including searching for increased nuchal fold thickness on US (Benacerraf and Frigoletto, 1987) and amniocentesis for karyotyping. Certain extraurinary diagnoses should prompt consideration of more careful urinary evaluation. Oligohydramnios has many etiologies, several of which are directly related to the urinary tract, including bladder outlet obstruction, dysplasia, and cystic kidneys. **The finding of a cardiac mass (rhabdomyosarcoma) is frequently associated with tuberous sclerosis and possible renal masses** (Becker, 2000).

Renal masses are unusual in the fetal urinary tract, and **the most common renal mass is congenital mesoblastic nephroma. This benign tumor typically replaces the entire kidney with a homogeneous round mass** (Fung et al, 1995; Shibahara et al, 1999; Irsutti et al, 2000). **It may be associated with polyhydramnios** (Geirsson et al, 1985). However, these masses must be considered potentially malignant, and early postnatal removal is recommended, although there is little justification for early delivery. Wilms' tumor has only rarely been described prenatally (Applegate et al, 1999). **Neuroblastoma has been detected prenatally and may appear as a renal mass** (Ho et al, 1993; Acharya et al, 1997; Granata et al, 2000). **Neuroblastomas have also been seen as cystic suprarenal masses** (Kozakewich et al, 1998; Hamada et al, 1999) (Fig. 51–15). **Metastatic neuroblastoma may also be present, and careful total body examination is needed** (Toma et al, 1994). Metabolic effects of excessive norepinephrine secretion by a neuroblastoma have been documented in fetuses, including maternal effects of tachycardia and hypertension (Newton et al, 1985).

Several **potential diagnostic pitfalls** are important to consider. The severity of hydronephrosis may be variable. This often reflects reflux, and the complete resolution of significant hydronephrosis in a short period is a strong indicator of VUR. This should prompt appropriate postnatal evaluation. Hydronephrosis may vary in the short term also, reflecting peristalsis of the pelvis and ureter (Persutte et al, 2000), but this is not seen with severe degrees of dilation. **A very difficult differentiation is between PUV and severe VUR in male fetuses.** In the absence of oligohydramnios, there is little prenatal clinical impact of an ambiguous diagnosis, and a VCUG is needed in either case. In this situation, the VCUG should be performed early, on the assumption that PUV is the diagnosis. **Clues**

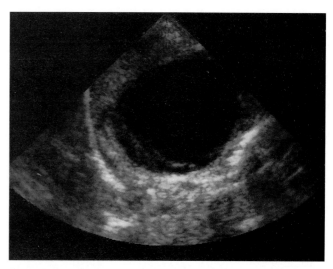

Figure 51–15. Ultrasound image of a suprarenal cystic structure with an irregularly thickened wall. This was found to be a cystic neuroblastoma at exploration shortly after birth. There may be more noticeable solid areas associated with the cystic elements.

that the diagnosis is obstruction, rather than VUR, include **bladder wall thickening, echogenic renal parenchyma, and a dilated posterior urethra** (Kaefer et al, 1997; Oliveira et al, 2000). All of these are subjective features of a prenatal US, but, if present, they indicate PUV. **The diagnosis of an upper pole renal cyst in a fetus indicates the presence of a duplication anomaly with hydronephrosis rather than a cyst.** Examination for a dilated upper pole ureter and possible ureterocele or ectopic ureter will usually reveal the actual diagnosis.

PATHOPHYSIOLOGY OF CONGENITAL OBSTRUCTION

The largest group of prenatally detected uropathies are manifest by hydronephrosis and represent the spectrum of congenital obstruction. This categorization deserves some analysis. Hydronephrosis is a manifestation or sign of obstruction in its broadest sense, and it exists in a wide spectrum. Any "threshold" of hydronephrosis that is considered diagnostic of obstruction is arbitrary and serves to confuse thinking about congenital obstructive processes. Not all obstruction is clinically significant, but all obstruction of the urinary tract produces hydronephrosis and, as noted earlier, all primary hydronephrosis not caused by reflux indicates some degree of obstruction. The term "physiologic hydronephrosis" has emerged in recent years in reference to those degrees of mild dilation that resolve spontaneously, and whose etiology is unclear. A lack of understanding of etiology and spontaneous resolution should not imply a "physiologic" process. **Furthermore, the term "physiologic hydronephrosis" begs the question as to when the condition becomes nonphysiologic** (Adra et al, 1995). This produces attempts to set absolute divisions within an entity that has a variety of presentations and probably represents multiple underlying causes. Hydronephrosis ranges from simple minimal pelvic dilation to extreme dilation of the pelvis and calyces. These issues become critical when clinical yes/no decisions must be made. Those decisions therefore should be based on the potential negative effects of a particular condition, and, to be able to determine those effects, some understanding of the pathophysiology of congenital obstruction, as a spectrum, is essential.

Congenital obstruction is different from postnatal obstruction. The affected kidney is not only undergoing rapid growth and differentiation (development), but it is not acting as the essential filtration system of the fetus (Peters 1995, 1997). **That function is taken up by the maternal placenta and urinary tract.** The responses of the developing kidney are distinct from those of the postnatal kidney. Although some of the pathophysiologic mechanisms acting in postnatal obstruction are likely to be acting in the fetus, others are even more important, and understanding of these mechanisms is rapidly improving. The obstructed fetal kidney undergoes alterations in its developmental patterns, and these changes are the basis for any functional abnormalities in postnatal life. **In broad terms, the patterns of response may be seen as affecting growth, differentiation, and induction of injury responses.**

A readily apparent feature of the severely obstructed kidney is that it is smaller than normal, suggesting reduced growth or hypoplasia (Chevalier et al, 1999c). This has been shown to occur with experimental fetal obstruction and may be related to the vigorous growth activity of the early fetal kidney (Peters et al, 1992b; Carr et al, 1995b). Reduced growth may be caused by decreased activity of growth factors, leading to less growth for each cell, but it may also be caused by increased cell death, producing a net reduction in growth rate (Chevalier, 1996; Winyard et al, 1996). Individual cell growth activity and cell death rates are regulated by growth factors, and several are altered in congenital obstruction, both in animals and in humans (Table 51–2). Those growth factors affected by obstruction may be useful as indicators of the growth effects of obstruction and as an aid in diagnosis and prognosis. Ultimately, they may be used with gene therapy techniques to reverse the negative effects of obstruction.

Closely tied to growth is differentiation, the process by which tissues develop their specific functional characteristics (Chevalier, 1998). This is a complex process, particularly in the kidney, in which multiple cell types have very specific and distinct functions in maturity. The basic processes of differentiation involve alteration of cell behavior based on genetic messages from within and on cell-to-cell signals from the surroundings (Woolf and Cale, 1997). The well-known process of induction of the primitive renal tissue, the metanephric mesenchyme, by the ureteral bud is a differentiation process involving cell-to-cell signaling. The signals act to turn on specific genes that produce alterations in the behavior of cells. Obstruction can affect these signals from the very earliest stages of induction of the nephron structure, altering the pattern of gene expression and differentiation (Attar et al, 1998). This disrupts the normal sequence that should lead to the mature kidney and obviously can lead to altered function. Obstruction has been shown to alter the expression of a variety of genes and proteins that are known to be important signals in renal differentiation. With impaired differentiation may come reduced nephron number in the kidney (Peters et al, 1992b). This has profound implications in terms of function, and once the opportunity for nephronogenesis is lost, it is not likely to be restored. **Obstruction can therefore produce altered structure of the kidney, presumably by changing the patterns of expression of various cell signals.** The net result may be termed "dysplasia" (Bernstein, 1968), although this term has various definitions. The key feature is that to understand obstruction, the specific patterns of altered cell signaling that disrupt differentiation need to be understood (Woolf and Winyard, 2000).

The sensitivity of the developing kidney to obstructive effects changes through the developmental process, and the same obstruction induced late in gestation will not create the same disordered structure as it would if induced early in gestation (Beck 1971; Peters et al, 1992b). The kidney at that point has already passed through certain developmental phases and they cannot be disordered, just as an adult kidney will never develop dysplasia in the face of obstruction. Nephron number may be significantly affected by early severe obstruction, but it will be less impaired

Table 51–2. GROWTH FACTORS IN CONGENITAL OBSTRUCTIVE UROPATHY

Growth Factor	Possible Effect	Model System	Reference
Epidermal growth factor (EGF)	Reduces tubular and interstitial effects of obstruction	Rodent	Chevalier et al, 1999a
	Reduces tubular apoptosis	Rodent	Kennedy et al, 1993
Insulin-like growth factor II (IGF II)	Predictive role in fetal obstruction	Human	Bussieres et al, 1995
	Protect renal development in obstruction	Opossum	Steinhardt et al, 1995
Transforming growth factor–β (TGF-β)	Fibrosis	Rodent	Chung et al, 1995
	Fibrosis	Sheep	Gobet et al, 1999a
	Inhibition of nephrogenesis	Sheep	Medjebeur et al, 1997
	Fibrosis	Rodent	Kaneto et al, 1993
	Correlation with obstruction	Human	Furness et al, 1999
Heparin-binding (HB) EGF	Antiapoptotic	Rodent	Nguyen et al, 2000b
Angiotensin II	Fibrosis, renovascular regulation	Rodent	Yoo et al, 1997
	Growth factor regulation	Rodent	Chung et al, 1995
	Direct role in development of obstruction	Rodent (knock-out)	Nishimur et al, 1999
	Fibrosis	Sheep	Gobet et al, 1999c
Platelet-derived growth factor A (PDGF-A)	Expression altered in obstruction	Opossum	Liapis et al, 1994

with later or lesser degrees of obstruction. In terms of growth effect, the early kidney is differentially sensitive to obstruction relative to the late gestation kidney, in which obstruction may produce a growth acceleration rather than impairment (Peters et al, 1992a). Multiple factors influence the response of the developing kidney to obstruction, and some reflect neurohumoral and vascular regulation. Obstruction of one kidney, with an intact contralateral kidney, produces a much more severe effect than does obstruction of both kidneys to the same degree. The cross-talk between kidneys is an important but incompletely understood process that is likely to involve renal innervation and hormonal factors (Chevalier, 1990).

The development of the regulatory characteristics of the kidney is no less susceptible to obstructive effects and has been studied closely. The most important of these characteristics are the renin-angiotensin system and renal vascular regulation (Chevalier and Gomez, 1988; Yoo et al, 1997). Congenital obstruction alters the developmental pattern of renin expression and the activity level of the renin-angiotensin system (Gomez et al, 1989; el-Dahr et al, 1990). This is likely to have direct functional effects, but it also illustrates an important principle of congenital obstructive nephropathy. **Obstruction during development changes the physiologic ability of the kidney to respond to stress (e.g., obstruction). The responses of the developing kidney are distinct from those of an otherwise normal postnatal kidney with obstruction imposed on it.** This fact may act to protect the developing kidney in that its responses are likely to have a compensatory role (Chevalier, 1999). Increased activity of the renin-angiotensin system, for example, may permit normal function of the congenitally obstructed kidney by increasing glomerular blood flow. If the degree of compensation is physiologic, this may permit stable growth and development and, therefore, adequate function. However, compensatory responses can become pathologic in time, as illustrated by cardiac compensation, which leads to cardiac insufficiency, or diabetic renal hyperfiltration, which ultimately ends in renal insufficiency through glomerulosclerosis. The determinants of this progression from physiologic to pathologic compensation in the developing kidney remain to be identified (Chevalier et al, 1999b).

In addition to the effect of obstruction on renal growth and differentiation, **the obstructed kidney shows patterns that may be characterized as injury responses. These include fibrosis, inflammation, and altered growth** (Klahr and Morrissey, 1998). Renal fibrosis is a common condition with a variety of underlying causes, including diabetes, hypertension, and immunologic causes, as well as obstruction (Diamond et al, 1998). The fibrosis may be within the glomerulus (glomerulosclerosis) or within the interstitium. The abnormal deposits of extracellular matrix (made up of collagens, fibronectin, and a variety of other proteins) produce functional impairment by disrupting normal cell-to-cell communication and fluid movement. As noted earlier, normal differentiation depends on cell-to-cell signaling, and fibrosis may affect this process as well. The mechanisms of tissue fibrosis have been studied actively, although for congenital obstruction there is a limited amount of information. It seems likely that several factors influence the balance of connective tissue synthesis and

breakdown. With less matrix breakdown, there is increased accumulation. Transforming growth factor-β (TGF-β) is well known to promote tissue fibrosis in many systems and is expressed at higher levels in obstructed developing kidneys. TGF-β is regulated by angiotensin and may be activated in this manner. Studies have shown coordinate increases in expression of these factors in the obstructed fetal kidney with increased fibrosis. In vitro studies of mechanically stretched renal epithelium support the role of TGF-β and its regulation by the renin-angiotensin system (Miyajima et al, 2000). TGF-β acts in several ways, both to promote the synthesis of collagens and to decrease their breakdown. The latter effect occurs through increased expression of the inhibitors of connective tissue degradation (tissue inhibitors of metalloproteinases, or TIMPs). **It has also been observed that primitive interstitial cells remain in the obstructed kidney. These cells, termed "activated fibroblasts," may contribute significantly to several of the mechanisms induced by obstruction. They are characterized by the abnormal presence of smooth muscle α-actin, which is a marker of developmental obstruction** (Diamond et al, 1995; Matsell et al, 1996; Gobet et al, 1999a; Badid et al, 2000). Each of these factors involved in the renal response to obstruction may be useful as a marker of obstruction or as a target for therapy to reverse or halt the negative effects.

Inflammatory responses, known to be important in postnatal obstruction, have an uncertain role in fetal obstruction. **In models of fetal obstruction, there is a notable absence of inflammatory cells in the kidney** (Peters et al, 1992b), **yet postnatally they are readily apparent, suggesting that the processes are different, or that a new level of response develops postnatally in the congenitally obstructed kidney.** These mechanisms are likely to be important in any event. Inflammatory processes have been shown to induce expression of various cytokines that can induce cellular injury and death, alter growth rate, or affect normal vasoregulatory mechanisms (Klahr and Morrissey, 1998). Well-described factors include the prostaglandins (Yanagisawa et al, 1990), thromboxane (Felsen et al, 1990; Harris et al, 1991), the kallikrein-kinin system (el-Dahr et al, 1993), and macrophages (Rovin et al, 1990; Diamond et al, 1994; Diamond, 1995). Macrophages have been shown to induce expression of TGF-β, whose potential role has been reviewed, as well as osteopontin. **Modulation of inflammatory responses may hold significant promise for therapeutic intervention in the obstructed kidney** (Chevalier and Klahr, 1998).

The critical clinical factor in prenatal obstruction is the effect it has on postnatal renal function. As the spectrum of hydronephrosis and obstruction is broad, so is the range of functional consequences. The functional consequences of obstruction may be barely measurable, particularly in unilateral obstruction, but they may also be profound and require renal replacement. The most readily measured effect is on glomerular filtration and clearance, but it must be recognized that the kidney performs a variety of essential functions. One of the more challenging clinical consequences of obstruction is that of impaired concentrating ability, nephrogenic diabetes insipidus (NDI). Most often apparent in patients with PUV, NDI may also be present with other forms of obstruction. With a normal contralateral kidney, the clinical impact of NDI may be less apparent. **Loss of expression and activity of the mediators of water metabolism, the aquaporins, can be produced by obstruction and is the likely basis for impaired concentration** (Frokiaer et al, 1997), **although more severe obstruction is characterized by markedly impaired medullary development as well.** There may simply be too few collecting ducts to permit urinary concentration. Postobstructive renal tubular acidosis is also clinically important and may require specific therapy. Hypertension is a rare consequence of congenital obstruction except in the setting of profound renal insufficiency, but it can be seen with unilateral congenital obstruction. In the perinatal period, it is rare for overall renal function to be impaired except with PUV. In those cases, however, functional problems may be profound and should be anticipated. These boys may have severe acidosis, high urine output, and hyperkalemia. If complicated by sepsis, management becomes very complex. Historical mortality rates of PUV reflect the critical nature of this condition.

Renal function in utero is also impaired, although the consequences are unique to the fetal environment. Potter first identified the association between renal agenesis, oligohydramnios, and pulmonary hypoplasia in the syndrome that bears her name (Potter, 1972). The pathophysiology of pulmonary hypoplasia in the setting of severe renal impairment and oligohydramnios remains incompletely defined, but several clues have emerged. Reid characterized the pathologic basis of pulmonary hypoplasia and defined it as reflecting a developmental insult of the lung (Hislop et al, 1979). This is evidenced by impairment of the normal orderly sequence of lung development, in which the patterns of bronchial branching are established by 16 to 18 weeks of gestation in humans. This branching is the foundation for all subsequent lung development. If it is abnormal, all future development is affected and a small, insufficient lung is the product. As with renal nephron development, if normal branching has not occurred, there is little likelihood of reversing the process to permit catch-up. After bronchial branching, canalicular development occurs before actual alveolar development. Reduced canalicular growth precludes adequate alveolar development as well. **It has further been shown that pulmonary hypoplasia reflects both abnormal growth and immaturity** (Docimo et al, 1989).

The role of the kidney in lung development is difficult to define, and it remains unclear how the lung and kidney interact. It seems that early in gestation normal kidney function is needed, independent of AF volume, whereas later the role of the AF is to provide a mechanical stenting force for later alveolar development (Peters et al, 1991). There is some evidence of a renal-lung axis that regulates the growth of each, although this remains speculative (Glick et al, 1990, 1991; Hosoda et al, 1993). It is clear that mechanical forces play a role in normal lung development, and perhaps normal AF volume is important to permit this (Wilson et al, 1993; DiFiore et al, 1994; Nobuhara et al, 1998). The mechanism is somewhat counterintuitive, however. It had long been thought that oligohydramnios would involve elevated intrauterine pressures that compressed the fetal thorax, causing poor lung growth. Intrauterine pressures measured in humans with oligohydramnios were lower than normal, however, presumably because of tenting effects of the fetus and its limbs on the uterine wall (Nicolini et al, 1989). With reduced external pressures, lung fluid could drain more freely into the amniotic space, reducing the stenting pressure in the lung and impairing normal growth. Experimental data support this notion (Moessinger et al, 1986). When lung fluid is retained by tracheal ligation, even in the absence of the kidneys, lung growth is maintained and actually accelerated (Wilson et al, 1993). This has become the basis for fetal interventions to prevent pulmonary hypoplasia associated with diaphragmatic hernia (DiFiore et al, 1995; Harrison et al, 1996).

The timing of the onset of oligohydramnios is therefore important in assessing its potential consequences. As would be predicted from an understanding of the pathophysiology, late-onset oligohydramnios is not associated with pulmonary insufficiency, with a threshold at about 30 weeks (Mandell et al, 1992c). In the setting of presumed severe bladder outlet obstruction, if oligohydramnios has developed by 22 or 24 weeks, pulmonary insufficiency is highly likely. This has become the basis for in utero interventions for bladder obstruction. In contrast, if oligohydramnios develops after 30 weeks, there is little likelihood of pulmonary complications and therefore no rationale to intervene or deliver the child early from a pulmonary basis. If the lungs have been able to develop adequately up to that point, they do not reverse themselves and become hypoplastic.

The incidence of certain prenatally detected uropathies is markedly sex specific. Hydronephrosis of all causes is four to five times more common in male fetuses. VUR indicated by prenatal hydronephrosis is four times more common in boys than in girls (Elder, 1992). These observations are well recognized, although there is no definite explanation. A variety of data suggest the possibility that these differences reflect elevated male bladder pressure due to higher bladder outlet resistance. Homsy examined different developmental patterns of the male rhabdosphincter and noted variation in the development of the normal omega shape from a circular form (Kokoua et al, 1993). Persistence of the circular sphincter may produce more resistance. This would lead to higher bladder pressures and upper tract dilation or reflux. Postnatal human studies have shown that boys tend to have higher grades of reflux, elevated voiding pressures, and more bladder instability than girls do (Sillen et al, 1992; Yeung et al, 1997). High voiding pressures and instability are characteristic of an obstructed bladder. Experimental data support this hypothesis: In fetal sheep urachal ligation without any bladder neck manipulation caused upper tract dilation in males only (Gobet et al, 1998a). Experimental fetal reflux is of higher grade in males, and its persistence seems to be related to bladder dynamics (Gobet et al, 1999b). This suggests that the developing male sphincter/urethral complex is of higher resistance than in the female. This may be a result of urethral length, but may also be caused by differences in the sphincter or prostate, an organ with a large component of smooth muscle. In the sheep, the urachus remains patent until term to maintain normal pressures, a function that does not seem to be needed in the human. However, a certain fraction of children have evidence of upper tract dilation in the absence of any other pathology. In most cases this mild hydronephrosis resolves spontaneously, just as the altered patterns of bladder activity resolve. Why this occurs in only some children remains unclear, yet it raises the question of differences in sphincteric maturation as a basis for the male predominance in transient congenital uropathies.

MANAGEMENT OF FETAL UROPATHIES

Incidence

Fetal urinary tract anomalies are a common finding, occurring in 0.2% to 0.9% of all pregnancies, based on large population studies (Helin and Persson, 1986; Scott and Renwick, 1987, 1993). Well over half of these anomalies are the result of some form of hydronephrosis. UPJ obstruction is the largest single entity producing hydronephrosis, followed by reflux, PUV, and megaureter (Mandell et al, 1991). Evidence of severe obstruction that might warrant fetal intervention is uncommon, representing about 5% of all prenatally detected uropathies. The clinical impact of these conditions is out of proportion to their incidence because of the severity of potential outcomes in these patients.

Indications

The principal role of the perinatal urologist is to act as an educator for prospective parents. The need for prenatal intervention is rare and its precise role remains undefined. It is important to recognize the anxiety of prospective parents who have been told that there is something wrong with their future child's kidneys. There is little appreciation for the wide spectrum of severity and the likelihood of minimal postnatal complications. Often, the initial diagnosis is made by someone with little perspective as to the necessary urologic evaluation and appropriate interventions. Some parents have already been given recommendations about management that may not reflect reasonable practice. These recommendations may reflect a defensive attitude among obstetricians concerned about the ramifications of a serious congenital defect. Many parents have used the Internet to try to learn about their child's condition, often drawing erroneous conclusions. Although it is seldom possible to provide an exact prediction of the natural history of a particular condition, it is usually very possible to give a detailed description of what may need to be done to define the condition and to determine a management plan. In cases with severe obstruction or the risk for serious postnatal problems, the perinatal urologist is often in the best position to provide a detailed discussion of the pros and cons of various management approaches in utero.

In cases of mild hydronephrosis with normal-appearing renal parenchyma, further prenatal follow-up is seldom useful, although it is usually recommended by obstetricians. In the rare case of rapid increases in severity of hydronephrosis, prompt evaluation may be appropriate,

but it is unlikely to change acute postnatal management. There are no data to strictly correlate the US appearance or course of mild-to-moderate hydronephrosis in utero with postnatal outcomes sufficient to define management. **For the parents, however, a follow-up study may be very reassuring to verify that there has been no worsening, and perhaps improvement may be noted.** Whether such data should alter postnatal evaluation is controversial (see later discussion). In the setting of more severe unilateral hydronephrosis or bilateral hydronephrosis, prenatal follow-up is reasonable and may be helpful. **When severe bilateral hydronephrosis is present, with the suspicion for bladder outlet obstruction, regular follow-up is needed. The particular parameters to be followed include AF volume, renal echogenicity, and the presence of any extrarenal fluid collections.** Fetal growth is monitored as well. Changes in these factors may provide useful information on prognosis and on the need for in utero intervention.

Fetal Intervention

Recognition of the lethal outcome in neonates determined to have severe bladder outlet obstruction in utero is a strong impetus to attempt to prevent neonatal death through an in utero intervention. As maternal fetal US evolved and specific diagnoses were made, this association became evident. Initial animal experiments with models of bladder outlet obstruction provided the encouragement to attempt in utero drainage procedures to salvage lung development (Adzick et al, 1985b). The first attempted intervention for obstructive uropathy was reported in 1982, when bilateral cutaneous ureterostomies were performed (Harrison et al, 1982a). The child did not survive, but subsequent attempts demonstrated proof of principle with surviving children who would otherwise have been predicted to die. Initial reports of success prompted widespread interventions for a variety of conditions, but a review in 1986 of 73 fetal interventions for obstructive uropathy brought practitioners back to earth (Manning et al, 1986). Despite an initial enthusiasm and less than stringent criteria for intervention, outcomes were less than encouraging, with a higher than expected mortality rate (59%) and high procedural complication rates (7% mortality). This report brought on a moratorium of activity for about 10 years, during which slow progress in refining techniques and selection was made.

Part of the problem of early practice may be seen in the report. Seventy percent of the cases were from institutions reporting only one intervention. A large fraction (45%) of patients had no specific etiology identified for their hydronephrosis. More recently, however, there has been a revitalization of fetal interventions for obstructive uropathy. Some of the same questions as to selection, techniques, and outcomes analysis persist.

At present fetal intervention for obstructive uropathy is indicated when the life of the neonate is at risk. This occurs when oligohydramnios is present in the setting of presumed bladder outlet obstruction. It is also essential that no other life-threatening conditions, particularly cardiovascular or neurologic conditions, exist. **It is also necessary that there is a reasonable chance that the fetus will benefit from in utero decompression of the bladder.**

Table 51–3. INDICATIONS AND CONDITIONS FOR IN UTERO URINARY DECOMPRESSION

Indices	Comment
Evidence of bladder outlet obstruction	Dilated bladder, hydroureteronephrosis
Normal karyotype	By amniocentesis
No systemic anomalies	Central nervous system, cardiovascular system, others
Male fetus	—
Singleton	—
Oligohydramnios	Early onset: <25 wk
Noncystic kidneys	Degree of echogenicity is subjective; cysts are poor prognostic sign
Favorable urinary indices	Na < 100 mEq/L, Cl < 110 mEq/L, Osm < 210 mOsm/L; or serial samplings trending toward normal; β_2-microglobulin <10 to 20 mg/L
Informed consent	Risks of partial treatment must be included

This is the difficult issue at present, and several means of assessing the fetal kidneys are in use. Other factors that must be present include a singleton pregnancy, normal karyotype, and informed consent (Table 51–3).

Early studies recognized that fetal bladder decompression provided no benefit in some fetuses. In these cases, there was no return of AF and ultimately neonatal death occurred. The pathology was usually consistent with renal dysplasia and correlated with severely echogenic and cystic kidneys in utero. Biochemical analysis of the fetal urine was performed to assess potential renal function, and parameters of a "good" prognosis were established (Glick et al, 1985). These reflected fetal renal function in which there was sodium retention and free water excretion. Clinical assessment of these parameters was not always encouraging in terms of their validity, and false-positive and false-negative results have been reported (Elder et al, 1990). Part of the explanation for these inconsistencies is the lack of standardization of the gestational age at sampling in many cases. Normal ranges for various components of fetal urine depend on gestational age. **A further refinement of this approach employed serial sampling of the bladder urine over 3 days (Johnson et al, 1995). This provided a dynamic assessment of the response of the fetal kidneys to decompression and gave a good indication of the ability of the kidneys to continue to produce urine, essential for correction of pulmonary hypoplasia.** The long-term accuracy of these indicators remains imperfect, but they are the best available. Long-term postnatal prognostication has been attempted with a range of obstructive severity. Based on an index of several urinary parameters, identification of neonates with normal, moderate, or severe renal impairment can be made with some reliability (Muller et al, 1993). These methods use urinary electrolytes as well as proteins as indicators of glomerular and tubular function. Reports of serum indicators of fetal renal function hold further promise of improved prognostic precision. Because β_2-microglobulin is excreted by the kidney and does not cross the placenta, fetal serum levels reflect fetal renal capacity; they are elevated in renal dysplasia, and the elevation correlates with postnatal serum creatinine levels in obstructive uropathy (Dommergues et al, 2000).

There has been a trend to consider intervention for the fetus who is without oligohydramnios but in whom chronic renal insufficiency is likely. Although this requires greater accuracy in prognostication, the potential gain is significant. The neonate with early renal failure is extremely difficult to manage and keep alive, and early renal transplantation is challenging. If intervention could delay the need for renal replacement for 2 or 3 years, or perhaps eliminate the need, the benefit would be enormous. This group of children would perhaps benefit even more than those at risk for pulmonary hypoplasia. As yet, however, there are no data on such interventions.

The technique of fetal intervention for bladder outlet obstruction emerged from research at the University of California, San Francisco and is based on placement of a double pigtail vesicoamniotic shunt (Harrison et al, 1982b). Placed under US guidance over an introducing needle, these shunts bypass the obstructed urethra. The initial shunts were limited by frequent dislodgement, clogging with debris, and the need for replacement. Subsequently, a larger shunt was developed, which was positioned within a large-bore trocar and held in place by a pigtail oriented flat against the abdomen, limiting the possibility of the fetus' pulling the shunt out. These shunts (Rodeck shunt, Rocket, London) drained well and remained in position but were complicated because of their large size (Nicolini et al, 1987). Several cases of intestinal herniation through the shunt site were reported (Robichaux et al, 1991). Current practice for vesicoamniotic shunt placement uses the Rodeck shunt placed under US guidance. It is occasionally necessary to perform amnioinfusion to permit fetal visualization. This is limited in amount, because too great an infusion permits excessive fetal movement. Occasionally the fetus must be paralyzed to facilitate shunt placement. The large-bore trocar needle is placed, and the shunt passed within it until it is seen in the bladder (Fig. 51–16). A persistent problem with all vesicoamniotic shunts has been accurate placement. In the setting of a markedly enlarged bladder, the shunt may be placed high in the abdomen; as the bladder decompresses, it pulls away from the shunt. Some authors have investigated endoscopically controlled placement of the shunt to prevent this problem (Luks et al, 1994; Skarsgard et al, 1995; Calvano et al, 1997).

Endoscopic fetal intervention is emerging as a new element in the management of fetal disease. Reports have described fetal cystoscopy and valve ablation using endoscopic techniques (Quintero et al, 1995). This method is being used actively in a small number of centers. The rationale is to ablate the valves, as would be done postnatally, and to maintain "normal" bladder filling and emptying. Antegrade and retrograde methods have been attempted using rigid and flexible instrumentation. Limited reporting of results has occurred to date, but there has been some success in the technique with a high mortality rate of the fetus. Although it may be attractive to maintain near-normal anatomy, **it is very uncertain that this approach would provide the degree of decompression sought in a fetus with sufficiently severe urinary compromise to re-**

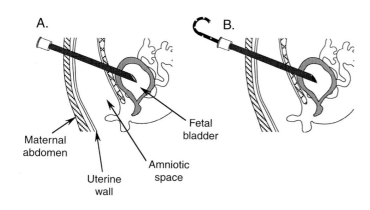

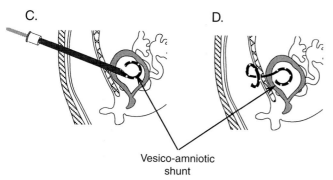

Figure 51–16. Diagram showing technique of fetal vesicoamniotic shunt placement. The fetal bladder is initially accessed by needle and a large-bore introducing sheath is passed into the bladder *(A)*. Within this sheath, the shunt is passed *(B* and *C)*. It is a double-pigtail shunt with holes at each end, allowing free drainage between the bladder and the amniotic space *(D)*. (From Peters CA: Surgical management of fetal uropathies. In Marshall FF: Textbook of Operative Urology. Philadelphia, WB Saunders, p 1063, 1996, with permission.)

quire intervention. Normal neonatal male bladder pressures are high without valves and will be high in the fetus whose bladder has been so severely obstructed. This condition, even with complete valve ablation, may not permit renal recovery that is adequate to allow for continued optimal development of the kidneys or lungs. **At present, in utero endoscopic valve ablation can be considered only experimental, yet no indication of any comparative trial is evident.**

The only outcome data available are for vesicoamniotic shunting, and this remains limited by variability in diagnosis and inadequate reporting as correlated with diagnosis. Most series include patients with the prune-belly syndrome, in whom the diagnosis of obstruction is controversial. Whether they benefit from in utero decompression is unclear. However, when all of the more recent reports are considered, there is evidence to support the benefits of fetal intervention for severe bladder outlet obstruction, although these benefits must be assessed carefully (Crombleholme et al, 1988; Johnson et al, 1994; Coplen et al, 1996; Freedman et al, 1996; Shimada et al, 1998).

Several aspects of the outcome assessment are important. Because the first priority is to save the life of the neonate, early survival is important, yet long-term renal function is critical as well. As seen in Fig. 51–17, for patients with a good prognosis survival is improved with in utero shunting, as is apparent in renal outcome. The duration of fol-

low-up is very important in considerations of renal functional outcome, because renal failure may take months or years to develop. In children with a poor prognosis at fetal urinary evaluation, the outcome is poor. Survival is increased, yet most of these patients have renal insufficiency, and they may have pulmonary impairment as well. These children may be alive, but the benefit of intervention is not certain. One study that reported on long-term outcomes of patients undergoing in utero shunting echoed the results of the initial reports (Freedman et al, 2000). A substantial fraction of children had renal insufficiency (57%), and many had growth impairment (86%). It is difficult to assess the real impact in this small series, however, as it included patients with both PUV and prune-belly syndrome. At present, the data suggest that the potential exists for in utero intervention to be effective in reducing the risk of a lethal neonatal outcome due to in utero bladder outlet obstruction. It is clear that the ability to identify patients with PUV who will benefit from in utero intervention has improved but remains limited.

The horizon of fetal intervention holds promise. It is anticipated that with a better understanding of the pathophysiology of congenital obstruction there will be increased ability to predict outcomes through markers of the relevant pathophysiologic processes. New technologies for in utero visualization, perhaps combining US and endoscopy, will facilitate placement of shunts or creation of a vesicostomy. Further refinements may permit rational shunting for chil-

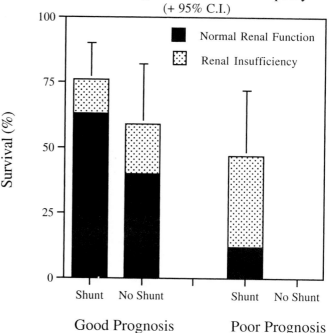

Figure 51–17. Chart showing relative outcomes of vesicoamniotic shunting for obstructive uropathy. In the good prognosis group, with bladder urine samples showing a good prognosis and no treatment, survival is about 59%, with 33% renal failure. With intervention, survival is increased slightly and the incidence of renal failure is reduced. In the poor prognosis group, survival without intervention is dismal. Although survival is increased to 47% with intervention, 75% of those children will be in renal failure.

dren at risk for renal failure in the early years of life, and thereby prevention of the multitude of complications associated with renal replacement in infancy.

POSTNATAL EVALUATION AND MANAGEMENT

The presumed diagnosis and severity of prenatally detected uropathies determine postnatal evaluation and management. This evaluation must account for the likely risk to the child from the specific condition and the nature of the postnatal evaluation needed. Structural conditions such as bladder exstrophy will be self-evident and are managed as if no prior diagnosis had been made. When a specific diagnosis has been made that must be confirmed by imaging studies, the timing and intensity of the examination is the critical issue, and this decision must be made in the context of the child's condition. A practical scheme to guide this process is shown in Table 51–4, which divides patients depending on their risk of complications.

Bilateral Hydronephrosis

Children who are at risk for severe bilateral obstruction, including PUV, should have early evaluation and initiation of treatment. Prenatally these children have bilateral, moderately severe to severe hydronephrosis, often with ureteral dilation and bladder distention or thickening. Evaluation should begin with US on the first day of life, recognizing that the findings may underestimate the severity of the hydronephrosis because of neonatal dehydration. In the presence of severe bilateral HUN in a boy, early VCUG is appropriate.

Posterior Urethral Valves

Bladder outlet obstruction from PUV in the newborn is now usually detected prenatally, but may also be identified in a boy with a palpable mass from a distended bladder, neonatal ascites in the setting of oligohydramnios and pulmonary insufficiency, or neonatal sepsis (see Chapter 63, Posterior Urethral Valves and Other Urethral Anomalies). The findings of a diminished urinary stream, although suggestive of PUV, are not common. In any of these situations in which a question of PUV is present, immediate US evaluation is needed to identify bladder distention, bladder wall thickening, HUN, and evidence of renal dysplasia. The bladder in boys with PUV is often not massively distended, as is more often seen with massive VUR. Wall thickening is a consistent finding. The dilated posterior urethra may also be visible when specifically sought. A VCUG establishes the diagnosis.

Immediate care of the neonate with PUV is dictated by the severity of the presentation and the overall clinical status. A bladder catheter is left in place until a decision is made as to appropriate initial therapy, usually valve ablation. A No. 5 Fr feeding tube is preferred over a Foley catheter. The retention balloon of the Foley may be compressed against the ureteral orifices with bladder spasm and cause ureteral obstruction. Bladder drainage usually permits upper urinary tract decompression and facilitates medical stabilization in the case of a child with respiratory compromise or acidosis. Antibiotics should be initiated as well. Initial creatinine levels reflect maternal levels but serve as a baseline. In boys who are clinically stable, valve ablation may be performed as the initial procedure, followed by careful assessment of any remnant valvular obstruction and the condition of the upper tracts.

In some boys the upper tracts do not drain well owing to ureteral obstruction by the thickened bladder wall. Failure of drainage is usually marked by persistent HUN, creatinine elevation, and acidosis. Definitive decompression should not be delayed more than 3 to 5 days in this setting. The various options for this situation include definitive ureteral reconstruction with tapering and reimplantation adjunctively with valve ablation, or temporary urinary diversion. The latter is usually achieved with the use of proximal loop ureterostomies or pyelostomies. Although

Table 51–4. POSTNATAL MANAGEMENT SCHEME FOR HYDRONEPHROSIS

Prenatal Findings	Early Antibiotics	Imaging	Timing	Possible Diagnoses	Surgery
Mild hydronephrosis	No	RUS VCUG (controversial)	2–3 mo	Mild UPJO Mild UVJO Reflux	Unlikely
Moderate-to-severe hydronephrosis	Yes	RUS VCUG	1–2 mo	Mod UPJO Mod UVJO Reflux PUV, mild	Unlikely
Severe unilateral hydronephrosis	Yes	RUS VCUG IVP/MAG-3	1 mo	UPJO UVJO Reflux PUV (unusual)	Possibly
Severe bilateral hydronephrosis	Yes	RUS VCUG	<1 wk	Reflux PUV Bilat UPJO Bilat UVJO	Probable
Intravesical cystic structure	Yes	RUS VCUG	<1 mo	Ureterocele	Likely

IVP/MAG-3, intravenous pyelogram or diuretic renogram; PUV, posterior urethral valves; RUS, renal ultrasound; UPJO, ureteropelvic junction obstruction; UVJO, ureterovesical junction obstruction; VCUG, voiding cystourethrogram.

this approach may be condemned by some, their attitude is in large part a result of a long history of misapplication. Proximal diversion, in the appropriate patient, offers efficient urinary drainage and does not necessarily hamper subsequent surgical reconstruction (Krueger et al, 1980). In performing any such diversion, however, plans for reconstruction should be made and carried out. Total early reconstruction is an option when the bladder is such that one may expect to be able to reimplant two ureters and achieve closure (Hendren, 1970). Careful follow-up of bladder function is essential in these boys.

Cutaneous vesicostomy is reserved for boys in whom primary valve ablation may not be achieved due to prematurity. A trial of bladder catheter drainage is best carried out in these patients, because they may require more proximal drainage for effective decompression of their urinary tracts. Vesicostomy should be used only as a temporary measure to permit clinical stabilization and growth. Closure of the vesicostomy and valve ablation are usually performed at 3 to 6 months of age. Controversy remains as to the long-term effects of early valve ablation, compared with diversion, on bladder function (Jayanthi et al, 1995; Kim et al, 1996; Smith et al, 1996; Close et al, 1997; Jaureguizar et al, 2000; Podesta et al, 2000).

Diligent follow-up of renal and bladder function is critical in all of these male children, including assessment of somatic growth, measured creatinine clearances, and imaging studies of the urinary tract. Aggressive early treatment may best serve to prevent the slow, often subtle progression of renal damage that can lead to end-stage renal failure (Merguerian et al, 1992).

Vesicoureteral Reflux and Megacystis-Megaureter

Some boys with bilateral HUN in utero have VUR only and do not need catheter drainage, but only antibiotics. The ability to differentiate between PUV and reflux in the fetus, however, remains limited except in the extremes.

The association of a massively dilated bladder, HUN, and bilateral VUR has been termed the megacystis-megaureter association (see Chapter 59, Vesicoureteral Reflux and Megaureter) (Willi and Lebowitz, 1979; Burbige et al, 1984). **The constant recycling of bladder urine into the upper tracts effectively prevents true bladder emptying.** The US appearance, both prenatally and postnatally, may mimic that of PUV, yet the bladders in these children are typically thin-walled and smooth. The association occurs most commonly in boys. Although prenatal diagnosis is common, boys may present early in life with sepsis. They may present with a clinical picture consistent with adrenal crisis, mimicking congenital adrenal hyperplasia with a salt-losing nephropathy, possibly because of renal aldosterone resistance caused by bacterial toxins (Vaid and Lebowitz, 1989).

In either presentation, antibiotic prophylaxis or treatment is needed and is often sufficient to stabilize the child. Although it may be of some merit to observe these children to permit spontaneous resolution of their reflux, many ultimately require surgery because of recurrent infection or deteriorating renal function. Surgical repair typically re-

quires formal excisional megaureter tailoring and ureteral reimplantation. There seems to be little indication for cutaneous vesicostomy.

With bilateral HUN in the absence of reflux or valves, bilateral obstructive megaureters are present. Evaluation for a neurogenic cause should be considered. If this is not present, management is usually elective with prophylactic antibiotics and delayed functional evaluation. If there is no ureteral dilation, the diagnosis is presumed to be bilateral UPJ obstruction, and the timing of evaluation can also be more elective. In the absence of a prenatal history of oligohydramnios, very few of these patients will have acute renal insufficiency. If the initial US shows profound hydronephrosis and renal parenchymal echogenicity, follow-up needs to be more aggressive. In girls, bilateral HUN suggests reflux or obstructive megaureters. Each of these can be managed more electively with prophylactic antibiotics and delayed VCUG.

Mild-to-moderate bilateral hydronephrosis may be managed more electively in boys and girls. Whether this condition is obstructive or refluxing, it is rarely necessary to intervene early in life so long as infection is prevented with prophylactic antibiotics. Postnatal US evaluation is deferred until 1 or 2 months and may be planned in combination with a VCUG. The decision regarding selection of patients for cystography is a difficult one, with conflicting recommendations in the literature (Anderson and Rickwood, 1991; Elder, 1992; Zerin et al, 1993; Walsh and Dubbins, 1996; Herndon et al, 1999; Horowitz et al, 1999). The same analysis applies to unilateral mild-to-moderate hydronephrosis.

Unilateral Hydronephrosis

There is rarely any indication to obtain urgent postnatal studies when unilateral hydronephrosis has been identified prenatally (in a child with a contralateral normal kidney). Even with the most severe unilateral obstruction, intervention is deferred for at least several weeks in current practice. There is often great pressure to obtain an early US study, but this will seldom prompt early intervention and, more importantly, the **normal oliguria of the neonate may under-represent the degree of obstruction or the likelihood of reflux.** Figure 51–18 illustrates the normal US obtained on day 2 of life from a child with prenatal unilateral, moderately severe hydronephrosis. With such findings, both parents and pediatrician have been known to determine that the condition had resolved and to resist recommendations for further evaluation. In this example, however, follow-up US demonstrated marked calicectasis resulting from significant UPJ obstruction. Docimo showed that an early US does not miss significant pathology in most cases but may cloud the issue and inappropriately guide follow-up (Docimo and Silver, 1997). In cases in which the perinatal urologist is not yet involved, the result may be neglect of a significant condition. We actively recommend against early US in these cases, because it serves little role in management.

The decision as to selecting patients in whom a VCUG is appropriate continues to evolve. Several studies have addressed this issue, and the conclusion seems

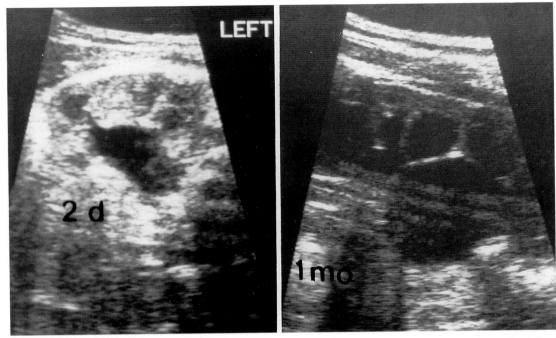

Figure 51–18. Postnatal renal ultrasound study of the same baby at 2 days of life and then again at 30 days. The baby had moderate hydronephrosis in utero. Early postnatal ultrasound findings may miss significant dilation and, more importantly, may lead to misguided recommendations regarding further evaluation. There is seldom a benefit to performing these studies early in life.

to be that if there has been any degree of prenatal hydronephrosis, reflux will be present in about 20% to 30% of the patients. Even when there is no hydronephrosis at birth, patients have a 23% chance of showing some degree of VUR (Zerin et al, 1993). In contrast, Mandell and colleagues (1991) concluded that routine cystography is not indicated if hydronephrosis is less than moderate (i.e., with calyceal dilation). In part, this was in recognition of the need to reduce the enormous number of cystograms being performed, because progressively greater numbers of infants with prenatal hydronephrosis were being identified. Other studies have identified thresholds of renal pelvic dilation as indicating the need for postnatal evaluation. Each threshold selects a level of tolerance for missing certain conditions. Most do not clearly separate between refluxing and nonrefluxing conditions, however.

Although it has been assumed that it is important to detect reflux in neonates, it is not established that all reflux will be clinically significant (Yerkes et al, 1999). The experience at our institution has also raised this question. Since 1992, VCUG has not been routinely performed in children with less than moderate hydronephrosis, except by individual physician preference. We have monitored a group of 270 patients with mild and mild-to-moderate hydronephrosis in whom no VCUG was performed and antibiotic prophylaxis was not used. Most have shown resolution of their hydronephrosis as expected. Based on reported data and our own recent experience, wherein cystography has been performed in similar degrees of hydronephrosis, between 20% and 30% of these patients may be presumed to have had reflux (Zerin et al, 1993). Seven of our patients developed infection, but none had reflux on subsequent evaluation. All others have been well, with up to 8 years of follow-up. It is unclear whether there is some

selection bias at work, or whether those children who have reflux but minimal upper tract dilation will not have complications of their reflux. Perhaps this reflects differences in bladder function.

We subsequently examined patients with mild-to-moderate hydronephrosis and attempted to select thresholds for cystography based on the incidence of reflux. **In order to identify 95% of patients with grade 3 reflux and higher, all levels of hydronephrosis would need to be evaluated with cystography.** Current practice varies around the country. Some centers chose to evaluate all patients with any history of prenatal hydronephrosis, whereas others use a cut-off at calyceal dilation or an AP pelvic diameter between 7 and 10 mm at term or immediately after birth. **The important issue in making a recommendation is that any cut-off point is arbitrary and some patients with reflux will not be diagnosed. The clinical significance of that misdiagnosis is not known. This information must be available to parents as they make their decisions regarding evaluation.**

Similar issues relating to selection of thresholds of risk are relevant to the selection of patients for renal functional evaluation of obstructive conditions. In profound bilateral obstruction, serum creatinine reflects renal functional impairment and is useful in the management of PUV; it is seldom useful in patients with bilateral megaureter or UPJ obstruction. In boys with PUV in whom it is apparent that renal function may be compromised based on the US appearance, it is useful to obtain a baseline creatinine level at day 1 or 2 of life. Although this measurement reflects the maternal creatinine concentration, it provides a starting point, and the significance of subsequent changes can be interpreted only with this knowledge. A creatinine concentration of 1.0 mg/dl at day 5 suggests very different degrees of functional impairment depending on whether the maternal creatinine at birth was 1.0 or 1.5 mg/dl. The rate of decline of neonatal creatinine is a useful guide to both renal function and efficacy of drainage.

For unilateral obstructive processes, functional imaging serves the purpose of determining the need for, and timing of, intervention. There is significant controversy as to the interpretation of functional imaging studies in cases of UPJ obstruction in infants (see Chapter 57, Anomalies and Surgery of the Uteropelvic Junction in Children). Therefore, it is impossible to establish absolute guidelines as to the selection of patients for these studies. All of the reports attempting to do so create arbitrary definitions of postnatal "obstruction" to permit creation of selection criteria. The study of Mandell and colleagues (1991) identified levels of AP diameter as indicating risk of having surgery. The selection criteria for surgery are controversial, so any threshold based upon them is of limited value. Those criteria have changed in the years since that report, as well.

A practical way of dealing with this difficulty is to select a threshold that is reproducible and identifies all patients in whom some consideration for surgery might be appropriate. Even if early surgery is not recommended, a baseline study will be available, and these children will need to be monitored closely. The specific functional study used is also controversial, although the intravenous pyelogram is falling away from use in this context, being replaced by diuretic renography. The advantage of the latter is that it makes longitudinal comparisons more practical using numerical parameters. Caution must be exercised, however, in the overinterpretation of those numbers. In our practice, the presence of generalized calyceal dilation is the selection threshold for a diuretic renogram. When patients with less than that level of dilation were studied, there was no evidence of any functional impairment, and the washout times were uniformly within normal ranges (i.e., less than 20 minutes).

When reflux is present, functional imaging as a baseline may be useful because there is a high incidence of abnormal renal scans in the absence of any infection (Nguyen et al, 2000a). Renal scan abnormalities in the absence of infection suggest either a prenatal effect of reflux on renal development or an underlying developmental defect that causes both reflux and abnormal renal development. This controversy remains unresolved, but it raises significant questions regarding the potential for ongoing postnatal renal impairment from uncorrected sterile reflux. **Several studies have identified markedly abnormal patterns of renal function in infants with dilating reflux, predominantly in boys** (Marra et al, 1994; Assael et al, 1998; Stock et al, 1998; Nguyen et al, 2000a; Polito et al, 2000). The incidence of renal abnormalities is heavily weighted toward male infants and toward higher degrees of reflux. Histologic studies of kidneys removed for nonfunction associated with reflux show heterogeneous patterns of structural abnormalities consistent with "dysplasia" (Risdon et al, 1993). This echoes the focal nature of reflux-induced pyelonephritic changes with infection. Experimental studies have shown renal abnormalities induced by fetal reflux in the absence of infection, particularly in males, and without the induction of bladder outlet obstruction (Gobet et al, 1998b, 1999b).

Associated with these observations have been several studies demonstrating markedly abnormal urodynamic patterns in boys with dilating reflux, in general showing a high incidence of bladder hypertonicity and instability. This raises the question of whether the high grades of reflux are a product of bladder dysfunction or simply associated with it (Sillen et al, 1992, 1996a, 1996b; Yeung et al, 1997). Some centers have begun intermittent catheterization in neonatal male infants with dilating reflux to reduce potential ongoing renal effects (Hjalmas, K., personal communication, 2000). Others have suggested temporary vesicostomy or early reimplantation. Although this debate continues, the frequency of renal abnormalities associated with neonatal reflux is high, and obtaining baseline data to permit interpretation of later studies is recommended. In some cases, severe reduction in function may prompt consideration of earlier intervention.

Renal Cystic Diseases

MCDK and ARPKD are the two principal cystic conditions identified prenatally (see Chapter 56, Renal Dysgenesis and Cystic Disease of the Kidney). **MCDK is usually a unilateral, isolated finding with a good prognosis, whereas ARPKD is typically bilateral and lethal.** It is important that the clinician be able to distinguish these two entities with certainty.

MCDK is usually detected prenatally, as described previously, having a typical US appearance characterized by multiple fluid-filled spaces of varying size, without interconnection or a central large cyst, and minimal associated parenchyma (Sanders and Hartman, 1984). Occasionally, MCDK is detected as an abdominal mass in an otherwise healthy newborn. Some are massive and impair pulmonary or gastrointestinal function. The principal responsibility of the urologist is to ensure that the contralateral kidney is entirely normal. An increased frequency of VUR and UPJ obstruction has been reported in association with contralateral MCDK. Appropriate evaluation and management of those conditions, if present, are of primary concern because they put the functionally solitary kidney at risk. Rarely, bilateral MCDK is identified, often prenatally, with a uniformly dismal postnatal outlook. These children die from the pulmonary hypoplasia associated with bilateral renal dysplasia.

When the diagnosis of MCDK is uncertain and severe hydronephrosis may be present, a dimercaptosuccinic acid (DMSA) renal scan is the most effective means to confirm the diagnosis. MCDK can be expected to demonstrate no uptake on DMSA scanning.

Urgent management of a patient with MCDK is seldom necessary. Controversy persists regarding the need for surgical removal; this should be a carefully considered decision between the clinician and parents (Wacksman and Phipps, 1993; Minevich et al, 1997).

ARPKD is now being identified prenatally, particularly in affected families. These children usually have a lethal outcome in the newborn period owing to pulmonary failure. If the diagnosis is made sufficiently early, prenatal termination is an option to some. **In the newborn, the classic US constellation of symmetrically large kidneys** with a reniform shape, multiple small cysts giving a uniformly bright echogenic sonotexture, and poor pulmonary and renal function is highly suggestive of ARPKD. Little specific therapy may be offered, although some centers have begun peritoneal dialysis in those children with sufficient pulmonary capacity. A small number of children with ARPKD present with large, echogenic cystic kidneys yet show a slower renal functional deterioration. They live long enough to develop evidence of hepatic and pancreatic cystic disease (Karoli's disease) (Cole et al, 1987; Hussman et al, 1991). It remains difficult to prognosticate about these children in the newborn period.

NEONATAL UROLOGIC EMERGENCIES

This section reviews the major and minor emergencies and urgencies that may be seen in the perinatal period, based on the presenting signs and symptoms (Table 51–5). Although an anatomic organization has been imposed on this review, disorders of one particular part of the urogenital system may affect the entire system and the entire well-being of the child. They may also be heralds of other aspects of congenital or acquired conditions. Therefore, it is often necessary to evaluate, to various degrees of intensity, the remainder of the genitourinary system. In this

Table 51–5. PRESENTING SIGNS OF NEONATAL UROLOGIC EMERGENCIES

Sign		Evaluation
Sepsis	Bladder outlet obstruction—valves, neurogenic	Urine and blood cultures
	Vesicoureteral reflux	Ultrasound
	Megaureter	VCUG
	Ectopic ureter	
	Ureterocele	
	Ureteropelvic junction obstruction	
	Fungal infection with secondary obstruction	
Hematuria	Urinary infection	Urine culture
	Renal vein thrombosis	Ultrasound
Hypertension	Renal vein thrombosis	Ultrasound
	Renal artery thrombosis	DMSA scan
Renal mass	Hydronephrosis	Ultrasound
	ARPKD	CT/DMSA/MRI
	MCDK	
	CMN	
	Neuroblastoma	
	Wilms' tumor	
Renal failure	Urinary obstruction	Urine culture
	Sepsis	Urine electrolytes
	Renal cortical necrosis	Ultrasound
	Renal dysplasia/agenesis	DMSA/MAG-3
Urinary ascites	Urinary obstruction	Ultrasound
Scrotal mass	Neonatal torsion	Examination
	Hydrocele	Ultrasound
	Tumor	

ARPKD, autosomal recessive polycystic kidney disease; CT, computed tomography; DMSA, dimercaptosuccinic acid; MAG-3, diuretic renogram; MCDK, multicystic dysplastic kidney; CMN, congenital mesoblastic nephroma; MRI, magnetic resonance imaging; VCUG, voiding cystourethrogram.

way, associated or secondary problems will not be neglected.

Genitalia

Ambiguous Genitalia

One of the most challenging clinical presentations in the newborn is that of ambiguous genitalia (see Chapter 68, Sexual Differentiation—Normal and Abnormal). This condition immediately produces anxiety, uncertainty, and embarrassment in parents and medical staff. It should always be considered an emergency, with the principal focus being parental education and determination of the most appropriate sex of rearing. The clinical findings are quite variable and may provide some clue as to the underlying etiology, yet a consistent clinical approach is the most prudent. Two important streams of effort should be initiated with the identification of such a baby. One is the medical evaluation and assessment of the most appropriate sex of rearing based on as much information as possible. The other is directed toward reassurance and education of the parents and family regarding the health of the baby (as appropriate) and providing information comprehensible by the parents and support staff in a consistent manner.

Medical evaluation begins with a careful history to identify possible drugs taken during pregnancy (suggesting exogenous virilization of a female fetus) or unexplained neonatal deaths in the family (suggesting virilizing adrenal hyperplasia). The physical examination may be particularly helpful in narrowing the diagnostic possibilities. Careful description of the phallic structure with measurements (stretched length and circumference), the development of scrotal structures, pigmentation, and the presence of gonads in the scrotum or inguinal canals should be noted. Palpation for abdominal masses and a rectal examination (with the fifth finger) to detect a uterus (the neonatal uterus should feel like a large match-head) should be carried out.

Initial laboratory studies should include chromosomal examination. This is one of the most important factors to use in evaluation, and it may now be obtained within 48 to 72 hours with good accuracy. Fluorescent in situ hybridization (FISH) analysis may permit identification of genetic sex even more rapidly. A buccal smear has too much uncertainty to be recommended. Serum studies for the by-products of disordered steroid synthesis are sent promptly yet may require several days to be reported. These may be supplemented by urine studies for 17-ketosteroid, 17-hydroxyprogesterone. **The principal aim of these studies is to rule in or rule out virilizing adrenal hyperplasia. This is the one condition that cannot be neglected, because it may produce life-threatening adrenal crisis at 7 to 10 days of life.** Children with virilizing adrenal hyperplasia are genetic females with almost normal reproductive capacity, yet they may appear markedly virilized. Pelvic US can identify the uterus that is present in these children. Radiologic evaluation of the internal genital structures should be performed within the first weeks of life. This may be best performed with a cone-shaped catheter adapter gently placed into the perineal opening. The aim of these studies is to assess the urethrovaginal anatomy, which may identify a cervix and uterus and provide important information for later reconstruction.

The decision regarding the sex of rearing is complex, and the many details and variations cannot be adequately presented in this format. In general, however, the priorities that influence this important choice are fertility potential, reconstructive potential (particularly in the male), and, to a lesser degree, genetic sex. Other issues that are critical for evaluation and management decisions include determination of the gonadal sex. This occasionally necessitates exploration and gonadal biopsy, which may now be performed laparoscopically (Lakshmanan and Peters, 2000).

The final recommendation regarding sex of rearing must be a team effort, involving the urologist, endocrinologist, geneticist, nursing staff, and, in some institutions, an ethical review committee working with the parents. Very often, no immediate therapy is appropriate, except in cases of congenital virilizing adrenal hyperplasia, yet plans must be laid for subsequent reconstruction, as needed.

On occasion, genital ambiguity is part of a more complex condition such as cloacal exstrophy or persistent cloaca. In most cases, this ambiguity represents a structural defect rather than a gonadal or chromosomal defect; nonetheless, chromosomal and basic endocrine evaluations are appropriate.

Undescended Testes

The testes of a normal full-term infant should be descended into the scrotum. The incidence of testicular maldescent is about 4% at term, and it is higher among premature children, proportionate to the degree of prematurity. Although little immediate action needs to be taken for undescended testes in the newborn, several exceptions must be borne in mind (see Chapter 67, Abnormalities of the Testes and Scrotum and Their Surgical Management). Undescended testes, including unilateral nonpalpable testis, in association with hypospadias must prompt an evaluation for intersex conditions, as with ambiguous genitalia (Kaefer et al, 1999a). In the unusual child with bilaterally nonpalpable testes and a normal penis, it is useful to obtain a determination of serum testosterone and follicle-stimulating hormone/luteinizing hormone levels to assess the pituitary gonadal axis, as well as a karyotype. This may eliminate the need for later evaluation using human chorionic gonadotropin to stimulate the testes. Because there is usually a surge of testosterone in the first weeks of life, its presence in such a child documents the presence of a hormonally functional testis, obviating subsequent stimulation tests. Parents should be counseled as to the fact that some testes will descend in the first months of life and that definitive treatment is best planned for 9 to 12 months of age.

Large Scrotum

The newborn male infant with a large scrotum should be evaluated promptly, and meticulous physical examination is critical. Principal causes include hydrocele, with or without associated hernia, neonatal testicu-lar torsion, and tumor (see Chapter 67, Abnormalities of the Testes and Scrotum and Their Surgical Management). Hydrocele is characterized by a transilluminating scrotum that feels fluid-filled. If this fluid readily communicates into the abdomen, a hernia is present and should be corrected on an elective basis, but without undue delay. In severely premature children, this is usually done before discharge home, or at 1500 g body weight. Noncommunicating hydroceles are often bilateral and moderate in size. In most cases these resolve spontaneously within the first year of life, and later repair of persistent large hydroceles may be elected.

Neonatal or perinatal testicular torsion often manifests as nontender unilateral scrotal enlargement, occasionally with ecchymosis or erythema, and a hard, smooth internal mass. The epididymis usually is not palpable. This finding is often detected on discharge examination in the absence of prior similar findings. Scrotal US may be useful in clarifying the condition of the testis. Typically the infarcted testis is enlarged uniformly, but there may be irregular areas of echolucency. Reactive hydrocele fluid may be present.

The definitive diagnostic test is exploration, and we believe that it is also the most appropriate therapeutic maneuver. Controversy exists regarding the urgency of surgical exploration. **It is unlikely that the infarcted testis will be salvaged; the primary aim is diagnosis and contralateral testicular fixation to prevent torsion of the now solitary testis.** The incidence of contralateral torsion is low, but it is not nil. Several reports have documented synchronous and metachronous contralateral neonatal torsion, and we have seen this within 6 hours after an initial presentation (LaQuaglia et al, 1987). The risk of preventable anorchia has prompted our group to perform urgent exploration in neonates with presumed neonatal torsion. Contralateral fixation is performed with permanent suture through the tunica albuginea, but the alternative of placement of the testis into a dartos pouch is probably equally effective.

Testicular prosthesis placement is elective, but concerns regarding the safety of silicone implants have curtailed its general use in neonates.

Circumcision Injury

The widespread application of neonatal circumcision in the United States is a fact of life, and on rare occasions problems arise. One problem is that of identification of a previously occult hypospadias during the procedure. In most cases this is a minor hypospadias, but an effort should be made to preserve as much foreskin as remains to be available for repair at a later date. Simple Vaseline gauze dressings are usually adequate for healing. What may appear as a markedly edematous and abnormal penis at the time of the urologist's examination will usually heal quite well.

Urethral injury is a far more serious complication and may require urgent repair. Incision of the urethra, usually at the coronal margin, may be repaired primarily, using conventional hypospadias surgical techniques involving multiple layers of coverage to prevent fistula formation. If there is significant tissue injury, proximal diversion or catheter drainage may be needed to permit healing before definitive reconstruction. Glanular transection occurs and requires acute repair. The amputated glans should be preserved in iced saline. Reanastomosis can be performed with direct urethral approximation and stenting. Results have been reported to be satisfactory, although secondary revisions may be needed (Gluckman et al, 1995). The robust vascularity of the glans seems to permit adequate healing of the graft.

In the event of a loss of penile shaft skin, often by electrocautery burns, the foreskin should be preserved and even grafted onto the area of the defect if possible. The aims of management are to prevent infection and to permit rapid healing. Urinary diversion may not be needed because the urethra is usually intact and regular dressing changes with Vaseline gauze will be effective. Subsequent reconstruction often requires release of contractures and skin grafting.

Hypospadias

Identification of hypospadias in the newborn is an opportunity to provide early counseling. Although little needs to be done physically in the newborn period, many questions and uncertainties may be settled (see Chapter 65, Hypospadias). Discussion of the timing and nature of surgical reconstruction, as well as the generally positive long-term outlook, is of enormous benefit to the family. A common cause for consultation in newborns with hypospadias is the inability to identify the urethral meatus. The meatus may be small and confused with accessory, distal pits, but it is not occlusive. Its location and patency may be easily demonstrated using a No. 5 Fr feeding tube with lubricant passed a few millimeters into the urethra. There is seldom a need for catheterization. When examining a neonate with hypospadias, palpation of the testes is important. In the setting of hypospadias, an undescended testis should prompt consideration of a possible intersex condition.

Epispadias

As with hypospadias, epispadias in the newborn provokes anxiety and uncertainty, even more so because of its infrequency. It is important to explain the condition, its anatomy, and its range of severity (see Chapter 61, Exstrophy, Epispadias, and Other Bladder Anomalies). In contrast to hypospadias, the urethral opening in epispadias is on the dorsal aspect of the penis and may be proximal (penopubic) or more distal (glanular). It may be impossible to predict ultimate continence in more proximal cases of epispadias, and the parents should be informed of the possible need for incontinence surgery and even bladder reconstruction. **An abnormally wide symphysis pubis suggests a defect in the bladder neck, and more pronounced distraction is associated with small bladder capacity. Review and planning for surgical repair are best begun early and reinforced over time.**

Urethral Duplication

Duplication of the urethra is a rare condition that often requires complex surgical reconstruction (see Chapter 63, Posterior Urethral Valves and Other Urethral Anomalies). **It may be seen as two distinct urethral meati on the penis, or as a second, functional urethral meatus anywhere below the normal position. The inferior urethra is the functional urethra, and it may exit as far posteriorly as the anal verge.** US and cystographic evaluation of the urinary tract is necessary to assess the concurrence of upper tract anomalies (Effmann et al, 1976) and to determine the relationship of the two urethras to the bladder and bladder neck. It is unusual that the functional urethra is obstructed, but if it is, temporary diversion should be instituted, with a concurrent plan for later refunctionalization and urethral reconstruction.

Perineal Mass in a Female Neonate

The appearance of a protuberant mass in the perineum of a newborn girl should suggest four principal diagnoses. The appearance usually indicates the most likely diagnosis. The most common entity producing this general finding in a newborn is a periurethral cyst. These are whitish and are covered by a delicate but normal epithelium. The urethral meatus is adjacent but uninvolved. Incision and drainage is usually curative. **Imperforate hymen with resulting hydrocolpos may manifest as a midline bulging of whitish tissue symmetrically between the labia and behind the urethra.** A palpable abdominal mass may be present because of uterine distention, and occasionally hydronephrosis is found on US. A separate fluid-filled cavity in the pelvis should be distinguishable from the bladder, yet it may also be confused for the bladder. Management of an imperforate hymen consists of incision and drainage, which is also appropriate for the less common vaginal stenosis. The substance drained is often milky white and may be of surprising volume. Subsequent intervention is seldom needed.

Prolapse of an ectopic ureterocele may have a similar appearance, distinguished by its often edematous, congested, or frankly necrotic appearance. With close examination the ureterocele may be seen emerging from the urethra in an eccentric fashion, usually posteriorly. A distended bladder may be palpable, and less often there is a palpable hydronephrotic kidney. US usually provides the diagnosis, which should be supplemented with VCUG and functional renal imaging. The most useful option is to incise the ureterocele sufficiently to allow reduction into the bladder and temporary catheter drainage. Further management of the ureterocele is dictated by the response of the bladder outlet obstruction and any associated obstruction of functional renal elements.

Urethral prolapse is uncommon in newborns but may be seen as a circumferential collar of edematous and ecchymotic tissue at the urethral meatus. Topical measures such as skin moisturizers, hot compresses, and relief of aggravating factors (urethral catheter, prolonged coughing, or straining) may relieve the prolapse. If tissue necrosis is evident, surgical resection is appropriate. Although uncommon in the neonatal period, botryoid sarcomata of the vagina may manifest as a protuberant vaginal mass, usually with a distinctive, multilobulated appearance. Evidence of a solid pelvic mass will be evident on examination and on US. This should prompt a thorough evaluation based on imaging, tissue diagnosis, and assessment of regional involvement.

Bladder

Bladder Exstrophy

The presence of classic bladder exstrophy is immediately apparent and requires prompt action, in terms of preparing for closure as well as providing reassurance and information to the parents. These children are usually full term and healthy, and associated severe anomalies are uncommon (see Chapter 61, Exstrophy, Epispadias, and Other Bladder Anomalies). **The initial examination should assess the genital structures, the location of the testes in boys, and the size of the exstrophic bladder. This may be apparent on inspection as the child cries and everts the bladder.** Some are large and protrude notably, while in other children the bladder may be a mere plate in the lower abdomen. The latter situation may preclude primary closure in extreme cases. A screening renal US is usually performed to document normal kidneys.

Immediate management should consist of protecting the bladder epithelium with a simple clear plastic (Saran wrap) dressing. Vaseline gauze should not be used. In most cases, primary closure is appropriate, but it should be performed only by a surgeon specifically experienced with both the early and long-term management of bladder exstrophy. Early closure may take advantage of the natural pliability of the neonate's pelvic bones to facilitate closure of the symphysis pubis. The details of surgical repair are well described in Chapter 61 (Exstrophy, Epispadias, and Other Bladder Anomalies) and Chapter 62 (Surgical Technique for One-Stage Reconstruction of the Exstrophy-Epispadias Complex). The principal aim is to anatomically close the bladder to permit more normal growth and protect the delicate epithelium. The concept of the staged functional repair is well established and validated by its results, although complete initial reconstruction has emerged as a possible viable alternative.

Patent Urachus

Urinary drainage from the umbilicus is often seen in association with the prune-belly syndrome, but it may also occur in isolation as a manifestation of a failure of closure of the urachus (see Chapter 61, Exstrophy, Epispadias, and Other Bladder Anomalies). It may become evident soon after birth or within the first weeks of life, and it may be associated with infection. **Urachal infection is usually associated with a urachal cyst that results from partial closure and formation of a closed space, and it is frequently caused by skin bacteria.** Although it is likely that spontaneous closure of a patent urachus would occur in some children, it is prudent to repair this defect to avoid later infectious complications. Because of its preperitoneal location, infections of the urachus have been reported to produce bacterial peritonitis. US imaging has been helpful to document a patent or cystic urachus. VCUG may also show the lesion and would serve to rule out associated bladder abnormalities, particularly obstruction. Umbilical

sinus injection may specifically define the patent urachus, but it is often difficult to achieve (Cilento et al, 1998).

Surgical repair depends on excision of the entire urachus, from the bladder dome to just below the umbilicus. This may be done through a small infraumbilical or umbilical incision.

Multisystem and Miscellaneous Conditions

Cloacal Exstrophy (see also Ch. 61)

The typical appearance of cloacal exstrophy should be recognized by any urologist who sees newborns (see Chapter 61, Exstrophy, Epispadias, and Other Bladder Anomalies). Although these children now usually survive, their care represents an enormous clinical challenge and requires a team effort over many years. A thorough understanding of the anatomy of the condition and its variants is essential to any surgeon undertaking any aspect of the care of these children, particularly in the early days. **The most critical element in the early management of these children rests in preserving all aspects of the gastrointestinal and urinary tracts** (Soffer et al, 2000). **Separation of the gastrointestinal and genitourinary tracts with the creation of an end colostomy (not ileostomy) permits the most efficient use of all levels of the gastrointestinal tract.** In this way, the bladder is in a configuration comparable to that of the classic exstrophic bladder. The surgical handling of the bladder is identical, with mobilization and closure in anticipation of a staged reconstruction. Because of the 50% incidence of myelomeningocele and subsequent neuropathic bladder dysfunction in patients with cloacal exstrophy, volitional voiding is rare. **Functionalization of the hindgut (colon) usually results in a remarkable enlargement. This colonic segment may later become a critical part of bladder reconstruction.** Its preservation and functionalization in the newborn period are of obvious significance. As with classic bladder exstrophy, **the initial management very often dictates the outcome of later reconstructions; early involvement in these cases should indicate a long-term commitment on the part of the surgeon** (Diamond and Jeffs, 1985; Hurwitz et al, 1987; Mathews et al, 1998).

Abdominal Mass

The diagnosis of an abdominal mass in a neonate has become greatly simplified with the availability of US imaging. In many cases the identity of the mass will have been suggested prenatally. **The principal entities to be considered include hydronephrosis, cystic renal disease, adrenal hemorrhage, a dilated bladder, gastrointestinal duplications, and tumor** (Hartman and Shochat, 1989; Schwartz and Shaul, 1989; McVicar et al, 1991) (Table 51–6). Physical examination should consider the location, size, texture, and mobility of the mass, as well as other abnormalities on examination, including limbs, cardiac, and central nervous system findings. US usually identifies the organ of origin, the cystic or solid nature of the mass, and the condition of the uninvolved elements of the genitourinary tract and permits a more focused and detailed subse-

Table 51–6. CAUSES OF ABDOMINAL MASS IN NEWBORNS

Etiology	Number	Percentage
Urinary tract	**186**	**68**
MCDK	65	35
Hydronephrosis (nonspecified)	38	20
Ureteropelvic junction obstruction	20	11
Posterior urethral valves	18	10
Ureteral duplication–ectopy complex	11	6
ARPKD	12	6
Wilms' tumor (also congenital mesoblastic nephroma)	8	4
Renal vein thrombosis	5	3
Miscellaneous	9	5
Other causes	**88**	**32**
Neuroblastoma	22	25
Gastrointestinal	16	18
Hydrometrocolpos	13	15
Ovarian cysts	9	10
Miscellaneous	28	32

ARPKD, autosomal recessive polycystic kidney disease; MCDK, multicystic dysplastic kidney.

McVicar M, Margouleff D, Chandra M: Diagnosis and imaging of the fetal and neonatal abdominal mass: An integrated approach. Adv Pediatr 1991;38: 135–149.

quent evaluation. It cannot be overemphasized that care must be taken to examine the entire abdomen, rather than immediately focusing attention on the usually obvious anomaly. In all instances, as with more specific genitourinary conditions, the aim of evaluation is to provide a detailed picture of the anatomy with an associated functional assessment.

The likelihood that any abdominal mass is of urinary tract origin is high, greater than 60%, with hydronephrosis and multicystic dysplastic kidneys being the most frequent causes (Schwartz and Shaul, 1989).

Cloacal Anomaly

The child with the cloacal anomaly may be mistaken for a female with a high imperforate anus, yet the condition will require the coordinated management of complex urinary and gastrointestinal anomalies (Hendren, 1988, 1998) (see Chapter 69, Surgical Management of Intersexuality, Cloacal Malformations, and Other Abnormalities of the Genitalia in Girls). These children, all female, may be recognized by their having a single perineal opening, the cloaca (from the Latin word *cloaca,* meaning sewer). The cloaca is the common channel of the colon, vagina, and urethra. Such patients may have an appearance similar to that of a girl with high imperforate anus, or there may be a more anomalous, undifferentiated perineal anatomy. We have seen one child with no perineal opening, although this is extremely unusual. **Urinary drainage may be impaired in children with cloaca, usually from distention of the vagina by urine, which causes obstruction of the bladder neck.** This situation should be sought with a careful examination to palpate a distended bladder or with a US examination to look for hydronephrosis, a distended vagina, and/or distended bladder. **Drainage is essential and may be readily achieved by decompression of the vagina, by use of a temporary indwelling cathe-**

ter, or by intermittent catheterization of the vagina. It may be difficult or impossible to actually catheterize the bladder, but this is seldom necessary. **Colonic decompression with a divided colostomy is necessary, and it is best performed in the transverse colon to avoid limiting later reconstructive options for rectal pull-through procedures.**

Precise definition of the urogenital anatomy is best performed with endoscopy and contrast studies, each of which may require extra time and patience to provide the needed information (Jaramillo et al, 1990). With adequate urinary drainage, definitive reconstructive genitourinary surgical management is seldom needed in the newborn period and is best deferred until later.

Imperforate Anus

The pediatric urologist should be familiar with the presentation and management of imperforate anus in light of the high frequency of associated genitourinary anomalies and the potential for functionally significant neurologic bladder dysfunction in these children. **Prenatally, the presence of imperforate anus may be suggested by punctate calcifications in the intestinal lumen resulting from the formation of meconium calcifications due to exposure to urine** (Mandell et al, 1992b). At initial presentation a routine US should be obtained to assess the urinary tract, as well as a VCUG. The latter may be of particular importance in assessing the level of the rectourethral-vesical fistula in boys. Complications caused by the confluence of the gastrointestinal and urinary tracts may occur, including infection and metabolic derangements. Initial management is usually with a diverting colostomy, which should be constructed using the transverse colon and with separation of the proximal and distal limbs. This limits the risk of fecal contamination of the urinary tract in boys in whom a rectourethral fistula is present. **Many children with imperforate anus have associated spinal cord abnormalities, particularly spinal cord tethering** (Warf et al, 1993; De Gennaro et al, 1994). This condition may be readily identified in the newborn by US of the distal spine before the vertebral column is fully ossified.

Prune-Belly Syndrome

The newborn with the prune-belly syndrome is readily recognized, and this is probably the only aspect of the management of these children that is straightforward. In general, a noninterventional approach with regard to the urinary tract of these children has had the most success (see Chapter 60, Prune-Belly Syndrome). Initially, one needs to closely monitor renal function, anticipating a slow drop of the serum creatinine concentration in the first 2 weeks of life. US evaluation usually reveals massive dilation, more so distally than proximally. This does not necessarily mean obstruction. **Bladder emptying will be inefficient at best, but any intervention should be justified only in terms of a renal functional impairment.** In cases of renal functional impairment early in life, the most efficacious intervention is cutaneous vesicostomy performed with a specific plan for undiversion and bladder management (Noh et al, 1999). Early orchiopexy has usually been advocated but should be tailored to the individual patient. Although many of these children have significant respiratory complications early in life, they may do surprisingly well despite their dramatically abnormal urinary tracts.

Myelomeningocele

Although the incidence of myelomeningocele seems to be declining, appropriate neonatal urologic management is critical for maintenance of long-term bladder and renal function (see Chapter 64, Voiding Dysfunction in Children—Neurogenic and Non-neurogenic). As soon as possible, a baseline renal and bladder US study should be obtained and an assessment of the patient's voiding pattern made. **The presence of hydronephrosis or high postvoid residuals is suggestive of bladder-sphincter dyssynergy and may require the institution of intermittent catheterization** (Kaefer et al, 1999b). Although it is usually not practical before closure of the myelomeningocele, urodynamic assessment of these children is necessary early in life. If no hydronephrosis is present and the bladder empties well, this assessment may be deferred until later in life (i.e., 6 months). **It is essential to introduce the concept to the parents of dynamic and somewhat unpredictable urinary tract function. Regular monitoring must be established early in life** (Spindel et al, 1987).

In children with evidence of bladder-sphincter dyssynergy, early institution of anticholinergic therapy and intermittent catheterization has been advocated with excellent results and a reduced need for subsequent bladder reconstruction (Kaefer et al, 1999b). Urethral dilation to produce incontinence has also been advocated, yet it seems contrary to the ultimate attainment of social continence.

Oligohydramnios/Potter's Syndrome/ Renal Agenesis

The anatomic features of Potter's syndrome should be familiar to all urologists. They include oligohydramnios, limb contractures (particularly club feet), and compressed facies with low-set ears. If Potter's syndrome is suspected, immediate US will permit confirmation of the diagnosis, as evidenced by absent, bilaterally dysplastic, or cystic kidneys. These children usually die from respiratory failure in the first hours of life, although survival for several days has been reported. The role of the urologist is largely one of confirming the diagnosis and providing counseling to parents and staff in these tragic cases. Little specific therapy is available.

Single Umbilical Artery

The presence of a single umbilical artery, occurring in about 0.3% to 0.55% of live births, was associated with an increased incidence of genitourinary anomalies in the past (Vlietinck et al, 1972). Many of these early studies included stillborn fetuses, among whom the incidence of renal anomalies was about 60% (Thummala et al, 1998). More recent examination of the incidence suggested that the degree of increase is relatively minimal, about 7.1% for all renal anomalies, including reflux with an incidence of

4.5% (Bourke et al, 1993). Routine screening for single umbilical artery was recommended, although the clinical significance of the anomalies identified is unclear. **A recent meta-analysis of 37 studies of single umbilical arteries indicated that it would require screening of 14 children with a single umbilical artery to identify 1 child with a renal anomaly, and such anomalies are of minimal significance** (Thummala et al, 1998). The authors did not recommend routine screening. If there is suspicion, renal US is an adequate screening tool.

Sepsis

The infant presenting with sepsis should be evaluated for a possible urinary source. A catheterized or suprapubically aspirated urine specimen for culture must be obtained before the institution of antibiotic therapy. If pyuria is present, urosepsis should be strongly considered. A screening US is an excellent means to quickly and accurately assess the urinary tract. In most cases of urosepsis, some sonographic abnormality is found and will permit directed evaluation. The most common causes are obstructive uropathy with anatomic abnormalities or massive VUR. A normal US does not rule out reflux, and in the presence of urosepsis a VCUG is essential. This should probably be obtained during the acute hospital admission. Further workup should be tailored to the findings of the initial examinations.

Infant boys with intact foreskins have a higher risk of urosepsis and may not have specific anatomic findings (Wiswell and Hachey, 1993). **These boys should undergo the usual evaluation in any event with a US and VCUG to rule out obstruction and reflux.**

Absence of Voiding

The pediatric urologist is often called to evaluate a newborn who has not voided. The normal time for the first postnatal void extends to 24 hours, and some normal children wait even longer (Clark, 1977). The most useful physical finding to determine is whether the bladder is distended. Physical examination may precipitate voiding. US examination may be obtained when there has been no void after 24 hours, when the bladder is distended, or when parental concern is high. Specific findings dictate management. The time to void after circumcision is predictable and depends in part on feeding times. Within 8 hours after circumcision, 75% of breast-fed and 100% of formula-fed infants had voided (Narchi and Kulaylat, 1998).

A common cause of concern is the pinpoint meatus often seen with hypospadias in conjunction with delayed first void. These are virtually never obstructed, as may readily be demonstrated with a feeding tube.

Hematuria

Hematuria in the newborn provokes anxiety yet often does not represent a significant process. One possible explanation is maternal hormonal withdrawal that produces urethral bleeding through an unspecified mechanism. Urine cultures, examination, and US evaluation are usually sufficient. Other causes include renal vein thrombosis (RVT), which will be identified on US examination, depending on the duration of the process, with an enlarged, echogenic kidney, and occasionally with a visible inferior vena caval thrombus (Hibbert et al, 1997).

Hypertension

Neonatal hypertension is rare and should prompt a careful evaluation of the infant's urinary tract. Iatrogenic renal injury from umbilical artery lines has been described to produce hypertension. Radioisotope renal scanning may be confirmatory by demonstrating focal or diffuse renal nonperfusion.

Urinary Ascites

The differential diagnosis of neonatal ascites includes urinary obstruction, which should be specifically sought, most efficiently with a US examination. PUV is probably the most common underlying etiology (Misra et al, 1987; Huang and Cheng, 1990; Ahmed et al, 1997; Sakai et al, 1998). Unusually, other obstructive processes may cause urinary ascites (Chun and Ferguson, 1997; Adams et al, 1998). Electrolyte analysis of the ascitic fluid may reveal a high creatinine concentration indicative of urine, but it may also have equilibrated with the serum across the peritoneum.

Specific Diagnoses

Renal Vein Thrombosis

RVT is suggested in the neonate who has enlarged kidneys, hematuria, anemia, thrombocytopenia, and often a history of a prolonged delivery (Keating and Althausen, 1985). Approximately 20% of infants with gross hematuria are found to have RVT, and about 20% of neonates with RVT have bilateral involvement. The presumed cause is impaired renal blood flow in the setting of a neonate with normally low blood pressure, polycythemia, and dehydration (Glassock et al, 1983). Conditions that aggravate those factors may predispose to RVT. Thrombosis is peripheral and does not usually propagate centrally.

The diagnosis of RVT is best made with the use of US; an enlarged kidney is evident, and the thrombus may be visualized directly (Hibbert et al, 1997). Management of RVT is directed initially at reversing any predisposing factors such as dehydration and secondary electrolyte imbalances. Specific treatment remains controversial but may include anticoagulation with heparin or fibrinolytic therapy with streptokinase. Each of these modalities can be associated with significant complications (Chevalier, 1991; Nuss et al, 1994; Bokenkamp et al, 2000). Bilateral RVT requires more aggressive therapy (Cozzolino and Cendron, 1997).

Adrenal Hemorrhage

Adrenal hemorrhage is a relatively common condition, estimated to occur in about 1% to 2% of healthy infants. More small adrenal hemorrhages are being detected with routine perinatal US. **Predisposing factors include prolonged labor, birth trauma, and large birth weight. RVT may be associated** (Suga et al, 2000). Clinically, the neonate with adrenal hemorrhage may have anemia, shock, and an abdominal mass. Gross hematuria is unusual. US is the most efficient diagnostic measure and usually reveals an echogenic suprarenal mass (Rubenstein et al, 1995; Schwarzler et al, 1999). This may appear similar to a neuroblastoma, and further evaluation, particularly magnetic resonance imaging, may be necessary. The imaging characteristics of an adrenal hemorrhage evolve with time, often providing a definitive diagnosis as the mass is seen to involute. Calcifications may later develop, reportedly as soon as 1 week (Smith and Middleton, 1979). **The late appearance of an adrenal hemorrhage is that of peripheral eggshell calcifications, in contrast to the stippled calcifications of neuroblastoma.** Management is almost always supportive and expectant, with rare need for intervention.

Renal Artery Thrombosis

Hypertension and hematuria in a neonate should suggest the possibility of renal artery thrombosis. The clinical setting is usually suggestive in that umbilical artery catheterization is the most common cause of this condition. Renal insufficiency may be a clinical feature of this condition, as may proteinuria and congestive heart failure. Thrombotic involvement of the aorta may be present as well. US examination usually reveals the diagnosis and the extent of the thrombus. Management depends on the clinical setting, and unilateral involvement is best managed expectantly, although thrombolytic therapy may be appropriate. Control of hypertension is the most important aspect of management and occasionally requires removal of a nonfunctional kidney.

REFERENCES

Abbott JF, Levine D, Wapner R: Posterior urethral valves: Inaccuracy of prenatal diagnosis. Fetal Diagn Ther 1998;13:179–283.

Acharya S, Jayabose S, Kogan SJ, et al: Prenatally diagnosed neuroblastoma. Cancer 1997;80:304–310.

Adams MC, Ludlow J, Brock JW 3rd, Rink RC: Prenatal urinary ascites and persistent cloaca: Risk factors for poor drainage of urine or meconium. J Urol 1998;160:2179–2181.

Adra AM, Mejides AA, Dennaoui MS, Beydoun SN: Fetal pyelectasis: Is it always "physiologic"? Am J Obstet Gynecol 1995;173:1263–1266.

Adzick NS, Harrison MR, Flake AW, deLorimier AA: Urinary extravasation in the fetus with obstructive uropathy. J Pediatr Surg 1985a;20:608–615.

Adzick N, Harrison M, Glick P, Flake A: Fetal urinary tract obstruction: Experimental pathophysiology. Semin Perinatol 1985b;9:79–90.

Ahmed S, Borghol M, Hugosson C: Urinoma and urinary ascites secondary to calyceal perforation in neonatal posterior urethral valves. Br J Urol 1997;79:991–992.

Anderson PA, Rickwood AM: Features of primary vesicoureteric reflux detected by prenatal sonography. Br J Urol 1991;67:267–271.

Applegate KE, Ghei M, Perez-Atayde AR: Prenatal detection of a Wilms' tumor [see comments]. Pediatr Radiol 1999;29:65–67.

Assael BM, Guez S, Marra G, et al: Congenital reflux nephropathy: A follow-up of 108 cases diagnosed perinatally. Br J Urol 1998;82:252–257.

Attar R, Quinn F, Winyard PJ, et al: Short-term urinary flow impairment deregulates PAX2 and PCNA expression and cell survival in fetal sheep kidneys. Am J Pathol 1998;152:1225–1235.

Austin PF, Homsy YL, Gearhart JP, et al: The prenatal diagnosis of cloacal exstrophy. J Urol 1998;160:1179–1181.

Avni EF, Thoua Y, Lalmand B, et al: Multicystic dysplastic kidney: Natural history from in utero diagnosis and postnatal followup. J Urol 1987;138:1420–1424.

Badid C, Mounier N, Costa AM, Desmouliere A: Role of myofibroblasts during normal tissue repair and excessive scarring: Interest of their assessment in nephropathies. Histol Histopathol 2000;15:269–280.

Bagolan P, Bilancioni E, Nahom A, et al: Prenatal diagnosis of a bronchogenic cyst in an unusual site. Ultrasound Obstet Gynecol 2000;15: 66–68.

Barakat AJ, Butler MG, Cobb CG, et al: Reliability of ultrasound in the prenatal diagnosis of urinary tract abnormalities. Pediatr Nephrol 1991; 5:12–14.

Barss VA, Benacerraf BR, Frigoletto FD Jr: Second trimester oligohydramnios: A predictor of poor fetal outcome. Obstet Gynecol 1984;64: 608–610.

Barth RA, Filly RA, Sondheimer FK: Prenatal sonographic findings in bladder exstrophy. J Ultrasound Med 1990;9:359–361.

Bauer SB, Dyro FM, Krarup C, et al: The unrecognized neuropathic bladder of infancy. J Urol 1989;142:589–591.

Bearman SB, Hine PL, Sanders RC: Multicystic kidney: A sonographic pattern. Radiology 1976;118:685–688.

Beck AD: The effect of intra-uterine urinary obstruction upon the development of the fetal kidney. J Urol 1971;105:784–789.

Becker AE: Primary heart tumors in the pediatric age group: A review of salient pathologic features relevant for clinicians. Pediatr Cardiol 2000; 21:317–323.

Bellinger MF, Comstock CH, Grosso D, Zaino R: Fetal posterior urethral valves and renal dysplasia at 15 weeks gestational age. J Urol 1983; 129:1238.

Benacerraf BR, Frigoletto FD Jr: Soft tissue nuchal fold in the second-trimester fetus: Standards for normal measurements compared with those in Down syndrome. Am J Obstet Gynecol 1987;157:1146–1149.

Benacerraf BR, Mandell J, Estroff JA, et al: Fetal pyelectasis: A possible association with Down syndrome. Obstet Gynecol 1990;76:58–60.

Benacerraf BR, Saltzman DH, Mandell J: Sonographic diagnosis of abnormal fetal genitalia. J Ultrasound Med 1989;8:613–617.

Bernstein J: Developmental abnormalities of the renal parenchyma: Renal hypoplasia and dysplasia. Pathol Annu 1968;3:213.

Bokenkamp A, von Kries R, Nowak-Gottl U, et al: Neonatal renal venous thrombosis in Germany between 1992 and 1994: Epidemiology, treatment and outcome. Eur J Pediatr 2000;159:44–48.

Borer JG, Glassberg KI, Kassner EG, et al: Unilateral multicystic dysplasia in 1 component of a horseshoe kidney: Case reports and review of the literature. J Urol 1994;152:1568–1571.

Bourke WG, Clarke TA, Mathews TG, et al: Isolated single umbilical artery: The case for routine renal screening. Arch Dis Child 1993;68: 600–601.

Bromley B, Mandell J, Gross G, et al: Masculinization of female fetuses with congenital adrenal hyperplasia may already be present at 18 weeks. Am J Obstet Gynecol 1994;171:264–265.

Burbige KA, Lebowitz RL, Colodny AH, et al: The megacystis-megaureter syndrome. J Urol 1984;131:1133–1136.

Bussieres L, Laborde K, Souberbielle JC, et al: Fetal urinary insulin-like growth factor I and binding protein 3 in bilateral obstructive uropathies. Prenat Diagn 1995;15:1047–1055.

Callan NA, Blakemore K, Park J, et al: Fetal genitourinary tract anomalies: Evaluation, operative correction, and follow-up. Obstet Gynecol 1990;75:67–74.

Calvano CJ, Moran ME, Mehlhaff BA, et al: Assessment of access strategies for fetoscopic urologic surgery: Preliminary results. J Endourol 1997;11:49–53.

Cardwell MS: Bilateral renal agenesis: Clinical implications. South Med J 1988;81:327–328.

Carr MC, Benacerraf BR, Estroff JA, Mandell J: Prenatally diagnosed bilateral hyperechoic kidneys with normal amniotic fluid: Postnatal outcome. J Urol 1995a;153:442–444.

Carr MC, Schlussel RN, Peters CA, et al: Expression of cell growth regulated genes in the fetal kidney: Relevance to in utero obstruction. J Urol 1995b;154:242–246.

Ceccherini I, Lituania M, Cordone MS, et al: Autosomal dominant polycystic kidney disease: Prenatal diagnosis by DNA analysis and sonography at 14 weeks. Prenat Diagn 1989;9:751–758.

Chevalier RL: Counterbalance in functional adaptation to ureteral obstruction during development. Pediatr Nephrol 1990;4:442–444.

Chevalier RL: What treatment do you advise for bilateral or unilateral renal thrombosis in the newborn, with or without thrombosis of the inferior vena cava? Pediatr Nephrol 1991;5:679.

Chevalier RL: Growth factors and apoptosis in neonatal ureteral obstruction. J Am Soc Nephrol 1996;7:1098–1105.

Chevalier RL: Pathophysiology of obstructive nephropathy in the newborn. Semin Nephrol 1998;18:585–593.

Chevalier RL: Molecular and cellular pathophysiology of obstructive nephropathy. Pediatr Nephrol 1999;13:612–619.

Chevalier RL, Gomez RA: Response of the renin-angiotensin system to relief of neonatal ureteral obstruction. Am J Physiol 1988;255:F1070.

Chevalier RL, Goyal S, Thornhill BA: EGF improves recovery following relief of unilateral ureteral obstruction in the neonatal rat. J Urol 1999a; 162:1532–1536.

Chevalier RL, Kim A, Thornhill BA, Wolstenholme JT: Recovery following relief of unilateral ureteral obstruction in the neonatal rat. Kidney Int 1999b;55:793–807.

Chevalier RL, Klahr S: Therapeutic approaches in obstructive uropathy. Semin Nephrol 1998;18:652–658.

Chevalier RL, Thornhill BA, Wolstenholme JT, Kim A: Unilateral ureteral obstruction in early development alters renal growth: Dependence on the duration of obstruction. J Urol 1999c;161:309–313.

Chun KE, Ferguson RS: Neonatal urinary ascites due to unilateral vesicoureteric junction obstruction. Pediatr Surg Int 1997;12:455–457.

Chung KH, Gomez RA, Chevalier RL: Regulation of renal growth factors and clusterin by AT1 receptors during neonatal ureteral obstruction. Am J Physiol 1995;268:F1117–F1123.

Cilento BG Jr, Bauer SB, Retik AB, et al: Urachal anomalies: Defining the best diagnostic modality. Urology 1998;52:120–122.

Cilento BG Jr, Benacerraf BR, Mandell J: Prenatal diagnosis of cloacal malformation. Urology 1994;43:386–388.

Clark DA: Times of first void and first stool in 500 newborns. Pediatrics 1977;60:457–459.

Close CE, Carr MC, Burns MW, Mitchell ME: Lower urinary tract changes after early valve ablation in neonates and infants: Is early diversion warranted? [see comments]. J Urol 1997;157:984–988.

Cole BR, Conley SB, Stapleton FB: Polycystic kidney disease in the first year of life. J Pediatr 1987;111:693.

Coplen DE, Hare JY, Zderic SA, et al: 10-Year experience with prenatal intervention for hydronephrosis. J Urol 1996;156:1142–1145.

Corteville JE, Gray DL, Crane JP: Congenital hydronephrosis: Correlation of fetal ultrasonographic findings with infant outcome. Am J Obstet Gynecol 1991;165:384–388.

Cozzolino DJ, Cendron M: Bilateral renal vein thrombosis in a newborn: A case of prenatal renal vein thrombosis. Urology 1997;50:128–131.

Crombleholme TM, Harrison MR, Longaker MT, Langer JC: Prenatal diagnosis and management of bilateral hydronephrosis. Pediatr Nephrol 1988;2:334–342.

De Gennaro M, Rivosecchi M, Lucchetti MC, et al: The incidence of occult spinal dysraphism and the onset of neurovesical dysfunction in children with anorectal anomalies. Eur J Pediatr Surg 1994;4(Suppl 1): 12–14.

Diamond DA, Jeffs RD: Cloacal exstrophy: A 22-year experience. J Urol 1985;133:779–782.

Diamond JR: Macrophages and progressive renal disease in experimental hydronephrosis. Am J Kidney Dis 1995;26:133–140.

Diamond JR, Kees-Folts D, Ding G, et al: Macrophages, monocyte chemoattractant peptide-1, and TGF-beta 1 in experimental hydronephrosis. Am J Physiol 1994;266:F926–F933.

Diamond JR, Ricardo SD, Klahr S: Mechanisms of interstitial fibrosis in obstructive nephropathy. Semin Nephrol 1998;18:594–602.

Diamond JR, van Goor H, Ding G, Engelmyer E: Myofibroblasts in experimental hydronephrosis. Am J Pathol 1995;146:121–129.

DiFiore JW, Fauza DO, Slavin R, et al: Experimental fetal tracheal ligation reverses the structural and physiological effects of pulmonary hypoplasia in congenital diaphragmatic hernia. J Pediatr Surg 1994;29: 248–256; discussion, 256–257.

DiFiore JW, Fauza DO, Slavin R, Wilson JM: Experimental fetal tracheal ligation and congenital diaphragmatic hernia: A pulmonary vascular morphometric analysis [see comments]. J Pediatr Surg 1995;30:917–923; discussion, 923–924.

Dinneen MD, Dhillon HK, Ward HC, et al: Antenatal diagnosis of posterior urethral valves [see comments]. Br J Urol 1993;72:364–369.

Docimo SG, Luetic T, Crone RK, et al: Pulmonary development in the fetal lamb with severe bladder outlet obstruction and oligohydramnios: A morphometric study. J Urol 1989;142:657–660.

Docimo SG, Silver RI: Renal ultrasonography in newborns with prenatally detected hydronephrosis: Why wait? J Urol 1997;157:1387–1389.

Dommergues M, Muller F, Ngo S, et al: Fetal serum beta2-microglobulin predicts postnatal renal function in bilateral uropathies. Kidney Int 2000;58:312–316.

Dorenbaum D, Reid WD, Natale R: Fetal megaureters masquerading as bowel obstruction. Urology 1986;28:297–298.

Eble JN, Bonsib SM: Extensively cystic renal neoplasms: Cystic nephroma, cystic partially differentiated nephroblastoma, multilocular cystic renal cell carcinoma, and cystic hamartoma of renal pelvis. Semin Diagn Pathol 1998;15:2–20.

Edwards OP, Baldinger S: Prenatal onset of autosomal dominant polycystic kidney disease. Urology 1989;34:265–270.

Effmann EL, Lebowitz RL, Colodny AH: Duplication of the urethra. Radiology 1976;119:179–185.

el-Dahr SS, Gomez RA, Gray MS, et al: In situ localization of renin and its mRNA in neonatal ureteral obstruction. Am J Physiol 1990;258: F854.

el-Dahr SS, Gee J, Dipp S, et al: Upregulation of renin-angiotensin system and downregulation of kallikrein in obstructive nephropathy. Am J Physiol 1993;264:F874–F881.

Elder JS: Commentary: Importance of antenatal diagnosis of vesicoureteral reflux. J Urol 1992;148:1750–1754.

Elder JS, O'Grady JP, Ashmead G, et al: Evaluation of fetal renal function: Unreliability of fetal urinary electrolytes. J Urol 1990;144:574.

Felsen D, Loo MH, Marion DN, Vaughan ED Jr: Involvement of platelet activating factor and thromboxane A2 in the renal response to unilateral ureteral obstruction. J Urol 1990;144:141–145.

Felson B, Cussen LJ: The hydronephrotic type of congenital multicystic disease of the kidney. Semin Roentgenol 1975;10:113.

Fernbach SK, Maizels M, Conway JJ: Ultrasound grading of hydronephrosis: Introduction to the system used by the Society for Fetal Urology. Pediatr Radiol 1993;23:478–480.

Fitzsimons PJ, Frost RA, Millward S, et al: Prenatal and immediate postnatal ultrasonographic diagnosis of ureterocele. Can Assoc Radiol J 1986;37:189–191.

Freedman AL, Bukowski TP, Smith CA, et al: Fetal therapy for obstructive uropathy: Diagnosis specific outcomes. J Urol 1996;156:720–723; discussion, 723–724.

Freedman AL, Johnson MP, Gonzalez R: Fetal therapy for obstructive uropathy: Past, present, future? Pediatr Nephrol 2000;14:167–176.

Frokiaer J, Christensen BM, Marples D, et al: Downregulation of aquaporin-2 parallels changes in renal water excretion in unilateral ureteral obstruction. Am J Physiol 1997;273:F213–F223.

Fung TY, Fung YM, Ng PC, et al: Polyhydramnios and hypercalcemia associated with congenital mesoblastic nephroma: Case report and a new appraisal. Obstet Gynecol 1995;85:815–817.

Furness PD 3rd, Maizels M, Han SW, et al: Elevated bladder urine concentration of transforming growth factor-beta1 correlates with upper urinary tract obstruction in children. J Urol 1999;162:1033–1036.

Gearhart JP, Ben-Chaim J, Jeffs RD, Sanders RC: Criteria for the prenatal diagnosis of classic bladder exstrophy. Obstet Gynecol 1995;85:961–964.

Geirsson RT, Ricketts NE, Taylor DJ, Coghill S: Prenatal appearance of a mesoblastic nephroma associated with polyhydramnios. J Clin Ultrasound 1985;13:488–490.

Glassock RJ, Duffee J, Kodroff MB, Chan JC: Dehydration, renal vein thrombosis and hyperkalemic renal tubular acidosis in a newborn. Am J Nephrol 1983;3:329–337.

Glick PL, Harrison MR, Golbus MS, et al: Management of the fetus with congenital hydronephrosis II: Prognostic criteria and selection for treatment. J Pediatr Surg 1985;20:376–387.

Glick PL, Siebert JR, Benjamin DR: Pathophysiology of congenital diaphragmatic hernia: I. Renal enlargement suggests feedback modulation by pulmonary derived renotropins: A unifying hypothesis to explain pulmonary hypoplasia, polyhydramnios, and renal enlargement in the fetus/newborn with congenital diaphragmatic hernia. J Pediatr Surg 1990;25:492–495.

Glick PL, Siebert JR, Benjamin DR: Possible trophic relationship between the growth of the lungs and kidneys in congenital diaphragmatic hernia (CDH) [letter; comment]. J Pediatr Surg 1991;26:643–644.

Gluckman GR, Stoller ML, Jacobs MM, Kogan BA: Newborn penile

glans amputation during circumcision and successful reattachment. J Urol 1995;153:778–779.

Gobet R, Bleakley J, Cisek L, et al: Fetal partial urethral obstruction causes renal fibrosis and is associated with proteolytic imbalance. J Urol 1999a;162:854–860.

Gobet R, Bleakley J, Peters CA: Premature urachal closure induces hydroureteronephrosis in male fetuses. J Urol 1998a;160:1463–1467.

Gobet R, Cisek LJ, Chang B, et al: Experimental fetal vesicoureteral reflux induces renal tubular and glomerular damage, and is associated with persistent bladder instability. J Urol 1999b;162:1090–1095.

Gobet R, Cisek LJ, Zotti P, Peters CA: Experimental vesicoureteral reflux in the fetus depends on bladder function and causes renal fibrosis. J Urol 1998b;160:1058–1062; discussion, 1079.

Gobet R, Park JM, Nguyen HT, et al: Renal renin-angiotensin system dysregulation caused by partial bladder outlet obstruction in fetal sheep. Kidney Int 1999c;56:1654–1661.

Gomez RA, Lynch KR, Sturgill BC, et al: Distribution of renin mRNA and its protein in the developing kidney. Am J Physiol 1989;257:F850–858.

Granata C, Fagnani AM, Gambini C, et al: Features and outcome of neuroblastoma detected before birth. J Pediatr Surg 2000;35:88–91.

Gunn TR, Mora JD, Pease P: Antenatal diagnosis of urinary tract abnormalities by ultrasonography after 28 weeks' gestation: Incidence and outcome. Am J Obstet Gynecol 1995;172:479–486.

Hamada Y, Ikebukuro K, Sato M, et al: Prenatally diagnosed cystic neuroblastoma. Pediatr Surg Int 1999;15:71–74.

Harris KP, Yanagisawa H, Schreiner GF, Klahr S: Evidence for two distinct and functionally important sites of enhanced thromboxane production after bilateral ureteral obstruction in the rat. Clin Sci 1991;81: 209–213.

Harrison MR, Adzick NS, Flake AW, et al: Correction of congenital diaphragmatic hernia in utero: VIII. Response of the hypoplastic lung to tracheal occlusion. J Pediatr Surg 1996;31:1339–1348.

Harrison MR, Golbus MS, Filly RA, et al: Fetal surgery for congenital hydronephrosis. N Engl J Med 1982a;306:591–593.

Harrison MR, Nakayama DK, Noall RA, deLorimier AA: Correction of congenital hydronephrosis in utero: II. Decompression reverses the effects of obstruction on the fetal lung and urinary tract. J Pediatr Surg 1982b;17:965.

Hartman GE, Shochat SJ: Abdominal mass lesions in the newborn: Diagnosis and treatment. Clin Perinatol 1989;16:123–135.

Helin I, Persson PH: Prenatal diagnosis of urinary tract abnormalities by ultrasound. Pediatrics 1986;78:879–883.

Hendren WH: A new approach to infants with severe obstructive uropathy: Early complete reconstruction. J Pediatr Surg 1970;5:184.

Hendren WH: Urological aspects of cloacal malformations. J Urol 1988; 140:1207–1213.

Hendren WH: Cloaca, the most severe degree of imperforate anus: Experience with 195 cases. Ann Surg 1998;228:331–346.

Herndon CD, McKenna PH, Kolon TF, et al: A multicenter outcomes analysis of patients with neonatal reflux presenting with prenatal hydronephrosis. J Urol 1999;162:1203–1208.

Hibbert J, Howlett DC, Greenwood KL, et al: The ultrasound appearances of neonatal renal vein thrombosis. Br J Radiol 1997;70:1191–1194.

Hislop A, Hey E, Reid LM: The lungs in congenital bilateral renal agenesis and dysplasia. Arch Dis Child 1979;54:32.

Ho PT, Estroff JA, Kozakewich H, et al: Prenatal detection of neuroblastoma: A ten-year experience from the Dana-Farber Cancer Institute and Children's Hospital [see comments]. Pediatrics 1993;92:358–364.

Hoffman CK, Filly RA, Callen PW: The "lying down" adrenal sign: A sonographic indicator of renal agenesis or ectopia in fetuses and neonates. J Ultrasound Med 1992;11:533–536.

Holmes LB: Prevalence, phenotypic heterogeneity and familial aspects of bilateral renal agenesis/dysgenesis. Prog Clin Biol Res 1989;305:1–11.

Horowitz M, Gershbein AB, Glassberg KI: Vesicoureteral reflux in infants with prenatal hydronephrosis confirmed at birth: Racial differences. J Urol 1999;161:248–250.

Hosoda Y, Rossman JE, Glick PL: Pathophysiology of congenital diaphragmatic hernia: IV. Renal hyperplasia is associated with pulmonary hypoplasia. J Pediatr Surg 1993;28:464–469; discussion, 469–470.

Huang CJ, Cheng YR: Urinary ascites in young infants: Report of 9 cases. J Singapore Paediatr Soc 1990;32:121–124.

Hurwitz RS, Manzoni GAM, Ransley PG, Stephens FD: Cloacal exstrophy: A report of 34 cases. J Urol 1987;138:1060–1064.

Hussman KL, Friedwald JP, Gollub MJ, Melamed J: Caroli's disease associated with infantile polycystic kidney disease: Prenatal sonographic appearance. J Ultrasound Med 1991;10:235–237.

Hutton KA, Thomas DF, Arthur RJ, et al: Prenatally detected posterior urethral valves: Is gestational age at detection a predictor of outcome? J Urol 1994;152:698–701.

Irsutti M, Puget C, Baunin C, et al: Mesoblastic nephroma: Prenatal ultrasonographic and MRI features. Pediatr Radiol 2000;30:147–150.

Jaramillo D, Lebowitz RL, Hendren WH: The cloacal malformation: Radiologic findings and imaging recommendations. Radiology 1990;177: 441–448.

Jaureguizar E, Lopez Pereira P, Martinez Urrutia MJ, et al: Does neonatal pyeloureterostomy worsen bladder function in children with posterior urethral valves? J Urol 2000;164:1031–1033; discussion, 1033–1034.

Jayanthi VR, McLorie GA, Khoury AE, Churchill BM: The effect of temporary cutaneous diversion on ultimate bladder function. J Urol 1995;154:889–892.

Johnson MP, Bukowski TP, Reitleman C, et al: In utero surgical treatment of fetal obstructive uropathy: A new comprehensive approach to identify appropriate candidates for vesicoamniotic shunt therapy. Am J Obstet Gynecol 1994;170:1770–1776; discussion, 1776–1779.

Johnson MP, Corsi P, Bradfield W, et al: Sequential urinalysis improves evaluation of fetal renal function in obstructive uropathy [see comments]. Am J Obstet Gynecol 1995;173:59–65.

Kaefer M, Diamond D, Hendren WH, et al: The incidence of intersexuality in children with cryptorchidism and hypospadias: Stratification based on gonadal palpability and meatal position. J Urol 1999a;162: 1003–1006; discussion, 1006–1007.

Kaefer M, Pabby A, Kelly M, et al: Improved bladder function after prophylactic treatment of the high risk neurogenic bladder in newborns with myelomeningocele. J Urol 1999b;162:1068–1071.

Kaefer M, Peters CA, Retik AB, Benacerraf BB: Increased renal echogenicity: A sonographic sign for differentiating between obstructive and nonobstructive etiologies of in utero bladder distension. J Urol 1997; 158:1026–1029.

Kaneto H, Morrissey J, Klahr S: Increased expression of TGF-beta 1 mRNA in the obstructed kidney of rats with unilateral ureteral ligation. Kidney Int 1993;44:313–321.

Kaya H, Oral B, Dittrich R, Ozkaya O: Prenatal diagnosis of cloacal exstrophy before rupture of the cloacal membrane. Arch Gynecol Obstet 2000;263:142–144.

Keating MA, Althausen AF: The clinical spectrum of renal vein thrombosis. J Urol 1985;133:938–945.

Kennedy WA II, Buttyan R, Sawczuk IS: Epidermal growth factor suppresses renal tubular apoptosis following ureteral obstruction. J Am Soc Nephrol 1993;4:738.

Kim YH, Horowitz M, Combs A, et al: Comparative urodynamic findings after primary valve ablation, vesicostomy or proximal diversion. J Urol 1996;156:673–676.

Klahr S, Morrissey JJ: The role of growth factors, cytokines, and vasoactive compounds in obstructive nephropathy. Semin Nephrol 1998;18: 622–632.

Kokoua A, Homsy Y, Lavigne JF, et al: Maturation of the external urinary sphincter: A comparative histotopographic study in humans. J Urol 1993;150:617–622.

Kozakewich HP, Perez-Atayde AR, Donovan MJ, et al: Cystic neuroblastoma: Emphasis on gene expression, morphology, and pathogenesis. Pediatr Dev Pathol 1998;1:17–28.

Krueger RP, Hardy BE, Churchill BM: Growth in boys and posterior urethral valves: Primary valve resection vs upper tract diversion. Urol Clin North Am 1980;7:265–272.

Lakshmanan V, Peters CA: Laparoscopy in the management of intersex anomalies. Pediatr Endosurg Innov Tech 2000;4:201–206.

LaQuaglia MP, Bauer SB, Eraklis A, et al: Bilateral neonatal torsion. J Urol 1987;138:1051–1054.

Liapis H, Nag M, Steinhardt G: Effects of experimental ureteral obstruction on platelet-derived growth factor-A and type I procollagen expression in fetal metanephric kidneys. Pediatr Nephrol 1994;8:548.

Liu HYA, Dillon HK, Yeung CK, et al: Clinical outcome and management of prenatally diagnosed primary megaureters. J Urol 1994;152: 614–617.

Lonergan GJ, Rice RR, Suarez ES: Autosomal recessive polycystic kidney disease: Radiologic-pathologic correlation. Radiographics 2000;20:837–855.

Luks FI, Deprest JA, Vandenberghe K, et al: A model for fetal surgery through intrauterine endoscopy. J Pediatr Surg 1994;29:1007–1009.

Mandell J, Blyth BR, Peters CA, et al: Structural genitourinary defects detected in utero. Radiology 1991;178:193–196.

Mandell J, Bromley B, Peters CA, Benacerraf BR: Prenatal sonographic detection of genital malformations. J Urol 1995;153:1994–1996.

Mandell J, Lebowitz RL, Peters CA, et al: Prenatal diagnosis of the megacystis-megaureter association. J Urol 1992a;148:1487–1489.

Mandell J, Lillehei CW, Greene M, Benacerraf BR: The prenatal diagnosis of imperforate anus with rectourinary fistula: Dilated fetal colon with enterolithiasis [see comments]. J Pediatr Surg 1992b;27:82–84.

Mandell J, Paltiel HJ, Peters CA, Benacerraf BR: Prenatal findings associated with a unilateral nonfunctioning or absent kidney. J Urol 1994; 152:176–178.

Mandell J, Peters CA, Estroff JA, Benacerraff BR: Late onset severe oligohydramnios associated with genitourinary abnormalities. J Urol 1992c;148:515–518.

Manning FA, Harrison MR, Rodeck C: Catheter shunts for fetal hydronephrosis and hydrocephalus: Report of the International Fetal Surgery Registry. N Engl J Med 1986;315:336–340.

Manning FA, Hill LM, Platt LD: Qualitative amniotic fluid volume determination by ultrasound: Antepartum detection of intrauterine growth retardation. Am J Obstet Gynecol 1981;139:254.

Marra G, Barbieri G, Dell'Agnola CA, et al: Congenital renal damage associated with primary vesicoureteral reflux detected prenatally in male infants. J Pediatr 1994;124:726–730.

Mathews R, Jeffs RD, Reiner WG, et al: Cloacal exstrophy—improving the quality of life: The Johns Hopkins experience. J Urol 1998;160: 2452–2456.

Matsell DG, Bennett T, Bocking AD: Characterization of fetal ovine renal dysplasia after mid-gestation ureteral obstruction. Clin Invest Med 1996;19:444–452.

McHugo JM, Shafi MI, Rowlands D, Weaver JB: Pre-natal diagnosis of adult polycystic kidney disease. Br J Radiol 1988;61:1072–1074.

McVicar M, Margouleff D, Chandra M: Diagnosis and imaging of the fetal and neonatal abdominal mass: An integrated approach. Adv Pediatr 1991;38:135–149.

Medjebeur AA, Bussieres L, Gasser B, et al: Experimental bilateral urinary obstruction in fetal sheep: Transforming growth factor-$\beta1$ expression. Am J Physiol 1997;273:F372–F379.

Meglin AJ, Balotin RJ, Jelinek JS, et al: Cloacal exstrophy: Radiologic findings in 13 patients. AJR Am J Roentgenol 1990;155:1267–1272.

Merguerian PA, McLorie GA, Churchill BM, et al: Radiographic and serologic correlates of azotemia in patients with posterior urethral valves. J Urol 1992;148:1499–1503.

Minevich E, Wacksman J, Phipps L, et al: The importance of accurate diagnosis and early close followup in patients with suspected multicystic dysplastic kidney. J Urol 1997;158:1301–1304.

Misra MC, Sethi RS, Kumar R: Neonatal ascites: A clinical manifestation of obstructive uropathy. J Indian Med Assoc 1987;85:240–241.

Miyajima A, Chen J, Kirman I, et al: Interaction of nitric oxide and transforming growth factor-BETA1 induced by angiotensin II and mechanical stretch in rat renal tubular epithelial cells. J Urol 2000;164: 1729–1734.

Moessinger AC, Collins MH, Blanc WA, et al: Oligohydramnios-induced lung hypoplasia: The influence of timing and duration in gestation. Pediatr Res 1986;20:951.

Muller F, Dommergues M, Mandelbrot L, et al: Fetal urinary biochemistry predicts postnatal renal function in children with bilateral obstructive uropathies. Obstet Gynecol 1993;82:813–820.

Narchi H, Kulaylat N: Neonatal circumcision: When can infants reliably be expected to void? Pediatrics 1998;102:150–152.

Newton ER, Louis F, Dalton ME, Feingold M: Fetal neuroblastoma and catecholamine-induced maternal hypertension. Obstet Gynecol 1985;65: 49S–52S.

Nguyen HT, Bauer SB, Peters CA, et al: 99m Technetium dimercaptosuccinic acid renal scintigraphy abnormalities in infants with sterile high grade vesicoureteral reflux. J Urol 2000a;164:1674–1679.

Nguyen HT, Bride SH, Badawy AB, et al: Heparin-binding EGF-like growth factor is up-regulated in the obstructed kidney in a cell- and region-specific manner and acts to inhibit apoptosis. Am J Pathol 2000b;156:889–898.

Nicolaides KH, Cheng HH, Abbas A, et al: Fetal renal defects: Associated malformations and chromosomal defects. Fetal Diagn Ther 1992;7: 1–11.

Nicolini U, Fisk N, Talbert D, et al: Intrauterine manometry: Technique and application to fetal pathology. Prenat Diagn 1989;9:243–254.

Nicolini U, Rodeck CH, Fisk NM: Shunt treatment for fetal obstructive uropathy. (Letter.) Lancet 1987;2:1338–1339.

Nishimura H, Yerkes E, Hohenfellner K, et al: Role of the angiotensin type 2 receptor gene in congenital anomalies of the kidney and urinary tract, CAKUT, of mice and men. Mol Cell 1999;3:1–10.

Nobuhara KK, Fauza DO, DiFiore JW, et al: Continuous intrapulmonary distension with perfluorocarbon accelerates neonatal (but not adult) lung growth. J Pediatr Surg 1998;33:292–298.

Noh PH, Cooper CS, Winkler AC, et al: Prognostic factors for long-term renal function in boys with the prune-belly syndrome. J Urol 1999;162:1399–1401.

Novelli G, Frontali M, Baldini D, et al: Prenatal diagnosis of adult polycystic kidney disease with DNA markers on chromosome 16 and the genetic heterogeneity problem. Prenat Diagn 1989;9:759–767.

Nuss R, Hays T, Manco-Johnson M: Efficacy and safety of heparin anticoagulation for neonatal renal vein thrombosis. Am J Pediatr Hematol Oncol 1994;16:127–131.

Oliveira EA, Diniz JS, Cabral AC, et al: Predictive factors of fetal urethral obstruction: A multivariate analysis. Fetal Diagn Ther 2000;15:180–186.

Persutte WH, Hussey M, Chyu J, Hobbins JC: Striking findings concerning the variability in the measurement of the fetal renal collecting system. Ultrasound Obstet Gynecol 2000;15:186–190.

Peters CA: Urinary obstruction in children. J Urol 1995;154:1874–1884.

Peters CA: Obstruction of the fetal urinary tract. J Am Soc Nephrol 1997;8:653–663.

Peters CA, Carr MC, Lais A, et al: The fetal kidney: An ovine model of partial ureteral obstruction. J Urol 1992a;147:224A.

Peters CA, Carr MC, Lais A, et al: The response of the fetal kidney to obstruction. J Urol 1992b;148:503.

Peters CA, Mandell J: The multicystic dysplastic kidney. AUA Update Series 1989;8:Lesson 7

Peters CA, Reid LM, Docimo S, et al: The role of the kidney in lung growth and maturation in the setting of obstructive uropathy and oligohydramnios. J Urol 1991;146:597–600.

Podesta ML, Ruarte A, Gargiulo C, et al: Urodynamic findings in boys with posterior urethral valves after treatment with primary valve ablation or vesicostomy and delayed ablation [see comments]. J Urol 2000;164:139–144.

Polito C, La Manna A, Rambaldi PF, et al: High incidence of a generally small kidney and primary vesicoureteral reflux. J Urol 2000;164:479–482.

Potter EL: Normal and Abnormal Development of the Kidney. Chicago: Year Book Medical Publishers, 1972.

Queenan JT, Thompson W, Whitfield C: Amniotic fluid volumes in normal pregnancies. Am J Obstet Gynecol 1972;114:34.

Quintero RA, Hume R, Smith C, et al: Percutaneous fetal cystoscopy and endoscopic fulguration of posterior urethral valves [see comments]. Am J Obstet Gynecol 1995;172:206–209.

Reeders ST, Zerres K, Gal A, et al: Prenatal diagnosis of autosomal dominant polycystic kidney disease with a DNA probe. Lancet 1986;2:6–8.

Reuter KL, Lebowitz RL: Massive vesicoureteral reflux mimicking posterior urethral valves in a fetus. J Clin Ultrasound 1985;13:584–587.

Risdon RA, Yeung CK, Ransley PG: Reflux nephropathy in children submitted to unilateral nephrectomy: A clinicopathological study. Clin Nephrol 1993;40:308–314.

Robichaux AI, Mandell J, Greene M, et al: Fetal abdominal wall defect: A new complication of vesicoamniotic shunting. Fetal Diagn Ther 1991;6:11–13.

Rovin BH, Harris KP, Morrison A, et al: Renal cortical release of a specific macrophage chemoattractant in response to ureteral obstruction. Lab Invest 1990;63:213–220.

Rubenstein SC, Benacerraf BR, Retik AB, Mandell J: Fetal suprarenal masses: Sonographic appearance and differential diagnosis. Ultrasound Obstet Gynecol 1995;5:164–167.

Sakai K, Konda R, Ota S, et al: Neonatal urinary ascites caused by urinary tract obstruction: Two case reports. Int J Urol 1998;5:379–382.

Sanders RC, Hartman DS: The sonographic distinction between neonatal multicystic kidney and hydronephrosis. Radiology 1984;151:621–625.

Schoenecker SA, Cyr DR, Mack LA, et al: Sonographic diagnosis of bilateral fetal renal duplication with ectopic ureteroceles. J Ultrasound Med 1985;4:617–618.

Schwartz MZ, Shaul DB: Abdominal masses in the newborn. Pediatr Rev 1989;11:172–179.

Schwarzler P, Bernard JP, Senat MV, Ville Y: Prenatal diagnosis of fetal adrenal masses: Differentiation between hemorrhage and solid tumor by color Doppler sonography. Ultrasound Obstet Gynecol 1999;13:351–355.

Scott J, Renwick M: Antenatal diagnosis of congenital abnormalities in the urinary tract. Br J Urol 1987;62:295–300.

Scott JE, Renwick M: Urological anomalies in the Northern Region Fetal Abnormality Survey. Arch Dis Child 1993;68:22–26.

Share JC, Lebowitz RL: Ectopic ureterocele without ureteral and calyceal dilatation (ureterocele disproportion): Findings on urography and sonography. AJR Am J Roentgenol 1989;152:567–571.

Sherer DM, Thompson HO, Armstrong B, Woods JRJ: Prenatal sonographic diagnosis of unilateral fetal renal agenesis. J Clin Ultrasound 1990;18:648–652.

Shibahara H, Mitsuo M, Fujimoto K, et al: Prenatal sonographic diagnosis of a fetal renal mesoblastic nephroma occurring after transfer of a cryopreserved embryo. Hum Reprod 1999;14:1324–1327.

Shimada K, Hosokawa S, Tohda A, et al: Follow-up of children after fetal treatment for obstructive uropathy. Int J Urol 1998;5:312–316.

Sillen U, Bachelard M, Hansson S, et al: Video cystometric recording of dilating reflux in infancy. J Urol 1996a;155:1711–1715.

Sillen U, Bachelard M, Hermanson G, Hjalmas K: Gross bilateral reflux in infants: Gradual decrease of initial detrusor hypercontractility. J Urol 1996b;155:668–672.

Sillen U, Hjalmas K, Aili M, et al: Pronounced detrusor hypercontractility in infants with gross bilateral reflux. J Urol 1992;148:598–599.

Skarsgard ED, Bealer JF, Meuli M, et al: Fetal endoscopic ("Fetendo") surgery: The relationship between insufflating pressure and the fetoplacental circulation. J Pediatr Surg 1995;30:1165–1168.

Smedley MG, Bailey RR: Autosomal dominant polycystic kidney disease diagnosed in utero using ultrasonography. (Letter,) N Z Med J 1987;100:606.

Smith GH, Canning DA, Schulman SL, et al: The long-term outcome of posterior urethral valves treated with primary valve ablation and observation. J Urol 1996;155:1730–1734.

Smith JA Jr, Middleton RG: Neonatal adrenal hemorrhage. J Urol 1979;122:674–677.

Soffer SZ, Rosen NG, Hong AR, et al: Cloacal exstrophy: A unified management plan. J Pediatr Surg 2000;35:932–937.

Spindel MR, Bauer SB, Dyro FM, et al: The changing neurourologic lesion in myelodysplasia. JAMA 1987;258:1630–1633.

Steinhardt GF, Liapis H, Phillips B, et al: Insulin-like growth factor improves renal architecture of fetal kidneys with complete ureteral obstruction. J Urol 1995;154:690–693.

Stiller RJ, Pinto M, Heller C, Hobbins JC: Oligohydramnios associated with bilateral multicystic dysplastic kidneys: Prenatal diagnosis at 15 weeks' gestation. J Clin Ultrasound 1988;16:436–439.

Stock JA, Wilson D, Hanna MK: Congenital reflux nephropathy and severe unilateral fetal reflux. J Urol 1998;160:1017–1018.

Suga K, Hara A, Motoyama K, et al: Coexisting renal vein thrombosis and bilateral adrenal hemorrhage: Renoscintigraphic demonstration. Clin Nucl Med 2000;25:263–267.

Takeuchi H, Koyanagi T, Yoshizato T, et al: Fetal urine production at different gestational ages: Correlation to various compromised fetuses in utero. Early Hum Dev 1994;40:1–11.

Thummala MR, Raju TN, Langenberg P: Isolated single umbilical artery anomaly and the risk for congenital malformations: A meta-analysis. J Pediatr Surg 1998;33:580–585.

Toma P, Lucigrai G, Marzoli A, Lituania M: Prenatal diagnosis of metastatic adrenal neuroblastoma with sonography and MR imaging. AJR Am J Roentgenol 1994;162:1183–1184.

Townsend RR, Goldstein RB, Filly RA, et al: Sonographic identification of autosomal recessive polycystic kidney disease associated with increased maternal serum/amniotic fluid alpha-fetoprotein. Obstet Gynecol 1988;71:1008–1012.

Vaid YN, Lebowitz RL: Urosepsis in infants with vesicoureteral reflux masquerading as the salt-losing type of congenital adrenal hyperplasia. Pediatr Radiol 1989;19:548–550.

Vergani P, Ceruti P, Locatelli A, et al: Accuracy of prenatal ultrasonographic diagnosis of duplex renal system. J Ultrasound Med 1999;18:463–467.

Vlietinck RF, Thiery M, Orye E, et al: Significance of the single umbilical artery: A clinical, radiological, chromosomal, and dermatoglyphic study. Arch Dis Child 1972;47:639–642.

Wacksman J, Phipps L: Report of the multicystic kidney registry: Preliminary findings. J Urol 1993;150:1870–1872.

Walsh G, Dubbins PA: Antenatal renal pelvis dilatation: A predictor of vesicoureteral reflux? AJR Am J Roentgenol 1996;167:897–900.

Warf BC, Scott RM, Barnes PD, Hendren WH: Tethered spinal cord in patients with anorectal and urogenital malformations. Pediatr Neurosurg 1993;19:25–30.

Willi UV, Lebowitz RL: The so-called megaureter-megacystis syndrome. AJR Am J Roentgenol 1979;133:409–416.

Wilson JM, DiFiore JW, Peters CA: Experimental fetal tracheal ligation prevents the pulmonary hypoplasia associated with fetal nephrectomy: Possible application for congenital diaphragmatic hernia. J Pediatr Surg 1993;28:1433–1439; discussion, 1439–1440.

Winyard PJ, Nauta J, Lirenman DS, et al: Deregulation of cell survival in cystic and dysplastic renal development. Kidney Int 1996;49:135–146.

Wiswell TE, Hachey WE: Urinary tract infections and the uncircumcised state: An update. Clin Pediatr (Phila) 1993;32:130–134.

Woolf AS, Cale CM: Roles of growth factors in renal development. Curr Opin Nephrol Hypertens 1997;6:10–14.

Woolf AS, Winyard PJ: Gene expression and cell turnover in human renal dysplasia. Histol Histopathol 2000;15:159–166.

Yanagisawa H, Morrissey J, Morrison AR, Klahr S: Eicosanoid production by isolated glomeruli of rats with unilateral ureteral obstruction. Kidney Int 1990;37:1528–1535.

Yerkes EB, Adams MC, Pope JC, Brock JW: Does every patient with prenatal hydronephrosis need voiding cystourethrography? J Urol 1999;162:1218–1220.

Yeung CK, Godley ML, Dhillon HK, et al: The characteristics of primary vesico-ureteric reflux in male and female infants with pre-natal hydronephrosis. Br J Urol 1997;80:319–327.

Yoo KH, Norwood VF, el-Dahr SS, et al: Regulation of angiotensin II AT1 and AT2 receptors in neonatal ureteral obstruction. Am J Physiol 1997;273:R503–R509.

Zerin JM, Ritchey ML, Chang AC: Incidental vesicoureteral reflux in neonates with antenatally detected hydronephrosis and other renal abnormalities [see comments]. Radiology 1993;187:157–160.

Zerres K, Hansmann M, Mallmann R, Gembruch U: Autosomal recessive polycystic kidney disease: Problems of prenatal diagnosis. Prenat Diagn 1988;8:215–229.

52
EVALUATION OF THE PEDIATRIC UROLOGIC PATIENT

Douglas A. Canning

Triage of the Pediatric Urologic Patient
  Emergencies
  Urgencies
  Semiurgencies
  Routine Evaluations

The Pediatric Urology Office Visit

History
Signs of Illness in the Pediatric Urologic Patient—
  The Physical Examination
The Laboratory Examination
Radiologic Examination
Office Procedures

Pediatric urology encompasses a spectrum of disorders, from complex reconstructive puzzles such as the repair of bladder or cloacal exstrophy to more routine but often pressing difficulties such as daytime wetting in a school-aged child. Because of the pioneering work of the past generation of pediatric urologists, most of these problems are readily identified and treated. Despite the dramatic progress made over the last 50 years, new discoveries are made each year that continue to streamline care. More than 80% of patients can now be cared for expediently with outpatient office visits or in outpatient surgical centers (Sampietro Crespo et al, 1995; Hoebeke et al, 1997; Valero Puerta et al, 1999). These impressive figures underscore the importance of rapid diagnosis and treatment in the child with a congenital or acquired pediatric urologic problem.

TRIAGE OF THE PEDIATRIC UROLOGIC PATIENT

In most cases, the initial contact with the child and family is made through a referring phone call from the parent, the pediatrician, the family practitioner, or, if prenatal evaluation is desired, the obstetrician. In many cases, the family is calling from a distance and the urologist needs to decide with the referring clinician whether the child is healthy enough to be transferred or must first be stabilized. Usually, even in remote areas, skilled general pediatric support is available. With coaching from the accepting team, most clinicians are able to manage even

complex problems in the stabilization phase of the triage process.

We try to triage all children into four categories (Table 52–1): those who need to be seen immediately (emergent), those who can be seen in the next 24 hours (urgent), those who must be seen in the next 72 hours (semiurgent), and those who require more routine evaluation (routine).

Emergencies

Children with acute problems related to recent surgical procedures, certain patients with neonatal hydronephrosis, acutely ill infants with urinary tract infection (UTI), and infants with gross hematuria, ambiguous genitalia, major abdominal defects, imperforate anus, or spina bifida may suffer further injury if not immediately evaluated. Children of all ages with acute abdominal pain, genitourinary trauma including spermatic cord torsion, or evidence of physical abuse should also be seen as soon as possible. In most cases, these children should be evaluated initially in the emergency department.

Patients who have developed acute problems such as pain, fever, or bleeding after a surgical procedure should also be evaluated immediately. Many problems that threaten success of the procedure can be averted if the child is evaluated and treated quickly.

Infants with severe bilateral hydronephrosis should be

1812

Table 52–1. A TRIAGE SYSTEM FOR PEDIATRIC UROLOGIC PATIENTS

Diagnosis	Triage Category*	Location
Trauma: renal, abdominal, or genital, including suspected sexual abuse, circumcision injuries	Emergent	Emergency department
Newborns with gross hematuria, urinary tract infection (UTI), myelomeningocele, intersex disorders, posterior urethral valves, prune-belly syndrome, bladder or cloacal exstrophy, imperforate anus, and variants including cloaca	Emergent	Direct admission to neonatal nursery or intensive care nursery
Bilateral hydronephrosis or hydronephrosis with thickened bladder wall on postnatal ultrasound, acute abdominal pain, ambiguous genitalia, acute scrotum, abdominal masses including masses associated with hernia or hydrocele, testicular masses, vaginal masses, febrile UTI except newborns	Emergent	Pediatric urology offices
UTI without fever except newborns, renal or ureteral stones, gross hematuria outside the newborn period, sexually transmitted diseases	Urgent	Pediatric urology offices
Initial postnatal evaluation of antenatal hydronephrosis with normal bladder; urinary frequency, urgency, or stranguria; hernia or hydrocele if changing in size or symptomatic; failure to thrive evaluation (in conjunction with pediatric team); amenorrhea in the adolescent girl	Semiurgent	Pediatric urology offices
Completion of antenatal hydronephrosis evaluation, asymptomatic hernia or hydrocele, undescended or absent testis, circumcision complications if no bleeding and child is voiding normally, hypospadias, varicocele, UTI follow-up, vesicoureteral reflux, microscopic hematuria, daytime and nighttime wetting, all other diagnoses	Routine	Pediatric urology offices

*Emergent, appointment as soon as possible; urgent, appointment within 24 hours; semiurgent, appointment within 1–3 days; routine, appointment at family's convenience.

evaluated immediately after delivery. Boys with an abnormally thickened bladder wall or dilated bladder outlet on the newborn ultrasound examination may have posterior urethral valves, the prune-belly syndrome, or urethral atresia. Many will develop compromised renal function. A few need direct admission to the newborn intensive care unit or to a similar inpatient step-down unit. These infants need to be stabilized immediately and may require surgery within 48 hours to improve urinary drainage. A few girls with urethral atresia need similar therapy.

UTI in the newborn is an emergency because newborns are particularly susceptible to significant renal damage if the infection is not treated promptly. These babies need intravenous antibiotics as early as possible after the diagnosis is made. Appropriate antibiotic therapy, administered without delay, has been shown to reduce the incidence of scarring (Ransley and Risdon, 1981).

Gross hematuria in the newborn is also an emergency because it may indicate renal venous or arterial thrombosis, both of which can be life-threatening. These infants require resuscitation and occasionally anticoagulant or operative therapy (Bokenkamp et al, 2000).

Infants with **ambiguous genitalia** also need immediate evaluation, and many require direct transfer from a referring hospital. **Because congenital adrenal hyperplasia (CAH) may result in salt wasting, which can be life-threatening in the infant, babies with ambiguous genitalia must be evaluated quickly and stabilized** (Glatzl, 1987). **If CAH is suspected, the infant should not be discharged home from the nursery before appropriate testing is complete.** In some cases, a genotypic female with CAH may be incorrectly identified as a male. The correct diagnosis should be made as quickly as possible to ensure the appropriate sex of rearing. Infants with ambiguous genitalia may also have other syndromes and may require further evaluation (Tables 52–2 and 52–3).

Patients with **major abdominal defects such as bladder**

or cloacal exstrophy require direct admission to the neonatal nursery for stabilization and surgical planning. Patients with imperforate anus and variants such as a cloacal anomaly require decompression of the intestinal tract, usually within the first 24 to 48 hours (Chen, 1999). At the time of the colostomy, the urologist may evaluate the perineum and perform endoscopy to further assess the urinary anomalies. Procedures to correct these major defects must be planned by surgeons who are familiar with the potential risks and complications associated with reconstruction of the urethra, vagina, and colon. In many cases, a team is assembled that provides orthopedic, general surgical, and urologic care during the surgery (Jeffs, 1978; Lattimer et al, 1979; Gearhart, 1999). The anesthesia team must be skillful in the management of complex metabolic changes that may occur in infants who are under anesthesia for long periods. The neonatologists must be expert in the management of infants who have undergone major surgical procedures.

One third of **infants with prune-belly syndrome or posterior urethral valves develop pulmonary insufficiency.** Care for these newborns may require intubation with assisted ventilation or extensive pulmonary therapy (Freedman et al, 1999; Noh et al, 1999). Surgical procedures to decompress the urinary tract or to reconstruct the urinary tract must follow the initial stabilization in these infants.

Today, many **newborns with spina bifida** are diagnosed in utero (Babcook et al, 1995). These infants are referred by direct admission to the neonatal intensive care nursery. Most of these children are not in urinary retention initially, but a few develop spinal shock after neurosurgery in the newborn period and have a transient period of overflow urinary drainage (Kaplan, 1985). As soon as possible after the back closure, these infants need an evaluation to assess the kidneys and bladder for evidence of hydronephrosis and to determine whether the bladder is emptying at suita-

Table 52–2. SYNDROMES ASSOCIATED WITH MULTISYSTEMIC DISEASE

Syndrome	Inheritance	Renal Anomaly	Genital Anomaly	Anomalies in Other Systems
Aarskog-Scott			Shawl scrotum, cryptorchidism	Broad facies, short stature
Beckwith-Wiedemann		Wilms' tumor		Macroglossia, gigantism, hepatoblastoma
Carpenter	AR		Small genitalia	Acrocephaly, polydactyly
Caudal regression		Hydronephrosis, renal agenesis	Vaginal and uterine agenesis	Imperforate anus, LS spine abnormality
Cerebro-oculo-facial	AR	Renal agenesis	Cryptorchidism	Arthrogryposis, microcephaly, cataracts
CHARGE			Small genitalia	Coloboma, heart defects, ear anomalies
Cornelia de Lange			Small genitalia, cryptorchidism	Micromelia, bushy eyebrows
Curran		Renal agenesis		Acral anomalies
Donohue			Enlarged penis or clitoris	Hirsutism, elfin face, thick lips, low-set ears
Drash		Wilms' tumor, glomerulonephritis	Mixed gonadal dysgenesis	
Dubowitz	AR		Hypospadias, cryptorchidism	Eczema, small stature, peculiar facies
Ehlers-Danlos	AR	Hydroureter		Skin hyperextensibility, poor wound healing
Fraser			Hypospadias, cryptorchidism	Cryptophthalmos
G			Hypospadias	Esophageal defect, low-set ears, abnormal facies
Holt-Oram		Renal anomalies		Defects of upper limb
Laurence-Moon-Biedl			Small genitalia	Obesity, retinal pigmentation, polydactyly
Marfan	AD	Renal duplication, hydroureter	Cryptorchidism	Aortic aneurysm, arachnodactyly
Mayer-Rokitansky		Renal agenesis	Duplex uterus, vaginal atresia	
Meckel-Gruber	AR	Renal cysts	Ambiguous genitalia, cryptorchidism	Microcephaly, polydactyly
Menkes		Hydronephrosis, reflux	Cryptorchidism	Kinky hair, CNS abnormality
Ochoa		Neurogenic bladder, hydronephrosis	Cryptorchidism	Aortic aneurysm, arachnodactyly
Opitz	AR		Hypospadias, cryptorchidism	Hypertelorism, mental retardation
Prader-Willi			Cryptorchidism	Hypotonia, obesity, mental retardation
Prune-belly		Hydronephrosis	Cryptorchidism	Hypoplastic abdominal muscle
Robert	AR	Hydroureter	Hypospadias, large penis, cryptorchidism	Hypomelia, growth retardation
Robinow	AD		Small genitalia, cryptorchidism	Flat face, short forearms
Rubenstein-Taybi	AR		Chordee	Hypoplastic maxilla, broad thumbs and toes
Rudiger	AR	Hydroureter	Small penis	Bicornuate uterus, coarse facies, stub nose
Russell-Silver	AR	Nonspecific renal anomalies	Small penis, hypospadias, cryptorchidism	Short stature, café-au-lait spots, skeletal asymmetry
Seckel	AR		Small genitalia, cryptorchidism	Small head, beak nose
Smith-Lemli-Opitz	AR		Hypospadias, cryptorchidism	Pernicious anemia, mental retardatic syndactyly, microcephaly
VATER		Hydronephrosis, renal dysplasia	Hypospadias	Vertebral anomalies, anal atresia, VSD, TE fistula, radial dysplasia
von Hippel-Lindau		Renal cyst, renal tumor		Pancreatic cyst, cerebral tumor, ichthyosis
Wolfram	AR	Hydroureter		Optic atrophy, deafness, diabetes
Zellweger	AR	Hydroureter	Hypospadias, cryptorchidism	Hypotonia, hepatomegaly

AD, Autosomal dominant; AR, autosomal recessive; CHARGE, coloboma, heart anomaly, choanal atresia, retardation, and genetic and ear anomalies; CNS, central nervous system; LS, lumbosacral; TE, tracheoesophageal fistula; VATER, vertebral, anal atresia, tracheoesophageal, renal; VSD, ventriculoseptal defect.

Data from Barakat AY, Seikaly MG, Perkaloustian VM: Urogenital abnormalities in genetic disease. J Urol 1987: 136:778–785; Walker RD: Familial and genetic urologic disorders in childhood. AUA Update Series 1987; 6:1–6; Mininberg D: The genetic basis of urologic disease. AUA Update Series 1992; 9:218–223.

bly low pressures (McGuire et al, 1977, 1983; Bauer, 1998). If the ultrasound shows evidence of hydronephrosis or dilation of the ureters, then a voiding cystourethrogram (VCUG) and conventional urodynamics study, or a video urodynamics study, should be done to ensure that bladder storage pressures are not excessive. Clean intermittent catheterization may then be started.

Children with acute abdominal pain should be seen immediately. In addition to a thorough abdominal examination designed to rule out surgical abdominal disease, these children should be evaluated for UTI, constipation, and spermatic cord torsion. Usually an acute abdominal series is ordered, which will show considerable amounts of stool throughout the colon if constipation is the problem. Other,

Table 52–3. CHROMOSOMAL SYNDROMES ASSOCIATED WITH GENITOURINARY ANOMALIES

Chromosome Number	Clinical Features	Renal Anomalies	Genital Anomalies
4 Autosome Wolf-Hirschhorn syndrome 4-P Trisomy 4-Q	Microcephaly Hemangiomas Hypertelorism Cleft lip/palate Low-set ears	Hydronephrosis	Hypospadias Undescended testicle
8 Autosome Trisomy 8	Large, square head Prominent forehead Widely spaced eyes Slender body and limbs	Hydronephrosis Horseshoe kidney Reflux	Hypospadias Undescended testicle
9 Autosome 9-P Trisomy, 9-P tetrasomy 9-P Monosomy	Small cranium Strabismus Large nose Webbed neck	Renal hypoplasia Pancake kidney	Hypospadias Undescended testicle Infantile male genitalia
10 Autosome 10-Q Syndrome 10-P Syndrome	Microcephaly Oval, flat face Miocropthalmia Short neck	Cystic kidney Hydronephrosis	Undescended testicle Small penis
11 Autosome 11-Q Syndrome	 Flat nose Wide glabella Cleft lip/palate	High forehead Micropenis	
13 Autosome Patau's syndrome Trisomy 13	Microcephaly Hypertelorism Polydactyly Congenital heart disease	Horseshoe kidney Hydronephrosis Cystic kidney	Undescended testicle
15 Autosome Monosomy 15-Q Prader-Willi syndrome	Obesity Hypotonia Retardation		Hypogonadism Cryptorchidism
18 Autosome Trisomy 18 Edwards' syndrome	Micrognathia Hypertonia Congenital heart disease	Horseshoe kidney Hydronephrosis	Undescended testicle Small penis
20 Autosome 20-P Syndrome	Round face Short nose Dental abnormalities Vertebral abnormalities	Hydronephrosis Polycystic kidney	Hypospadias
21 Autosome Trisomy 21 Down's syndrome	Brachycephalic skull Congenital heart disease Nasal hypoplasia Broad, short hands		Undescended testicle Small penis
22 Autosome Trisomy 22	Microcephaly Preauricular skin tags Low-set ears Beaked nose Cleft palate		Undescended testicle Small penis
Cat's eye syndrome Possibly from both 13 and 22 autosomes	Coloboma Anal atresia Low-set ears Hemivertebrae Congenital heart disease	Renal agenesis Horseshoe kidney Reflux	
Sex chromosome Y Klinefelter's syndrome XXY, XXXY XXXXY	Elongated legs Gynecomastia Eunuchoid body build Sparse body hair		Small penis Small testes
Sex chromosome X Turner's syndrome XO	Short stature Primary amenorrhea Webbed neck Broad chest Coarctation of aorta	Horseshoe kidney	Infantile genitalia

Data from Barakat AY, Seikaly MG, Derkaloustian VM: Urogenital anomalies in genetic diseases. J Urol 1986;136:778–785; Walker RD: Familial and genetic urologic disorders in childhood. AUA Update Series 1987;6:1–6; Mininberg D: The genetic basis of urologic disease. AUA Update Series 1992;9:218–223.

more unusual causes for abdominal pain should also be considered (Table 52–4). Occasionally, spermatic cord torsion is missed in the diagnosis of acute abdominal pain. Some children with spermatic cord torsion complain of abdominal pain and have surprisingly few complaints referring to the scrotum. Conversely, constipation may result in pain in the scrotum and perineum (Fein et al, 2001). **If spermatic cord torsion cannot be definitively excluded with the physical examination, surgical exploration should be performed. Occasionally, if the physical examination suggests a diagnosis other than spermatic cord torsion, then Doppler ultrasound or testicular scin-**

Table 52-4. RECURRENT ABDOMINAL PAIN IN CHILDREN

Disorder	Characteristics	Key Evaluations
Nonorganic		
Recurrent abdominal pain syndrome (functional abdominal pain)	Nonspecific pain, often periumbilical	History and PE; tests as indicated
Irritable bowel syndrome	Intermittent cramps, diarrhea, and constipation	History and PE
Nonulcer dyspepsia	Peptic ulcer-like symptoms without abnormalities on evaluation of the upper GI tract	History; esophagogastroduodenoscopy
Gastrointestinal tract		
Chronic constipation	History of stool retention, evidence of constipation on examination	History and PE; plain x-ray of abdomen
Lactose intolerance	Symptoms may be associated with lactose ingestion; bloating, gas, cramps, and diarrhea	Trial of lactose-free diet; lactose breath hydrogen test
Parasite infection (especially *Giardia*)	Bloating, gas, cramps, and diarrhea	Stool evaluation for ova and parasites; specific immunoassays for *Giardia*
Excess fructose or sorbitol ingestion	Nonspecific abdominal pain, bloating, gas, and diarrhea	Large intake of apples, fruit juice, or candy-chewing gum sweetened with sorbitol
Crohn's disease		
Peptic ulcer	Burning or gnawing epigastric pain; worse on awakening or before meals; relieved with antacids	Esophagogastroduodenoscopy or upper contrast x-rays
Esophagitis	Epigastric pain with substernal burning	Esophagogastroduodenoscopy
Meckel's diverticulum	Periumbilical or lower abdominal pain; may have blood in stool	Meckel scan or enteroclysis
Recurrent intussusception	Paroxysmal severe cramping abdominal pain; blood may be present in stool with episode	Identify intussusception during episode or lead point in intestine between episodes with contrast studies of GI tract
Internal, inguinal, or abdominal wall hernia	Dull abdomen or abdominal wall pain	PE, CT of abdominal wall
Chronic appendicitis or appendiceal mucocele	Recurrent RLQ pain; often incorrectly diagnosed, may be rare cause of abdominal pain	Barium enema, CT
Gallbladder and pancreas		
Cholelithiasis	RUQ pain, may worsen with meals	Ultrasound of gallbladder
Choledochal cyst	RUQ pain ± elevated bilirubin	Ultrasound or CT of RUQ
Recurrent pancreatitis	Persistent boring pain, may radiate to back, vomiting	Serum amylase and lipase ± serum trypsinogen; ultrasound of pancreas
Genitourinary tract		
Urinary tract infection	Dull suprapubic pain, flank pain	Urinalysis and urine culture; renal scan
Hydronephrosis	Unilateral abdominal or flank pain	Ultrasound of kidneys
Urolithiasis	Progressive, severe pain: flank to inguinal region to testicle	Urinalysis, ultrasound, IVP, spinal CT
Other genitourinary disorders	Suprapubic or lower abdominal pain; genitourinary symptoms	Ultrasound of kidneys and pelvis; gynecologic evaluation
Miscellaneous causes		
Abdominal migraine	Nausea, family history of migraine	History
Abdominal epilepsy	May have seizure prodrome	EEG (may require more than one study, including sleep-deprived EEG)
Gilbert's syndrome	Mild abdominal pain (causal or coincidental?); slightly elevated unconjugated bilirubin	Serum bilirubin
Familial Mediterranean fever	Paroxysmal episodes of fever, severe abdominal pain, and tenderness with other evidence of polyserositis	History and PE during an episode, DNA diagnosis
Sickle cell crisis	Anemia	Hematologic evaluation
Lead poisoning	Vague abdominal pain ± constipation	Serum lead level
Henoch-Schönlein purpura	Recurrent, severe crampy abdominal pain, occult blood in stool, characteristic rash, arthritis	History, PE, urinalysis
Angioneurotic edema	Swelling of face or airway, crampy pain	History, PE, upper GI contrast x-rays, serum C1 esterase inhibitor
Acute intermittent porphyria	Severe pain precipitated by drugs, fasting, or infections	Spot urine for porphyrins

From Ulshen M: Major symptoms and signs of digestive tract disorders. In Behrman R, Kliegman R, Jenson H (eds). Nelson Textbook of Pediatrics, 16th ed. Philadelphia, WB Saunders, 2000, p 1106.

CT, computed tomography; EEG, electroencephalogram; GI, gastrointestinal; IVP, intravenous pyelography; PE, physical examinations; RLQ, right lower quadrant; RUQ, right upper quadrant.

Table 52–5. DISTRIBUTION OF ABDOMINAL MASSES OF 280 PATIENTS IN THE NEONATAL PERIOD*

Type	Number
Kidney (65%)	
Hydronephrosis (UPJ obstruction, UVJ obstruction, ureterocele, etc.)	80 (28%)
Multicystic kidney	63 (22%)
Polycystic kidney disease	18
Renal vein thrombosis	5
Solid tumor	13
Ectopy	4
Total	183
Retroperitoneum (9%)	
Neuroblastoma	17
Teratoma	3
Hemangioma	1
Abscess	4
Total	25
Bladder (1%)	
Posterior urethral valves	2
Female genital system (10%)	
Hydrocolpos	16
Ovarian cyst	13
Total	31
Gastrointestinal (12%)	
Duplication	17
Giant cystic meconium ileus	4
Mesenteric cyst	3
Ileal atresia	2
Volvulus (ileum)	2
Teratoma (stomach)	1
Leiomyosarcoma (colon)	1
Meconium peritonitis with ascites	1
Ascites	1
Total	32
Hepatic or biliary (3%)	
Hemangioma (liver)	3
Solitary cyst (liver)	2
Hepatoma	1
Distended gallbladder	1
Choledochal cyst	1
Adenomatoid malformation of the lung	1
Total	9

*Distended bladder, hepatomegaly, and splenomegaly were excluded in most series.

UPJ, ureteropelvic junction; UVJ, ureterovesical junction.

Modified from Griscom, 1965; Raffensperger and Abousleiman, 1968; Wedge et al, 1971; Wilson, 1982; Emanuel and White, 1968.

tigraphy can be performed to help rule out torsion. If there is any doubt, the boy should be taken to the operating room for surgical exploration (Van Glabeke et al, 1998).

The majority of abdominal masses originate in genitourinary organs (Raffensperger and Abousleiman, 1968; Wedge et al, 1971; Wilson, 1982). A child with a mass should be evaluated immediately (Griscom, 1965) (Table 52–5). If an abdominal mass is suspected, an abdominal ultrasound examination should be ordered. If the mass is solid, a computed tomography (CT) scan is almost always required. **Testicular masses should be evaluated immedi-** ately. Testicular tumors occur in the newborn and in early childhood as well as after adolescence. The peak incidence of childhood testicular tumor is at age 2 years. The incidence tapers after about age 4 but then begins to rise again at puberty (Li and Fraumeni, 1972; Levy et al, 1994).

Vaginal masses may be palpable or may protrude from the introitus. The differential diagnosis of these masses includes benign periurethral cysts, skin tags, ureteroceles, prolapsed urethra, and malignancies (e.g., rhabdomyosarcoma). An adolescent with amenorrhea may present late with abdominal pain and a bulging introitus associated with an imperforate hymen. **Suspected child abuse must be evaluated immediately. Sexual abuse** victims may sometimes suffer trauma and initially be evaluated in the emergency room, but they may also present in the urologist's office with symptoms of urinary frequency or urgency, dysfunctional voiding, or constipation. The incidence of **sexually transmitted diseases** is declining but remains relatively high, with the peak ages for women with gonorrhea in the United States being 15 to 19 years. Pelvic inflammatory disease rates are highest in women age 15 to 25 years. Thirty-three per cent of those infections are in women younger than 19 years of age (Jenkins, 2000).

Urgencies

Gross hematuria outside of the newborn period, although not life-threatening, should be evaluated without delay. Many children have an easily recognized source such as UTI, urethral prolapse, trauma, meatal stenosis with ulceration, coagulation abnormalities, or urinary tract stones. Less obvious sources include acute nephritis, ureteropelvic junction obstruction, cystitis cystica, epididymitis, and tumor (Diven and Travis, 2000).

Febrile urinary infections in children older than newborns should be evaluated acutely. Children of all ages with a severe UTI may be subject to renal scarring (Ransley and Risdon, 1981; Dacher et al, 1993; van der Voort et al, 1997) and should be seen within 24 hours or sooner.

Infants and children with an inguinal hernia or a hydrocele that changes in volume should be seen within 24 hours and sooner if there is a history of inguinal or scrotal pain. Not all of these children need emergency surgery, but a few need surgery within a short period. If there is a history of scrotal or inguinal pain, the child's parents should be taught to recognize the signs of an incarcerated inguinal hernia and instructed to go to the emergency room if symptoms occur before the planned surgical correction.

Boys with painful priapism must be evaluated immediately. Pain may suggest ischemia of the corporal bodies, which may progress to corporal fibrosis if left untreated.

Semiurgencies

For infants with a normal bladder, we begin the **postnatal evaluation of prenatally diagnosed hydronephrosis** within the first few days of life. Families are concerned about the diagnosis and are anxious to make a management plan.

Children older than newborns with UTI should be

seen acutely. Children with a severe UTI may be subject to renal scarring and should be seen within 24 hours or sooner. In practice, many of these patients are seen by their pediatrician and are seen in follow-up by the pediatric urologist. Almost all children with culture-proven UTI should be evaluated with a VCUG and an ultrasound (Downs, 1999).

A few infants undergoing evaluation for **failure to thrive** are referred for suspected renal or ureteral disease. The child's pediatrician coordinates the diagnostic plan. The process is extensive and may require a complicated sequence of examinations that can be time-consuming and frustrating for the family. These children should be scheduled quickly to expedite the work-up and minimize the inconvenience to the child and family.

We see **adolescent girls who have not menstruated** in whom there is concern about ureteral or vaginal anomaly within 3 days. Many of these patients have an imperforate hymen or uterine anomaly that results in poor uterine drainage, which may be uncomfortable. If the condition is left untreated, retrograde drainage of the uterus may place these patients at risk of endometriosis and infertility (Rock et al, 1982).

Routine Evaluations

The remaining children are scheduled at the family's convenience. These include infants with a history of prenatal hydronephrosis with no evidence of bladder outlet obstruction on the postnatal ultrasound. The ultrasound study must not show bilateral hydronephrosis or a thickened bladder wall. The infant must be thriving and have normal electrolytes and normal blood urea nitrogen (BUN) and creatinine values. The additional tests include a repeat ultrasound, a renal scan, or a VCUG to evaluate the relative drainage and percentage of function of the kidneys and to evaluate for vesicoureteral reflux (VUR).

Children with **asymptomatic hydrocele** rarely require surgery initially. In most cases the hydrocele resolves during the first year. An exception is the hydrocele that is particularly large or palpable in the inguinal region. A large hydrocele with a palpable inguinal component or one that is increasing in size may indicate the presence of an abdominal perineal hydrocele. These do not spontaneously resolve; they usually increase in size and should be corrected, usually at 6 to 12 months (Luks et al, 1993). We operate on patients with **undescended or absent testes** at about 6 months of age. Very few of these testes will descend after 3 months of age (Berkowitz et al, 1993). If the testis has not descended by the age of 3 months, we recommend orchiopexy as soon as the anesthetic risk is reduced (usually between age 4 and 6 months in a term infant). Some infants with impalpable testes may require laparoscopic evaluation, and this examination may be done at 6 months as well.

As long as there is no active bleeding, the child is voiding normally, and there has been no injury to the penile shaft or shaft skin, we evaluate children who have developed a complication after circumcision at the convenience of the family. Narrowing of the preputial ring after circumcision may result in a trapped penis (Bergeson et al,

1993; Casale et al, 1999). This condition usually can be managed with the application of petroleum jelly to the penis for 4 to 6 weeks as healing continues. As long as voiding remains normal during this period, the revision of the circumcision may be postponed until age 4 to 6 months, when a day surgical procedure can be performed. A more common complication, **urethral meatal stenosis,** may be present as early as 6 months of age in circumcised infants (Upadhyay et al, 1998; Ahmed et al, 1999). This problem can be corrected easily in the office (Smith and Smith, 2000).

Boys with **hypospadias** are seen routinely. Normally, we initiate the evaluation in the newborn period, because most parents of a child with a birth defect, even a relatively minor one such as hypospadias, desire an early opportunity to speak with a specialist.

Boys develop **varicocele** usually just before adolescence (Niedzielski et al, 1997). We normally try to document the size of the varicocele with an ultrasound examination. From the three-dimensional measurements on ultrasound, the relative testicular volumes may be calculated (Diamond et al, 2000). We then repeat the examination at 6-month intervals through puberty to assess testicular growth. We normalize the relative volume of each side and compare the results with the combined total testicular volume. We do not recommend surgery unless the volume of the left side provides less than 40% of total testicular volume on two separate ultrasound examinations separated by 6 months.

The **completion of the evaluation for UTI** is done at the parents' convenience after the initial infection has been treated. In most cases, radiologic studies after a UTI in a child include a VCUG and occasionally renal scintigraphy. We monitor patients with known VUR with yearly or biennial VCUG while awaiting resolution of the reflux.

Microscopic hematuria in the absence of other symptoms is not an emergency in children. In more than 30% of cases, the source is never definitively identified. Our algorithm for a practical evaluation is discussed later in this chapter.

Children with daytime or nighttime wetting are evaluated routinely in the absence of other complicating problems. The care of children with nocturnal enuresis is individualized. Although some recommend treatment in children after the age of 5 years, we often wait to treat until the child seems bothered by the problem. If the child does not perceive nighttime wetting as a problem, there is usually little to be gained by treatment with medications or alarms. In our experience, only a few children younger than 6 or 7 years of age are bothered emotionally by nocturnal enuresis. Daytime wetting is of more concern. Wetting during the day may indicate incomplete or infrequent voiding, which may lead to a UTI that may exacerbate wetting.

An increasing number of **pregnant mothers carrying a fetus with hydronephrosis seek prenatal evaluation with the urologist. These visits are scheduled within the week unless the following conditions exist: (a) there is bilateral hydronephrosis, (b) there is oligohydramnios, or (c) there is evidence of significant cystic renal disease in a fetus of less than 22 weeks' gestation.** In a few instances, termination of pregnancy may be considered. In these cases, fetal intervention may be indicated. Because the decision for discontinuation of the pregnancy may depend on gestational age of the fetus, prompt evaluation may be required.

THE PEDIATRIC UROLOGY OFFICE VISIT

In most cases the primary care provider has identified a problem that requires review by the pediatric urologist. However, because other processes may coexist, the urologist must be alert for evidence of disease in other organ systems. Although few children are severely ill when evaluated in the urologist's office, it is important to develop the skills to recognize an infant or child who requires hospitalization. The ability to determine when an infant requires an inpatient admission is particularly important because the metabolic reserve is less abundant in the newborn (Park, 2000).

The risk for serious illness in a child with a fever varies depending on the child's age (Escobar et al, 2000). **Because of an immature immunologic system, the infant in the first 3 months is particularly susceptible to sepsis and meningitis caused by group B streptococcus or gram-negative organisms** (Waisman et al, 1999; Lin et al, 2000). UTIs are more frequent in uncircumcised male infants (Schoen et al, 2000; Wiswell, 2000). Infants with UTI carry a higher risk of underlying anatomic anomaly of the urinary tract than do older children with UTI. After infancy, UTIs are seen more often in girl children. Serious acute illnesses documented in a series of children in the first 3 years of life who presented with fever are shown in Table 52–6 (McCarthy, 1988). **Observation of the child and a careful history from the parent may be more important than the vital signs or the physical examination when attempting to determine the severity of illness, particularly in an infant or small child. The child's color (pale or cyanotic), level of alertness, response to the parent's comforting, quality of interaction with the examiner, and quantity of tearing while crying may provide considerable information about mental status and level of hydration.** If the child's response in any of these areas suggests severe illness, the child should be transferred to the emergency department, where appropriate resuscitation can be delivered while the diagnostic evaluation continues.

History

An important first question when taking the history of a pediatric patient with a urologic problem is, **"Why is the child here?"** In some cases, the child can begin to answer these questions, and it is worthwhile early in the interview to ask the child a few questions directly. This shows respect for the child, who may be an excellent historian despite young age. Children who realize that the interview is directed to them, rather than the parent, will concentrate harder. If future therapy requires behavioral training that involves cooperation from the child, he or she may be more receptive. **What goals do the patient and family have?** Does the family expect treatment at the facility, or do they seek a second opinion to confirm or refute another treatment plan? Do they prefer a reconstructive surgical procedure or the most appropriate nonsurgical therapy? In many children, the treatment must be tailored to the family's social condition or geographic location. Families in the foreign service or in the military who may be mobile may require a different approach to a surgical problem than families who live near a major center. In some cases, there is more than one possible therapy for a given problem, and the clinician should be prepared to offer more than one approach in order to provide the most appropriate care.

Generalized Symptoms in the Pediatric Patient

The term "failure to thrive" (FTT) may be used to describe an infant or child whose physical growth is significantly less than that of his or her peers. Often associated with poor developmental and socioemotional functioning, the prevalence of FTT depends on the population sampled (Wright et al, 2000). From 5% to 10% of low-birth-weight children and children living in poverty may have FTT. Family discord, maternal depression, and neonatal problems other than low birth weight are also associated with FTT. In the United States, psychosocial FTT is far more common than organic FTT. Psychosocial FTT is usually a result of poverty or of the poor child-parent interaction that sometimes occurs with severe stress (e.g., child abuse). The causes of insufficient growth include (a) failure of the parent to offer adequate calories, (b) failure of the child to take in sufficient calories, and (c) failure of the child to retain sufficient calories. Major organic causes of FTT and an approach to the work-up based on age are listed in Tables 52–7 and 52–8. Urologists must be alert to common urologic sources of FTT such as UTI, renal tubular acidosis, diabetes insipidus, and chronic renal insufficiency. But we must also be wary of psychosocial or abusive issues that may exist and be ready to alert the pediatrician and to play a supportive role in the analysis of this often serious problem (Bauchner, 2000).

In children, as in adults, normal body temperature varies

Table 52–6. DIAGNOSIS OF SERIOUS ILLNESSES DURING 996 EPISODES OF ACUTE INFECTIOUS ILLNESS IN FEBRILE CHILDREN YOUNGER THAN 36 MO

Diagnosis	Cases No.	Cases %
Bacterial meningitis	9	0.9
Aseptic meningitis	12	1.2
Pneumonia	30	3.0
Bacteremia	10	1.0
Focal soft tissue infection	10	1.0
Urinary tract infection	8	0.8
Bacterial diarrhea	1	0.1
Abnormal electrolytes, abnormal blood gases	9	0.9
Total	89	8.9

From McCarthy PL: Acute infectious illness in children. Comp Ther 1988; 14:51.

Table 52–7. MAJOR ORGANIC CAUSES OF FAILURE TO THRIVE

System	Cause
Gastrointestinal	Gastroesophageal reflux, celiac disease, pyloric stenosis, cleft palate/cleft lip, lactose intolerance, Hirschsprung's disease, milk protein intolerance, hepatitis, cirrhosis, pancreatic insufficiency, biliary disease, inflammatory bowel disease, malabsorption
Renal	Urinary tract infection, renal tubular acidosis, diabetes insipidus, chronic renal insufficiency
Cardiopulmonary	Cardiac diseases leading to congestive heart failure, asthma, bronchopulmonary dysplasia, cystic fibrosis, anatomic abnormalities of the upper airway, obstructive sleep apnea
Endocrine	Hypothyroidism, diabetes mellitus, adrenal insufficiency or excess, parathyroid disorders, pituitary disorders, growth hormone deficiency
Neurologic	Mental retardation, cerebral hemorrhages, degenerative disorders
Infectious	Parasitic or bacterial infections of the gastrointestinal tract, tuberculosis, human immunodeficiency virus disease
Metabolic	Inborn errors of metabolism
Congenital	Chromosomal abnormalities, congenital syndromes (fetal alcohol syndrome), perinatal infections
Miscellaneous	Lead poisoning, malignancy, collagen vascular disease, recurrently infected adenoids and tonsils

From Bachner H: Failure to thrive. In Behrman R, Kliegman R, Jenson HB (eds): Nelson Textbook of Pediatrics. Philadelphia, WB Saunders, 2000, p 120.

Table 52–8. APPROACH TO FAILURE TO THRIVE BASED ON AGE

Age at Onset	Major Diagnostic Consideration
Birth to 3 mo	Psychosocial failure to thrive, perinatal infections, gastroesophageal reflux, inborn errors of metabolism, cystic fibrosis
3–6 mo	Psychosocial failure to thrive, human immunodeficiency virus infection, gastroesophageal reflux, inborn errors of metabolism, milk protein intolerance, cystic fibrosis, renal tubular acidosis
7–12 mo	Psychosocial failure to thrive (autonomy struggles), delayed introduction of solids, gastroesophageal reflux, intestinal parasites, renal tubular acidosis
12+ mo	Psychosocial failure to thrive (coercive feeding, new psychologic stressor), gastroesophageal reflux

Adapted from Frank D, Silva M, Needlman R: Failure to thrive: Mystery, myth and method. Contemp Pediatr 1993; 10:114.

urologic sources for fever, the urologist should be aware of other causes of fever, particularly in children from compromised or at-risk groups (Table 52–9).

The evaluation and relief of **pain** is as old as the profes-

Table 52–9. FEBRILE PATIENTS AT INCREASED RISK FOR SERIOUS BACTERIAL INFECTIONS

Condition	Comment
Immunocompetent patients	
Neonates (<28 days)	Sepsis and meningitis caused by group B streptococci, Escherichia coli, Listeria monocytogenes, herpes simplex virus
Infants <3 mo	Serious bacterial disease (10–15%); bacteremia in 5% of febrile infants
Infants and children 3–36 mo	Occult bacteremia in 4%; increased risk with temperature >39°C and white blood cell count >15,000/μl
Hyperpyrexia (>41°C)	Meningitis, bacteremia, pneumonia, heatstroke, hemorrhagic shock-encephalopathy syndrome
Fever with petechiae	Bacteremia and meningitis caused by Neisseria meningitidis, Haemophilus influenzae type b, Streptococcus pneumoniae
Immunocompromised patients	
Sickle cell anemia	Pneumococcal sepsis, meningitis
Asplenia	Encapsulated bacteria
Complement/properdin deficiency	Meningococcal sepsis
Agammaglobulinemia	Bacteremia, sinopulmonary infection
Acquired immunodeficiency syndrome	S. pneumoniae, H. influenzae type b, Salmonella
Congenital heart disease	Increased risk of endocarditis
Central venous line	Staphylococcus aureus, coagulase-negative staphylococci, Candida
Malignancy	Gram negative enteric bacteria, S. aureus coagulase-negative staphylococci, Candida

From Powell KR: Fever. In Behrman R, Kliegman R, Jenson H (eds): Nelson Textbook of Pediatrics, 16th ed. Philadelphia, WB Saunders, 2000, p 74.

in a regular pattern each day. This circadian temperature rhythm results in lower body temperatures in the early morning and temperatures approximately 1°C higher in the later afternoon or early evening. Fevers with temperatures lower than 39°C in healthy children generally do not require treatment. If the temperatures becomes higher, administration of antipyretics usually makes the child more comfortable. Other than providing symptomatic relief, antipyretic therapy does not change the course of infectious diseases in normal children. Antipyretic therapy can be beneficial, however, in higher-risk patients with chronic pulmonary disease, metabolic disorders, or neurologic diseases. **Hyperpyrexia (temperature greater than 41°C) places patients at higher risk than do normal temperature responses.** This high temperature elevation is associated with severe infection, hypothalamic disorders, or central nervous system hemorrhage and always requires antipyretic therapy (Powell, 2000). **Aspirin has been associated with Reye's syndrome in children and adolescents and is not recommended for the treatment of fever in children.** Acetaminophen, 10 to 15 mg/kg every 4 hours, or ibuprofen, 5 to 10 mg/kg every 6 hours, is not associated with significant adverse effects. However, prolonged use of acetaminophen may result in renal injury. Massive overdoses can cause hepatic failure. Ibuprofen can cause dyspepsia, gastrointestinal bleeding, reduced renal blood flow, or, rarely, aseptic meningitis. Aplastic anemia has been associated with ibuprofen use. However, both of these drugs are normally well tolerated in children and should be used if the temperature is high. Although the focus must be on

Table 52–10. DISTINGUISHING FEATURES OF ACUTE GASTROINTESTINAL TRACT PAIN IN CHILDREN

Disease	Onset	Location	Referral	Quality	Comments
Pancreatitis	Acute	Epigastric, left upper quadrant	Back	Constant, sharp, boring	Nausea, emesis, tenderness
Intestinal obstruction	Acute or gradual	Periumbilical—lower abdomen	Back	Alternating cramping (colic) and painless periods	Distention, obstipation, emesis, increased bowel sounds
Appendicitis	Acute	Periumbilical, localized to lower right quadrant; generalized with peritonitis	Back or pelvis if retrocecal	Sharp, steady	Anorexia, nausea, emesis, local tenderness, fever with peritonitis
Intussusception	Acute	Periumbilical—lower abdomen	None	Cramping, with painless periods	Hematochezia, knees in pulled-up position
Urolithiasis	Acute, sudden	Back (unilateral)	Groin	Sharp, intermittent, cramping	Hematuria
Urinary tract infection	Acute, sudden	Back	Bladder	Dull to sharp	Fever, costochondral tenderness, dysuria, urinary frequency

From Ulshen M: Major symptoms and signs of digestive tract disorders. In Behrman R, Kliegman R, Jenson H (eds): Nelson Textbook of Pediatrics, 16th ed. Philadelphia, WB Saunders, 2000, p 1107.

sion of medicine. As primarily abdominal and retroperitoneal surgeons, we focus on abdominal and perineal sources of pain. **Abdominal pain** commonly suggests pyelonephritis, hydronephrosis, or constipation, but it may also be the result of sickle cell crisis. **An accurate history of the character of the pain may be the best indicator of its source.** Details about the character of the pain, time and acuteness of onset, and radiation or migration are important and should, if possible, be elicited directly from the child. Associated loss of appetite, nausea, vomiting, or a change in bowel pattern may help to distinguish gastrointestinal from genitourinary sources (Table 52–10).

A child with acute scrotal pain must be presumed to have spermatic cord torsion regardless of age until proven otherwise (Van Glabeke et al, 1999). However, in some cases, an accurate history may save the child an unnecessary surgical exploration. It is particularly important to interview the child as well as the parent. Gradual onset of the pain is more consistent with epididymitis, whereas abrupt pain suggests spermatic cord torsion or torsion of one of the testicular appendices. Associated scrotal wall swelling, erythema, or superior displacement of the testis is suggestive of spermatic cord torsion. **Perineal or rectal pain** may be associated with chronic constipation or bladder spasm. The pain of constipation or of bladder spasm may be referred to the penis, the testicles, the scrotum, or the perineum, as well as to the groin (Fein et al, 2001).

Voiding Symptoms

A large number of children are referred with voiding complaints. **The ability to place children in categories based on the voiding history will help to focus the rest of the evaluation and guide further therapy.** The time and duration of the voiding disorder must be identified early in the interview. Did symptoms begin before or after potty training? Is wetting associated with pain, urgency, or frequency? What is the character of the voiding? Is the urinary stream steady from beginning to end, or is it a "staccato" or stop-and-start pattern suggestive of dysfunctional voiding? Are the symptoms worse at a particular time of the day? Does the child void frequently during the day yet sleep through the night without wetting? Is wetting confined to the nighttime, suggesting primary nocturnal enuresis?

The voiding history is incomplete without a record of the child's eating and drinking pattern. Does the child consume small amounts of water during the day and large amounts of alternative liquids such as soft drinks and juices, which tend to be laden with salt and sugar and low on free water? What is the stooling pattern? Does the child have firm, chunky or pebble-like bowel movements, which suggest a retentive pattern of stooling, or does the child have soft, well-formed bowel movements more suggestive of a normal stooling pattern? Very few children hold the urine and not the stool. Conversely, children who retain stool almost always retain urine. All of these are indicators of a dysfunctional voiding pattern, which may lead to UTI.

Signs of Illness in the Pediatric Urologic Patient—The Physical Examination

We record vital signs on every new patient and, for children with a history of renal anomalies or VUR, on all subsequent visits. **Because the blood pressure and heart rate change as a function of age**, reference ranges for blood pressure and pulse rates for boys and girls should be posted in the clinic near where the vital signs are taken (Bernstein, 2000). Assistants taking the blood pressure should all be aware of the variation with age and should notify the team of blood pressure readings greater than the 90th percentile.

In the infant, **generalized edema** may occur with prematurity or hypoproteinemia. Localized edema suggests a congenital malformation of the lymphatic system. **When confined to one or more extremities, edema may be a presenting sign of coarctation of the aorta in association with Turner's syndrome.** Vasomotor instability and decreased peripheral circulation are revealed by red or purple color in a crying infant, whose color may darken profoundly with closure of the glottis preceding a vigorous cry. **Harmless cyanosis** of the hands and feet may be present, especially when the infant is cool. **Mottling,** another example of general circulatory instability, may be associated with serious illness or related to a transient fluctuation in skin temperature (Stoll and Kliegman, 2000). **Scattered petechiae** in the infant may be present in the scalp and face after a difficult delivery. **Light blue, well-demarcated areas of pigmentation** are seen over the buttocks, back, and sometimes other parts of the body in more than 50% of African American, Native American, and Asian American infants and occasionally in white babies. These have no known anthropologic significance despite their name, "**Mongolian spots.**" They tend to disappear within the first year. **Café-au-lait spots** are uniformly hyperpigmented, sharply demarcated, macular lesions, the hues of which vary within the normal degree of pigmentation of the individual. They may be dark brown in African American children. They may vary in size and may be large, covering a significant proportion of the trunk or limb. One to three lesions are common in normal children. Approximately 10% of normal children have café-au-lait macules. They may be present at birth or develop during childhood. If there are **five or more spots, each more than 5 mm in diameter, in a prepubertal patient, or six or more spots greater than 15 mm in diameter in a postpubertal child, neurofibromatosis type 1 (von Recklinghausen's disease) should be suspected.**

The **skin, hair, and nails** should be evaluated with special focus on congenital or metabolic problems that may be associated with **brittle or abnormal hair and nails or abnormal skin dryness** (see Tables 52–2 and 52–3). **Supernumerary nipples** may occur in a unilateral or bilateral distribution along a line from the anterior axillary fold to the inguinal area. They are more common in African American infants (3.5%) than in white children (0.6%). Accessory nipples may not have an associated areola and may be mistaken for congenital nevi. They may be excised if desired to improve appearance. Renal or urinary tract anomalies may be present.

An **exceptionally large head** suggests hydrocephaly, a storage disease, achondroplasia, cerebral gigantism, neurocutaneous syndromes, or inborn errors of metabolism, or it may be familial. Dysmorphic features such as **broadened epicanthal folds, widely spaced eyes, micrognathia, and low-set ears often are associated with congenital syndromes that may suggest a genitourinary problem.** Preauricular sinuses and pits may be the result of imperfect fusion of the tubercles of the first and second branchial arches. These anomalies may be unilateral or bilateral, may be familial, are more common in female children and in blacks, and at times are associated with other anomalies of the ears and face. **Preauricular pits are present in bronchio-oto-renal dysplasia, an autosomal dominant** disorder that consists of external ear malformations, bronchial fistulas, hearing loss, and renal anomalies. When the tracts become chronically infected, retention cysts may form and drain intermittently. Such lesions require excision. **Macroglossia can be associated with the Beckwith-Wiedemann syndrome, which also includes hepatosplenomegaly, nephromegaly, and hypoglycemia secondary to pancreatic beta cell hyperplasia in a large-for-gestational-age infant.** These children are predisposed to a specific subset of childhood neoplasms, including Wilms' tumor and adrenocorticocarcinoma. **Webbing of the neck in a female infant** suggests intrauterine lymphedema in Turner's syndrome, as do the widely spaced nipples with a shield-shaped chest (Stoll and Kliegman, 2000).

The abdomen is protuberant in boys with the prune-belly syndrome. Occasionally, children with other types of bladder outlet obstruction or profound antenatal hydronephrosis also have considerable laxity of the abdominal muscles. The abdomen should be inspected for other abnormalities, such as ventral hernia, flaring of the rib cage, umbilical leakage, mass, or hernia. When examining the abdomen, the examiner's hand should be placed behind the flank to help palpate the kidney on either side. If the abdomen is supple, the approximate size and location of each kidney may be determined with deep palpation. An attempt should be made to feel the liver edge and spleen as well as the colon, particularly the descending colon. In the newborn, the liver may be palpable, sometimes as much as 2 cm below the ribs on the left. When examining the left lower quadrant, an estimate should be made of the volume of stool in the descending colon. In infants, a large amount of gas may be present within the gastrointestinal tract. The abdominal wall is normally weak, especially in premature infants. Separation of the rectus muscles and umbilical hernia are common in the newborn. Unusual masses should be investigated immediately with ultrasonography. **Renal pathology is the source of up to two thirds of neonatal abdominal masses** (Raffensperger and Abousleiman, 1968; Wedge et al, 1971; Pinto and Guignard, 1995). **Cystic abdominal masses include hydronephrosis, multicystic dysplastic kidneys, adrenal hemorrhage, hydrometrocolpos, intestinal duplication, and choledochal ovarian omental or pancreatic cysts. Solid masses include neuroblastoma, congenital mesoblastic nephroma, hepatoblastoma, and teratoma.** A solid flank mass may be caused by **renal venous thrombosis,** which becomes apparent with signs of hematuria, hypertension, and thrombocytopenia. Renal venous thrombosis in infants is associated with polycythemia, dehydration, diabetic mother, asphyxia, sepsis, and coagulopathies such as antithrombin 3 or protein C deficiencies. **Abdominal distention at birth or shortly afterward suggests either obstruction or perforation of the gastrointestinal tract, often due to meconium ileus. Later distention suggests bowel obstruction, sepsis, or peritonitis.** Abdominal wall defects may be present, either through the umbilicus (omphalocele) or lateral (gastroschisis). Omphaloceles are associated with other anomalies and syndromes, such as the Beckwith-Wiedemann syndrome, conjoined twins, trisomy 18, meningomyelocele, and imperforate anus (Hassink et al, 1996; Chen et al, 1997; Kallen et al, 2000).

The **inguinal canal** should be inspected on each side for signs of asymmetry or mass. To begin the **examination**, the examiner's left hand closes the internal inguinal ring. This maneuver prevents an intracanalicular testis from migrating into the abdomen. The inguinal canal is then palpated to identify a fullness or mass suggestive of a hernia or hydrocele of the spermatic cord. The examiner may feel a "silk glove" sign, which is suggestive of a thickened patent processus vaginalis that may be present if a hernia is intermittent. The examiner's right hand is then brought down to the scrotal area, and the testis is palpated. The testis should be examined with consideration of the anatomy of the testis, the epididymis, and the vas deferens, which can be palpated even in some newborns. **Particular attention to the symmetry of the examination is important if intersex conditions are thought to exist. A symmetric gonadal examination (gonads palpable on each side or impalpable on both sides) suggests a global disorder such as CAH or androgen insensitivity. Asymmetry in the gonadal examination suggests a localized problem such as mixed gonadal dysgenesis or true hermaphroditism.**

Undescended testes can be palpated if they are in the scrotum or outside the external inguinal ring. Occasionally, the testis in a newborn can be palpated if it is in the inguinal canal, but in many cases the testis moves in and out of the canal into the abdomen, which makes palpation of the testis inconsistent. Retractile testes may in some cases be difficult to distinguish from a low, undescended testis. Pressure on the femoral artery sometimes helps to relax the cremasteric reflex in boys older than 2 years of age. Placing the child in a squatting or legs-crossed position sometimes relaxes the reflex and facilitates palpation of the testis. A testis is descended if it can be manipulated to the base of the scrotum and remain there after release, at least for a moment. Testes that feel tethered during manipulation and cannot be manipulated to the base of the scrotum are at risk for becoming ascending testes. If doubt exists, a second examination 6 to 18 months later may be helpful to distinguish a retractile testis from a tethered testis. As the child ages, an ascending or tethered testis (both cryptorchid testes) will be more and more difficult to manipulate into the bottom of the scrotum (Eardley et al, 1994; Clarnette and Hutson, 1997; Davey, 1997)

The normal newborn scrotum is relatively large. Its size may be increased with the trauma of breech delivery or by a newborn hydrocele, which can be distinguished from hernia by palpation and transillumination and by the absence of a mass in the inguinal canal. **A hydrocele that changes in volume suggests a patent processus vaginalis. These infants are at risk for inguinal hernia.** The processus vaginalis is not likely to close after birth. If a hernia has been symptomatic, it should be corrected in the newborn period. In boys who have not had a symptomatic hernia, surgery to correct a patent processus vaginalis may be postponed until an outpatient surgery can be performed, usually at age 4 to 6 months. In the absence of volume changes within the hydrocele, the processus vaginalis is usually not patent and the newborn hydrocele resolves by the age of 1 year without surgery. Persistence of a hydrocele beyond 12 to 18 months even in the absence of volume changes usually indicates a patent processus vaginalis

and is an indication for surgical ligation of the processus vaginalis and incision of the scrotal component of the hydrocele.

In the newborn, the foreskin is adherent to the glans. These glanular adhesions should not be separated, and the glans need not be inspected if the parents do not desire a circumcision. Glanular preputial adhesions usually separate before the age of 4 years, but they may persist longer in some boys. In the absence of balanitis or UTI, the prepuce should not be retracted but allowed to separate naturally (Imamura, 1997). The position of the urethral meatus is almost never abnormal in the uncircumcised penis with a circumferential foreskin. If the ventral foreskin is short or absent, or if ventral or dorsal chordee is present, the boy should not be circumcised and should be re-examined at a later date, when hypospadias or epispadias correction may be performed on an outpatient basis with the child under a general anesthetic. We describe the severity of **hypospadias** based on the position of the urethral meatus, the presence or absence of chordee, and the degree of ventral penile shaft skin coverage. Occasionally, when the foreskin is pulled back before a circumcision, the distal urethra and urethral meatus are found to be enlarged. If a **megameatus** is identified before a newborn is circumcised, the circumcision should be cancelled. The foreskin may be removed at the time of the urethral repair. However, because normal spongiosum is present on the ventral surface of the penis, repair of the urethra is usually not difficult even after a circumcision has been performed (Duckett and Keating, 1989).

Stretched penile length and girth should be measured. If the penis in a term baby is less than 1.9 cm, micropenis should be suspected; a karyotype should be performed, and the hypothalamic-pituitary-testicular axis should be assayed. The penis should be examined in relation to the scrotum for evidence of **penile concealment, buried penis, or webbed penis.** In these conditions, the penis is normal sized but is buried or concealed beneath a prominent pubic fat pad; trapped by a narrowed, more proximal preputial ring; or tethered to the scrotum. If the penile shaft skin is shortened, correction may require a rotational flap of inner preputial skin to provide additional coverage for the ventrum of the penis after release of the narrowed preputial ring. If a newborn clamp circumcision is performed, more penile shaft than indicated is often removed, resulting in a scar and sometimes a secondary trapped penis. If there is encroachment of the scrotum onto the penile shaft (webbed penis), circumcision should be deferred until it can be done freehand in the main operating room with the child under general anesthesia, usually at 4 to 6 months (Casale et al, 1999; Williams et al, 2000).

Varicoceles (varicosities of the internal spermatic vein) are found in 10% of adolescent boys but are rare in boys younger than 10 years of age. They occur almost always on the left side and are bilateral in about 10% of cases. Varicoceles are palpable when the boy is standing, but drain when supine. If only the right side is involved or if the varicocele does not decompress when supine, there exists a possibility that a retroperitoneal tumor is present and compressing the vein. Testicular size should be documented in the preadolescent or adolescent boy with a varicocele. We monitor these boys with ultrasound examina-

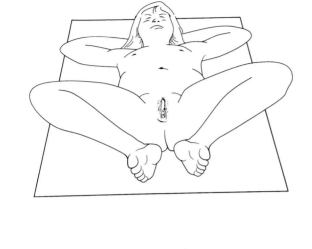

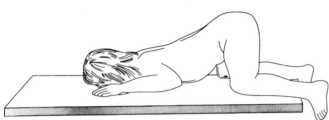

Figure 52–1. Frog-leg position *(top)* and knee-chest position *(bottom)*.

tions to observe testicular growth. If the testicular volume contribution from the left side normalized to total testicular volume drops to less than 40%, surgery may be indicated to correct the varicocele (Fideleff et al, 2000).

The **perineal examination in the female child** is similar to that in the male. In a teenaged girl, the examination should be performed in the absence of the father, but the mother may be present as long as the adolescent agrees. In general, bimanual examination in an adolescent is best performed in the operating room. The girl is placed in a frog-leg position or in a knee-chest position (Fig. 52–1). The clitoris is examined for evidence of hypertrophy that may be suggestive of an intersex condition. Gently spreading the labia majora in an inferior direction will allow for inspection of the clitoral area and usually of the introitus. The vestibule is assessed for any evidence of discharge. An easy way of examining the perineum is to gently grasp the labia majora and pull inferiorly. This maneuver tends to better define the various perineal folds and provide for a consistent examination in almost all cases (Redman, 1982). The hymen should be inspected, as well as the introitus. An **imperforate hymen** may result in hydrometrocolpos and a lower abdominal mass. In older girls, a small speculum may be used to evaluate the cervix and interior of the vagina. Palpation of the vaginal walls and cervix and bimanual examination of the uterus complete the examination. A Valsalva maneuver may allow adequate assessment of the introital vaginal area. **Vaginal discharge** is frequently associated with vaginal voiding and is particularly common in children who hold the urine and subsequently dribble urine into the vagina. Treatment of dysfunctional voiding results in reduced vaginal drainage. Vaginal bleeding in the preadolescent may result from foreign bodies

such as wadded toilet paper trapped in the vagina. Occasionally other foreign bodies may have been inserted intentionally or accidentally.

Urethral prolapse is relatively common, particularly in African American girls. The prolapse is through the meatus and forms a hemorrhagic, often sensitive mass that bleeds with palpation or with contact by the undergarments. Girls may have difficulty with urination depending on the size of the prolapse and whether it includes the urethral meatus. Urethral prolapse may respond to topical application of estrogen and may be managed expectantly as long as voiding is normal (Redman, 1982).

Although genital injuries may be accidental, the possibility of physical or sexual abuse must be considered in all cases of genital trauma in girls or boys.

Sexual abuse includes any activity with a child before the age of legal consent that is for sexual gratification of an adult or a significantly older child. Sexual abuse includes oral-genital, genital-genital, genital-rectal, hand-genital, hand-rectal, or hand-breast contact; exposure of sexual anatomy; forced viewing of sexual anatomy; and showing of pornography to a child or use of a child in the production of pornography. Sexual intercourse includes vaginal, oral, or rectal penetration. Penetration is entry into an orifice with or without tissue injury. Younger perpetrators tend to have younger victims, but they are more likely to have intercourse with older victims. Sex acts perpetrated by young children are learned behaviors and are associated with experiencing sexual abuse or exposure to adult sex or pornography. Without detection and intervention, sexual abuse may progress from touching to intercourse. Sexual play, on the other hand, may be defined as viewing or touching of the genitals, buttocks, or chest by preadolescent children separated by not more than 4 years in age where there has been no force or coercion. Sexual abuse is surprisingly common. **Twelve percent to 38% of adult women are sexually abused by the age of 18 years. The incidence of sexual abuse of boys range from 3% to 9% of the population; male victims account for up to 20% of the reports. About one third of sexual abuse victims are younger than 6 years of age, one third are between 6 and 12 years of age, and one third are 12 to 18 years of age. Ninety-seven percent of reported offenders are male** (Johnson, 2000).

The abuse of daughters by fathers and stepfathers is the most common form of reported incest, although brother-sister incest is considered to be the most common type. Pedophiles have indicated that they seek positions and opportunities where they can be in contact with potential victims. The vulnerable children they describe include those with mental and physical handicaps, unloved and unwanted children, previously abused children, and children in single-parent families. Children of drug abusers and children with low self-esteem and poor achievement are also at risk. A father's desire for sexual gratification and a daughter's need for affection and nurturing may lead to incest when the mother is unavailable and there is longing to maintain the family unit. Violence is not common in sexual abuse; however, its incidence increases with the age and size of the victim.

The possibility of sexual abuse should be considered in the presence of associated physical symptoms, includ-

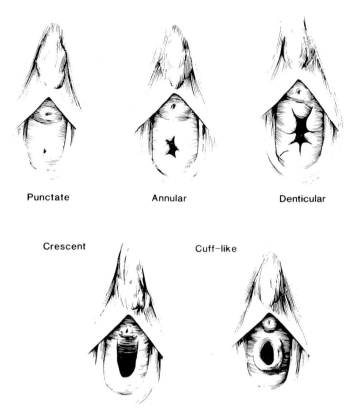

Punctate   Annular   Denticular

Crescent   Cuff-like

Figure 52–2. Normal hymenal configurations in older children and adolescents. (From Herman-Giddens ME, Frothingham TE: Prepubertal female genitalia: Examination for evidence of sexual abuse. Reproduced by permission of Pediatrics, vol 80, pages 203–208, copyright 1987.)

ing **(a) vaginal, penile, or rectal pain, discharge, or bleeding, and (b) chronic dysuria, enuresis, constipation, or encopresis.** Behaviors likely to be associated with sexual abuse include sexualized activity with peers, animals, or objects; seductive behavior; and age-inappropriate sexual knowledge and curiosity. Investigating the possibility of sexual abuse requires supportive, sensitive, and detailed history taking. Many hospitals have a sexual abuse team that can be readily consulted if sexual abuse is suspected. The key is to be aware of the possibilities when they might exist and to invite the team in early. The pediatric urologist will probably be asked to evaluate the child's abdomen and perineum (Johnson, 2000). Examination of the female genitalia with the patient in the frog-leg position for young children or the knee-chest position for older children expedites the examination with minimal touching (see Fig. 52–1). Normal hymenal configurations described by Herman-Giddens and Frothingham are shown in Figure 52–2. Sexual abuse should be considered when the vaginal mucosa is bruised or injected, the vaginal opening is dilated, or the hymen is damaged, showing a V notch or cleft (Walker, 1998). Despite these guidelines, the diagnosis of sexual abuse is made by the history and not by the physical examination. In one review of 157 children referred to a sexual abuse clinic with only a physical complaint and no history of abuse, only 16% had examination findings suggestive of sexual abuse (Kellogg et al, 1998). **If abuse is suspected, it must be reported to the police. If the perpetrator is a caregiver of the child or a par-**

ent, the state child welfare team must be contacted as well.

Blunt injury to the perineum may result in hematoma beneath the perineal skin. The presence of hematoma or contusion alone does not usually require treatment. Penetrating injuries of the vaginal area warrant further careful evaluation, including radiologic evaluation of the urethra and bladder. **Benign and malignant tumors of the vaginal area** should be considered when vaginal bleeding occurs in young girls. A broad spectrum of entities including capillary hemangioma, rhabdomyosarcoma, neuroblastoma, and carcinoma may be associated with vaginal bleeding. **Labial masses** may be associated with hernia or hydrocele of the canal of Nuck (Kizer et al, 1995). **Adhesions of the labia minora** are common; in most cases, they are not symptomatic. Occasionally, a girl with labial adhesions complains of vaginal irritation from pooled urine. If the labia are not separated, the irritation may progress to irregular voiding, which may exacerbate the problem. In some girls, a short course of estrogen creme applied to the labia may be effective. In many, however, separation of the adhesions in the office with local anesthetic creme may be required. After separation, the child or her mother must apply a barrier ointment within the labia minora to prevent recurrence until the inflammation of the labial membranes has resolved. **Labial fusion** may be associated with CAH, gonadal dysgenesis, or cloaca (Powell et al, 1995). A genitosinogram is indicated in cases where the urethra cannot be distinguished from the vaginal orifice.

Passage of meconium usually occurs within the first 12 hours after birth; 99% of term infants and 95% of premature infants pass meconium within 48 hours after birth. The presence of an imperforate anus is not always obvious. Gentle insertion of the small finger or a rectal tube to the anal dimple may be necessary to confirm the diagnosis. Imperforate anus or a variant must be suspected in any child with an early and consistent history of constipation (Kim et al, 2000).

The lower back should be examined for any evidence of presacral dimpling. The dimple or irregularity of skin fold that is normally present in the sacrococcygeal midline may be mistaken for an actual or potential neurocutaneous sinus. **A presacral dimple may indicate spina bifida or cord tethering if the dimple is off center, more than 2.5 cm from the anal verge at birth, or deeper than 0.5 cm** (Soonawala et al, 1999). **Tufts of hair over the lumbosacral spine suggest an underlying abnormality such as spina bifida occulta, sinus tract, or tumor.** We recommend an ultrasound of the lumbosacral spine in the newborn if any of these conditions exist (Unsinn et al, 2000). A brief evaluation of the upper and lower extremities and of the back is performed for any evidence of asymmetry, length discrepancy, or misalignment of the spine.

The Laboratory Examination

The **urine specimen** may be obtained in a number of different ways. In the child who is not potty trained, a bagged specimen, although the most susceptible to contamination, is the easiest and least invasive to obtain. To minimize contamination with fecal or skin flora, a hole is cut in the diaper and the perineal bag is brought through the hole in the diaper. A parent is instructed to watch the bag and to remove the bag as soon as urine is noted. If the specimen is collected in the office, the bag is immediately drained and the urine is plated and sent to the laboratory for culture. In this way, skin contamination of the urine specimen is minimized and the trauma of catheterization is avoided (Falcao et al, 1999).

Older children usually can provide a clean midstream urine. Most studies have failed to show any benefit to formally cleansing the introitus before obtaining the specimen. Only the midstream of the urine is collected and sent to the laboratory for urinalysis and culture. **Pyuria** is defined as more than 5 white blood cells (WBCs) per high-powered field for girls and more than 3 WBCs per high-powered field for boys. Infection can occur without pyuria, and pyuria may be present without UTI. Consequently pyuria as an isolated finding is more confirmatory than diagnostic for UTI. Nitrate and leukocyte esterase assays are usually positive in infected urine. However, if the urine has not remained in the bladder for more than 1 hour, the conversion of nitrates to nitrites may not be complete and the chemical strip may read negative despite the presence of nitrogen-splitting bacteria in the bladder. If the culture grows more than 100,000 colonies of a single pathogen, or if there are 10,000 colonies and the child is symptomatic, we consider a UTI to be present. **White blood cell casts and urinary sediment suggest renal involvement,** but these are rarely identified. If the child is not symptomatic and the urinalysis is normal, it is unlikely that the urine is infected. However, if the child is symptomatic, a UTI is possible regardless of the results of the urinalysis (Bonadio, 1987). **Microscopic hematuria** is common in acute bacterial as well as viral cystitis. Gross hematuria may be present in viral cystitis but is less common in acute bacterial cystitis.

If the child is symptomatic, the urinalysis is suggestive of UTI, and the culture grows more than one organism or fewer than 100,000 colonies, the clinician has the option of treating with an antibiotic that is effective based on the sensitivities or repeating the culture. We repeat the culture but start the child on a treatment dose of antibiotics at that time. If a second catheterized culture is negative, then the antibiotics are discontinued and close follow-up is provided. This is particularly important in infants, who may not demonstrate the usual signs and symptoms of infection that would be present in an older child.

Hematuria

Microscopic hematuria is common in children. Routine office screening with urinalysis for urinary abnormalities is no longer recommended. For this reason, the actual time of onset for microscopic hematuria is often unknown. Children with hematuria present in one of three ways: **(a) gross hematuria, (b) urinary or other symptoms with the incidental finding of microscopic hematuria, or (c) the discovery of microscopic hematuria during a visit for which a urinalysis is required (e.g., precamp or presports physical examination).** Normally the first indicator is a positive urine strip test for blood. Most strips can detect concentrations of 5 to 10 intact red blood cells

(RBCs) per microliter. This corresponds to 2 to 5 RBCs per high-powered field. Improper interpretation of the dipstick, such as delayed reading or cross-contamination of urine from other chemically impregnated pads, may cause a false-positive result. The urine should be dipped, the excess urine tapped off, and the strips read immediately at the recommended time. **Confirmation of microscopic hematuria after a positive dipstick examination requires a microscopic examination of the urine for the presence of RBCs.** Microscopic hematuria may be defined as more than 5 RBCs per high-powered field in three of three consecutive fresh urine specimens obtained at least 1 week apart. Therefore, the positive dipstick result on a single specimen with microscopic confirmation should be viewed as an indication for further urine testing rather than as diagnostic until persistence is confirmed on subsequent studies (Fig. 52–3).

Gross hematuria is uncommon in children. The prevalence of gross hematuria was reported as 0.13% based on a retrospective review of children seen in emergency walk-in clinics. Most children have an easily recognized cause of the gross hematuria. The most common diagnoses are UTI (26%), perineal irritation (11%), trauma (7%), meatal stenosis with ulceration (7%), coagulation abnormalities (3%), and urinary tract stones (2%). Fewer than half of the children have a source that is either not obvious or requires additional or more sophisticated examinations. These include acute nephritis (4%), ureteropelvic junction obstruction (1%), and tumor (1%) (Ingelfinger et al, 1977). Adenoviral infection, hypocalciuria, and hyperuricosuria are other sources to consider. A few patients with hypocalciuria have a positive family history of urolithiasis (Stapleton et al, 1984). We perform an ultrasound of the kidneys, ureters, and bladder for children who have gross hematuria, although the yield is low (Fernbach, 1992).

Our recommendation for patients who have microscopic hematuria with unrelated clinical symptoms is to treat the affiliated illness (pulmonary or immunologic condition, glomerular and interstitial disease, lower urinary tract disease, stones, tumors, vascular disease, or acute abdominal condition) and ignore the hematuria until the treatment for the underlying illness is underway.

If microscopic hematuria persists, hematologic disorders, drugs and medications, or a host of other, less obvious sources may also be responsible. If microscopic hematuria without proteinuria is present in an asymptomatic patient, the urinalysis is repeated two to three times over 2 to 3 weeks. If the hematuria resolves, no follow-up is recommended. If it persists, then a urine culture is obtained. If the culture is positive, the child is treated and then evaluated as appropriate. If proteinuria develops, the patient is referred to the pediatric nephrologist. If the hematuria without proteinuria persists, then a urine calcium-to-creatinine ratio is obtained. If this value is elevated, the patient is prescribed an increased free water program to reduce the risk of stone disease.

If the child has microscopic hematuria and proteinuria, the amount of protein in the urine should be measured. If there is more than 4 mg/m^2/hr in the urine, or if the protein-to-creatinine ratio is greater than 0.2, the child should be referred to a nephrologist for evaluation. If the

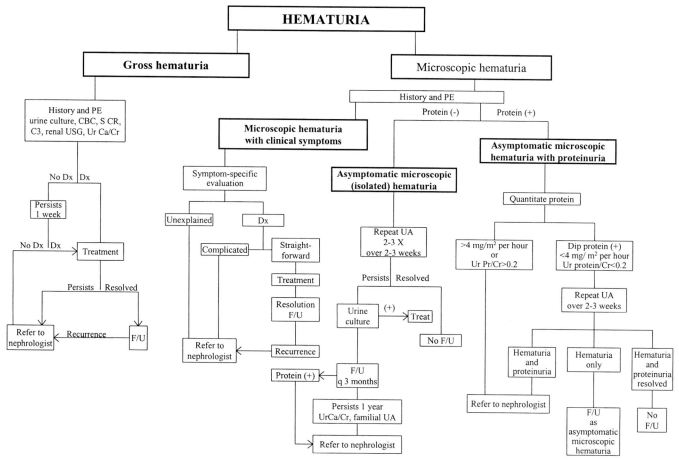

Figure 52–3. An algorithm for the practical evaluation of a child with hematuria. CBC, complete blood count; Dx, diagnosis; F/U, follow-up; PE, physical examination; SCr, serum creatinine; UA, urinalysis; Ur Ca/Cr, urinary calcium/creatinine ratio; USG, ultrasonography. (From Diven SC, Travis LB. A practical primary care approach to hematuria in children. Pediatr Nephrol 2000;14:65–72.)

urinary protein is less than 4 mg/m^2/hr, or if the urine protein-to-creatinine ratio is less than 0.2, then a repeat urinalysis over 2 to 3 weeks is performed. If hematuria is absent or the proteinuria resolves, no further follow-up is performed. If it is persistent in the face of normal renal function, absence of proteinuria, and normal blood pressure, the child is screened at the pediatrician's office with urinalyses and blood pressure checks every 3 months for the first year, every 6 months for the next year, and yearly thereafter. Further evaluation occurs with the nephrologist only if proteinuria or hypertension develops or if the hematuria worsens. **The large majority of children with microscopic hematuria are evaluated, and the source of the hematuria is never identified** (Diven and Travis, 2000).

Radiologic Examination

The ultrasound study of the kidneys, ureters, and bladder is an extension of the physical examination. Palpable masses within the abdomen can be localized and even diagnosed with the aid of ultrasonography performed by a uroradiologist with an interest in pediatrics. The examination should evaluate not only the genitourinary system but also adjacent organs such as the adrenals, liver, and spleen.

The image of the parenchyma of the liver and spleen should be used as a comparison to assess the parenchyma of the right and left kidney, respectively. The density of the kidney and of the renal medullary pyramids, the wall thickness and configuration of the collecting system, and the presence or absence of caliectasis, pelviectasis, or ureterectasis are all important indicators of renal and ureteral pathophysiology (Hulbert et al, 1992). The luminal diameter of the ureters, thickness of the bladder wall, and volume of the bladder both before and after voiding should be recorded. If hydronephrosis or ureterectasis is present before voiding, the kidneys and ureters should be rescanned after voiding. A skillful ultrasonographer can provide anatomic detail about the insertion of the ureters and the degree of dilation of the ureter and can identify the jet of urine as it enters the bladder (Kirby and Rosenberg, 1992).

Ultrasound is sensitive in detecting solid renal masses, particularly those that measure at least 1.5 cm in largest dimension. For smaller renal masses, the ultrasound findings should be considered preliminary and confirmation should be sought with CT or MRI (Jamis-Dow et al, 1996). Ultrasonography may also be used to accurately measure postvoid residual urine (Coombes and Millard, 1994). Increased thickness of the bladder wall may be suggestive of bladder outlet obstruction from posterior urethral valves or urethral atresia. Trabeculation within the bladder, bladder diverticulum, and ureteral duplication or ureterocele are all easily identified with ultrasound (Gylys-Morin et al, 2000). **Ultrasound in the absence of comparison studies or an appropriate history cannot by itself distinguish obstructive from nonobstructive hydronephrosis.** Therefore, a functional study (e.g., renal scan) is usually required for diagnosis.

Ultrasound is also frequently used to examine the scrotum to assess testicular volume in boys with varicocele (Diamond et al, 2000). It may also be used to assess blood flow if spermatic cord torsion is suspected, and to distinguish between epididymitis and torsion of the appendix testis in cases where tenderness is localized to the upper pole of the testis. We have also found it useful in distinguishing hernia from hydrocele, or identifying abdominoperineal hydroceles (Finkelstein et al, 1986; Uehling and Richards, 1992; Luks et al, 1993).

With very few exceptions, children with a proven UTI should undergo VCUG to identify VUR, to evaluate the anatomy of the bladder outlet during bladder filling and voiding, and to assess the presence of residual urine after micturition. Additional information regarding trabeculation of the bladder, bladder diverticula, and presence or absence of urachal abnormalities may be identified with a fluoroscopic VCUG (Fernbach, 2000; Goldman et al, 2000; Lin et al, 2000; McDonald et al, 2000). The VCUG begins with a plain film, followed by placement of a feeding tube rather than a Foley catheter. The balloon on a Foley catheter may obscure the anatomy of the bladder neck and trigone, particularly at the beginning of the study. On the plain film, abnormalities of the spine, ribs, and pelvis and the presence or absence of stones within the kidneys, ureters, or bladder should be noted. The gas pattern and volume of stool are particularly important in infants and in children with dysfunctional voiding, in whom constipation may be an important part of the clinical pattern. Gas should normally be present in the rectum on plain film by 24 hours of age. The bladder should be drained, and contrast should be gently infused. For children with suspected ureterocele, the first few images during filling of the bladder best demonstrate the ureterocele. The bladder is then filled slowly, and the child voids.

Voiding views must be obtained in all cases, but particularly if bladder outlet obstruction (e.g., posterior urethral valves) is suspected. For children with suspected VUR and those with an ectopic ureter, a cyclic VCUG must be performed in which at least two voiding cycles are completed. In some cases, the ectopic ureter that is draining to the bladder neck must empty in order for additional contrast material to reflux. If a second voiding cycle is not performed, the reflux into the ectopic system might be missed (Hellstrom and Jacobsson, 1999; Polito et al, 2000). It is important to image the bladder neck during voiding in the female as well as the male patient. The presence of a "spinning top" urethra in a school-aged girl may be an important indicator of dysfunctional voiding (Saxton et al, 1988; Kondo et al, 1994; Batista et al, 1998). Vaginal voiding should also be noted; it may be seen on the postvoid views.

In patients with a genitourinary sinus, the VCUG is modified to image the urethra and vagina simultaneously. In this study, the genitourinary sinus is intubated with a blunt-tipped catheter (which can be made by trimming the cone-shaped end of a feeding tube) that is placed against the perineal opening. Contrast material is injected retrograde to identify the point where the vaginal introitus meets the urethra to form the genitourinary sinus. The genitourinary sinogram helps to differentiate a cervix from a prostatic utricle. If a cloaca is present, the sinogram provides detail about the positions of rectum, vagina, and urethra; the point of confluence; and the distance to the perineum (Parrott and Woodard, 1979; Shaul and Harrison, 1997; De Filippo et al, 1999).

We use the **nuclear cystogram** as part of the follow-up examinations for children with VUR. We also use it as the first examination to screen for VUR in sisters of children with VUR. The nuclear cystogram may be quantitated by measuring the percentage of bladder volume refluxing into the ureters during bladder filling. The percentage of bladder filling when the reflux is first identified may also be an indicator of potential resolution of VUR. On subsequent examinations, improvement in VUR may be assumed if a smaller percentage of total bladder volume refluxes into the ureter or if the reflux occurs after a greater percentage of total bladder filling (Mozley et al, 1994).

The **radionuclide renal scan** is measured in two phases, the cortical imaging and the tubular imaging phase. Most radionuclide agents demonstrate renal tubular as well as renal cortical binding. Radionuclide studies are best suited to demonstrate changes in tubular or cortical transit that result from abnormalities of renal perfusion, secretion, and filtration. In most cases, the radionuclide study is inferior to CT scanning, MRI, or ultrasound for demonstration of morphologic alterations. When a glomerular filtration excreted agent such as **technetium 99m diethylenetriaminepentaacetic acid (DTPA)** is given, an approximate estimation of the glomerular filtration rate may be calculated, either in vivo by computer-aided scanning or in vitro with the collection of one or two blood samples at predetermined time intervals. In addition, an "extraction factor" can be calculated which estimates the single-kidney glomerular filtration rate during minutes 1 and 2 of the clearance of the radiotracer (Heyman and Duchett, 1988). The newest tracer, **technetium 99m mercaptoacetyltriglycine (MAG-3)** is secreted in part by renal tubular function and may also be used to approximate relative renal plasma flow. If detailed imaging of the renal cortex is required to identify renal scarring, **technetium 99m dimercaptosuccinic acid (DMSA)** may be given, with the kidneys imaged 3 to 4 hours after the injection.

Despite the newer imaging techniques that are now available, the intravenous pyelogram (IVP) is useful in selected cases. The plain film of the abdomen should be inspected for calculi, spinal abnormalities, and an abnormal intestinal gas pattern. The nephrogram phase of the IVP identifies mass effects within the kidney and the presence or absence of scarring after pyelonephritis. Subsequent views can sequentially assess the anatomy of the renal cortex, calyces, fornices, renal pelvis, ureters, bladder, and urethra (Smellie, 1995). Subtle anatomic variations in normal anatomy of the renal calyces or of the ureteropelvic junction that are confusing on ultrasound or CT may be clarified with the IVP. The contrast agent may persist in the collecting system for longer than 24 hours.

The spiral CT scan has in most cases replaced the IVP as the first-line study in children with suspected stone disease. In addition, a CT scan with or without contrast is particularly important as an adjunct in children with suspected focal segmental bacterial pyelonephritis. CT scans are also particularly important in the diagnosis and staging of solid tumors of the chest and abdomen. **Contrast-enhanced CT scanning is particularly useful in cases of nephroblastomatosis,** where the ultrasound shows little displacement of the renal capsule.

Gadolinium-enhanced MRI and magnetic resonance angiography (MRA) may provide the best three-dimensional image of the kidneys, ureters, and bladder in children. MRI has been used to assess ureteral obstruction (Borthne et al, 2000). MRI has improved the imaging of the pelvic organs in children as in adults (Liu et al, 1998; Lang et al, 1999) Although not routine, MRA is used more frequently now in the evaluation and identification of the impalpable testis (Lam et al, 1998; Yeung et al, 1999).

Inflammation-seeking isotopes (gallium 67 citrate, indium 111–labeled WBCs) may be helpful to isolate the presence or absence of infection (Yen et al, 1999). These techniques may be used to identify and guide therapy for children with focal segmental bacterial pyelonephritis in whom the duration of therapy is uncertain. They are particularly useful in patients with abnormal renal anatomy and in those with diminished renal function, in whom the DMSA scan may be less specific.

Office Procedures

The well-equipped urology office has a **urodynamic suite** as part of the overall complex. Modern urodynamic systems allow accurate measurements of intraluminal bladder pressures before, during, and after bladder contraction. From these measurements, estimates of bladder compliance as well as the bladder outlet resistance may be made. With this information, the pediatric urologist may assess whether the bladder stores at pressures low enough to prevent renal damage and empties well enough to prevent UTI. **Biofeedback training,** designed to help the child to improve bladder emptying, may also be performed in the office. Biofeedback sessions should be done in a room that is separate from the urodynamic suite, because in most cases a different population of patients require biofeedback training than will undergo urodynamic study (Schulman et al, 1999; Yamanishi et al, 2000). Biofeedback, if done properly, is time-consuming. The child must be relaxed for the session to be effective. Our biofeedback suite is equipped with stereo and video and low lighting to help make the child feel more comfortable.

Office Surgical Procedures

Successful outpatient surgery with local anesthesia depends on cooperation from the parent as well as the child. Parents must believe that the convenience of having the procedure in the office outweighs the advantages of a general anesthetic in the main operating room.

We believe that many babies who weigh less than 10 pounds may easily undergo an office **circumcision** with an anesthetic cream combined with injected local anesthetic (Hoebeke et al, 1997; Taddio et al, 2000). We rarely provide for office circumcision in older children. Infants older than 3 months are too big to be easily restrained, and the risk of bleeding postoperatively if the skin edges are not sutured is considerable.

A number of **techniques** may be used in the clinic for circumcision. Most of these are clamp procedures. We use the Gomco clamp, which is a three-component device that includes a bell, which fits over the glans of the penis and separates the glans from the inner preputial skin (Guazzo, 1999; Amir et al, 2000). The clamp is applied, and the foreskin is trimmed away from the clamp. If the clamp is left in place for a considerable amount of time (usually about 10 minutes), then there is very little separation of the skin postoperatively. If desired, a small, nonstick bandage may be placed beneath a transparent adhesive dressing. The bandage is removed the next day. The boy's parents are instructed to apply Vaseline to the incision during the healing period.

Complications after neonatal circumcision include bleeding, wound infection, meatal stenosis, and secondary phimosis resulting from removal of insufficient foreskin or removal of insufficient inner preputial skin. Potentially serious complications include sepsis, amputation of the distal part of the glans, removal of excessive foreskin, and urethrocutaneous fistula (Baskin et al, 1997; Moses et al, 1998).

Meatal stenosis is common after circumcision. It may result from contraction of the meatus after healing of the inflamed, denuded glans tissue that occurs following retraction of the foreskin or from damage to the frenular artery at the time of circumcision (Persad et al, 1995; Upadhyay et al, 1998). If the narrowing is pronounced enough to cause deflection of the urinary stream or dysuria, a **meatotomy** is indicated. This procedure is easily performed in the office of the pediatric urologist.

To perform a meatotomy in the office setting, an anesthetic creme is applied. After 45 minutes, lidocaine with 1% epinephrine is injected with a 26-gauge needle to provide a small wheal at the ventrum of the urethral meatus. The ventral edge of the urethral meatus is clamped, and a small wedge of the scarred tissue is crushed with a straight hemostat and sharply excised. After the procedure, the parents are advised to apply a fine petroleum ointment to the cut edges of the urethral meatus. A small meatal dilator is used twice a day for 4 to 6 weeks. Postoperatively, these children are seen 2 to 3 months later to assess the result.

The adhesions that are present between the glans penis and the inner surface of the prepuce in an uncircumcised boy should never be forcefully separated. These filmy preputial-glanular adhesions rarely result in symptoms and often re-adhere after they are separated. As the child ages, these adhesions will spontaneously separate (Imamura, 1997). However, after a circumcision, the cut edge of the preputial surface may occasionally graft to the inflamed glans tissue, forming a preputial-glanular bridge, which may be incised in the office with application of local anesthetic cream and subsequent injection of local anesthetic. After the injection, the skin bridge is clamped, the clamp is removed, and the skin bridge is sharply incised. No suturing is required in most cases. This procedure is easy and virtually painless. After the procedure, the parents apply petroleum jelly to the incised edges to prevent them from re-adhering.

If a VCUG is required, or if dysuria associated with vaginal pooling of urine contributes to a dysfunctional voiding pattern, we have occasionally separated labial adhesions in the office. These membranous adhesions are easy to separate on the midline with a probe or the tip of a curved hemostat. We apply a local anesthetic cream to the labia to ease the discomfort, which is minimal. After lysis of the adhesions, the child's parent must separate the labia and apply a barrier cream (e.g., petroleum jelly) at least twice a day for 4 to 6 weeks while the labial tissue matures. With diligent postoperative care, recurrence is rare.

SUMMARY

The final goal of the surgical care of children is to ensure as normal an adult life as possible. **Children born with complicated problems may require lifelong follow-up by a skilled urologist.** The pediatric urologist should continue to act as consultant even after the child enters adulthood for boys with prune-belly syndrome or posterior urethral valves and for children of either sex born with bladder or cloacal exstrophy. **As the children grow into adults, the pediatric team must develop a liaison with a skilled, interested adult team. In this way, a lifetime plan of care may be designed and carried out to ensure well-coordinated urologic therapy that is capable of addressing the complicated problems unique to this special group of patients.**

REFERENCES

American Academy of Pediatrics, Committee on Quality Improvement, Subcommittee on Urinary Tract Infection: Practice parameter: The diagnosis, treatment, and evaluation of the initial urinary tract infection in febrile infants and young children. Pediatrics 1999;103:843–852.

Ahmed A, Mbibi NH, et al: Complications of traditional male circumcision. Ann Trop Paediatr 1999; 19:113–117.

Amir M, Raja MH, et al: Neonatal circumcision with Gomco clamp: A hospital-based retrospective study of 1000 cases. J Pak Med Assoc 2000;50:224–227.

Babcook CJ, Goldstein RB, et al: Prenatally detected fetal myelomeningocele: Is karyotype analysis warranted? Radiology 1995;194:491–494.

Baskin LS, Canning DA, et al: Surgical repair of urethral circumcision injuries. J Urol 1997;158:2269–2271.

Batista JE, Caffaratti J, et al: The reliability of cysto-urethrographic signs in the diagnosis of detrusor instability in children. Br J Urol 1998;81: 900–904.

Bauchner H: Failure to thrive. In Behrman R, Kliegman R, Jenson HB (eds): Nelson Textbook of Pediatrics, 16th ed. Philadelphia, WB Saunders, 2000, pp 120–121.

Bauer SB: The challenge of the expanding role of urodynamic studies in the treatment of children with neurological and functional disabilities. (Editorial; comment.) J Urol 1998;160:527–528.

Bergeson PS, Hopkin RJ, et al: The inconspicuous penis. Pediatrics 1993; 92:794–799.

Berkowitz GS, Lapinski RH, Dolgin SE, et al: Prevalence and natural history of cryptorchidism. Pediatrics 1993;92:44–49.

Bernstein D: History and physical examination. In Behrman R, Kliegman R, Jenson H (eds): Nelson Textbook of Pediatrics, 16th ed. Philadelphia, WB Saunders, 2000, 1343–1351.

Bokenkamp A, von Kries R, et al: Neonatal renal venous thrombosis in Germany between 1992 and 1994: Epidemiology, treatment and outcome. Eur J Pediatr 2000;159:44–48.

Bonadio WA: Urine culturing technique in febrile infants. Pediatr Emerg Care 1987;3:75–78.

Borthne A, Pierre-Jerome C, et al: MR urography in children: Current status and future development. Eur Radiol 2000;10:503–511.

Casale AJ, Beck SD, et al: Concealed penis in childhood: A spectrum of etiology and treatment. J Urol 1999;162:1165–1168.

Chen CJ: The treatment of imperforate anus: Experience with 108 patients. J Pediatr Surg 1999;34:1728–1732.

Chen CP, Shih SL, et al: Perinatal features of omphalocele-exstrophy-imperforate anus-spinal defects (OEIS complex) associated with large meningomyeloceles and severe limb defects. Am J Perinatol 1997;14: 275–279.

Clarnette TD, Hutson JM: Is the ascending testis actually "stationary"? Normal elongation of the spermatic cord is prevented by a fibrous remnant of the processus vaginalis. Pediatr Surg Int 1997;12:155–157.

Coombes GM, Millard RJ: The accuracy of portable ultrasound scanning in the measurement of residual urine volume. J Urol 1994;152:2083–2085.

Dacher JN, Boillot B, et al: Rational use of CT in acute pyelonephritis: Findings and relationships with reflux. Pediatr Radiol 1993;23:281–285.

Davey RB: Undescended testes: Early versus late maldescent. Pediatr Surg Int 1997;12:165–167.

De Filippo RE, Shaul DB, et al: Neurogenic bladder in infants born with anorectal malformations: Comparison with spinal and urologic status. J Pediatr Surg 1999;34:825–827; discussion, 828.

Diamond DA, Paltiel HJ, et al: Comparative assessment of pediatric testicular volume: Orchidometer versus ultrasound. J Urol 2000;164: 1111–1114.

Diven SC, Travis LB: A practical primary care approach to hematuria in children. Pediatr Nephrol 2000;14:65–72.

Downs SM: Technical report: Urinary tract infections in febrile infants and young children. The Urinary Tract Subcommittee of the American Academy of Pediatrics Committee on Quality Improvement. Pediatrics 1999;103:E54.

Duckett JW, Keating MA: Technical challenge of the megameatus intact prepuce hypospadias variant: The pyramid procedure. J Urol 1989;141: 1407–1409.

Eardley I, Saw KC, et al: Surgical outcome of orchidopexy: II. Trapped and ascending testes. Br J Urol 1994;73:204–206.

Escobar GJ, Li DK, et al: Neonatal sepsis workups in infants ≥2000 grams at birth: A population-based study. Pediatrics 2000;106:256–263.

Falcao MC, Leone CR, et al: Urinary tract infection in full-term newborn infants: Value of urine culture by bag specimen collection. Rev Hosp Clin Fac Med Sao Paulo 1999;54:91–96.

Fein J, Donoghue A, et al: Constipation as a cause of scrotal pain in children. Am J Emerg Med 2001; 19(4):290–292.

Fernbach SK: The dilated urinary tract in children. Urol Radiol 1992;14: 34–42.

Fernbach SK: Towards an understanding of urinary tract infection in children: A model for the future of paediatric radiology and urology. BJU Int 2000;86(Suppl 1):80–83.

Fideleff HL, Boquete HR, et al: Controversies in the evolution of paediatric-adolescent varicocele: Clinical, biochemical and histological studies. Eur J Endocrinol 2000;143:775–781.

Finkelstein MS, Rosenberg HK, et al: Ultrasound evaluation of scrotum in pediatrics. Urology 1986;27:1–9.

Freedman AL, Johnson MP, Smith CA, et al: Long-term outcome in children after antenatal intervention for obstructive uropathies. Lancet 1999;354:374–377.

Gearhart JP: Bladder exstrophy: Staged reconstruction (review). Curr Opin Urol 1999;9:499–506.

Glatzl J: Forms of intersexuality in childhood (pathogenesis—clinical aspects—diagnosis—therapy). Wien Klin Wochenschr 1987;99:295–306.

Goldman M, Lahat E, et al: Imaging after urinary tract infection in male neonates. Pediatrics 2000;105:1232–1235.

Griscom N: The roentgenology of abdominal masses. AJR Am J Roentgenol 1965;93:447–463.

Guazzo E: Gomco circumcision. Am Fam Physician 1999;59:2730–2732.

Gylys-Morin VM, Minevich E, et al: Magnetic resonance imaging of the dysplastic renal moiety and ectopic ureter. J Urol 2000;164:2034–2039.

Hassink EA, Rieu PN, et al: Additional congenital defects in anorectal malformations. Eur J Pediatr 1996;155:477–482.

Hellstrom M, Jacobsson B: Diagnosis of vesico-ureteric reflux. Acta Paediatr Suppl 1999;88:3–12.

Heyman SH, Duchett JW: The extraction factor: An estimate of single kidney function in children during routine radionuclide renography with 99m-technetium diethylene triamine pentaacetic acid. J Urol 1988;140: 780–783.

Hoebeke P, Depauw P, et al: The use of Emla cream as anaesthetic for minor urological surgery in children. Acta Urol Belg 1997;65:25–28.

Hulbert WC, Rosenberg HK, et al: The predictive value of ultrasonography in evaluation of infants with posterior urethral valves. J Urol 1992; 148:122–124.

Imamura E: Phimosis of infants and young children in Japan. Acta Paediatr Jpn 1997;39:403–405.

Ingelfinger JR, Davis AE, et al: Frequency and etiology of gross hematuria in a general pediatric setting. Pediatrics 1977;59:557–561.

Jamis-Dow CA, Choyke PL, et al: Small (≤3-cm) renal masses: Detection with CT versus US and pathologic correlation. Radiology 1996;198: 785–788.

Jeffs RD: Exstrophy and cloacal exstrophy. Urol Clin North Am 1978;5: 127–140.

Jenkins R: Sexually transmitted diseases. In Behrman R, Kliegman R, Jenson H (eds): Nelson Textbook of Pediatrics, 16th ed. Philadelphia, WB Saunders, 2000, pp 583–586.

Johnson C: Sexual abuse. In Behrman R, Kliegman R, Jenson H (eds): Nelson Textbook of Pediatrics, 16th ed. Philadelphia, WB Saunders, 2000, pp 115–117.

Kallen K, Castilla EE, et al: OEIS complex: A population study. Am J Med Genet 2000;92:62–68.

Kaplan WE: Management of myelomeningocele. Urol Clin North Am 1985;12:93–101.

Kellogg ND, Parra JM, et al: Children with anogenital symptoms and signs referred for sexual abuse evaluations. Arch Pediatr Adolesc Med 1998;152:634–641.

Kim HL, Gow KW, et al: Presentation of low anorectal malformations beyond the neonatal period. Pediatrics 2000;105:E68.

Kirby CL, Rosenberg HK: Ultrasound shows masses in pediatric abdomen. Diagn Imaging (San Francisco) 1992;14:168–173.

Kizer JR, Bellah RD, et al: Meconium hydrocele in a female newborn: An unusual cause of a labial mass. J Urol 1995;153:188–190.

Kondo A, Kapoor R, et al: Functional obstruction of the female urethra: Relevance to refractory bed wetting and recurrent urinary tract infection. Neurourol Urodyn 1994;13:541–546.

Lam WW, Tam PK, et al: Gadolinium-infusion magnetic resonance angiogram: A new, noninvasive, and accurate method of preoperative localization of impalpable undescended testes. J Pediatr Surg 1998;33:123–126.

Lang IM, Babyn P, et al: MR imaging of paediatric uterovaginal anomalies. Pediatr Radiol 1999;29:163–170.

Lattimer JK, Hensle TW, et al: The exstrophy support team: A new concept in the care of the exstrophy patient. J Urol 1979;121:472–473.

Levy DA, Kay R, Elder JS: Neonatal testis tumors: A review of the Prepubertal Testis Tumor Registry. J Urol 1994;151:715–717.

Li FP, Fraumeni JF: Testicular cancers in children: Epidemiologic characteristics. J Natl Cancer Inst 1972;48:1575–1581.

Lin DS, Huang SH, et al: Urinary tract infection in febrile infants younger than eight weeks of age. Pediatrics 2000;105:E20.

Liu PF, Krestin GP, et al: MRI of the uterus, uterine cervix, and vagina: Diagnostic performance of dynamic contrast-enhanced fast multiplanar gradient-echo imaging in comparison with fast spin-echo T2-weighted pulse imaging. Eur Radiol 1998;8:1433–1440.

Luks FI, Yazbeck S, et al: The abdominoscrotal hydrocele. Eur J Pediatr Surg 1993;3:176–178.

McCarthy P: Acute infectious illness in children. Compr Ther 1988;14:51.

McDonald A, Scranton M, et al: Voiding cystourethrograms and urinary tract infections: How long to wait? Pediatrics 2000;105:E50.

McGuire EJ, Woodside JR, et al: Upper urinary tract deterioration in patients with myelodysplasia and detrusor hypertonia: A followup study. J Urol 1983;129:823–826.

McGuire EJ, Diddel G, Wagner F: Balanced bladder function in spinal cord injury patients. J Urol 1977;118:626–628.

Moses S, Bailey RC, et al: Male circumcision: Assessment of health benefits and risks. Sex Transm Infect 1998;74:368–373.

Mozley PD, Heyman S, Duckett JW, et al: Direct vesicoureteral scintigraphy: Quantifying early outcome predictors in children with primary reflux. J Nucl Med 1994;35:1602–1608.

Niedzielski J, Paduch D, et al: Assessment of adolescent varicocele. Pediatr Surg Int 1997;12:410–413.

Noh PH, Cooper CS, Winkler AC, et al: Prognostic factors for long-term renal function in boys with the prune-belly syndrome. J Urol 1999;162: 1399–1401.

Park JW: Fever without source in children: Recommendations for outpatient care in those up to 3. Postgrad Med 2000;107:259–262,265–266.

Parrott TS, Woodard JR: Importance of cystourethrography in neonates with imperforate anus. Urology 1979;13:607–609.

Persad R, Sharma S, et al: Clinical presentation and pathophysiology of meatal stenosis following circumcision. Br J Urol 1995;75:91–93.

Pinto E, Guignard JP: Renal masses in the neonate. Biol Neonate 1995; 68:175–184.

Polito C, Moggio G, et al: Cyclic voiding cystourethrography in the diagnosis of occult vesicoureteric reflux. Pediatr Nephrol 2000;14:39–41.

Powell DM, Newman KD, et al: A proposed classification of vaginal anomalies and their surgical correction. J Pediatr Surg 1995;30:271–275; discussion, 275–276.

Powell KR: Fever. In Behrman R, Kliegman R, Jenson H (eds): Nelson Textbook of Pediatrics, 16th ed. Philadelphia, WB Saunders, 2000;742–747.

Raffensperger J, Abousleiman A: Abdominal masses in children under one year of age. Surgery 1968;63:770–775.

Ransley PG, Risdon RA: Reflux nephropathy: Effects of antimicrobial therapy on the evolution of the early pyelonephritic scar. Kidney Int 1981;20:733–742.

Redman JF: Conservative management of urethral prolapse in female children. Urology 1982;19:505–506.

Rock JA, Zacur HA, et al: Pregnancy success following surgical correction of imperforate hymen and complete transverse vaginal septum. Obstet Gynecol 1982;59:448–451.

Sampietro Crespo A, Vaquerizo Gareta A, et al: Major outpatient surgery in urology: Our experience. Arch Esp Urol 1995;48:343–346.

Saxton HM, Borzyskowski M, et al: Spinning top urethra: Not a normal variant. Radiology 1988;168:147–150.

Schoen EJ, Colby CJ, et al: Newborn circumcision decreases incidence and costs of urinary tract infections during the first year of life. Pediatrics 2000;105:789–793.

Schulman SL, Quinn CK, et al: Comprehensive management of dysfunctional voiding. Pediatrics 1999;103:E31.

Shaul DB, Harrison EA: Classification of anorectal malformations: Initial approach, diagnostic tests, and colostomy. Semin Pediatr Surg 1997;6: 187–195.

Smellie JM: The intravenous urogram in the detection and evaluation of renal damage following urinary tract infection. Pediatr Nephrol 1995;9: 213–219; discussion, 219–220.

Smith C, Smith DP: Office pediatric urologic procedures from a parental perspective. Urology 2000;55:272–276.

Soonawala N, Overweg-Plandsoen WC, et al: Early clinical signs and symptoms in occult spinal dysraphism: A retrospective case study of 47 patients. Clin Neurol Neurosurg 1999;101:11–14.

Stapleton FB, Roy SD, et al: Hypercalciuria in children with hematuria. N Engl J Med 1984;310:1345–1348.

Stoll BJ, Kliegman RM: The newborn infant. In Behrman R, Kliegman R, Jenson H (eds): Nelson Textbook of Pediatrics, 16th ed. Philadelphia, WB Saunders, 2000;454–460.

Taddio A, Ohlsson K, et al: Lidocaine-prilocaine cream for analgesia during circumcision in newborn boys. Cochrane Database Syst Rev 2000;93:496.

Uehling DT, Richards WH: Abdominoscrotal hydrocele: Diagnosis by herniogram and ultrasound. Urology 1992;40:147–148.

Unsinn KM, Geley T, et al: US of the spinal cord in newborns: Spectrum of normal findings, variants, congenital anomalies, and acquired diseases. Radiographics 2000;20:923–938.

Upadhyay V, Hammodat HM, et al: Post circumcision meatal stenosis: 12 years' experience. N Z Med J 1998;111:57–58.

Valero Puerta JA, Medina Perez M, et al: Results of ambulatory major surgery in urology, within an integrated unit. Actas Urol Esp 1999;23: 523–526; discussion, 526–527.

van der Voort J, Edwards A, et al: The struggle to diagnose UTI in children under two in primary care. Fam Pract 1997;14:44–48.

Van Glabeke E, Khairouni A, et al: Spermatic cord torsion in children. Prog Urol 1998;8:244–248.

Van Glabeke E, Khairouni A, et al: Acute scrotal pain in children: Results of 543 surgical explorations. Pediatr Surg Int 1999;15:353–357.

Waisman Y, Lotem Y, et al: Management of children with aseptic meningitis in the emergency department. Pediatr Emerg Care 1999;15:314–317.

Walker R: Evaluation of the pediatric urologic patient. In Walsh P, Retik A, Vaughan E, Wein A (eds): Campbell's Urology, 7th ed. Philadelphia, WB Saunders, 1998, pp 1619–1628.

Wedge JJ, Grosfeld JL, et al: Abdominal masses in the newborn: 63 cases. J Urol 1971;106:770–775.

Williams CP, Richardson BG, et al: Importance of identifying the inconspicuous penis: Prevention of circumcision complications. Urology 2000;56:140–142.

Wilson DA: Ultrasound screening for abdominal masses in the neonatal period. Am J Dis Child 1982;136:147–151.

Wiswell TE: The prepuce, urinary tract infections, and the consequences. Pediatrics 2000;105:860–862.

Wright C, Loughridge J, et al: Failure to thrive in a population context: Two contrasting studies of feeding and nutritional status. Proc Nutr Soc 2000;59:37–45.

Yamanishi T, Yasuda K, et al: Biofeedback training for detrusor overactivity in children. J Urol 2000;164:1686–1690.

Yen TC, Tzen KY, et al: The value of Ga-67 renal SPECT in diagnosing and monitoring complete and incomplete treatment in children with acute pyelonephritis. Clin Nucl Med 1999;24:669–673.

Yeung CK, Tam YH, et al: A new management algorithm for impalpable undescended testis with gadolinium enhanced magnetic resonance angiography. J Urol 1999;162:998–1002.

53
RENAL DISEASE IN CHILDHOOD

Shane Roy, III, M.D.
H. Norman Noe, M.D.

History and Physical Examination

Laboratory Data
    Urinalysis
    Creatinine Clearance
    Urinary Calcium Excretion

Hematuria
    Etiology
    Algorithm for Hematuria Evaluation

Proteinuria
    Isolated Proteinuria
    Proteinuria with Glomerular Diseases
    Proteinuria with Tubulointerstitial Diseases

Renal Tubular Disorders
    Nephrogenic Diabetes Insipidus
    Miscellaneous Tubular Disorders

Disease of the renal parenchyma in a child requires interaction and efficient communication between the pediatric urologist and nephrologic colleagues. Prompt recognition of such renal disorders can lead to appropriate evaluation and management, which can decrease unnecessary testing and avoid costly or invasive procedures. Close cooperation in this area will lead to the maximum treatment outcome as well as cost-effective management.

Although in many urban areas and medical centers all specialties are represented, many primary care physicians, because of well-established referral patterns, continue to send all children with any form of urinary finding or complaint to the urologist for initial evaluation. Such trust demands skill on the part of the urologist in distinguishing medical renal disease from purely urologic disorders. This differentiation requires a thorough knowledge of the signs and symptoms of renal parenchymal diseases and the normal development of renal function during childhood as well as an ability to interpret laboratory data correctly. In these circumstances, the urologist must not only be concerned with abnormal urologic anatomy but also understand the pathophysiology and potential histopathology pertaining to renal parenchymal disorders.

The purpose of this chapter is to review the renal disorders of childhood from a clinical perspective and to provide guidelines for their evaluation and management. The fundamentals of the history and physical examination as well as basic laboratory studies are discussed, and

certain specific renal diseases are defined in relation to children.

HISTORY AND PHYSICAL EXAMINATION

The history often provides enough information to make a presumptive diagnosis or at least to allow a targeted evaluation. The symptoms expressed by the parents or the child may be nonspecific and may include fatigue, malaise, or even abdominal pain and nausea and vomiting. A general sense of ill health may be marked by a history of weight loss or failure to thrive. A prior recent streptococcal illness may be suggestive of glomerulonephritis, or a prior viral illness might precede hematuria with immunoglobulin A (IgA) nephropathy. The child may have a concurrent illness that could give rise to a renal parenchymal abnormality or may be receiving medications that have nephrotoxic effects. It is especially important to emphasize a family history to uncover diseases that are genetic or familial in nature. During the physical examination, certain clues may suggest a renal parenchymal disorder. In many cases, renal disease is asymptomatic and somewhat insidious, with failure to thrive or small stature the only indicator of disease. Height and weight should be determined; these data, when plotted to allow assessment of any changes in rate of growth of the child, can be critical. Other findings, such as

Table 53–1. CLASSIFICATION OF HYPERTENSION BY AGE GROUP

Age Group	Significant Hypertension (mm Hg)		Severe Hypertension (mm Hg)	
	Systolic	*Diastolic*	*Systolic*	*Diastolic*
Newborn				
7 days	96	—	106	—
8–30 days	104	—	110	—
Infant (<2 yr)	112	74	118	82
Children (3–5 yr)	116	76	124	84
Children (6–9 yr)	122	78	130	86
Children (10–12 yr)	126	82	134	90
Adolescents (13–15 yr)	136	86	144	92
Adolescents (16–18 yr)	142	92	150	98

Reproduced with permission from Report of the Second Task Force on Blood Pressure Control in Children. Pediatrics, 1987;79:1–25.

flank pain, abdominal tenderness, renal enlargement, edema, or the presence of a rash, may be equally nonspecific. In many cases, edema can suggest certain disease processes—for example, dependent edema; labial and scrotal edema, which may be seen more with the nephrotic syndrome; periorbital edema, which may occur in both the nephrotic syndrome and acute nephritis; and edema of the scalp, forehead, and lower back, which occurs more often in Henoch-Schönlein purpura. The chest should be examined for signs of fluid overload such as rales, pleural effusions, murmur, or gallops. Funduscopic examination may reveal retinal edema or vascular spasm, particularly in the presence of acute nephritis and hypertension.

An important aspect of the physical examination in children with suspected renal parenchymal disease is the blood pressure measurement. The 1987 report of the Second Task Force on Blood Pressure includes revised blood pressure standards for children grouped by age and sex. Attention to detail must be paid when obtaining the blood pressure in a child. **Cuff size is a major variable, and the appropriate size cuff should be used in all instances.** The inflatable bladder within the blood pressure cuff should be long enough to encircle the arm completely, and the cuff should cover three quarters of the upper arm between the elbow and the proximal end of the humerus. The Task Force designation for significant hypertension is a reading above the 95th percentile for age (Table 53–1). Elevation of blood pressure above this level has been found to be a major contributor to the progressive nature of certain renal diseases (Still and Cottom, 1967; Mimran, 1988).

LABORATORY DATA

Laboratory evaluation of the patient with suspected renal disease should be based on the differential diagnosis suggested by the history and physical examination as well as the findings on urinalysis. The main findings that suggest renal parenchymal disease are hematuria and proteinuria. Additional laboratory studies include the complete blood count (CBC), serum electrolytes, serum creatinine, blood urea nitrogen (BUN), C3 and C4 complement, fluorescent antinuclear antibody (FANA), hepatitis B serology, sickle cell prep or hemoglobin electrophoresis (in African-American patients), quantitative urinary protein excretion, and a creatinine clearance measurement. Renal ultrasound with or without Doppler flow study of the renal vessels may also be performed in patients with suspected renal disease. The number of diagnostic studies as well as the rapidity of their performance are determined by the child's symptoms and clinical presentation. In some cases, renal biopsy is indicated depending on the specific disease or the clinical course of the patient.

Urinalysis

The one laboratory test required for *every* patient in whom a renal parenchymal disorder is suspected is a urinalysis. The urine must be collected carefully by either clean or sterile technique and examined in the fresh state, **preferably by a physician or an experienced technician** to ensure maximum accuracy. The urinalysis consists of a gross inspection of the urine, including its volume, concentration, and color, as well as dipstick and microscopic examination of the urinary sediment. A red or brown hue suggests either fresh or old bleeding associated with nephritis. However, the urine may be discolored for a number of reasons other than hematuria.

Dipstick examination of urine can be easily and quickly performed with any of the commercially available reagent strips. These strips are impregnated with individual reagents that give information about urinary constituents such as red blood cells (RBCs), hemoglobin, protein, nitrites, pH, specific gravity, glucose, bilirubin, ketones, and so on.

Hematuria

Hematuria is the abnormal presence of RBCs in the urine. It is typically described as either gross or microscopic, the latter being much more common in children. **The presence of blood in any quantity in the urine must always be confirmed by both dipstick reading and microscopic examination.** This is especially important in the evaluation of grossly discolored urine. It should be remembered that many conditions can produce a red urine that may not involve the presence of RBCs (Table 53–2).

Table 53–2. CAUSES OF RED URINE MIMICKING HEMATURIA

Heme positive (dipstick)
  Hemoglobinuria
    Hemolysis
    Sepsis
    Dialysis
  Myoglobinuria
    Ketoacidosis
    Myositis
    Trauma
Heme negative (dipstick)
  Drugs
    Sulfa drugs
    Nitrofurantoin
    Salicylates
  Foods
    Beets
    Food coloring
  Metabolites
    Homogentisic acid
    Porphyrin

Although microscopic hematuria is more common than gross hematuria in children, it is more arbitrarily defined. Both adults and children normally excrete erythrocytes in their urine, and although the excretion rate in children has not been well established, most practitioners probably agree that rates of up to 50,000 RBCs/hr (24-hour collection) are normal (Vehaskari et al, 1979). Because quantitative measurement techniques to determine the excretion rate of RBCs are not practical for office use, we rely on qualitative measurements with impregnated reagent strips (dipsticks). The dipsticks are very sensitive and can detect as few as 5 to 20 RBCs/ml (50 or more RBCs/ml are required for an abnormal finding) (Norman, 1987).

Dipsticks can actually detect blood in the urine in the physiologic range. Most dipsticks test for hemoglobin on the basis of a pseudoperoxidase reaction in the reagent strip. In addition, some dipsticks test for intact erythrocytes, which are hemolyzed on a specific reagent strip that releases the hemoglobin, which then provides the indicator reaction for blood. Dipsticks are so sensitive that they can detect insignificant amounts of hematuria, necessitating microscopic examination of any urinary sediment in which blood is suspected.

Microscopy of the urinary sediment can be performed on either an unspun or a centrifuged specimen. The number of intact erythrocytes present per high-powered field determines the significance of hematuria. Although some disagreement exists about the number of RBCs that is significant, most would agree that the presence of more than 5 RBCs per high-powered field in a spun specimen or 2 RBCs per high-powered field in an unspun specimen defines significant microscopic hematuria.

The presence of RBC casts on microscopy also strongly suggests glomerular disease in children. These casts are fragile, and low-speed centrifugation or even gravity sedimentation for 30 minutes will enhance the detection rate. Although RBC casts strongly support a diagnosis of glomerular bleeding, they are not always found. **Attention to RBC morphology in patients with sus-** pected renal parenchymal disease has been used to enhance the accuracy of diagnosis.

RED BLOOD CELL MORPHOLOGY

Traditionally, localization of the site of hematuria has relied heavily on routine urine microscopy. **The hallmark of glomerular bleeding has been the presence of RBC casts with or without proteinuria.** However, many children with glomerular or renal parenchymal disease have neither RBC casts nor proteinuria. Examination of the morphology of the RBCs in the urine has been shown to be very helpful in determining whether these cells have a glomerular or a nonglomerular origin (Birch and Fairley, 1979; Rizzoni et al, 1983; Crompton et al, 1993; Roth et al, 1991). **Specifically, RBCs that retain their normal biconcave disc shape or are crenated (eumorphic) indicate nonglomerular bleeding, whereas dysmorphic RBCs are most often associated with glomerular bleeding (Fig. 53–1). Dysmorphic cells have distorted, irregular outlines as well as variable cell size when examined under high-power magnification (Fig. 53–2).** One particular cell type, a doughnut-shaped cell with cytoplasmic extrusions, has been said to be especially associated with glomerular bleeding.

The original reports of urinary RBC morphology relied exclusively on phase-contrast microscopy. Alternatives to this method for determining RBC morphology include Wright staining of a dry smear of urinary sediment or simple light microscopy performed by an experienced examiner. Although no rigid criteria have been established for correlating RBC dysmorphism with a specific diagnosis, it can be a reliable tool in distinguishing glomerular bleeding. **One study indicated that a rate of 10% dysmorphism was diagnostic of glomerulonephritis and found a diagnostic specificity of 94% and a sensitivity of 92% in such cases** (Stapleton, 1987).

Although RBC morphology has proved to be a valuable adjunct to urine microscopy, the presence or absence of dysmorphic cells is not an absolute diagnostic finding. In some conditions the RBC morphology is inconsistent with

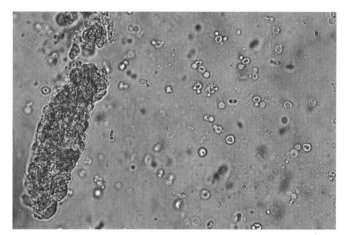

Figure 53–1. Urine from a patient who has poststreptococcal glomerulonephritis demonstrating a red blood cell cast and predominantly dysmorphic red blood cells.

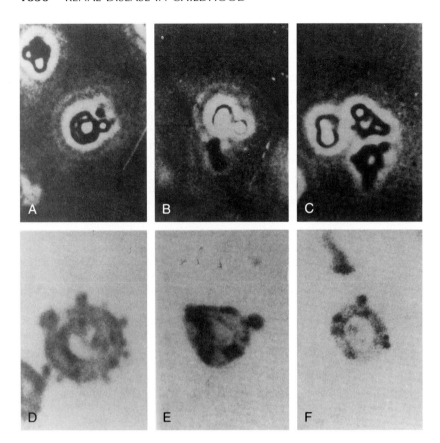

Figure 53–2. *A* through *C,* Dysmorphic red blood cells viewed by phase microscopy. *D* through *F,* Dysmorphic red blood cells with Wright stain.

the clinical diagnostic finding. Examples include dysmorphic RBCs seen in nonglomerular disorders such as urinary tract infections, reflux nephropathy, and urolithiasis. However, RBC morphology considered along with other urinary sediment findings (e.g., proteinuria, casts, bacteria) is frequently all that is needed to localize the bleeding to a glomerular or nonglomerular source. This is especially true in the presence of the appropriate clinical history and physical findings suggestive of renal parenchymal disease. However, if dysmorphic urinary erythrocytes are identified in children with asymptomatic isolated hematuria (without protein or cellular casts), an appropriate evaluation for glomerulonephritis should still be initiated, but in addition an examination of the upper urinary tract with renal ultrasound is indicated to exclude urologic causes of hematuria, especially urolithiasis. On the other hand, if all urinary RBCs are eumorphic, the initial diagnostic studies should be directed toward discovering a nonglomerular or urologic cause of the hematuria. Such studies involve a urine culture, renal ultrasound, and possibly a voiding cystourethrogram. **If these studies are all normal, particularly in patients with gross eumorphic hematuria, cystoscopy is indicated.**

Proteinuria

QUALITATIVE DETECTION OF PROTEINURIA

Detection of proteinuria is most commonly made by dipstick (Albustix, Labstix, Multistix). The dye indicator turns a pale to dark green as the urine protein concentration varies from 0 to more than 2000 mg/dl. Only urine with a specific gravity greater than 1.018 should be tested, because the dipstick reading for proteinuria is affected by the urine concentration. A strongly alkaline urine can produce a falsely positive dipstick reading for protein.

QUANTITATIVE MEASUREMENT OF PROTEINURIA

In the evaluation of persistent proteinuria or follow-up of parenchymal renal diseases, quantitation of urinary protein excretion in a timed urine collection is recommended. Normal urinary protein excretion is less than 4 mg/m^2/hr, abnormal urinary protein excretion is between 4 and 40 mg/m^2/hr, and nephrotic range proteinuria is greater than 40 mg/m^2/hr.

URINARY PROTEIN/URINARY CREATININE RATIO

Measurement of a urinary protein/urinary creatinine (Upr/Ucr) ratio in a random (preferably early morning) urine sample is a reasonably accurate way of assessing and monitoring patients with renal disease. **Upr/Ucr ratios correlate very closely with timed quantitative urinary protein measurements. The normal range is between 0 and 20 mg of protein per millimole of creatinine, or a Upr/Ucr ratio of 0 to 0.18 (mg/mg).** Further estimation of the protein excretion in children with nephrosis also reveals that a Upr/Ucr ratio of less than 0.1 is physiologic and that nephrotic range proteinuria is identified by a ratio greater than 1.0. When necessary, quantitation of urine protein excretion can be estimated from the linear regression equation: Total protein in $(g/m^2/day) = 0.63 \times (Upr/Ucr)$.

Creatinine Clearance

Clinical estimation of the glomerular filtration rate (GFR) is accomplished with the use of timed urinary creatinine excretion and plasma creatinine concentration measurements to calculate the creatinine clearance (Ccr). Ccr is less accurate than inulin, ethylenediaminetetra-acetic acid (EDTA), or iothalamate clearance measurements, which require infusion of these markers. GFR corrected for body surface area can also be estimated by the following formula:

$$GFR = K \times HE \div Pcr$$

where K is an empirically derived constant, HE represents body height in centimeters, and Pcr equals the plasma creatinine concentration in milligrams per deciliter (Schwartz et al, 1976). K for infants younger than 1 year of age is 0.45, for children it is 0.55, for adolescent boys it is 0.7, and for preterm infants it is 0.33. This estimate of Ccr obviates the collection of a timed urine sample with the inherent mistakes associated with its collection.

Urinary Calcium Excretion

Quantitative Urinary Calcium Excretion

The normal value for urinary calcium excretion in 24 hours is less than 4 mg/kg in children (Ghazali and Barratt, 1974; Stapleton et al, 1982).

Urinary Calcium/Urinary Creatinine Ratio

Screening for hypercalciuria is performed on a random, preferably fasting, urine sample. A urinary calcium/urinary creatinine (Uca/Ucr) ratio of less than 0.21 is normal in infants and children (Stapleton et al, 1982).

HEMATURIA

Etiology

Gross Hematuria

Among all renal findings, gross hematuria seems to be the most anxiety producing for parents, patients, and physicians. Although hematuria is always alarming, its cause is most often benign, and its course is usually limited. Nonetheless, it is important to ascertain a specific diagnosis in each case to alleviate both family and physician worry that a serious disorder may be overlooked. In the general pediatric population, gross hematuria is uncommon, occurring in approximately 1 of every 1000 visits (Ingelfinger et al,

1977). Among children presenting with acute onset of gross hematuria, the causes of such hematuria are most readily detectable. **In Ingelfinger's study (1977), 49% of such patients had either confirmed or suspected urinary tract infections, and only 4% were found to have renal parenchymal disease.** Routine urine cultures are always necessary in any child with hematuria in which white blood cells or bacteria are present on urinalysis. It must be remembered that white blood cells can also suggest inflammation resulting solely from nephritis; if there is a question, a urine culture should always be obtained. A positive culture would most likely occur in a child with a purely urologic or congenital disorder as opposed to a renal parenchymal disease.

Microscopic Hematuria

Microscopic hematuria is more difficult to define and has a prevalence of 1.5% in children and adolescents (Dodge et al, 1976). As mentioned earlier, the presence of hematuria must be confirmed by both dipstick and microscopic examination of the urinary sediment. Microscopic hematuria is defined as the presence in a spun urine specimen of 5 or more RBCs per high-powered field in two of three urinalyses in an otherwise asymptomatic child. In the symptomatic child in the appropriate clinical situation, however, blood in a single urine sample is sufficient to require an evaluation.

Algorithm for Hematuria Evaluation

There are many causes of hematuria in children. An understanding of the causes allows one to formulate an approach not only to the differential diagnosis of hematuria but also to the most efficient method of evaluation. Figures 53–3 and 53–4 offer a differential diagnostic approach to the causes of hematuria in children and a planned evaluation designed to find the source of the hematuria (Fitzwater and Wyatt, 1994). These plans are based on documentation of blood in the urine, urinary RBC morphology, and the presence or absence of proteinuria, all taking into account the history, physical findings, and family history.

Hematuria with Eumorphic Red Blood Cells

When hematuria with eumorphic RBCs is observed, an investigation for a nonglomerular cause of bleeding is necessary. Causes such as hypercalciuria, nephrolithiasis, nephrocalcinosis, cystitis, trauma, cystic kidney disease, tumors, and urinary tract infections must be considered (see Fig. 53–3). Sickle cell hematuria is listed under the eumorphic RBC category because the RBC distortion arises from deoxygenation of sickle hemoglobin within the RBC, rather than from external distortion of the cell resulting from its being squeezed through the glomerular basement membrane. The RBCs in patients with sickle cell disease are otherwise normal or eumorphic except in sickle cell crisis, which is determined by the history and physical examination and confirmed by hemoglobin electrophoresis.

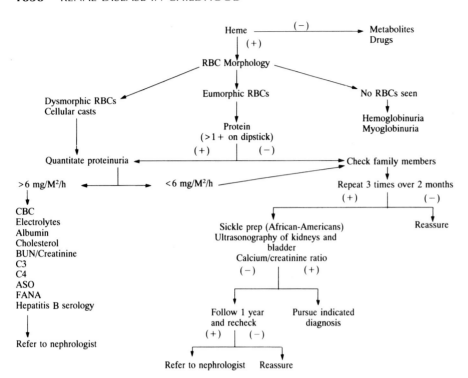

Figure 53–3. Evaluation of hematuria.

The sickled appearance of the RBCs is also unique to this disease.

HYPERCALCIURIA AND NEPHROLITHIASIS

Hypercalciuria is a common condition and a frequent cause of hematuria in otherwise healthy children. Hypercalciuria is present in approximately 5% of healthy white children and is the most frequent cause of isolated hematuria in this group. Approximately 30% of children in whom hematuria is isolated (i.e., the urine is noninfected and the hematuria is nonglomerular) are found to be hypercalciuric (Moore, 1981; Stapleton et al, 1984). Hypercalciuria may be associated with episodic gross hematuria in an absence of demonstrated renal stones, but there are potential long-term implications for the development of stone disease in a child who has hematuria but has not yet manifested urolithiasis (Roy et al, 1981; Kalia et al, 1981; Noe et al, 1984).

Hypercalciuria may be associated with certain conditions such as immobilization, vitamin D intoxication, and the use of loop diuretics, but in most children it is idiopathic. The mechanism causing the hematuria is unclear but may involve irritation or actual tubular cell injury by calcium-containing crystals. The percentage of children with hypercalciuria who later develop stones is not clear, but it has been shown that two thirds of children with urolithiasis have associated hypercalciuria (Noe et al, 1983).

Urinary findings in the child with hypercalciuria usually are nonspecific, with predominantly eumorphic red cells being noted in the urinary sediment. Calcium oxalate crystals may be present, but their presence is inconsistent. Occasionally, dysmorphic cells are seen in the child with established urolithiasis, as previously discussed. **Screening for hypercalciuria is performed with a random urine Uca/Ucr ratio. A ratio greater than 0.21 indicates hy-**

percalciuria in infants and children. Definitive diagnosis of hypercalciuria is established by quantitative measurement of calcium in a 24-hour collection. A urinary calcium excretory rate of more than 4 mg/kg/day is abnormal in children (Ghazali and Barratt, 1974; Stapleton et al, 1982).

Management of hypercalciuria depends on the clinical symptoms. Simple dietary measures include avoidance of dietary excesses of calcium and sodium and increases in fluid intake. Specific therapy with hydrochlorothiazide is reserved for those with clinically significant stone formation. A short course of hydrochlorothiazide often results in the disappearance of microscopic hematuria and can serve as a diagnostic test.

Hematuria with Dysmorphic Red Blood Cells

POSTINFECTIOUS GLOMERULONEPHRITIS

Hematuria with symptoms and signs of acute glomerulonephritis, including edema, hypertension, oliguria, and the presence of dysmorphic RBCs and RBC casts on urine microscopy, requires an investigation to determine the cause. Postinfectious glomerulonephritis, usually occurring after group A beta-hemolytic streptococcal sore throat or pyoderma, is the most common cause of glomerulonephritis in children. There is a latency period of 7 to 10 days after a group A beta-hemolytic streptococcal sore throat or 21 to 30 days after streptococcal pyoderma before the appearance of the common presenting symptoms of edema and brownish, cola-colored urine. **A positive anti-streptolysin-O or streptozyme titer and a decreased serum complement (C3) concentration are usually present.** Varying degrees of acute renal insufficiency with oliguria or even anuria requiring intermittent dialysis may be seen.

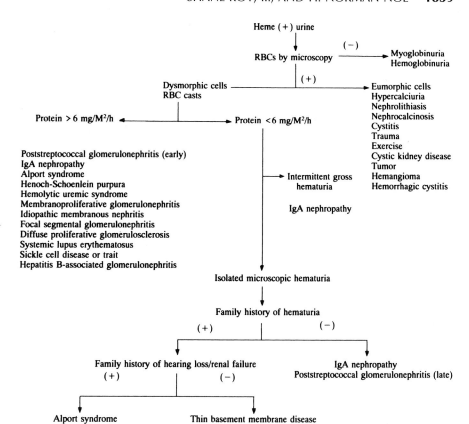

Figure 53–4. Differential diagnosis of hematuria.

Control of hypertension, management of electrolyte and fluid balance, and treatment of renal functional impairment are necessary during the acute phase of the illness. **Complete recovery of renal function can be expected in more than 90% of cases, even in those who have a protracted clinical course requiring peritoneal dialysis or hemodialysis.** Microscopic hematuria and minimal proteinuria may persist for 3 to 6 months. C3 concentrations usually become normal within 2 months after disease onset. **Proteinuria that persists for 12 months after disease onset may require a renal biopsy to assess the degree of renal histologic damage.**

IMMUNOGLOBULIN A NEPHROPATHY

IgA nephropathy is a common cause of glomerulonephritis that is defined immunohistologically by the presence of mesangial deposits of IgA in renal biopsy tissue in the absence of a systemic disease. Patients usually present with recurrent macroscopic hematuria during the course of an upper respiratory tract infection. IgA nephropathy is most often confused with postinfectious glomerulonephritis. **However, the prodromal period between infection and the appearance of symptoms of nephritis is 7 to 10 days or longer in patients with postinfectious glomerulonephritis. Gross hematuria in patients with IgA nephropathy usually appears during an acute infection.** A poor prognosis in patients with IgA nephropathy is indicated by the presence of renal histologic findings of glomerulosclerosis, severe mesangial proliferation, glomerular crescents, and significant interstitial fibrosis associated with renal

function impairment, hypertension, male gender, older age at the time of biopsy, and more than 2 g/day of proteinuria (Hogg et al, 1994). **Progressive renal failure may be expected in 30% to 50% of patients after 10 to 20 years of follow-up. No treatment has proved to be of benefit.** Prednisone treatment protocols are currently being evaluated at several centers.

HENOCH-SCHÖNLEIN PURPURA

Henoch-Schönlein purpura is a vasculitic syndrome observed primarily in boys between the ages of 2 and 11 years. It is manifested by nonthrombocytopenic purpura, colicky abdominal pain, joint pain and swelling, and glomerulonephritis. The diagnosis is confirmed by clinical findings. Renal involvement occurs in 20% to 50% of patients, persistent nephropathy is seen in 1% of all cases, and progression to end-stage renal disease (ESRD) occurs in fewer than 1%. **Children with hematuria alone do not develop chronic renal failure,** but 15% of those who have both hematuria and proteinuria develop renal failure. **Approximately 50% of patients who develop nephrotic syndrome with Henoch-Schönlein purpura will develop ESRD within 10 years. Patients with either a nephritic or a nephrotic clinical presentation should be considered for renal biopsy.** No specific treatment is available for Henoch-Schönlein purpura. Steroids can produce favorable results in patients with soft tissue swelling, joint disease, scrotal swelling, and abdominal colic or gastrointestinal hemorrhage. **Neither prednisone nor other immunosuppressants have been proved in a controlled study** to benefit patients with Henoch-Schönlein purpura nephritis, but they continue to be used clinically in patients with severe nephritis or nephrotic syndrome.

HEMOLYTIC-UREMIC SYNDROME

The hemolytic-uremic syndrome (HUS) is a heterogeneous group of disorders manifested by microangiopathic hemolytic anemia, thrombocytopenia, and acute renal failure. It is the most frequent cause of acute renal failure in children. The vasculopathy involves endothelial damage in small- to medium-sized arteries with fibrin deposition and thrombotic microangiopathy. There are diarrheal and nondiarrheal forms of HUS. The diarrheal form is most common and is associated with cytotoxin-producing organisms such as verotoxin-producing *Escherichia coli* or *Shigella dysenteriae*, which produce the Shiga toxin. Nondiarrheal forms of HUS may be related to infections with *Streptococcus pneumoniae* or many viruses or to autosomal dominant or recessive inheritance, malignancy, renal transplantation, or drugs such as cyclosporin A, oral contraceptives, and chemotherapeutic agents (Kaplan et al, 1990).

Treatment of HUS includes dialysis for renal failure, management of acute renal insufficiency, maintenance of the hemoglobin level at 8 g/dl or higher, and administration of platelet transfusions for symptomatic bleeding. Plasma transfusion for hereditary, prolonged, or recurrent HUS may be considered but should be avoided in patients with pneumococcal-associated HUS (Siegler, 1988). Plasmapheresis, if technically feasible, may be beneficial in patients with recurrent, inherited, or drug-induced HUS.

The prognosis of HUS is poor in patients who have nondiarrheal forms of the disease, are less than 1 year of age, or have prolonged anuria, severe hypertension, or severe central nervous system disease. Renal transplantation may be necessary after dialysis, but HUS can recur in the transplanted kidney. Recovery of renal function occurs in 65% to 85% of patients with HUS excluding the hereditary and recurrent forms.

ALPORT'S SYNDROME

Alport's syndrome consists of hereditary nephritis, high-frequency hearing loss, and ocular abnormalities. Children may present with recurrent or persistent hematuria and proteinuria. A family history of nerve deafness is usually obtained, and one or more family members may have died from renal failure, undergone dialysis, or received a renal transplant. Gene-mapping studies suggest that clinical subtypes of juvenile-onset ESRD with deafness and adult-onset ESRD with normal hearing are caused by allelic mutations of a single genetic locus on the X chromosome. Also, there is strong evidence that a genetic defect in type IV collagen is responsible for the glomerular basement membrane defects found in renal biopsy tissue from these patients (Kashtan et al, 1990). The nephritis is progressive in nature, especially in male patients, and leads to renal failure in the second or third decade of life.

SYSTEMIC LUPUS ERYTHEMATOSUS

Systemic lupus erythematosus (SLE) is a multisystem autoimmune disease characterized by widespread inflammation that most often affects women in the second or third decade of life. SLE affects Asian Americans, African Americans, Hispanic Americans, and white Americans in decreasing order of prevalence. The classic disease onset is marked by fever, rash, arthritis, varying degrees of renal involvement, and decreased C3 and C4 complement. Renal involvement is a major cause of morbidity and mortality. Eighty percent of pediatric patients with SLE are female, and the peak age at onset is 12 years. Between 60% and 80% of children have renal involvement at the time of diagnosis, and renal involvement occurs in most of the rest within 2 years.

The histologic forms of SLE nephropathy are mesangial lupus nephritis (or minimal glomerular involvement), membranous lupus nephropathy, focal glomerulonephritis (FGN), and diffuse proliferative glomerulonephritis (DPGN), which is the most severe form. Hematuria and proteinuria are almost always observed at diagnosis in children with DPGN (88%), and at least half of these patients have massive proteinuria leading to the nephrotic syndrome. Renal insufficiency is most often seen in patients with DPGN. Membranous nephropathy is usually associated with the nephrotic syndrome, and 50% of patients have microscopic hematuria. Children with FGN have hematuria and mild proteinuria.

SLE may be treated with prednisone, azathioprine, chlorambucil, or cyclophosphamide. Patients with DPGN are treated with an initial course of methylprednisolone followed by high doses of prednisone. Patients with changes in renal function, urinary protein excretion, C3 and C4, and anti-DNA antibody concentration receive follow-up care. If clinical or laboratory improvement after several weeks of treatment fails to occur, or if unacceptable steroid side effects appear, intravenous cyclophosphamide therapy can be considered. Studies in both adults and children demonstrate gratifying improvement in renal function after treatment with low-dose oral prednisone, seven monthly doses of intravenous cyclophosphamide, and additional intravenous cyclophosphamide every 3 months for 18 to 24 months. Longer follow-up observations of patients receiving treatment with this latter protocol are ongoing.

CRESCENTIC GLOMERULONEPHRITIS

Crescentic glomerulonephritis may be associated with most forms of primary glomerulonephritis or with systemic diseases such as SLE, Henoch-Schönlein purpura, and systemic vasculitis. Patients with a rapidly progressive clinical course usually have large epithelial crescents in more than 50% of their glomeruli on renal biopsy. Children with poststreptococcal crescentic glomerulonephritis usually recover after only symptomatic therapy. However, systemic vasculitis carries a worse prognosis, which may be favorably influenced by treatment with plasmapheresis, corticosteroids, or alkylating agents.

Anti-neutrophil cytoplasmic autoantibodies (ANCA) are found in the circulation of patients with necrotizing systemic vasculitis (polyarteritis nodosa, Wegener's gran-

ulomatosis) **or idiopathic pauci-immune glomerulonephritis.** Few if any immune deposits are observed by immunofluorescence microscopy in these patients.

The presence of anti-glomerular basement membrane
(GBM) antibodies in patients with lung hemorrhage (Good-
pasture's syndrome) and in those without lung hemorrhage
(anti-GBM disease) aid in diagnosing anti-GBM–mediated
glomerulonephritis. Anti-DNA autoantibodies, anti-strepto-
coccal antibodies, and serum cryoglobulins differentiate lupus glomerulonephritis, poststreptococcal glomerulonephritis, and cryoglobulinemic glomerulonephritis, respectively,
as forms of immune complex glomerulonephritis.

SICKLE CELL NEPHROPATHY

**Specific renal functional abnormalities, such as in-
creased total renal blood flow, decreased flow in the
vasa recta, decreased maximum urine osmolality in response to water deprivation, abnormal lowering of
urine pH in response to acid loading, and increased
tubular secretion of uric acid, occur in patients with
sickle cell disease. The features of the clinical entity
referred to as sickle cell nephropathy include hematuria, papillary necrosis, glomerulopathy, nephrogenic diabetes insipidus, incomplete renal tubular acidosis, hyperuricemia, and asymptomatic bacteriuria.**

**Hematuria is a common renal abnormality in patients
with sickle cell anemia. Dysmorphic RBCs similar to
those seen in other forms of glomerulonephritis are usually seen in patients with sickle cell nephropathy, but
sickled forms of RBCs may or may not be observed
microscopically in this condition.** Heterozygotes are affected more frequently than homozygotes, probably because there are many more heterozygotes in the population.
**Boys are affected more often than girls, and the hema-
turia most frequently arises from the left kidney. Bed
rest and hydration should be tried first as treatment. If
hematuria is prolonged for 1 to 2 weeks or if transfusion is necessary, alkalinization, aminocaproic acid, or
intravenous diuresis should be tried.**

Patients with sickle cell disease may develop the nephrotic syndrome, which can progress to renal failure. Glomerular pathology includes reduplication of the basement
membrane with mild mesangial proliferation, focal glomerulosclerosis, or immune complex glomerulonephritis. We
(Roy et al, 1976) and others have reported acute poststreptococcal glomerulonephritis in several patients with sickle
cell disease.

THIN GLOMERULAR BASEMENT MEMBRANE DISEASE

Recurrent or permanent microhematuria may occur in a
familial form. This finding has also been referred to as
benign recurrent hematuria or benign familial hematuria to
differentiate it from Alport's syndrome, which has a much
worse prognosis. In some children benign familial hematuria is accompanied by thin glomerular basement membranes and lamina densa (1233 ± 51 Å and 682 ± 31 Å,
respectively, as opposed to the normal dimensions of
1863 ± 31 Å and 1402 ± 40 Å). In one study of 43
patients with isolated microhematuria and abnormal find-

ings on renal biopsy, the only abnormality in 17 patients
was thin glomerular capillary basement membranes
(Trachtman et al, 1984). The presence of microhematuria
in other family members who do not have a history of
renal disease or neurosensory deafness (or did not die from
renal disease) is usual, but urinalyses must be performed
on these family members. RBC casts are common, but
proteinuria is usually absent or minimal.

The results of one well-designed and -performed study
(Trachtman et al, 1984) in children suggest that a renal
biopsy is necessary in patients with microhematuria only if
there is a positive family history of hematuria in a first-
degree relative or if the child has had at least one episode
of gross hematuria. In this study, the findings in almost
75% of renal biopsy specimens were abnormal, and IgA
nephropathy and Alport's syndrome were present in 60%
of cases. The renal biopsy in a child with isolated microscopic hematuria almost always shows a normal morphology or nonspecific alterations of unknown clinical relevance.

PROTEINURIA

Isolated Proteinuria

Transient Proteinuria

Proteinuria on a routine screening urinalysis is not uncommon in the pediatric population. It may be related to a
febrile illness, exercise, congestive heart failure, seizures,
or exposure to cold. **In a study of 8954 schoolchildren
between the ages of 8 and 15 years, proteinuria was
present in one of four urine specimens in 10.5% of the
children and in at least two of four specimens in 2.5%**
(Vehaskari and Rapola, 1982). Proteinuria may indicate a
completely benign condition, or it may be the first clue to
a significant renal parenchymal disease such as the nephrotic syndrome or glomerulonephritis. Proteinuria is initially detected most often by a semiquantitative dipstick
analysis or by the turbidimetric sulfosalicylic acid method.
In an otherwise asymptomatic child, the test for proteinuria
should be repeated two or more times. If only the first
urine sample is positive for protein, routine medical care is
recommended, and the proteinuria is considered isolated or
transient.

Orthostatic Proteinuria

If two or more urine samples are positive for protein,
testing to demonstrate orthostatic proteinuria is recommended. The child voids at bedtime and the sample is
discarded. A urine sample is then obtained before the patient arises in the morning or after as little ambulation as
possible; this is labeled specimen number 1. A second
sample is collected later in the day and labeled specimen
number 2. The specific gravity of the first urine sample
should be 1.018 or greater. If specimen 1 is free of protein
and specimen 2 is positive for protein, the orthostatic test
is positive. This test should be repeated to confirm the
presence of orthostatic proteinuria. If both samples of urine

contain protein, a systematic evaluation for other causes of proteinuria is necessary.

Persistent Asymptomatic Proteinuria

Persistent proteinuria exists when at least 80% of urine specimens contain excessive amounts of protein. The first step in evaluating a child with persistent proteinuria is to quantitate the urinary protein excretion by means of a timed urine sample (12- or 24-hour collection) or with a random urine Upr/Ucr ratio. Urinary protein excretion of more than 4 mg/m²/hr is abnormal, and a level greater than 40 mg/m²/hr is in the nephrotic range. A Upr/Ucr ratio (mg/mg) in a random urine sample that is greater than 0.18 is abnormal, and a ratio greater than 1.0 is in the nephrotic range.

In patients with a confirmatory test for orthostatic proteinuria and more than 1.0 g/day of urinary protein excretion and in those with a nonconfirmatory test for orthostatic proteinuria, the following studies should be performed: serum electrolytes, BUN, serum creatinine, serum albumin, serum complement (C3), urine culture, and renal ultrasound. A renal biopsy may also be considered, depending on the results of this evaluation.

Studies in children with persistent asymptomatic proteinuria have reported either a good prognosis, minimal histologic changes on renal biopsy, or significant renal histologic changes associated with the possibility of progressive renal failure. Among 53 children who underwent renal biopsy because of persistent asymptomatic proteinuria, significant glomerular abnormalities were observed in 47% (Yoshikawa et al, 1991). Focal segmental glomerulosclerosis (FSGS) was observed in 15 patients, with chronic renal failure in 7 of them. A worse prognosis in children with FSGS plus the nephrotic syndrome than in those with FSGS and persistent asymptomatic proteinuria has been reported (Roy and Stapleton, 1987). However, patients in the latter category occasionally progress to chronic renal failure during follow-up. Effective treatment in many patients with persistent asymptomatic proteinuria may not be possible. It is reasonable to recommend a renal biopsy when excessive asymptomatic proteinuria has persisted for longer than 6 to 12 months. This allows a more accurate prognosis to be made in anticipation of potential specific treatment in the future.

Proteinuria with Glomerular Diseases

Nephrotic Syndrome

The nephrotic syndrome in children is defined as the presence of edema, hypoalbuminemia (<2.5 g/dl), hypercholesterolemia, and urinary protein excretion greater than 40 mg/m²/hr or a Upr/Ucr ratio greater than 1.0 (mg/mg). Other laboratory abnormalities, such as hyponatremia, hypocalcemia (low albumin-bound calcium with normal ionized calcium concentration), and coagulation abnormalities, are commonly present. Recognized histologic forms of childhood nephrotic syndrome are minimal change disease (MCNS), FSGS, membranoproliferative glomerulonephritis

(MPGN), membranous glomerulonephritis (MEMB-GN), and mesangial proliferative glomerulonephritis (MESP-GN) (Kelsch and Sedman, 1993).

MINIMAL CHANGE NEPHROTIC SYNDROME

Children with the nephrotic syndrome present with edema or with proteinuria discovered during a routine office visit. MCNS accounts for 60% to 90% of children with the nephrotic syndrome. Evaluation of these patients should include measurements of serum electrolytes, BUN, creatinine, C3 and C4 complement, streptozyme titer, antinuclear antibody titer, and hepatitis B antibody titer. **Children with MCNS almost always have a normal C3. A renal biopsy is necessary in children with the nephrotic syndrome who are younger than 1 year or older than 10 years of age, children who have a low C3 level or a positive antinuclear antibody test, and those in whom the disease has a major "nephritic" component.** Recommended treatment consists of daily prednisone (60 mg/m²/day) for 4 to 6 weeks, followed by a dose of 40 mg/m² on alternate days for 4 to 6 weeks and tapering doses for 4 weeks thereafter (Brodehl, 1991). Approximately 93% of children with MCNS respond to prednisone, 71% have a subsequent relapse, and 44% have multiple relapses. Steroid-resistant patients should have a renal biopsy, and patients with multiple relapses may require a biopsy before a course of either cyclophosphamide or chlorambucil.

FOCAL SEGMENTAL GLOMERULOSCLEROSIS

Children with the nephrotic syndrome who fail to respond to a 2-month course of prednisone require a renal biopsy. **Many of these nephrotic children are found to have FSGS, especially those who are older than 8 to 10 years of age.** FSGS discovered on renal biopsy generally carries a poor prognosis and may progress to renal failure. Up to 30% of patients with FSGS who receive a renal transplant may develop a recurrence of FSGS in the transplanted organ.

MEMBRANOPROLIFERATIVE GLOMERULONEPHRITIS

MPGN is diagnosed most often during the initial evaluation of patients with nephrotic syndrome because 70% to 80% have a low C3 concentration and are candidates for renal biopsy. They tend to have a nephritic clinical picture rather than the typical nephrotic syndrome at initial presentation. Approximately half of these patients will progress to ESRD after 10 years of follow-up. Prednisone (40 mg/m² on alternate days) is usually recommended for children with MPGN and is continued for years.

MEMBRANOUS NEPHROPATHY

Idiopathic membranous nephropathy is rarely seen in children. The secondary form of MEMB-GN may be seen in patients with SLE, hepatitis B infection, or gold therapy for severe rheumatoid arthritis; on rare occasions it appears de novo in patients who have undergone renal transplantation. As many as half of children with primary membranous nephropathy sustain a spontaneous remission. A course of prednisone is indicated for patients with membranous nephropathy and clinically overt nephrotic syndrome or renal insufficiency.

Membranous nephropathy in North American children secondary to hepatitis B surface antigenemia is not common. In one report (Southwest Pediatric Nephrology Study Group, 1985) 7 of 11 children were male and black, and the mean age of 5.3 years was somewhat less than that of children with idiopathic membranous nephropathy. Eight of 10 patients had elevated aspartate aminotransferase concentrations, all 11 children at some stage of their illness had low serum C3 concentrations, and 10 of 11 had the nephrotic syndrome.

MESANGIAL PROLIFERATIVE GLOMERULONEPHRITIS

MESP-GN has an unpredictable clinical course. Some patients respond to prednisone in a manner similar to those with MCNS, but others fail to respond to steroids or alkylating agents and progress to renal insufficiency. Some patients undergo a remission of the nephrotic syndrome without any treatment.

CONGENITAL NEPHROTIC SYNDROME

If the nephrotic syndrome is diagnosed in a child who is younger than 1 year of age, a renal biopsy is indicated. If edema and proteinuria are noted during the first 3 months of life, the congenital nephrotic syndrome should be suspected. Cytomegalic inclusion disease and syphilis must be excluded. Congenital nephrotic syndrome does not respond to steroids and must be managed conservatively. Long-term management may include daily intravenous albumin infusion, bilateral nephrectomy, dialysis, and early renal transplantation. These children are prone to pneumococcal sepsis, peritonitis, clotting abnormalities, and malnutrition. On rare occasions a spontaneous remission occurs, so aggressive therapy such as bilateral nephrectomy, dialysis, and transplantation should be delayed until a serious, life-threatening complication of congenital nephrotic syndrome occurs.

Proteinuria with Tubulointerstitial Diseases

Reflux Nephropathy

Proteinuria in a child with a history of a urinary tract infection or unexplained febrile illness treated with antibiotics should alert the physician to the possibility of reflux nephropathy. These children are usually hypertensive. Renal ultrasound may not demonstrate cortical scarring, and therefore a dimercaptosuccinic acid (DMSA) scan should be obtained. Especially in older children, vesicoureteral reflux may have resolved by the time renal scarring is demonstrated.

Acute Tubulointerstitial Nephritis

Acute tubulointerstitial nephritis (ATIN) is characterized by diffuse or focal inflammation and edema of the renal interstitium with secondary involvement of the tubules and minimal or no glomerular changes. **Clinically, patients may have mild to severe renal failure, normal or decreased urinary output, mild hematuria, decreased urinary concentration, proteinuria, pyuria, white blood cell casts, and, in up to 86% of patients with drug-induced ATIN, eosinophiluria as documented by Hassel stain. Eosinophiluria is evident in fewer than 5% of patients with ATIN induced by use of nonsteroidal anti-inflammatory drugs.**

IMMUNE-MEDIATED ACUTE TUBULOINTERSTITIAL NEPHRITIS

The major clinical manifestations of immune-mediated ATIN are those of tubular dysfunction, including proteinuria with glomerular dysfunction, proximal renal tubular acidosis or Fanconi's syndrome with proximal tubular dysfunction, distal renal tubular acidosis, hyperkalemia or sodium wasting with distal tubular dysfunction, and decreased concentrating capacity with medullary and papillary dysfunction. A histologic form of ATIN showing linear immunofluorescence of the tubular basement membrane with IgG and complement is known as anti-tubular basement membrane disease. Sarcoidosis, Sjögren's syndrome, and tubulointerstitial nephritis-uveitis syndrome are other examples of immune-mediated ATIN. **When findings are inconclusive for prerenal azotemia, the clinical picture is not characteristic of ATIN, and obstructive nephropathy has been excluded, a renal biopsy may be required for diagnosis.**

DRUG-RELATED ACUTE TUBULOINTERSTITIAL NEPHRITIS

Systemic manifestations of an allergic process—such as rash, fever, and eosinophilia—may accompany ATIN in patients with drug-induced ATIN. The drugs most commonly associated with ATIN are antibiotics (methicillin, penicillin, ampicillin, cephalosporins, sulfonamides, rifampin); nonsteroidal anti-inflammatory drugs (fenoprofen, naproxen, ibuprofen); and diuretics.

INFECTION-RELATED ACUTE TUBULOINTERSTITIAL NEPHRITIS

Streptococcal diseases, diphtheria, toxoplasmosis, brucellosis, syphilis, rickettsia, Epstein-Barr virus infections, and other conditions have also been implicated in the etiology of ATIN. Resolution of ATIN often occurs with removal of the inciting factors (e.g., drugs) or with treatment of the causative infections. **In biopsy-proven ATIN in which renal failure has persisted for longer than 1 week after removal of the inciting factors or when no inciting factors can be found, a short course of high-dose prednisone therapy is recommended** (Neilson, 1989). If the biopsy already shows significant interstitial scarring, less chance of benefit from steroid therapy can be expected. Lack of response to steroids after 3 to 4 weeks is an indication to discontinue therapy. Cyclophosphamide is very effective in animal models of ATIN. **In patients who fail to respond to steroids and have minimal or no fibrosis on biopsy, cyclophosphamide is suggested for 3 to 4 months if the GFR improves.**

RENAL TUBULAR DISORDERS

Nephrogenic Diabetes Insipidus

The inability of a male child to form concentrated urine after receiving the antidiuretic hormone arginine vasopressin suggests a diagnosis of X-linked nephrogenic diabetes insipidus (NDI). In neonates the symptoms of NDI are seen during the first weeks of life and include polyuria, polydipsia, irritability, poor feeding, poor weight gain, fever, and dehydration. Later in childhood obstipation, nocturia, enuresis, poor growth, and mental retardation are seen. Long-standing polyuria may lead to the development of megaureter and hydronephrosis, which can mimic lower urinary tract obstruction. Plasma vasopressin levels are usually normal or slightly elevated in affected children.

Two genetically recessive forms of NDI are recognized. Defects in the X-linked gene encoding the type 2 vasopressin receptor, AVPR2, are responsible for most cases. Congenital NDI may also be caused by homozygous defects in AQP2, a gene on chromosome 12 encoding the water channel protein aquaporin-2. Genetic testing for NDI may be used to confirm a clinical diagnosis in an affected male or female, to establish the carrier status of a female relative, to test a newborn in a family with known NDI, or to establish an X-linked inheritance pattern.

Secondary forms of NDI must be excluded. These include drug-induced disease (lithium and tetracyclines), analgesic nephropathy, sickle cell disease, hypokalemia, hypercalcemia, obstructive uropathy, renal dysplasia, chronic hydronephrosis, amyloidosis, sarcoidosis, and chronic uremic nephropathy.

A combination of hydrochlorothiazide and amiloride will decrease urine volume, increase urine osmolality, and conserve potassium in patients with NDI. The efficiency of this therapy in patients with NDI is attributed to reduction of the extracellular sodium concentration with enhancement of sodium reabsorption.

Miscellaneous Tubular Disorders

Cystinosis

Low serum bicarbonate, potassium, and phosphate concentrations associated with glucosuria, aminoaciduria, hyperchloremic metabolic acidosis, and rickets characterize the proximal tubulopathy known as Fanconi's syndrome. In the past the most common cause of Fanconi's syndrome in children was infantile nephropathic cystinosis. These children have blond hair, photophobia, depigmentation of the retina, short stature, rickets,

and renal insufficiency by 10 years of age. The syndrome is caused by an abnormal efflux of cystine out of the lysosome of most cells of the body. In addition to bicarbonate, phosphate, and vitamin D (calcitriol) supplementation, cysteamine, a cystine-depleting agent, may slow the eventual progression to renal failure.

Ifosfamide Toxicity

Acquired forms of Fanconi's syndrome may occur after exposure to heavy metals (lead, cadmium, mercury); antibiotics (gentamicin, outdated tetracycline, cephalosporin); or ifosfamide or during the final stages of the nephrotic syndrome secondary to FSGS. Ifosfamide has been used with increasing frequency in the treatment of solid tumors, especially Wilms' tumor, in children. One report (Burk et al, 1990) described five children with Wilms' tumor who developed Fanconi's syndrome after a total ifosfamide dose of 70 to 108 g/m². In addition to the tubulopathy a marked decline in glomerular filtration was observed in these patients. **Appropriate monitoring before each course of ifosfamide and close attention to the total drug dose given during treatment are recommended.**

Renal Glucosuria

Renal glucosuria is defined by the presence of glucosuria when the plasma glucose concentration is less than 120 mg/dl. The loss of a glucose transport system is the cause of the glucosuria. The glucose threshold is significantly reduced. Glucosuria is usually found unexpectedly by a glucose-specific dipstick urine test. Because isolated glucosuria is frequently familial, siblings and parents should also be tested with a glucose-specific urinary test. Glucosuria may also be caused by an overflow mechanism secondary to hyperglycemia that occurs in patients with diabetes mellitus who are receiving intravenous dextrose solutions, epinephrine injections, or glucocorticoid administration. **Treatment is not indicated for isolated glucosuria.**

Bartter's Syndrome

A distal renal tubular syndrome that is caused by disordered sodium chloride reabsorption and is characterized by hyper-reninemic hypokalemic metabolic alkalosis is known as Bartter's syndrome. **Signs and symptoms associated with the syndrome are usually the consequence of hypokalemia. Patients initially present with weakness, fatigue, neuromuscular irritability, muscle cramps, polyuria, polydipsia, and failure to thrive in infancy.** Three genetic and clinical entities have been recognized: neonatal Bartter's syndrome (type 1), "classic" Bartter's syndrome (type 2), and Gitelman's syndrome (type 3). Two molecular defects at the gene coding for the renal bumetanide-sensitive Na-K-2Cl cotransporter (NKCC2) or at the gene coding for the inwardly rectifying K channel (ROMK) have been described for type 1 Bartter's syndrome. Either deletions or mutations at the gene coding for a renal chloride channel gene (ClC-Kb) have been identified for the type 2 "classic" syndrome. Mutations at the gene coding for the thiazide-sensitive NaCl cotransporter (NCCT) have been identified for type 3 Gitelman's syndrome. Bartter's syndrome must be distinguished from surreptitious vomiting and diuretic use and abuse. Therapy consists of potassium chloride replacement in conjunction with either spironolactone or amiloride.

REFERENCES

History and Physical Examination

Mimran A: Renal function in hypertension. Am J Med 1988;84(Suppl 1B):69–75.
Still JL, Cottom D: Severe hypertension in childhood. Arch Dis Child 1967;42:34–39.

Laboratory Data

Birch DF, Fairley KF: Hematuria: Glomerular or nonglomerular? Lancet 1979;2:845–846.
Crompton CH, Ward PB, Hewitt JK: The use of urinary red cell morphology to determine the source of hematuria in children. Clin Nephrol 1993;39:44–49.
Ghazali S, Barratt TM: Urinary excretion of calcium and magnesium in children. Arch Dis Child 1974;49:97–101.
Norman ME: An office approach to hematuria and proteinuria. Pediatr Clin North Am 1987;34:545–560.
Rizzoni G, Braggion F, Zacchelo G: Evaluation of glomerular and nonglomerular hematuria by phase-contrast microscopy. J Pediatr 1983;103:370–374.
Roth S, Renner E, Rathert P: Microscopic hematuria: Advances in identification of glomerular dysmorphic erythrocytes. J Urol 1991;146:680–684.
Schwartz GJ, Haycock G, Edelmann CM Jr, Spitzer A: A simple estimate of glomerular filtration rate in children derived from body length and plasma creatinine. Pediatrics 1976;58:258–263.
Stapleton FB: Morphology of urinary red blood cells: A simple guide to localizing the site of hematuria. Pediatr Clin North Am 1987;34:561–569.
Stapleton FB, Noe HN, Jerkins GR, Roy S III: Urinary excretion of calcium following an oral calcium loading test in healthy children. Pediatrics 1982;69:594–597.
Vehaskari VM, Rapola J, Koskimies O, et al: Microscopic hematuria in school children: Epidemiology and clinicopathologic evaluation. J Pediatr 1979;95:676–684.

Hematuria

Dodge WF, West EF, Smith EH, Bunce H: Proteinuria and hematuria in school children: Epidemiology and early natural history. J Pediatr 1976;88:327–347.
Fitzwater DS, Wyatt RJ: Hematuria. Pediatr Rev 1994;15:102–109.
Ghazali S, Barratt TM: Urinary excretion of calcium and magnesium in children. Arch Dis Child 1974;49:97–101.

Hogg RJ, Silva FG, Wyatt RJ, et al: Prognostic indicators in children with IgA nephropathy: Report of the Southwest Pediatric Nephrology Study Group. Pediatr Nephrol 1994;8:15–20.
Ingelfinger JR, Davis AE, Grupe WE: Frequency and etiology of gross hematuria in a general pediatric setting. Pediatrics 1977;59:557–561.
Kalia A, Travis LB, Brouhard BH: The association of idiopathic hypercalciuria and asymptomatic gross hematuria in children. J Pediatr 1981;99:716–719.
Kaplan BS, Cleary TG, Obrig TG: Recent advances in understanding the pathogenesis of the hemolytic uremic syndromes. Pediatr Nephrol 1990;4:276–283.
Kashtan CE, Kleppel MM, Bukowski RJ, et al: Alport syndrome, basement membranes and collagen. Pediatr Nephrol 1990;4:523–532.
Moore ES: Hypercalciuria in children. Contrib Nephrol 1981;27:20–32.
Noe HN, Stapleton FB, Jerkins GR, Roy S III: Clinical experience with pediatric urolithiasis. J Urol 1983;129:1166–1168.
Noe HN, Stapleton FB, Roy S III: Potential surgical implications of unexplained hematuria in children. J Urol 1984;132:737–738.
Roy S III, Murphy WM, Pitcock JA, Rimer RL: Sickle-cell disease and poststreptococcal acute glomerulonephritis. Am J Clin Pathol 1976;66:986–990.
Roy S III, Stapleton FB, Noe HN, Jerkins GR: Hematuria preceding renal calculus formation in children with hypercalciuria. J Pediatr 1981;99:712–715.
Siegler RL: Management of hemolytic uremic syndrome. J Pediatr 1988;112:1014–1020.
Stapleton FB, Noe HN, Jerkins GR, Roy S III: Urinary excretion of calcium following an oral calcium loading test in healthy children. Pediatrics 1982;69:594–597.
Stapleton FB, Roy S III, Noe HN, Jerkins GR: Hypercalciuria in children with hematuria. N Engl J Med 1984;310:1345–1348.
Trachtman H, Weiss RA, Bennett B, Griefer I: Isolated hematuria in children: Indications for a renal biopsy. Kidney Int 1984 25:94–99.

Proteinuria

Brodehl J: Conventional therapy for idiopathic nephrotic syndrome in children. Clin Nephrol 1991;35:58–65.
Kelsch R, Sedman AB: Nephrotic syndrome. Pediatr Rev 1993;14:30–38.
Neilson EG: Pathogenesis and therapy of interstitial nephritis. Kidney Int 1989;35:1257–1270.
Roy S III, Stapleton FB: Focal segmental glomerulosclerosis in children: Comparison of nonedematous and edematous patients. Pediatr Nephrol 1987;1:281–285.
Southwest Pediatric Nephrology Study Group: Hepatitis B surface antigenemia in North American children with membranous glomerulonephropathy. J Pediatr 1985;106:571–578.
Vehaskari VM, Rapola J: Isolated proteinuria: Analysis of a school-age population. J Pediatr 1982;101:661–668.
Yoshikawa N, Kitagawa K, Ohta K, et al: Asymptomatic constant isolated proteinuria in children. J Pediatr 1991;119:375–379.

Renal Tubular Disorders

Burk CK, Restaino I, Kaplan BS, Meadows AT: Ifosfamide-induced renal tubular dysfunction and rickets in children with Wilms tumor. J Pediatr 1990;117:331–335.

54
URINARY TRACT INFECTIONS IN INFANTS AND CHILDREN

Linda M. Dairiki Shortliffe, MD

Recognition that evaluating for risk factors of urinary tract infections (UTIs) in children may prevent bacteriuria and subsequent renal parenchymal and functional loss has prompted recommendations for rapid diagnosis and evalua-tion of UTIs and the development of new genitourinary imaging techniques and tests. In infants UTIs are a com-mon cause of fever and are probably the most common cause of renal parenchymal loss. For this reason the goal of managing UTIs in children is based on identifying and modifying, if possible, those factors that may increase the risk of renal parenchymal and functional loss beginning at the time of the index infection. This chapter focuses on the host and bacterial mechanisms by which bacteria gain access to the bladder and kidney, the management and evaluation of first and recurrent UTIs, the short- and long-term complications of UTI, and possible means of preventing or limiting renal damage.

EPIDEMIOLOGY OF PEDIATRIC URINARY TRACT INFECTIONS

More boys than girls get UTIs during the first year of life (Asscher et al, 1973; Winberg et al, 1974), and during that period uncircumcised boys have as high as 10 times the risk of circumcised boys of having a UTI (Rushton and Majd, 1992a; Wiswell and Hachey, 1993). By 1 year of age, 2.7% of boys and 0.7% of girls have had bacteriuria (Wettergren et al, 1980). Although this incidence falls below 1% in school-age boys (ranging between 0.03% and 1.2% during the school years), it rises to 1% to 3% in school-age girls (Asscher, 1975; Savage, 1975; Bailey, 1979), and sexually active females have more UTIs than sexually inactive females do (Kunin and McCormack, 1968).

DIAGNOSIS OF URINARY TRACT INFECTION

Clinical Symptoms

Rapid and early diagnosis of UTIs is essential to initiating prompt antimicrobial treatment and preventing renal damage. Among infants and young children who have no source for their fever from the history or physical findings, more than 5% have a UTI (American Academy of Pediatrics, 1999). Among febrile infants (younger than 8 weeks of age), the prevalence of UTI has been found to be 13.6%, with the majority of infections occurring in male infants (Lin et al, 2000).

UTI in infants may be vague and without localization. Young children may show only signs of generalized illness—fever, irritability, poor feeding, vomiting, and diarrhea. In seriously ill infants and young children, one must suspect UTI and obtain a urinary specimen even if signs may point elsewhere (Hoberman and Wald, 1997; American Academy of Pediatrics, 1999). Older children may describe symptoms that localize to the urinary tract, such as dysuria, suprapubic pain, intermittent voiding dysfunction, and incontinence.

Physical Examination

There are no signs specific for UTI in the infant. If there is a gross genitourinary anatomic abnormality, a renal mass may be palpable, as found in children with xanthogranulomatous pyelonephritis or infected severe hydronephrosis.

Palpation in the suprapubic and flank areas may cause pain in the older child, but generalized abdominal or upper quadrant pain may also be present. Perineal examination rarely shows an ectopic ureteral opening, ureterocele, or urethral discharge in girls. Signs such as back scars, sacral fat pads, or sacral dimples or pits may suggest a neurogenic bladder and may require further investigation. In boys the testes may be abnormal if affected by epididymitis or epididymo-orchitis, and in girls labial adhesions and vaginal abnormalities should be noted.

Diagnostic Tests

Urinary Specimens

Good urinary specimens with which to make the diagnosis of UTI may be hard to obtain in children, and the reliability of the diagnosis is related to the quality of the specimen. Routinely there are four ways that urinary specimens are obtained in children. They are listed in order of least to most reliable for UTI diagnosis (Hardy et al, 1976): (1) plastic bag attached to the perineum—"a bagged specimen," (2) midstream void, (3) catheterized, or (4) suprapubic bladder aspirate. Even after extensive skin cleansing, a plastic bag specimen usually reflects the perineal and rectal flora and often leads to indeterminate results. Although a midstream-voided specimen in a circumcised boy, older girl, or older uncircumcised boy who can retract his foreskin may reliably reflect bacteriuria, such specimens obtained in young girls and uncircumcised boys usually reflect periurethral and preputial organisms and cells. A catheterized specimen is reliable if the first portion of urine that may contain urethral organisms is discarded and the specimen is taken from later flow through the catheter, but it has the disadvantages of being traumatic and of potentially introducing urethral organisms into a sterile bladder (Dele Davies et al, 1992; Lohr et al, 1994).

The most reliable urinary specimen for culture is obtained by suprapubic bladder aspiration. This can be performed safely in children and even in premature infants with a full bladder by cleansing the skin and percutaneously introducing a 21- or 22-gauge needle 1 to 2 cm above the pubic symphysis until urine is obtained by aspiration into a sterile syringe (Barkemeyer, 1994). Although it is unnecessary in most instances, in infants and young children suprapubic aspiration may be simplified with ultrasound guidance (Buys et al, 1994) and use of topical and local anesthesia. Because the urine does not cross the urethra, urethral and periurethral organisms are absent; skin contamination should be nil. Organisms that are present in a suprapubic aspirate are pathognomonic of bacteriuria, and low bacterial counts are routine (Buys et al, 1994). The main drawback of suprapubic aspiration is that needle aspiration may be distasteful or inconvenient to the older child, parent, or physician, and these considerations may be important (Kramer et al, 1994a).

Generally, if a UTI is suspected in a child who is not yet toilet-trained, only a catheterized or needle-aspirated specimen is acceptable for diagnosis because "bagged" urinary specimens have an unacceptably high false-positive rate. Under special collection circumstances when the perineum is cleaned well and the bag is removed and processed promptly after voiding, a "bagged" specimen or even a diaper specimen showing no growth may be useful in eliminating bacteriuria as a possibility (Ahmad et al, 1991). Plastic bag specimens are unreliable and unacceptable for diagnosis of UTI in high-risk populations and in infants younger than 2 months old (Crain and Gershel, 1990).

Urinalysis

The gold standard for the diagnosis of UTI is quantitative urinary culture. This requires that known quantity of urine to be plated onto a culture plate and the number of bacterial colony-forming units (cfu) that grow to be counted and determined as number of units per milliliter. The interpretation of the culture result defining a UTI diagnosis is, however, debatable and is dependent on specimen quality. Because it may take 24 hours or longer before bacterial colony-forming units grow and the culture is complete, indirect urinary tests that may be performed with routine urinalysis to detect the presence of bacteria or byproducts have been sought for more rapid diagnosis. Four determinations from the urinalysis have been advocated to support a diagnosis of UTI: (1) microscopic urinary examination for white blood cells (WBCs)—"pyuria"—usually defined as more than 5 WBCs per high-powered field in a centrifuged specimen; (2) microscopic urinary examination for bacteria, defined as any number of bacteria per high-powered field in the unstained, centrifuged urinary sediment; (3) urinary leukocyte esterase; and (4) urinary nitrite. The finding of red blood cell (RBC) and WBC casts in the urinary sediment is unreliable.

Microscopic Examination

Although there are many confounding factors, the microscopic identification of bacteria in the urine is more sensitive and specific for diagnosing UTI than identification of pyuria (Hallender et al, 1986; Lohr, 1991). Identification of bacteria under high dry magnification (450× to 570×) represents about 30,000 bacteria per milliliter. In a meta-analysis of screening tests, microscopic identification of any bacteria on Gram staining of uncentrifuged urine had the best combination of sensitivity and false-positive rate (Gorelick and Shaw, 1999). The use of either of these tests separately has such low sensitivity in this high-risk population, however, that neither can be relied on.

In febrile children younger than 2 years of age, Hoberman and associates found that catheter-collected specimens had a positive predictive value for UTI diagnosis of 84.6% if microscopic examination showed bacteria (any bacteria on 10 oil-immersion fields in a Gram-stained specimen) and at least 10 WBCs/mm³ (*not* per high-powered field—enhanced urinalysis) (Hoberman and Wald, 1997). Although these two parameters may offer the best predictive value, neither test as described (quantitative WBC count and Gram-stained bacteria on unspun specimen) can be easily and rapidly performed by the office practitioner without further instruction. Moreover, the investigators emphasized that UTI in these children is still best defined by

a urinary leukocyte count of at least 10 WBCs/mm³ and at least 50,000 cfu/ml bacteria on culture (Hoberman et al, 1994; Hoberman and Wald, 1997).

Urinary Leukocyte Esterase, Nitrite, and Other Chemical Tests

Several other "quick" tests that may be performed on urinalysis have been popular for trying to predict UTI. The **urinary leukocyte esterase** test detects urinary enzymes produced by the breakdown of WBCs in the urine and, as such, is dependent on the presence of WBCs that may or may not be present with the infection. The test may be less reliable in infants (Hoberman et al, 1994). Dietary nitrates that are reduced to nitrite by many gram-negative urinary bacteria are measured by the **urinary nitrite test**. The facts that a first morning voided urinary specimen should be used for this test (because bacterial reduction of nitrate may take several hours) and that most gram-positive bacteria do not perform this reduction are serious drawbacks. The test for **urinary catalase**, an enzyme commonly produced by bacteria infecting the urinary tract, although sensitive, has too high a false-positive rate for reliability (Waisman et al, 1999). Although these tests may be performed by urinary dipstick or rapid screening, they are even less reliable when the bacterial count is less than 100,000 cfu/ml.

In a general pediatric population it has been shown that when urinary specimens are properly collected and promptly processed, the combination of positive leukocyte esterase and nitrite testing with microscopic confirmation of bacteria has almost 100% sensitivity for detection of UTI and, when all (or the leukocyte esterase and nitrite tests) are negative, the negative predictive value approaches 100% (Wiggelinkhuizen et al, 1988; Lohr et al, 1993). The arguments for and against relying on urinalysis characteristics for presumptive diagnosis of a UTI are well summarized (Lohr, 1991; American Academy of Pediatrics, 1999; Gorelick and Shaw, 1999).

Although there is no test or combination of urinary tests that meets the gold standard of culture, combinations of these tests may help suggest patients in whom culture will be positive and in whom presumptive treatment might be started. However, the urinalysis cannot replace urinary culture (American Academy of Pediatrics, 1999).

When a risk-benefit analysis based on the current literature on febrile children aged 3 to 24 months was performed with the goal of preventing the majority of cases of end-stage renal disease (ESRD) and hypertension, both urinalysis and culture were needed to optimize prevention (Kramer et al, 1994b).

Urinary Culture

What constitutes a "significant" UTI is unclear. It is controversial whether "colonization" of the urinary tract occurs (i.e., benign bacteriuria) or whether "colonization" represents specimen contamination or asymptomatic benign infection. As already discussed, **the technique by which the urinary specimen is collected is related to its reli-**

Table 54–1. CULTURE CRITERIA FOR DIAGNOSIS OF URINARY TRACT INFECTION

Method of Collection	Colony Count (Pure Culture)	Probability of Infection (%)
Suprapubic aspiration	Gram-negative bacilli: any number	
	Gram-positive cocci: more than a few thousand	>99
Catheterization	>10^5	95
	10^4–10^5	Infection likely
	10^3–10^4	Suspicious; repeat
	<10^3	Infection unlikely
Clean-voided (male)	>10^4	Infection likely
Clean-voided (female)	3 specimens: >10^5	95
	2 specimens: >10^5	90
	1 specimen: >10^5	80
	5×10^4–10^5	Suspicious; repeat
	10^4–5×10^4	Symptomatic; suspicious; repeat
	10^4–5×10^4	Asymptomatic; infection unlikely
	<10^4	Infection unlikely

From Hellerstein S: Recurrent urinary tract infections in children. Pediatr Infect Dis 1982;1:271–281.

ability for UTI diagnosis (Table 54–1) (Hellerstein, 1982). Although at least 100,000 cfu/ml of voided urine is the traditional definition for a clinically significant UTI (Kass and Finland, 1956), other studies have shown that 10,000 or fewer organisms on a voided specimen may indicate a significant UTI (Stamm et al, 1982; Bollgren et al, 1984). In febrile children younger than 2 years of age, Hoberman and associates showed that 50,000 or more colony-forming units per milliliter in catheterized specimens constituted a significant UTI (Hoberman et al, 1994). It should be noted, however, that in most of these studies only 0.001 ml of urine was cultured, so that the minimal limit of detection was 1000 cfu. Occasionally low numbers of bacteria may indicate a significant UTI, especially when the specimen is obtained by suprapubic aspiration, a circumstance under which any number of organisms might be significant. The number of cultured colony-forming units per milliliter may be low because of hydrational dilution, frequent voiding that prevents bacterial multiplication in the bladder, or bacterial growth characteristics.

Tests Indicating Renal Involvement

Complete blood counts (Kramer et al, 1993), erythrocyte sedimentation rate (ESR), C-reactive protein (CRP), urinary concentrating ability (Åbyholm and Monn, 1979), urinary tubular enzymes (Johnson et al, 1990; Tomlinson et al, 1994), antibody coated bacteria, urinary antibodies, and interleukin 6 (Il-6) (Benson et al, 1994) have been examined as possible simple and noninvasive markers of renal infection (Buyan et al, 1993). Although the host urinary tract responds to bacterial infections with the production of cytokines, and Il-6 is secreted in response to *Escherichia coli* attachment, it appears that this local response is then followed by a systemic increase in CRP and fibrinogen, which suggests that fever, CRP, and ESR are all part of the same host response to bacterial attachment (de Man et al, 1991). Reduced urinary concentrating ability is usually associated with pyelonephritis, but this appears to be unassociated with the acute febrile response in pyelonephritis and is probably not a reliable sign for early detection of pyelonephritis (de Man et al, 1991). None of these tests has proven reliable enough for early detection, differentiation between upper and lower tract infections, or determination of the severity of infection to become used routinely. They are performed primarily on experimental bases.

CLASSIFICATION OF URINARY TRACT INFECTIONS

UTIs have been classified in many ways: complicated versus uncomplicated, upper versus lower tract, persistent infections versus reinfections, and symptomatic versus asymptomatic. For practical purposes, **pediatric UTIs may be simply categorized into two types: initial (first) infections and other (recurrent) infections. Recurrent infections may then be classified as (1) unresolved bacteriuria during therapy, (2) bacterial persistence at an anatomic site, or (3) reinfection** (Stamey, 1975). The reason for categorizing infections in children as first or other is related to their evaluation and management. In infants and children first UTIs are "complicated" because of the evaluation and management implications (Fig. 54–1).

UTIs may be *unresolved* because of inadequate therapy related to bacterial resistance to the selected therapeutic agent, inadequate antimicrobial urinary concentration due to poor renal concentration or gastrointestinal malabsorption, or infection by multiple organisms. Unresolved infections can usually be treated successfully once proper culture and antimicrobial sensitivity patterns are obtained.

In infants and children, sources of urinary tract bacterial *persistence* are usually found early because radiologic evaluation is performed after the first UTI. The discovery of urinary tract sources of bacterial persistence that are surgically correctable are obviously important (Table 54–2). Most recurrent UTIs are, however, reinfections with the same or a different organism.

Infections that are asymptomatic or "covert," as designated by Savage (1975) and found only on screening urinary culture when a child is being examined for reasons unrelated to urinary infection, can still be classified among these types.

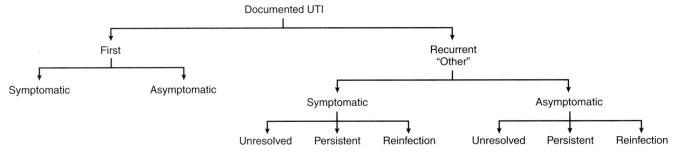

Figure 54–1. Functional classification of urinary tract infections in children.

BACTERIA

The most common bacteria infecting the urinary tract are the gram-negative Enterobacteriaceae, usually *E. coli* (Kunin et al, 1964; Bergström, 1972; Winberg et al, 1974). Specific cell wall O-antigens that can be identified by serotyping have shown that specific *E. coli* serotypes (e.g., O1, O2, O4, O6, O7, and O75) are associated with pediatric UTIs (Kunin et al, 1964; Winberg et al, 1974).

Another bacterial trait that may increase virulence for the urinary tract are surface structures called *pili* or *fimbriae*. The bacterial fimbriae mediate bacterial adherence to uroepithelial cells and RBC agglutination, both of which can be used to characterize virulence. RBC agglutinating characteristics of the *E. coli*, called hemagglutination, can be blocked by various sugars (Duguid et al, 1978; Svanborg Edén and Hanson, 1978). Using this characteristic, Källenius and associates (1981) discovered that pyelonephritogenic *E. coli* cause mannose-resistant hemagglutination (MRHA) of human RBCs. Characterization of this reaction showed that the terminal glycolipid of the human RBC P blood-group antigen is a receptor that binds P fimbriae on these *E. coli*. Therefore, two important markers for *E. coli* virulence are MRHA characteristics and P blood-group-specific adhesins (P fimbriae or P pili) (Källenius et al, 1981; Väisänen et al, 1981).

The importance of these two virulence markers has been supported by research examining their association with clinically diagnosed pyelonephritis and cystitis. In one study, most *E. coli* strains causing pediatric clinical pyelonephritis had both MRHA (29/32 or 91%) and P fimbriae (81%), and P fimbriae were absent on less virulent strains (Väisänen et al, 1981). Similarly, Källenius and associates (1981) found P fimbriae on 94% (33/35) of *E. coli* causing acute pyelonephritis, on 19% (5/26) of *E. coli* causing

acute cystitis, on 14% (5/36) of *E. coli* causing asymptomatic bacteriuria, and on 7% (6/82) of *E. coli* from the feces of healthy children.

More recently, when pyelonephritis and cystitis were defined by findings of renal inflammation on technetium 99m dimercaptosuccinic acid (^{99m}Tc-DMSA) renal scanning, the distinctions between upper and lower tract bacteria were less clear. When pyelonephritis was defined by inflammation as determined by ^{99m}Tc-DMSA scanning, P-fimbriated *E. coli* were more likely to cause fever than non–P-fimbriated *E. coli*, whether or not the kidney was involved (Majd et al, 1991; Jantausch et al, 1992). This characteristic of P fimbriation was supported by the finding that the urinary Il-6 response is higher in children infected with P-fimbriated *E. coli* than in those infected by other organisms (Benson et al, 1994). It has been suggested, moreover, that UTIs caused by P-fimbriated strains may need longer antimicrobial courses than those caused by other strains (Tambic et al, 1992). Other, less well characterized virulence factors may involve the hydrophobic properties of *E. coli* and an iron-binding capability of the bacteria associated with Aerobactin production (Jacobson et al, 1988, 1989b).

There is some evidence that covert or asymptomatic UTIs are caused by bacteria that have less virulent characteristics (e.g., self-agglutination) and are less likely to have fimbriae.

PATHOGENESIS OF URINARY TRACT INFECTION IN CHILDREN

The natural history of the pediatric UTI is unpredictable and incompletely understood. Although a child's risk factors and the bacterial virulence may partially predict the course of a UTI, these factors alone have not been useful in predicting an individual's susceptibility for pyelonephritis, renal scarring, or parenchymal and functional loss from a single or recurrent UTI. About 3% of girls and 1% of boys will get a prepubertal UTI (Winberg et al, 1974), and of these children 17% or more will get infection-related renal scarring. Of those with scarring, 10% to 20% will become hypertensive, and a rare child will get progressive renal dysfunction culminating in ESRD (Fig. 54–2).

Although it has been recognized that the course of UTIs in adults and children may differ, UTIs in children have often been studied en bloc without regard for age and other pediatric-specific factors. For this reason, the course of pediatric UTIs is still elusive. Research has shown, how-

Table 54–2. SURGICALLY CORRECTABLE CAUSES OF BACTERIAL PERSISTENCE IN CHILDREN

Infection stones
Infected nonfunctioning or poorly functioning kidneys or renal segments
Infected ureteral stumps after nephrectomy
Vesicointestinal or urethrorectal fistula
Vesicovaginal fistula
Infected necrotic papillae in papillary necrosis
Unilateral medullary sponge kidney
Infected urachal cyst
Infected urethral diverticulum or periurethral gland

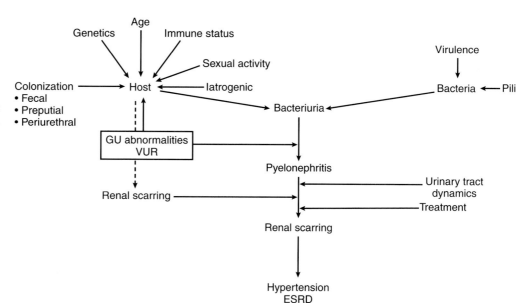

Figure 54–2. Factors that affect the development of bacteriuria and subsequent pyelonephritis, renal scarring, hypertension, and end-stage renal disease (ESRD). Urinary tract urodynamics reflects urinary tract pressures and related factors.

ever, that host factors such as genetics, immune status, gender, circumcision status, diet, and gut and periurethral colonization may alter susceptibility to UTIs in children.

Cystitis and Pyelonephritis

Bacterial clonal studies have shown that common entry into the urinary tract occurs through a fecal-perineal-urethral route with retrograde ascent of periurethral bacteria (Kaijser and Larsson, 1982; Tullus et al, 1984; Mitsumori et al, 1997). Once bacteria have reached the bladder, ascent to the kidneys may be affected by factors such as impaired ureteral peristalsis, vesicoureteral reflux (VUR), or the specific organism. Although hematogenous dissemination of infection can occur, it usually occurs in infants with incompletely developed immunity, from staphylococcal skin or systemic infections, or from specific organisms, such as tuberculosis. In these situations renal, perirenal, or epididymal abscesses may be occur.

Although the importance of pyelonephritis is emphasized because of its potential for causing renal damage, bacterial infection of the collecting system also causes bladder and ureteral inflammation with changes that alter the dynamics of the entire urinary tract (Hinman, 1971; Boyarsky and Labay, 1972; Issa and Shortliffe, 1992; Johnson et al, 1992). Although the full cause of ureteral dilation observed during acute infection is unclear, it is in part related to the effect of bacterial toxins and smooth muscle compliance changes associated with inflammation. Animal studies have shown that UTIs cause abnormally elevated renal pelvic pressures even if (or especially if) VUR is absent (Issa and Shortliffe, 1992; Angell et al, 1998), thus giving increased pressure as a further explanation for the ureteral dilation observed in children with acute pyelonephritis and otherwise normal upper tract collecting systems (Mårild et al, 1989a).

Clinically, determining the progression from cystitis to pyelonephritis or differentiating between these entities is difficult because simple techniques with which to localize the level and extent of urinary tract bacteria are lacking. Although ureteral catheterization has been the gold standard for localizing upper and lower tract bacteriuria, this requires invasive cystoscopy and is an impractical way of monitoring the course of infection (Stamey, 1980). It cannot, moreover, reveal the extent of renal inflammation. The Fairley bladder washout localization technique requires urethral catheterization during acute infection and washing of the bladder with sterile water to determine whether the source of bacteria is from the bladder or supravesical. This technique also cannot be performed or repeated easily during the course of a UTI. In localization studies that have used the Fairley or ureteral catheterization techniques, however, clinical symptoms have correlated poorly with location of bacteria. In one such study, fewer than half the patients (the majority children) with fever and flank pain had upper tract bacteria (34/73), whereas almost 20% (83/473) who were asymptomatic had upper tract bacteria (Busch and Huland, 1984).

UTI is a common cause of pediatric bacterial infection (Crain and Gershel, 1990; Bonadio et al, 1993; Hoberman et al, 1993). Fever accounts for about 20% of pediatric office visits (Eggli and Tulchinsky, 1993), and UTI causes 4.1% to 7.5% of these febrile episodes (American Academy of Pediatrics, 1999). In children younger than 2 years of age, symptoms of UTI are vague and generalized—fever, irritability, poor feeding, vomiting, diarrhea, and ill appearance (Ginsburg and McCracken, 1982) (Table 54–3). Specifically, in febrile infants from birth to 8 to 10 weeks, neither clinical symptoms nor laboratory tests can be used to predict a presumptive UTI, nor to eliminate the likelihood of a UTI, even if other sites of infection are suggested clinically (Crain and Gershel, 1990). The prevalence of UTI in febrile infants (younger than 8 weeks) has been found to be about 13.6% with the majority of UTIs occurring in male infants (Lin et al, 2000). Furthermore, it

Table 54–3. SYMPTOMS OF URINARY TRACT INFECTION IN 100 INFANTS WITH ACUTE URINARY TRACT INFECTIONS

Symptom	Percentage
Fever	67
≥38°C	100
≥39°C	57
Irritable	55
Poor feeding	38
Vomiting	36
Diarrhea	36
Abdominal distention	8
Jaundice	7

Modified from Ginsburg CM, McCracken GHJ: Urinary tract infections in young infants. Pediatrics 1982;69:409–412.

is important that **febrile infants in whom UTI is unsuspected are as likely to have a urinary source of infection as those with suspected UTI (5.1% versus 5.9%), and 3.5% of infants with another possible source (e.g., otitis media) also had a UTI** (Hoberman et al, 1993)

The older, toilet-trained, talking child may indicate signs that better localize to the urinary tract, such as dysuria, suprapubic pain, voiding dysfunction, incontinence, or flank and/or abdominal pain, but many of these children still do not describe urinary tract symptoms. In children without localizing signs or with symptoms only vaguely referable to the urinary tract, suspicion must be high to avoid missing the diagnosis.

The clinical course of pyelonephritis depends on the severity of the disease and the rapidity of treatment. Among 288 children age 2 years or younger (median age, 5.6 months) who were hospitalized with a diagnosis of febrile UTI, 89% became afebrile within 48 hours after treatment with parenteral antimicrobial agents was started, even if bacteremia or a significant genitourinary abnormality was found (Bachur, 2000). The median time to attain a normal temperature was 13 to 16 hours.

Acute and Focal Pyelonephritis (Lobar Nephronia or Focal Bacterial Nephritis)

Symptoms and Signs

Children with pyelonephritis have the classic symptoms of fever, chills, and unilateral or bilateral flank pain with or without accompanying lower tract symptoms of dysuria, frequency, and urgency. They may not localize symptoms to their flanks and may complain of nonspecific abdominal discomfort. Physical examination reveals fever, usually accompanied by abdominal discomfort and pain over the costovertebral area.

The urine is usually cloudy and malodorous. Urinary sediment usually shows pyuria, WBC casts, and RBCs. Bacterial rods are often present. Bacterial infection of the urinary tract causes bladder, ureteral, renal pelvic, and renal inflammation that alters urinary tract urodynamics and causes ureterectasis, elevated renal pelvic pressures, and renal inflammatory changes that may be associated with renal swelling (Hinman, 1971; Boyarsky and Labay, 1972; Issa and Shortliffe, 1992; Johnson et al, 1992).

Radiologic Findings

The discoveries that early renal cortical lesions from pyelonephritis can be detected by ^{99m}Tc-DMSA nuclear scanning and that these lesions correlate with histopathologic areas of acute renal inflammation in animal models have advanced knowledge of the natural history of urinary tract bacteriuria (Parkhouse et al, 1989; Wikstad et al, 1990; Rushton and Majd, 1992a; Giblin et al, 1993). Radiologic findings in acute pyelonephritis depend on the imaging modality used. When intravenous urography was the main urinary tract imaging modality, the majority of patients had normal studies. Other modalities now show that findings commonly include renal enlargement related to inflammation and edema, focal renal enlargement (acute lobar nephronia or focal bacterial pyelonephritis), impaired or delayed excretion, and dilation of the urinary collecting system.

Focal or general renal enlargement or swollen kidneys may be found in acute pyelonephritis. Renal ultrasonography, nuclear scans, and computed tomography (CT) may show generalized renal enlargement or focal hypoechoic or hyperechoic areas representing focal pyelonephritis (lobar nephronia). The latter represents a localized, severe, nonliquefactive infection of one or more renal lobules (Greenfield and Montgomery, 1987; Klar et al, 1996; Wallin et al, 1997; Uehling et al, 2000). Other findings on ultrasonography include thickening of the renal pelvis, hypoechogenicity, and focal or diffuse hyperechogenicity and ureteral dilation (Mårild et al, 1989a; Morin et al, 1999). CT or power Doppler studies may show areas of decreased perfusion (Dacher et al, 1996). High-resolution renal ultrasonography has been suggested to be almost as sensitive as DMSA for diagnosing renal involvement in pyelonephritis (Dacher et al, 1996; Morin et al, 1999).

When DMSA-defined lesions are used as the standard for diagnosis of acute pyelonephritis, about 50% to 86% of children with febrile UTI and other clinical signs (about 60% of kidneys) have renal involvement or pyelonephritis (Verber and Meller, 1989; Rushton and Majd, 1992b; Benador et al, 1994; Jakobsson et al, 1994). About half (38% to 75%) of these lesions persist on DMSA scans performed 2 months to 2 years later (Rushton and Majd, 1992b; Benador et al, 1994; Stokland et al, 1996), with fewer lesions persisting at longer intervals of follow-up. **This suggests that as many as 40% to 50% of young children who have febrile UTIs suffer renal scarring.** Among children older than 1 year of age with their first symptomatic UTI, 38% had DMSA evidence of renal damage after 1 year, and almost half of these (47%) had reflux. Children who presented with an elevated CRP, fever, and dilating reflux had a 10 times higher risk of renal damage than children with UTI who had a normal or slightly elevated CRP, no or mild fever, and no VUR (Stokland et al, 1996; Yen et al, 1999).

Pyonephrosis

Pyonephrosis is characterized by the accumulation of purulent debris and sediment in the renal pelvis and urinary collecting system. Children with pyonephrosis have symptoms similar to those of acute pyelonephritis but have additional obstructive hydronephrosis. This situation usually implies bacterial infection and obstruction, and rapid diagnosis and treatment are essential to avoid sepsis and parenchymal loss.

Most often renal ultrasonography is diagnostic. The majority of obstructed pyonephrotic kidneys are either nonfunctioning or poorly functioning (Colemen et al, 1981). The renal sonogram may show shifting fluid–debris levels with changes in the patient's position, persistent echoes from the lower collecting system, air in the collecting system, or weak echoes secondary to pus in a dilated, poorly transonic renal collecting system (Colemen et al, 1981). If performed, retrograde pyelography shows ureteral obstruction and irregular renal pelvic filling defects caused by purulent sediment. When it is possible to pass a ureteral catheter past the obstruction, drainage becomes both diagnostic and therapeutic.

Pyonephrosis is treated by administration of appropriate antimicrobial drugs and prompt drainage of the infected pelvis by either retrograde catheterization or nephrostomy placement. When the acute infection is treated and the patient is taking appropriate antimicrobial agents, further evaluation may be needed to identify and treat the obstruction.

Perinephric or Renal Abscess

Improvements in radiologic imaging of the genitourinary tract and widespread use of powerful antimicrobial agents have changed the diagnosis and natural history of perinephric and renal abscesses (Shortliffe and Stamey, 1986a). In the past the high mortality rate from perinephric abscesses related in part to the diagnostic delay. Perinephric and renal abscesses are uncommon in children.

These abscesses arise from either hematogenous seeding from extragenitourinary sites of infection or renal extension of ascending urinary infection. Since the introduction of broad-spectrum and powerful antimicrobial agents in the 1940s, the percentage of perirenal abscesses caused by staphylococci decreased from 45% before 1940 to 6% after 1940, and the percentage attributed to *E. coli* and *Proteus* rose from 8% to 30% and from 4% to 44% percent, respectively (Thorley et al, 1974). This large decrease in perirenal and renal abscesses due to staphylococci is thought to be related to the wide use of antimicrobial agents to treat skin and wound abscesses (Thorley et al, 1974; Shortliffe and Stamey, 1986a).

Clinically, patients with these renal and perirenal abscesses present with symptoms of severe pyelonephritis—fever, flank pain, leukocytosis, and occasionally sepsis. With the frequent use of renal ultrasonography for evaluation of such symptoms, this is the most common diagnostic modality. Because most abscesses have a fluid component, perinephric collections usually appear sonolucent, and diagnostic aspiration of this area usually carries minimal morbidity. The extent of the abscess may be better assessed by CT, which may show perirenal fluid or gas, renal distortion, and involvement of the retroperitoneum (Hoddick et al, 1983).

Although *Staphylococcus aureus* with antecedent skin

lesions may have been the most common cause of renal abscesses in children and adults more than 2 decades ago (Rote et al, 1978), gram-negative organisms (*E. coli*) are now more common proportionately and are more likely to be associated with retrograde extension of ascending infection in relation to genitourinary anomalies (Rote et al, 1978; Steele et al, 1990; Barker and Ahmed, 1991; Vachvanichsanong et al, 1992). Anaerobic bacteria may cause perinephric or renal abscesses in association with previous abdominal surgery, renal transplantation, malignancy, or oral or dental infection (Brook, 1994).

Newer, powerful antimicrobial agents have occasionally allowed successful treatment of abscesses in children with antimicrobial agents alone, without surgical drainage (Steele et al, 1990; Vachvanichsanong et al, 1992). In many cases, however, a combination of percutaneous or surgical drainage with appropriate antibiotic therapy is eventually required for treatment (Rote et al, 1978; Steele et al, 1990; Vachvanichsanong et al, 1992).

Chronic Pyelonephritis, Renal Scarring, and Function

Previously coarse renal scarring detected radiologically by calyceal deformity and renal parenchymal thinning over localized or multiple calyces was called "reflux nephropathy." Now that it is clear that such scarring is as likely to occur with or without reflux, this kind of scarring would probably be better termed "pyelonephritogenic scarring."

The reason that children's kidneys scar and adult's rarely do is not known. Renal scarring appears to be affected by at least five factors: intrarenal reflux, urinary tract pressure, host immunity, age, and treatment. In 1974 Rolleston and associates found that areas of renal scarring were associated with foci of intrarenal reflux (pyelotubular backflow) observed on voiding cystourethrography in children younger than 4 years of age who had VUR (Rolleston et al, 1974). Calyces allowing reflux contained papillae fused with adjacent papillae such that the papillary ducts opened at right angles, rather than at oblique angles more resistant to reflux (Ransley and Risdon, 1974). These compound papillae were found most commonly at the renal poles, the areas in which renal scarring is most commonly observed clinically (Hannerz et al, 1987). Common patterns of scarring are shown in Figure 54–3.

In pigs with VUR and even intrarenal reflux, however, renal scarring occurred only when both VUR and bacteriuria are present (Ransley and Risdon, 1978). Reflux alone without bacteriuria resulted in renal scarring only if the urethra was partially obstructed, causing abnormally high voiding pressures (Hodson et al, 1975; Ransley et al, 1984). Experimentally, therefore, the "water-hammer" effect of vesicoureteral and intrarenal reflux caused renal scarring only if reflux occurred with abnormally high bladder and renal pressures. Renal infection stimulates both humoral and cellular immune responses. In rat models of pyelonephritis, maximal renal suppuration and exudation with inflammatory infiltration occurs 3 to 5 days after the infection starts, and collagen infiltration and scarring follow (Glauser et al, 1978; Miller et al, 1979; Miller and Phillips, 1981; Roberts et al, 1981; Shimamura, 1981; Slotki and Asscher, 1982). During the acute inflammatory infiltration,

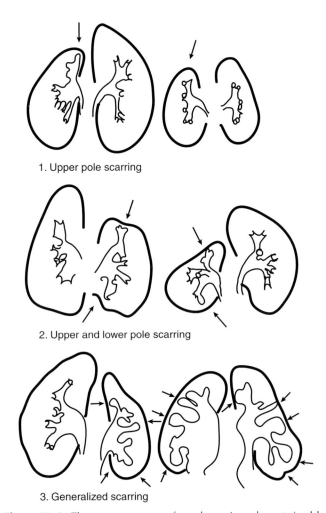

1. Upper pole scarring

2. Upper and lower pole scarring

3. Generalized scarring

Figure 54–3. The common areas of renal scarring, characterized by parenchymal thinning over a deformed calyx, as examined from intravenous pyelograms. The extent of scarring may be related to single polar scars; multiple areas of upper, lower, and medial scars; or generalized scarring, as depicted. (Reproduced by permission from Hodson CJ: Natural history of chronic pyelonephritic scarring. Br Med J 1965;2:191–194.)

granulocytic aggregation may cause vascular occlusion and ischemia with elevation in renin (Kaack et al, 1986; Ivanyi and Thoenes, 1987). Bactericidal activity of the neutrophils and the release of enzymes, superoxide, and oxygen radicals may cause the renal tubular damage observed in pyelonephritis (Roberts et al, 1982). The resulting proximal and distal tubular dysfunction causes reduced urinary concentrating ability (Walker, 1990) with increased fractional sodium excretion, decreased phosphate reabsorption, and increased excretion of low-molecular-weight proteins (Tulassy et al, 1986). Clinical studies have correlated decreased renal concentrating capacity with severity of renal scarring (bilateral worse than unilateral) (Åbyholm and Monn, 1979). Other studies have correlated increased excretion of urinary retinol-binding protein (RBP, a tubular protein giving evidence of tubular dysfunction) with the type and severity of renal scarring and have linked elevated excretion of N-acetyl-β-D-glucosaminidase (NAG, an excretory protein indicating tubular damage) and albumin mainly to children with bilateral scarring. These data sug-

gest that tubular dysfunction occurs before glomerular dysfunction and that it commonly occurs in children with bilateral renal scarring (Tomlinson et al, 1994).

If antimicrobial treatment is started within the first days of infection, the acute suppurative response to the bacteria may be minimized and renal scarring may be decreased or prevented (Glauser et al, 1978; Miller and Phillips, 1981; Shimamura, 1981; Slotki and Asscher, 1982). Inhibition of superoxide production may decrease renal inflammation and tubular damage (Roberts et al, 1982). Other animal studies suggest that supplementing antimicrobial treatment with anti-inflammatory agents—such as ibuprofen, which decreases neutrophil chemotaxis and blocks the cyclooxygenase pathways, or other glucocorticoid anti-inflammatory agents—may decrease renal scarring (Huang et al, 1999; Pohl et al, 1999). **Clinical studies have shown that the larger cortical defects correlate with longer delay to treatment and longer length of illness** (Jakobsson et al, 1992). **Moreover, the likelihood of renal scarring correlates directly with the number of occurrences of UTI** (Jodal, 1987; American Academy of Pediatrics, 1999) (Fig. 54–4).

Other **clinical reports confirm the kidney in the young child to be at greatest risk of renal scarring from bacterial pyelonephritis.** Several factors contribute to this situation. First, the neonatal kidney may respond to urinary backpressure, the "water-hammer" effect, in different ways and at different thresholds than the adult kidney. Autopsy studies on normal neonates (younger than 1 month) reveal that intrarenal reflux into compound calyces may be created at low pressures of 2 mm Hg, whereas the same reflux in a child 1 year old occurs at 20 mm Hg. Furthermore, in autopsy studies of children younger than 12 years of age, intrarenal reflux was found to occur in all calyces, even simple ones, at 50 mm Hg (Funston and Cremin, 1978). This suggests that physiologically normal urinary intrapelvic pressures in adults or older children may be abnormally high in neonates. This effect may be augmented by increased renal pelvic pressures that may result from ureteral and pelvic smooth muscle dysfunction (Issa and Shortliffe,

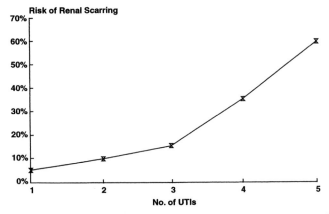

Figure 54–4. The relationship between risk of renal scarring and number of urinary tract infections. (Reproduced with permission from American Academy of Pediatrics Committee on Quality Improvement, Subcommittee on Urinary Tract Infection: Practice parameter: The diagnosis, treatment, and evaluation of the initial urinary tract infection in febrile infants and young children. Pediatrics 1999;103:845.)

1992). Moreover, it is known that renal scarring may occur with or without VUR. Animal models of bacterial urinary infection have shown that infection elevates renal pelvic pressures whether or not reflux is present and, in fact, renal pelvic pressures may even be higher when reflux is absent. This may also account for further parenchymal damage with severe infection (Issa and Shortliffe, 1992; Angell et al, 1998).

Second, **very young children have an incompletely developed immune and neurologic system.** A depressed or incompletely mature immune system may allow easier colonization of the bladder and kidney by bacteria because of decreased local and systemic defenses. It may also kill or eliminate bacteria less efficiently once bacteriuria occurs. Moreover, neurologic immaturity of the bladder may allow frequent uninhibited bladder contractions to transmit these pressures to the upper tracts in even the apparently normal child (Koff and Murtagh, 1984). Bacteriuria combined with reflux in such a child may result in greater susceptibility to renal damage.

Third, **neonatal symptoms of urinary infection and pyelonephritis are often vague and nonspecific, resulting in delayed or inadequate treatment.** This may result in a kidney that responds to bacterial invasion with an inflammatory response characterized by vascular granulocytic aggregation and hypoperfusion with subsequent scarring and loss of renal parenchyma (Winberg et al, 1974).

Small, scarred kidneys must not be confused with congenitally small, dysplastic, poor, or nonfunctioning kidneys. This distinction, one that is difficult and sometimes impossible to make radiologically, is important because dysplastic kidneys are congenitally histologically abnormal. Dysplastic kidneys and atrophic, scarred kidneys are histologically different. Although gross renal changes may be detected radiologically, lesser lesions that may be related to infectious insult (e.g., cortical pitting, mild global renal shrinkage) may not be detected by radiologic tests and yet may affect renal function.

With the older imaging techniques used before DMSA, about 17% of school children with screening bacteriuria (i.e., bacteriuria found on cultures performed for screening rather than for symptoms) were shown to have renal scarring (Asscher et al, 1973; Newcastle Asymptomatic Bacteriuria Research Group, 1975; Savage, 1975). This correlates with Winberg's observation that 4.5% of children had radiologic renal scars after their first symptomatic UTI, and 17% had scars after the second symptomatic UTI (Winberg et al, 1974). The percentage of scars in these reports may underestimate actual scarring, because **current studies using DMSA scintigraphy suggest that the incidence of scarring after symptomatic UTI could be almost twice this rate. These data emphasize that children with both covert and symptomatic UTI risk significant renal scarring.** By definition the natural history and pathogenesis of scarring in covert or asymptomatic bacteriuria cannot be known, but these scars may really reflect injury from previous undiagnosed bacteriuric episodes and the child's predisposition for recurrent infections.

In most children with UTI in whom renal scars are found, the scars are found on the first set of imaging studies and remain unchanged regardless of the child's future clinical course (Verber and Meller, 1989). It has

been hypothesized that the young kidney is more prone to damage and that the initial UTI in the neonate or young child (before 4 or 5 years of age) causes whatever renal damage will occur, this initial response determining the kidney's future course. This theory is supported by the higher prevalence of early cortical DMSA defects observed in children younger than 2 years of age who have UTIs, compared with those who are older (Ditchfield et al, 1994b).

Although older children may have less risk of scarring from infection than those younger than 5 years of age, vulnerability for scarring persists at least until puberty (10 to 15 years) (Smellie et al, 1985; Shimada et al, 1989). Studies of DMSA-detected renal scarring suggest that new or progressive scarring may be more common than previously thought; that up to 7.3% of children with recurrent or persistent bacteriuria and reflux may scar (Shimada et al, 1989; Verber and Meller, 1989; Jakobsson et al, 1994); and that almost all young children with recurrent pyelonephritis suffer renal scarring (Jakobsson et al, 1994). Earlier studies also linked new or progressive renal scarring to uncontrolled recurrent UTIs and VUR (Filly et al, 1974; Smellie et al, 1985). Filly and associates found that in girls younger than 10 years of age who had recurrent UTIs and VUR, renal scars progressed (i.e., developed clubbing or scarring in an area that was previously normal or developed a focal parenchymal decrease of at least 3 mm between examinations) in 43% (17/40) of kidneys, and 2 of 16 normal kidneys developed new scars (Filly et al, 1974). Some of the scars took up to 2 years from the episode of pyelonephritis to evolve maximally.

Conversely, radiologic evaluation of girls with nonobstructive reflux grade 2 to 4/5 (International Grading) without recurrent infections showed no renal damage for up to 10 years (Holland et al, 1990). This supports earlier animal and clinical data that, given normal urinary tract urodynamics, VUR alone (sterile reflux) does not cause renal damage or impaired renal growth (Ransley and Risdon, 1978; Smellie et al, 1981; Ransley et al, 1984). If no infections occur, no association between severity of VUR and impaired renal growth has been demonstrated in an otherwise normal urinary tract (Smellie et al, 1981). Moreover, adults who have acute nonobstructive pyelonephritis and normal urinary tracts rarely develop focal renal cortical scarring, and papillary and/or calyceal distortion or measurable generalized renal shrinkage rarely occurs (Davison and Lindheimer, 1978).

Pyelonephritogenic Hypertension

The incidence of hypertension in childhood depends on age and sex and has been reported to be between 1% and 11%. Renal-related hypertension is most common (Dillon, 1979). **Children with gross pyelonephritogenic nephropathy (reflux nephropathy) have at least a 10% to 20% risk of future hypertension** (Holland et al, 1975; Wallace et al, 1978; Smellie and Normand, 1979; Jacobson et al, 1989a) with risks of later progressive deterioration in renal function and other complications of hypertension.

Wallace and associates (1978) found that 12.8% of 141 patients with urinary infections and surgically corrected

VUR developed hypertension during the first 10 years of follow-up. Of those with renal scarring, 17% became hypertensive during follow-up. In another series, Smellie and Normand (1979) monitored 83 children with scars, of whom 11 had initial hypertension (6 with malignant hypertension) and another 14 (19%) became hypertensive over the next 4 to 20 years, making a total of 30% who developed infection-related hypertension. In Sweden, Jacobson and associates (1989a) found that 7 (23%) of 30 children with nonobstructive focal renal scarring developed hypertension after 27 years, and of these 10% developed ESRD. Eleven of the children studied by Smellie and Normand had hypertension initially but none of Wallace's or Jacobson's did, probably indicating that the group monitored by Smellie and Normand had more severe initial renal damage. In both series, however, **hypertension occurred whether renal scarring was segmental, focal, unilateral, or bilateral and was, therefore, independent of the degree of scarring.**

The etiology of pyelonephritogenic hypertension is poorly understood. It is likely that the renin-angiotensin system is involved. In 1978 at Great Ormand Street in London the plasma renin activity was measured in children with reflux nephropathy that had been corrected surgically 1 to 10 years before (Savage et al, 1978). Among 15 children who were hypertensive when studied, all had plasma renin activities above the normal mean, and 9 were above normal for their age, whereas plasma renin levels were above the normal range for age in 8 of 100 children who were normotensive after the surgery. When 85 of these 100 children were traced 5 years later, it was found that 4 had developed serious hypertension and 4 others had borderline hypertension (Savage et al, 1987). A single elevated plasma renin activity level in 1978 did not, however, predict hypertension 5 years later, and by 1987 19% (16/85) of the children had elevated plasma renin activity. In this study, moreover, the normal tendency for the plasma renin activity to decrease with increasing age was not seen and instead the opposite was observed: plasma renin activity increased with age and the standard deviation increased. On further follow-up the percentage of children with elevated peripheral plasma renin activity continued to increase during the teenage years after age 15 but appeared to plateau by 25 years of age, and blood pressure had leveled by 15 years of age (Goonasekera et al, 1996). Peripheral plasma renin elevation did not predict future hypertension during the 15 years of follow-up.

The value of selective renal vein renin measurements in the management of hypertension from reflux nephropathy in children is controversial (Holland et al, 1975; Stecker et al, 1977; Bailey et al, 1978, 1984a; Dillon et al, 1984) even though segmental renal vein renins have been useful in some for localizing sources of renin production (Dillon et al, 1984). Further indirect evidence of the role of renin in pyelonephritogenic nephropathy has been the successful treatment of hypertension with agents specifically aimed at blocking the renin-angiotensin system. In those children who were examined with renal arteriography, normal main renal arteries were found to proceed into scarred kidneys, with vascular changes limited to small interlobular arterial branches (Holland et al, 1975; Stecker et al, 1977).

Renal Function After Pyelonephritis

Although renal failure associated with acute pyelonephritis occurs rarely, after recurrent pyelonephritis, especially that associated with pyelonephritogenic nephropathy, some children develop delayed hypertension and progressive renal dysfunction without further known UTIs. Generally, when measured years after UTI, overall renal function is well preserved but the individual glomerular filtration rate (GFR) of scarred kidneys is decreased; this decrease correlates inversely with the original degree of VUR when associated with reflux (higher-grade reflux = lower GFR) (Jacobson et al, 1989a; Wennerström et al, 2000). As might be expected with long-term follow-up, individuals with small kidneys, whether scarred or not, had a lower GFR than those with normal kidneys, and those with bilaterally small or scarred kidneys had the lowest GFRs (Berg, 1992). Most long-term studies suggest that early detection of complications of renal scarring, such as hypertension, renal insufficiency, and proteinuria, is useful in minimizing progressive deterioration in renal function (Jacobson et al, 1989a; Berg, 1992; Martinell et al, 1996; Smellie et al, 1998; Wennerström et al, 2000). When renal scarring is found in children or bilateral renal scarring is found in adults with a history of UTI, it appears to be a risk factor for further decrease in renal function (Smellie, 1991; Smellie et al, 1998; Wennerström et al, 2000).

For more than a decade glomerular lesions and progressive proteinuria have been observed in patients with renal scarring (Kincaid-Smith, 1975; Torres et al, 1980). Significant proteinuria (>1 g/24 hr) has been a routine finding in patients with VUR and progressive deterioration in renal function (Torres et al, 1980). Certain investigators, moreover, have found glomerular sclerosis in the nonscarred, radiologically normal kidney in cases of unilateral reflux nephropathy (Kincaid-Smith, 1975, 1984; Bailey et al, 1984b). Two theories—one involving progressive renal damage from hyperfiltration of remaining nephrons and the other involving progressive immunologic damage to the kidney—have been postulated to explain this finding.

Micropuncture studies of rat renal tubules allow measurement of single-nephron GFRs. These investigations show that removal of a kidney or loss of a majority of its functioning nephrons results in hyperfiltration in the remaining nephrons and increased glomerular plasma flow. From rat studies in which one kidney and two-thirds of the other kidney were removed (a five-sixths nephrectomy model), increases in glomerular plasma flow, mean net glomerular transcapillary hydraulic pressure, and single-nephron GFR were measured in the remnant nephrons. Later, as an apparent consequence, these rats developed focal segmental glomerulosclerosis (FSGS) (Hostetter et al, 1981, 1982). The glomerulosclerosis was thought to have resulted from vascular injury caused by renal hyperfiltration. Rats maintained on a low-protein diet failed to show the pressure or pathologic changes, and indeed, rats maintained on a high-protein diet had greater degrees of glomerular sclerosis and more rapid renal death than those fed normal diets (Brenner et al, 1982).

FSGS has been found in children with reflux nephropathy and proteinuria even when renal function (measured by GFR) is relatively well preserved. In these children glomerular involvement correlates with degree of proteinuria. Because most children with renal scarring and loss of parenchyma have adequate renal function, the glomerular and vascular changes may be an evolving response to hyperfiltration injury (Morita et al, 1990).

Another explanation for the progressive renal dysfunction involves a chronic inflammatory response that develops as an autoimmune phenomenon. Tamm-Horsfall protein is produced in the renal tubular cells of the loop of Henle and distal convoluted tubules and is secreted into the urine. Whether it has any specific physiologic role is unknown, but it does appear to affect bacterial adherence to the mucosa and may serve some protective role (Duncan, 1988). Although Tamm-Horsfall protein is usually found only in the urine and on the luminal side of the tubules, both clinically and experimentally the protein has been detected in interstitial deposits in kidneys that have been subject to infection or reflux, and it has been associated with mononuclear cell infiltrates and renal scarring (Andriole, 1985). In addition, even though antibodies (autoantibodies) to Tamm-Horsfall protein are widespread, the immunologic response to Tamm-Horsfall protein after a UTI may be disturbed in children with renal scarring (Fasth et al, 1980). This protein may account for findings of renal dysfunction or scarring associated with urinary VUR without known infections, and the autoimmune response related to it may also provide a reason why chronic or progressive renal damage occurs long after cessation of reflux or active infection (Andriole, 1985).

End-Stage Renal Disease

ESRD related to UTI alone is probably rare, but ESRD related to reflux nephropathy is commonly associated with UTI and is estimated to account for 7% to 17% of ESRD cases worldwide (Craig et al, 2000), although only about 2% in the United States. A retrospective analysis of ESRD caused by reflux nephropathy was unable to show that treatment of VUR with long-term antimicrobial prophylaxis or surgery has improved the natural history of reflux nephropathy (Craig et al, 2000). Whether this can be explained by the finding that about one third of renal scarring diagnosed may be detected on antenatal ultrasonography and represents congenital renal dysplasia or hypoplasia related to antenatal VUR rather than postnatal pyelonephritogenic scarring is unclear (Craig et al, 2000).

Xanthogranulomatous Pyelonephritis

Under certain circumstances chronic bacterial pyelonephritis and obstruction are associated with a distinct severe inflammatory process known as xanthogranulomatous pyelonephritis (XGP). Although this complication occurs in only about 1% of cases of renal inflammation (Malek and Elder, 1978), it is important because the entity has been confused with childhood renal tumors (Wilms' tumor, multilocular cystic nephroma, congenital mesoblastic nephroma, malignant rhabdoid, and clear cell sarcoma). Al-

though the cause is unknown, the process is almost always associated with both infection and obstruction.

XGP mainly affects adults, but pediatric cases have been reported. Symptoms in children are similar to those in adults, with flank pain, fever, chills, and chronic bacteriuria associated with more vague symptoms of malaise, malnutrition, weight loss, and failure to thrive. Lower tract irritative symptoms are uncommon. Symptoms are often chronic, and the majority of patients with XGP are symptomatic for longer than 1 month (Brown et al, 1996). The most common infecting organisms are *Proteus* and *E. coli*. Urinalysis usually shows pus and protein, and blood counts often show anemia, reflecting the chronic nature of the disease.

The process is usually unilateral and may involve pericalyceal tissue alone (focal) or the kidney diffusely (diffuse), with extension into the perinephric fat, and even into the retroperitoneum with encasement of the great vessels (Malek and Elder, 1978; Eastham et al, 1994). The clinical presentation in children differs from that in adults. In children XGP often affects those younger than 8 years of age and affects the kidney focally more frequently than diffusely (17% to 25% of cases in children). Boys are affected more frequently (Brown et al, 1996), and contralateral renal hypertrophy may occur (Quinn et al, 1999). Although obstructive calculi are found in children as well as adults, obstruction in children may also involve obstructive genitourinary abnormalities. It has also been noted that focal XGP is seldom associated with obstruction (Brown et al, 1996).

Radiologic findings include renal calculi in 38% to 70% of cases, nonfunctioning renal segments 27% to 80%, and a mass in as many as 62% (Anhalt et al, 1971; Malek and Elder, 1978). Ultrasonography may show an enlarged kidney with hypoechoic areas that represent areas of necrosis and pus-filled calyces. CT with contrast shows areas of low attenuation that do not enhance and may show extension of the mass into the perinephric fat. The "bear paw" sign with areas of low-attenuation, nonenhancing dilated calyces and abscesses within areas of high-attenuation, enhancing renal parenchyma may be present (Cousins et al, 1994; Goodman et al, 1998). No radiologic feature of XGP is diagnostic, but CT has allowed correct preoperative diagnosis and planning in some patients (Cousins et al, 1994; Eastham et al, 1994; Goodman et al, 1998).

Grossly, the kidney shows yellow-white nodules and evidence of pyonephrosis. The histologic diagnostic feature is the xanthoma cell—a foamy, lipid-laden histiocyte that may simulate the renal carcinoma cell. These xanthoma cells may also appear in other conditions of chronic inflammation and obstruction, such as obstructive pneumonia (Moller and Kristensen, 1980).

If the diagnosis is made preoperatively, localized XGP may be treated with partial nephrectomy, but diffuse and extensive disease associated with a nonfunctioning kidney usually requires removal of the involved kidney and perinephric fat. Rare instances of successful medical treatment of focal XGP have been reported (Brown et al, 1996; Quinn et al, 1999). Amyloidosis has been reported as a remote complication in the remaining kidney (Brown et al, 1996; Quinn et al, 1999).

ASSOCIATED PROBLEMS

Urinary Tract Abnormalities

As stated previously, **epidemiologic data show that 5% to 10% of children with UTIs have obstructive urinary tract lesions, and an additional 21% to 57% have VUR** (Kunin et al, 1964; Abbott, 1972; Asscher et al, 1973; Winberg et al, 1974; Newcastle Asymptomatic Bacteriuria Research Group, 1975). When only children with pyelonephritis diagnosed by DMSA are examined, 25% to 83% have VUR; many studies show reflux absent in more than half the children with pyelonephritis (Tappin et al, 1989; Jakobsson et al, 1992; Rushton and Majd, 1992b; Ditchfield et al, 1994a).

Children with febrile UTI and reflux have a high incidence of acute DMSA defects. Which of these acute defects results in scar is still debatable, but the risk of scarring increases with grade of reflux (Jakobsson et al, 1992). Older investigations documented scars in 5% to 20% of kidneys with grade 1 reflux and in 50% or more of kidneys with grade 5 reflux (Govan et al, 1975; Ozen and Whitaker, 1987; Skoog et al, 1987). Conversely, when renal scarring is used as the index and children with renal scarring are examined, about 60% have VUR (Asscher et al, 1973; Newcastle Asymptomatic Bacteriuria Research Group, 1975; Savage, 1975). In at least 25% of children the urinary tract is normal except for the scarring (Jodal, 1987). These data confirm that **VUR is only one factor involved in the ascent of bacteria into the kidney and the subsequent risk of renal scarring. There is no documented association between VUR and risk of bacteriuria.**

Normal Genitourinary System and Recurrent Urinary Tract Infections

Recurrent UTIs are common, and the natural history was well documented by Winberg and colleagues (Winberg et al, 1974). Among boys who became infected before they were 1 year old, 18% got a recurrent infection, but recurrences more than 1 year after the initial infection were rare. In contrast, if the initial infection occurred in an older boy, 32% became reinfected. About 26% of girls who had an initial neonatal infection got a recurrence, and, as with infant boys, recurrences after 1 year from the neonatal infection were rare. Girls who had their first infection after the neonatal period had a 40% recurrence rate, with the majority of recurrences occurring within the first 3 months and two thirds occurring within the first year. Although the risk of recurrent infection in these girls dropped with each infection-free subsequent year, 8% had their first recurrence more than 4 years after their original infection, so the risk never totally disappeared. For a girl who has had UTIs, Winberg found **the risk of occurrence of another UTI within 1 year after the last UTI was proportional to the number of previous infections** (i.e., the more infections a girl had had, the more likely she was to get another). His data showed that the risk of getting another UTI within 1 year was greater than 25% with one previous UTI, greater than 50% with two previous UTIs, and almost 75% after three previous UTIs (Winberg et al, 1974). **This recurrence rate did not change, whether the initial infection was symptomatic or asymptomatic, or pyelonephritis or cystitis; in fact, about one third of the recurrences were asymptomatic.**

The low rate of recurrence of UTI in neonates and young boys and higher recurrence rates for older girls and boys support the importance of variable host risk factors. First, neonates may be affected by hematogenous infection and age-related factors such as an immature immune system or unstable gut flora. Second, when a UTI occurs after the immune system attains maturity and fecal flora are stable, the child may have other biologic factors that influence the risk for UTI.

Voiding Dysfunction and Constipation

Symptoms of nocturnal and diurnal incontinence are common in children with recurrent UTIs. Epidemiologic studies have shown that nocturnal enuresis alone is not associated with UTIs, but diurnal enuresis or a combination of diurnal and nocturnal enuresis are associated with pediatric UTIs even when the enuretic episodes are as infrequent as once a week (Hansson, 1992). The same study also revealed that 7-year-old girls who were 3 years or older when they had their first UTI were more likely to have symptoms associated with voiding dysfunction than those who had UTIs when younger than 3 years (Hansson, 1992). Furthermore, when followed prospectively, almost 20% of children who experienced a recurrent UTI developed new diurnal enuresis with the onset of the recurrent UTI, and this persisted for as long as 12 months even though the urine remained clear (Sørensen et al, 1988).

Urodynamic testing in neurologically normal children with recurrent UTIs and incontinence has shown abnormal cystometry and voiding patterns (Kass et al, 1979; Koff et al, 1979; Bauer et al, 1980; Koff, 1982; Kondo et al, 1983; Qvist et al, 1986; Hansson, 1992; Passerini-Glazel et al, 1992; vanGool et al, 1992a). In 35 such children, Bauer and associates found that 12 (34%) had normal filling cystometry; 9 (26%) had large, hypotonic bladders; 9 (26%) had small-capacity, hypertonic bladders with increased intravesical filling pressure and sustained, uncontrolled detrusor contraction at a low volume; and 5 (14%) had hyperreflexic bladders showing uninhibited detrusor contractions during filling (Bauer et al, 1980). Voiding dysfunction has also been described, with staccato (interrupted) urinary flows during voiding showing increased pelvic floor activity during voiding, with resulting incomplete bladder emptying (Bauer et al, 1980; Hansson, 1992; Passerini-Glazel et al, 1992; vanGool et al, 1992a; Kjølseth et al, 1993).

In addition to bladder filling and voiding dysfunction, recurrent UTIs are associated with bowel dysfunction with constipation (O'Regan et al, 1985; Loening-Baucke, 1997). When 47 girls with normal urinary tracts but recurrent UTIs (with or without incontinence) and cystometry-proven bladder instability were studied by digital rectal examination and rectal manometry, all had signs of functional constipation (O'Regan et al, 1985). Diurnal and nocturnal urinary incontinence (29% and 34%, respectively) and UTIs (11%) were found in children older than 5 years of age who had chronic constipation (as defined by stool retention on rectal examination) and encopresis at least once a week (Loening-Baucke, 1997). These findings were present even when constipation or encopresis was specifically denied.

Although these findings do not establish causality between UTIs and constipation and/or voiding dysfunction, it can be seen that UTIs may initiate symptoms of bladder and sphincter (urethral and rectal) dysfunction with variable persistence. In some situations, treatment of constipation and/or voiding abnormalities has resulted in decreased frequency of UTIs (Kass et al, 1979; Koff et al, 1979; Bauer et al, 1980; Koff, 1982; O'Regan et al, 1985; vanGool et al, 1992a, 1992b; Kjølseth et al, 1993; Loening-Baucke, 1997), and **this relationship should be considered in the management of VUR as well** (Koff et al, 1998). This suggests that bacteriuria or constipation may provoke abnormal detrusor/sphincter activity or vice-versa.

FACTORS AFFECTING RISK OF BACTERIURIA AND RENAL DAMAGE FROM URINARY TRACT INFECTIONS IN CHILDREN

Although bacterial virulence characteristics may increase the likelihood of any periurethral bacterial strain's entering the urinary tract, there are specific host characteristics that alter the risk of bacteriuria and others that alter the risk of subsequent renal damage once bacteriuria occurs. Moreover, any infant or young child with an untreated or inadequately treated UTI that involves renal inflammation risks renal damage. Some of these host characteristics are discussed (Table 54–4).

Age

Age affects the incidence of bacteriuria. Bacteriuria appears to be more common at the extremes of life—in the neonates and in the elderly. The incidence of bacteriuria for both boys and girls before the age of 1 year is higher than at other times during childhood. There may be many

Table 54–4. HOST FACTORS AFFECTING BACTERIURIA

Age
Gender
Colonization
   Periurethral
   Preputial
   Fecal
Genetics (uroepithelial receptors)
Renal scarring
Native immunity
Sexual activity
Genitourinary abnormalities
   Vesicoureteral reflux
   Pregnancy
   Neurogenic bladder
Iatrogenic factors

causes of this age-dependent relationship, some of which involve interactions with other host factors, such as periurethral colonization, breast-feeding, or immature immune status.

Genetics

Genetic factors that may affect the risk of bacteriuria and others that affect subsequent morbidity are multifactorial and incompletely investigated. Most known at present fall into categories related to gender, race or ethnicity, and other factors that have been related to genetic influences.

Gender

As discussed previously, the ratio of UTIs by sex shows a preponderance of infections in boys during the first year of life. Thereafter, more girls than boys have UTIs. Many factors, including urethral length, prostate, and foreskin, have been hypothesized to account for this difference, but the reasons are not entirely known.

Race and Ethnicity

Although UTIs occur in all races, epidemiologic studies show varying prevalence and complications of infection in different races. These factors are incompletely studied. Various studies show that African Americans have fewer UTIs, lower incidence of VUR, and perhaps less likelihood of reflux nephropathy (Kunin and McCormack, 1968; Kunin, 1970; Lohr et al, 1994; Hoberman and Wald, 1997).

Other Genetic and Familial Factors

Other factors that appear to have genetic links by formal genetic studies or epidemiology relate to familial occurrence of UTI, adherence and blood group antigens, VUR, and potential of renal parenchymal damage.

The factors causing increased colonization were unclear until bacterial adherence was recognized to be related to colonization. **When bacterial P fimbriae were identified as a virulence factor, it was realized that glycolipids characterizing the P blood group system are found on host uroepithelial cells and that these serve as bacterial receptors.** Because hosts with these receptors (i.e., P blood group phenotype) might have special susceptibility for infection, children with recurrent infections were examined for the P blood group phenotype (Lomberg et al, 1983). The P1 blood group phenotype was found in 97% (35/36) of girls with recurrent pyelonephritis with minimal (grade 1) or no reflux but in only 75% (63/84) of control subjects without infections. Eighty-four percent (27/32) of girls with pyelonephritis and reflux (grades 2 through 5) had the P1 blood group phenotype; this was not significantly different from the incidence in individuals without infection. Moreover, bacteria binding to glycolipid receptors (bacteria with P fimbriae) were more likely to be found in the girls with P1 blood group and no reflux than in those with the P1 blood group with reflux, further suggesting in this instance that host VUR contributes more to getting bacteria into the kidney than virulence does. In children with minimal or no reflux, P fimbriae may be a major contributing factor.

Other blood group antigens on the urothelial surface (ABO, Lewis, and secretor phenotypes) appear to also influence susceptibility to UTIs. Adult women with Le(a−b−) and Le(a+b−) blood phenotypes have a three times greater risk of recurrent UTIs than Le(a−b+) women do, and epithelial cells from nonsecretors have more bacterial receptors than cells from secretors (Sheinfeld et al, 1989). Similarly, in children with UTIs the frequency of Le(a−b−) phenotype is higher and the relative risk of infection in these children is 3.2 (Jantausch et al, 1994).

Immunohistochemical analysis to characterize H, A, B, Le^a, and Le^b was performed in 72 children with various anatomic abnormalities (ureteropelvic junction obstruction, VUR, ureteroceles, and primary obstruction) (Sheinfeld et al, 1990). Children with anatomic abnormalities and presumed nonsecretor phenotype (minimal or undetectable ABO and Le^b immunoreactivity) were more likely to have had a history of UTIs (16/17, 94.1%) than were secretors whose tissue had intense ABO and Le^b staining (16/30, 53.3%). Twenty-three (95.8%) of 24 children without UTIs were secretors and had intense ABO and Le^b immunoreactivity. In summary, nonsecretor status may allow structures that serve as bacterial receptors to be more available for binding and result in greater susceptibility to UTI.

Clinical studies support familial risk factors for UTI. Sisters of girls who have recurrent UTIs have a higher incidence of significant bacteriuria on screening cultures than expected for the normal population (Fennell et al, 1977).

The possible genetic relationship of renal scarring and UTI is discussed in the following section.

Renal Scarring

Renal scarring is a risk factor for further complications such as hypertension, renal insufficiency, progressive renal scarring, and renal functional deterioration (Berg, 1992). This notion that renal scarring begets renal scarring was supported by clinical studies that examine the association of recurrent bacteriuria and new renal scarring or progressive renal scarring (Newcastle Asymptomatic Bacteriuria Research Group, 1975; Savage, 1975; Cardiff Oxford Bacteriuria Study Group, 1978; Newcastle Covert Bacteriuria Research Group, 1981). Long-term follow-up also showed that kidneys that were initially normal after UTI tended to remain normal, whereas those that were initially scarred were more likely to suffer subsequent damage (Smellie, 1991; Smellie et al, 1998).

Angiotensin-converting enzyme (ACE) gene polymorphism has been implicated in renal scarring. The ACE gene is located on chromosome 17, and a specific 287 base pair deletion (D) polymorphism is associated with increased renin-angiotensin system activity and increased angiotensin II levels. Increased DD genotype has been associated with increased risk of progressive renal failure in immunoglobulin A (IgA) nephropathy, diabetic nephropathy, autosomal dominant polycystic kidney disease, and focal glomerulosclerosis (Brock et al, 1998). Several series suggest that the DD genotype may also be associated with patients with congenital urologic abnormalities who have evidence of renal parenchymal damage and reflux nephropathy (Brock et al, 1997; Ozen et al, 1999).

Colonization

Periurethral Colonization

Host factors causing susceptibility to UTIs have also been examined (see Table 54–4). From epidemiologic data, it is known that the incidence of UTIs for all infants is higher during the first few weeks to months than at any subsequent time in the next few years. During this period, the periurethral area of healthy girls and boys is massively colonized with aerobic bacteria (especially E. coli, enterococci, and staphylococci) (Bollgren and Winberg, 1976a). This colonization decreases during the first year and is unusual in children who do not get recurrent infections after the age of 5 years. After this time, only those women and children who have repeated UTIs remain more colonized by periurethral gram-negative bacteria than those who do not get infections (Stamey and Sexton, 1975; Bollgren and Winberg, 1976a, 1976b). Times and conditions of increased periurethral colonization are, therefore, associated with increased risk of UTI.

Preputial Skin

During the first few months of life there appears to be a connection between the foreskin, periurethral and preputial colonization, and UTIs. During the last decade, however, the association of the foreskin and neonatal UTIs has caused controversy regarding the advantages and disadvantages of circumcision (Hallett et al, 1976). This has resulted in numerous editorials and recommendations by the American Academy of Pediatrics (King, 1982; Cunningham, 1986; Roberts, 1986; Lohr, 1989; Schoen et al, 1989; Winberg et al, 1989; Poland, 1990; Schoen, 1990; American Academy of Pediatrics, 1999).

In a group of mainly uncircumcised normal boys, Bollgren and Winberg (1976a) documented that **preputial aerobic bacterial colonization is highest during the first months after birth, decreases after 6 months, and is uncommon after 5 years of age.** Subsequently, Wiswell and associates compared the periurethral bacterial flora (using intraurethral and glandular cultures) during the first year of life in circumcised and uncircumcised boys and found that for the first 6 months periurethral uropathogenic organisms were cultured more frequently from the former group (Wiswell et al, 1988). They and others have concluded that the foreskin is responsible for this finding (Hallett et al, 1976; Glennon et al, 1988; Wiswell et al, 1988).

The reasons for neonatal bacterial colonization of the foreskin may be related to multiple factors, including immature immune status, unusual nosocomial colonization, breast-feeding (Winberg et al, 1989), and other characteristics mediating bacterial adherence (Fussell et al, 1988). This higher colonization is associated with a greater number of neonatal UTIs. In a series of retrospective reviews of 55 worldwide U.S. Army Hospitals, Wiswell and Roscelli (1986) examined the incidence of UTI diagnosed by catheterization or suprapubic aspirate in male infants hospitalized from 1974 through 1983. They found that the incidence of UTI was 0.11% (193/175,317) in circumcised male infants, 1.12% (468/41,799) in uncircumcised male infants, and 0.57% (1164/205,212) in female infants. **Overall, the incidence of UTI in infant boys is 2.2% to 4.1%, with the majority (70% to 86%) occurring in uncircumcised infants** (Wiswell et al, 1985; Schoen et al, 2000; Wiswell, 2000). **Uncircumcised male infants, moreover, have an increased relative risk for UTI of 3 to 12 compared with circumcised boys;** in one study, this risk decreased from 3.7 at 1 year to 3.0 at 3 years (Wiswell and Hachey, 1993; To et al, 1998; Wiswell, 2000). The majority of infections occurred during the first 3 months of life. When the incidence of UTIs during the first and the final years of the study were compared, the total number of infections increased as the circumcision rate decreased (Wiswell and Roscelli, 1986; Wiswell et al, 1987). Wiswell concluded that UTIs were more frequent in uncircumcised boys. Although there may be difficulties with these data related to retrospective analysis and selection bias, periurethral colonization is associated with increased risk of UTI in girls and women also.

The natural history of an infection in an uncircumcised male child can be determined from the study of Winberg and coworkers in which the majority of boys were uncircumcised. They found that boys who had a UTI during the first year after birth had an 18% recurrence rate, but recurrences later than 1 year were rare. If a boy had a UTI when he was older than 1 year of age (when the incidence is lower), the recurrence rate was 32%. This suggests that boys who have UTIs after the neonatal period are more likely to have a biologic predisposition for urinary infections (Winberg et al, 1974).

At this time there is no way of predicting whether a male infant with a normal urinary tract who gets a UTI has a genetic or familial predisposition for infection. Because few infant boys who get a neonatal UTI risk a recurrent UTI after 1 year if they remain clear in the interim, prophylactic antibiotics for 6 months may be helpful in these boys. There is no evidence that prophylactic circumcision after a neonatal UTI will prevent future infections in a boy. Present data do not support routine neonatal circumcision for medical benefits (American Academy of Pediatrics, 1999).

Fecal Colonization

Because most UTIs result from fecal-perineal-urethral ascent of bacteria, fecal colonization is an important consideration. The human fecal flora is dependent on the surrounding microbial ecology, native immunity, and microbe-altering drugs and foods. The importance of abnormal fecal colonization in neonates is emphasized by studies showing that fecal colonization with specific pyelonephritogenic bacteria may occur in a neonatal nursery or hospital with subsequent bacteriuria or pyelonephritis occurring several months later (Tullus, 1986).

The creation of and selection for organisms resistant to multiple antimicrobial agents in the gut through antimicrobial use is well recognized. **Because the fecal flora are commonly responsible for perineal and periurethral colonization, the importance of responsible antimicrobial use cannot be underestimated.** In one study, antibiotic treatment of school-aged girls with phenoxymethylpenicillin for intercurrent infections, usually otitis media, caused recolonization and bacteriuria with strains more likely to be symptomatic (Hansson et al, 1989b).

Immune Status

The complete influence of host native cellular and humoral immunity on the risk of UTI is unknown, but in all human disease decreased or lacking native immunity relates to increased risk of bacterial infection. In children, the infection risk related to immune status may vary during normal development of immunity, with lack of transmission of immunity, and routinely in congenital or acquired situations of immunodeficiency.

UTIs are common in infants and young children during a time that their immune system is incompletely developed. For instance, serum IgG is lowest between 1 and 3 months of age (Robbins, 1972), when periurethral colonization is high in normal children. Secretory IgA is an important human immunoglobulin at the secretory and mucosal surface and may be transferred to the newborn in colostrum if the child is breast-fed. Serum IgA is found in diminished concentrations for the first several months; it is either absent or almost absent at the secretory surfaces of the nasopharynx, gut, and urothelium during this time (Svanborg Edén et al, 1985; Fliedner et al, 1986; Yoder and Polin, 1986) and is undetectable in the urine at birth (James-Ellison et al, 1997). **Urinary secretory IgA and total IgA concentrations rise during the first year and then plateau; concentrations are higher in children who are breast-fed** (James-Ellison et al, 1997).

The role that urinary IgA plays in children with UTIs has not been examined extensively. In infants and children with acute UTI or pyelonephritis, urinary excretion of IgA is greater than in those without UTI, and these levels are still far below those found in adults (Svanborg Edén et al, 1985; James-Ellison et al, 1997). Urinary IgA in infants, moreover, occurs in the monomeric rather than the secretory form normally found in adults, suggesting that urinary IgA in infants may be a systemic immunoglobulin that reaches the urine as a result of infection-related tubular dysfunction rather than by secretion (Svanborg Edén et al, 1985). Children with recurrent UTIs are also reported to have lower urinary secretory IgA concentrations than children without infections (Fliedner et al, 1986).

The benefits of breast milk in preventing infection in infancy have been expounded for some time, but whether its effect is related to colostral IgA or other factors is unclear (Hanson, 1998). **Case-control studies suggest that the duration of breast-feeding may be related to its protective effect against UTI during the first 6 months of life.** These studies showed the duration of breast-feeding to be shorter in children who had UTIs (9 versus 16 weeks in children who were exclusively breast-fed) (Mårild et al, 1989b), but also that full or partial breast-feeding may confer a protective effect against UTIs for the first 6 months of life (Pisacane et al, 1990, 1992). Although the mechanism of the protective effect is unknown, the oligosaccharide content of the mother's breast milk and urine are the same as the breast-fed infant's, and these oligosaccharides may inhibit the adherence of pathogenic *E. coli* to the uroepithelium (Coppa et al, 1990). Other studies have now shown that exclusive breast-feeding for 4 months or longer may protect against single or recurrent episodes of otitis media in children (Duncan et al, 1993) or in infants with cleft palate (Paradise et al, 1994).

As expected, children with specific immune deficiency syndromes have altered immunity and often have increased risk of bacteriuria and progression of infection. About 20% of children infected with the human immunodeficiency virus (HIV) get bacterial UTIs with both common and opportunistic organisms (Grattan-Smith et al, 1992).

Sexual Activity

Epidemiologic studies have shown that sexual activity may also be a risk factor for UTI. In one study, sexually active women were shown to have more UTIs than sexually inactive women (nuns) (Kunin and McCormack, 1968). Whether this relates to colonization or other factors is unclear.

Genitourinary Anatomic Abnormalities

Historically, UTIs have been a marker for genitourinary tract anatomic abnormalities in children. **Specific genitourinary abnormalities, especially nonfunctioning segments, may serve as a nidus of bacterial infection and cause bacterial persistence because of the difficulty in achieving urinary antimicrobial concentrations adequate to treat UTIs in a poorly concentrating renal segment.** Similarly, conditions of genitourinary partial obstruction or renal functional impairment may create an increased risk of renal damage because of poor or inadequate treatment. Although usually rare in children, the particularly severe sequela of chronic UTI and inflammation, XGP, may occur in young children with obstruction and UTI, especially when associated with genitourinary abnormalities and renal nonfunction (Stamey et al, 1977; Zafaranloo et al, 1990; Cousins et al, 1994; Hammadeh et al, 1994).

Several special conditions that may alter a child's risk for UTI are discussed in the following sections.

Vesicoureteral Reflux

VUR is discussed fully in Chapter 59, Vesicoureteral Reflux and Megaureter. It is common in children with UTIs, but no correlation between reflux and susceptibility to UTIs has been found (Winberg et al, 1974). Epidemiologic surveys have shown that 21% to 57% of children who have had bacteriuria are subsequently found to have VUR (Kunin et al, 1964; Abbott, 1972; Asscher et al, 1973; Newcastle Asymptomatic Bacteriuria Research Group, 1975). Reflux may resolve spontaneously (Bellinger and Duckett, 1984; Skoog et al, 1987). In one study when UTIs were prevented, 87% of grade 1, 63% of grade 2, 53% of grade 3, and 33% of grade 4 reflux resolved over

about 3 years (Bellinger and Duckett, 1984). In groups in which reflux resolves, the rate of spontaneous resolution is about 30% to 35% each year (Skoog et al, 1987).

Peripubertal Girls with Persistent Vesicoureteral Reflux (Pregnancy)

The question of whether girls approaching puberty who have persistent VUR risk increased renal damage is problematic. If primary VUR persists as a girl approaches puberty, it becomes statistically less likely each year to resolve spontaneously. For this reason, some have recommended that girls approaching puberty undergo surgical correction of reflux to avoid the risks of pyelonephritis during future pregnancies. Whether the female patient with persistent VUR but no predisposition for UTIs is actually at increased risk of morbidity during pregnancy and should undergo routine correction of reflux is unclear.

Although the prevalence of bacteriuria in pregnant women is the same as in nonpregnant women (Shortliffe and Stamey, 1986b; Shortliffe, 1991), **the likelihood that the bacteriuria will progress to pyelonephritis is greatly increased.** Between 13.5% and 65% of pregnant women who are bacteriuric on a screening urinary culture will develop pyelonephritis during pregnancy if left untreated (Sweet, 1977), whereas an uncomplicated cystitis in a nonpregnant woman rarely progresses to pyelonephritis. The reason for this increased risk of pyelonephritis may be related to the hydronephrosis of pregnancy that occurs as a result of hormonal and mechanical changes. There is increased compliance of the bladder and collecting system that together with bladder enlargement and an enlarging uterus may cause some anatomic displacement of the bladder and ureters (Hsia and Shortliffe, 1995).

There are no data to suggest that pregnancy causes VUR (Shortliffe and Stamey, 1986b). In one series in which 321 women had a single-film voiding cystourethrogram during the third trimester of pregnancy or immediately postpartum, only 9 (2.8%) had VUR (Heidrick et al, 1967). Although 6.2% (20/321) of these women had asymptomatic bacteriuria, only 1 of those 20 had VUR. Therefore, few of the pregnant women with bacteriuria who developed pyelonephritis had reflux. On the other hand, of the 9 women who had reflux, 3 had experienced pyelonephritis during a pregnancy. In another series, 21 of 100 pregnant women with asymptomatic bacteriuria (27 refluxing renal units in 21 patients) were found to have VUR postpartum, mostly of low grade (67% into the ureter only), and 17% of these women also had renal scarring (Williams et al, 1968). Although some have inferred that this scarring was caused by the bacteriuria during pregnancy, this percentage is similar to the percentage of children with screening bacteriuria who have renal scarring (Asscher et al, 1973; Newcastle Asymptomatic Bacteriuria Research Group, 1975; Savage, 1975). Because the women were not evaluated radiologically before their pregnancy, it is unknown when they developed the scars, and it is most likely that the scars were present since childhood. These data suggest that **postpubertal girls who have VUR and a predisposition for frequent UTIs will continue to have this predisposition for infections into adulthood and pregnancy.** Moreover, those women who were prone to UTIs before pregnancy will continue to be more likely to develop UTI during and after pregnancy whether or not they have VUR (Mansfield et al, 1995; Bukowski et al, 1998).

Even though spontaneous resolution of VUR or ureteral reimplantation may decrease the likelihood of ascending pyelonephritis under normal circumstances, under the physiologic changes that occur during pregnancy the nonrefluxing orifice may not offer the expected protection from pyelonephritis should bacteriuria occur. Unless the postsurgical nonrefluxing ureteral orifice is less likely to allow pyelonephritis during pregnancy than the normal nonrefluxing ureteral orifice, which seems unlikely, correction of the reflux would not protect a woman from pyelonephritis. Therefore, both the persistent reflux and the girl's predisposition for bacteriuria should be assessed before surgical correction of reflux is considered. **If VUR is surgically corrected, these girls should not be assured that pyelonephritis during pregnancy is impossible or even unlikely,** because most episodes of pyelonephritis occurring during pregnancy occur in women with nonrefluxing kidneys. The urine of these women should be screened routinely for bacteriuria during pregnancy.

Finally, **before a woman with known reflux nephropathy and possible renal insufficiency is counseled about pregnancy, her renal function should be evaluated carefully.** Although data on the outcome of pregnancies in women with varying degrees of renal insufficiency are limited, **when there is either moderate (initial serum creatinine, 1.4 to 2.4 mg/dl) or severe ($\geq$2.5 mg/dl) renal insufficiency, both maternal and obstetrical complications are high** even though infant survival may be greater than 90% (Bear, 1976; Davison and Lindheimer, 1978; Jones and Hayslett, 1996). Among such high-risk women in one study, 43% had a pregnancy-related deterioration in creatinine clearance of at least 25% that occurred either during pregnancy (20%) or immediately postpartum (23%), and in the majority this drop was irreversible (Epstein, 1996; Jones and Hayslett, 1996). This accelerated renal insufficiency was associated with increased hypertension and high-grade proteinuria (Jones and Hayslett, 1996). Almost 60% of these pregnancies ended in preterm delivery with cesarean section, and the majority of infants were below the 50% in birth weight (Jones and Hayslett, 1996). These data have been interpreted to indicate that when the serum creatinine exceeds 2.0 mg/dl in a pregnant woman, she has a 1 in 3 risk of progressing to ESRD either during or just after delivery (Epstein, 1996).

Neurogenic Bladder

Children who have neurogenic bladders with abnormally elevated bladder pressures risk increased renal damage from UTIs because of the elevated urinary tract pressures and the increased instrumentation common with neurogenic bladders. A neurogenic bladder with chronically or intermittently elevated bladder pressures may cause secondary VUR from decompensation of the ureterovesical junction due to the elevated pressure (Hutch, 1952). If this does not occur, the elevated bladder pressures associated with a neurogenic bladder may also cause effective ureterovesical obstruction. This obstruction increases the risk of renal dam-

age associated with UTIs. As discussed earlier, intermittent elevations in bladder pressure associated with physiologic bladder dynamics in the immature bladder may exacerbate VUR and the risks associated with it.

Children with neurogenic bladder may be more likely to risk the effects of bacteriuria and possible renal damage because of their lack of ability to spontaneously clear the urinary tract of bacteria. Clean intermittent catheterization programs are useful for emptying the neurogenic bladder, but these catheterizations may introduce bacteria. Although conclusions from previous studies involving clean intermittent catheterization in these children are limited because they combined sexes, wide age ranges, different types of neurogenic bladders, short follow-up, different prophylactic regimens, and differing definitions of bacteriuria, they all agree that bacteriuria and even pyuria occurs in most children and in 40% to 80% of the urinary specimens sampled (Taylor et al, 1985; de la Hunt et al, 1989; Joseph et al, 1989; Gribble and Puterman, 1993; Johnson et al, 1994; Schlager et al, 1995, 1998). Few of these children had fever or symptoms, however (Geraniotis et al, 1988; Joseph et al, 1989; Schlager et al, 1995). One study with more than 5 years of follow-up noted several episodes of urinary calculi and epididymitis (de la Hunt et al, 1989), so the long-term natural history of children on clean intermittent catheterization programs deserves further study. Although prophylactic antibiotics administered during clean intermittent catheterization may delay and possibly decrease bacteriuria in the short term (Johnson et al, 1994), the actual efficacy of such antibiotic use is unproven.

Iatrogenic Factors

There are no good data regarding the risk of catheter-induced infections in children, but in adult women the incidence of catheter-induced UTI ranges from 1% to 20% depending on the circumstances of catheterization (Stamey, 1980). It has been documented that nosocomial UTIs frequently complicate hospitalization in children, especially when urethral catheterization has taken place (Dele Davies et al, 1992; Lohr et al, 1994). This may be a reason why antimicrobial prophylaxis should be given when urethral manipulation occurs. Children who get hospital-acquired UTIs, have urinary tract abnormalities, have recently been instrumented, or have had recent antimicrobial treatment are more likely to have infections caused by unusual and more antibiotic-resistant organisms (Ashkenazi et al, 1991b).

In school-age boys, urethral self-manipulation with water injection or self-instrumentation has been reported to cause UTIs (Labbé, 1990). About 25% of children who are victims of sexual abuse complain of dysuria and urinary frequency, but these children rarely have UTIs (Klevan and DeJong, 1990).

MANAGEMENT OF PEDIATRIC URINARY TRACT INFECTIONS

The therapeutic strategy in managing pediatric UTIs is first to minimize renal damage during the acutely diagnosed UTI, and second to minimize risk of future

renal damage from subsequent infections. Early recognition of a UTI and rapid, appropriate antimicrobial treatment are keys to preventing renal damage. As discussed previously, clinical and experimental data show that early antimicrobial treatment appears to be the most effective means of preventing renal scarring and subsequent complications.

Treatment of Acute Urinary Tract Infections

Treatment depends on the child's age and severity of illness. The child younger than 2 to 3 months with a presumptive UTI who is severely systemically ill, has a fever and flank or abdominal pain, or is unable to take fluids and the immune compromised child should be treated with parenteral broad-spectrum antimicrobial agents (e.g., aminoglycoside and ampicillin, a third-generation cephalosporin, aminoglycoside and cephalosporin) (Table 54–5). Whether this child requires hospitalization or outpatient parenteral or oral treatment depends on the clinical status.

In appropriate infants and young children with presumptive febrile UTI who are taking fluids, who have cooperative and reliable parents, and with whom daily contact is possible, some of the newer third-generation cephalosporins (e.g., ceftriaxone) allow once-daily outpatient parenteral therapy (Gordon, 1991; Baskin et al, 1992). Most of these third-generation cephalosporins have a broad spectrum, treat even *Enterobacter* species and some *Pseudomonas aeruginosa*, and conveniently require only once- or twice-daily dosing, but *Enterococcus* is still resistant to most.

Because the antimicrobial spectrum varies slightly for each of these drugs, the environment and local ecology (e.g., community-acquired outpatient versus hospital-acquired UTI) should determine drug selection. National and local antimicrobial resistance to organisms that commonly infect the urinary tract should be considered in the selection of both the agent for initial treatment and that for prophylaxis. Generally, parenteral treatment is continued for 2 to 4 days until bacterial sensitivities are available to allow treatment with a drug with a narrower spectrum and the child is clinically improved (afebrile and able to take adequate fluids with sterile urine). The treatment may then be switched to an appropriate oral antimicrobial agent that attains adequate serum levels. Although the duration of treatment is debatable, in most studies involving treatment of febrile UTIs in young children the total duration of therapy has extended from 7 to 10 days. When culture and sensitivity information is available, the antimicrobial agent should be re-evaluated and changed if necessary, with treatment continuing for 7 to 10 days. In most cases a drug to which the organism is sensitive with the narrowest spectrum can be continued.

Less ill older infants and young children who have presumptive febrile UTIs and are capable of taking fluids and oral medicines may be treated with an antimicrobial agent that has a broad spectrum for genitourinary pathogens (Table 54–6). Although the newer oral cephalosporins have good gram-positive and gram-negative treatment spectrums and most often can be given only once or twice daily, many *Enterococcus, Pseudomonas,* and *Enterobacter* species may be resistant to treatment (Fennell et al, 1980; Ginsburg et al, 1982; Dagan et al, 1992; Stutman, 1993). In a multicenter randomized clinical trial, oral cefixime appeared to be as effective as initial intravenous cefotaxime in children 1 to 24 months of age with febrile UTI (Hoberman et al, 1999). In adults the newer quinolones are useful because of their broader antimicrobial spectrum and special activity against *P. aeruginosa*, but in children use of this drug has been limited because of studies showing quinolone-induced cartilage toxicity in young animals. With careful monitoring, limited use of quinolone has resulted in no cartilage-related toxicities, and an abnormal urinary tract with upper UTI with *P. aeruginosa* may be a potential indication for its use (Schaad, 1991). To date (2002) the quinolones are not approved for the treatment of pediatric UTIs, but clinical trials are examining pediatric safety and efficacy issues.

In school-age children who do not appear systemically ill and have a "clinically uncomplicated bladder infection," **many oral broad-spectrum antimicrobial agents that are well tolerated will cure the "uncomplicated" UTI in a course of 3 to 5 days and there are no advantages to longer therapy** (Lohr et al, 1981; Copenhagen Study Group of Urinary Tract Infections in Children, 1991; Jójárt, 1991; Gaudreault et al, 1992). In some of these children single-dose treatment, particularly with intramuscular aminoglycoside, may be curative and cause less fecal antimi-

Table 54–5. PARENTERAL ANTIMICROBIAL DRUGS USEFUL FOR TREATING PEDIATRIC URINARY TRACT INFECTIONS

Drug	Daily Dosage	Frequency	Maximum
Aminoglycosides			
Gentamicin	7.5 mg/kg/day*	q 8h (>1 wk)	
Tobramycin	7.5 mg/kg/day*	q 8h (>1 wk)	
Penicillins			
Ampicillin	50–100 mg/kg/day	q 6h	
Ticarcillin	50–200 mg/kg/day	q 4–8h (>1 mo)	
Cephalosporins			
Cefazolin	25–50 mg/kg/day*	q 6–8h (>1 mo)	
Cefotaxime	50–180 mg/kg/day*	q 4–6h (>1 mo)	12 g/day
Ceftriaxone	50–75 mg/kg/day*	q 12–24h	2 g/day
Ceftazidime	90–150 mg/kg/day*	q 8–12h (>1 mo)	6 g/day

*Dosage change refined for azotemia.

Table 54–6. ORAL ANTIMICROBIAL DRUGS USEFUL IN TREATING PEDIATRIC URINARY TRACT INFECTIONS

Drug	Daily Dosage	Frequency
Penicillins		
Ampicillin	50–100 mg/kg/day	q 6h
Amoxicillin	20–40 mg/kg/day	q 8h
Augmentin (amoxicillin/clavulanate)	20–40 mg/kg/day	q 8h
Sulfonamides		
Sulfisoxazole	120–150 mg/kg/day*	q 6h (>2 mo)
Trimethoprim-sulfamethoxazole	8 mg/kg/day*	q 12h (>2 mo)
Cephalosporins		
Cephalexin	25–50 mg/kg/day	q 6h
Cefaclor	20 mg/kg/day	q 8h (>1 mo)
Cefixime	8 mg/kg/day*	q 12–24h (>6 mo)
Cefadroxil	30 mg/kg/day*	q 12–24h
Cefpodoxime	10 mg/kg/day*	q 12h (>6 mo)
Cefprozil	30 mg/kg/day*	q 12h (>6 mo)
Loracarbef	15–30 mg/kg/day*	q 12h (>6 mo)
Other		
Nitrofurantoin	5–7 mg/kg/day	q 6h (>1 mo)
Nalidixic acid	55 mg/kg/day	q 6h (>mo)

*Dose adjustment required with azotemia.

crobial resistance (Grimwood, 1988; Khan, 1994), but in unselected children single doses may not be quite as effective as 3 to 5 days of treatment (Madrigal et al, 1988; Khan, 1994). Nitrofurantoin attains high urinary concentrations and low serum concentrations; as such, it may be a poor choice to treat a severe systemic and renal infection, but is ideal for treating a bladder UTI when there is a normal urinary tract. Resistance rates to nitrofurantoin have changed little over the past decade.

Common uropathogens are increasingly resistant to trimethoprim-sulfamethoxazole (TMP-SMX) and ampicillin. This should be considered when prescribing initial antimicrobial therapy for UTI. The prevalence of uropathogen resistance to TMP-SMX rose from 8% in 1992 to more than 16% in 1996 (Gupta et al, 1999), with *E. coli* resistance as high as 32% (range, 0% to 46%) in the western United States (Talan et al, 2000). Resistance to ampicillin has been reported to range from 25% to 45% in recent years (Dyer et al, 1998; Gupta et al, 1999). Predictors of situations in which uropathogens will be more likely to be resistant to commonly used agents are diabetes, recent hospitalization, recent use of antibiotics (especially TMP-SMX) (Wright et al, 1999), presence of urinary malformations, urethral catheters, and antimicrobial prophylaxis (Ashkenazi et al, 1991a).

After the therapeutic regimen for acute UTI, the child should be given a daily prophylactic antimicrobial agent until full radiologic evaluation of the urinary tract may be conveniently performed in the next days to weeks.

Prophylactic Antimicrobial Agents

Urinary prophylactic antimicrobial agents are effective, with varying degrees of supporting evidence, in preventing bacteriuria under certain circumstances. In children these agents are most commonly used to prevent UTI in the situations listed in Table 54–7. Although urinary tract prophylaxis is accepted and has been shown to decrease infec-

tions over a limited period in some groups such as children with VUR (Hanson et al, 1989), long-term efficacy has not been studied in all situations in which prophylaxis has been recommended. In some of these situations, such as partially obstructive hydronephrosis, the efficacy of prophylaxis has not been established. The use of antimicrobial prophylaxis with clean intermittent catheterization is controversial, and some of the related considerations have been discussed in the section on neurogenic bladder.

Once urinary tract antimicrobial prophylaxis is initiated, the time for discontinuing prophylaxis is unclear. Prophylaxis is usually stopped when resolution of the urinary tract abnormality for which prophylaxis is being given occurs (e.g., spontaneous resolution of VUR or obstruction). When resolution does not occur within a few months to years, however, a time for stopping prophylaxis has not been determined. Because evidence exists that renal scarring in girls with pyelonephritis may be less likely after 5 to 6 years of age, and may occur less frequently until age 15 to 16 years (see previous discussion of renal scarring), it may be reasonable to perform a trial of stopping prophylaxis when the child reaches age 5 to 8 years or older if there is no history of UTI and no renal scarring. Although selected groups of children have been monitored for a few years after stopping prophylaxis and have generally done well without evidence of UTIs or new scars, these studies have

Table 54–7. REASONS FOR URINARY TRACT PROPHYLAXIS

Vesicoureteral reflux
Unstable urinary tract abnormality (e.g., partial urinary tract obstruction)
Normal urinary tract but frequent reinfections
After acute UTI awaiting radiologic evaluation
Urethral instrumentation
Immunosuppressed or immunocompromised status
Infants with first UTI before 8–12 weeks of age
Clean intermittent catheterization and vesicoureteral reflux (?)

UTI, urinary tract infection.

Table 54–8. ORAL ANTIMICROBIAL AGENTS USEFUL FOR PEDIATRIC URINARY TRACT PROPHYLAXIS

Drug	Daily Dosage	Age Limitations
Useful and tested		
Nitrofurantoin	1–2 mg/kg/day	>1 mo
Trimethoprim-sulfamethoxazole	(trimethoprim) 1–2 mg/kg/day	>2 mo
Cephalexin	2–3 mg/kg/day	
Possibly useful		
Amoxicillin	5 mg/kg/day	
Sulfisoxazole	20–30 mg/kg/day	>2 mo
Trimethoprim	2 mg/kg/day	>2 mo ?

?, little data.

been limited by lack of randomization, short follow-up, and small numbers (Cooper et al, 2000).

Many agents may be used for treatment of a UTI, but fewer agents have been studied for low dose prophylaxis in children. The ideal prophylactic agent should have low serum levels, high urinary levels, and minimal effect on the normal fecal flora; be well tolerated; and be cheap. The potency of these antimicrobial agents is based on the general susceptibility of most fecal Enterobacteriaceae at urinary levels. Because these agents are generally concentrated in the urine, the urinary drug levels should be much higher than the drug levels found simultaneously in serum, gut, or tissue; if they are sufficiently low, antimicrobial resistance patterns should not develop in the gut. In some instances this characteristic of the prophylactic antimicrobial agents may be dose-related, so that inappropriately high dosing for prophylaxis is less rather than more effective because bacterial resistance is created (Martinez et al, 1985). The parent who doubles or triples the dose of prophylactic antimicrobial agent each time the child develops the slightest symptom or cold may be destroying the prophylactic value of the agent. Another consideration is that long-term patient compliance with daily prophylaxis may be difficult (Smyth and Judd, 1993).

Because urinary prophylaxis is usually initiated after treatment of an infection for which long-term (10 days) high-dose treatment was given, the fecal flora is usually resistant to the treating drug and to many of the prophylactic agents. The child who is very susceptible to UTIs may then become reinfected with a bacteria resistant to the prophylactic agent before the gut is repopulated with more normal flora. This accounts for frustrating "breakthrough" infections that occur soon after the child is placed on prophylactic antimicrobial agents or after treatment of other frequent infections such as otitis media. The period of greatest risk of recurrent infection is usually the first few weeks after any full-dose treatment. For this reason the treating antimicrobial agent should not necessarily be the prophylactic agent.

In children with normal urinary function, useful agents for urinary prophylaxis that have been studied are nitrofurantoin, cephalexin, and TMP-SMX (Brendstrup et al, 1990). Amoxicillin, sulfisoxazole, and TMP alone may also be useful urinary tract prophylactic antimicrobial agents, but they have not been as well studied in children. In continent children, urinary tract prophylactic antimicrobial drugs may best be given once nightly, when they will be excreted into and remain in the urine overnight (Table 54–8). The long-term microbial effects of prophylactic antimicrobial agents have been incompletely studied. Although there is some evidence that agents that lack systemic absorption result in less overall bacterial resistance and change to human microbial ecology than systemic agents do, long-term studies are lacking (Gribble and Puterman, 1993; Johnson et al, 1994; Sandock et al, 1995; Schlager et al, 1998).

Nitrofurantoin

Nitrofurantoin is an effective urinary prophylactic agent because its serum levels are low; its urinary levels are high; and it produces minimal effect on the fecal flora (Winberg et al, 1973). Its effectiveness is based on urinary excretion of antimicrobial once a day, and it has been found to be effective in girls at doses of 1.2 to 2.4 mg/kg each evening (Lohr et al, 1977). When renal function is reduced to less than half normal, the efficacy of nitrofurantoin may be reduced.

Although the majority of nitrofurantoin drug reactions occur in adults, it has caused acute allergic pneumonitis, neuropathy, and liver damage (Holmberg et al, 1980). Long-term treatment has been associated with rare cases of pulmonary fibrosis. It should not be used in children with glucose-6-phosphate dehydrogenase deficiencies because it is an oxidizing agent and can cause hemolysis. About 10% of blacks in the United States, Sardinians, non-Ashkenazi Jews, Greeks, Eti-Turks, and Thais have a glucose-6-phosphate deficiency, and in these people the regeneration of glutathione, which is partially responsible for maintaining RBC integrity, is impaired by the enzyme deficiency. When nitrofurantoin is given, it oxidizes the hemoglobin to methemoglobin, which is degraded (Thompson, 1969).

Cephalexin

Cephalexin has been studied in adults as a prophylactic agent (Martinez et al, 1985). Although resistance has developed in fecal Enterobacteriaceae in many patients taking full-dose cephalexin (500 mg four times daily), patients taking low-dose cephalexin (one quarter to one eighth of the adult daily dose: 250 to 125 mg/day) do not appear to develop resistance. Cephalexin at one quarter or less of the treatment dose per weight may then be a useful pediatric prophylactic agent.

Trimethoprim-Sulfamethoxazole

TMP-SMX has been a successful combination drug in the treatment of UTIs and has been useful for prophylaxis at a dose of approximately 2 mg/kg of TMP (Grüneberg et al, 1976; Stamey et al, 1977). TMP is unusual in that it is diffuses into the vaginal fluid, and therefore it also decreases vaginal bacterial colonization (Stamey and Condy, 1975). Because the TMP-SMX contains a sulfonamide, it probably should not be used for the first few months of life, because sulfonamides may compete for bilirubin binding sites on albumin and cause neonatal hyperbilirubinemia and kernicterus. As previously mentioned, an increased rate of bacterial resistance to this drug has been seen over the past decade.

Trimethoprim

Initial studies performed in adult women found TMP (dose approximately 2 mg/kg once nightly) to be as effective as TMP-SMX or nitrofurantoin in preventing recurrent UTIs (Stamm et al, 1980), but **other studies showed rapid emergence of significant TMP-resistant *E. coli* during either treatment or prophylaxis** (Huovinen and Toivanen, 1980; Brogden et al, 1982; Murray et al, 1982; Murray and Rensimer, 1983; Brumfitt et al, 1985; Brendstrup et al, 1990). Studies examining the emergence of resistance are controversial. In one study, after 14 days of TMP 200 mg daily, 96% of the TMP-resistant *E. coli* isolated from the fecal flora were resistant to at least four other antimicrobial agents (Murray et al, 1982), emphasizing the need for concern regarding resistance and the spread of multidrug resistance. A more recent clinical trial in children examined the efficacy of nitrofurantoin and TMP prophylaxis in preventing recurrent UTI and showed nitrofurantoin to be more effective as prophylaxis when used in association with urinary tract abnormalities or VUR (Brendstrup et al, 1990). Nitrofurantoin prophylaxis did not change the resistance pattern in uropathogens causing subsequent UTI, whereas

TMP prophylaxis led to breakthrough UTI with an organism resistant to the drug in 76% of patients (Brendstrup et al, 1990). With the recent distribution of liquid TMP approved for treatment of acute otitis media in children and possible wider usage, the drug should be used judiciously to prevent a repetition of previous antimicrobial resistance.

Nalidixic Acid

Nalidixic acid was used to treat children before the advent of more powerful quinolones; however, testing of the newer quinolones (norfloxacin, cinoxacin, ciprofloxacin) has shown that these drugs may be contraindicated in prepubertal children because they have caused cartilage erosion in weight-bearing joints and arthropathy in immature animals. In limited groups of children treated with quinolones, no such effects have been noted (Schaad, 1991).

Future Treatments

At this time the most powerful therapies for UTI are antimicrobial agents. On the horizon are promising trials of vaccines that prevent mucosal adherence of uropathogenic *E. coli* in animals by using common bacterial antigens or the FimH subunit of type 1 pili (Langermann et al, 1997; Thankavel et al, 1997; Uehling et al, 1999). Future studies will need to examine whether these vaccines will be clinically useful in children.

RADIOLOGIC EVALUATION

Imaging studies are basic to urinary tract evaluation for infection. The goal of management in UTI is to minimize renal damage from the acute infection and minimize future risk of renal damage. With the multiple imaging modalities available, the most efficient and rational order and selection of studies must be made with this goal in mind. **Radio-**

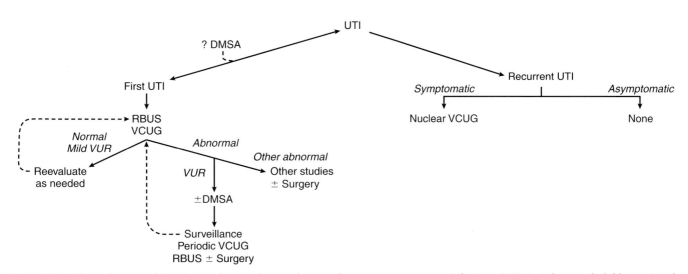

Figure 54–5. Flow diagram of imaging studies used to evaluate and manage urinary tract infections (UTI) in infants and children using the functional classification of UTI from Figure 54–1. DMSA, technetium 99m dimercaptosuccinic acid renal scanning; RBUS, renal and bladder ultrasonography; VCUG, voiding cystourethrogram; VUR, vesicoureteral reflux.

logic imaging can be used to (1) evaluate and localize the acute urinary infection, (2) detect renal damage from the acute infection, (3) identify genitourinary anatomy that increases the risk of future renal damage from infection, and (4) evaluate changes in the urinary tract over time. Deciding which studies are necessary in a child with a presumptive or diagnosed UTI should depend on whether potential radiologic findings would change the clinical management (Fig. 54–5).

Acute Imaging

Early urinary tract imaging is important in a seriously ill or febrile child in whom the site of infection is unclear, or where there are unusual circumstances. Circumstances such as newly diagnosed azotemia, a poor response to appropriate antimicrobial drugs after 3 to 4 days, an unusual infecting organism (tuberculosis or a urea-splitting organism such as *Proteus*), known partial obstruction (e.g., ureterocele), ureteropelvic junction obstruction, megaureters, nonfunctioning or poorly functioning renal units, or a history of diabetes, papillary necrosis, or a neuropathic bladder may warrant acute or early upper and lower urinary tract imaging.

If treatment depends on localizing the infection to the kidney, an acute imaging study should be performed. This is particularly important in the severely ill hospitalized child who improves on initial parenteral treatment but has urinary cultures that are inadequate or indeterminate for bacterial infection. An acute DMSA scan may show whether acute renal inflammation is present and justify a decision to treat or not to treat. If, on the other hand, UTI appears highly likely and antimicrobial treatment will be started regardless of radiologic findings, early DMSA scintigraphy may be unnecessary.

Definition of Renal Morphology and Identification of Urinary Tract Abnormalities

Because UTIs in infants and young children may serve as a marker for anatomic abnormalities, after the initial UTI has been adequately treated the child should be maintained on antimicrobial prophylaxis and radiologic studies should be performed to delineate the urinary tract. Although there is controversy as to whether such studies should be performed after the first or a recurrent episode, if obstructive lesions are found in 5% to 10% of children and reflux occurs in 21% to 57% (Kunin et al, 1964; Abbott, 1972; Asscher et al, 1973; Newcastle Asymptomatic Bacteriuria Research Group, 1975), **early detection of these abnormalities merits full radiologic urinary tract evaluation after the first documented UTI in all young children and infants. This consists of some form of renal and upper collecting system evaluation (usually renal and bladder ultrasound) and a voiding cystourethrogram (VCUG).**

As previously emphasized, the child's kidney is prone to renal scarring, and evaluation of the renal morphology and documentation of any anomalies or scarring may be important to management. Although the American Academy of Pediatrics Practice Parameter limited their recommendations for first UTI imaging evaluation of the upper and lower urinary tract to children between 2 months and 2 years of age (American Academy of Pediatrics, 1999), others support such evaluation in even younger infants (Goldman et al, 2000). However, acute studies of the kidney may cause overestimation of renal size, because of initial edema, or lack of appreciation of renal scarring, because mature renal scars can take up to 2 years to be seen by certain imaging techniques (Filly et al, 1974; Troell et al, 1984; Gordon, 1986; Conway, 1988; Johansson et al, 1988b). As a result, later studies may show smaller or scarred kidneys that may be misinterpreted and cause inappropriate changes in patient management.

Obviously, obstruction and other anatomic abnormalities demonstrated by radiologic evaluation may require further evaluation specific to their diagnosis before definitive management decisions can be made. These situations need to be evaluated and treated individually.

Follow-up Radiologic Evaluation

When a child who has a UTI has no abnormality found after urinary tract radiologic evaluation, no routine further studies are prescribed. If the collecting systems were normal but one or both kidneys showed massive generalized or focal edema with areas of possible hypoperfusion during the acute infection, a subsequent study should be performed to examine the kidney for signs of renal scarring or shrinkage. In this way children who need to be reexamined for later hypertension and renal dysfunction may be identified.

If a child has recurrent symptomatic pyelonephritis and no reflux found on previous fluoroscopic VCUG, a nuclear VCUG may be more sensitive at revealing reflux, although less likely to define it (Kogan et al, 1986; Macpherson and Gordon, 1986).

Imaging Techniques in Pediatric Urinary Tract Infection

Imaging techniques that are useful for evaluating children with UTIs are discussed. The radiologic follow-up of children diagnosed with VUR is discussed in Chapter 59, Vesicoureteral Reflux and Megaureter.

Voiding Cystourethrography

The VCUG is the most important examination in assessing VUR in children, and as such, is important for assessing UTIs. The VCUG may be performed either with fluoroscopy and iodinated contrast or with nuclear imaging agents (usually ^{99m}Tc-pertechnetate) using similar techniques (direct radionuclide cystography), but these studies give different information. The traditional fluoroscopic VCUG can show urethral and bladder abnormalities and vesicourethral reflux. The radionuclide VCUG may be more sensitive for reflux detection, but it offers poorer spatial resolution so that urethral lesions, degree of reflux, and details of the collecting system may not be realized. In both fluoroscopic and radionuclide VCUG, detection of VUR depends on the child's voiding and the technical performance of the study (Fairley and Roysmith, 1977; Lebowitz, 1986; Macpherson and Gordon, 1986).

The main advantage of radionuclide VCUG has been the lower radiation exposure of 1 to 5 mrad (ovarian dose), compared with 27 to 1000 mrad for fluoroscopic VCUG (reported ovarian exposure depending on equipment) (Cleveland et al, 1992; Lebowitz, 1992). With modern imaging technology and a tailored examination, however, the fluoroscopic VCUG has been done with exposure of 1.7 to 5.2 mrad (Kleinman et al, 1994); if available, this may offer advantages of anatomic resolution compared with the radionuclide VCUG. In general the radionuclide VCUG may be most useful for VUR screening, for evaluating the UTI in older children who have lower risk of reflux, and for periodic reflux reevaluation (Lebowitz, 1992). The radionuclide VCUG should not be used to evaluate infections in infant or young boys in whom risk of genitourinary abnormality is high and urethral visualization important, nor in any child in whom high-resolution imaging of the lower urinary tract is important.

Indirect radionuclide VCUG is performed as part of a renal imaging study. The radionuclide is injected intravenously, and the study is performed when the kidneys and upper collecting systems are cleared of the radiopharmaceutical agent and bladder is filled maximally with it. The child is then asked to void. Although this method avoids catheterization, when compared with the direct radionuclide VCUG there is increased radiation exposure and decreased resolution because of body radionuclide background. Because it detects only about 60% of the reflux compared with the direct VCUG, there are few reasons to perform this test (Eggli and Tulchinsky, 1993).

The VCUG may be performed as soon as the urine is sterile, and evaluation compliance may be greater when it is performed within 1 week after diagnosis (McDonald et al, 2000). Studies have shown that UTIs do not cause reflux, and there is no reason to wait 3 to 6 weeks to perform the study as long as voiding and bladder volumes have returned to normal (Lebowitz, 1986; McDonald et al, 2000). **Whether the VCUG is done during treatment, immediately afterward, or a few weeks afterward is not important as long as the child has normal renal function, responds rapidly to antimicrobial treatment, and is maintained on prophylactic antimicrobial treatment to keep the urine sterile in the interval between the herald infection and the radiologic evaluation.**

If the VCUG is performed as the initial radiologic study, subsequent imaging may be planned depending on the VCUG results (Hellström et al, 1989). If the VCUG is normal, shows a ureterocele, or shows VUR, an ultrasound examination of the kidney and bladder will usually demonstrate other urinary tract structural abnormalities or anomalies, such as dysplasia or obstruction, should they exist. In general renal and bladder ultrasound examination will identify children who may need urgent urologic surgery (Alon et al, 1986; Honkinen et al, 1986; Lindsell and Moncrieff, 1986; Macpherson, 1986; Alon et al, 1989). If, however, VUR appears to be the primary diagnosis, DMSA scinti-

graphy may be the most useful study with which to detect renal scars.

Renal and Bladder Ultrasonography

Routine renal ultrasonography is not as sensitive as DMSA at detecting the subtle changes associated with acute UTI (Verboven et al, 1990; Björgvinsson et al, 1991; Eggli and Tulchinsky, 1993; MacKenzie et al, 1994; Mucci and Maguire, 1994). Ultrasonography may show enlarged swollen kidneys, focal enlargement from edema and inflammation (focal pyelonephritis or lobar nephronia), and ureteral widening (Silver et al, 1976; Hellström et al, 1987; Conway, 1988; Johansson et al, 1988a); high-resolution power and color Doppler ultrasonography may also detect small areas of inflammation and resulting hypoperfusion that are seen on DMSA (Dacher et al, 1996; Morin et al, 1999). Renal and bladder sonography is, moreover, more likely to detect perinephric fluid collections or anatomic abnormalities, especially those involving urinary tract dilation, than either DMSA or intravenous urography (MacKenzie et al, 1994). However, pediatric renal and bladder ultrasonography may be more dependent on the skill and experience of the ultrasonographer with children than DMSA scintigraphy (Patel et al, 1993).

Nuclear Renography

The fact that nuclear scintigraphy can accurately detect areas of acute renal inflammation and chronic scarring has changed the imaging of pediatric UTIs since the mid-1990s. Because about 60% of injected ^{99m}Tc-DMSA is bound to the proximal renal tubular cells and excreted only slowly in the urine, it is a good cortical imaging agent (Jakobsson et al, 1992). Radionuclide technology using pinhole images and high-resolution CT (single-photon emission computed tomography, or SPECT) provides greater renal anatomic detail, resolution, and scar detection (Eggli and Tulchinsky, 1993). DMSA imaging is the common agent when cortical definition alone is needed (Björgvinsson et al, 1991; Eggli and Tulchinsky, 1993).

On the other hand, ^{99m}Tc-glucoheptonate is partially concentrated and excreted and partially bound to the renal tubule, so some collecting system visualization and cortical definition is observed. Similarly, ^{99m}Tc-mertiatide (MAG3), a tubular renal imaging agent that is primarily used to assess renal parenchymal flow and function and drainage, also has renal cortical imaging characteristics (planar or SPECT), and this agent or ^{99m}Tc-glucoheptonate may be almost as effective as DMSA in detecting changes of acute pyelonephritis (Traisman et al, 1986; Sreenarasimhaiah and Alon, 1995; Sfakianakis and Georgiou, 1997; Laguna et al, 1998). MAG3 imaging has advantages over DMSA in that it is more rapid, gives a lower radiation dose to most organs and the urinary bladder and gonads, and can be used to evaluate urinary tract drainage (Sfakianakis and Georgiou, 1997).

In acute pyelonephritis nuclear scintigraphy usually shows either uptake defects or renal swelling (Wallin and Bajc, 1993; Wallin et al, 1997). The uptake defects may appear as wedge-shaped polar or lateral renal defects or as scattered uptake defects within the kidney (Wallin and

Bajc, 1993). Later, after the acute episode is healed, the scans will show either (1) normal pattern; (2) generally diminished uptake and small kidney volume; (3) diminished uptake in the medial kidney; or (4) polar defects with diminished uptake in the renal poles (Wallin and Bajc, 1994). **DMSA is clearly more sensitive than routine renal ultrasonography or even intravenous urography at detecting renal scarring, but newer high-resolution ultrasonography is almost as sensitive as DMSA in diagnosing acute renal involvement** (Morin et al, 1999). Because recurrent pyelonephritis appears to occur in the same areas, however, it may be difficult to differentiate new from old or progressive renal scarring unless serial studies have been performed (Björgvinsson et al, 1991; Rushton and Majd, 1992b).

In cases in which severe renal scarring has occurred and the GFR may need to be estimated, the radionuclide renogram has been found to give an accurate estimate of GFR even in young children (Gates, 1982; Shore et al, 1984; Rehling et al, 1989).

Intravenous Urography

Although the traditional means of evaluating the upper urinary tract and documenting renal scarring was intravenous urography with renal tomography, in most situations DMSA scintigraphy has replaced the role of intravenous urography. DMSA scintigraphy is more sensitive for detecting renal scars but shows less resolution in defining the scars. Intravenous urography still defines collecting system abnormalities in more detail than either DMSA or ultrasonography. It is probably most useful in defining the collecting system in patients with confusing situations or in whom calyceal detail may be important.

Computed Tomography and Magnetic Resonance Imaging

No studies have directly compared the sensitivity and specificity of DMSA and CT or magnetic resonance imaging for detecting renal lesions in acute or chronic pyelonephritis. For the routine evaluation of UTI neither modality is practical, but in children with complicated infections either CT or magnetic resonance imaging may be highly useful in defining renal abnormalities and extent of disease when other modalities do not, and they are probably as sensitive or more sensitive than DMSA scintigraphy in detecting renal scars (June et al, 1985; Montgomery et al, 1987; Rodriguez et al, 2001) (Fig. 54–6).

MANAGEMENT OF SPECIFIC PROBLEM SITUATIONS

Covert or Asymptomatic Urinary Tract Infection

When covert or asymptomatic infections are diagnosed on screening urinary cultures, children often have symptoms related to the lower urinary tract when carefully interviewed. They may have nocturnal and/or diurnal enuresis, squatting, and urgency, and at least 20% have a history of previous UTI (Kunin et al, 1962; Savage et al, 1975); these symptoms were not the reason they had the urinalysis or culture, however.

About 50% of these children have normal urinary tracts as defined by an intravenous urogram and VCUG (Kunin et al, 1962; Savage et al, 1975). Although a majority of infants who had covert bacteriuria in one study were found to clear their bacteriuria without treatment (Jodal, 1987), other investigators found that only about 30% of school-age girls cleared their infections spontaneously without treatment (Verrier-Jones et al, 1975; Lindberg et al, 1978). **Whether the infection is treated when diagnosed or not, the majority of these girls have or will have persistent infections or reinfections** (Savage, 1975; Verrier-Jones et al, 1975; Jodal, 1987).

Whether the UTI is symptomatic or asymptomatic may not be important for the first UTI, because the UTI marks host susceptibility. For this reason the first UTI should be evaluated and managed the same as any first UTI in children. Once the urinary tract has been evaluated and found to be normal, treatment of subsequent asymptomatic or covert UTI is debatable (Shortliffe, 1995).

Because covert bacteriuria is rarely totally asymptomatic, if potentially associated symptoms such as incontinence are elicited they may be troublesome enough to warrant treatment. Treatment of the infection alone, however, may not obviate symptoms of voiding dysfunction. Controlled studies involving older children with treated and untreated covert bacteriuria show that treatment makes little difference in the rate of future reinfections: more than half will have recurrent infections whether treated or not, and the risk of any renal damage in these older children is very low (Savage, 1975; Verrier-Jones et al, 1975; Lindberg et al, 1978; Jodal, 1987). There is little evidence, therefore, that the natural history of asymptomatic UTI is changed by treatment; the UTI event, whether symptomatic or asymptomatic, marks a susceptible host.

In several series in which girls with UTIs were randomly assigned to receive antimicrobial treatment or nontreatment, subsequent renal scars rarely occurred when the kidney started out without scarring; conversely, new or increased scarring usually occurred in previously scarred kidneys in which VUR was present and was independent of antimicrobial treatment (Newcastle Asymptomatic Bacteriuria Research Group, 1975; Savage, 1975; Cardiff Oxford Bacteriuria Study Group, 1978; Newcastle Covert Bacteriuria Research Group, 1981).

There is evidence that E. coli causing covert bacteriuria may belong to strains of E. coli that show self-agglutination, loss of surface antigens, and less overall pathogenicity (Lindberg et al, 1975; Hansson et al, 1989b). Some studies have suggested that urinary tract colonization with a strain of E. coli causing asymptomatic bacteriuria may prevent colonization with a strain of E. coli causing symptoms, and that treatment may actually lead to later acute symptomatic pyelonephritis (Hansson et al, 1989a, 1989b). For this reason, **in difficult cases of recurrent asymptomatic infection without other urinary tract abnormalities, follow-up without further antimicrobial treatment should be considered.**

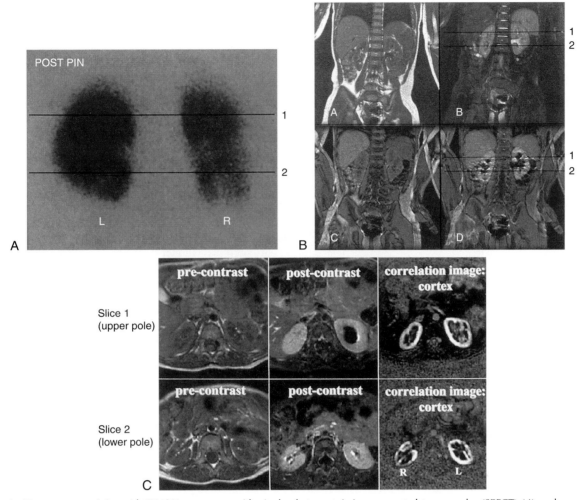

Figure 54–6. Dimercaptosuccinic acid (DMSA) renogram with single-photon emission computed tomography (SPECT) (*A*) and magnetic resonance imaging (MRI) (*B* and *C*), showing renal scars in a 3-year-old girl with reflux nephropathy. Comparative coronal levels of DMSA (*A*) and MRI (*B*) are shown. Approximate levels of transverse MRI images with correlation images are shown for comparison (*C*). (From Rodriguez L, Spielman D, Herfkens R, Shortliffe L: Magnetic resonance imaging (MRI) for the evaluation of hydronephrosis, reflux, and renal scarring in children. J Urol 2001;166:1023–1027.)

Treatment of Recurrent Urinary Tract Infections in Children with a Normal Urinary Tract

Because host uroepithelial characteristics are probably independent of gross urinary tract abnormalities or reflux, recurrent UTIs will occur regardless of whether the urinary tract is normal. Children with urinary tract anatomic abnormalities or VUR may be treated with prophylactic antimicrobial agents in an attempt to minimize the risk of infections. However, there are no routinely available tests to predict which children with a normal urinary tract may have a biologic predisposition for UTIs. Routine bacterial biotyping and sensitivity data obtained from culture, moreover, will not necessarily give data relating to bacterial virulence. For this reason, management of the possibility of recurrences in these patients depends on the child's age and severity of symptoms.

In the majority of children with normal urinary tracts who have mainly bladder irritative symptoms with their UTIs (so-called uncomplicated infections), there is evidence

that 3 to 5 days of treatment with an appropriate antimicrobial agent to which the organism is sensitive (Lohr et al, 1981; Madrigal et al, 1988; Copenhagen Study Group of Urinary Tract Infections in Children, 1991; Jójárt, 1991), or even a single dose of a parenteral antimicrobial agent (e.g., aminoglycoside), is an effective treatment (Principi et al, 1977; Vigano et al, 1985; Grimwood, 1988). Longer antimicrobial courses of 10 to 14 days have not proved to be more effective in these cases and may cause increased side effects and antimicrobial resistance in the fecal bacteria (Hansson et al, 1989b; Copenhagen Study Group of Urinary Tract Infections in Children, 1991).

If the child gets frequent recurrent UTIs (two or more infections over a 6-month period), a urinary prophylactic antimicrobial treatment over a limited period may be worthwhile, because the child is then established to have a biologic predisposition for infections. Antimicrobial agents taken at a prophylactic dosage will usually successfully decrease the rate of infections during the period of prophylaxis. When the antimicrobial agent is stopped, the child may extend into a period of remission from infection but often eventually returns to an increased basic susceptibility for urinary infections (Winberg et al, 1974; Kraft and Stamey, 1977).

Management of Urinary Incontinence Associated with Urinary Tract Infections and a Normal Urinary Tract

When symptoms of voiding dysfunction accompany recurrent UTIs, it is probably worth observing the child during treatment with prophylactic antimicrobial agents to look for any change in voiding pattern while the urine is sterile. If symptoms of incontinence persist, addition of an anticholinergic agent such as oxybutynin and/or bladder rehabilitation that includes timed voidings and biofeedback techniques may help to improve incontinence and decrease the frequency of UTIs (Kass et al, 1979; Koff et al, 1979; Qvist et al, 1986; Passerini-Glazel et al, 1992; vanGool et al, 1992b; Kjølseth et al, 1993; Shortliffe, 1995). In addition, **if constipation is found or even suspected, there may be an improvement in voiding and reduction in UTIs if the constipation is treated** (O'Regan et al, 1985); Loening-Baucke, 1997. With the acute onset of bowel and bladder dysfunction in the previously continent child, the possibility of tethered cord or other neurologic abnormalities must be eliminated.

OTHER GENITOURINARY TRACT INFECTIONS AND SYNDROMES

Acute Hemorrhagic Cystitis

Acute hemorrhagic cystitis accompanied by frequency, urgency, and dysuria in children has been associated with UTIs caused by adenovirus 11 (Numazaki et al, 1968; Manolo et al, 1971; Mufson et al, 1973; Numazaki et al, 1973) or occasionally by *E. coli* (Loghman-Adham et al, 1988–89). **Adenovirus is the most common cause of viral acute hemorrhagic cystitis in children.** In a series of 69 infants and children with acute hemorrhagic cystitis, adenovirus 11 was recovered from the urine of 10 patients (14.5%), adenovirus 21 from 2 (2.9%), and *E. coli* from 12 (17.4%), but the remainder (more than 60%) had no infectious agents isolated from the urine (Mufson et al, 1973).

Polyomaviruses have caused both hemorrhagic and non-hemorrhagic cystitis in children. In addition, **BK, a DNA virus of the polyomavirus genus, has been found in the urine of bone marrow transplantation and other immunosuppressed patients with hemorrhagic cystitis** (0.5 to 5 months after transplantation) causing both symptomatic (hematuria and dysuria) and asymptomatic infections (Apperley et al, 1987; Bedi et al, 1995). It is hypothesized that immunosuppression may relate to reactivation of BK virus. In several series hemorrhagic cystitis was associated with persistent BK viruria the majority of the time, and shedding of BK virus was usually correlated with onset of hemorrhagic cystitis (Bedi et al, 1995).

Because viral cultures are rarely done, children with symptoms of acute hemorrhagic cystitis most often have no growth on routine urinary culture. Although no antimicrobial treatment is indicated in healthy individuals with viral cystitis, radiologic evaluation should still be performed to eliminate other causes for hematuria as well. It has been suggested that ribavirin may be useful for adenovirus cystitis after bone marrow transplantation (Cassano, 1991).

Interstitial Cystitis

Although individuals with interstitial cystitis often have a history of possible UTI, there is no evidence that the condition results from infection. Initial symptoms of frequency, suprapubic pain, nocturia, and urgency may be confused with UTI but must be differentiated in children from either voiding dysfunction or urinary frequency syndrome. When strict diagnostic criteria of interstitial cystitis—such as Hunner's ulcers, pain on bladder filling relieved with emptying, suprapubic pain, and urinary urgency or frequency—are applied, this is a rare condition in children (Farkas et al, 1977; Close et al, 1996). This is primarily a diagnosis of exclusion, but the diagnosis is usually based on finding bladder glomerulations on cystoscopy and decreased compliance on cystometrogram. Urodynamic findings of instability and involuntary bladder contractions are incompatibile with this diagnosis (Close et al, 1996). When culture and sensitivity information is available, the antimicrobial agent should be re-evaluated and changed if necessary, with treatment continuing for 7 to 10 days.

Epididymitis, Epididymo-orchitis, and Orchitis

Epididymitis is an important clinical syndrome because of its differential diagnosis and management. Although in earlier series prepubertal epididymitis was diagnosed rarely (Anderson and Giacomantonio, 1985), **more recent series using newer imaging modalities have diagnosed epididymitis almost as frequently as acute testicular torsion.** Epididymitis is often difficult to distinguish from other pediatric acute scrotal processes, especially acute testicular torsion, and it occurs almost as frequently (15% to 45%) (Caldamone et al, 1984; Knight and Vassy, 1984; Mendel et al, 1985; Yazbeck and Patriquin, 1994). Although the differential diagnosis and evaluation of the acute scrotum is discussed in the chapter on testicular torsion, the etiology and evaluation of epididymitis is related to UTI in many of these cases.

Although there is some overlap, pediatric epididymitis occurs in somewhat of a bimodal age distribution. It occurs in very young boys and again in greater numbers postpubertally (Gierup et al, 1975; Knight and Vassy, 1984; Anderson and Giacomantonio, 1985; Likitnukul et al, 1987; Siegel et al, 1987; Melekos et al, 1988). This is a useful distinction clinically because the etiologies and management differ.

Symptoms and Signs

The symptoms and signs of acute epididymitis cannot be differentiated from those of any other acute scrotal condition. Characteristics that may be useful for comparison to acute torsion of the testes are a history of more gradual onset, dysuria, urethral discharge, and a history of urethral manipulation, recent urinary tract surgery (hypospadias, ureteral reimplantation), catheterization, neurogenic bladder, imperforate anus, or known lower tract genitourinary anatomic abnormalities (e.g., ureteral or vasal ectopia, bladder exstrophy) (Mandell et al, 1981; Knight and Vassy, 1984; Umeyama et al, 1985; Siegel et al, 1987; de la Hunt, 1989; Stein et al, 1994).

The scrotum is usually inflamed and swollen, and there may be localized epididymal pain. Between 18% and 33% of affected boys have fever (Doolittle et al, 1966; Gierup et al, 1975; Knight and Vassy, 1984; Siegel et al, 1987), 24% to 73% have pyuria (Doolittle et al, 1966; Siegel et al, 1987), and 17% to 73% have a peripheral leukocytosis (Doolittle et al, 1966; Gierup et al, 1975; Gislason et al, 1980; Knight and Vassy, 1984; Anderson and Giacomantonio, 1985; Siegel et al, 1987). Although these symptoms are more likely to be associated with epididymitis than acute testicular torsion, none is diagnostic. Pyuria and bacteriuria are rarely found in torsion, however (Doolittle et al, 1966; Gierup et al, 1975; Knight and Vassy, 1984; Anderson and Giacomantonio, 1985; Siegel et al, 1987).

Scrotal color flow Doppler ultrasound and radionuclide testes scans have been helpful to confirm or monitor epididymitis (Mendel et al, 1985; Mueller et al, 1988; McAlistar and Sisler, 1990; Atkinson et al, 1992; Yazbeck and Patriquin, 1994). Ultrasonography may show an enlarged epididymis of mixed echogenicity surrounded by reactive fluid. Color flow Doppler sonography usually shows increased testicular flow except when there is such extensive swelling that ischemia occurs. Similarly, nuclear scintigraphy usually shows increased perfusion and increased radiotracer deposition in the affected side of the scrotum. Although nuclear scintigraphy may be somewhat more sensitive in detecting flow, especially in prepubertal boys (Atkinson et al, 1992), sonography has better anatomic resolution and may also indicate epididymal or testicular abscesses (McAlistar and Sisler, 1990).

Pathogenesis

In young boys and infants, epididymitis is more likely to be related to genitourinary abnormalities (abnormal connections) or systemic hematogenous dissemination than in older boys (Williams et al, 1979). Urethral and urinary cultures from the prepubertal male child are likely to show either nothing or gram-negative organisms and thus be referred to as "nonspecific epididymitis," whereas in postpubertal, sexually active boys the cause may involve sexually transmitted organisms (*Neisseria gonorrhoeae, Chlamydia trachomatis*). As with the pathogenesis of renal abscess, data support two means of bacterial access to the epididymitis and testes: hematogenous dissemination and urinary tract—related infection. In young boys and infants, hematogenous pathogenesis is supported by reports in which *Haemophilus influenzae* type b has been cultured from epididymal abscesses concurrent with other sites of infection (e.g., otitis media) while the urinalysis remains normal (Weber, 1985; Greenfield, 1986; Lin et al, 1988). The fact that organisms such as *H. influenzae* require spe-

cial culture techniques that may not ordinarily be used for urinary cultures may also account for the 40% to 84% of cultures from boys diagnosed as having epididymitis without an identifiable organism (Knight and Vassy, 1984; Cabral et al, 1985; Likitnukul et al, 1987). The fact that ascending UTI or bacteriuria may cause epididymitis and epididymo-orchitis is supported by the observation that the boys who have pyuria and bacteriuria are more likely to have a urinary tract abnormality and to present at a younger age (Siegel et al, 1987).

Management

Epididymitis should be treated according to the likelihood of the causative organism. Specifically, in the young child who has pyuria and possible bacterial epididymitis, initial broad-spectrum antimicrobial coverage similar to that used to treat a UTI in an ill child should be used. Once the culture results and antimicrobial sensitivities are available, the most specific, most cost-effective agent with few side effects that achieves good tissue and urinary levels should be selected. **During or after treatment of the acute urinary and epididymal infections, radiologic evaluation of the urinary tract should be performed, as with any UTI.** Two studies report high likelihood of genitourinary anatomic abnormalities, in particular abnormal connections between the urinary tract and bowel or genital duct system, when a child has bacterial epididymitis and a UTI (Siegel et al, 1987; Anderson et al, 1989). In both studies boys with negative urinary cultures had normal urinary tracts. Whether all boys with epididymitis (including those with negative urethral and urinary cultures) need a full radiologic evaluation of the urinary tract is unclear from current data. It does appear prudent, however, to perform a VCUG and renal and bladder ultrasound for prepubertal boys with documented urinary infections, and perhaps for those in whom epididymal abscesses are found, although the latter may be related to hematogenous spread.

Epididymitis Associated with Unusual Organisms

Whenever scrotal masses are considered, tuberculous epididymitis must also be considered as the most common form of urogenital tuberculosis (Cabral et al, 1985). Whereas this form of epididymitis is more likely to be confused with a malignancy rather than a cause of an acute scrotal mass (because it usually involves painless swelling), it can be an important cause of epididymitis when dealing with patients from areas in which tuberculosis is endemic. Although there is evidence for both local urinary spread and hematogenous spread of tuberculosis to the epididymis, in the reported pediatric cases of tuberculous epididymitis there were usually other signs of hematogenous involvement, and the urine may or may not be positive for the organism (Cabral et al, 1985).

Funguria

Fungal UTIs are an increasing health care–associated infection, especially in individuals who have received antimicrobial agents and have urinary drainage catheters (Kauffman et al, 2000). Candidemia in one neonatal intensive care unit increased more than 11-fold between 1985 and 1995 (Kossoff et al, 1998). In children, predisposing factors may include antimicrobial therapy, prematurity, intravenous or umbilical artery catheterization, parenteral nutrition, and immunocompromised status (Keller et al, 1977). The urinary tract may serve both as a primary portal of entry and as a site of disseminated infection.

In children and adults with disseminated candidiasis, the kidney is the most commonly involved organ (Keller et al, 1977). *Candida* species are the most common cause of fungal UTI, with *C. albicans* the most common species and responsible for about a half of these cases. The second most common organism is *Torulopsis glabrata* (also known as *Candida glabrata*), an important species to recognize because of its common resistance to fluconazole (Kauffman et al, 2000; van't Wout, 1996).

Fungal bezoars may form in the renal pelvis, causing obstruction and anuria in infants with bilateral involvement (Keller et al, 1977; Eckstein and Kass, 1982; Robinson et al, 1987; Bartone et al, 1988; Rehan and Davidson, 1992; Hitchcock et al, 1995). For this reason, renal ultrasonography may be helpful in evaluating the extent of fungal infection when funguria is persistent (Bartone et al, 1988). Although urinary alkalinization and oral and intravenous antifungal chemotherapy may dissolve some of these fungus balls, in infants they may totally obstruct the small urinary tract, and percutaneous or surgical removal of the bezoars or drainage may be required so that both local irrigation and systemic therapy can be given.

The decision whether to treat asymptomatic funguria related to an indwelling urethral catheter remains controversial. A surveillance study involving 861 patients showed that progression to disseminated candidemia is relatively uncommon (Kauffman et al, 2000). When repeated cultures grow more than 10,000 to 15,000 cfu/ml, treatment is usually recommended (Wise, 1998).

Although stopping unnecessary antimicrobial agents, changing or removing the indwelling catheter, and urinary alkalinization may be helpful, these interventions do not clear many cases of funguria. Prospective studies with intravesical amphotericin B bladder irrigation and oral fluconazole appear to show that either drug may clear funguria, although fungal recurrences are common (Gubbins et al, 1994, 1999). Optimal dosage, length of treatment, and, for amphotericin, mode of delivery (intermittent versus continuous) are indeterminant and controversial, but amphotericin B (50 mg/L) infused continuously at 42 ml/hr for 72 hours is effective (Trinh et al, 1995; Nesbit et al, 1999). Fluconazole has been used successfully in children, although it is not approved for those younger than 6 months of age (Hitchcock et al, 1995; Zia-ul-Miraj and Miraz, 1997).

Fungal bezoars in the collecting system require treatment of obstruction when present with a percutaneous nephrostomy tube for drainage and potential local irrigation. In these situations both local and systemic therapy with amphotericin B or oral fluconazole or both may be useful for management (Bartone et al, 1988; Eckstein and Kass, 1982; Hitchcock et al, 1995; Keller et al, 1977; Rehan and Davidson, 1992; Robinson et al, 1987; Zia-ul-Miraj and Miraz, 1997). Should the fungal balls persist, surgical removal is necessary.

RENAL FUNCTION AND ESTIMATION OF GLOMERULAR FILTRATION RATE

Plasma creatinine cannot give the same estimation of renal function in a child that it can in an adult, because

Table 54–9. DISTRIBUTION OF PLASMA CREATININE CONCENTRATIONS FOR BOYS AND GIRLS BY AGE

| Age | Females | | | Males | | | |
	n	$\bar{x}$	s	n	$\bar{x}$	s	p
1	8	0.35	0.05	9	0.41	0.10	<0.2
2	13	0.45	0.07	18	0.43	0.12	<0.7
3	24	0.42	0.08	30	0.46	0.11	<0.1
4	28	0.47	0.12	49	0.45	0.11	<0.5
5	44	0.46	0.11	50	0.50	0.11	<0.1
6	44	0.48	0.11	62	0.52	0.12	<0.1
7	50	0.53	0.12	59	0.54	0.14	<0.9
8	61	0.53	0.11	60	0.57	0.16	<0.1
9	61	0.55	0.11	52	0.59	0.16	<0.1
10	46	0.55	0.13	58	0.61	0.22	<0.1
11	57	0.60	0.13	56	0.62	0.14	<0.5
12	54	0.59	0.13	67	0.65	0.16	<0.1
13	41	0.62	0.14	53	0.68	0.21	<0.2
14	30	0.65	0.13	44	0.72	0.24	<0.2
15	22	0.67	0.22	40	0.76	0.22	<0.2
16	16	0.65	0.15	24	0.74	0.23	<0.2
17	12	0.70	0.20	22	0.80	0.18	<0.2
18–20	15	0.72	0.19	19	0.91	0.17	<0.005

n, Sample number: $\bar{x}$, mean plasma creatinine concentration (mg/dl); s, standard deviation: p, significance of difference between male and female means.
Reproduced by permission from Schwartz G, Haycock MB, Spitzer A: Plasma creatinine and urea concentration in children: Normal values for age and sex. J Pediatr 1976;88: 830.

Table 54–10. DISTRIBUTION OF PLASMA UREA CONCENTRATIONS FOR BOYS AND GIRLS BY AGE

Age	Females			Males			
	n	$\bar{x}$	s	n	$\bar{x}$	s	p
1	8	4.91	1.23	9	4.82	1.71	<0.9
2	13	6.23	2.47	18	4.93	2.12	<0.2
3	24	5.08	1.29	30	5.07	1.58	<0.9
4	28	4.57	2.02	49	4.78	1.40	<0.6
5	44	4.68	1.36	50	5.52	1.74	<0.02
6	44	4.81	1.63	62	5.23	1.56	<0.2
7	50	4.67	1.39	59	5.44	1.74	<0.02
8	61	5.02	1.61	60	4.84	1.69	<0.6
9	61	5.16	1.85	52	5.60	2.68	<0.4
10	46	4.67	1.82	58	5.55	3.00	<0.1
11	57	4.51	1.62	56	5.04	1.73	<0.1
12	54	4.23	1.18	67	5.18	1.46	<0.001
13	41	4.82	1.71	53	5.24	1.65	<0.3
14	30	5.38	2.18	44	5.11	1.90	<0.7
15	22	4.87	2.11	40	5.35	1.62	<0.4
16	16	4.77	1.59	24	5.18	1.48	<0.5
17	12	4.56	1.64	12	5.67	1.59	<0.1
18–20	15	5.41	1.46	19	5.48	1.26	<0.9

n, Sample number: $\bar{x}$, mean plasma urea concentration (mM/1): s, standard deviation: p, significance of difference between male and female means.
Reproduced by permission from Schwartz GJ, Haycock MB, Spitzer A: Plasma creatinine and urea concentration in children: Normal values for age and sex. J Pediatr 1976;88: 830.

the plasma creatinine concentration changes with age and size (Donckerwolcke et al, 1970; Schwartz et al, 1976b). GFR, on the other hand, when corrected for body surface area, does not change appreciably after 2 years of age (Counahan et al, 1976). For this reason, several estimates of GFR from plasma creatinine and body height have been developed for use in serial monitoring of renal function in children and for calculating drug doses of nephrotoxic agents (Schwartz et al, 1976a; Counahan et al, 1976; Morris et al, 1982). By one formula, GFR in children (in milliliters per minute per 1173 m²) can be estimated as 0.55 times the body length (in centimeters) divided by the plasma creatinine concentration (in milligrams per deciliter) (Schwartz et al, 1976a). This formula has compared favorably with inulin and creatinine clearance measurements performed simultaneously. Normal values for plasma creatinine and urea for children of various ages are presented in Tables 54–9 and 54–10.

CONSIDERATIONS IN TREATING CHILDREN WITH URINARY TRACT INFECTIONS

Rational treatment of infants and children with UTIs is based on an understanding of bacterial and host risk factors with rapid detection and evaluation of these to modify them when possible. Moreover, judicious use of antimicrobial agents allows effective treatment and limits organism selection and bacterial resistance. Antimicrobial use should be limited to the shortest effective duration and narrowest spectrum. When a child with bacteriuria and renal scarring has been identified, management should minimize the chance of future bacteriuria and assess potential risk factors to prevent further renal infection–related renal damage. In some instances, awareness of predisposing risk

factors may help select children for urinary tract antimicrobial prophylaxis or further evaluation.

When renal scarring is identified, the child and parents need to be educated about possibilities of future hypertension, proteinuria, and progressive nephropathy. In moderate to severe renal scarring with renal insufficiency, early nephrologic consultation for evaluation and surveillance for hypertension, proteinuria, acid-base balance, and dietary counseling (low protein intake) may improve or stabilize renal function and improve body growth. In addition, the young female patient with renal insufficiency due to pyelonephritogenic nephropathy and recurrent UTIs may desire pregnancy counseling.

Although familial screening for VUR may not be routine in all situations, families in whom a member has VUR or renal scarring must be made aware of the familial risk of VUR, consequences of UTIs, and the need for early diagnosis, treatment, and evaluation of UTIs in family members.

REFERENCES

Epidemiology, Diagnosis, Classification, and Bacteria

Åbyholm G, Monn E: Intranasal DDAVP test in the study of renal concentrating capacity in children with recurrent urinary tract infections. Eur J Pediatr 1979;130:149–154.

Ahmad T, Vickers D, Campbell S, et al: Urine collection from disposable nappies. Lancet 1991;338:674–676.

American Academy of Pediatrics, Committee on Quality Improvement and Subcommittee on Urinary Tract Infection: Practice parameter: The diagnosis, treatment, and evaluation of the initial urinary tract infection in febrile infants and young children. Pediatrics 1999;103:843–852.

Asscher AW: Urinary tract infection: The value of early diagnosis. Kidney Int 1975;7:63–67.

Asscher AW, McLachlan MSF, Verrier-Jones R, et al: Screening for asymptomatic urinary-tract infection in schoolgirls. Lancet 1973;2:1.

Bailey RR: A overview of reflux nephropathy. In Hodson JJ, Kincaid-

Smith P (eds): Reflux Nephropathy. New York, Masson, 1979, pp 3–13.

Barkemeyer B: Suprapubic aspiration of urine in very low birth weight infants. Pediatrics 1994;92:457–459.

Benson M, Jodal U, Andreasson A, et al: Interleukin 6 response to urinary tract infection in childhood. Pediatr Infect Dis J 1994;13:612–616.

Bergström T: Sex differences in childhood urinary tract infection. Arch Dis Child 1972;47:227–232.

Bollgren I, Engström CF, Hammarlind M, et al: Low urinary counts of P-fimbriated *Escherichia coli* in presumed acute pyelonephritis. Arch Dis Child 1984;59:102–106.

Buyan N, Bircan Z, Hasanoglu E, et al: The importance of 99m Tc DMSA scanning in the localization of childhood urinary tract infections. Int Urol Nephrol 1993;25:11–17.

Buys H, Pead L, Hallett R, Maskell R: Suprapubic aspiration under ultrasound guidance in children with fever of undiagnosed cause. BMJ 1994;308:690–692.

Crain E, Gershel J: Urinary tract infections in febrile infants younger than 8 weeks of age. Pediatrics 1990;86:363–367.

de Man P, Jodal U, Svanborg C: Dependence among host response parameters used to diagnose urinary tract infection. J Infect Dis 1991;163:331–335.

Dele Davies H, Ford Jones E, Sheng R, et al: Nosocomial urinary tract infections at a pediatric hospital. Pediatr Infect Dis J 1992;11:349–354.

Duguid JP, Clegg S, Wilson MI: The fimbrial and nonfimbrial hemagglutinins of *Escherichia coli*. J Med Microbiol 1978;12:213.

Gorelick M, Shaw K: Screening tests for urinary tract infection in children: A meta-analysis. Pediatrics 1999;104:e54. Available at http://www.pediatrics.org/cgi/content/full/104/5/e54.

Hallender HO, Kallner A, Lundin A, Österberg E: Evaluation of rapid methods for the detection of bacteriuria (screening) in primary health care. Acta Pathol Microbiol Immunol Scand 1986;94:39–49.

Hardy J, Furnell P, Brumfitt W: Comparison of sterile bag, clean catch and suprapubic aspiration in the diagnosis of urinary infection in early childhood. Br J Urol 1976;48:279–283.

Hellerstein S: Recurrent urinary tract infections in children. Pediatr Infect Dis 1982;1:271–281.

Hoberman A, Wald E: Urinary tract infections in young febrile children. Pediatr Infect Dis J 1997;16:11–17.

Hoberman A, Wald E, Reynolds E, et al: Pyuria and bacteriuria in urine specimens obtained by catheter from young children with fever. J Pediatr 1994;124:513–519.

Jacobson SH, Hammarlind M, Lidefeldt KJ, et al: Incidence of aerobactin-positive *Escherichia coli* strains in patients with symptomatic urinary tract infection. Eur J Clin Microbiol Infect Dis 1988;7:630–634.

Jacobson SH, Tullus K, Brauner A: Hydrophobic properties of *Escherichia coli* causing acute pyelonephritis. J Infect 1989b;19:17–23.

Jantausch B, Widermann B, Hull S, et al: *Escherichia coli* virulence factors and 99m Tc-dimercaptosuccinic acid renal scan in children with febrile urinary tract infection. Pediatr Infect Dis J 1992;11:343–349.

Johnson C, Vacca C, Fattlar D, Fulton D, Hall P: Urinary *N*-acetyl-β-glucosaminidase and the selection of children for radiologic evaluation after urinary tract infection. Pediatrics 1990;86:211–216.

Källenius G, Möllby R, Svenson SB, et al: Occurrence of P-fimbriated *Escherichia coli* in urinary tract infections. Lancet 1981;2:1369–1372.

Kass EH, Finland M: Asymptomatic infections of the urinary tract. Trans Assoc Am Physicians 1956;69:56–64.

Kramer M, Etezadi-Amoli J, Ciampi A, et al: Parents' versus physicians' values for clinical outcomes in young febrile children. Pediatrics 1994a;93:697–702.

Kramer M, Tange S, Drummond K, Mills E: Urine testing in young febrile children: A risk-benefit analysis. J Pediatr 1994b;125:6–13.

Kramer M, Tange S, Mills E, et al: Role of the complete blood count in detecting occult focal bacterial infection in the young febrile child. J Clin Epidemiol 1993;46:349–357.

Kunin C, McCormack R: An epidemiologic study of bacteriuria and blood pressure among nuns and working women. N Engl J Med 1968;278:635–642.

Kunin CM, Deutscher R, Paquin A: Urinary tract infection in school children: An epidemiologic, clinical and laboratory study. Medicine (Baltimore) 1964;43:91–130.

Lin D-S, Huang S-H, Lin C-C, et al: Urinary tract infection in febrile infants younger than eight weeks of age. Pediatrics 2000;105:e20. Available at http://www.pediatrics.org/cgi/content/full/105/2/e20.

Lohr J: Use of routine urinalysis in making a presumptive diagnosis of urinary tract infection in children. Pediatr Infect Dis J 1991;10:646–650.

Lohr J, Downs S, Dudley S, Donowitz L: Hospital-acquired urinary tract infections in the pediatric patient: A prospective study. Pediatr Infect Dis J 1994;13:8–12.

Lohr J, Portilla M, Geuder T, et al: Making a presumptive diagnosis of urinary tract infection by using a urinalysis performed in an on-site laboratory. J Pediatr 1993;122:22–25.

Majd M, Rushton H, Jantausch B, Wiedermann B: Relationship among vesicoureteral reflux, P-fimbriated *Escherichia coli*, and acute pyelonephritis in children with febrile urinary tract infection. J Pediatr 1991;119:578–585.

Rushton H, Majd J: Pyelonephritis in male infants: How important is the foreskin? J Urol 1992a;148:733–736.

Savage DCL: Natural history of covert bacteriuria in schoolgirls. Kidney Int 1975;8:S90–S95.

Stamey TA: A clinical classification of urinary tract infections based upon origin. (Editorial.) South Med J 1975;68:934.

Stamm WE, Counts GW, Running KR, et al: Diagnosis of coliform infection in acutely dysuric women. N Engl J Med 1982;307:463–468.

Svanborg Edén C, Hanson LA: *Escherichia coli* pili as possible mediators of attachment to human urinary tract epithelial cells. Infect Immun 1978;21:229.

Tambic T, Oberiter V, Delmis J, Tambic A: Diagnostic value of a P-fimbriation test in determining duration of therapy in children with urinary tract infections. Clin Ther 1992;14:667–671.

Tomlinson P, Smellie J, Prescod N, et al: Differential excretion of urinary proteins in children with vesicoureteric reflux and reflux nephropathy. Pediatr Nephrol 1994;8:21–25.

Väisänen V, Elo J, Tallgren LG, et al: Mannose-resistant haemagglutination and P antigen recognition are characteristic of *Escherichia coli* causing primary pyelonephritis. Lancet 1981;2:1366–1369.

Waisman Y, Zerem E, Amir L, Mimouni M: The validity of the Uriscreen test for early detection of urinary tract infection in children. Pediatrics 1999;104:e41. Available at http://www.pediatrics.org/cgi/content/full/104/4/e41.

Wettergren B, Fasth A, Jacobsson B, et al: UTI during the first year of life in a Göteborg area 1977–79. Pediatr Res 1980;14:981.

Wiggelinkhuizen J, Maytham D, Hanslo D: Dipstick screening for urinary tract infection. S Afr Med J 1988;74:224–228.

Winberg J, Anderson HJ, Bergström T, et al: Epidemiology of symptomatic urinary tract infection in childhood. Acta Paediatr Scand 1974;S252:1–20.

Wiswell T, Hachey W: Urinary tract infections and the uncircumcised state: An update. Clin Pediatr 1993;32:130–134.

Pathogenesis of Urinary Tract Infections

Åbyholm G, Monn E. Intranasal DDAVP test in the study of renal concentrating capacity in children with recurrent urinary tract infections. Eur J Pediatr 1979;130:149–154.

American Academy Pediatrics, Committee on Quality Improvement and Subcommittee on Urinary Tract Infection: Practice parameter: The diagnosis, treatment, and evaluation of the initial urinary tract infection in febrile infants and young children. Pediatrics 1999;103:843–852.

Andriole VT: The role of Tamm-Horsfall protein in the pathogenesis of reflux nephropathy and chronic pyelonephritis. Yale J Biol Med 1985;58:91–100.

Angell S, Pruthi R, Shortliffe L: The urodynamic relationship between renal pelvic and bladder pressure with varying urinary flow rates in rats with congenital vesicoureteral reflux. J Urol 1998;160:150–156.

Anhalt M, Cawood D, Scott R: Xanthogranulomatous pyelonephritis: A comprehensive review with report of 4 additional cases. J Urol 1971;105:10.

Asscher AW, McLachlan MSF, Verrier-Jones R, et al: Screening for asymptomatic urinary-tract infection in schoolgirls. Lancet 1973;2:1.

Bachur R: Nonresponders: Prolonged fever among infants with urinary tract infections. Pediatrics 2000;105:e59.

Bailey RR, Lynn KL, McRae CU: Unilateral reflux nephropathy and hypertension. In Hodson CJ, Heptinstall TH, Winberg J (eds): Reflux Nephropathy Update: 1983. New York, S. Karger, 1984a; pp 116–125.

Bailey RR, McRae CU, Maling TMJ, et al: Renal vein renin concentration in the hypertension of unilateral reflux nephropathy. J Urol 1978;120:21–23.

Bailey RR, Swainson CP, Lynn KL, Burry AF: Glomerular lesions in the "normal" kidney in patients with unilateral reflux nephropathy. In Hodson CJ, Heptinstall RH, Winberg J (eds): Reflux Nephropathy Update: 1983. New York, 1984b, pp 126–131.

Barker A, Ahmed S: Renal abscess in childhood. Aust N Z J Surg 1991; 61:217–221.

Benador D, Benador N, Slosman D, et al: Cortical scintigraphy in the evaluation of renal parenchymal changes in children with pyelonephritis. J Pediatr 1994;124:17–20.

Berg U: Long-term followup of renal morphology and function in children with recurrent pyelonephritis. J Urol 1992;148:1715–1720.

Bonadio W, Webster H, Wolfe A, Gorecki D: Correlating infectious outcome with clinical parameters of 1130 consecutive febrile infants aged zero to eight weeks. Pediatr Emerg Care 1993;9:84–86.

Boyarsky S, Labay P: Ureteral Dynamics: Pathophysiology, Drugs, and Surgical Implications. Baltimore, Williams & Wilkins, 1972.

Brenner BM, Meyer TW, Hostetter TH: Dietary protein intake and the progressive nature of kidney disease. N Engl J Med 1982;307:652–659.

Brook I: The role of anaerobic bacteria in perinephric and renal abscesses in children. Pediatrics 1994;93:261–264.

Brown P, Dodson M, Weintrub P: Xanthogranulomatous pyelonephritis: Report of nonsurgical management of a case and review of the literature. Clin Infect Dis 1996;1996:308–314.

Busch R, Huland H: Correlation of symptoms and results of direct bacterial localization in patients with urinary tract infections. J Urol 1984; 132:282–285.

Colemen BG, Arger PH, Mulhern CB, et al: Pyonephrosis: Sonography in the diagnosis and management. AJR Am J Roentgenol 1981;137:939–943.

Cousins C, Somers J, Broderick N, et al: Xanthogranulomatous pyelonephritis in childhood: Ultrasound and CT diagnosis. Pediatr Radiol 1994; 24:210–212.

Craig M, Irwig L, Knight J, Roy L: Does treatment of vesicoureteric reflux in childhood prevent end-stage renal disease attributable to reflux nephropathy? Pediatrics 2000;105:1236–1241.

Crain E, Gershel J: Urinary tract infections in febrile infants younger than 8 weeks of age. Pediatrics 1990;86:363–367.

Dacher JN, Pfister C, Monroc M, et al: Power Doppler sonographic pattern of acute pyelonephritis in children: Comparison with CT. AJR Am J Roentgenol 1996;166:1451–1455.

Davison JM, Lindheimer MD: Renal disease in pregnant women. Clin Obstet Gynecol 1978;21:411.

Dillon MJ: Recent advances in evaluation and management of childhood hypertension. Eur J Pediatr 1979;132:133–139.

Dillon JM, Gordon I, Shah V: Tc(99m)-DMSA scanning and segmental renal vein renin estimations in children with renal scarring. In Hodson CJ, Heptinstall RH, Winberg J (eds): Reflux Nephropathy Update: 1983. New York, 1984, pp 28–35.

Ditchfield M, de Campo J, Nolan T, et al: Risk factors in the development of early renal cortical defects in children with urinary tract infection. AJR Am J Roentgenol 1994b;162:1393–1397.

Duncan JL: Differential effect of Tamm-Horsfall protein on adherence of *Escherichia coli* to transitional epithelial cells. J Infect Dis 1988;158: 1379–1382.

Eastham J, Ahlering T, Skinner E: Xanthogranulomatous pyelonephritis: Clinical findings and surgical considerations. Urology 1994;43:295–299.

Eggli D, Tulchinsky M: Scintigraphic evaluation of pediatric urinary tract infection. Semin Nucl Med 1993;23:199–218.

Fasth A, Bjure J, Hellström M, et al: Autoantibodies to Tamm-Horsfall glycoprotein in children with renal damage associated with urinary tract infections. Acta Paediatr Scand 1980;69:709–715.

Filly R, Friedland GW, Govan DE, Fair WR: Development and progression of clubbing and scarring in children with recurrent urinary tract infections. Pediatr Radiol 1974;113:145–153.

Funston MR, Cremin BJ: Intrarenal reflux: Papillary morphology and pressure relationships in children's necropsy kidneys. Br J Urol 1978; 51:665–670.

Giblin J, O'Connor K, Fildes R, et al: The diagnosis of acute pyelonephritis in the piglet using single photon emission computerized tomography dimercaptosuccinic acid scintigraphy: A pathological correlation. J Urol 1993;150:759–762.

Ginsburg CM, McCracken GHJ: Urinary tract infections in young infants. Pediatrics 1982;69:409–412.

Glauser MP, Lyons JM, Braude AI: Prevention of chronic experimental pyelonephritis by suppression of acute suppuration. J Clin Invest 1978; 61:403.

Goodman T, McHugh K, Lindsell D: Paediatric xanthogranulomatous pyelonephritis. Int J Clin Pract 1998;52:43–45.

Goonasekera C, Shah V, Wade A, et al: 15-year follow-up of renin and blood pressure in reflux nephropathy. Lancet 1996;347:640–643.

Greenfield SP, Montgomery P: Computerized tomography and acute pyelonephritis in children: A clinical correlation. Urology 1987;29:137–140.

Hannerz L, Kikstad I, Johansson L, et al: Distribution of renal scars and intrarenal reflux in children with a past history of urinary tract infection. Acta Radiol 1987;28:443–446.

Hinman F: Peristalsis in the diseased ureter: A brief summary of current knowledge. In Boyarsky S, Gottschalk C, Tanagho E, Zimskind P (eds): Urodynamics: Hydrodynamics of the Ureter and Renal Pelvis. New York, Academic Press, 1971, pp 359.

Hoberman A, Chao H, Keller D, et al: Prevalence of urinary tract infection in febrile infants. J Pediatr 1993;123:17–23.

Hoddick W, Jeffrey R, Goldberg H, et al: CT and sonography of severe renal and perirenal infections. AJR Am J Roentgenol 1983;140:517.

Hodson J, Maling TMJ, McManamon PJ, Lewis MG: Reflux nephropathy. Kidney Int 1975;8:S50–S58.

Holland N, Jackson E, Kazee M, et al: Relation of urinary tract infection and vesicoureteral reflux to scars: Follow-up and thirty-eight patients. J Pediatr 1990;116:S65–S71.

Holland NH, Kotchen T, Bhathena D: Hypertension in children with chronic pyelonephritis. Kidney Int 1975;Suppl:S243–S251.

Hostetter TH, Olson JL, Rennke HG, et al: Hyperfiltration in remnant nephrons: A potentially adverse response to renal ablation. Am J Physiol 1981;10:F85–F93.

Hostetter TH, Rennke HG, Brenner BM: Compensatory renal hemodynamic injury: A final common pathway of residual nephron destruction. Am J Kidney Dis 1982;5:310–314.

Huang A, Palmer L, Hom D, et al: Ibuprofen combined with antibiotics suppresses renal scarring due to ascending pyelonephritis in rats. J Urol 1999;162:1396–1398.

Issa M, Shortliffe L: Effect of bacteriuria on bladder and renal pelvic pressures in the rat. J Urol 1992;148:559–563.

Ivanyi B, Thoenes W: Microvascular injury and repair in acute human bacterial pyelonephritis. Virchows Arch 1987;411:257–265.

Jacobson SH, Eklöf O, Eriksson CG, et al: Development of hypertension and uraemia after pyelonephritis in childhood: 27 year follow up. BMJ 1989a;299:703–706.

Jakobsson B, Berg U, Svensson L: Renal scarring after acute pyelonephritis. Arch Dis Child 1994;70:111–115.

Jakobsson B, Nolstedt L, Svensson L, et al: ^{99m}Technetium-dimercaptosuccinic acid scan in the diagnosis of acute pyelonephritis in children: Relation to clinical and radiological findings. Pediatr Nephrol 1992;6: 328–334.

Jodal U: The natural history of bacteriuria in childhood. Infect Dis Clin North Am 1987;1:713–729.

Johnson JR, Vincent LM, Wang K, et al: Renal ultrasonographic correlates of acute pyelonephritis. Clin Infect Dis 1992;14:15–22.

Kaack M, Dowling K, Patterson G, Roberts J: Immunology of pyelonephritis: VIII. *E. coli* causes granulocytic aggregation and renal ischemia. J Urol 1986;136:1117–1122.

Kaijser B, Larsson P: Experimental acute pyelonephritis caused by enterobacteria in animals: A review. J Urol 1982;127:786.

Kincaid-Smith P: Glomerular lesions in atrophic pyelonephritis and reflux nephropathy. Kidney Int 1975;8:S81–S83.

Kincaid-Smith PS: Diffuse parenchymal lesions in reflux nephropathy and the possibility of making a renal biopsy diagnosis in reflux nephropathy. In Hodson CJ, Heptinstall RH, Winberg J (eds): Reflux Nephropathy Update: 1983. New York, 1984, pp 111–115.

Klar A, Hurvitz H, Berkun Y, et al: Focal bacterial nephritis (lobar nephronia) in children. J Pediatr 1996;128:850–853.

Koff SA, Murtagh D: The uninhibited bladder in children: Effect of treatment on vesicoureteral reflux resolution. In Hodson CJ, Heptinstall RH, Winberg J (eds): Reflux Nephropathy Update: 1983. New York, 1984, pp 211–220.

Lin DS, Huang SH, Lin CC, et al: Urinary tract infection in febrile infants younger than eight weeks of age. Pediatrics 2000;105:e20. Available at http://www.pediatrics.org/cgi/content/full/105/2/e20.

Malek R, Elder J: Xanthogranulomatous pyelonephritis: A critical analysis of 26 cases and the literature. J Urol 1978;119:589–593.

Mårild S, Hellström M, Jacobsson B, et al: Influence of bacterial adhesion on ureteral width in children with acute pyelonephritis. J Pediatr 1989a; 115:265–268.

Martinell J, Lidin-Janson G, Jagenburg R, et al: Girls prone to urinary infections followed into adulthood: Indices of renal disease. Pediatr Nephrol 1996;10:139–142.

Miller T, Phillips S: Pyelonephritis: The relationship between infection, renal scarring, and antimicrobial therapy. Kidney Int 1981;19:1981.

Miller TE, Stewart E, North JDK: Immunobacteriological aspects of pyelonephritis. Contrib Nephrol 1979;16:11–15.

Mitsumori K, Terai A, Yamamoto S, Yoshida O: Virulence characteristics and DNA fingerprints of *Escherichia coli* isolated from women with acute uncomplicated pyelonephritis. J Urol 1997;158:2329–2332.

Moller J, Kristensen I: Xanthogranulomatous pyelonephritis. Acta Pathol Microbiol Scand 1980;88:89.

Morin D, Veyrac C, Kotzki P, et al: Comparison of ultrasound and dimercaptosuccinic acid scintigraphy changes in acute pyelonephritis. Pediatr Nephrol 1999;13:219–222.

Morita M, Yoshiara S, White R, Raafat F: The glomerular changes in children with reflux nephropathy. J Pathol 1990;162:245–253.

Newcastle Asymptomatic Bacteriuria Research Group: Asymptomatic bacteriuria in schoolchildren in Newcastle upon Tyne. Arch Dis Child 1975;50:90.

Parkhouse H, Godley M, Cooper J, et al: Renal imagining with 99Tcm-labelled DMSA in the detection of acute pyelonephritis: An experimental study in the pig. Nucl Med Commun 1989;10:63–70.

Pohl H, Rushton H, Park J-S, et al: Adjunctive oral corticosteroids reduce renal scarring: The piglet model of reflux and acute experimental pyelonephritis. Urology 1999;162:815–820.

Quinn F, Dick A, Corbally M, et al: Xanthogranulomatous pyelonephritis in childhood. Arch Dis Child 1999;81:483–486.

Ransley PG, Risdon RA: Renal papillae and intrarenal reflux in the pig. Lancet 1974;2:1114.

Ransley PG, Risdon RA: Reflux and renal scarring. Br J Radiol 1978;51: 1–35.

Ransley PG, Risdon RA, Godley ML: High pressure sterile vesicoureteral reflux and renal scarring: An experimental study in the pig and minipig. In Hodson CJ, Heptinstall RH, Winberg J (eds): Reflux Nephropathy Update: 1983. New York, 1984, pp 320–343.

Roberts JA, Domingue GJ, Martin LN, et al: Immunology of pyelonephritis in the primate model: Live versus heat-killed bacteria. Kidney Int 1981;19:297.

Roberts JA, Roth JK, Domingue GJ: Immunology of pyelonephritis in the primate model: V. Effect of superoxide dismutase. J Urol 1982;128: 1394.

Rolleston GL, Maling TMJ, Hodson CJ: Intrarenal reflux and the scarred kidney. Arch Dis Child 1974;49:531–539.

Rote A, Bauer S, Retik A: Renal abscess in children. J Urol 1978;119: 254–258.

Rushton H, Majd J: Pyelonephritis in male infants: How important is the foreskin? J Urol 1992a;148:733–736.

Rushton H, Majd M: Dimercaptosuccinic acid renal scintigraphy for the evaluation of pyelonephritis and scarring: A review of experimental and clinical studies. J Urol 1992b;148:1726–1732.

Savage DCL: Natural history of covert bacteriuria in schoolgirls. Kidney Int 1975;8:S90–S95.

Savage JM, Dillon MJ, Shah V, et al: Renin and blood pressure in children with renal scarring and vesicoureteric reflux. Lancet 1978;2: 441–444.

Savage JM, Koh CT, Barratt TM, Dillon MJ: Five year prospective study of plasma renin activity and blood pressure in patients with longstanding reflux nephropathy. Arch Dis Child 1987;62:678–682.

Shimada K, Matsui T, Ogino T, Ikoma F: New development and progression of renal scarring in children with primary VUR. Int Urol Nephrol 1989;21:153–158.

Shimamura T: Mechanisms of renal tissue destruction in an experimental acute pyelonephritis. Exp Mol Pathol 1981;34:34.

Shortliffe LD, Stamey T: Infections of the urinary tract: Introduction and general principles. In Walsh PC, Gittes RF, Perlmutter AD, Stamey TA (eds): Campbell's Urology. Philadelphia, WB Saunders, 1986a, pp 738–796.

Slotki IN, Asscher AW: Prevention of scarring in experimental pyelonephritis in the rat by early antibiotic therapy. Nephron 1982;30:262.

Smellie J: Reflections on 30 years of treating children with urinary tract infections. J Urol 1991;146:665–668.

Smellie J, Prescod N, Shaw P, et al: Childhood reflux and urinary infection: A follow-up of 10–41 years in 226 adults. Pediatr Nephrol 1998; 12:727–736.

Smellie JM, Edwards D, Normand ICS, Prescod N: Effect of vesicoureteric reflux on renal growth in children with urinary tract infection. Arch Dis Child 1981;56:593–600.

Smellie JM, Normand ICS: Reflux nephropathy in childhood. In Hodson J, Kincaid-Smith P (eds): Reflux Nephropathy. New York, Masson, 1979, pp 14–20.

Smellie JM, Ransley PG, Norman ICS, et al: Development of new renal scars: A collaborative study. BMJ 1985;290:1957–1960.

Stamey TA: Pathogenesis and Treatment of Urinary Tract Infections. Baltimore, Williams & Wilkins, 1980.

Stecker JF, Read BP, Poutasse EF: Pediatric hypertension as a delayed sequela of reflux-induced chronic pyelonephritis. J Urol 1977;118:644–646.

Steele B, Petrou C, deMaria J: Renal abscess in children. Urology 1990; 36:325–328.

Stokland E, Hellström M, Jacobsson B, et al: Early 99m Tc dimercaptosuccinic acid (DMSA) scintigraphy in symptomatic first-time urinary tract infection. Acta Paediatr 1996;85:430–436.

Thorley J, Jones S, Sanford J: Perinephric abscess. Medicine (Baltimore) 1974;53:441.

Tomlinson P, Smellie J, Prescod N, et al: Differential excretion of urinary proteins in children with vesicoureteric reflux and reflux nephropathy. Pediatr Nephrol 1994;8:21–25.

Torres VE, Velosa JA, Holley KE, et al: The progression of vesicoureteral reflux nephropathy. Ann Intern Med 1980;92:776–784.

Tulassy T, Miltényi M, Dobos M: Alterations of urinary carbon dioxide tension, electrolyte handling and low molecular weight protein excretion in acute pyelonephritis. Acta Scand 1986;75:415–419.

Tullus K, Hörlin K, Svenson SB, Källenius G: Epidemic outbreaks of acute pyelonephritis caused by nosocomial spread of P-fimbriated *Escherichia coli* in children. J Infect Dis 1984;150:728–736.

Uehling D, Hahnfeld L, Scanlan K: Urinary tract abnormalities in children with acute focal bacterial nephritis. Br J Urol 2000;85:885–888.

Vachvanichsanong P, Dissaneewate P, Patrapinyokul S, et al: Renal abscess in healthy children: Report of three cases. Pediatr Nephrol 1992; 6:273–275.

Verber I, Meller S: Serial 99mTc dimercaptosuccinic acid (DMSA) scans after urinary infections presenting before the age of 5 years. Arch Dis Child 1989;64:1533–1537.

Walker RD: Renal functional changes associated with vesicoureteral reflux. Urol Clin North Am 1990;17:307–316.

Wallace DMA, Rothwell DL, Williams DI: The long-term follow-up of surgically treated vesicoureteric reflux. Br J Urol 1978;50:479–484.

Wallin L, Helin I, Bajc M: Kidney swelling: Findings on DMSA scintigraphy. Clin Nucl Med 1997;22:292–299.

Wennerström M, Hansson S, Jodal U, et al: Renal function 16–26 years after the first urinary tract infection in childhood. Arch Pediatr Adolesc Med 2000;154:339–345.

Wikstad I, Hannerz L, Karlsson A, et al: 99m Tc DMSA renal cortical scintigraphy in the diagnosis of acute pyelonephritis in rats. Pediatr Nephrol 1990;4:331–334.

Winberg J, Anderson HJ, Bergström T, et al: Epidemiology of symptomatic urinary tract infection in childhood. Acta Paediatr Scand 1974; S252:1–20.

Yen TC, Tzen KY, Chen WP, Lin CY: The value of Ga-67 renal SPECT in diagnosing and monitoring complete and incomplete treatment in children with acute pyelonephritis. Clin Nucl Med 1999;24:669–673.

Associated Problems

Abbott GD: Neonatal bacteriuria: A prospective study in 1460 infants. BMJ 1972;1:267.

Asscher AW, McLachlan MSF, Verrier-Jones R, et al: Screening for asymptomatic urinary-tract infection in schoolgirls. Lancet 1973;2:1.

Bauer SB, Retik AB, Colodny AH, et al: The unstable bladder of childhood. Urol Clin North Am 1980;7:321–336.

Ditchfield M, De Campo J, Cook DJ, et al: Vesicoureteral reflux: An accurate predictor of acute pyelonephritis in childhood urinary tract infection? Radiology 1994a;190:413–415.

Govan DE, Fair WR, Friedland GW, Filly RA: Management of children with urinary tract infections: The Stanford experience. Urology 1975;6: 273–286.

Hansson S: Urinary incontinence in children and associated problems. Scand J Urol Nephrol 1992;141:47–55.

Jakobsson B, Nolstedt L, Svensson L, et al: ^{99m}Technetium-dimercaptosuccinic acid scan in the diagnosis of acute pyelonephritis in children: Relation to clinical and radiological findings. Pediatr Nephrol 1992;6: 328–334.

Jodal U: The natural history of bacteriuria in childhood. Infect Dis Clin North Am 1987;1:713–729.

Kass EJ, Diokno AC, Montealegre A: Enuresis: Principles of management and result of treatment. J Urol 1979;121:794–796.

Kjølseth D, Knudsen LM, Jadsen B, et al: Urodynamic biofeedback training for children with bladder-sphincter dyscoordination during voiding. Neurourol Urodyn 1993;12:211–221.

Koff SA: Bladder-sphincter dysfunction in childhood. Urology 1982;19: 457–461.

Koff SA, Lapides J, Piazza DH: Association of urinary tract infection and reflux with uninhibited bladder contractions and voluntary sphincteric obstruction. J Urol 1979;122:373–376.

Koff S, Wagner T, Jayanthi V: The relationship among dysfunctional elimination syndromes, primary vesicoureteral reflux and urinary tract infections in children. J Urol 1998;160:1019–1022.

Kondo A, Kobayashi M, Otani T, et al: Children with unstable bladder: Clinical and urodynamic observation. J Urol 1983;129:88–91.

Kunin CM, Deutscher R, Pacquin A: Urinary tract infection in school children: An epidemiologic, clinical and laboratory study. Medicine (Baltimore) 1964;43:91–130.

Loening-Baucke V: Urinary incontinence and urinary tract infection and their resolution with treatment of chronic constipation of childhood. Pediatrics 1997;100:228–232.

Newcastle Asymptomatic Bacteriuria Research Group: Asymptomatic bacteriuria in schoolchildren in Newcastle upon Tyne. Arch Dis Child 1975;50:90.

O'Regan S, Yazbeck S, Schick E: Constipation, bladder instability, urinary tract infection syndrome. Clin Nephrol 1985;23:152–154.

Ozen HA, Whitaker RH: Does the severity of presentation in children with vesicoureteric reflux relate to the severity of the disease or the need for operation? Br J Urol 1987;60:110–112.

Passerini-Glazel, G, Cisternino A, Camuffo MC, et al: Video-urodynamic studies of minor voiding dysfunctions in children: An overview of 13 years' experience. Scan J Urol Nephrol 1992;141:70–84.

Qvist N, Kristensen ES, Nielsen KK, et al: Detrusor instability in children with recurrent urinary tract infection and/or enuresis. Urol Int 1986;41: 196–198.

Rushton H, Majd M: Dimercaptosuccinic acid renal scintigraphy for the evaluation of pyelonephritis and scarring: A review of experimental and clinical studies. J Urol 1992b;148:1726–1732.

Savage DCL: Natural history of covert bacteriuria in schoolgirls. Kidney Int 1975;8:S90–S95.

Skoog SJ, Belman AB, Majd M: A nonsurgical approach to the management of primary vesicoureteral reflux. J Urol 1987;138:941–946.

Sørensen K, Lose G, Nathan E: Urinary tract infections and diurnal incontinence in girls. Eur J Pediatr 1988;148:146–147.

Tappin D, Murphy A, Mocan H, et al: A prospective study of children with first acute symptomatic E. coli urinary tract infection: Early 99m-technetium dimercaptosuccinic acid scan appearances. Acta Paediatr Scand 1989;78:923–929.

vanGool JD, Vijverberg MAW, deJong TPVM: Functional daytime incontinence: Clinical and urodynamic assessment. Scand J Urol Nephrol 1992a;141:58–69.

vanGool JD, Vijverberg MAW, Messer AP, et al: Functional daytime incontinence: Non-pharmacological treatment. Scand J Urol Nephrol 1992b;141:93–103.

Winberg J, Anderson HJ, Bergström T, et al: Epidemiology of symptomatic urinary tract infection in childhood. Acta Paediatr Scand 1974; S252:1–20.

Factors Affecting Risk of Bacteriuria and Renal Damage

Abbott GD: Neonatal bacteriuria: A prospective study in 1460 infants. BMJ 1972;1:267.

American Academy of Pediatrics, Task Force on Circumcision: Circumcision policy statement. Pediatrics 1999;103:686–693.

Ashkenazi S, Even-Tov S, Samra Z, Dinari G: Uropathogens of various childhood populations and their antibiotic susceptibility. Pediatr Infect Dis J 1991b;10:742–746.

Asscher AW, McLachlan MSF, Verrier-Jones R, et al: Screening for asymptomatic urinary-tract infection in schoolgirls. Lancet 1973;2:1.

Bear RA: Pregnancy in patients with renal disease: A study of 44 cases. Obstet Gynecol 1976;48:13–18.

Bellinger MF, Duckett JW: Vesicoureteral reflux: A comparison of non-surgical and surgical management. Contrib Nephrol 1984;39:81–93.

Berg U: Long-term followup of renal morphology and function in children with recurrent pyelonephritis. J Urol 1992;148:1715–1720.

Bollgren I, Winberg J: The periurethral aerobic bacterial flora in healthy boys and girls. Acta Paediatr Scand 1976a;65:74–80.

Bollgren I, Winberg J: The periurethral aerobic flora in girls highly susceptible to urinary infections. Acta Paediatr Scand 1976b;65:81–87.

Brock J, Adams M, Hunley T, et al: Potential risk factors associated with progressive renal damage in childhood urological diseases: The role of angiotensin-converting enzyme gene polymorphism. J Urol 1997;158: 1308–1311.

Brock J, Hunley T, Adams M, Kon V: Role of the renin angiotensin system in disorders of the urinary tract. J Urol 1998;160:1812–1819.

Bukowski T, Betrus G, Aqulina J, Perlmutter A: Urinary tract infections and pregnancy in women who underwent antireflux surgery in childhood. J Urol 1998;159:1286–1289.

Cardiff Oxford Bacteriuria Study Group: Sequelae of covert bacteriuria in schoolgirls: A four-year follow-up study. Lancet 1978;1:889–893.

Coppa G, Gabrielli O, Giorgi P, et al: Preliminary study of breastfeeding and bacterial adhesion to uroepithelial cells. Lancet 1990;335:569–571.

Cousins C, Somers J, Broderick N, et al: Xanthogranulomatous pyelonephritis in childhood: Ultrasound and CT diagnosis. Pediatr Radiol 1994; 24:210–212.

Cunningham N: Circumcision and urinary tract infections. Pediatrics 1986;77:267–269.

Davison JM, Lindheimer MD: Renal disease in pregnant women. Clin Obstet Gynecol 1978;21:411.

de la Hunt M, Deegan S, Scott J: Intermittent catheterisation for neuropathic urinary incontinence. Arch Dis Child 1989;64:821–824.

Dele Davies H, Ford Jones E, Sheng R, et al: Nosocomial urinary tract infections at a pediatric hospital. Pediatr Infect Dis J 1992;11:349–354.

Duncan B, Ey J, Holberg C, et al: Exclusive beast-feeding for at least 4 months protects against otitis media. Pediatrics 1993;91:867–872.

Epstein F: Pregnancy and renal disease. N Engl J Med 1996;335:277–278.

Fennell, R, Wilson S, Garin E, et al: Bacteriuria in families of girls with recurrent bacteriuria. Clin Pediatr 1977;16:1132–1135.

Fliedner M, Mehls O, Rauterberg EW, Ritz E: Urinary sIgA in children with urinary tract infection. J Pediatr 1986;109:416–421.

Fussell EN, Kaack MB, Cherry R, Roberts JA: Adherence of bacteria to human foreskins. J Urol 1988;140:997–1001.

Geraniotis E, Koff S, Enrile B: The prophylactic use of clean intermittent catheterization in the treatment of infants and young children with myelomeningocele and neurogenic bladder dysfunction. J Urol 1988; 139:85–86.

Glennon J, Ryan PJ, Keane CT, Rees JPR: Circumcision and periurethral carriage of Proteus mirabilis in boys. Arch Dis Child 1988;63:556–557.

Grattan-Smith D, Harrison L, Singleton E: Radiology of AIDS in the pediatric patient. Curr Probl Diagn Radiol 1992;79–109.

Gribble J, Puterman M: Prophylaxis of urinary tract infection in persons with recent spinal cord injury: A prospective, randomized, double-blind, placebo-controlled study of trimethoprim-sulfamethoxazole. Am J Med 1993;95:141–152.

Hallett RJ, Pead L, Maskell R: Urinary infection in boys: A three-year prospective study. Lancet 1976;2:1107–1110.

Hammadeh M, Nicholls G, Calder C, et al: Xanthogranulomatous pyelonephritis in childhood: Pre-operative diagnosis is possible. Br J Urol 1994;73:83–86.

Hanson L: Breastfeeding provides passive and likely long-lasting active immunity. Ann Allergy Asthma Immunol 1998;81:523–533.

Hansson S, Jodal U, Lincoln K, Svanborg-Edén C: Untreated asymptomatic bacteriuria in girls: II. Effect of phenoxymethylpenicillin and erythromycin given for intercurrent infections. BMJ 1989b;298:856–859.

Heidrick WP, Mattingly RF, Amberg JR: Vesicoureteral reflux in pregnancy. Obstet Gynecol 1967;29:571–578.

Hoberman A, Wald E: Urinary tract infections in young febrile children. Pediatr Infect Dis J 1997;16:11–17.

Hsia TY, Shortliffe L: The effect of pregnancy on the rat urinary tract. J Urol 1995;154:684–689.

Hutch JA: Vesico-ureteral reflux in the paraplegic: Cause and correction. J Urol 1952;68:457–467.

James-Ellison M, Roberts R, Verrier-Jones K, et al: Mucosal immunity in the urinary tract: Changes in sIgA, FSC and total IgA with age and in urinary tract infection. Clin Nephrol 1997;48:69–78.

Jantausch T, Criss V, O'Donnell R, et al: Association of Lewis blood group phenotypes with urinary tract infection in children. J Pediatr 1994;124:863–868.

Johnson H, Anderson J, Chambers G, et al: A short-term study of nitrofurantoin prophylaxis in children managed with clean intermittent catheterization. Pediatrics 1994;5:752–755.

Jones D, Hayslett J: Outcome of pregnancy in women with moderate or severe renal insufficiency. N Engl J Med 1996;335:226–232.

Joseph D, Bauer S, Colodny A, et al: Clean, intermittent catheterization of infants with neurogenic bladder. Pediatrics 1989;84:78–82.

King LR: Neonatal circumcision in the United States in 1982. J Urol 1982;128:1135–1136.

Klevan J, DeJong A: Urinary tract symptoms and urinary tract infection following sexual abuse. Am J Dis Child 1990;144:242–244.

Kunin C: Natural history of recurrent bacteriuria in school girls. N Engl J Med 1970;282:1443.

Kunin CM, Deutscher R, Paquin A: Urinary tract infection in school children: An epidemiologic, clinical and laboratory study. Medicine (Baltimore) 1964;43:91–130.

Kunin CM, McCormack RC: An epidemiologic study of bacteriuria and blood pressure among nuns and working women. N Engl J Med 1968; 278:635–642.

Labbé J: Self-induced urinary tract infection in school-age boys. Pediatrics 1990;86:703–706.

Lohr JA: The foreskin and urinary tract infections. J Pediatr 1989;114: 502–504.

Lohr J, Downs S, Dudley S, Donowitz L: Hospital-acquired urinary tract infections in the pediatric patient: A prospective study. Pediatr Infect Dis J 1994;13:8–12.

Lomberg H, Hanson LÅ, Jacobsson B, et al: Correlation of P blood group, vesicoureteral reflux, and bacterial attachment in patients with recurrent pyelonephritis. N Engl J Med 1983;308:1189–1192.

Mansfield J, Snow B, Cartwright P, Wadsworth K: Complications of pregnancy in women after childhood reimplantation for vesicoureteral reflux: An update with 25 years of followup. J Urol 1995;154:787–790.

Mårild S, Jodal U, Mangelus L: Medical histories of children with acute pyelonephritis compared with controls. Pediatr Infect Dis J 1989b;8: 511–515.

Newcastle Asymptomatic Bacteriuria Research Group: Asymptomatic bacteriuria in schoolchildren in Newcastle upon Tyne. Arch Dis Child 1975;50:90.

Newcastle Covert Bacteriuria Research Group: Covert bacteriuria in school girls in Newcastle upon Tyne: a 5-year followup. Arch Dis Child 1981;56:585–592.

Ozen S, Alikasifoglu M, Saatci U, et al: Implications of certain genetic polymorphisms in scarring in vesicoureteric reflux: Importance of ACE polymorphism. Am J Kidney Dis 1999;34:140–145.

Paradise J, Elster B, Tan L: Evidence in infants with cleft palate that breast milk protects against otitis media. Pediatrics 1994;94:853–860.

Pisacane A, Graziano L, Mazzarella G, et al: Breast-feeding and urinary tract infection. J Pediatr 1992;120:87–89.

Pisacane A, Graziano L, Zona G: Breastfeeding and urinary tract infection. Lancet 1990;336:50.

Poland RL: The question of routine neonatal circumcision. N Engl J Med 1990;322:1312–1315.

Robbins JB: Immunologic mechanisms. In Barnett HL (ed): Pediatrics. New York, Appleton-Century-Crofts, 1972, Chapter 10.

Roberts JA: Does circumcision prevent urinary tract infection. J Urol 1986;135:991–992.

Savage DCL: Natural history of covert bacteriuria in schoolgirls. Kidney Int 1975;8:S90–S95.

Schlager T, Anderson S, Trudell J, Hendley J: Nitrofurantoin prophylaxis for bacteriuria and urinary tract infection in children with neurogenic bladder on intermittent catheterization. J Pediatr 1998;132:704–708.

Schlager T, Dilks S, Trudell J, et al: Bacteriuria in children with neurogenic bladder treated with intermittent catheterization: Natural history. J Pediatr 1995;126:490–496.

Schoen E, Colby C, Ray G: Newborn circumcision decreases incidence and costs of urinary tract infections during the first year of life. Pediatrics 2000;105:789–793.

Schoen EJ: The status of circumcision of newborns. N Engl J Med 1990; 322:1308–1312.

Schoen EJ, Anderson G, Bohon C, et al: Report of the Task Force on Circumcision. Pediatrics 1989;84:388–391.

Sheinfeld J, Cordon-Cardo C, Fair W, et al: Association of type 1 blood group antigens (BGA) with urinary tract infections in children with genitourinary structural abnormalities. J Urol 1990;143:189A.

Sheinfeld J, Schaeffer AJ, Cordon-Cardo C, et al: Association of the Lewis blood-group phenotype with recurrent urinary tract infections in women. N Engl J Med 1989;320:773–777.

Shortliffe L: Pregnancy changes the rules when treating UTI. Contemp Urol 1991;3:57–67.

Shortliffe LMD, Stamey TA: Urinary infections in adult women. In Walsh PC, Gittes RF, Perlmutter AD, Stamey TA (eds): Campbell's Urology. Philadelphia, WB Saunders, 1986b, pp 797–830.

Skoog SJ, Belman AB, Majd M: A nonsurgical approach to the management of primary vesicoureteral reflux. J Urol 1987;138:941–946.

Smellie J: Reflections on 30 years of treating children with urinary tract infections. J Urol 1991;146:665–668.

Smellie J, Prescod N, Shaw P, et al: Childhood reflux and urinary infection: A follow-up of 10–41 years in 226 adults. Pediatr Nephrol 1998; 12:727–736.

Stamey TA: Pathogenesis and treatment of urinary tract infections. Baltimore, Williams & Wilkins, 1980.

Stamey TA, Condy M, Mihara G: Prophylactic efficacy of nitrofurantoin macrocrystals and trimethoprim-sulfamethoxazole in urinary infections. N Engl J Med 1977;296:780.

Stamey TA, Sexton CC: The role of vaginal colonization with Enterobacteriaceae in recurrent urinary infections. J Urol 1975;113:214–217.

Svanborg Edén C, Kulhavy R, Mårild S, et al: Urinary immunoglobulins in healthy individuals and children with acute pyelonephritis. Scand J Immunol 1985;21:305–313.

Sweet RL: Bacteriuria and pyelonephritis during pregnancy. Semin Perinatol 1977;1:25–40.

Taylor C, Hunt G, Matthews I: Bacterial study of clean intermittent catheterisation in children. Br J Urol 1985;58:64–69.

To T, Agha M, Dick P, Feldman W: Cohort study on circumcision of newborn boys and subsequent risk of urinary-tract infection. Lancet 1998;352:1813–1816.

Tullus K: Fecal colonization with P-fimbriated *Escherichia coli* in newborn children and relation to development of extraintestinal *E. coli* infections. Acta Paediatr Scand 1986;334:1–35.

Williams GL, Davies DKL, Evans KT, Williams JE: Vesicoureteric reflux in patients with bacteriuria in pregnancy. Lancet 1968;2:1202–1205.

Winberg J, Anderson HJ, Bergström T, et al: Epidemiology of symptomatic urinary tract infection in childhood. Acta Paediatr Scand 1974; S252:1–20.

Winberg J, Bollgren I, Gothefors L, et al: The prepuce: A mistake of nature? Lancet 1989;1:598–599.

Wiswell T: The prepuce, urinary tract infections, and the consequences. Pediatrics 2000;105:860–861.

Wiswell T, Hachey W: Urinary tract infections and the uncircumcised state: An update. Clin Pediatr 1993;32:130–134.

Wiswell TE, Enzenauer RW, Holton ME, et al: Declining frequency of circumcision: Implications for changes in the absolute incidence and male to female sex ratio of urinary tract infections in early infancy. Pediatrics 1987;79:338–342.

Wiswell TE, Miller GM, Gelston HM, et al: Effect of circumcision status on periurethral bacterial flora during the first year of life. J Pediatr 1988;113:442–446.

Wiswell TE, Roscelli JD: Corroborative evidence for the decreased incidence of urinary tract infections in circumcised male infants. Pediatrics 1986;78:96–99.

Wiswell TE, Smith FR, Bass JW: Decreased incidence of urinary tract infections in circumcised male infants. Pediatrics 1985;75:901–903.

Yoder MC, Polin RA: Immunotherapy of neonatal septicemia. Pediatr Clin North Am 1986;33:481–501.

Zafaranloo S, Gerard P, Bryk D: Xanthogranulomatous pyelonephritis in children: Analysis by diagnostic modalities. Urol Radiol 1990;12:18–21.

Management

Ashkenazi S, Even-Tov S, Samra Z, Dinari G: Uropathogens of various childhood populations and their antibiotic susceptibility. Pediatr Infect Dis J 1991a;10:742–746.

Baskin M, O'Rourke E, Fleisher G: Outpatient treatment of febrile infants 28 to 89 days of age with intramuscular administration of ceftriaxone [see comments]. J Pediatr 1992;120:22–27.

Brendstrup L, Hjelt K, Petesen K, et al: Nitrofurantoin versus trimethoprim prophylaxis in recurrent urinary tract infection in children. Acta Paediatr Scand 1990;79:1225–1234.

Brogden R, Carmine A, Heel R, et al: Trimethoprim: A review of its antibacterial activity, pharmacokinetics and therapeutic use in urinary tract infections. Drugs 1982;23:405–340.

Brumfitt W, Smith G, Hamilton-Miller J, Gargan R: A clinical comparison between Macrodantin and trimethoprim for prophylaxis in women with recurrent urinary infections. J Antimicrob Chemother 1985;16:111–120.

Cooper C, Chung B, Kirsch A, et al: The outcome of stopping prophylactic antibiotics in older children with vesicoureteral reflux. J Urol 2000;163:269–273.

Copenhagen Study Group of Urinary Tract Infections in Children. Short-term treatment of acute urinary tract infection in girls. Scand J Infect Dis 1991;23:213–220.

Dagan R, Einhorn M, Lang R, et al: Once daily cefixime compared with twice daily trimethoprim/sulfamethoxazole for treatment of urinary tract infection in infants and children. Pediatr Infect Dis J 1992;11:198–203.

Dyer I, Sankary T, Dawson J: Antibiotic resistance in bacterial urinary tract infections 1991–1997. West J Med 1998;169:265–268.

Fennell R, Luengnaruemitchai M, Iravani A, et al: Urinary tract infections in children. Clin Pediatr 1980;19:121–124.

Gaudreault P, Beland M, Girodias J, Thivierge R: Single daily doses of trimethoprim/sulphadiazine for three or 10 days in urinary tract infections. Acta Paediatr 1992;81:695–697.

Ginsburg C, McCracken G, Petruska M: Once-daily cefadroxil versus twice-daily cefaclor for treatment of acute urinary tract infections in children. J Antimicrob Chemother 1982;10:53–56.

Gordon P: Serious bacterial infections in children: When can outpatient treatment be used? Postgrad Med 1991;90:87–90.

Gribble J, Puterman M: Prophylaxis of urinary tract infection in persons with recent spinal cord injury: A prospective, randomized, double-blind, placebo-controlled study of trimethoprim-sulfamethoxazole. Am J Med 1993;95:141–152.

Grimwood K: Single dose gentamicin treatment of urinary infections in children. N Z Med J 1988;101:539–41.

Grüneberg RN, Smellie JM, Leaky A, et al: Long-term low-dose cotrimoxazole in prophylaxis of childhood urinary tract infection: Bacteriological aspects. BMJ 1976;2:206.

Gupta K, Scholes D, Stamm W: Increasing prevalence of antimicrobial resistance among uropathogens causing acute uncomplicated cystitis in women. JAMA 1999;281:736–738.

Hanson G, Hansson S, Jodal U: Trimethoprim-sulphadiazine prophylaxis in children with vesico-ureteric reflux. Scand J Infect Dis 1989;21:201–204.

Hoberman A, Wald E, Hickey R, Baskin M: Oral versus initial intravenous therapy for urinary tract infections in young febrile children. Pediatrics 1999;104:79–86.

Holmberg L, Boman G, Bottiger LE, et al: Adverse reactions to nitrofurantoin: Analysis of 921 reports. Am J Med 1980;69:733–738.

Huovinen P, Toivanen P: Trimethoprim resistance in Finland after five years' use of plain trimethoprim. BMJ 1980;280:72–74.

Johnson H, Anderson J, Chambers G, et al: A short-term study of nitrofurantoin prophylaxis in children managed with clean intermittent catheterization. Pediatrics 1994;5:752–755.

Jójárt G: Comparison of 3-day versus 14-day treatment of lower urinary tract infection in children. Int Urol Nephrol 1991;23:129–134.

Khan A: Efficacy of single-dose therapy of urinary tract infection in infants and children: A review. J Natl Med Assoc 1994;86:690–696.

Langermann S, Palaszynski S, Barnhart M, et al: Prevention of mucosal Escherichia coli infection by FimH-adhesin-based systemic vaccination. Science 1997;276:607–611.

Lohr JA, Hayden GF, Kesler RW, et al: Three-day therapy of lower urinary tract infections with nitrofurantoin macrocrystals: A randomized clinical trial. Pediatrics 1981;99:980–983.

Lohr JA, Nunley DH, Howards SS, Ford RF: Prevention of recurrent urinary tract infections in girls. Pediatrics 1977;59:562–565.

Madrigal G, Odio CM, Mohs E, et al: Single dose antibiotic therapy is not as effective as conventional regimens for management of acute urinary tract infections in children. Pediatr Infect Dis J 1988;7:316–319.

Martinez FC, Kindrachuk RW, Thomas E, Stamey TA: Effect of prophylactic, low dose cephalexin on fecal and vaginal bacteria. J Urol 1985;133:994–996.

Murray B, Rensimer E: Transfer of trimethoprim resistance from fecal Escherichia coli isolated during a prophylaxis study in Mexico. J Infect Dis 1983;147:724–728.

Murray B, Rensimer E, DuPont H: Emergence of high-level trimethoprim resistance in fecal Escherichia coli during oral administration of trimethoprim or trimethoprim-sulfamethoxazole. N Engl J Med 1982;306:130–135.

Sandock D, Gothe B, Bodner D: Trimethoprim-sulfamethoxazole prophylaxis against urinary tract infection in the chronic spinal cord injury patient. Paraplegia 1995;33:156–160.

Schaad UB: Use of quinolones in pediatrics. Eur J Clin Microbiol Infect Dis 1991;10:355–360.

Schlager T, Anderson S, Trudell J, Hendley J: Nitrofurantoin prophylaxis for bacteriuria and urinary tract infection in children with neurogenic bladder on intermittent catheterization. J Pediatr 1998;132:704–708.

Smyth A, Judd B: Compliance with antibiotic prophylaxis in urinary tract infection. Arch Dis Child 1993;68:235–236.

Stamey TA, Condy M: The diffusion and concentration of trimethoprim in human vaginal fluid. J Infect Dis 1975;131:261.

Stamey TA, Condy M, Mihara G: Prophylactic efficacy of nitrofurantoin macrocrystals and trimethoprim-sulfamethoxazole in urinary infections. N Engl J Med 1977;296:780.

Stamm WE, Counts GW, Wagner KF, et al: Antimicrobial prophylaxis of recurrent urinary tract infections. Ann Intern Med 1980;92:770–775.

Stutman H: Cefprozil. Pediatr Ann 1993;22:167–176.

Talan D, Stamm W, Hooton T, et al: Comparison of ciprofloxacin (7 days) and trimethoprim-sulfamethoxazole (14 days) for acute uncomplicated pyelonephritis in women: A randomized trial. JAMA 2000;283:1583–1590.

Thankavel K, Madison B, Ikeda T, et al: Localization of a domain in the FimH adhesin of Escherichia coli type 1 fimbriae capable of receptor recognition of use of a domain-specific antibody to confer protection against experimental urinary tract infection. J Clin Invest 1997;100:1123–1136.

Thompson RB: A Short Textbook of Haematology. Philadelphia, JB Lippincott, 1969.

Uehling D, Johnson D, Hopkins W: The urinary tract response to entry of pathogens. World J Urol 1999;17:351–358.

Winberg J, Bergström T, Lidin-Janson G, Lincoln K: Treatment trials in urinary tract infection (UTI) with special reference to the effect of antimicrobials on the fecal and periurethral flora. Clin Nephrol 1973;1:142.

Wright S, Wrenn K, Haynes M: Trimethoprim-sulfamethoxazole resistance among urinary coliform isolates [see comments]. J Gen Intern Med 199914:606–609.

Radiologic Evaluation

Abbott GD: Neonatal bacteriuria: A prospective study in 1460 infants. Br Med J 1972;1:267.

Alon U, Berant M, Pery M: Intravenous pyelography in children with urinary tract infection and vesicoureteral reflux. Pediatrics 1989;83:332–336.

Alon U, Pery M, et al: Ultrasonography in the radiologic evaluation of children with urinary tract infection. Pediatrics 1986;78:58–64.

American Academy Pediatrics, Committee on Quality Improvement, Subcommittee on Urinary Tract Infection: Practice parameter: The diagnosis, treatment, and evaluation of the initial urinary tract infection in febrile infants and young children. Pediatrics 1999;103:843–852.

Asscher AW, McLachlan MSF, Verrier-Jones R, et al: Screening for asymptomatic urinary-tract infection in schoolgirls. Lancet 1973;2:1.

Björgvinsson E, Majd M, Eggli K: Diagnosis of acute pyelonephritis in children: Comparison of sonography and 99mTc-DMSA scintigraphy. AJR Am J Roentgenol 1991;157:539–543.

Cleveland R, Constantinou C, Blickman J, et al: Voiding cystourethrography in children: Value of digital fluoroscopy in reducing radiation dose. AJR Am J Roentgenol 1992;158:137–142.

Conway JJ: The role of scintigraphy in urinary tract infection. Semin Nucl Med 1988;18:308–319.

Dacher JN, Pfister C, Monroc M, et al: Power Doppler sonographic pattern of acute pyelonephritis in children: Comparison with CT. AJR Am J Roentgenol 1996;166:1451–1455.

Eggli D, Tulchinsky M: Scintigraphic evaluation of pediatric urinary tract infection. Semin Nucl Med 1993;23:199–218.

Fairley KF, Roysmith J: The forgotten factor in the evaluation of vesicoureteric reflux. Med J Aust 1977;2:10–12.

Filly R, Friedland GW, Govan DE, Fair WR: Development and progression of clubbing and scarring in children with recurrent urinary tract infections. Pediatr Radiol 1974;113:145–153.

Gates GF: Glomerular filtration rate: Estimation from fractional renal accumulation of 99m Tc-DTPA (stannous). AJR Am J Roentgenol 1982;138:565–570.

Goldman M, Lahat E, Strauss S, et al: Imaging after urinary tract infection in male neonates. Pediatrics 2000;105:1232–1235.

Gordon I: Use of Tc-99m DMSA and Tc-99m DTPA in Reflux. Semin Urol 1986;4:99–108.

Hellström M, Jacobsson B, Mårild S, Jodal U: Voiding cystourethrography as a predictor of reflux nephropathy in children with urinary-tract infection. AJR Am J Roentgenol 1989;152:801–804.

Hellström M, Jodal U, Mårild S, Wettergren B: Ureteral dilatation in children with febrile urinary tract infection or bacteriuria. AJR Am J Roentgenol 1987;148:483–486.

Honkinen O, Ruuskanen O, et al: Ultrasonography as a screening procedure in children with urinary tract infection. Pediatr Infect Dis 1986;5:633–635.

Jakobsson B, Nolstedt L, Svensson L, et al: 99mTechnetium-dimercaptosuccinic acid scan in the diagnosis of acute pyelonephritis in children: Relation to clinical and radiological findings. Pediatr Nephrol 1992;6:328–334.

Johansson B, Troell S, Berg U: Renal parenchymal volume during and after acute pyelonephritis measured by ultrasonography. Arch Dis Child 1988a;63:1309–1314.

Johansson B, Troell S, Berg U: Urographic renal size in acute pyelonephritis in childhood. Acta Radiol 1988b;29:155–158.

June C, Browning M, Smith P, et al: Ultrasonography and computed tomography in severe urinary tract infection. Arch Intern Med 1985;145:841–845.

Kleinman P, Diamond D, Karellas A, et al: Tailored low-dose fluoroscopic voiding cystourethrography for the reevaluation of vesicoureteral reflux in girls. AJR Am J Roentgenol 1994;162:1151–1154.

Kogan SJ, Sigler L, Levitt SB, et al: Elusive vesicoureteral reflux in children with normal contrast cystograms. J Urol 1986;136:325–328.

Kunin CM, Deutscher R, Paquin A: Urinary tract infection in school children: An epidemiologic, clinical and laboratory study. Medicine (Baltimore) 1964;43:91–130.

Laguna R, Silva F, Orduña E, et al: Technetium-99m-MG3 in early identification of pyelonephritis in children. 1998.

Lebowitz R: The detection of vesicoureteral reflux in the child. Invest Radiol 1986;21:519–531.

Lebowitz R: The detection and characterization of vesicoureteral reflux in the child. J Urol 1992;148:1640–1642.

Lindsell D, Moncrieff M: Comparison of ultrasound examination and intravenous urography after a urinary tract infection. Arch Dis Child 1986;61:81–82.

MacKenzie J, Fowler K, Hollman A, et al: The value of ultrasound in the child with an acute urinary tract infection. Fr J Urol 1994;74:240–244.

Macpherson RI, Gordon L: Vesicoureteric reflux: Radiologic aspects. Semin Urol 1986;4:89–98.

McDonald A, Scranton M, Gillespie R, et al: Voiding cystourethrograms and urinary tract infections: How long to wait? Pediatrics 2000;105:951–952. Available at http://www.pediatrics.org/cgi/content/full/105/4/350.

Montgomery P, Kuhn J, Afshani E: CT evaluation of severe renal inflammatory disease in children. Pediatr Radiol 1987;17:216–222.

Morin D, Veyrac C, Kotzki P, et al: Comparison of ultrasound and dimercaptosuccinic acid scintigraphy changes in acute pyelonephritis. Pediatr Nephrol 1999;13:219–222.

Mucci B, Maguire B: Does routine ultrasound have a role in the investigation of children with urinary tract infection? Clin Radiol 1994;49:324–325.

Newcastle Asymptomatic Bacteriuria Research Group: Asymptomatic bacteriuria in schoolchildren in Newcastle upon Tyne. Arch Dis Child 1975;50:90.

Patel K, Charron M, Hoberman A, et al: Intra- and interobserver variability in interpretation of DMSA scans using a set of standardized criteria. Pediatr Radiol 1993;23:506–509.

Rehling M, Jensen JJ, Scherling B, et al: Evaluation of renal function and morphology in children by 99m Tc-DTPA gamma camera renography. Acta Paediatr Scand 1989;78:601–607.

Rodriguez L, Spielman D, Herfkens R, Shortliffe L: Magnetic resonance imaging (MRI) for the evaluation of hydronephrosis, reflux, and renal scarring in children. J Urol 2001;166:1023–1027.

Rushton H, Majd M: Dimercaptosuccinic acid renal scintigraphy for the evaluation of pyelonephritis and scarring: A review of experimental and clinical studies. J Urol 1992b;148:1726–1732.

Sfakianakis G, Georgiou M: MAG3 SPECT: A rapid procedure to evaluate the renal parenchyma. J Nucl Med 1997;38:478–483.

Shore RM, Koff SA, Mentser M, et al: Glomerular filtration rate in children: Determination from the Tc-99m-DTPA renogram. Radiology 1984;151:627–633.

Silver TM, Kass EJ, Thornbury JR, et al: The radiological spectrum of acute pyelonephritis in adults and adolescents. Radiology 1976;118:65–71.

Sreenarasimhaiah V, Alon U: Uroradiologic evaluation of children with urinary tract infection: Are both ultrasonography and renal cortical scintigraphy necessary? J Pediatr 1995;127:373–377.

Traisman E, Conway J, Traisman H, et al: The localization of urinary tract infection with 99mTc glucoheptonate scintigraphy. Pediatr Radiol 1986;16:403–406.

Troell S, Berg U, Johansson B, Wikstad I: Ultrasonographic renal parenchymal volume related to kidney function and renal parenchymal area in children with recurrent urinary tract infections and asymptomatic bacteriuria. Acta Radiol Diagn (Stockh) 1984;25:411–416.

Verboven M, Ingels M, Delree M, Piepsz A: 99mTc-DMSA scintigraphy in acute urinary tract infection in children. Pediatr Radiol 1990;20:540–542.

Wallin L, Bajc M: Typical technetium dimercaptosuccinic acid distribution patterns in acute pyelonephritis. Acta Paediatr 1993;82:1061–1065.

Wallin L, Bajc M: The significance of vesicoureteric reflux on kidney development assessed by dimercaptosuccinate renal scintigraphy. Br J Urol 1994;73:607–611.

Wallin L, Helin I, Bajc M: Kidney swelling: Findings on DMSA scintigraphy. Clin Nucl Med 1997;22:292–299.

Management of Specific Problems

Cardiff Oxford Bacteriuria Study Group: Sequelae of covert bacteriuria in schoolgirls: A four-year follow-up study. Lancet 1978;1:889–893.

Copenhagen Study Group of Urinary Tract Infections in Children: Short-term treatment of acute urinary tract infection in girls. Scand J Infect Dis 1991;23:213–220.

Grimwood K: Single dose gentamicin treatment of urinary infections in children. N Z Med J 1988;101:539–541.

Hansson S, Caugant D, Jodal U, Svanborg-Edén C: Untreated asymptomatic bacteriuria in girls: I. Stability of urinary isolates. BMJ 1989a;298:853–855.

Hansson S, Jodal U, Lincoln K, Svanborg-Edén C: Untreated asymptomatic bacteriuria in girls: II. Effect of phenoxymethylpenicillin and erythromycin given for intercurrent infections. BMJ 1989b;298:856–859.

Jodal U: The natural history of bacteriuria in childhood. Infect Dis Clin North Am 1987;1:713–729.

Jójárt G: Comparison of 3-day versus 14-day treatment of lower urinary tract infection in children. Int Urol Nephrol 1991;23:129–134.

Kass EJ, Diokno AC, Montealegre A: Enuresis: Principles of management and result of treatment. J Urol 1979;121:794–796.

Kjølseth D, Knudsen LM, Jadsen B, et al: Urodynamic biofeedback training for children with bladder-sphincter dyscoordination during voiding. Neurourol Urodyn 1993;12:211–221.

Koff SA, Lapides J, Piazza DH: Association of urinary tract infection and reflux with uninhibited bladder contractions and voluntary sphincteric obstruction. J Urol 1979;122:373–376.

Kraft JK, Stamey TA: The natural history of symptomatic recurrent bacteriuria in women. Medicine (Baltimore) 1977;56:55.

Kunin CM, Zacha E, Paquin A: Urinary-tract infections in schoolchildren: I. Prevalence of bacteriuria and associated urologic findings. N Engl J Med 1962;266:1287–1296.

Lindberg U, Claesson I, Hanson LÅ, Jodal U: Asymptomatic bacteriuria in schoolgirls: VIII. Clinical course during a 3-year follow-up. J Pediatr 1978;92:194–199.

Lindberg U, Hanson LÅ, Jodal U, et al: Asymptomatic bacteriuria in schoolgirls. Acta Paediatr Scand 1975;64:432–436.

Loening-Baucke V: Urinary incontinence and urinary tract infection and their resolution with treatment of chronic constipation of childhood. Pediatrics 1997;100:228–232.

Lohr JA, Hayden GF, Kesler RW, et al: Three-day therapy of lower urinary tract infections with nitrofurantoin macrocrystals: A randomized clinical trial. Pediatrics 1981;99:980–983.

Madrigal G, Odio CM, Mohs E, et al: Single dose antibiotic therapy is not as effective as conventional regimens for management of acute urinary tract infections in children. Pediatr Infect Dis J 1988;7:316–319.

Newcastle Asymptomatic Bacteriuria Research Group: Asymptomatic bacteriuria in schoolchildren in Newcastle upon Tyne. Arch Dis Child 1975;50:90.

Newcastle Covert Bacteriuria Research Group: Covert bacteriuria in school girls in Newcastle upon Tyne: A 5-year followup. Arch Dis Child 1981;56:585–592.

O'Regan S, Yazbeck S, Schick E: Constipation, bladder instability, urinary tract infection syndrome. Clin Nephrol 1985;23:152–154.

Passerini-Glazel G, Cisternino A, Camuffo MC, et al: Video-urodynamic studies of minor voiding dysfunctions in children: An overview of 13 years' experience. Scand J Urol Nephrol 1992;141:70–84.

Principi N, Gervasoni A, Reali E, Tagliabue P: Treatment of urinary tract infections in children with a single daily dose of gentamicin. Helv Paediatr Acta 1977;32:343–350.

Qvist N, Kristensen ES, Nielsen KK, et al: Detrusor instability in children with recurrent urinary tract infection and/or enuresis. Urol Int 1986;41:196–198.

Savage DCL: Natural history of covert bacteriuria in schoolgirls. Kidney Int 1975;8:S90–S95.

Savage DCL, Howie G, Adler K, Wilson MI: Controlled trial of therapy in covert bacteriuria of childhood. Lancet 1975;1:358–361.

Shortliffe LD: The management of urinary tract infections in children without urinary tract abnormalities. In Kaplan G (ed): Urol Clin North Am 1995;22(1):67–74.

vanGool JD, Vijverberg MAW, Messer AP, et al: Functional daytime incontinence: Non-pharmacological treatment. Scand J Urol Nephrol 1992b;141:93–103.

Verrier-Jones ER, Meller ST, McLachlan MSF, et al: Treatment of bacteriuria in schoolgirls. Kidney Int 1975;4(Suppl):S85–S89.

Vigano A, Dalla-Villa A, Bianchi C, et al: Single-dose netilmicin therapy of complicated and uncomplicated lower urinary tract infections in children. Acta Paediatr Scand 1985;74:584–588.

Winberg J, Anderson HJ, Bergström T, et al: Epidemiology of symptomatic urinary tract infection in childhood. Acta Paediatr Scand 1974²52:1–20.

Other Genitourinary Infections and Syndromes

Anderson P, Giacomantonio J: The acutely painful scrotum in children: Review of 113 consecutive cases. Can Med Assoc J 1985;132:1153–1155.

Anderson P, Giacomantonio J, Schwarz R: Acute scrotal pain in children: Prospective study of diagnosis and management. Can J Surg 1989;32:29–32.

Apperley J, Rice S, Bishop J, et al: Late-onset hemorrhagic cystitis associated with urinary excretion of polyomaviruses after bone marrow transplantation. Transplantation 1987;43:108–112.

Atkinson G, Patrick L, Ball T, et al: The normal and abnormal scrotum in children: Evaluation with color Doppler sonography. AJR Am J Roentgenol 1992;158:613–617.

Bartone F, Hurwitz R, Rojas E, et al: The role of percutaneous nephrostomy in the management of obstructing candidiasis of the urinary tract in infants. J Urol 1988;140:338–341.

Bedi A, Miller C, Hanson J, et al: Association of BK virus with failure of prophylaxis against hemorrhagic cystitis following bone marrow transplantation. J Clin Oncol 1995;13:1103–1109.

Cabral D, Johnson H, Coleman G, et al: Tuberculous epididymitis as a cause of testicular pseudomalignancy in two young children. Pediatr Infect Dis 1985;4:59–62.

Caldamone A, Valvo J, Altebarmakian V, Rabinowitz R: Acute scrotal swelling in children. J Pediatr Surg 1984;19:581–584.

Cassano W: Intravenous ribavirin therapy for adenovirus cystitis after allogeneic bone marrow transplantation. Bone Marrow Transplant 1991;7:247–248.

Close C, Carr M, Burns M, et al: Interstitial cystitis in children. J Urol 1996;156:860–862.

de la Hunt, Deegan S, Scott J, et al: Intermittent catheterisation for neuropathic urinary incontinence. Arch Dis Child 1989;64:821–824.

Doolittle KH, Smith JP, Saylor ML: Epididymitis in the prepubertal boy. J Urol 1966;96:364–366.

Eckstein C, Kass E: Anuria in a newborn secondary to bilateral ureteropelvic fungus balls. J Urol 1982;127:109–110.

Farkas A, Waisman J, Goodwin W: Interstitial cystitis in adolescent girls. J Urol 1977;118:837–839.

Gierup J, von Hedenberg C, Osterman A: Acute nonspecific epididymitis in boys: A survey based on 48 consecutive cases. Scand J Urol Nephrol 1975;9:5–7.

Gislason T, Noronha F, Gregory J: Acute epididymitis in boys: A five-year retrospective study. J Urol 1980;124:533–534.

Greenfield S: Type b *Haemophilus influenzae* epididymo-orchitis in the prepubertal boy. J Urol 1986;136:1311–1313.

Gubbins P, McConnell S, Penzak S: Current management of funguria. Am J Health Syst Pharm 1999;56:1929–1938.

Gubbins P, Occhipinti D, Danziger L: Surveillance of treated and untreated funguria in a university hospital. Pharmacotherapy 1994;14:463–470.

Hitchcock R, Pallett A, Hall M, Malone P: Urinary tract candidiasis in neonates and infants. Br J Urol 1995;76:252–256.

Kauffman C, Vazquez J, Sobel J, et al: Prospective multicenter surveillance study of funguria in hospitalized patients. Clin Infect Dis 2000;30:14–18.

Keller M, Sellers B, Melish M, et al: Systemic candidiasis in infants: A case presentation and literature review. Am J Dis Child 1977;131:1260–1263.

Knight P, Vassy L: The diagnosis and treatment of the acute scrotum in children and adolescents. Ann Surg 1984;200:664–673.

Kossoff E, Buescher E, Karlowicz M: Candidemia in a neonatal intensive care unit: Trends during fifteen years and clinical features of 111 cases. Pediatr Infect Dis J 1998;17:504–508.

Likitnukul S, McCracken GJ, Nelson J, Votteler T: Epididymitis in children and adolescents: A 20-year retrospective study. Am J Dis Child 1987;141:41–44.

Lin YC, King D, Birken G, Barson W: Acute scrotum due to *Haemophilus influenzae* type b. J Pediatr Surg 1988;23:183–184.

Loghman-Adham M, Tejero HT, London R: Acute hemorrhagic cystitis due to *Escherichia coli*. Child Nephrol Urol 1988–89;9:29–32.

Manolo D, Mufson MA, Zollar LM, Mankad VN: Adenovirus infection in acute hemorrhagic cystitis: A study of 25 children. Am J Dis Child 1971;121:281–285.

McAlistar W, Sisler C: Scrotal sonography in infants and children. Curr Probl Diagn Radiol 1990;19:201–242.

Melekos J, Asbach H, Markou S: Etiology of acute scrotum in 100 boys with regards to age distribution. J Urol 1988;139:1023–1025.

Mandell J, Bauer S, et al: Ureteral ectopia in infants and children. J Urol 1981;126:219–222.

Mendel J, Taylor G, Cheng T, et al: Testicular torsion in children: Scintigraphic assessment. Pediatr Radiol 1985;15:110–115.

Mueller D, Amundson G, Rubin S, Wesenberg R: Acute scrotal abnormalities in children: Diagnosis by combined sonography and scintigraphy. AJR Am J Roentgenol 1988;150:643–646.

Mufson MA, Belshe RB, Horrigan TJ, Zollar LM: Cause of acute hemorrhagic cystitis in children. Am J Dis Child 1973;126:605–609.

Nesbit S, Katz L, McClain B, Murphy D: Comparison of two concentrations of amphotericin B bladder irrigation in the treatment of funguria in patients with indwelling urinary catheters. Am J Health Syst Pharm 1999;56:872–875.

Numazaki Y, Kumasaka T, Yano N, et al: Further study on acute hemorrhagic cystitis due to adenovirus type 11. N Engl J Med 1973;289:344–347.

Numazaki Y, Shigeta S, Kumasaka T, et al: Acute hemorrhagic cystitis in children: Isolation of adenovirus type 11. N Engl J Med 1968;278:700–704.

Rehan V, Davidson D: Neonatal renal candidal bezoar. Arch Dis Child 1992;67:63–64.

Robinson P, Pocock R, Frank J: The management of obstructive renal candidiasis in the neonate. Br J Urol 1987;59:380–2.

Siegel A, Snyder H, Duckett J: Epididymitis in infants and boys: Underlying urogenital anomalies and efficacy of imaging modalities. J Urol 1987;138:1100–1103.

Stein R, Stöckle M, et al: The fate of the adult exstrophy patient. J Urol 1994;152:1413–1416.

Trinh T, Simonian J, Vigil S, et al: Continuous versus intermittent bladder irrigation of amphotericin B for the treatment of candiduria. J Urol 1995;154:2032–2034.

Umeyama T, Kawamura T, Hasegawa A, Ogawa O: Ectopic ureter presenting with epididymitis in childhood: Report of 5 cases. J Urol 1985; 134:131–133.

van't Wout J: Fluconazole treatment of candidal infections caused by non-albicans *Candida* species. Eur J Clin Microbiol Infect Dis 1996;15: 238–242.

Weber T: *Haemophilus influenzae* epididymo-orchitis. J Urol 1985;133: 487.

Williams C, Litvak A, McRoberts J: Epididymitis in infancy. J Urol 1979; 121:125–126.

Wise G: Fungal infections of the urinary tract. In Walsh P, Wein A, Vaughan D, Retik A (eds): Campbell's Urology, 7th ed. Philadelphia, WB Saunders 1998, pp 789–806.

Yazbeck S, Patriquin H: Accuracy of Doppler sonography in the evaluation of acute conditions of the scrotum in children. J Pediatr Surg 1994;29:1270–1272.

Zia-ul-Miraj M, Miraz I: Fluconazole for treatment of fungal infections of the urinary tract in children. Pediatr Surg Int 1997;12:414–416.

Renal Function

Counahan R, Chantler C, Ghazali S, et al: Estimation of glomerular filtration rate from plasma creatinine concentration in children. Arch Dis Child 1976;51:875–878.

Donckerwolcke RAMG, Sander PC, Van Stekelenburg GJ, et al: Serum creatinine values in healthy children. Acta Paediatr Scand 1970;59:399–402.

Morris MC, Allanby CW, Toseland P, et al: Evaluation of a height/plasma creatinine formula in the measurement of glomerular filtration rate. Arch Dis Child 1982;57:611–615.

Schwartz GJ, Haycock MB, Edelmann CM, Spitzer A: A simple estimate of glomerular filtration rate in children derived from body length and plasma creatinine. Pediatrics 1976a;58:259–263.

Schwartz GJ, Haycock MB, Spitzer A: Plasma creatinine and urea concentration in children: Normal values for age and sex. J Pediatr 1976b; 88:828–830.

55
ANOMALIES OF THE UPPER URINARY TRACT

Stuart B. Bauer, M.D.

Anomalies of Number
   Agenesis
   Supernumerary Kidney

Anomalies of Ascent
   Simple Renal Ectopia
   Cephalad Renal Ectopia
   Thoracic Kidney

Anomalies of Form and Fusion
   Crossed Renal Ectopia With and Without Fusion
   Horseshoe Kidney

Anomalies of Rotation

Anomalies of Renal Vasculature
   Aberrant, Accessory, or Multiple Vessels
   Renal Artery Aneurysm
   Renal Arteriovenous Fistula

Anomalies of the Collecting System
   Calyx and Infundibulum
   Pelvis

Congenital anomalies of the upper urinary tract comprise a diversity of abnormalities, ranging from complete absence to aberrant location, orientation, and shape of the kidney as well as aberrations of the collecting system and blood supply. This wide range of anomalies results from a multiplicity of factors that interact to influence renal development in a sequential and orderly manner. Abnormal maturation or inappropriate timing of these processes at critical points in development can produce any number of deviations in the development of the kidney and ureter.

The embryology of the urinary tract is described in Chapter 49, Normal and Anomalous Development of the Urogenital System. The reader is encouraged to review this material in order to appreciate the complexity of renal and ureteral development and the factors involved in the formation of an abnormality.

The classification of renal and ureteral anomalies used in this chapter is based on structure rather than function. The anomalies of volume and structure are discussed in Chapter 49, Normal and Anomalous Development of the Urogenital System.

   I. Anomalies of number
      A. Agenesis
         1. Bilateral
         2. Unilateral
      B. Supernumerary kidney
  II. Anomalies of volume and structure
      A. Hypoplasia
      B. Multicystic kidney
      C. Polycystic kidney
         1. Infantile
         2. Adult
      D. Other cystic disease
      E. Medullary cystic disease
 III. Anomalies of ascent
      A. Simple ectopia
      B. Cephalad ectopia
      C. Thoracic kidney
 IV. Anomalies of form and fusion
      A. Crossed ectopia with and without fusion
         1. Unilateral fused kidney (inferior ectopia)
         2. Sigmoid or S-shaped kidney
         3. Lump kidney
         4. L-shaped kidney
         5. Disc kidney
         6. Unilateral fused kidney (superior ectopia)
      B. Horseshoe kidney
  V. Anomalies of rotation
      A. Incomplete
      B. Excessive
      C. Reverse
 VI. Anomalies of renal vasculature
      A. Aberrant, accessory, or multiple vessels
      B. Renal artery aneurysm
      C. Arteriovenous fistula
VII. Anomalies of the collecting system

A. Calyx and infundibulum
  1. Calyceal diverticulum
  2. Hydrocalyx
  3. Megacalycosis
  4. Unipapillary kidney
  5. Extrarenal calyces
  6. Anomalous calyx (pseudotumor of the kidney)
  7. Infundibulopelvic dysgenesis
B. Pelvis
  1. Extrarenal pelvis
  2. Bifid pelvis

ANOMALIES OF NUMBER

Agenesis

Bilateral Renal Agenesis

Of all the anomalies of the upper urinary tract, **bilateral renal agenesis (BRA) has the most profound effect on the individual.** Fortunately, it occurs infrequently when compared with other renal abnormalities. Although BRA was first recognized in 1671 by Wolfstrigel, it was not until Potter's eloquent and extensive description of the constellation of associated defects that the full extent of the syndrome could be appreciated and easily recognized (Potter, 1946a, 1946b, 1952). Subsequently, many investigators have attempted to understand all of the facets of this syndrome and to explain them by employing a single unifying etiology (Fitch and Lachance, 1972). However, there is no unanimity regarding this topic, and controversy still exists concerning the exact mechanism of formation.

Incidence. The anomaly is quite rare, with only slightly more than 500 cases having been cited in the literature. Potter (1965) estimated that BRA occurs once in 4800 births, but in British Columbia the incidence is one in 10,000 births (Wilson and Baird, 1985). Davidson and Ross (1954) noted a 0.28% incidence in autopsies of infants and children whereas **Stroup and associates (1990) detected an incidence of 3.5 per 100,000** in the Centers for Disease Control (CDC) Birth Defects Monitoring Program. As with most anomalies, there is **significant male predominance (almost 75%).** Neither maternal age, nor any specific complication of pregnancy, nor any maternal disease appears to influence its development (Davidson and Ross, 1954). The anomaly was reported in two infants of an insulin-dependent diabetic mother (Novak and Robinson, 1994). It has been observed in several sets of siblings (Rizza and Downing, 1971; Dicker et al, 1984) and even in monozygotic twins (Thomas and Smith, 1974; Cilento et al, 1994). In two pairs of monozygotic twins, one sibling was anephric while the other had normal kidneys (Kohler, 1972; Mauer et al, 1974; Cilento et al, 1994). **It has been suggested that an autosomal recessive inheritance pattern exists** (Dicker et al, 1984). There is a genetic predisposition to this syndrome with a high level of penetrance (Stella, 1998): **when siblings and parents of an index child with BRA were screened, 4.5% had unilateral renal agenesis** (Roodhooft et al, 1984), **and 3.5% had BRA** (McPherson et al, 1987). This is 1000 times higher than what has been reported in the general population

(Stroup et al, 1990). Other investigators have suggested this is an autosomal dominant trait with variable penetrance (Kovacs et al, 1991; Murugasu et al, 1991; Moerman et al, 1994).

Embryology. Complete **differentiation of the metanephric blastema into adult renal parenchyma requires the presence and orderly branching of a ureteral bud. This occurs normally between the 5th and 7th weeks of gestation,** after the ureteral bud arises from the mesonephric or wolffian duct. It is theorized that induction of ureteral branching into major and minor calyces depends on the presence of a normal metanephric blastema (Davidson and Ross, 1954). **The absence of a nephrogenic ridge on the dorsolateral aspect of the celomic cavity or the failure of a ureteral bud to develop from the wolffian duct will lead to agenesis of the kidney. The absence of both kidneys, therefore, requires a common factor causing renal or ureteral maldevelopment on both sides of the midline.**

It is impossible to say which of these two factors is most important. Certainly no kidney can form in the absence of a metanephric blastema, but the presence of a ureteral bud and orderly branching are also necessary for the renal anlage to attain its potential. In an extensive autopsy analysis, Ashley and Mostofi (1960) found many clues to the multifactorial nature of this developmental process and shed some light on the causes of BRA. Most anephric children in their series had at least a blind-ending ureteral bud of varying length. Therefore, the embryologic insult in such cases was thought to affect the ureteral bud just as or shortly after it arose from the mesonephric duct. Even with complete ureteral atresia, structures of wolffian duct origin (vas deferens, seminal vesicle, and epididymis) were usually present and normally formed, suggesting that the injury occurred at about the time the ureteral bud formed (the 5th or 6th week of gestation). With complete absence of the ureter, a rudimentary kidney was discovered in only a few instances, supporting the concept of the interdependency of the two processes. Conversely, in some instances, the ureter was normal in appearance up to the level of the ureteropelvic junction (UPJ), where it ended abruptly. In those cases, no recognizable renal parenchyma could be identified. In a small number of autopsies the gonads were absent as well, indicating an abnormality or insult that took place before the 5th week and involved the entire urogenital ridge (Carpentier and Potter, 1959). Although the nephric and genital portions of the urogenital ridge are closely aligned on the dorsal aspect of the celomic cavity, an extensive lesion affecting the entire area is necessary to produce both conditions in the developing fetus. **Therefore, absence of one or both kidneys may result from any of several etiologies.**

Description. The kidneys are completely absent on gross inspection of the entire retroperitoneum. Occasionally, there may be a small mass of poorly organized mesenchymal tissue, containing primitive glomerular elements. Tiny vascular branches from the aorta penetrate this structure, but no identifiable major renal artery is present (Ashley and Mostofi, 1960) (Fig. 55–1).

Besides the absence of functioning kidneys, each ureter may be either wholly or partially absent. **Complete ureteral atresia is observed in slightly more than 50% of**

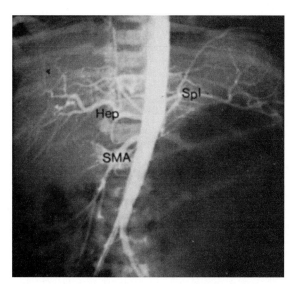

Figure 55–1. Aortogram obtained via an umbilical artery catheter in a newborn with Potter's facies outlines major branches of the aorta but fails to demonstrate either renal artery or kidney. (Hep = Hepatic artery, SMA = superior mesenteric artery, Spl = splenic artery.)

affected individuals (Ashley and Mostofi, 1960). **The trigone,** if developed, **is poorly formed** owing to failure of mesonephric duct structures to be incorporated into the base of the bladder. **The bladder,** when present (about 50% of cases), **is usually hypoplastic from the lack of**

stimulation by fetal urine production. Alternatively, it has been postulated that ureteral bud and wolffian duct structures migrating into the ventral cloacal region are needed to initiate bladder development; their absence, and not the *lack* of urine, is the cause of arrested development (Katz and Chatten, 1974; Levin, 1952).

Associated Anomalies. Other findings associated with BRA were extensively described by Dr. Potter. **The infants have low birth weights,** ranging from 1000 to 2500 g, and intrauterine growth retardation due in part to low iron stores in the liver (Georgieff et al, 1996). At birth, **oligohydramnios (absent or minimal amniotic fluid) is present.** In addition, the characteristic facial appearance and deformity of the extremities sets these children apart from normal newborns. **The infants generally look prematurely senile and have "a prominent fold of skin that begins over each eye, swings down in a semi-circle over the inner canthus and extends onto the cheek"** (Potter, 1946a, 1946b). It is Dr. Potter's contention that this facial feature is a sine qua non of nonfunctioning renal parenchyma. She even suggests that its absence confirms the presence of kidneys (Fig. 55–2A). In addition to this finding, the nose is blunted, and a prominent depression between the lower lip and chin is evident. The ears appear to be somewhat low set, are drawn forward, and are often pressed against the side of the head, making the lobes seem unusually broad and exceedingly large (see Fig. 55–2B). The ear canals are not dislocated, but the appearance of the ear lobes gives the impression that the ears are

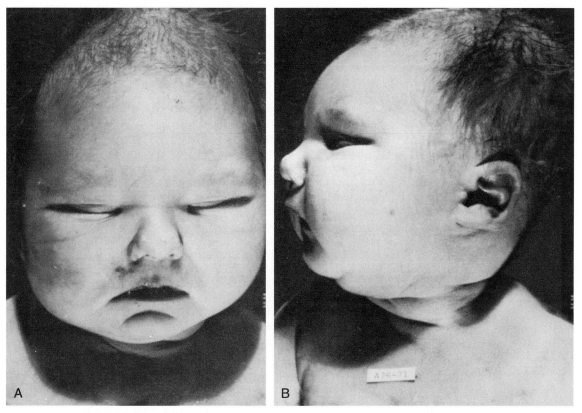

Figure 55–2. An anephric child who lived 2 days has typical Potter's facial appearance. *A,* Note the prominent fold and skin crease beneath each eye, blunted nose, and depression between lower lip and chin. *B,* The ears give an impression of being low-set because lobes are broad and drawn forward, but actually the ear canals are located normally.

displaced downward. The legs are often bowed and clubbed, with excessive flexion at the hip and knee joints. Occasionally, the lower extremities are completely fused as well (sirenomelia) (Bain et al, 1960).

The skin can be excessively dry and appears too loose for the body. This may be secondary to severe dehydration or loss of subcutaneous fat. The hands are relatively large and clawlike.

It is thought that these characteristic facial abnormalities and limb features are caused by the effects of oligohydramnios rather than by multiple organ system defects (Fitch and Lachance, 1972; Thomas and Smith, 1974). This observation was confirmed by an experiment in nature in which one twin with bilateral agenesis did not have the characteristic Potter facies because it shared the same amniotic sac, containing adequate amniotic fluid, with the second twin (Klinger et al, 1997). Therefore, **compression of the fetus against the internal uterine walls without any cushioning effect from amniotic fluid could explain all of the findings of this syndrome. Urine from the developing kidney is the major source of amniotic fluid, accounting for more than 90% of its volume by the third trimester** (Thomas and Smith, 1974), but the skin, gastrointestinal tract, and central nervous system also contribute small amounts, particularly before urine production begins at 14 weeks. Therefore, the absence of kidneys reduces severely the amount of amniotic fluid produced during the latter stages of pregnancy.

Pulmonary hypoplasia and a bell-shaped chest are common associated conditions. Originally, these findings were thought to be secondary to uterine wall compression of the thoracic cage as a result of the oligohydramniotic state (Bain and Scott, 1960). Subsequently, it was thought that the amniotic fluid itself is responsible for pulmonary development (Fitch and Lachance, 1972). However, this theory was discounted when it was discovered there is a significant reduction in the number of airway generations as well as a decrease in acini formation in these fetuses (Hislop et al, 1979). Pulmonary airway divisioning occurs between the 12th and 16th weeks of gestation (Reid, 1977). A reduction in the number of divisions implies an interference with this process before the 16th week of gestation. The contribution from the kidneys to the amniotic fluid volume before that time is small, if any. Therefore, the oligohydramnios seen in cases of BRA is a later finding in pregnancy, occurring long after the structural groundwork of the lung has been laid out. **Hislop and colleagues (1979) suggested that the anephric fetus fails to produce proline, which is needed for collagen formation in the bronchiolar tree. The kidney is the primary source of proline** (Clemmons, 1977). **Thus pulmonary hypoplasia may result from the absence of renal parenchyma and not from diminished amniotic fluid.** This hypothesis is supported by the finding of normal lungs in two babies with prolonged leakage of amniotic fluid beginning at a time when pulmonary hypoplasia would have been expected if the amniotic fluid alone were responsible for the defect (Perlman et al, 1976; Cilento et al, 1994).

In the male, **penile development is usually normal,** but a few cases of penile agenesis have occurred (O'Connor et al, 1993). **Hypospadias is rare,** but its occurrence is not related to the presence or absence of the testes. **In 43% of** the cases, however, the testes are undescended (Carpentier and Potter, 1959). They did not find any infants without testes, but Ashley and Mostofi (1960) noted testicular agenesis in 10%. **The vas deferens is normal in most cases. The presence of vasa implies that whatever caused the renal agenesis influenced the ureteral bud only after it formed or that the insult affected just the nephrogenic ridge.**

Although this syndrome occurs uncommonly in females, they have a relatively high incidence of genitourinary anomalies when it does appear in them (Carpentier and Potter, 1959). The ovaries are frequently hypoplastic or absent. The uterus is usually either rudimentary or bicornuate; occasionally, it is absent entirely, as in sirenomelia. Finally, the vagina is either a short, blind pouch or completely absent.

The adrenal glands are rarely malpositioned or absent (Davidson and Ross, 1954), but they can appear flattened or "lying down" on ultrasonography (Hoffman et al, 1992). Anomalies of other organ systems are not unusual. **The legs are frequently abnormal, with clubbed or even fused feet producing sirenomelia.** A lumbar meningocele with or without the Arnold-Chiari malformation is not infrequently observed (Davidson and Ross, 1954; Ashley and Mostofi, 1960). Other malformations include abnormalities of the cardiovascular and gastrointestinal systems, which are present in up to 50% of infants.

Diagnosis. The characteristic Potter facies and the presence of oligohydramnios are pathognomonic and should alert the practitioner to this severe urinary malformation. Amnion nodosum—small white, keratinized nodules found on the surface of the amniotic sac—may also suggest this anomaly (Bain et al, 1960; Thompson, 1960). Ninety percent of newborns void during the first day of life (Clarke, 1977; Sherry and Kramer, 1955). Failure to urinate in the first 24 hours is not uncommon and should not arouse suspicion. **Anuria after the first 24 hours without distention of the bladder should suggest renal agenesis** (D.I. Williams, personal communication, 1974). **However, most infants who are born alive experience severe respiratory distress** within the first 24 hours of life. When this becomes the focus of attention, the anuria may go unnoticed, with the renal anomaly being thought of only secondarily.

When the association is made, excretory urography may be attempted, but it is usually fruitless. **Renal ultrasonography is probably the easiest way to identify the kidneys and bladder in order to confirm the presence or absence of urine within these structures.** The advent of power Doppler ultrasonography to diagnose renal agenesis when renal arteries are not detectable has been highly accurate, even in fetuses with oligohydramnios and suspected BRA (Sepulveda et al, 1998). A clue to an absent kidney (or kidneys) is a flattened adrenal gland which lies in its normal location (Hoffman et al, 1992). **If abdominal ultrasonography is inconclusive, a renal scan can be performed.** The absence of uptake of the radionuclide in the renal fossa above background activity confirms the diagnosis of BRA. Umbilical artery catheterization and an aortogram can be undertaken if other modalities are unavailable or not diagnostic. This defines the absence of renal arteries and kidneys. (See Fig. 55–1.)

As the use of maternal ultrasonic screening becomes more pervasive, babies with this condition are being diagnosed in the second and third trimesters, when severe oligohydramnios is noted and no kidney tissue can be detected. Termination of the pregnancy has been considered when the clinician is certain of the diagnosis (Rayburn and Laferla, 1986).

Prognosis. Almost 40% of the affected infants are stillborn. Most of the children who are born alive do not survive beyond the first 24 to 48 hours because of respiratory distress associated with pulmonary hypoplasia. Those infants who do not succumb early remain alive for a variable period, depending on the rate at which renal failure develops. The longest-surviving child lived 39 days (Davidson and Ross, 1954).

Unilateral Renal Agenesis

Complete absence of one kidney occurs more commonly than does BRA. In general, **there are no telltale signs** (as with BRA) **that suggest an absent kidney** (Campbell, 1928). The diagnosis usually is not suspected, and the condition remains undetected unless careful examination of the external and internal genitalia uncovers an abnormality that is associated with renal agenesis or an imaging study done for other reasons reveals only one kidney. Prenatal ultrasonography has increased the detection rate of this condition and has revealed that some cases are caused by involution of a multicystic or dysplastic kidney before birth (Mesrobian et al, 1993; Hitchcock and Burge, 1994).

Incidence. The clinically silent nature of this anomaly precludes a completely accurate account of its incidence. Most autopsy series, however, suggest that **unilateral agenesis occurs once in 1100 births** (Doroshow and Abeshouse, 1961). In a survey of excretory urograms performed at the Mayo Clinic, the clinical incidence approached 1 in 1500 (Longo and Thompson, 1952), but Wilson and Baird (1985) noted a 1 in 5000 occurrence rate in British Columbia. With the increased use of prenatal and postnatal ultrasonic screening, the incidence of unilateral renal agenesis (URA) may actually be higher than previously reported. **Ultrasonic screening** of 280,000 school children in Taipei **revealed the incidence of unilateral agenesis to be 1 in 1200** (Sheih et al, 1990), and in the Czech Republic a similar incidence was found on prenatal screening (Sipek et al, 1997).

The higher incidence of BRA noted in male children is not nearly as striking in the unilateral condition, but **males still predominate in a ratio of 1.8:1** (Doroshow and Abeshouse, 1961). This is not surprising considering the timing of embryologic events. Wolffian duct differentiation occurs earlier in the male fetus than does müllerian duct development in the female, taking place closer to the time of ureteral bud formation. Therefore, it is postulated that the ureteral bud is influenced more by abnormalities of the wolffian duct than by those of the müllerian duct.

Absence of one kidney occurs somewhat more frequently on the left side. A familial tendency has been noted (Arfeen et al, 1993; Selig et al, 1993). Siblings within a single family and even monozygotic twins have been affected (Kohn and Borns, 1973; Uchida et al, 1990). In a study of several families, McPherson and associates

(1987) noted a familial pattern of inheritance and concluded in this study group that **an autosomal dominant transmission with a 50% to 90% penetrance exists.** This inheritance pattern has been confirmed by others who evaluated families with more than one affected individual (Biedel et al, 1984; Roodhooft et al, 1984; Battin et al, 1993).

Embryology. The embryologic basis for URA does not differ significantly from that described for the bilateral type. **The fault lies most probably with the ureteral bud.** Complete absence of a bud or aborted ureteral development prevents maturation of the metanephric blastema into adult kidney tissue.

It is unlikely that the metanephros is responsible, because the ipsilateral gonad (derived from adjacent mesenchymal tissue) is rarely absent, malpositioned, or nonfunctioning (Ashley and Mostofi, 1960). The high incidence of absent or malformed proximal mesonephric duct structures in the male and müllerian duct structures in the female strengthens the argument that the embryologic insult affects the ureteral bud primarily early in its development and even influences its precursor, the mesonephric duct. **The abnormality most likely occurs no later than the 4th or 5th week of gestation,** when the ureteral bud forms and the mesonephric or wolffian duct in the male begins to develop into the seminal vesicle, prostate, and vas deferens. The müllerian duct in the female fetus at this time starts its medial migration, crossing over the degenerating wolffian duct (6th week) on its way to differentiating into the fallopian tube, uterine horn and body, and proximal vagina (Woolf and Allen, 1953; Yoder and Pfister, 1976).

Magee and coworkers (1979) proposed an embryologic classification based on the timing of the faulty differentiation. If the insult occurs before the 4th week (type I URA, Fig. 55–3A), nondifferentiation of the nephrogenic ridge with retardation of the mesonephric and müllerian components results, leading to complete unilateral agenesis of genitourinary structures. The individual has a solitary kidney and a unicornuate uterus. In type II anomalies (Fig. 55–3B), the defect occurs early in the 4th week of gestation, affecting both the mesonephric duct and the ureteral buds. The maldeveloped mesonephric duct prevents crossover of the müllerian duct and subsequent fusion. As a consequence a didelphys uterus with obstruction of the ipsilateral horn and the vagina is produced. If the insult occurs after the 4th week (type III, Fig. 55–3C), the mesonephric and müllerian ducts develop normally; only the ureteral bud and metanephric blastema are affected. Normal genital architecture is present despite the absence of one kidney.

With the discovery that multicystic and dysgenetic kidneys can involute completely before birth, it is clear that **the cause of every case of URA cannot be attributed to one of the mechanisms cited previously.** In fact, the presence of the splenic flexure of the bowel in its normal location and not in the left renal fossa suggests that a dysplastic or multicystic kidney may have started to form in the proper location but involuted before delivery.

Associated Anomalies. The ipsilateral ureter is completely absent in slightly more than half of the patients (Fortune, 1927; Collins, 1932; Ashley and Mostofi, 1960). **Many of the remaining individuals have only a partially developed ureter.** In no instance is the ureter totally nor-

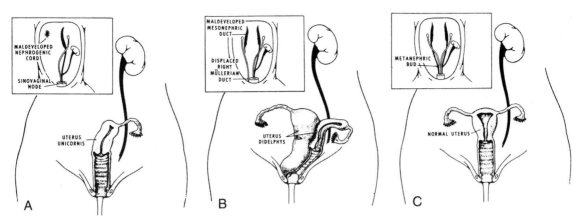

Figure 55–3. A proposed categorization of genital and renal anomalies in females. See text for details. (From Magee MC, Lucey DT, Fried FA: A new embryologic classification for uro-gynecologic malformations: The syndromes of mesonephric duct induced müllerian deformities. J Urol 1979;121:265.)

mal. Partial ureteral development is associated with either complete luminal atresia or patency of a variable degree. A hemitrigone (in association with complete ureteral agenesis) or an asymmetric trigone (in the presence of a partially developed ureter) is recognizable at cystoscopy. Segmental ureteral atresia on one side has been associated with contralateral ureteral or renal ectopia (Limkakeng and Retik, 1972). **Except for ectopia or malrotation, anomalies of the contralateral kidney are very infrequently encountered** (Longo and Thompson, 1952). **However, abnormalities of the contralateral collecting system are not uncommon,** including ureteropelvic and ureterovesical junction obstruction in 11% and 7%, respectively (Cascio et al, 1999), and vesicoureteral reflux in 30% (Atiyeh et al, 1993).

Ipsilateral adrenal agenesis is rarely encountered with URA: it is noted in fewer than 10% of autopsy reports (Fortune, 1927; Collins, 1932; Ashley and Mostofi, 1960) and in 17% of affected individuals evaluated by computed tomography (Kenney et al, 1985). This is not surprising in view of the different embryologic derivations of the adrenal cortex and medulla, which arise separately from the metanephros.

Genital anomalies are much more frequently observed. Despite the predominance of male infants with URA, reproductive organ abnormalities seem to occur with more regularity in females, occurring in at least 25% to 50% of cases, compared with 10% to 15% in males. Although a genital anomaly is easier to detect in the female, which may account for the difference in incidence between the two sexes, a more plausible explanation is related to the difference in timing and interaction of the male and female genital ducts in relation to the developing mesonephric duct and ureteral bud. The incidence of a genital organ malformation for both sexes varies from 20% to 40% (Smith and Orkin, 1945; Doroshow and Abeshouse, 1961; Thompson and Lynn, 1966).

Regardless of the sex, **both the ipsilaterally and contralaterally positioned testes are normal, and the gonad is usually normal. But structures derived from the müllerian or wolffian duct are most often anomalous. In the male, the testis and globus major,** which contains the efferent ductules and which arises from mesonephric tu-

bules, **are invariably present; all structures proximal to that point which develop from the mesonephric duct** (the globus minor, vas deferens, seminal vesicle, ampulla, and ejaculatory duct) **are frequently absent, with an incidence approaching 50%** (Radasch, 1908; Collins, 1932; Charny and Gillenwater, 1965; Ochsner et al, 1972). In a review of the literature (Donohue and Fauver, 1989) **of adult males with absence of the vas deferens, 79% were found to have an absent kidney on the ipsilateral side; left-sided lesions predominated in a ratio of 3.5:1.** Occasionally, the mesonephric duct structures are rudimentary or ectopic rather than absent (Holt and Peterson, 1974). Seminal vesicle cysts are being diagnosed with increasing frequency as pelvic ultrasound examinations are performed more often (Lopez-Garcia et al, 1998): 6 cases (5%) were noted among 119 boys who were found to have URA during ultrasonic screening of schoolchildren (Shieh et al, 1990). Rarely has ipsilateral cryptorchidism been noted.

In the female, a variety of anomalies may result from incomplete or altered müllerian development caused by mesonephric duct maldevelopment. **Approximately one third of women with URA have an abnormality of the internal genitalia** (Thompson and Lynn, 1966). Conversely, 43% of women with genital anomalies have URA (Semmens, 1962). **Most common of these is a true unicornuate uterus with complete absence of the ipsilateral horn and fallopian tube or a bicornuate uterus with rudimentary development of the horn on the affected side** (Candiani et al, 1997). The fimbriated end of the fallopian tube, however, is usually fully formed and corresponds in its development to the globus major in the male (Shumacker, 1938).

Partial or complete midline fusion of the müllerian ducts may result in a double (didelphys) or septate uterus with either a single or a duplicated cervix (Radasch, 1908; Fortune, 1927). Complete duplication or separation of the vagina, proximal vaginal atresia associated with a small introital dimple, and even complete absence of the vagina have been reported (Woolf and Allen, 1953; D'Alberton et al, 1981). **Obstruction of one side of a duplicated system is not uncommon, and unilateral hematocolpos or hydrocolpos associated with a pelvic mass and/or pain has been described** in the pubertal girl (Weiss and Dykhuizen, 1967;

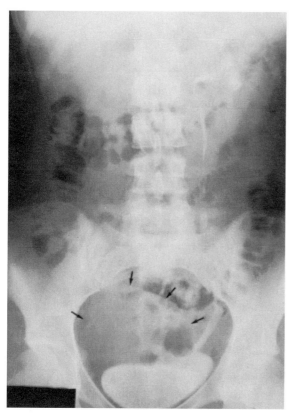

Figure 55–4. A 16-year-old girl with a solitary left kidney had abdominal pain and a pelvic mass that proved to be an obstructed duplicate vagina with hematocolpos. (Arrows outline the obstructed vaginal segment.)

uel et al, 1974) (Fig. 55–5). They include septal and valvular cardiac defects; imperforate anus and anal or esophageal strictures or atresia; and vertebral or phalangeal abnormalities (Jancu et al, 1976). **Several syndromes are associated with URA**—Turner's syndrome, Poland's syndrome (Mace et al, 1972), DiGeorge anomaly when associated with insulin-dependent diabetes mellitus in the mother (Wilson et al, 1993; Novak and Robinson, 1994), dysmorphogenesis, and more recently, Kallmann's syndrome. Abnormalities of the *KAL1* locus at Xp22 in the X-linked autosomal dominant disorder have a high frequency of URA: 40% (Say and Gerald, 1968; Colquhoun-Kerr et al, 1999; Zenteno et al, 1999). Twenty percent to 30% of children with the VACTERL association (vertebral, imperforate anus, cardiac, tracheo-esophageal atresia, renal, and limb anomalies) have URA (Barry and Auldist, 1974; Kolon et al, 2000). Therefore, **a comprehensive review of all organ systems should be undertaken when more than one anomaly is discovered** or when specific complexes of anomalies associated with renal agenesis are present. In a small number of children the constellation of defects is incompatible with life and gestational or neonatal death ensues.

Diagnosis. In general, **there are no specific symptoms heralding an absent kidney.** Most reports are composed of surveys from autopsy series. **The contralateral kidney does not appear to be more prone to disease** from being solitary unless the absent kidney is truly secondary to a multicystic dysplastic organ that went unrecognized at birth, in which case there may be a mild UPJ obstruction in the remaining functioning kidney. **The demands placed**

Vinstein and Franken, 1972; Gilliland and Dick, 1976; Wiersma et al, 1976; Yoder and Pfister, 1976) (Fig. 55–4). In rare instances, this anomalous condition has been mistaken for a large or infected Gartner's duct cyst. Sometimes a true Gartner's duct cyst has been found in a prepubertal girl in association with an ectopic ureter that is blind-ending at its proximal end or one that is connected to a rudimentary kidney (Currarino, 1982). Six percent of girls with URA were found to have a Gartner's cyst on mass screening of school children (Shieh et al, 1990). Infertility occurs in as many as 33% of affected women with renal agenesis and unicornuate uterus (Heinonen, 1997).

Radiologic investigation of the upper urinary tract in individuals with anomalies of the internal genitalia often leads to the discovery of an absent kidney on the affected side (Bryan et al, 1949; Phelan et al, 1953). In fact, because URA is so frequently associated with anomalies of the internal female genitalia, **the clinician should evaluate the entire genitourinary system in any girl with one or more of the above-mentioned abnormalities.** It is just as reasonable to investigate the pelvic area with ultrasound in boys diagnosed with URA because of its association with seminal vesicle abnormalities (Van den Ouden et al, 1998).

In addition, **anomalies of other organ systems are found frequently in affected individuals. The more common sites involve the cardiovascular (30%), gastrointestinal (25%), and musculoskeletal (14%) systems** (Eman-

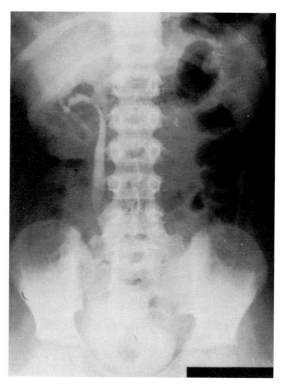

Figure 55–5. A 4-year-old girl had an excretory urogram because of imperforate anus and duplicate vagina. Note absence of left kidney and medial placement of the splenic flexure. At cystoscopy, a hemitrigone was noted.

on the solitary kidney lead to compensatory enlargement (hyperplasia), which can then raise the specter of contralateral agenesis because the kidney is larger than normal.

The diagnosis should be suspected during a physical examination when the vas deferens or body and tail of the epididymis is missing, or when an absent, septate, or hypoplastic vagina is associated with a unicornuate or bicornuate uterus (Bryan et al, 1949). **Radiologically, an absent left kidney can be surmised when a plain film of the abdomen demonstrates the gas pattern of the splenic flexure of the colon in a medial position because the colon now occupies the area normally reserved for the left kidney** (Mascatello and Lebowitz, 1976) (see Fig. 55–5). When this characteristic gas pattern is present, it is a very reliable sign. A similar finding showing the hepatic flexure positioned in the right renal fossa suggests congenital absence of the right kidney (Curtis et al, 1977). **The diagnosis of agenesis usually can be confirmed by renal ultrasonography or excretory urography, which reveals an absent kidney or nephrogram on that side and compensatory hypertrophy of the contralateral kidney** (Hynes and Watkin, 1970; Cope and Trickey, 1982). However, a multicystic kidney can easily be mistaken for true agenesis in an older individual, because the cysts involute as the fluid gets absorbed during the first several months of life. The colonic gas pattern will not occupy a position closer to the midline if a multicystic kidney was present during gestation, so this provides an excellent clue to the diagnosis when no kidney can be detected by ultrasonography later on in life. Prenatal and perinatal ultrasonography examinations are being performed more routinely today, and URA is being detected with increased frequency (Sipek et al, 1997). The kidney may be larger than normal due to compensatory hypertrophy, which may occur even in utero (Mesrobian, 1998), providing a clue to the absence of the opposite kidney. In addition, the ipsilateral adrenal gland may have a characteristic appearance—flattened or lying down—when the kidney never formed, alerting the clinician to URA (Hoffman et al, 1992).

Failure of one kidney to "light up" during the total body image phase of a radionuclide technetium scan is compatible with the diagnosis of an absent kidney, but this may not be infallible. **Radionuclide imaging of the kidney** using an isotope that traces renal blood flow **will clearly differentiate URA** from other conditions in which the renal function may be severely impaired (e.g., severe obstruction, high-grade reflux). Isotope scanning and ultrasonography have largely replaced arteriography in defining agenesis. Fluoroscopic monitoring of the renal fossa at the end of a cardiac catheterization or renal ultrasonography at the end of echocardiography has demonstrated an absent kidney on occasion. **The relatively high incidence of contralateral reflux** (Cascio et al, 1999) **warrants cystography, either conventional or nuclear, in these individuals.**

Cystoscopy, if performed, usually reveals an asymmetric trigone or hemitrigone, suggesting either partial or complete ureteral atresia and renal agenesis. Cystoscopy has been relegated to a minor diagnostic tool since the development of other, more sophisticated, noninvasive radiographic studies (Kroovand, 1985).

Prognosis. There is no clearcut evidence that patients with a solitary kidney have an increased susceptibility to other diseases. Most reviews dealing with this subject were conducted in the preantibiotic era, and they reported a high incidence of "pyelitis," nephrolithiasis and ureterolithiasis, tuberculosis, and glomerulonephritis. The increased ability to prevent infection and its sequelae has reduced the incidence of morbidity and mortality among patients with a solitary kidney. In Ashley and Mostofi's series (1960), only 15% of the patients died as a result of renal disease, the nature of which in almost every case would have been bilateral had two kidneys been present initially. Renal trauma resulted in death for 5%; some patients in this group might have lived had there been two kidneys (however, because the source of the autopsy material included many military personnel, the potential risk of injury was accentuated). In other words, **URA with an otherwise normal contralateral kidney is not incompatible with normal longevity and does not predispose the remaining contralateral kidney to greater than normal risks** (Gutierrez, 1933; Dees, 1960). One should be prudent, however, in advising individuals to participate in contact sports or strenuous physical exertion.

Rugui and associates (1986) found an increased occurrence of hypertension, hyperuricemia, and decreased renal function but no proteinuria in a small group of patients with congenital absence of one kidney. Only one patient had a renal biopsy, and this showed focal glomerular sclerosis, similar to what has been found in the remaining kidney in patients with the hyperfiltration syndrome noted after unilateral nephrectomy. The authors concluded that URA may carry the same potential factor. Focal glomerulosclerosis has been confirmed in six other individuals with URA (Nomura and Osawa, 1990). **Argueso and colleagues (1992) assessed 157 middle-aged patients with congenital URA and noted hypertension and proteinuria in 47% and in 19%, respectively, as well as mild renal insufficiency in 13%.** Despite these findings, survival was not impaired in this group of people. In addition, the ability of the kidney to excrete increased loads of protein was not impaired, even in patients with renal insufficiency or proteinuria (DeSanto et al, 1997).

Supernumerary Kidney

Parenchymal development is controlled, in part, by an unidentified substance that acts to limit the amount of functioning renal tissue. It is, therefore, interesting to find that nature has created, albeit rarely, a condition in which the individual has three separate kidneys and an excessive amount of functioning renal parenchyma. In such instances, the two main kidneys are usually normal and equal in size whereas the third is small. **The supernumerary kidney is truly an accessory organ with its own collecting system, blood supply, and distinct encapsulated parenchymal mass.** It may be either totally separate from the normal kidney on the same side or connected to it by loose areolar tissue (Geisinger, 1937). **The ipsilateral ureters may be bifid or completely duplicated.** The condition is not analogous to a single kidney with ureteral duplication, in which each collecting system drains portions of one parenchymatous mass surrounded by a single capsule.

Incidence. The true incidence of this anomaly cannot be calculated because of its very infrequent occurrence. **Approximately 80 cases have been reported since it was**

first described in 1656; it represents a very rare anomaly of the urinary system (Sasidharan et al, 1976; McPherson, 1987). It affects males and females equally but has a higher predilection for the left side (N'Guessan and Stephens, 1983). Campbell (1970) recorded one case involving bilateral supernumerary kidneys, an anomaly that has been observed in other animal species (i.e., cow and pig).

Embryology. The sequence of interdependent events involved in ureteral bud formation and metanephric blastema development, which is required for the maturation of the normal kidney, probably also allows for the occurrence of a supernumerary kidney. **It is postulated that a deviation involving both of these processes must take place to create the anomaly. A second ureteral outpouching off the wolffian duct or a branching from the initial ureteral bud appears as a necessary first step. Next, the nephrogenic anlage may divide into two metanephric tails, which separate entirely** when induced to differentiate by the separate or bifid ureteral buds (N'Guessan and Stephens, 1983). The twin metanephroi develop only when the bifid or separate ureteral buds enter them. N'Guessan and Stephens do not accept that this condition is the result of widely divergent bifid or separate ureteral buds. Geisinger (1937) proposed that the separate kidneys may have been caused either by fragmentation of a single metanephros or by linear infarction producing separate viable fragments that develop only when a second ureteral bud is present.

Description. The **supernumerary kidney is a distinct parenchymatous mass that may be either completely separate or only loosely attached to the major kidney on the ipsilateral side.** In general, it is located somewhat caudad to the dominant kidney, which is in its correct position in the renal fossa. Occasionally, the supernumerary kidney lies either posterior or craniad to the main kidney, or it may even be a midline structure anterior to the great vessels and loosely attached to each of the other two kidneys (Fig. 55–6).

The supernumerary kidney is reniform in shape but generally smaller than the main ipsilateral organ. In

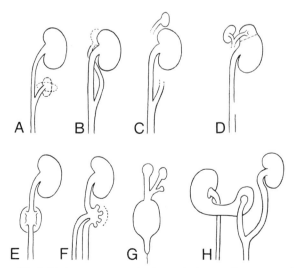

Figure 55–6. Various patterns of urinary drainage when ureters form a common stem. All kidney positions are relative only and are depicted on the left side for ease of interpretation. Dashed lines indicate that detail was not defined. (From N'Guessan G, Stephens FD: Supernumerary kidney. J Urol 1983;130:649.)

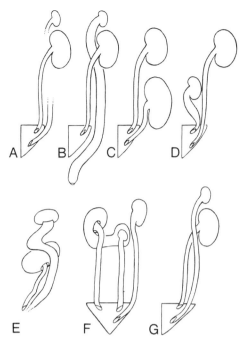

Figure 55–7. Various patterns of urinary drainage of supernumerary and ipsilateral kidneys when ureters are completely separated. All kidney positions are relative only and are depicted on the left side for ease of interpretation. Dashed lines indicate that detail was not defined. (From N'Guessan G, Stephens FD: Supernumerary kidney. J Urol 1983;130:649.)

about one third of cases, the kidney or its collecting system is abnormal. In almost half of the reported cases, the collecting system is severely dilated with thinned parenchyma, indicating an obstructed ureter.

The ureteral interrelationships on the side of the supernumerary kidney are quite variable (Kretschmer, 1929). Convergence of the ipsilateral ureters distally to form a common stem and a single ureteral orifice occurs in 50% of the cases (Exley and Hotchkiss, 1944; N'Guessan and Stephens, 1983). Two completely independent ureters, each with its own entrance into the bladder, is seen in the other 50% of cases. **The Weigert-Meyer principle** (see Chapter 58) **usually is obeyed,** but in 10% the caudal kidney has a ureter that does not follow the rule and enters the trigone below the ipsilateral ureter (Tada et al, 1981) (Fig. 55–7). Rarely, the supernumerary kidney has a completely ectopic ureter opening into the vagina or introitus (Rubin, 1948; Carlson, 1950). Individual case reports have described calyceal communications between the supernumerary and the dominant kidney, or fusion of the dominant kidney's ureter with the pelvis of the supernumerary kidney (Kretschmer, 1929) to create a single distal ureter, which then enters the bladder (see Fig. 55–6). **The vascular supply to the supernumerary kidney is, as might be expected, anomalous** and depends on its position in relation to the major ipsilateral kidney. Although some investigators believe that the blood supply to the individual parenchymal masses should be separate to consider this a true supernumerary kidney (Kaneoya et al, 1989), this view is not held universally.

Associated Anomalies. Usually the ipsilateral and contralateral kidneys are normal. Except for an occasional ectopic orifice from the ureter draining the supernumerary kidney, no genitourinary abnormalities are present in any consistent pattern. **Few of the case reports describe anomalies of other organ systems.**

Symptoms. Although this anomaly is obviously present at birth, **it is rarely discovered in childhood. It may not produce symptoms until early adulthood, if at all.** The average age at diagnosis in all reported cases was 36 years. Pain, fever, hypertension, and a palpable abdominal mass are the usual presenting complaints. Urinary infection or obstruction, or both, are the major conditions that lead to an evaluation. Ureteral ectopia from the supernumerary kidney may produce urinary incontinence, but this is extremely rare because of the hypoplastic nature of the involved renal element (Shane, 1942; Hoffman and McMillan, 1948).

A palpable abdominal mass secondary to development of carcinoma in the supernumerary kidney has been noted in two patients. In 25% of all reported cases, however, the supernumerary kidney remains completely asymptomatic and is discovered only at autopsy (Carlson, 1950).

Diagnosis. If the supernumerary kidney is normal and not symptomatic, it is usually diagnosed when excretory urography or abdominal ultrasonography is performed for other reasons. The kidney may be inferior and distant enough from the ipsilateral kidney that it does not disturb the latter's architecture (Conrad and Loes, 1987). If it is in close proximity, its mere presence may displace the predominant kidney or its ureter very slightly.

If the supernumerary organ is hydronephrotic, it may distort the normal ipsilateral kidney and ureter, a condition that is detectable by ultrasonography. If the collecting system is bifid, the dominant kidney on that side is usually involved in the same disease process. If the ureters are separate, the ipsilateral kidney may show the effects of an abnormal supernumerary kidney. Voiding cystourethrography, ultrasonography, computed tomography with contrast, and even retrograde pyelography may be needed to help delineate the pathologic process. Radionuclide imaging provides information about relative function in the supernumerary as well as normal kidneys (Conrad and Loes, 1987). Cystoscopy reveals one or two ureteral orifices on the ipsilateral side, depending on whether the ureters are completely duplicated and, if so, to what extent ureteral ectopia exists in or outside of the bladder. Occasionally a supernumerary kidney is not accurately diagnosed until the time of surgery or at autopsy.

ANOMALIES OF ASCENT

Simple Renal Ectopia

When the mature kidney fails to reach its normal location in the "renal" fossa, the condition is known as *renal ectopia*. The term is derived from the Greek words *ek* ("out") and *topos* ("place") and literally means "out of place." It is to be differentiated from renal ptosis, in which the kidney initially is located in its proper place (and has normal vascularity) but moves downward in relation to body position. The ectopic kidney has never resided in the appropriate location.

An ectopic kidney can be found in one of the following positions: pelvic, iliac, abdominal, thoracic, and contralat-

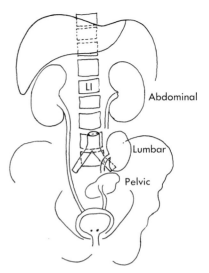

Figure 55–8. Incomplete ascent of kidney: The kidney may halt at any level of its ascent from the pelvis. (From Gray SW, Skandalakis JE: The kidney and ureter. In Gray SW, Skandalakis JE: Embryology for Surgeons. Philadelphia, W. B. Saunders Company, 1972.)

eral or crossed (Fig. 55–8). Only the ipsilateral retroperitoneal location of the ectopic kidney is discussed here. Thoracic kidney and crossed renal ectopia (with and without fusion) are described later.

Incidence. Renal ectopia has been known to exist since it was described by 16th century anatomists, but it did not achieve clinical interest until the mid-19th century. In recent times, with greater emphasis on diagnostic acumen and uroradiologic visualization including prenatal imaging, this condition has been noted with increasing frequency.

The actual incidence among autopsy series varies from 1 in 500 (Campbell, 1930) **to 1 in 1200** (Stevens, 1937; Thompson and Pace, 1937; Anson and Riba, 1939; Bell, 1946), but the average occurrence is about 1 in 900 (Abeshouse and Bhisitkul, 1959). With increasing clinical detection, the incidence among hospitalized patients has approached the autopsy rate (Abeshouse and Bhisitkul, 1959). **Autopsy studies reveal no significant difference in incidence between the sexes.** Clinically, renal ectopia is more readily recognized in females because they undergo uroradiologic evaluation more frequently than males as a result of their higher rate of urinary infection and/or associated genital anomalies (Thompson and Pace, 1937).

The left side is favored slightly over the right. Pelvic ectopia has been estimated to occur in 1 of 2100 to 3000 autopsies (Stevens, 1937). **A solitary ectopic kidney occurs in 1 of 22,000 autopsies** (Stevens, 1937; Hawes, 1950; Delson, 1975); by 1973, only **165 cases of a solitary pelvic kidney had been recorded** (Downs et al, 1973). **Bilateral ectopic kidneys are even more rarely observed and account for only 10% of all patients with renal ectopia** (Malek et al, 1971).

Embryology. The ureteral bud first arises from the wolffian duct at the end of the 4th week of gestation. It then grows craniad toward the urogenital ridge and acquires a cap of metanephric blastema by the end of the 5th week. At this point, the nephrogenic tissue is opposite the upper sacral somites.

As elongation and straightening of the caudal end of the

embryo commence, the developing reniform mass either migrates on its own, is forcibly extruded from the true pelvis, or appears to move as the tail uncurls and differential growth between the body and tail of the embryo occurs. **Whatever the mechanism or driving force for renal ascent, it is during this migration that the upper ureteral bud matures into a normal collecting system and medial rotation of the renal pelvis takes place. This process of migration and rotation is completed by the end of the 8th week of gestation. Factors that may prevent the orderly movement of kidneys include ureteral bud maldevelopment** (Campbell, 1930), **defective metanephric tissue that by itself fails to induce ascent** (Ward et al, 1965), **genetic abnormalities, and maternal illnesses or teratogenic causes,** because genital anomalies are common (Malek et al, 1971). A vascular barrier that prevents upward migration secondary to persistence of the fetal blood supply has also been postulated (Baggenstoss, 1951), but the existence of an "early" renal blood supply does not prevent the affected kidney's movement to its ultimate position. More probably it is the end result, not the cause, of renal ectopia.

Description. The classification of ectopia is based on the position of the kidney within the retroperitoneum: the *pelvic* kidney is opposite the sacrum and below the aortic bifurcation; the *lumbar* kidney rests near the sacral promontory in the iliac fossa and anterior to the iliac vessels; and the *abdominal* kidney is so named when it is above the iliac crest and adjacent to the second lumbar vertebra (see Fig. 55–8). **No single location is most preferred for the ectopic kidney** (Dretler et al, 1971).

The ectopic kidney is usually smaller than normal, and it may not conform to the usual reniform shape, owing to the presence of fetal lobulations. The axis of the kidney is slightly medial or vertical, but it may be tilted as much as 90 degrees laterally, so that it lies in a true horizontal plane. **The renal pelvis is usually anterior (instead of medial) to the parenchyma because the kidney has incompletely rotated. As a result, 56% of ectopic kidneys have a hydronephrotic collecting system. Half of these cases result from obstruction at either the ureteropelvic or the ureterovesical junction (70% and 30%, respectively); 25% from reflux grade 3 or greater, and 25% from the malrotation alone** (Gleason et al, 1994).

The length of the ureter usually conforms to the position of the kidney, but occasionally it is slightly tortuous. It is rarely redundant, in contrast to the ptotic kidney, in which the ureter has achieved its full length before the kidney drops (Fig. 55–9). **The ureter usually enters the bladder on the ipsilateral side with its orifice situated normally.** Therefore, cystoscopy will not distinguish renal ectopia from a normal kidney. **The arterial and venous network is predictable only by the fact that it is anomalous;** its vascular pattern depends on the ultimate resting place of the kidney (Anson and Riba, 1939). There may be one or two main renal arteries arising from the distal aorta or from the aortic bifurcation, with one or more aberrant arteries coming off the common or external iliac or even the

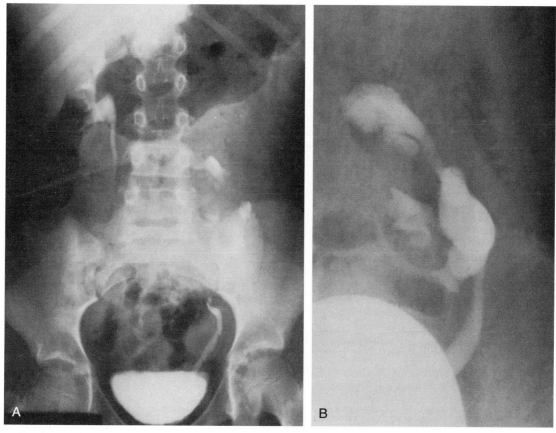

Figure 55–9. *A,* Excretory urography in a 9-year-old girl investigated for recurrent urinary tract infection shows a left lumbar kidney. *B,* Voiding cystourethrography demonstrates reflux to the ectopic kidney. At cystoscopy, the ureteral orifice was found to be located at the bladder neck.

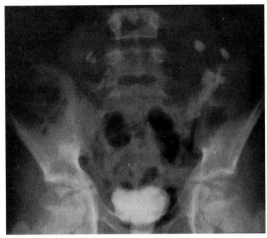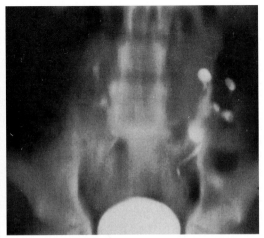

Figure 55–10. A palpable abdominal mass in an 8-year-old girl proved to be bilateral pelvic kidneys.

inferior mesenteric artery. The kidney may be supplied entirely by multiple anomalous branches, none of which arises from the aorta. **In no instance has the main renal artery arisen from that level of the aorta that would be its proper origin if the kidney were positioned normally.**

Associated Anomalies. Although the contralateral kidney is usually normal, it is associated with a number of congenital defects. Malek and colleagues (1971) and Thompson and Pace (1937) found **the incidence of contralateral agenesis to be rather high,** suggesting that a teratogenic factor affecting both ureteral buds and/or metanephric blastemas may be responsible for the two anomalies (see Fig. 55–9). Bilateral ectopia is seen in a very small number of patients (Fig. 55–10). **Hydronephrosis secondary to obstruction or reflux may be seen in as many as 25% of nonectopic contralateral kidneys** (Gleason et al, 1994).

The most striking feature is the association of genital anomalies in the patient with ectopia. The incidence varies from 15% (Thompson and Pace, 1937) **to 45%** (Downs et al, 1973), depending on how carefully the patient is evaluated. **Twenty percent to 66% of females have one or more of the following abnormalities** of the reproductive organs: bicornuate or unicornuate uterus with atresia of one horn (McCrea, 1942); rudimentary or absent uterus and proximal and/or distal vagina (Tabisky and Bhisitkul, 1965; D'Alberton et al, 1981); and duplication of the vagina. **Among male patients, 10% to 20% have a recognizable associated genital defect;** undescended testes, duplication of the urethra, and hypospadias are the most common (Thompson and Pace, 1937).

Rarely, the adrenal gland is absent or abnormally positioned. Twenty-one percent of patients have anomalies of other organ systems (Downs et al, 1973); **most of these involve the skeletal or cardiac systems.**

Diagnosis. With the increasing use of radiography, ultrasonography, and radionuclide scanning to visualize the urinary tract, the incidence of fortuitous discovery of an asymptomatic ectopic kidney is also increasing. The steady rise in reported cases in recent years attests to this fact.

Most ectopic kidneys are clinically asymptomatic. Vague abdominal complaints of frank ureteral colic sec-

ondary to an obstructing stone is still the most frequent symptom leading to discovery of the misplaced kidney. The abnormal position of the kidney results in a pattern of direct and referred pain that is atypical for colic and may be misdiagnosed as acute appendicitis or as pelvic organ inflammatory disease in female patients. It is rare to find symptoms of compression from organs adjacent to the ectopic kidney. Patients with renal ectopia may also present initially with a urinary infection or a palpable abdominal mass. Several cases of a rare association of renal and ureteral ectopia causing urinary incontinence have been reported (Borer et al, 1993, 1998). The difficulty in diagnosing this condition is related to the poor function of the ectopic kidney. Dimercaptosuccinic acid (DMSA) scintigraphy or computed tomography with contrast will delineate these unusual cases (Borer et al, 1998; Leitha, 1998).

Malposition of the colon (as discussed earlier in regard to renal agenesis) **may be a clue to the ectopic position of a lumbar or pelvic kidney.** The diagnosis is easily made when the excretory urogram or renal ultrasound study fails to reveal a kidney in its proper location. **The fact that many of these kidneys overlie the bony pelvis, which obscures the collecting system, can lead to a misdiagnosis with failure to recognize the true position of the kidney.**

Nephrotomography during an excretory urogram (if the diagnosis is suspected early enough), ultrasonography, radionuclide scanning, or retrograde pyelography will usually satisfy the diagnostician. Cystoscopy alone is rarely useful, because the trigone and ureteral orifices are invariably normal unless the ureteral orifice is also ectopic—a rare event. Arteriography may be helpful in delineating the renal vascular supply in anticipation of surgery on the ectopic kidney. This is especially important in cases of solitary ectopia.

Prognosis. The ectopic kidney is no more susceptible to disease than the normally positioned kidney except for the development of hydronephrosis or urinary calculus formation (Gleason et al, 1994). This is in part a result of the anteriorly placed pelvis and malrotation of the kidney, which may lead to impaired drainage of urine from a high insertion of the ureter to the pelvis or an anomalous vasculature that partially blocks one of the major calyces or the upper ureter. In addition, there may be an increased risk of injury from blunt abdominal trauma because the low-lying kidney is not protected by the rib cage.

Renovascular hypertension secondary to an anomalous blood supply has been reported, but a higher than normal incidence is yet to be proved. Anderson and Harrison (1965), in a review of pregnant women with renal ectopia, could find no increased occurrence of difficult deliveries or maternal or fetal complications related to the ectopic kidney (Anderson and Harrison, 1965; Delson, 1975). Dystocia from a pelvic kidney is a very rare finding, but when it does occur, early recognition is mandatory and cesarean section is indicated. Although two cases of cancer in an ectopic kidney have been reported, **there does not appear to be an increased risk for malignant transformation.** No deaths have been directly attributable to the ectopic kidney, but in at least five instances a solitary ectopic kidney has been mistakenly removed, with disastrous results, because the kidney was thought to represent a pelvic malignancy (Downs et al, 1973). This should not happen today, with the multiplicity of imaging techniques available to accurately diagnose the condition.

Cephalad Renal Ectopia

The mature kidney may be positioned more craniad than normal in patients who have had a history of omphalocele (Pinckney et al, 1978). When the liver herniates into the omphalocele sac with the intestines, the kidneys continue to ascend until they are stopped by the diaphragm. In all reported cases, both kidneys were affected and lay immediately beneath the diaphragm at the level of the 10th thoracic vertebra (Fig. 55–11). The ureters are excessively long but otherwise normal. An angiogram in these patients demonstrates that the origin of each renal artery is more cephalad than normal, but no other abnormality of the vascular network is present. Patients with this anomaly usually have no symptoms referable to the malposition, and urinary drainage is not impaired.

Thoracic Kidney

A very rare form of renal ectopia exists when the kidney is positioned considerably higher than normal. **Intrathoracic ectopia denotes either a partial or a complete protrusion of the kidney above the level of the diaphragm into the posterior mediastinum. Fewer than 5% of all patients with renal ectopia have an intrathoracic kidney** (Campbell, 1930). This condition is to be differentiated from a congenital or traumatic diaphragmatic hernia, in which other abdominal organs as well as the kidney have advanced into the chest cavity.

Incidence. Before 1940, all reports of this condition were noted as part of autopsy series (DeCastro and Shumacher, 1969). Since that time, however, **at least 140 patients have been reported** in the literature (Donat and Donat, 1988), 4 of whom had bilateral thoracic kidneys (Berlin et al, 1957; Hertz and Shahin, 1969; Lundius, 1975; N'Guessan and Stephens, 1984; Liddell et al, 1989).

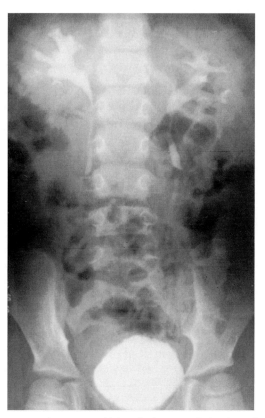

Figure 55–11. This 6-year-old boy had an omphalocele at birth. At the time, the liver was noted to be in the sac. An excretory urogram after a urinary tract infection revealed the kidneys to be located more cephalad than usual and opposite the 10th thoracic vertebra.

There appears to be a slight left-sided predominance of 1.5:1, and the sex ratio favors males by 2:1 (Lozano and Rodriguez, 1975). This entity has been discovered in all age groups, from a neonate (Shapira et al, 1965) to a 75 year-old man evaluated for prostatic hypertrophy (Burke et al, 1967).

Embryology. The kidney reaches its adult location by the end of the 8th week of gestation. At this time, the diaphragmatic leaflets are formed as the pleuroperitoneal membrane separates the pleural from the peritoneal cavity. Mesenchymal tissues associated with this membrane eventually form the muscular component of the diaphragm. **It is uncertain whether delayed closure of the diaphragmatic anlage allows for protracted renal ascent above the level of the future diaphragm, or whether the kidney overshoots its usual position because of accelerated ascent before normal diaphragmatic closure** (Burke et al, 1967; N'Guessan and Stephens, 1984; Spillane and Prather, 1952). Delayed involution of mesonephric tissue has been proposed as a causative factor (Angulo et al, 1992), because intrathoracic kidneys occur in only 0.25% of patients with a diaphragmatic hernia (Donat and Donat, 1988). Renal angiography has demonstrated either a normal site (Lundius, 1975) or a more cranial origin (Franciskovic and Martincic, 1959) for the renal artery take-off from the aorta supplying the thoracic kidney.

Description. The kidney is situated in the posterior mediastinum and usually has completed the normal ro-

tation process (Fig. 55–12). The renal contour and collecting system are normal. **The kidney usually lies in the posterolateral aspect of the diaphragm in the foramen of Bochdalek.** The diaphragm at this point thins out, and a flimsy membrane surrounds the protruding portion of kidney. **Therefore the kidney is not within the pleural space, and there is no pneumothorax** (N'Guessan and Stephens, 1984). The lower lobe of the adjacent lung may be hypoplastic secondary to compression by the kidney mass. The renal vasculature and the ureter enter and exit from the pleural cavity through the foramen of Bochdalek.

Associated Anomalies. The ureter is elongated to accommodate the excessive distance to the bladder, **but it never enters ectopically into the bladder or other pelvic sites.** The adrenal gland has been mentioned in only two reports; in one it accompanied the kidney into the chest (Barloon and Goodwin, 1957), and in the other it did not (Paul et al, 1960). However, N'Guessan and Stephens (1984) analyzed 10 cases and determined that **the adrenal gland is below the kidney in its normal location in most of the patients. In unilateral cases the contralateral kidney is usually normal.** No consistent anomalies have been described in other organ systems; however, one child did have trisomy-18 (Shapira et al, 1965), and another patient had multiple pulmonary and cardiac anomalies in addition to the thoracic kidney (Fusonie and Molnar, 1966).

Symptoms. The vast majority of affected individuals have remained asymptomatic. Pulmonary symptoms are exceedingly rare, and urinary ones are even more infrequent. Most cases are discovered on routine chest radiogra-

phy or at the time of thoracotomy for a suspected mediastinal tumor (DeNoronha et al, 1974).

Diagnosis. The diagnosis is most commonly made after a routine chest radiograph in which the affected hemidiaphragm is found to be elevated slightly. A smooth, rounded mass is seen extending into the chest near the midline on an anteroposterior film and along the posterior aspect of the diaphragmatic leaflet on a lateral view. Excretory urography or renal scintigraphy (Williams et al, 1983) usually suffices to clarify the diagnosis. In some instances, retrograde pyelography may be needed. Rarely, when arteriography has been employed to delineate a cardiac or pulmonary anomaly, it has revealed a thoracic kidney at the same time (Fusonie and Molnar, 1966).

Prognosis. Neither autopsy series nor clinical reports suggest that a thoracic kidney can cause serious urinary or pulmonary complications. Because most patients are discovered fortuitously and have no specific symptoms referable to the misplaced kidney, no treatment is necessary once the diagnosis has been confirmed.

ANOMALIES OF FORM AND FUSION

Crossed Renal Ectopia With and Without Fusion

When a kidney is located on the side opposite from which its ureter inserts into the bladder, the condition is known as *crossed ectopia*. Ninety percent of crossed

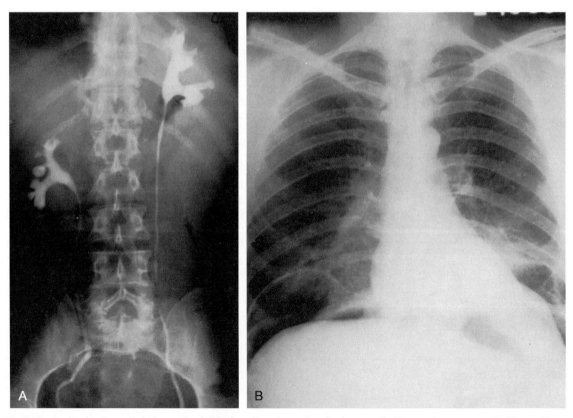

Figure 55–12. Radiograph of a thoracic kidney. The left kidney lies above the diaphragm. *A,* Diagnostic urogram. *B,* Diagnostic pneumoperitoneum. (From Hill JE, Bunts RC: Thoracic kidney: Case reports. J. Urol 1960;84:460.)

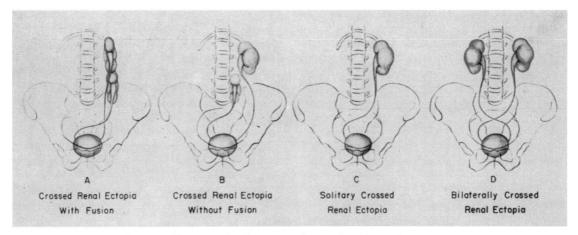

Figure 55–13. Four types of crossed renal ectopia.

ectopic kidneys are fused to their ipsilateral mate. Except for the horseshoe anomaly, they account for the majority of fusion defects. The various renal fusion anomalies associated with ectopia are discussed in this section; horseshoe kidney, the most common form of renal fusion, is described later.

Fusion anomalies of the kidney were first logically categorized by Wilmer (1938), but McDonald and McClellan (1957) refined and expanded that classification to include crossed ectopia with fusion, crossed ectopia without fusion, solitary crossed ectopia, and bilaterally crossed ectopia (Fig. 55–13A through D, respectively). The fusion anomalies have been designated as (1) unilateral fused kidney with inferior ectopia; (2) sigmoid or S-shaped; (3) lump or cake; (4) L-shaped or tandem; (5) disc, shield, or doughnut; and (6) unilateral fused kidneys with superior ectopia (Fig. 55–14A through F, respectively). Although this classification has little clinical significance, it does lend some order to understanding the embryology of renal ascent and rotation.

Incidence. The first reported case of crossed ectopia was described by Pamarolus in 1654. Abeshouse and Bhisitdul, in 1959, conducted the last significant review of the subject and collected exactly 500 cases of crossed ectopia with and without fusion. Subsequently, numerous case reports have been published.

Sixty-two patients with crossed ectopia without fusion have been reported (Diaz, 1953; Winram and Ward-Mc-Quaid, 1959). This represents approximately 10% of all

Figure 55–14. Six forms of crossed renal ectopia with fusion.

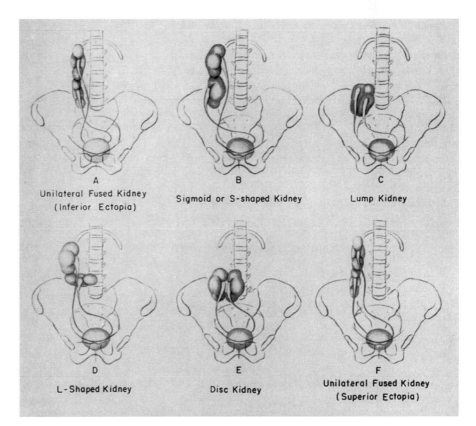

crossed ectopic kidneys (Lee, 1949). **The anomaly occurs more commonly in males in a ratio of 2:1, and left-to-right ectopia is seen three times more frequently than right-to-left** (Lee, 1949).

Solitary crossed ectopia has been reported in 34 patients (Miles et al, 1985; Gu and Alton, 1991). **Males predominate in a ratio of 2:1. The crossed ectopia involves migration of the left kidney to the right side with absence of the right kidney, rather than the reverse, in a ratio of almost 2:1** (Kakei et al, 1976). In most cases the kidney fails to ascend and rotate completely. Bilateral crossed renal ectopia has been described in five patients (Abeshouse and Bhisitkul, 1959; McDonald and Mc-Clelland, 1957) and is considered the rarest form.

Abeshouse and Bhisitkul (1959) compiled 443 reports of crossed ectopia with fusion and estimated its occurrence at 1 in 1000 live births. This figure varies with the type of fusion anomaly; **the unilaterally fused kidney with inferior ectopia is the most common variety, whereas fusion with superior ectopia is the least common.** The autopsy incidence has been calculated at 1 in 2000 (Baggenstoss, 1951). Crossed ectopia with fusion has been discovered in newborns (S.B. Bauer, unpublished observation, 1977) but also was reported in a 70-year-old man undergoing urologic evaluation for benign prostatic hypertrophy. **There is a slight male predominance (3:2), and a left-to-right crossover occurs somewhat more frequently than its counterpart.**

Embryology. The ureteral bud enters the metanephric blastema while the latter is situated adjacent to the anlage of the lumbosacral spine. During the next 4 weeks the developing kidney comes to lie at the level of the L1–L3 vertebrae. Because the factors responsible for the change in kidney position during gestation are still undetermined, **the reasons for crossed ectopia are similarly uncertain.** Wilmer (1938) suggested that crossover occurs as a result of pressure from abnormally placed umbilical arteries that prevent cephalad migration of the renal unit, which then follows the path of least resistance to the opposite side.

Potter (1952) and Alexander and coworkers (1950) theorized that crossed ectopia is strictly a ureteral phenomenon, with the developing ureteral bud wandering to the opposite side and inducing differentiation of the contralateral nephrogenic anlage. Ashley and Mostofi (1960) deduced that strong but undetermined forces are responsible for renal ascent and that these forces attract one or both kidneys to their final place on the opposite side of the midline.

Cook and Stephens (1977) postulated that crossover is the result of malalignment and abnormal rotation of the caudal end of the developing fetus, with the distal curled end of the vertebral column being displaced to one side or the other. As a result, either the cloaca and wolffian duct structures lie to one side of the vertebral column, allowing one ureter to cross the midline and enter the opposite nephrogenic blastema, or the kidney and ureter are transplanted to the opposite side of the midline during "normal" renal ascent Hertz et al, 1977; Maizels and Stephens, 1979).

Kelalis and coworkers (1973) implicated teratogenic factors after they noted an increased incidence of associated genitourinary and other organ system anomalies. Finally, genetic influences may play a role, because similar anomalies have occurred within a single family (Greenberg and Nelsen, 1971; Hildreth and Cass, 1978).

Fusion of the metanephric masses may occur when the renal anlagen are still in the true pelvis before or at the start of cephalad migration, or it may occur during the latter stages of ascent. The extent of fusion is determined by the proximity of the developing renal anlagen to one another. After fusion, advancement of the kidneys toward their normal location is impeded by midline retroperitoneal structures—the aortic bifurcation, the inferior mesenteric artery, and the base of the small bowel mesentery (Joly, 1940).

Description. Fusion of a crossed ectopic kidney is related to the time at which it comes in contact with its mate. The crossed kidney usually lies caudad to its normal counterpart on that side. It is likely that migration of each kidney begins simultaneously but ascent of the ectopic renal unit lags behind because of crossover time. Therefore, **it is the superior pole of the ectopic kidney that usually joins with the inferior aspect of the normal kidney. Ascent continues until either the uncrossed kidney reaches its normal location or one of the retroperitoneal structures prevents further migration of the fused mass. The final shape of the fused kidneys depends on the time and extent of fusion and the degree of renal rotation that has occurred.** No further rotation is likely once the two kidneys have joined (Fig. 55–15). Therefore, **the**

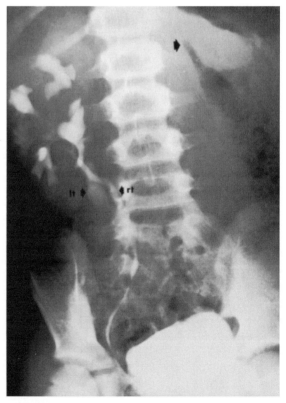

Figure 55–15. An 8-year-old boy with a left-to-right crossed, fused ectopia, in which the two kidneys lie abreast of one another (arrows marked Lt and Rt refer to both kidneys and their collecting systems on the right side of the abdomen). Splenic flexure lies in empty right renal fossa (larger black arrow accentuates gas pattern of splenic flexure in empty left renal fossa).

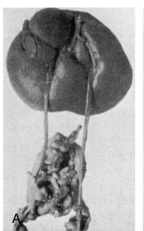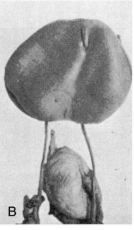

Figure 55–16. *A,* Lump kidney showing the unusual anatomy, with the anterior blood supply coming from above and the ureters leaving from below. *B,* Posterior view of *A,* with the blood supply entering from above and a deep grooving of the parenchyma indicating where the kidney pressed against the spine. (Courtesy of Dr. H. S. Altman.)

position of each renal pelvis may provide a clue as to the chronology of the congenital defect. An anteriorly placed pelvis suggests early fusion, whereas a medially positioned renal pelvis indicates that fusion probably occurred after rotation was completed.

Ninety percent of crossed ectopic kidneys are fused with their mate. When they are not fused, the uncrossed kidney usually resides in its normal dorsolumbar location and with proper orientation, while the ectopic kidney is inferior and in either a diagonal or a horizontal position with an anteriorly placed renal pelvis. The two kidneys are usually separated by a variable but definite distance, and each is surrounded by its own capsule of Gerota's fascia. In every case of crossed ectopia without fusion, the ureter from the normal kidney enters the bladder on the same side and that of the ectopic kidney crosses the midline at the pelvic brim and enters the bladder on the contralateral side.

In cases of solitary crossed ectopia, the kidney is usually located somewhat low but in the opposite renal fossa at the level of L1–L3 and is oriented anteriorly, having incompletely rotated on its vertical axis (Alexander et al, 1950; Purpon, 1963). When the kidney remains in the pelvis or ascends only to the lower lumbar region, it may assume a horizontal lie with an anteriorly placed pelvis because it has failed to rotate fully (Tabrisky and Bhisitkul, 1965). Here, too, the ureter crosses the midline above the S2 vertebra and enters the bladder on the opposite side (Gu and Alton, 1991). The contralateral ureter, if present, is often rudimentary (Caine, 1956). The patient with bilateral crossed ectopia may have perfectly normal-appearing kidneys and renal pelves, but the ureters cross the midline at the level of the lower lumbar vertebrae (Abeshouse and Bhisitkul, 1959).

Inferior Ectopic Kidney. Two thirds of all unilaterally fused kidneys involve inferior ectopia. The upper pole of the crossed kidney is attached to the inferior aspect of the normally positioned mate. Both renal pelves are anterior, so fusion probably occurs relatively early.

Sigmoid or S-Shaped Kidney. The sigmoid or S-shaped kidney is the second most common anomaly of fusion. The crossed kidney is again inferior, with the two kidneys fused at their adjacent poles. Fusion of the two kidneys occurs relatively late, after complete rotation on the vertical axis has taken place. Therefore, each renal pelvis is oriented correctly, and they face in opposite directions from one another. The lower convex border of one kidney is directly opposite the outer border of its counterpart, and there is an S-shaped appearance to the entire renal outline. The ureter from the normal kidney courses downward anterior to the outer border of the inferior kidney, and the ectopic kidney's ureter crosses the midline before entering the bladder.

Lump Kidney. The lump or cake kidney is a relatively rare form of fusion (Fig. 55–16). Extensive joining has taken place over a wide margin of maturing renal anlage. The total kidney mass is irregular and lobulated. Usually ascent progresses only as far as the sacral promontory, but in many instances the kidney remains within the true pelvis. Both renal pelves are anterior, and they drain separate areas of parenchyma. The ureters do not cross.

L-*Shaped Kidney.* The L-shaped or tandem kidney occurs when the crossed kidney assumes a transverse position at the time of its attachment to the inferior pole of the normal kidney (Fig. 55–17). The crossed kidney lies in the midline or in the contralateral paramedian space anterior to the L4 vertebra. Rotation about the long axis of the kidney may produce either an inverted or a reversed pelvic position. The ureter from each kidney enters the bladder on its respective side.

Disc Kidney. Disc, shield, doughnut, or pancake kidneys are kidneys that have joined at the medial borders of each pole to produce a doughnut- or ring-shaped mass; when there is more extensive fusion along the entire medial aspect of each kidney, a disc or shield shape is created. The lateral aspect of each kidney retains its normal contour. This type of fusion differs from the lump or cake kidney in that the reniform shape is better preserved owing to the

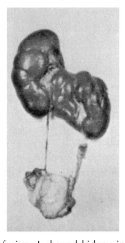

Figure 55–17. Renal fusion. L-shaped kidney in a 1-year-old child in whom a considerable portion of the left renal segment lies across the lower lumbar spine. On each side, the pelvic outlet faces anteriorly. (From Campbell MF: Anomalies of the kidney. In Campbell MF, Harrison JH [eds]: Urology, vol 2, 3rd ed. Philadelphia, WB Saunders, 1970.)

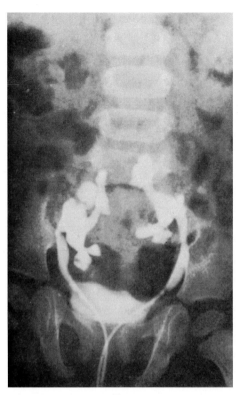

Figure 55-18. Pelvic fused kidney in a 2-year-old girl examined because of the low abdominal mass thought to be an ovarian cyst. (From Campbell MF: Anomalies of the kidney. In Campbell MF, Harrison JH [eds]: Urology, vol 2, 3rd ed. Philadelphia, WB Saunders Company, 1970.)

somewhat less extensive degree of fusion. The pelves are anteriorly placed, and the ureters remain uncrossed. Each collecting system drains its respective half of the kidney and does not communicate with the opposite side (Fig. 55-18).

Superior Ectopic Kidney. The least common variety of renal fusion is the crossed ectopic kidney that lies superior to the normal kidney. The lower pole of the crossed kidney is fused to the upper pole of the normal kidney. Each renal unit retains its fetal orientation, with both pelves lying anteriorly, suggesting that fusion occurred very early.

Regardless of the type of fusion encountered, the vascular supply to each kidney is variable and unpredictable. The crossed ectopic kidney is supplied by one or more branches from the aorta or common iliac artery (Rubinstein et al, 1976). The normal kidney frequently has an anomalous blood supply, with multiple renal arteries originating from various levels along the aorta. In one rare instance, Rubinstein (1976) discovered that one renal artery had crossed the midline to supply the tandem ectopic kidney. The solitary crossed ectopic kidney is found to receive its blood supply generally from that side of the aorta or iliac artery on which it is positioned (Tanenbaum et al, 1970).

Associated Anomalies. In all the types of fusion anomalies, the ureter from each kidney usually is not ectopic. Except for solitary crossed ectopia, in which there may be a hemitrigone or a poorly developed trigone with a rudimentary or absent ureter on the side of the ectopic kidney, most patients with crossed ectopia have a normal trigone with no indication that an anomaly of the upper urinary tract is present (Magri, 1961; Tanenbaum et al, 1970; Yates-Bell and Packham, 1972). An ectopic ureteral orifice from the crossed renal unit has been observed about 3% of the time (Abeshouse and Bhisitkul, 1959; Hendren et al, 1976; Magri, 1961). Occasionally, the ureter from the uncrossed renal segment of a fusion anomaly has an ectopic orifice (Hendren et al, 1976). In one instance, Malek and Utz (1970) discovered an ectopic ureterocele associated with the uncrossed kidney. **Vesicoureteral reflux is noted frequently into the collecting system of the ectopic kidney** (Kelalis et al, 1973). Currarino and Weisbruch (1989) collected 10 cases of midline renal fusion in which a single ureter divided into two pelves that stretched across the midline to drain one respective half of the total parenchymatous mass. In 4 of the 10 cases, a second ureter was present that drained a separate duplex system on either the right or left side. Most of the affected individuals had an imperforate anus or abnormal vertebrae, or both.

Most orthotopic renal units are normal. If an abnormality exists, it usually involves the ectopic kidney and consists of cystic dysplasia, UPJ obstruction (29%), reflux (15%), or carcinoma (Abeshouse and Bhisitkul, 1959; Gerber et al, 1980; Caldamone and Rabinowitz, 1981; Macksood and James, 1983; Nussbaum et al, 1987; Gleason et al, 1994).

The highest incidence of associated anomalies occurs in children with solitary renal ectopia and involves both the skeletal system and genital organs (Miles et al, 1985; Gleason et al, 1994). This seems to be related more to renal agenesis than to the ectopic anomaly per se. **Fifty percent of patients with solitary crossed renal ectopia have a skeletal anomaly, and 40% have a genital abnormality** (Gu and Alton, 1991). The most common of the latter in the male is either cryptorchidism or absence of the vas deferens; in the female, it is vaginal atresia or a unilateral uterine abnormality (Kakei et al, 1976; Yates-Bell and Packham, 1972). Imperforate anus has also been observed in 20% of the patients with solitary crossed ectopia.

In general, the occurrence of an associated anomaly in crossed renal ectopia, excluding solitary crossed ectopia, is low; the most frequent such conditions are imperforate anus (4%), orthopedic anomalies (4%), skeletal abnormalities, and septal cardiovascular defects.

Symptoms. Most individuals with crossed ectopic anomalies have no symptoms. The defects are often discovered incidentally at autopsy, during routine perinatal ultrasound screening, or after bone scanning. If manifestations do occur, signs and symptoms usually develop in the third or fourth decades of life and include vague lower abdominal pain, pyuria, hematuria, and urinary tract infection (Gleason et al, 1994). Hydronephrosis and renal calculi have been discovered in conjunction with some of these symptoms. It is believed that the abnormal kidney position and the anomalous blood supply may impede drainage from the collecting system, creating a predisposition to urinary tract infection and calculus formation.

In one third of patients, an asymptomatic abdominal mass is the presenting sign (Abeshouse and Bhisitkul, 1959; Nussbaum et al, 1987). In a few individuals, hypertension has led to the discovery of an ectopic fusion anomaly (Abeshouse and Bhisitkul, 1959), and in one case this was attributable to a vascular lesion in one of the anomalous vessels (Mininberg et al, 1971).

Diagnosis. In the past, the usual method of detection was by excretory urography, but ultrasonography and radionuclide scanning have revealed more asymptomatic cases recently (for unrelated reasons). Nephrotomography can be used when necessary to further define the renal outlines (Dretler et al, 1971). Cystoscopy and retrograde pyelography are useful in mapping out the collecting system and pattern of drainage. Renal angiography may be required before performing extensive surgery on the ectopic or normal kidney due to the anomalous blood supply to both kidneys. Ultrasound evaluation of the pelvic kidney may demonstrate absence of renal sinus echoes, a normal finding associated with the extrarenal position of the pelvis and calyces (Barnewolt and Lebowitz, 1996).

Prognosis. Most individuals with crossed renal ectopia have a normal longevity and prognosis. However, some patients with an obstructive-appearing collecting system are at risk for development of urinary tract infection or renal calculi, or both (Kron and Meranze, 1949). Boatman and associates (1972) noted that one third of their symptomatic patients required a pyelolithotomy for an obstructing stone. More recently, extracorporeal shock wave lithotripsy therapy has rendered most of these unusual patients stone free (Semerci et al, 1997). Stubbs and Resnick (1977) reported a struvite staghorn calculus in a patient with crossed renal ectopia. Urinary infection in association with either vesicoureteral reflux or hydronephrosis has been implicated in the formation of these calculi.

Horseshoe Kidney

The horseshoe kidney is probably the most common of all renal fusion anomalies. It should not be confused with asymmetric or off-center fused kidneys, which may give the impression of being horseshoe-shaped. **The anomaly consists of two distinct renal masses lying vertically on either side of the midline and connected at their respective lower poles by a parenchymatous or fibrous isthmus that crosses the midplane of the body.** It was first recognized during an autopsy by DeCarpi in 1521, but Botallo in 1564 presented the first extensive description and illustration of a horseshoe kidney (Benjamin and Schullian, 1950). In 1820 Morgagni described the first diseased horseshoe kidney and since then more has been written about this condition than about any other renal anomaly. Almost every renal disease has been described in the horseshoe kidney.

Incidence. Horseshoe kidney occurs in 0.25% of the population, or about 1 in 400 persons (Dees, 1941; Nation, 1945; Bell, 1946; Glenn, 1959; Campbell, 1970). **As with other fusion anomalies, it is found more commonly in males by a 2:1 margin.** The abnormality has been discovered clinically in all age groups ranging from fetal life to 80 years, but in autopsy series it is more prevalent in children (Segura et al, 1972). **This early age prevalence is related to the high incidence of multiple congenital anomalies associated with the horseshoe kidney, some of which are incompatible with long-term survival.**

Horseshoe kidneys have been reported in identical twins (Bridge, 1960) and among several siblings within the same family (David, 1974). From the rarity of these reports and the relative frequency of the anomaly, it is doubtful that these observations represent a particular genetic predisposition, but they might be the result of a genetic expression with a low degree of penetrance (Leiter, 1972).

Embryology. The abnormality occurs between the 4th and 6th week of gestation, after the ureteral bud has entered the renal blastema. In view of the ultimate spatial configuration of the horseshoe kidney, the entrance of the ureteral bud had to have taken place before rotation and considerably before renal ascent ensued. Boyden (1931) described a 6-week-old embryo with a horseshoe kidney, the youngest fetus ever discovered with this anomaly. He postulated that at the 14-mm stage (4.5 weeks), the developing metanephric masses lie close to one another; any disturbance in this relationship might result in joining at their inferior poles. A slight alteration in the position of the umbilical or common iliac artery could change the orientation of the migrating kidneys, leading to contact and fusion (Fig. 55–19). It has been postulated that an abnormality in the formation of the tail of the embryo or another pelvic organ could account for the fusion process (Cook and Stephens, 1977). Domenech-Mateu and Gonzales-Compta (1988), after studying a 16-mm human embryo, suggested that posterior nephrogenic cells migrate abnormally to form an isthmus or connection between the two developing kidneys to create the horseshoe shape.

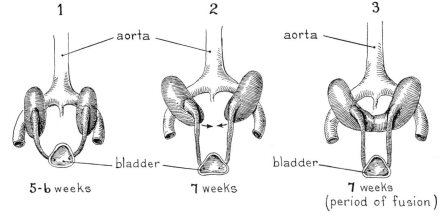

Figure 55–19. Embryogenesis of horseshoe kidney. The lower poles of the two kidneys touch and fuse as they cross the iliac arteries. Ascent is stopped when the fused kidneys reach the junction of the aorta and interior mesenteric artery. (From Benjamin JA, Schullian DM: Observation on fused kidneys with horseshoe configuration: The contribution of Leonardo Botallo (1564). J Hist Med Allied Sci 1950;5:315, after Gutierrez, 1931.)

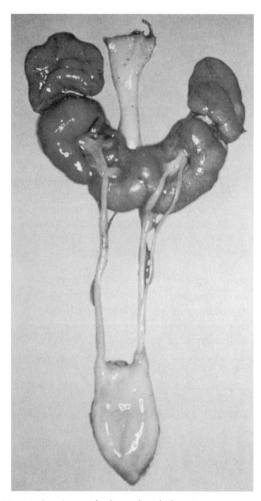

Figure 55–20. Specimen of a horseshoe kidney in a neonate who had multiple anomalies, including congenital heart disease. Note the thick parenchymatous isthmus.

Whatever the actual mechanism responsible for horseshoe kidney formation, the joining occurs before the kidneys have rotated on their long axis. In its mature form, the pelves and ureters of the horseshoe kidney are usually anteriorly placed, crossing ventrally to the isthmus (Fig. 55–20). Very rarely, the pelves are anteromedial, suggesting that fusion occurred somewhat later, after some rotation had taken place. In addition, **migration is usually incomplete, with the kidneys lying lower in the abdomen than normal. It is presumed that the inferior mesenteric artery prevents full ascent by obstructing the movement of the isthmus.**

Description. There are several variations in the basic shape of the horseshoe kidney. **In 95% of patients, the kidneys join at the lower pole; in a small number, an isthmus connects both upper poles instead** (Love and Wasserman, 1975).

Generally, the isthmus is bulky and consists of parenchymatous tissue with its own blood supply (Glenn, 1959; Love and Wasserman, 1975). Occasionally it is just a flimsy midline structure composed of fibrous tissue that tends to draw the renal masses close together. **It is located adjacent to the L3 or L4 vertebra just below the origin of the inferior mesenteric artery from the aorta.** As a

result, the paired kidneys tend to be somewhat lower than normal in the retroperitoneum. In some instances, the anomalous kidneys are very low, anterior to the sacral promontory or even in the true pelvis behind the bladder (Campbell, 1970). **The isthmus most often lies anterior to the aorta and vena cava,** but it is not unheard of for it to pass between the inferior vena cava and the aorta or even behind both great vessels (Jarmin, 1938; Meek and Wadsworth, 1940; Dajani, 1966).

The calyces, normal in number, are atypical in orientation. Because the kidney fails to rotate, the calyces point posteriorly, and the axis of each pelvis remains in the vertical or obliquely lateral plane (on a line drawn from lower to upper poles). **The lowermost calyces extend caudally or even medially** to drain the isthmus and may overlie the vertebral column.

The ureter may insert high on the renal pelvis and lie laterally, probably as the result of incomplete renal rotation. It courses downward and has a characteristic bend as it crosses over and anterior to the isthmus, a deviation that is proportionate to the thickness of the midline structure. Despite upper ureteral angulation, the lower ureter usually enters the bladder normally and rarely is ectopic.

The blood supply to the horseshoe kidney can be quite variable (Fig. 55–21). In 30% of cases, it consists of one renal artery to each kidney (Glenn, 1959), but it may be atypical with duplicate or even triplicate renal arteries supplying one or both kidneys. The blood supply to the isthmus and lower poles is also variable. The isthmus and adjacent parenchymal masses may receive a branch from each main renal artery, or they may have their own arterial supply from the aorta originating either above or below the level of the isthmus. Not infrequently this area is supplied by branches from the inferior mesenteric,

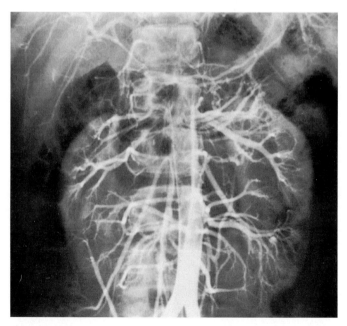

Figure 55–21. Arteriogram in a patient with a horseshoe kidney showing a multiplicity of arteries supplying kidney arising from aorta and common iliac arteries. (From Kelalis PP: Anomalies of the urinary tract: The kidney. In Kelalis PP, King LR [eds]: Clinical Pediatric Urology. Philadelphia, WB Saunders, 1976, p 492.)

common or external iliac, or sacral arteries (Boatman et al, 1971; Kolln et al, 1972). Three cases of retrocaval ureter and isthmus have been reported (Eidelman et al, 1978; Hefferman et al, 1978).

Associated Anomalies. The horseshoe kidney, even though it produces no symptoms, **is frequently found in association with other congenital anomalies.** Boatman and coworkers (1972) discovered that **almost one third of the 96 patients they studied had at least one other abnormality.** Many newborns and young infants with multiple congenital anomalies have a horseshoe kidney. Judging from autopsy reports, the incidence of other anomalies is certainly greater in patients who die at birth or in early infancy than in those who reach adulthood (Zondek and Zondek, 1964). This implies that a horseshoe kidney may occur more often in patients with other serious congenital anomalies. The organ systems most commonly affected include the skeletal, cardiovascular (primarily ventriculoseptal defects [Voisin et al, 1988]), and central nervous systems. Horseshoe kidney is found in 3% of children with neural tube defects (Whitaker and Hunt, 1987). Anorectal malformations are frequently encountered in these patients. **Horseshoe kidney may also be seen in** 20% of patients with trisomy 18 and **as many as 60% of females with Turner's syndrome** (Smith, 1970; Lippe et al, 1988).

Boatman and his colleagues (1972) **also discovered an increased occurrence of other genitourinary anomalies in patients with a horseshoe kidney.** Hypospadias and undescended testes each occurred in 4% of males, and a bicornuate uterus or septate vagina (or both) were noted in 7% of the females.

Duplication of the ureter occurs in 10% of patients (Zondek and Zondek, 1964; Boatman et al, 1972); in some cases this has been associated with an ectopic ureterocele. Vesicoureteral reflux has been noted in more than half of affected individuals (Segura et al, 1972; Pitts and Muecke, 1975). Cystic disease, including multicystic dysplasia in one half (the upper pole) of one side (Novak et al, 1977; Boullier et al, 1992) and adult polycystic kidney disease, has been reported in patients with horseshoe kidney (Gutierrez, 1934; Campbell, 1970; Pitts and Muecke, 1975; Correa and Paton, 1976).

Symptoms. Almost one third of all patients with horseshoe kidney remain asymptomatic (Glenn, 1959; Kolln et al, 1972). In most instances, the anomaly is an incidental finding at autopsy (Pitts and Muecke, 1975). **When symptoms are present, however, they are related to hydronephrosis, infection, or calculus formation.** The most common symptom that reflects these conditions is vague abdominal pain that may radiate to the lower lumbar region. Gastrointestinal complaints may be present as well. The so-called Rovsing sign—abdominal pain, nausea, and vomiting on hyperextension of the spine—has been infrequently observed. Signs and symptoms of urinary tract infection occur in 30% of patients, and calculi have been noted in 20% to 80% (Glenn, 1959; Kolln et al, 1972; Pitts and Muecke, 1975; Evans and Resnick, 1981; Sharma and Bapna, 1986). Five percent to 10% of horseshoe kidneys are detected after palpation of an abdominal mass (Glenn, 1959; Kolln et al, 1972). Horseshoe kidneys have been detected after angiography for evaluation of an abdominal aortic aneurysm (Huber et al, 1990; deBrito et al, 1991).

UPJ obstruction causing significant hydronephrosis occurs in as many as one third of individuals (Whitehouse, 1975; Das and Amar, 1984). The high insertion of the ureter into the renal pelvis, its abnormal course anterior to the isthmus, and the anomalous blood supply to the kidney may individually or collectively contribute to this obstruction.

Diagnosis. Except for the possibility of a palpable midline abdominal mass (Grandone et al, 1985), the horseshoe kidney does not by itself produce symptoms. The clinical features from a diseased kidney, however, are often vague and nonspecific. The anomalies, therefore, may not be suspected until a renal ultrasound or an excretory urogram is obtained. Prenatal ultrasonography is detecting horseshoe kidneys before birth (Sherer and Woods, 1992; Van Every, 1992). The classic radiologic features are easily recognized and a diagnosis is readily made (Fig. 55–22). Findings that suggest a horseshoe kidney singly or collectively include the following: kidneys that are somewhat low lying and close to the vertebral column; a vertical or outward axis, so that a line drawn through the midplane of each kidney bisects the midline inferiorly; a continuation of the outer border of the lower pole of each kidney toward and across the midline; the characteristic orientation of the collecting system, which is directly posterior to each renal pelvis, with the lowermost calyx pointing caudally or even medially; and the high insertion of the ureter into the pelvis as well as the anteriorly displaced upper ureter that appears to

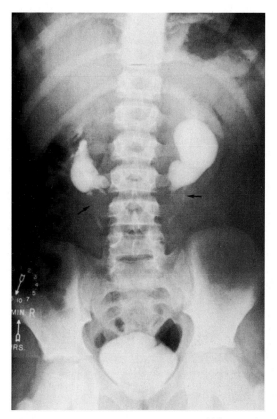

Figure 55–22. Excretory urogram in an 11-year-old boy evaluated for nocturnal incontinence reveals a horseshoe kidney. Note vertical renal axes and medial orientation of the collecting systems. The ureters (*arrows*) are laterally displaced and bow over the isthmus.

drape over a midline mass. However, obstruction from either a calculus or a UPJ stricture may obscure the radiologic picture (Love and Wasserman, 1975; Christoffersen and Iversen, 1976). Other studies, such as retrograde pyelography or computed tomography, may be necessary to confirm the diagnosis.

Prognosis. Although Smith and Orkin (1945) believed that horseshoe kidneys are almost always associated with disease, subsequent investigators have not found this to be so. **Glenn (1959) observed patients with horseshoe kidneys for an average of 10 years after discovery and found that almost 60% remained symptom-free.** Only 13% had persistent urinary infection or pain, and 17% developed recurrent calculi. Operations to remove these stones or relieve obstruction were necessary in only 25%. Today ESWL therapy has rendered 68% of these patients stone free and markedly reduced the stone burden in another 21% (Kupeli et al, 1999). In Glenn's series, no patients benefitted from division of the isthmus for relief of pain; as a result, this idea has now been largely repudiated (Glenn, 1959; Pitts and Muecke, 1975).

Many patients with a horseshoe kidney have other congenital anomalies, some of which are incompatible with life beyond the neonatal period or early infancy. Excluding that group, survival is not reduced merely by the presence of this anomaly. Often a horseshoe kidney is found incidentally, and it is rarely a cause for mortality (Dajani, 1966; Boatman et al, 1972).

Many disease processes have been described with a horseshoe kidney, but this only reflects the relative frequency of the congenital defect. **Renal carcinoma has been reported in 114 patients within a horseshoe kidney** (Buntley, 1976; Hohenfellner et al, 1992); **more than half of these cancers were hypernephromas.** However, **renal pelvic tumors and Wilms' tumor each accounted for 25% of the total.** Overall, 13 of 2961 Wilms' tumors in the National Wilms' Tumor study occurred in horseshoe kidneys, mostly on the left side, rarely in the isthmus, and practically all with favorable histology. This incidence of Wilms' tumor in horseshoe kidneys is more than twice that expected in the general population (Mesrobian et al, 1985). Except for renal pelvic tumors, a surprisingly high number of these cancers appear to have arisen in the isthmus (Blackard and Mellinger, 1968). For this reason, it has been suggested that teratogenic factors are responsible for abnormal migration of nephrogenic cells to form an isthmus, which then leads to the horseshoe shape and the increased potential of carcinoma development in this portion of the kidney (Domenech-Mateu and Gonzales-Compta, 1988; Hohenfellner et al, 1992).

It has been suggested that the increased occurrence of chronic infection, obstruction, and stone formation may be instrumental in producing a higher than expected incidence of renal pelvic tumors in this group (Shoup et al, 1962; Castor and Green, 1975). Wilms' tumor frequently originates in the isthmus as well (Beck and Hlivko, 1960), often creating a very bizarre radiologic picture (D. Walker, personal communication, 1977). The incidence of tumors within horseshoe kidneys seems to be increasing when compared with the occurrence of tumors in the general population (Dische and Johnston, 1979). Survival from these tumors is related to the pathology and stage of the tumor at diagnosis and not to the renal anomaly (Murphy and Zincke, 1982).

Because it is located above the pelvic inlet, a horseshoe kidney should not adversely affect pregnancy or delivery (Bell, 1946). Glomerulocystic disease has been reported in children before 1 year of age but does not appear to be related specifically to the horseshoe anomaly (Craver et al, 1993). The development of renal failure associated with adult polycystic kidney disease is not any greater in the presence of a horseshoe kidney (Correa and Paton, 1976). Finally, the North American Pediatric Renal Transplant Cooperative Study (NAPRTCS, McDonald et al, 2000) and the Department of Health and Human Services 2000 Annual Report (the US Scientific Registry of Transplant Recipients and the Organ Procurement and Transplant Network, 2000) each failed to reveal any patient with a horseshoe kidney receiving a renal transplant.

ANOMALIES OF ROTATION

The adult kidney, as it assumes its final position in the "renal" fossa, orients itself so that the calyces point laterally and the pelvis faces medially. When this alignment is not exact, the condition is known as *malrotation*. Most often, this inappropriate orientation is found in conjunction with another renal anomaly, such as ectopia with or without fusion or horseshoe kidney. This discussion centers on malrotation as an isolated renal entity. It must be differentiated from other conditions that mimic it and are caused by extraneous forces such as an abnormal retroperitoneal mass.

Incidence. The true incidence of this developmental anomaly cannot be accurately calculated because minor degrees of malrotation are never reported and generally do not cause much concern. Campbell (1963) found renal malrotation in 1 of 939 autopsies, and Smith and Orkin (1945) noted 1 case per 390 admissions. **It is frequently observed in patients with Turner's syndrome** (Gray and Skandalakis, 1972). **Males are affected twice as often as females, but there does not appear to be any predilection for one side or the other.** In other animals (e.g., reptiles, birds), the "malrotated kidney" is actually properly oriented for these individual species.

Embryology. It is thought that **medial rotation of the collecting system occurs simultaneously with renal migration.** The kidney starts to turn during the 6th week, just when it is leaving the true pelvis, and it completes this process, having rotated 90 degrees toward the midline, by the time ascent is complete, at the end of the 9th week of gestation.

It has been postulated (Felix, 1912) that rotation is actually the result of unequal branching of successive orders of the budding ureteral tree, with two branches extending ventrally and one dorsally during each generation or division. Each ureteral branch then induces differentiation of the metanephrogenic tissue surrounding it to encase it as a cap. More parenchyma develops ventrally than dorsally, and the pelvis seems to rotate medially. Weyrauch (1939) accepted this theory of renal rotation as the result of excessive ventral versus dorsal branching of the ureteral tree and concluded that the fault of malrotation lies entirely with the ureter. A late-appearing ureteral bud may insert into an atypical portion of the renal blastema, leading to a lessened propensity for the developing nephric tissue to shift. Late appearance of the ureteral bud is almost always associated with an aberrant origin from the wolffian duct; this translates into ureteral ectopia at the level of the lower urinary tract. Mackie and colleagues (1975), however, did not describe any malrotation anomalies in their study of renal ectopia. The renal blood supply does not appear to be the cause or a limiting factor in malrotation but rather follows the course of renal hyporotation, hyper-rotation, or reverse rotation.

Description. The kidney and renal pelvis normally rotate 90 degrees ventromedially during ascent. Weyrauch (1939), in an exhaustive and detailed study, outlined the various abnormal phases of medial and reverse rotation and labeled each according to the position of the renal pelvis (Fig. 55–23).

Ventral Position. The pelvis is ventral and in the same anteroposterior plane as the calyces, which point dorsally, since they have undergone no rotation at all. This is the most common form of malrotation. Very rarely, this position may represent excessive medial rotation, in which a complete 360-degree turn has occurred. In one such presumed case reported by Weyrauch (1939), the vasculature had rotated with the kidney and passed around dorsally and laterally to it before entering the anteriorly placed hilus.

Ventromedial Position. The pelvis faces ventromedially because of an incompletely rotated kidney. Excursion probably stops during the 7th week of gestation, when the

kidney and pelvis normally reach this position. The calyces thus point dorsolaterally.

Dorsal Position. Renal excursion of 180 degrees occurs to produce this position. The pelvis is dorsal to the parenchyma, and the vessels pass behind the kidney to reach the hilum. This is the rarest form of malrotation.

Lateral Position. When the kidney and pelvis rotate more than 180 degrees but less than 360 degrees, or when reverse rotation of up to 180 degrees takes place, the pelvis faces laterally and the kidney parenchyma resides medially. The renal vascular supply provides the only clue to the actual direction of excursion. Vessels that course ventral to the kidney to enter a laterally or dorsolaterally placed hilum suggest reverse rotation, whereas a path dorsal to the kidney implies excessive ventral rotation. Both types of anomalous turning were cited in Weyrauch's series (1939).

In cases of isolated malrotation, certain other characteristic features may be present. The kidney shape may be discoid, elongated, oval, or triangular, with flattened anterior and posterior surfaces. Fetal lobulations are invariably present and accentuated beyond normal limits. A dense amount of fibrous tissue encases the hilar area, possibly even distorting and fixing the pelvis. The ureteropelvic junction (UPJ) may be distorted as well. The upper ureter initially courses laterally, and it too may be encased in this fibrous matting. The pelvis is elongated and narrow, and calyces, especially the superior calyx, may be stretched. The blood supply, as previously described, may vary widely, depending on the direction and degree of rotation. The vasculature may consist of a single vessel with or without multiple additional branches entering the parenchyma along the course of the renal artery. In addition, there may be a polar vessel in conjunction with the main renal artery. **The vascular orientation around the kidney provides the only clue to the type and extent of renal rotation (i.e., whether medial or lateral rotation has occurred).**

Symptoms. Rotation anomalies per se do not produce any specific symptoms. The excessive amount of fibrous tissue encasing the pelvis, UPJ, and upper ureter, however, may lead to a relative or actual obstruction of the upper collecting system. Vascular compression from an accessory or main renal artery or distortion of the upper ureter or UPJ may contribute to impaired drainage. Symptoms of hydronephrosis (namely, dull, aching flank pain) may be experienced during periods of increased urine production. This is the most frequent cause of symptoms. Hematuria, which occurs occasionally within a hydronephrotic collecting system from jostling of sidewalls, may be noted as well. Infection and calculus formation, each with its attendant symptoms, may also occur secondary to poor urinary drainage.

Diagnosis. The diagnosis may be surmised when a renal calculus is detected in an abnormal location, but confirmation should be obtained only from a renal ultrasound, excretory urogram, or retrograde pyelogram (Fig. 55–24). These studies should reveal the abnormal orientation of the renal pelvis and calyces, a flattened and elongated pelvis, a stretched superior calyx with blunting of the remaining calyces, and a laterally displaced upper third of the ureter. Bilateral malrotation is not uncommon and may

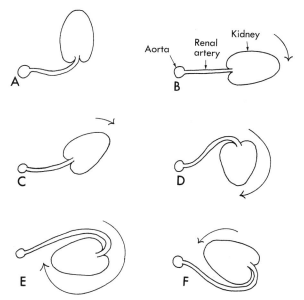

Figure 55–23. Rotation of the kidney during its ascent from the pelvis. The left kidney with its renal artery and the aorta are viewed in transverse section to show normal and abnormal rotation during its ascent to the adult site. *A*, Primitive embryonic position; hilus faces ventrad (anterior). *B*, Normal adult position; hilus faces mediad. *C*, Incomplete rotation. *D*, Hyper-rotation; hilus faces dorsad (posterior). *E*, Hyper-rotation; hilus faces laterad. *F*, Reverse rotation; hilus faces laterad. (From Gray SW, Skandalakis JE: Embryology for Surgeons. Philadelphia, WB Saunders, 1972.)

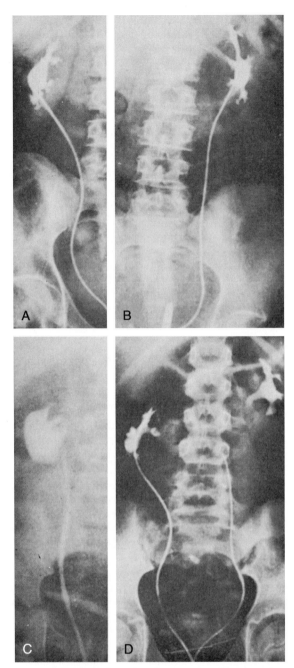

Figure 55–24. Congenital renal malrotation. *A,* Complete, the pelvis faces median, *B,* Pelvis faces posteriorly. *C,* Complete renal rotation in a 20-month-old girl with abnormally high insertion of the ureter into the pelvis. *D,* Diminutive malrotated pelvis in a 5-year-old girl. Urinary infection was the indication for urologic examination in all four cases. (From Campbell MF: Anomalies of the kidney. In Campbell MF, Harrison JH [eds]: Urology, vol 2, 3rd ed. Philadelphia, WB Saunders, 1970.)

lead to the diagnosis of a horseshoe kidney. However, careful inspection for an isthmus and observation of the lower pole renal outline should help to distinguish the two entities.

Prognosis. No abnormality of function of the kidney has been detected secondary to malrotation, and this anomaly is therefore compatible with normal longevity. Hydro-

nephrosis resulting from impaired urinary drainage may lead to infection and calculus formation with their sequelae.

ANOMALIES OF RENAL VASCULATURE

Aberrant, Accessory, or Multiple Vessels

Knowledge of the anatomy of the renal blood supply is important to every urologic surgeon, and fortunately this subject lends itself to easy investigation. Anatomists were keenly interested in renal vascular patterns before the end of the 19th century, but the advent of aortography in the 1940s and 1950s spearheaded a systematic clinical approach to this topic. Most of the classic work was performed by investigators in the middle to late 1950s and early 1960s (Graves, 1954, 1956; Anson and Kurth, 1955; Merklin and Michele, 1958; Anson and Daseler, 1961; Geyer and Poutasse, 1962).

The kidney is divided into various segments, each supplied by a single "end" arterial branch that usually courses from one main renal artery. "Multiple renal arteries" is the correct term to describe any kidney supplied by more than one vessel. The term "anomalous vessels" or "aberrant vessels" should be reserved for those arteries that originate from vessels other than the aorta or main renal artery. The term "accessory vessels" denotes two or more arterial branches supplying the same renal segment.

Incidence. Between 71% (Merklin and Michele, 1958) **and 85%** (Geyer and Poutasse, 1962) **of kidneys have one artery that supplies the entire renal parenchyma. A slightly higher percentage of right-sided kidneys (87%) have a single renal artery compared with left-sided organs** (Geyer and Poutasse, 1962). This figure does not seem to be influenced significantly by either sex or race. True aberrant vessels are rare except in patients with renal ectopia, with or without fusion, and in individuals with a horseshoe kidney.

Embryology. The renal arterial tree is derived from three groups of primitive vascular channels that coalesce to form the mature vascular pattern for all retroperitoneal structures. The cranial group consists of two pairs of arteries dorsal to the suprarenal gland that shift dorsally to form the phrenic artery. The middle group is made up of three pairs of vessels that pass through the suprarenal area. They retain the same lateral position and become the adrenal artery. Finally, the caudal group has four pairs of arteries that cross ventral to the suprarenal area and become the main renal artery. Sometimes they are joined by the most inferior pair from the middle group (Guggemos, 1962). It is believed that during renal migration this network of vessels selectively degenerates, and the remaining adjacent arteries assume a progressively more important function. **By a process of elimination, one primitive renal arterial pair eventually becomes the dominant vessel, the completed process being dependent on the final position of the kidney** (Graves, 1956). **Polar**

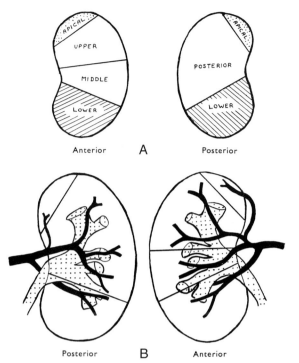

Figure 55–25. Usual pattern of arteries to the kidney. *A,* The five vascular lobes of Graves. *B,* Relationships of renal artery branch and renal pelvis to the five lobes. (From Graves FT: The anatomy of the intrarenal arteries and its application to segmental resection of the kidney. Br J Surg 1954;42:132. By permission of the publisher, Butterworth-Heinemann Ltd.)

arteries or multiple renal arteries to the normally positioned kidney represent a failure of complete degeneration of all primitive vascular channels. The multiple vessel pattern that has been described for renal ectopia should be considered as an arrested embryonic state for

that particular renal position (Gray and Skandalakis, 1972).

Description. On the basis of vascular supply, the renal parenchyma is divided into five segments—apical, upper, middle, lower, and posterior (Fig. 55–25). The main renal artery divides initially into an anterior and posterior branch. The anterior branch almost always supplies the upper, middle, and lower segments of the kidney. The posterior branch invariably nourishes the posterior and lower segments (Sampaio and Aragao, 1990a). The vessel to the apical segment has the greatest variation in origin; it arises from (1) the anterior division (43%), (2) the junction of the anterior and posterior divisions (23%), (3) the main stem renal artery or aorta (23%), or (4) the posterior division of the main renal artery (10%) (Graves, 1954). Rarely, the upper segment is supplied from a branch totally separate from the main renal artery (Merklin and Michele, 1958). The arterial and venous tree of the kidney and its relationship to the collecting system was beautifully depicted in endocasts by Sampaio and Aragao (1990a, 1990b). These investigations showed that the least likely areas to encounter vessels when entering the collecting system, either endourologically or with open surgery, is directly end-on through a fornix or inferiorly on the posterior aspect of the pelvis.

The lower renal segment, however, is often fed by an accessory vessel. This vessel is usually the most proximal branch when it arises from the main renal artery or its anterior division (Graves, 1954). However, it may originate directly from the aorta near the main renal artery, or it may be aberrant, arising from the gonadal vessel. **A summary of findings from Merklin and Michele (1958), who analyzed reports from almost 11,000 kidneys, is depicted in Table 55–1. The relationship of the main renal artery and its proximal branches to the renal vein can be seen**

Table 55–1. VARIATIONS IN THE ARTERIAL SUPPLY TO THE KIDNEY

	Condition	Percentage
	1 Hilar artery	71.1
	1 Hilar artery and 1 upper pole branch	12.6
	2 Hilar arteries	10.8
	1 Hilar artery and 1 upper pole aortic artery	6.2
	1 Hilar artery and 1 lower pole aortic artery	6.9
	1 Hilar artery and 1 lower pole branch	3.1
	3 Hilar arteries	1.7
	2 Hilar arteries, one with upper pole branch	2.7
	Other variations	—

From Gray SW, Skandalakis JE (eds): Embryology for Surgeons. Philadelphia, WB Saunders, 1972.

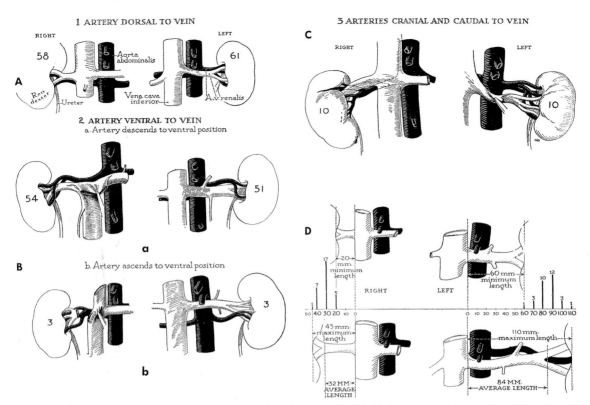

Figure 55–26. Relationships of renal arteries and veins. *A,* Artery dorsal to vein (47.6%). *B,* Artery ventral to vein (*Ba,* 42%; *Bb,* 2.4%). *C,* Artery cranial and caudal to vein (8.0%). *D,* Maximum, minimum, and average lengths of the renal pedicle in 30 successive specimens. (From Anson BJ, Daseler EH: Common variations in renal anatomy, affecting the blood supply, form and topography. Surg Gynecol Obstet 1961;112:439. By permission of Surgery, Gynecology, and Obstetrics.)

in Figure 55–26. The venous drainage of the kidney has been carefully restudied by Sampaio and Aragao (1990b), who noted a close association between the inferior branch to the main renal vein and the anterior inferior aspect of the renal pelvis in 40% of kidneys. They cautioned that an endourologic incision of an obstructed UPJ should be done laterally and posteriorly instead of anteriorly to avoid injury to this vessel.

Symptoms. Symptoms attributable to renal vascular anomalies are those that might result from inadequate urinary drainage. Multiple, aberrant, or accessory vessels may constrict an infundibulum (Fig. 55–27*A*), a major calyx, or the UPJ (Fig. 55–28). Pain, hematuria secondary to hydronephrosis, signs and symptoms of urinary tract infection, or calculus formation may result.

Diagnosis. Excretory urography may reveal multiple renal vessels or an aberrant artery (1) when a filling defect in the renal pelvis is consistent with an anomalous vascular pattern; (2) when hydronephrosis is noted along with a sharp cutoff in the superior infundibulum (see Fig. 55–27*B*) (Fraley, 1966, 1969); (3) when UPJ obstruction is seen in association with an angulated ureter near the renal pelvis and a kidney whose pole-to-pole axis is more vertical than normal; or (4) when differences are noted in the timing and concentration of one renal segment or in the entire kidney when compared with the opposite side (especially when hypertension is present). Renal angiography has been the gold standard for defining the vascular tree of the kidney, but less invasive imaging

studies have been developed that are as accurate in delineating the precise ating the precise anatomy with its variants and any disease states (Textor and Canzanello, 1996; Salcarga et al, 1999).

Prognosis. None of these variations in the vascular tree increases the kidney's susceptibility to disease. Hydronephrosis secondary to a vascular anomaly is a very rare finding, especially when one considers the relative frequency of all renal vascular variations. Hypertension is no more frequent in patients with multiple renal arteries than in those with a single vessel (Geyer and Poutasse, 1962). Nathan (1958) did report the development of orthostatic proteinuria in seven patients with a lower pole renal artery that wrapped around and compressed the main renal vein. He thought there might have been a causal relationship but did not prove it.

Renal Artery Aneurysm

Aneurysmal dilation was the first disease process of the renal artery to be recognized (Poutasse, 1957); it was considered a rare occurrence until selective renal angiography came into vogue. Since then, **the overall incidence has been calculated to be between 0.1% and 0.3%. Abeshouse (1951),** in a comprehensive review, **classified renal artery aneurysms as follows: saccular, fusiform, dissecting, and arteriovenous.** The saccular aneurysm, a localized outpouching that communicates with the arterial lu-

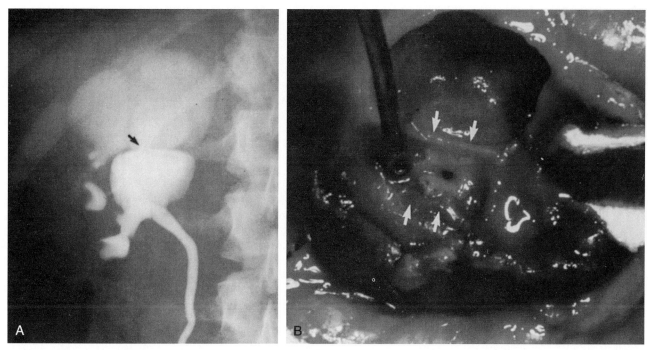

Figure 55–27. *A*, A 14-year-old girl with right flank pain underwent an excretory urogram, and this retrograde pyelogram revealed dilated upper calyces and a narrow upper infundibulum (*arrow*). *B*, At surgery, the infundibular channel was found sandwiched between two segmental arteries (*arrows*).

men by a narrow or wide opening, is the most common type, accounting for 93% of all aneurysms (McKeil et al, 1966; Stanley et al, 1975; Hageman et al, 1978; Zinman and Libertino, 1982). **Renal artery aneurysms have been associated with autosomal dominant polycystic kidney disease** (Schievink, 1998). When the aneurysm is located at the bifurcation of the main renal artery and its anterior and posterior divisions or at one of the more distal branchings, it is considered to be congenital in origin and is called the fusiform type (Poutasse, 1957). The presence of similar aneurysms at branching points in the vasculature of

other organ systems attests to this possible origin (Lorentz et al, 1984). Acquired aneurysms may be located anywhere and may result from inflammatory, traumatic, or degenerative factors. A localized defect in the internal elastic tissue and the media allows the vessel to dilate at that point. It is a true aneurysm because its walls are composed of most of the layers that make up the normal artery (Poutasse, 1957). The outpouchings may vary in size from 1 to 2 cm up to 10 cm (Garritano, 1957) but 90% are smaller than 2 cm.

Most renal artery aneurysms are silent, especially in

Figure 55–28. Accessory renal vessels demonstrated by celluloid corrosion preparation. *A*, In a full-term fetus. The renal pelves and ureters are shown in relationship to the main arterial distribution. On each side there are two accessory renal vessels above and one below, the lower one on the left being in proximity to the ureterovesical junction. *B*, In an 8-month-old fetus, the kidney on the right had one renal artery but the organ on the left had an accessory branch to the lower renal pole. Yet, the location of the lower accessory vessel on the left does not suggest that it might cause ureteral obstruction. On the right, there are early hydronephrosis, secondary kinking, and narrowing at the ureterovesical junction. (Courtesy of Dr. Duncan Morison.)

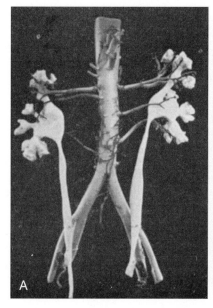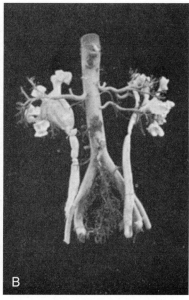

children (48%) (Sarker et al, 1991). Some produce symptoms at a later age in relation to their size because there is a tendency for them to enlarge with time. Pain (15%), hematuria (microscopic and macroscopic) (30%), and hypertension (55%) secondary to compression of adjacent parenchyma or to altered blood flow within the vascular tree can occur (Glass and Uson, 1967; Bulbul and Farrow, 1992). The hypertension is renin-mediated, secondary to relative parenchymal ischemia (Lorentz et al, 1984).

The diagnosis may be suspected when a pulsatile mass is palpated in the region of the renal hilum or when a bruit is heard on abdominal auscultation. A wreathlike calcification in the area of the renal artery or its branches (30%) is highly suggestive (Silvis et al, 1956), but this finding is often missed on a plain abdominal radiograph (Bulbul and Farrow, 1992). Excretory urography may suggest a vascular lesion in 60% of cases, and color Doppler (Bunchman et al, 1991) will demonstrate decreased flow, but selective renal angiography (Cerney et al, 1968), digital subtraction angiography, or, more recently, color Doppler ultrasound (Okamoto et al, 1992) or magnetic resonance angiography (Takebayashi et al, 1994) is needed to confirm the diagnosis.

Many asymptomatic renal artery aneurysms come to light after the discovery and workup of hypertension. Fifty percent are diagnosed when a renal arteriogram is performed for other reasons (Zinman and Libertino, 1982). Generally, **excision is recommended if (1) the hypertension cannot be easily controlled; (2) incomplete ringlike calcification is present; (3) the aneurysm is larger than 2.5 cm** (Poutasse, 1975); **(4) the patient is female and may become pregnant, because rupture during pregnancy is a likely possibility** (Cohen and Shamash, 1987); **(5) the aneurysm increases in size on serial angiograms; or (6) an arteriovenous fistula is present.** The likelihood of spontaneous rupture (about 10%), with its dire consequences, dictates attentive treatment in the foregoing situations. Recent improvements in endovascular techniques dictate early prophylactic treatment (Yamamoto et al, 1998).

Renal Arteriovenous Fistula

Although rare, renal arteriovenous fistulas have been discovered with increasing frequency since they were first described by Varela in 1928. **Two types exist, congenital and acquired** (Maldonado et al, 1964), **with the latter (secondary to trauma, inflammation, renal surgery, or percutaneous needle biopsy) accounting for the recent increased incidence.** Only the congenital variant is discussed here.

Fewer than 25% of all arteriovenous fistulas are of the congenital type. They are easily identifiable by their cirsoid configuration and multiple communications between the main or segmental renal arteries and venous channels (Crummy et al, 1965; Cho and Stanley, 1978). **Although they are considered congenital** (because similar arteriovenous malformations can be found elsewhere in the body), **they rarely present clinically before the** third or fourth decade. **Women are affected three times as often as men, and the right kidney is involved slightly more often than the left** (Cho and Stanley, 1978). **The lesion is usually located in the upper pole (45% of cases), but not infrequently it may be found in the midportion (30%) or in the lower pole (25%) of the kidney** (Yazaki et al, 1976). A total of 91 cases had been reported (Takaha et al, 1980) when the last review was conducted.

The exact cause remains an enigma, but the condition is thought to be either present at birth or the result of a congenital aneurysm that erodes into an adjacent vein and slowly enlarges (Thomason et al, 1972). **The pathophysiology involved in the shunting of blood,** which bypasses the renal parenchyma and rapidly joins the venous circulation and returns to the heart, **results in a varied clinical picture. The myriad of symptoms are based on the size of the arteriovenous malformation and how long it has existed** (Messing et al, 1976).

The hemodynamic derangement often produces a loud bruit (in 75% of cases). Diminished perfusion of renal parenchyma distal to the fistulous site leads to relative ischemia and renin-mediated hypertension (40% to 50%) (McAlhany et al, 1971). **The increased venous return and high cardiac output with concomitant diminution in peripheral resistance may result in left ventricular hypertrophy and eventually in high-output cardiac failure (50%)** (Maldonado et al, 1964). In addition, the arteriovenous fistula usually is located close to the collecting system. As a result, macroscopic and microscopic hematuria occurs in more than 75% of affected individuals (Messing et al, 1976; Cho and Stanley, 1978). Although flank or abdominal pain may be present, a mass is rarely felt (10%).

Excretory urography may reveal diminished or absent function either in one segment or in the entire portion of the involved kidney (DeSai and DeSautels, 1973), an irregular filling defect in the renal pelvis or calyces (secondary to either clot or encroachment by the fistula), or calyceal distortion or obstruction distal to the site of the lesion (Gunterberg, 1968). Despite these specific radiographic features, an abnormality may be noted in only 50% of excretory urograms. **Three-dimensional Doppler ultrasound is a more accurate and noninvasive test** (Mohaupt et al, 1999), **but selective renal arteriography or digital subtraction angiography is the most definitive method for diagnosing the lesion.** A cirsoid appearance with multiple small, tortuous channels; prompt venous filling; and an enlarged renal and possibly gonadal vein are pathognomonic for a renal arteriovenous fistula (DeSai and DeSautels, 1973).

The symptomatic nature of this lesion, which causes progressive alterations in the cardiovascular system, often dictates surgical intervention. The congenital variant rarely behaves like its acquired counterpart, which may disappear spontaneously after several months. Nephrectomy, partial nephrectomy, vascular ligation (Boijsen and Kohler, 1962), selective embolization (Bookstein and Goldstein, 1973), and balloon catheter occlusion (Bentson and Crandalls, 1972) have been employed to obliterate the fistula.

ANOMALIES OF THE COLLECTING SYSTEM

Calyx and Infundibulum

Calyceal Diverticulum

A calyceal diverticulum is a cystic cavity lined by transitional epithelium, encased within the renal substance, and situated peripheral to a minor calyx, to which it is connected by a narrow channel. This abnormality, first described by Rayer in 1841, may be multiple, with the upper calyx being most frequently affected.

An incidence of 4.5 per 1000 excretory urograms has been reported (Timmons et al, 1975). A similar incidence was noted in both children and adults, with no predilection for either side or sex. Most diverticula, labeled type I, occur adjacent to an upper- or occasionally a lower-pole calyx. Type II diverticula are larger and communicate with the renal pelvis directly; they tend to be the symptomatic ones (Wulfsohn, 1980).

Congenital and acquired factors have been suggested to explain the formation of calyceal diverticula. The similarity in incidence in children and adults is consistent with an embryologic etiology (Abeshouse, 1950; Mathieson, 1953; Devine et al, 1969; Middleton and Pfister, 1974). At the 5-mm stage of the embryo, some of the ureteral branches of the third and fourth generation, which ordinarily degenerate, may persist as isolated branches, resulting in the formation of a calyceal diverticulum (Lister and Singh, 1973).

A localized cortical abscess draining into a calyx has also been postulated as an etiologic factor. Other proposed causes include obstruction secondary to stone formation or infection within a calyx, progressive fibrosis of an infundibular stenosis, renal injury, achalasia, and spasm or dysfunction of one of the supposed sphincters surrounding a minor calyx. Small diverticula are usually asymptomatic and are found incidentally at excretory urography or renal ultrasonography. Over time these diverticula tend to progressively distend with trapped urine (Schneck et al, 1994). Infection, milk of calcium (crystallization of calcium salts without actual stone formation) (Patriquin et al, 1985), or true stone formation are complications of stasis or obstruction that can produce symptoms (Lister and Singh, 1973; Siegel and McAlister, 1979). Hematuria, pain, and urinary infection may be seen in the presence of stones. In the Mayo Clinic series (Timmons et al, 1975), 39% of patients with calyceal diverticula had calculi.

The diagnosis is made by excretory urography; one child in our series developed an abscess in her infected diverticulum that required percutaneous drainage (Ellis et al, 1990; Schneck et al, 1994). Delayed films are helpful in demonstrating pooling of contrast material in the diverticulum. Retrograde pyelography (Fig. 55–29) and, more recently, delayed imaging computed tomography with contrast and magnetic resonance imaging are sometimes useful in making the diagnosis and defining the precise anatomy. Ultrasonography delineates a fluid-filled area more centrally located near the collecting system than a simple renal cyst.

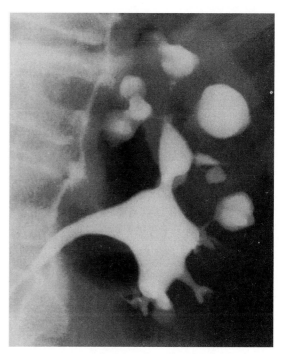

Figure 55–29. A 13-year-old girl with hematuria had a retrograde pyelogram demonstrating multiple calyceal diverticula.

When it is filled with microcalculi, ultrasound characteristically demonstrates a layering effect within the diverticulum between clear fluid above and echo-dense debris without shadowing below (Patriquin et al, 1985). In fact, ultrasonography may be more definitive because it is easier to image the milk of calcium within the diverticulum as the patient changes position. Milk of calcium appears on excretory urography as a crescent-shaped density that changes as the patient assumes different positions. **Reflux is found in as many as two thirds of the children,** which may explain why some children present with urinary infection (Amar, 1975).

In general, patients who are asymptomatic do not require treatment. Persistent pain, resistant urinary infections, hematuria, and milk of calcium or true calculus formation are indications for surgery (Siegel and McAlister, 1979). **Partial nephrectomy was the treatment of choice in the past, but now percutaneous removal of the stones and ablation of the mucosal surface** and communication with the collecting system (Goldfischer et al, 1998), ureteroscopic enlargement of the diverticular communication with removal of the stones (Baldwin et al, 1998), or extracorporeal laparoscopic stone removal with marsupialization of the diverticulum (Hoznek et al, 1998) **have been reported as successful kidney-sparing alternatives.**

Hydrocalycosis

Hydrocalycosis is a very rare cystic dilation of a major calyx with a demonstrable connection to the renal pelvis; it is lined by transitional epithelium. **It may be caused by a congenital or acquired intrinsic obstruction such as a parapelvic cyst** (Fig. 55–30).

Dilation of the upper calyx due to obstruction of the

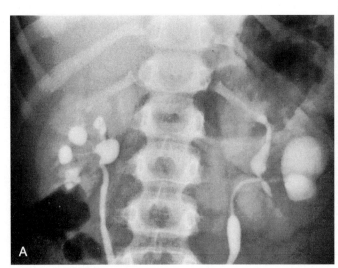
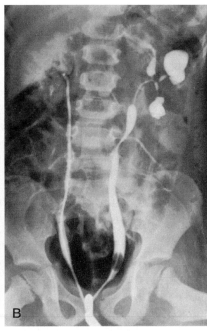

Figure 55–30. Hydrocalycosis of infundibulopelvic stenosis in a 3-year-old boy with bilaterally ectopic ureteral orifices (at the vesical neck) and other congenital anomalies, who presented with urinary infection. Reflux was not demonstrable, and the patient has remained uninfected on suppressive antibiotics. There has been no urographic change for 5 years. *A,* Long-term excretory urogram. Right infundibular and left infundibulopelvic stenosis. *B,* Retrograde ureteropyelogram (bilateral). Mildly dilated left ureter. Note diffuse tubular backflow on right. (From Malek RS: Obstructive uropathy: Calyx. In Kelalis PP, King LR [eds]: Clinical Pediatric Urology. Philadelphia, WB Saunders, 1976, p 235.)

upper infundibulum by vessels or stenosis has been described (see Fig. 55–27) (Fraley, 1966; Johnston and Sandomirsky, 1972). Cicatrization of an infundibulum may result from infection or trauma. Conversely, **hydrocalycosis has been reported to occur without an obvious cause** (Williams and Mininberg, 1968). It has been postulated that achalasia of a ring of muscle at the entrance of the infundibulum into the renal pelvis causes a functional obstruction (Moore, 1950; Williams and Mininberg, 1968).

Mild upper calyceal dilation caused by partial infundibular obstruction is relatively common but usually asymptomatic. The most frequent presenting symptom is upper abdominal or flank pain. On occasion a mass may be palpated. Stasis can lead to hematuria or urinary infection, or both.

Hydrocalycosis must be differentiated from multiple dilated calyces secondary to ureteral obstruction, calyceal clubbing as a result of recurrent pyelonephritis or medullary necrosis, renal tuberculosis, a large calyceal diverticulum, and megacalycosis. These entities can be differentiated by a combination of excretory urography, findings at surgery, histopathology of removed tissue, and bacteriology.

Hydrocalycosis due to vascular obstruction is usually treated by dismembered infundibulopyelostomy, which changes the relationship of the infundibulum to the vessel. If the cystic dilation is caused by an intrinsic stenosis of the infundibulum, an intubated infundibulotomy or partial nephrectomy may be performed. Percutaneous treatment of these narrowed areas has also been successful and is probably the approach of choice today (Lang, 1991).

Although clinical improvement is apparent in most instances, the radiologic appearance often is not altered significantly.

Megacalycosis

Megacalycosis is best defined as nonobstructive enlargement of calyces resulting from malformation of the renal papillae (Fig. 55–31). It was first described by Puigvert in 1963. **The calyces are generally dilated** and malformed and may be increased in number. The renal pelvis is not dilated, nor is its wall thickened, and the **UPJ is normally funneled without evidence of obstruction**. The cortical tissue around the abnormal calyx is normal in thickness and shows no signs of scarring or chronic inflammation. The medulla, however, is underdeveloped and assumes a falciform crescent appearance instead of its normal pyramidal shape. The collecting tubules are not dilated but are definitely shorter than normal, and they are oriented transversely rather than vertically from the corticomedullary junction (Puigvert, 1963). A mild disorder of maximum concentrating ability has been reported (Gittes and Talner, 1972), but acid excretion is normal after an acid load (Vela-Navarrete and Garcia Robledo, 1983). Other functions of the kidney—glomerular filtration, renal plasma flow, and isotope uptake—also are not altered (Gittes, 1984).

Megacalycosis is most likely to be congenital. It occurs predominantly in males in a ratio of 6:1 and has been found only in Caucasian patients. Bilateral disease has been seen almost exclusively in males, whereas segmental unilateral involvement occurs only in females

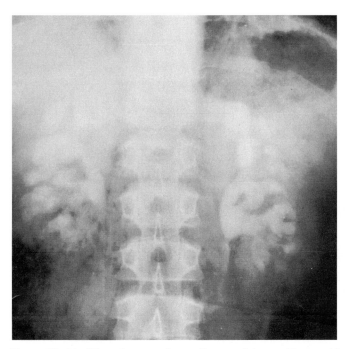

Figure 55–31. Bilateral megacalyces discovered in an 11-year-old boy with abdominal pain and hematuria. He had no history of urinary infection, and voiding cystography did not demonstrate vesicoureteral reflux.

(Cacciaguerra et al, 1996). **This suggests an X-linked partially recessive gene with reduced penetrance in females** (Gittes, 1984). Except for one report of two affected brothers, the entity has not been thought to be familial (Briner and Thiel, 1988).

It was theorized by Puigvert (1964) and endorsed by Johnston and Sandomirsky (1972) that there is transient delay in the recanalization of the upper ureter after the branches of the ureteral bud hook up with the metanephric blastema. This produces a short-lived episode of obstruction when the embryonic glomeruli start producing urine. The fetal calyces may dilate and then retain their obstructed appearance despite the lack of evidence of obstruction in postnatal life (Gittes and Talner, 1972). **The increased number of calyces frequently seen in this condition may be an aborted response by the branching ureteral bud to the obstruction.**

Primary hypoplasia of juxtamedullary glomeruli was suggested as an etiology by Galian and associates (1970); this theory nicely explains the reason for the lack of concentrating ability, but it has not been corroborated by others.

The abnormality is noticed in children, usually when x-ray studies are obtained after a urinary tract infection or as part of an evaluation when other congenital anomalies are present. Adults frequently present with hematuria secondary to renal calculi, which leads to excretory urographic investigation.

The calyces are dilated and usually increased in number, but the infundibuli and pelvis may not be enlarged. Although the UPJ does not appear obstructed, there may be segmental dilation of the distal third of the ureter (Kozakewich and Lebowitz, 1974). Megacalycosis associated with

an ipsilateral segmental megaureter was described in 12 children (Mandell et al, 1987), mostly boys, and predominantly left-sided. A normal-caliber ureter was interposed between the two entities (Fig. 55–32). Not frequently this anatomic picture has been mistaken for congenital ureteropelvic or ureterovesical junction obstruction, with surgery being performed to correct the suspected defect. Postoperatively, the calyceal pattern remains unchanged.

Diuretic renography reveals a normal pattern for uptake and washout of the isotope, whether or not the Whitaker test generates high pressure in the collecting system. Therefore, an obstructive picture cannot be proven. **Long-term follow-up of patients with this anomaly does not reveal any progression of the anatomic derangement or functional impairment of the kidney** (Gittes, 1984).

Unipapillary Kidney

The unipapillary kidney is an exceptionally rare anomaly in humans. Only 18 cases have been reported (Neal and Murphy, 1960; Sakatoku and Kitayama, 1964; Harrison et al, 1976; Morimoto et al, 1979; Toppercer, 1980; Kaneto et al, 1997). This anomaly is present not uncommonly in monkeys, rabbits, dogs, marsupials, insectivores, and monotremes. **The cause is thought to be a failure of progressive branching after the first three to five generations** (which create the pelvis) of the ureteral bud (Potter, cited by Harrison et al, 1976). **The solitary calyx drains a ridgelike papilla.** Nephrons attach to fewer collecting tubules, which then drain directly into the pelvis. **Biopsies of these kidneys reveal glomerulosclerosis, tubular atrophy, and increased fibrosis** (Bischel et al, 1978).

The kidney is smaller than normal but usually is in its correct location. Its function is often reduced (Smith et al, 1984; Kaneto et al, 1997). The arterial tree, although sparse, has a normal configuration. **The opposite kidney is frequently absent.** Genital anomalies are often present. The condition is frequently asymptomatic, being discovered fortuitously in most instances. More often than not there are abnormalities of the proximal ureter (i.e., megaureter, reflux, or ectopic insertion), suggesting an underlying ureteral bud defect as the cause (Smith et al, 1984; Kaneto et al, 1997). The anomaly has also come to light during a workup for urinary infection (Kaneto et al, 1997).

Extrarenal Calyces

Extrarenal calyces are an uncommon congenital anomaly in which the major calyces as well as the renal pelvis are outside the parenchyma of the kidney (Fig. 55–33). This entity was originally reviewed by Eisendrath in 1925 and then more extensively by Malament and co-workers in 1961. The kidney is usually discoid, with the pelvis and the major and minor calyces located outside the renal parenchyma. The renal vessels have an anomalous distribution into the kidney, usually at the circumferential edge of the flat, widened hilus. **Malament considered this condition to be the result of abnormal nephrogenic anlage or a too early and rapidly developing ureteral bud.**

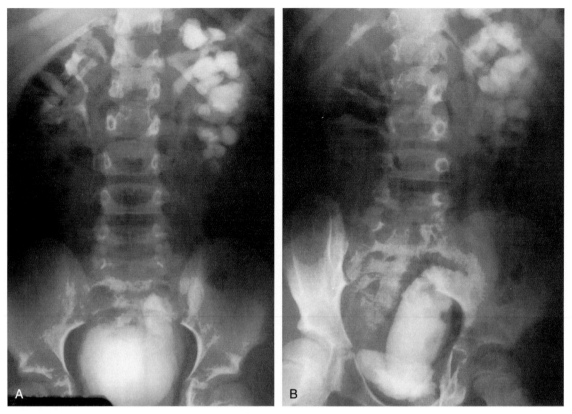

Figure 55–32. An 8-year-old boy with urinary infection was found to have left-sided megacalycosis and a distal megaureter (*A* and *B*). Note the normal caliber upper ureter. A voiding cystogram revealed no reflux, and a diuretic renogram did not demonstrate any obstruction.

Extrarenal calyces usually do not produce symptoms, although failure of normal drainage may lead to stasis, infection, and calculi. Sometimes, the calyces are blunted, mimicking the radiographic changes usually seen with pyelonephritis or obstruction, from which this condition should be distinguished. Surgery is reserved for those cases in which infection or obstruction is demonstrated.

Anomalous Calyx (Pseudotumor of the Kidney)

A number of normal variants of the pyelocalyceal system in the kidney have been described. One such entity manifests as **a localized mass, usually situated between the infundibula of the upper and middle calyceal**

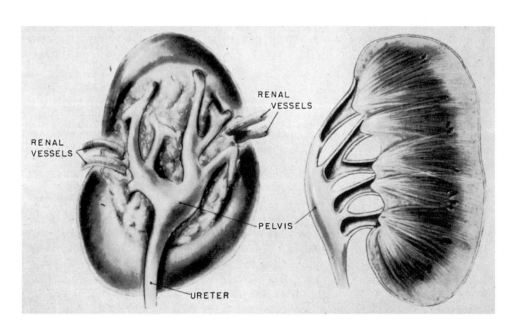

Figure 55–33. Extrarenal calyces. These represent delayed rather than insufficient ureteral growth. (From Malament M, Schwartz B, Nagamatsu GR: Extrarenal calyces: Their relationship to renal disease. AJR Am J Roentgenol 1961;86:823.)

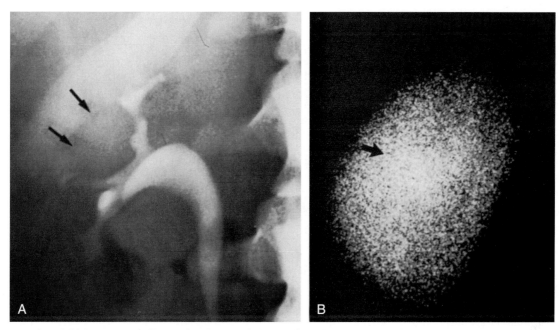

Figure 55–34. *A,* This child has a mass effect with splaying of the middle calyces. *B,* A renal scan demonstrates normal uptake in the area (*arrow*), suggesting the pseudotumor is really a hypertrophied column of Bertin.

groups, and is called a hypertrophied column of Bertin (Fig. 55–34). The column may be sufficiently large to compress and deform the adjacent pelvis and calyces, suggesting a mass on excretory urography; this is the so-called pseudotumor. The individual calyces, however, are normally shaped and developed.

It is important to differentiate this calyceal anomaly from true disease of the calyx and from a parenchymal tumor. **A renal scan shows normal uptake of the radioisotope in this area** (Parker et al, 1976), and **a renal ultrasound study shows a normal echogenic pattern** of parenchyma to the area in question.

Infundibulopelvic Dysgenesis

Infundibulopelvic stenosis most likely forms a link between cystic dysplasia of the kidney and the grossly hydronephrotic organ (Kelalis and Malek, 1981; Uhlenhuth et al, 1990). This condition includes a variety of roentgenographically dysmorphic kidneys with varying degrees of infundibular or infundibulopelvic stenosis that may be associated with renal dysplasia (Fig. 55–35). Although not called as such, the first case involving the entire pelvis and all the infundibuli of both kidneys was reported by Boyce and Whitehurst in 1976. Rayer had described a focal form of the disease in 1841, and several reports noting narrowing of one or two infundibuli appeared between 1949 and 1976 (Uhlenhuth et al, 1990). These authors tried to link the focal form to cystic dysplasia secondary to obstruction, in which multicystic kidney disease is the severest form in the spectrum. **Uhlenhuth and coworkers (1990) believed that this phenomenon is the result of extensive dysgenesis of the pyelocalyceal system but with preservation of renal function.** Reflux is not commonly observed in these patients.

Infundibulopelvic stenosis is usually bilateral and is

commonly associated with vesicoureteral reflux, suggesting an abnormality of the entire ureteral bud (Kelalis and Malek, 1981). Patients usually present with urinary infection, hypertension, or flank pain. Sometimes, an asymptomatic child with multiple anomalies is evaluated

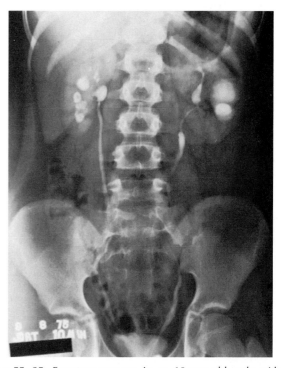

Figure 55–35. Excretory urogram in an 18-year-old male with one urinary tract infection shows severe stenosis of the infundibula and left ureteropelvic junction and a milder form of infundibulopelvic dysgenesis in the right kidney. Vesicoureteral reflux was absent on voiding cystourethrography. (Courtesy of Dr. Panos Kelalis.)

and found to have this condition. **Despite extensively dysmorphic kidney features, the function is either normal or only slightly affected** (Kelalis and Malek, 1981). **Long-term follow-up, however, reveals that progressive renal deterioration is common, leading to severe renal insufficiency or end-stage renal disease in all patients with bilateral involvement** (Husmann et al, 1994). **Biopsies in patients with renal failure demonstrate lesions consistent with hyperfiltration injury.** Progressive hydronephrosis is not thought to be responsible for the deterioration in renal function, based on histologic assessment of renal tissue adjacent to dilated calyces. Therefore, infundibulotomy is not recommended unless there is a specific need (i.e., caliceal stones) (Husman et al, 1994).

Pelvis

Extrarenal Pelvis

An extrarenal pelvis is of clinical importance only when drainage is impaired. This is sometimes associated with a variety of kidney abnormalities, including malposition and malrotation, that predispose to urinary stasis, infection, and calculous disease. UPJ obstruction causing dilation of only the renal pelvis and not the calyces has been reported (Johnson, 1999).

Bifid Pelvis

Approximately 10% of normal renal pelves are bifid, the pelvis dividing first at or just within its entrance to the kidney to form two major calyces. **A bifid pelvis should be considered a variant of normal.** No increased incidence of disease has been reported in patients with this entity. If further division of the renal pelvis occurs, triplication of the pelvis may result, but this is extremely rare.

REFERENCES

Anomalies of Number

Bilateral Renal Agenesis

Ashley DJB, Mostofi FK: Renal agenesis and dysgenesis. J Urol 1960;83: 211.

Bain AD, Scott JS: Renal agenesis and severe urinary tract dysplasia: A review of 50 cases, with particular reference to associated anomalies. Br Med J 1960;1:841.

Bain AD, Beath MM, Flint WF: Sirenomelia and monomelia with renal agenesis in amnion nodosum. Arch Dis Child 1960;35:250.

Carpentier PJ, Potter EL: Nuclear sex and genital malformation in 48 cases of renal agenesis with special reference to nonspecific female pseudohermaphroditism. Am J Obstet Gynecol 1959;78:235.

Cilento BG Jr, Benacerraf BR, Mandell J: Prenatal and postnatal findings in monochorionic, monoamniotic twins discordant for bilateral renal agenesis-dysgenesis (perinatal lethal renal disease). J Urol 1994;151: 1034–1035.

Clark DA: Times of first void and first stool in 500 newborns. Pediatrics 1977;60:457.

Clemmons JJW: Embryonic renal injury: A possible factor in fetal malnutrition. Pediatr Res 1977;11:404.

Davidson WM, Ross GIM: Bilateral absence of the kidneys and related congenital anomalies. J Pathol Bacteriol 1954;68:459.

Dicker D, Samuel N, Feldberg D, Goldman JA: The antenatal diagnosis of Potter syndrome: A lethal and not so rare malformation. Eur J Obstet Gynecol Reprod Biol 1984;18:17.

Fitch N, Lachance RC: The pathogenesis of Potter's syndrome of renal agenesis. Can Med Assoc J 1972;107:653.

Georgieff MK, Petry CD, Wobken JD, Oyer CE: Liver and brain iron deficiency in newborn infants with bilateral renal agenesis. Pediatr Pathol Lab Med 1996;16:509–519.

Hislop A, Hey EJ, Reid L: The lungs in congenital bilateral renal agenesis and dysplasia. Arch Dis Child 1979;54:32.

Hoffman CK, Filly RA, Allen PW: The "lying down" adrenal sign: A sonographic indicator of renal agenesis or ectopia in fetuses and neonates. J Ultrasound Med 1992;11:533.

Katz SH, Chatten J: The urethra in bilateral renal agenesis. Arch Pathol 1974;97:269.

Klinger G, Merlob P, Aloni D, et al: Normal pulmonary function in a monoamniotic twin discordant for bilateral renal agenesis. Am J Med Genet 1997;73:76–79.

Kohler HG: An unusual case of sirenomelia. Teratology 1972;6:659.

Kovacs T, Csecsei K, Toth L, Papp Z: Familial occurrence of bilateral renal agenesis. Acta Paediatr Hung 1991;31:13.

Levin H: Bilateral renal agenesis. J Urol 1952;67:86.

Mauer SM, Dobrin RS, Vernier RL: Unilateral and bilateral renal agenesis in nonamniotic twins. J Pediatr 1974;84:236.

McPherson E, Carey J, Kramer A, et al: Dominantly inherited renal adysplasia. Am J Med Genet 1987;26:863.

Moerman P, Fryns JP, Sastrowijoto SH, et al: Hereditary renal adysplasia: New observations and hypotheses. Pediatr Pathol 1994;14:405.

Murugasu B, Cole BR, Hawkins EP, et al: Familial renal dysplasia. Am J Kidney Dis 1991;18:490.

Novak RW, Robinson HB: Coincident DiGeorge anomaly and renal agenesis and its relation to maternal diabetes. Am J Med Genet 1994;50: 311.

O'Connor TA, LaCour ML, Friedlander ER, Thomas R: Penile agenesis associated with urethral and bilateral renal agenesis. Urology 1993;41: 564.

Perlman M, Williams J, Hirsh M: Neonatal pulmonary hypoplasia after prolonged leakage of amniotic fluid. Arch Dis Child 1976;51:349.

Potter EL: Bilateral renal agenesis. J Pediatr 1946a;29:68.

Potter EL: Facial characteristics in infants with bilateral renal agenesis. Am J Obstet Gynecol 1946b;51:885.

Potter EL: Pathology of the Fetus and the Newborn. Chicago, Year Book Medical Publishers, 1952.

Potter EL: Bilateral absence of ureters and kidneys: A report of 50 cases. Obstet Gynecol 1965;25:3.

Rayburn WF, Laferla JJ: Mid-gestational abortion for medical or genetic indications. Clin Obstet Gynecol 1986;13:71.

Reid L: The lung: Its growth and remodeling in health and disease. AJR Am J Roentgenol 1977;129:777.

Rizza JM, Downing SE: Bilateral renal agenesis in two female siblings. Am J Dis Child 1971;121:60.

Roodhooft AM, Birnholz JC, Holmes LD: Familial nature of congenital absence and severe dysgenesis of both kidneys. N Engl J Med 1984; 310:1341.

Sepulveda W, Corral E, Sanchez J, et al: Sirenomelia sequence versus renal agenesis: Prenatal differentiation with power Doppler ultrasound. Ultrasound Obstet Gynecol 1998;11:445–449.

Sherry SN, Kramer I: The time of passage of first stool and first urine by the newborn infant. J Pediatr 1955;46:158.

Stella A: Hereditary renal agenesis. Minerva Ginecol 1998;50:255–259.

Stroup NE, Edmonds L, O'Brien TR: Renal agenesis and dysgenesis: Are they increasing? Teratology 1990;42:383–395.

Thomas IT, Smith DW: Oligohydramnios, cause of the nonrenal features of Potter's syndrome, including pulmonary hypoplasia. J Pediatr 1974; 84:811.

Thompson VM: Amnion nodosum. J Obstet Gynaecol Br Commonw 1960;67:611.

Wilson RD, Baird PA: Renal agenesis in British Columbia. Am J Med Genet 1985;21:153.

Unilateral Renal Agenesis

Arfeen S, Rosborough D, Lugar M, Nolph KD: Familial renal agenesis and focal and segmental glomerulosclerosis. Am J Kidney Dis 1993;21: 663.

Argueso LR, Ritchey ML, Boyle ET Jr, et al: Prognosis of patients with unilateral renal agenesis. Pediatr Nephrol 1992;6:412.

Ashley DJB, Mostofi FK: Renal agenesis and dysgenesis. J Urol 1960;83:211.

Atiyeh B, Husmann D, Baum M: Contralateral renal anomalies in patients with renal agenesis and noncystic renal dysplasia. Pediatrics 1993;91:812.

Barry JE, Auldist AW: The VATER association. Am J Dis Child 1974;128:769.

Battin J, Lacombe D, Leng JJ: Familial occurrence of hereditary renal adysplasia with müllerian anomalies. Clin Genet 1993;43:23.

Biedel CW, Pagon RA, Zapata JO: Müllerian anomalies and renal agenesis: Autosomal dominant urogenital adysplasia. J Pediatr 1984;104:861.

Bryan AL, Nigro JA, Counseller VS: One hundred cases of congenital absence of the vagina. Surg Gynecol Obstet 1949;88:79.

Campbell MF: Congenital absence of one kidney: Unilateral renal agenesis. Ann Surg 1928;88:1039.

Candiani GB, Fedele L, Candiani M: Double uterus, blind hemivagina, and ipsilateral renal agenesis: 36 cases and long-term followup. Obstet Gynecol 1997;90:26.

Cascio S, Paran S, Puri P: Associated urological anomalies in children with unilateral renal agenesis. J Urol 1999;162:1081–1083.

Charny CW, Gillenwater JY: Congenital absence of the vas deferens. J Urol 1965;93:399.

Collins DC: Congenital unilateral renal agenesis. Ann Surg 1932;95:715.

Cope JR, Trickey SE: Congenital absence of the kidney: Problems in diagnosis and management. J Urol 1982;127:10.

Colquhoun-Kerr JS, Gu W-X, Jameson JL, et al: X-Linked Kallmann syndrome and renal agenesis occurring together and independently in a large Australian family. Am J Med Genet 1999;83:22–27.

Currarino G: Single vaginal ectopic ureter and Gartner's duct cyst with ipsilateral renal hypoplasia and dysplasia (or agenesis). J Urol 1982;128:988.

Curtis JA, Sadhu V, Steiner RM: Malposition of the colon in right renal agenesis, ectopia and anterior nephrectomy. AJR Am J Roentgenol 1977;129:845.

D'Alberton A, Reshini E, Ferrari N, Candiani P: Prevalence of urinary tract abnormalities in a large series of patients with uterovaginal atresia. J Urol 1981;126:623.

Dees JE: Prognosis of the solitary kidney. J Urol 1960;83:550.

DeSanto NG, Anastasio P, Spitali L, et al: Renal pressure is normal in adults born with unilateral renal agenesis and is not related to hyperfiltration or renal failure. Miner Electrolyte Metab 1997;23:283–286.

Donohue RE, Fauver HE: Unilateral absence of the vas deferens. JAMA 1989;261:1180.

Doroshow LW, Abeshouse BS: Congenital unilateral solitary kidney: Report of 37 cases and a review of the literature. Urol Surv 1961;11:219.

Emanuel B, Nachman RP, Aronson N, Weiss H: Congenital solitary kidney: A review of 74 cases. Am J Dis Child 1974;127:17.

Fortune CH: The pathological and clinical significance of congenital one-sided kidney defect with the presentation of three new cases of agenesis and one of aplasia. Ann Intern Med 1927;1:377.

Gilliland B, Dick F: Uterus didelphys associated with unilateral imperforate vagina. Obstet Gynecol 1976;48(Suppl 1):5s.

Gutierrez R: Surgical aspects of renal agenesis: With special reference to hypoplastic kidney, renal aplasia and congenital absence of one kidney. Arch Surg 1933;27:686.

Heinonen PK: Unicornuate uterus and rudimentary horn. Fertil Steril 1997;68:224–230.

Hitchcock R, Burge DM: Renal agenesis: An acquired condition. J Pediatr Surg 1994;29:454.

Hoffman CK, Filly RA, Callen PW: The "lying down" adrenal sign: A sonographic indicator of renal agenesis or ectopia in fetuses and neonates. J Ultrasound Med 1992;11:533.

Holt SA, Peterson NE: Ectopia of seminal vesicle: Associated with agenesis of ipsilateral kidney. Urology 1974;4:322.

Hynes DM, Watkin EM: Renal agenesis: Roentgenologic problem. AJR Am J Roentgenol 1970;110:772.

Jancu J, Zuckerman H, Sudarsky M: Unilateral renal agenesis associated with multiple abnormalities. South Med J 1976;69:94.

Kenny PJ, Robbins GL, Ellis DA, Spert BA: Adrenal glands in patients with congenital renal anomalies: Computed tomography appearance. Radiology 1985;155:181.

Kohn G, Borns PF: The association of bilateral and unilateral renal aplasia in the same family. J Pediatr 1973;83:95.

Kolon TF, Gray CL, Sutherland RW, et al: Upper urinary tract manifestations of the VACTERL association. J Urol 2000;163:1949–1951.

Kroovand RL: Cystoscopy. In Kelalis PP, King LR, Belman AB (eds): Clinical Pediatric Urology. Philadelphia, WB Saunders, 1985.

Limkakeng AD, Retik AB: Unilateral renal agenesis with hypoplastic ureter: Observations on the contralateral urinary tract and report of four cases. J Urol 1972;108:149.

Longo VJ, Thompson GJ: Congenital solitary kidney. J Urol 1952;68:63.

Lopez-Garcia JA, Azparren Echevarria J, Garmendia G, et al: Seminal vesicle cyst with renal agenesis. Arch Esp Urol 1998;51:419–426.

Mace JW, Kaplan JM, Schanberger JE, Gotlin RW: Poland's syndrome: Report of seven cases and review of the literature. Clin Pediatr 1972;11:98.

Magee MC, Lucey DT, Fried FA: A new embryologic classification for uro-gynecologic malformations: The syndromes of mesonephric duct induced müllerian deformities. J Urol 1979;121:265.

Mascatello V, Lebowitz RL: Malposition of the colon in left renal agenesis and ectopia. Radiology 1976;120:371.

McPherson E, Carey J, Kramer A, et al: Dominantly inherited renal adysplasia. Am J Med Genet 1987;26:863.

Mesrobian HG: Compensatory renal growth in the solitary kidneys of Danforth mice with genetic renal agenesis. J Urol 1998;160:146–149.

Mesrobian HG, Rushton HG, Bulas D: Unilateral renal agenesis may result from in utero regression of multicystic renal dysplasia. J Urol 1993;150:793.

Nomura S, Osawa G: Focal glomerular sclerotic lesions in a patient with urinary oligomeganephronia and agenesis of the contralateral kidney: A case report. Clin Nephrol 1990;33:7.

Novak RW, Robinson HB: Coincident DiGeorge anomaly and renal agenesis and its relation to maternal diabetes. Am J Med Genet 1994;50:311.

Ochsner MG, Brannan W, Goodier EH: Absent vas deferens associated with renal agenesis. JAMA 1972;222:1055.

Phelan JT, Counseller VS, Greene LF: Deformities of the urinary tract with congenital absence of the vagina. Surg Gynecol Obstet 1953;97:1.

Radasch HE: Congenital unilateral absence of the urogenital system and its relation to the development of the Wolffian and Muellerian ducts. Am J Med Sci 1908;136:111.

Roodhooft AM, Birnholz JC, Holmes LD: Familial nature of congenital absence and severe dysgenesis of both kidneys. N Engl J Med 1984;310:1341.

Rugui C, Oldrizzi L, Lupo A, et al: Clinical features of patients with solitary kidneys. Nephron 1986;43:10.

Say B, Gerald PS: A new polydactyly/imperforate-anus/vertebral anomalies syndrome? Lancet 1968;1:688.

Selig AM, Benacerraf B, Greene MF, et al: Renal dysplasia, megalocystis and sirenomelia in four siblings. Teratology 1993;47:65.

Semmens JP: Congenital anomalies of the female genital tract: Functional classification based on review of 56 personal cases and 500 reported cases. Obstet Gynecol 1962;19:328.

Shieh CP, Hung CS, Wei CF, Lin CY: Cystic dilatations within the pelvis in patients with ipsilateral renal agenesis or dysplasia. J Urol 1990;144:324.

Shumacker HB: Congenital anomalies of the genitalia associated with unilateral renal agenesis. Arch Surg 1938;37:586.

Sipek A, Gregor V, Horacek J, et al: Incidence of renal agenesis in the Czech Republic from 1961–1995. Ceska Gynekol 1997;62:340–343.

Smith EC, Orkin LA: A clinical and statistical study of 471 congenital anomalies of the kidney and ureter. J Urol 1945;53:11.

Thompson DP, Lynn HB: Genital anomalies associated with solitary kidney. Mayo Clin Proc 1966;41:538.

Uchida S, Akiba T, Sasaki S, et al: Unilateral renal agenesis associated with various metabolic disorders in three siblings. Nephron 1990;54:86.

Van den Ouden D, Blom JH, Bangma C, deSpiegeleer AH: Diagnosis and management of seminal vesicle cysts associated with unilateral renal agenesis: A pooled analysis of 52 cases. Eur Urol 1998;33:433–440.

Vinstein AL, Franken EA Jr: Unilateral hematocolpos associated with agenesis of the kidney. Radiology 1972;102:625.

Weiss JM, Dykhuizen RF: An anomalous vaginal insertion into the bladder: A case report. J Urol 1967;98:60.

Wiersma AF, Peterson LF, Justema EJ: Uterine anomalies associated with unilateral renal agenesis. Obstet Gynecol 1976;47:654.

Wilson RD, Baird PA: Renal agenesis in British Columbia. Am J Med Genet 1985;21:153.

Wilson TA, Blethen SL, Vallone A, et al: DiGeorge anomaly with renal agenesis in infants of mothers with diabetes. Am J Med Genet 1993;47: 1078.

Woolf RB, Allen WM: Concomitant malformations: The frequent simultaneous occurrence of congenital malformations of the reproductive and urinary tracts. Obstet Gynecol 1953;2:236.

Yoder IC, Pfister RC: Unilateral hematocolpos and ipsilateral renal agenesis: Report of two cases and review of the literature. AJR Am J Roentgenol 1976;127:303.

Zenteno JC, Mendez JP, Maya-Nunez G, et al: Renal anomalies in patients with Kallmann syndrome. Br J Urol Int 1999;83:383–386.

Supernumerary Kidney

Campbell MF: Anomalies of the kidney. In Campbell MF, Harrison JH (eds): Urology, vol 2, 3rd ed. Philadelphia, WB Saunders, 1970, p 1422.

Carlson HE: Supernumerary kidney: A summary of fifty-one reported cases. J Urol 1950;64:221.

Conrad GR, Loes DJ: Ectopic supernumerary kidney: Functional assessment using radionuclide imaging. Clin Nucl Med 1987;12:253.

Exley M, Hotchkiss WS: Supernumerary kidney with clear cell carcinoma. J Urol 1944;51:569.

Geisinger JF: Supernumerary kidney. J Urol 1937;38:331.

Hoffman RI, McMillan TE: Discussion. Trans South Central Sec, American Urology Assoc 1948;82.

Kaneoya F, Botoh B, Yokokawa M: Unusual duplication of renal collecting system mimicking supernumerary kidney. Nippon Hinyokika Bakkai Zasshi 1989;80:270.

Kretschmer HL: Supernumerary kidney: Report of a case with review of the literature. Surg Gynecol Obstet 1929;49:818.

McPherson RI: Supernumerary kidney: Typical and atypical features. Can Assoc Radiol J 1987;38:116.

N'Guessan G, Stephens FD: Supernumerary kidney. J Urol 1983;130:649.

Rubin JS: Supernumerary kidney with aberrant ureter terminating externally. J Urol 1948;61:405.

Sasidharan K, Babu AS, Rao MM, Bhat HS: Free supernumerary kidney. Br J Urol 1976;48:388.

Shane JH: Supernumerary kidney with vaginal ureteral orifice. J Urol 1942;47:344.

Tada Y, Kokado Y, Hashinaka Y, et al: Free supernumerary kidney: A case report and review. J Urol 1981;126:231.

Anomalies of Ascent

Simple Renal Ectopia

Abeshouse BS, Bhisitkul I: Crossed renal ectopia with and without fusion. Urol Int 1959;9:63.

Anderson EE, Harrison JH: Surgical importance of the solitary kidney. N Engl J Med 1965;273:683.

Anson BJ, Riba LW: The anatomical and surgical features of ectopic kidney. Surg Gynecol Obstet 1939;68:37.

Baggenstoss AH: Congenital anomalies of the kidney. Med Clin North Am 1951;35:987.

Bell ET: Renal Diseases. Philadelphia, Lea & Febiger, 1946.

Borer JG, Bauer SB, Peters CA, et al: Single system ectopic ureter draining an ectopic dysplastic kidney: Delayed diagnosis in the young female with continuous urinary incontinence. Br J Urol 1998;81:474–478.

Borer JG, Corgan FJ, Krantz R, et al: Unilateral single vaginal ectopic ureter with ipsilateral hypoplastic pelvic kidney and bicornuate uterus. J Urol 1993;149:1124.

Campbell MF: Renal ectopy. J Urol 1930;24:187.

D'Alberton A, Reschini E, Ferrari N, Candiani P: Prevalence of urinary tract abnormalities in a large series of patients with uterovaginal atresia. J Urol 1981;126:623.

Delson B: Ectopic kidney in obstetrics and gynecology. N Y State J Med 1975;75:2522.

Downs RA, Lane LW, Burns E: Solitary pelvic kidney: Its clinical implications. Urology 1973;1:51.

Dretler SP, Olsson CA, Pfister RC: The anatomic, radiologic and clinical characteristics of the pelvic kidney: An analysis of 86 cases. J Urol 1971;105:623.

Gleason PE, Kelalis PP, Husmann DA, Kramer SA: Hydronephrosis in renal ectopia: Incidence, etiology and significance. J Urol 1994;151:1660.

Hawes CJ: Congenital unilateral ectopic kidney: A report of two cases. J Urol 1950;64:453.

Leitha T: The usefulness of Tc99m-DMSA SPECT and three-dimensional surface rendering in an asymptomatic patient with a single kidney in the pelvis. Clin Nucl Med 1998;23:414–416.

Malek RS, Kelalis PP, Burke EC: Ectopic kidney in children and frequency of association of other malformations. Mayo Clin Proc 1971;46:461.

McCrea LE: Congenital solitary pelvic kidney. J Urol 1942;48:58.

Stevens AR: Pelvic single kidneys. J Urol 1937;37:610.

Tabisky J, Bhisitkul I: Solitary crossed ectopic kidney with vaginal aplasia: A case report. J Urol 1965;94:33.

Thompson GJ, Pace JM: Ectopic kidney: A review of 97 cases. Surg Gynecol Obstet 1937;64:935.

Ward JN, Nathanson B, Draper JW: The pelvic kidney. J Urol 1965;94:36.

Cephalad Renal Ectopia

Pinckney LE, Moskowitz PS, Lebowitz RL, Fritzsche P: Renal malposition associated with omphalocele. Radiology 1978;129:677.

Thoracic Kidney

Angulo JC, Lopez JI, Vilanova JR, Flores N: Intrathoracic kidney and vertebral fusion: A model of combined misdevelopment. J Urol 1992; 147:1351.

Barloon JW, Goodwin WEJ: Thoracic kidney: Case reports. J Urol 1957; 78:356.

Berlin HS, Stein J, Poppel MH: Congenital superior ectopia of the kidney. AJR Am J Roentgenol 1957;78:508.

Burke EC, Wenzl JE, Utz DC: The intrathoracic kidney: Report of a case. Am J Dis Child 1967;113:487.

Campbell MF: Renal ectopy. J Urol 1930;24:187.

DeCastro FJ, Shumacher H: Asymptomatic thoracic kidney. Clin Pediatr 1969;8:279.

DeNoronha LL, Costa MFE, Godinho MTM: Ectopic thoracic kidney. Am Rev Respir Dis 1974;109:678.

Donat SM, Donat PE: Intrathoracic kidney: A case report with a review of the world's literature. J Urol 1988;140:131.

Franciskovic V, Martincic N: Intrathoracic kidney. Br J Urol 1959;31:156.

Fusonie D, Molnar W: Anomalous pulmonary venous return, pulmonary sequestration, bronchial atresia, aplastic right upper lobe, pericardial defect and intrathoracic kidney: An unusual complex of congenital anomalies in one patient. AJR Am J Roentgenol 1966;97:350.

Hertz M, Shahin N: Ectopic thoracic kidney. Isr J Med Sci 1969;5:98.

Hill JE, Bunts RC: Thoracic kidney: Case reports. J Urol 1960;84:460.

Liddell RM, Rosenbaum DM, Blumhaen JD: Delayed radiologic appearance of bilateral thoracic ectopic kidneys. AJR Am J Roentgenol 1989; 152:120.

Lozano RH, Rodriguez C: Intrathoracic ectopic kidney: Report of a case. J Urol 1975;114:601.

Lundius B: Intrathoracic kidney. AJR Am J Roentgenol 1975;125:678.

N'Guessan G, Stephens FD: Congenital superior ectopic (thoracic) kidney. Urology 1984;24:219.

Paul ATS, Uragoda CG, Jayewardene FLW: Thoracic kidney with report of a case. Br J Surg 1960;47:395.

Shapira E, Fishel E, Levin S: Intrathoracic kidney in a premature infant. Arch Dis Child 1965;40:86.

Spillane RJ, Prather C: Right diaphragmatic eventration with renal displacement: Case report. J Urol 1952;68:804.

Williams AG, Christie JH, Mettler SA: Intrathoracic kidney on radionuclide renography. Clin Nucl Med 1983;8:408.

Anomalies of Form and Fusion

Crossed Renal Ectopia With and Without Fusion

Abeshouse BS, Bhisitkul I: Crossed renal ectopia with and without fusion. Urol Int 1959;9:63.

Alexander JC, King KB, Fromm CS: Congenital solitary kidney with crossed ureter. J Urol 1950;64:230.

Ashley DJB, Mostofi FK: Renal agenesis and dysgenesis. J Urol 1960;83: 211.

Baggenstoss AH: Congenital anomalies of the kidney. Med Clin North Am 1951;35:987.

Barnewolt CE, Lebowitz RL: Absence of a renal sinus echo complex in the ectopic kidney of a child: A normal finding. Pediatr Radiol 1996; 26:18–23.

Boatman DL, Culp DA Jr, Culp DA, Flocks RH: Crossed renal ectopia. J Urol 1972;108:30.

Caine M: Crossed renal ectopia without fusion. Br J Urol 1956;28:257.

Caldamone AA, Rabinowitz R: Crossed fused renal ectopia, orthotopic multicystic dysplasia and vaginal agenesis. J Urol 1981;126:105.

Campbell MF: Anomalies of the kidney. In Campbell MF, Harrison JH (eds): Urology, vol 2, 3rd ed. Philadelphia, WB Saunders, 1970, pp 1447–1452.

Cook WA, Stephens FD: Fused kidneys: Morphologic study and theory of embryogenesis. In Bergsma D, Duckett JW (eds): Urinary System Malformations in Children. New York, Allen R. Liss, 1977.

Currarino G, Weisbruch GJ: Transverse fusion of the renal pelves and single ureter. Urol Radiol 1989;11:88.

Diaz G: Renal ectopy: Report of a case with crossed ectopy without fusion, with fixation of kidney in normal position by the extraperitoneal route. J Int Coll Surg 1953;19:158.

Dretler SP, Olsson CA, Pfister RC: The anatomic, radiologic and clinical characteristics of the pelvic kidney: An analysis of eighty-six cases. J Urol 1971;105:623.

Gerber WL, Culp DA, Brown RC, et al: Renal mass in crossed-fused ectopia. J Urol 1980;123:239.

Gleason PE, Kelalis PP, Husmann DA, Kramer SA: Hydronephrosis in renal ectopia: Incidence, etiology and significance. J Urol 1994;151:1660.

Greenberg LW, Nelsen CE: Crossed fused ectopia of the kidneys in twins. Am J Dis Child 1971;122:175.

Gu L, Alton DJ: Crossed solitary renal ectopia. Urology 1991;38:556.

Hendren WH, Donahoe PK, Pfister RC: Crossed renal ectopia in children. Urology 1976;7:135.

Hertz M, Rabenstein ZJ, Shairin N, Melzer M: Crossed renal ectopia: Clinical and radiologic findings in 22 cases. Clin Radioli 1977;28:339.

Hildreth TA, Cass AS: Cross renal ectopia with familial occurrence. Urology 1978;12:59.

Joly JS: Fusion of the kidneys. Proc R Soc Med 1940;33:697.

Kakei H, Kondo A, Ogisu BI, Mitsuya H: Crossed ectopia of solitary kidney: A report of two cases and a review of the literature. Urol Int 1976;31:40.

Kelalis PP, Malek RS, Segura JW: Observations on renal ectopia and fusion in children. J Urol 1973;110:588.

Kron SD, Meranze DR: Completely fused pelvic kidney. J Urol 1949;62:278.

Lee HP: Crossed unfused renal ectopia with tumor. J Urol 1949;61:333.

Macksood MJ, James RE Jr: Giant hydronephrosis in ectopic kidney in a child. Urology 1983;22:532.

Magri J: Solitary crossed ectopic kidney. Br J Urol 1961;33:152.

Maizels M, Stephens FD: Renal ectopia and congenital scoliosis. Invest Urol 1979;17:209.

Malek RS, Utz DC: Crossed, fused, renal ectopia with an ectopic ureterocele. J Urol 1970;104:665.

McDonald JH, McClellan DS: Crossed renal ectopia. Am J Surg 1957;93:995.

Miles BJ, Moon MR, Bellville WD, Keesling VJ: Solitary crossed renal ectopia. J Urol 1985;133:1022.

Mininberg DT, Roze S, Yoon HJ, Parl M: Hypertension associated with crossed renal ectopia in an infant. Pediatrics 1971;48:454.

Nussbaum AR, Hartman DS, Whitley N, et al: Multicystic dysplasia and crossed renal ectopia. AJR Am J Roentgenol 1987;149:407.

Potter EL: Pathology of the Fetus and the Newborn. Chicago, Year Book Medical Publishers, 1952.

Purpon I: Crossed renal ectopy with solitary kidney: A review of the literature. J Urol 1963;90:13.

Rubinstein ZJ, Hertz M, Shahin N, Deutsch V: Crossed renal ectopia: Angiographic findings in six cases. AJR Am J Roentgenol 1976;126:1035.

Semerci B, Verit A, Nazli O, et al: The role of ESWL in the treatment of calculi with anomalous kidneys. Eur Urol 1997;31:302–304.

Stubbs AJ, Resnick MI: Struvite staghorn calculi in crossed renal ectopia. J Urol 1977;118:369.

Trabrisky J, Bhisitkul I: Solitary crossed ectopic kidney with vaginal aplasia. A case report. J Urol 1965;94:33.

Tanenbaum B, Silverman N, Weinberg SR: Solitary crossed renal ectopia. Arch Surg 1970;101:616.

Wilmer HA: Unilateral fused kidney: A report of five cases and a review of the literature. J Urol 1938;40:551.

Winram RG, Ward-McQuaid JN: Crossed renal ectopia without fusion. Can Med Assoc J 1959;81:481.

Yates-Bell AJ, Packham DA: Giant hydronephrosis in a solitary crossed ectopic kidney. Br J Surg 1972;59:104.

Horseshoe Kidney

Beck WC, Hlivko AE: Wilms' tumor in the isthmus of a horseshoe kidney. Arch Surg 1960–81:803.

Bell R: Horseshoe kidney in pregnancy. J Urol 1946;56:159.

Benjamin JA, Schulian DM: Observation on fused kidneys with horseshoe configuration: The contribution of Leonardo Botallo (1564). J Hist Med Allied Sci 1950;5:315.

Blackard CE, Mellinger GT: Cancer in a horseshoe kidney. Arch Surg 1968;97:616.

Boatman DL, Cornell SH, Kolln CP: The arterial supply of horseshoe kidney. AJR Am J Roentgenol 1971;113:447.

Boatman DL, Kolln CP, Flocks RH: Congenital anomalies associated with horseshoe kidney. J Urol 1972;107:205.

Boullier J, Chehval MJ, Purcell MH: Removal of a multicystic half of a horseshoe kidney: Significance of pre-operative evaluation in identifying abnormal surgical anatomy. J Pediatr Surg 1992;27:1244.

Boyden EA: Description of a horseshoe kidney associated with left inferior vena cava and disc-shaped suprarenal lands, together with a note on the occurrence of horseshoe kidneys in human embryos. Anat Rec 1931;51:187.

Bridge RAC: Horseshoe kidneys in identical twins. Br J Urol 1960;32:32.

Buntley D: Malignancy associated with horseshoe kidney. Urology 1976; 8:146.

Campbell MF: Anomalies of the kidney. In Campbell MF, Harrison JH (eds): Urology, vol 2, 3rd ed. Philadelphia, WB Saunders, 1970, pp 1447–1452.

Castor JE, Green NA: Complications of horseshoe kidney. Urology 1975; 6:344.

Christoffersen J, Iversen HG: Partial hydronephrosis in a patient with horseshoe kidney and bilateral duplication of the pelvis and ureter. Scand J Urol Nephrol 1976;10:91.

Cook WA, Stephens FD: Fused kidneys: Morphologic study and theory of embryogenesis. In Bergsma D, Duckett JW (eds): Urinary System Malformations in Children. New York, Allen R. Liss, 1977.

Correa RJ Jr, Paton RR: Polycystic horseshoe kidney. J Urol 1976;116:802.

Craver RD, Ortenberg J, Baliga R: Glomerulocystic disease: Unilateral involvement of a horseshoe kidney in trisomy 18. Pediatr Nephrol 1993;7:375.

Dajani AM: Horseshoe kidney: A review of twenty-nine cases. Br J Urol 1966;38:388.

Das S, Amar AD: Ureteropelvic junction obstruction with associated renal anomalies. J Urol 1984;131:872.

David RS: Horseshoe kidney: A report of one family. Br Med J 1974;4:571.

deBrito CJ, Silva LA, Fonseca Filho VL, Fernandes DC; Abdominal aortic aneurysm in association with horseshoe kidney. Int Angiol 1991; 10:122.

Dees J: Clinical importance of congenital anomalies of upper urinary tract. J Urol 1941;46:659.

Department of Health and Human Services: 2000 Annual Report: The US Scientific Registry of Transplant Recipients and the Organ Procurement and Transplantation Network, United Network for Organ Sharing, HRSA, 2000.

Dische MR, Johnston R: Teratoma in horseshoe kidneys. Urology 1979; 13:435.

Domenech-Mateu JM, Gonzales-Compta X: Horseshoe kidney: A new theory on its embryogenesis based on the study of a 16-mm human embryo. Anat Rec 1988;222:408.

Eidelman A, Yuval E, Simon D, Sibi Y: Retrocaval ureter. Eur Urol 1978;4:279.

Evans WP, Resnick MI: Horseshoe kidney and urolithiasis. J Urol 1981; 125:620.

Glenn JF: Analysis of 51 patients with horseshoe kidney. N Engl J Med 1959;261:684.

Gradone CH, Haller JO, Berdon WE, Friedman AP: Asymmetric horseshoe kidney in the infant: Value of renal nuclear scanning. Radiology 1985;154:366.

Gutierrez R: The Clinical management of Horseshoe Kidney: A Study of

Horseshoe Kidney Disease, Its Etiology, Pathology, Symptomatology, Diagnosis and Treatment. New York, Paul B. Hoeber, 1934.

Hefferman JC, Lightwood RG, Snell ME: Horseshoe kidney with retrocaval ureter: Second reported case. J Urol 1978;120:358.

Hohenfellner M, Schultz-Lampel D, Lampel A, et al: Tumor in the horseshoe kidney: Clinical implications and review of embryogenesis. J Urol 1992;147:1098.

Huber D, Griffin A, Niesche J, et al: Aortic aneurysm in the presence of a horseshoe kidney. Aust N Z J Surg 1990;60:963.

Jarmin WD: Surgery of the horseshoe kidney with a postaortic isthmus: Report of two cases of horseshoe kidney. J Urol 1938;40:1.

Kelalis PP: Anomalies of the urinary tract: The kidney. In Kelalis PP, Kin LR (eds): Clinical Pediatric Urology. Philadelphia, WB Saunders, 1976, p 492.

Kolln CP, Boatman DL, Schmidt JD, Flocks RH: Horseshoe kidney: A review of 105 patients. J Urol 1972;107:203.

Kupeli B, Isen K, Biri H, et al: Extracorporeal shockwave lithotripsy in anomalous kidneys. J Endourol 1999;13:349–352.

Leiter E: Horseshoe kidney: Discordance in monozygotic twins. J Urol 1972;108:683.

Lippe B, Geffner ME, Dietrich RB, et al: Renal malformations in patients with Turner syndrome: Imaging in 141 patients. Pediatrics 1988;82:852.

Love L, Wasserman D: Massive unilateral nonfunctioning hydronephrosis in horseshoe kidney. Clin Radiol 1975;26:409.

McDonald R, Donaldson L, Emmett L, Tejani A: A decade of living donor transplantation in North American children: The 1998 Annual Report of the North American Pediatric Renal Transplant Cooperative Study (NAPRTCS). Pediatric Transplantation 2000;4:221–234.

Meek JR, Wadsworth GH: A case of horseshoe kidney lying between the great vessels. J Urol 1940;43:448.

Mesrobian H-GJ, Kelalis PP, Hrabovsky E, et al: Wilms' tumor in horseshoe kidneys: A report from the National Wilms' Tumor Study. J Urol 1985;133:1002.

Murphy DM, Zincke H: Transitional cell carcinoma in the horseshoe kidney: Report of 3 cases and review of the literature. Br J Urol 1982;54:484.

Nation EF: Horseshoe kidney: A study of thirty-two autopsy and nine surgical cases. J Urol 1945;53:762.

Noval ME, Baum NH, Gonzales ET: Horseshoe kidney with multicystic dysplasia associated ureterocele. Urology 1977;10:456.

Pitts WR, Muecke EC: Horseshoe kidneys: A 40 year experience. J Urol 1975;113:743.

Segura JW, Kelalis PP, Burke EG: Horseshoe kidney in children. J Urol 1972;108:333.

Sharma SK, Bapna BC: Surgery of the horseshoe kidney: An experience of 24 patients. Aust N Z J Surg 1986;56:175.

Sherer DM, Woods JR Jr: Antenatal diagnosis of horseshoe kidney. J Ultrasound Med 1992;11:274.

Shoup GD, Pollack HM, Dou JH: Adenocarcinoma occurring in a horseshoe kidney. Arch Surg 1962;84:413.

Smith DW: Recognizable patterns of human malformation: Genetic embryologic and clinical aspects. In Smith DW: Major Problems in Clinical Pediatrics, vol 7. Philadelphia, WB Saunders, 1970, p 50.

Smith EC, Orkin LA: A clinical and statistical study of 471 congenital anomalies of the kidney and ureter. J Urol 1945;53:11.

Van Every MJ: In utero detection of horseshoe kidney with unilateral multicystic dysplasia. Urology 1992;40:435.

Voisin M, Djernit A, Morin D, et al: Cardiopathies congenitales et malformations urinaires. Arch Mal Coeur Vaiss 1988;81:703.

Whitaker RH, Hunt GM: Incidence and distribution of renal anomalies in patients with neural tube defects. Eur Urol 1987;13:322.

Whitehouse GH: Some urographic aspects of the horseshoe kidney anomaly: A review of 59 cases. Clin Radiol 1975;26:107.

Zondek LH, Zondek T: Horseshoe kidney in associated congenital malformations. Urol Int 1964;18:347.

Anomalies of Rotation

Campbell MF: Anomalies of the kidney. In Campbell MF (ed): Urology, vol 2, 2nd ed. Philadelphia, WB Saunders, 1963, p 1589.

Felix W: The development of the urogenital organs. In Keibel F, Mall FP (eds): Manual of Human Embryology, vol 2. Philadelphia, JB Lippincott, 1912, p 752.

Gray SW, Skandalakis JE: The kidney and ureter. In Gray SW, Skandalakis JE (eds): Embryology for Surgeons. Philadelphia, WB Saunders, 1972, p 480.

Mackie GG, Awang H, Stephens FD: The ureteric orifice: The embryologic key to radiologic status of duplex kidneys. J Pediatr Surg 1975;10:473.

Smith EC, Orkin LA: A clinical and statistical study of 471 congenital anomalies of the kidney and ureter. J Urol 1945;53:11.

Weyrauch HM Jr: Anomalies of renal rotation. Surg Gynecol Obstet 1939;69:183.

Anomalies of the Renal Vasculature

Aberrant, Accessory, or Multiple Vessels

Anson BJ, Daseler EH: Common variations in renal anatomy, affecting the blood supply, form and topography. Surg Gynecol Obstet 1961;112:439.

Anson BJ, Kurth LE: Common variations in the renal blood supply. Surg Gynecol Obstet 1955;100:157.

Fraley EE: Vascular obstruction of superior infundibulum causing nephralgia: A new syndrome. N Engl J Med 1966;275:1403.

Fraley EE: Dismembered infundibulopyelostomy: Improved technique for correcting vascular obstruction of the superior infundibulum. J Urol 1969;101:144.

Geyer JR, Poutasse EF: Incidence of multiple renal arteries on aortography. JAMA 1962;183:118.

Graves FT: The aberrant renal artery. J Anat 1956;90:553.

Graves FT: The anatomy of the intrarenal arteries and its application to segmental resection of the kidney. Br J Surg 1954;42:132.

Gray SW, Skandalakis JE: Anomalies of the kidney and ureter. In Gray SW, Skandalakis JE (eds): Embryology for Surgeons. Philadelphia, WB Saunders, 1972, p. 485.

Guggemos E: A rare case of an arterial connection between the left and right kidneys. Ann Surg 1962;156:940.

Merklin RJ, Michele NA: The variant renal and suprarenal blood supply with data on the inferior phrenic, ureteral and gonadal arteries: A statistical analysis based on 185 dissections and review of the literature. J Int Coll Surg 1958;29:41.

Nathan J: Observation on aberrant renal arteries curving around and compressing the renal vein: Possible relationship to orthostatic proteinuria and to orthostatic hypertension. Circulation 1958;18:1131.

Salcarga ME, Arslan H, Unal O: The role of power Doppler sonography in the renal evaluation of fetal renal vasculature. Clin Imaging 1999;23:32.

Sampaio FJB, Aragao AHM: Anatomical relationship between the intrarenal arteries and the kidney collecting system. J Urol 1990a;143:679.

Sampaio FJB, Aragao AHM: Anatomical relationship between the renal venous arrangement and the kidney collecting system. J Urol 1990b;143:679.

Textor SC, Canzanello VJ: Radiologic evaluation of the renal vasculature. Curr Opin Nephrol Hypertens 1996;5:541.

Renal Artery Aneurysm

Abeshouse BS: Renal aneurysm: Report of two cases and review of the literature. Urol Cutan Rev 1951;55:451.

Bulbul MA, Farrow GA: Renal artery aneurysms. Urology 1992;40;124.

Bunchman TE, Walker HS, Joyce PF, et al: Sonographic evaluation of renal artery aneurysm in childhood. Pediatr Radiol 1991;21:312.

Cerny JC, Chang CY, Fry WJ: Renal artery aneurysms. Arch Surg 1968;96:653.

Cohen JR, Shamash FS: Ruptured renal artery aneurysms during pregnancy. J Vasc Surg 1987;6:51.

Garritano AP: Aneurysm of the renal artery. Am J Surg 1957;94:638.

Glass PM, Uson AC: Aneurysms of the renal artery: A study of 20 cases. J Urol 1967;98:285.

Hageman JH, Smith RF, Szilagyi DE, Elliot JP: Aneurysms of the renal artery: Problems of prognosis and surgical management. Surgery. 1978;84:563.

Lorentz WB Jr, Browning MC, D'Souza VJ, et al: Intrarenal aneurysm of the renal artery in children. Am J Dis Child 1984;138:751.

McKeil CF Jr, Graf EC, Callahan DH: Renal artery aneurysms: A report of 16 cases. J Urol 1966;96:593.

Okamato M, Hashimoto M, Sueda T, et al: Renal artery aneurysm: The significance of abdominal bruit and use of color Doppler. Intern Med 1992;31:1217.

Poutasse EF: Renal artery aneurysm: Report of 12 cases, two treated by excision of the renal aneurysma and repair of renal artery. J Urol 1957; 77:697.

Poutasse EF: Renal artery aneurysms. J Urol 1975;113:443.

Sarker R, Coran AG, Cilley RE, et al: Arterial aneurysms in children: Clinicopathologic classification. J Vasc Surg 1991;13:47.

Schievink WI: Genetics and aneurysm formation. Neurosurg Clin North Am 1998;9:485–495.

Silvis RS, Hughes WF, Holmes FH: Aneurysm of the renal artery. Am J Surg 1956;91:339.

Stanley JC, Rhodes EL, Gewertz GL, et al: Renal artery aneurysms: Significance of macroaneurysms exclusive of dissections and fibrodysplastic mural dilations. Arch Surg 1975;110:1327.

Takebayashi S, Ohno T, Tanaka K, et al: MR angiography of renal vascular malformations. J Comp Assist Tomo 1994;18:596.

Yamamoto N, Ishihara S, Yoshimura S, et al: Endovascular embolization of a renal artery aneurysm using interlocking coils. Scand J Urol Nephrol 1998;32:143.

Zinman L, Libertino JA: Uncommon disorders of the renal circulation: Renal artery aneurysm. In Breslin DJ, Swinton NW, Libertino JA, Zinman L (eds): Renovascular Hypertension. Baltimore, Williams & Wilkins, 1982, pp 110–114.

Renal Arteriovenous Fistula

Bentson JR, Crandall PH: Use of the Fogarty catheter in arteriovenous malformations of the spinal cord. Radiology 1972;105:65.

Boijsen E, Kohler R: Renal arteriovenous fistulae. Acta Radiol 1962;57: 433.

Bookstein JJ, Goldstein HM: Successful management of post biopsy arteriovenous fistula with selective arterial embolization. Radiology 1973; 109:535.

Cho KJ, Stanley JC: Non-neoplastic congenital and acquired renal arteriovenous malformations and fistula. Radiology 1978;129:333.

Crummy AB Jr, Atkinson RJ, Caruthers SB: Congenital renal arteriovenous fistulas. J Urol 1965;93:24.

DeSai SG, DeSautels RE: Congenital arteriovenous malformation of the kidney. J Urol 1973;110:17.

Gunterberg B: Renal arteriovenous malformation. Acta Radiol 1968;7:425.

Maldonado JE, Sheps SG, Bernatz PE, et al: Renal arteriovenous fistula. Am J Med 1964;37:499.

McAlhany JC Jr, Black HC, Hanback LD Jr, Yarbrough DR III: Renal arteriovenous fistulas as a cause of hypertension. Am J Surg 1971;122: 117.

Messing E, Kessler R, Kavaney RB: Renal arteriovenous fistula. Urology 1976;8:101.

Mohaupt MG, Perrig M, Vogt B: 3D ultrasound imaging: A useful noninvasive tool to detect A-V fistulas in transplanted kidneys. Nephrol Dial Transplant 1999;14:943.

Takaha M, Matsumoto A, Ochi K, et al: Intrarenal arteriovenous malformation. J Urol 1980;124:315.

Thomason WB, Ross M, Radwin HM, et al: Intrarenal arteriovenous fistulas. J Urol 1972;108:526.

Yazaki T, Tomita M, Akimoto M, et al: Congenital renal arteriovenous fistula: Case report, review of Japanese literature and description of nonradical treatment. J Urol 1976;116:415.

Anomalies of the Collecting System

Calyx and Infundibulum

Abeshouse BS: Serous cysts of the kidney and their differentiation from other cystic diseases of the kidney. Urol Cutan Rev 1950;54:582.

Amar A: The clinical significance of renal caliceal diverticulum in children: Relation to vesicoureteral reflux. J Urol 1975;113:255.

Baldwin DD, Beaghler MA, Ruckle HC, et al: Ureteroscopic treatment of symptomatic caliceal diverticular calculi. Tech Urol 1998;4:92.

Bischel MD, Blustein WC, Kinnas NC, et al: Solitary renal calix. JAMA 1978;240:2467–2468.

Boyce WH, Whitehurst AW: Hypoplasia of the major renal conduits. J Urol 1976;116:352.

Briner V, Thiel G: Hereditares Poland syndrom mit megacalicose der rechten niere. Schweitz Med Wochenschr 1988;118:898.

Cacciaguerra S, Bagnara V, Arena C, et al: Megacalycosis on duplex system upper moiety. Eur J Pediatr Surg 1996;6:42.

Devine CJ Jr, Guzman JA, Devine PC, Poutasse EF: Calyceal diverticulum. J Urol 1969;101:8.

Eisendrath DN: Report of case of hydronephrosis in kidney with extrarenal calyces. J Urol 1925;13:51.

Ellis JH, Patterson SK, Sonda LP, et al: Stones and infection in renal caliceal diverticula: Treatment with percutaneous procedures. AJR Am J Roentgenol 1990;156:995.

Fraley EE: Vascular obstruction of superior infundibulum causing nephralgia: New syndrome. N Engl J Med 1966;275:1403.

Galian P, Forest M, Aboulker P: La megacaliose. Nouv Presse Med 1970; 78:1663.

Gittes RF: Congenital megacalices. Monogr Urol 1984;5:1.

Gittes RF, Talner LB: Congenital megacalyces vs. obstructive hydronephrosis. J Urol 1972;108:833.

Goldfischer ER, Stravodimos KG, Jabbour ME, et al: Percutaneous removal of stone from caliceal diverticulum in patient with nephroptosis. J Endourol 1998;12:356.

Hoznek A, Herard A, Ogiez N, et al: Symptomatic caliceal diverticula treated with extraperitoneal laparoscopic marsupialization, fulguration and gelatin resorcinol formaldehyde glue obliteration. J Urol 1998;160:352.

Harrison RB, Wood JL, Gillenwater JY: A solitary calyx in a human kidney. Radiology 1976;121:310.

Husmann DA, Kramer SA, Malek RS, Allen TD: Infundibulopelvic stenosis: A long-term follow-up. J Urol 1994;152:837.

Imamoglu T, Balkanci F, Unsal M, Ozturk MH: One calyx one ureter. Int Urol Nephrol 1998;30:429.

Johnston JH, Sandomirsky SK: Intrarenal vascular obstruction of the superior infundibulum in children. J Pediatr Surg 1972;7:318.

Kaneto H, Metoki R, Fukuzaki A, et al: Unicalyceal kidney associated with ureteral anomalies. Eur Urol 1997;32:328.

Kelalis PP, Malek RS: Infundibulopelvic stenosis. J Urol 1981;125:568.

Kozakewich HPW, Lebowitz FL: Congenital megacalices. Pediatr Radiol 1974;2:251.

Lang EK: Percutaneous infundibuloplasty: Management of calyceal diverticula and infundibular stenosis. Radiology 1991;181:871.

Lister J, Singh H: Pelvicalyceal cysts in children. J Pediatr Surg 1973;8: 901.

Malament M, Schwartz B, Nagamatsu GR: Extrarenal calyces: Their relationship to renal disease. AJR Am J Roentgenol 1961;86:823.

Malek RS: Obstructive uropathy: Calyx. In Kelalis PP, King LR (eds): Clinical Pediatric Urology. Philadelphia, WB Saunders, 1976, p 235.

Mandell GA, Snyder HM 3rd, Haymen SK, et al: Association of congenital megacalycosis and ipsilateral segmental megaureter. Pediatr Radiol 1987;17:28.

Mathieson AJM: Calyceal diverticulum: A case with a discussion and a review of the condition. Br J Urol 1953;25:147.

McMillan PJ, Gingell JC, Penry JB: Bilateral unipapillary kidneys and hematuria. J R Soc Med 1987;80:456–457.

Middleton AW Jr, Pfister RC: Stone-containing pyelocaliceal diverticulum: Embryogenic, anatomic, radiologic and clinical characteristics. J Urol 1974;111:1.

Moore T: Hydrocalycosis. Br J Urol 1950;22:304.

Morimoto S, Sangen H, Takamatsu M, et al: Solitary calix in siblings. J Urol 1979;122:690.

Neal A, Murphy L: Unipapillary kidney: An unusual developmental abnormality of the kidney. J Coll Radiol Aust 1960;4:81.

Parker JA, Lebowitz R, Mascatello V, Treves S: Magnification renal scintigraphy in differential diagnosis of septa of Bertin. Pediatr Radiol 1976;4:157.

Patriquin H, Lafortune M, Filiatrault D: Urinary milk of calcium in children and adults: Use of gravity-dependent sonography. AJR Am J Roentgenol 1985;144:407.

Puigvert A: Megacaliosis: Diagnostico diferencial con la hidrocaliectasia. Med Clin (Barc) 1963;41:294.

Puigvert A: Megacalicose: Diagnostic differential avec l'hydrocaliectasia. Helv Chir Acta 1964;31:414.

Sakatoku J, Kitayama T: Solitary unipapillary kidney: Presentation of a case. Acta Urol Jpn 1964;10:349.

Schneck FX, Bauer SB, Peters CA, Kavoussi LR: Natural history and management of calyceal diverticula in children [Abstract No. 185]

Presented at the annual meeting of the American Urological Association, San Francisco, May 15, 1994.

Siegel MJ, McAlister WH: Calyceal diverticula in children: Unusual features and complications. Radiology 1979;131:79.

Smith SJ, Cass AS, Aliabadi H, et al: Unipapillary kidney: A case report and review of the literature. Urol Radiol 1984;6:43–47.

Timmons JW Jr, Malek RS, Hattery RR, DeWeerd J: Caliceal diverticulum. J Urol 1975;114:6.

Toppercer A: Unipapillary human kidney associated with urinary and genital abnormalities. Urology 1980;16:194.

Uhlenhuth E, Amin M, Harty JI, Howerton LW: Infundibular dysgenesis: A spectrum of obstructive renal disease. Urology 1990;35:334.

Vela Navarrete R, Garcia Robledo J: Polycystic disease of the renal sinus: Structural characteristics. J Urol 1983;129:700.

Williams DI, Mininberg DT: Hydrocalycosis: Report of three cases in children. Br J Urol 1968;40:541.

Wulfsohn M: Pyelocaliceal diverticula. J Urol 1980;123:1.

Pelvis

Johnson JF: Ureteropelvic junction obstruction associated with extrarenal pelvis: A potential cause of cystic abdominal mass anterior to a normal appearing kidney in the newborn. J Clin Ultrasound 1999; 27:474.

56
RENAL DYSGENESIS AND CYSTIC DISEASE OF THE KIDNEY

Kenneth I. Glassberg, M.D.

Not so long ago the student of urology thought of normal kidney development simply in terms of a ureteric bud developing from the wolffian duct at 4 weeks of gestation and growing toward a cluster of mesenchymal cells, where it would induce metanephric development. Today, a basic knowledge of molecular genetics is required to better understand normal renal development, absence of renal development, and the effects of genetic mutations and abnormal signaling proteins on renal maldevelopment and cystic diseases. This chapter begins with a simplified interpretation of the molecular genetics of renal development. The remainder of the chapter is devoted to renal maldevelopment in terms of dysgenesis and cystic disease. Understanding the molecular genetics of renal development will help the reader to understand the genetic and molecular defects of many of the conditions discussed.

1925

MOLECULAR GENETICS OF RENAL DEVELOPMENT

If a mutant gene is responsible for maldevelopment of an organ in utero, that gene in its normal form is likely to play an integral role in normal organogenesis. Likewise, if a mutant gene is responsible for the development of a tumor in an organ later in life, that gene in its normal state most likely acts as a tumor suppressor gene postnatally and may play a role in regulating the growth of cells in utero. This section discusses a number of gene defects that are responsible for renal disease or maldevelopment and how some of these same genes, when normal, play a part in normal renal development.

Classic Genetics

Typically, geneticists follow a sequence to identify a gene that causes a specific disease. The sequence starts with mapping the area of a chromosome where a gene is located. This is facilitated by finding common flanking genetic markers in a specific chromosomal area in multiple affected family members. The genetic markers will be the same in all affected members within a family but will be different from the markers in unaffected family members. An effort is made to find closer flanking genetic markers that are "linked" to the disease gene, progressively leading to a very small area. Once the gene site is identified, the gene can be cloned. Geneticists then create defects in that gene in animal models and observe whether a similar malfunction, disease, or tumor results. When sporadic cases exist, the geneticist must determine whether the same gene defect is involved. For example, **von Hippel–Lindau disease (VHL) is inherited in 70% of patients, but in 30% the disease is sporadic and is not present in other family members. However, whether inherited or sporadic, the same gene is defective in both, although the defect may differ from patient to patient** (Zbar et al, 1996; Neumann and Zbar, 1997).

Genes and Their Products

The protein product of a gene often has the same name as the gene. When that is the case, a lower case "p" precedes the name of the protein product. For example, the WNT4 gene produces the glycoprotein pWNT4. Whether the WNT4 gene is normal or abnormal, it is still called WNT4. In general, when a gene is normal its protein product is normal as well. When a gene is abnormal, it produces an abnormal protein that can lead to maldevelopment or disease. When a defective gene is responsible for a disease, that gene, when normal or even when abnormal, often is named after the disease. For example, the gene responsible for the entity von Hippel–Lindau disease (VHL) is called the VHL gene either in its normal state performing its normal activities or in its mutant state causing the disease to manifest. When normal, VHL is a tumor suppressor gene; when abnormal, it can play a role in mitogenesis.

Sometimes more than one gene is responsible for a specific disease. For example, an abnormality of one of two genes is responsible for the entity tuberous sclerosis. One tuberous sclerosis gene, TSC1, is located on chromosome 2 and the second, TSC2, on chromosome 16. In autosomal dominant polycystic kidney disease (ADPKD), an abnormality in any one of three genes is responsible for manifestation of the disease. The PKD1 gene is located on chromosome 16 and the PKD2 gene on chromosome 4; a PKD3 gene is believed to exist, but its location has not yet been identified.

Polycystin-1 is a long-chain glycoprotein produced by the ADPKD gene PKD1 on chromosome 16. Polycystin-2 is produced by the PKD2 gene on chromosome 4. These two genes seem to play a role, along with the signaling molecule WNT4, in normal tubulogenesis in the developing metanephrenic kidney. When either the PKD1 or the PKD2 gene is abnormal, cystic kidneys can develop. Because defects of PKD1 and PKD2 manifest similarly, Qian and associates (1996) suggested that the gene product of each is involved in the same pathway and that an abnormality of either product results in similar manifestation of the disease.

Murcia and colleagues (1999) hypothesized that a macromolecular complex involving polycystin-1 and -2 and a protein called pTg737 work together to form the nephron tubule. The latter protein is produced by the Tg737 gene and, when abnormal, is associated with a form of recessive polycystic kidney disease in mice. It was originally thought that this Tg737 gene was also the gene responsible for autosomal recessive polycystic kidney disease (ARPKD) in humans. However, Tg737 in humans is located on chromosome 13, whereas the gene responsible for ARPKD is located on chromosome 6. pTg737 in yeast has the potential to interact with polycystin, which is one reason why Murcia and colleagues (1999) chose to include it in their hypothesized macromolecular complex. This example shows that similar genes with similar functions may be present in different species, but the location of the gene may vary greatly between species.

Two-Hit Theory

Each gene within a cell is one of a set of two, each called an allele. One defective allele may be the carrier for the defect. Its normal allele is referred to as the "wild type." In Knudson's (1991) two-hit theory, the first hit in an inherited mutation is found in all cells of an individual (i.e., a germ-line mutation). The second hit occurs when the wild-type allele spontaneously mutates within a specific organ, although it may be a different mutation than in the primarily affected allele (Knudson, 1993).

For example, the typical somatic cells in the kidney and all other cells of a patient with VHL typically are heterozygous for the VHL gene located on chromosome 3; that is, the mutant VHL allele is inherited and its mate is the normal wild-type allele. However, the configuration of the wild-type VHL gene makes it prone to spontaneous mutation. If the wild-type allele develops a defect within the cells of a specific organ, those cells no longer are able to produce wild-type pVHL with its suppressor properties.

That organ then has the propensity to develop a tumor. In kidney cells of individuals with VHL, for example, heterozygosity is lost when the wild-type allele mutates, and there is a propensity to develop a clear cell renal cell carcinoma. To determine whether cysts lined with epithelial cells are predisposed to renal cell carcinoma (RCC), Lubensky and coworkers (1996) studied partial nephrectomy specimens of two patients with familial VHL with RCC who underwent renal-sparing surgery. The makeup of 26 cysts was studied with microdissection techniques. Each cyst was found to be lined with a single layer of clear epithelial cells. Twenty-five of the 26 cysts had a mutation of the wild-type allele; in only one case was the usual heterozygosity of the disease maintained. This finding supports the two-hit theory. Once the heterozygosity for VHL is lost in a specific organ, in this case the kidney, the cyst can progress into a tumor. However, the progression to RCC in VHL typically is slow.

The variability in manifestations of ADPKD may be related to a two-hit phenomenon as well. For example, ADPKD is a heterozygous condition in which one allele of the PKD1 or PKD2 set is responsible for the genetic transmission of the disease but may not be enough for cystogenesis. A spontaneous mutation of the wild-type allele may be responsible for cystogenesis or for other manifestations of the disease. Qian and associates (1996) suggested that the PKD1 gene has an unusual genomic structure that makes it readily mutable for a second hit, and the timing of this second hit may account for the phenotypic variability within one family. The second hit itself may occur only in a few cells, possibly accounting for the fact that fewer than 1% of nephrons in ADPKD eventually develop cysts (Qian et al, 1996). Within a cyst, many but not all of the lining cells have lost their heterozygosity (Brazier and Henske, 1997; Qian et al, 1999).

Signaling Molecules

Signaling molecules are protein products of genes whose appearance during development signals the initiation of a particular phase of development. The family of signaling genes referred to as the WNT family are defined by a similarity to the original Wnt-1 gene found in the mouse by Nusse and Varmus (1982). A mutation of Wnt-1 acts as an oncogene and induces mouse mammary tumors. Other WNT genes have been found in other animals. WNT genes encode glycoproteins that usually consist of a chain of 350 to 450 amino acids. In vertebrates, they are largely expressed in the nervous system and mesoderm. WNT genes are in part responsible for embryonic induction of cells to form an organ, for cell polarity, and for cell axis development. For example, another WNT gene is wg (wingless). This gene signals during the development of the wings in the *Drosophila melanogaster,* and if it is abnormal the result will be defective wings. Wnt-4 and Wnt-11 have been found to be involved with embryonic differentiation of the mouse kidney. Wnt-4 stimulates transcription processes within epithelial cells as well as the development of cell adhesion molecules that allow the kidney epithelial cells to adhere to one another in such a fashion as to take on the shape of a tubule. Wnt-11 activity

is present at a site in the wolffian duct adjacent to the site where the metanephric mesenchyme is located and is involved in ureteric branching. **The presence of Wnt-11 activity in the mouse precedes the formation of the ureteric bud, and it, along with other genes such as tyrosine kinase c-ret, induces a cascade of molecular events leading to ureteric bud formation and branching morphogenesis** (Pepicelli et al, 1997).

Another group of signaling genes involved with organogenesis is the paired box (PAX) family. Its member, PAX2, is expressed in epithelial derivatives of intermediate mesoderm such as the wolffian ducts, in branching ureteric bud ampullae, and in the metanephric blastema at the time of conversion of mesenchymal (blastemal) cells into epithelial cells. Its expression in the metanephric kidney persists in utero until nephron formation is completed. Overexpression of PAX2 in mice models can lead to renal cyst development (Dressler et al, 1993).

Wilms' Tumor Gene

The Wilms' tumor gene (WT1) is a protooncogene located on chromosome 11 (Pritchard-Jones et al, 1990). A protooncogene in its normal form is a gene that suppresses cell proliferation. In the developing metanephric blastema, insulin-like growth factor−2 (IGF-2) is present at high levels. It inhibits mesenchymal cell apoptosis, thus allowing mesenchymal cell proliferation. WT1 expression coincides with suppression of IGF-2 activity and a cascade of events that it possibly initiates, including development of the ureteric bud from the wolffian duct, ascent of the ureteric bud into the metanephric blastema, PAX2 expression, and conversion of mesenchymal cells into epithelial cells, the precursors of the nephron (Kriedberg et al, 1993). In 10% of sporadic Wilms' tumors and most familiar Wilms' tumors, the WT1 gene is defective and acts as an oncogene in accordance with the two-hit theory. In such situations, IGF-2 is not suppressed. Instead, IGF-2 levels rise and blastemal cell rests proliferate (Drummond et al, 1992). In the mouse fetus, WT1 malfunction is associated with absent ureteric bud formation, lack of PAX2 expression, and absence of mesenchymal to epithelial cell conversion.

Renal Development

At 4 weeks' gestation, the ureteric bud derived from the wolffian duct grows to adjacent mesenchymal cells that cluster and become the future metanephric kidney. **Signals from the mesenchymal cells induce ureteric bud formation from the wolffian duct as well as ureteric bud branching. Reciprocal signals from the ureteric bud and later from its branching tips induce mesenchymal cells to condense, proliferate, and convert into epithelial cells.**

The presence of a signaling agent produced by mesenchymal cells, glial cell line−derived neurotrophic factor (GDNF), precedes the branching process. The receptor for GDNF is called tyrosine kinase c-ret, and it is located on the wolffian duct, later on the tip of the ureteric bud and still later at the branching ureteric tips. In mice, either a deficiency in GDNF or an abnormality of c-ret occasionally

Table 56-1. STEPS IN RENAL DEVELOPMENT

1. GDNF from mesenchyme cells binds to tyrosine kinase c-ret receptors on the wolffian duct, signaling ureteric bud formation and subsequent ureteric bud branching.
2. pPAX2 induces mesenchyme cells to change into epithelial cells.
3. pWNT4 helps to activate β-catenin, a protein that binds epithelial cells in such a fashion as to produce a tubule, the precursor to a nephron.
4. A cleft forms at the proximal end of the tubule that will surround a cluster of capillaries to form a glomerulus.
5. The nephron tubules link distally to collecting ducts, the most peripheral branches of the branching ureteric tips.

GDNF, glial cell line–derived neurotrophic factor.

can result in renal agenesis or, in some cases, severe dysgenesis (Pichel et al, 1996). Once GDNF binds to its receptor, c-ret, WNT11 becomes activated and its protein product induces ureteric branching. The branches become future infundibuli, calyces, and collecting ducts. The tips of the branches induce the adjacent mesenchyme cells to condense around them and convert into pretubular clusters of epithelial cells. This conversion process is facilitated and modulated by PAX2. When PAX2 protein levels are reduced, mesenchymal cells fail to cluster and fail to change into epithelial cells (Rothentieler and Dressler, 1993). With normal signaling, the epithelial cells eventually form single simple tubules. A tubule, together with a proximal cluster of vessels (the glomerulus), forms the future nephron. For these epithelial cells to orient in such a way as to form a tube-like structure requires other signaling protein molecules, including pWNT4.

pWNT4 induces transcription processes within epithelial cells as well as the development of cell adhesion molecules, which in turn orient the cells to adhere to one another in such a fashion as to take on the shape of a tubule. One such adhesion molecule is β-catenin. It is located at the cytoplasmic side of the cell membrane and forms a link between the transmembrane intercellular adhesion molecule cadherin and intracellular α-catenin, binding one epithelial cell to the next to orient them in such a fashion as to form a tubule. β-catenin also binds with transcription proteins, and together these migrate to the nucleus to influence transcription processes. Mice lacking Wnt-4 have hypoplastic or absent kidneys (Stark et al, 1994). Polycystin, the protein product of PKD genes, seems to play a role in WNT4 signaling, and its presence has been localized to the ureteric tips and mesenchymal cells at a time that WNT4 can also be localized to the mesenchymal cells (Kim et al, 1997). Kim and coworkers (1997) suggested that polycystin activates the WNT4 signaling mechanism, resulting in the attachment of WNT4 to a frizzled protein membrane receptor on a tubular precursor epithelial cell. This sets up a chain of events that leads to the activation of β-catenin and increases its amount in the cytoplasm and in the nucleus (Table 56–1).

Glycogen synthetase kinase-3 (GSK-3) destabilizes or inhibits the β-catenin molecule by attaching to it. APC (adenomatous polyposis coli), a protein produced by a gene that, when abnormal in the colon, can induce adenocarcinoma, also can destabilize β-catenin by bonding with it. WNT4 blocks the destabilizing effect of GSK-3 on β-

catenin, resulting in increased levels of active β-catenin. pVHL has an opposite effect and helps the binding of the APC protein as well as GSK-3 to β-catenin, thus reducing the levels of active β-catenin (Fig. 56–1). One can theorize that pVHL later on in life, as during development, slows the transcription process of cells by enhancing APC binding of β-catenin, a transcription activating agent. In its mutant form in VHL and in some non-VHL patients who carry a mutant VHL gene line in kidney cells, renal tumors manifest because the mutant VHL gene has lost its ability to slow the transcription process (i.e., it has lost its tumor suppressive quality).

In summary, polycystin activates WNT4. WNT4 blocks the inhibitory affect of GSK-3 on β-catenin, which in turn increases the levels of β-catenin. β-catenin then becomes available to increase the speed of transcription and to help in the configuration and binding of epithelial cells so that they align in such a manner as to form a tubule (Pollack et al, 1997).

Kim and colleagues (1999) suggested that, although polycystin-1 may be required to activate WNT4 for normal tubulogenesis, it may also be required later in life "to maintain tubular structure, polarity, and integrity." Mutant mice embryos lacking both PKD1 alleles have timely tubulogenesis but soon thereafter develop proximal tubular cysts (Kim et al, 1999). One can postulate that when PKD1 heterozygosity is lost in ADPKD patients normal polycystin is not made, epithelial cells lose their ability to maintain a tubular orientation, and cysts subsequently develop.

If the PKD1 gene is prone to spontaneous mutation with age, one can consider this a possible cause for simple renal cysts in normal individuals and why their incidence increases with age. For example, theoretically a loss of normal function in both wild-type alleles could occasionally

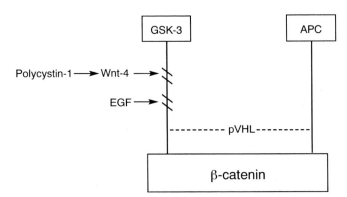

Figure 56–1. β-Catenin seems to play at least two significant roles in renal development: (1) as a transcription activator and (2) as an intercellular binding molecule necessary for aligning kidney epithelial cells in tubular fashion. When it is bound to glycogen synthetase-3 (GSK-3) or APC (adenomatous polyposis coli), it is inactivated. When it is not bound to GSK-3 or APC, it becomes activated. Polycystin-1, the normal product of the gene PKD1 (when PKD-1 is abnormal, autosomal dominant polycystic kidney disease develops), activates the signaling protein WNT-4. WNT-4 blocks the binding of GSK-3 to β-catenin, allowing more free β-catenin. Epidermal growth factor (EGF) also plays a role in activating β-catenin, also by blocking the binding of GSK-3 to β-catenin. pVHL, the normal protein product of the von Hippel–Lindau gene, may play a role in destabilizing β-catenin by strengthening the inhibitory bonds of GSK-3 and APC with it.

occur with age in a kidney epithelial cell, and one or more of these cells could lose their normal orientation and initiate the formation of a cyst (Brazier and Henske, 1997).

Elongin is a protein that stimulates the transcription process (the process by which a gene's DNA sequence is converted into a corresponding messenger RNA molecule). Elongin helps in the elongation of the RNA chain by reducing the pause in the time of the process. Elongin is made of three subunits—Elongin A, B, and C. Elongin A is the activating subunit, B stabilizes the complex, and C activates A. Normal pVHL, the protein product of the wild-type or nonmutated VHL gene, competes with Elongin A for binding to the B and C subunits and thereby regulates, inhibits, or slows the transcription process (Kibel et al, 1995; Neumann and Zbar, 1997). For example, large amounts of vascular endothelial growth factor (VEGF) are secreted by VHL ophthalmologic and central nervous system tumors (Neumann and Zbar, 1997). The normal VHL gene is referred to as a tumor suppressor gene, and it seems to play this role by reducing levels of both active β-catenin and active Elongin. In the former case it works to repress a transcriptional activator (i.e., Elongin), and in the latter inhibits development of the active form of a transcriptional activator (i.e., β-catenin).

Epidermal growth factor (EGF) and its fetal form, transforming growth factor–α (TGF-α), are both mitogens necessary for nephrogenesis (Rogers et al, 1992). When not modulated, they induce epithelial hyperplasia and cyst formation (Pugh et al, 1995). **Epidermal growth factor receptor (EGFR) is the receptor for both EGF and TGF-α.** Tyrosine kinase activity of EGFR receptors sets off intracellular phosphorylation events that result in increased cellular activity (Pugh et al, 1995; Sweeney et al, 1999, 2000). By inhibiting EGFR–tyrosine kinase activity with a blocking antibody, Pugh and colleagues (1995) were able to abolish the mitogenic and cystogenic effects of TGF-α and EGF in a murine metanephric organ culture. Binding EGFR activity in mice models not only abolishes its cystogenic and hyperplastic effects; more aggressive blocking can inhibit the conversion of mesenchymal cells into epithelial cells (Pugh et al, 1995) and lead to poor renal differentiation and the development of nodules of blastema cells (Table 56–2). For further information on EGF and EGFR, see the discussions of etiology and management of ADPKD.

Defects in any of the signaling activities could cause a kidney not to form (i.e., renal agenesis), to differentiate abnormally (i.e., renal dysgenesis), or to develop cysts. For example, in experimental mouse models, absence of Wnt-4, deficient production of GDNF, abnormal c-ret, and absent or reduced levels of PAX2 protein have been associated with a range of renal dysgenetic outcomes including agenesis, aplasia, hypoplasia, and dysplasia. A PAX2 mutation is the only one of these potential genetic defects that has so far been documented in humans (in whom it causes a condition called renal-colomba syndrome). The syndrome is associated with a heterozygous PAX2 mutation and includes blindness secondary to an optic nerve malformation called a colomba, unilateral hypoplastic kidney (i.e., small kidneys with a reduced number of nephrons), and in some cases vesicoureteral reflux (Woolf, 2000). Homozygous PAX2 loss in mice is associated with bilateral renal agenesis (Woolf, 2000).

Just as PAX2 seems to have incremental defects in mice depending on whether the gene defect is heterozygous or homozygous, I believe that other examples of the spectrum

Table 56–2. SIGNAL INDUCTION OF THE KIDNEY*–DEFINITIONS

Term	Definition
Insulin-like growth factor–2 (IGF-2)	A growth factor that inhibits mesenchymal cell apoptosis.
WT1	The Wilms' tumor gene; its expression is essential for suppression of IGF-2 and the cascade of events that leads to ureteric bud formation, ureteric bud ascent into the renal blastema, and mesenchymal to epithelial cell conversion.
PAX2 protein	Induces mesenchymal cells to differentiate into epithelial cells.
GDNF (glial cell line–derived neurotrophic factor)	Produced by mesenchymal cells; stimulates ureteric bud formation and branching.
C-ret	The receptor for GDNF located at branching ureteric tips.
β-Catenin	Binds with cadherin and α-catenin, providing adherence between epithelial cells, and orients the cells to develop into tubules, the precursors of nephrons; probably plays a role in speeding up intranuclear transcription processes.
GSK-3 (glycogen synthetase kinase-3)	Inhibits β-catenin activity.
WNT4 protein	Product of WNT-4 gene that blocks GSK-3 and increases β-catenin levels; signals tubule formation.
EGF (epidermal growth factor)	Inhibits GSK-3 activity.
Polycystin-1 and -2	Products of the polycystic kidney disease genes PKD1 and PKD2 that activate WNT-4 signaling.
Tg737	A gene that in its mutated form causes a type of autosomal recessive polycystic kidney disease in mice.
Adenomatous polyposis coli (APC) protein	Serves as bridging molecule between GSK-3 and β-catenin.
pVHL	Product of von Hippel–Lindau gene that facilitates binding of APC and GSK-3 to β-catenin and inhibits binding of Elongin A to Elongin. As a result it down-regulates transcription activity.
Transforming growth factor–α (TGF-α)	Fetal form of EGF
EGFR–tyrosine kinase	Induces intracellular phosphorylation events resulting in increased mitotic activity; receptor for EGF and TGF-α.

*In experimental mouse models, absence of Wnt-4, deficient production of GDNF, abnormal tyrosine kinase c-ret, and reduced PAX2 protein levels have been associated with renal agenesis or dysgenesis. (Schuchardt et al, 1994; Stark et al, 1994; Torres et al, 1995; Pepicelli et al, 1996; Pichel et al, 1996).

of renal dysgenesis will be found to be associated in humans with defects such as WNT4, GDNF, c-ret, and host of other genes yet to be identified. One such recently identified gene, KAL1, is located on the short arm of the X-chromosome; when defective, it is known to be associated with Kallmann's syndrome. This X-linked condition is associated with anosmia and unilateral renal agenesis in 37% of affected patients (Kirk et al, 1994). There also are reports of stillborns in Kallmann families with bilateral renal agenesis, but it is not known whether both alleles were affected in these patients (Woolf, 2000). KAL1 activity is present at 11 weeks' gestation in the olfactory bulbs and metanephric blastema, corresponding to the sites of its clinical manifestations (Duke et al, 1995; Woolf, 2000). The actual role that KAL1 plays in renal organogenesis has yet to be determined.

RENAL AGENESIS

Renal agenesis, or absent kidney development, can occur secondary to a defect of the wolffian duct, ureteric bud, or metanephric blastema. Bilateral agenesis occurs in 1 of every 4000 births and has a male predominance (Potter, 1965). Because the placenta filters the fetus's blood, it is not the lack of kidney tissue that causes early death but rather the lack of urine production and oligohydramnios. Affected babies are born with immature lungs and pneumothorax, Potter's facies (hypertelorism, prominent inner canthal folds, and recessive chin), and orthopedic defects secondary to intrauterine compression. The actual incidence of agenesis cannot be determined by imaging studies because aplastic kidneys can be misinterpreted as agenesis because they lack function and are too small to be visualized on any study. Most cases of bilateral agenesis are sporadic, and many are associated with other congenital anomalies including urogenital sinus defects.

Bilateral renal agenesis or severe bilateral renal disease is associated with oligohydramnios. However, if severe oligohydramnios is present, the kidneys may not be able to be seen because the window provided by the fluid is not present. Other nonrenal causes of oligohydramnios might then exist, such as a cord accident, ruptured membranes, or intrauterine growth retardation caused by placental insufficiency (Latini et al, 1998).

Unilateral agenesis is more common, with an incidence of 1 in 450 to 1000 births (Kass and Bloom, 1992). Because it may be secondary to a wolffian duct abnormality and the wolffian duct lies adjacent to the müllerian duct, renal agenesis may be associated with malformation of the ipsilateral uterine horn or fallopian tube or absence of the ipsilateral ovary in the female, or with absence of the ipsilateral testicle, vas deferens, or seminiferous tubules in the male. **The pseudonym Mayer-Rokitansky-Küster-Hauser syndrome refers to a group of associated findings that include unilateral renal agenesis or renal ectopia, ipsilateral müllerian defects, and vaginal agenesis.** Cystic dysplasia of the rete testis, a rare benign tumor, often is associated with ipsilateral renal agenesis. The association suggests a wolffian duct induction abnormality common to both conditions (Wojcik et al, 1997).

Cascio and associates (1999) found **unilateral renal agenesis to be associated with other urologic abnormalities in 48% of patients, including primary vesicoureteral reflux (28%), obstructive megaureter (11%), and ureteropelvic junction obstruction (3%). These findings are similar to those associated with unilateral multicystic kidney disease, suggesting the possibility that some of these "agenetic" kidneys represent involuted multicystic dysplastic kidneys.** Furthermore, it implies that unilateral renal agenesis and unilateral multicystic kidney may have similar etiologies.

On rare occasions, when either unilateral or bilateral agenesis is associated with a group of other renal abnormalities within a family, the term *familial renal adysplasia* is used. Additional reading on renal agenesis may be found in Chapter 55, Anomalies of the Kidney.

DYSPLASIA

Precise definitions as adopted in 1987 by the American Academy of Pediatrics (AAP) Section on Urology (Glassberg et al, 1987) are employed in this chapter. *Renal dysgenesis* **is maldevelopment of the kidney that affects its size, shape, or structure. Dysgenesis is of three principal types: dysplastic, hypoplastic, and cystic.** Although dysplasia is always accompanied by a decreased number of nephrons (i.e., hypoplasia), the converse is not true; hypoplasia may occur in isolation. When both conditions are present, the term *hypodysplasia* is preferred (Schwarz et al, 1981a).

A dysplastic kidney contains focal, diffuse, or segmentally arranged primitive structures, specifically primitive ducts, as a result of abnormal metanephric differentiation. "Dysplasia" is, therefore, a histologic diagnosis. The condition may affect all or only part of the kidney, and in a duplex system one segment may be normal and the other dysplastic. The kidney may be of normal size or small, and it may be grossly normal or deformed. **Cysts of various sizes may or may not be present. When they are present, the condition is called** *cystic dysplasia.* **When the entire kidney is dysplastic with a preponderance of cysts, that kidney is referred to as a** *multicystic dysplastic kidney.* This condition is discussed later in this chapter. Aplastic dysplasia is represented by a nubbin of nonfunctioning tissue, not necessarily of reniform shape, that meets the histologic criteria for dysplasia. In utero and postnatal follow-up by ultrasound has shown that some multicystic kidneys shrink with time into such nubbins. Therefore, **some instances of aplasia may represent the involuted stage of a multicystic kidney.**

Dysplasia may be associated with an absent renal pelvis or ureter; with atresia, stenosis, or tortuosity of the ureter; or with a normal, atretic, or absent ureterovesical junction. The appearance of a grossly abnormal collecting system with or without ureteral anomalies on intravenous urography is sometimes described as renal dysplasia, but such features may occur in the absence of dysplasia. Williams (1974) suggested that the term *renal dysmorphism,* rather than renal dysplasia, be applied to abnormalities noted radiographically or grossly without histologic proof of primitive structures.

Etiology

The origin of renal dysplasia is unclear. Normal renal development is initiated by penetration of metanephric blastema by a ureteric bud at the proper time and place. **According to the Mackie and Stephens (1975) "bud" theory, abnormal ureteric budding can lead not only to an ectopic orifice but also to inappropriate penetration of the blastema, causing renal dysplasia.** These investigators provided supportive evidence from studies of duplex systems that showed a high correlation between the degree of lateral ectopia of the lower pole orifice and the extent of dysplasia of the lower pole segment. Recent molecular genetic evidence has provided additional support for the bud theory (Pope et al, 1999).

Once renal function begins, obstruction can distort development secondary to the physical and chemical effects of poor drainage. It was long assumed that obstruction is a significant factor in dysplasia (Beck, 1971; Bernstein, 1971). Certainly, some evidence exists for the role of obstruction. For example, when both kidneys drain poorly, as in patients with posterior urethral valves, both kidneys may be dysplastic, whereas only the ipsilateral kidney is affected in cases of unilateral obstruction. Also in favor of a role for obstruction is the dysplasia observed in the upper pole of duplex systems when there is an associated obstructed ectopic ureter or ureterocele. The ipsilateral lower pole in such cases is not dysplastic, but the upper pole orifice is ectopic.

According to Mackie and Stephens (1975), an ectopic orifice is a sign of abnormal ureteric budding and metanephric development (i.e., dysplasia). However, some of these findings could also be explained as an embryologic abnormality that causes both obstruction and dysplasia. Moreover, one form of widespread dysplasia, namely the type associated with multicystic disease, usually develops before urine formation. Potter suggested in 1972 that a teratogenic force acts at various sites to produce the combination of ureteral atresia and multicystic renal disease.

Growing awareness of the importance of the interactions between epithelial cells and mesenchyme in the control of normal development and growth has shed light on the origin of renal dysgenesis. In the chick embryo, simple ureteral ligation alone does not induce renal dysplasia (Berman and Maizel, 1982), whereas reduction of the condensed metanephrogenic mesenchyme is likely to lead to dysplasia (Maizel and Simpson, 1983). Moreover, ligation of the ureter seems to facilitate the dysplastic development of blastemas already deficient in mesenchyme (Maizel and Simpson, 1986). Spencer and Maizel (1987) found that inhibition of the glycosylation of extracellular matrix, which alters the interaction of epithelial and mesenchymal cells, can lead to dysplasia in the absence of obstruction. The role of abnormal signaling molecules and receptors in the persistence of primitive structures was discussed earlier in this chapter.

The question of the etiology of dysplasia has assumed more than theoretical importance since the advent of fetal surgery. If obstruction is an epiphenomenon of dysplasia rather than its cause, then operations on a fetus to relieve obstruction are unlikely to be of value in preventing severe renal dysplasia or aplasia.

Histology

The histologic definition of renal dysplasia has evolved since the seminal work by Ericsson and Ivemark (1958a, 1958b), who sought to identify the structures that could arise only from embryonic maldevelopment, not from secondary events. They concluded that primitive ducts and cartilage were such unique features. Although the first part of their definition is still accepted, the second part is not. Ericsson and Ivemark (1958b), like some other investigators (Biglar and Killingsworth, 1949; Bernstein, 1971), considered all renal cartilage to be representative of aberrant development of the metanephric blastema and therefore dysplastic. However, foci of hyaline cartilage have been found in normal kidneys (Potter, 1972) and in otherwise normal kidneys with chronic inflammation (Taxy and Filmer, 1975). The present definition, therefore, does not specify nests of metaplastic cartilage as an absolute criterion for dysplasia.

Primitive ducts, which are lined by cuboidal or tall columnar epithelium (often ciliated) and surrounded by concentric rings of connective tissue containing collagen and a few smooth muscle cells but no elastin, are undeniable evidence of dysplasia (Fig. 56–2) (Ericsson and Ivemark, 1958b; Bernstein, 1971). The ducts are of various sizes and can be found in many sites, principally in the medulla and sometimes in the medullary rays. As a rule, the more severely deformed the kidney, the more extensive the primitive ducts (Ericsson, 1974), and in less severe cases only the peripelvic area may be affected. These structures resemble the aberrant ductules of the fallopian tube and may be remnants of the mesonephric duct (Eisendrath, 1935; Ericsson, 1954).

Several other histologic findings may (but need not) accompany the primitive ducts. Primitive ductules, which are smaller than the primitive ducts, are surrounded by connective tissue devoid of smooth muscle cells. Primitive tubules and glomeruli may be seen also; these resemble structures seen in human kidneys that are regenerating after neonatal renal necrosis (Bernstein and Meyer, 1961), in scars from renal biopsies (Bernstein, 1971), and in animal kidneys after trauma (Bernstein, 1966). Cysts and loose, disorganized mesenchyme and fibrous tissue are other possible features.

Familial Adysplasia

Renal agenesis, renal dysplasia, multicystic dysplasia, and renal aplasia usually appear as isolated, sporadic occurrences. On rare occasions, this group of anomalies may appear in many family members but heterogeneously. In other words, one family member may have renal agenesis while another has renal dysplasia and still another has a multicystic dysplastic or aplastic kidney. When all or part of this group of anomalies is seen in one family, an encompassing term for these four entities is used: *familial renal adysplasia.*

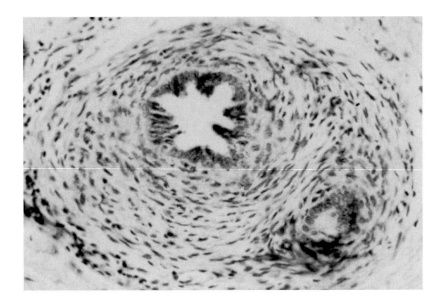

Figure 56–2. Primitive duct lined with columnar epithelial cells. Note concentric arrangement of spindle mesenchymal cells around the duct. Special staining is required to demonstrate smooth muscle cells.

When the disorder is familial, it usually is transmitted as an autosomal dominant disease (Buchta et al, 1973; McPherson et al, 1987). The fact that all of the entities of renal adysplasia can appear in one family suggests that one primary defect leads to this spectrum of anomalies. That primary defect may be either a ureteric bud abnormality or a defect of the metanephric blastema. Curry and associates (1984) made a case for investigating by ultrasound family members and subsequent pregnancies when there is a history of bilateral renal adysplasia and Potter's syndrome. Bernstein (1991) went further and suggests giving parents an option for investigative studies of family members when a child with even one adysplastic kidney is identified. Incidentally, noncystic dysplastic kidneys not associated with reflux are associated with a 14% incidence of vesicoureteral reflux into the contralateral ureter (Atiyeh et al, 1993).

HYPOPLASIA AND HYPODYSPLASIA

Hypoplasia and hypodysplasia have been subclassified as shown in Table 56–3. The subdivision according to the nature of the ureteral orifice acknowledges the bud theory but is not necessarily intended to be an endorsement of that theory. **Hypodysplastic kidneys most often occur in conjunction with ectopic ureteral orifices, with the extent of dysplasia correlating with the degree of ectopia** (Schwarz et al, 1981a, 1981b, 1981c). However, hypodysplastic kidneys are seen in a few patients with normal ureteral orifices. In such cases, obstruction may or may not be present.

Renal Hypoplasia

To avoid perpetuating the confusion that has attended the use of the term "hypoplasia," I restrict its use to kidneys that have less than the normal number of calyces and nephrons but are not dysplastic or embryonic. The truly hypoplastic kidney may have a normal nephron density despite its small size.

Hypoplasia is not a specific condition; rather, it is a group of pathologic conditions with the same feature—an abnormally small kidney. It should be distinguished from renal aplasia, in which the kidney is rudimentary and the ureter atretic, and from renal agenesis, in which the kidney does not develop at all.

Hypoplasia may be bilateral or unilateral. In unilateral cases, the other kidney usually shows greater compensatory growth than is characteristic in patients with renal atrophy caused by acquired disease. Hypoplasia can be associated with reflux, and the term *reflux nephropathy* is now applied to all types of abnormality associated with reflux. Segmental hypoplasia (Ask-Upmark kidney) probably is a type of reflux nephropathy.

Because of the similarity of the word *oligonephronia* (literally translated as a decreased number of nephrons) to *oligomeganephronia*, which is a specific clinical entity (see following discussion), the former term should not be used.

Table 56–3. CLASSIFICATION OF HYPOPLASIA AND HYPODYSPLASIA

Hypoplasia
  True ("oligonephronia")
    With normal ureteral orifice
    With abnormal ureteral orifice
  Oligomeganephronia
  Segmental (Ask-Upmark kidney)
Hypodysplasia
  With normal ureteral orifice
    With obstruction
    Without obstruction
  With abnormal ureteral orifice
    Lateral ectopia
    Medial or caudal ectopia with ureterocele
  With urethral obstruction
  Prune-belly syndrome

True Hypoplasia

True hypoplasia is a congenital condition with no apparent familial tendency or gender predilection. The incidence is unknown because many investigators fail to distinguish among the various causes of a small kidney. In a series of 2153 consecutive autopsies, Rubenstein and coworkers (1961) found a 2.5% incidence of true hypoplasia.

Clinical Features

Clinical manifestations of true renal hypoplasia may be severe or absent. In patients with bilateral true hypoplasia or unilateral true hypoplasia with contralateral aplasia or agenesis, renal insufficiency, dehydration, or failure to thrive may be present. Often, these patients are premature infants who have developmental abnormalities of other organs, particularly the central nervous system. Respiratory problems are a common cause of death in these infants. At the other extreme, in patients with unilateral hypoplasia and contralateral hypertrophy, the diagnosis usually is made incidentally during an evaluation for some other urinary problem or for hypertension.

The urine is of low specific gravity when the condition is bilateral.

Histopathology

For the diagnosis of hypoplasia to be made, the renal parenchyma must be normal and without dysplasia, although Bernstein (1968) has described tubular degeneration, focal cortical scarring, and healed focal necrosis. The characteristic feature is the size of the kidney.

Evaluation

Ultrasound may be useful in demonstrating the presence and site of these kidneys, although it does not reveal the type of hypoplasia (Goldberg et al, 1975). Intravenous urography shows nonappearance or a small shadow; retrograde pyelography reveals a normal-caliber ureter and a reduced number of calyces. Reports by Porstman (1970) and by Templeton and Thompson (1968) indicated the finding of a uniformly narrow renal artery on arteriography, in contrast to the tapered vessel seen in acquired atrophy, such as that secondary to pyelonephritis.

Differential diagnosis must take into account solid dysplasia (Potter's type IIB), segmental hypoplasia (Ask-Upmark kidney), oligomeganephronia, and acquired disease (chronic atrophic pyelonephritis, renal ischemia, and glomerulonephritis). Renal biopsy is the only way of proving the diagnosis.

Oligomeganephronia

The combination of a marked reduction in the number of nephrons and hypertrophy of each nephron was described in 1962 (Habib et al, 1962; Royer et al, 1962) **and termed** *oligomeganephronia.* It is usually a bilateral condition, although a few instances of unilateral oligomeganephronia associated with contralateral renal agenesis have been reported (Griffel et al, 1972; Lam et al, 1982; Forster and Hawkins, 1994).

There are probably two types of oligomeganephronia: one that appears in association with variable malformation defects and the other a solitary sporadic entity that comprises the majority of cases. Among the multiple defects

that have been reported with oligomeganephronia are ocular, auditory, and skeletal anomalies (e.g., lobster-claw deformity of the hands and feet) and mental retardation. Park and Chi (1993) reported on two such patients, both of whom had a 4p deletion-type chromosomal anomaly, and suggested that perhaps many other cases with multiple malformations associated with oligomeganephronia may actually be part of a similar 4p deletion-type syndrome.

Clinical Features

Oligomeganephronia is a congenital but nonfamilial disorder that affects boys more often than girls (3:1). It frequently is associated with low birth weight (<2500 g). The condition usually is discovered soon after the child's birth or, if not, then usually by age 2 years. Infants most frequently are brought to medical attention because of vomiting, dehydration, intense thirst, and polyuria. The creatinine clearance is abnormal (10 to 50 ml/minute per 1.73 m²), and the maximum specific gravity of the urine is 1.007 to 1.012. Moderate proteinuria may be present, but this is more likely to be a later finding.

Renal function remains below normal (although stable) for many years, but polydipsia and polyuria can worsen, and growth is severely retarded in many cases. As the patient enters his or her teens, the creatinine clearance begins to drop rapidly. Marked proteinuria (2 g/24 hours) is common, and the characteristic metabolic features of renal failure—disturbed acid-base balance and abnormal calcium and phosphorus metabolism—are seen. The blood pressure usually is normal. At this point, hemodialysis is required to maintain the patient's life.

Histopathology

The kidneys are smaller than normal (average weight at autopsy, 20 to 25 g) and are not always the same size. Van Acker and colleagues (1971) suggested that because of the reduced number of nephrons, those that do exist increase in size to compensate for the deficiency in number. The kidneys are pale and firm with a granular cortical surface and no clear distinction between the cortex and the medulla. The number of renal segments is reduced, usually to five or six, although unirenicular and birenicular kidneys have been described (Bernstein, 1968). The renal artery is small.

The particular histologic features of a case depend on the duration of the disease. In patients 2 to 3 years of age, the characteristic findings are a reduced number of nephrons, enormously enlarged glomeruli (seven to ten times the normal volume), juxtaglomerular bodies, and proximal tubules elongated to four times their normal length, often with multiple diverticula (Fig. 56–3). In older children, interstitial fibrosis and atrophy become more prominent, and the glomeruli become increasingly hyalinized until they are destroyed. The end-stage kidney closely resembles that observed in glomerulonephritis except for persisting enlargement of the glomeruli. Dysplasia is not seen.

Evaluation

The kidneys may concentrate contrast medium adequately for an intravenous urogram, producing a picture of small kidneys, usually with normally formed calyces,

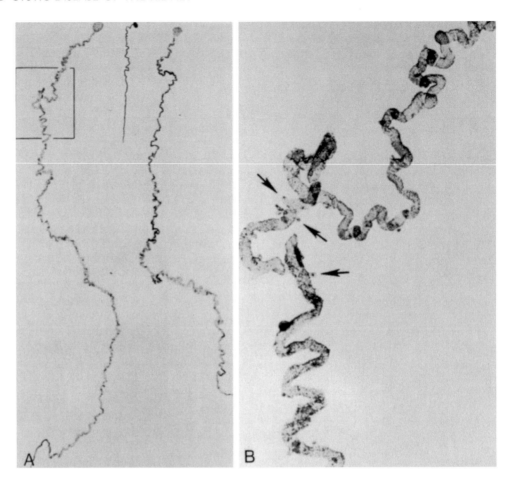

Figure 56–3. *A,* Mosaic photograph of two typical proximal tubules dissected from the kidney of a patient with oligomeganephronia. The silhouette in the top center is a diagrammatic representation to scale of an average proximal tubule from a kidney of an age-matched control. *B,* Enlargement of the inset in *A,* showing the diverticula along the course of the nephron *(arrows).* (From Fetterman GH, Habib R: Congenital bilateral oligonephronic renal hypoplasia with hypertrophy of nephrons (oligomeganephronic). Am J Clin Pathol 1969;52:199–207. Reproduced with permission of the American Society of Clinical Pathologists.)

although Morita and associates (1973) described a patient with dysmorphic calyces. The small kidneys also can be identified by sonography (Scheinman and Abelson, 1970).

Oligomeganephronia may resemble juvenile nephronophthisis–medullary cystic disease complex in its clinical features, but the latter condition generally appears later in life, and defects of tubular function precede glomerular insufficiency (Herdman et al, 1967). Moreover, juvenile nephronophthisis–medullary cystic disease is familial; other cases are found in the relatives of 50% to 80% of affected persons (Habib, 1974). The kidneys in juvenile nephronophthisis are small but not as small as those seen in oligomeganephronia.

Simple bilateral renal hypoplasia may be confused with oligomeganephronia (Carter and Lirenman, 1970). Segmental hypoplasia (Ask-Upmark kidney) is almost always accompanied by severe hypertension, which is not seen in oligomeganephronia.

Treatment

High fluid intake and correction of salt loss and acidosis are the initial steps. Daily dietary protein should be limited to 1.5 g/kg during the stable phase (Royer et al, 1962). Frank renal failure is managed by dialysis and transplantation. The allograft may come from a living related donor because the disease is not familial.

Ask-Upmark Kidney (Segmental Hypoplasia)

In 1929, Ask-Upmark described distinctive small kidneys in eight patients, seven of whom had malignant hypertension; six of these patients were adolescents.

Etiology

Although the Ask-Upmark kidney was originally thought to be a developmental lesion because of the youth of the first patients, findings suggest otherwise. The presence of fibrotic glomeruli and chronic inflammatory cells, as described by Habib and associates (1965) and by Rauber and Langlet (1976), led both Johnston and Mix (1976) and Shindo and coworkers (1983) to **suggest that the Ask-Upmark kidney is the result of reflux and ascending pyelonephritis. This hypothesis is supported by the data of Arant and coworkers (1979), who found that 16 of 17 affected patients had vesicoureteral reflux and that signs of reflux had been present in more than 50% of the previously described cases in which appropriate studies were done.**

Chronic pyelonephritis secondary to reflux may be the cause even if no inflammatory cell infiltrates are found. For example, Heptinstall (1979) showed that such cells may disappear from the tissues with time. Hodson (1981) demonstrated in pigs that acute lesions of pyelonephritis may be followed by a histologic picture similar to that of Ask-Upmark kidney, in which glomeruli, collecting ducts, and inflammatory cells have disappeared. Hodson was able to produce histologically similar lesions with sterile high-pressure reflux. The presence of glomerular traces in periodic acid–Schiff (PAS)–stained sections of Ask-Upmark kidneys in areas grossly without glomeruli is further evidence of an acquired rather than a developmental lesion.

Despite these data, the etiology of Ask-Upmark kidney is not yet clear. Some of these kidneys do contain dysplastic elements, indicating a developmental contribution (Bernstein, 1975).

Clinical Features

Most patients are 10 years of age or older at diagnosis, although the lesion has been reported in a premature infant (Valderrama and Berkman, 1979) and in a 13-month-old infant (Mozziconacci et al, 1968). Girls are twice as likely as boys to be affected (Royer et al, 1971; Arant et al, 1979).

Severe hypertension is a prominent symptom. Headache is common, either alone or together with hypertensive encephalopathy (Rosenfeld et al, 1973). Retinopathy is discovered in half of the patients (Royer et al, 1971).

Proteinuria and some degree of renal insufficiency may be present if the disease is bilateral. Approximately half of the patients in the series described by Royer and associates (1971) had these signs at diagnosis.

Histopathology

The Ask-Upmark kidney is smaller than normal—12 to 35 g (Royer et al, 1971). **Its distinctive feature is one or more deep grooves on the lateral convexity, underneath which the parenchyma consists of tubules resembling those in the thyroid gland.** Usually, the hypoplastic segments are easily distinguished from adjacent areas. The medulla consists of a thin band, and remnants of the corticomedullary junction and arcuate arteries are seen. Arteriosclerosis is common, and juxtaglomerular hyperplasia may be seen (Bernstein, 1968; Meares and Gross, 1972; Kaufman and Fay, 1974; Arant et al, 1979).

Treatment

In patients with unilateral disease, partial or total nephrectomy may control the hypertension (Royer et al, 1971; Meares and Gross, 1972). Failure of this measure suggests an unrecognized scar or generalized arteriosclerosis in the remaining kidney (Arant et al, 1979). Bilateral disease with renal insufficiency usually is managed medically, although dialysis and transplantation may be needed. Correction of reflux may prevent further renal damage but probably will have no effect on the hypertension.

Renal Hypodysplasia

Hypodysplasia may be associated with a normal or abnormal ureteral orifice, ureterocele, urethral obstruction, or prune-belly syndrome.

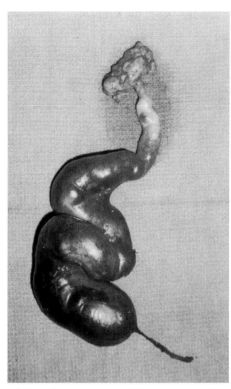

Figure 56–4. Small hypodysplastic kidney found in association with a severely obstructed primary megaureter. (From Glassberg KI, Filmer RB: Renal dysplasia, renal hypoplasia and cystic disease of the kidney. In Kelalis P, King LR, Belman AB [eds]: Clinical Pediatric Urology. Philadelphia, WB Saunders, 1985, pp 922–971.)

Hypodysplasia with Normal Ureteral Orifice

WITH OBSTRUCTION

Primary obstructive megaureter and ureteropelvic junction obstruction usually are associated with small but normal-appearing and normally situated ureteral orifices. In general, this kidney has suffered diffuse damage because of hydronephrosis, although in a few cases small areas or even the entire kidney is hypodysplastic or shows multicystic dysplasia (Fig. 56–4).

WITHOUT OBSTRUCTION

The "dwarf" kidney, although usually described as hypoplastic, is in fact usually hypodysplastic. The calyces are normally cupped but generally fewer in number than would be expected from the size of the kidney. According to the bud theory, the dwarf kidney is the result of deficient metanephric blastema rather than a budding abnormality (Stephens, 1983).

Hypodysplasia with Abnormal Ureteral Orifice

The small kidney associated with an abnormally positioned orifice usually is thin with ectatic calyces. The thin parenchyma is thought to reflect insufficient divisions of the ureteral bud, with a consequent reduction in the num-

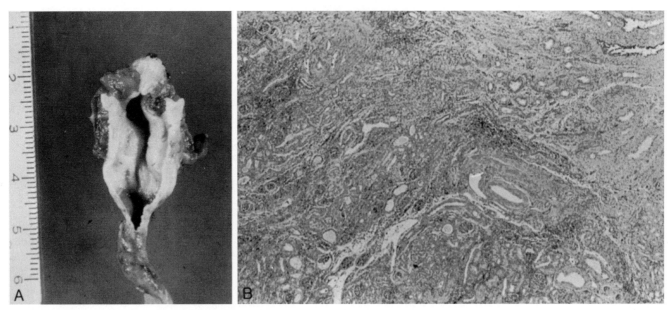

Figure 56–5. Upper pole of a duplex kidney associated with an ectopic ureterocele. *A,* Gross specimen has visible tiny cysts. *B,* On histology, primitive glomeruli are seen on left side and primitive ducts are seen in upper right corner (×40).

ber of nephrons induced (Stephens, 1983). The calyces generally are rounded, a picture characteristic of an earlier stage of development, before proliferating nephrons and papillary bulging indent the calyces to create the mature cup shape (Sommer and Stephens, 1981).

The radiographic appearance of rounded calyces should not be mistaken for the clubbing associated with reflux nephropathy, which is caused by parenchymal scars overlying the calyces rather than by the premature termination of calyceal development. On the basis of the view that abnormal budding leads to an ectopic ureteral orifice with thin renal parenchyma and ectatic calyces, Sommer and Stephens (1981) designated the condition the "pan-bud anomaly." Their theory seems particularly applicable in duplex systems in which the thin renal segment with ectatic calyces is associated with a ureter draining ectopically into either a medial (often obstructed) or a lateral ureteric orifice.

LATERAL ECTOPIA

Lateral ectopia usually is associated with reflux. If the pan-bud theory is correct, the rounded calyces found in the newborn infant with no history of infection are the result of premature termination of calyceal development rather than of ballooning under the constant high-pressure assault by refluxing urine. Of course, infection leading to scarring and clubbing can confuse the picture, although pyelonephritic scars often create a characteristic indentation of the renal outline over the clubbed calyx (Hodson, 1981).

MEDIAL OR CAUDAL ECTOPIA AND URETEROCELES

When the ureterovesical junction is displaced medially, the ureter and renal pelvis usually are dilated. The renal cortex may be thin, as in hydronephrosis, or severely dysplastic, perhaps with numerous small cysts (Fig. 56–5). When obstruction is complete, as in blind ureterocele, the upper pole segment may mimic the multicystic kidney histologically (Stephens, 1983).

Hypodysplasia with Urethral Obstruction

According to Osathanondh and Potter (1964), posterior urethral valves may be associated with two types of renal hypodysplasia. In the less severe form, there are small, usually subcapsular cysts and nearly normal renal function, a picture that could be caused by increased pressure secondary to urinary outflow obstruction. In the second form, the cysts are larger and more widely distributed, and numerous islands of cartilage are present. This form usually is associated with earlier onset and more severe obstruction and reflux (Fig. 56–6). Osathanondh and Potter (1964) believed that this highly abnormal condition has etiologic factors beyond urethral obstruction, and here again abnormal budding appears to be involved.

In patients with posterior urethral valves, the position of the ureteral orifice correlates well with the extent of hypodysplasia, as shown by Henneberry and Stephens (1980) and by Schwarz and colleagues (1981b). When the orifice is normally positioned, the kidney is histologically good but hydronephrotic, whereas a laterally placed orifice is associated with hypoplasia and an extremely lateral orifice with hypodysplasia. This correlation is present regardless of the presence or absence of reflux or the degree of urethral obstruction, suggesting that obstruction is not the only factor involved in creating the histologic picture. Further evidence of the role of factors beyond obstruction comes from cases of congenital ureteropelvic junction ob-

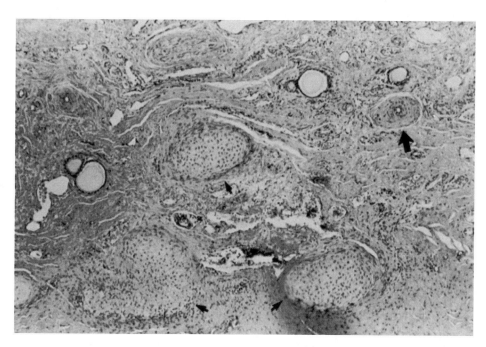

Figure 56–6. Histologic specimen of a nonfunctioning reflux kidney in a patient with posterior urethral valves. Note presence of nests of cartilage *(small arrows)*. Primitive ducts are scattered throughout the specimen *(large arrow)* (×100). The findings are compatible with dysplasia.

struction or primary obstructive megaureter, in which the ureteral orifices are almost always normally positioned and the kidneys are rarely dysplastic.

Hypodysplasia Associated with Prune-Belly Syndrome

The features of the prune-belly syndrome (absent abdominal musculature, triad syndrome) include grossly deformed kidneys, which may have various degrees of dysplasia. The ureters are wide and tortuous, often with large and laterally placed orifices. The dysplasia in the kidneys of these patients is explainable by the abnormal budding theory of Mackie and Stephens (1975). Urethral obstruction or atresia may be present in the most severe cases, but usually there is no lower urinary tract obstruction.

CYSTIC DISEASE

The kidney is one of the most common sites in the body for cysts. Although the lesions themselves in the various cystic conditions are histologically similar (i.e., microscopic or macroscopic sacs lined with epithelium), their number, location, and clinical features are different. Some renal cysts are actually ectatic tubules or collecting ducts that are continuous with the nephron. Because any dilated duct or tubule within the kidney can be potentially referred to as a renal cyst, criteria have been suggested for specifying when a dilatation is appropriately called a cyst. Gardner (1988) suggested that ducts dilated to four times their normal diameter (i.e., 200 μm) be called cysts. Some cysts are saccular or fusiform structures that resemble diverticula and are located at various sites along the nephron. Other cysts may or may not communicate with a glomerulus, tubule, collecting duct, or calyx, or they may initially have communicated only to become isolated later on. Cysts may be located diffusely throughout the kidney or in one segment only. They may appear unilaterally or bilaterally. In some entities cysts may represent a form of dysplasia and may be accompanied by other findings of dysplasia.

When cysts are part of an inherited disorder, they may be present at birth or may develop sometime thereafter, perhaps even in adulthood. Some very different entities have similar features. For example, in ADPKD, tuberous sclerosis, VHL, and acquired renal cystic disease (ARCD), the cysts have a hyperplastic lining, sometimes with nodules of hyperplasia or polyps that project into the cyst lumen. However, these hyperplastic conditions are very different from each other. Another example of such similarities is the ectatic collecting ducts seen in two very different clinical entities, ARPKD and medullary sponge kidney.

Most renal cystic conditions—congenital, sporadic, and acquired—arise from the nephrons and collecting ducts after they have formed, whether normally or abnormally. Multicystic dysplasia is an exception in that it arises before formation of the nephron, from abnormal induction of metanephric development, a primary abnormality of the nephrogenic blastema, or obstruction occurring early in renal development. Another exception, benign multilocular cyst, represents a neoplastic growth. The origin of simple cysts is not clear because they develop in kidneys that have apparently been normal throughout life.

Classification

Several classifications have been proposed based on the clinical presentation, the supposed time of cyst appearance, the radiographic appearance, or the microscopic anatomy (Osthanondh and Potter, 1964; Spence and Singleton, 1972;

Table 56–4. CYSTIC DISEASES OF THE KIDNEY

Genetic
  Autosomal recessive (infantile) polycystic kidney disease
  Autosomal dominant (adult) polycystic kidney disease
  Juvenile nephronophthisis–medullary cystic disease complex
  Juvenile nephronophthisis (autosomal recessive)
  Medullary cystic disease (autosomal dominant)
  Congenital nephrosis (familial nephrotic syndrome) (autosomal recessive)
  Familial hypoplastic glomerulocystic disease (autosomal dominant)
  Multiple malformation syndromes with renal cysts (e.g., tuberous sclerosis, von Hippel-Lindau disease)
Nongenetic
  Multicystic kidney (multicystic dysplastic kidney)
  Benign multilocular cyst (cystic nephroma)
  Simple cysts
  Medullary sponge kidney
  Sporadic glomerulocystic kidney disease
  Acquired renal cystic disease
  Calyceal diverticulum (pyelogenic cyst)

Bernstein, 1973, 1976; Bernstein and Gardner, 1979a). The best known classification may be that of Potter (1972), which is based on microdissection studies and considers principally the location of the cysts within the uriniferous tubule. Unfortunately, this system is difficult to apply clinically, and it groups together clearly dissimilar conditions, such as ADPKD and medullary sponge kidney.

In this chapter, the system used is based on one proposed in 1987 by the Committee on Classification, Nomenclature and Terminology of the AAP Section on Urology, in which **the primary distinction is between genetic and nongenetic disease** and the various disorders are further classified according to their clinical, radiologic, and pathologic features (Table 56–4). A similar classification was offered by Stephens and Cussen (1983) and by Glassberg and Filmer (1985). Two discrete glomerulocystic entities have been added to the AAP classification; these are included in Table 56–4.

Although I have chosen to continue to employ the two broad categories, genetic and nongenetic cystic disease, it is likely that specific genes will eventually be identified as the cause of most of the entities included in the nongenetic category. If that becomes the case, the ninth edition of *Campbell's Urology* would more appropriately employ the terms "heritable" and "nonheritable" for these two broad categories.

The terms *multicystic* and *polycystic* should not be confused, even though both terms literally mean "many cysts." Multicystic refers to a dysplastic entity, and polycystic refers to a number of separate entities, most inherited, all without dysplasia and all with nephrons throughout the kidney (Table 56–5). The term "polycystic kidney disease" traditionally leads the student to think predominantly of two conditions, ARPKD and ADPKD. Many of the polycystic kidney disease entities progress to renal failure as the nephrons become more diseased. Other polycystic conditions include a number of diseases with "glomerulocystic" pathology. In tuberous sclerosis and VHL, there are hyperplastic cysts and the individual nephrons are normal. Only occasionally do the nephrons become compressed by the cysts or by associated tumors, and only in such situations does renal failure ensue.

Among the nongenetic cystic diseases, benign multilocular cysts and other variants are considered neoplasms. Medullary sponge kidney is a disease principally of dilated ectatic collecting ducts, with cysts playing a lesser role, although the size of the ducts by definition makes them cysts. The nephrons initially are normal.

It will be helpful to the reader to refer back to the genetic and nongenetic entities listed in Table 56–4, as well as to Table 56–5, which summarizes many of the entities encountered later in the chapter.

Genetic Cystic Disease

Genetic cystic diseases can be broadly classified as autosomal dominant and autosomal recessive forms of polycystic kidneys, autosomal dominant and autosomal recessive forms of medullary cystic kidneys, the autosomal recessive disorder congenital nephrosis, the autosomal dominant disorder familial hypoplastic glomerulocystic disease, and a group of rare disorders that have multiple systemic anomalies.

The genetically determined renal cystic diseases range from the very common to the very rare. Some of these disorders are caused by a single gene defect, some by an X-linked gene defect, and others by chromosomal defects. The specific gene or gene locus has been identified for almost every single-gene (mendelian) disorder (see Table 56–5).

AUTOSOMAL RECESSIVE ("INFANTILE") POLYCYSTIC KIDNEY DISEASE

When polycystic kidney disease is diagnosed in the neonate, it is most often of the recessive type (Cole et al, 1987). The autosomal recessive type in the past has been referred to as the "infantile" form. This confusing and inaccurate age designation should be discarded, because the disease can become manifest initially in adolescents and young adults, although significantly less frequently.

ARPKD has been reported as a rare disease affecting about 1 of every 40,000 live births (Zerres et al, 1988), as a not so rare disease occurring in 1 of 10,000 births in Finland (Kääriäiren, 1987), and even as frequently as 1 in 5000 to 10,000 live births (Bernstein and Slovis, 1992). However, as many as 50% of affected newborns die in the first few hours or days of life, making for a significantly lower incidence among children who live for at least 1 year. Of those infants who survive the neonatal period, approximately 50% are alive at 10 years of age (Kaplan et al, 1989b).

ARPKD has a spectrum of severity, the most severe forms appearing earliest in life. If it is not apparent at birth, the disease will become apparent later in childhood (up to age 13 years or, rarely, up to age 20 years) and is bilateral. All patients have varying degrees of congenital hepatic fibrosis as well.

Table 56–5. CHARACTERISTICS OF VARIOUS FORMS OF CYSTIC KIDNEYS

Entity	Site of Chromosomal Defect	Characteristic Renal Findings	Associated Anomalies	Incidence
Genetic Cystic Disease				
Autosomal recessive polycystic kidney disease (ARPKD)	6	In newborn usually large, homogeneous, echogenic kidneys; predominantly cysts of collecting ducts	Congenital hepatic fibrosis biliary dysgenesis	1:5,000 to 40,000
Autosomal dominant polycystic kidney disease (ADPKD)		Scattered renal cysts throughout parenchyma; if presenting in infancy may have glomerular cysts; large kidneys	Diverticulitis; liver, spleen and pancreatic cysts; mitral valve regurgitation; intracranial aneurysms; rare association with congenital hepatic fibrosis in neonatal cases	1:500 to 1000
PKD1	16			~90% of cases
PKD2	4			~10% of cases
PKD3	Not mapped			<1% of cases
Juvenile nephronophthisis–medullary cystic disease complex				
Juvenile nephronophthisis (autosomal recessive)	2	Cysts at corticomedullary junction; develop after onset of renal failure; always thickened tubular basement membrane	80% of families have no extra renal lesions	1:50,000
Senior-Loken syndrome (autosomal recessive)	Not mapped	Cyst at corticomedullary junction	Retinitis pigmentosa	1:200,000
Medullary cystic disease (autosomal dominant)	Not mapped	Cysts at corticomedullary junction; develop before onset of renal failure; tubular basement membrane may not be thickened	None	1:100,000
Congenital nephrosis Finnish type	19	Dilatation of proximal convoluted tubules; diffuse hypertrophy of podocytes; interstitial fibrosis	Enormously enlarged and edematous placenta; high amniotic alphafetoprotein	1:8200 in Finland; very rare elsewhere; reported in Minnesota
Diffuse mesangial sclerosis	Occasionally inherited	Dilatation of proximal convoluted tubules; diffuse hypertrophy of podocytes; interstitial fibrosis	Drash syndrome: nephrotic syndrome, Wilms' tumor, and male pseudohermaphroditism	Rare; more common worldwide than Finnish type
Familial glomerulocystic kidney disease	Not mapped	Small or normal size kidneys with glomerular cysts	None	Very rare
Tuberous sclerosis (autosomal dominant)				1:6,000 to 14,500
TSC1	9	Cysts and angiomyolipomas throughout kidney; cysts even present in utero; 3% incidence of renal cell carcinoma	Adenoma sebaceum; epilepsy; mental retardation; cranial tumors	
TSC2	16			
von Hippel–Lindau disease (autosomal dominant)	3	Cysts, adenomas, and clear cell renal carcinoma (35%–38% of cases)	Cerebellar hemangioblastoma; retinal angiomas; pheochromocytoma; cysts of pancreas and epididymis	1:30,000 to 50,000

Table continued on following page

Table 56–5. CHARACTERISTICS OF VARIOUS FORMS OF CYSTIC KIDNEYS *Continued*

Entity	Site of Chromosomal Defect	Characteristic Renal Findings	Associated Anomalies	Incidence
Nongenetic Cystic Disease				
Multicystic dysplastic kidney	No genetic predisposition	Renal maldevelopment with diffuse cysts and remnants of early metanephric development; minimal if any nephron development	Not usual	Most frequent cystic disease in newborn
Benign multilocular cyst	No genetic predisposition	Benign cystic tumor of the kidney; remainder of kidney has normal nephrons that may become crushed by the expanding tumor	None	When present more often in males when younger than age 4 and females when older than age 30
Simple cysts	Rare genetic predisposition	Single or multiple cysts; normal nephrons throughout kidney	None	Very common in normal kidneys with increasing age
Medullary sponge kidney	Rare genetic predisposition	Ectactic collecting ducts; nephrons fairly normal	None	1:5000 to 20,000
Sporadic glomerulocystic kidney disease	No genetic predisposition	Large kidneys, predominantly glomerular cysts; when seen in infancy, indistinguishable from ADPKD with glomerular cystic kidney disease	10% biliary dysgenesis; heptic cysts	Very rare
Acquired renal cystic disease	No genetic predisposition (seen with end-stage renal disease)	Diffuse cysts; adenomas; occasionally renal cell carcinoma	None	Incidence increases with duration of end-stage renal disease

Genetics

Once the diagnosis of ARPKD is strongly suspected, referral for genetic evaluation and counseling is appropriate. A detailed history should be taken of at least three generations. **Because the disease is transmitted as an autosomal recessive trait, siblings of either sex have a 1 in 4 chance of being affected, and neither parent should show evidence of the disease.**

Through linkage studies, an area of chromosome 6 has been identified as the genetic locus for both the milder forms (Zerres et al, 1994) **and the more severe forms of ARPKD, including severe perinatal disease** (Guay-Woodford et al, 1995). **In other words, despite the clinical variability of ARPKD, it appears that a single gene is responsible for all forms.** In utero genetic testing for ARPKD should be readily available in the near future.

Clinical Features

Blyth and Ockenden (1971) subdivided ARPKD into four types according to age at presentation and severity of the renal abnormality (Table 56–6). The earlier the age at which the disease is identified, the more severe the disease.

Table 56–6. BLYTH AND OCKENDEN CLASSIFICATION OF AUTOSOMAL RECESSIVE POLYCYSTIC KIDNEY DISEASE

Feature	Perinatal	Neonatal	Infantile	Juvenile
Number of cases	9	6	5	5
Age at presentation	Birth	<1 mo	3–6 mo	6 wk (1); 1–5 y
Mode of presentation	Huge abdominal masses, normal liver	Large kidneys, hepatic enlargement	Large kidneys, hepatosplenomegaly	Variable renal enlargement, hepatomegaly
Typical course	Early death or rapid progression of uremia	Progressive renal failure	Chronic renal failure, systemic and portal hypertension	Portal hypertension, often necessitating portocaval shunt
Length of survival	All dead by 6 wk	Five dead by 8 mo	Two dead by 8 y; three alive at 18 mo; four alive at 10 y	One dead at 9 mo and another at 20 y; three alive after 12 y
Proportion of kidney affected*	>90%	60%	25%	<10%
Periportal fibrosis	Minimal	Mild	Moderate	Marked

*Dilated tubules; all patients had dilated and infolded bile ducts in the liver.
Adapted from Blyth H, Ockenden BG: Polycystic disease of kidneys and liver presenting in childhood. J Med Gene 1971;8:257.

These investigators thought that only one of the various types—perinatal, neonatal, infantile, or juvenile—is present in a given family. However, numerous instances were subsequently described that contradict this hypothesis. However, the four clinical types in the Blyth and Ockenden classification correlate reasonably well with what might be expected when the disease manifests in different age groups. A fifth, milder group of patients who present as teenagers or young adults could be added. **In general, the younger the patient at presentation with ARPKD, the milder the liver disease; and, conversely, the younger the patient who presents with congenital hepatic fibrosis, the milder the renal cystic disease.** One must keep in mind that there are many clinical examples of patients that do not fit this generalization, but no matter what the severity of the renal disease, all patients with ARPKD have liver involvement in the form of congenital hepatic fibrosis and vary in the degree of biliary ectasia and periportal fibrosis (Habib, 1974; Kissane and Smith, 1975).

The affected newborn usually has enormous, kidney-shaped, nonbosselated flank masses that are hard and do not transilluminate. In some cases, the kidneys are large enough to impede delivery. Oligohydramnios is common because of the lack of normal urine production by the fetus. The infant often displays Potter's facies and deformities of the limbs and may have respiratory distress as a consequence of pulmonary hypoplasia. Oliguria is to be expected. Because of in utero "dialysis" by the placenta, the infant's serum creatinine and blood urea nitrogen (BUN) concentrations are normal at birth but soon begin to rise.

For infants in whom ARPKD is evident at birth, the usual clinical course is death within the first 2 months as a result of uremia or respiratory failure. However, infants who survive their first 31 days have a good chance of living at least 1 year if they receive proper supportive therapy. Cole and associates (1987) monitored 17 such children for a mean of 6.1 years and found that 8 were doing well with glomerular filtration rates greater than 40 ml/minute per 1.73 m², although most were hypertensive. Moreover, three of the five patients who required hemodialysis had needed it before 7 years of age. In such survivors, the kidneys atrophy and shrink (Lieberman et al, 1971).

Children whose disease appears later in life develop renal failure and hypertension more slowly than those in whom ARPKD is manifest at birth. In general, their clinical problems are the consequence of liver disease rather than the renal condition, with hepatic fibrosis leading to portal hypertension, esophageal varices, and hepatosplenomegaly.

Some patients have an intermediate type of disease in which both hepatic and renal failure appear between the ages of 5 and 20 years (McGonigle et al, 1981). Neumann and associates (1988) described two sisters whose disease did not appear until their teens. The similarity of the clinical findings supports the view of Blyth and Ockenden that the type of disease tends to be similar within a family. The first case was identified as a result of abdominal pain when the girl was 14 years old. None of the cysts was larger than 3 to 4 cm. Blood pressure was 150/95 mm Hg, and all laboratory values were normal. When the patient was

18 years old, her serum creatinine level was 1.3 mg/dl, and at age 21 years it was 1.6 mg/dl. Cystic kidneys were identified in the patient's 18-year-old sister as a result of family screening, and her serum creatinine level was found to be 2.8 mg/dl. A liver biopsy revealed congenital hepatic fibrosis.

In contrast, Kaplan and coworkers (1988) described a family in which the index case was an infant who died at the age of 18 hours. Both ARPKD and congenital hepatic fibrosis were found in an asymptomatic 16-year-old sister. This girl and the two described by Neumann and associates (1988) may provide evidence for a fifth type of ARPKD in the Blyth and Ockenden system.

Histopathology

The kidneys retain their fetal lobulation. Small subcapsular cysts, representing generalized fusiform dilations of the collecting tubules, are grossly visible when the capsule is removed. In the sectioned kidney, the dilated tubules can be seen in a radial arrangement from the calyx outward to the capsule. The cortex is crowded with minute cysts. The renal pedicle is normal, as are the renal pelvis and ureter. In older children whose disease has been evident since birth, the cysts are large and spherical, similar to those seen in the dominantly inherited disease (see later discussion). The nephron configuration is normal except for small dilatations, leading Potter (1972) to suggest that the abnormality appears late in gestation, with the dilatations of the collecting ducts and nephrons resulting from hyperplasia. Guay-Woodford and colleagues (1998) made similar observations and believed that medullary duct dilatation occurs first and then is followed by cortical collecting duct dilatation. Among patients who survive into childhood, cortical cysts may be the principal finding (Guay-Woodford et al, 1998).

All children with ARPKD have lesions in the periportal areas of the liver (Habib, 1974; Kissane and Smith, 1975). Proliferation, dilatation, and branching of well-differentiated bile ducts and ductules accompany some degree of periportal fibrosis. Gross cysts are not found. Some have suggested that, just as all children with ARPKD have liver disease, all children with congenital hepatic fibrosis have ARPKD; however, it is not certain that this is the case. Darmis and associates (1970) found a 100% incidence of ARPKD in children with congenital hepatic fibrosis; however, there are reports of children with hepatic but not renal disease. Kerr and colleagues (1962) found evidence of ARPKD in 60% of children with congenital hepatic fibrosis using excretory urography. The kidneys were not studied histologically, however, so the true incidence of ARPKD in this series is unknown. **Confusing the issue further is the fact that a small number of infants with ADPKD have been found to have congenital hepatic fibrosis** (Cobben et al, 1990).

Evaluation

The diagnosis may be suspected from in utero ultrasound examination and may be associated with oligohydramnios, a finding secondary to low urinary output. **In both fetus and newborn, sonography identifies very enlarged, ho-**

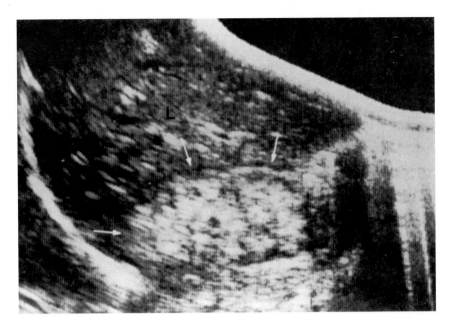

Figure 56–7. Sonogram of left kidney *(arrows)* in an infant with autosomal recessive polycystic kidney disease. Note homogeneously hyperechogenic kidneys, especially in comparison with the less echogenic liver (L). Increased echogenicity is caused by the multiple interphases created by the dilated medullary ducts. (From Grossman H, Rosenberg ER, Bowie JD, et al: Sonographic diagnosis of renal cystic diseases. AJR Am J Roentgenol 1983;140:81.)

mogeneously hyperechogenic kidneys, especially when compared with the echogenicity of the liver. The increased echogenicity is a result of the return of sound waves from the enormous number of interfaces created by tightly compacted, dilated collecting ducts. In the normal newborn, the kidneys have an equal or slightly increased echogenicity compared with the liver. Within the normal newborn kidney, hypoechogenic areas are seen circumferentially and are very typical of newborn renal pyramids. In comparison, in ARPKD the pyramids are hyperechogenic because they blend in with the rest of the kidney (Fig. 56–7). This appearance differs from that of severe bilateral hydronephrosis, in which the kidneys are enlarged with hypoechogenic calyces, or of multicystic kidney, in which hypoechogenic cysts lie within a nonreniform mass that has very little parenchyma. Bilateral mesoblastic nephroma–Wilms' tumor does not appear as homogeneous masses, and the infant has functioning kidneys. Bilateral renal vein thrombosis produces renal enlargement but hypoechogenic medullary areas. If the diagnosis remains in doubt, computed tomography (CT) is valuable because it is more sensitive to inhomogeneity (and therefore to tumor) within abdominal masses. Macrocysts are rare in newborns but increase in frequency as the child gets older.

Occasionally a newborn with severe ADPKD also has enlarged, homogeneously hyperechogenic kidneys. More often, cysts are apparent and predominate on the sonographic image in ADPKD. Macrocysts are rare in newborns with ARPKD but do increase in frequency as the child gets older, producing an appearance similar to that of the dominant disease. However, with time and prolonged renal failure, the kidneys tend to become smaller, whereas in the dominant disease the kidneys usually remain enlarged. **Fetuses with sporadic glomerulocystic kidney disease also can have enlarged, hyperechogenic kidneys** (Table 56–7).

Intravenous urography with delayed films may show functioning kidneys with characteristic radial or medul- lary streaking (sunburst pattern) caused by dilated collecting tubules filled with contrast medium. This picture can persist for as long as 48 hours after the study (Fig. 56–8). The calyces, renal pelvis, and ureter usually are not visible. In a few cases, the kidneys are already so dysfunctional that no opacification or only an increasingly dense nephrogram is apparent.

Some investigators have reported cases of transient neonatal nephromegaly that mimicked ARPKD. Avner and associates (1982) described a case in which an excretory urogram at the age of 2 days showed findings typical of ARPKD, whereas repeat studies at 6 weeks and 1 year showed normal renal architecture and size. They postulated that the radiographic findings were produced by transient intratubular obstruction. Berdon and coworkers (1969) presented a case of transient renal enlargement simulating ARPKD after an excretory urogram. Stapleton and colleagues (1981) described a similar case in which the sonographic findings were those expected in ARPKD. Therefore, one must remain aware of the possibility of transient nephromegaly, especially if a contrast study has been per-

Table 56–7. SONOGRAPHIC DIFFERENTIAL DIAGNOSIS OF A NEWBORN WITH BILATERAL, LARGE, CYSTIC KIDNEYS

Homogenous, Hyperechogenic Kidneys Without Macrocysts	With Diffuse Macrocysts
Autosomal recessive polycystic kidney disease (characteristic appearance)	Autosomal recessive polycystic kidney disease (atypical appearance)
Autosomal dominant polycystic kidney disease (atypical appearance)	Autosomal dominant polycystic kidney disease (characteristic appearance)
Sporadic glomerulocystic kidney disease	Sporadic glomerulocystic kidney disease
Contrast nephropathy	Tuberous sclerosis
Renal vein thrombosis	

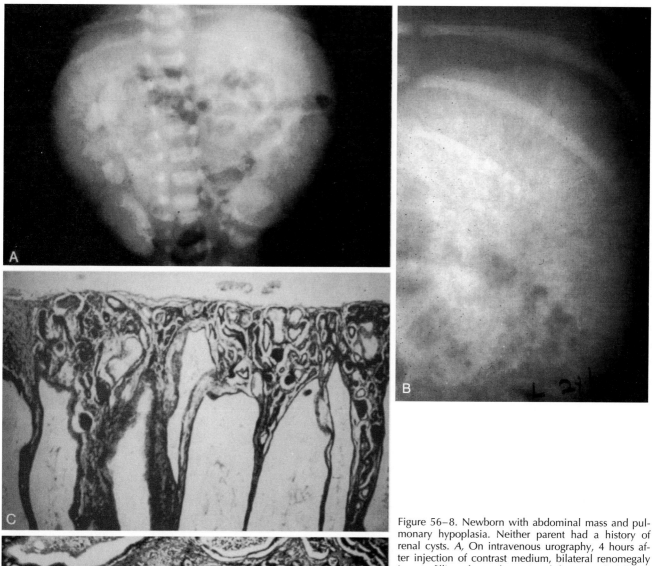

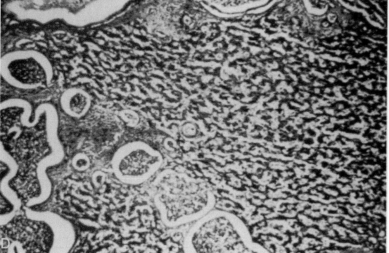

Figure 56–8. Newborn with abdominal mass and pulmonary hypoplasia. Neither parent had a history of renal cysts. *A,* On intravenous urography, 4 hours after injection of contrast medium, bilateral renomegaly is seen filling almost the entire abdomen with full and splayed out calyceal systems. Contrast medium can also be seen in the right kidney as rays stretching from the calyces to the periphery of the kidney. *B,* Twenty-four hours later, contrast medium still is seen within the left kidney in radially oriented dilated ducts. *C,* Renal histology also demonstrates dilated ducts radiating out to the periphery of the kidney. *D,* On liver histology, ectatic biliary ducts are seen in the left half of the figure, and periportal fibrosis is seen at the upper edge. The final diagnosis was autosomal recessive polycystic disease.

formed, and should not make a diagnosis of ARPKD prematurely. If necessary, a liver biopsy may be performed.

A detailed family history covering at least three generations is needed when ARPKD is suspected. Once the diagnosis is confirmed, referral for genetic counseling is appropriate. Because this condition is transmitted in an autosomal recessive fashion, siblings of either sex have 1 chance in 4 of being affected.

Zerres and coworkers (1988) attempted to make prenatal diagnoses of ARPKD in 11 at-risk pregnancies and concluded that early identification was possible only in severe cases. In one instance, ultrasound scans at 18 and 22 weeks yielded normal findings, yet the child was born with enormous kidneys and soon died.

Treatment

No cure has been found for ARPKD. Respiratory care can ease or extend the child's life. Patients who survive may require treatment for hypertension, congestive heart failure, and renal and hepatic failure. Portal hypertension may be dealt with by end-to-side anastomosis of the left renal vein to the splenic vein. Esophageal varices may be managed at least temporarily by gastric section and reanastomosis. Transcatheter sclerotherapy has been employed in adults with chronically bleeding varices, but I am not aware of the use of this measure in children with ARPKD. Hemodialysis and renal transplantation must eventually be considered in many patients.

AUTOSOMAL DOMINANT ("ADULT") POLYCYSTIC KIDNEY DISEASE

The autosomal dominant form of polycystic kidney disease (ADPKD) is an important cause of renal failure, accounting for 10% to 15% of patients who receive hemodialysis (Hildenbrandt, 1995). **Its incidence is approximately 1 in 500 to 1000, and approximately 500,000 Americans have been diagnosed with the disease** (Gabow, 1993). **Two genes for ADPKD have been localized, PKD1 on chromosome 16** (Reeders et al, 1986a) **and PKD2 on chromosome 4** (Peters et al, 1993). **A third but rare genetic locus, PKD3, is thought to exist but has not yet been identified. The trait theoretically has a 100% penetrance, and on average, because it is transmitted in an autosomal dominant fashion, 50% of an affected individual's offspring will likewise be affected. According to Gabow (1991), 96% of affected persons will manifest the disease clinically by age 90 years.**

The traditional descriptor of "adult" polycystic disease is inaccurate. Although most cases are identified when the patients are between 30 and 50 years of age, **the condition has been recognized in newborns.** Presumably, the typical age at diagnosis will decline as more members of families at risk for the trait are screened by genetic testing and by ultrasound examination. All affected individuals manifest the disease (although not necessarily symptomatically) if they live long enough, but renal failure is seldom seen before the age of 40 years—**unless the disease manifests during infancy, in which case it is much more aggressive.**

A number of associated anomalies are common, including cysts of the liver, pancreas, spleen, and lungs; aneurysms of the circle of Willis (berry aneurysms); colonic diverticula; and mitral valve prolapse (Table 56–8).

Etiology

The genetically encoded defect responsible for ADPKD is the subject of several theories. **One of these suggests that a defect in the basement membrane of the tubules accounts for cyst development.** This theory is supported by the finding of abnormal basement membrane antigens (Carone et al, 1988). It is hypothesized that an abnormal basement membrane leads to increased compliance, allowing outpockets to develop from tubules or expansion of tubules. However, this theory is somewhat negated by the finding that both normal and cystic basement membranes are equally compliant (Grantham et al, 1987a, 1987b).

A second theory, suggested by Grantham and co-workers (1987a), holds that epithelial hyperplasia is an integral part of cyst formation. This theory is supported by the frequency of hyperplasia and adenomas in ADPKD. Hyperplasia might cause tubular obstruction, resulting in weakening of the basement membrane and secondary proximal outpouching. In addition, EGF has been identified in cyst fluid (Ye et al, 1986), **and the receptors for EGF have been identified ectopically on the apical side of cells adjacent to the cyst fluid as well as in their normal basolateral location** (Du and Wilson, 1991).

A third theory postulates a defect in one of the proteins of the supportive extracellular connective tissue matrix. Such an abnormality could account for both the basement membrane abnormalities (Gabow and Schrier, 1989) **and the cysts found in other organs** (Dalgaard and Norby, 1989). **Support for this theory is provided by the**

Table 56–8. COMPARISON OF AUTOSOMAL RECESSIVE AND AUTOSOMAL DOMINANT POLYCYSTIC KIDNEY DISEASE

Item	Autosomal Recessive Polycystic Kidney Disease (ARPKD)	Autosomal Dominant Polycystic Kidney Disease (ADPKD)
Gene defect	Chromosome 6	Chromosomes 4 and 16
Incidence	1:5000 to 1:40,000	1:500 to 1:1000
Usual age of clinical presentation	Perinatal	Third to fifth decades
Typical sonographic appearance of kidneys	Symmetrically enlarged, homogeneous, hyperechogenic kidneys	Large cystic kidneys, sometimes asymmetrical
Histology	Collecting duct ectasia; cysts derived principally from collecting duct	Microcysts and macrocysts derived from entire nephron
Liver	Always congenital hepatic fibrosis but of varying severity	Cysts, mostly in adults (on very rare occasions a newborn may have congenital hepatic fibrosis)
Other system involvement	None	Intracranial aneurysms; colonic diverticuli; mitral valve regurgitation; cysts of other organs

association of ADPKD with mitral valve prolapse, colonic diverticula, and hepatic cysts (Gabow and Schrier, 1989), **because similar constellations are seen in conditions that are known to involve defects of matrix proteins.** Diverticulosis, mitral valve prolapse, and berry aneurysms are common in patients with Ehlers-Danlos syndrome, and diverticulosis and mitral valve prolapse are seen in Marfan's syndrome.

A fourth theory involves the location of Na⁺-K⁺-ATPase in the cystic epithelium. Wilson and associates (1991) found that Na⁺-K⁺-ATPase in polycystic epithelial cells was located in the apical position in cells lining the cyst rather than in the usual basolateral position. In this case, fluid would preferably enter the cyst lumen rather than leave it (Gabow, 1993). This theory is supported by the finding that when in vitro cysts are exposed to ouabain (a sodium pump inhibitor), cyst enlargement is slowed down (Grantham et al, 1989; Avner et al, 1989).

From a review of a number of these theories, **it appears that tubular epithelial cell hyperplasia is the major component of cyst development, although possibly not the first.** The identity of the prime mover in initiating the epithelial hyperplasia process is not yet clear. Perhaps it is an injury to the tubular basement membrane or to tubular epithelial lining cells that occurs first, and the healing process becomes a hyperplastic one. Maybe the gene defect leads to the production of a protein or lack of production of a protein that causes the injury.

What is apparent is that tubular cell growth depends on a balance between cell growth inhibitors and cell growth stimulators. Factors inhibiting or stimulating cell growth are located in the cell, in the cell membrane, in the basement membrane, and in the extracellular matrix. A change in the balance of these factors results in cell growth or growth suppression. Extracellular matrix lays down a substance called heparan sulfate proteoglycan (HSPG) to form part of the tubular basement membrane. HSPG and another substance, TGF-β, inhibit cell growth. EGF is a growth stimulator whose activity is increased when there is an increase in EGF receptor activity or a decrease in HSPG or TGF-β inhibitory activity. In cystic disease in mice and in early cystic disease in humans, it has been shown that the dynamic balance between stimulators and inhibitors of cell growth changes in favor of the stimulators. First, EGF activity is increased in the lumens of cysts. In addition, EGF receptor activity is localized ectopically at the apical position (lumen side) of the tubular cells, as well as at its normal basolateral position, enhancing by proximity the activity of the intraluminal EGF. At the same time, inhibitor TGF-β and HSPG activity seem to diminish as well. The net effect favors cell growth (Wilson and Sherwood, 1991).

As the cells proliferate, the tubules expand, coil, or form diverticula to preserve a monolayer epithelial lining. Sometimes dilated tubules or diverticula separate from the rest of the nephron to form an isolated sac. Aided by the apical location of Na⁺-K⁺-ATPase (fourth theory, described earlier), solute and water are pumped into the lumen of the isolated sacs (cysts), causing cyst expansion.

In ARPKD, Avner and Sweeney (1992) found cyst epithelial cells derived from proximal tubule cells to have apical mislocation of neither EGFR or Na⁺-K⁺-ATPase.

Although collecting duct–derived cyst epithelial cells had apical EGFR, apical mislocation of Na⁺-K⁺-ATPase was not found. Because ARPKD is predominantly a collecting duct disease, the apical EGFR location in collecting duct epithelial cells seems to correlate with pathologic findings.

Genetics

Two genes have been identified as the culprits for ADPKD: (1) the polycystic kidney disease (PKD1) gene localized on the short arm of chromosome 16 (Reeders et al, 1985; Breuning et al, 1987; Ryynanen et al, 1987; Pieke et al, 1989), **which accounts for approximately 85% to 90% of cases, and (2) the PKD2 gene localized to chromosome 4** (Peters et al, 1993), **which accounts for approximately 5% to 10% of cases.** The PKD1 gene itself has now been isolated (European Polycystic Disease Consortium, 1994); the PKD2 gene has yet to be isolated. **The presence of a third locus (PKD3) is now accepted as the cause of disease in a very small percentage of patients who have been found to have neither a PKD1 nor a PKD2 gene defect** (Dauost et al, 1993).

The means to make an early diagnosis of ADPKD (before cyst development) by identifying the mutated gene, particularly in PKD1 disease, is still not easy or readily available. The more conventional approach is to use linkage analysis instead, but this also is difficult and requires the availability of at least two affected family members (Watson, 1997). Flanking genetic markers on either side of the PKD1 or PKD2 gene need to be identified. The closer a flanking marker is to the gene of interest, the more likely it is to be transmitted with that gene. Flanking genetic markers may differ from one family to the next. Therefore, one must find two affected individuals in the same family with the same linkages before one can say that an individual has either the PKD1 or the PKD2 gene. Chorionic villus samplings are employed to make the diagnosis of ADPKD in utero (Reeders et al, 1986b; Turco et al, 1992). However, only a few families have sought in utero genetic diagnosis, and even fewer have elected abortion.

In general, although families with PKD1 and PKD2 gene defects share the same major manifestations, those with the PKD2 defect usually (but not uniformly) have a later onset of clinical symptoms and a slower progression of disease (Dauost et al, 1993). **In addition, Bear and associates (1992) suggested that the disease in general is more severe and manifests earlier when it is inherited from the mother rather than from the father.** This phenomenon is referred to as *genetic imprinting.* The phenomenon of *genetic anticipation* is seen as well; it is manifested by progressively earlier presentation and increased severity in subsequent generations of patients with ADPKD (Fick et al, 1994; Zerres and Rudnick-Schöeheborn, 1995). (Additional information on the genetics of ADPKD was presented earlier, in the section on molecular genetics.)

Clinical Features

Neonates present mostly on the basis of renomegaly. When the disease is severe, stillbirth or significant respiratory distress can occur. For example, of the first 29 reported cases in newborns, 7 were stillborn infants, 4 of whom died of dystocia (McClean et al, 1964; Mebrizi et al, 1964; Blyth and Ockenden, 1971; Kaye and Lewy, 1974; Bengtsson et al, 1975; Ross and Trovers, 1975; Stickler and Kelales, 1975; Stillaert et al, 1975; Fellows et al, 1976; Ritter and Siafarikas, 1976; Begleiter et al, 1977; Kaplan et al, 1977; Loh et al, 1977; Euderink and Hogewind, 1978; Wolf et al, 1978; Shokeir, 1978; Fryns and van den Berghe, 1979; Proesmans et al, 1982). Of the 20 patients who survived the neonatal period, 13 died within 9 months, 8 of renal failure, usually in association with hypertension. Nevertheless, five of the seven patients who were alive at the time they were reported, at the ages of 3 months to 9 years, had good renal function.

In children who present after 1 year of age, the principal signs and symptoms are related to hypertension and enlarged and impaired kidneys (e.g., proteinuria, hematuria). Now that the families of ADPKD patients are being screened by sonography, large numbers of asymptomatic children with renal cysts are being identified before full-blown disease develops.

Typically, symptoms or signs first occur between the ages of 30 and 50 years (Glassberg et al, 1981). **These include microscopic and gross hematuria, flank pain, gastrointestinal symptoms (perhaps secondary to renomegaly or associated colonic diverticula), and renal colic secondary either to clots or stone and hypertension. Microscopic or gross hematuria is seen in 50% of patients, and in 19% to 35% it is the presenting symptom** (Milutinovic, 1984; Delaney et al, 1985; Zeier et al, 1988; Gabow et al, 1992). In the series of Gabow and associates (1992), 42% of patients had at least one episode of gross hematuria, the mean age at first episode being 30 ± 1 year. Only in 10% of patients did the first episode occur before the age of 16 years. In general, they found that increased episodes of gross hematuria were associated with higher serum creatinine levels. Because these patients with ADPKD have increased renal mass, erythropoietin levels are increased, making anemia unusual even when end-stage renal disease (ESRD) is present (Gabow, 1993).

Twenty percent to 30% of patients with ADPKD develop stones (Fick and Gabow, 1994), and these are treated by conservative means (i.e., urine alkalinization and extracorporal shock wave lithotripsy). However, the finding of hydronephrosis, which helps make the diagnosis of stones, may not be as useful in ADPKD patients because of the number of cysts camouflaging the findings (Choyke, 1996).

As blood pressure screening has become more widespread, hypertension more than hematuria has become the principal form of presentation. For example, in a series from Heidelberg, Germany (Zeier et al, 1988), as many as 81% of patients with ADPKD presented with hypertension. Among the Heidelberg patients who had a normal serum creatinine concentration, 30% were found to be hypertensive. Antihypertensive medication instituted early resulted in fewer complications, particularly with regard to the incidence of cerebral hemorrhage. Other series suggest that the incidence of hypertension is about 60% before the onset of renal failure (Nash, 1977; Gabow et al, 1984, 1990; Valvo et al, 1985). The hypertension seems to be renin mediated and secondary to stretching of the intrarenal vessels around cysts, causing distal ischemia (Gabow, 1993).

As noted earlier, the polycystic condition in ADPKD is not confined to the kidneys. **Hepatic cysts, usually identified incidentally by sonography, help in making the diagnosis of ADPKD and usually appear later than renal cysts. These cysts are more likely to be found in adults than in children and more frequently in females** (Fick and Gabow, 1994). Such cysts were found by CT scanning in almost 60% of one series of adults (mean age, 49 years) (Thomsen and Thaysen, 1988). Hepatic cysts often grow, but they seldom produce any clinically important effects. New ones may appear as the patient grows older (Thomsen and Thaysen, 1988). In rare instances, enlargement of hepatic cysts leads to portal hypertension and bleeding esophageal varices (Campbell et al, 1958). When secondary portal hypertension appears, differentiating ADPKD from ARPKD can be difficult. In ARPKD portal hypertension is seen much more frequently and is always secondary to congenital hepatic fibrosis. However, **congenital hepatic fibrosis on very rare occasions may accompany ADPKD as well, particularly when the diagnosis is made perinatally.** When congenital hepatic fibrosis accompanies ADPKD, the clinical course is quite variable, just as it is in ARPKD. In three ADPKD families in which at least one family member had congenital hepatic fibrosis, the genetic defect was localized to PKD1 on chromosome 16, clearly supporting a diagnosis of ADPKD rather than ARPKD (Cobben et al, 1990). In these three families, congenital hepatic fibrosis was not transmitted vertically with ADPKD but instead was found only in siblings.

Approximately 10% to 40% of patients have berry aneurysms, and approximately 9% of these patients die because of subarachnoid hemorrhages (Hartnett and Bennett, 1976; Grantham, 1979; Wakabayashi et al, 1983; Sedmon and Gabow, 1984; Ryu, 1990). Now with magnetic resonance imaging (MRI), even small berry aneurysms can be detected. Using MRI, Huston and associates (1993) found that families with a previous history of intracranial aneurysms had a higher incidence of berry aneurysms than families without a positive history. In their series, 6 (27%) of 27 patients with a family history and 3 (5%) of 56 patients without a family history were found to have aneurysms. The problem is what to do with these aneurysms when they are diagnosed, because they average only 6.1 mm in size. Although small aneurysms (<1 cm) have a lower risk of rupture, patients with small aneurysms have a greater risk of rupture when there is a positive family history of ruptured intracranial aneurysms or the presence of ADPKD (Huston et al, 1993).

However, not all intracranial hemorrhages in patients with ADPKD represent subarachnoid bleeding secondary to berry aneurysms; in some patients, hemorrhage follows the rupture of intracerebral arteries, which is the usual type of intracranial hemorrhage seen in patients with hypertension who do not have ADPKD. For example, in Ryu's series (1990), a cerebral artery rupture accounted for the hemorrhage in eight patients and a ruptured berry aneurysm in only three. In 10 of these 11 patients, hypertension was present, and funduscopy suggested previous hypertension in the remaining patient also. A 17.4% incidence of conventional cerebrovascular accidents was suggested in Choyke's review (1996). Now, with earlier detection and treatment of hypertension, one can expect fewer deaths from intracranial hemorrhage.

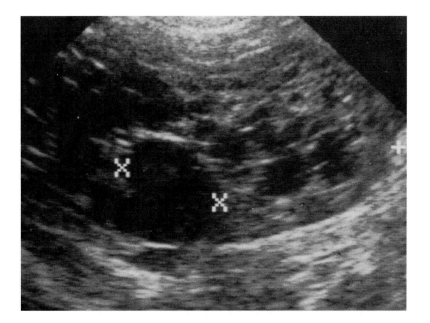

Figure 56–9. Asymmetric presentation of autosomal dominant polycystic kidney disease in a 9-year-old boy with hematuria. Sonogram demonstrates right kidney with multiple cysts. No cysts were identified in the left kidney. Subsequently, the diagnosis was made in the patient's brother and mother. Cysts can be expected to develop in the right kidney with time.

Intracerebral bleeding has been reported in at least one child with ADPKD. This child also had hypertrophic pyloric stenosis (Proesmans et al, 1982), a condition that was reported in association with ADPKD in a set of identical twins and their father (Loh et al, 1977). Hypertrophic pyloric stenosis also has accompanied ARPKD (Gaisford and Bloor, 1968; Lieberman et al, 1971; McGonigle et al, 1981). **Other abnormalities associated with ADPKD are mitral valve prolapse and colonic diverticulosis** (Scheff et al, 1980; Hossack et al, 1986; Kupin et al, 1987). Patients who have diverticulosis are more likely to have hepatic cysts and symptomatic berry aneurysms (Kupin et al, 1987).

When patients with ADPKD present clinically, they usually are found to have bilateral cysts. However, the disease can manifest asymmetrically, with cysts on only one side at first or with a unilateral renal mass (Fig. 56–9).

A variant form of ADPKD probably exists in which the renal cysts are located primarily in Bowman's space. The cytogenetic study of Reeders and associates (1985) provided evidence that such a condition is a form of ADPKD. They found that a fetus with cystic disease predominantly of the glomeruli had the same genetic linkages on chromosome 16 as did its ADPKD-affected mother. Bernstein and Landing (1989) suggested that glomerulocystic kidneys in members of families with ADPKD are variants; the glomerular cysts may be an early stage of ADPKD gene expression (Fig. 56–10). One caution: this condition should not be referred to as "glomerulocystic kidney disease," to avoid confusing it with sporadic glomerulocystic kidney disease, a condition that seems to be histologically identical to ADPKD in infants except for the absence of affected family members (Bernstein, 1993), or with other disorders associated with glomerular cysts, which are discussed later in this chapter. Both of these forms of glo-

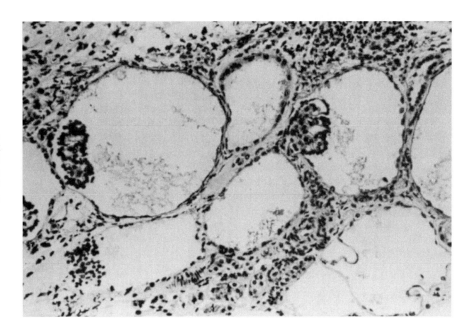

Figure 56–10. Glomerular cysts with a pattern compatible with that of autosomal dominant polycystic kidney disease in early childhood (×190). (From Bernstein J, Gardner KD: Cystic disease and dysplasia of the kidneys. In Murphy WM [ed]: Urological Pathology. Philadelphia, WB Saunders, 1989, pp 483–524.)

merulocystic kidneys, sporadic glomerulocystic kidney disease and ADPKD with glomerular cysts, when diagnosed in neonates, are associated with about a 10% incidence of biliary dysgenesis (Bernstein, 1993).

Histopathology

The renal cysts range from a few millimeters to a few centimeters in diameter and appear diffusely throughout the cortex and medulla with communications at various points along the nephron (Kissane, 1974). Frequently, the epithelial lining resembles the segment of the nephron from which the cyst is derived (Kaplan and Miller, unpublished data), and it often is active in secretion and reabsorption (Gardner, 1988).

In affected fetuses the renal abnormality may develop earlier in ARPKD because the cortical cysts develop simultaneously with abnormal medullary differentiation, rather than as a subsequent event as in ADPKD, where the kidneys are more normally differentiated (Guay-Woodford, 1998). The first pathologic finding in fetuses is focal tubular dilatation, which may occur anywhere along the nephron (Choyke, 1996).

Epithelial hyperplasia or even adenoma formation in the cyst wall is common, and the basement membrane of the wall is thickened. Arteriosclerosis is present in more than 70% of patients with preterminal or terminal renal failure, and interstitial fibrosis, with or without infiltrates, is common (Zeier et al, 1988). This fibrosis may be secondary to infection or to an inflammatory reaction set off by spontaneously rupturing cysts.

Apoptosis may play a role in the development of renal failure. It appears in the epithelial lining of the cysts and to a lesser degree in the cells lining nondilated nephrons (Winyard et al, 1996).

Gregoire and coworkers (1987) found a 91% incidence of hyperplastic polyps in kidneys removed from ADPKD patients either at autopsy or before transplantation. Some of the autopsies were performed on patients with normal renal function, yet polyps were still found. However, there was a greater predominance of polyps in patients with renal failure and in those receiving dialysis therapy. Because hyperplastic epithelium is seen in both chronic renal failure and ADPKD, a uremic toxin not removed by dialysis may be involved.

Association with Renal Cell Carcinoma

The incidence of renal adenomas is almost as high in ADPKD as in ESRD associated with ARCD (i.e., one in four to five patients). However, whereas ESRD is associated with an increased incidence of RCC, especially when associated with ARCD (three to six times the incidence seen in the general population), the incidence of RCC in patients with ADPKD is no higher than that in the general population. That the incidence of RCC is not increased in ADPKD is also surprising in view of the frequent finding of epithelial hyperplasia. For example, two other conditions, tuberous sclerosis and VHL, are associated with epithelial hyperplasia (and adenomas as well) and are associated with an increased incidence of RCC (tuberous sclerosis, 2%; VHL, 35% to 38%). Although it is

recognized that there is no increased incidence of RCC in ADPKD patients, it is hard to account for certain findings considered typical of a predisposition to RCC that are seen more frequently in patients with ADPKD than in the general population. For example, RCC in ADPKD is more often concurrently bilateral (12%, versus 1% to 5% in the general population), multicentric (28% versus 6%), and sarcomatoid in type (33% versus 1% to 5%) (Keith et al, 1994).

Three factors may have contributed to the impression of a higher incidence of RCC in ADPKD. First, the chance association of these two rather common lesions is expected to be frequent. Second, some cases of simultaneous ADPKD and RCC may actually represent cancers in patients with VHL or tuberous sclerosis. Third, the epithelial hyperplasia of ADPKD, which is a precancerous lesion in other conditions, may have been considered precancerous in ADPKD as well, although available data do not at present justify this view (Jacobs et al, 1979; Zeier et al, 1988).

Evaluation

To make the diagnosis, it is important to have a history of the patient's family spanning at least three generations. Questions should be asked about renal disease, hypertension, and strokes. Abdominal sonography may reveal renal cysts as well as cysts in other organs. When there is no family history to support a diagnosis of ADPKD, a presumptive diagnosis can be made if bilateral renal cysts are present and two or more of the following symptoms are present as well: bilateral renal enlargement; three or more hepatic cysts; cerebral artery aneurysm; and a solitary cyst of the arachnoid, pineal gland, pancreas, or spleen (Grantham, 1993).

When ADPKD is manifested in utero or in infancy, 50% of affected kidneys are large with identifiable macrocysts (Pretorius et al, 1987). However, the kidneys may appear identical to those seen in ARPKD, having no apparent macrocysts and showing only enlargement and homogeneous hyperechoic features. In such situations, one must look for a parent with ADPKD to confirm the diagnosis.

On intravenous urography, the calyces may be stretched by cysts. However, the picture may simulate that of ARPKD, with medullary streaking of contrast medium. In adults, intravenous urography usually reveals bilateral renal enlargement, calyceal distortion, and a bubble or Swiss cheese appearance in the nephrogram phase. A CT scan or MRI (or both) may be helpful in some cases and often is superior to sonography for detecting cysts in organs other than the kidney (Fig. 56–11; see Fig. 56–10). CT is helpful in making the diagnosis of hemorrhage within a cyst. More acute hemorrhage has a higher density (50 to 90 Hounsfield units [HU]) than old hemorrhage (Choyke, 1996). **MRI also may be helpful, particularly in patients with compromised renal function, because no contrast agent is needed** (Fig. 56–12).

According to Gabow and associates (1989b), patients with ADPKD have a reduced maximum urine osmolality (680 $\pm$ 14 mOsm) after overnight water deprivation and administration of vasopressin, a finding that may be helpful

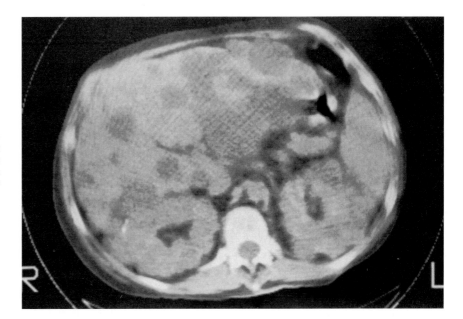

Figure 56–11. Computed tomographic scan of an adult male patient with autosomal dominant polycystic kidney disease. Bilateral renal cysts are seen in enlarged kidneys with calcification. Large asymptomatic cysts are seen throughout the liver as well.

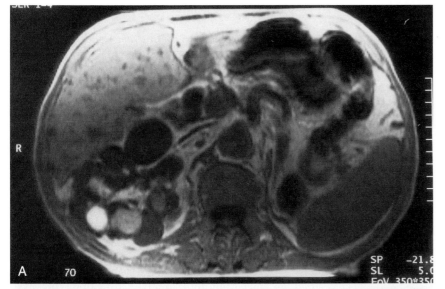

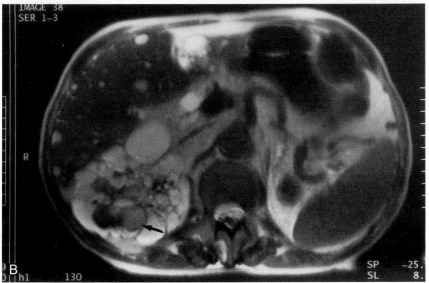

Figure 56–12. Magnetic resonance cholangiogram in a 55-year-old female with autosomal dominant polycystic kidney disease done for evaluation of biliary distention. Patient has had a left nephrectomy for pain. Right renal and hepatic cysts are seen on both T1 and T2 coronal images. *A,* T1 image demonstrates renal cysts with low and high *(white)* signals. High-signal cysts correlate with intracystic hemorrhage. *B,* On T2, hemorrhagic cysts are dark and cysts without hemorrhage are white. On T2 imaging with the patient in the supine position, cysts with blood tend to get darker more posteriorly *(arrow).* (Courtesy of H. Zinn, M.D.)

in identifying other family members with the disease. However, within the next few years cytogenetic screening should be readily available to identify the gene defects on chromosomes 4 and 16.

Examination of Family Members and Genetic Counseling

Because ADPKD is an autosomal dominant condition, 50% of the children of affected adults will also be affected. Therefore, when the disease is diagnosed, the patient's children should be examined by ultrasound. Before 1970, diagnosis of ADPKD before the age of 25 years was rare. With ultrasound, the possibility of making the diagnosis in affected individuals before this age is at least 85% (Table 56–9). **When genetic studies are used, the diagnostic accuracy approaches 100%.**

Gabow and coworkers (1989a) identified ADPKD in 16 of 59 children before the age of 12 years, and the disease was suspected in another 10. Bear and colleagues (1984), who studied 61 children sonographically, found ADPKD in only 2 of 18 children younger than age 10 but in 14 of 43 children between 10 and 19 years of age. Similarly, Sahney and associates (1983) found the disease in only one of five children younger than age 15 but in 16 of 19 children aged 16 to 25 years. This last figure points out the fact that the 50% incidence of affected offspring is an average, not a guarantee.

Bear and coworkers (1984) calculated that the chance that an asymptomatic relative between the ages of 10 and 19 years has ADPKD is 28% if an ultrasound scan is negative and that, for a similar individual aged 20 to 29 years, the risk is 14%. Other investigators have found rates of 32% to 50% in siblings and children younger than 20 years of age (Walker et al, 1984; Sedman et al, 1987; Taitz et al, 1987). **When patients with a known PKD1 defect were selected for renal sonographic screening, 40 (83%) of 48 individuals were found to have cysts before the age of 30 years, and all 48 had them after age 30** (Parfrey et al, 1990). Because the number of simple cysts increases with age, criteria to make the diagnosis need to change with increasing patient age. For example, Ravine and colleagues (1994) suggested that, in patients with a family history, only two cysts (either unilateral or bilateral) are required in patients 30 years of age or younger to make the diagnosis of ADPKD, whereas in those between 31 and 59 years of age, at least two cysts in each kidney are required, and in those older than 60 years, more than four cysts are required in each kidney for diagnosis.

At present, family members of an individual with ADPKD cannot obtain insurance before the age of 25 years because of the possibility of the disease (Dalgaard and Norby, 1989). Between the ages of 25 and 35 years, insurance is available but at higher rates, and after the age of 35 years insurance can be obtained at normal rates if a sonogram has been negative. Now, with definitive cytogenetic diagnosis available, it may be time for insurance companies to revise their criteria of insurability.

Treatment and Prognosis

Men tend to have more renal involvement than women, manifesting with hypertension and renal insufficiency earlier than in women (Grantham, 1993). However, women seem to have more severe cystic involvement of the liver, which causes pain and requires treatment more often than that in men (Grantham, 1993).

More than 60% of patients with ADPKD who do not yet have renal impairment have hypertension (Gabow et al, 1984), **which can worsen renal function, cause cardiac disease, and predispose the patient to intracranial hemorrhage. The complications of ADPKD can be reduced significantly by controlling the blood pressure.**

The rate of renal deterioration seems to correlate with the rate of cyst growth, supposedly because the enlarging cysts cause pressure atrophy. However, histologic studies by Zeier and coworkers (1988) revealed no evidence of pressure atrophy, nor did these investigators find evidence of glomerular hyperperfusion, which had been thought to damage the remaining glomeruli after some had been destroyed.

Fifty percent to 70% of patients with ADPKD at some time have loin or back pain (Grantham, 1992). **The pain can be colicky, acute, or chronic. Colicky pain occurs secondary to the passage of either stones or clots. Acute pain may be secondary to infection or hemorrhage into a cyst or to subcapsular bleeding.** Chronic loin pain requiring narcotics is probably related to distention of cysts and the renal capsule. **Rovsing in 1911 described an operation that involved unroofing the cysts to relieve the pain. The procedure fell into some dispute because of reports that renal function could deteriorate after such a procedure.** More recent reports, however, are repopularizing the procedure. Ye and associates (1986) reported that the incidence of relief of pain after Rovsing's operation was 90.6% after 6 months and 77.1% after 5 years, whereas Elzinga and colleagues (1992) found that 80% of patients were pain free at 1 year and 62% at 2 years. Of significance was the finding that renal function did not deteriorate after the procedure in either series; in fact, in the former study there was a significant improvement in renal function in some patients. When pain did return after an unroofing procedure, it often was less severe than it was preoperatively and required narcotics infrequently (Elzinga et al, 1992). Percutaneous cyst aspiration with or without instillation of a sclerosing agent such as alcohol (Bennett et al, 1987; Everson et al, 1990) also can play a therapeutic role. However, aspiration alone is more likely to be associated with reaccumulation of cyst fluid. **In 1993, Elzinga and associates suggested laparo-**

Table 56–9. INCIDENCE OF RENAL CYSTS IN SIBLINGS AND OFFSPRING OF PATIENTS WITH AUTOSOMAL DOMINANT POLYCYSTIC KIDNEY DISEASE

Reference	Age at Study (Yr)	No. with Cysts/No. Studied (%)
Bear et al, 1984	<10	2/18 (11)
Gabow et al, 1989a	<12	26/59 (40)
Taitz et al, 1987	<14	10/22 (45)
Sahney et al, 1983	<15	1/5 (20)
Walker et al, 1984	5–17	11/22 (50)
Bear et al, 1984	10–19	14/43 (34)
Sedman et al, 1987	<19	49/154 (32)
Bear et al, 1984	<20–29	26/62 (42)
Sahney et al, 1983	<26	17/24 (70)

scopic unroofing of cysts as an alternative to an open procedure in order to reduce the incidence of morbidity. Within 2 years after that report, four more studies appeared (Rubenstein et al, 1993; Chehval and Neilsen, 1995; Segura et al, 1995; Teichman and Hubert, 1995). **More recently, Dunn and colleagues (2001) reported on 15 patients, 6 with bilateral cysts, who had undergone laparoscopic unroofing of cysts for the management of pain. With time, these authors have become more aggressive in their treatment, extending the number of cysts unroofed in some patients to more than 300 and the time of procedure to more than 5 hours. At a mean follow-up of 2.2 years, subjective pain was reduced by 62% in 11 of the 15 patients, and those with bilateral unroofing faired better. The remaining 4 patients had less impressive results. The effect of laparoscopic unroofing in those patients with hypertension was quite variable.**

Because only 1% of nephrons develop cysts in ADPKD, it is not clear why renal failure develops. Possible causes include compression of nondilated nephrons by the cysts; prominence of apoptosis in epithelial cells—not only in the cells lining the cysts but also in the nondilated nephrons (Winyard et al, 1996); and secondary effects of hypertension. The fact that unroofing of cysts does not dramatically improve renal function makes one question the role that compression plays.

Upper tract urinary tract infections are common in patients with ADPKD, especially women. Schwab and coworkers (1987) divided these cases into parenchymal and cyst infections. In their series, **87% of cyst infections and 91% of parenchymal infections occurred in women.** When a gram-negative enteric organism was the cause, 100% of the infections were seen in women. Presumably, in women the infection is an ascending one. Schwab and coworkers (1987) found that parenchymal infections responded better than cyst infections to treatment, even when the organism causing the cyst infection was proved to be sensitive to the antibiotic used. **In their experience, the only dependable antibiotics were those that were lipid soluble, namely, trimethoprim-sulfamethoxazole and chloramphenicol. Chloramphenicol produced better results. The fluoroquinolones, which are also lipid soluble, are likewise proving useful** (Bennett et al, 1990). **If a patient with suspected pyelonephritis does not respond to an antibiotic and if the antibiotic used is not lipid soluble, one must consider whether the infection may be present in a noncommunicating cyst** (Gabow, 1993).

Symptomatic children usually are in the terminal stages of the disease, but their survival may be extended by supportive care for complications. As in affected adults, dialysis and transplantation may be appropriate. In the past, allografts from siblings were ruled out because of the frequency of ADPKD in such donors. However, now that siblings can be screened, this ban may no longer be appropriate.

Presymptomatic patients with ADPKD should be monitored with blood pressure measurements and tests of renal function. The advantages of such monitoring include the abilities to prevent or control infection and hypertension, to identify potential kidney donors from among the family, to offer advice on marriage and childbearing, and to provide prenatal diagnosis. The question of abortion of an affected fetus is an issue that the parents and the physician must consider in view of the improved prognosis for such patients.

In earlier reports of ADPKD, the prognosis was quite poor, the mean life expectancy ranging from 4 to 13 years after clinical presentation. Life expectancy was even shorter if the disease became apparent after the age of 50 years (Braasch and Schacht, 1933; Rall and Odell, 1949; Dalgaard, 1957). Death usually was attributable to uremia, heart failure, or cerebral hemorrhage (Dalgaard, 1957). **Churchill and associates (1984) calculated that patients with sonographically identifiable ADPKD have a 2% chance of developing end-stage renal failure by age 40 years, a 23% chance by age 50, and a 48% chance by age 73.** Because of enhanced ability to deal with problems such as urinary infection, calculi, hypertension, and renal failure, the outlook for patients with ADPKD appears to be improving dramatically.

Emerging Therapeutics

Because EGF and its receptor (see previous discussion) are thought to play an important role in the genesis of ADPKD, some investigators have taken this knowledge into account in developing medications that have the potential to control the disease. For example, Sweeney and coworkers (2000) developed an EGFR–tyrosine kinase inhibitor, EKI-785, and used it to treat an ARPKD entity in postnatal mice between days 7 and 14. Untreated mice died by day 24 with collecting duct cysts, renal failure, and severe biliary abnormalities. Those treated until day 48 were alive and well, with normal renal function, much less cyst formation, and significantly fewer biliary abnormalities. If the EGFR of these mice is the same or similar to that in humans with ARPKD and ADPKD, EKI-785 or a similar agent may be useful in the treatment of these diseases. By using such an agent that enters the urine through the nephron, apical EGFR–tyrosine kinase activity and subsequent cyst development could be inhibited. Such inhibition of EGFR is already being used in the treatment of psoriasis, a condition in which there is sustained activation of TGF-α on keratinocytes. In psoriasis, the EGFR blocker tryphostin inhibits the proliferation of keratinocytes. Decreased DNA synthesis and EGF-induced tyrosine phosphorylation parallels the decreased proliferation (Dvir et al, 1991). Because the EGFRs in ADPKD are located at the apical side of tubular cells, the receptors would be exposed to any blocking agent or receptor antibody that passes through the nephron tubular lumen. If almost all of an administered EGFR blocking agent were eliminated through the kidney, that agent would reach its site of need (i.e., at the apical luminal side of tubular epithelial cells) rapidly and with little likelihood of side effects to other tissues.

Because polycystic kidney disease entities represents hyperplastic cystic conditions, Grantham (2000) suggested that it is time to treat polycystic kidney diseases like the neoplastic disorders they are. One such method would be to block the action of growth factors or their receptors. Another would be to consider chemotherapeutic agents. For example, Woo and associates (1994) found taxol to be effective in limiting a form of recessive polycystic kidney disease in mice with homozygous loss of the cpk gene. Martinez and colleagues (1997) confirmed those findings, but found no benefit in the use of taxol for a form of polycystic kidney disease in rats nor for another form of polycystic kidney disease in mice.

JUVENILE NEPHRONOPHTHISIS– MEDULLARY CYSTIC DISEASE COMPLEX

Juvenile nephronophthisis was first described by Fanconi and colleagues in 1951. Medullary cystic disease was first reported by Smith and Graham in 1945. Although the two conditions are similar anatomically and clinically, they have a different mode of transmission and a different clinical onset.

Although juvenile nephronophthisis is the more common condition and is responsible for approximately 10% to 20% of cases of renal failure occurring in children (Cantani et al, 1986), this relatively high incidence does not appear to correlate with the low incidence (1 in 50,000 births) reported by Lirenman and associates (1974). A frequency of less than 1 in 100,000 was reported for medullary cystic disease by Reeders (1990). Both conditions have been known by other names, such as uremic medullary cystic disease, salt-losing enteropathy, and uremic sponge kidney.

Genetics

Although either condition can occur sporadically, juvenile nephronophthisis usually is inherited as an autosomal recessive trait and becomes manifest between the ages of 6 and 20 years. Renal failure develops at a mean age of 13 years and almost always before 25 years (Neumann et al, 1997). **Medullary cystic disease usually is inherited in an autosomal dominant fashion and manifests in early adulthood, with ESRD most often developing in the third or fourth decade.** The recessive transmission of juvenile nephronophthisis is supported by the frequency of consanguineous marriages among the parents of affected children (Bernstein and Gardner, 1979b; Cantani et al, 1986). Antignac and associates (1993) demonstrated by linkage analysis and Hildebrandt and coworkers (1993) confirmed that the gene defect for juvenile nephronophthisis is located on chromosome 2. The chromosomal locus for medullary cystic disease is unknown. Because it is transmitted in an autosomal dominant fashion, 50% of all offspring will have the disease. It will manifest in all by 50 years of age (Bernstein and Gardner, 1979b). Because patients with either condition theoretically can be fertile in their early childbearing years, the risk of transmitting the condition to offspring must be acknowledged— 1% for juvenile nephronophthisis and 50% for medullary cystic disease (Neumann et al, 1997).

Clinical Features

Juvenile nephronophthisis and medullary cystic disease both cause polydipsia and polyuria in more than 80% of cases, but not to the extent observed in patients with diabetes insipidus (Gardner, 1984a; Cantani et al, 1986). **The polyuria is attributable to a severe renal tubular defect associated with an inability to conserve sodium. The polyuria is resistant to vasopressin, and a large dietary salt intake frequently is necessary. Hypertension is not associated with juvenile nephronophthisis, because these patients have a salt-losing nephropathy. On the other hand, medullary cystic disease nephropathy is associated with hypertension, because these patients do not have a salt-losing problem. Proteinuria and hematuria usually are absent.** In children, growth gradually slows, and malaise and pallor may appear in advanced disease. These latter findings are secondary to anemia, which may be attributable to a deficiency of erythropoietin production by the failing kidneys (Gruskin, 1977). Renal failure usually ensues 5 to 10 years after initial presentation (Cantani et al, 1986).

Juvenile nephronophthisis often is associated with disorders of the retina (particularly retinitis pigmentosa), skeletal abnormalities, hepatic fibrosis, and Bardet-Biedl syndrome—a combination of obesity, mental retardation, polydactyly, retinitis pigmentosa, and hypogenitalism. **Sixteen percent of patients with juvenile nephronophthisis have associated retinitis pigmentosa** (Hildebrandt et al, 1993). **When the two entities coexist, the condition is referred to as renal-retinal or Senior-Løken syndrome.** However, if one member in a family with juvenile nephronophthisis has retinal disease, that does not mean that others in the family with nephronophthisis necessarily also have retinal disease. Alstrom's syndrome, a nephropathy accompanied by blindness, obesity, diabetes mellitus, and nerve deafness, may be a form of juvenile nephronophthisis (Bernstein, 1976). Eighty percent of families have no extrarenal lesions (Neumann et al, 1997).

Extrarenal abnormalities classically have been associated only with juvenile nephronophthisis. However, Green and coworkers (1990) described two sisters who presented with medullary cystic disease when they were in their mid-30s. Both had a history of congenital spastic quadriparesis.

Histopathology

Early in the disease course, the kidneys may be of normal size (Cantani et al, 1986). **In clinically manifest cases, the kidneys almost always demonstrate interstitial nephritis, with round cell infiltrates and tubular dilatation with atrophy. The corticomedullary junction is poorly defined. Atrophy begins in the cortex, but later the entire organ becomes very small and has a granular surface.**

Cysts are present in the kidneys of many patients, particularly those with medullary cystic disease (incidence, 85%, versus 40% for patients with juvenile nephronophthisis) (Mongeau and Worthen, 1967). **These cysts, which range in diameter from 1 mm to 1 cm, appear usually at the corticomedullary junction and less often in the medulla, generally within the distal convolutions and the collecting ducts** (Fig. 56–13) (Cantani et al, 1986). Biopsies do not always reveal cysts, however, both because affected areas may be missed and because **cysts tend to appear only with renal failure in the recessive disease. In the dominant disorder, medullary cysts are sometimes seen before the development of re-**

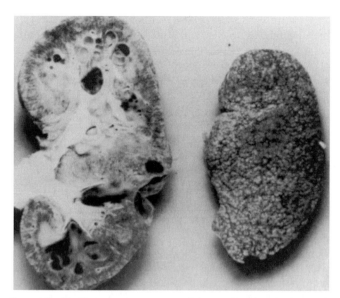

Figure 56–13. The gross appearance of the sectioned and subcapsular surface of a kidney from a patient with medullary cystic disease. Note that the cysts are concentrated at the corticomedullary junction, not at the papillae as in medullary sponge kidney. (From Kissane JM: Pathology of Infancy and Childhood, 2nd ed. St. Louis, CV Mosby, 1975.)

nal failure (Lirenman et al, 1974; Steele et al, 1980; Garel et al, 1984; Cantani et al, 1986; Kleinknecht and Habib, 1992). Similar findings of tubulointerstitial nephritis with medullary cysts have been reported in Bardet-Biedl syndrome (or Laurence-Moon-Bardet-Biedl syndrome)—namely, obesity, mental retardation, hypogenitalism, polydactyly, and retinitis pigmentosa—as well as in Jeune's syndrome.

Some have suggested that the primary defect in juvenile nephronophthisis and medullary cystic disease is a defect of the tubular basement membrane. On histopathology, alternating areas of thickening and thinning of the tubular basement membrane are seen (Cohen and Hoyer, 1986). **However, this finding is seen more consistently in juvenile nephronophthisis than in medullary cystic disease** (Kleinknecht and Habib, 1992) (Table 56–10). Cohen and Hoyer (1986) reported no abnormalities in the glomerular capillaries or Bowman's capsule and theorized that the interstitial damage was secondary to leakage of Tamm-Horsfall protein through the thin areas of the basement membrane. Kelly and Neilson (1990) were impressed by the number of inflammatory cells seen in the interstitium with medullary cystic disease. Particularly in the early stages, a heavy infiltrate of mononuclear cells is seen. The role of these cells is not clear. They may represent a response to tubular leakage, antigen, or tissue damage, or they may play a primary role in the development of the cysts. Renal failure may be associated with a large mononuclear cell infiltrate and little evidence of cysts (Bernstein and Gardner, 1983; Neilson et al, 1985).

In some patients with juvenile nephronophthisis, especially those with hepatic disease, glomerular cysts have been detected. These lesions are rarely seen in other forms of nephronophthisis (Bernstein and Landing, 1989). Therefore, if glomerular cysts are discovered in a renal biopsy from a patient with juvenile nephronophthisis, hepatic biopsy is advisable. Hepatic biopsy is particularly important

if renal transplantation is being considered, because hepatic fibrosis may lead to portal hypertension (Bernstein and Landing, 1989).

Evaluation

In the early stages of the disease, intravenous urography may show a normal or slightly shrunken kidney (Habib, 1974; Chamberlin et al, 1977). Homogeneous streaking of the medulla may be found, presumably secondary to retention of contrast medium within dilated tubules, or ring-shaped densities at the bases of papillae may be seen, again perhaps representing contrast-filled tubules (Olsen et al, 1988). In the late stages of the disease, intravenous urography is of little value. Calcifications are not seen.

Sonography may show smaller than normal kidneys in juvenile nephronophthisis. Cysts may be seen on imaging studies if they are large enough (Rosenfeld et al, 1977), but early in the disease cysts are rarely visible. For example, Garel and associates (1984) demonstrated medullary cysts in 17 of 19 patients with end-stage disease but not in twins who had only mild uremia. The parenchyma may appear hyperechogenic secondary to tubulointerstitial fibrosis (Resnick and Hartman, 1990) (Fig. 56–14).

McGregor and Bailey (1989) described the CT appearance of juvenile nephronophthisis in a 19-year-old patient. In this case, cysts approximately 0.5 cm in diameter were apparent throughout the medulla, although no cysts were visible by sonography. These investigators recommended CT rather than sonography for examining relatives of known cases. Even though the cysts may be prominent and may help in diagnosis, renal failure probably results not from the cysts but from the tubulointerstitial changes. However, as Wise and colleagues (1998) pointed out, CT may require the use of a contrast agent, which often is contraindicated in renal failure. They see a future for MRI for this entity, especially with such new advances as fast spin echo and breath-hold sequences, which overcome

Table 56–10. JUVENILE NEPHRONOPHTHISIS–MEDULLARY CYSTIC DISEASE COMPLEX*

Item	Juvenile Nephronophthisis	Medullary Cystic Disease
Inheritance	Autosomal recessive (chromosome 2)	Autosomal dominant (chromosome ?)
Incidence	1:50,000	1:100,000
End-stage renal disease	By age 13 yr	20–40 yr
Medullary cysts	Develop after renal failure	May develop before onset of renal failure
Tubular basement membrane	Thickened	May not be thickened
Symptoms	Polyuria, polydipsia, anemia, growth retardation (usually after age 2)	Polyuria, polydipsia, anemia; may have hematuria and proteinuria (symptoms usually appear after patient is fully grown)

*Both have tubulointestinal nephritis and small kidneys with granular surface; medullary cysts are not essential for diagnosis and are not present in all cases.

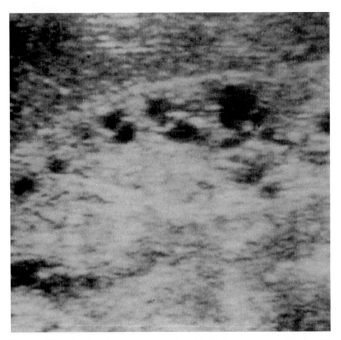

Figure 56–14. Renal sonogram of right kidney in a patient with medullary cystic disease. Note small to medium-size cysts located predominantly at outer edge of medulla and a few well within the medulla. The hyperechogenicity is secondary to the tubulointerstitial fibrosis. (From Resnick JS, Hartman DS: Medullary cystic disease. In Pollack HM [ed]: Clinical Urography. Philadelphia, WB Saunders, 1990, pp 1178–1184.)

breathing and motion artifact. It remains to be seen whether MRI will be more useful than ultrasound in demonstrating small cysts and whether gadolinium will demonstrate communication between the collecting duct and the cysts.

Treatment

Sodium replacement is indicated early in the course of the disease. Later, dialysis and transplantation must be considered. Allografts apparently are not susceptible to the same process that destroyed the native kidney, because there is no evidence of serum antibodies to the basement membrane or other renal structural proteins (Cantani et al, 1986; Cohen and Hoyer, 1986).

CONGENITAL NEPHROSIS

Congenital nephrosis is predominantly of two types. The more common variety, referred to as the **Finnish type** (CNF), has, as the name suggests, been reported principally in Finland, where the incidence is 1 in 8200 (Norio, 1966; Lanning et al, 1989). It has also been reported in other areas, including Minnesota (Kestilä et al, 1994). The other type, described by Habib and Bois in 1973, is referred to as diffuse mesangial sclerosis (DMS). The Finnish type is recessive (Norio, 1966) and has been localized to chromosome 19 (Kestilä et al, 1994), but only 10 of the 30 reported cases of DMS were familial (Habib et al, 1989).

More recently, Kestilä (1998) cloned the gene (NPHSI), which encodes a protein called nephrin that plays a significant role in functional renal development (Ruotsalainen et al, 1999). Both conditions are associated with dilatation of the proximal convoluted tubules. The term "microcystic disease" is now rarely used.

Clinical Features

CNF usually is discovered because of an enormously enlarged and edematous placenta, which accounts for more than 25% of the birth weight (Norio and Rapola, 1989). In DMS, the placenta usually is not enlarged.

In infants with CNF, proteinuria is present in the first urinalysis. Edema usually develops within the first few days, and always by the age of 3 months. Essentially, these infants starve because of their severe loss of protein in the urine; without treatment, they probably would die from sepsis before renal failure killed them. Without dialysis, half of the patients die by the age of 6 months, and the rest before their fourth birthday (Huttunen, 1976).

In DMS, the onset of symptoms is variable and the diagnosis is usually made by the age of 1 year. All children have terminal renal failure by the age of 3 years.

Habib and colleagues (1985) demonstrated that the nephropathy of Drash syndrome (nephrotic syndrome and Wilms' tumor with or without male pseudohermaphroditism) is, in fact, DMS. Of the 35 cases of DMS diagnosed by Habib and coworkers (1989), 13 were associated with Drash syndrome.

Histopathology

CNF and DMS are both characterized by normal-sized kidneys, initially with pronounced proximal tubular dilatation. DMS is distinctive in that the glomeruli have an accumulation of PAS-positive and silver phosphate–staining mesangial fibrils. With advanced disease, the glomerular tufts sclerose and contract (Norio and Rapola, 1989; Habib et al, 1989). Diffuse hypertrophy of the podocytes is also found.

CNF is characterized by a proliferation of the glomerular mesangial cells. In both DMS and CNF, as in all types of nephrosis, there is fusion of the glomerular podocytes. Interstitial fibrosis is present in both conditions but is more pronounced in DMS (Norio and Rapola, 1989).

Evaluation

The diagnosis of CNF can be made at about 6 weeks of gestation because of the greatly elevated concentrations of amniotic α-fetoprotein (AFP) secondary to fetal proteinuria. The use of AFP to diagnose DMS in utero has not been demonstrated.

In the later stages of disease postnatally, ultrasonography reveals enlarged kidneys with cortices that are more echogenic than those of the liver or spleen. The pyramids are small and hazy, and the corticomedullary junction is indistinct or absent. In one study, the kidneys continued to enlarge and the corticomedullary junction became more effaced as the disease become worse (Lanning et al, 1989).

Treatment

After the kidneys have failed, transplantation is curative. Neither type of disease responds to steroids.

FAMILIAL HYPOPLASTIC GLOMERULOCYSTIC KIDNEY DISEASE (CORTICAL MICROCYSTIC DISEASE)

In 1982, Rizzoni and coworkers described two families in which a mother and two daughters were affected by what these investigators called hypoplastic glomerulocystic disease. Melnick and associates (1984) described the same condition under the name cortical microcystic disease, and Kaplan and colleagues (1989a) reported it in a mother and son. This condition is autosomal dominant.

The diagnosis of familial hypoplastic glomerulocystic disease requires four features. First, stable or progressive chronic renal failure must be present. Second, the kidneys must be small or of normal size with irregular calyceal outlines and abnormal papillae. Third, the condition must by present in two generations of a family. Last, histologic evidence of glomerular cysts must be found. These cysts are thin-walled and tend to be subcapsular. Tubular atrophy with some normal glomeruli and tubules in the deeper cortex is also observed. Marked prognathism is present in some patients (Kaplan et al, 1989a; Rizzoni et al, 1982).

MULTIPLE MALFORMATION SYNDROMES WITH RENAL CYSTS

Renal cysts are a feature of several syndromes characterized by multiple malformations (Table 56–11). Tuberous sclerosis and VHL are autosomal dominant disorders and are the ones most likely to be encountered by urologists. Meckel's syndrome, Jeune's asphyxiating thoracic dystrophy, and Zellweger's cerebrohepatorenal syndrome are some of the more common autosomal recessive syndromes. Many of these conditions involve glomerular cysts, and some have cystic dysplasia as a feature. The most frequently encountered syndromes are listed in Table 56–11.

Tuberous Sclerosis

Bourneville described tuberous sclerosis in 1880. The incidence seems to be rising with each report, now ranging between 1 in 6000 and 1 in 14,500 (Webb et al, 1991; O'Hagan et al, 1996). The rise is the result not of an increased incidence but rather of an increased awareness of the disease and its manifestations.

Classically, tuberous sclerosis is described as part of a triad of epilepsy (80% of cases), mental retardation (60% of cases), and adenoma sebaceum (75% of cases) (Lagos and Gomez, 1967; Pampigliana and Moynahan, 1976). **The lesions of adenoma sebaceum are flesh-colored papules of angiofibroma and are especially preva-**lent in the malar area. An earlier skin lesion that is a white papule in the shape of an "ash leaf" is sometimes identified (Shepherd et al, 1991). **An examination of the skin with ultraviolet light may reveal cutaneous lesions earlier and should be part of a diagnostic evaluation.**

The hallmark lesion of the central nervous system is a superficial cortical hamartoma of the cerebrum, which sometimes looks like hardened gyri, creating the appearance of a tuber (root). Hamartomas often affect other organs as well, especially the kidneys and eyes. Periventricular subependymal nodules also occur frequently.

The kidneys of these patients may be free of lesions (Stillwell et al, 1987) or may display cysts, angiomyolipomas, or both (Fig. 56–15).

Genetics

Although it is transmitted as an autosomal dominant trait in 25% to 40% of cases, in the remainder tuberous sclerosis occurs either sporadically or as an example of the genetic condition with variable or incomplete penetrance.

Two genes, TSC1 on chromosome 9 and TSC2 on chromosome 16, have been identified as being responsible for the autosomal dominant transmission of tuberous sclerosis (Kandt et al, 1992; Brook-Carter et al, 1994). However, in a review of 10 previously reported cases (in addition to 1 new patient in whom severe bilateral cystic disease was diagnosed by the age of 4 months), 6 of the infants had no family history of tuberous sclerosis, in 3 no family history was available, and in only 1 was the disease found to be familial (Campos et al, 1993). In another study (Brook-Carter et al, 1994) **of six patients with tuberous sclerosis and a known history of diffuse bilateral cystic disease in early infancy, all were found to have deletions not only at the TSC2 gene site on chromosome 16 but also in the adjacent PKD1 gene, the gene responsible for ADPKD.** There were no signs of tuberous sclerosis in parents or other family members, suggesting that in these six patients the disease probably represented a new mutation. It is interesting that of the 11 cases reviewed by Campos and colleagues (1993) and the 6 studied by Brook-Carter and associates (1994) with diffuse bilateral cystic disease in early infancy, the disease was identified as familial in only one child (Fig. 56–16).

In summary, when severe polycystic kidneys are present in patients, particularly infants, with tuberous sclerosis, the condition probably represents a contiguous gene syndrome (i.e., defects in both TSC2 and PKD1). Such contiguous gene syndromes are relatively rare phenomena. In an infant with polycystic kidney disease, other findings associated with tuberous sclerosis should be investigated to exclude the diagnosis of tuberous sclerosis (Gillis et al, 1997).

Histopathology

The renal cysts are of a unique histologic type in that they have a lining of hypertrophic, hyperplastic eosinophilic cells (Bernstein and Meyer, 1967; Stapleton et al, 1980). These cells have large, hyperchromatic nuclei, and mitoses are seen occasionally. The cells often aggregate into masses or tumorlets (Bernstein and Gardner, 1986;

Table 56–11. MULTIPLE MALFORMATION SYNDROMES ASSOCIATED WITH RENAL CYSTS

Genetics	Syndrome	Features	Cyst Characteristics	Other Renal Lesions	Renal Sequelae
Mendelian (single gene disorders)					
Autosomal dominant	Tuberous sclerosis	Adenoma sebaceum, elipepsy, mental retardation, cranial calcifications	Variable size, eosinophilic hyperplastic lining*	Angiomyolipomas (more common than cysts), renal cell carcinoma (2% incidence)	Occasionally masses compress or obstruct kidney leading to renal failure.
	von Hippel–Lindau disease	Cerebellar hemangioblastomas, retinal angiomatosis, pheochromocytoma, cysts of pancreas and epididymis	Variable size; hyperplastic lining	Clear cell carcinoma (35%–38% incidence)	Rarely, masses compress or obstruct kidney leading to renal failure
Autosomal recessive	Meckel's syndrome	Microcephaly, polydactyly, posterior encephalocele	Large with fibromuscular collars that probably arise from collecting ducts	Dysplasia, hypoplasia	Possible renal failure
	Jeune's asphyxiating thoracic dystrophy	Small chest, respiratory failure	From subcapsular cortical microcysts to dysplasia with cystic component; generalized dilatation of various segments of nephron (similar to ADPKD)	Dysplasia	Possible renal failure or chronic nephritis
	Zellweger's cerebrohepatorenal syndrome	Hypotonia, high forehead, hepatomegaly	From glomerular microcysts to 1-cm cortical cysts	—	Rarely, mild azotemia; usually no manifestations
	Ivemark's syndrome (renal-hepatic-pancreatic dysplasia)	Bilary dysgenesis, dilated intrahepatic ducts, pancreatic dysplasia	Diffuse, microscopic to large	Dysplasia	Possible renal failure
X-linked dominant disorders	Orofaciodigital syndrome I	Hypertrophic lingular and buccal frenula; cleft lip, palate, and tongue; hypoplasia of alinasal cartilage, brachydactyly, syndactyly, alopecia	Develop with age	—	Hypertension, renal failure
Chromosomal disorders	Trisomy 13 (Patau's syndrome) Trisomy 18 (Edwards' syndrome) Trisomy 21 (Down's syndrome)		Any cystic changes usually are not clinically significant. Findings are variable, but cysts generally are microscopic (dysplastic cysts, subcortical cysts, glomerular cysts)		

ADPKD, autosomal dominant polycystic kidney disease.
*May resemble ADPKD in imaging studies.
Adapted from Glassberg KI: Cystic disease of the kidney. Probl Urol 1988;2:157 and Glassberg KI: Renal cystic diseases. Curr Probl Urol 1991;1:137.

Bernstein and Gardner, 1989). Later in the disease, the cyst walls may atrophy into a thickened, unidentifiable lining (Mitnick et al, 1983). In a few patients, predominantly glomerular cells have been seen (Bernstein and Gardner, 1989). **The cystic disease can lead to renal failure with or without the presence of angiomyolipomas. The probable mechanism is compression of the parenchyma by the expanding cysts.** Hypertension may also be present.

Angiomyolipomas occur in 40% to 80% of patients (Chonko et al, 1974; Gomez, 1979). They are rarely identified before the age of 6 years but are common after age 10 (Bernstein et al, 1986). By themselves, these lesions probably do not cause renal failure (Okada et al, 1982; Bernstein et al, 1986). Also, belying their aggressive histologic ap-

pearance, which is characterized by pleomorphism and mitoses, no evidence of metastases has been presented.

Evaluation

The rising incidence of identified tuberous sclerosis is in part the result of full investigation of patients with seizure disorders, of children with hypomelanotic macules, and of some infants and young children misdiagnosed as having ADPKD who actually have tuberous sclerosis. The most significant primary diagnostic finding is multiple calcified subepdidymal nodules penetrating into the ventricle by CT or MRI (Roach et al, 1992).

Sometimes both renal cysts and angiomyolipomas can

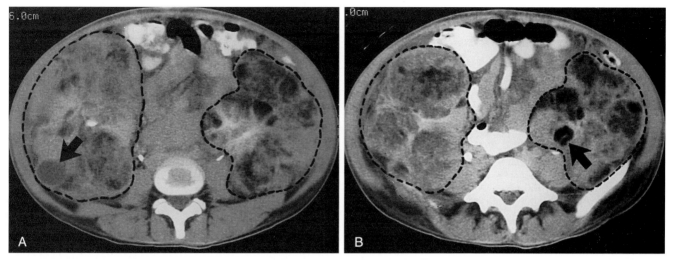

Figure 56–15. A 24-year-old woman known to have tuberous sclerosis since early childhood. Enhanced computed tomographic (CT) scan demonstrates bilateral renomegaly with multiple renal cysts and angiomyolipomas. *A,* Arrow points to a cyst with a CT value of +10 HU. *B,* The arrow points to an angiomyolipoma with a negative CT value (−50 HU) secondary to its high fat content.

be identified by sonography in tuberous sclerosis, the former lesions being sonolucent and the latter having a fluffy, white appearance. When renal cysts are present without angiomyolipomas, the sonographic appearance of the kidneys in tuberous sclerosis is very similar to that in ADPKD. Therefore, it is not that unusual for a patient in whom cysts typical of ADPKD are identified to be diagnosed as having ADPKD, only to develop the stigmata of tuberous sclerosis a few years later. To help make the diagnosis, abdominal CT scans can be useful in demonstrating angiomyolipomas that may be present in the kidney or other organs (findings that are compatible with tuberous sclerosis) and in revealing cysts in other organs (compatible with ADPKD). MRI or CT of the head may demonstrate the classic cranial calcifications associated with tubers or gliosis (Okada et al, 1982). Ultraviolet light examination of the skin may reveal cutaneous lesions before they become manifest grossly and should be part of the differential diagnosis.

Clinical Features and Prognosis

Renal cysts develop in approximately 20% of patients and most often manifest before 3 years of age; one third of children are younger than 1 year of age at presentation. Patients with large cysts or polycystic kidney disease may be identified by in utero ultrasound or may present with an abdominal mass and distended abdomen in

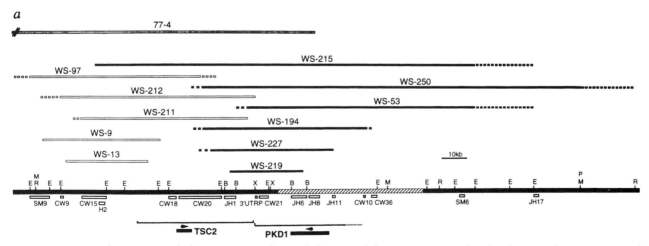

Figure 56–16. A map of a segment of chromosome 16 that includes one of the genes associated with tuberous sclerosis (TSC2) and one associated with autosomal dominant polycystic kidney disease (PKD1). The positions of DNA probes *(open boxes)* and of the TSC2 and PKD1 genes *(solid boxes)* are illustrated below the chromosomal segment map. Above the segment map, the open boxes represent deletions in patients who have tuberous sclerosis without evidence of perinatal polycystic kidneys. The six closed boxes represent deletions in patients with tuberous sclerosis who have evidence of perinatal polycystic kidneys but not autosomal dominant polycystic kidney disease. Because there were no signs of tuberous sclerosis in parents or other family members of the six patients, the condition might represent a new mutation. The gray bar represents patient 77–4, who has both tuberous sclerosis and autosomal dominant polycystic kidney disease. (From Brook-Carter PA, Peral B, Ward CJ, et al: Deletion of the TSC 2 and PKD 1 gene associated with severe infantile polycystic kidney disease—a contiguous gene syndrome. Nature Genet 1994;8:328.)

the first year of life. Most patients with renal cysts do not develop any serious renal compromise, but when the disease is more widespread within the kidney and large cysts are present, renal failure may develop in the milder form with polycystic kidney disease. **If any renal failure develops, it is uncommon before the fourth decade** (Glazier et al, 1996). The cysts probably originate from nephrons lined with hyperplastic cells that may be present even at birth (Bernstein, 1993).

Because more patients with tuberous sclerosis now survive their central nervous system lesions than in the past, the urologist is more likely to be called on for management of the renal problems (Stillwell et al, 1987). Shepherd and associates (1991) found that renal disease was the leading cause of death (11 of 40 deaths). Of 355 patients they observed at the Mayo Clinic, 49 had died, 9 from disease not related to tuberous sclerosis, 10 from brain tumors, 4 from lymphangiomatosis of the lung, 13 from causes secondary to status epilepticus or bronchopneumonia, and 11 from renal disease. Of these 11 patients, 2 died from metastatic RCC, 2 from massive hemorrhage associated with renal angiomyolipomas, and 6 from renal failure secondary to the cysts, angiomyolipomas, or both.

Large angiomyolipomas are more likely to bleed. Van Baal and coworkers (1994) have recommended careful monitoring of the size of angiomyolipomas and prophylactic embolization or surgical excision if they enlarge to greater than 4 cm.

Association with Renal Cell Carcinoma

The numerous reports of RCC in patients with tuberous sclerosis make it clear that this association is more than coincidental and may be as frequent as 2% (Bernstein et al, 1986; Bernstein, 1993). **However, the incidence of RCC is considerably less than that seen in other conditions involving hyperplastic epithelial cells, specifically VHL and ARCD of chronic renal failure (although it is more frequent than that seen in another condition with hyperplastic cells, ADPKD, which may not even have an increased incidence).**

These cancers appear in patients who are younger than would be expected (7 to 39 years); they may be single or multiple and unilateral or bilateral (Bernstein and Gardner, 1989). The karyotype of the cells near the tumor is similar to that of the tumor itself, and it is reasonable to suspect that the lining of the cysts evolves into the cancer (Ibrahim et al, 1989).

Von Hippel–Lindau Disease

von Hippel, a German ophthalmologist, published two articles describing retinal angiomatosis in 1904 and 1911. One of his patients developed renal cancer and was reported on in 1921. Four years later, Lindau published a series of patients with retinal and cerebellar tumors, with four of his patients also having renal cysts and renal cancer.

VHL is an autosomal dominant condition manifested by cerebellar hemangioblastomas; retinal angiomas; cysts of the pancreas, kidney, and epididymis; epididymal cystadenoma; pheochromocytoma; and clear cell RCC. It has an incidence of approximately 1 in 35,000 (Neumann and Wiestler, 1991).

Genetics

The gene associated with the transmission of VHL is located on chromosome 3 (Latif et al, 1993). **The penetrance probably is 100%** (Jennings and Gaines, 1988), **and therefore the condition can be expected to appear in 50% of the offspring or siblings of affected persons.** The VHL mutation has been demonstrated in only 70% of families investigated (Zbar et al, 1996).

The gene for VHL is characterized as a recessive tumor-suppressor gene, and its gene product is referred to as pVHL. Many different mutations of the VHL gene have been identified, five of which are most frequently seen (Zbar et al, 1996). Three of these mutations are each associated with one of the following three specific phenotypes: type 1, renal carcinoma without pheochromocytoma; type 2, renal carcinoma with pheochromocytoma; and type 3, pheochromocytoma without RCC (Zbar et al, 1996). This differs from ADPKD, in which two or three distinct genes are responsible. **In non-VHL patients with sporadic clear cell RCC, 50% of cell lines are associated with a mutational form of the VHL gene.**

The genetic nature of VHL mandates careful screening. However, because of molecular genetic advances, the screening process for the disease in family members can now be more selective. Previously, asymptomatic relatives required routine ophthalmoscopic examination to rule out retinal angiomas, as well as frequent abdominal CT scans. Now only genetically affected family members require screening.

The recommendations of Levine and colleagues (1990) for all asymptomatic relatives now applies only to those with genetic evidence of the disease. For example, ophthalmoscopic examination for retinal angiomas is useful, and an abdominal CT scan should be obtained when an asymptomatic genetically effected relative is between the ages of 18 and 20 years. If no disease is found, re-evaluation is recommended at 4-year intervals (Levine et al, 1990). If cysts or small indeterminate lesions are identified, CT examination should be repeated every 2 years, perhaps with narrow-screen collimation (Levine et al, 1990). The goal is to diagnose the disease early so that malignancies can be identified before they metastasize.

The diagnosis can be made without a family history if a patient has two cardinal manifestations. In such families, germline mutations may be present without clinical manifestations and should be screened for.

Neumann and Zbar (1997), as well as Maher and Kaelin (1997), have published thorough molecular reviews of VHL. (Additional discussion of the genetics of von Hippel–Lindau disease is included in the earlier discussion of molecular genetics.)

Histopathology

When present, renal cysts and tumors often are multiple and bilateral. The cysts usually simulate simple

benign cysts, with flattened epithelium that some investigators consider precancerous. When Poston and associates (1993) studied cysts that were surgically removed along with specimens of RCC, they found that **cysts larger than 2 cm were more likely than smaller cysts to have components of RCC. Frank cancer usually appears between the ages of 20 and 50 years** (Jennings and Gaines, 1988). Loughlin and Gittes (1986) found that the hyperplastic lining cells frequently resembled the clear cell type of RCC, the most common type in these patients. Ibrahim and coworkers (1989) studied the cysts adjacent to carcinomas and found, much as in tuberous sclerosis, that the karyotype resembled that of the tumors. This similarity is evidence that the hyperplastic cells of the cyst lining are precursors of the carcinomas.

Solomon and Schwartz (1988) believed that a spectrum of pathology is found within the kidneys of patients with VHL. At one extreme is a simple cyst with a single layer of bland epithelium. The next step is a typical proliferative cyst with layers of epithelial cells. In the ensuing step, there are complex neoplastic projections into the cyst lumen. If one agrees with the arbitrary distinction between adenoma and carcinoma on the basis of size, the next stage would be adenoma. Finally, there is the full-blown RCC. In some cases, one might stretch the spectrum two steps further: sclerosing RCC with residual foci of malignant epithelium, and completely hyalinized fibrotic nodules lacking epithelial foci. The latter condition may represent the end point of evolution of the RCC. All of these stages may be found within a single kidney (Solomon and Schwartz, 1988). More recently, Lubensky and associates (1996) presented molecular evidence supporting the concept that benign-appearing cysts are indeed representative precursors to RCC in individuals with VHL.

Evaluation

Sonography is useful in diagnosing the typical benign cystic features of VHL: absence of internal echoes, well-defined margins, and acoustic enhancement. On CT scans, sharp, thin walls are seen around homogeneous contents without enhancement after contrast injection. Because multiple lesions (cysts, tumors, or both) are often present, CT frequently is more useful than sonography. CT often is useful in examining the adrenal glands for pheochromocytomas.

When the lesions are small, it is impossible to distinguish tumors from cysts. In such cases, patients should have regular CT scans with narrow-screen collimation (Levine et al, 1982). With larger lesions, and whenever RCC is suspected, renal angiography with magnification or subtraction is advisable (Kadir et al, 1981; Loughlin and Gittes, 1986). This type of study helps to reveal any additional tumors and indicates the appropriateness of conservative surgery (Kadir et al, 1981; Loughlin and Gittes, 1986). Intra-arterial administration of epinephrine is sometimes helpful because it causes vasoconstriction of the normal vessels but has no effect on tumor neovasculature.

MRI has not been very useful for small tumors of the kidney unless the shape of the kidney is altered. The lesions on MRI have a signal intensity that is similar to that of normal renal parenchyma on T1- and T2-weighted images. However, gadolinium is useful because it enhances RCC. The heterogenous nature of the larger tumors makes them more readily diagnosed (Rominger et al, 1992).

Clinical Features: Association with Renal Cell Carcinoma

The mean age at presentation is 35 to 40 years (Neumann and Zbar, 1997). **There is no sex preference for the disease or for RCC development.** (Sporadic RCC in individuals without VHL occurs more often in males.)

Renal cysts, the most common and often earliest manifestation, are seen in 76% of patients (Levine et al, 1982). **The cysts are bilateral 75% of the time and multifocal in 87%** (Reichard et al, 1998). **Diagnosis of the RCC usually occurs in the fourth or fifth decade of life, whereas in the general population it more often manifests in the sixth decade** (Reichard et al, 1998). **RCC occurs in 35% to 38% of affected individuals** (Fill et al, 1979; Levine et al, 1982). The renal cysts as well as the tumors usually are asymptomatic, although large tumors may cause pain or a mass. Hematuria may occur after rupture of the tumor into the pelvicalyceal system. When cysts are present, typically they are large. Only rarely do images typify ADPKD and even less often do cysts cause renal failure.

Pheochromocytoma occurs in 10% to 17% of affected individuals and appears to be confined to specific families (Horton et al, 1976; Levine et al, 1982). Patients may present with seizures or dizziness secondary to hemangioblastomas of the central nervous system. Cerebellar hemangioblastomas usually become symptomatic between 15 and 40 years of age (Jennings and Gaines, 1988). Retinal angiomas (hemangiomas) frequently manifest early. Bleeding may cause blurred vision, retinal detachment, and blindness. Early diagnosis is important because these tumors respond to laser therapy or cryotherapy.

Because of the high incidence of RCC in patients with VHL, the urologist's primary role is careful surveillance so that small tumors can be identified and treated before they metastasize. Annual or perhaps biannual CT examinations are advised. Although central nervous system hemangioblastomas account for more than half of the deaths, RCC causes its own share, approximately 30% (Reichard et al, 1998).

Treatment

Frydenberg and associates (1993) recommended conservative surgery—that is, excision or partial nephrectomy—for small low-grade tumors but more aggressive surgery for tumors that are larger than 5 cm. The outlook is poorer with bilateral tumors. Low-grade bilateral tumors can be treated cautiously like unilateral tumors with close monitoring. Patients with bilateral high-grade tumors are probably served best with bilateral nephrectomy (Frydenberg et al, 1993). Between 1977 and 1997, approximately 20 patients with VHL received a kidney transplant. However, it is not known whether the immunosuppressive drugs required for transplantation increase the growth rate of other lesions associated with VHL (Neumann and Zbar, 1997). The most important need in improving survival is careful surveillance to identify tumors early and even more careful surveillance after surgery because of the multicentric characteristics of the tumor.

Classically, the survival rate after nephrectomy has been only 50%. However, in the closely monitored series of seven patients treated by Loughlin and Gittes (1986), six patients were monitored for 4 months to 8 years, and only one death from metastatic disease was reported. With renal-sparing surgery, there is a 75% incidence of recurrence in the same or opposite kidney (Malek et al, 1987).

MULTICYSTIC DYSPLASTIC KIDNEY

Historically, the terms multicystic and polycystic were used interchangeably in discussing the kidney. However, in 1955, Spence stressed that these terms designated completely different entities. He included them separately in his classification, and subsequent investigators have done likewise.

The multicystic kidney represents a severe form of nongenetic dysplasia that is sometimes described as multicystic dysplasia. The kidney does not have a reniform configuration, and no calyceal drainage system is present. Typically, the kidney has the appearance of "a bunch of grapes," with little stroma between the cysts (Fig. 56–17A). Renal size is highly variable, from slightly less than normal to enormous, filling most of the abdomen. When the cysts are small, even microscopic, and stroma predominates, the condition is referred to as solid cystic dysplasia (Fig. 56–17B). And when an identifiable renal pelvis is associated with what appears to be a multicystic dysplastic kidney, the condition is referred to as the hydronephrotic form of multicystic kidney (Fig. 56–17C) (Felson and Cussen, 1975).

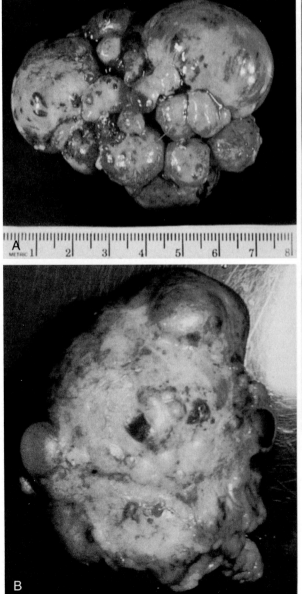

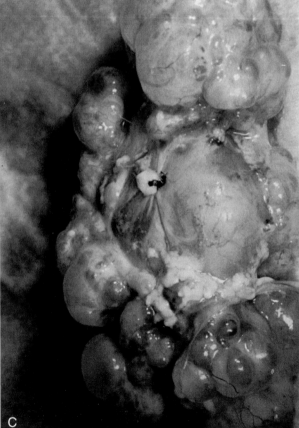

Figure 56–17. Three forms of multicystic dysplastic kidney. *A,* A typical multicystic kidney having the appearance of a bunch of grapes. The kidney was composed almost entirely of cysts with very little stroma. *B,* Nonfunctioning solid cystic dysplastic kidney, which differs from classic multicystic kidney in that it has smaller and fewer cysts and is composed predominantly of stroma. *C,* Hydronephrotic form of multicystic kidney, which has a medial pelvis that typically is larger than any of the cysts in its associated kidney.

Etiology

In the view of Felson and Cussen (1975), the multicystic kidney is an extreme form of hydronephrosis that occurs secondary to atresia of the ureter or renal pelvis, which is a frequent concomitant condition. The fact that the left kidney is the one more often affected supports this view, because this is the kidney more often associated with primary obstructive megaureter (Glassberg, 1977) and ureteropelvic junction obstruction (Johnston et al, 1977). In testing this hypothesis, several investigators have attempted to establish an animal model by ligating the ureter at various points in gestation (Beck, 1971; Tanagho, 1972; Fetterman et al, 1974). This approach is not effective in middle or late gestation; early ligation of the fetal lamb ureter produces renal dysplasia but not multicystic dysplasia (Beck, 1971). However, Berman and Maizel (1982) were unable to obtain similar results in the chick. Similarly, other investigators have been able to induce dysplasia, but no one as yet has been able to induce a multicystic dysplastic kidney.

Other theories have been offered by Hildebrandt (1894) and by Osathanondh and Potter (1964). Hildebrandt (1894) suggested that failure of the union between the ureteric bud and the metanephric blastema leads to cystic dilatation in the latter; this hypothesis, like the obstructive view, is supported by the high incidence of concomitant ureteral atresia. Osathanondh and Potter (1964) postulated that Potter type IIA kidneys, the type with large cysts, result from an ampullary abnormality in which the ampullae stop dividing early and therefore produce fewer generations of tubules. In this view, the last generation of tubules produced is cystic and does not induce metanephric differentiation, and the occasional normal or near-normal nephron is the result of a rare normal ampulla and collecting tubules.

Clinical Features

Multicystic dysplasia is the most common type of renal cystic disease, and it is one of the most common causes of an abdominal mass in infants (Longino and Martin, 1958; Melicow and Uson, 1959; Griscom et al, 1975). Widespread prenatal ultrasound evaluation has greatly increased the frequency with which the condition is identified. Although the pathogenetic process leading to a multicystic kidney probably is operative by the 8th week in utero, the mean age at the time of antenatal diagnosis is about 28 weeks, with a range of 21 to 35 weeks (Avni et al, 1987). The reason is not apparent. In less severely affected patients, the condition may be an incidental finding during evaluation of an adult for abdominal pain, hematuria, hypertension, or an unrelated condition. At any age, the condition is more likely to be found on the left (Friedman and Abeshouse, 1957; Fine and Burns, 1959; Parkkulainen et al, 1959; Pathak and Williams, 1964; Griscom et al, 1975). **Males are more likely to have unilateral multicystic dysplastic kidneys (2.4:1), whereas bilateral multicystic kidneys appear twice as often in females** (Lazebnick et al, 1999). Unilateral multicystic kidneys, when not associated with other renal or nonrenal anomalies, rarely involve a chromosomal disorder. Bilateral disease, however, is associated with other anomalies as well as chromosomal anomalies. Such information may be important for genetic counseling (Lazebnick et al, 1999).

The contralateral system frequently is abnormal as well. For example, contralateral ureteropelvic junction obstruction is found in 3% to 12% of infants with multicystic kidney, and contralateral vesicoureteral reflux is seen even more often, in 18% to 43% of infants (Heikkinen et al, 1980; Atiyeh et al, 1992; Flack and Bellinger, 1993; Wacksman and Phipps, 1993; Al-Khaldi et al, 1994). **The high incidence of reflux makes voiding cystourethrography advisable in the evaluation of these children, especially because the reflux affects the only functioning kidney.**

When a diagnosis of multicystic kidney is made in utero by ultrasound, the disease is found to be bilateral in 19% to 34% of cases (Kleiner et al, 1986; Al-Khaldi et al, 1994). Those with bilateral disease often have other severe deformities or polysystemic malformation syndromes (Al-Khaldi et al, 1994). In bilateral cases, the newborn has the classic abnormal facies and oligohydramnios characteristic of Potter's syndrome. The bilateral condition is incompatible with survival, although one infant reportedly survived for 69 days (Kishikawa et al, 1981). Another association, between multicystic kidney and contralateral renal agenesis, likewise is incompatible with life. The association of any of several entities—renal agenesis, renal dysplasia, multicystic dysplastic kidney, and renal aplasia—within one family has been referred to as *familial renal adysplasia* (see earlier discussion).

Involution sometimes occurs in the multicystic kidney, either antenatally or postnatally (Hashimoto et al, 1986; Avni et al, 1987). **This involution may be so severe that the affected kidney disappears from subsequent sonograms. In such cases, the kidney may be only a "nubbin," and the condition is referred to as "renal aplasia" or "aplastic dysplasia"** (Bernstein and Gardner, 1989; Glassberg and Filmer, 1992). **Previously, aplastic kidneys, which often are associated with atretic ureters, were thought to be a separate entity. Now, with the experience of monitoring multicystic kidneys sonographically, it is apparent that most aplastic kidneys represent involuted multicystic organs.**

In a few cases, multicystic dysplasia involves a horseshoe kidney (Greene et al, 1971; Walker et al, 1978; Borer et al, 1994) or one pole of a duplex kidney.

Cystic dysplasia of the testes, a benign rare lesion of the rete testis, may be associated with an ipsilateral multicystic dysplastic kidney, although more often with renal agenesis. Some of the cases of unilateral agenesis probably represent involuted multicystic dysplastic kidney. The common etiology in such cases would seem to be abnormalities of the ipsilateral wolffian duct that cause anomalies in both the testis and kidney (Wojcik et al, 1997; Lane et al, 1998).

Histopathology

Multicystic kidneys with large cysts tend to be large with little stroma, whereas those with small cysts generally are smaller and more solid. The blood supply likewise is variable, ranging from a pedicle with small vessels to no pedicle at all (Parkkulainen et al, 1959). Usually the ureter is partly or totally atretic, and the renal pelvis may be absent. Griscom and associates (1975) referred to the form without a renal pelvis as "pyeloinfundibular atresia" and reported finding no evidence of communication between the cysts. However, others have shown distribution of contrast medium among the cysts by means of connecting tubules (Saxton et al, 1981). My colleagues and I have found these tubules by probing gross specimens and by injecting contrast medium into one of the cysts and visualizing the connections between the cysts radiographically (Fig. 56–18). Felson and Cussen (1975) referred to the variety with a renal pelvis as the "**hydronephrotic type**" and demonstrated connections between the cysts and the renal pelvis. Thirty-three multicystic kidneys, including 7 of our own cases and 11 of Dewan and Goh's cases, were injected with contrast intracystically. Seven of the 33 kidneys were of the hydronephrotic type (Dewan and Goh, 1994; Glassberg and Kassner, 1998). **Connections between cysts were identified in 30 of the 33 kidneys injected. In other words, the vast majority of multicystic dysplastic kidneys, including both the hydronephrotic and nonhydronephrotic variants, had communication between cysts.** We found, as did Griscom and coworkers (1975) previously, the presence of one or more pits or orifices at the hilum side of each cyst. These pits were found to communicate with the tubular structures that are seen on radiographic examination between the cysts.

Microscopically, the cysts are lined by low cuboidal epithelium. They are separated by thin septa of fibrous tissue and primitive dysplastic elements, especially primitive ducts. Frequently immature glomeruli are present, and on occasion a few mature glomeruli are seen.

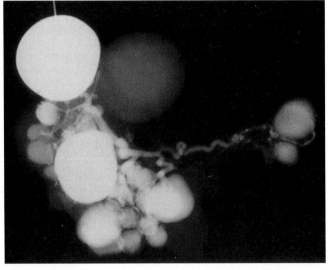

Figure 56–18. Contrast study of a multicystic kidney representing one component of a horseshoe kidney removed at surgery. Contrast medium injected into one cyst demonstrates communication between the cysts by tubular structures. (From Borer JG, Glassberg KI, Kassner G, et al: Unilateral multicystic dysplasia in one component of a horseshoe kidney: Case report and review of the literature. J Urol 1994; 152:1568.)

Evaluation

Renal masses in infants most often represent either multicystic kidney disease or hydronephrosis, and it is important to distinguish between the two, especially if the surgeon wishes to remove a nonfunctioning hydronephrotic kidney or repair a ureteropelvic junction obstruction while leaving a multicystic organ in situ. In newborns, ultrasonography usually is the first study performed. In a few cases, it is difficult to differentiate multicystic kidney disease from severe hydronephrosis (Gates, 1980; Hadlock et al, 1981). **In general, however, the multicystic kidney has a haphazard distribution of cysts of various sizes without a larger central or medial cyst and without visible communications between the cysts. Frequently, very small cysts appear between the large cysts. In comparison, in ureteropelvic junction obstruction the cysts or calyces are organized around the periphery of the kidney, connections usually can be demonstrated between the peripheral cysts and a central or medial cyst that represents the renal pelvis, and there is absence of small cysts between the larger cysts** (Fig. 56–19). **When there is an identifiable renal sinus, the diagnosis is more likely to be hydronephrosis than multicystic kidney.**

A particular diagnostic problem arises in the unusual hydronephrotic form of multicystic kidney disease. Among 14 patients with multicystic kidneys, Felson and Cussen (1975) retrospectively identified 4 who, on intravenous urography, were found to have the calyceal crescents typical of severe hydronephrosis. This feature is thought to represent contrast medium in tubules compressed and displaced by dilated calyces (Dunbar and Nogrady, 1970). All four of these kidneys had small amounts of parenchyma and glomeruli, but no correlation could be made between the parenchymal tissue and the appearance of crescents. In all four kidneys communications between the cysts were found, and communications with the renal pelvis were found in the three kidneys in which this structure was present.

In these difficult cases, radioisotope studies may be helpful. **Hydronephrotic kidneys usually show some function on a dimercaptosuccinic acid (DMSA) scan, whereas renal concentration is seldom seen in multicystic kidneys.** Angiography reveals an absent or small renal artery in the multicystic kidney, but this study is rarely indicated. Cystoscopy may reveal a hemitrigone and absent ureteral orifice on the affected side; more often, however, an orifice is present but retrograde urography demonstrates ureteral atresia. Again, this study is seldom performed.

In a few cases, diagnostic studies are not performed until the patient is older. In these instances, the plain abdominal film often reveals renal calcifications. These deposits usually appear as annular or arcuate shadows (Felson and Cussen, 1975).

As mentioned previously, voiding cystourethrography is indicated in the work-up because of the high incidence of reflux into the single functioning kidney.

Treatment and Prognosis

It has often been stated that the multicystic kidney can be ignored unless its bulk is inconvenient (Pathak and

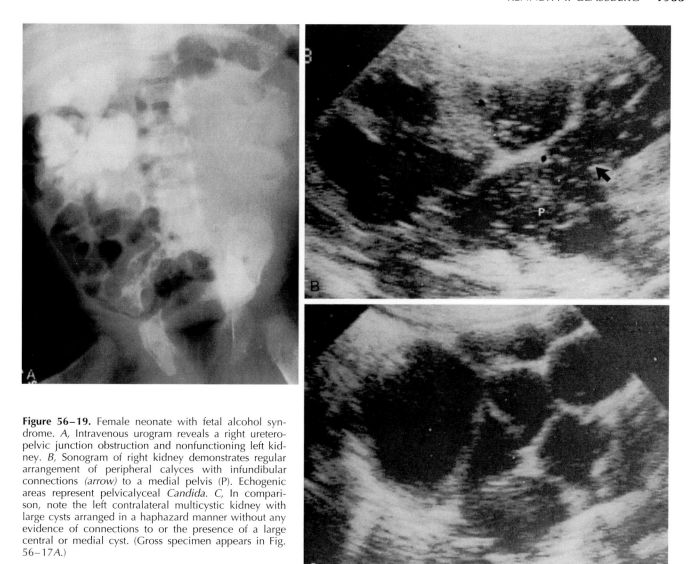

Figure 56–19. Female neonate with fetal alcohol syndrome. *A,* Intravenous urogram reveals a right ureteropelvic junction obstruction and nonfunctioning left kidney. *B,* Sonogram of right kidney demonstrates regular arrangement of peripheral calyces with infundibular connections *(arrow)* to a medial pelvis (P). Echogenic areas represent pelvicalyceal *Candida. C,* In comparison, note the left contralateral multicystic kidney with large cysts arranged in a haphazard manner without any evidence of connections to or the presence of a large central or medial cyst. (Gross specimen appears in Fig. 56–17*A.*)

Williams, 1964; Griscom et al, 1975) and that attention should be directed instead to identifying any abnormalities of the contralateral urinary tract. Certainly, the need in the past to explore some multicystic kidneys to rule out malignancy (e.g., cystic Wilms' tumor, congenital mesoblastic nephroma) has largely been erased by new diagnostic tools. Kidneys that do contain malignancies are likely to be explored because of the retention of some function as seen by excretory urography or nuclear medicine studies (Walker et al, 1984); therefore, routine exploration solely to rule out malignancy is inappropriate.

A nonfunctioning hydronephrotic kidney could be mistaken for a multicystic kidney, although complete nonfunction on a nuclear medicine study is unusual in kidneys affected by ureteropelvic junction obstruction. Even if the correct diagnosis is missed in such a case, however, there are unlikely to be significant consequences, because a totally nonfunctioning hydronephrotic kidney is rarely salvageable and probably will cause no problems other than a predisposition to infection or hyperkalemia.

Of greater concern is the potential for malignant degeneration in a multicystic kidney. In very few reports has the diagnosis of multicystic kidney been made before the diagnosis of an associated cancer (Oddone et al, 1994).

Most case reports have been of a Wilms' tumor and less often an RCC that developed in a previously "unrecognized" multicystic dysplastic kidney. Because many tumors have cystic components (e.g., cystic partially differentiated nephroblastoma), one cannot absolutely conclude that such a kidney was a multicystic dysplastic one at birth. Beckwith (1997) cited examples of reports in the literature of Wilms' tumor in a multicystic dysplastic kidney which, on his review of the photomicrographs, were not Wilms' tumor but nephrogenic rests.

Two reports in the literature might be interpreted as reinforcing the arguments in favor of prophylactic surgical removal. Dimmick and coworkers (1989) and Noe and coworkers (1989) described a total of 120 patients, of whom 5 had nephrogenic rests of nodular renal blastema. In addition, one of the patients in the series of Dimmick and coworkers (1989) had Wilms' tumorlets in the hilar region. Although these findings suggest a hazard in leaving a multicystic kidney in situ, it is unusual for nodular renal blastema or even Wilms' tumorlets to develop into frank Wilms' tumor. For example, nodular renal blastema has been reported in 0.25% to 0.5% of normal kidneys (Bennington and Beckwith, 1975; Bove and McAdams, 1976; Beckwith, 1986), yet the incidence of Wilms' tumor in the general population is much lower. Therefore, although nodular renal blastema and Wilms' tumorlets may be part of a nephroblastomatosis–Wilms' tumor spectrum, the majority of these lesions involute in time without ever becoming malignant.

Trying to predict what percentage of multicystic kidneys will develop Wilms' tumors, Noe and associates (1989) used Beckwith's estimated 1% incidence of Wilms' tumor development in nodular renal blastema. They then calculated, using a 5% incidence of nodular renal blastema in multicystic kidneys, that 2000 nephrectomies for multicystic kidney disease would have to be performed to prevent 1 Wilms' tumor. Accordingly, the risk of surgery must be weighed against that of Wilms' tumor. If one elects to monitor without surgery, the cost-benefit ratio or even the effectiveness of long-term follow-up must be considered. Because nodular renal blastema occurs most often in the hilum (Dimmick et al, 1989), and because most kidneys that shrink lose only cyst fluid, leaving the dysplastic tissue, follow-up by sonography may not be helpful (Colodny, 1989).

In an effort to determine whether there is a relationship between multicystic dysplasia and neoplasia, Jung and coworkers (1990) performed flow cytometric analyses on specimens from 30 patients. No evidence of tetraploidy or aneuploidy, as would be expected in a preneoplastic condition, was found. This report is comforting to the surgeon who does not routinely remove multicystic kidneys. Still, one must be aware that some malignant cells retain a diploid karyotype. In a more recent study, Perez and colleagues (1998) identified only five reported cases in the United States of Wilms' tumor developing in a multicystic dysplastic kidney over the preceding 14 years. They estimated the incidence of this progression to be 3 to 10 times greater than in the general population. This number corresponds with Beckwith's report of a fivefold incidence of nephrogenic rests in persons with multicystic kidney compared with the general population.

Of the 7500 Wilms' tumor specimens reviewed by Beckwith (1997) over 18.75 years, only 5 cases had oc-

curred in a multicystic dysplastic kidney. Beckwith thought it unlikely that the incidence of Wilms' tumor developing in multicystic dysplastic kidneys is greater than fourfold, citing an incidence of 1 in 8000 in the general population and 1 in 2000 in the multicystic dysplastic population. He concluded that this fourfold increase does not make a case for prophylactic nephrectomy. He further pointed out that if a Wilms' tumor does develop, the condition is not as severe as in the past, because the survival rate is now greater than 90%.

Homsy and associates (1997) reported perhaps the two best documented cases of previously diagnosed multicystic dysplastic kidneys that went on to develop Wilms' tumor.

Another management question in multicystic kidney disease is the frequency of hypertension. Gordon and associates (1988) reviewed this topic in a thoughtful article. They noted that since 1966 only nine well-documented cases of hypertension in association with multicystic kidneys in situ had been published. In three of these cases, the hypertension resolved after nephrectomy (Javadpour et al, 1970; Burgler and Hauri, 1983; Chen et al, 1985).

In more recent reports, hypertension resolved after nephrectomy in two of three hypertensive patients studied by Webb and colleagues (1997) and in two of four children studied by Snodgrass (2000). Of 887 patients in the AAP Multicystic Kidney Disease Registry, only 6 (0.7%) had hypertension, and the etiology of the hypertension was questionable in most.

In a series of 20 patients older than 11 years who had multicystic kidney disease, Ambrose (1976) found that 2 had hypertension, and in neither of these patients was the blood pressure controlled by nephrectomy. **In summary, hypertension occurs infrequently with multicystic dysplastic kidney, and it may or may not normalize after nephrectomy. The role of peripheral vein renin is not clear (Snodgrass, 2000). Nevertheless, the incidence of hypertension is not high enough to warrant nephrectomy, although it certainly is a finding warranting routine blood pressure monitoring.** Other reports suggest that the incidence of hypertension may actually be greater than that reported in the literature (Emmert and King, 1994; Hanna, 1995; Webb et al, 1997).

A large number of patients have now been monitored for longer than 5 years by the National Multicystic Kidney Registry (Table 56–12). When the status of neonatal multicystic kidneys is monitored over a period of time, the vast majority either become smaller or stay the same size, and only a very small percentage become larger. If the kidney

Table 56–12. NATIONAL MULTICYSTIC KIDNEY REGISTRY: SONOGRAPHIC FOLLOW-UP

Follow-up	No. of Children	Not Identifiable	Smaller	Larger	Unchanged
1–3 mo	140	7 (5.0%)	64 (45.7%)	16 (11.4%)	53 (37.9%)
4–6 mo	181	13 (7.2%)	119 (65.7%)	9 (5.0%)	40 (22.1%)
7–9 mo	134	13 (9.7%)	73 (54.5%)	4 (3.0%)	44 (32.0%)
10–12 mo	96	14 (14.6%)	41 (42.7%)	5 (5.2%)	36 (37.5%)
1–3 yr	622	99 (15.9%)	286 (46.0%)	26 (4.2%)	211 (33.4%)
3–5 yr	183	42 (22.9%)	63 (34.4%)	10 (5.5%)	68 (37.2%)
>5 yr	159	38 (23.9%)	60 (37.7%)	2 (1.3%)	59 (37.1%)

Data supplied by J. Wacksman and L. Phipps, National Multicystic Kidney Registry, American Academy of Pediatrics, October, 2000.

becomes larger, depending on the surgeon's inclinations, consideration can be given to removal. When the kidney stays the same size, it actually becomes smaller in proportion to the size of the child as he or she gets older. Most kidneys that become smaller do so during the first year of follow-up, and an increasing number of those that become smaller disappear from view with time on ultrasound examination. None of the multicystic kidneys in the Registry has developed a tumor during follow-up. However, a number of kidneys were removed at the time of entry into the study by decision of the individual surgeon, and a smaller number were removed later because of increasing size during follow-up. As a result, it cannot be determined whether the kidneys that were selected for nephrectomy had a greater potential for malignancy or hypertension. Hypertension has developed in only five of the patients in the Registry, and it is not clear from the data how many of these cases of hypertension were thought to be secondary to the multicystic kidney. Occasional urinary tract infections have been seen, but it is unclear whether the multicystic kidney had anything to do with them, particularly because many of these patients also have contralateral reflux.

Questions still must be answered. Does the disappearance of a multicystic kidney on imaging studies mean that there is no longer a potential risk? When these kidneys disappear from view, it means only that the fluid within the cysts has disappeared; the cells still remain. How necessary is it to follow those patients who are not operated on, since many inevitably will be lost to follow-up? Perez and co-workers (1998) recommended renal ultrasound every 3 months until 8 years of age, when the incidence of Wilms' tumor is almost nil. From the experience of Ambrose (1976), it appears that flank pain as an adult is the chief risk of a multicystic kidney that is left in situ, and in such cases the pain usually responds to nephrectomy.

Elder and coworkers (1995) reported on 30 multicystic kidneys that were removed in an ambulatory setting within an operative time of 20 to 70 minutes, making the case for an alternative approach to nonsurgical management. In the clinical setting, however, parents will respond differently to the suggestion that surgery provides less risk than long-term follow-up of a disease that has a low association with development of malignancy. Certainly the prejudices of the individual surgeon presenting the choice of surgery or conservative follow-up plays a significant role in a parent's decision.

If we use the recommendations of Perez and colleagues (1997) for conservative management including a renal ultrasound study every 3 months until 8 years of age, the cost ($2,000–$5,000) is still not more than for a simple nephrectomy ($5,000–$7,000). In summary, although the incidence of Wilms' tumor developing in a multicystic dysplastic kidney may be higher than in a normal kidney (3- to 10-fold), the numbers do not make a strong case for either prophylactic nephrectomy or conservative nonsurgical follow-up.

BENIGN MULTILOCULAR CYST (CYSTIC NEPHROMA)

A multilocular cystic lesion in a child's kidney may be a benign multilocular cyst, a multilocular cyst with partially differentiated Wilms' tumor, a multilocular cyst with nodules of Wilms' tumor, or a cystic Wilms' tumor (Fig. 56–20). **These four lesions form a spectrum, with the benign multilocular cyst at one extreme and the cystic Wilms' tumor at the other.** There has been some debate as to whether these represent a spectrum of one disease with one etiology lying between a benign multilocular cyst and a cystic adenocarcinoma or some other cystic renal tumor.

A multilocular cyst is not a renal segment affected by multicystic kidney disease; these conditions differ clinically, histologically, and radiographically. However, controversy continues about whether the multilocular cyst is a segmental form of renal dysplasia (Powell et al, 1951; Osathanondh and Potter, 1964; Johnson et al, 1973); a hamartomatous malformation (Arey, 1959); or a neoplastic

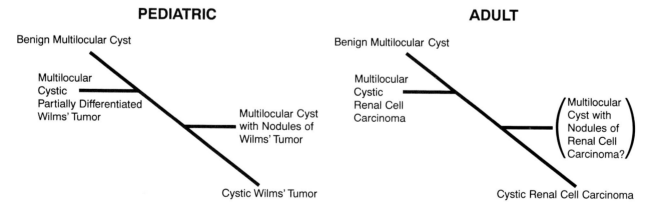

Figure 56–20. The spectrum of multilocular cystic lesions in children and adults. There is no evidence that one lesion can convert into the other. Benign cystic partially differentiated Wilms' tumor and multilocular cystic renal cell carcinoma act as benign lesions. When nodules of tumor are present the lesion should be considered malignant, although the prognosis of this lesion as well as cystic Wilms' tumor and cystic renal cell carcinoma seems to be better than that of the corresponding solid lesions. It is not clear whether clinical examples of "multilocular cyst with nodules of renal cell carcinoma" actually exist, but this entity is placed in the spectrum for consideration. For simplicity, the multilocular-appearing lesions of other cystic tumors (e.g., cystic oncocytoma, cystic hamartoma of the renal pelvis) are not included in the figure.

disease (Boggs and Kimmelsteil, 1956; Christ, 1968; Fowler, 1971; Gallo and Penchansky, 1977). The confusion arises in part from the variability of the histologic picture: the appearance of the primitive stroma, the maturity of tubular and even on occasion of muscle elements, and the degree of epithelial atypia differ not only from patient to patient but also within the same lesion.

Past use of many nonspecific terms—such as lymphangioma, partial or focal polycystic kidney, multicystic kidney, and cystic adenoma—makes it difficult to identify relevant published cases for review (Aterman et al, 1973). Edmunds used the term "cystic adenoma" in 1892 in what was probably the first published description of this lesion. I favor the term *benign multilocular cyst* because the descriptor "benign" separates this lesion from other multilocular cystic lesions and the term "multilocular cyst" clearly describes the gross appearance of the lesion. Joshi and Beckwith (1989) prefer the term *cystic nephroma* because it implies a benign but neoplastic lesion. Some refer to the spaces within the lesion as "loculi," and others use the term "cysts."

Clinical Features

The great majority of patients present before the age of 4 years or after 30 years. Five percent present between 4 and 30 years. The patient is twice as likely to be male if younger than 4 years and eight times as likely to be female if older than 30 years of age (Eble and Bonsib, 1998).

The signs and symptoms differ according to the age at presentation. In children an asymptomatic flank mass is the most common finding, whereas most adults present with either a flank mass, abdominal pain, or hematuria. The bleeding is secondary to herniation of the cyst through the transitional epithelium into the renal pelvis (Uson and Melicow, 1963; Aterman et al, 1973; Madewell et al, 1983).

Seven cases of bilateral benign multilocular cysts of the kidney have been described (Castillo et al, 1991); in one of these patients, the lesion recurred after excision (Geller et al, 1979). Also, at least two instances are known in which multilocular cysts arose in kidneys known to have been normal previously (Uson and Melicow, 1963; Chatten and Bishop, 1977). Such cases support a neoplastic theory of the origin of this lesion.

Histopathology

These lesions are bulky and are circumscribed by a thick capsule. Normal renal parenchyma adjacent to the lesion frequently is compressed by it. The lesion may extend beyond the renal capsule into the perinephric space or renal pelvis. The loculi, which range from a few millimeters to centimeters in diameter, do not intercommunicate. They contain clear, straw-colored or yellow fluid and are lined by cuboidal or low columnar epithelial cells. In some cases, eosinophilic cuboidal cells project into the cyst lumen, creating a hobnail appearance (Madewell et al, 1983). The definitions of multilocular cystic kidney given by Powell and coworkers (1951) and by Boggs and Kimmelsteil

(1956) require a normal epithelial lining for the diagnosis. **Joshi and Beckwith (1989) also defined the septa of a benign multilocular cyst as being composed of fibrous tissue in which well-differentiated tubules may be present but poorly differentiated tissues and blastemal cells are not present.**

When Castillo and associates (1991) reviewed the literature on multilocular cysts, they included lesions that had interlocular septa containing tissue of two different types: (1) fibrous tissue only or (2) embryonic-type tissue. Adults in general have only the first type, whereas children, principally those younger than 3 years of age, have either type. Joshi and Beckwith (1989) referred to the embryonic type as an immature form. They prefer the term "cystic partially differentiated nephroblastoma" (Joshi, 1980), **because histologically this form is different from the first group, which they believe is the typical benign multilocular cyst. To make the diagnosis of a cystic partially differentiated nephroblastoma, blastemal cells must be present. Often varying amounts of poorly differentiated tissues such as tubules, glomeruli, mesenchyme, skeletal muscle, and, rarely, cartilage are admixed with the blastemal cells** (Joshi and Beckwith, 1989). **These elements are not present in benign multilocular cysts.** Supportive evidence that the second variety should not be called a benign multilocular cyst lies in the histories of Joshi and Beckwith's (1989) 18 patients with cystic partially differentiated nephroblastoma: 1 patient had a contralateral anaplastic Wilms' tumor, and another had two local recurrences after nephrectomy.

Eble and Bonsib (1998) believe that cystic nephroma in children is a different entity than in adults. They believe that benign multilocular cyst and cystic partially differentiated Wilms' tumor are the same disease in childhood. Because neither metastasizes, they prefer to call both conditions in childhood "cystic partially differentiated nephroblastoma" and to leave the term "cystic nephroma" to the adult variety.

As noted earlier, benign multilocular cysts **can be considered as part of a spectrum. Within that spectrum lies cystic partially differentiated nephroblastoma (see Fig. 56–19). I prefer the term "multilocular cystic partially differentiated Wilms' tumor" to "cystic partially differentiated nephroblastoma," because two of the other entities within the spectrum are described with the category Wilms' tumor. For example, when nodules of Wilms' tumor are present, Joshi (1980) designates the lesion as a "multilocular cyst with nodules of Wilms' tumor." The term "cystic Wilms' tumor" is reserved for the rare cases of tumor in which cysts are lined by epithelial cells. This entity should not be confused with Wilms' tumors that have sonolucent or radiolucent cyst-like spaces attributable to tumor necrosis.**

Although in children there may be a continuum from benign multilocular cyst to cystic Wilms' tumor, and although all of these lesions may be derived from similar cells or tissues, no evidence suggests that one entity transforms into another. Furthermore, **none of the genetically determined conditions associated with Wilms' tumor (e.g., hemihypertrophy, aniridia) has accompanied a benign multilocular cyst** (Banner et al, 1981).

In adults there also is a spectrum of multilocular cystic lesions. For example, **if an adult is identified with a multilocular cystic lesion, it can be either a multilocular cystic RCC, a cystic RCC, a cystic oncocytoma, or some rare tumor such as cystic hamartoma of the renal pelvis.** Eble and Bonsib (1998) found 44 reported adult cases of "multilocular cystic RCC." One year later, Kirsh et al (1999) added four of their own cases, but they preferred the term "benign adenomatous multicystic kidney tumor" because of the lesion's benign nature. This tumor has also been referred to as Perlmann's tumor, because Perlmann (1928) was the first to describe the lesion. Perlmann, however, interpreted his findings as representing a cystic lymphoangioma (Perlmann, 1928; Kirsh et al, 1999). **Just as cystic partially differentiated Wilms' tumor in children falls in the spectrum between benign multilocular cyst and cystic Wilms' tumor, so does multilocular cystic RCC in adults fall in the spectrum between a benign multilocular cyst and a cystic RCC. Also, just as in partially differentiated Wilms' tumor there are blastema cells lying in the septa between loculi and sometimes lining the loculi, so too in multilocular cystic RCC, clear cells and clear epithelial cells lie between the loculi and line the loculi. Neither condition has expansile nodules, and neither condition metastasizes** (Eble and Bonsib, 1998). It is not clear whether there is a condition in adults that resembles the next lesion in the pediatric spectrum—multilocular cyst with nodules of Wilms' tumor. **The cystic component of the tumor at the carcinomatosis end of the spectrum in both children and adults (i.e., cystic Wilms' tumor and cystic RCC) improves the prognosis of the malignant lesion** (Kirsh et al, 1999). **In adults, as in children, there is no evidence that one lesion can convert into another.** As an education tool, the spectrum of multilocular cystic lesions in children and adults may be considered in a parallel fashion. I therefore suggest use of the parallel terms, "multilocular cystic partially differentiated Wilms' tumor" and "multilocular cystic RCC" (Fig. 56–21).

An even rarer tumor in adults, cystic hamartoma of the renal pelvis, also cannot be differentiated from other multilocular cystic tumors on imaging studies. Although the tumor arises centrally within the kidney, its proximity to the pelvis and often herniation into the pelvis give it its name. The benign tumors are composed of microcysts and tubules. The stroma consists of spindle cells. Mitotic figures do not appear (Eble and Bonsib, 1998).

Evaluation

A number of tests may be useful, including intravenous urography, sonography, CT, MRI, cyst puncture with aspiration and double-contrast cystography, and arteriography. **Ultrasound and CT can distinguish multicystic kidney and multilocular cyst, but neither study is sufficiently reliable to distinguish multilocular cyst, multilocular cyst with foci of Wilms' tumor or adenocarcinoma, mesoblastic nephroma, cystic Wilms' tumor, and clear cell sarcoma.** Typically, the septa are highly echogenic with sonolucent loculi, although if there is debris in a loculus, it may appear more solid. On CT, the septa are less dense than normal parenchyma; when myxomatous material is present, the density is equal to that of solid structures (Wood et al, 1982). Calcification is rarely visible in such lesions in children (Madewell et al, 1983).

In the few cases in which angiography was performed, vascular, hypovascular, and hypervascular patterns were seen (Davides, 1976; Madewell et al, 1983; DeWall et al, 1986). A tumor blush and neovascularity that sometimes was extensive were apparent in some cases (Madewell et al, 1983).

Clear to yellow fluid is recovered by cyst puncture. Contrast agents opacify only those loculi through which the needle has passed, because the loculi do not communicate (Madewell et al, 1983).

Treatment

The treatment for benign multilocular cyst, multilocular cystic partially differentiated Wilms' tumor, and multilocular cystic RCC is nephrectomy. If the lesion is localized enough and there is well preserved normal tissue, excision of the lesion or partial nephrectomy is feasible. Children who have a multilocular cyst with nodules of Wilms' tumor or a cystic Wilms' tumor should be treated as for Wilms' tumor, recognizing their generally favorable outlook. Similarly, cystic RCC in adults should be managed as a malignant lesion, again, however, recognizing its better prognosis. In adults, benign multilocular cysts more often are associated with larger amounts of normal renal tissue, making partial nephrectomy more often feasible. In a report by Castillo and associates (1991), 24 of 29 patients underwent renal-sparing surgery, including 2 who were children. The treatment for multilocular cystic lesions in most children is nephrectomy, because the lesion usually is associated with little preserved tissue. In children, two questions must be answered in selecting the treatment for a multilocular cystic lesion: (1) Is the contralateral urinary tract normal? and (2) Is the abnormal kidney involved with Wilms' tumor? At least four of the cystic tumors in the National Wilms' Tumor Study (NWTS) metastasized (Beckwith and Palmer, 1978); therefore, these lesions clearly have malignant potential, although they appear to be less aggressive than classic Wilms' tumor.

The treatment for a multilocular cyst in most children is nephrectomy. If pathologic review shows cystic Wilms' tumor, further treatment should be given according to the NWTS recommendations for the appropriate stage of disease. However, if the focus of tumor does not exceed 2 cm, nephrectomy alone may be sufficient. If enucleation or partial nephrectomy is chosen, recurrence is possible. However, with more Wilms' tumors being treated by local excision, the case for enucleation or partial nephrectomy combined with close follow-up by sonography and CT is stronger, even if malignancy is found within the lesion. In comparison, if a clear cell sarcoma is found after enucleation, the remaining ipsilateral renal tissue should be removed because of the aggressiveness of this cancer. The recurrence of a multilocular cyst not containing malignancy probably reflects inadequate excision of the initial lesion.

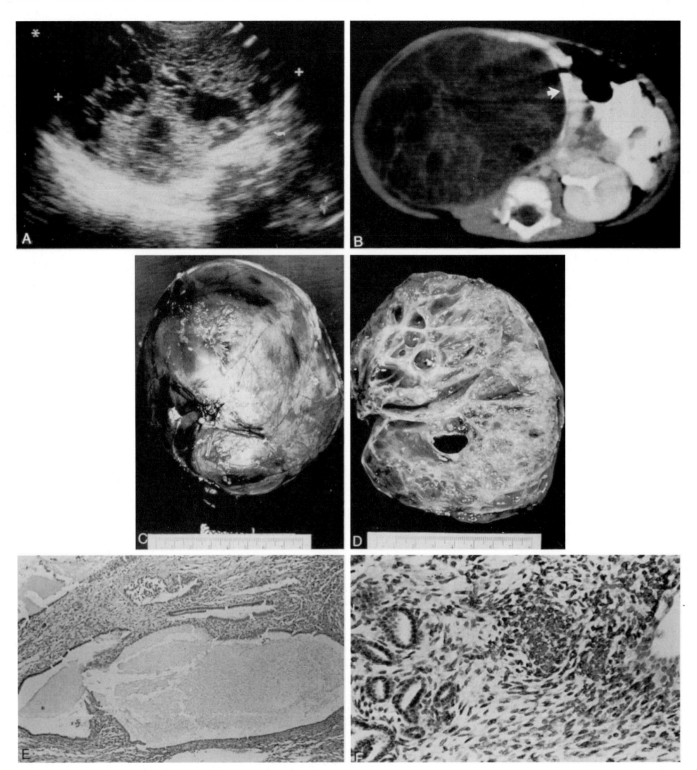

Figure 56–21. A 4-year-old girl with a right-sided abdominal mass. *A,* Renal sonogram shows multiple cysts throughout the left kidney. *B,* On contrast-enhanced computed tomographic scan, a large, smoothly outlined left renal mass is seen with fine septa throughout the mass. Residual preserved parenchyma and the pelvicalyceal system are compressed medially and pushed to the contralateral side *(arrow)*. *C,* Uncut gross specimen reveals a smooth-walled, encapsulated renal mass. *D,* Cross section of mass reveals multiple noncommunicating loculations. *E,* On histology, a hypocellular cystic area is seen with monotonous stroma (×100). *F,* Between loculi, nests of blastematous cells are visualized along with tubular elements *(left)*, making the diagnosis of multilocular cyst with partially differentiated Wilms' tumor (×200).

SIMPLE CYSTS

A simple cyst is a discrete finding that may occur well within a kidney or on its surface. It is usually oval to round in shape, has a smooth outline bordered by a single layer of flattened cuboidal epithelium, and is filled with transudate-like clear or straw-colored fluid. It is not connected to any part of the nephron, although it may originate initially from a portion of the nephron. Simple cysts may be singular or multiple, unilateral or bilateral.

Simple cysts may manifest at any time in utero and have been diagnosed as early as 14 weeks of gestation. **Sonography done on 29,984 fetuses in succession revealed (0.09%) of 11,000 pregnancies to have renal cysts** (Blazer et al, 1999). **In 25 fetuses the cysts resolved before birth. Of two cysts that remained postnatally, one was the first sign of a multicystic kidney.** All 28 children were healthy postnatally without genitourinary system anomalies and with no chromosomal anomalies (Blazer et al, 1999). Between birth and 18 years of age, the incidence of simple renal cysts is fairly stable, ranging from 0.1% to 0.45% with an average incidence of 0.22% (McHugh et al, 1991). **However, in adults the frequency rises with age. Using CT, Laucks and McLachlan (1981) demonstrated that the incidence of cysts was 20% by age 40 years and approximately 33% after age 60. On autopsy, Kissane and Smith (1975) identified a 50% incidence of simple renal cysts after age 50.** Most reports show no gender predilection; however, in at least two studies, men were affected more frequently than women (Bearth and Steg, 1977; Tada et al, 1983).

Clinical Features

In both children and adults, cysts rarely call attention to themselves. Instead, they are discovered incidentally on sonography, CT, or urography performed for a urinary tract or other pelvic or abdominal problem. However, cysts can produce an abdominal mass or pain, hematuria secondary to rupture into the pyelocalyceal system, and hypertension secondary to segmental ischemia (Rockson et al, 1974; Lüscher et al, 1986; Papanicolaou et al, 1986). Cysts can cause calyceal or renal pelvic obstruction as well (Wahlqvist and Grumstedt, 1966; Evans and Coughlin, 1970; Hinman, 1978; Barloon and Vince, 1987). They may or may not increase in size with time. Of 23 cysts in 22 children who underwent sonographic follow-up for up to 5 years, McHugh and associates (1991) found that 17 cysts (74%) remained unchanged in size.

Over an 18-year period, Papanicolaou and coworkers (1986) treated 25 patients who had spontaneous or traumatic rupture of a known cyst, a large number of cases considering the rarity of cyst rupture. Most of these ruptures (21) were spontaneous; 3 occurred after blunt trauma, and 1 was iatrogenic. The cyst ruptured into a calyx in 12 patients. In one patient, the rupture was into the renal pelvis, through the parenchyma but not the capsule. In another, the cyst ruptured through the parenchyma and capsule. In five patients, the rupture was both calyceal and perinephric, and in the remaining four patients, the site of

rupture could not be determined. In 21 patients hematuria was present, and in 17 patients flank pain was present. The diagnosis was made by high-dose drip infusion nephrotomography in 22 patients, by CT in 2, and by retrograde pyelography in 1. In 11 patients the cyst communication closed spontaneously, and in 8 the cyst cavity was obliterated on follow-up studies. Two patients had persistent calyceal communication with 2 months or less of follow-up.

Cysts can rupture into the pelvicalyceal system, maintain a communication, and become a pseudocalyceal diverticulum. The reverse is also possible: closure of the communication of a diverticulum can create a simple cyst (Mosli et al, 1986; Papanicolaou et al, 1986). These two sequences of events can be distinguished only by histologic examination. **Theoretically, diverticula should have linings of transitional epithelium, whereas simple cysts should be lined by a single layer of flattened or cuboidal epithelium.**

Hypertension caused by cysts has been confirmed in several reports. For example, in two children with simple cysts and hypertension, the blood pressure normalized after surgical decompression of the cysts (Babka et al, 1974; Hoard and O'Brien, 1976). Also, Lüscher and coworkers (1986) identified 22 published cases of renal cysts and hypertension. Surgical removal or aspiration of the cyst was therapeutic in 10 patients and yielded improvement in 2 others with a mean follow-up of 1 year. Ten of the 15 patients who were studied by renal vein renin assays had elevated activity, suggesting local tissue or arterial compression by the cyst. This hypothesis is easily believable if one realizes that a simple cyst can have a pressure as high as 57 cm H_2O and that the lesions in this series of cases generally were large, most exceeding 6 cm in diameter and containing several hundred milliliters of fluid (Amis et al, 1982; Lüscher et al, 1986).

Histopathology

Simple cysts vary considerably in size, ranging from less than 1 cm to greater than 10 cm. The majority are less than 2 cm in diameter, however (Tada et al, 1983). **The wall is fibrous and of varying thickness and has no renal elements. The cyst lining is a single layer of flattened or cuboidal epithelium.**

Because cysts are increasingly common with age, they have been considered an acquired lesion. Bearth and Steg (1977) found greater ectasia and cystic dilatation of the distal tubules and collecting ducts in patients older than 60 years of age and considered these changes to be precursors of macroscopic cysts.

Evaluation

One can safely make the diagnosis of a classic benign simple cyst by sonography when the following criteria are met: (1) absence of internal echoes; (2) sharply defined, thin, distinct wall with a smooth and distinct margin; (3) good transmission of sound waves through the cyst with consequent acoustic enhancement behind the cyst; and (4) spherical or slightly ovoid shape (Goldman and Hartman, 1990). **If all of these criteria are satisfied, the chance that malignancy is present is negligible**

(Fig. 56–22) (Lingard and Lawson, 1979; Livingston et al, 1981).

When some of these criteria are not met—for example, when there are septations, irregular margins, calcifications, or suspect areas—further evaluation by CT or perhaps needle aspiration or MRI is indicated (Bosniak, 1986). A cluster of cysts is another indication for further study, because they may be hiding a small carcinoma. CT is better than sonography in defining such a camouflaged lesion (Bosniak, 1986). Peripelvic cysts often require CT confirmation because they frequently are interspersed between structures of the collecting system and hilum, which can create artificial echoes (Bosniak, 1986).

The CT criteria for a simple cyst are similar to those used in sonography: (1) sharp, thin, distinct, smooth walls and margins; (2) spherical or ovoid shape; and (3) homogeneous content. The density ranges from −10 to +20 HU, similar to the density of water, and no enhancement should occur after the intravenous injection of contrast medium. Bosniak (1986) stated that he had not seen a tumor with a density of less than 20 HU on a contrast-enhanced scan, but a truly benign cyst can have fluid with a density greater than 20 HU. In these cases, intravenous contrast injection is particularly helpful.

When the cyst fluid is hyperdense (i.e., between 20 and 90 HU), it still is likely to be a simple cyst if no enhancement occurs when intravenous contrast agent is injected and if the other criteria of CT and sonography are met. Hyperdense cysts must be evaluated with narrow window settings to make sure that they are homogeneous. Other criteria that must be met to avoid further evaluation of hyperdense cysts (e.g., cyst puncture or exploration) include size (the lesion should be 3 cm or smaller) and location (at least one fourth of the cyst's circumference should extend beyond the renal contour so that the smoothness of a good portion of the cyst can be evaluated) (Bosniak, 1991a, 1991b; Hartman et al, 1992). When reviewing the CT study of a hyperdense cyst with the radiologist, the urologist must be reassured that the Hounsfield units were calibrated by using fluid in the gallbladder or unopacified urine. Still, on rare occasions, although all criteria for a benign hyperdense cyst are carefully met, a cystic RCC may be missed (Hartman et al, 1992). Technical factors can affect the results—for example, injecting too little contrast or waiting too long to scan after injection (Macari and Bosniak, 1999).

Because cysts have no blood vessels and do not communicate directly with nephrons, they should not enhance; enhancement therefore implies vascular tissue or contrast medium mixing with fluid. However, for several days after the injection of contrast medium, the fluid in a benign cyst may enhance (Hartman, 1990). Despite the diagnostic utility of contrast enhancement, the first scan should always be performed without enhancement because contrast medium may obscure calcification, small amounts of fat, or recent hemorrhage (Bosniak, 1986). When the aforementioned criteria are respected, the accuracy of diagnosis of a simple cyst by CT approaches 100% (Figs. 56–23 and 56–24) (McClennan et al, 1979). Occasionally, a high-density (>30 HU), well-marginated lesion may be noticed on a postcontrast CT when no record of density of the previously unrecognized lesion was obtained (Macari and Bosniak, 1999). In such situations one can look for "de-enhancement," a finding that occurs after the initial flow of contrast to an organ and that offers proof of vascularity (i.e., neoplasm). Macari and Bosniak (1999) found 15 minutes to be a sufficient period of delay to detect de-enhancement. If there is still a question of de-enhancement, the patient can be taken off the table and returned 30 or more minutes later.

When sonographic or CT criteria are not met, such as when there is a thick wall, calcification, septation, nonhomogeneous or hyperdense fluid, or fluid with internal echoes, conditions other than simple cyst must be considered. Other possibilities are complicated cysts (i.e., those containing blood, pus, or calcification) and cystic neoplasms. One of the more common sources of confusion is the parenchymal beak classically seen on intravenous urogra-

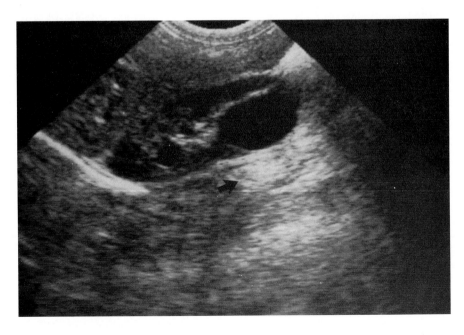

Figure 56–22. Two renal cysts in an 8-year-old boy. Note evidence of enhancement of sound wave transmission through the larger oval cyst by the hyperechogenicity (whiteness) of the image behind the cyst. Family history or even sonographic evaluation of family should be considered to rule out autosomal dominant polycystic kidney disease, especially when more than one cyst is present. In children, it is not unusual for autosomal dominant polycystic kidney disease to first manifest with one or two cysts.

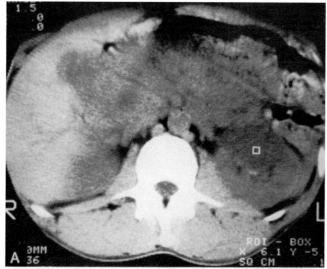

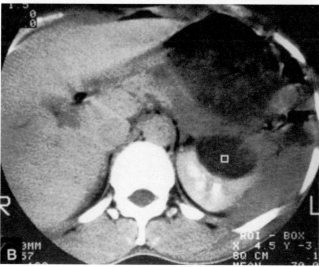

Figure 56–23. *A,* Hyperdense renal cysts on precontrast computed tomographic (CT) scan measuring +33 HU. *B,* After contrast administration, CT scan values were +30 HU. Absence of enhancement, spherical shape, and fine outline are findings compatible with the diagnosis of a simple cyst despite CT values greater than +20 HU.

phy when the tissue partially engulfs the cyst margin. When seen in cross section on sonography or CT, this beak can create the appearance of a thick wall (Segal and Spitzer, 1979). Cyst puncture and aspiration with or without contrast medium injection was popular in the 1960s and 1970s. Fluid from cystic RCC may be hemorrhagic or may contain elevated levels of protein, lactic dehydrogenase, or fat (Marotti et al, 1987). Today, with the improvements in sonography and CT, cyst puncture is less likely to be needed. The remaining indications for cyst puncture are (1) suspected infection, in which case puncture may be therapeutic as well as diagnostic; (2) the presence of low-level echoes on sonography but a classic cyst on CT; and (3) a borderline lesion in a poor surgical candidate.

Bosniak (1986) believed that hyperdense cysts larger than 3 cm in diameter require further evaluation or close follow-up because there are few data on the nature of hyperdense lesions of this size. In such cases, the following

options might be considered, depending on the patient's age and general health: (1) cyst puncture with aspiration for cytologic study, (2) puncture and injection of contrast medium, or (3) follow-up by sonography or CT at progressively longer intervals.

When evaluating a possibly infected cyst, one must be aware that the wall may be thickened and sometimes calcified. Debris is often present (Hartman, 1990). Calcification may also be present in the absence of infection or malignancy; 1% to 3% of renal cysts are calcified (Daniel et al, 1972; Bree et al, 1984). Such calcification is dystrophic and usually occurs secondary to hemorrhage, infection, or ischemia (Hartman, 1990). Also, 6% of simple cysts can hemorrhage (Jackman and Stevens, 1974; Pollack et al, 1979). In 1971, 31% of hemorrhagic cysts were reported to be malignant (Gross and Breach, 1971), but it was deemed necessary at that time to explore the majority of such cysts. Today, even if blood is present, the decision to operate usually can be made on the basis of sonographic or CT findings.

MRI offers little information beyond that available from sonography and CT, although it is more specific in identifying the nature of the cyst fluid. Marotti and coworkers (1987) found that if the fluid has low signal intensity (similar to that of urine) on T1-weighted images, the cyst is benign even if the wall is thick or septa are present. If this report is substantiated by additional studies, MRI may prove valuable in deciding which indeterminate cysts are benign and which should be considered for exploration. **The T2-weighted images identify bloody fluid with an extremely bright image** (Fig. 56–25).

Technical points need to be made about the evaluation of simple cysts by each of these imaging methods. First, when poor acoustic enhancement or low-level internal echoes are identified by real-time sonography, the findings may be an artifact of the method. Weinreb and coworkers (1986) suggested that, in these cases, a static ultrasound scan should be obtained to see whether the findings are reproducible before performing CT. If no internal echoes are seen or if acoustic enhancement is clearly demonstrable, the contrary findings on the real-time scan can be considered artifactual and CT can be avoided. Second, problems may occur in judging the density of cyst fluid by CT if the scanner is not regularly calibrated against gallbladder fluid or urine without contrast medium in the renal pelvis or bladder. These fluids should have densities near that of water (−10 to +20 HU). Third, it must be remembered with MRI that ventilatory and bowel motions can degrade the signal intensity of cyst fluid as well as lesion definition (Marotti et al, 1987).

To summarize, in most cases of simple cysts, the diagnosis is readily made. **When the cyst is indeterminate, the most important diagnostic question is whether the cyst is a manifestation of malignancy. When the cysts are diffuse, multiple, or bilateral, the possibility of ADPKD must be considered. The sonographic and CT appearance of these two types of lesions can be identical. Diagnosis then depends on identifying other family members with ADPKD or finding reduced renal function or other signs of ADPKD, such as hepatic cysts. In its early stages, ADPKD is not always represented by multiple bilateral cysts; it may initially appear sono-**

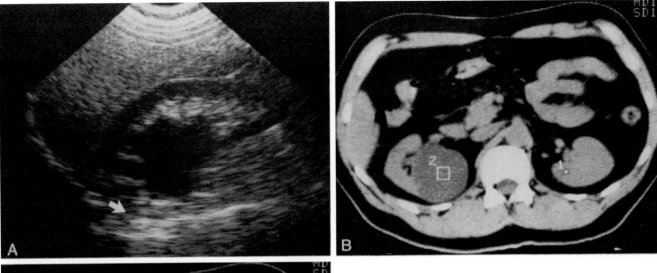

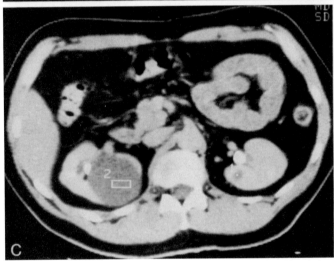

Figure 56–24. A 56-year-old man with an indeterminate, left renal cyst on renal sonography. *A,* Note the nonspherical, non-smoothly outlined sonolucent mass in left kidney. However, there is good sound wave transmission through the cysts (acoustic enhancement), which is illustrated by the intensity (whiteness) of the sonogram image behind the cyst *(arrow). B,* On precontrast CT scan, a very small cyst (1) is seen in the left kidney. The right renal cyst (2) that was identified on sonography measures 17 HU. *C,* Following contrast administration, the CT value (2) was 16 HU, signifying no enhancement. CT values between −10 and +20 HU are characteristic of cysts. No enhancement with contrast confirms the diagnosis of a simple renal cyst. The small cyst (1) was not large enough for determining accurate CT values. (Courtesy of G. Laungani, M.D.)

graphically as a single renal cyst, multiple unilateral cysts, or cysts localized to one portion of the kidney.

Simple Cyst Variations

Two variations of simple cysts must be considered: unilateral renal cystic disease and autosomal dominant simple cyst disease.

UNILATERAL RENAL CYSTIC DISEASE

Large renal cysts of varying size appearing side by side, often more numerous at one pole, have been referred to as *unilateral renal cystic disease.* Evidence from Levine and Huntrakoon (1989) strongly supports the view that this condition is a discrete unilateral, nongenetic entity. On sonography the appearance is that of multiple simple cysts lying side by side; on CT normal parenchyma separates the cysts (Levine and Huntrakoon, 1989). These cysts do not seem to be separated into one encapsulated mass lesion. Because the entity seems to represent nothing more than multiple simple cysts lying side by side within a kidney, I prefer, for the present, to include it as a variation of the presentation of simple cysts.

It is important not to overdiagnose unilateral simple cyst disease, because the entity itself is rare and when first identified in an individual it is more likely to represent a unilateral asymmetric presentation of ADPKD (Glassberg, 1991). **Such a diagnosis therefore requires long-term follow-up demonstrating absence of cyst development in the contralateral kidney and no family members with cystic disease** (Glassberg, 1999). In previous reports, cysts have not been identified in other organs. The term "unilateral polycystic kidney disease" (Lee et al, 1978; Kossow and Meek, 1982) should not be employed because it confuses the diagnosis with ADPKD. If warranted, studies to rule out VHL and tuberous sclerosis should be considered. Now that genetic studies are becoming available for ADPKD, tuberous sclerosis, and VHL, the diagnosis of unilateral renal cystic disease can more readily be confirmed.

AUTOSOMAL DOMINANT SIMPLE CYST DISEASE

Our group studied the families of five children with simple cysts sonographically to determine whether simple cysts in children might in some cases be inherited. In two of the five families, several members were found

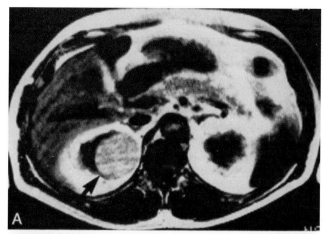

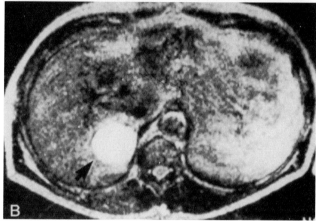

Figure 56–25. Magnetic resonance image of a hemorrhagic cyst. *A,* Blood is seen on T1-weighted images *(arrow)*. *B,* Blood appears extremely white *(arrow)* on T2-weighted image because of the presence of methemoglobin.

to have simple cysts (Schulsinger et al, 1994). In one of the families four siblings, the father, and the paternal grandmother also had renal cysts. In the second affected family the mother, but not the father or siblings, had simple cysts. Genetic linkage studies were unable to identify ADPKD in these two families. In addition, neither family had findings associated with tuberous sclerosis or VHL. The evidence so far leads us to conjecture that we might be identifying a new entity, *autosomal dominant simple cyst disease.* Until there is further genetic proof that it is a new entity, I prefer not to include autosomal simple cyst disease as a formal separate entity in this classification.

Treatment and Prognosis

The propensity of simple cysts to enlarge is not clear. Laucks and McLachlan (1981) found that cyst diameter increases with age. Contrary data were reported by Richter and associates (1983), who found an increase in cyst size in only 2 of 31 patients who were observed for as long as 10 years. Also, Dalton and coworkers (1986) monitored 59 patients by sonography and found no significant changes in cyst size, although they did see an increase in the number of cysts in 20% of cases.

Before 1970, most simple cysts in children were treated surgically. However, a number of large series published in the 1970s indicated that cysts could be managed much like those in adults because they are the same type of lesion. Once malignancy has been ruled out, unroofing or removal of an asymptomatic cyst is not indicated (Gordon et al, 1979; Bartholomew et al, 1980; Ravden et al, 1980; Siegel and McAlister, 1980).

When a benign simple cyst causes pyelocalyceal obstruction or hypertension, the problem may be corrected either surgically, by unroofing the cyst, or percutaneously, by aspirating the fluid and perhaps injecting a sclerosing agent, particularly if fluid has reaccumulated after an earlier aspiration. Several sclerosing agents have been used, including glucose, phenol, iophendylate (Pantopaque), and absolute ethanol, but none has been sufficiently impressive for its use to become dominant (Holmberg and Hietala, 1989).

Holmberg and Hietala (1989) managed simple cysts in 156 patients in one of three ways. In one group, no treatment was given; in 25% of these patients, the cysts grew during a mean follow-up period of 3 years. In a second group, cyst aspiration was performed. In this group, the cysts disappeared in 10% of patients, and the mean size of the cysts in the remainder declined to 90% of the original volume after 24 months. In the third group, cyst aspiration was followed by sclerotherapy with bismuth phosphate. In this group, the cysts disappeared in 44% of patients, and the mean size of the cysts in the remainder was only 21% of the original size after 3 to 4 years.

On the basis of this study and another study by Westberg and Zachrisson (1975), in which all bismuth-treated cysts shrank, it appears that, when treatment is needed for a simple cyst because of pain or compression effects, sclerosis of the cyst lining with instilled bismuth phosphate is a method worthy of consideration. Newer approaches to recalcitrant cysts are percutaneous resection and intrarenal marsupialization (Hubner et al, 1990; Hulbert and Hunter, 1990; Meyer and Jonas, 1990) and laparoscopic unroofing, either transperitoneally (Morgan and Rader, 1992) or retroperitoneally (Raboy et al, 1994).

Plas and Hübner (1993) investigated the long-term results (median follow-up, 45.7 months) in 10 patients who underwent percutaneous resection of a renal cyst. There was no evidence of renal cyst in 50% of the patients at follow-up, a recurrence in 30%, and a 45% decrease in size in 20%. In all 10 patients the symptoms that made the cyst resection necessary disappeared, and in none of the patients were there any late complications.

In an attempt to sort out the difficult cases into surgical and nonsurgical ones, Bosniak (1986) suggested a classification (Table 56–13). The main problem in deciding a borderline case that falls between the nonsurgical category II (which requires no surgery) and category III (which requires exploration) is that there is no specific number that determines when septa are too thick or when there is too much calcium. Much of the decision process is left to experience (Bosniak, 1997).

Type II cysts are benign cystic lesions that are minimally complicated, such as by septations, small calcifications, infection, or high density, and do not require

Table 56–13. BOSNIAK'S CLASSIFICATION OF SIMPLE AND COMPLEX CYSTS

Category I	Simple benign cyst with (1) good through transmission (i.e., acoustic enhancement), (2) no echoes within the cyst, (3) sharply, marginated smooth wall, **requires no surgery.**
Category II	Looks benign with some radiologic concerns including septation, minimal calcification, and high density; **requires no surgery.**
Category III	More complicated lesion that cannot confidently be distinguished from malignancy, having more calcification, more prominent septation of a thicker wall than a category II lesion; more likely to be benign than malignant; **requires surgical exploration and/or removal.**
Category IV	Clearly a malignant lesion with large cystic components, irregular margins; solid vascular elements; **requires surgical removal.**

surgery. For example, when all the criteria for a simple cyst are met except that a fine line of calcium is seen in the wall, the lesion should be considered a benign cyst, and exploration is not required. Another example is the cyst with fine traversing strands, perhaps containing calcium. In this case, exploration is not required unless the septa are numerous, irregular, or thick.

Type III cysts are more complicated lesions with radiologic features that also are seen in malignancy. One example is the lesion with more extensive calcification, especially if the wall is not pencil-point thin or is irregular. Other type III cysts are those with septations, suggesting a multilocular cystic lesion, or chronic infection with a thickened wall. These lesions are more problematic and require a surgical approach that is individualized. In some cases, one might consider violating Gerota's fascia to expose the kidney for examination of the lesion or partial nephrectomy.

Bosniak type IV lesions are cystic malignant tumors and are dealt with as such—namely, by radical nephrectomy.

MEDULLARY SPONGE KIDNEY

The condition known as medullary sponge kidney was recognized by Beitzke in 1908, and its radiographic features were described by Lenarduzzi in 1939. The name of this disorder dates from a 1949 publication by Cacchi and Ricci. **The characteristic features of medullary sponge kidney are dilatation of the distal portion of the collecting ducts with numerous associated cysts and diverticula. The dilated ducts can be counted individually on an intravenous pyelogram and have the appearance of the bristles on a brush. At times the collecting ducts are more ectatic and are filled with calcifications, giving an appearance suggestive of a "bouquet of flowers."** The term "precalyceal canalicular ectasia" sometimes is used for this entity, especially in Europe, because it describes a condition in which dilatation is predominantly of the papillary portion of the collecting ducts (Fig. 56–26).

A significant number of patients with medullary sponge kidney are asymptomatic, and their condition is never diagnosed. As a result, the true incidence of the condition is unknown. Among patients undergoing intravenous urography for various indications, 1 in 200 were found to have medullary sponge kidney (Palubinskas, 1961; Myall, 1970). Bernstein and Gardner (1986), on the basis of a literature review, estimated the incidence in the general population to be between 1 in 5000 and 1 in 20,000 persons.

Clinical Features

Any clinical presentation usually occurs after age 20, although Hamberger and colleagues (1968) found, in more

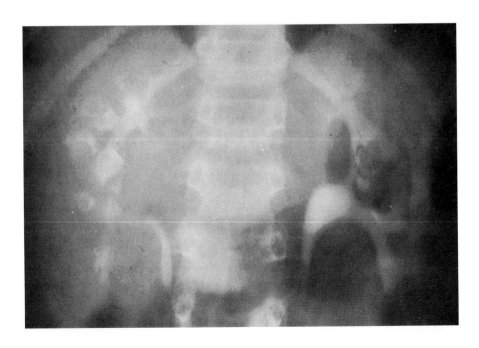

Figure 56–26. Intravenous urogram in a 9-year-old girl with hematuria. Characteristic puddling of contrast medium in the ectatic papillary collecting ducts makes the diagnosis of medullary sponge kidney. (From Glassberg KI, et al: Congenital anomalies of kidney, ureter, and bladder. In Kendall AR, Karafin L [eds]: Harry S. Goldsmith's Practice of Surgery: Urology. New York, Harper & Row, 1981, pp 1–82.)

than 100 cases, that the first symptoms appeared at ages ranging from 3 weeks to 71 years. **The most common presentation is renal colic (50% to 60%), followed by urinary tract infection (20% to 33%) and gross hematuria (10% to 18%)** (Kuiper, 1976b). In many cases, the diagnosis is made when a patient is evaluated by intravenous urography for some unrelated problem, such as a renal mass, benign prostatic hyperplasia, or hypertension. Rarely is such hypertension attributable to the medullary sponge kidney unless there is pyelonephritis.

Another possible sign is the formation of urinary stones. Yendt (1990) found the incidence of medullary sponge kidney in patients who formed stones before age 20 to be twice as high as that in all other age groups combined. The incidence of medullary sponge kidney in stone-formers differs widely in the reported series, ranging from 2.6% to 21%. The incidence appears to be higher in female than in male stone-formers (Palubinskas, 1961; Lavan et al, 1971; Parks et al, 1982; Sage et al, 1982; Wikstrom et al, 1983; Vagelli et al, 1988; Yendt, 1990). Urinary tract infections likewise seem to be more common in female patients with medullary sponge kidney (Parks et al, 1982).

One third to one half of the patients with medullary sponge kidney have hypercalcemia (Ekstrom et al, 1959; Harrison and Rose, 1979; Parks et al, 1982; Yendt, 1990). The etiology does not appear to be the same in all cases. Maschio and coworkers (1982) found a renal calcium leak in eight patients and increased calcium absorption in two. Yendt (1990) found increased parathyroid hormone levels in 2 of 11 patients with medullary sponge kidney.

In the absence of infection, the stones passed by patients with medullary sponge kidney are composed of calcium oxalate either alone or in combination with calcium phosphate.

Although medullary sponge kidney is not considered a genetic disease, there are a small number of isolated reports of autosomal dominant and autosomal recessive inheritance. In addition, medullary sponge kidney has been reported in association with rare congenital anomalies such as hemihypertrophy, Beckwith-Wiedemann syndrome (macroglossia, omphalocele, and gigantism), Ehler-Danlos syndrome, anodontia, and Caroli's disease. Beetz and associates (1991) reported on a case of bilateral medullary sponge kidney in a 14-year-old girl with Beckwith-Wiedemann syndrome, hemihypertrophy, and Wilms' tumor. Twenty other patients have been reported with congenital hemihypertrophy and fewer with Beckwith-Wiedemann syndrome (Gardner, 1992).

Histopathology

The principal finding is dilated intrapapillary collecting ducts and small medullary cysts, which range in diameter from 1 to 8 mm and give the cross-sectioned kidney the appearance of a sponge. The cysts are lined by collecting duct epithelium (Bernstein, 1990) and usually communicate with the collecting tubules. The cysts and the dilated collecting ducts may have concretions adherent to their walls. Ekstrom and coworkers (1959) found these concretions to be composed of pure apatite (calcium phosphate) in 7 of 10 patients and of apatite and calcium

oxalate in the remaining 3. The cysts contain a yellow-brown fluid and desquamated cells or calcified material.

Diagnosis

In general, intravenous urography is more sensitive than CT in detecting mild cases of medullary sponge kidney. In 75% of patients the disease is bilateral (Kuiper, 1976a), but in some only one pyramid is affected. **The urographic features of the disorder are as follows: (1) enlarged kidneys, sometimes with calcification, particularly in the papillae; (2) elongated papillary tubules or cavities that fill with contrast medium; and (3) papillary contrast blush and persistent medullary opacification** (Gedroyc and Saxton, 1988). **In some cases the papillae resemble bunches of grapes or bouquets of flowers, and in others discrete linear stripes appear that can be counted readily.**

On occasion, the intravenous urogram of an older child or young adult with one of the milder forms of ARPKD mimics the appearance of medullary sponge kidney (Yendt, 1990). In these instances, the liver should be evaluated before a diagnosis is made.

When nephrocalcinosis is found, other hypercalciuric states, such as hyperparathyroidism, sarcoidosis, vitamin D intoxication, multiple myeloma, tuberculosis, and milk alkali syndrome, must be ruled out. In these conditions the calcium deposits are in collecting ducts of normal caliber, whereas in medullary sponge kidney the calcifications occur in dilated ducts (Levine and Grantham, 1990).

Given that the cysts are small, sonography is not expected to be helpful. However, because children have less renal sinus fat and overlying muscle than adults, sonographic resolution is better, and hyperechoic papillae are seen on occasion (Patriquin and O'Regan, 1985). The hyperechogenicity is secondary to the multiple interfaces created by the dilated ducts and small cysts and to any intraductal calcification.

Gedroyc and Saxton (1988) described two groups of patients in whom additional renal anomalies were detected by ultrasound examination. One group had multiple cortical cysts; the other had cavities deep in the medulla, which often communicated with the calyces.

Although at present urography generally is more sensitive in detecting medullary sponge kidney than CT, newer scanners can identify the tubular ectasia with the use of bone-detail algorithms and window settings (Boag and Nolan, 1988). Therefore, CT may be advantageous when bowel gas obscures the kidneys on urography or when renal function is poor.

Treatment and Prognosis

It is the complications of medullary sponge kidney—calculus formation and infection—that require management. As noted earlier, many of these patients have hypercalciuria. **Thiazides are effective for lowering hypercalciuria and limiting stone formation. If thiazides cannot be used, inorganic phosphates may be appropriate. For those patients with renal lithiasis, thiazides should be administered even if hypercalciuria is not present**

(Yendt, 1990). Yendt (1990) reported that these drugs prevent calcium stones and arrest the growth of stones already present. If thiazides are ineffective or not tolerated, inorganic phosphates should be tried. However, they should not be used in patients with urinary tract infections caused by urease-producing organisms because of the risk of struvite stones (Yendt, 1990).

Because infections are not unusual in patients with medullary sponge kidney, especially if stones are present, cultures should be obtained frequently, and long-term prophylaxis should be considered in some cases. Infections by coagulase-positive staphylococci are common in patients with stones and should be treated even when the colony count in the cultures is less than 100,000/ml (Yendt, 1990).

Stones can now be removed by extracorporeal lithotripsy and percutaneous nephrolithotomy. Therefore, open surgery is rarely necessary.

Kuiper (1976b) estimated that 10% of symptomatic patients with medullary sponge kidney have a poor long-term prognosis because of nephrolithiasis, septicemia, and renal failure. However, this figure is probably lower now because of the more effective treatment available for hypercalciuria and renal lithiasis and because of the better antibiotics available and the selective use of prophylaxis.

SPORADIC GLOMERULOCYSTIC KIDNEY DISEASE

Glomerulocystic disease is a specific entity, but the term has often been applied as a catchall to include all conditions in which there are glomerular cysts. **The term *glomerulocystic* means that cysts of the glomeruli or Bowman's space are present diffusely and bilaterally. However, cysts of the glomeruli are present in many forms of renal cystic disease, and they may or may not be the predominant pathology. Therefore, the presence of glomerular cysts does not prove that the patient has glomerulocystic disease.**

Table 56–14 shows the Bernstein and Landing classification of conditions with glomerular cysts, as modified by Glassberg and Filmer (1992) to make it compatible with the AAP classification. The diagnosis of sporadic glomerulocystic disease should be made only when the disorder conforms to the 1941 definition of Roos and the 1976

Table 56–14. CONDITIONS ASSOCIATED WITH GLOMERULAR CYSTS

Sporadic glomerulocystic kidney disease
Familial hypoplastic glomerulocystic disease
Autosomal dominant polycystic disease
Juvenile nephronophthisis in association with hepatic fibrosis
Multiple malformation syndromes
 Zellweger's syndrome
 Trisomy 13
 Meckel's syndrome
 Short-rib polydactyly (Majewski type)
 Tuberous sclerosis
 Orofaciodigital syndrome type I
 Brachymesomelia renal syndrome
 Renal-hepatic-pancreatic dysplasia

definition of Taxy and Filmer. That is, glomerulocystic disease is a noninheritable condition producing bilaterally enlarged kidneys containing small cysts, predominantly of Bowman's space. Characteristically, no other family members are affected, and no associated anomalies are present, although in the case described by Taxy and Filmer (1976), subcapsular hepatic cysts were present. Sporadic glomerulocystic disease clearly is different from familial hypoplastic glomerulocystic disease. It is not an inherited disorder, and the kidneys are larger.

The patients evaluated by Bernstein and Landing (1989) after referral and those they found described in the literature differed in age of presentation, clinical course, and renal morphology. These investigators suggested that, in some of the published cases, features of other syndromes were overlooked or family members were inadequately screened for ADPKD. They recommended the use of the term "sporadic glomerulocystic disease" to show that the condition is not genetic.

Bernstein (1993) believed that sporadic glomerulocystic kidney disease in young infants is indistinguishable from ADPKD when the latter is seen in infants and glomerular cysts are a major histologic finding. The only difference clinically or histologically between the two is that no family history can be identified in the sporadic entity. Bernstein went so far as to question whether sporadic glomerulocystic kidney disease represented a new mutation of classic ADPKD rather than a different disease. He concluded that the question was at that time unanswerable.

ACQUIRED RENAL CYSTIC DISEASE

In 1977, Dunhill and coworkers described ARCD in patients in renal failure. **At first, ARCD was thought to be confined to patients receiving hemodialysis. However, it shortly became apparent that the disorder is almost as common in patients receiving peritoneal dialysis** (Thompson et al, 1986) **and that it may develop in patients with chronic renal failure who are being managed medically without any type of dialysis** (Fisher and Horvath, 1972; Ishikawa et al, 1980; Kutcher et al, 1983; Miller et al, 1989). **Therefore, ARCD appears to be a feature of end-stage kidneys rather than a response to dialysis.** Ishikawa (1985) suggested that the term "uremic acquired cystic disease" be applied to this entity (Fig. 56–27).

The incidence of ARCD differs among institutions, perhaps as a result of population differences or diagnostic criteria. Some reports include patients with only one cyst, but Thompson and coworkers (1986) grade ARCD according to the number of cysts involved, from grade 1 (less than 5 cysts bilaterally) to grade 4 (more than 14 cysts bilaterally). Levine and associates (1991) suggested that the presence of five cysts on CT is consistent with the diagnosis, whereas Heinz-Peer and colleagues (1995) suggested that three cysts should be present on ultrasound to make the diagnosis, because this modality is less sensitive. Reichard and associates (1998) thought that at least three to five cysts must be visible on either CT or MRI.

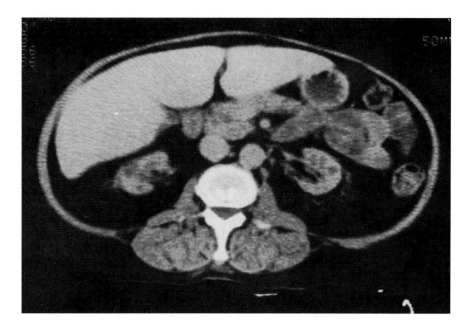

Figure 56–27. Small kidneys with multiple small cysts in a hemodialysis patient with acquired renal cystic disease.

The significance of ARCD lies in two areas: (1) the symptoms it may produce (pain and hematuria), and (2) the high incidence of benign and malignant renal tumors that accompany the condition. The incidence of renal tumors warrants special consideration.

Incidence: Association With Renal Cell Carcinoma

In 1984, Gardner identified 160 patients with ARCD among 430 patients receiving long-term hemodialysis, an incidence of 34% (Gardner, 1984b). This incidence represents an overall figure, because the incidence of ARCD rises with time on dialysis and perhaps also with the duration of chronic renal failure and the age of the patient. For example, Ishikawa and coworkers (1980) found ARCD in 44% of patients who had been receiving hemodialysis for less than 3 years but in 79% of those who had been receiving hemodialysis for a longer time. In a later study, the same group found a higher incidence of ARCD with age, particularly in men (Ishikawa et al, 1985). They suggested that a sex-related endogenous growth factor combined with a uremic metabolite was important. Hughson and coworkers (1986) found a 2.9:1 male-to-female ratio for ARCD, which is striking when one considers that the number of male patients undergoing dialysis only slightly exceeds the number of female patients. **When ARCD is present in men, it usually is more advanced.** African Americans, and perhaps Japanese, are more prone than European Americans to develop ARCD (Reichard et al, 1998).

ARCD can occur in children as well. Hakim and associates (1994) found a 23% incidence of ARCD in a group of 22 children with ESRD who had been receiving dialysis for a period of 7 to 49 months. Because simple cysts in children are rare, they thought that the presence of ARCD should be considered even when there are only one or two cysts. A Japanese study group investigated the incidence of ARCD in 56 children undergoing continuous ambulatory peritoneal dialysis. The patients were grouped according to length of time on dialysis: 0 to 4 years (n = 33), 5 to 9 years (n = 16), and longer than 10 years (n = 5). The corresponding incidences of ARCD were 9.1%, 50%, and 80%. In general, the number and size of cysts increased with the duration of dialysis (Kyushu Pediatric Nephrology Study Group, 1999).

The incidence of ARCD appears to be higher in patients with end-stage kidneys secondary to nephrosclerosis than in those in whom renal failure was the result of diabetes (Fallon and Williams, 1989; Miller et al, 1989). However, the lower incidence of ARCD in diabetic patients may well be a result of their shorter survival time on dialysis (Fallon and Williams, 1989).

Renal neoplasms, principally adenomas, occur in 10% of patients receiving chronic hemodialysis, and when ARCD is present the incidence of neoplasms is even higher, ranging from 20% to 25% (Gardner and Evan, 1984). **When RCC develops in ESRD, 80% of the time it is associated with ARCD; and, when RCC is associated with ARCD, it frequently occurs at an earlier age than in the general population, often in the third or fourth decade. In these cases, the cysts are pronounced. When RCC appears after the age of 60 years in a patient with ARCD, there usually are fewer cysts** (Hughson et al, 1986).

In Japan, the incidence of RCC among dialysis patients is several times to 20 times higher than it is in the general population (Ishikawa, 1993), whereas in the United States it is three to six times higher based on an annual incidence of 8 per 100,000 among the general population (Resseguie et al, 1978; Levine et al, 1991). In Michigan a fivefold increase of RCC among dialysis patients was reported, correlating well with the overall U.S. statistic (Port et al, 1989). Perhaps the difference in incidence of RCC in Japan and the United States is a result of the stronger push in Japan toward routine screening of the kidneys by CT after 3 years of dialysis. According to Levine and associates (1991), CT screening at approximately $600 per study would amount to a cost of $36 million a year, making the cost of such mass screening almost prohibitive.

RCC occurring in ESRD is different biologically in a number of ways from classic RCC: (1) the age at occurrence averages 5 years younger in patients with ESRD; (2) the male-to-female ratio is significantly greater in ESRD patients with RCC than in the general population with RCC (7:1 and 2:1, respectively); and (3) the incidence of RCC in ESRD is 3 to 6 times that of the general population and may be as high as 10 times the incidence in blacks (Matson and Cohen, 1990; Cohen, 1993). **These differences probably reflect the high incidence of epithelial hyperplasia, renal cysts, and adenomas seen in patients with ESRD.**

A 15-year follow-up report on 39 ARCD patients found that if no RCC had developed before 10 years of chronic dialysis, development after 10 to 15 years was unusual. The study also found that kidney size tended to plateau in males after 13 years of dialysis, but significant enlargement of cysts occurred in females after 18 years of dialysis (Ishikawa et al, 1997).

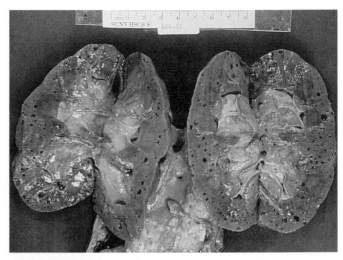

Figure 56–28. Kidneys on autopsy from a 55-year-old man who was receiving chronic hemodialysis demonstrate acquired renal cystic disease with numerous small, diffuse renal cysts.

Etiology

As noted earlier, the initial view that ARCD is a consequence of hemodialysis per se has been shown to be incorrect. However, if uremic toxins are the principal risk factor, why are there different incidences of ARCD at various institutions? It is possible that different durations of predialysis medical therapy or different dialysis regimens are important, but no data have been collected on this point.

A number of findings suggest a role for toxins. First, the cysts, adenomas, and carcinomas usually are multiple and bilateral, as are the carcinomas induced experimentally in rats by toxins. Second, there is a regression of the cysts after successful transplantation (Ishikawa et al, 1983), **suggesting that some cystogenic or carcinogenic toxin of uremia is being eliminated by the allo-**

graft. Third, if transplantation fails and dialysis is resumed, the cysts return.

Another theory suggests that loss of renal tissue functioning leads to the production of renotrophic agents that induce hyperplasia of remaining glomeruli, cyst development, and, in extreme cases, renal tumors (Harris et al, 1983; Yamamoto et al, 1983).

Clinical Features

The most common presentation of ARCD is loin pain, hematuria, or both. Bleeding occurs in as many as 50% of patients (Levine, 1996). When it occurs, whether into the kidney or into the retroperitoneum, it may be secondary to renal cysts or to RCC. Feiner and coworkers (1981)

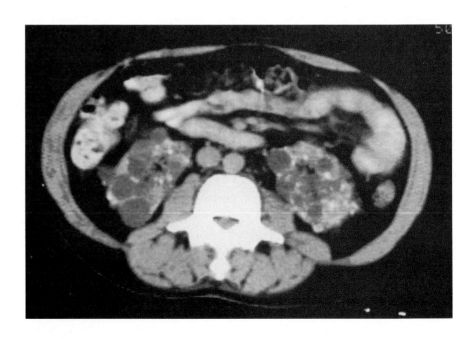

Figure 56–29. Bilateral multiple renal cysts and diffuse calcification in enlarged kidneys in a patient undergoing chronic hemodialysis. The findings simulate those of autosomal dominant polycystic kidney disease. However, cystic disease was not the cause of the uremia, and the diagnosis of acquired renal cystic disease was made. (Courtesy of D. Gordon, M.D.)

suggested that cystic bleeding is secondary to rupture of unsupported sclerotic vessels in the wall. If the cyst communicates with the nephron, hematuria may result. In some patients, bleeding occurs after heparinization during dialysis. Also, in some cases, the serum hemoglobin concentration is elevated secondary to increased renal production of erythropoietin (Shalhoub et al, 1982; Ratcliffe et al, 1983; Mickisch et al, 1984).

Histopathology

The cysts develop predominantly in the cortex, although the medulla may be affected, and usually they are bilateral (Fig. 56–28). They average 0.5 to 1.0 cm in diameter, but some have been reported to reach 5.0 cm (Miller et al, 1989). The cysts are filled with clear, straw-colored or hemorrhagic fluid and often contain calcium oxalate crystals (Miller et al, 1989). Some resemble simple retention cysts, with a flat epithelial lining.

The nuclei of the epithelial cells in these cases are round and regular, without prominent nucleoli (Hughson et al, 1980). However, some cysts (atypical or hyperplastic) are lined by epithelial cells with larger, irregular nuclei that contain prominent nucleoli and may show mitotic activity. This hyperplastic lining is thought by some to be a precursor of renal tumors. Moreover, some hyperplastic cysts have papillary projections, and to some observers the distinction between cyst and neoplasm becomes blurred when papillary hyperplasia predominates.

Feiner and coworkers (1981) found that the cysts begin as dilatations or outpouchings of the nephrons. One theory suggests that calcium oxalate crystals precipitate along the nephron lining, disrupting it and causing outpouchings that dilate as they become obstructed by further crystallization (Rushton et al, 1981; Hughson et al, 1986). That oxalate crystals may be a factor in cyst formation is conceivable because crystals have been implicated in the development of cysts in rats given ethylene glycol (Rushton et al, 1981).

The renal adenomas usually are multiple and often are bilateral. Miller and colleagues (1989) performed autopsies on 155 patients with ESRD and found 25 to have small renal cortical nodules (adenomas). These nodules were multiple, and all were smaller than 2.5 cm in diameter. They usually arose from the walls of the atypical (hyperplastic) cysts.

The cells were either oriented into papillary projections or arranged as solid nodules with tubule formation. The cells were smaller than those found in RCC, with cytoplasm that was either granular and eosinophilic (oncocytes) or pale staining. The nuclei typically appeared small, rounded, and uniform with insignificant nucleoli. Anaplasia and mitosis were absent. In three of these cases, lesions of 3.0 to 3.5 cm were found, all of which were RCC. The cells in these lesions were usually of the clear cell type, with wrinkled nuclei and prominent nucleoli. They were arranged in solid or tubular patterns.

Differentiating these renal tumors into adenomas and carcinomas is arbitrary at times. In Bell's classic 1935 article, renal tumors larger than 3 cm in diameter were considered carcinomas, whereas the smaller ones were considered adenomas. However, even in Bell's work, tumors

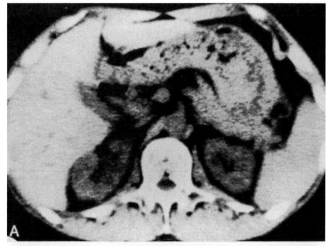

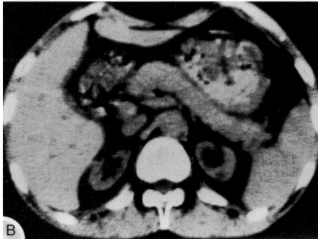

Figure 56–30. Effect of renal transplantation on acquired cystic kidney disease. *A,* Computed tomographic scan obtained 1 month before renal transplantation in a patient who had been receiving dialysis for 7.5 years. Numerous bilateral renal cysts are present. *B,* Ten months after successful renal transplantation, almost all cysts, except one in the left kidney, have regressed. The kidney size has decreased considerably. (From Ishikawa I, et al: Regression of acquired cystic disease of the kidney after successful renal transplantation. Am J Nephrol 1983;3:310. S. Karger AG, Basel.)

as small as 1 cm were associated with metastases in a few cases. Also, although the majority of RCCs in patients with ARCD are larger than 2.0 to 3.0 cm, some have measured only 1.0 to 1.5 cm (Feiner et al, 1981; Chung-Park et al, 1983; Hughson et al, 1986). The smallest RCC associated with known metastases was 1.2 cm in diameter (Ishikawa, 1988a, 1988b). In sum, most renal nodules that are smaller than 1 cm in diameter are adenomas, and most that are larger than 3 cm in diameter are carcinomas. Tumors between 1 and 3 cm in diameter must be considered a gray zone.

It is not clear whether renal adenomas undergo malignant transformation. The large incidence of renal adenomas in the general population and the even larger incidence in uremic patients, combined with the low incidence of RCC in both populations, suggest that the frequency of malignant transformation is low if it occurs at all. However, because of the higher incidence of both RCC and adeno-

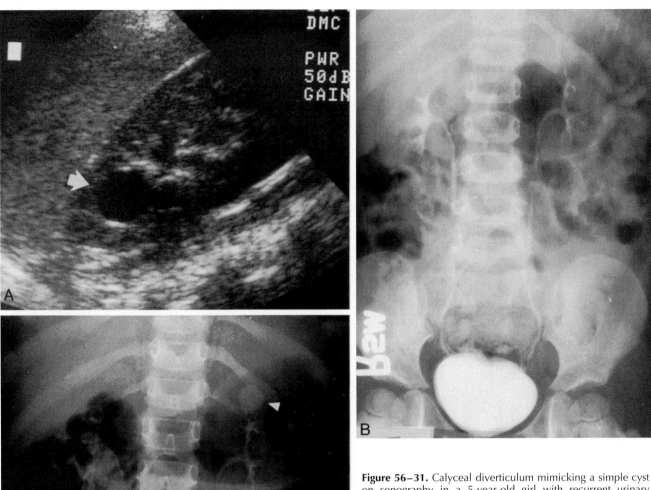

Figure 56–31. Calyceal diverticulum mimicking a simple cyst on sonography in a 5-year-old girl with recurrent urinary tract infections and no vesicoureteral reflux. *A,* Renal sonogram demonstrates a spherical mass in upper pole of left kidney *(arrow)* having the characteristics of a renal cyst. *B,* Early exposure on intravenous urography reveals normal kidneys bilaterally. *C,* Exposure obtained 2 hours after injection reveals contrast-filled upper pole calyceal diverticulum *(arrowhead).*

mas in patients with ARCD, one cannot rule out malignant transformation.

Bretan and associates (1986) postulated a continuum ranging from simple cysts to epithelial hyperplasia to carcinoma. In support of their hypothesis, they offered the finding of renal tumors in the hyperplastic epithelial lining of some cysts. However, no study to my knowledge has demonstrated such a continuum. A curiosity is the morphologic similarity of the nuclei in the hyperplastic cells to those of RCC and the lack of similarity of the nuclei of the adenoma cells to those seen in either of the other lesions.

Hughson and coworkers (1986) believed that atypical hyperplastic epithelium occurs even without cyst formation and that it is these cells that are the precursors of both atypical cysts and adenomas. This theory accounts for the finding of end-stage kidneys containing multiple adenomas without cysts. These investigators also believed that either hyperplastic cysts or adenomas can become RCCs. Therefore, one must not ignore the native kidney left in situ during a renal transplantation. Whereas the cysts as precursors of RCC may disappear, the cells lining the cysts and the small adenomas probably persist, and these, too, may be premalignant lesions. Hyperplastic cyst epithelium has been considered a possible precursor of RCC in other cystic diseases, in particular, VHL and tuberous sclerosis (Fayemi and Ali, 1980).

Evaluation

In uremic patients with fever, one should consider the diagnosis of ARCD and the possibility of an infected cyst (Bonal et al, 1987). Sonography usually shows small, hyperechoic kidneys with cysts of various sizes. Cyst wall

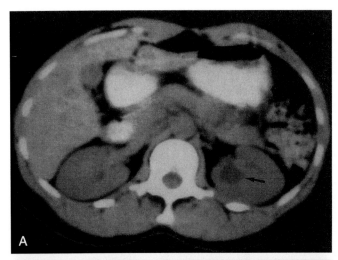

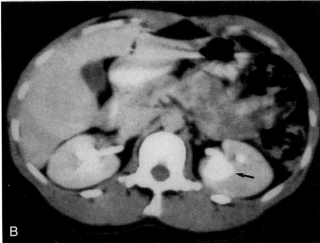

Figure 56–32. Computed tomographic scan of pyelogenic cyst *(arrows). A,* Precontrast scan. *B,* Postcontrast scan demonstrating communication to renal pelvis.

calcification may be visible, but it is more readily seen on CT. Infection should be suspected if sonographic examination shows internal echoes or a thickened wall. Cyst puncture can be used to confirm the diagnosis and to identify the infecting microorganism.

Ultrasound has been the most common modality used to diagnose and monitor patients with ARCD. CT and MRI identify more cysts, and MRI is probably better at demonstrating and characterizing small lesions in particular (Heinz-Peer et al, 1998).

CT examination may identify cyst wall thickening in cases with infection. If the patient is receiving dialysis, contrast medium can be given safely to see whether it causes enhancement (Levine et al, 1984). In some cases, one can identify a metastatic retroperitoneal RCC but cannot identify the primary lesion in the kidney.

In the differential diagnosis of ARCD, the etiology of the renal failure must be considered, and in particular, the possibility of ADPKD. Usually, patients with ARCD have smaller kidneys and smaller cysts and are free of the extrarenal manifestations of ADPKD. In patients receiving hemodialysis, kidneys affected by ARCD usually are less than 300 g; ADPKD kidneys usually are larger than 800 g (Feiner et al, 1981) (Fig. 56–29).

The chief presentations of both cysts and tumors in patients receiving hemodialysis are abdominal or flank pain and gross hematuria. Gehrig and coworkers (1985) found that 11 of 24 patients with ARCD and symptomatic bleeding had renal tumors; 8 of these 11 proved to have RCCs. The tumors themselves may be asymptomatic, revealing their presence only by metastases. The most common manifestation is loin pain, sometimes secondary to a retroperitoneal mass rather than to the primary tumor.

Treatment

If heparinization is associated with hematuria during hemodialysis, peritoneal dialysis may be substituted. Other options are embolization and nephrectomy.

Figure 56–33. Computed tomographic scan of the kidneys demonstrates a calyceal diverticulum *(arrow)* in the right kidney with contrast material precipitating posteriorly because the patient is lying on his back. (Courtesy of D. Gordon, M.D.)

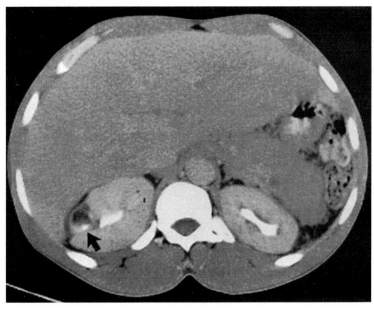

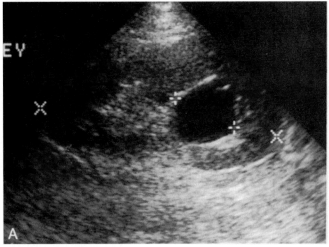
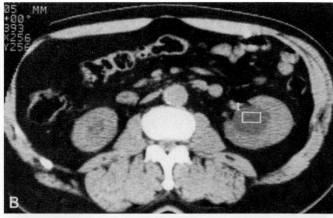
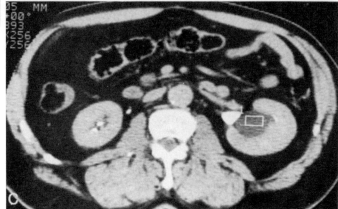

Figure 56–34. Simple cyst with peripelvic location. *A,* Renal sonogram reveals a centrally located left renal cyst. *B,* On precontrast CT scan, the cyst measures 3 HU. *C,* After contrast, the cyst is calibrated to 2 HU. Note how the cyst is situated between a calyx and the renal pelvis. This is a simple parenchymal cyst in a peripelvic location and should not be confused with a renal sinus cyst.

For an infected cyst, percutaneous drainage may be effective. When it is not, surgical drainage or nephrectomy should be considered.

Neumann and associates (1988) recommended that patients who have been receiving hemodialysis for longer than 3 years be screened by ultrasound and CT and then monitored by ultrasonography every 6 months if the kidneys are without cysts and tumors or by both ultrasonography and CT on the same schedule if cysts or tumors smaller than 2 cm are identified. However, more recently a less aggressive approach has been taken in the United States toward routine CT screening because of the high cost attached to such a program.

Reichard and associates (1998) suggested that screening of patients should be considered when known risk factors exist, such as prolonged dialysis, presence of ARCD, and male gender.

A number of investigators have found that the cysts of ARCD regress after renal transplantation (Fig. 56–30) (Ishikawa et al, 1983; Thompson et al, 1986; Kutcher et al, 1983). **Tajima and colleagues (1998) found improvement in regard to number and size of cysts in 16 (64%) of 25 ARCD patients 1 year after transplantation.** Therefore, it was considered that the incidence of RCC might fall after transplantation as well. However, Ishikawa and associates (1991) found that although the majority of cysts either disappeared or became smaller, 18% of patients developed new cysts after transplantation. And more recently, Levine and Gburek (1994) reported

four cases of renal carcinoma occurring in the native kidney 3 to 8 years after transplantation and **suggested that the risk of carcinoma does not lessen after transplantation.** In a series of 96 transplantation patients, Heinz-Peer and coworkers (1995) found that RCC had developed in 6 patients and that 5 of the 6 had associated ARCD. **They suggested that the malignant potential of ARCD persists for many years after transplantation.** They also found a higher incidence of RCC in older transplantation patients and in men. In must be kept in mind that, although the native kidneys may become smaller after transplantation and although the cysts may disappear from view on ultrasound follow-up, it does not necessarily mean that the cells that previously surrounded these cysts have disappeared.

The immunosuppression received by these patients in itself makes them vulnerable to carcinoma. Native kidneys account for 4.5% of all malignancies in renal transplantation recipients (Penn, 1979).

CALYCEAL DIVERTICULUM (PYELOGENIC CYST)

A calyceal diverticulum is a smoothly outlined, intrarenal sac that communicates with the pelvicalyceal system by means of a narrow neck. Diverticula usually arise from the fornix of a calyx and most often affect upper pole calyces (Fig. 56–31). **Some investigators reserve the term** *calyceal diverticulum* **for those lesions that commu-**

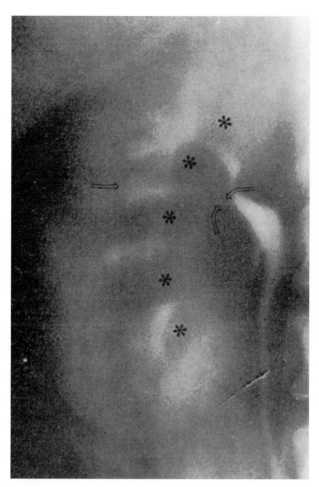

Figure 56–35. "Polycystic disease of the renal sinus" simulating renal pelvic lipomatosis. Nephrotomography demonstrates multiple renal lucencies in the renal sinus *(asterisks)* with medial displacement of the renal pelvis and elongation and stretching of infundibuli *(arrows)*. (From Vela-Navarrete R, Robledo AG: Polycystic disease of the renal sinus: Structural characteristics. J Urol 1983;129:700.)

nicate with a calyx or infundibulum and use the term *pyelogenic cyst* **to designate lesions that communicate with the renal pelvis** (Fig. 56–32). Other workers employ the term *pyelocal calyceal diverticulum* to encompass both entities (Fig. 56–33) (Friedland et al, 1990).

Diverticula are lined by a smooth layer of transitional epithelium and are covered by a thin patch of renal cortex. Most affected patients are adults. Timmons and colleagues (1975) found the incidence of calyceal diverticula on intravenous urograms in children to be 3.3 per 1000.

The etiology of these diverticula is unknown. Beneventi (1943) suggested that they are caused by achalasia of the calyceal neck, whereas Anderson (1963) thought that they arise from an inflammatory stricture of the infundibulum. Starer (1968) suggested that they are generated by anomalous vessels impinging on the infundibulum, and Amesur and Roy (1963) postulated rupture of a solitary cyst. However, solitary cysts are lined by a flat layer of epithelium, whereas diverticula have a transitional epithelial lining.

It is not clear how often a calyceal diverticulum becomes a simple cyst, although the possibility of such a transformation was suggested by Gordon and coworkers (1979). Only three confirmed cases of the sealing of a diverticulum into a simple cyst have been published (Nicholas, 1975; Mosli et al, 1986). Because of the possibility of cyst formation, Mosli and associates (1986) recommended long-term ultrasound follow-up of patients with diverticula. However, such management is costly and is unlikely to be tolerated by the patient.

Calyceal diverticula usually are asymptomatic and are discovered incidentally on an intravenous urogram. Any symptoms are often the result of a stone or infection.

Operation is seldom necessary. Either a partial nephrectomy or a wedge resection was often used in the past. Williams and associates (1969) described six cases treated by unroofing, ligation of the diverticular neck, and filling of the cavity with fat. Noe and Raghavaiah (1982) excised a diverticulum in toto through a nephrotomy incision.

More recently, some workers have described management of diverticula containing stones by a percutaneous procedure (Hulbert et al, 1986; Eshghi et al, 1987). The stone is removed with a nephroscope by way of a nephrostomy tract, and the infundibulum is incised with a cold knife or dilated. The lining of the diverticulum is fulgurated in some cases. Usually, the calyx is stented postoperatively. This essentially closed procedure probably is the best choice today in those few patients who require treatment.

PARAPELVIC AND RENAL SINUS CYSTS

Definitions

A number of terms have been used for cysts adjacent to the renal pelvis or within the hilum: peripelvic cysts, parapelvic cysts, renal sinus cysts, parapelvic lymphatic cysts, hilus cysts, cysts of the renal hilum, and peripelvic lymphangiectasis. Some peripelvic cysts are, in fact, simple cysts that arise from the renal parenchyma but happen to abut the renal pelvis, with or without obstruction. Clearly, these are not cysts of the renal sinus. **The terms peripelvic and parapelvic generally describe cysts around the renal pelvis or renal sinus. Cysts derived from the renal sinus have no parenchymal etiology.**

To avoid confusion, the terms peripelvic and parapelvic should be used only to describe location. The author prefers to use these terms only as adjectives to describe simple parenchymal cysts adjacent to the renal pelvis or hilum, i.e., a peripelvic simple parenchymal cyst (Fig. 56–34). The term *renal sinus cyst* should be reserved for all other cysts in the hilum, i.e., those that are not derived from the renal parenchyma but rather from the other structures of the sinus, such as arteries, lymphatics, and fat.

Renal Sinus Cysts

The predominant type of renal sinus cyst appears to be one derived from the lymphatics. Most often, these

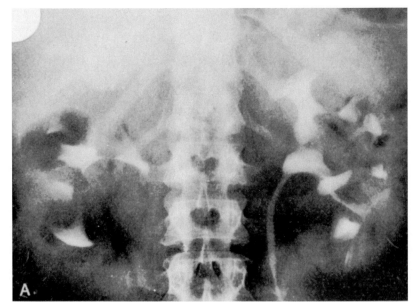

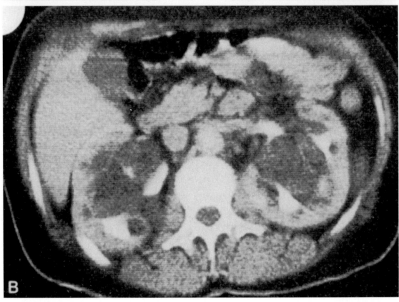

Figure 56–36. "Polycystic disease of the renal sinus," a form of renal sinus cysts. *A,* Intravenous urogram with enlargement of both kidneys, stretching of infundibuli, and trumpet-shaped calyces. *B,* Computed tomographic scan in midportion of kidneys demonstrates multiple sinus cysts with peripheral displacement of renal pelvis and calyces. (From Vela-Navarrete R, Robledo AG: Polycystic disease of the renal sinus: Structural characteristics. J Urol 1983;129:700.)

cysts are multiple, and often they are bilateral. The majority appear after the fifth decade, and they may be associated with inflammation, obstruction, or a calculus (Jordan, 1962; Kutcher et al, 1982).

One etiologic theory suggests that lymphatic cysts are secondary to obstruction. Kutcher and associates (1982) noted that lymphatic cysts or ectasia also is found in other abdominal organs; these investigators refer to the condition in the renal sinus as "peripelvic multicystic lymphangiectasia." In their patient, the cysts were lined by endothelial cells, and the fluid contained lymphocytes. The intrarenal lymphatics also were dilated, with focal cyst formation. These cysts can cause obstruction or even extravasation of contrast medium during urography (Kutcher et al, 1982).

A condition previously described in the Spanish literature (Paramo and Segura, 1972; Vela-Navarrete et al, 1974; Paramo, 1975), but only recently described in the English literature has been called **polycystic disease of the renal sinus** (Vela-Navarrete and Robledo, 1983)—a problematic term because of the possible confusion with polycystic disease of the kidney. Vela-Navarrete and Robledo (1983) described 32 patients with this condition, some in multiple generations of a family (Vela-Navarrete, personal communication, 1990). This entity sounds very much like the case reported by Kutcher and colleagues (1982) and is similar to others reported in association with renal calculi.

Vela-Navarrete and Robledo (1983) found nephrotomography and CT to be particularly useful in defining the lesions. Sonography was less helpful, perhaps because of the limitations of the equipment then available. On nephrotomography, radiolucencies are identifiable in the renal sinus, along with stretching of the infundibula. Therefore, the appearance is similar to that of renal sinus lipomatosis, a fact that led Vela-Navarrete and Robledo (1983) to suggest that many cases of lipomatosis would be identified as polycystic disease of the renal sinus if CT were used (Fig.

56–35). On CT, the cysts can be seen within the renal sinus as they displace the calyces peripherally (Fig. 56–36). The columns of Bertin may appear attenuated. In the Spanish series, 9 of the 32 patients had small renal calculi visible on plain film.

In five patients in the Spanish series, the lesions were explored. Multiple cysts were found, ranging from 2 to 4 cm in diameter and intertwined with stretched infundibula. The fluid was clear, with a plasma-like chemical composition. Histologically, the cyst walls were suggestive of a lymphatic vessel.

This entity has a benign natural history except for the small calculi. These concretions may be secondary to stasis.

Serous cysts have also been reported in the renal sinus. Barrie (1953) suggested that these lesions are secondary to fatty tissue wasting in the renal sinus. Because the space left by the atrophied fat cannot collapse, it fills with transudate. However, no recent reports of serous cysts have been published, and I suspect that earlier cases were, in fact, lymphatic cysts.

Androulakakis and coworkers (1980) reported eight patients with parapelvic cysts, which they described as extraparenchymal. However, it is not clear how the cysts were identified as such. All lesions were said to be single cysts, but the description suggests that multiple cysts were present in some cases.

From a review of the literature, including CT findings in current cases, it appears that most multiple cystic structures in the area of the renal sinus will turn out to be lymphatic cysts, whereas most singular cysts will be found to be derived from the renal parenchyma. Continued study of cases by CT should clarify the nature of parapelvic and renal sinus cysts.

CONCLUSION

Bilateral renal cystic disease creates a dilemma in diagnosis at any age. The differential diagnosis includes ARPKD, ADPKD, tuberous sclerosis, VHL, bilateral simple cysts, and ARCD (Table 56–15). The cysts in ARPKD can manifest at any time from in utero to the age of 20 years, those in ADPKD from in utero to autopsy, those in tuberous sclerosis from in utero to anytime in life but usually before the age of 30, and those in VHL infrequently in the first few years of life but almost always by the age of 30. Bilateral simple cysts can manifest at any age but particularly after age

35 years, and ARCD may become evident after ESRD develops.

REFERENCES

Al-Khaldi N, Watson AR, Zuccollo J, et al: Outcome of antenatally detected cystic dysplastic kidney disease. Arch Dis Child 1994;70:520.

Ambrose SS: Unilateral multicystic renal disease in adults. Birth Defects 1976;13:349.

Amesur NR, Roy HG: Para-pelvic cyst of the kidney. Indian J Surg 1963;25:45.

Amis ES Jr, Cronan JJ, Yoder IC, et al: Renal cysts: Curios and caveats. Urol Radiol 1982;4:199.

Anderson JC: Hydronephrosis. Springfield, IL, Charles C Thomas, 1963.

Androulakakis PA, Kirayiannis B, Deliveliotis A: The parapelvic renal cyst: A report of 8 cases with particular emphasis on diagnosis and management. Br J Urol 1980;52:342.

Antignac C, Arduy CH, Beckman JS, et al: A gene for familial juvenile nephronophthisis (recessive medullary cystic disease) maps to chromosome 2p. Nat Genet 1993;3:342.

Arant BS, Sotero-Avila C, Bernstein J: Segmental hypoplasia of the kidney (Ask-Upmark). J Pediatr 1979;95:931.

Arey JB: Cystic lesions of the kidney in infants and children. J Pediatr 1959;54:429.

Ask-Upmark E: Über juvenile maligne Nephrosklerose und ihre Verhaltnis zu Störungen in der Nierenentwicklung. Acta Pathol Microbiol Scand 1929;6:383.

Aterman K, Boustani P, Gillis DA: Solitary multilocular cysts of the kidney. J Pediatr Surg 1973;8:505.

Atiyeh B, Husmann D, Baum M: Contralateral renal abnormalities in multicystic-dysplastic kidney disease. J Pediatr 1992;121:65.

Atiyeh B, Husmann D, Baum M: Contralateral renal abnormalities in patients with renal agenesis and noncystic renal dysplasia. Pediatrics 1993;9:812.

Avner ED, Ellis D, Jaffe R, et al: Neonatal radiocontrast nephropathy simulating infantile polycystic kidney disease. Pediatrics 1982;100:85.

Avner ED, Sweeney WE Jr, Ellis D: In vitro modulation of tubular cyst regression in murine polycystic kidney disease. Kidney Int 1989;36:960.

Avner ED, Sweeney WE: Epidermal growth factor receptor (EGFR), but not Na-K-ATPase is mislocated to the cell surfaces of collecting tubule cysts in human autosomal recessive polycystic kidney disease (ARPKD). J Am Soc Nephrol 1992;3:292.

Avni E, Thova Y, Lalmand B, et al: Multicystic dysplastic kidney: Natural history from in utero diagnosis and postnatal followup. J Urol 1987;138:1420.

Babka JC, Cohen MS, Sode J: Solitary intrarenal cyst causing hypertension. N Engl J Med 1974;291:343.

Banner MP, Pollack HM, Chatten J, et al: Multilocular renal cysts: Radiological-pathologic correlation. AJR Am J Roentgenol 1981;136:239.

Barloon JT, Vince SW: Caliceal obstruction owing to a large parapelvic cyst: Excretory urography, ultrasound and computerized tomography findings. J Urol 1987;137:270.

Barrie JH: Paracalyceal cysts of the renal sinus. Am J Pathol 1953;29:985.

Bartholomew TH, Solvis TL, Kroovand RL, et al: The sonographic evaluation and management of simple renal cysts in children. J Urol 1980;123:732.

Bear JC, McManamon P, Morgan J, et al: Age at clinical onset and at ultrasonographic detection of adult polycystic disease. Am J Med Genet 1984;18:45.

Bear JC, Parfrey PS, Morgan JM, et al: Autosomal dominant polycystic kidney disease: New information for genetic counselling. Am J Med Genet 1992;43:548.

Bearth K, Steg A: On the pathogenesis of simple cysts in the adult: A microdissection study. Urol Res 1977;5:103.

Beck AD: The effect of intra-uterine urinary obstruction upon the development of the fetal kidney. J Urol 1971;105:784.

Beckwith JB: Editorial comment. J Urol 1997;158:2259.

Beckwith JB: Wilms tumor and other renal tumors in childhood: An update. J Urol 1986;136:320.

Beckwith JB, Palmer NF: Histopathology and prognosis of Wilms' tumor:

Table 56–15. DIFFERENTIAL DIAGNOSIS: BILATERAL RENOMEGALY AND RENAL CYSTS

Autosomal recessive polycystic kidney disease
Autosomal dominant polycystic kidney disease
Tuberous sclerosis
von Hippel-Lindau disease
Bilateral simple cysts
Sporadic glomerulocystic kidney disease
Acquired renal cystic disease

Results from First National Wilms' Tumor Study. Cancer 1978;41: 1937.

Beetz R, Schofer O, Riedmiller H, et al: Medullary sponge kidneys and unilateral Wilms' tumour in a child with Beckwith-Wiedemann syndrome. Eur J Pediatr 1991;150:489.

Begleiter ML, Smith TH, Harris DJ: Ultrasound for genetic counselling in polycystic kidney disease. Lancet 1977;2:1073.

Beitzke H: Über Zysten in Nierenmark. Charite Ann 1908;32:285.

Bell ET: Cystic disease of the kidneys. Am J Pathol 1935;11:373.

Beneventi FA: Hydrocalyx: Its relief by retrograde dilatation. Am J Surg 1943;61:244.

Bengtsson U, Hedman L, Svalander C: Adult type of polycystic kidney disease in a newborn child. Acta Med Scand 1975;197:447.

Bennett WM, Elzinga LW, Barry JM: Management of cystic kidney disease. In Gardner KD Jr, Bernstein J (eds): The Cystic Kidney. Boston, Kluwer Academic, 1990, pp 247–275.

Bennett WM, Elzinga L, Golper TA, et al: Reduction of cyst volume for symptomatic management of autosomal dominant polycystic kidney disease. J Urol 1987;137:620.

Bennington JL, Beckwith JB: Tumors of the kidney, renal pelvis and ureter. In Atlas of Tumor Pathology, Series 2, Fascicle 12. Washington, DC, Armed Forces Institute of Pathology, 1975, p 33.

Berdon WE, Schwartz RH, Becker J, et al: Tamm-Horsfall proteinuria. Radiology 1969;92:714.

Berman DJ, Maizel M: Role of urinary obstruction in the genesis of renal dysplasia: A model in the chick embryo. J Urol 1982;128:1091.

Bernstein J: Experimental study of renal parenchymal maldevelopment (renal dysplasia). Presented at the 3rd International Congress of Nephrology. Washington, DC, September, 1966.

Bernstein J: Developmental abnormalities of the renal parenchyma: Renal hypoplasia and dysplasia. Pathol Annu 1968;3:213.

Bernstein J: The morphogenesis of renal parenchymal maldevelopment (renal dysplasia). Pediatr Clin North Am 1971;18:395.

Bernstein J: The classification of renal cysts. Nephron 1973;11:91.

Bernstein J: Developmental abnormalities of the renal parenchyma: Renal hypoplasia and dysplasia. In Sommers SC (ed): Kidney Pathology Decennial 1966–1975. New York, Appleton-Century-Crofts, 1975, pp 11–17, 36–37.

Bernstein J: A classification of renal cysts. In Gardner KD Jr (ed): Cystic Disease of the Kidney. New York, John Wiley & Sons, 1976, p 7.

Bernstein J: A classification of renal cysts. In Gardner KD, Bernstein J (eds): The Cystic Kidney. Dordrecht, Kluwer Academic, 1990, p 163.

Bernstein J: The multicystic kidney and hereditary renal adysplasia. Am J Kidney Dis 1991;18:495.

Bernstein J: Glomerolocystic kidney disease nosological considerations. Pediatr Nephrol 1993;7:464.

Bernstein J, Gardner KD Jr: Cystic disease of the kidney and renal dysplasia. In Harrison JH, Gittes RF, Perlmutter AD, et al (eds): Campbell's Urology, 4th ed. Philadelphia, WB Saunders, 1979a, p 1399.

Bernstein J, Gardner KD Jr: Familial juvenile nephronophthisis: Medullary cystic disease. In Edelman CM Jr (ed): Pediatric Kidney Disease. Boston, Little, Brown, 1979b, p 580.

Bernstein J, Gardner KD: Hereditary tubulointerstitial nephropathies. In Cotran R, Brenner B, Stein J (eds): Tubulointerstitial Nephropathies. New York, Churchill Livingstone, 1983, pp 335–357.

Bernstein J, Gardner KD Jr: Cystic disease of the kidney and renal dysplasia. In Walsh PC, Gittes RF, Perlmutter AD, et al (eds): Campbell's Urology, 5th ed. Philadelphia, WB Saunders, 1986, p 1760.

Bernstein J, Gardner KD: Cystic disease and dysplasia of the kidneys. In Murphy WM (ed): Urological Pathology. Philadelphia, WB Saunders, 1989, p 483.

Bernstein J, Landing BH: Glomerulocystic kidney disease. Prog Clin Biol Res 1989;305:27.

Bernstein J, Meyer R: Congenital abnormalities of the urinary system: II. Renal cortical and medullary necrosis. J Pediatr 1961;59:657.

Bernstein J, Meyer R: Parenchymal maldevelopment of the kidney. In Kelley VC (ed): Brenneman-Kelley, Practice of Pediatrics, vol 3. New York, Harper & Row, 1967, pp 1–30.

Bernstein J, Robbins TO, Kissane JM: The renal lesion of tuberous sclerosis. Semin Diagn Pathol 1986;3:97.

Bernstein J, Slovis TL: Polycystic diseases of the kidney. In Edelman CM (ed): Pediatric Kidney Disease, 2nd ed. Boston, Little, Brown, 1992, pp 1139–1153.

Biglar JA, Killingsworth WP: Cartilage in the kidney. Arch Pathol 1949; 47:487.

Blazer S, Zimmer EZ, Blumefeld Z, et al: Natural history of fetal simple renal cysts detected in pregnancy. J Urol 1999;162:812.

Blyth H, Ockenden BG: Polycystic disease of kidneys and liver presenting in childhood. J Med Genet 1971;8:257.

Boag GS, Nolan R: CT visualization of medullary sponge kidney. Urol Radiol 1988;9:220.

Boggs LK, Kimmelsteil P: Benign multilocular cystic nephroma: Report of two cases of so-called multilocular cyst of the kidney. J Urol 1956; 76:530.

Bonal J, Caralps A, Lauzurica R, et al: Cyst infection in acquired renal cystic disease. Br Med J 1987;295:25.

Borer JG, Glassberg KI, Kassner G, et al: Unilateral multicystic dysplasia in one component of a horseshoe kidney: Case report and review of literature. J Urol 1994;152:1568.

Bosniak MA: The current radiological approach to renal cysts. Radiology 1986;158:1.

Bosniak MA: Difficulties in classifying cystic lesions of the kidney. (Commentary.) Urol Radiol 1991a;13:91.

Bosniak MA: The small (≤3.0 cm) renal parenchymal tumor: Detection, diagnosis and controversies. Radiology 1991b;179:307.

Bosniak MA: The use of the Bosniak classification system for renal cysts and cystic tumors. J Urol 1997;157:1852.

Bourneville DM: Sclérose tubereuse des circonvolutions cérébrales idote et épilepsie hémiplegique. Arch Neurol (Paris) 1880;1:81.

Bove KE, McAdams AJ: The nephroblastomatosis complex and its relationship to Wilms' tumor: A clinicopathologic treatise. Perspect Pediatr Pathol 1976;3:185.

Braasch WF, Schacht FW: Pathological and clinical data concerning polycystic kidney. Surg Gynecol Obstet 1933;57:467.

Brazier JL, Henske EP: Loss of the polycystic kidney disease (PKD1) region of chromosome 16 p13 in renal cyst cells supports a loss-of-function model for cyst pathogenesis. J Clin Invest 1997;99:194.

Bree BL, Raiss GJ, Schwab RE: The sonographically ambiguous renal mass: Can surgery be avoided? Radiology 1984;153(Suppl.):212.

Bretan PN, Busch MP, Hricak H, et al: Chronic renal failure: A significant risk factor in the development of acquired renal cysts and renal cell carcinoma. Cancer 1986;57:1871.

Breuning MH, Reeder ST, Brunner H, et al: Improved early diagnoses of adult polycystic kidney disease with flanking DNA markers. Lancet 1987;2:1359.

Brook-Carter PT, Peral B, Ward CJ, et al: Deletion of the TSC2 and PKD1 genes associated with severe infantile polycystic kidney disease—a contiguous gene syndrome. Nat Genet 1994;8:328.

Buchta RM, Viseskul C, Gilbert EF, et al: Familial bilateral renal agenesis and hereditary renal adysplasia. Z Kinderheilkd 1973;115:111.

Burgler W, Hauri D: Vitale Komplikationen bei multizystischer Nierende Generation (multizystischer Dysplasie). Urol Int 1983;38:251.

Cacchi R, Ricci V: Sur une rare maladie kystique multiple des pyramides rénales le "rein en éponge." J Urol Nephrol (Paris) 1949;55:497.

Campbell GS, Bick HD, Paulsen EP: Bleeding esophageal varices with polycystic liver: Report of three cases. N Engl J Med 1958;259:904.

Campos A, Figueroa ET, Gunaselcaran S, et al: Early presentation of tuberous sclerosis as bilateral renal cysts. J Urol 1993;149:1077.

Cantani A, Bamonte G, Ceccoli D, et al: Familial nephronophthisis: A review and differential diagnosis. Clin Pediatr 1986;25:90.

Carone FA, Maiko H, Kanwar YS: Basement membrane antigens in renal polycystic disease. Am J Pathol 1988;130:466.

Carter JE, Lirenman DS: Bilateral renal hypoplasia with oligomeganephronia: Oligomeganephronic renal hypoplasia. Am J Dis Child 1970; 120:537.

Cascio S, Paran S, Prori P: Associated urological anomalies in children with unilateral renal agenesis. J Urol 1999;162:1081.

Castillo O, Boyle ET, Kramer SA: Multilocular cysts of the kidney: A study of 29 patients and review of the literature. Urology 1991;37:156.

Chamberlin BC, Hagge WW, Stickler GB: Juvenile nephronophthisis and medullary cystic disease. Mayo Clin Proc 1977;52:485.

Chatten J, Bishop HC: Bilateral multilocular cysts of the kidney. J Pediatr Surg 1977;12:749.

Chen YH, Stapleton FB, Roy S, et al: Neonatal hypertension from a unilateral multicystic dysplastic kidney. J Urol 1985;133:664.

Chehval M, Neilsen C: Laparoscopic cyst decompression of polycystic kidney disease. J Endourol 1995;9:281.

Chonko AM, Weiss JM, Stein JH, et al: Renal involvement in tuberous sclerosis. Am J Med 1974;56:124.

Choyke PL: Inherited cystic diseases of the kidney: Advances in uroradiology. Radiology Clin North Am 1996;34,925–946.

Christ ML: Polycystic nephroblastoma. J Urol 1968;98:570.

Chung-Park M, Ricanati E, Lankerani M, et al: Acquired renal cysts and multiple renal cell and urothelial tumors. Am J Clin Pathol 1983;141:238.

Churchill DN, Bear JC, Morgan J, et al: Prognosis of adult onset polycystic kidney disease re-evaluated. Kidney Int 1984;26:190.

Cobben JM, Breuning MH, Schoots C, et al: Congenital hepatic fibrosis in autosomal-dominant polycystic kidney disease. Kidney Int 1990;38:880.

Cohen AH, Hoyer JR: Nephronophthisis: A primary tubular basement membrane defect. Lab Invest 1986;55:564.

Cohen EP: Epidemiology of acquired cystic kidney disease. In Gabow PA, Grantham JJ (eds): Proceedings of the Fifth International Workshop on Polycystic Kidney Disease. Kansas City, MO, The PKR Foundation, 1993, pp 81–84.

Cole BR, Conley SB, Stapleton FB: Polycystic kidney disease in the first year of life. J Pediatr 1987;111:693.

Colodny AH: Comments in discussion. J Urol 1989;142:489.

Curry CJR, Jensen K, Holland J, et al: The Potter sequence: A clinical analysis of 80 cases. Am J Med Genet 1984;19:679.

Dalgaard OZ: Bilateral polycystic disease of the kidneys: A follow-up of two hundred eighty-four patients and their families. Acta Med Scand Suppl 1957;38:1.

Dalgaard OZ, Norby S: Autosomal dominant polycystic kidney disease in the 1980's. Clin Genet 1989;36:320.

Dalton D, Neiman H, Grayhack JJ: The natural history of simple renal cysts: A preliminary study. J Urol 1986;135:905.

Daniel WW Jr, Hartman GW, Witten DM, et al: Calcified renal masses: A review of 10 years' experience at the Mayo Clinic. Radiology 1972;103:503.

Darmis F, Nahum H, Mosse A, et al: Fibrose hépatique congénitale à progression clinique renal. Presse Med 1970;78:885.

Dauost MC, Bichet DG, Somlo S: A French-Canadian family with autosomal dominant polycystic kidney disease (ADPKD) unlinked to ADPKD1 or ADPKD2. J Am Soc Nephrol 1993;4:262.

Davides KC: Multilocular kidney disease. J Urol 1976;116:246.

Delaney VB, Adler S, Bruns FJ, et al: Autosomal dominant polycystic kidney disease: Presentation, complications and progression. Am J Kidney Dis 1985;5:104.

DeWall JG, Schroder FH, Scholmeijer RJ: Diagnostic work up and treatment of multilocular cystic kidney: Difficulties in differential diagnosis. Urology 1986;28:73.

Dewan PA, Goh DW: A study of the radiologic anatomy of the multicystic kidney. Pediatr Surg Int 1994;9:368.

Dimmick J, Johnson HW, Coleman GU, et al: Wilms tumorlet, nodular renal blastema and multicystic renal dysplasia. J Urol 1989;142:484.

Dressler GR, Wilkinson JE, Rothenpieler UW, et al: Deregulation of PAX-2 expression in transgenic mice generates severe kidney abnormalities. Nature 1993;362:65.

Drummond IA, Madden SL, Rohwer-Nutter P, et al: Repression of the insulin-like growth factor II gene by the Wilms' tumor suppressor WT1. Science 1992;257:674.

Du J, Wilson PD: Abnormal polarization of EGF receptors and autocrine stimulation of cyst epithelial growth in human ADPKD. Am J Physiol 1995;269:C487.

Duke VM, Winyard PJD, Thorogood P, et al: KAL, a gene mutated in Kallman's syndrome, is expressed in the first trimester of human development. Cell Endocrinol 1995;110:73.

Dunbar JS, Nogrady MG: The calyceal crescent: A roentgenographic sign of obstructive hydronephrosis. AJR Am J Roentgenol 1970;110:520.

Dunhill MS, Milard PR, Oliver DO: Acquired cystic disease of the kidneys: A hazard of long-term intermittent maintenance hemodialysis. J Clin Pathol 1977;30:368.

Dunn MD, Elbahnasy AM, Naughton C, et al: Laparoscopic marsupialization in patients with autosomal dominant polycystic kidney disease. J Urol 2001;165:1888.

Dvir A, Milner Y, Chomsky O, et al: The inhibition of EGF-dependent proliferation of keratincysts by trophostin tyrosin kinase blockers. J Cell Biol 1991;113:857.

Edmunds W: Cystic adenoma of kidney. Trans Pathol Soc Lond 1892;43:89.

Eisendrath DN: Clinical importance of congenital renal hypoplasia. J Urol 1935;33:331.

Eble JN, Bonsib SM: Extensively cystic renal neoplasms: Cystic nephroma, cystic partially differentiated nephroblastoma, multilocular cystic renal cell carcinoma and cystic hamartoma of the renal pelvis. Semin Diagn Path 1998;15:2.

Ekstrom T, Engfeldt B, Langergren C, et al: Medullary Sponge Kidney. Stockholm, Almquist and Wiksells, 1959.

Elder JS, Hladky D, Selzman AA: Outpatient nephrectomy for non-functioning kidneys. J Urol 1995;154:712.

Elzinga LW, Barry JM, Torres VT, et al: Cyst decompression surgery for autosomal dominant polycystic kidney disease. J Am Soc Nephrol 1992;2:1219.

Elzinga LW, Barry JM, Bennett WM: Surgical management of painful polycystic kidneys. Am J Kidney Dis 1993;22:532.

Emmert GK Jr, King LR: The risk of hypertension is underestimated in the multicystic dysplastic kidney: A personal perspective. Urology 1994;44:404.

Ericsson NO: Ectopic ureterocele in infants and children: Clinical study. Acta Chir Scand Suppl 1954;97:1.

Ericsson NO: Renal dysplasia. In Johnston JH, Goodwin WE (eds): Reviews in Paediatric Urology. Amsterdam, Excerpta Medica, 1974, p 25.

Ericsson NO, Ivemark BI: Renal dysplasia and pyelonephritis in infants and children I. Arch Pathol 1958a;66:255.

Ericsson NO, Ivemark BI: Renal dysplasia and pyelonephritis in infants and children: II. Primitive ductules and abnormal glomeruli. Arch Pathol 1958b;66:264.

Eshghi M, Tuong W, Fernandez R, et al: Percutaneous (endo) infundibulotomy. J Endourol 1987;1:107.

Euderink F, Hogewind BL: Renal cysts in premature children: Occurrence in a family with polycystic kidney disease. Arch Pathol Lab Med 1978;102:592.

European Polycystic Disease Consortium: The polycystic kidney disease 1 gene encodes a 14kb transcipt and lies within a duplicated region of chromosome 16. Cell 1994;77:881.

Evans AT, Coughlin JP: Urinary obstruction due to renal cysts. J Urol 1970;103:277.

Everson GT, Emmett M, Brown WR, et al: Functional similarities of hepatic cysts and biliary epithelium: Studies of fluid constituents and in vivo secretion in response to secretin. Hepatology 1990;11:557.

Fallon B, Williams RD: Renal cancer associated with acquired cystic disease of the kidney and chronic renal failure. Semin Urol 1989;7:228.

Fanconi G, Hanhart E, Ailbertini A, et al: Die familiäre juvenile Nephronophtise (die idiopathische parenchymatose Schrumptniere). Helv Paediatr Acta 1951;6:1.

Fayemi AD, Ali M: Acquired renal cysts and tumor superimposed on chronic primary diseases: An autopsy study of 24 patients. Pathol Res Pract 1980;68:73.

Feiner HD, Katz LA, Gallo GR: Acquired renal cystic disease of kidney in chronic hemodialysis patients. Urology 1981;17:260.

Fellows RA, Leonidas JC, Beatty EC Jr: Radiologic features of "adult type" polycystic kidney disease in the neonate. Pediatr Radiol 1976;4:87.

Felson B, Cussen LJ: The hydronephrotic type of congenital multicystic disease of the kidney. Semin Roentgenol 1975;10:113.

Fetterman GH, Ravitch MM, Sherman FE: Cystic changes in fetal kidneys following ureteral ligation: Studies of microdissection. Kidney Int 1974;5:111.

Fick GM, Gabow PA: Heredity and acquired cystic disease of the kidney. Kidney Int 1994;46:951.

Fick GM, Johnson AM, Gabow PA: Is there evidence for anticipation in autosomal-dominant polycystic kidney disease. Kidney Int 1994;43:1153.

Fill WL, Lamiel JM, Polk NO: The radiographic manifestations of von Hippel-Lindau disease. Radiology 1979;133:289.

Fine MG, Burns E: Unilateral multicystic kidney: Report of six cases and discussion of the literature. J Urol 1959;81:42.

Fisher ER, Horvath B: Comparative ultrasound study of so-called renal adenoma and carcinoma. J Urol 1972;108:382.

Flack CE, Bellinger MF: The multicystic dysplastic kidney and contralateral reflex: Protection of the solitary kidney. J Urol 1993;150:1873.

Forster SV, Hawkins EP: Deficient metanephric blastema: A cause of oligomeganephronia. Pediatr Pathol 1994;14:935.

Fowler M: Differentiated nephroblastoma: Solid, cystic or mixed. J Pathol 1971;105:215.

Friedland GW, deVries PA, Nino-Murcin M, et al: Congenital anomalies of the papillae, calyces, renal pelvis, ureter and ureteral orifice. In Pollack HM (ed): Clinical Urography. Philadelphia, WB Saunders, 1990, p 653.

Friedman H, Abeshouse BS: Congenital unilateral multicystic kidney: A review of the literature and a report of three cases. Sinai Hosp J (Baltimore) 1957;6:51.

Frydenberg M, Malek R, Zincke H: Conservative renal surgery for renal cell carcinoma in von Hippel-Lindau disease. J Urol 1993;149:461.

Fryns JP, van den Berghe H: "Adult" form of polycystic kidney disease in neonates. Clin Genet 1979;15:205.

Gabow PA: Autosomal dominant polycystic kidney disease. N Engl J Med 1993;329:332.

Gabow PA: Polycystic kidney disease: Clues to pathogenesis. Kidney Int 1991;40,989.

Gabow PA, Chapman AB, Johnson AM, et al: Renal structure and hypertension in autosomal dominant polycystic kidney disease. Kidney Int 1990;38:1177.

Gabow PA, Duley I, Johnson AM: Clinical profiles of gross hematuria in autosomal polycystic kidney disease. Am J Kidney Dis 1992;20:140.

Gabow PA, Grantham JJ, Bennett WN, et al: Gene testing in autosomal dominant polycystic kidney disease: Results of National Kidney Foundation Workshop. Am J Kidney Dis 1989a;13:85.

Gabow PA, Ikle W, Holmes JH: Polycystic kidney disease: Prospective analysis of non-azotemic patients and family members. Ann Intern Med 1984;101:238.

Gabow PA, Kaehny WD, Johnson AM, et al: The clinical utility of renal concentrating capacity in polycystic kidney disease. Kidney Int 1989b; 35:675.

Gabow PA, Schrier RW: Pathophysiology of adult polycystic kidney disease. Adv Nephrol 1989;18:19.

Gaisford W, Bloor K: Congenital polycystic disease of kidney and liver: Portal hypertension, portacaval anastomosis. Proc R Soc Med 1968;61:304.

Gallo GE, Penchansky L: Cystic nephroma. Cancer 1977;39:1322.

Gardner KD Jr: Juvenile nephronophthisis–renal medullary cystic disease. Dialogues Pediatr Urol 1984a;7:3.

Gardner KD Jr: Acquired renal cystic disease and renal adenocarcinoma in patients on long-term hemodialysis. N Engl J Med 1984b;310:390.

Gardner KD Jr: Pathogenesis of human cystic renal disease. Annu Rev Med 1988;39:185.

Gardner KD Jr: Medullary sponge kidney. In Edelman CM (ed): Pediatric Kidney Disease. Boston, Little, Brown, 1992, pp 1641–1646.

Gardner KD, Evan AP: Cystic kidneys: An enigma evolves. Am J Kidney Dis 1984;3:403.

Garel LA, Habib R, Pariente D, et al: Juvenile nephronophthisis: Sonographic appearance in children with severe uremia. Radiology 1984; 151:93.

Gates GF: Ultrasonography of the urinary tract in children. Urol Clin North Am 1980;7:215.

Gedroyc WMW, Saxton HM: More medullary sponge variants. Clin Radiol 1988;39:423.

Gehrig JJ, Gottheiner TI, Swenson RS: Acquired cystic disease of the end-stage kidney. Am J Med 1985;79:609.

Geller RA, Pataki KI, Finegold RA: Bilateral multilocular renal cysts with recurrence. J Urol 1979;121:808.

Gillis D, Picard E, Herz A, Bar-Ziv J: Tuberous sclerosis with polycystic kidneys in an infant. Clin Pediat 1997;36:603.

Glassberg KI: The dilated ureter: Classification and approach. Urology 1977;9:1.

Glassberg KI: Unilateral renal cystic disease. (Editorial comment.) Urology 1999;53:1227.

Glassberg KI, Filmer RB: Renal dysplasia, renal hypoplasia and cystic disease of the kidney. In Kelalis PP, King LR, Belman AB (eds): Clinical Pediatric Urology, 3rd ed. Philadelphia, WB Saunders, 1992.

Glassberg KI, Hackett RE, Waterhouse K: Congenital anomalies of the kidney, ureter and bladder. In Kendall AR, Karafin L (eds): Harry S. Goldsmith's Practice of Surgery: Urology. Hagerstown, Harper & Row, 1981, p 1.

Glassberg KI, Kassner EG: Ex vivo intracystic contrast studies of multicystic dysplastic kidney. J Urol 1998;160(Suppl.):1204.

Glassberg KI, Stephens FD, Lebowitz RL, et al: Renal dysgenesis and cystic disease of the kidney: A report of the Committee on Terminology, Nomenclature and Classification, Section on Urology, American Academy of Pediatrics. J Urol 1987;138:1085.

Glazier DB, Fleischer MH, Cummings KB, Barone JG: Cystic renal disease and tuberous sclerosis in infants. Urology 1996;48:613.

Goldberg BB, Kotler MM, Ziskin MC, et al: Diagnostic Uses of Ultrasound. New York, Grune & Stratton, 1975.

Goldman SM, Hartman DS: The simple renal cysts. In Pollack HM (ed): Clinical Urography. Philadelphia, WB Saunders, 1990, p 1603.

Gomez MR: Tuberous Sclerosis. New York, Raven Press, 1979.

Gordon AC, Thomas DFM, Arthur RJ, et al: Multicystic dysplastic kidney: Is nephrectomy still appropriate? J Urol 1988;140:1231.

Gordon RL, Pollack HM, Popky GL, et al: Simple serous cysts of the kidney in children. Radiology 1979;131:357.

Grantham JJ: Polycystic renal disease. In Early LE, Gottschalk CW (eds): Strauss and Welt's Diseases of the Kidney, 3rd ed. Boston, Little, Brown, 1979, p 1123.

Grantham JJ: Renal pain in polycystic kidney disease: When the hurt won't stop. J Am Soc Nephrol 1992;2:1161.

Grantham JJ: Polycystic kidney disease: Hereditary and acquired. Adv Intern Med 1993;38:409.

Grantham JJ: Time to treat polycystic kidney diseases like the neoplastic disorders they are. (Editorial.) Kidney Int 2000;57:339.

Grantham JJ, Dunoso VS, Evan AP, et al: Viscoelastic properties of tubule basement membranes in experimental renal cystic diseases. Kidney Int 1987;32:187.

Grantham JJ, Geiser JL, Evan AP: Cyst formation and growth in autosomal dominant polycystic kidney disease. Kidney Int 1987;31:1145.

Grantham JJ, Uchic M, Cragoe EJ Jr, et al: Chemical modification of cell proliferation and fluid secretion in renal cysts. Kidney Int 1989;35:1379.

Gregoire JR, Torres VE, Holley KE, et al: Renal epithelial hyperplastic and neoplastic proliferation in autosomal dominant polycystic kidney disease. Am J Kidney Dis 1987;9:27.

Green A, Kinirons M, O'Meara Y, et al: Familial adult medullary cystic disease with spastic quadriparesis: A new disease association. Clin Nephrol 1990;33:231.

Greene LF, Feinzaig W, Dahlin DC: Multicystic dysplasia of the kidney: With special reference to the contralateral kidney. J Urol 1971;105:482.

Griffel B, Pewzner S, Berandt M: Unilateral "oligomeganephronia" with agenesis of the contralateral kidney, studied by microdissection. Virchows Arch [Pathol Anat] 1972;357:179.

Griscom NT, Vawter FG, Fellers FX: Pelvoinfundibular atresia: The usual form of multicystic kidney; 44 unilateral and two bilateral cases. Semin Roentgenol 1975;10:125.

Gross M, Breach PD: The simultaneous occurrence of renal carcinoma and cyst: Problems in management. South Med J 1971;64:1059.

Gruskin AB: Pediatric nephrology for the urologist. In Kendall AR, Karafin L (eds): Harry S. Goldsmith's Practice of Surgery: Urology. Hagerstown, Harper & Row, 1977, p 1.

Guay-Woodford LM, Galliani CA, Musulman-Mroczek EM, et al: Diffuse renal cystic disease in children: Morphologic and genetic correlations. Pediatr Nephrol 1998;12:173.

Guay-Woodford LM, Muecher G, Hopkins SD, et al: The severe perinatal form of autosomal recessive polycystic kidney disease maps to chromosome 6p21.1-p12: Implications for genetic counseling. Am J Hum Genet 1995;56:110.

Habib R: Renal dysplasia, hypoplasia and cysts. In Strauss J (ed): Pediatric Nephrology: Current Concepts in Diagnosis and Management. New York, Intercontinental Medical Book Corp, 1974, p 209.

Habib R, Bois E: Heterogeneite des syndromes nephrotiques a debut precoce de nourisson (syndrome nephrotique "infantile"): Etude anatomoclinique et genetique de 37 observations. Helv Paediatr Acta 1973; 28:91.

Habib R, Courtecuisse V, Ehrensperger J, et al: Hypoplasie segmentaire du rein avec hypertension arterielle chez l'enfant. Ann Pediatr (Paris) 1965;12:262.

Habib R, Courtecuisse V, Mathieu H, et al: Un type anatomoclinique particular, d'insuffisance renale chronique de l'enfant: l'Hypoplasieoligonephronique congenitale bilaterale. J Urol Nephrol (Paris) 1962;68:139.

Habib R, Gubler M, Niavdet P, Gagnadoux M: Congenital/infantile nephrotic syndrome with diffuse mesangial sclerosis: Relationships with Drash syndrome. In Bartsocas CS (ed): Genetics of Kidney Disorders: Progress in Clinical and Biological Research, vol 305. New York, Alan R. Liss, 1989, p 193.

Habib R, Loirat C, Gubler MD, et al: The nephropathy associated with male pseudohermaphroditism and Wilson's tumor (Drash syndrome): A distinctive glandular lesion—report of 10 cases. Clin Nephrol 1985;24:269.

Hadlock FP, Deter RL, Carpenter P, et al: Sonography of fetal urinary tract abnormalities. AJR Am J Roentgenol 1981;137:261.

Hakim LS, Adler H, Glassberg KI: Acquired renal cystic disease (ARCD) in the pediatric patient. J Urol 1994;151:330A.

Hamberger J, Richet G, Crosnier J, et al: Nephrology. Philadelphia, WB Saunders, 1968, p 1087.

Hanna MK: The multicystic dysplastic kidney. (Letter to the editor.) Urology 1995;45:171.

Harris RH, Wise MK, Best CF: Renotrophic factors in urine. Kidney Int 1983;23:616.

Harrison AR, Rose GA: Medullary sponge kidney. Urol Res 1979;7:197.

Hartman DS: Cysts and cystic neoplasms. Urol Radiol 1990;12:7.

Hartman DS, Weatherby E III, Laskin WB, et al: Cystic renal cell carcinoma: CT findings simulating a benign hyperdense cyst. AJR Am J Roentgenol 1992;159:1235.

Hartnett M, Bennett W: External manifestations of cystic renal disease. In Gardner KD Jr (ed): Cystic Disease of the Kidney. New York, John Wiley & Sons, 1976, pp 201–219.

Hashimoto B, Filly R, Cullen P: Multicystic dysplastic kidney in utero: Changing appearance on US. Radiology 1986;159:107.

Heikkinen ES, Herva R, Lanning P: Multicystic kidney: A clinical and histologic study of 13 patients. Ann Chir Gynaecol 1980;69:15.

Heinz-Peer G, Maier A, Eibenberger K, et al: Role of magnetic resonance imaging in renal transplant recipients with acquired cystic kidney disease. Urology 1998;51:534.

Heinz-Peer G, Schoder M, Rand T, et al: Prevalence of acquired cystic kidney disease and tumors in native kidneys of renal transplant recipients: A prospective US study. Radiology 1995;667.

Henneberry MO, Stephens FD: Renal hypoplasia and dysplasia in infants with posterior urethral valves. J Urol 1980;123:912.

Heptinstall RH: Discussion. In Hodson J, Kincaid-Smith P (eds): Reflux Nephropathy. New York, Masson, 1979, p 253.

Herdman RC, Good RA, Vernier RL: Medullary cystic disease in two siblings. Am J Med 1967;43:335.

Hildebrandt F: Genetic renal diseases in children. Curr Opin Pediatr 1995;7:182.

Hildebrandt F, Singh-Sawhney I, Schnieders B, et al: Mapping of a gene for familial juvenile nephronophthisis: Refining the map and defining flanking markers on chromosome 2. Am J Hum Genet 1993;53:1256.

Hildebrandt O: Weiterer Beitrag zur patologischen Anatomie der Nierengeschwulste. Arch Klin Chir 1894;48:343.

Hinman JAF: Obstructive renal cysts. J Urol 1978;119:681.

Hoard TD, O'Brien DP III: Simple renal cyst and high renin hypertension cured by cyst decompression. J Urol 1976;115:326.

Hodson CR: Reflux nephropathy: A personal historical review. AJR Am J Roentgenol 1981;137:451.

Holmberg G, Hietala S: Treatment of simple renal cysts by percutaneous puncture and instillation of bismuth-phosphate. Scand J Urol Nephrol 1989;23:207.

Homsy YL, Anderson JH, Oudjhane K, Russo P: Wilms' tumor and multicystic dysplastic kidney disease. J Urol 1997;158:2256.

Horton WA, Wong V, Eldridge R: Von Hippel-Lindau disease: Clinical and pathological manifestations in nine families with 50 affected members. Arch Intern Med 1976;136:769.

Hossack KF, Leddy CL, Schrier RW, et al: Incidence of cardiac abnormalities associated with autosomal dominant polycystic kidney disease (ADPKD). (Abstract.) Am Soc Nephrol 1986;19:46A.

Hubner W, Pfaf R, Porpaczy P, et al: Renal cysts: Percutaneous resection with standard urologic instruments. J Endourol 1990;4:61.

Hughson MD, Buckwald D, Fox M: Renal neoplasia and acquired cystic kidney disease in patients receiving long term dialysis. Arch Pathol Lab Med 1986;110:592.

Hughson MD, Henniger GR, McManus JF: Atypical cysts, acquired renal cystic disease, and renal cell tumors in end stage dialysis kidneys. Lab Invest 1980;42:475.

Hulbert JC, Hunter D: Percutaneous techniques for intrarenal marsupialization of difficult symptomatic renal cysts. Presented at the 85th Annual Meeting of the American Urological Association. New Orleans, May, 1990.

Hulbert JC, Reddy PK, Hunter DW, et al: Percutaneous techniques for the management of caliceal diverticula containing calculi. J Urol 1986;135:225.

Huston J, Torres VE, Wiebers DO: Value of magnetic resonance angiography for detection of intracranial aneurysms in autosomal dominant polycystic kidney disease. J Am Soc Nephrol 1993;3:1871.

Huttunen JR: Congenital nephrotic syndrome of Finnish type: Study of 75 patients. Arch Dis Child 1976;51:344.

Ibrahim RE, Weinberg DS, Weidner N: Atypical cysts and carcinomas of the kidneys in the phacomatoses: A quantitative DNA study using static and flow cytometry. Cancer 1989;63:148.

Ishikawa I: Development of adenocarcinoma and acquired cystic disease of the kidney in hemodialysis patients. In Miller RW, et al (eds): Unusual Occurrences as Clues to Cancer Etiology. Tokyo, Japan Scientific Society Press, 1988a, p 77.

Ishikawa I: Adenocarcinoma of the kidney in chronic hemodialysis patients. Int J Artif Organs 1988b;11:61.

Ishikawa I: Letter to the editor. J Urol 1993;149:1146.

Ishikawa I: Uremic acquired cystic disease. Urology 1985;26:101.

Ishikawa I, Onouchi Z, Saito Y, et al: Sex differences in acquired cystic disease of the kidney on long term dialysis. Nephron 1985;39:336.

Ishikawa I, Saito Y, Nakamura M, et al: Fifteen year follow up of acquired renal cystic disease: A gender difference. Nephron 1997;75:315.

Ishikawa I, Saito Y, Onouchi Z, et al: Development of acquired cystic disease and adenocarcinoma of the kidney in glomerulonephrotic chronic hemodialysis patients. Clin Nephrol 1980;14:1.

Ishikawa I, Snikura N, Shinoda A: Cystic transformation in native kidneys in renal allograft recipients with long-standing good function. Am J Nephrol 1991;11:217.

Ishikawa I, Yuri T, Kitada H, et al: Regression of acquired cystic disease of the kidney after successful renal transplantation. Am J Nephrol 1983;3:310.

Jackman RJ, Stevens JM: Benign hemorrhagic renal cyst: Nephrotomography, renal arteriography and cyst puncture. Radiology 1974;110:7.

Jacobs C, Reach I, Degoulet P: Cancer in patients on hemodialysis. N Engl J Med 1979;300:1279.

Javadpour N, Chelouhy E, Moncada L, et al: Hypertension in a child caused by a multicystic kidney. J Urol 1970;104:918.

Jennings CM, Gaines PA: The abdominal manifestations of von Hippel-Lindau disease and a radiological screening protocol for an affected family. Clin Radiol 1988;39:363.

Johnson DE, Ayala AG, Medellin H, et al: Multilocular renal cystic disease in children. J Urol 1973;109:101.

Johnston JH, Evans JP, Glassberg KI, et al: Pelvic hydronephrosis in children: A review of 219 personal cases. J Urol 1977;117:97.

Johnston JH, Mix LW: The Ask-Upmark kidney: A form of ascending pyelonephritis? Br J Urol 1976;48:393.

Jordan WP Jr: Peripelvic cysts of the kidney. J Urol 1962;87:97.

Joshi VV: Cystic partially differentiated nephroblastoma: An entity in the spectrum of infantile renal neoplasia. Perspect Pediatr Pathol 1980;5:217.

Joshi VV, Beckwith JB: Multilocular cyst of the kidney (cystic nephroma) and cystic partially differentiated nephroblastoma. Cancer 1989;64:466.

Jung WH, Peters CA, Mandell JA, et al: Flow cytometric evaluation of multicystic dysplastic kidneys. J Urol 1990;144:413.

Kääriäinen H: Polycystic kidney disease in children: A genetic and epidemiological study of 82 Finnish patients. J Med Genet 1987;24:474.

Kadir S, Kerr WS, Athanasoulis CA: The role of arteriography in the management of renal cell carcinoma associated with von Hippel-Lindau disease. J Urol 1981;126:316.

Kandt RS, Haines JL, Smith M, et al: Linkage of an important gene locus for tuberous sclerosis to a chromosome 16 member for polycystic kidney disease. Nat Genet 1992;2:37.

Kaplan BS, Gordon I, Pincott J, et al: Familial hypoplastic glomerulocystic kidney disease: A definite entity with dominant inheritance. Am J Med Genet 1989a;34:569.

Kaplan BS, Kaplan P, de Chadarevian JP, et al: Variable expression of autosomal recessive polycystic kidney disease and congenital hepatic fibrosis within a family. Am J Med Genet 1988;29:639.

Kaplan BS, Kaplan P, Rosenberg HK, et al: Polycystic kidney disease in childhood. J Pediatr 1989b;115:867.

Kaplan BS, Rabin I, Nogrady MG, et al: Autosomal dominant polycystic renal disease in children. J Pediatr 1977;90:782.

Kass EJ, Bloom D: Anomalies of the urinary tract. In Edelman CM (ed): Pediatric Kidney Disease. Boston, Little, Brown, 1992, pp 2023–2035.

Kaufman J, Fay R: Renal hypertension in childhood. In Johnston JH, Goodwin WE (eds): Reviews in Pediatric Urology. Amsterdam, Excerpta Medica, 1974, p 201.

Kaye C, Lewy P: Congenital appearance of adult type (autosomal dominant) polycystic kidney disease. J Pediatr 1974;85:807.

Keith DS, Torres VE, King BF, et al: Renal cell carcinoma in autosomal dominant polycystic kidney disease. J Am Soc Nephrol 1994;4:1661.

Kelly CJ, Neilson EG: The interstitium of the cystic kidney. In Gardner KD Jr, Bernstein J (eds): The Cystic Kidney. The Netherlands, Kluwer Academic Publishers, 1990, pp 43–53.

Kerr DNS, Warrick CK, Hart-Mercer J: A lesion resembling medullary sponge kidney in patients with congenital hepatic fibrosis. Clin Radiol 1962;13:85.

Kestilä M, Männikä M, Holmberg C, et al: Congenital nephrotic syndrome of the Finnish type maps to the long arm of chromosome 19. Am J Hum Genet 1994;54:757.

Kestilä M, Lenkkeri U, Männikkö M, et al: Positionally cloned gene for a novel glomerular protein—nephrin is mutated in congenital nephrotic syndrome. Mol Cell 1998;1:575.

Kibel A, Iliopulos O, DeCaprio JA, Kaelin WG Jr: Binding of von Hippel-Lindau tumor suppressor protein to Elongin B and C. Science 1995;269:1444.

Kim E, Arnould T, Walz G: Isolation of polycystic-interacting proteins. J Am Soc Nephrol 1997;8:357A.

Kim E, Arnould T, Sellin LK, et al: The polycystic kidney disease 1 gene product modulates Wnt signaling. J Biol Chem 1999;274:4947.

Kirk JMW, Grant DB, Besser GM, et al: Unilateral renal aplasia in X-linked Kallman's syndrome. Clin Genet 1994;46:260.

Kirsh EJ, Strauss FH II, Goldfischer ER, et al: Benign adenomatous kidney tumor (Perlmann's tumor) and renal cortical carcinoma with adenomatous multicystic features: 12 cases. Urology 1999;53:65.

Kishikawa T, Toda T, Ito H, et al: Bilateral congenital multicystic dysplasia of the kidney. Jpn J Surg 1981;11:198.

Kissane JM: Congenital malformations. In Heptinstall RH (ed): Pathology of the Kidney, 2nd ed: Boston, Little, Brown, 1974, p 69.

Kissane JM, Smith MG: Pathology of Infancy and Childhood, 2nd ed. St. Louis, CV Mosby, 1975, p 587.

Kleiner B, Filly R, Mack L, et al: Multicystic dysplastic kidney: Observations of contralateral disease in the fetal population. Radiology 1986; 161:27.

Kleinknecht C, Habib R: Nephronophthisis. In Cameron S, Davison AM, Grünfeld JP, et al (eds): Oxford Textbook of Clinical Nephrology. New York, Oxford University Press, 1992, pp 2188–2197.

Knudson A: Mutation and cancer: Statistical study of retinoblastoma. Proc Natl Acad Sci U S A 1991;68:820.

Knudson AG: All in the (cancer) family. Nat Genet 1993;5:103.

Kossow AS, Meek JM: Unilateral polycystic kidney disease. J Urol 1982; 127:297.

Kriedberg JA, Sariola H, Loring JM, et al: WT-1 is required for early kidney development. Cell 1993;74:679.

Kuiper JJ: Medullary sponge kidney. Perspect Nephrol Hypertens 1976a; 4:151.

Kuiper JJ: Medullary sponge kidney. In Gardner KD (ed): Cystic Diseases of the Kidney. New York, John Wiley & Sons, 1976b, p 151.

Kupin W, Norris C, Levin NW, et al: Incidence of diverticular disease in patients with polycystic kidney disease (PCKD). Presented at the 10th International Congress of Nephrology, London, July, 1987.

Kutcher R, Amodio JR, Rosenblatt R: Uremic renal cystic disease: Value of sonographic screening. Radiology 1983;147:833.

Kutcher R, Manadevia P, Nussbaum MK, et al: Renal peripelvic multicystic lymphangiectasia. Urology 1982;30:177.

Kyushu Pediatric Nephrology Study Group: Acquired cystic kidney disease in children undergoing continuous ambulatory peritoneal dialysis. Am J Kidney Dis 1999;34:242.

Lagos JC, Gomez MR: Tuberous sclerosis: Reappraisal of a clinical entity. Mayo Clin Proc 1967;42:26.

Lam M, Halverstadt D, Altshuler G, et al: Congenital oligomeganephronia in a solitary kidney: Report of a case. Am J Kidney Dis 1982;1:300.

Lane WM, Robson M, Thomason MA, Minette L: Cystic dysplasia of the testis associated with multicystic dysplasia of the kidney. Urology 1998;51(3):477.

Lanning P, Uhari M, Kouvalainen K, et al: Ultrasonic features of the congenital nephrotic syndrome of the Finnish type. Acta Paediatr Scand 1989;78:717.

LaSalle MD, Stock JA, Hanna MK: Insurability of children with congenital urological anomalies. J Urol 1997;158:1312.

Latif F, Tory K, Gnarra J, et al: Identification of the von Hippel-Lindau disease tumor suppressor gene. Science 1993;260:317.

Latini JM, Curtis MR, Cendron M, et al: Prenatal failure to visualize kidneys: A spectrum of disease. Urology 1998;52:36.

Laucks SP Jr, McLachlan MSF: Aging and simple renal cysts of the kidney. Br J Radiol 1981;54:12.

Lavan JN, Neale FC, Posen S: Urinary calculi: Clinical, biochemical and radiological studies in 619 patients. Med J Aust 1971;2:1049.

Lazebnik N, Bellinger MF, Ferguson JE II, et al: Insights into the pathogenesis and natural history of fetuses with multicystic dysplastic kidney disease. Prenat Diagn 1999;19:48.

Lee JKT, McLennan BL, Kissane JM: Unilateral polycystic kidney disease. AJR Am J Roentgenol 1978;130:1165.

Lenarduzzi G: Repert pielografico poco commune (dilatazione delle vie urinarie intrarenali). Radiol Med 1939;26:346.

Levine E: Acquired cystic kidney disease: Radiol Clin North Am 1996; 34:947.

Levine E, Collins DL, Horton WA, et al: CT screening of the abdomen in von Hippel-Lindau disease. AJR Am J Roentgenol 1982;139:505.

Levine E, Grantham JJ: Radiology of cystic kidneys. In Gardner KD Jr, Bernstein J (eds): The Cystic Kidney. The Netherlands, Kluwer Academic Publishers, 1990, p 171.

Levine E, Grantham JJ, Slusher SL, et al: CT of acquired cystic disease and renal tumors in long-term dialysis patients. AJR Am J Roentgenol 1984;142:125.

Levine E, Hartmann DS, Smirnidtopoulos JG: Renal cystic disease associated with renal neoplasms. In Pollack HM (ed): Clinical Urography. Philadelphia, WB Saunders, 1990, pp 1126–1150.

Levine E, Huntrakoon M: Unilateral renal cystic disease. J Comput Assist Tomogr 1989;13:273.

Levine E, Slusher SL, Grantham JJ, et al: Natural history of acquired renal cystic disease in dialysis patients: A prospective longitudinal CT study. AJR Am J Roentgenol 1991;156:501.

Levine LA, Gburek BM: Acquired cystic disease and renal adenocarcinoma following renal transplantation. J Urol 1994;151:129.

Lieberman E, Salinas-Madrigal L, Gwinn JL, et al: Infantile polycystic disease of the kidneys and liver: Clinical, pathological and radiological correlations and comparison with congenital hepatic fibrosis. Medicine (Baltimore) 1971;50:277.

Lingard DA, Lawson TI: Accuracy of ultrasound in predicting the nature of renal masses. J Urol 1979;122:724.

Lirenman DS, Lowry RB, Chase WH: Familial juvenile nephronophthisis: Experience with eleven cases. Birth Defects 1974;10:32.

Livingston WD, Collins TL, Novick DE: Incidental renal masses. Urology 1981;17:257.

Loh JP, Haller JO, Kassner EG, et al: Dominantly inherited polycystic kidneys in infants: Association with hypertrophic pyloric stenosis. Pediatr Radiol 1977;6:27.

Longino LA, Martin LW: Abdominal masses in the newborn infant. Pediatrics 1958;21:596.

Loughlin KR, Gittes RF: Urological management of patients with von Hippel-Lindau disease. J Urol 1986;136:789.

Lubensky IA, Gnarra JR, Bertheau P, et al: Allelic deletions of the VHL gene detected In multiple microscopic clear cell renal lesion in von Hippel-Lindau disease patients. Am J Pathol 1996;149:2089.

Lüscher TF, Wanner C, Siegenthaler W, et al: Simple renal cyst and hypertension: Cause or coincidence? Clin Nephrol 1986;26:91.

Macari M, Bosniak MA: Delayed CT to evaluate renal masses accidentally discovered at contrast-enhanced CT: Demonstration of vascularity with deenhancement. Radiology 1999;213:674.

Mackie GG, Stephens FD: Duplex kidneys: A correlation of renal dysplasia with position of the ureteral orifice. J Urol 1975;114:274.

Madewell JE, Goldman SM, Davis CJ Jr: Multilocular cystic nephroma: A radiographic pathologic correlation of 58 patients. Radiology 1983; 146:309.

Maher ER, Kaelin WG Jr: von Hippel-Lindau disease. Medicine 1997;76: 381.

Maizel M, Simpson SB Jr: Primitive ducts in renal dysplasia induced by culturing ureteral buds denuded of condensed renal mesenchyme. Science 1983;209:509.

Maizel M, Simpson SB Jr: Ligating the embryonic ureter facilitates the induction of renal dysplasia. Dev Biol Part B 1986;445.

Malek R, Omess P, Benson R, et al: Renal cell carcinoma in Von Hippel-Lindau disease. Am J Med 1987;82:236.

Marotti M, Hricak H, Fritzche P, et al: Complex and simple cysts: Comparative evaluation with MR imaging. Radiology 1987;162:679.

Martinez JR, Lowley BD Jr, Gattone VHIII, et al: The effect of paclitaxel on the progression of polycystic kidney disease in rodents. Am J Kidney Dis 1997;29:435.

Maschio G, Tessitore N, D'Angelo A: Medullary sponge kidney and hyperparathyroidism: A puzzling association. Am J Nephrol 1982;2:77.

Matson MA, Cohen EP: Acquired kidney cystic disease: Occurrence, prevalence, and renal cancers. Medicine (Baltimore) 1990;69:217.

McClean RH, Goldstein G, Conrad FU, et al: Myocardial infarctions and endocardial fibro-elastosis in children with polycystic kidneys. Bull Johns Hopkins Hosp 1964;115:92.

McClennan BL, Stanley RJ, Melson GL, et al: CT of the renal cyst: Is a cyst puncture necessary? AJR Am J Roentgenol 1979;133:671.

McGonigle RJS, Mowat AP, Benwick M, et al: Congenital hepatic fibrosis and polycystic kidney disease: Role of portacaval shunting and transplantation in three patients. Q J Med 1981;50:269.

McGregor AI, Bailey R: Nephronophthisis-cystic medulla complex: Diagnosis by computerized tomography. Nephron 1989;53:70.

McHugh K, Stringer DA, Hebert D, et al: Simple renal cysts in children: Diagnosis and follow-up with US. Radiology 1991;178:383.

McPherson E, Carey J, Kramer A, et al: Dominantly inherited renal adysplasia. Am J Med Genet 1987;26:863.

Meares EM Jr, Gross DM: Hypertension owing to unilateral renal hypoplasia. J Urol 1972;108:197.

Mebrizi A, Rosenstein BJ, Pusch A, et al: Myocardial and endocardial fibro-elastosis in children with polycystic kidneys. Bull Johns Hopkins Hosp 1964;115:92.

Melicow MM, Uson AC: Palpable abdominal masses in infants and children: A report based on a review of 653 cases. J Urol 1959;81:705.

Melnick SC, Brewer DB, Oldham JS: Cortical microcystic disease of the kidney with dominant inheritance: A previously undescribed syndrome. J Clin Pathol 1984;37:494.

Meyer WM, Jonas D: Endoscopic percutaneous resection of renal cysts. Presented at the Eighth World Congress on Endourology and ESWL, Washington, DC, August–September, 1990.

Mickisch O, Bommer J, Blackman J, et al: Multicystic transformation of kidneys in chronic renal failure. Nephron 1984;38:93.

Miller LR, Soffer O, Nasser VH, et al: Acquired renal cystic disease in end stage renal disease: An autopsy study of 155 cases. Am J Nephrol 1989;9:322.

Milutinovic J, Fialkow PJ, Agoda LY, et al: Autosomal dominant polycystic kidney disease: Symptoms and clinical findings. Am J Med 1984;53:511.

Mitnick JS, Bosniak MA, Hilton S: Cystic renal disease in tuberous sclerosis. Radiology 1983;147:85.

Mongeau JG, Worthen HG: Nephronophthisis and medullary cystic disease. Am J Med 1967;43:345.

Morgan C Jr, Rader D: Laparoscopic unroofing of a renal cyst. J Urol 1992;148:1835.

Morita T, Wenzl J, McCoy J, et al: Bilateral renal hypoplasia with oligomeganephronia: Quantitative and electron microscopic study. Am J Clin Pathol 1973;59:104.

Mosli H, MacDonald P, Schillinger J: Caliceal diverticulum developing into simple renal cyst. J Urol 1986;136:658.

Mozziconacci P, Attal C, Boisse J, et al: Hypoplasie segmentaire du rein avec hypertension artérielle. Ann Pediatr 1968;15:337.

Murcia NS, Sweeney WE Jr, Avner ED: New insights into molecular pathophysiology of polycystic kidney disease. Kidney Int 1999;55:1187.

Myall GF: The incidence of medullary sponge kidney. Clin Radiol 1970;21:171.

Nash DA Jr: Hypertension in polycystic kidney disease without renal failure. Arch Intern Med 1977;137:1571.

Neilson EG, McCafferty E, Mann R, et al: Murine interstitial nephritis III. J Immunol 1985;134:2375.

Neumann HPH, Wiestler OD: Clustering of features of Von Hippel-Lindau syndrome: Evidence for a complex genetic locus. Lancet 337:1052,1991.

Neumann HPH, Zauner I, Strahm B, et al: Late occurrence of cysts in autosomal dominant medullary cystic kidney disease. Nephrol Dial Transplant 1997;12:1242.

Neumann HPH, Zbar B: Renal cysts, renal cancer and Von Hippel-Lindau disease. Kidney Int 1997;51:16.

Neumann HPH, Zerres K, Fischer CL, et al: Late manifestations of autosomal-recessive polycystic kidney disease in two sisters. Am J Nephrol 1988;8:194.

Nicholas JL: An unusual complication of calyceal diverticulum. Br J Urol 1975;47:370.

Noe HN, Marshall JH, Edwards OP: Nodular renal blastema in the multicystic kidney. J Urol 1989;127:486.

Noe HN, Raghavaiah NV: Excision of pyelocalyceal diverticulum under renal hypothermia. J Urol 1982;127:294.

Norio R: Heredity in the congenital nephrotic syndrome: A genetic study of 57 Finnish families with a review of reported cases. Ann Paediatr (Finn) 1966;12(Suppl. 27):1.

Norio R, Rapola J: Congenital and infantile nephrotic syndromes. In Bartsocas CS (ed): Genetics of Kidney Disorders: Progress in Clinical and Biological Research, vol 305. New York, Alan R. Liss, 1989, pp 179–192.

Nusse R, Varmus HE: Many tumors induced by the mouse mammary tumor virus contain a provirus integrated in the same region of the host genome. Cell 1982;31:99.

Oddone M, Marino C, Sergi C, et al: Wilms' tumor arising in a multicystic kidney. Pediatr Radiol 1994;24:236.

O'Hagan AR, Ellsworth R, Secic MS, et al: Renal manifestations of tuberous sclerosis complex. Clin Pediatr 1996;183.

Okada RD, Platt MA, Fleischman J: Chronic renal failure in patients with tuberous sclerosis: Association with renal cysts. Nephron 1982;30:85.

Olsen A, Hansen Hojhus J, Steffensen G: Renal medullary cystic disease. Acta Radiol 1988;29(Fasc 5):527.

Osathanondh V, Potter EL: Pathogenesis of polycystic kidneys: Historical survey. Arch Pathol 1964;77:459.

Palubinskas AJ: Medullary sponge kidney. Radiology 1961;76:911.

Pampigliana G, Moynahan EJ: The tuberous sclerosis syndrome: Clinical and EEG studies in 100 children. J Neurol Neurosurg Psychiatry 1976;39:666.

Papanicolaou N, Pfister RC, Yoder IC: Spontaneous and traumatic rupture of renal cysts: Diagnosis and outcome. Radiology 1986;160:99.

Paramo PG: Patologia quística renal. Acta Assoc Esp Urol 1975;7:1.

Paramo PG, Segura A: Hilioquisosis renal. Rev Clin Esp 1972;126:387.

Parfrey SP, Bear JC, Morgan J, et al: The diagnosis and prognosis of autosomal dominant polycystic kidney disease. N Engl J Med 1990;323:1085.

Park SH, Chi JGP: Oligomeganephronia associated with 4p deletion type chromosomal anomaly. Pediatr Pathol 1993;13:731.

Parkkulainen KV, Hjeldt L, Sirola K: Congenital multicystic dysplasia of kidney: Report of nineteen cases with discussion on the etiology, nomenclature and classification of cystic dysplasia of the kidney. Acta Chir Scand Suppl 1959;244:5.

Parks JH, Coe FL, Strauss AL: Calcium nephrolithiasis and medullary sponge kidney in women. N Engl J Med 1982;306:1088.

Pathak IG, Williams DI: Multicystic and cystic dysplastic kidneys. Br J Urol 1964;36:318.

Patriquin HB, O'Regan S: Medullary sponge kidney in childhood. AJR Am J Roentgenol 1985;145:315.

Penn I: Tumor incidence in renal allograft recipients. Transplant Proc 1979;11:1047.

Pepicelli CV, Kispert A, Rowitch DH, McMahon AP: GDNF induces branching and increased cell proliferation in the ureter of the mouse. Dev Biol 1997;192:193.

Perez LM, Naidu SI, Joseph DB: Outcome and cost analysis of operative versus non-operative management of neonatal multicystic dysplastic kidneys. J Urol 1998;160:1207.

Perlmann S: Uber einen Fall von Lymphangioma cysticum der Niere. Virchows Arch [Pathol Anat] 1928;268:524.

Peters DJM, Spruit L, Saris JJ, et al: Chromosome 4 localization of a second gene for autosomal dominant polycystic kidney disease. Nat Genet 1993;5:359.

Pichel JG, Shen L, Sheng HZ, et al: Defects in enteric intervention and kidney development in mice lacking GDNF. Nature 1996;382:73.

Pieke SA, Kimberling WJ, Kenyon KG, et al: Genetic heterogenicity of polycystic kidney disease: An estimate of the proportion of families unlinked to chromosome 16. Am J Hum Genet 1989;45:458.

Plas EG, Hübner WA: Percutaneous resection of renal cysts: A long-term follow-up. J Urol 1993;149:703.

Pollack AL, Barth AIM, Altschuler Y, et al: Dynamics of beta-catenin interactions with APC protein regulate epithelial tubulogenesis. J Cell Biol 1997;137:1651.

Pollack HM, Banner MP, Arger PH, et al: Comparison of computed tomography and ultrasound in the diagnosis of renal masses. In Rosenfeld AT (ed): Genitourinary Ultrasonography. New York, Churchill Livingstone, 1979, p 25.

Pope JC, Brock JW, Adams MC, et al: How they begin and how they end: Classic and new theories for the development and deterioration of congenital anomalies of the kidney and urinary tract, CAKUT. J Am Soc Nephrol 1999;10:2018.

Porstman W: Renal angiography in children. Prog Pediatr Radiol 1970;3:51.

Port FK, Ragheb NE, Schwartz SH, et al: Neoplasms in dialysis patients: A population-based study. Am J Kidney Dis 1989;14:199.

Poston DO, Jaffes GS, Lubensky IA, et al: Characterization of the renal pathology of a familial form of renal cell carcinoma associated with von Hippel Lindau's disease. J Urol 1993;153:22.

Potter EL: Bilateral absence of ureters and kidneys: A report of 50 cases. Obstet Gynecol 1965;25:3.

Potter EL: Normal and Abnormal Development of the Kidney. Chicago, Year Book Medical Publishers, 1972.

Powell T, Schackman R, Johnson HD: Multilocular cysts of the kidney. Br J Urol 1951;23:142.

Pretorius DH, Lee ME, Manco-Johnson ML, et al: Diagnosis of autosomal dominant polycystic kidney disease in utero and in the young infant. J Ultrasound Med 1987;6:249.

Pritchard-Jones K, Fleming S, Davidson D, et al: The candidate Wilms' tumour gene is involved in genitourinary development. Nature 1990; 346:194.

Proesmans W, Van Damme B, Basaer P, et al: Autosomal dominant polycystic kidney disease in the neonatal period: Association with a cerebral arteriovenous malformation. Pediatrics 1982;70:971.

Pugh JL, Sweeney WE Jr, Avner EO: Tyrosine kinase activity of EGF receptor in murine metanephric organ culture. Kidney Int 1995;47:774.

Qian F, Watnick TJ, Onuchic LF, Germino GG: The molecular basis of focal cyst formation in human autosomal dominant polycystic kidney disease type I. Cell 1996;87:979.

Raboy A, Hakim LS, Ferzli G, et al: Extraperitoneal endoscopic surgery for benign renal cysts. In Das S, Crawford EW (eds): Urologic Laparoscopy. Philadelphia, WB Saunders, 1994, pp 145–149.

Rall JE, Odell HM: Congenital polycystic disease of the kidney: Review of the literature and the data on 207 cases. Am J Med Sci 1949;298: 394.

Ratcliffe PJ, Dunhill MS, Oliver DO: Clinical importance of acquired cystic disease of the kidneys in patients undergoing dialysis. Br Med J 1983;287:1855.

Rauber G, Langlet ML: Hypoplasies segmentaires du rein: Distinction de deux formes histologiques. Nouv Presse Med 1976;5:1759.

Ravden MI, Zuckerman HL, Kay CJ, et al: Evaluation of solitary simple renal cysts in children. J Urol 1980;124:904.

Ravine D, Gibson RN, Walker RG, et al: Evaluation of ultrasonographic diagnostic criteria for autosomal dominant polycystic kidney diesease. 1. Lancet 1994;343:824.

Reeders ST: The genetics of renal cystic disease. In Gardner KD Jr, Bernstein J (eds): The Cystic Kidney. The Netherlands, Kluwer Academic Publishers, 1990, pp 117–146.

Reeders ST, Breuning MH, Comey G, et al: Two genetic markers closely linked to adult polycystic kidney disease on chromosome 16. Br Med J 1986a;292:851.

Reeders ST, Bruening MH, Davies KE, et al: A highly polymorphic DNA marker linked to adult polycystic kidney disease on chromosome 16. Nature 1985;317:542.

Reeders ST, Keeres K, Gal A, et al: Prenatal diagnosis of autosomal dominant polycystic kidney disease with a DNA probe. Lancet 1986b; 2:6.

Reichard EAP, Robidoux MA, Dunnick NR: Renal neoplasms in patients with renal cystic disease. Abdom Imaging 1998;23:237.

Resnick JS, Hartman DS: Medullary cystic disease of the kidney. In Pollack HM (ed): Clinical Urography. Philadelphia, WB Saunders, 1990, pp 1178–1184.

Ressequire LJ, Nobrega FT, Farrow GM, et al: Epidemiology of renal and ureteral cancer in Rochester, Minnesota 1950–1978, with special reference to clinical and pathologic features. Mayo Clin Proc 1978;53:503.

Richter S, Karbel G, Bechar L, et al: Should a benign renal cyst be treated? Br J Urol 1983;55:457.

Ritter R, Siafarikas K: Hemihypertrophy in a boy with renal polycystic disease: Varied patterns of presentation of renal polycystic disease in his family. Pediatr Radiol 1976;5:98.

Rizzoni G, Loirat C, Levy M, et al: Familial hypoplastic glomerulocystic kidneys: A new entity? Clin Nephrol 1982;18:263.

Roach ES, Smith M, Huttenlocker P, et al: Diagnostic criteria: Tuberous sclerosis complex. Report of the Diagnostic Criteria Committee of the National Tuberous Sclerosis Association. J Child Neurol 1992;7:221.

Rockson SG, Stone RA, Gunnels JC Jr: Solitary renal cyst with segmental ischemia and hypertension. J Urol 1974;112:550.

Rogers SA, Ryan G, Hammerman MR: Metanephric transforming growth factor is required for renal organogenesis in vitro. Am J Physiol 1992; 262:F533.

Rominger M, Kenney P, Morgan D, et al: Gandolinium-enhanced MR imaging of renal masses. Radiographics 1992;12:1097.

Roos A: Polycystic kidney: Report of a case. Am J Dis Child 1941;61: 116.

Rosenfeld AT, Siegel NJ, Kappleman MB: Grey scale ultrasonography in medullary cystic disease of the kidney and congenital hepatic fibrosis with tubular ectasia: New observations. AJR Am J Roentgenol 1977; 129:297.

Rosenfeld JB, Cohen L, Garty I, et al: Unilateral renal hypoplasia with hypertension (Ask-Upmark kidney). Br Med J 1973;2:217.

Ross DG, Travers H: Infantile presentation of adult-type polycystic kidney disease in a large kindred. J Pediatr 1975;87:760.

Rothentieler UW, Dressler GR: Pax-2 is required for mesenchyme to epithelium conversion during kidney development. Development 1993; 119:711.

Ruotsalainen V, Ljungberg P, Wartiovaara J, et al: Nephrin is specifically located at the slit diaphragm of glomerular podocytes. Proc Natl Acad Sci USA 1999;96:1962.

Royer P, Habib R, Broyer M, et al: Segmental hypoplasia of the kidney in children. Adv Nephrol 1971;1:145.

Royer P, Habib R, Mathieu H, et al: L'Hypoplasie renale bilaterale congenitale avec reduction du nombre et hypertrophie des nephrons chez l'enfant. Ann Pediatr (Paris) 1962;38:133.

Rubenstein M, Meyer R, Bernstein J: Congenital abnormalities of the urinary system: I. A postmortem survey of developmental anomalies and acquired congenital lesions in a children's hospital. J Pediatr 1961; 58:356.

Rubenstein SC, Hulbert JG, Pharand D, et al: Laparoscopic ablation of symptomatic renal cysts. J Urol 1993;150:1103.

Rushton GH, Spector M, Rogers AL, et al: Developmental aspects of calcium oxalate tubular deposits and calculi induced in rat kidneys. Invest Urol 1981;19:52.

Ryu S: Intracranial hemorrhage in patients with polycystic kidney disease. Stroke 1990;21:291.

Ryynanen M, Dolata MM, Lampainen E, et al: Localization of mutation producing autosomal dominant polycystic kidney disease without renal failure. J Med Genet 1987;24:462.

Sage MR, Lawson AD, Marshall VR, et al: Medullary sponge kidney and urolithiasis. Clin Radiol 1982;33:435.

Sahney S, Sandler MA, Weiss L, et al: Adult polycystic disease: Presymptomatic diagnosis for genetic counseling. Clin Nephrol 1983;20: 89.

Saxton HM, Golding SJ, Chantler C, et al: Diagnostic puncture in renal cystic dysplasia (multicystic kidney). Evidence on the aetiology of the cysts. Br J Urol 1981;54:555.

Scheff RT, Zuckerman G, Harter H, et al: Diverticular disease in patients with chronic renal failure due to polycystic kidney disease. Ann Intern Med 1980;92:202.

Scheinman JI, Abelson HT: Bilateral renal hypoplasia with oligonephronia. J Pediatr 1970;76:369.

Schuchardt A, D'Agatl V, Larsson-Blomberg L, et al: Defects in the kidney and enteric nervous system of mice lacking the tyrosine kinase receptor Ret. Nature 1994;367:380.

Schulsinger DA, Rachlin S, Huller JO, et al: Simple cysts in childhood: An early expression of autosomal dominant polycystic kidney disease? J Urol 1994;151:273A.

Schwab SJ, Bander SJ, Klahr S: Renal infection in autosomal dominant polycystic kidney disease. Am J Med 1987;82:714.

Schwarz RD, Stephens FD, Cussen LJ: The pathogenesis of renal hypodysplasia: I. Quantification of hypoplasia and dysplasia. Invest Urol 1981a;10:94.

Schwarz RD, Stephens FD, Cussen LJ: The pathogenesis of renal hypodysplasia: II. The significance of lateral and medial ectopy of the ureteric orifice. Invest Urol 1981b;19:97.

Schwarz RD, Stephens FD, Cussen LJ: The pathogenesis of renal hypodysplasia: III. Complete and incomplete urinary obstruction. Invest Urol 1981c;19:101.

Sedman A, Bell P, Manco-Johnson M, et al: Autosomal dominant polycystic kidney disease in childhood: A longitudinal study. Kidney Int 1987;31:1000.

Sedman A, Gabow PA: Autosomal dominant polycystic kidney disease. Dialogues Pediatr Urol 1984;7:4.

Segal AJ, Spitzer RM: Pseudo thick-walled renal cyst by CT. AJR Am J Roentgenol 1979;132:827.

Segura J, Torres V, Braun F, Rochester M: Laparoscopic marsupialization of multiple renal cysts: A high rate of persistent and recurrent cyst and symptoms. J Urol 1995;153:513A.

Shalhoub RJ, Rajan U, Kim VV, et al: Erythrocytosis in patients on long-term hemodialysis. Ann Intern Med 1982;97:686.

Shepherd CW, Scahill SJ, Stephenson JBP, et al: Tuberous sclerosis complex in Olmsted County, Minnesota, 1950–1989. Arch Neurol 1991;48:400.

Shindo S, Bernstein J, Arant BS Jr: Evolution of renal segmental atrophy (Ask-Upmark kidney) in children with vesico-ureteral reflux: Radiographic and morphologic studies. J Pediatr 1983;102:847.

Shokeir MHK: Expression of "adult" polycystic renal disease in the fetus and newborn. Clin Genet 1978;14:61.

Siegel MJ, McAlister WH: Simple renal cysts in children. J Urol 1980; 123:75.

Smith CH, Graham JB: Congenital medullary cysts of the kidneys with severe refractory anemia. Am J Dis Child 1945;69:369.

Snodgrass WT: Hypertension associated with multicystic dysplastic kidney in children. J Urol 2000;164:472.

Solomon D, Schwartz A: Renal pathology in von Hippel-Lindau disease. Hum Pathol 1988;19:1072.

Sommer JT, Stephens FD: Morphogenesis of nephropathy with partial ureteral obstruction and vesicoureteral reflux. J Urol 1981;125:67.

Spence HM: Congenital unilateral multicystic kidney: An entity to be distinguished from polycystic kidney disease and other cystic disorders. J Urol 1955;74:893.

Spence HM, Singleton R: Cysts and cystic disorders of the kidney: Types, diagnosis, treatment. Urol Surv 1972;22:131.

Spencer JR, Maizel M: Inhibition of protein glycosylation causes renal dysplasia in the chick embryo. J Urol 1987;138:94.

Stapleton FB, Hilton S, Wilcox J, et al: Transient nephromegaly simulating infantile polycystic disease of the kidneys. Pediatrics 1981;67:554.

Stapleton FB, Johnson D, Kaplan GW, et al: The cystic renal lesion in tuberous sclerosis. J Pediatr 1980;97:574.

Starer F: Partial hydronephrosis due to pressure from normal renal arteries. Br Med J 1968;1:98.

Stark K, Vainio S, Vassiliera G, McMahon AP: Epithelial transformation of metanephric mesenchyme in the developing kidney regulated by Wnt-4. Nature 1994;372:679.

Steele BT, Lirenman DS, Beattie CW: Nephronophthisis. Am J Med 1980;68:531.

Stephens FD: Congenital Malformations of the Urinary Tract. New York, Praeger Publishers, 1983.

Stephens FD, Cussen LG: Renal dysgenesis: A "urologic" classification. In Stephens FD (ed): Congenital Malformations of the Urinary Tract. New York, Praeger Publishing, 1983, pp 463–475.

Stickler GB, Kelalis PP: Polycystic kidney disease: A recognition of the "adult" form (autosomal dominant) in infancy. Mayo Clin Proc 1975; 50:547.

Stillaert J, Baert A, Van Damme B, et al: A propos du rein polykystique. In Kuss R, Legrain M (eds): Seminaries d'Uronephrologie in Pitiere-Salpetriere, 1975. Paris, Masson et Cie, 1975, p 159.

Stillwell TJ, Gomez MR, Kelalis PP: Renal lesions in tuberous sclerosis. J Urol 1987;138:477.

Sweeney WE, Futey L, Frost P, Avner ED: In vitro modulation of cyst formation by a novel tyrosine kinase inhibitor. Kidney Int 1999;56:406.

Sweeney WJ, Chen Y, Nakanishi K, et al: Treatment of polycystic kidney disease with a novel tyrosine kinase inhibitor. Kidney Int 2000;57:33.

Tada S, Yamagishi J, Kobayashi H, et al: The incidence of simple renal cyst by computed tomography. Clin Radiol 1983;150:207.

Taitz LS, Brown CB, Blank CE, et al: Screening for polycystic kidney disease: Importance of clinical presentation in the newborn. Arch Dis Child 1987;62:45.

Tajima E, Aikawa A, Ohara T, et al: Effect of kidney transplantation on acquired cystic lesions in native kidneys. Transpl Proc 1998;30:3060–3061.

Tanagho EA: Surgically induced partial urinary obstruction in the fetal lamb: III. Ureteral obstruction. Invest Urol 1972;10:35.

Taxy JB, Filmer RB: Metaplastic cartilage in nondysplastic kidneys. Arch Pathol 1975;99:101.

Taxy JB, Filmer RB: Glomerulo-cystic kidney. Arch Pathol Lab Med 1976;100:186.

Teichman JMH, Hubert JC: Laparoscopic marsupialization of the painful polycystic kidney. J Urol 1995;153:1105.

Templeton AW, Thompson IM: Aortographic differentiation of congenital and acquired small kidneys. Arch Surg 1968;97:114.

Thompson BJ, Jenkins DAS, Allan PL, et al: Acquired cystic disease of the kidney: An indication for transplantation? Br Med J 1986;293:209.

Thomsen HS, Thaysen JH: Frequency of hepatic cysts in adult polycystic kidney disease. Acta Med Scand 1988;224:381.

Timmons JW Jr, Malek RS, Hattery RR, et al: Calyceal diverticulum. J Urol 1975;114:6.

Torres M, Gomez-Pardo E, Dressler GR, et al: Pax-2 is required for mesenchyme-to-epithelium conversion during kidney development. Development 1995;121:4057.

Turco A, Peissel B, Quaia P, et al: Prenatal diagnosis of autosomal dominant polycystic kidney disease using flanking DNA markers and the polymerase chain reaction. Prenatal Diag 1992;6:513.

Uson AC, Melicow MM: Multilocular cysts of the kidney with intrapelvic herniation of a "daughter" cyst: Report of 4 cases. J Urol 1963;89:341.

Vagelli G, Ferraris V, Calbrese G, et al: Medullary sponge kidney and calcium nephrolithiasis. (Abstract.) Urol Res 1988;16:201.

Valderrama E, Berkman JI: The Ask-Upmark kidney in a premature infant. Clin Nephrol 1979;11:313.

Valvo E, Gammaro L, Tessitore N, et al: Hypertension of polycystic kidney disease: Mechanisms and hemodynamic alterations. Am J Nephrol 1985;5:176.

Van Acker KJ, Vincke H, Quatacker J, et al: Congenital oligonephronic renal hypoplasia with hypertrophy of nephrons (oligonephronia). Arch Dis Child 1971;46:321.

Van Baal JG, Smits NJ, Keeman JN, et al: The evolution of renal angiomyolipomas in patients with tuberous sclerosis. J Urol 1994;152:35.

Vela-Navarrete R, Garcia de la Péna E, Alverez Villalobos C, et al: Quistes nonefrogénicos del seno renal: Expreividad radiográphica y consideraciones diagnóticas. Rev Clin Esp 1974;132:29.

Vela-Navarrete R, Robledo AG: Polycystic disease of the renal sinus: Structural characteristics. J Urol 1983;129:700.

Wacksman J, Phipps L: Report of the multicystic kidney registry: Preliminary findings. J Urol 1993;150:1870.

Wahlqvist L, Grumstedt B: Therapeutic effect of percutaneous puncture of simple renal cyst: Follow-up investigation of 50 patients. Acta Chir Scand 1966;132:340.

Wakabayashi T, Fujita S, Onbora Y, et al: Polycystic kidney disease and intracranial aneurysms: Early angiographic diagnosis and early operation for the unruptured aneurysm. J Neurosurg 1983;58:488.

Walker FC, Loney LC, Rout ER, et al: Diagnostic evaluation of adult polycystic disease in childhood. AJR Am J Roentgenol 1984;142:1273.

Walker RD, Fennell R, Garin E, et al: Spectrum of multicystic renal dysplasia: Diagnosis and management. Urology 1978;11:433.

Watson ML: Complications of polycystic kidney disease. Kidney Int 1997;51:353.

Webb DW, Osborne JP, Fryer AE: On the incidence of mental retardation in tuberous sclerosis. J Med Genet 1991;28:385.

Webb NJA, Lewis MA, Bruce J, et al: Unilateral multicystic dysplastic kidney: The case for nephrectomy. Arch Dis Child 1997;76:31.

Weinreb JC, Arger PH, Coleman BG, et al: Cystic renal mass evaluation: Real-time versus static imaging. J Clin Ultrasound 1986;14:29.

Westberg G, Zachrisson L: Proceedings of the Swedish Society of Medical Radiology, 1975, p 4.

Wikstrom B, Backman U, Danielson BG: Ambulatory diagnostic evaluation of 38 recurrent renal stone formers: A proposal for clinical classification and investigation. Klin Wochenschr 1983;61:85.

Williams DI: Urology in Childhood. New York, Springer-Verlag, 1974, p 79.

Williams G, Blandy JP, Tressider GC: Communicating cysts and diverticula of the renal pelvis. Br J Urol 1969;41:163.

Wilson PD, Sherwood AC: Tubulocystic epithelium. Kidney Int 1991;39:450.

Wilson PD, Sherwood AG, Palla K, et al: Reversed polarity of Na^+-K^+-ATPase: Mislocation to apical plasma membranes in polycystic kidney disease epithelia. Am J Physiol 1991;260(3pt2):F420.

Winyard PJD, Nauta J, Lirenman DS, et al: Deregulation of cell survival in cystic and dysplastic renal development. Kidney Int 1996;49:135.

Wise SW, Hartman DS, Hardesty LA, Mosher TJ: Renal medullary cystic disease: Assessment by MRI. Abdom Imaging 1998;23:649.

Wojcik LJ, Hansen K, Diamond DA, et al: Cystic dysplasia of the rete testis: A benign congenital lesion associated with ipsilateral urological anomalies. J Urol 1997;158:600.

Wolf B, Rosenfield AT, Taylor KJW, et al: Presymptomatic diagnosis of adult onset polycystic kidney disease by ultrasonography. Clin Genet 1978;14:1.

Woo DDL, Miao SYP, Pelayo SC, Woolf AS: Taxol limits progression of congenital polycystic kidney disease. Nature 1994;368:750.

Wood BP, Muurahainen N, Anderson VM, et al: Multicystic nephroblastoma: Ultrasound diagnosis (with a pathologic-anatomic commentary). Pediatr Radiol 1982;12:43.

Woolf AS: A molecular and genetic view of human renal and urinary tract malformations. Kidney Int 2000;58:500.

Yamamoto N, Kanetake H, Yamara J: In vitro evidence from tissue cultures to prove existence of rabbit and human renotropic growth factor. Kidney Int 1983;23:624.

Ye M, An SY, Jiang HM: Clinical analysis of 141 cases of adult polycystic kidney disease. Chinese J Surg 1986;24:73.

Yendt ER: Medullary sponge kidney. In Gardner KD Jr, Bernstein J (eds): The Cystic Kidney. The Netherlands, Kluwer Academic Publishers, 1990, p 379.

Zbar B, Kishida T, Chen F, et al: Germline mutations in the von Hippel-Lindau disease (VHL) gene in families from North America, Europe and Japan. Hum Mutat 1996;8:348.

Zeier M, Geberth S, Ritz E, et al: Adult dominant polycystic kidney disease: Clinical problems. Nephron 1988;49:177.

Zerres K, Hansmann M, Mallman R, et al: Autosomal recessive polycystic kidney disease: Problems of prenatal diagnosis. Prenat Diagn 1988; 8:215.

Zerres K, Mucher G, Bachner L, et al: Mapping of the gene for autosomal recessive polycystic kidney diesease (ARPKD) to chromosome 6p21-cen. Nat Genet 1994;7:429.

57
ANOMALIES AND SURGERY OF THE URETEROPELVIC JUNCTION IN CHILDREN

Michael C. Carr, M.D., Ph.D.

Evidence

Etiology
    Intrinsic
    Extrinsic
    Secondary Ureteral Pelvic Junction Obstruction
    Associated Anomalies

Symptoms/Presentation

Diagnosis
    Ultrasonography

Magnetic Resonance Imaging
Radionuclide Renography
Pressure-Flow Studies
Biochemical Parameters

Surgical Repair
    Dismembered Pyeloplasty
    Alternative Techniques

Outcome

There is ongoing debate as to whether a hydronephrotic kidney is obstructed, primarily because the tools we use to measure or define obstruction are less than precise. A ureteropelvic junction (UPJ) obstruction can be thought of as a restriction to flow of urine, from the renal pelvis to the ureter, which, if left uncorrected, will lead to progressive renal deterioration (Whitaker, 1975; Koff et al, 1986; Koff, 1990). The response to obstruction is the development of renal pelvic hypertrophy, in which the kidney compensates to maintain adequate urinary flow. Eventually, there are further changes to the renal pelvis and pressure-induced injury that leads to irreversible renal damage.

This chapter considers only congenital UPJ obstruction. Other conditions that delay drainage of the proximal urinary tract and secondarily affect the UPJ are discussed elsewhere in this text.

EVIDENCE

UPJ obstruction occurs in all pediatric age groups, but there tends to be a clustering in the neonatal period because of the detection of antenatal hydronephrosis and again later in life because of symptomatic occurrence. At one point about 25% of cases were discovered within the first year of life (Williams and Kenawi, 1976), but today the majority of cases are identified and diagnosed in the perinatal period (Brown et al, 1987). **UPJ obstruction is the most common cause of significant dilation of the collecting system in the fetal kidney,** accounting for 48% of all dilation of the collecting system and far exceeding the incidence of multicystic dysplastic kidney (Colodny et al, 1980; Brown et al, 1987). The problem that exists today is that the diagnosis of UPJ is "made" at the time of prenatal ultrasonography, so that expectant parents are often informed that their fetus will most likely require surgical intervention as a neonate. This has contributed to ongoing anxiety and altered parental enjoyment during pregnancy (Harding et al, 1999).

Beyond the neonatal period, UPJ obstruction is seen during childhood and adolescence but to a lesser degree. Often, the cause is an aberrant lower-pole parenchymal vessel that crosses over the UPJ (Lowe and Marshall, 1984). **Obstruction occurs more commonly in boys than in girls** (Williams and Karlaftis, 1966, Kelalis et al, 1971; Johnston et al, 1977), especially in the newborn period, when the ratio exceeds 2:1 (Robson et al, 1976; Williams and Kenawi, 1976; Johnston et al, 1977). **Left-sided lesions predominate,** particularly in the neonate (approximately 67%). Bilateral UPJ obstruction is present in 10% to 40% of cases (Nixon, 1953; Uson et al, 1968; Robson et al, 1976; Williams and Kenawi, 1976; Johnston et al, 1977; Lebowitz and Griscom, 1977), with both synchronous and asynchronous occurrences. This tends to occur in infants younger than 6 months of age (Perlmutter et al, 1980; Snyder et al, 1980), and it has been known to affect members of more than one generation (Cohen et al, 1978).

ETIOLOGY

The precise cause of UPJ obstruction remains elusive despite investigation along a number of lines: embryologic (Osathanondh and Potter, 1963; Allen, 1973; Ruano-Gil et al, 1975), anatomic (Nixon, 1953; Johnston, 1969), functional (Whitaker, 1975), and histologic (Murnaghan, 1958; Notley, 1968; Hanna et al, 1976). A narrowing of the UPJ is often found (Allen, 1973; Lebowitz and Griscom, 1977), but whether this is a result of developmental arrest (Osathanondh and Potter, 1963; Allen, 1973) or of incomplete recanalization of the ureter (Ruano-Gil et al, 1975) is not yet known.

Intrinsic

The typical finding at the time of pyeloplasty is a narrowed segment of the ureter at the UPJ that is probe patent (Fig. 57–1). This finding may be the result of an **interruption in the development of the circular musculature of the UPJ** (Murnaghan, 1958) **or an alteration of the collagen fibers and composition between and around the muscle cells** (Notley, 1968; Hanna et al, 1976; Hanna, 2000). The muscle fibers become widely separated and attenuated, leading to a functional discontinuity of the muscular contractions and ultimately to insufficient emptying. Further characterization of the UPJ by Starr and colleagues (1992) noted a significant increase in the lamina muscularis and in the number of inner longitudinal muscular bundles of the UPJ complex of obstructed kidneys in infants younger than 1 year of age, compared with age-matched normal infants. These findings suggest a dramatic response by the muscular layers to obstruction. Further work has shown that the expression of transforming growth factor–β (TGF-β) is increased in the pelvis of partially obstructed kidneys (Seremetis and Maizels, 1996), which may help explain some of the histologic and electron microscopic findings that were described by Notley and Hanna and their colleagues.

Other causes of intrinsic UPJ obstruction include valvular mucosal folds (Maizels and Stephens, 1980), persistent fetal convolutions (Leiter, 1979), and upper ureteral polyps (Colgan et al, 1973; Gup, 1975; Williams and Kenawi, 1976; Williams et al, 1980; Thorup et al, 1981).

Congenital folds are a common finding in the upper ureter of fetuses after the fourth month of development and may persist until the newborn period. Such folds are mucosal infolds with an axial offshoot and adventitia that does not flatten out when the ureter is distended or stretched. The epithelial folds are secondary to differential growth rates of the ureter and the body of the child, with excessive ureteral length occurring early in gestation. This provides a

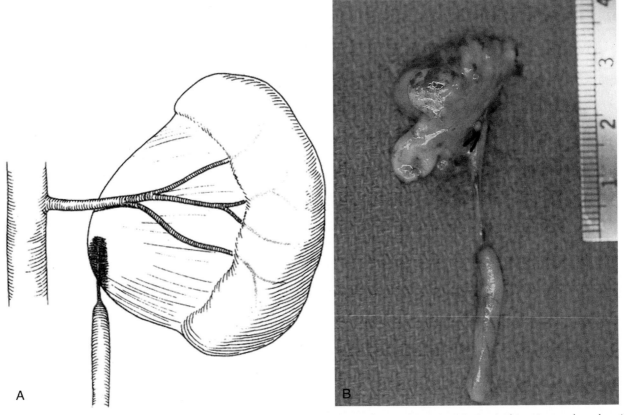

Figure 57–1. *A,* Intrinsic narrowing of upper ureter contributing to ureteropelvic junction obstruction. *B,* Surgical specimen of nonfunctioning kidney with significant proximal ureteral narrowing.

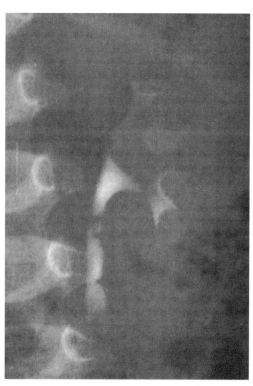

Figure 57–2. Early image of left kidney from intravenous urogram of 4-month-old girl with prenatal hydronephrosis, depicting Östling's folds.

"length reserve" for the ureter, which traverses a shorter distance in the newborn than in the adult (Östling, 1942). Östling thought that these folds were a precursor of UPJ obstruction because they frequently were discovered in babies who had a contralateral UPJ obstruction. This concept has evolved, and **"Östling's folds" are now considered folds that are not obstructive and disappear with a person's linear growth** (Leiter, 1979) (Fig. 57–2). They are rarely seen in an older child or adult. On the other hand, persistent fetal folds containing muscle and high insertion of a valvular leaflet at the UPJ may become obstructive (Maizels and Stephens, 1980). This type of obstruction sometimes can be relieved by dissection of the folds and elimination of the kinking (Johnston, 1969), but more commonly the ureteral portion containing the valve must be excised.

Extrinsic

An aberrant, accessory, or early-branching lower-pole vessel is the most common cause of extrinsic UPJ obstruction (Fig. 57–3). These vessels pass anteriorly to the UPJ or proximal ureter and contribute to mechanical obstruction. Nixon (1953) reported that 25 of 78 cases of UPJ obstruction were secondary to vascular compression; other reported incidences have varied between 15% and 52% (Ericsson et al, 1961; Williams and Kenawi, 1976, Johnston et al, 1977; Stephens, 1982; Lowe and Marshall, 1984). This is a major cause of UPJ obstruction in adults.

Whether the aberrant vessel causes obstruction or is a covariable that exists along with an intrinsic narrow-

ing is unclear. Stephens (1982) theorized that when an aberrant or accessory renal artery to the lower pole of the kidney is present and the ureter courses behind it, the ureter may angulate at both the UPJ and the point at which it traverses over the vessel as the pelvis fills and bulges anteriorly. Further angulation of the ureter occurs as it becomes adherent to the UPJ secondary to an inflammatory process. A two-point obstruction ensues, with kinking of the ureter at the UPJ and at the point where the ureter drapes over the vessel. Stephens (1982) could find no evidence of stricture or fibrosis at these points when the ureter was freed of its adhesions and lifted off the vessel. However, he suggested that, over time, these areas may become ischemic, fibrotic, and finally stenotic.

Secondary Ureteral Pelvic Junction Obstruction

UPJ obstruction may also be seen with severe vesicoureteral reflux (VUR); these conditions coexist in 10% of cases. The ureter elongates and develops a tortuous course in response to the obstructive element of reflux. A kink may develop in the UPJ area, a point of relative fixation, and may cause obstruction secondarily (Lebowitz and Blickman, 1983). In such a situation the obstructive lesion needs to be corrected initially, even though the VUR contributed to the initial problem (Fig. 57–4).

Associated Anomalies

Congenital renal malformations are commonly seen in association with UPJ obstruction. Other urologic abnormal-

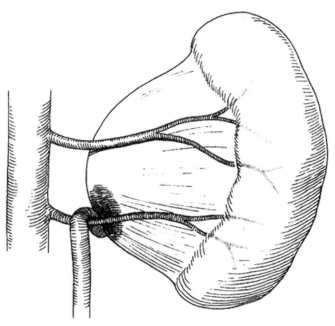

Figure 57–3. A lower-pole–crossing vessel contributes to significant kinking at the ureteropelvic junction and resultant intermittent obstruction. Often, when the ureter is mobilized, no evidence of intrinsic narrowing is found. Insertional anomaly and peripelvic fibrosis may also be present as secondary obstructive factors.

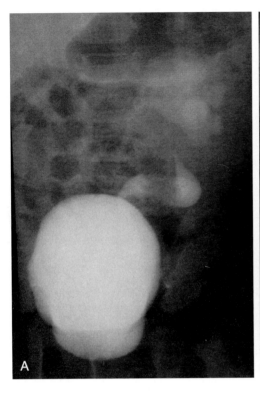
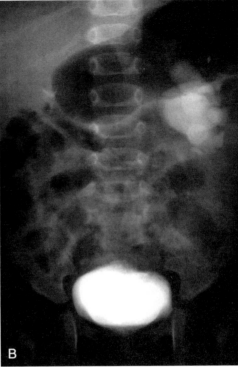

Figure 57–4. *A*, Voiding cystourethrogram demonstrating left vesicoureteral reflux. Note dilutional effect of contrast in renal pelvis. *B*, Postvoid view demonstrating right grade II vesicoureteral reflux and significant retained contrast in left renal pelvis. Patient developed worsening left hydronephrosis, which was observed on subsequent ultrasound imaging, and underwent a left dismembered pyeloplasty. There was evidence of a lower-pole–crossing vessel contributing to intermittent kinking of the ureter.

ities may be found in 50% of affected infants (Uson et al, 1968; Robson et al, 1976; Lebowitz and Griscom, 1977). **UPJ obstruction is the most common anomaly encountered in the opposite kidney;** it occurs in 10% to 40% of cases. Renal dysplasia and multicystic dysplastic kidney are the next most frequently observed contralateral lesions (Williams and Karlaftis, 1966). In addition, unilateral renal agenesis has been noted in almost 5% of children (Robson et al, 1976; Williams and Kenawi, 1976; Johnston et al, 1977). UPJ obstruction may also occur in either the upper or the lower half (usually the latter) of a duplicated collecting system (Amar, 1976; Joseph et al, 1989) (Fig. 57–5) or of a horseshoe or ectopic kidney (Fig. 57–6).

VUR has been found in as many as 40% of affected children (Williams and Kenawi, 1976; Juskiewenski et al, 1983; Lebowitz and Blickman, 1983). This degree of reflux is often low grade, not contributing to upper urinary tract obstruction, and with a high likelihood of spontaneous resolution. In certain situations, high-grade VUR can have a profound effect on the UPJ, as previously noted. Anomalies of other organ systems are frequently observed but without any consistent pattern of inheritance. UPJ obstruction was noted in 21% of children with the VATER (*v*ertebral defects, imperforate *a*nus, *t*racheo*e*sophageal fistula, and *r*adial and *r*enal dysplasia) association (Uehling et al, 1983), and a more recent review showed a high percentage of hydronephrosis, UPJ obstruction, or VUR in such patients (Kolon et al, 2000).

SYMPTOMS/PRESENTATION

The dichotomy of presentation of infants and children with UPJ obstruction is that **most infants are asympto-**

matic and most children are discovered because of their symptoms. Previously, infants were discovered to have UPJ obstruction because of a palpable mass (Williams and Karlaftis, 1966; Robson et al, 1976; Johnston et al, 1977). Now, the almost universal use of prenatal sonography has made discovery of UPJ obstruction a common occurrence. It has changed our approach to evaluation, because now we are attempting to prove that a problem exists in an otherwise asymptomatic infant. There are still occasionally infants who present with failure to thrive, feeding difficulties, sepsis secondary to urinary tract infection, or pain or he-

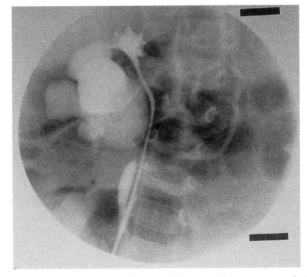

Figure 57–5. Retrograde pyelogram demonstrating anatomy of right incomplete renal duplication with lower-pole ureteropelvic junction obstruction.

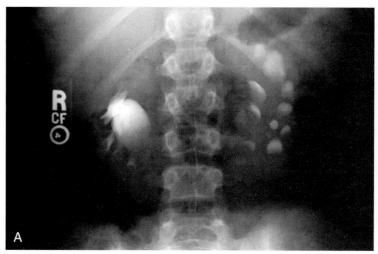

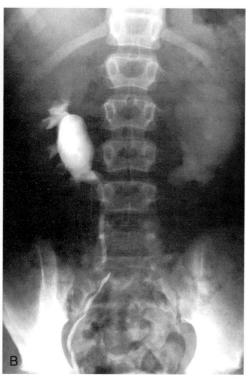

Figure 57–6. *A,* Intravenous urogram (10-minute image) showing delayed uptake and excretion of contrast from left kidney. *B,* Thirty-minute image demonstrating horseshoe kidney and wisp of contrast in proximal left ureter. Patient was found to have high insertion and intermittent kinking of the ureter, which was contributing to periodic abdominal pain. He presented with gross hematuria after being struck by a soccer ball.

maturia related to nephrolithiasis. Urinary tract infection is the presenting sign in 30% of affected children beyond the neonatal period (Snyder et al, 1980).

In the older child, episodic flank or upper abdominal pain, sometimes associated with nausea and vomiting due to intermittent UPJ obstruction, is a prominent symptom (Kelalis et al, 1971; Williams and Kenawi, 1976)

(Fig. 57–7). At other times, cyclic vomiting alone is caused by intermittent UPJ obstruction. The pathology may be manifested only during the episode of cyclic vomiting and/or abdominal pain. Hematuria, which is seen in 25% of children, may occur after minor abdominal trauma (Kelalis et al, 1971; Williams and Kenawi, 1976). This hematuria is believed to be caused by disruption and rupture of

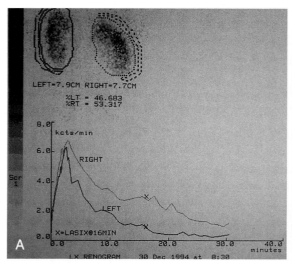

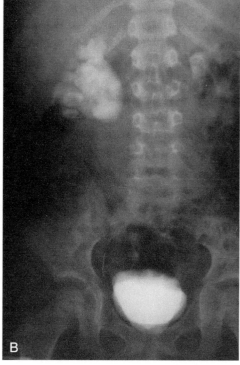

Figure 57–7. *A,* MAG-3 Lasix renogram of patient with mild to moderate right hydronephrosis and a history of intermittent abdominal pain. *B,* Intravenous urogram obtained after the patient developed right flank pain and hematuria following a fall from bicycle, consistent with ureteropelvic junction obstruction.

mucosal vessels in the dilated collecting system (Kelalis et al, 1971). In the young adult, episodic flank or abdominal pain, particularly during diuresis, is a common manifestation. Occasionally, a patient with the UPJ obstruction presents with hypertension (Squitieri et al, 1974; Johnston et al, 1977; Munoz et al, 1977; Grossman et al, 1981). The pathophysiology is thought to be a functional ischemia with reduced blood flow caused by the enlarged collecting system that produces a renin-mediated hypertension (Belman et al, 1968).

DIAGNOSIS

In the evaluation of prenatal hydronephrosis, a number of different recommendations and algorithms have been devised (Homsey et al, 1990; Blyth et al, 1993; Cendron et al, 1994). Postnatal ultrasound imaging is usually deferred until day 3 of life, to allow for improvement in the relative oliguria, which could lead to underestimation of the degree of hydronephrosis. The fetal and neonatal kidney may appear to be hydronephrotic on ultrasonography secondary to the sonolucent appearance of the medullary area and pyramids. This appearance tends to resolve after parenchymal maturation, which occurs at 3 months of age. Further evaluation includes a voiding cystourethrogram or nuclear voiding cystourethrogram study to rule out the presence of VUR, which is reported to occur in 13% to 42% of infants studied (Anderson et al, 1997; Zerin et al, 1993). Some investigations have reported a predominance of boys detected with VUR (Bouachrine et al, 1996), whereas others are evenly divided between boys and girls (Anderson et al, 1997). Each instance underscores the need for postnatal investigation of infants with a renal pelvic measurement of 5 mm or greater and reinforces the notion that a normal postnatal ultrasound scan does not preclude the presence of VUR (Jaswon et al, 1999).

A number of diagnostic studies have been and are still used to define whether a kidney is obstructed. They have generally been used in adult patients and then applied to the pediatric/neonatal population. The neonatal kidney is undergoing considerable growth and development. Ongoing obstruction may lead not only to functional deterioration but to impairment of the functional potential of the kidney (Peters, 1995). Some of the diagnostic tests that have been used and some of the newer methods that complement these studies are briefly presented here.

Ultrasonography

Ultrasonography is the standard method for identifying hydronephrosis in infancy. The size of the renal pelvis (anteroposterior diameter) can correlate with the likelihood of obstruction, but this **does not diagnose obstruction, nor can it answer whether the hydronephrosis will improve or worsen.** This is particularly true in the newborn, in whom hydronephrosis may transiently disappear after birth or fluctuate significantly with time, hydration, and bladder fullness. Sequential studies become meaningful, because they define a trend with regard to the hydronephro-

sis. Worsening hydronephrosis usually indicates obstruction, and improved hydronephrosis suggests the opposite.

To further improve the diagnostic accuracy of ultrasonography, the renal parenchyma/pelvicaliceal area has been measured and compared with the result of conventional diuretic renography. A ratio of less than 1.6 correlates well with an obstructive process and need for pyeloplasty, whereas patients with a ratio greater than 1.6 can be safely observed (Cost et al, 1996). These measurements are more stringent than measurements of anteroposterior diameter but are certainly more operator dependent. On the other hand, they reflect the amount of pelvocaliectasis that exists, which is more meaningful than pelvic diameter alone.

Serial ultrasound measurements can provide another useful parameter in helping to confirm the presence or absence of obstruction by monitoring changes in the growth rate of the normal kidney opposite the hydronephrosis (Koff et al, 1994; Koff and Peller, 1995). Obstruction of one kidney can lead to functional changes in its contralateral mate, affecting its rate of growth. A renal growth–renal function chart was generated with four reproducible, clinically relevant diagnostic patterns derived. Obstruction of one kidney manifests as a decrease of overall function as well as an increase in the growth rate of its contralateral mate. Application of this technique at other institutions did not reveal a significant correlation between unilateral hydronephrosis and contralateral renal length (Brandell et al, 1996).

Renal duplex Doppler ultrasound has also shown promise as a means of identifying obstruction. A resistive index (RI) is defined as the peak systolic velocity minus the lowest diastolic velocity divided by the peak systolic velocity. Infants younger than 1 year of age had a greater resistive index (0.66) than did children older than 1 year of age (0.57). In hydronephrotic kidneys, the **RI values were much higher in those kidneys that had an obstructive pattern on diuretic renography** (RI $\geq$ 0.75) (Gilbert et al, 1993). When these Doppler studies were modified by the addition of furosemide, the differences between obstructed and nonobstructed kidneys were further accentuated. In addition, follow-up of these patients also demonstrated that the RI normalized after successful pyeloplasty (average preoperative RI, 0.87; average postoperative RI, 0.63) (Ordorica et al, 1993).

Magnetic Resonance Imaging

New, ultrafast magnetic resonance imaging (MRI) offers unique advantages for evaluating renal blood flow, anatomy, and urinary excretion. Anatomic analysis of MRI noncontrast studies showed precise dilatation of the hydronephrotic pelvis and cortical medullary junction in a rat model with unilateral congenital hydronephrosis (Fichtner et al, 1994). After injection of contrast gadolinium–diethylenetriamine-pentaacetic acid (DTPA), signal intensity from the region of interest of hydronephrotic kidneys differed from that of nonhydronephrotic kidneys by showing less cortical decrease, suggesting decreased blood flow, less medullary decrease, and delayed contrast excretion. These techniques are beginning to gain acceptance and hold the promise for a single study that can provide information on both perfusion and function. The evaluation of renal perfusion with MRI has become feasible with the development of rapid data acquisition techniques, which provide adequate temporal resolution to monitor the rapid signal changes during the first passage of contrast agents in the kidneys (Bennett and Li, 1997). More recently, magnetically labeled water protons in blood flowing into kidneys have been used to noninvasively quantitate regional measurement of cortical and medullary perfusion. Other techniques being investigated with MRI for assessment of renal function include diffusion imaging glomerular filtration rate (GFR) estimation and blood oxygenation level–dependent imaging to evaluate intrarenal oxygenation levels.

Radionuclide Renography

Intravenous urography was in the past the primary radiographic study used to define UPJ obstruction. In most institutions, this has been supplanted by **radionuclide renography, which provides differential renal function data and an assessment of washout from the individual kidney.** Several radiopharmaceuticals have been used, each with slightly different properties. DTPA is eliminated entirely by glomerular filtration, with an extraction efficiency of 20%. Because it is excreted only by glomerular filtration, this agent provides an indirect means of measuring the GFR. Differential GFR can be determined by comparing the amount of uptake in each kidney during the first 1 to 3 minutes after intravenous injection (Rowell et al, 1986).

Mercaptoacetyltriglycine (MAG-3) is cleared by the kidneys primarily by tubular secretion and to a lesser extent by glomerular filtration. Therefore, MAG-3 is an excellent agent for estimating the effective renal plasma flow. Differential renal plasma flow measured with MAG-3 correlates reasonably well with differential renal function. Because it is not retained in the parenchyma of the normal kidney for very long, MAG-3 also provides excellent imaging characteristics. In addition, it may be more effective than other radiopharmaceutical agents in cases of renal functional impairment because of its relatively high degree of renal tubular secretion.

Pressure-Flow Studies

Whitaker (1978) defined obstruction in the kidney as impedance to flow such that proximal pressure must be raised to transmit the usual flow rate through it. His study involved placing catheters into the renal pelvis and bladder, infusing fluid at a rate of 10 ml/sec into the kidney, and measuring the intrapelvic pressure of the kidney. A differential pressure between kidney and bladder could then be indicative of obstruction to the kidney. Whitaker studies are usually not performed in pediatric patients, but the concept of measuring intrapelvic pressure to help delineate whether obstruction exists remains. For example, infusion of the renal pelvis of hydronephrotic kidneys is performed, and the decrease in pressure with time is determined as a pressure decay curve (Fung et al, 1996). As might be

expected, renal units without elevated pelvic pressure during infusion at a high physiologic flow rate have relatively rapid pressure decay, whereas those with elevated renal pelvic pressure during infusion are associated with much slower pressure decay. The diuretic nuclear renography half-lives ($T_{1/2}$) have no correlation with collecting system pressure dynamics. The pressure decay half-life reflects both efficient urine transport and the relative compliance and volume of the collecting system. Further refinements with this technique of antegrade nephrostomy have included measurement of the ureteral opening pressure, which is defined as the pressure at which contrast material is first seen beyond the suspected site of obstruction (Fung et al, 1998). In all patients with a renal pelvic pressure greater than 14 cm H_2O, the pressure-flow study also demonstrated evidence of obstruction. In contrast, negative ureteral opening pressure had a much lower specificity or negative predictive value.

Biochemical Parameters

Various biochemical markers have been used as indicators of renal tubular injury in the setting of obstructive uropathy. Such markers could be assessed to determine the need for intervention, based on a detrimental change. N-acetyl-β-D-glucosaminidase (NAG) was measured in patients who were thought to have a UPJ obstruction (Carr et al, 1994). Urinary NAG levels were consistently elevated in urine obtained directly from the kidney, although bladder urines did not provide a significant discriminator when compared with control urinary NAG levels. A similar observation was made when urinary TGF-β1 was measured in children with UPJ obstruction (Palmer et al, 1997). The presence of TGF-β mRNA was noted in the renal pelvis after both clinical and experimental UPJ obstruction and may relate to the adaptive molecular responses that increase muscle and collagen in the renal pelvis (Seremetis and Maizels, 1996). A biochemical or molecular marker that is found in the urine and is easily assayed would hold the greatest promise of improving diagnostic ability in obstructive uropathy.

SURGICAL REPAIR

The evolution in the surgical correction of UPJ obstruction has occurred on a number of fronts, with open surgical techniques yielding way to endoscopic and laparoscopic approaches. The open techniques that have had the greatest applicability can be classified into three main groups: the flap type, the incisional-incubated type, and the dismembered type. The Anderson-Hynes pyeloplasty (1949) has become the most commonly employed "open" surgical procedure for the repair of UPJ. This repair had as its underpinnings both the Foley Y-V plasty (1937) and the Davis intubated ureterotomy (1943).

The Foley operation was designed for the correction of UPJ with a high ureteral insertion. As such, this technique cannot be used in conjunction with transposition of a lower-pole vessel, nor does it allow for any significant reduction of the renal pelvic size. The Davis intubated ureterotomy depends on secondary epithelialization from the incised ureter. It is applicable when multiple or extensive strictures of the proximal ureter are present but cannot be bridged by a pelvic flap. Its use requires maintenance of ureteral continuity on at least one side and the presence of an indwelling ureteral stent for 6 weeks, the time needed for full circumferential regeneration of all layers of the ureter.

Culp and DeWeerd's (1951) spiral flap is created from the renal pelvis, which is used to repair the defect at the UPJ. Such a flap is able to bridge the gap between the pelvis and healthy ureter over a distance of several centimeters. Scardino and Prince (1953) described a vertical flap that can be used in the situation of a dependent UPJ with a large, square-shaped extrarenal pelvis. The rare cases of giant hydronephrosis that may be associated with a completely atretic ureter can be corrected by reconstructing the entire ureter using redundant pelvic tissue (Kheradpir, 1983).

Dismembered Pyeloplasty

The technique of dismembering the ureter was borne out of necessity in the repair of a retrocaval ureter (Anderson and Hynes, 1949). This technique was embraced by English surgeons in the repair of UPJ obstruction, but there was reluctance on the part of surgeons elsewhere because of concerns about severing the neural continuity between pelvis and ureter. Later work, however, demonstrated that the bolus of urine is the peristaltic stimulus. Furthermore, injection studies (Douville and Hollingshead, 1955) demonstrated that the arborization of blood vessels in the renal pelvis would ensure appropriate healing even with dismembering.

The principal reasons for the universal acceptance of the dismembered pyeloplasty are (1) broad applicability, including preservation of anomalous vessels; (2) excision of the pathologic UPJ and appropriate repositioning; and (3) successful reduction pyeloplasty. This operation is generally easy to perform and can be accomplished by a number of surgical approaches, including anterior subcostal, flank, and posterior lumbotomy.

A dismembered pyeloplasty may be problematic if there is inadequate ureteral length. A spiral flap from the renal pelvis can overcome this problem. Alternatively, excision of all scar tissue along with a dismembered technique is often possible when the kidney is completely mobilized and brought down as a "reverse" nephropexy. This can provide an additional 5 cm of length, avoiding such maneuvers as bowel interposition, ureterocalicostomy, or autotransplantation.

The age and size of the patient and the position of UPJ are factors that must be considered when choosing a surgical approach. A posterior lumbotomy affords good exposure in the neonate but may not be a good choice in a muscular adolescent. The position of the UPJ can be determined from an intravenous urogram, but most surgeons now perform renal scans instead. Therefore, retrograde pyelography can be used for making this determination. Cockrell and Hendren (1990) noted the benefits of performing retrograde pyelography at the time of pyeloplasty. Findings included a discrete area of narrowing, a long segment of narrowing, tortuosity of the upper ureter, more than one area of narrowing, high insertion of the ureter on the renal pelvis, and compression of the ureter by the lower pole of the kidney. Rushton and colleagues (1994) noted that their surgical findings confirmed obstruction at the UPJ in all patients. Undiagnosed distal ureteral obstruction was not seen, and therefore routine retrograde pyelography is not necessary.

The actual repair for the modified Anderson-Hynes dismembered pyeloplasty, as performed through an anterior subcostal incision, is as follows:

1. The anterior subcostal incision is a muscle-splitting incision that is made with the patient supine and a roll placed transversely beneath the patient to elevate the flank.

2. Each muscle layer encountered is split in the direction of the muscle fibers until Gerota's fascia is identified by sweeping the peritoneum medially. The fascia is then incised posteriorly over the lateral aspect of the kidney.

3. The renal pelvis is identified by medial retraction of the peritoneum and lateral traction of the kidney. If the renal pelvis is significantly dilated, an angiocath can be inserted to decompress the pelvis and facilitate identification of the UPJ.

4. Anterior exposure is usually better when a dismembered pyeloplasty is being performed. **Once the ureter and UPJ are identified, a traction suture is displaced anteriorly through the proximal ureter** to minimize subsequent handling.

5. The area of UPJ is dissected free to allow for a clear area in which to perform the anastomosis. **Traction sutures may be placed in the renal pelvis superiorly, medially, laterally, and inferiorly to the UPJ.** Once adequate ureteral length is confirmed and the pathology of UPJ identified, the ureter can be transected at the UPJ. If the ureter is short, the kidney is completely mobilized to determine whether it can be brought down sufficiently to allow for a primary tension-free anastomosis.

6. After transection of the UPJ, the renal pelvis may not spontaneously drain until it is incised. This should be done after the site for anastomosis is chosen.

7. The **ureter is spatulated on the side opposite to the traction suture** using Potts tenotomy scissors. The distance over which the ureter is opened is variable, until healthy ureter is encountered, which springs open when forceps are placed into it.

8. The **portion of pelvis is excised,** usually a diamond-shaped segment that is present within the traction sutures that were placed in the renal pelvis. It is better to leave too much renal pelvis than too little, especially when resecting along the medial aspect of the renal pelvis. Infundibula can be encountered if one is not careful.

9. The ureter and renal pelvis are aligned to ensure that the anastomosis can be accomplished without tension. If a nephrostomy tube is to be used, it is placed at this time. An inferior calix is chosen, preferably where the overlying parenchyma is not too thick. A Malecot catheter works well and is positioned away from the repair to minimize the chance of the catheter's causing urinary blockage through the reconstructed UPJ.

10. The anastomosis is started by placing the first suture at the apex of the "V" in the ureter and into the tip of the inferior pelvic flap. As the suture is tied down, the ureter and renal pelvis are brought together to minimize tension on the repair. A small feeding tube is placed into the ureter; it can be used to stabilize the ureter during the anastomosis. **A "no-touch" technique is employed with the ureter to minimize trauma and edema** to the ureteral tissue. Either interrupted sutures or a running closure may be used, depending on the surgeon's preference. The area of the initial anastomosis is critical to ensuring a watertight closure.

11. Before the repair is completed, the renal pelvis is irrigated to remove any blood clots or debris that could obstruct the UPJ. If an indwelling JJ ureteral stent is employed, it should be placed now, with care taken to place the stent into the bladder and renal pelvis without kinking it.

12. A Penrose drain is placed adjacent to the repair and brought out through a separate stab wound.

13. The kidney is returned to its native position, and perinephric fat, if available, is placed over the anastomosis.

14. Closure of the three fascia is readily accomplished, followed by closure of Scarpa's fascia and subcuticular skin.

15. A Foley catheter, which was placed at the beginning of the procedure, may be left in place for 24 to 48 hours postoperatively. The Penrose drain usually can be removed before discharge or, if left in place, it can easily be removed in the office 7 to 10 days postoperatively.

Posterior Lumbotomy

The patient is placed in a prone position with a roll under the chest, pelvis, and knees. After the skin incision, Scarpa's fascia is sharply incised and a vertical incision is made through the lumbodorsal fascia (posterior lamella). The lateral edge of the lumbodorsal fascia is elevated, and the sacrospinalis muscle is medially retracted. An incision is made through the middle and anterior lamella of the lumbodorsal fascia, taking care not to injure the ileohypogastric nerve. The quadratus lumborum muscle is retracted, exposing Gerota's fascia beneath the paranephric fat, and then this fascia is opened. The renal pelvis is identified, and several holding stitches are placed in the pelvis. The ureter is identified, a holding stitch is placed in the ureter, and the surgeon proceeds with the dismembered pyeloplasty.

Flank Approach

The patient is placed over the kidney rest in a flank position; the kidney rest is elevated and the operating room table is flexed. The skin incision is made off the tip of the 12th rib, or, if necessary, a supracostal 12th rib incision is made. The external oblique and latissimus dorsi muscles are divided. Next the internal oblique and serratus posterior inferior muscle are divided. The transversalis muscle is often thin and can be divided with digital dissection. The peritoneum is identified and retracted medially. Gerota's fascia is then encountered and opened longitudinally to gain exposure to the perinephric space. After identification of the renal pelvis and the ureter, a dismembered pyeloplasty can be performed as described earlier.

Alternative Techniques

Minimally invasive approaches in the repair of UPJ obstruction include pyeloplasties performed laparoscopically (Schuessler, 1993; Chen et al, 1998; Tan, 1999) and endoscopic approaches. A thorough description of laparoscopic pyeloplasties can be found elsewhere in this text.

Endoscopic Approaches

The endoscopic approach to the UPJ has been successful in both an anterograde and retrograde fashion. The initial attempts at balloon dilatation (Tan et al, 1995) have been superseded by the use of an Acucise device (Applied Medical, ureteral cutting balloon catheter, No. 5 Fr) (Bolton et al, 1994). Postoperative stenting is required for 6 weeks, with a 100% success rate being reported in a small series of patients. In a much larger series of adult patients, Kim et al (1998) reported an overall success rate of 78%. Two patients required angiographic studies and embolization of lower-pole branching arteries because they developed gross hematuria after Acucise endopyelotomy.

Antegrade endopyelotomy can readily be accomplished in both adults and preadolescent or adolescent patients. Figenshau and Clayman (1998) recommended this procedure for any patient with a reasonably functioning kidney, mild to moderate hydronephrosis, and no evidence of a crossing vessel. Computed tomography or MRI can be used for preoperative assessment of a crossing vessel, or an endoluminal ultrasonography can be performed before the procedure. The antegrade endopyelotomy requires access to the kidney via a midpole posterior calix. Direct visualization of UPJ obstruction allows for use of a cold knife, electrocautery, and even contact laser fiber to achieve the endopyelotomy (Renner et al, 1998). After fluoroscopic documentation of successful incision and/or dilation of the UPJ, a double-pigtail ureteral stent is placed under direct vision in the renal collecting system and fluoroscopically positioned into the bladder.

The need for fluoroscopy for urologic intervention along with two and sometimes three anesthetics for preoperative stent placement (nephrostomy tube placement), endopyelotomy, and subsequent stent removal must be weighed against the more invasive open dismembered pyeloplasty. Older pediatric patients may be managed with the less invasive procedures, with the expectation of good results (80% to 85% success) and improved postoperative convalescence. The ideal situation exists in the case of a failed pyeloplasty, because the UPJ should be in a dependent location (Fig. 57–8). A nephrostomy tube may already be in place and a stricture or stenosis is most likely to be encountered at the UPJ. After a successful endopyelotomy, a double-pigtail ureteral stent is maintained for 6 weeks. Unlike the adult endopyelotomy stent (No. 14 Fr/7 Fr), a pediatric endopyelotomy stent does not exist. The ideal stent would be a biodegradable stent that would not require removal (Lumiaho et al, 2000).

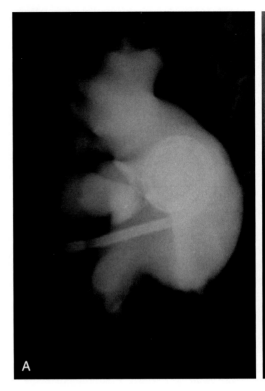 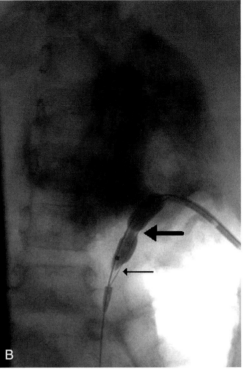

Figure 57–8. *A,* Right antegrade nephrostogram performed 2 months after dismembered pyeloplasty, demonstrating persistent obstruction at the ureteropelvic junction. A nephrostomy tube was placed 2 weeks after surgery, after the patient developed flank pain, fever, and *Staphylococcus aureus* urinary tract infection. *B,* Acucise balloon being inflated across the ureteropelvic junction narrowing. Note waist present in balloon *(upper arrow)* and cutting wire positioned laterally *(lower arrow).*

OUTCOME

Adherence to sound surgical principles, minimal handling of the ureter at the time of repair, and judicious use of internal stenting or nephrostomy tube drainage ensure a successful outcome. Success is defined as improvement in hydronephrosis and stabilization or improvement in function on renal scan along with a decrease in washout time. In those situations in which symptomatic presentation occurred, resolution of flank/abdominal pain or vomiting should also occur.

Imaging of the kidneys postoperatively depends on whether a nephrostomy tube has been used. A nephrostogram performed 10 to 14 days after surgery allows for visualization of the anastomosis. Others have simply clamped the nephrostomy tube for 24 hours and checked the residual in the renal pelvis. If the residual is less than 15 ml, then the nephrostomy tube is removed (Flint et al, 1998). If a double-pigtail ureteral stent is left indwelling, it is removed 6 to 8 weeks after the initial procedure. A renal ultrasound is obtained 6 weeks after pyeloplasty or after stent removal to ensure that the hydronephrosis (pelvocal-

iectasis) is improving. A renal scan is obtained 1 year after the pyeloplasty to provide a relative assessment of the overall renal function. Long-term imaging at 3 years may be obtained to look for that rare situation of delayed cicatrization and restenosis of the UPJ. Table 57–1 lists the results from a number of contemporary series of pyeloplasties.

Early complications of pyeloplasty are uncommon and usually involve prolonged urinary leakage from the Penrose drain. Depending on the amount of drainage, observation is generally the best approach. If it persists beyond 10 to 14 days, placement of a retrograde ureteral stent can often rectify the situation. Spontaneously delayed opening of the anastomosis has occurred as late as several months after the repair. If a patient presents postoperatively with fever, flank pain, and significant hydronephrosis, a nephrostomy tube may be necessary to decompress the kidney. Lack of drainage for a prolonged period would necessitate further intervention, including an endopyelotomy, redo pyeloplasty, or even ureterocalicostomy. It is not advisable to embark on such a procedure before 2 months postoperatively.

Future surgical progress will be made in understanding the underlying factors that contribute to the formation of UPJ obstruction, along with continuing improvements in successful surgical approaches. The day will come when biological modifiers are used to facilitate appropriate wound healing and further reduce the already low incidence of complications.

REFERENCES

Allen TD: Congenital ureteral strictures. In Lutzeyer W, Melchior H (eds): Urodynamic: Upper and Lower Urinary Tract. Berlin, Springer-Verlag, 1973, pp 137–147.

Table 57–1. PYELOPLASTY

Author and Year	Patients/Kidneys	Success (%)
Poulsen et al, 1987	35	100
O'Reilly, 1989	30	83–93
MacNeily et al, 1993	75	85
Shaul et al, 1994	32/33 (<2 mo old)	97
	30/33 (>2 mo old)	93
Salem et al, 1995	100	98
McAleer and Kaplan, 1999	79	90
Austin et al, 2000	135/137	91
Houben et al, 2000	186/203	93

Amar AD: Congenital hydronephrosis of lower segment in duplex kidney. Urology 1976;7:480–485.

Anderson JC, Hynes W: Retrocaval ureter: A case diagnosed preoperatively and treated successfully by a plastic operation. Br J Urol 1949; 21:209.

Anderson NG, Abbott GD, Mogridge N, et al: Vesicoureteric reflux in the newborn: Relationship of fetal renal pelvic diameter. Pediatr Nephrol 1997;11:610–616.

Austin PF, Cain MP, Rink RC: Nephrostomy tube drainage with pyeloplasty: Is it necessarily a bad choice? J Urol 2000;163:1528–1530.

Belman AB, Kropp KF, Simon NM: Renal pressor hypertension secondary to unilateral hydronephrosis. N Engl J Med 1968;278:1133.

Bennett HF, Li D: MR imaging of renal function. Magn Reson Imaging Clin North Am 1997;5:107–126.

Blyth B, Snyder HM, Duckett JW: Antenatal diagnosis and subsequent management of hydronephrosis. J Urol 1993;149:693–698.

Bolton DM, Bogaert GA, Mevorach RA, et al: Pediatric ureteropelvic junction obstruction treated with retrograde endopyelotomy. Urology 1994;44:609–613.

Bouachrine H, Lemelle JL, Didier F, Schmitt M: A follow-up study of prenatally detected primary vesicoureteric reflux: A review of 61 patients. Br J Urol 1996;78:936–939.

Brandell RA, Brock JW III, Hamilton BD, et al: Unilateral hydronephrosis in infants: Are measurements of contralateral renal length useful? J Urol 1996;156:188–189.

Brown T, Mandell J, Lebowitz RL: Neonatal hydronephrosis in the era of ultrasonography. AJR Am J Roentgenol 1987;148:959–963.

Carr MC, Peters CA, Retik AB, Mandell J: Urinary levels of the renal tubular enzyme N-acetyl-beta-D-glucosaminidase in unilateral obstructive uropathy. J Urol 1994;151:442–445.

Cendron M, D'Alton ME, Crombleholme TM: Prenatal diagnosis and management of the fetus with hydronephrosis. Semin Perinatol 1994;18:163–181.

Chen RN, Moore RG, Kavoussi LR: Laparoscopic pyeloplasty: Indications, technique and long-term outcome. Urol Clin North Am 1998;25:323–330.

Cockrell SN, Hendren WH: The importance of visualizing the ureter before performing a pyeloplasty. J Urol 1990;144:588–592.

Cohen B, Goldman SM, Kopilnick M, et al: Ureteropelvic junction obstruction: Its occurrence in 3 members of a single family. J Urol 1978; 120:361–364.

Colgan JR III, Skaist L, Morrow JW: Benign ureteral tumors in childhood: A case report and a plea for conservative management. J Urol 1973;109:308–310.

Colodny AH, Retik AB, Bauer SB: Antenatal diagnosis of fetal urologic abnormalities by intrauterine ultrasonography: Therapeutic implications. Presented at Annual Meeting of the American Urological Association, San Francisco, May 18, 1980.

Cost GA, Merguerian PA, Cheerasarn SP, Shortliffe LM: Sonographic renal parenchymal and pelvicaliceal areas: New quantitative parameters for renal sonographic follow-up. J Urol 1996;145:725–729.

Culp OS, DeWeerd JH: A pelvic flap operation for certain types of ureteropelvic obstruction: Preliminary report. Mayo Clinic Proc 1951; 26:483.

Davis DM: Intubated ureterotomy: A new operation for ureteral and ureteropelvic stricture. Surg Gynecol Obstet 1943;76:513.

Douville H, Hollingshead WH: Blood supply of normal renal pelvis. J Urol 1955;73:906–909.

Ericsson NO, Rudhe U, Livaditis A: Hydronephrosis associated with aberrant renal vessels in infants and children. Surgery 1961;50:687–690.

Fichtner J, Spielman D, Herfkens R, et al: Ultrafast contrast enhanced resonance imaging of congenital hydronephrosis in a rat model. J Urol 1994;152:682–687.

Figenshau RS, Clayman RV: Endourologic options for management of ureteropelvic junction obstruction in the pediatric patient. Urol Clin North Am 1998;25:199–210.

Flint LD, Libertino JA, Doyle DE: Ureteropelvic junction obstruction. In Libertino JA (ed): Reconstructive Urologic Surgery, 3rd ed. St. Louis, Mosby, 1998, pp 155–177.

Foley FEB: New plastic operation for stricture at the ureteropelvic junction. J Urol 1937;38:643.

Fung LCT, Khoury AE, McLorie GA, et al: Pressure decay half life: A method for characterizing upper urinary tract urine transport. J Urol 1996;155:1045–1049.

Fung LCT, Churchill BM, McLorie GA, et al: Ureteral opening pressure: A novel parameter for the evaluation of pediatric hydronephrosis. J Urol 1998;159:1326–1330.

Gilbert R, Garra B, Gibbons MD: Renal duplex Doppler ultrasound: An adjunct in the evaluation of hydronephrosis in the child. J Urol 1993; 150:1192–1194.

Grossman IC, Cromie WJ, Wein AJ, Duckett JW: Renal hypertension secondary to ureteropelvic junction obstruction. Urology 1981;17:69–72.

Gup A: Benign mesodermal polyp in childhood. J Urol 1975;114:619–620.

Hanna MK, Jeffs RD, Sturgess JM, Barkin M: Ureteral structure and ultrastructure: Part II. Congenital ureteropelvic junction obstruction and primary obstructive megaureter. J Urol 1976;116:725–730.

Hanna JK: Antenatal hydronephrosis and ureteropelvic junction obstruction: The case for early intervention. Urology 2000;55:612–615.

Harding LJ, Malone PSJ, Wellesley DG: Antenatal minimal hydronephrosis: Is its follow-up an unnecessary cause of concern? Prenat Diagn 1999;19:701–705.

Homsey YL, Saad F, Laberge I, et al: Transitional hydronephrosis of the newborn and infant. J Urol 1990;144:579–583.

Houben CH, Wischermann A, Borner G, Slaney E: Outcome analysis of pyeloplasty in infants. Pediatr Surg Int 2000;16:189–193.

Jaswon MS, Dibble L, Puri S, et al: Prospective study of outcome in antenatally diagnosed renal pelvis dilatation. Arch Dis Child Fetal Neonatal Ed 1999;80:F135–F138.

Johnston JH: The pathogenesis of hydronephrosis in children. Br J Urol 1969;41:724–734.

Johnston JH, Evans JP, Glassberg KI, Shapiro SR: Pelvic hydronephrosis in children: A review of 219 personal cases. J Urol 1977;117:97–101.

Joseph DB, Bauer SB, Colodny AH, et al: Lower pole ureteropelvic junction obstruction and incomplete duplication. J Urol 1989;141:896–899.

Juskiewenski S, Moscovici J, Bouissou F, et al: Le syndrome de la junction pyelo-ureterale chez l'enfant: A propos de 178 observations. J d'Urologie 1983;89:173–182.

Kelalis PP, Culp OS, Stickler GB, Burke EC: Ureteropelvic obstruction in children: Experiences with 109 cases. J Urol 1971;106:418–422.

Kheradpir MH: Neo-ureter made from renal pelvis: A new method for treatment of giant hydronephrosis. Z Kinderchir 1983;38:361–362.

Kim FJ, Herrell SD, Jahoda AE, Albala DM: Complications of Acucise endopyelotomy. J Endourol 1998;12:433–436.

Koff SA: Pathophysiology of ureteropelvic junction obstructions. Urol Clin North Am 1990;17:263–272.

Koff SA, Hayden LJ, Cirulli C, Shore R: Pathophysiology of ureteropelvic junction obstruction: Experimental and clinical observations. J Urol 1986;136:336–338.

Koff SA, Peller PA: Diagnostic criteria for assessing obstruction in the newborn with unilateral hydronephrosis using the renal growth–renal function chart. J Urol 1995;154:662–666.

Koff SA, Peller PA, Young DC, Pollifrome DL: The assessment of obstruction in the newborn with unilateral hydronephrosis by measuring the size of the opposite kidney. J Urol 1994;152:596–599.

Kolon TF, Gray CL, Sutherland RW, et al: Upper urinary tract manifestations of the VACTERL association. J Urol 2000;163:1949–1951.

Lebowitz RL, Blickman JG: The coexistence of ureteropelvic junction obstruction and reflux. AJR Am J Roentgenol 1983;140:231–238.

Lebowitz RI, Griscom NT: Neonatal hydronephrosis: 146 cases. Radiol Clin North Am 1977;15:49–59.

Leiter E: Persistent fetal ureter. J Urol 1979;122:251–254.

Lowe FC, Marshall SF: Ureteropelvic junction obstruction in adults. Urology 1984;23:331–335.

Lumiaho J, Heino A, Pietiläinen T, et al: The morphological, in situ effects of a self-reinforced bioabsorbable polylactide (SR-PLA 96) ureteric stent: An experimental study. J Urol 2000;164:1360–1363.

MacNeily AE, Maizels M, Kaplan WE, et al: Does early pyeloplasty really avert loss of renal function? A retrospective review. J Urol 1993; 150:769–773.

Maizels M, Stephens FD: Valves of the ureter as a cause of primary obstruction of the ureter: Anatomic, embryologic and clinical aspects. J Urol 1980;123:742–747.

McAleer IM, Kaplan GW: Renal function before and after pyeloplasty: Does it improve? J Urol 1999;162:1041–1044.

Munoz AI, Pascual y Baralt JF, Melendez MT: Arterial hypertension in infants with hydronephrosis. Am J Dis Child 1977;131:38–40.

Murnaghan GF: The dynamics of the renal pelvis and ureter with reference to congenital hydronephrosis. Br J Urol 1958;30:321–324.

Nixon HH: Hydronephrosis in children: A clinical study of seventy-eight cases with special reference to the role of aberrant renal vessels and the results of conservative operations. Br J Surg 1953;40:601–604.

Notley RG: Electron microscopy of the upper ureter and the pelviureteric junction. Br J Urol 1968;40:37–52.

Ordorica RC, Lindfors KK, Palmer JM: Diuretic Doppler sonography following successful repair of renal obstruction in children. J Urol 1993;150:774–777.

O'Reilly PH: Functional outcome of pyeloplasty for ureteropelvic junction obstruction: Prospective study in 30 consecutive cases. J Urol 1989;142:273–276.

Osathanondh V, Potter EL: Development of the kidney as shown by microdissection. Arch Pathol 1963;76:271–277.

Östling K: The genesis of hydronephrosis. Acta Chir Scand 1942;86(Suppl.):72.

Palmer LS, Maizels M, Kaplan WE, et al: Urine levels of transforming growth factor-beta 1 in children with ureteropelvic junction obstruction. Urology 1997;50:769–773.

Perlmutter AD, Kroovand RL, Lai YW: Management of ureteropelvic obstruction in the first year of life. J Urol 1980;123:535–537.

Peters CA: Urinary tract obstruction in children. J Urol 1995;154:1874–1884.

Renner C, Frede T, Seemann O, Rassweiler J: Laser endopyelotomy: Minimally invasive therapy of ureteropelvic junction stenosis. J Endourol 1998;12:537–540.

Robson WJ, Rudy SM, Johnston JH: Pelviureteric obstruction in infancy. J Pediatr Surg 1976;11:57–61.

Rowell KL, Kontzen F, Stutzman M: Technical aspects of a new technique for estimating glomerular filtration rate using technetium-99m-DTPA. J Nucl Med Technol 1986;14:196.

Ruano-Gil D, Coca-Payeras A, Tejedo-Mateu A: Obstruction and normal recanalization of the ureter in the human embryo: Its relation to congenital ureteric obstruction. Eur Urol 1975;1:287–293.

Rushton HG, Salem Y, Belman AB, Majd M: Pediatric pyeloplasty: Is routine retrograde pyelography necessary? J Urol 1994;152:604–606.

Salem YH, Majd M, Rushton HG, Belman AB: Outcome analysis of pediatric pyeloplasty as a function of patient age, presentation and differential renal function. J Urol 1995;154:1889–1893.

Scardino PL, Prince CL: Vertical flap ureteropelvioplasty: Preliminary report. South Med J 1953;46:325.

Schuessler WW, Grune MT, Tecuanhuey LV, Preminger GM: Laparoscopic dismembered pyeloplasty. J Urol 1993;150:1795–1799.

Seremetis GM, Maizels M: TGF-beta mRNA expression in the renal pelvis after experimental and clinical ureteropelvic junction obstruction. J Urol 1996;156:261–266.

Shaul DB, Cunningham JA, Lowe P, et al: Infant pyeloplasty is a low-risk procedure. J Pediatr Surg 1994;29:343–347.

Snyder HM III, Lebowitz RL, Colodny AH, et al: Ureteropelvic junction obstruction in children. Urol Clin North Am 1980;7:273–290.

Squitieri AP, Ceccarelli FE, Wurster JC: Hypertension with elevated renal vein renins secondary to ureteropelvic junction obstruction. J Urol 1974;111:284–287.

Starr NT, Maizels M, Chou P, et al: Microanatomy of and morphometry of the hydronephrotic "obstructed" renal pelvis in asymptomatic infants. J Urol 1992;148:519–524.

Stephens FD: Ureterovascular hydronephrosis and the "aberrant" renal vessels. J Urol 1982;128:984–987.

Tan HL, Roberts JP, Grattan-Smith D: Retrograde balloon dilation of ureteropelvic obstructions in infants and children: Early results. Urology 1995;46:89–91.

Tan HL: Laparoscopic Anderson-Hynes dismembered pyeloplasty in children. J Urol 1999;162:1045–1048.

Thorup J, Pederson PV, Clausen N: Benign ureteral polyps as a cause of hydronephrosis in a child. J Urol 1981;126:796–797.

Uehling DT, Gilbert E, Chesney R: Urologic implications of the VATER association. J Urol 1983;129:352–354.

Uson AC, Cox LA, Lattimer JK: Hydronephrosis in infants and children: I. Some clinical and pathological aspects. JAMA 1968;205:327–332.

Whitaker RH: Some observations and theories on the wide ureter and hydronephrosis. Br J Urol 1975;47:377–385.

Whitaker RH: Clinical assessment of pelvis and ureteral function. Urology 1978;12:146–150.

Williams DI, Karlaftis CM: Hydronephrosis due to pelviureteric obstruction in the newborn. Br J Urol 1966;38:138–144.

Williams DI, Kenawi MM: The prognosis of pelviureteric obstruction in childhood: A review of 190 cases. Eur Urol 1976;2:57–63.

Williams PR, Fegetter J, Miller RA, Wickham JEA: The diagnosis and management of benign fibrous ureteric polyps. Br J Urol 1980;52:253–256.

Zerin JM, Ritchey ML, Chang AC: Incidental vesicoureteral reflux in neonates with antenatally detected hydronephrosis and other renal abnormalities. Radiology 1993;187:157–160.

58
ECTOPIC URETER, URETEROCELE, AND OTHER ANOMALIES OF THE URETER

Richard N. Schlussel, MD
Alan B. Retik, MD

TERMINOLOGY

Ureteral anomalies are some of the most significant anomalies in all of pediatric urology because they directly affect overall renal function. These congenital problems may manifest acutely or insidiously. Similarly, if they are incorrectly treated, the adverse outcome may not be appreciated for years. Appropriate management is predicated on knowledge of the relevant embryology, anatomy, and physiology, as well as all the variants thereof. Finally, the urologist entrusted with the care of these children must be familiar with the many reconstructive techniques available so that an optimal outcome can be achieved.

The study of ureteral anomalies has yielded a rich array of terms and descriptions. Many of these terms and categories were put forth by some of the founders of pediatric urology. Because all of medicine is predicated on effective communication, this chapter summarizes classifications used in the past, defines current common usages, and proposes a standard rational nomenclature that, it is hoped, will allow accurate communication.

Because ureteral anomalies are at times associated with duplications of the kidney, it is prudent to review renal terminology. **A *duplex kidney* is one that has two separate pelvicalyceal systems. A duplex kidney has an upper pole and a lower pole. The ureters may join at any point. If they join at the level of the ureteropelvic junction, the configuration is termed a *bifid system*. If the ureters join more distally but are still proximal to the bladder level, the configuration is termed *bifid ureters*** (Fig. 58–1A). ***Double ureters* are ureters that drain their respective poles and empty separately into the genitourinary tract.** This represents a complete duplication (Fig. 58–1B). A ureter that drains the upper or lower pole should be referred to respectively as the "upper pole ureter" and the "lower pole ureter."

The word *ectopia* is derived from the Greek *ex* ("out") and *topos* ("place"); any ureter whose orifice terminates anywhere other than the normal trigonal position is considered ectopic. *Lateral ectopia* implies an orifice more cranial and lateral than normal. *Caudal ectopia* implies that the orifice is more medial and distal than the normal position. Such an orifice may theoretically be found between the normal orifice position and the bladder neck. However,

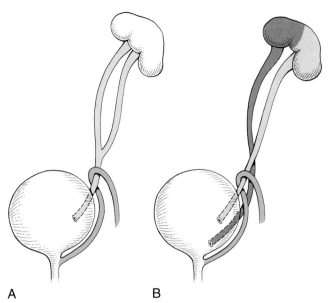

Figure 58–1. *A,* A bifid ureter is depicted; the upper pole and lower pole ureters join proximal to the bladder. *B,* Double ureters are seen when the upper pole ureter and lower pole ureter empty separately into the bladder.

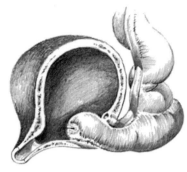

Figure 58–2. The orifice of a stenotic ectopic ureterocele may be located at the tip or at the superior or inferior surface of the ureterocele.

in general practice, **the term *ectopic ureter* is meant to imply a ureter whose orifice terminates even more caudally, such as in the urethra or outside of the urinary tract.**

Ericsson (1954) characterized ureteroceles as either simple or ectopic. A "simple ureterocele" was defined as one that lies completely within the bladder, whereas those that extended to the bladder neck or distally to the urethra were considered to be "ectopic." Stephens (1958, 1964, 1971, 1983) described ureteroceles as either stenotic, sphincteric, or sphincterostenotic, or as a cecoureterocele. A stenotic ureterocele is one whose narrowed or pinpoint opening is found inside the bladder (Fig. 58–2). **If a ureterocele has an orifice distal to the bladder neck, it is termed *sphincteric* (Fig. 58–3). If a ureterocele has an orifice that was both stenotic and distal to the bladder neck, it is considered a *sphincterostenotic ureterocele* (Fig. 58–4A). A *cecoureterocele* has an intravesical orifice and a submucosal extension that dips into the urethra.** This type of ureterocele can distend with urine and obstruct the urethra (Fig. 58–4B).

Several terms for ureteroceles in common use are confusing. They are listed here not to encourage their use but to clarify their intended meaning. A "simple ureterocele" is frequently used to mean a single-system ureterocele. The "adult ureterocele" has the same implication. An "orthotopic ureterocele" is a ureterocele contained within the bladder. Often, the phrase "ectopic ureterocele" is used to explain a ureterocele associated with a duplicated system.

Obviously, these terms are not completely clear because they are nondescriptive and sometimes inaccurate. In an effort to eliminate this ambiguity and confusion, the Committee on Terminology, Nomenclature and Classification of the Section of Urology of the American Academy of Pediatrics proposed standardized terms that are both descriptive and accurate (Glassberg et al, 1984). According to this classification, **a ureterocele is *intravesical* if the ureterocele is contained in the bladder in its entirety, and it is *ectopic* if any portion of the ureterocele extends to the bladder neck or the urethra** (Fig. 58–5). Ureteroceles are classified further according to the number of systems (single or duplex) and the type of orifice involved (e.g., stenotic, sphincteric, sphincterostenotic, or as a cecoureterocele). Therefore, by way of example, the ureterocele seen in Figure 58–6 would be categorized as an intravesical ureterocele of a left single system with a stenotic orifice, and the ureterocele shown in Figure 58–4A would be categorized as an ectopic ureterocele of a duplicated left system. Such classifications lead to little doubt, and their use should be encouraged.

EMBRYOLOGY

An understanding of normal renal development is critical to an appreciation of how ureteral anomalies evolve and whether they are clinically significant. At 4 weeks' gestation, an outpouching arises from the distal mesonephric duct. This outpouching is the ureteric bud, and it interacts with a mass of mesenchyme that is the metanephric blastema. This interaction results in the ureteric bud's branching and developing into the calyces, renal pelvis, and ureter. The metanephric blastema is induced to form all elements of the nephron, including the collecting duct, distal convoluted tube, loop of Henle, proximal convoluted tubule, and glomerulus. **The segment of mesonephric duct distal to the ureteric bud is the common excretory**

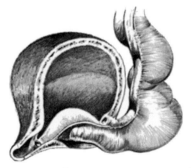

Figure 58–3. Sphincteric ectopic ureteroceles.

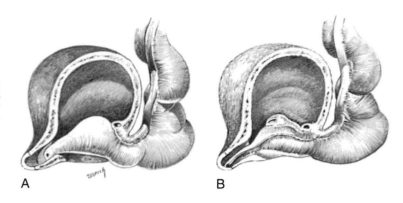

Figure 58–4. *A,* Sphincterostenotic ectopic ureterocele. *B,* Cecoureterocele lumen extends distal to the orifice as a long tongue beneath the ureteral submucosa. The orifice communicates with the lumen of the bladder and is large and incompetent.

A   B

duct (Fig. 58–7). **This duct eventually is absorbed into the developing bladder and becomes part of the trigone. The point of origin of the ureteric bud is the ureteral orifice.** When the common excretory duct is absorbed into the bladder, the ureteral orifice begins to migrate in the bladder in a cranial and lateral direction (Moore, 1988) (Fig. 58–8).

If the ureteric bud arises off the mesonephric duct more distally than normally, the ureteral orifice enters the bladder earlier than usual and hence has a greater period for cranial and lateral migration (Mackie and Stephens, 1975; Tanagho, 1976; Schwartz et al, 1981). This results in lateral ectopia. **If the ureteric bud arises more proximally on the mesonephric duct than normally, the ureteral orifice has less time in the bladder to undergo its normal migration and results in a ureteral orifice more medial and caudal than is usual** (Fig. 58–9). **An even further proximal ureteric bud position on the mesonephric duct may result in the ureteral orifice's remaining on the mesonephric duct, with the end result being that the orifice terminates outside the bladder altogether.** In the male, the embryologic equivalents of the mesonephric duct are the epididymis, vas deferens, seminal vesicles, and prostate. In the female, the mesonephric duct proximal to the ureteric bud becomes the epoöphoron,

oophoron, and Gartner's duct. An ectopic ureter draining into any of these female structures can rupture into the adjoining fallopian tube, uterus, upper vagina, or vestibule.

The interaction of the ureteric bud with the metanephric blastema is critical to the correct ontogeny of the ureter and collecting system and the future kidney. Examination of the developing kidney reveals close cell-to-cell interactions between the ureteric bud and the metanephric blastema (Saxen, 1987). Experimental models have shown that if these interactions are altered or disrupted, the blastema fails to differentiate into normal nephrons (Grobstein, 1956; Kirrilova et al, 1982; Sariola et al, 1988).

In clinical practice, it appears that renal units drained by ureters that terminate in positions other than the trigone do, in fact, have problems with proper development. Recalling the embryology of the trigone and ureteral orifice, it is likely that an abnormal ureteral orifice position reflects an abnormal point of origin of the ureteric bud from the mesonephric duct. This ureteric bud would be poorly positioned for the necessary interactions with the metanephric blastema. Therefore, these clinical and experimental observations combine to support the commonly held notion that dysplasia is the product of inadequate ureteric bud-to-blastema interaction (Mackie and Stephens, 1975).

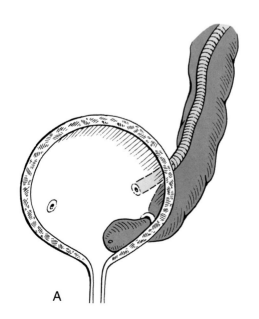
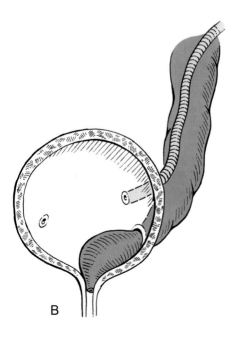

Figure 58–5. *A,* An intravesical ureterocele located entirely within the bladder. *B,* The distal portion of an ectopic ureterocele extends outside the bladder and into the urethra.

A   B

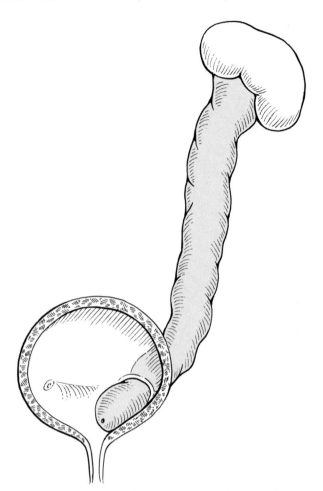

Figure 58–6. A single-system intravesical ureterocele.

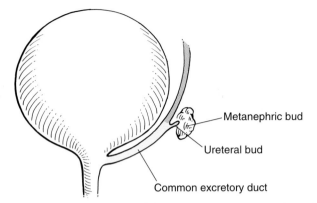

Figure 58–7. The structures of the urinary tract originate from the primitive metanephric blastema and the ureteral bud, which arises from the mesonephric duct. The common excretory duct is the portion of the mesonephric duct that is distal to the ureteral bud.

After its emergence from the mesonephric duct, the ureteric bud can become a split or bifid structure. The splitting creates two separate collecting systems that join eventually in a common ureter (Fig. 58–10). As mentioned previously, this anatomic arrangement is termed a duplex kidney with a bifid ureter. The ureter distal to the bifurcation has arisen from a normal position on the mesonephric duct, and therefore its single ureteral orifice is in the normal trigonal location.

If two separate ureteric buds originate from the mesonephric duct, two complete and separate interac-tions will develop between the ureter and the metaneph-ric blastema. The result is two separate renal units and collecting systems, ureters, and ureteral orifices. Using our earlier terminology, this complete duplication is synonymous with a duplex system drained by double ureters (Fig. 58–11). The final position of the ureteral orifices has important clinical implications. Both Weigert (1877) and Meyer (1946) noted that there is a constant trigonal relationship between the upper and lower pole orifices. When performing a cystoscopic examination, it is important to remember this counterintuitive concept: the so-called lower or distally placed orifice is in fact the orifice of the upper pole, and the so-called higher or cranial orifice is the lower pole orifice. **The lower pole orifice is more cranial and lateral to the caudad, medial upper pole orifice.** To achieve these positions, the two ureters and orifices rotate 180 degrees clockwise on their longitudinal axes (Fig. 58–12). The Weigert-Meyer rule of complete duplicated systems yields a fairly constant anatomy that is important for radiologic, cystoscopic, and reconstructive considerations.

All congenital anomalies of the ureter can be considered as falling into one of the categories in which we have organized this chapter: anomalies of termination, anomalies of structure, anomalies of number, and anomalies of position.

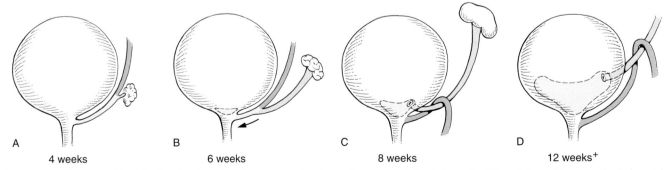

A	B	C	D
4 weeks	6 weeks	8 weeks	12 weeks[+]

Figure 58–8. The ureteral bud further develops into the ureter and induces the metanephric blastema to differentiate and become the kidney. The common excretory duct is progressively absorbed into the bladder and becomes the trigone. The mesonephric duct will become the vas deferens in the male.

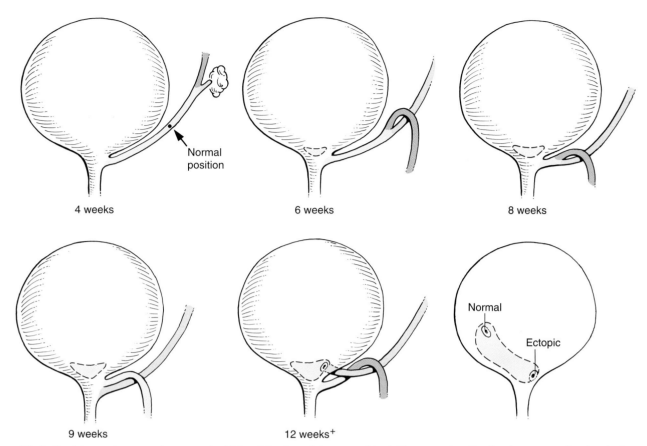

Figure 58–9. Caudal ectopia occurs because of a high origination of the ureteral bud. The ureteral orifice has less time to be absorbed into the bladder and has a caudal, medial trigone location or is extravesically located along the path of the mesonephric duct remnants.

ANOMALIES OF TERMINATION

Lateral Ectopia

Primary reflux is defined as reflux that occurs in the absence of predisposing associated conditions, such as myelomeningocele, detrusor-sphincter dyssynergia, posterior urethral valves, or ureteroceles. This reflux is caused in large part by the abnormal development noted previously that results in lateral ectopia (Cussen, 1979).

The laterally placed ureteral orifice is a result of the ureteric bud's originating from a more caudal point on the mesonephric duct than is usual. As the portion of the mesonephric duct that is distal to the ureteric bud (i.e., the common excretory duct) begins to be absorbed into the bladder, it brings the ureteric bud with it. The ureteral orifice begins its cranial and lateral migration on entering the bladder. If the orifice has a prolonged period during which to undergo such migration (e.g., when the ureteric bud originates closer to the bladder), the orifice will ultimately reside more cranially and laterally than is normal. Eventually, there will be a ureter whose submucosal course is short and almost perpendicular to the bladder wall, as opposed to the normally long and oblique submucosal

Figure 58–10. Branching of the ureteral bud *(gray)* after it arises from the mesonephric duct *(red)* creates a bifid ureter.

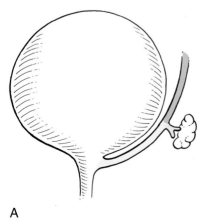

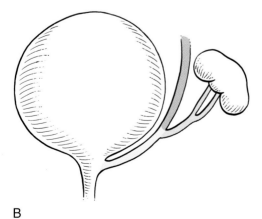

A   B

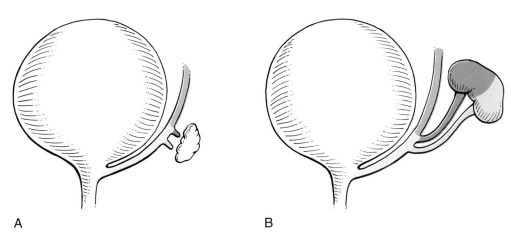

A

B

Figure 58-11. When two separate ureteral buds come off the mesonephric duct, they develop into an upper pole and its ureter *(black)* and a lower pole and its ureter *(gray)*, each having distinct ureteral orifices in the bladder.

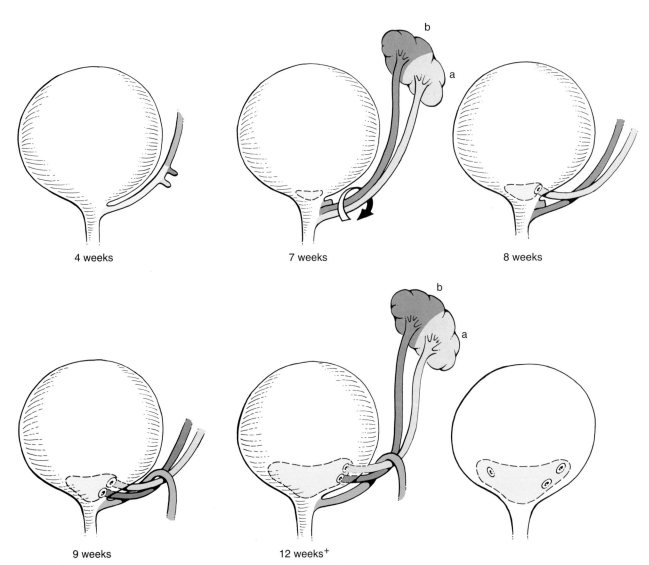

4 weeks

7 weeks

8 weeks

9 weeks

12 weeks⁺

Figure 58-12. The Weigert-Meyer rule is depicted. The upper pole ureter *(black)* and the lower pole ureter *(gray)* rotate on their long axes to yield an upper pole orifice (b) that is medial and caudal to the lower pole orifice (a).

course (Ambrose and Nicolson, 1962; Stephens and Lenaghan, 1962). A decreased, shorter submucosal course prevents the normal operation of the so-called flap valve mechanism, and vesicoureteral reflux ensues (Fig. 58–13). The degree of reflux correlates with the degree of laterality and inversely with the length of the submucosal ureter.

Another factor in primary reflux is the frequently found abnormality of a poorly developed trigone. As previously stated, in primary reflux the ureteric bud arises from the mesonephric duct more caudally than is normal, resulting in a short common excretory duct. Because the common excretory duct was shortened, its mesenchymal contribution to the muscular development of the trigone was decreased. Therefore, the trigone is not only large but also poorly muscularized. Because there has been less time for the common mesenchyme to accumulate around the developing ureteric bud, the intramural ureter is also deficient in musculature. The normal arrangement has been compared to a hammer and anvil, with the intravesical urine being the hammer that compresses the ureter against the bladder wall musculature, which is the anvil. This altered development also affects the flap valve mechanism by denying the ureter sufficient muscular backing against which it can be compressed.

In addition, because there has been less time for the common mesenchyme to accumulate around the developing

ureteric bud, the intramural ureter is likewise deficient in musculature. Because of the altered trigonal development and the poor attachments of the ureter, the orifice can be patulous or gaping. It is because of the combined effects of the lateral ureteral orifice position, the ureter's shortened submucosal course, the poorly developed trigone, and the abnormal morphology of the ureteral orifice that primary vesicoureteral reflux develops (Tanagho et al, 1965).

Ectopic Ureters

As mentioned previously, in the strictest sense, a ureter whose orifice is laterally and cranially located in the bladder could be considered ectopic. However, the term "ectopic ureter" has universally been used to describe a ureter that terminates at the bladder neck or distally into one of the aforementioned mesonephric duct structures. We employ this general terminology in the following discussion.

The true incidence of an ectopic ureter is uncertain, because many cause no symptoms. Campbell (1970) noted 10 examples in 19,046 autopsies in children (an incidence of 1 in 1900) but thought that some had been overlooked. **Of all ectopic orifices, 80% are associated with a duplicated collecting system. In females, more than 80% are duplicated, but in males, most ectopic ureters drain single systems** (Schulman, 1976; Ahmed and Barker, 1992). This is particularly true when ectopic ureteroceles are excluded from consideration.

Ectopic ureters appear more commonly in females clinically, from 2 to 12 times more frequently, with the lesser frequency probably reflecting the incidence more accurately (Eisendrath, 1938; Mills, 1939; Burford et al, 1949; Lowsley and Kerwin, 1956). Ellerker (1958) noted 366 females and 128 males in his review of 494 ectopic ureters, including autopsies, for a female-to-male ratio of 2.9:1. Between 5% and 17% of ectopic ureters appear bilaterally (Eisendrath, 1938; Ellerker, 1958; Ahmed and Barker, 1992; Malek et al, 1972; Mandell et al, 1981). A small percentage involve a solitary kidney. With unilateral ectopic ureter, a contralateral ureteral duplication is not uncommon. Various other abnormalities, including imperforate anus and tracheoesophageal fistula, may be found in association with the ectopic ureter (Ahmed and Barker, 1992).

The distribution of ectopic ureters is itemized by location in Table 58–1. **In the male, the posterior urethra is the most common site of termination of an ectopic ureter. Drainage into the genital tract involves the seminal vesicle three times more often than the ejaculatory duct and vas deferens combined** (Riba et al, 1946; Ellerker, 1958; Lucius, 1963; Sullivan et al, 1978; Squadrito et al, 1987). **In the female, the urethra and vestibule are the most common sites.** The age at diagnosis ranges widely, with many examples not detected during life (Ellerker, 1958).

The earlier reports failed to provide adequate descriptions of the upper tracts, but later reports emphasized that **the more remote the ureteral opening, the greater the degree of renal maldevelopment** (Schulman, 1976). **With duplicated systems, this means hypoplasia or dysplasia of the upper pole segment.** Of 10 cases involving an

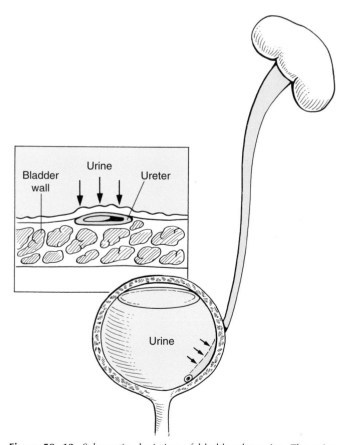

Figure 58–13. Schematic depiction of bladder dynamics. The urine compresses the ureter between the bladder mucosa and the bladder wall muscle, which creates the flap valve mechanism that prevents reflux.

Table 58–1. LOCATION OF 494 ECTOPIC URETERS (INCLUDING AUTOPSIES)

Type	Number	Percentage
128 male subjects		
Posterior urethra	60	47
Prostatic utricle	13	10
Seminal vesicle	42	33
Ejaculatory duct	7	5
Vas deferens	6	5
366 female subjects		
Urethra	129	35
Vestibule	124	34
Vagina	90	25
Cervix or uterus	18	5
Gartner's duct	3	<1
Urethral diverticulum	2	<1

From Ellerker AG: The extravesical ectopic ureter. Br J Surg 1958;45:344.

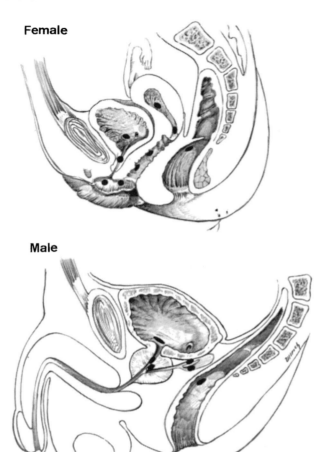

Female

Male

Figure 58–14. Sites of ectopic ureteral orifices in girls and boys.

ectopic ureter that drained a single system and opened into the male seminal tracts, the kidney was not visualized radiographically in any (Rognon et al, 1973). Of 16 single renal ducts drained by an ectopic ureter, renal dysplasia was present in 7 (Prewitt and Lebowitz, 1976). The kidney drained by an ectopic ureter may be in an abnormal position as well (Borer et al, 1998; Bozorgi et al, 1998; Utsunomiya et al, 1984; Moores et al, 1997). This kidney is often quite small and difficult to localize on imaging studies. Ectopic ureters draining single systems appear to be seen more frequently in Japan (Moores et al, 1997; Gotoh et al, 1983; Wakhlu et al, 1998; Suzuki et al, 1993). In Borer's report of single-system ectopic ureters, each child was initially believed to have a solitary hypertrophied kidney, and all had received erroneous diagnoses and undergone multiple diagnostic investigations (average 10) before the correct diagnosis was made. In seven of their eight patients, the single-system ectopic ureter terminated in the vagina.

The ectopic ureter itself is also abnormal, usually to a greater degree in the single system than in the duplicated system. Usually, the ureter is variably dilated and drainage is impaired (Williams and Royle, 1969). Muscle cells may show severe alterations on ultrastructure studies. Whether these changes are developmental or acquired is not yet known (Hanna et al, 1977).

Clinical presentation of an ectopic ureter usually differs in males and females, reflecting the differing termination of the ectopic ureters in the two genders. Recalling the embryology of ureteral ectopia, when the ureteric bud arises more proximally on the mesonephric duct than it normally should, the ureteral orifice remains on the mesonephric duct caudally and is not absorbed in the bladder. **In the female, these parts of the mesonephric duct become the epoöphoron, oophoron, and Gartner's duct. If an ectopic ureter drains into any of these respective female structures, they can rupture or be incorporated into any of the nearby müllerian duct structures, such as the vagina, uterus, cervix, or fallopian tubes** (Fig. 58–14). Therefore, in the female patient, an ectopic ureteral orifice may be within (e.g., bladder neck, proximal urethra) or outside the realm of the urinary sphincter, making ectopic

ureters one of the more important causes of urinary incontinence in girls (Freedman and Rickwood, 1994). **Continuous incontinence in a girl with an otherwise normal voiding pattern after toilet training is the classic symptom of an ectopic ureteral orifice.**

On occasion, incontinence becomes apparent at a later age and may be confused with stress incontinence, incontinence associated with neurogenic bladder dysfunction, or psychogenic incontinence. A persistent vaginal discharge from an ectopic orifice located in the vagina is another clinical sign (Acien et al, 1990; See and Mayo, 1991; Gharagozloo and Lebowitz, 1995). Most ectopic ureters are associated with acute or recurrent urinary tract infection. A patient may also present with abdominal pain, failure to thrive, and chronic infection (Fig. 58–15). **Patients with ectopic ureters draining into the proximal urethra often experience reflux, and urge incontinence is common. An ectopic ureter may be severely obstructed, causing massive hydronephrosis and hydroureter**, and it may manifest as an abdominal mass (Uson et al, 1972) or be detected on prenatal ultrasonographic evaluation.

In males, the mesonephric duct structures eventually form the epididymis, vas deferens, and seminal vesicles. Therefore, an ectopic ureter in the male patient can drain into the bladder neck, the prostatic urethra, or the aforementioned wolffian duct structures (see Fig. 58–14). All of

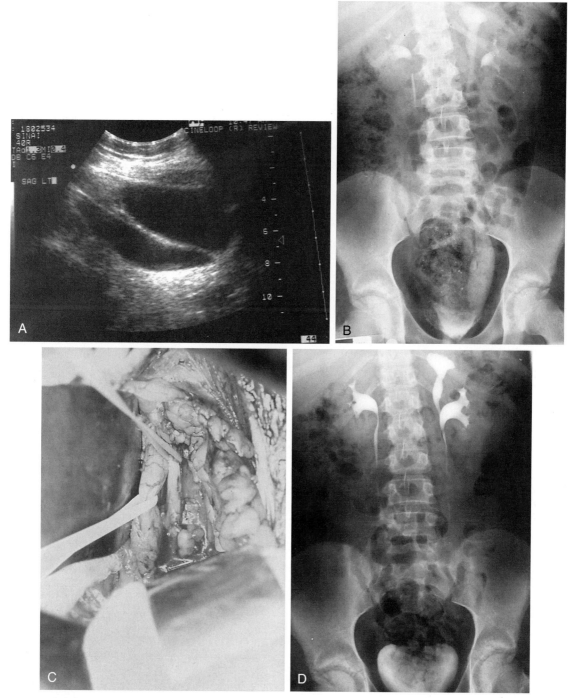

Figure 58–15. Ectopic left upper pole ureter in a teenage girl with chronic abdominal pain. *A,* Sonogram of dilated ureter entering bladder neck. *B,* Intravenous pyelogram demonstrating severe upper pole hydroureteronephrosis with dilated ureter entering the bladder neck. *C,* Intraoperative photograph of dilated medial upper pole ureter and normal-caliber lateral lower pole ureter. *D,* Intravenous pyelogram after upper pole to lower pole ureteroureterostomy. The patient was free of symptoms immediately after the procedure.

these locations are proximal to the external sphincter. Therefore, males with ectopic ureters do not suffer from urinary incontinence as females do.

Because their ectopic ureters drain most commonly into the prostatic urethra and bladder neck, **males most often present with urinary tract infection.** They may also experience urgency and frequency. In some instances, the

ureter ends in the wolffian duct remnants (seminal vesicles, vas deferens, or epididymis), predisposing the individual to epididymitis (Williams and Sago, 1983; Umeyama et al, 1985). Therefore, **epididymitis in a prepubertal boy should prompt the physician to consider the presence of an ectopic ureter.** In males, the symptoms may not be as obvious as incontinence in females; males may complain of

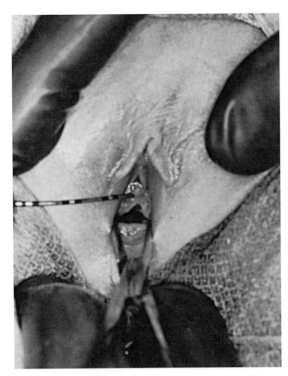

Figure 58–16. Photograph at the time of cystoscopy of an ectopic ureteral orifice in the urethrovaginal septum. A ureteral catheter is in the orifice.

constipation, abdominal pain, pelvic pain, or discomfort during ejaculation, and they may even be infertile (Squadrito et al, 1987). A stone may form in the ectopic ureter. It is most important to remember that boys will be continent because the ectopic ureter always drains proximal to the external sphincter. Urgency and frequency in a male patient, caused by the ectopic ureter's draining into the prostatic fossa, should not be mistaken for incontinence.

Diagnosis

Prenatal sonographic diagnosis of ectopic ureters has become common. The condition is identifiable by virtue of the hydronephrosis produced by the obstruction. If this is isolated to the upper pole of a duplex system and the bladder is normal, the diagnosis is relatively straightforward. In other situations, prenatal findings serve to initiate a postnatal evaluation that will specifically identify the condition.

In a girl, sometimes the diagnosis of an ectopic ureter can be made by physical examination. Direct visualization of the vulva may reveal continuous urinary dribbling or wetness. In the absence of neurogenic vesical dysfunction or a urethral sphincter defect, an ectopic ureter is likely. Often, a punctum or orifice is apparent in the urethrovaginal septum (Fig. 58–16). Perineal and genital skin erythema or maceration may reflect the irritating effect of the urine that continually bathes this area.

The ultrasonographic findings of an ectopic ureter include the dilated pelvis and collecting system of the upper pole and a dilated ureter behind an otherwise normal bladder (Fig. 58–17). A large ectopic ureter may

press against the bladder and create an indentation that appears much like a ureterocele and is termed a *pseudoureterocele* (Diard et al, 1987; Sumfest et al, 1995). The difference is that an ectopic ureter is clearly extravesical, with a thick septum of bladder muscle between the ureteral lumen and bladder lumen. In contrast, in a ureterocele the septum is thin and delicate and the ureteral lumen is partially intravesical. Sumfest and associates (1995) noted that their patients had ectopic ureteral drainage into mesonephric duct cysts; these mesonephric duct cysts can rupture into the vagina or bladder. The renal parenchyma associated with a ectopic ureter is often thinner than that of a normally draining lower pole (Nussbaum et al, 1986).

In most instances, the diagnosis of an ectopic ureter is confirmed by excretory urography (Figs. 58–18 and 58–19). The usual radiographic feature is a nonvisualizing or poorly visualizing upper pole of a duplex system that may be massively hydronephrotic. **The upper pole displaces the lower pole downward and outward, the so-called drooping lily appearance.** When the upper pole does not excrete contrast and make the duplicated system readily apparent, there are several other clues to suggest that a duplicated system is present. First, the calyces of a lower pole are fewer in number than in the normal kidney. Second, the axis of the lowest to uppermost calyx does not point toward the midline. Third, the uppermost calyx of the **lower pole** unit is usually farther from the **upper pole** border than is the lowest calyx from the corresponding **lower pole** limit. **In addition, the lower pole pelvis and the upper portion of its ureter may be farther from the spine than on the contralateral side, and the lower pole ureter may also be scalloped and tortuous secondary to its wrapping around a markedly dilated upper pole ureter** (similar to the findings of upper pole hydroureteronephrosis in the child with a ureterocele in Figure 58–33). When an ectopic ureter drains a nonvisualizing, diminutive, dysplastic renal unit, these typical radiologic features may not be demonstrated. Care must be taken to identify exactly which kidney is responsible for the ectopic ureter and

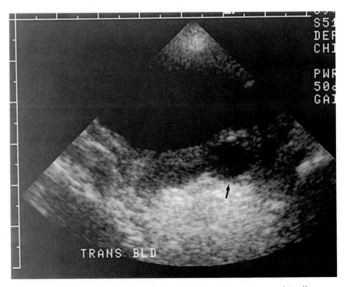

Figure 58–17. Distal ureteral dilatation is seen sonographically as a round, hypoechoic area behind the bladder (*arrow*).

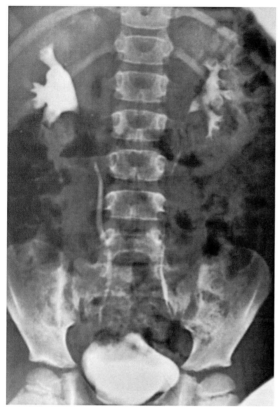

Figure 58–18. Excretory urogram in a 5-year-old girl with urinary incontinence shows a nonvisualizing upper pole on the right side that is displacing the lower pole downward and outward. Also, note that the right renal pelvis and upper ureter are farther from the spine than are the structures on the left.

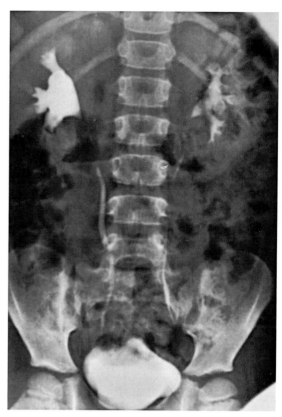

Figure 58–19. Excretory urogram in a 4-month-old girl with a urinary tract infection reveals a left renal duplication with hydronephrosis and hydroureter of the upper pole system.

the incontinence, because there may be bilateral duplicated systems. Failure to make the correct identification may result in removing the wrong upper pole and the patient's experiencing the same symptoms postoperatively! Particular attention should be paid to the contralateral kidney on excretory urography to avoid missing bilateral ureteral ectopia. This is reported to occur in 5% to 17% of cases but was noted in 25% of cases in one series (Campbell, 1951).

The functional status of the upper pole renal segment of duplex systems may be evident on excretory urography, but more precise assessment may become important if upper pole salvage is considered. Isotopic renal scanning using technetium 99m–dimercaptosuccinic acid (^{99m}Tc-DMSA) has proved to be the most adequate, although differentiating between the function of the upper and lower poles may be difficult.

Voiding cystourethrography demonstrates reflux into the lower pole ureter in at least half of the cases. More importantly, reflux into the ectopic ureter may be demonstrated at different phases of voiding, providing evidence of the location of the orifice (Fig. 58–20). If the reflux into the ectopic ureter is seen before voiding, the orifice is proximal to the bladder neck; reflux only with voiding suggests an orifice in the urethra. The latter finding may be evident only with several cycles of voiding monitored fluoroscopically (Wyly and Lebowitz, 1984). Sphincteric orifices may not produce reflux at all.

Occasionally, the renal parenchyma is difficult to locate

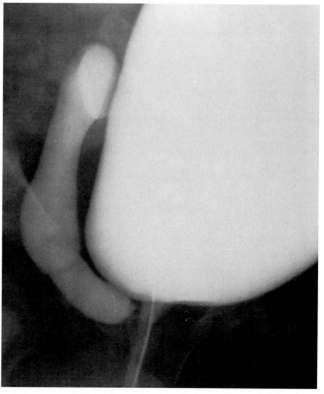

Figure 58–20. A cystogram demonstrates reflux into an ectopic ureter that enters the urethra immediately distal to the bladder neck.

and may be identified only by alternative imaging studies (Giles et al, 1982; Gharagozloo and Lebowitz, 1995). In such cases, in which an ectopic ureter is strongly suspected because of incontinence yet no definite evidence of the upper pole renal segment is found (Simms and Higgins, 1975), computed tomography (CT) or magnetic resonance imaging has demonstrated the small, poorly functioning upper pole segment (Braverman and Lebowitz, 1991) (Fig. 58–21).

If ^{99m}Tc-DMSA scanning and CT are done in a delayed fashion, small, poorly functioning kidneys that are unapparent on other studies or renal upper poles may be visualized for the first time. (Borer et al, 1998; Pantuck et al, 1996; Moores et al, 1997; Utsunomiya et al, 1984; Bozorgi et al, 1998; Komatsu et al, 1999). The position of the ectopic

kidney on a nuclear scan can direct the radiologist to order thin cuts of the CT scan through the suspected ectopic renal location.

Ectopic ureteral orifices may be identified at the time of cystourethroscopy and vaginoscopy. Careful inspection of the vestibule, urethra, and vagina sometimes reveals the ectopic orifice. Often, the orifice is difficult to identify amidst the various mucosal folds of these structures. If an orifice is identifiable, a ureteral catheter can be passed into it and a retrograde pyelogram can be performed to better delineate the anatomy. If there is a single-system ectopic ureter, the characteristic features are a hypertrophied contralateral kidney and the cystoscopic findings of an absent ureteral orifice and absent ipsilateral hemitrigone.

We have not found the intravenous injection of indigo carmine to be particularly helpful because of the delayed function of the segment drained by the ectopic ureter. It has been suggested that two oral doses of phenazopyridine (Pyridium) given the night before and the morning of cystoscopy improve visualization of the ectopic ureter (Weiss et al, 1984). Filling the bladder with a dye solution, such as methylene blue or indigo carmine, is sometimes helpful in detecting the elusive ectopic orifice. If a clear fluid continues to drain into the vulva, one can be certain that an ectopic orifice is present. Deep flank palpation at the time of the examination may result in expression of urine and thereby reveal the orifice location.

Sometimes, the diagnosis must be made by exclusion—that is, the vestibule is damp, no orifice is found, the excretory urogram shows subtle changes suggesting a tiny dysplastic upper segment of a duplex system, and the patient is cured by an upper pole nephrectomy. With current imaging techniques and an appropriate degree of suspicion, the diagnosis is invariably made before surgery.

Treatment

Most ectopic ureters drain renal moieties (either an upper pole or a single-system kidney) that have minimal function. Therefore, upper pole nephrectomy (or nephrectomy in a single system) is often recommended (Sullivan et al, 1978; Plaire et al, 1997). In some cases, particularly with single-system ectopic ureters, renal function is worth salvaging. This may become more commonplace as antenatal sonography brings such patients to medical attention at an earlier stage and possibly before the damaging long-term effects of obstruction. Either ureteropyelostomy or common sheath ureteral reimplantation for a duplicated system, or solitary reimplantation for a single system, will achieve the goal of relief of obstruction. In our experience, many of these reconstructive procedures have resulted in decreased dilatation of the upper urinary tract and improved function (Fig. 58–22).

Heminephrectomy and ureteropyelostomy are well described elsewhere (Mor et al, 1994), but several technical points deserve emphasis (Fig. 58–23). A flank approach for heminephrectomy usually offers better exposure to the upper pole vessels. Of primary concern is the need to avoid damaging the viable lower pole. The kidney should be retracted gently so as not to cause any vascular embarrassment. **Transecting the upper pole ureter and placing a traction stitch on the proximal portion of this ureter**

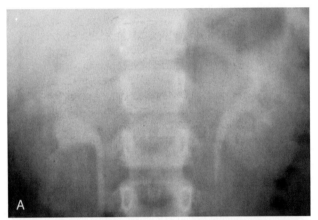
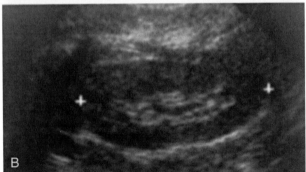
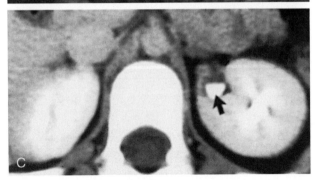

Figure 58–21. *A,* Excretory urogram in 10-year-old girl with constant wetting. No definite evidence for an upper pole segment is present. *B,* Left renal ultrasound in the same patient, also without a clear indication of the presence of an upper pole segment. *C,* Contrast-enhanced computed tomographic image in the same girl specifically demonstrates the small upper pole segment *(arrow)* associated with the ectopic ureter. Upper pole nephrectomy cured the wetting.

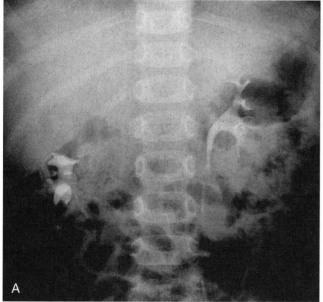

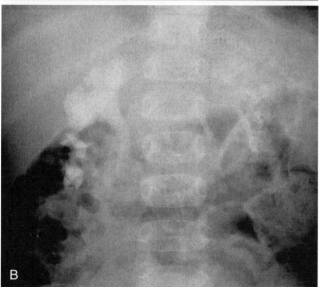

Figure 58–22. Preoperative *(A)* and postoperative *(B)* intravenous pyelograms demonstrate relief of the right upper pole obstruction after ureteroureterostomy between the upper and lower pole ureters.

affords the surgeon a good method of retraction and manipulation of the upper pole. The ureter is passed behind the main renal vessels. The dissection around the renal vessels should be done carefully to avoid damage to the lower pole. The **upper pole** vessels (most often two to three in number) are sequentially ligated. **Demarcation of the upper pole parenchyma becomes apparent after the upper pole vessels are ligated. Stripping the capsule off the upper pole in continuity allows it to be used in the closure. During upper pole nephrectomy, we have favored atraumatic clamping of the renal pedicle.** This approach enables us to work in a bloodless field. Administration of an intravenous osmotic diuretic (e.g., mannitol) moments before and after clamping of the pedicle helps avert acute tubular necrosis. Topical vasodilating agents (e.g., papaverine) should be available in case vasospasm

occurs. **When performing the upper pole ureterectomy, it is of utmost importance to maintain the dissection immediately on the wall of the upper pole ureter as much as possible to preserve the blood supply to the remaining lower pole ureter.**

If, in addition to obstruction, there is concomitant reflux into the ectopic ureter, a second incision is necessary (i.e., a Gibson incision) to resect the ureter in its entirety. Care must be taken to avoid injury to the vas deferens in male patients. As mentioned previously, dissection should be performed strictly along the wall of the upper pole ureter. To prevent complications that may arise from dissection within a common sheath of two ureters (especially distally), the back wall of the upper pole ureter should be left attached to the lower pole ureter. The remainder of the upper pole ureter should be removed (Fig. 58–24). Such a maneuver prevents damage to the lower pole ureteral blood supply, which courses between both ureters. Resection is carried out to the level of the bladder, where several vesicle sutures are placed to close the upper pole ureteral hiatus.

A Penrose drain (brought through a separate stab wound) is placed in such a fashion as to drain the renal fossa and the area of the ureteral dissection. Postoperative evaluation includes an upper urinary tract study (intravenous pyelogram or nuclear renal scan) to demonstrate the anatomy and function in the lower pole.

The procedure of ureteropyelostomy can be done either through a flank incision or via a dorsal lumbotomy approach, which is both effective and less morbid than a muscle-dividing flank incision.

Another surgical option is laparoscopic nephrectomy or heminephrectomy (Fig. 58–25). This can be done by either a transabdominal or a retroperitoneal approach. Laparoscopic procedures putatively offer reduced morbidity in regard to less postoperative pain, earlier return of gastrointestinal function, sooner discharge home, and presumably a quicker return to work for the parents (Yao and Poppas, 2000; Janetschek et al, 1997; Prabhakaran and Lingaraj, 1999; Kobashi e al, 1998; El-Ghoneimi et al, 1998). Other advantages include direct lighting and increased magnification of the operative field, improved cosmesis, and avoidance of a second incision that is often needed for the distal ureterectomy of a nephroureterectomy. Laparoscopic renal procedures can be performed in children as young as 2 to 4 months of age (Yao and Poppas, 2000; El-Ghoneimi et al, 1998) with a minimum of blood loss.

These procedures have been performed by our group as well as others (Jordan and Winslow, 1993; Rassweiler et al, 1993; Suzuki et al, 1993; Figenshau et al, 1994), and they may be used more frequently as laparoscopy experience grows in the urologic community.

Operative time for transperitoneal laparoscopic heminephrouterectomy is approximately 4 hours, which is significantly longer than the same procedure done via a laparoscopic retroperitoneal approach (average time, 153 minutes) (El-Ghoneimi et al, 1998).

Some authors believe that cystoscopic placement of a ureteral catheter allows for easier identification of the ureter at the time of laparoscopy (Yao and Poppas, 2000; Prabhakaran and Linaraj, 1999). The laparoscopic heminephrouretectomy commences similarly to the open procedure

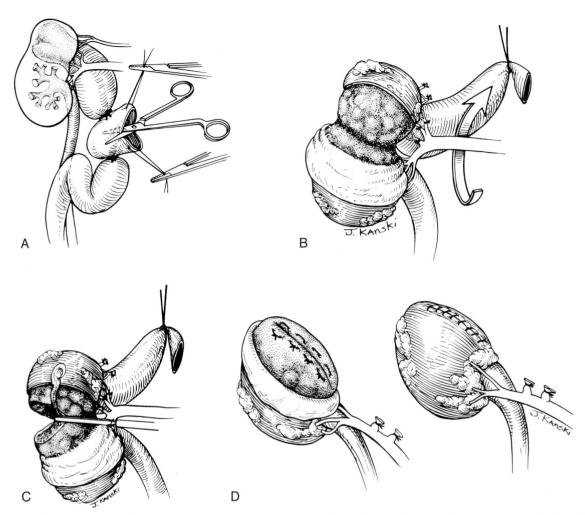

Figure 58–23. Technique of upper pole nephrectomy. *A,* The upper pole ureter is usually very dilated and tortuous and can be identified readily at the lower pole of the kidney. It is separated carefully from the lower pole ureter, divided, and used to improve access to the upper pole moiety. *B,* The upper pole ureter is passed beneath the hilar renal vessels and retracted upward. Small feeding vessels to the upper pole are individually ligated and divided. Any larger vessels that may be supplying the upper pole can be temporarily clamped to determine the extent of their distribution. The capsule of the upper pole is bluntly stripped away, exposing the often coarse and cystic parenchyma of the upper pole. This can usually be distinguished from the smooth texture of the normal lower pole. Often, an indented demarcation is seen between the two poles. *C,* While traction is applied to the lower pole ureter, the upper pole is excised with the use of electrocautery. Vascular control is achieved by temporary clamping of the lower pole vessels. This may also be accomplished by gentle finger compression of the lower pole. Individual vessels are identified and ligated during this part of the procedure. *D,* The parenchyma of the lower pole is approximated at the site of removal of the upper pole with the use of broad mattress sutures. The redundant capsule is then brought over the site of repair and sewn together with a running suture.

in that the pathologic ureter is grasped as a handle and dissected closely to its wall to avoid compromise of the blood supply to the normal ureter. The polar renal vessels are then ligated with clips or divided with electrocautery; this allows for a more discernible demarcation of the affected upper pole. After the polar element is removed with electrocautery, one can check for collecting system leakage with intravenous injection of methylene blue (Yao and Poppas, 2000). Janetschek and colleagues (1997) place fibrin glue and hemostatic agents on the cut surface and then cover it with Gerota's fascia to aid in hemostasis.

Laparoscopic complications are inversely related to surgeon experience (Peters, 1996). In the above-cited reports, complications were uncommon but included inferior vena cava laceration; duodenal perforation and total nephrectomy; and peritoneal tears (if done via the retroperitoneum).

Bilateral single-system ectopic ureters are fortunately rare, because they present a complex therapeutic problem (Koyanagi et al, 1977; Ahmed and Barker, 1992). In this condition, the ureters usually drain into the prostatic urethra in the male and into the distal urethra in the female. Embryologically, the portion of the urogenital sinus between the orifices of the wolffian duct and the ureter develops into the bladder neck musculature. This development does not occur if both ureters remain in the position of the wolffian duct orifice. **Because there is no formation of the trigone and base plate, a very wide, poorly defined, incompetent vesical neck results.** In rare instances, bilateral single ectopic ureters are associated with agenesis of the bladder and urethra. This condition is usually, but not always, incompatible with life (Glenn, 1959)

Commonly, the involved kidneys are dysplastic or display varying degrees of hydronephrosis (Fig. 58–26). The

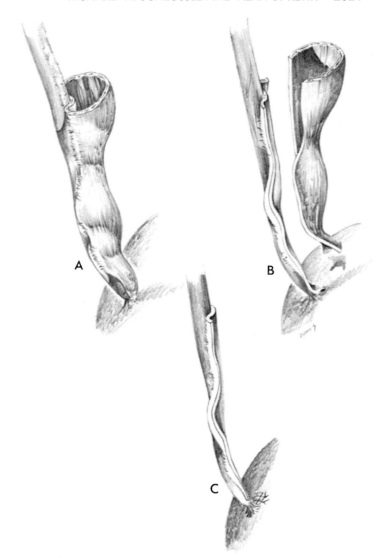

Figure 58–24. Surgical management of the refluxing ureteral stump. *A,* It is difficult to completely separate the distal 2 to 3 cm of the upper pole ureter from the lower pole ureter. The ectopic ureter is excised to this point. *B,* The outer wall of the ectopic ureter is excised to the bladder level. *C,* A transfixing suture obliterates its lumen, with care being taken not to injure the orthotopic ureter.

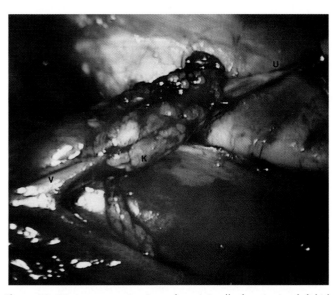

Figure 58–25. Laparoscopic view of a minimally functioning left kidney that was drained by an ectopic ureter in a 16-year-old incontinent girl. Laparoscopic nephrectomy resulted in immediate continence. U, ureter; K, kidney; V, vessels.

ureters are usually dilated, and reflux is often present. The bladder neck is incompetent, so the child dribbles continuously. Because there is poor resistance, the bladder does not have the opportunity to distend with urine and has a small capacity (Fig. 58–27). In the male, incontinence is not as severe as in the female, and bladder capacity may be greater because the external sphincter provides a variable degree of control.

At cystoscopy, the ureteral orifices can be identified in the male, usually just distal to the bladder neck. The lax bladder neck and small bladder are clearly evident. In the female, it can be difficult to find both ureteral orifices, which usually are located in the distal urethra but occasionally enter the genital tract.

The abnormality is akin to epispadias, with the basic defect being a short urethra and incompetent bladder neck. However, in contrast to epispadias, there is a high incidence of renal and urethral abnormalities in addition to the small bladder capacity.

Treatment usually consists of ureteral reimplantation and reconstruction of the bladder neck for continence by one of the tubularization procedures, such as the Young-Dees-Leadbetter (Leadbetter, 1985), Kropp (Kropp and Angwafo,

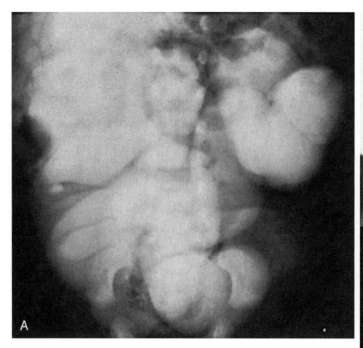

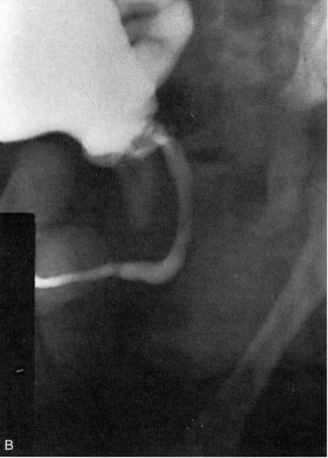

Figure 58–26. *A,* Excretory urogram in a 6-day-old boy shows severe bilateral hydronephrosis and hydroureter. *B,* A voiding cystourethrogram demonstrates refluxing ectopic ureters draining into the prostatic urethra.

1986), or Salle (Rink et al, 1994) procedures. It is often helpful to employ vesicourethral suspension at the same time. Increased exposure through symphyseal splitting has been helpful during these reconstructions (Peters and Hendren, 1989). The success rate is higher in boys than in girls. Bladder capacity often increases in the child who gains satisfactory control. Enterocystoplasty to increase bladder capacity may be necessary in selected cases.

ANOMALIES OF STRUCTURE

Ureteroceles

Few entities in pediatric urology present as great a clinical challenge as ureteroceles. Ureteroceles have varied effects in regard to obstruction, reflux, continence, and renal function; hence, each ureterocele must be managed on an individual basis and not by a simple algorithm. It is imperative for the treating physician to be acquainted with the multiple presentations, radiologic appearances, and treatment options of ureteroceles, as well as the complications to avoid. Such knowledge yields the best possible clinical results.

Embryology

A ureterocele is a cystic dilatation of the terminal ureter. How this develops has been the subject of several discus-

sions. At 37 days' gestation, Chwalle's membrane, a two-layered cell structure, transiently divides the early ureteric bud from the urogenital sinus (Chwalle, 1927). The stenotic orifice commonly seen in the ureterocele has led several researchers to postulate that this dilatation results from incomplete dissolution of Chwalle's membrane. Others have theorized that the affected intravesical ureter suffers from abnormal muscular development; without the appropriate muscular backing, the distal ureter assumes a balloon morphology (Tokunaka et al, 1981). A third theory implicates a developmental stimulus responsible for bladder expansion acting simultaneously on the intravesical ureter (Stephens, 1971). Incontrovertible evidence does not exist to uphold any of these theories, which, in fact, have very little effect on clinical practice.

Diagnosis

As with ectopic ureters, ureteroceles are increasingly diagnosed by prenatal ultrasound studies. Prenatal ultrasonography is capable of demonstrating both the hydronephrosis and the intravesical cystic dilatation. Shekarriz and associates (1999) reported that 30% of their ureteroceles were diagnosed prenatally; however, this series began in 1979, when obstetric sonography was performed less commonly than today. More recent series reveal a high proportion of prenatally diagnosed ureteroceles. Pfister and colleagues (1998) reported that 31 of their 35 patients with

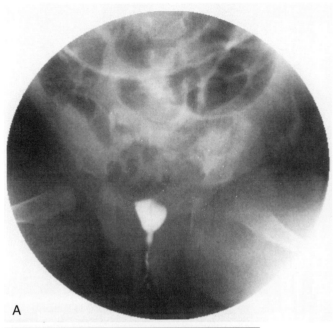

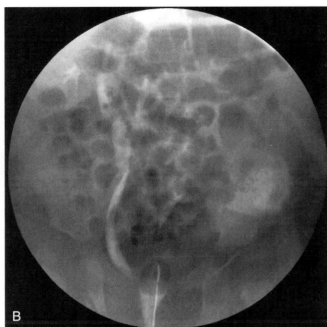

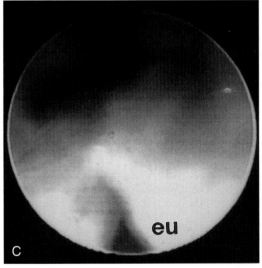

Figure 58–27. A 6-month-old girl was diagnosed with a solitary right kidney drained by an ectopic ureter entering the urethra. *A,* Diminutive bladder was seen on voiding cystourethrogram (VCUG). *B,* Reflux seen on VCUG. *C,* Cystoscopic image of wide bladder neck anteriorly and ectopic ureter (eu) entering just below it into the urethra.

ureteroceles were diagnosed prenatally. In the latter half of their study, Husmann and coworkers (1995) reported a median age at diagnosis of ureterocele of 3 months, with the implication that many of these cases were diagnosed prenatally. Di Benedetto and Monfort (1997) reported that all 25 of their patients with ureteroceles presenting between 1980 and 1994 were diagnosed in utero. If ureteroceles are diagnosed prenatally, the physician is alerted to perform a more comprehensive postnatal evaluation and to administer prophylactic antibiotics at birth.

Ureteroceles have a particular predilection for race and gender (Brock and Kaplan, 1978; Mandell et al, 1980; Cobb et al, 1982; Caldamone and Duckett, 1984; Scherz et al, 1989; Monfort et al, 1992; Rickwood et al, 1992). **They occur most frequently in females (4:1 ratio) and almost exclusively in Caucasians. Approximately 10% are bilateral. Eighty percent of all ureteroceles arise from the upper poles of duplicated systems.** Single-system ureteroceles are sometimes called simple ureteroceles and are usu-

ally found in adults. These single-system ureteroceles are less prone to the severe obstruction and dysplasia associated with duplicated systems.

However, many ureteroceles are still diagnosed clinically. The most common presentation is that of an infant who has a urinary tract infection or urosepsis (Gonzales, 1992; Monfort et al, 1992; Retik and Peters, 1992; Coplen and Duckett, 1995). We have seen patients whose ultrasound and intraoperative findings revealed frank pus in the obstructed upper pole collecting system, and this has also been noted by others (Glazier and Packer, 1997). For this reason, all children with a ureterocele (or, less specifically, any significant hydronephrosis) should be given prophylactic antibiotics. Of 33 patients prescribed prophylactic antibiotics after their prenatal diagnosis, only 1 developed a urinary tract infection (Husmann et al, 1995). Stasis of urine in this obstructed system can lead not only to infection but also to calculus formation (Thornbury et al, 1977; Rodriguez, 1984; Moskovitz et al, 1987). Some children

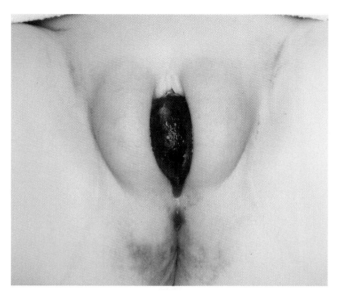

Figure 58–28. A prolapsed ureterocele presented as an interlabial mass in a 3-week-old girl.

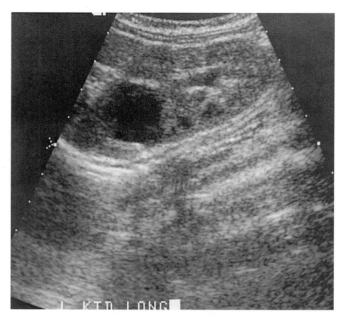

Figure 58–29. Sonographic appearance of upper pole hydronephrosis caused by a ureterocele.

present with a palpable mass in their abdomen, which is a hydronephrotic kidney. The ureterocele, if ectopic, can prolapse out of the urethra as a vaginal mass (Fig. 58–28).

If the ureterocele is large enough, it can obstruct the bladder neck or even the contralateral ureteral orifice and result in hydronephrosis of that collecting system. The bladder outlet obstruction causing bilateral hydronephrosis can even be diagnosed prenatally (Gloor et al, 1996; Austin et al, 1998).

Ectopic ureteroceles can cause incontinence by hindering the normal sphincteric function at or distal to the bladder neck. Infrequently, a child with a ureterocele can present with hematuria. Ureteroceles may have an insidious clinical course, resulting in no specific urologic symptoms but manifesting only as a failure to thrive or as abdominal or pelvic pain. Usually, lengthy evaluation of other organ systems ensues before the problem is correctly localized to the urinary tract.

Imaging studies that are now available afford a great deal of insight into the effects of the ureterocele on normal anatomy and physiology. **The first study obtained in these evaluations is usually an ultrasound** (Geringer et al, 1983b; Cremin, 1986; Teele and Share, 1991). Most commonly, the ureterocele is associated with a duplicated collecting system. Sonographically, two separate renal pelves surrounded by their echogenic hila can be seen. This duplex kidney is larger than a kidney associated with a single collecting system. **A dilated ureter emanates from a hydronephrotic upper pole** (Fig. 58–29). This finding should signal the examiner to image the bladder to determine whether a ureterocele is present. If the lower pole is associated with reflux, or if the ureterocele has caused delayed emptying from the ipsilateral lower pole, this lower pole may likewise be hydronephrotic. Similarly, the ureterocele may impinge on the contralateral ureteral orifice or obstruct the bladder neck and cause hydronephrosis in the opposite kidney. **The upper pole parenchyma drained by the ureterocele will exhibit varying degrees of thickness and echogenicity. Increased echogenicity**

correlates with dysplastic changes. **The bladder frequently displays a thin-walled cyst that is the ureterocele** (Fig. 58–30).

However, there are several pitfalls in ultrasound diagnosis. If the bladder is overdistended, the ureterocele may be effaced and go unnoticed. At times the bladder may be empty, in which case it is difficult to discriminate between the wall of the ureterocele and the wall of the bladder. In such instances, the empty bladder with a ureterocele may be interpreted as simply a partially filled bladder. The dilated ureter should be seen posterior to the bladder. On occasion, a large ureterocele is associated with a diminutive ureter and collecting system. The corresponding upper pole parenchyma can be so small as to be nonvis-

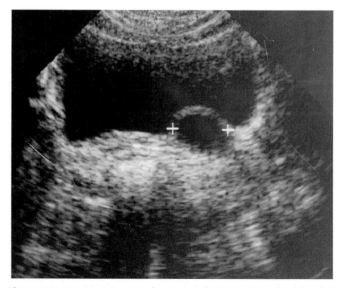

Figure 58–30. An intravesical ureterocele in a 2-month-old girl is outlined by the two crosshatches on an ultrasound image.

ualized. The diagnosis of ureterocele may be overlooked because the duplicated collecting system cannot be identified. This entity has been termed both nonobstructive ectopic ureterocele (Bauer and Retik, 1978) and ureterocele disproportion (Share and Lebowitz, 1989) (Fig. 58–31).

On occasion, the dilated ectopic ureter may be seen immediately posterior to the bladder and may impinge on the bladder wall, giving the appearance that the dilated ureter is intravesical. This may give the false impression of a ureterocele—the pseudoureterocele referred to previously (Diard et al, 1987; Sumfest et al, 1995). The difference between the two entities is that a ureterocele is separated from the bladder space by its thin wall, whereas an ectopic ureter has the thicker bladder wall separating it from the intravesical space. A mesonephric duct cyst that communicates with an ectopic ureter can open into the bladder and mimic a ureterocele on radiographic studies (Sumfest et al, 1995).

Intravenous pyelography is a valuable imaging study in the evaluation of a ureterocele. There are several hallmarks of a urogram in a patient with a ureterocele (Geringer et al, 1983a; Muller et al, 1988), and these findings are similar to those mentioned in the discussion on ectopic ureters. **In the great majority of cases, the upper pole functions poorly and excretes contrast in a delayed fashion or not at all. This upper pole is deviated laterally from the spine because of its hydronephrosis.** This same upper

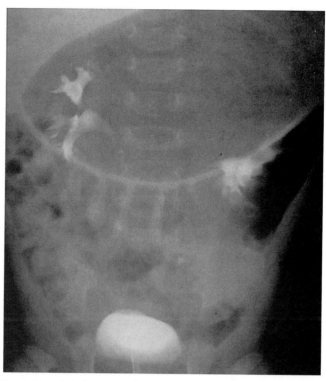

Figure 58–32. Left upper pole hydronephrosis causes lower pole displacement inferiorly and laterally, which is referred to as the drooping lily sign.

pole hydronephrosis is responsible for pushing the lower pole laterally and inferiorly (Fig. 58–32). Because only the lower pole calyces are seen, the number of calyces is less than the complement of a normal kidney.

Whereas the upper pole ureter is infrequently seen on the intravenous pyelogram because of the lack of contrast excretion, its presence may be inferred from its effect on the lower pole ureter. **The lower pole ureter can be seen as laterally deviated, taking a serpiginous course, and notched. These characteristics all result from its association with the dilated, tortuous upper pole ureter** (Fig. 58–33). As mentioned earlier in the section on ultrasonography, hydronephrosis may be seen in the contralateral kidney as a result of obstruction by the ureterocele.

Voiding cystourethrography can demonstrate the size and location of the ureterocele as well as the presence or absence of vesicoureteral reflux. Assessing the severity of such reflux is critical to future management. **Reflux into the ipsilateral lower pole is commonly seen** (Feldman and Lome, 1981; Caldamone and Duckett, 1984) (Fig. 58–34). Pfister and colleagues (1998) noted an incidence of reflux of 49%. Shekarriz and coworkers (1999) reported an overall incidence of reflux of 59% (intravesical ureteroceles 44% and extravesical ureteroceles 63%). In Husmann's series (Husmann et al, 1999), the incidence of reflux was 67%. Sen and associates (1992) reported reflux in 80 (54%) of 148 ipsilateral lower pole ureters. Rickwood and coworkers (1992) noted that 15 (65%) of 23 patients had ipsilateral lower pole reflux. Forty percent of patients with ureteroceles in Monfort's series had reflux (Monfort et al, 1992). Reflux may also be seen in the contralateral system if the ureterocele is large enough to distort the trigone and

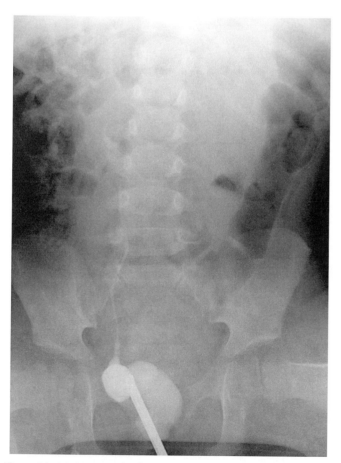

Figure 58–31. Ureterocele disproportion demonstrated via retrograde pyelography. Note the disparity between the large ureterocele and the thin ureter and nondilated collecting system.

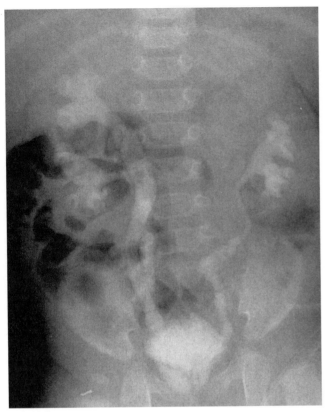

Figure 58–33. An intravenous pyelogram reveals the effects of left upper pole hydronephrosis caused by its obstructing ureterocele. The left upper pole is not visualized, the left lower pole ureter takes a serpiginous course around the dilated upper pole ureter, and there is contralateral hydronephrosis owing to obstruction of the bladder neck by the ureterocele.

the opposite ureteral submucosal tunnel. Pfister and colleagues (1998) noted that 9% of their patients had reflux into the contralateral kidney. In Sen's series, 35 (28%) of 127 patients had reflux in the contralateral unit. Reflux into the ureterocele and its ureter may be present but is uncommon and should alert the physician to the possibility of an ectopic ureterocele whose open mouth in the urethra is allowing reflux.

Images should be obtained from early in the filling phase, because some ureteroceles may efface later in filling and may not be seen. The ureterocele may evert into the ureter and appear to be a diverticulum (Fig. 58–35). Bellah and coworkers (1995) reported on 12 children who were noted to have vesicoureteral reflux and an ipsilateral bladder diverticulum. At surgery, each of these children had a ureterocele associated with a duplex system, and in five the ureterocele was not correctly identified preoperatively. These authors made the point that the lower pole ureter actually enters into a bladder diverticulum that is present because of attenuation of the bladder musculature by the ureterocele. They believed that in these cases the ureterocele is not everting into its own ureter but is rather everting through a weakened bladder wall and dragging the lower pole ureteral orifice along with this segment of herniated bladder mucosa. This description may explain the clinical finding of infrequent resolution of reflux associated with a ureterocele.

When it is performed diligently, cystography demonstrates the ureterocele in the bladder. It **appears as a smooth, broad-based filling defect located near the trigone.** It is frequently eccentrically located, and the superior portion of the ureterocele may be angled to one side, thereby giving a clue as to which side the ureterocele is associated with (Fig. 58–36). However, on cystography,

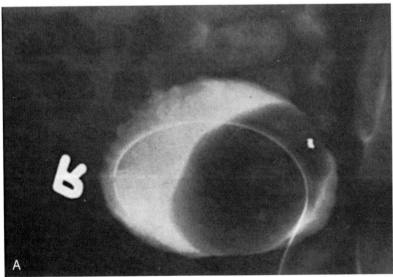

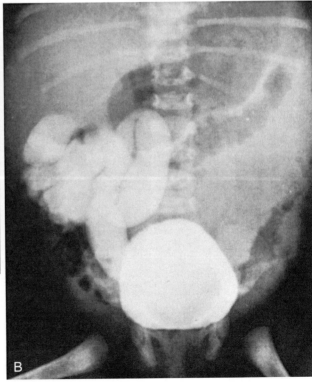

Figure 58–34. *A,* Cystogram outlines a *left* ureterocele. *B,* Postvoiding film shows reflux to the *right* lower pole. This girl had *bilateral* ureteroceles, with the right one being a small subtrigonal ureterocele that was not demonstrated on the cystogram.

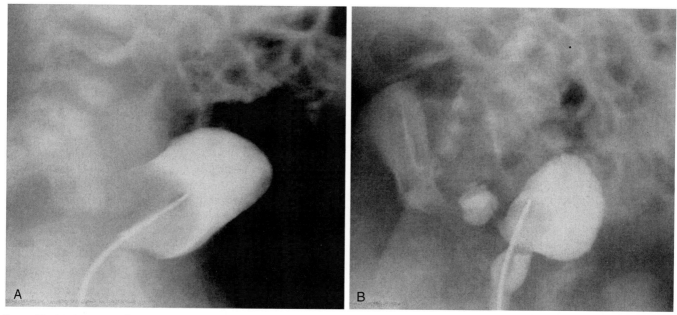

Figure 58–35. A ureterocele seen on a cystogram during early filling *(A)* may be mistaken during late filling for a diverticulum as the ureterocele everts into its own ureter *(B)*.

the ureterocele is often centrally placed, and it may not be helpful in this regard. In such instances, cystoscopy may shed light on the issue. If the cystoscopic findings are inconclusive, the answer can be obtained by injecting contrast material into the ureterocele; this method should define the side from which the ureterocele emanated (Fig. 58–37). Injection of contrast into the ureterocele can verify the diagnosis of ureterocele disproportion when the upper

tract findings are difficult to interpret. Such information is obviously necessary in planning the surgical approach.

Nuclear scans with agents such as DMSA and diethyl-enetriaminepentaacetic acid (DTPA) or mercaptoacetyl triglycine (MAG3) can give valuable estimates of upper pole

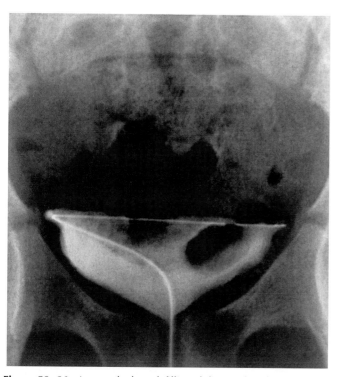

Figure 58–36. A smooth, lateral filling defect is the classic appearance of a ureterocele on a cystogram.

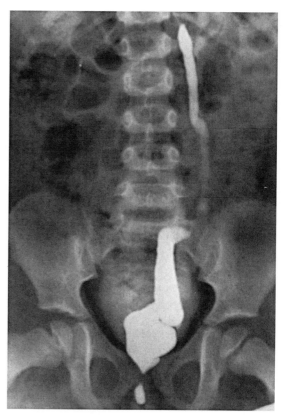

Figure 58–37. Endoscopic injection of a ureterocele outlines the upper pole and the distal extent of the ureterocele.

contribution to overall renal function as well as degrees of obstruction (Arap et al, 1984). It is important to trace the regions of interest correctly and consistently to obtain accurate information. This information is often helpful in determining whether the upper pole moiety is worth saving.

Treatment

It should once again be stressed that, before any surgical intervention, the surgeon must obtain as much information as possible regarding the patient's altered anatomy and physiology. Only then can a rational treatment plan be devised.

Because ureteroceles have a broad spectrum of presentation, anatomy, and pathophysiology, each child must be treated individually. No single method of surgical repair suffices for all cases. The goals of therapy should be clearly defined and factored into the clinical decisions. **These goals are preservation of renal function; elimination of infection, obstruction, and reflux; and maintenance of urinary continence. Minimizing surgical morbidity is a goal that must be included in this consideration.** The management of a ureterocele associated with an upper pole of a duplicated system has generated much debate. Although the goals of treatment could certainly generate a consensus, the means to achieving those goals have not necessarily been agreed on.

A primary concern is the preservation of renal parenchyma if at all possible. This goal is achieved by correcting obstruction and preventing reflux with its risks of renal parenchymal damage from infection. At times, it is necessary to balance one against the other, because relieving the obstruction of a ureterocele may induce reflux in either or both poles of the involved duplication. In other instances, the same action may cause existing lower pole reflux to resolve. Several means of achieving these goals of therapy are available. Because there are a sizable number of permutations when one considers all the possible combinations and degrees of ipsilateral and contralateral reflux, ipsilateral and contralateral obstruction, varying degrees of salvageable function, infection, and age, one can easily see why most people believe that when dealing with ureteroceles each case must be managed on an individual basis.

In most instances, the upper pole contributes little, if at all, to overall renal function. The aim therefore is to deal with this offending unit in a manner that is geared not only toward alleviating obstruction and its potential for recurrent infection but also toward the cessation of reflux that is present in about half of the cases.

There is a diversity of opinion in this regard. One group of surgeons advocates the so-called upper tract approach; this approach consists of upper pole nephrectomy and partial ureterectomy, or, less commonly, when significant upper pole function is present, a ureteropyelostomy (Mandell et al, 1980; Cendron et al, 1981; Feldman and Lome, 1981; Caldamone et al, 1984; Reitelman and Perlmutter, 1990). With either of these procedures, the ureterocele should decompress and, with return of the trigone to a more normal configuration, resolution of the ipsilateral lower pole reflux may occur. The advantages of this approach are avoidance of the morbidity of a sec-

ond surgical procedure and, it is hoped, elimination of a potentially difficult bladder neck and urethral dissection. If a second procedure is eventually required, it can be performed when the child is older on an elective basis (King et al, 1983). **Mandell and associates (1980) treated 18 patients in this manner. In 14 of these patients, a one-stage procedure was planned; only 3 patients (21%) required reoperation** (the indications being persistent lower pole reflux, reflux into the ureteral stump, and failure of ureterocele decompression). They are proponents of the upper pole approach because it meets the goals of a low reoperative rate and resolution of the problems described earlier. They do state, however, that if a patient has high-grade reflux into the ipsilateral lower pole ureter, a combination of upper pole nephroureterectomy, ureterocele excision, and lower pole ureteral reimplantation may be necessary. This combined approach would be recommended because these severe degrees of reflux are less likely to disappear spontaneously and would probably require a second procedure.

Another scenario that should prompt consideration for a single-stage repair at the kidney and bladder level is the case of lower pole reflux associated with a large everting ureterocele and a poorly functioning upper pole. This, too, is unlikely to result in reflux resolution, because the muscular backing necessary for ureteral compression is usually lacking in everting ureteroceles.

Caldamone and associates (1984) had a similar rate for secondary procedures using the upper tract approach. Of 36 patients managed in this way (including 4 who underwent ureteropyelostomy), only 7 (19%) needed secondary procedures. Four had bladder outlet obstruction, and three had persistent reflux associated with poor renal growth, renal scarring, or recurrent urinary tract infections. Ten of their patients had delayed reflux (i.e., reflux that appeared after an upper tract procedure in a patient with no preoperative reflux), and only 3 of these 10 patients had spontaneous resolution of the reflux. The authors concluded that most patients can be managed with an upper urinary tract approach alone.

Likewise, Perlmutter and associates (Kroovand and Perlmutter, 1979; Reitelman and Perlmutter, 1990) directed their attention to removal of the upper pole of the kidney. They combined this procedure with a total ureterectomy to the level of the bladder to prevent possible problems from a retained stump (e.g., pyoureter, diverticulum). When the upper pole merited salvage, they performed either an ipsilateral ureteropyelostomy or a distal ureteroureterostomy. In most instances, there was a reasonable chance for resolution of the reflux after decompression of the ureterocele.

One of the more extensive experiences in the literature is that of Scherz and colleagues (1989). They reported their clinical observations in 60 patients with ectopic ureteroceles (defined as either a ureterocele associated with an upper pole of a duplicated system or a ureterocele in an ectopic position). They also compared the need for further surgery in patients treated with the upper urinary tract approach alone and in those who had a combined upper and lower urinary tract approach. The combined approach uses two incisions to achieve upper pole heminephrectomy, partial ureterectomy, and intravesical excision and marsupialization of the ureterocele, along with correction of reflux when present. **Of 19 evaluable patients who had the upper urinary tract approach alone, 9 (47%) required reoperation for recurrent reflux or infection. In contrast, of 28 patients who were treated with the combined approach, only 4 (14%) required reoperation, all for reflux.** These authors believed that marsupialization of the ureterocele was less likely to cause sphincter damage than enucleation. They also emphasized the need for passing a large catheter antegrade through the bladder neck to ascertain that all mucosal lips that might act as obstructing valves had been removed. They believed that the combined approach is a superior one because of its lower reoperative rate. **With the exception of the acutely ill child with urosepsis, Hendren and Mitchell (1979) also advocated a complete repair, namely, upper pole nephrectomy, ureterocele excision, and ureteral reimplantation.**

Gotoh and colleagues (1988) reported use of the presence or absence of radiographic eversion of the ureterocele, the separation between the upper and lower orifices, and the upper pole function to determine the means of correction. In cases with eversion and separation of the orifices, upper pole function was always absent. When the orifices were adjacent, function was absent in one third of cases. Upper pole nephrectomy was performed with an extravesical resection of the ureterocele and repair of the bladder wall, without lower pole reimplantation.

The reports of Decter and associates (1989) and Gonzales (1992) reiterated the need to consider each case individually. Essentially, they proceeded with an upper tract approach in infants who had low-grade or no reflux in the ipsilateral lower pole. In those infants who were likely to need a secondary procedure (such as those with high-grade reflux or a prolapsed ureterocele) and in septic patients not responding to antibiotic therapy, they advocated initial decompression of the ureterocele via endoscopic incision.

A body of evidence has begun to emerge from the literature delineating the difference in success of treatment based on whether the ureteroceles were intravesical versus ectopic and whether there was associated reflux. In regard to upper pole nephrectomy for the treatment of a ureterocele, Shekarriz and associates (1999) noted that of their 41 extravesical ureteroceles treated with an upper tract approach, 17 (41%) required reoperation. The reoperation rate varied based on the degree of preoperative reflux. If there was no reflux, only 20% required reoperation. Low-grade reflux required reoperation in 30% of cases, and high-grade reflux in 53%. The same upper tract approach in intravesical ureteroceles resulted in two of six patients' requiring a second operation.

Husmann and colleagues (1999) similarly noted a high reoperative rate when upper pole nephrectomy was performed for an ectopic ureterocele associated with reflux. Their overall need for a second procedure after a partial nephrectomy for an ectopic ureterocele was 65%. A partial nephrectomy was the definitive procedure for 85% of patients if there was no reflux, but for only 16% of those with grade III or greater reflux.

Churchill and coworkers (1992) divided their 43 patients into three groups based on the number and severity of the renal units jeopardized by hydronephrosis and reflux. Group 1 was defined as those patients with an ectopic ureterocele whose only renal unit with significant hydronephrosis was the upper pole that drained into the ureterocele. This group was successfully treated with an upper tract approach 89% of the time. Group 2 (ipsilateral lower pole significant hydronephrosis and/or reflux) and group 3 (ipsilateral lower pole significant hydronephrosis and/or reflux and a contralateral kidney with significant hydronephrosis and/or reflux) required a second surgical procedure 71% and 60% of the time, respectively.

The technique of upper pole nephrectomy for nonfunctioning upper poles due to ureteroceles is the same technique as upper pole nephrectomy described previously in this chapter for ectopic ureters (see Fig. 58–23).

Our intravesical approach to the ureterocele begins with a transverse incision of the ureterocele between two stay sutures (Fig. 58–38). Proximally, a plane is obtained between the ureterocele wall and the wall of the bladder. The ureterocele is dissected off the bladder to the point at which it joins the lower pole ureter. Then the ureters are dissected as a unit, the upper pole ureter is tapered as needed, and both ureters are reimplanted submucosally. Amar (1978) advocated submucosal saline injection to facilitate creation of the submucosal tunnel. The distal portion of the ureterocele is dissected in the same plane to the level of the bladder neck, where it is resected. **The detrusor muscle is plicated if it is attenuated and it appears that it may offer insufficient backing.** Bladder mucosal flaps are raised to cover the area of the removed ureterocele.

Once again, several technical points regarding ureterocele excision and common sheath reimplantation deserve mention. **Separation of the duplicated ureters during intravesical dissection should be discouraged, because it can lead to sacrifice of the common blood supply running longitudinally between the two ureters. Plication of the detrusor muscle underlying the ureterocele may be necessary to shore up any areas of muscle deficiency. Further, the distal portion of the ureterocele may extend below the bladder neck. Extreme care must be taken in this part of the dissection to avoid injury to the sphincter mechanisms.**

A commonly held belief is that an upper pole drained by a ureterocele is compromised by atrophy and dysplasia to such an extent that it rarely has any significant function. However, **with the increased use of prenatal sonography, more ureteroceles are coming to clinical attention at an earlier stage and potentially at a time when upper pole function can be salvaged** (Monfort et al, 1992). Treatment options to effect salvage are either upper pole to lower pole ureteropyelostomy or ureteroureterostomy, ureterocele excision with common sheath reimplantation, or transurethral incision of the ureterocele.

Upper pole biopsy at the time of renal exploration may aid in assessing whether the tissue is dysplastic or viable (Coplen and Duckett, 1995). Before that procedure, radiographic imaging can provide information regarding the presence of function. An intravenous pyelogram that demonstrates an upper pole that excretes contrast, either *parri passu* with the lower pole or even in only a slightly delayed fashion, is suggestive of parenchyma with recoverability. Similarly, a nuclear medicine renal scan with an agent such as ^{99m}Tc-DMSA, which binds to the functional

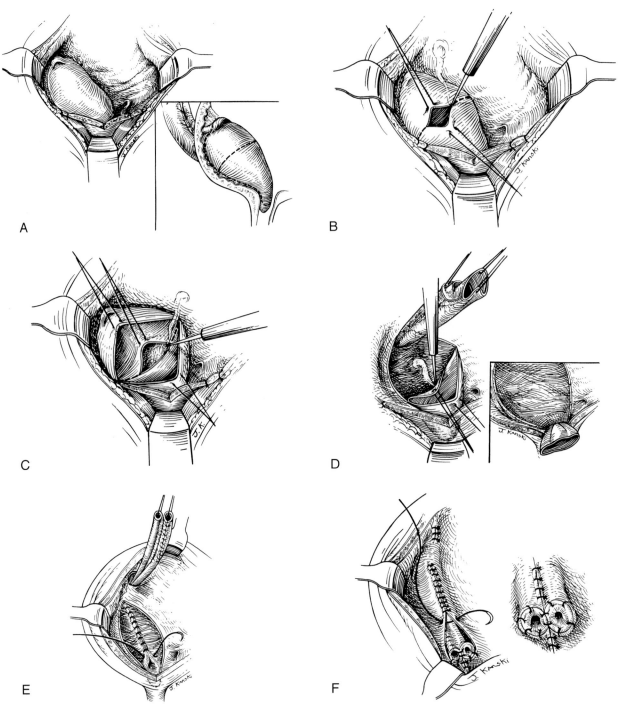

Figure 58–38. Technique for excision of ectopic ureterocele and common sheath reimplantation of upper and lower pole ureters. *A,* Appearance of right-sided ureterocele with open bladder, viewed from below. Note proximity of the contralateral ureteral orifice. *Inset,* Cutaway side view demonstrating the close association of the two polar ureters with a common vascular supply. The dotted line indicates the planned initial incision of the ureterocele. *B,* After stay sutures are placed, the ureterocele is incised with electrocautery in a transverse direction, exposing the inner cavity of the ureterocele. *C,* The posterior mucosal wall of the ureterocele is incised transversely, revealing the often thinned posterior muscular wall of the bladder. This incision will then be continued around the bladder mucosal edge of the ureterocele, including the orifice of the lower pole ureter. Stay sutures are important to provide adequate exposure. *D,* The upper and lower pole ureters have been mobilized and are retracted into the bladder. The distal aspect of the ureterocele is being mobilized in a similar fashion. The bladder mucosal surface will also be incised around the edge of the ureterocele to permit complete removal of the ureterocele. *Inset,* The fully mobilized distal ureterocele is retracted caudally, revealing its narrowing attachment at the bladder neck. *E,* The dilated upper pole ureter associated with the ureterocele has been tapered and remains in continuity with the lower pole ureter. Both have been brought into the bladder through a newly formed muscular hiatus to provide adequate tunnel length for the ureteral reimplantation. The thinned-out posterior bladder wall has been repaired with multiple interrupted sutures to provide adequate muscular backing for the ureters. The bladder mucosa surrounding the ureterocele defect has been mobilized to permit covering of the ureters. *F, left,* The ureters have been reimplanted into the new ureteral tunnel, have been sutured distally after spatulation, and are being covered with bladder mucosa. The lower pole orifice is medial. *Right,* Final appearance of the ureteral tunnel following completion of the reimplantation.

nephron tubules, can demonstrate an upper pole that may have salvageable renal parenchyma despite obstruction. The goal in these cases is to create effective drainage of the upper pole collecting system.

One option used to achieve this goal is the upper urinary tract anastomotic techniques of ureteroureterostomy or ureteropyelostomy. This results in the upper pole system's draining into the lower pole system. Such high anastomoses are preferable to a distal ureteroureterostomy, because the latter is prone to the travel of urine boluses down one ureter and then, at the ureteral-ureteral junction, retrograde up the other ureter. This phenomenon is sometimes referred to as the yo-yo effect. It can detrimentally affect urinary drainage and lead to stasis, infection, and ureteral dilatation.

When performing the upper tract anastomoses, dissection should be limited to an absolute minimum, especially medially, to prevent disruption of either ureter's blood supply. The upper pole ureter may be considerably larger than the lower pole ureter. A generous longitudinal ureterotomy made in the lower pole ureter is performed to overcome such disproportion, and the anastomosis is performed in an end-to-side fashion. The distal portion of the upper pole ureter should be aspirated with a fine feeding tube to decompress the ureterocele. The distal upper pole ureter is resected as far inferiorly as possible, with care taken to stay directly on this ureter's wall and avoid the vasculature of the adjacent lower pole ureter. If the ureterocele does not reflux, the resection is taken as distally as the wound allows and the remnant lower portion of ureter may be left open.

Ureterocele excision with common sheath reimplantation also achieves the goal of upper tract drainage. The technical aspects of this approach were described earlier. The disadvantage of this approach compared with the flank upper pole to lower pole anastomoses just described is that the bladder approach has the added morbidity of hematuria, bladder spasm, and several days of bladder drainage with a catheter. In addition, the dissection of the ureterocele bed may be a more involved one and has the potential problems of bladder neck injury.

Descriptions of ureterocele incisions date back to Zielinski's technique of a low transverse incision (Zielinski, 1962) and a longitudinal ureterocele incision proposed by Hutch and Chisholm (1966). These so-called meatotomies were performed via open surgery. **There has been an increased interest in the endoscopic treatment of ureteroceles** (Cobb et al, 1982; Monfort et al, 1992; Blythe et al, 1993; Coplen and Duckett, 1995). Although transurethral resection was satisfactory in achieving decompression (Wines and O'Flynn, 1972; Tank, 1986), it often led to massive reflux of the involved system. As a result, this procedure fell out of favor, except in cases of sepsis when urgent relief of obstruction was needed. However, improvements in equipment and refinements in technique have led to a re-evaluation of the role of ureterocele incision. **Blythe and coauthors** (1993) **described their technique of using a No. 3 Fr Bugbee electrode to puncture the ureterocele near its base and proximal to the bladder neck.** The new opening should have an intravesical position while the bladder is empty, to avoid obstruction by the bladder neck. With the use of

such a technique, obstruction is relieved, and the roof of the ureterocele presumably should collapse onto the floor of the bladder and act as a flap valve mechanism to prevent reflux. With this technique, 73% of their patients needed no further procedures. However, **when analyzing their data further, they concluded that intravesical ureteroceles fared better than ectopic ureteroceles with regard to decompression (93% versus 75%), preservation of upper pole function (96% versus 47%), newly created reflux (18% versus 47%), and need for secondary procedures (7% versus 50%).** Based on these findings, they recommended ureterocele incision in all neonates as well as in older children with either an intravesical ureterocele, a ureterocele associated with a functioning upper pole, or a single-system ureterocele.

Hagg and associates (2000) presented a more recent compilation of patients from the same group; in this series, they used a slightly modified method of endoscopic ureterocele decompression. With endoscopic ureterocele puncture, rather than incision, 19 (37%) of 51 patients with a ureterocele associated with a duplicated system required a secondary open procedure. Twenty-two of these patients had an intravesical ureterocele, and 5 of them (23%) required a secondary open procedure. Of the 29 patients with an ectopic ureterocele, 14 (48%) required a secondary open procedure. For ectopic ureteroceles, these authors recommended puncture of the intravesical component just proximal to the bladder neck and omission of the puncture of the urethral component of the ureterocele. Of note, none of the nine intravesical single-system ureteroceles that were endoscopically punctured required a secondary open procedure. Nineteen of the 51 patients had iatrogenic reflux, and 7 went on to ureteral reimplantation.

However, there is an opposing school of thought that perhaps ureterocele incision is not quite as effective and should not be employed as the initial approach in the majority of ureteroceles. This disaffection with transurethral incision appears to be directed more toward the ectopic ureterocele than the intravesical ureterocele. Husmann and associates (1999) treated 25 patients with intravesical ureteroceles with endoscopic decompression; only 3 required a second procedure (2 for failed decompression and 1 for reflux into the ureterocele). Two patients were treated with repeat endoscopy, and the patient with reflux was treated with ureteral reimplantation. There appeared to be no difference in the success rate whether the decompression was achieved via ureterocele puncture or via ureterocele incision. However, in regard to ectopic ureteroceles, the incision was markedly less successful. If the ectopic ureterocele was associated with no reflux, only 36% of the patients were spared a second procedure. If the ureterocele was associated with grade III reflux or greater, then only 16% required no further surgery. The upper pole nephrectomy had no better success in this group of patients with high-grade preoperative reflux.

Pfister and associates (1998) also observed a difference in the success of ureterocele incision based on the type of ureterocele, (i.e., intravesical versus ectopic). Of the 16 intravesical ureteroceles incised, only 1 required a second procedure. Of the 21 patients with ectopic ureteroceles, 4 required a second procedure for incomplete decompression, 7 required reoperative surgery for preoperative reflux that

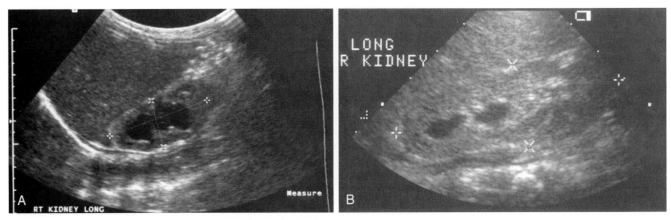

Figure 58–39. *A,* Sonographic appearance of right upper pole hydronephrosis secondary to a ureterocele. *B,* Same patient 3 months after cystoscopic incision of ureterocele; the upper pole has been significantly decompressed.

persisted in all 7 patients, and 8 patients required ureteral reimplantation for reflux into the ureterocele that did not resolve in follow-up ranging from 12 to 36 months. Therefore, although incision of the ectopic ureterocele appeared to be mostly successful in regard to decompression, it did not achieve the goal of correcting preexisting reflux, and it resulted in a significant incidence of reflux into the ureterocele itself (30%). The authors did note, however, that there were 14 patients whose upper pole was subtended by a ureterocele that was presumed to have no preoperative function. Of these, 10 had return of function to the upper pole (as seen by intravenous pyelogram) after ureterocele incision.

Husmann and coauthors (1999) concluded that neither transurethral incision nor upper pole nephrectomy adequately addresses the needs of patients with an ectopic ureterocele and significant reflux, and lower tract complete reconstruction may be the optimal approach. Shekarriz and associates (1999) also expressed a lack of enthusiasm for the transurethral incision of ectopic ureteroceles. The intravesical ureteroceles that were incised in their series had an acceptable reoperative rate of only 23%. All 13 patients with ectopic ureteroceles that were cystoscopically incised

needed secondary procedures. The reoperative rate in the literature for ectopic ureteroceles treated with upper pole nephrectomy varies but can be as high as 62% (Husmann et al, 1995; Caldemon et al, 1984; Rickwood et al, 1992). Their success rate with upper pole nephrectomy for the ectopic ureterocele associated with preoperative high-grade reflux was only 47%. They therefore concluded that endoscopic incision has a limited application and should be used only in cases of intravesical ureteroceles, or ectopic ureteroceles causing bladder outlet obstruction and sepsis. However, for the ectopic ureterocele with significant preoperative reflux, they believed that patients are best served by complete lower tract reconstruction. This is defined as ureterocelectomy and ureteral reimplantation. They treated 18 patients who had an ectopic ureterocele with this approach (of whom 83% had preoperative reflux), and none required secondary surgery. Approximately half of their patients were operated on before 1 year of age, and all of the patients were continent on follow-up. They believed that their experience refuted the commonly held notion that lower tract reconstruction for ureterocele in the young child is fraught with complications and should be avoided.

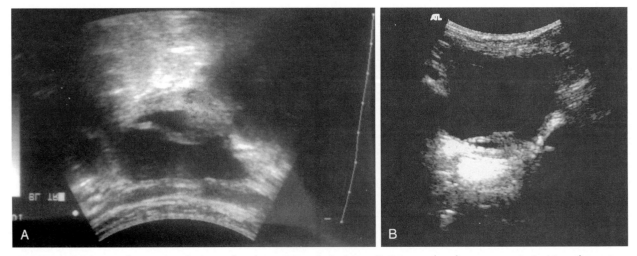

Figure 58–40. *A,* Sonogram of a ureterocele 3 months after cystoscopic incision. *B,* Ten months after cystoscopic incision, the ureterocele is collapsed. (Bladder volume is the same in both images.)

We have endoscopically incised ureteroceles in selected cases. In our experience, ureterocele incision resulted in partial or complete decompression of all ureteroceles (Fig. 58–39). More importantly, the radiographic appearance of the upper tract improved in 20 of 22 cases (Fig. 58–40). Five of 12 children who had reflux into the ipsilateral lower pole had their reflux resolve after ureterocele incision, and three others had their reflux decrease in grade. Transurethral incision of the ureterocele resulted in reflux into the ureterocele ureter in 44% of the cases; this induced reflux was equivalent for ectopic and intravesical ureteroceles as well as single and duplicated systems. One third of the patients underwent a second operative procedure, primarily for reflux. One could argue that this minimally invasive outpatient procedure is of benefit to the remainder of the patients who require no further surgery. If future reimplantation surgery is performed, the ureter is less dilated and easier to manipulate.

We have made several observations based on our experience with transurethral incisions of ureteroceles. When performing routine cystoscopy in a female patient, it is acceptable to blindly pass the cystoscope sheath and obturator into the bladder via the urethra. However, blind passage of a cystoscope in a child with a ureterocele may result in a tearing of the ureterocele. Therefore, we pass the cystoscope under direct vision. In addition, we try to instill a minimum of irrigation so as not to collapse the ureterocele. The entire bladder is inspected to ascertain the position of the ipsilateral lower pole ureteral orifice and the contralateral ureteral orifice.

Our preferred method of incising the ureterocele is similar to the one described by Rich and colleagues (1990): a transverse incision through the full thickness of the ureterocele wall using the cutting current. Making the incision as distally on the ureterocele and as close to the bladder floor as possible lessens the chance of postoperative reflux into the ureterocele. One can either use a Bugbee electrode or the metal stylet of a ureteral catheter, which is extended just beyond the catheter. We favor the latter instrument because it has a finer tip and allows for more precision. The No. 3 Fr straight and angle-tipped wires are also acceptable for ureterocele incision. We prefer to perform the incision under video projection because the magnification enhances accuracy.

The ureterocele should be incised deeply, because ureteroceles are often thick walled. Adequacy of ureterocele incision is confirmed either by the escape of a jet of urine from the ureterocele or by viewing the urothelium of the inside of the ureterocele (Fig. 58–41). For the ectopic ureterocele that extends into the urethra, several people advocate either a longitudinal incision that extends down from the intravesical portion into the urethral portion or two separate punctures, one in the intravesical portion of the ureterocele and one in the urethral portion of the ureterocele.

In institutions where suburetic Teflon injections are an accepted means of treating reflux, an entirely endoscopic approach has been tried whereby the ureterocele is incised with electrocautery; if reflux occurs in the upper pole or persists in the lower pole, it is managed with Teflon injections (Diamond and Boston, 1987; Yachia, 1993).

Single-System Ureteroceles

Although the single-system ureterocele usually manifests in adults, it is sometimes seen in children. The ureterocele in these cases is almost always intravesical and occupies the proper trigonal position. Although most simple ureteroceles have obstructing pinpoint orifices, unobstructed ureteroceles do exist. The degree of obstruction is probably not significant in most adult cases and likewise tends to be less severe than the obstruction seen in duplicated systems in children (Sen et al, 1992).

The ureterocele may vary in size from a tiny cystic dilatation of the submucosal ureter to a large balloon that fills the bladder. Histologically, the wall of the ureterocele contains varying degrees of attenuated smooth muscle bundles and fibrous tissue. The ureterocele is covered by vesical mucosa and lined with ureteral mucosa.

Most children with simple ureteroceles present with symptoms of urinary tract infection. Prenatal ultrasonography has detected other, asymptomatic cases. Stasis and

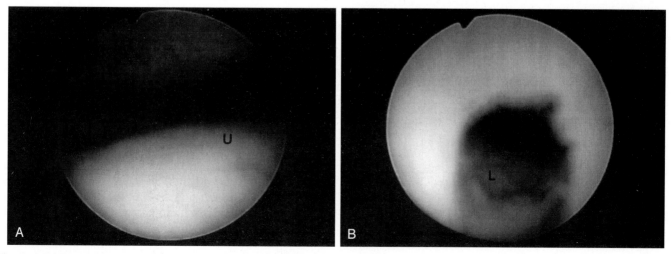

Figure 58–41. *A,* Cystoscopic view of the smooth-walled dome of a ureterocele (u) with the bladder cavity in the distance. *B,* Magnified cystoscopic view of the ureterocele and its lumen (L) after endoscopic puncture of the ureterocele.

infection predispose the patient to stone formation in the ureterocele and upper urinary tract. Rarely, large simple ureteroceles prolapse through the bladder neck, causing urinary obstruction.

Excretory urography often demonstrates the characteristic cobra-head (or spring-onion) deformity, an area of increased density similar to the head of a cobra with a halo or less dense shadow around it (Fig. 58–42). The halo represents a filling defect, which is the ureterocele wall, and the oval density is contrast excreted into the ureterocele from the functioning kidney. Larger ureteroceles often fail to fill early with contrast material, resulting in a sizable filling defect in the bladder. These findings are associated with varying degrees of hydronephrosis and hydroureter. The upper urinary tract changes associated with a simple ureterocele are usually not as severe as those associated with an ectopic ureterocele. At cystoscopy, the ureterocele usually expands rhythmically with each peristaltic wave that fills it and then shrinks as a thin jet of urine drains, usually continuously, through the small orifice.

Single-system ureteroceles more readily lend themselves to transvesical excision and reimplantation, with any muscular defect corrected as necessary. **These ureteroceles are also more amenable to endoscopic incision (Rich et al, 1990) and are less likely to exhibit postoperative reflux into the incised ureterocele.**

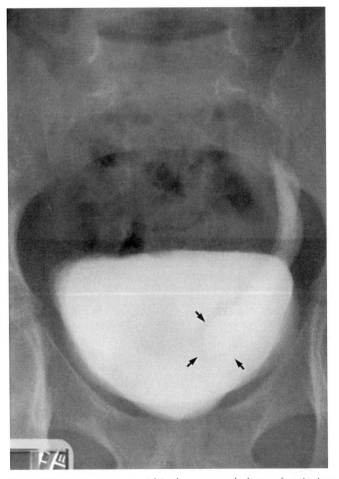

Figure 58–42. Contrast material in the ureterocele from a functioning renal unit looks like a cobra head on the intravenous pyelogram because of the filling defect of the ureterocele wall.

Prolapsing Ureteroceles

A ureterocele that extends through the bladder neck and the urethra and presents as a vaginal mass in girls is termed a prolapsing ureterocele (Orr and Glanton, 1953). This mass can be distinguished from other interlabial masses (e.g., rhabdomyosarcoma, urethral prolapse, hydrometrocolpos, periurethral cysts) by virtue of its appearance and location (Witherington and Smith, 1979; Nussbaum and Lebowitz, 1983). The prolapsed ureterocele has a smooth, round wall in contrast to the grapelike cluster that typifies rhabdomyosarcoma (see Fig. 58–28). The color may vary from pink to bright red to the necrotic shades of blue, purple, or brown. The ureterocele usually slides down the posterior wall of the urethra, and therefore it can be demonstrated anterior to the mass and can be catheterized. The vagina (and the corresponding masses that emanate from it, such as hydrometrocolpos) is posterior to the ureterocele.

The prolapse can be intermittent and may cause vesical obstruction and, consequently, bilateral renal obstruction. Alternatively, the child may be able to void around the ureterocele. In the former scenario, the patient may have varying degrees of hydronephrosis and azotemia and may be septic.

The short-term goal is to decompress the ureterocele. The prolapsing ureterocele may be manually reduced back into the bladder, but, even if this is successful, the prolapse is likely to recur. Upper pole nephrectomy (as previously described) combined with aspiration of the ureterocele from above is usually effective in achieving decompression. However, this decompression may not occur rapidly enough in the acutely ill child. In an effort to decompress the ureterocele rapidly, one can make a transverse incision in the ureterocele at the level of the vagina. Because the wall of the ureterocele may be thick, the incision should be appropriately deep. This maneuver is not uniformly successful because the bladder neck in its resting state is closed and this may keep the intravesical ureterocele, which is proximal to the point of incision and proximal to the bladder neck, distended.

Therefore, if incision at the level of the vagina is not effective, endoscopic incision of the ureterocele in its intravesical portion may be necessary. If all these measures fail and the child remains in extremis, open surgical unroofing or marsupialization of the ureterocele is indicated. Common sheath ureteral reimplantation to correct the ensuing reflux can be carried out on an elective basis when the child is older.

Ureteral Stenosis and Stricture

Congenital anatomic narrowing or narrowing of the ureteral lumen as detected by calibration is referred to as congenital ureteral stenosis or congenital ureteral stricture, but developmentally the term "stricture" should refer only to obstructions involving a histologic lesion in the ureter. Cussen (1971), in his series of 147 ureteral lesions, noted 81 (55%) with ureteral stenosis. His histologic studies of the stenotic zone revealed normal transitional epithelium, a diminished population of otherwise normal-appearing smooth

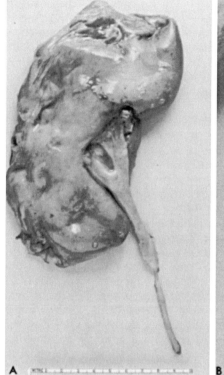
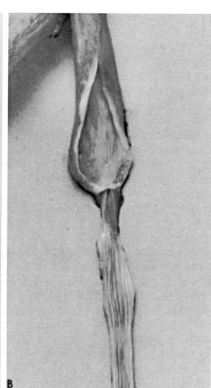

Figure 58–43. Congenital ureteral valve. *A,* Extended view. *B,* Long section showing greatly dilated ureter above the valve and normal size below. (From Simon HB, et al: J Urol 1955;74:336.)

muscle cells, and no increase in fibrous tissue in the wall of the stenotic zone. Ultrastructural studies were not conducted.

The cause of congenital ureteral stenosis is not certain, but ultrastructural studies such as those of Notley (1972) and Hanna and associates (1976, 1977) may provide the answer. Developmentally, simple narrowing probably re-

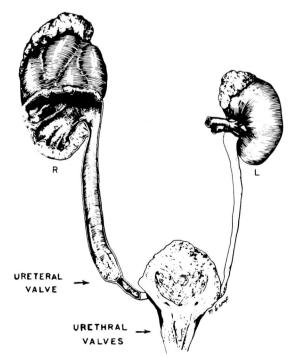

Figure 58–44. Complete diaphragm obstructing the right ureter, with hydroureter and hydronephrosis above. (From Roberts RR: J Urol 1956;76:62.)

sults from a disturbance in embryogenesis around the 11th to 12th weeks, with disturbed development of the mesenchyme contributing to the ureteral musculature (Allen, 1977). A spectrum of histologic abnormalities, with or without demonstrable anatomic narrowing, may occur at the zone of obstruction (Hanna et al, 1976). (See the discussion of megaureter in Chapter 59, Vesicoureteral Reflux and Megaureter, for a description of the reported ultrastructural abnormalities.) Three areas of the ureter are particularly liable to ureteral stenosis. In order of decreasing frequency, they are the distal ureter just above the extravesical junction, the ureteropelvic junction and, rarely, the midureter at the pelvic brim (Allen, 1970; Campbell, 1970). More than one area of segmental stenosis may be present in the same ureter, with a widened length of ureter between the segments, suggesting a developmental defect that affects the entire ureteric bud.

The clinical manifestations and treatment of ureteral stenosis and stricture involving the ureteropelvic junction are included in the section on ureteropelvic junction obstruction.

Ureteral Valves

Ureteral valves are uncommon causes of ureteral obstruction, consisting of transverse folds of redundant mucosa that contain smooth muscle (Wall and Wachter, 1952). These are single annular or diaphragmatic lesions with a pinpoint opening (Figs. 58–43 and 58–44). The ureter is dilated above the obstruction and normal below it. As determined in a review of 40 congenital ureteral valves, **the valves are distributed throughout the length of the ureter, although least commonly in the middle third or**

the pelviureteral junction (Dajani et al, 1982). Presenting symptoms include flank pain, urinary tract infection, incontinence, hypertension, and hematuria. The valves appear to **occur equally in boys and girls, and equally on the right and left sides** (Sant et al, 1985).

Transverse, nonobstructing mucosal folds are present in 5% of ureters in newborns and gradually disappear with growth (Wall and Wachter, 1952). They may be one of the normal findings described by Östling (1942) and by Kirks and associates (1978). Cussen (1971, 1977) identified what he termed ureteral valves in 46 of 328 abnormal ureters from infants and children at surgery or at autopsy. Unlike the diaphragmatic valves described previously, these are cusps that can be demonstrated by perfusing the upper ureter with fixative, dilating the lumen, flattening the mucosa, and accentuating the valves. In a patient with valvular obstruction, Cussen noted that the long axis of the distal ureter was eccentric relative to the long axis of the dilated proximal segment, with the fold being an eccentric cusp (Fig. 58–45). He also noted that these flaps could be found in the presence of a normal or stenotic distal ureter. In Cussen's series of 328 intrinsic ureteral lesions, there were 24 primary valves with no distal obstruction. A total of 19 valves were reported to be associated with a more distal obstruction.

Others have observed ureteral obstructions from eccentric cusps, believed to be distinct from secondary folds and kinks associated with ureteral dilation and elongation (Maizels and Stephens, 1980; Gosalbez et al, 1983). The cusp need not contain smooth muscle (Gosalbez et al, 1983; Reinberg et al, 1987). However, Williams (1977) believed that eccentric obstructing valves may be more infrequent than Cussen reported. Many of the apparent valves may be artifacts of distention because the dilated ureter at its junction with the undilated segment assumes a kinked and eccentric position resulting from elongation and pull of the surrounding adventitia.

In summary, diaphragmatic annular valves are a rare, although definite, form of ureteral obstruction. Eccentric, cusplike flaps or folds can be obstructing, but

they can also be secondary to the elongation and tortuosity that occurs with ureteral distention at the site of an underlying anatomic or functional obstruction. It has been postulated that several of these anomalies may appear transiently in utero and may be responsible for the milder forms of hydronephrosis that are found postnatally to be nonobstructive. If the lesion is in fact obstructive, an intravenous pyelogram and a retrograde pyelogram should be obtained, because these studies deliver the most complete anatomic information about the ureter. Resection of this obstructing lesion with primary reanastomosis is then curative. The involved kidney may be devoid of significant function and require nephrectomy (Sant et al, 1985).

Spiral Twists and Folds of the Ureter

Campbell (1970) observed this anomaly only twice in 12,080 autopsies of children (Fig. 58–46). He ascribed it to failure of the ureter to rotate with the kidney. This explanation may be simplistic, because the illustration shows more than one twist. Obstruction and hydronephrosis may result from spiral twists. The condition may arise from one of a number of possible persistent manifestations of normal fetal upper ureteral development, as described by Östling (1942) (Fig. 58–47; see Fig. 58–46). These manifestations include ureteral mucosal redundancy and apparent folds and convolutions that may have a spiral appearance. Radiographic evidence of such findings is often present in the excretory urograms of otherwise normal newborns. However, most of these folds gradually disappear with normal growth of the infant. Occasionally, ureteral convolutions that are enclosed by investing fascia persist as a form of ureteropelvic obstruction (Gross, 1953).

Persistent fetal folds were described in a previous paragraph. An isolated single fold or kink demonstrated radiographically with an otherwise normal upper urinary tract may be acquired, nonobstructing, and reversible and represents acute or intermittent elongation of the ureter with distal obstruction or reflux. Campbell (1970) believed that isolated primary obstructing congenital kinks could occur as an uncommon disorder, but the example he presented did not demonstrate convincing obstruction. Nevertheless, this sort of deformity is often one manifestation of ureteropelvic junction obstruction in association with ensheathment by dense fibrous bands (Gross, 1953).

Ureteral Diverticula

Diverticula of the ureter have been classified by Gray and Skandalakis (1972) into three categories: (1) abortive ureteral duplications (blind-ending bifid ureters), discussed later; (2) true congenital diverticula containing all tissue layers of the normal ureter; and (3) acquired diverticula representing mucosal herniations. Congenital diverticula are very uncommon and have been reported as arising from the distal ureter above the ureterovesical junction, midureter, and ureteropelvic junction (Culp, 1947; McGraw and Culp, 1952). These diverticula can become very large, and secondary hydronephrosis can ensue. The patient may present with abdominal pain or

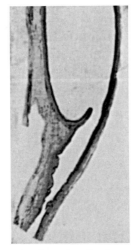

Figure 58–45. A 12-year-old girl with obstructing distal congenital ureteral valve in an ectopic, duplicated ureter. (Courtesy of Dr. Laurence R. Wharton.)

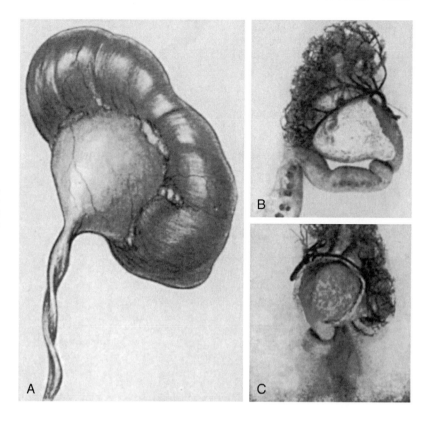

Figure 58–46. Torsion (spiral twists) of the ureter. *A,* Torsion observed in an infant at autopsy. There is secondary hydronephrosis. *B* and *C,* Corrosion specimens from late fetal life: anterior view *(B)* and lateral view from pelvic aspect. (Courtesy of Dr. Karl Östling.)

renal colic and a palpable cystic mass. McGraw and Culp's patient, a 64-year-old woman, had a cystic lesion at surgery, extending from under the right costal margin to the pelvic brim.

A typical diverticulum in a 20-year-old man is shown in Figure 58–48. Even small diverticula may be symptomatic.

Sharma and coworkers (1980) reported on two patients with repeated infections and a girl with intermittent colic. Fluoroscopy in the second patient demonstrated stasis and peristaltic dysfunction with back-and-forth ureter-to-diverticulum reflux. She was cured by diverticulectomy.

As discussed in the section on blind-ending duplications,

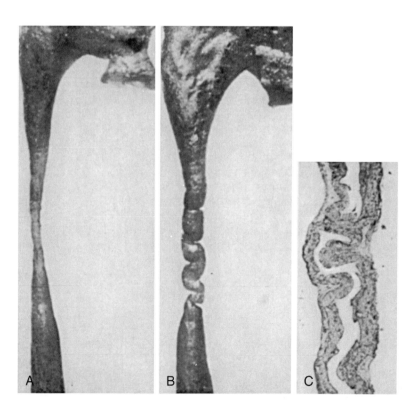

Figure 58–47. Embryologic considerations in the genesis of ureteral folds, kinks, and strictures. *A,* Cast of the ureter and the renal pelvis in a newborn. There is physiologic narrowing of the upper ureter, below which is the normal main spindle of the ureter. No ureteral folds are present. *B,* Cast of the ureter and the renal pelvis in the newborn. The ureteral folds proceed alternately from the opposite sides. *C,* Ureteral kinks that appear as muscular folds with axial offshoots of the loose adventitia. (Courtesy of Dr. Karl Östling.) (From Campbell MF: In Campbell MF, Harrison JH (eds): Urology, vol 2, 3rd ed. Philadelphia, WB Saunders, 1970.)

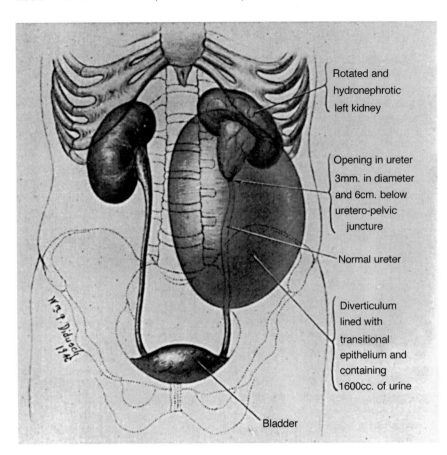

Figure 58–48. Congenital diverticulum of left ureter containing 1600 ml of urine. The kidney was hydronephrotic. (From Culp OS: Ureteral diverticulum: Classification of the literature and report of an authentic case. J Urol 1947; 58:309.)

congenital diverticula below the level of the ureteropelvic junction arise from premature cleavage of the ureteric bud with abortive development of the accessory limb. Those from the ureteropelvic junction region arise from primitive calyceal formation that similarly failed to encounter metanephric tissue (Gray and Skandalakis, 1972).

Single acquired diverticula may be associated with strictures or calculi and may occur after trauma (Culp, 1947). Multiple diverticula that are small (<5 mm) have been ascribed to the effect of chronic infection (Holly and Sumcad, 1957; Rank et al, 1960). However, Norman and Dubowy (1966) reported two cases of multiple diverticula that were demonstrable by retrograde ureteropyelography. Such lesions, demonstrable only by supraphysiologic pressures, may be congenital variants with weaknesses of the ureteral wall rather than acquired conditions (Hansen and Frost, 1978). However, the published reports do not contain histologic observations to support either hypothesis. Large diverticula usually can be removed without sacrificing the kidney.

Congenital High Insertion of the Ureter

This rare malformation may drain an otherwise normal and unobstructed kidney (Fig. 58–49). Most high insertions, however, are encountered with ureteropelvic junction obstruction, as discussed elsewhere in this textbook.

ANOMALIES OF NUMBER

The reported incidence of ureteral duplication varies widely in different series, depending in part on whether the survey was based on autopsy or clinical data and on the composition of patient material, and on whether bifid pelves were separately recorded (Fig. 58–50). Because it is generally recognized that clinical series usually contain a disproportionate number of duplication anomalies, unselected autopsy data are more accurate in predicting the true incidence. At least two large autopsy series have provided data not too dissimilar regarding partial and complete ureteral duplication (Nation, 1944; Campbell, 1970) (Table 58–2). Nation (1944) reviewed 230 cases of duplication; 121 of these were clinical. He identified 109 cases in approximately 16,000 autopsies, an incidence of 1 in 147, or 0.68%. Campbell's personal series of 51,880 autopsies in adults, infants, and children included 342 ureteral duplications (1 in 152, or 0.66%), but only 61 of the 19,046 children in the series had this abnormality (1 in 312, or 0.32%). Because the anomaly should be found with equal frequency in unselected autopsies of adults or children, Campbell concluded that some of the duplications in children had been overlooked. **Combining Nation's autopsy series and Campbell's adult series, the projected incidence of duplication is 1 in 125, or 0.8%.**

Despite a wealth of information about gender differences in the incidence of duplication in clinical series (the anomaly is identified in women at least two times more frequently than in men), there are no reliable data on gender

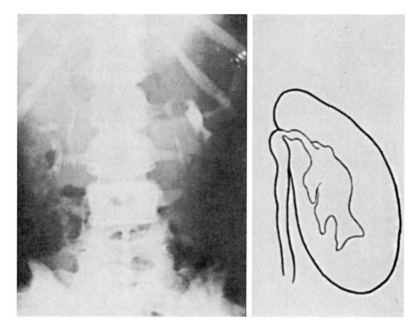

Figure 58-49. A 4-year-old girl with high ureteropelvic insertion and no obstruction.

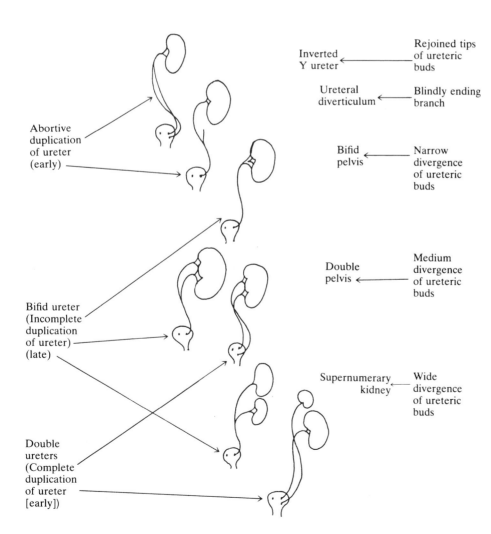

Abortive
duplication
of ureter
(early)

Bifid ureter
(Incomplete
duplication
of ureter)
(late)

Double
ureters
(Complete
duplication
of ureter
[early])

Inverted
Y ureter ← Rejoined tips
of ureteric
buds

Ureteral
diverticulum ← Blindly ending
branch

Bifid
pelvis ← Narrow
divergence
of ureteric
buds

Double
pelvis ← Medium
divergence
of ureteric
buds

Supernumerary
kidney ← Wide
divergence
of ureteric
buds

Figure 58-50. Gradations in ureteral and kidney duplications. (From Gray SW, Skandalakis JE (eds): Embryology for Surgeons. Philadelphia, WB Saunders, 1972.)

Table 58–2. URETERAL DUPLICATION: CLINICAL, RADIOGRAPHIC, AND AUTOPSY STUDIES

Author, Year	Database		No. Duplications	Female	Male	Unilateral	Bilateral	Complete	Partial	Unilateral Complete/ Partial	Bilateral Complete/ Partial	Bilateral Mixed
Archangelskj, 1926	110	R	619			502 (80%)	117 (20%)					
		A	3 (2.7%)									
Colosimo, 1938	1500	X	50 (3.3%)	88 (68%)								
Nation, 1944	16,000	A	109 (0.68%)	*(63%)	*							
		C	121	88 (73%)	33	177 (77%)	53 (23%)	102 (44%)	118 (51)	78 (44%)/99 (56%)	35 (45%)/19 (36%)	10 (4.3%)
			230 total									
Nordmark, 1948	4744	X	138 (2.8%)			119 (86%)	19 (14%)	70 (51%)	65 (47%)	59/60	11/5	3 (2.1%)
Payne, 1959		C	141	87 (62%)	54	120 (85%)	21 (15%)	45	78 + 18 bifid pelvis			
Johnston, 1961	5000	X	83									
		C	73					63 (77%)	19 (33%)			
		A	9	57 (70%)	25							
			82 total									
Kaplan and Elkin, 1968	(Partial duplications only)	X	51	33 (65%)	18	43 (84%)	8 (16%)					
Campbell, 1970	51,880	A	342 (0.65%)			293 (85%)	53 (15%)	101 (30%)			4	"one in five cases"
	(19,046 children)		61 (0.32%)									
	(32,834 adults)		281 (0.85%)									
Timothy et al, 1971		C	46	39 (85%)	7			24 (52%)	16 (35%)	13/15	11/1	6 (13%)
Privett et al, 1976	5196 (1716 children)	X	91 (1.8%)	63 (66%)	32	79 (85%)	16 (15%)	33 (29%)	57 (52%)			
	(3480 adults)							(but 21 not known)				
	(2896 male)											
	(2300 female)											

A, autopsy; C, clinical; R, review; X, X-ray; *, see text.

differences in unselected series. Campbell's autopsy data do not document such a difference. Of Nation's 109 autopsy cases, 56 were female and 53 male. However, only 40% of the 16,000 autopsies were performed in women. Calculating a correction for this difference, one could project a female-to-male ratio of 1.6:1. These statistics, however, may not be reliable in view of the small number of cases recorded.

Nevertheless, clinical and autopsy data are in substantial agreement about other aspects of duplication (see Table 58–3). **Unilateral duplication occurs about six times more often than bilateral duplication, with the right and left sides being involved about equally.** Excluding bifid pelvis, there does not appear to be a difference in the literature in the incidence of bifid ureter versus double ureters. A small percentage of individuals with bilateral duplications have a mixed condition, such as bifid ureter on one side and double ureters on the other.

Genetics

Evidence exists that duplication may be genetically determined by an autosomal dominant trait with incomplete penetrance (Cohen and Berant, 1976). **In parents and siblings of probands with duplication, the incidence of duplication increases from the predicted 1 in 125 to 1 in 8** (Whitaker and Danks, 1966) or 1 in 9 (Atwell et al, 1974).

Two reports of geographic foci suggest that environmental factors can also play a role (Philips et al, 1987; Barnes and McGeorge, 1989).

Position of Orifices

In double ureters, the two orifices are characteristically inverted in relation to the collecting systems they drain. The orifice to the lower pole ureter occupies the more cranial and lateral position, and that of the upper pole ureter has a caudal and medial position (see Fig. 58–12). As mentioned previously, this relationship is so consistent that it has been termed the Weigert-Meyer law. When the two orifices are not immediately adjacent, the orifice from the upper pole can be found anywhere along a predictable pathway, which Stephens (1958, 1963) called the ectopic pathway (Fig. 58–51).

Rare exceptions to the Weigert-Meyer law have been observed, in which the upper pole orifice is cranial, although it is still medial to the orthotopic orifice. Stephens (1958) collected four examples from the literature and added seven more. Stephens studied the positional relationship between the lower portions of the ureters and noted that it, too, varies according to the terminal position of the upper pole orifice. With the rare cranially placed upper pole orifice, the ureter lies anterior to the lower pole ureter, with the ureters being uncrossed. With a medial orifice the

URETER DUPLICATION
normal development

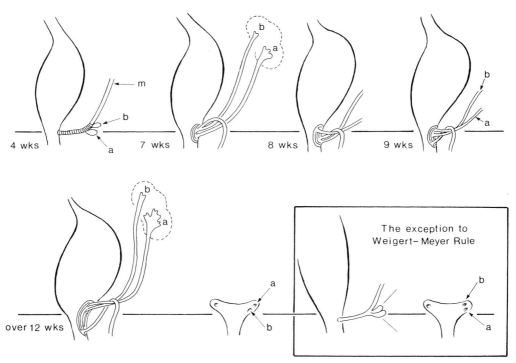

Figure 58–51. Simplified diagram of the changing position of the ureters and mesonephric duct in the development of complete duplication. a, lower pole ureter; b, upper pole ureter; m, mesonephric duct. (Redrawn from Tanagho EA: Embryologic basis for lower ureteral anomalies: A hypothesis. Urology 1976;7:451.)

upper pole ureter lies medially, and with a caudally placed orifice it spirals in an anterior-to-medial direction around the lower pole ureter as it descends, terminating posterior to the lower pole orifice. Ahmed and Pope (1986) documented a case of uncrossed complete ureteral duplication and reflux into the upper pole, which fits this pattern.

An embryonic hypothesis to explain the exception to the Weigert-Meyer law was proposed by Stephens (1958) and is based on the premise that an upper pole orifice located craniomedially arises from a junctional ureteric bud, one that bifurcated immediately, rather than from a second bud. The embryology is diagrammed in Figure 58–51.

Associated Findings

The distribution of the renal mass drained by each ureter in duplication varies somewhat. On average, about one third of the renal parenchyma is served by the upper collecting system. In a detailed radiographic review, Privett and associates (1976) reported a number of observations about duplication. **The mean total number of calyces for single-system kidneys was 9.4, and for duplex units it was 11.3, with a mean of 3.7 calyces in the upper collecting system and 7.6 in the lower collecting system.** These investigators also observed that 97% of the single-system kidneys in their series were radiographically normal, whereas 29% of the duplex units had scarring or dilatation, or both. **Reflux also was more common in the duplex units in patients who had voiding cystograms.**

Two (12%) of 17 nonduplex units generated reflux, compared with 13 (42%) of 31 duplex units.

Hydronephrosis of the lower pole segment is not infrequent and is generally associated with severe reflux into that unit. However, primary ureteropelvic junction obstruction can involve the lower pelvis (Dahl, 1975; Christofferson and Iversen, 1976; Privett et al, 1976).

Other anomalies are encountered with increased frequency. In Nation's (1944) series, 27 (12%) had other urinary tract anomalies, with just over half of these being on the same side. The anomalies included renal hypoplasia and aplasia (today these conditions would probably be termed *dysplasia*) and various ureteral anomalies, among them ectopic insertion of the upper pole ureter in four cases (3% of the complete duplications). Coexisting urologic anomalies were encountered in 29 of Campbell's (1970) series of 342 duplications. Nonurologic anomalies were found in 63 cases. These were not recorded in detail, but most of the urologic anomalies were, as in Nation's series, a variety of ipsilateral renal and ureteral lesions; 22 were anomalies of the contralateral kidney. The nonurologic lesions mainly involved the gastrointestinal tract plus a few cardiopulmonary lesions. However, both of these were autopsy series. Rarely, the pelvicalyceal systems communicate, presumably from later fusion of the ureteric buds during pelvicalyceal expansion (Braasch, 1912; Beer and Mencher, 1938).

The increased incidence of duplications in investigations of childhood urinary infections is well established. Campbell (1970) reported a personal series of 1102 children with pyuria, 307 of whom proved to have ureteropelvic anomalies. Of these, 82 (27%) had duplications, or 7.5% of the total group. Kretschmer (1937) reviewed 101 cases of hydronephrosis in infancy and childhood, and noted 24 nonureteral anomalies, more than half of which were duplications.

Based on three cases of duplication with some form of ureteral ectopy, coexistent renal dysplasia, and nodular renal blastema, Cromie and colleagues (1980) raised the possibility that this pattern of findings might be more than a coincidental association, accounting for an increased risk of neoplasm (Pendergrass, 1976). This concept deserves further investigation.

Bifid ureter is often clinically unimportant, but stasis and pyelonephritis do occur. When the Y junction is extravesical, free to-and-fro peristalsis of urine from one collecting system to the other may appear, with preferential retrograde waves passing into slightly dilated limbs instead of down the common stem. This results in stasis that is more marked when the Y junction is more distal, when the bifid limbs are wide, or when the Y junction is large. Increased urinary reprocessing from vesicoureteral reflux may enhance this phenomenon, and loin pain can result. About one quarter of the patients studied with nuclear renography by O'Reilly and coworkers (1984) had significant urodynamic abnormalities. Treatment by ureteroneocystostomy is effective when the junction is sufficiently close to the vesical wall that resection of the common sheath or common stem permits placement of both orifices within the bladder. Reimplantation of the common stem may be effective when vesicoureteral reflux is severe and the Y junction is higher up. In the absence of reflux, ureteropyelostomy or pyelopyelostomy with resection of one ureteral limb, preferably the upper limb, down to the Y junction is effective in eliminating regurgitation of urine (Lenaghan, 1962; Kaplan and Elkin, 1968).

Blind-Ending Duplication of the Ureter

Rarely, a ureteral duplication does not drain a renal segment; hence, the term "blind-ending." Fewer than 70 of these anomalies have been reported, although they occur considerably less infrequently than the published data indicate. Most blind-ending ureteral duplications involve one limb of a bifid system; even more unusual is one involving complete duplication (Szokoly et al, 1974; Jablonski et al, 1978). Although the Y junction in the bifid type may be at any level, most are found in the midureter or distal ureter. Blind-ending segments are diagnosed three times more frequently in women than in men, and twice as often on the right side (Schultze, 1967; Albers et al, 1971). The condition has been reported in twins (Bergman et al, 1977) and in sisters (Aragona et al, 1987). Many of these blind segments cause no problems. Symptomatic patients most often complain of vague abdominal or chronic flank pain, sometimes complicated by infection or calculi, or both (Marshall and McLoughlin, 1978). The majority of cases are not diagnosed until the third or fourth decade of life.

Because the blind segment does not always fill on excretory urography, retrograde pyelography may be required for diagnosis (Fig. 58–52). At times, however, urinary

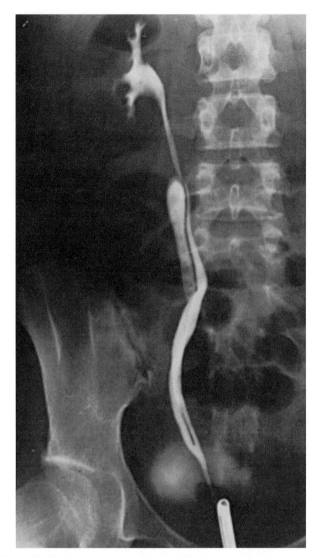

Figure 58–52. Retrograde pyelogram. Blind-ending duplication in an 18-year-old girl was noted in evaluation of transitory hematuria. Only the distal portion of this blind-ending duplication has been visualized on intravenous pyelogram.

stasis from disordered peristalsis (ureteroureteral reflux) may be demonstrated (Lenaghan, 1962), with secondary dilatation of the branch. This may be the cause of the pain (van Helsdingen, 1975). Because the lesion is more common in women and on the right side, the propensity for dilation of the right urinary tract with pregnancy might explain the relatively late onset of symptoms.

The embryogenesis of blind-ending ureteral duplication is similar to that for duplications in general. It is postulated that the affected ureteric bud is abortive and fails to make contact with the metanephros. Histologically, the blind segment contains all normal ureteral layers. The blind end tends to have a bulbous dilation. Most of these blind segments are not surrounded by any abortive renal tissue, but in a few segments there is a fibrous stalk (ureteral atresia) extending into a dysplastic renal segment. The blind limb may vary from a short stump of a few centimeters to one extending all the way into the renal fossa.

The area of union between the two limbs is invested in a common sheath that may be attenuated proximally. The blind segment and the adjacent normal ureter share a common blood supply (Albers et al, 1968; Peterson et al, 1975). When surgery is necessary, excision of the blind segment is indicated. Because the ensheathment is less dense at the upper or proximal end, the dissection should start there. Care should be taken to denude only the blind segment and not to enter the normal ureter. Some investigators suggest leaving a short stump at the junction with the common stem (Peterson et al, 1975; Rao, 1975).

Diverticula of the ureter have also been described. Controversy exists in the literature about the distinction between some diverticula and blind-ending duplications. In most cases, it may simply be a matter of terminology. For example, Campbell (1936) described a case of a finger-like extension from the lower ureter that he called a ureteral diverticulum, but he ascribed it developmentally to an abortive duplication. Similarly, Youngen and Persky (1965) labeled as a diverticulum a tubular, finger-like appendage from the pelvis but also ascribed its origin to an abortive budding. Rank and coworkers (1960) and Gray and Skandalakis (1972) agreed that congenital ureteral diverticula have the same embryogenesis as blind duplications. Gray and Skandalakis specifically noted that a diverticulum from the ureteropelvic area represents a primitive calyx that has failed to meet nephrogenic mesenchyme. Sarajlic and colleagues (1989) believed that all of these lesions could be described as congenital diverticula.

For some investigators, the distinction between a diverticulum and a blind-ending ureter is one of morphology. The typical blind-ending ureteral segment of a Y ureter joins the normal ureter at an acute angle and extends upward parallel to the normal ureter. It is at least twice as long as it is wide (Culp, 1947). A congenital diverticulum, in comparison, has a ballooned appearance. Histologically, both are similar, and both arise from disordered ureteric budding. Additional descriptions of ureteral diverticula were presented in a previous section.

Inverted Y Ureteral Duplication

This is the rarest of the anomalies of ureteral branching. It consists of two ureteral limbs distally that fuse proximally to become a single channel draining the kidney. This condition is more common in females than in males. **One of the distal ureteral limbs not uncommonly ends in an ectopic ureter or ureterocele** (Klauber and Reid, 1972; Beasley and Kelly, 1986; Harrison and Williams, 1986; Mosli et al, 1986; Ecke and Klatte, 1989). In several cases, one distal segment was atretic (Britt et al, 1972; Suzuki et al, 1977). In one case of bilateral inverted Y duplication in a 12-year-old girl, there was an atretic distal limb on each side, each with a calculus (Suzuki et al, 1977).

The embryology of inverted Y ureteral duplication is ascribed to two separate ureteric buds whose tips coalesce and fuse into a single duct before joining the metanephros. The frequently ectopic position of one limb is caused by widely separated buds on the mesonephric duct, with the second bud relatively cephalad. To explain the distal atresia of the ectopic limb in their case, Britt

and associates (1972) offered two possibilities. One was failure of Chwalle's membrane to rupture. The second, also postulated by Hawthorne (1936), was atresia of the wolffian duct's normal regression in the female before absorption of the too cephalad second ureteric bud into the urogenital sinus distally. Bingham (1986) reported on a woman with a single right ureter that divided into two segments and then rejoined, showing the features of a bifid ureter distally and an inverted Y proximally. He postulated that the ureteric bud split after migration began and then re-fused before entering the metanephros. Treatment, usually resection of the accessory channel, is directed toward any problems that result from an ectopic limb.

Ureteral Triplication and Supernumerary Ureters

Just as two buds from the mesonephric duct or premature fission of a single bud can explain double and bifid ureters, so the presence of three buds from the mesonephric duct or two with early fission of one of them can explain the rarely encountered complete and partial triplications (Marc et al, 1977). Most investigators use the classification of Smith (1946), who distinguished four varieties of triplicate ureter:

1. Complete triplication: three ureters from the kidney, with three draining orifices to the bladder, urethra, or elsewhere.
2. Incomplete triplication: a bifid ureter plus a single ureter, with three ureters from the kidney and two orifices draining below.
3. **Trifid ureter: all three ureters unite and drain through a single orifice; this appears to be the most common form encountered.**
4. Two ureters from the kidney, one becoming an inverse Y bifurcation, resulting in three draining orifices below.

In one apparently unique case, Fairchild and associates (1979) reported a typical bifid system with a third, lateral ureter that appeared to communicate with the lower pole calyx.

Triplication has been reported with renal fusion anomalies (Pode et al, 1983; Golomb and Ehrlich, 1989). Patients with triplication also may, of course, present with symptoms and signs of reflux and obstruction, ureterocele (Arap et al, 1982; Finkel et al, 1983; Rodo Salas et al, 1986; Juskiewinski et al, 1987), or ectopia, as in duplication anomalies. Treatment is based on the same principles as for duplication anomalies.

ANOMALIES OF POSITION

Vascular Anomalies Involving the Ureter

A variety of vascular lesions can cause ureteral obstruction. With these lesions, the vascular system rather than the urinary system is anomalous. With the exception of accessory renal blood vessels, all of these lesions are relatively uncommon, although all have clinical relevance.

Accessory Renal Blood Vessel

Accessory or aberrant vessels to the lower pole of the kidney can cross ventral to the ureteropelvic junction, causing obstruction. These vessels are described elsewhere in this text.

Preureteral Vena Cava

ANATOMY

This anomaly is commonly known to urologists as circumcaval or retrocaval ureter, terms that are anatomically descriptive but misleading in regard to development. Of the two terms, *circumcaval ureter* is preferred, because rarely a ureter may lie behind (dorsal to) the vena cava for some portion of its lumbar course without encircling the cava, and this form of retrocaval ureter appears to be developmentally different (Lerman et al, 1956; Dreyfuss, 1959; Peisojovich and Lutz, 1969). In the case reported by Dreyfuss, there was also a small branch vein between the vena cava and right iliopsoas muscle, over which (cephalad to it) the ureter coursed to enter the retrocaval area. **The term *preureteral vena cava* emphasizes that the circumcaval ureter results from altered vascular, rather than ureteral, development.**

This disorder involves the right ureter, which typically deviates medially behind (dorsal to) the inferior vena cava, winding about and crossing in front of it from a medial to a lateral direction, to resume a normal course, distally, to the bladder. The renal pelvis and upper ureter are typically elongated and dilated in a "J" or fishhook shape before passing behind the vena cava (Fig. 58–53). However, the collecting system is not inevitably obstructed. Bateson and Atkinson (1969), Crosse and associates (1975), and Kenawi and Williams (1976) classified circumcaval ureters into two clinical types: (1) the more common type I has hydronephrosis and a typically obstructed pattern demonstrating some degree of fishhook-shaped deformity of the ureter to the level of the obstruction, and (2) type II has a lesser degree of hydronephrosis or none at all. Here, the upper ureter is not kinked but passes behind the vena cava at a higher level, with the renal pelvis and upper ureter lying almost horizontal before encircling the vena cava in a smooth curve. In type I, the obstruction appears to occur at the edge of the iliopsoas muscle, at which point the ureter deviates cephalad before passing behind the vena cava. In type II, the obstruction, when present, appears to be at the lateral wall of the vena cava as the ureter is compressed against the perivertebral tissues.

EMBRYOLOGY

The definitive inferior vena cava develops on the right side from a plexus of fetal veins (Fig. 58–54). Initially, the venous retroperitoneal pathways consist of symmetrically placed vessels, both central and dorsal. The posterior cardinal and supracardinal veins lie dorsally, and the sub-

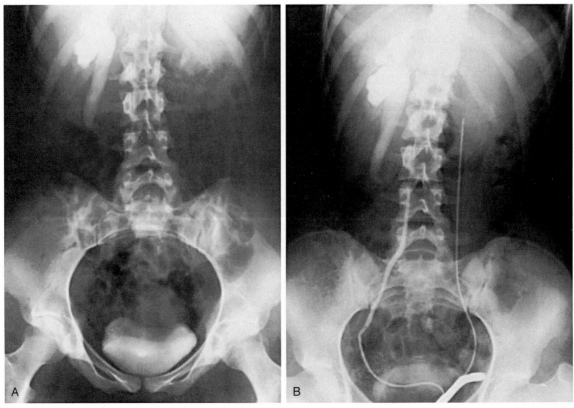

Figure 58–53. Circumcaval ureter in a 20-year-old woman with intermittent flank pain. *A,* Intravenous pyelogram. *B,* Retrograde ureteropyelogram.

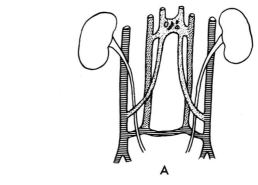

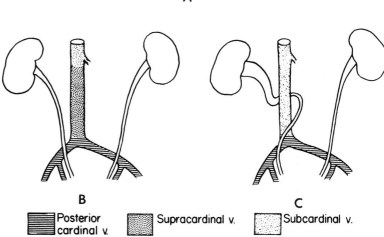

Figure 58–54. Fetal venous ring *(A)*, normal vena cava *(B)*, and preureteric vena cava *(C)*. (Redrawn from Hollinshead WH: Anatomy for Surgeons, vol 2. New York, Hoeber Medical Division of Harper and Row, 1956.)

⬛ Posterior cardinal v.   ⬛ Supracardinal v.   ⬛ Subcardinal v.

cardinal veins lie ventrally. These channels, with their anastomoses, form a collar on each side through which the ascending kidneys pass. Normally, the left supracardinal veins and the lumbar portion of the right posterior cardinal vein atrophy. The subcardinal veins become the internal spermatic veins. The definitive right-sided inferior vena cava forms from the right supracardinal vein. **If the subcardinal vein in the lumbar portion fails to atrophy and becomes the primary right-sided vein, the ureter is trapped dorsal to it.**

When the definitive vena cava forms normally and the ventral portion of the primitive ring also persists, a double right vena cava is formed because of the persistence of both the right subcardinal vein dorsally and the right subcardinal vein ventrally. This double vena cava traps the right ureter between its limbs (Fig. 58–55) (Gruenwald and Surks, 1943; Sasai et al, 1986).

Although bilateral vena cava or left-sided vena cava can occur (Clements et al, 1978; Mayo et al, 1983), a bilateral circumcaval ureter has been described in a case of situs inversus (Brooks, 1962). In cases of bilateral vena cava associated with a circumcaval ureter, the circumcaval ureter has been reported only on the right side, denoting that the right vena cava developed abnormally from a persistent subcardinal vein, whereas the left vena cava developed from the left supracardinal vein but otherwise normally (Pick and Anson, 1940).

INCIDENCE

The incidence of preureteral vena cava at autopsy is about 1 in 1500 (Heslin and Mamonas, 1951), and the anomaly is three to four times more common in male than in female cadavers. Gray and Skandalakis (1972) considered this frequency to be too high because of the preponderance of male autopsies performed, but **the 4:1 male-female ratio appears to be seen clinically as well** (Xiaodong et al, 1990).

Kenawi and Williams (1976), in reviewing the literature, recorded 114 male and 41 female patients, with 7 not known. The symptoms of preureteral vena cava are those of obstruction. **Although the lesion is congenital, most patients do not present until the third or fourth decade of life** (Kenawi and Williams, 1976).

DIAGNOSIS

Excretory urography often fails to visualize the portion of the ureter beyond the J hook (i.e., extending behind the vena cava), but retrograde ureteropyelography demonstrates an S curve to the point of obstruction (see Fig. 58–53), **with the retrocaval segment lying at the level of L3 or L4** (Kenawi and Williams, 1976). Cavography is no longer a necessary diagnostic test.

Ultrasound (Schaffer et al, 1985; Murphy et al, 1987) and CT or magnetic resonance imaging also have been useful in defining the vascular malformation. When necessary, CT may be the procedure of choice to confirm the diagnosis and avoid retrograde ureteropyelography (Hattori et al, 1986; Sasai et al, 1986; Murphy et al, 1987; Kellman et al, 1988). Helical CT (which is quite useful in visualizing ureteral stones) can demonstrate the course of the ureter. Nuclear renal Lasix scanning can categorize the anomaly as obstructed or nonobstructed (Pienkny, 1999).

Briefly, surgical correction involves ureteral division, with relocation and ureteroureteral or ureteropelvic

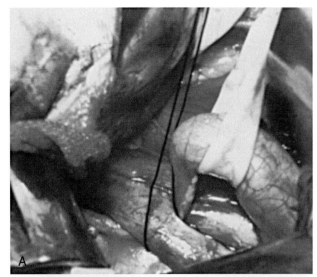

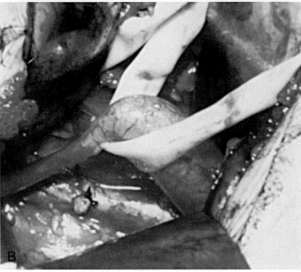

Figure 58–55. A 4-year-old boy with right ureteral obstruction from a double right vena cava. The site of obstruction is apparent distally, because the ureter lies between the ventral and dorsal limbs of the double cava. Intraoperative photographs were taken before *(A)* and after *(B)* division of the ventral limb.

reanastomosis, **usually with excision or bypass of the retrocaval segment, which can be aperistaltic.** It is important to be mindful of the ureter's blood supply from the renal artery and aorta superiorly and the iliac vessels inferiorly (Hellsten et al, 1980). This blood supply must be preserved during the ureteral dissection. As stated earlier, the preferred approach for the obstructed ureter is ureteral division and relocation; however, in the case of a solitary kidney, division of the anomalous inferior vena cava and its reposition behind the ureter may be contemplated.

Other Anomalies of Position

Several instances of horseshoe kidney have been reported (Cukier et al, 1969; Cendron and Reis, 1972; Eidelman et al, 1978; Heffernan et al, 1978; Kumeda et al, 1982; Taguchi et al, 1986). Anomalies include a variety of

left renal anomalies, such as agenesis, hydronephrosis, malrotation, and hypoplasia (Kenawi and Williams, 1976). There has been one case of left hydronephrosis with ensheathing of both ureters by a single fibrous membrane below the level of the venous anomaly (Salem and Luck, 1976). An obstructing branch of the right spermatic vein has mimicked circumcaval ureteral obstruction (Psihramis, 1987), as has an anomalous tendon of the iliopsoas muscle (Guarise et al, 1989).

PREURETERAL ILIAC ARTERY (RETROILIAC URETER)

A ureter coursing behind the common iliac artery is rare (Dees, 1940; Corbus et al, 1960; Seitzman and Patton, 1960; Hanna, 1972; Iuchtman et al, 1980; Radhkrishnan et al, 1980). Either side can be involved; in two cases, the condition was bilateral (Hanna, 1972; Radhrishnan et al, 1980). Obstruction occurs at the level of L5 or S1 as the ureter is compressed behind the artery. Coexisting anomalies are common (Nguyen et al, 1989).

Gray and Skandalakis (1972) believed that this condition was vascular in origin. Normally, the primitive ventral root of the umbilical artery is replaced by development of a more dorsal branch between the aorta and the distal umbilical artery. Persistence of the ventral root as the dorsal root fails to form traps the ureter dorsally (Fig. 58–56). Dees (1940) also considered the possibility that aberrant upward migration of the kidney in the case he reported might have placed it dorsal to the iliac artery, which was redundant.

Ureteral or mesonephric duct ectopia is often present. In Dees' case, there was evidence, although not definite proof, that the ureteral orifice was ectopic in the vesical neck, supporting the concept of anomalous renoureteral development. The case of Seitzman and Patton (1960) involved an ectopic ureter that emptied, along with the ipsilateral vas deferens, via a persistent common mesonephric duct into the proximal posterior urethra. In the case of Radhrishnan and colleagues (1980), bilateral retroiliac ureters also involved bilateral ectopic termination of the vasa deferentia into the ureters. Iuchtman and associates (1980) described ectopic vaginal termination of the involved ureter, with urometrocolpos from an imperforate hymen.

Taibah and coworkers (1987) reported the unusual finding of left ureteral obstruction from a retrointernal iliac artery ureter in an otherwise normal young woman.

VASCULAR OBSTRUCTION OF THE DISTAL URETER

Obstruction of the distal ureter from uterine, umbilical, obturator, and hypogastric vessels close to the bladder has been described (Hyams, 1929; Campbell, 1933, 1936, 1970; Greene et al, 1954; Young and Kiser, 1965; Scultety and Varga, 1975). However, it is not always clear that vascular impressions on a dilated ureter are the cause of the obstruction. At times, these findings may be an artifact, as when a dilated ureter from an intrinsic obstruction is secondarily compressed against the adjacent vessel (Campbell, 1970). Judging from the paucity of contemporary reports describing this lesion, it is likely that primary termi-

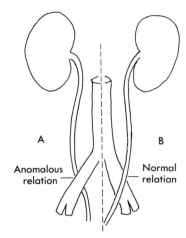

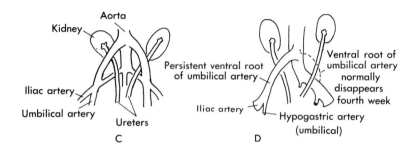

Figure 58–56. Preureteral iliac artery (postarterial ureter). *A,* Anomalous relationship of ureter and artery. *B,* Normal relationship of ureter and artery. *C,* Relationships between the ureter and the iliac and umbilical arteries in the embryo. *D,* Development of a normal iliac channel on the right and an anomalous iliac channel (persistence of proximal umbilical artery) on the left. (From Gray SW, Skandalakis JE (eds): Embryology for Surgeons. Philadelphia, WB Saunders, 1972.)

nal ureteral obstruction by vascular lesions is a rare occurrence.

HERNIATION OF THE URETER

Herniation of the ureter is another extremely rare condition. Dourmashkin (1937) searched the literature and tabulated a series of inguinal, scrotal, and femoral herniations of the ureter. Most of these were paraperitoneal, that is, a loop of herniated ureter extended alongside a peritoneal hernial sac. Only a minority were extraperitoneal (i.e., with no hernial sac present). In paraperitoneal ureteral hernias, the ureteral loop is always medial to the peritoneal sac. Of six scrotal hernias, four did not have peritoneal sacs. When the ureter extended into the scrotum, it was more likely to be dilated, causing upper tract obstruction.

Watson (1948) collected 102 cases of inguinal or femoral hernia involving the ureter. Jewett and Harris (1953) described a case of left ureteral hernia into the scrotum in a 9-year-old boy with left hydronephrosis (Fig. 58–57). This hernia was of the extraperitoneal type: a mesentery-like blood source supplied two loops of ureter within the scrotum that were adherent to the cord structures. Powell and Kapila (1985) reported a unique case of a 1-week-old male infant with bilateral megaureters presenting as a left inguinal hernia. The loop of the dilated left ureter was lateral, in the inguinal canal, to an incomplete hernial sac.

Dourmashkin (1937) believed that herniation of the ureter could be acquired or congenital, with the acquired form being a so-called sliding hernia and the congenital form being present since birth. In the latter form, he proposed that the loop of ureter had been drawn down with the descent of the testis and the developing ureter had adhered to the migrating vas.

Internal hernias of the ureter are even more exceptional. Reports have been published of a sciatic hernia containing

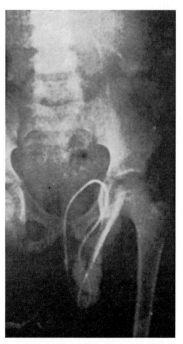

Figure 58–57. A 9-year-old boy with herniation of the left ureter into the scrotum. No hernial sac is present. The obstructed system was treated by ureteral resection and reanastomosis. (Courtesy of Dr. Hugh J. Jewett.)

a ureter—one of which was diagnosed by CT in an elderly woman (Lindblom, 1947; Beck et al, 1952; Oyen et al, 1987)—and of herniation between the psoas muscle and iliac vessels (Page, 1955).

REFERENCES

Terminology and Embryology

Ericsson NO: Ectopic ureterocele in infants and children. Acta Chir Scand Suppl 1954;197:8.

Glassberg KI, Braren V, Duckett JW, et al: Suggested terminology for duplex systems, ectopic ureters and ureteroceles. J Urol 1984;132:1153.

Grobstein C: Trans-filter induction of tubules in mouse metanephrogenic mesenchyme. Exp Cell Res 1956;10:424.

Kirrilova IA, Kulazhenko VP, Kulazhenko LG, et al: Cystic kidney in an eight week human embryo. Acta Anat 1982;114:68.

Mackie GG, Awang H, Stephens FD: The embryologic key to radiologic status of duplex kidneys. J Pediatr Surg 1975;10:473.

Mackie GG, Stephens FD: Duplex kidneys: A correlation of renal dysplasia with position of the ureteral orifice. J Urol 1975;114:274.

Meyer R: Normal and abnormal development of the ureter in the human embryo: A mechanistic consideration. Anat Rec 1946;96:355.

Moore KL: The urogenital system. In Moore KL (ed): The Developing Human, vol 1, 4th ed. Philadelphia, WB Saunders, 1988, p 258.

Sadler TW: Urogenital system. In Langman J (ed): Medical Embryology, 7th ed. Baltimore, Williams & Wilkins, 1995, p 272.

Sariola H, Aufderheide E, Bernhard H, et al: Antibodies to cell surface ganglioside GD3 perturb inductive epithelial-mesenchymal interactions. Cell 1988;54:235.

Saxen L: Organogenesis of the kidney. In Barlow PW, Green PB, Wylie CC (eds): Development and Cell Biology Series. Cambridge, Cambridge University Press, 1987.

Schwartz RD, Stephens FD, Cussen LJ: The pathogenesis of renal dysplasia II: The significance of lateral and medial ectopy of the ureteric orifice. Invest Urol 1981;19:97.

Stephens FD: Ureterocele in infants and children. Aust N Z J Surg 1958; 27:288.

Stephens FD: Congenital Malformations of the Rectum, Anus and Genitourinary Tracts. London, E & S Livingstone, 1963.

Stephens FD: Intramural ureter and ureterocele. Postgrad Med J 1964;40: 179.

Stephens FD: Caecoureterocele and concepts on the embryology and aetiology of ureteroceles. Aust N Z J Surg 1971;40:239.

Stephens FD: Congenital Malformations of the Urinary Tract. New York, Praeger, 1983.

Tanagho EA: Embryologic basis for lower ureteral anomalies: A hypothesis. Urology 1976;7:451.

Weigert C: Uebeteinige bil dunfehter der uretern. Virchows Arch 1877; 70:490.

Anomalies of Termination

Acien P, Garcia-Lopez F, Ferrando J, et al: Single ectopic ureter opening into blind vagina, with renal dysplasia and associated utero-vaginal duplication. Int J Gynaecol Obstet 1990;31:179.

Ahmed S, Barker A: Single-system ectopic ureters: A review of 12 cases. J Pediatr Surg 1992;27:491.

Ambrose SS, Nicolson WP III: The causes of vesicoureteral reflux in children. J Urol 1962;87:688.

Borer JG, Corgan FJ, Krantz R, et al: Unilateral single vaginal ectopic ureter with ipsilateral hypoplastic pelvic kidney and bicornuate uterus. J Urol 1993;149:1124–1127.

Borer JG, Bauer SB, Peters CA, et al: A single-system ectopic ureter draining an ectopic dysplastic kidney: Delayed diagnosis in the young female with continuous urinary incontinence. Br J Urol 1998;81:474–478.

Bozorgi F, Connolly LP, Bauer SB, et al: Hypoplastic dysplastic kidney with a vaginal ectopic ureter identified by technetium-99m-DMSA scintigraphy. J Nucl Med 1998;39:113–115.

Braverman RM, Lebowitz RL: Occult ectopic ureter in girls with urinary incontinence: Diagnosis by using CT. AJR Am J Roentgenol 1991;156: 365.

Burford CE, Glenn JE, Burford EH: Ureteral ectopia: A review of the literature and 2 case reports. J Urol 1949;62:211.

Campbell M: Ureterocele: A study of 94 instances in 80 infants and children. Surg Gynecol Obstet 1951;93:705.

Campbell MF: Anomalies of the ureter. In Campbell MF, Harrison JH (eds): Urology, 3rd ed. Philadelphia, WB Saunders, 1970, p 1512.

Cussen LJ: Normal position of the ureteral orifice in infancy and childhood: A quantitative study. J Urol 1979;121:646.

Diard F, Chateil JF, Bondonny JM, et al: "Pseudo-ureterocele": Buckling of an ectopic megaureter imprinting the urinary bladder. J Radiol 1987; 68:177.

Eisendrath DN: Ectopic opening of the ureter. Urol Cutan Rev 1938;42: 401.

El-Ghoneimi A, Valla JS, Steyaert H, Aigrain Y: Laparoscopic renal surgery via a retroperitoneal approach in children. J Urol 1998;160: 1138–1141.

Ellerker AG: The extravesical ectopic ureter. Br J Surg 1958;45:344.

Figenshau RS, Clayman RV, Kerbl K, et al: Laparoscopic nephroureterectomy in the child: Initial case report. J Urol 1994;151:740.

Freedman ER, Rickwood AM: Urinary incontinence due to unilateral vaginally ectopic single ureters [see comments]. Br J Urol 1994;73:716.

Gharagozloo AM, Lebowitz RL: Detection of a poorly functioning malpositioned kidney with single ectopic ureter in girls with urinary dribbling: Imaging evaluation in five patients. AJR Am J Roentgenol 1995; 164:957.

Giles DJ, Nixon GW, Middleton AW Jr, et al: Vaginal ectopic ureter: A continuing diagnostic challenge. West J Med 1982;136:436.

Glenn JF: Agenesis of the bladder. JAMA 1959;169:2016.

Gotoh T, Morita H, Tokunaka S, et al: Single ectopic ureter. J Urol 1983; 129:271–274.

Hanna MK, Jeffs RD, Sturgess JM, et al: Ureteral structure and ultrastructure: Part III. The congenitally dilated ureter (mega-ureter). J Urol 1977;117:24.

Janetschek G, Seibold J, Radmayr C, Bartsch G: Laparoscopic heminephrourreterectomy in pediatric patients. J Urol 1997;158:1928–1930.

Jordan GH, Winslow BH: Laparoendoscopic upper pole partial nephrectomy with ureterectomy. J Urol 1993;150:940.

Kobashi KC, Chamberlin DA, Rajpoot D, Shanberg AM: Retroperitoneal laparoscopic nephrectomy in children. J Urol 1998;160:1142–1144.

Komatsu K, Niikura S, Maeda Y, et al: Single ectopic vaginal ureter diagnosed by computed tomography. Urol Int 1999;63:147–150.

Koyanagi T, Tsuji I, Orikasa S, Hirano T: Bilateral single ectopic ureter: Report of a case. Int Urol Nephrol 1977; 9:123.

Kropp KA, Angwafo FF: Urethral lengthening and reimplantation for neurogenic incontinence in children. J Urol 1986;135:533.

Leadbetter GW Jr: Surgical reconstruction for complete urinary incontinence. J Urol 1985;133:205.

Lowsley OS, Kerwin TJ: Clinical Urology, vol 1, 3rd ed. Baltimore, Williams & Wilkins, 1956.

Lucius GF: Klinik und Therapie der dystopen Hernleitermundungen in die Samenwege. Urologe 1963;2:360.

Malek RS, Kelalis PP, Stickler GB, et al: Observations on ureteral ectopy in children. J Urol 1972;107:308.

Mandell J, Bauer SB, Colodny AH, et al: Ureteral ectopia in infants and children. J Urol 1981;126:219–222.

Mills JC: Complete unilateral duplication of ureter with analysis of the literature. Urol Cutan Rev 1939;43:444.

Moores D, Cohen R, Hayden L: Laparoscopic excision of pelvic kidney with single vaginal ectopic ureter. J Pediatr Surg 1997;32:634–635.

Mor Y, Goldwasser B, Ben-Chaim J, et al: Upper pole heminephrectomy for duplex systems in children: A modified technical approach. Br J Urol 1994;73:584.

Nussbaum AR, Dorst JP, Jeffs RD, et al: Ectopic ureter and ureterocele: Their varied sonographic manifestations. Radiology 1986;159:227.

Pantuck AJ, Barone JG, Rosenfeld DL, Fleisher MH: Occult bilateral ectopic vaginal ureters causing urinary incontinence: Diagnosis by computed tomography. Abdom Imaging 1996;21:78–80.

Peters CA, Hendren WH: Splitting the pubis for exposure in difficult reconstructions for incontinence. J Urol 1989;142:527.

Peters CA: Complications in pediatric urological laparoscopy: Results of a survey. J Urol 1996;155:1070–1073.

Plaire JC, Pope JCt, Kropp BP, et al: Management of ectopic ureters: Experience with the upper tract approach. J Urol 1997;158:1245–1247.

Prabhakaran K, Lingaraj K: Laparoscopic nephroureterectomy in children. J Pediatr Surg 1999;34:556–558.

Prewitt LH, Lebowitz RL: The single ectopic ureter. AJR Am J Roentgenol 1976;127:941.

Rassweiler JJ, Henkel TO, Joyce AD, et al: The technique of transperitoneal laparoscopic nephrectomy, adrenalectomy and nephroureterectomy. Eur Urol 1993;23:425.

Riba LW, Schmidlapp CJ, Bosworth NL: Ectopic ureter draining into the seminal vesicle. J Urol 1946;56:332.

Rink RC, Adams MC, Keating MA: The flip flap technique to lengthen the urethra (Salle procedure) for treatment of neurogenic urinary incontinence. J Urol 1994;152:799.

Rognon L, Brueziere J, Soret JY, et al: Abouchement ectopique de l'ureter dans le tractus seminal: A propos de 10 cas. Chirurgie 1973;99:741.

Schulman CC: The single ectopic ureter. Eur Urol 1976;2:64.

See WA, Mayo M: Ectopic ureter: A rare cause of purulent vaginal discharge. Obstet Gynecol 1991;78:552.

Simms MH, Higgins PM: Diagnosis of the occult ectopic ureter in a duplex kidney. J Urol 1975;114:697.

Squadrito J Jr, Rifkin MD, Mulholland SG, et al: Ureteral ectopia presenting as epididymitis and infertility. Urology 1987;30:67.

Stephens FD, Lenaghan D: The anatomical basis and dynamics of vesicoureteral reflux. J Urol 1962;87:669.

Sullivan M, Halpert L, Hodges CV: Extravesical ureteral ectopia. Urology 1978;11:577.

Sumfest JM, Burns MW, Mitchell ME, et al: Pseudoureterocele: Potential for misdiagnosis of an ectopic ureter as a ureterocele. Br J Urol 1995;75:401.

Suzuki K, Ihara H, Kurita Y, et al: Laparoscopic nephrectomy for atrophic kidney associated with ectopic ureter in a child. Eur Urol 1993;23:463.

Tanagho EA, Hutch JA, Meyers FH, et al: Primary vesicoureteral reflux: Experimental studies of its etiology. J Urol 1965;93:165.

Umeyama T, Kawamura T, Hasegawa A, et al: Ectopic ureter presenting with epididymitis in childhood: Report of 5 cases. J Urol 1985;134:131.

Uson AC, Womack CD, Berdon WE: Giant ectopic ureter presenting as an abdominal mass in a newborn infant. J Pediatr 1972;80:473.

Utsunomiya M, Itoh H, Yoshioka T, et al: Renal dysplasia with a single vaginal ectopic ureter: The role of computerized tomography. J Urol 1984;132:98–100.

Wakhlu A, Dalela D, Tandon RK, et al: The single ectopic ureter. Br J Urol 1998;82:246–251.

Weiss JP, Duckett JW, Snyder H McC III: Single unilateral vaginal ectopic ureter: Is it really a rarity? J Urol 1984;132:1177.

Williams DI, Royle M: Ectopic ureter in the male child. Br J Urol 1969;41:421.

Williams JL, Sago AL: Ureteral ectopia into seminal vesicle: Embryology and clinical presentation. Urology 1983;22:594.

Wyly JB, Lebowitz RL: Refluxing urethral ectopic ureters: Recognition by the cyclic voiding cystourethrogram. AJR Am J Roentgenol 1984;142:1263.

Yao D, Poppas DP: A clinical series of laparoscopic nephrectomy, nephroureterectomy and heminephroureterectomy in the pediatric population. J Urol 2000;163:1531–1535.

Anomalies of Structure

Allen TD: Congenital ureteral strictures. J Urol 1970;104:196.

Allen TD: Discussion. In Bergsma D, Duckett JW Jr (eds): Urinary System Malformations in Children. Birth Defects: Original Article Series, vol 13, No. 5. New York, Alan R. Liss, 1977, p 39.

Amar AD: Operative technique for treatment of ureterocele of single ureter in children. Urology 1978;12:197.

Arap S, Nahas WC, Alonso G, et al: Assessment of hydroureteronephrosis by renographic evaluation under diuretic stimulus. Urol Int 1984;39:170.

Austin PF, Cain MP, Casale AJ, et al: Prenatal bladder outlet obstruction secondary to ureterocele. Urology 1998;52:1132–1135.

Bauer SB, Retik AB: The nonobstructive ectopic ureterocele. J Urol 1978;119:804.

Bellah RD, Long FR, Canning DA: Ureterocele eversion with vesicoureteral reflux in duplex kidneys: Findings at voiding cystourethrography. AJR Am J Roentgenol 1995;165:409–413.

Blythe B, Passerini GG, Camuffo C, et al: Endoscopic incision of ureteroceles: Intravesical versus ectopic. J Urol 1993;149:556.

Brock WA, Kaplan GW: Ectopic ureteroceles in children. J Urol 1978;119:800.

Caldamone AA, Duckett JW: Update on ureteroceles in children. AUA Update Series 1984;3:Lesson 36.

Caldamone AA, Snyder HM III, Duckett JW: Ureteroceles in children: Follow-up of management with upper tract approach. J Urol 1984;131:1130.

Campbell MF: Anomalies of the ureter. In Campbell MF, Harrison JH (eds): Urology, 3rd ed. Philadelphia, WB Saunders, 1970, p 1512.

Cendron J, Melin Y, Valayer J: Simplified treatment of ectopic ureterocele in 35 children. Eur Urol 1981;7:321.

Churchill BM, Abara EO, McLorie GA: Ureteral duplication, ectopy and ureteroceles. Pediatr Clin North Am 1987;34:1273–1289.

Churchill BM, Sheldon CA, McLorie GA: The ectopic ureterocele: A proposed practical classification based on renal unit jeopardy. J Pediatr Surg 1992;27:497–500.

Chwalle R: The process of formation of cystic dilatations of the vesical end of the ureter and of diverticula at the ureteral ostium. Urol Cutan Rev 1927;31:499.

Cobb LM, Desai PG, Price SE: Surgical management of infantile (ectopic) ureteroceles: Report of a modified approach. J Pediatr Surg 1982;17:745.

Coplen DE: Neonatal ureterocele incision. (Editorial; comment.) J Urol 1998;159:1010.

Coplen DE, Duckett JW: The modern approach to ureteroceles. J Urol 1995;153:166.

Cremin BJ: A review of the ultrasonic appearances of posterior urethral valve and ureteroceles. Pediatr Radiol 1986;16:357.

Culp OS: Ureteral diverticulum: Classification of the literature and report of an authentic case. J Urol 1947;58:309.

Cussen LJ: The morphology of congenital dilatation of the ureter: Intrinsic ureteral lesions. Aust N Z J Surg 1971;41:185.

Cussen LJ: Valves of the ureter. In Bergsma D, Duckett JW Jr (eds): Urinary System Malformations in Children. Birth Defects: Original Article Series, vol 13, No. 5. New York, Alan R. Liss, 1977, p 19.

Dajani AM, Dajani YF, Dahabrah S: Congenital ureteric valves: A cause of urinary obstruction. Br J Urol 1982;54:98.

Decter RM, Roth DR, Gonzales ET: Individualized treatment of ureteroceles. J Urol 1989;142:535.

Diamond T, Boston VE: Reflux following endoscopic treatment of ureteroceles: A new approach using endoscopic subureteric Teflon injection. Br J Urol 1987;60:279.

Diard F, Eklöf O, Leibowitz R, Maurseth K: Urethral obstruction in boys caused by prolapse of simple ureterocele. Pediatr Radiol 1981;11:139.

Diard F, Chateil JF, Bondonny JM, et al: "Pseudo-ureterocele": Buckling of an ectopic megaureter imprinting the urinary bladder. J Radiol 1987;68:177.

Di Benedetto V, Monfort G: How prenatal ultrasound can change the treatment of ectopic ureterocele in neonates. Eur J Pediatr Surg 1997;7:338–340.

Feldman S, Lome LG: Surgical management of ectopic ureterocele. Urology 1981;17:252.

Geringer AM, Berdon WE, Seldin DW, et al: The diagnostic approach to ectopic ureterocele and the renal duplication complex. J Urol 1983a;129:539.

Geringer AM, Berdon WE, Seldin DW, et al: Ultrasonic demonstration of ectopic ureterocele. Pediatrics 1983b;71:568.

Glazier DB, Packer MG: Infected obstructive ureterocele. Urology 1997;50:972–973.

Gloor JM, Ogburn P, Matsumoto J: Prenatally diagnosed ureterocele presenting as fetal bladder outlet obstruction. J Perinatol 1996;16:285–287.

Gonzales ET: Anomalies of the renal pelvis and ureter. In Kelalis PP, King LR, Belman AB (eds): Clinical Pediatric Urology, vol 1. Philadelphia, WB Saunders, 1992, p 530.

Gosalbez R, Garat JM, Piro C, et al: Congenital ureteral valves in children. Urology 1983;21:237.

Gotoh T, Koyanagi T, Matsuno T: Surgical management of ureteroceles in children: Strategy based on the classification of ureteral hiatus and the eversion of ureteroceles. J Pediatr Surg 1988;23:159.

Gray SW, Skandalakis JE (eds): Embryology for Surgeons. Philadelphia, WB Saunders, 1972.

Gross RE: Uretero-pelvic obstruction. In Gross RE (ed): The Surgery of Infancy and Childhood. Philadelphia, WB Saunders, 1953, p 635.

Hagg MJ, Mourachov PV, Snyder HM, et al: The modern endoscopic approach to ureterocele. J Urol 2000;163:940–943.

Hanna MK, Jeffs RD, Sturgess JM, et al: Ureteral structure and ultrastructure. Part II. Congenital ureteropelvic junction obstruction and primary obstructive megaureter. J Urol 1976;116:725.

Hanna MK, Jeffs RD, Sturgess JM: Ureteral structure and ultrastructure. Part III. The congenitally dilated ureter (mega-ureter). J Urol 1977;117:24.

Hansen EI, Frost B: Multiple diverticula of the ureter. Scand J Urol Nephrol 1978;12:93.

Hendren WH, Mitchell ME: Surgical correction of ureterocele. J Urol 1979;121:590.

Hertle L, Nawrath H: In vitro studies on human primary obstructed megaureters. J Urol 1985;133:884.

Holly LE, Sumcad B: Diverticular ureteral changes: A report of four cases. AJR Am J Roentgenol 1957;78:1053.

Hutch JA, Chisholm ER: Surgical repair of ureterocele. J Urol 1966;96:445.

Husmann DA, Ewalt DH, Glenski WJ, Bernier PA: Ureterocele associated with ureteral duplication and a nonfunctioning upper pole segment: Management by partial nephroureterectomy alone. J Urol 1995;154:723–726.

Husmann D, Strand B, Ewalt D, et al: Management of ectopic ureterocele associated with renal duplication: A comparison of partial nephrectomy and endoscopic decompression. J Urol 1999;162:1406–1409.

King LR, Kozlowski JM, Schacht MJ: Ureteroceles in children: A simplified and successful approach to management. JAMA 1983;249:1461.

Kirks DR, Currarino G, Weinberg AG: Transverse folds in the proximal ureter: A normal variant in infants. AJR Am J Roentgenol 1978;130:463.

Kroovand RL, Perlmutter AD: A one stage surgical approach to ectopic ureterocele. J Urol 1979;122:367.

Maizels M, Stephens FD: Valves of the ureter as a cause of primary obstruction of the ureter: Anatomic, embryologic and clinical aspects. J Urol 1980;123:742.

Mandell J, Colodny A, Lebowitz RL, et al: Ureteroceles in infants and children. J Urol 1980;123:921.

McGraw AB, Culp OS: Diverticulum of the ureter: Report of another authentic case. J Urol 1952;67:262.

Monfort G, Guys JM, Coquet M, et al: Surgical management of duplex ureteroceles. J Pediatr Surg 1992;27:634.

Monfort G, Morisson-Lacombe G, Coquet M: Endoscopic treatment of ureteroceles revisited. J Urol 1985;133:1031–1033.

Moskovitz B, Bolkier M, Levin DR: Ureterocele containing calcified stone. J Pediatr Surg 1987;22:1047.

Muller LC, Troger J, Notscher KS: Ureterocele in childhood: Clinical and radiologic picture. Radiologe 1988;28:29.

Norman CH Jr, Dubowy J: Multiple ureteral diverticula. J Urol 1966;96:152.

Notley RG: Electron microscopy of the primary obstructive megaureter. Br J Urol 1972;44:229.

Nussbaum AR, Lebowitz RL: Interlabial masses in little girls: Review and imaging recommendations. AJR Am J Roentgenol 1983;141:65.

Orr LM, Glanton JB: Prolapsing ureterocele. J Urol 1953;70:180.

Östling K: The genesis of hydronephrosis. Acta Chir Scand 1942;86(Suppl 72):10.

Pfister C, Ravasse P, Barret E, et al: The value of endoscopic treatment for ureteroceles during the neonatal period. J Urol 1998;159:1006–1009.

Rank WB, Mellinger GT, Spiro E: Ureteral diverticula: Etiologic considerations. J Urol 1960;83:566.

Reinberg Y, Aliabadi H, Johnson P, Gonzalez R: Congenital ureteral valves in children: Case report and review of the literature. J Pediatr Surg 1987;22:379.

Reitelman C, Perlmutter AD: Management of obstructing ectopic ureteroceles. Urol Clin North Am 1990;17:317.

Retik AB, Peters CA: Ectopic ureter and ureterocele. In Walsh PC (ed): Campbell's Urology, vol 2. Philadelphia, WB Saunders, 1992, p 1743.

Rich MA, Keating MA, Snyder HM III, et al: Low transurethral incision of single-system intravesical ureteroceles in children. J Urol 1990;144:120.

Rickwood AM, Reiner I, Jones M, Pournaras C: Current management of duplex-system ureteroceles: Experience with 41 patients. Br J Urol 1992;70:196.

Rodo Salas RJ, Bishara F, Claret I: Triplication ureteral con reflujo y ureterocele. Arch Esp Urol 1986;39:343.

Rodriguez JV: Endoscopic surgery of calculi in ureteroceles. Eur Urol 1984;10:36.

Sant GR, Barbalias GA, Klauber GT, et al: Congenital ureteral valves: An abnormality of ureteral embryogenesis? J Urol 1985;133:427.

Scherz HC, Kaplan GW, Packer MG, et al: Ectopic ureteroceles: Surgical management with preservation of continence: Review of 60 cases. J Urol 1989;142:538.

Sen S, Beasley SW, Ahmed S, et al: Renal function and vesicoureteral reflux in children with ureteroceles. Pediatr Surg Int 1992;7:192.

Share JC, Lebowitz RL: Ectopic ureterocele without ureteral and calyceal dilatation (ureterocele disproportion): Findings on urography and sonography. AJR Am J Roentgenol 1989;152:567.

Sharma SK, Malik N, Kumar S, Bapna BC: Bilateral incomplete ureteric duplication with a ureteric diverticulum. Aust N Z J Surg 1980;51:204.

Shekarriz B, Upadhyay J, Fleming P, et al: Long-term outcome based on the initial surgical approach to ureterocele. J Urol 1999;162:1072–1076.

Stephens D: Caecoureterocele and concepts on the embryology and aetiology of ureteroceles. Aust N Z J Surg 1971;40:239.

Sumfest JM, Burns MW, Mitchell ME, et al: Pseudoureterocele: Potential for misdiagnosis of an ectopic ureter as a ureterocele. Br J Urol 1995;75:401.

Tank ES: Experiences with endoscopic incision and open unroofing of ureteroceles. J Urol 1986;136:241.

Tatu W, Brennan RE: Primary megaureter in a mother and daughter. Urol Radiol 1981;3:185.

Teele RL, Share JC: Ultrasonography of Infants and Children. Philadelphia, WB Saunders, 1991, p 234.

Thornbury JR, Silver TM, Vinson RK: Management of urinary calculous disease in patients with ureterocele. J Urol 1977;117:34.

Tokunaka S, Gotoh T, Koyanagi T, et al: Morphological study of the ureterocele: A possible clue to its embryogenesis as evidenced by a locally arrested myogenesis. J Urol 1981;126:726.

Wall B, Wachter HE: Congenital ureteral valve: Its role as a primary obstructive lesion. Classification of the literature and report of an authentic case. J Urol 1952;68:684.

Williams DI: Discussion. In Bergsma D, Duckett JW Jr (eds): Urinary System Malformations in Children. Birth Defects: Original Article Series, vol 13, No. 5. New York, Alan R. Liss, 1977, p 39.

Wines RD, O'Flynn JD: Transurethral treatment of ureteroceles. Br J Urol 1972;44:207.

Witherington R, Smith AM: Management of prolapsed ureterocele: Past and present. J Urol 1979;121:813.

Yachia D: Endoscopic treatment of ureterocele in a duplex system. Br J Urol 1993;71:105.

Zielinski J: Avoidance of vesicoureteral reflux after transurethral meatotomy for ureterocele. J Urol 1962;88:386.

Anomalies of Number

Ahmed S, Pope R: Uncrossed complete ureteral duplication with upper system reflux. J Urol 1986;135:128.

Albers DD, Geyer JR, Barnes SD: Clinical significance of blind-ending branch of bifid ureter: Report of 3 additional cases. J Urol 1971;105:634.

Albers DD, Geyer JR, Barnes SD: Blind-ending branch of bifid ureter: Report of 3 cases. J Urol 1968;99:160.

Aragona F, Passerini-Glazel G, Zacchello G, Andreetta B: Familial occurrence of blind-ending bifid and duplicated ureters. Int Urol Nephrol 1987;19:137.

Arap S, Lopes RN, Mitre AI, Menezes De Goes G: Triplicité ureterale complete associée a une ureterocele ectopique. J Urol 1982;88:167.

Atwell JD, Cook PL, Howell CJ, et al: Familial incidence of bifid and double ureters. Arch Dis Child 1974;49:390.

Barnes DG, McGeorge AM: The duplex ureter in Burnley, Pendle and Rossendale. Br J Urol 1989;64:345.

Beasley SW, Kelly JH: Inverted Y duplication of the ureter in association with ureterocele and bladder diverticulum. J Urol 1986;136:899.

Beer E, Mencher WH: Heminephrectomy in disease of the double kidney: Report of fourteen cases. Ann Surg 1938;108:705.

Bergman B, Hansson G, Nilson AEV: Duplication of the renal pelvis and blind-ending bifid ureter in twins. Urol Int 1977;32:49.

Bingham JG: Duplicate segment within a single ureter. J Urol 1986;135:1234.

Braasch WF: The clinical diagnosis of congenital anomaly in the kidney and ureter. Ann Surg 1912;56:756.

Britt DB, Borden TA, Woodhead DM: Inverted Y ureteral duplication with a blind-ending branch. J Urol 1972;108:387.

Campbell MF: Anomalies of the ureter. In Campbell MF, Harrison JH (eds): Urology, 3rd ed. Philadelphia, WB Saunders, 1970, p 1512.

Campbell MF: Diverticulum of the ureter. Am J Surg 1936;34:385.

Christofferson J, Iversen HG: Partial hydronephrosis in a patient with horseshoe kidney and bilateral duplication of the pelvis and ureter. Scand J Urol Nephrol 1976;10:91.

Cohen N, Berant M: Duplications of the renal collecting system in the hereditary osteo-onychodysplasia syndrome. J Pediatr 1976;89:261.

Cromie WJ, Engelstein MS, Duckett JW Jr: Nodular renal blastema, renal dysplasia and duplicated collecting systems. J Urol 1980;123:100.

Culp OS: Ureteral diverticulum: Classification of the literature and report of an authentic case. J Urol 1947;58:309.

Dahl DS: Bilateral complete renal duplication with total obstruction of both lower pole collecting systems. Urology 1975;6:727.

Ecke M, Klatte D: Inverted Y-ureteral duplication with a uterine ectopy as cause of ureteric enuresis. Urol Int 1989;44:116–118.

Fairchild WV, Solomon HD, Spence CR, Gangai MP: Case profile: Unusual ureteral triplication. Urology 1979;14:95.

Finkel LI, Watts FB Jr, Corbett DP: Ureteral triplication with a ureterocele. Pediatr Radiol 1983;13:346.

Golomb J, Ehrlich RM: Bilateral ureteral triplication with crossed ectopic fused kidneys associated with the VACTERL syndrome. J Urol 1989; 141:1398.

Gray SW, Skandalakis JE (eds): Embryology for Surgeons. Philadelphia, WB Saunders, 1972.

Harrison GSM, Williams RE: Inverted Y ureter in the male. Br J Urol 1986;58:564.

Hawthorne AB: Embryologic and clinical aspects of double ureter. JAMA 1936;106:189.

Jablonski JP, Voldman C, Brueziere J: Duplication totale de la voie excretrice dont un uretere est borgne. J Urol Nephrol 1978;84:837.

Juskiewenski S, Soulie M, Baunin C, et al: Ureteral triplication. Chir Pediatr 1987;28:314.

Kaplan N, Elkin M: Bifid renal pelves and ureters: Radiographic and cinefluorographic observations. Br J Urol 1968;40:235.

Klauber GT, Reid EC: Inverted Y reduplication of the ureter. J Urol 1972;107:362.

Kretschmer HL: Hydronephrosis in infancy and childhood: Clinical data and a report of 101 cases. Surg Gynecol Obstet 1937;64:634.

Lenaghan D: Bifid ureters in children: An anatomical and clinical study. J Urol 1962;87:808.

Marc J, Drouillard J, Bruneton JN, Tavernier J: La triplication ureterale. J Radiol Electrol Med Nucl 1977;58:427.

Marshall FF, McLoughlin MG: Long blind ending ureteral duplications. J Urol 1978;120:626.

Meyer R: Development of the ureter in the human embryo: A mechanistic consideration. Anat Rec 1946;96:355.

Mosli HA, Schillinger JF, Futter N: Inverted Y duplication of the ureter. J Urol 1986;135:126.

Nation EF: Duplication of the kidney and ureter: A statistical study of 230 new cases. J Urol 1944;51:456.

O'Reilly PH, Shields RA, Testa J, et al: Ureteroureteric reflux: Pathological entity or physiological phenomenon? Br J Urol 1984;56:159.

Pendergrass TW: Congenital anomalies in children with Wilms' tumor: A new survey. Cancer 1976;37:403.

Peterson LJ, Grimes JH, Weinerth JL, et al: Blind-ending branches of bifid ureters. Urology 1975;5:191.

Philips DIW, Divall JM, Maskell RM, Barker JP: A geographical focus of duplex ureter. Br J Urol 1987;60:329.

Pode D, Shapiro A, Lebensart P: Unilateral triplication of the collecting system in a horseshoe kidney. J Urol 1983;130:533.

Privett JT, Jeans WD, Roylance J: The incidence and importance of renal duplication. Clin Radiol 1976;27:521.

Rank WB, Mellinger GT, Spiro E: Ureteral diverticula: Etiologic considerations. J Urol 1960;83:566.

Rao KG: Blind-ending bifid ureter. Urology 1975;6:81.

Rodo Salas RJ, Bishara F, Claret I: Triplication ureteral con reflujo y ureterocele. Arch Esp Urol 1986;39:343.

Sarajlic M, Durst-Zivkovic B, Svoren E, et al: Congenital ureteric diverticula in children and adults: Classification, radiological and clinical features. Br J Radiol 1989;62:551.

Schultze R: Der blind endende Doppelureter. Z Urol 1967;4:27.

Smith I: Triplicate ureter. Br J Surg 1946;34:182.

Stephens FD: Anatomical vagaries of double ureters. Aust N Z J Surg 1958;28:27.

Stephens FD: Congenital Malformations of the Rectum, Anus and Genitourinary Tracts. London, E & S Livingstone, 1963.

Suzuki S, Tsujimura S, Suguira H: Inverted Y ureteral duplication with a ureteral stone in atretic segment. J Urol 1977;117:248.

Szokoly V, Veradi E, Szporny G: Blind ending bifid and double ureters. Int Urol Nephrol 1974;6:174.

van Helsdingen PJRO: A case of bifid ureter with blind-ending segment as the cause of chronic pain in the flank. Arch Chir Nederl 1975;27: 277.

Weigert C: Uebeteinige bil dunfehter der uretern. Virchows Arch 1877; 70:490.

Whitaker J, Danks DM: A study of the inheritance of duplication of the kidney and ureters. J Urol 1966;95:176.

Youngen R, Persky P: Diverticulum of the renal pelvis. J Urol 1965;94: 40.

Anomalies of Position

Bateson EM, Atkinson D: Circumcaval ureter: A new classification. Clin Radiol 1969;20:173.

Beck WC, Baurys W, Brochu J, et al: Herniation of the ureter into sciatic foramen ("curlicue ureter"). JAMA 1952;149:441.

Brooks RJ: Left retrocaval ureter associated with situs inversus. J Urol 1962;88:484.

Campbell MF: Vascular obstruction of the ureter in juveniles. Am J Surg 1933;22:527.

Campbell MF: Vascular obstruction of the ureter in children. J Urol 1936; 36:366.

Campbell MF: Anomalies of the ureter. In Campbell MF, Harrison JH (eds): Urology, 3rd ed. Philadelphia, WB Saunders, 1970.

Cendron J, Reis CF: L'uretere retro-cave chez l'infant, A propos de 4 cas. J Urol Nephrol 1972;78:375.

Clements JC, McLeod DG, Greene WR, Stutzman RE: A case report: Duplicated vena cava with right retrocaval ureter and ureteral tumor. J Urol 1978;119:284.

Corbus BC, Estrem RD, Hunt W: Retro-iliac ureter. J Urol 1960;84:67.

Crosse JEW, Soderdahl DW, Teplick SK, et al: Nonobstructive circumcaval (retrocaval) ureter. Radiology 1975;116:69.

Cukier J, Aubert J, Dufour B: Uretere retrocave et rein en fer a cheval chez un garcon hypospade de 6 ans. J Urol Nephrol 1969;75:749.

Dees JE: Anomalous relationship between ureter and external iliac artery. J Urol 1940;44:207.

Dourmashkin RL: Herniation of the ureter. J Urol 1937;38:455.

Dreyfuss W: Anomaly simulating a retrocaval ureter. J Urol 1959;82:630.

Eidelman A, Yuval E, Simon D, Sibi Y: Retrocaval ureter. Eur Urol 1978;4:279.

Gray SW, Skandalakis JE (eds): Embryology for Surgeons. Philadelphia, WB Saunders, 1972.

Greene LF, Priestley JT, Simon HB, et al: Obstruction of the lower third of the ureter by anomalous blood vessels. J Urol 1954;71:544.

Gruenwald P, Surks SN: Pre-ureteric vena cava and its embryological explanation. J Urol 1943;49:195.

Guarise P, Cimaglia ML, Spata F, et al: Uretere retrotendineo: Una causa eccezionale di ostruzione del tratto urinario superiore. Pediatr Med Chir 1989;11:85.

Hanna MK: Bilateral retro-iliac artery ureters. Br J Urol 1972;44:339.

Hattori N, Fujikawa J, Kubo K, et al: CT diagnosis of periureteric venous ring. J Comput Assist Tomogr 1986;10:1078.

Heffernan JC, Lightwood RG, Snell ME: Horseshoe kidney with retrocaval ureter: Second reported case. J Urol 1978;120:358.

Hellsten S, Grabe M, Nylander G: Retrocaval ureter. Acta Chir Scand 1980;146:225–228.

Heslin JE, Mamonas C: Retrocaval ureter: Report of four cases and review of literature. J Urol 1951;65:212.

Hyams JA: Aberrant blood vessels as factor in lower ureteral obstruction. Surg Gynecol Obstet 1929;48:474.

Iuchtman M, Assa J, Blatnoi I, et al: Urometrocolpos associated with retroiliac ureter. J Urol 1980;124:283.

Jewett HJ, Harris AP: Scrotal ureter: Report of a case. J Urol 1953;69: 184.

Kellman GM, Alpern MB, Sandler MA, Craig BM: Computed tomography of vena caval anomalies with embryologic correlation. Radiographics 1988;8:533.

Kenawi MM, Williams DI: Circumcaval ureter: A report of four cases in children with a review of literature and a new classification. Br J Urol 1976;48:183.

Kumeda K, Takamatsu M, Sone M, et al: Horseshoe kidney with retrocaval ureter: A case report. J Urol 1982;128:361.

Lerman I, Lerman S, Lerman F: Retrocaval ureter: Report of a case. J Med Soc N J 1956;53:74.

Lindblom A: Unusual ureteral obstruction by herniation of ureter into sciatic foramen: Report of a case. Acta Radiol 1947;28:225.

Mayo J, Gray R, St. Louis E, et al: Anomalies of the inferior vena cava. AJR Am J Roentgenol 1983;140:339.

Murphy BJ, Casillas J, Becerra JL: Retrocaval ureter: Computed tomography and ultrasound appearance. J Comput Assist Tomogr 1987;11:89.

Nguyen DH, Koleilat N, Gonzalez R: Retroiliac ureter in a male newborn with multiple genitourinary anomalies: Case report and review of literature. J Urol 1989;141:1400.

Oyen R, Gielen J, Baert L, et al: CT demonstration of a ureterosciatic hernia. Urol Radiol 1987;9:174.

Page BH: Obstruction of ureter in internal hernia. Br J Urol 1955;27:254.

Peisojovich MR, Lutz SJ: Retrocaval ureter: A case report and successful repair with a new surgical technique. Mich Med 1969;68:1137.

Pick JW, Anson BJ: Retrocaval ureter: Report of a case, with a discussion of its clinical significance. J Urol 1940;43:672.

Pienkny AJ, Herts B, Streem SB: Contemporary diagnosis of retrocaval ureter. J Endourol 1999;13:721–722.

Powell MC, Kapila L: Bilateral megaureters presenting as an inguinal hernia. J Pediatr Surg 1985;20:175.

Psihramis KE: Ureteral obstruction by a rare venous anomaly: A case report. J Urol 1987;138:130.

Radhrishnan J, Vermillion CD, Hendren WH: Vasa deferentia inserting into retroiliac ureters. J Urol 1980;124:746.

Salem RJ, Luck RJ: Midline ensheathed ureters. Br J Urol 1976;48:18.

Sasai K, Sano A, Imanaka K, et al: Right periureteric venous ring detected by computed tomography. J Comput Assist Tomogr 1986;10:349.

Schaffer RM, Sunshine AG, Becker JA, et al: Retrocaval ureter: Sonographic appearance. J Ultrasound Med 1985;4:199.

Scultety S, Varga B: Obstructions of the lower ureteral segment caused by vascular anomalies. (Author's translation.) Urologe A 1975;14:144.

Seitzman DM, Patton JF: Ureteral ectopia: Combined ureteral and vas deferens anomaly. J Urol 1960;84:604.

Taguchi K, Shimada K, Mori Y, Ikoma F: A case of combined anomaly of horseshoe kidney, retrocaval ureter and pelviureteric stenosis. Hinyokika Kiyo 1986;32:745.

Taibah K, Roney PD, McKay DE, Wellington JL: Retro-internal iliac artery ureter. Urology 1987;30:159.

Watson LF: Hernia, 3rd ed. London, Henry Kimpton, 1948.

Xiaodong Z, Shukun H, Jichuan Z, et al: Diagnosis and treatment of retrocaval ureter. Eur Urol 1990;18:207.

Young JD Jr, Kiser WS: Obstruction of the lower ureter by aberrant blood vessels. J Urol 1965;94:101.

59
VESICOURETERAL REFLUX AND MEGAURETER

Anthony Atala, MD
Michael A. Keating, MD

Vesicoureteral reflux (VUR), the retrograde flow of urine from the bladder to the upper urinary tract, is one of the most common problems encountered by urologists who care for children. It is also one of the most perplexing. Although the surgical solutions to the anomaly have withstood scrutiny for years, the indications for its correction are continually changing. The natural history of reflux continues to be rewritten by its perinatal detection, an evolving understanding of the clinical implications of urinary tract infections (UTIs), and the reports of prospective randomized clinical studies of affected children. Recommendations for management have been altered accordingly and will undoubtedly continue to change in the future, especially because, as with much of medicine, new data often raise more questions than they answer. In this regard, it is notable that VUR is the focus of more than 150 manuscripts in the literature each year. As a consequence, treating physicians are cautioned to keep abreast of this logarithmically expanding body of knowledge and, when necessary, to search beyond the distillation presented here.

HISTORICAL PERSPECTIVES

Galen in the first century AD (Polk, 1965) and later Leonardo da Vinci were the first to allude to the importance of a competent ureterovesical junction (UVJ) in the unidirectional flow of urine from the kidney. It was not until 1883 that Semblinow experimentally demonstrated reflux as a normal finding in rabbits and dogs (Semblinow, 1907). A decade later, Pozzi reported the first case of VUR in humans after a ureter was divided during a gynecologic procedure (Pozzi, 1893). Studies by Sampson (1903) defined the valvular "ureterovesical lock" mechanism created by the obliquity of the ureter at its intersection with the bladder. He also suggested that reflux from an incompetent junction could conceivably lead to renal infections. Young (1898), working under a similar premise, was unable to cause reflux in cadavers after filling their bladders with significant volumes of fluid. A few decades later, detailed studies by Gruber (1929) defined the anatomic relationships of the UVJ and noted that the incidence of VUR varied with the length of intravesical ureter and the muscular development of its surrounding trigone. In the interim operations were devised for reconstructing the UVJ and cystography was introduced, but the clinical implications of reflux remained unclear (Kretschmer, 1916), especially because the finding, which was present in a number of other mammals, was considered normal.

The modern era in our understanding of the functional significance of this anomaly was ushered in by Hutch, who, in 1952, described the causal relationship between reflux and chronic pyelonephritis in paraplegics. Hodson (1959), applying Hutch's observations of adults to the pediatric population, noted that reflux was more common in children with UTIs and renal parenchymal scarring. Anatomic correlates in animal models were provided by Tanagho and colleagues (1965), who created reflux by incising the trigone distal to the ureteral orifice, thus weakening the muscular backing of the ureter. Ransley and Risdon (1975) were also able to demonstrate reflux after resecting the roof of the ureter's submucosal tunnel in pigs.

DEMOGRAPHICS

Incidence

General

The overall incidence of reflux is probably best estimated at greater than 10%. Kollerman (1974) reported an incidence of reflux of 18.5% in 161 children. Sargent (2000) reviewed 250 articles from the literature to determine the prevalence of VUR in children undergoing a cystogram. The prevalence of VUR in children without a history of a UTI was 17.2%. **In contrast to studies in normal subjects, reflux is found in up to 70%** (Baker, 1966) **of infants who present with UTIs** (Smellie and Normand, 1966; Scott and Stansfeld, 1968; Walker et al, 1977). Reflux is also a common finding (37%) in fetuses with antenatally diagnosed hydronephrosis (Zerin et al, 1993). The postnatal evaluation of 130 neonates and young infants with abnormal prenatal ultrasound studies found reflux in 49 (37%) as the single most common urologic diagnosis (Zerin et al, 1993).

Sexual Dichotomy

Gender differences do exist. **Infants with antenatally detected reflux show a male preponderance in contrast to that diagnosed in the evaluation of UTIs later in development, where females predominate** (Ring et al, 1993). **Although the vast majority (85%) of reflux detected later in life occurs in females, males who present with UTI have a higher likelihood of having the anomaly.** This association was amplified by the results of a study by Shopfner (1970), who found reflux in 29% of 523 boys with infection but only 14% of 1695 girls with a similar presentation (Shopfner, 1970). Boys tend to present at a younger age, 25% during the first 3 months of life (Decter et al, 1988), and they often arrive with more severe degrees of reflux, especially if diagnosed in infancy or during the postnatal workup of antenatal hydronephrosis (Yeung et al, 1997). **Circumcision practices also appear to influence the predisposition to infection. During the first few months of life, uncircumcised males are 10 times more likely to have a UTI than those who are circumcised** (Wiswell and Roscelli 1986; Wiswell et al, 1987). Not surprisingly, this same propensity affects the detection of reflux. In the International Reflux Study in Children (IRSC), 10% of the children entered from the United States were boys, as opposed to 24% of those from the European arm. Notably, circumcision had been performed in 62% of the American boys, in contrast to only 5% of the European boys ($P < .001$) (Weiss et al, 1992b).

Fetal Reflux

Reflux is a common finding in neonates with prenatally diagnosed hydronephrosis. The postnatal evaluation of 130 neonates and young infants with abnormal prenatal ultrasound results found reflux in 49 infants (37%) as the single most common urologic diagnosis (Zerin et al, 1993). Although the anteroposterior renal pelvis diameter during prenatal sonography has been used as a guideline for predicting the occurrence of reflux (Persutte et al, 1997; Jaswon et al, 1999), this value varies depending on the timing of the study and the experience of the individual performing it (Brown et al, 1987; Walsh and Dubbins, 1996; Persutte et al, 2000).

Most studies of neonates cite as much as 80% of prenatally diagnosed reflux as occurring in boys (Scott, 1987; Marra et al, 1994a). **The reflux is usually high grade and bilateral in boys, compared with girls** (Gordon et al, 1990; Yeung et al, 1997; Herndon et al, 1999). A transient urethral obstruction has been proposed to explain this finding (Marra et al, 1994b). Recent work has also implicated a difference in urodynamic patterns in which hypercontractile bladders that generate high voiding pressures and have small functional capacity are more common in infant boys (Sillen, 1999).

Renal scans in newborns with reflux who have been given prophylactic drugs and have been infection free have demonstrated the presence of renal damage (17% to 51%), supporting the belief that renal impairment is frequently present at birth and probably caused by congenital dysplasia (Crabbe et al, 1992; Oliveira et al, 1998; Stock et al, 1998). These findings also have been confirmed with the use of animal models of fetal reflux, wherein tubular function is altered and there is a mild decrease in glomerular filtration and excess matrix deposition (Gobet et al, 1998, 1999; Dewan et al, 1999).

Fetal reflux has also been associated with a significant degree of resolution, even with high grades (Burge et al, 1992; Herndon et al, 1999). However, prospective long-term studies are needed to ascertain actual resolution rates like those already defined for older patients.

Age

The detection of reflux is also influenced by the age of the child being evaluated, with the highest incidence found in younger children. Table 59–1 summarizes the findings of a study by Baker and associates (1966), who found the presence of reflux to be inversely related to age in patients with UTIs. This association was also borne out by similar studies of children with infections and with asymptomatic bacteriuria (Smellie et al, 1975; Walker et al,

Table 59–1. INCIDENCE OF REFLUX IN PATIENTS WITH URINARY TRACT INFECTIONS

Age (Yr)	Incidence (%)
<1	70
4	25
12	15
Adults	5.2

From Baker R, Maxted W, Maylath J, et al: Relation of age, sex, and infection to reflux: Data indicating high spontaneous cure rate in pediatric patients. J Urol 1966;95:27.

1977). An explanation for this finding has its basis in the spontaneous resolution of reflux that occurs in many children with interval growth of the bladder and elongation of ureteral tunnel length (see later discussion).

Race

It should be noted that the majority of studies on reflux come from North America, northern Europe, and Scandinavia. **Caucasian girls were 10 times more likely to have reflux than their black American counterparts, when evaluated for asymptomatic bacteriuria** (Kunin, 1976). Black girls are also less likely to have reflux when evaluated for UTI (12%, vs. 41% in white girls) (Askari and Belman, 1982). **However, once reflux is discovered, its grade and chance of spontaneous resolution are similar for both races** (Skoog and Belman, 1991). Others have suggested an increased risk among fair-skinned children with blue eyes and blond hair (Manley, 1981) or among red-haired children alone (Urrutia and Lebowitz, 1983). The prevalence of reflux in many other countries and races has not been defined.

Species Specificity

Reflux is a common finding in other animals. Rabbits, rats, and other rodents are almost uniformly affected yet never suffer any measurable loss of renal function (Gruber, 1929). A high incidence (80%) is seen in puppies, although resolution by adulthood is the rule (Christie, 1971). Reflux also occurs in other primates at variable rates that are both species- and age-specific. Interestingly, resolution occurs in rhesus monkeys, who are phylogenetically neighbors of humans, at rates that are similar to those seen in children with UTIs (Roberts, 1974; Walker, 1991).

Inheritance and Genetics

Like most genitourinary anomalies, VUR appears to have a multifactorial etiology, although a genetic component undoubtedly exists. **Reflux is the most common inherited anomaly of the genitourinary tract, and siblings of patients with reflux are at much greater risk of having reflux than the normal population. Up to 45% of siblings have been noted to have reflux in some studies** (Van den Abbeele et al, 1987; Noe, 1992). **The large majority (75%) are asymptomatic.** Contrary to the findings in some earlier studies, **there appears to be no relation between the grade of reflux in index patients and that in their siblings.** The presence of renal scars in the index case is probably also less important than was once supposed. There is a slightly higher incidence among sisters of female patients with reflux, although this difference is not statistically strong enough to suggest an X-linked mode of transmission (Noe et al, 1992).

The first large study to address this issue was performed by Dwoskin and coworkers (1976), who found reflux in 26% of siblings from 125 families of probands with reflux. A subsequent report by Jerkins and Noe (1982) cited a 33% incidence in more than 100 siblings of 78 index cases. In the largest study to date, reflux was found in 144 (27%) of 622 siblings (Wan et al, 1996a). The majority had low-grade reflux, but nuclear scintigraphy showed reflux nephropathy in 14%. The incidence of reflux decreased after 7 years of age but was still occasionally present in older siblings. The age at the time of screening also played a role in a study by Connolly and coworkers (1997), who reported decreasing yields in studies of children 24 months of age or younger (46%), compared with those age 25 to 72 months (33%) and those older than 72 months (7%). In a similar study examining the natural history of reflux detected in asymptomatic siblings (mean age at detection, 21 months), more than 50% of cases resolved after 18 months of follow-up; these findings were believed to support observational management and periodic imaging in most siblings (Connolly et al, 1996).

Two follow-up studies by Noe were revealing. The first (Noe, 1988) noted **a greater incidence of sibling reflux in probands without bladder dysfunction (38%) compared to those with bladder dysfunction (20%),** suggesting a secondary etiology when bladder dynamics are abnormal (see later discussion). The second placed a greater emphasis on **parent-to-child transmission** than on that of sibling-to-sibling. For a selected group of 23 parents with a known history of reflux, 24 (66%) of 36 progeny were also found to have the problem. The mother was primarily affected 69% of the time, while reflux was discovered in 77% of females and 43% of males (Noe et al, 1992). **Although a polygenic mode of transmission was favored by earlier investigators** (Burger and Smith, 1971), **a variety of data suggest a dominant inheritance pattern having variable penetrance.** These include an approximate 50% incidence of sibling reflux in the first 2 years of life and the high incidence of parent-to-child transmission (66%) (Noe, 1992; Wan et al, 1996a). Perhaps most suggestive of autosomal dominant transmission is the incidence of sibling reflux found in multiple-gestation births. One study demonstrated **reflux in 80% of identical twins and 35% of fraternal twins** (Kaefer et al, 2000).

An autosomal dominant mode of transmission is also suggested by experimental work involving the PAX family of transcriptional regulatory factors (Wilson, 1996). PAX genes are responsible for cell specification and body segmentation (Gruss and Walther, 1992). They also appear to play a role in the interplay between the ureter and the developing kidney (Torres et al, 1995). PAX mutations are also implicated in syndromes that involve reflux, renal anomalies, and colobomas and are inherited in an autosomal dominant manner (Sanyanusin et al, 1995). However, PAX mutations have not been demonstrated clinically in patients with familial VUR (Choi et al, 1998).

Clinical Correlates

The innocuous nature of sibling reflux amplifies the need for some form of screening. In Noe's study (1992) of 119 children with sibling reflux, 15 (13%) showed renal damage by excretory urography, many of whom were asymptomatic. In a smaller group of 16 children diagnosed with the condition who had never had UTIs, renal scintigraphy using dimercaptosuccinic acid (DMSA) showed scarring in 6 (38%) (Buonomo et al, 1993). **A voiding cystourethrogram (VCUG) is recommended as a screening test for reflux in babies and young children, especially those younger than 5 years of age. In older siblings, urinary ultrasonography is recommended. If the ultrasound shows a discrepancy in renal size, any renal scarring, a dilated ureter, hydronephrosis, or a change in size of the renal pelvis during the study, further investigation with a VCUG is recommended.** Although this study may not detect lower grades of reflux, families can be reassured that the kidneys are not grossly abnormal. Periodic checks of the blood pressure and urine are also appropriate. **The appearance of UTIs also warrants further evaluation with standard or radionuclide cystography, which remain the only definitive tests for reflux** (Van den Abbeele et al, 1987). When VUR is detected in symptomatic siblings, it is often of high grade and associated with renal scarring (Puri et al, 1998).

ETIOLOGY AND PATHOGENESIS

Anatomic Considerations

The normal ureter propels boluses of urine into the bladder in an antegrade fashion. To achieve this, certain criteria must be met. First, the three muscular layers (inner longitudinal, middle circular, and outer longitudinal) of the ureter must respond with effective peristalsis to a stretch reflex caused by the bolus. Secondly, the pressures in the recipient bladder must be low enough to allow for the free egress of urine. Finally, the UVJ must occlude the distal ureter with the increases in pressure that inevitably occur with bladder filling or contraction. **To achieve this "flap-valve" effect, the intravesical ureter ideally has an oblique course as it enters the bladder, proper muscular attachments to provide fixation and posterior support to enable its occlusion, and adequate submucosal length** (Harrison, 1888; Johnson, 1962; King et al, 1974) (Fig. 59–1).

As the ureter penetrates the bladder, its muscular layers disperse. The circular layer and ureteral adventitia meld into the detrusor in the upper part of the hiatus to form Waldeyer's sheath, which attaches the ureter to the bladder and is in continuity with the deep trigone (Hutch, 1972). Distally, the inner longitudinal muscles continue along a medial course with the submucosal intravesical ureter. Along this route the muscle fibers decussate and intersperse with the detrusor musculature to form the borders of the superficial trigone. Some longitudinal fibers project beyond the ureteral orifice to meet those of the contralateral ureter, creating Bell's muscle of the posterior urethra. Others pass medially to form Mercier's bar and the intraureteric ridge (Mathisen, 1964). The area is replete with autonomic innervation that undoubtedly plays a role in smooth muscle interactions at the junction (Dixon et al, 1998).

Functional Correlates

The ureterovesical complex functions as a single unit that exhibits both passive and active components. When a bolus of urine approaches the hiatus, the intravesical

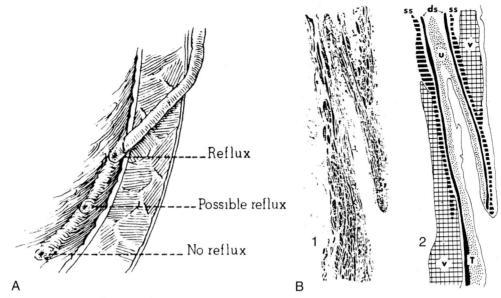

Figure 59–1. *A,* Refluxing ureterovesical junction has same anatomic features as nonrefluxing orifice, except for inadequate length of intravesical submucosal ureter. Some orifices with marginal submucosal tunnels may reflux intermittently. (From Glenn J [ed]: Urologic Surgery, 2nd ed. New York, Harper & Row, 1975.) *B,* Ureterovesical junction in longitudinal section. 1, Photomicrograph. 2, Diagrammatic representation. The ureteral muscularis (u) is surrounded by superficial (ss) and deep (ds) periureteral sheaths, which extend in the roof of the submucosal segment and continue beyond the orifice into the trigonal muscle (t). The relationship of superficial sheath to the vesical muscularis (v) is clearly seen. Transverse fascicles in the superior lip of the ureteral orifice belong to the superficial and deep sheaths. No true space separates ureter from bladder. (From Elbadawi A: Anatomy and function of the urethral sheath. J Urol 1972;107:224.)

longitudinal muscles contract. This action pulls the orifice toward the hiatus to shorten and widen the intravesical ureter, thus reducing resistance. The peristaltic pressures of the ureter (usually between 20 and 35 mm Hg) sufficiently propel the bolus into the bladder, which typically has low resting pressures (8 to 12 mm Hg). After the ureter relaxes it returns to its normal position beneath the bladder mucosa. Here a passive "flap-valve" mechanism prevents reflux during bladder filling (Hinman, 1990). The intravesical ureter, a delicate and supple structure sandwiched between mucosa and muscle, coapts with resting bladder pressures. An active component that increases the intraluminal pressure of the distal ureter with bladder filling and can be eliminated by anesthetizing the UVJ may also be contributory (Shafik, 1996). During micturition, the longitudinal muscles of the UVJ close the meatus and submucosal tunnel to provide an "active" component, especially during bladder contraction. Disrupting the trigone causes lateral and upward migration of the ureteral orifice and reflux. In contrast, prolonged electrical stimulation can cause resistance to flow as it draws the orifice inferomedially (Tanagho et al, 1968).

Primary Reflux

Primary reflux is a congenital anomaly of the UVJ wherein a deficiency of the longitudinal muscle of the intravesical ureter results in an inadequate valvular mechanism. The factor most critical to a competent UVJ is the length of submucosal ureter relative to its diameter. Large-caliber ureters and those having short intravesical segments cannot be effectively shut by the junction's valvular mechanisms. Rigid ureters that have been chronically scarred by repeated infection and cannot coapt pose a similar problem. **In Paquin's novel study, a 5:1 ratio of tunnel length to ureteral diameter was found in normal children without reflux; in contrast, children with reflux had a ratio of 1.4:1** (Paquin, 1959). The relation between intravesical (intramural and submucosal) ureteral length and ureteral diameter in normal children is shown in Table 59–2. Hutch estimated the average intravesical ureter length to be 0.5 cm in neonates and 1.3 cm in adults (Hutch, 1962). Although the 5:1 ratio sets the standard for reimplantation surgery, it may not be absolutely necessary to obviate reflux.

Secondary Reflux

Anatomic and Functional Causes

Secondary reflux is caused by bladder obstruction and the elevated pressures that accompany it. Such ob-

Table 59–2. MEAN URETERAL TUNNEL LENGTHS AND DIAMETERS IN NORMAL CHILDREN (IN MILLIMETERS)

Age (Yr)	Intravesical Ureteral Length	Submucosal Ureteral Length	Ureteral Diameter at Ureterovesical Junction
1–3	7	3	1.4
3–6	7	3	1.7
6–9	9	4	2.0
9–12	12	6	1.9

From Paquin AJ: Ureterovesical anastomosis: The description and evaluation of a technique. J Urol 1959;82:573.

structions are either *anatomic* or *functional*, although the outcomes can be the same. The chronicity and degree of obstruction undoubtedly influence the severity of secondary reflux. **The most common anatomic cause is posterior urethral valves, which are associated with reflux in approximately 50% of affected boys** (Henneberry and Stevens, 1980; Scott, 1985). Anatomic obstructions in girls are extremely rare, although ureteroceles can block the bladder outlet and distort the anatomic relationships of the trigone in both sexes. Urethral stenosis remains commonly (although incorrectly) implicated by some urologists. **Meatal stenosis causing urinary symptoms and reflux in either sex is rare. Instead, functional causes are far more common. These include neurogenic bladder, non-neurogenic neurogenic bladder, and bladder instability or dysfunction.**

Any child with altered bladder dynamics is at risk for reflux. A poorly compliant bladder or its abnormal interplay with the urinary sphincters can result in increased intravesical pressures. These can gradually weaken and overcome the ureteral sphincter mechanism at the UVJ and cause reflux in patients with previously normal studies. **Patients with spina bifida and other types of neurogenic bladder are particularly susceptible in this regard** (Bauer et al, 1982). A thorough physical examination should be completed in any child with a UTI. Children with sacral agenesis or external signs of occult spinal dysraphism, including a hair patch, sacral dimple, aberrant gluteal cleft, or decreased rectal tone or perineal sensation, are at risk. The lower extremities should also be checked for orthopedic or neurologic deficits. If a spinal dysraphism is suspected, magnetic resonance imaging (MRI) studies should be obtained.

Transient urodynamic abnormalities have been identified as the cause of UTIs and reflux in the first year of life. One study identified abnormalities, including detrusor hyperreflexia and elevated filling pressures, in 97% of boys and 77% of girls who presented in infancy with reflux (Chandra et al, 1996). The pressures in boys were usually higher, a finding noted by others (Sillen, 1996; Yeung et al, 1998) that may account for the difference in degree of reflux seen in infancy between the sexes. **In older children, bladder dysfunction is apparently an acquired phenomenon resulting from abnormal voiding patterns in neurologically normal children.** Young children commonly demonstrate a labile, infantile-type response to bladder filling in the form of uninhibited contractions. The child, who is typically in the early stages of toilet training and attempting to maintain continence, responds to this instability by contracting the external sphincter (Allen, 1979). Variable degrees of incontinence result, depending on the threshold volume for contractions and effectiveness of the sphincter control. **Continence can be maintained, but at the expense of abnormally increased intravesical pressures. Complete emptying is seen, at least initially, but gradually incomplete emptying occurs.** The residual that remains becomes an obvious risk factor for UTIs. **On the far end of this spectrum are children with *non-neurogenic neurogenic bladders*. Here, constriction of the urinary sphincter occurs during voiding in a voluntary form of detrusor-sphincter dyssynergia. Gradual bladder decompensation and myogenic failure result**

from incomplete emptying and increasing amounts of residual urine. In addition, as many as 75% of children with this syndrome also have bladder instability (Hinman, 1986; Mayo and Burns, 1990).

The intravesical pressures seen with bladder dysfunction can be impressive and have VUR as their common sequela. Reflux is a common finding at presentation in children with non-neurogenic neurogenic bladders (Fig. 59–2). Koff and Murtaugh (1983) noted reflux in almost 50% of children who were urodynamically evaluated for voiding dysfunction. **Conversely, the most common urodynamic abnormality in patients with reflux is uninhibited bladder contractions** (Homsy et al, 1985). These were found in 75% of girls with reflux in one series (Taylor et al, 1982). Both reflux and bladder dysfunction peak between the ages of 3 and 5 years, and many children present soon after the onset of toilet training. The normal UVJ is extremely resistant to reflux, even in the face of the intermittently exceptional pressures that occur with normal voiding (greater than 100 cm H_2O in some young boys). Yet the sustained effects of chronically elevated intravesical pressures take their toll. **Decreased bladder wall compliance, detrusor decompensation, and incomplete emptying gradually damage the complex anatomic relationships required of the UVJ.** The development of reflux further impairs bladder emptying and amplifies resting and filling pressures, thus initiating a self-perpetuating cycle of upper and lower urinary tract damage (Koff, 1992). Immature bladders and ureters are especially susceptible in this regard, although a similar scenario sometimes occurs in adults with bladder outlet obstruction.

Clinical Correlates

The identification and treatment of secondary causes of reflux often brings about its spontaneous resolution, unless the UVJ has been irreparably damaged. In addition, failure to do so significantly jeopardizes any surgery that might inadvertently be done in an attempt to correct the problem. The importance of identification is emphasized by the findings of the European arm of the IRSC, in which more frequent breakthrough UTIs, greater variability in follow-up reflux grade, and increased persistence of reflux were noted in patients with untreated bladder dysfunction (Van Gool et al, 1992). **The initial management of functional causes of reflux is medical. It is imperative that clinicians inquire about and determine the voiding patterns of children with reflux.** Otherwise, bladder dysfunction presents increased risks of delay in the spontaneous resolution expected of reflux and breakthrough UTIs, which lead to reimplantation surgery and adverse outcomes after that surgery (Koff et al, 1998).

In addition to a careful physical examination, signs or symptoms of voiding dysfunction include dribbling, urgency, and incontinence. Little girls often exhibit curtseying behavior, and boys may squeeze the penis in an attempt to suppress bladder contractions. Encopresis and constipation also suggest abnormal toilet behavior and altered dynamics of the pelvic sphincters. Constipation poses a significant risk of recurrent UTIs (O'Regan et al, 1985). The urinary symptoms in many children resolve once bowel function is improved. In one series, for exam-

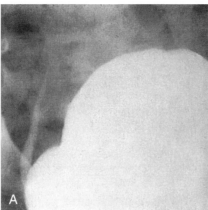

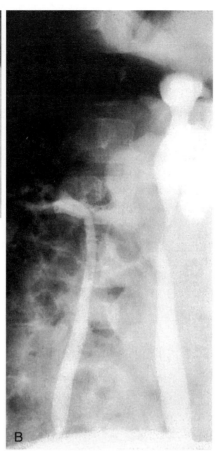

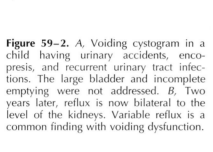

Figure 59–2. *A,* Voiding cystogram in a child having urinary accidents, encopresis, and recurrent urinary tract infections. The large bladder and incomplete emptying were not addressed. *B,* Two years later, reflux is now bilateral to the level of the kidneys. Variable reflux is a common finding with voiding dysfunction.

ple, 89% of daytime incontinence, 63% of nocturnal enuresis, and all UTIs, where no abnormalities were present, resolved with treatment of the constipation (Loening-Baucke, 1997). This constellation of symptoms should probably be better termed *toilet dysfunction* in recognition of its global implications for the bladder and bowel. Incomplete evacuation, residual urine on voiding studies or ultrasonography, and a thick bladder wall or multiple diverticula are other suspicious findings.

Treatment of bladder dysfunction and instability, regardless of its severity or cause, is directed at dampening uninhibited contractions and lowering intravesical pressures. Neurologically normal children with reflux, whose uninhibited bladder contractions were treated with anticholinergics, showed statistically different rates of resolution when compared to age-matched controls with normal bladder function (44% vs. 17%) and also had higher rates of resolution when compared to similar children with bladder instability who were not treated with anticholinergics (33%) (Koff and Murtaugh, 1983). Other series have since documented the efficacy of medication in neurologically normal children who have the combination of reflux and bladder hyperreflexia and/or some degree of abnormal urinary sphincter activity. Oxybutynin contributed to the resolution or downgrading of reflux in 62% of ureters in 37 children in one report (Homsy et al, 1985). Although a control arm was not included, this is a higher rate of improvement than that expected of the population as a whole. In another study of 53 children

using diazepam, baclofen, or other muscle relaxing agents aimed at lessening sphincter contractions, reflux resolved in 92% of ureters and decreased in the remainder (Seruca, 1989).

There is a strong association between intravesical pressures greater than 40 cm H_2O and the presence of reflux in patients with myelodysplasia and neuropathic bladders. If pressures at the typical capacity (average catheterization volume) or leak point are kept below this standard, reflux often resolves even when it is significant (Flood et al, 1994). High-grade reflux (grade III to V) either ceased or was downgraded in 18 (55%) of 33 patients with myelodysplasia after lowering of intravesical pressures and facilitation of emptying with intermittent catheterization. In a larger series of 200 myelodysplastics with neurogenic bladder, reflux lessened or resolved in 124 (62%) (Kaplan and Firlit, 1983). These same pressure relationships form the basis of reflux seen with bladder dysfunction and non-neurogenic neurogenic bladder. When medical management is unsuccessful in correcting abnormal bladder dynamics (regardless of cause) and resolving secondary reflux, enterocystoplasty, vesicostomy, or some other form of urinary diversion becomes a necessary option in management.

When residual urine is present, a finding that can be amplified by the yo-yo effect of high-grade reflux, treatment is directed at facilitating emptying. In normal children without bladder dysfunction, this includes double voiding. Otherwise, relaxation techniques or biofeedback aimed at lessening constriction of the external sphincter is sometimes successful for patients with a non-neurogenic neurogenic picture (Hellstrom, 1987a). Occasionally, intermittent catheterization combined with medication becomes the key to management for the most severely affected normal subjects (Lapides et al, 1972).

Lower Urinary Tract Infection

Bladder infections (UTIs) and their accompanying inflammation can also cause reflux by lessening compliance, elevating intravesical pressures, and distorting and weakening the UVJ (Van Gool and Tanagho, 1977; Roberts et al, 1988). The ureteral atony caused by gram-negative endotoxins can also be a contributing factor (Jeffs and Allen, 1962). For the same reasons, the spontaneous resolution of reflux normally expected of some ureters can be delayed (Roberts and Riopelle, 1978). In some patients transient reflux occasionally occurs during episodes of acute cystitis and resolves with treatment and dissipation of inflammation (Kaplan, 1980). The immature or damaged UVJ may be particularly prone to this phenomenon. The cystitis that results from the chemotherapeutic agent Cytoxan (cyclophosphamide) can have a similar effect (Jerkins et al, 1988).

Clinical Correlates

Because of the bladder changes that occur with cystitis, the recommendation for the timing of VCUG remains open to debate. Some clinicians defer the study for a few weeks to allow for inflammation to resolve and to avoid patient discomfort and so-called false-positive studies. This approach, however, risks overlooking reflux that occurs only with infection. Instead, other clinicians now obtain the study during its active phases. When parenteral antibiotics have been taken for a few days, the latter approach seems reasonable because cystography itself poses little risk in the presence of reflux, with or without bacteriuria. When reflux cannot be documented but the clinical presentation or radiographic results (or both) suggest an upper UTI, the patient should be prescribed a short course of prophylactic antibiotics while therapy is directed at underlying risk factors. Bladder dysfunction and its residual urine are prime offenders. The latter acts as a fertile medium for bacteria and also potentially alters bladder dynamics. Timed voids and relaxation therapy directed at bladder emptying are initiated in any patient with recurrent UTIs, whether reflux is present or not. Dietary alterations and cathartics are also commonly prescribed to treat constipation.

CLASSIFICATION AND GRADING

Several systems for grading VUR have been proposed in the past several decades. Their role is to classify the severity of the disease process so that clinicians are better able to predict the likelihood of spontaneous resolution and the risk of reflux-associated complications. Early classifications graded reflux in relation to the physiologic state of the bladder. The terms "high-pressure" and "low-pressure"

Table 59–3. INTERNATIONAL CLASSIFICATION OF VESICOURETERAL REFLUX

Grade	Description
I	Into the nondilated ureter
II	Into the pelvis and calyces without dilatation
III	Mild to moderate dilatation of the ureter, renal pelvis, and calyces with minimal blunting of the fornices
IV	Moderate ureteral tortuosity and dilatation of the pelvis and calyces
V	Gross dilatation of the ureter, pelvis, and calyces; loss of papillary impressions; and ureteral tortuosity

were introduced to describe reflux that occurred during bladder emptying or on bladder filling (Hinman and Hutch, 1962; Melick et al, 1962; Lattimer et al, 1963; Smellie and Normand, 1968). Reflux that occurs during the filling phase may represent an intrinsic defect that is perhaps less likely to spontaneously resolve. Later classifications relied on the degree of pelvicalyceal dilatation caused by the reflux as well as the ureteral diameter (Howerton and Lich, 1963; Heikel and Parkkulainen, 1966; Bridge and Roe, 1969; Dwoskin and Perlmutter, 1973; Rolleston et al, 1975). The Heikel and Parkkulainen system gained popularity in Europe a few years before the Dwoskin and Perlmutter system became widely accepted in the United States. **The International Classification System,** devised in 1981 by the IRSC, represents a melding of the two. It **provides the current standard for grading reflux based on the appearance of contrast material in the ureter and upper collecting system during VCUG** (International Reflux Study Committee, 1981) (Table 59–3 and Fig. 59–3). Because reflux appears as a continuum on cystography, any grading system suffers from being somewhat arbitrary (Lebowitz, 1992). However, a classification system that is widely accepted allows for a common understanding of the natural history of the disease, sequential comparisons of individual patients, and comparisons between patients or groups of patients despite this and its other drawbacks.

One shortcoming of the International Classification System and other systems based primarily on calyceal appearance is that the degree of ureteral dilatation may not correlate with the degree of pyelocalyceal dilatation. Some lower ureteral segments are impressively dilated yet associ-

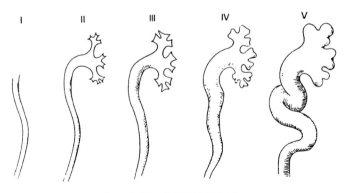

GRADES OF REFLUX

Figure 59–3. International classification of vesicoureteral reflux.

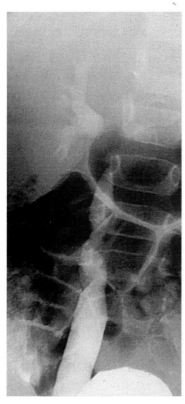

Figure 59–4. The refluxing ureter with significant dilatation of the lower segment but no distortion of the collecting system may be different from the typical system with grade II reflux.

ated with little if any proximal reflux. Whether their rates of resolution are similar to those of ureters that have a luminal caliber typically found with similar grades of reflux remains unclear (Fig. 59–4). In addition, inconsistencies occur because the degree of ureteral dilatation can vary with bladder pressure and filling at the time of each film. Finally, **accurately grading reflux is impossible when there is coexistent ipsilateral obstruction.** If obstruction goes unrecognized, the grade of reflux can be falsely elevated by contrast filling the hydronephrotic kidney. **The permanent calyceal distortion associated with postinfection scarring or nonobstructive dilatation can also lead to overestimations of the severity of reflux.** To be completely accurate, grading systems must reflect the degree of primary reflux, unaltered by associated pathology (Lebowitz, 1992).

Other problems arise when comparing standard VCUG

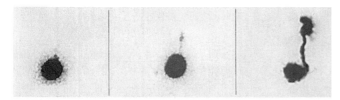

Figure 59–5. Nuclear voiding cystography showing right-sided reflux. Radionuclide tracer can be quantitated (from left to right) as grade 1 (grade I International Grading System); grade 2 (grade II–III International Grading System); and grade 3 (grade IV–V International Grading System).

and radionuclide cystography (RNC), which is commonly used for follow-up screening (see later discussion). **Classifying reflux with RNC is difficult because it is impossible to accurately assess ureteral and pelvicalyceal anatomy with radionuclide tracer.** In response to this dilemma, Willi and Treves (1983) devised a system for grading RNC that correlates closely with the International Classification System. The three degrees of reflux identified within this schema are shown (Fig. 59–5). Nevertheless, when management decisions depend on comparisons of grade and trends in the degree of reflux, it is preferable to revert to standard cystography.

DIAGNOSIS AND EVALUATION

Clinical Presentations

Most patients with reflux present initially with some symptom or symptoms that suggest a UTI, although the findings in newborns typically are nonspecific. Failure to thrive and lethargy are worrisome signs in newborns, while high fevers are uncommon. Infants and younger children arrive with fever, malodorous urine, dysuria and urinary frequency, lethargy, and gastrointestinal symptoms including nausea and vomiting. Pyelonephritis often causes vague abdominal discomfort rather than localized flank pain. Even in the absence of an infection, children and adults with VUR sometimes describe abdominal or flank discomfort, usually associated with a full bladder or immediately after voiding. When reflux has gone undetected and renal scarring has occurred, children of any age can arrive with renal insufficiency, hypertension, and impaired somatic growth.

Most importantly, a urine culture should be included in the evaluation of any infant or child who presents with fever or malaise. Unfortunately, UTIs and reflux are often overlooked, and their ill-defined presentations are mistakenly attributed to otitis media, viral gastroenteritis, respiratory infection, or fever of unknown origin. Until a proper diagnosis is made, severe renal damage can be incurred. **The presence of fever may be an indicator of upper urinary tract involvement, but it is not always a reliable sign** (Farnsworth et al, 1991). **However, if fever (and presumably pyelonephritis) is present, the likelihood of discovering VUR is significantly increased** (Govan and Palmer, 1969; Woodard and Holden, 1976; Smellie et al, 1981b). In one study of 919 girls with UTI, reflux was present in 56% of those younger than 6 months of age with a temperature higher than 38.5°C. Girls older than 10 years of age arriving with similar fevers were less likely to have the problem (13%) (Gelfand et al, 2000). A variety of laboratory tests have been used to localize infections to the kidneys, including β_2-macroglobulin, lactate dehydrogenase, and antibody-coated bacteria, but have given equivocal results (Neal, 1989). Elevated cytokines including interleukin-6 (IL-6) and IL-8 have also been observed with acute UTI, and the latter may provide a marker of renal scarring (Haraoka et al, 1996). Antibodies to Tamm-Horsfall protein, urinary proteins including N-acetyl-D-glucosaminidase (NAG), and serum intracellular adhesion molecule (ICAM-1) and epidermal growth factor have also been studied as markers of pyelonephritis or scarring

(Miyakita et al, 1995; Jelakovic et al, 1996; Goonasekera et al, 1996a; Konda et al, 1997). Their current clinical applicability remains unclear.

Documenting Urinary Tract Infections

When a UTI is suspected from the clinical history, a urine culture is essential to making the diagnosis. Microscopy alone may not provide a valid assessment of the urine, although the combined use of dipsticks increases sensitivity. Specimens should be refrigerated immediately at 4°C until they can be cultured. The method of collection also is extremely important. **In toilet-trained children, a midstream voided specimen is adequate. The first portion of urine, which contains the bulk of bacterial contaminant of the periurethral region, should be discarded. Any growth beyond 100,000 colonies per high-power field per milliliter of urine (CFU/ml) is considered significant.** Approximately 10% of samples yield growths of between 10 and 50,000 CFU/ml that have no correlation whatsoever with actual UTI (Wettergren, 1985).

Catheterization is also an excellent way of obtaining a urine sample with minimal contamination and is the preferred method in infants and in older children when contamination is suspected in specimens collected otherwise. Catheterized specimens with bacterial counts greater than 10,000 CFU/ml are considered significant. Finally, suprapubic aspiration is the most sensitive but also most challenging means of assessing bacteriuria in children. Suprapubic specimens with bacterial counts greater than 10,000 CFU/ml are considered significant. Uncircumcised boys, whose prepuce makes valid specimen collection difficult, are occasionally candidates. Many void during the technique because of anxiety or pain, making collection difficult, although squeezing the penis beforehand helps. In addition, needle trauma can cause microscopic hematuria that clouds the diagnostic picture. When the bladder is not extremely full, ultrasonic needle guidance is helpful. **Collection of urine specimens by means of adhesive bags is the most widely used yet least reliable technique. These specimens carry a high risk of contamination and should probably be deferred in the symptomatic infant. Bagged specimens can also be unreliable despite yielding pure growths of more than 100,000 CFU/ml, although specimens whose culture result is negative provide useful information.**

Evaluating Urinary Tract Infections

VUR is found in 29% to 50% of children with UTI (International Reflux Study Committee, 1981). Approximately 30% of these already have some evidence of renal parenchymal scarring that is usually proportional to the severity of reflux (Bellinger and Duckett, 1984; Blickman et al, 1985). Baker and associates (1966) found that reflux was more commonly associated with UTI in younger children. In contrast, Smellie and coworkers did not find any age-related difference in the incidence of reflux in children with UTI (Smellie et al, 1981b). In addition, there were thought to be no reliable clinical features that distinguished

children with reflux from those without (Smellie et al, 1981b; Johnson et al, 1985). Renal scarring can occur after a single UTI, even in the absence of fever (Ransley and Risdon, 1981; Smellie et al, 1985; Rushton et al, 1992). These types of data amplify the need for a thorough evaluation of any child with suspected UTI.

The diagnostic work-up is tailored to the individual according to age, gender, and clinical history. **Complete evaluations that include VCUG and ultrasonography are required of three groups: any child younger than 5 years of age with a documented UTI; any child with a febrile UTI, regardless of age; and any boy with a UTI unless the child is sexually active or has a past urologic history** (Burbige et al, 1984). Younger children who have had one UTI are highly prone (80% to 85%) to have another, whether an anomaly or voiding dysfunction was its cause. As many as half of these children will be asymptomatic. Therefore, **a work-up is recommended after the first UTI to rule out anatomic risk factors.** If none are present, parents can be reassured that the urinary tract is normal and that further UTIs should generally remain confined to the lower urinary tract and not pose a serious health threat. Therapeutic efforts are then directed at improving the child's toilet behavior (e.g., timed voids, relaxation to facilitate emptying, treatment of constipation). **Older children who present with asymptomatic bacteriuria or UTI that manifests solely with lower tract symptoms can be screened initially with ultrasonography alone, reserving cystorrhaphy for those with abnormal upper tracts or recalcitrant infections.** Full radiographic evaluations of black children are usually reserved for those with recurrent or febrile UTI, because of their low incidence of the anomaly (Askari and Belman, 1982).

Finally, the detection of asymptomatic reflux is becoming increasingly common, especially since the anomaly is the predisposing cause of many cases of antenatally diagnosed hydronephrosis (Fig. 59–6). **Newborns with moderate to severe degrees of upper tract dilatation should be fully evaluated with VCUG, as should any baby who had intermittent hydronephrosis as a fetus, another common presentation of the problem.** Postnatal ultra-

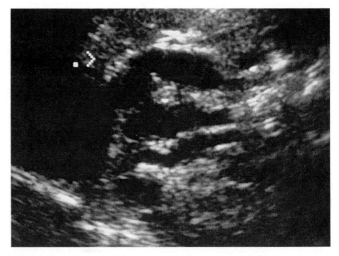

Figure 59–6. Antenatal ultrasound demonstrates bilateral ureteropelvic dilatation. Reflux is a common cause of such a finding.

sound alone is a poor screening technique for reflux in the neonate. In one study the results of postnatal ultrasound were normal in 25% of patients with antenatal hydronephrosis who were shown to have reflux on VCUG (Lebowitz, 1993). The significance of such reflux, most of which is of low grade and spontaneously resolves, remains open to question. However, attempts to modify the work-up depending on the degree of antenatal hydronephrosis may leave some children at risk. In one study of 60 infants with mild hydronephrosis (less than Society for Fetal Urology grade II), reflux was detected in 15%, yet none developed significant renal problems after as long as 4.5 years of follow-up (Yerkes et al, 1999). Other studies using pelvic diameter as the criterion for VCUG reported a similar yield with even minor degrees of dilatation (4 mm) (Walsh and Dubbins, 1996; Anderson et al, 1997). Counseling and careful follow-up are mandatory. Racial differences may allow some modification, because reflux in black girls being evaluated for antenatal hydronephrosis is reportedly rare (Horowitz et al, 1999).

Lower Urinary Tract Assessment: Cystography

The presence of VUR can be established with either fluoroscopic or radionuclide voiding cystography, although certain factors affect the diagnostic yield. **Some reflux can be appreciated only during detrusor contractions and active voiding, causing reflux to be easily missed in the anxious or stubborn child who is unable to void** (Poznanski and Poznanski, 1969). **Cystograms done with a Foley catheter or while the child is under anesthesia are static studies that inaccurately screen for reflux or sometimes exaggerate its degree because of bladder overfilling.** In addition, general anesthesia can influence the severity of reflux by reducing glomerular filtration and urinary output (Mazze et al, 1963). As a result, studies done during general anesthesia are of equivocal value. **Conversely, excessive hydration may mask low grades of reflux, because diuresis can blunt the retrograde flow of urine** (Ekman et al, 1966). **Finally, some reflux is demonstrated only during active infection, when cystitis weakens the UVJ through edema or through increasing intravesical pressures** (Van Gool and Tanagho, 1977; Kaplan, 1980). **In addition, cystograms obtained during active infection can overestimate the grade of reflux, because the endotoxins produced by some gram-negative organisms can paralyze ureteral smooth muscle and exaggerate ureteral dilatation** (Roberts, 1975; Boyarsky et al, 1978; Hellstrom et al, 1987a). Most pediatric centers are now performing VCUG soon after the diagnosis of a UTI, sometimes within 1 week, in order to maximize patient compliance (Craig et al, 1997; McDonald et al, 2000).

Fluoroscopic voiding cystourethrography is an outpatient procedure that should provide more information than mere anatomic detail. Children who are old enough are asked to void in the bathroom. After the perimeatal area is cleansed, a small-caliber lubricated feeding tube (No. 5 Fr in newborns, No. 8 Fr in others) is placed through the urethra into the bladder. The postvoid residual urine is measured, and a sample is sent for culture. Dilute contrast agent is then instilled via gravity (not to exceed 100 cm H_2O) under fluoroscopic control. Given the small catheter sizes used, the intravesical pressure generated during gravity filling is independent of the height of the bottle (Koff et al, 1979a). Once the contrast agent ceases to drip, the bladder capacity can also be calculated from the end point of infusion. Intermittent fluoroscopic scans assess the presence of reflux during filling and while voiding. A complete VCUG also includes views of the UVJs and urethra during voiding, while a film of the bladder after voiding provides a useful assessment of emptying. **When reflux is present, delayed films are obtained to assess upper tract drainage. Contrast material that is refluxed proximally should return readily to the bladder. Its hangup may implicate a coexisting obstruction in the renal moiety.** Leibovic and Lebowitz (1980) showed that a comprehensive voiding study can be completed using a minimal duration of fluoroscopy (average, 36 seconds). Similar findings were noted by Diamond and colleagues (1996a). The accuracy of cystography is improved by repeating several cycles of filling and voiding. With cyclic cystography, an increase of up to 12% in incidence of reflux or change in grading may be seen by repeating the procedure (Paltiel et al, 1992; Polito et al, 2000). Cyclic VCUG is time-intensive and requires more fluoroscopic exposure, but it is indicated in patients when there is a strong suspicion of reflux that is not appreciated on a single-sequence study (Jequier and Jequier, 1989; Paltiel et al, 1992; Polito et al, 2000).

Nuclear cystography (RNC) is the scintigraphic equivalent of conventional cystography. **Although the technique does not provide the anatomic detail of fluoroscopic studies, it is an accurate method for detecting and monitoring reflux.** Technetium Tc99m pertechnetate, instilled into the bladder in saline, provides doses of radiation 100-fold less than a standard VCUG (Blaufox et al, 1971). **In addition to minimizing radiation exposure, the technique allows for prolonged observation under the gamma camera, which enhances sensitivity** (Fig. 59–7). **These advantages make RNC an effective means of screening for reflux, of monitoring reflux after its initial grading and anatomic detail are obtained by standard VCUG, and of making sure that the reflux has resolved after corrective surgery.** When reflux is initially discovered by RNC, VCUG often becomes necessary to more accurately grade the reflux and better delineate lower urinary tract anatomy (Willi and Treves, 1983).

Indirect cystography uses intravenously injected ^{99m}Tc-diethylenetriamine penta-acetic acid (^{99m}Tc-DTPA) (Pollet et al, 1981). This agent is cleared by glomerular filtration and excreted into the bladder within 20 minutes. The child can then be scanned for reflux, thus avoiding catheterization (Conway et al, 1975). Unfortunately, the method produces a high percentage of false-negative studies and is particularly unreliable with milder grades of reflux.

Ultrasonic cystography offers an ideal screening tool for reflux, because there is no exposure to radiation. Sonicated human serum albumin, composed of 3 to 5×10^8 air-filled echogenic spheres per milliliter, can be detected by ultrasound and has been used successfully to detect reflux in animal models (Fig. 59–8) (Atala et al, 1993c) and humans (Atala et al, 1998). A galactose-based echogenic con-

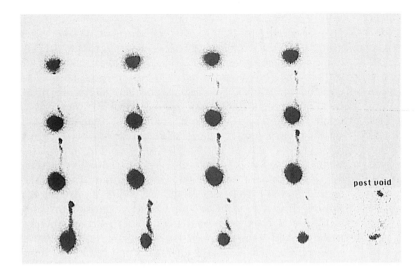

Figure 59–7. Radionuclide cystogram shows right-sided reflux that worsens with bladder filling. The upper collecting system drains fully with voiding.

post void

trast medium has also been used with good success in children (Bosio, 1998). Until these procedures are standardized, this modality must be considered a research tool.

Diagnostic Drawbacks

It is important to know whether reflux is present before completing upper tract functional studies (excretory urogram, renal scintigraphy), because reflux can cause both underestimations and overestimations of renal function (Lebowitz and Avni, 1980; Blickman et al, 1985). For example, contrast material or a radionuclide agent excreted from one kidney can reflux into a nonfunctioning contralateral partner to mimic function. Conversely, the reflux of nonopaque or unlabeled urine into the collecting system of a kidney with good function can dilute excreted material, causing underestimation of function. **To avoid such artifacts, catheter drainage of the bladder is required for any renal functional studies in patients with known reflux.** To avoid multiple manipulations, catheters are also placed before functional studies that precede the VCUG in patients being initially evaluated.

Upper Tract Assessment

Ultrasonography **has replaced the excretory urogram (intravenous pyelogram, IVP) as the diagnostic study of choice to initially evaluate the upper urinary tracts of patients with suspected or proven VUR. Ultrasound alone cannot effectively rule out reflux, especially with lower grades that do not cause renal pelvic dilatation, and VCUG is required for children with suspected reflux** (Scott et al, 1991; Blane et al, 1993). However, the information gleaned from the study can be invaluable. Urinary ultrasound includes views of the bladder as well as kidneys and offers baseline assessments of overall renal size, parenchymal thickness, and the presence of scars, hydronephrosis, or other renal and ureteral anomalies (Fig. 59–9). Information on postvoid residuals and bladder wall thickness also becomes useful in children with suspected bladder dysfunction. Although mild renal pelvic dilatation is not predictive of reflux (Davey et al, 1997), intermittent dilatation of the renal pelvis or ureter suggests the presence of reflux (Hiraoka et al, 1996; Weinberg and Yeung, 1998). A yearly ultrasound is recommended for patients with reflux who are medically managed to monitor interval

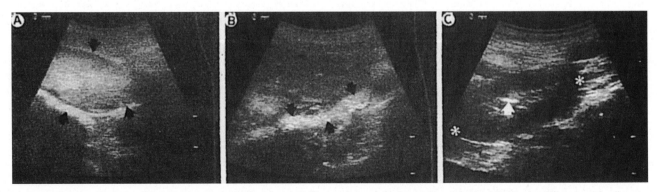

Figure 59–8. Sonographic visualization of sonicated albumin. *A,* Diffuse echogenicity is produced in the bladder by filling it with albumin and saline (*arrows* outline bladder). *B,* Sonicated albumin that refluxes into the ureter produces a bright echogenic band *(arrows). C,* Echogenic area is caused by albumin that has refluxed into the renal pelvis.

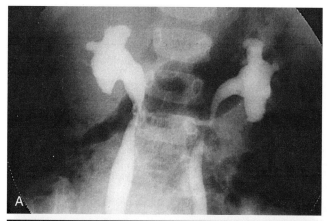

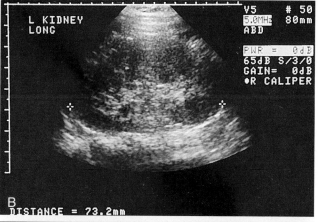

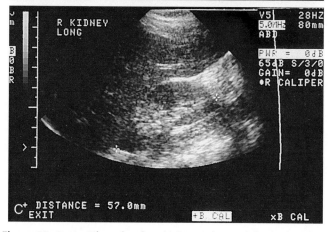

Figure 59–9. *A,* Bilateral reflux (right, grade IV; left, grade III). *B,* Sonogram shows normal left kidney, 73 mm in length. *C,* Small, scarred right kidney (57 mm) with significant thinning of the upper pole.

renal growth and detect grossly evident renal scarring, although the study does not provide the sensitivity of scintigraphy to define subtleties of the latter (see later discussion).

Doppler ultrasound allows visualization of the ureteric jet that is created by the passage of a urine bolus through the UVJ. Usually, two to six peristaltic waves occur per minute (Elejalde and DeElejalde, 1983). Color Doppler ultrasound facilitates visualization of the anteromedially directed jet in the bladder. Although severe renal parenchymal scarring reduces the frequency and amplitude of jets,

Doppler analysis fails to allow the diagnosis or exclusion of reflux (Jequier et al, 1990; Marshall et al, 1990; Haberlik, 1997).

Functional studies are required of the severely scarred kidney when the question of salvageability is raised. A baseline functional study is also usually obtained in anticipation of reimplantation surgery, but it is probably unnecessary with a normal renal ultrasound.

Excretory urography (IVP) once provided the gold standard for the imaging of kidneys associated with reflux. Rough measures of function and assessment of scars and parenchymal thinning are gradually being displaced by the more sophisticated information provided by scintigraphy (Fig. 59–10). Several findings on excretory urography suggest the presence of reflux. These include pyelonephritic scarring without obstruction (Claesson and Lindberg, 1977), renal growth retardation (Ginalski et al, 1985), and the presence of a retrograde ureteral jet on the bladder phase of an IVP (Kuhns et al, 1977). Any of these findings, whether present in a patient with or without suspected reflux, should prompt further evaluation with VCUG.

Renal scintigraphy using ^{99m}Tc-labeled DMSA is the best study to detect pyelonephritis and the cortical renal scarring that sometimes results. Radionuclide uptake is directly proportional to functional proximal tubular mass and correlates well with glomerular filtration rates (Taylor, 1982). Pyelonephritis impairs tubular uptake and causes areas of photon deficiency in the cortical outline. Many completely resolve, especially with prompt medical treatment, whereas others persist as actual scars from irreparable tubular damage (Rushton et al, 1988). A 98% specificity and 92% sensitivity in detecting renal scars was shown in a study of 79 children monitored for 1 to 4 years after a proven UTI (Merrick et al, 1980). The role of scintigraphy is changing with the altered understanding of upper UTIs. Contrary to historical beliefs, most pyelonephritis does not result from infection that relies on reflux as its delivery system but from infection alone (Bjorgvinsson et al, 1991; Stockland et al, 1996). This was shown in a prospective study by Majd and colleagues, who found that 63% of children (mean age, 3 years) with DMSA-proven pyelonephritis did not have VUR, even when evaluated at the same admission (Majd et al, 1991). A similar prevalence of cortical defects in the absence of reflux was also noted by Ditchfield and Nadel (1998).

High-resolution single-photon emission computed tomography (SPECT), which involves 360-degree imaging and computer reconstruction, may provide greater renal cortical detail (Joseph et al, 1990). This technology, which has the capacity of providing coronal, sagittal, and transaxial imaging, has been applied to DMSA scans in an effort to enhance the detection of acute pyelonephritis. Tarkington and colleagues (1990) compared the findings of SPECT and standard pinhole imaging in 33 children with various acute and chronic pathologic renal conditions. They found that SPECT imaging improved the ability to identify cortical defects, compared with the more commonly used imaging mode. Other investigators also reported that SPECT scintigraphy was more effective than planar scintigraphy in demonstrating anatomic damage to the renal parenchyma in

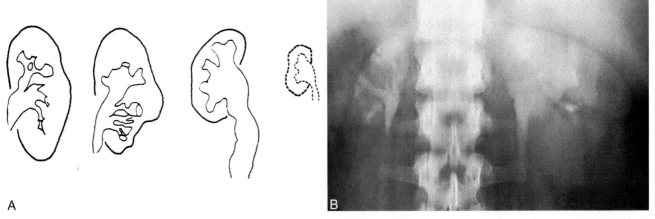

A

B

Figure 59-10. *A,* Classification of renal scarring based on alterations in renal size and contour seen on excretory urography. (From Smellie J, Edwards D, Hunter N, et al: Vesicoureteral reflux and renal scarring. Kidney Int 1975;8[Suppl 4]:65.) *B,* Excretory urogram demonstrates bilateral renal scarring.

patients with various urologic disorders (Fig. 59–11) (Itoh et al, 1995; Yen et al, 1998).

Because scan results do not alter treatment or the need for further work-up, the role of DMSA scanning in the evaluation of any child who presents clinically with acute pyelonephritis remains unclear. However, because of the nonspecific presentation of UTIs in many children, the study is an invaluable aid to diagnosis when pyelonephritis is suspected but has not been proven (Verber et al, 1988). In addition, because of its sensitivity for detecting scars, DMSA scans are now being used by some clinicians to periodically (every 2 years) screen patients with known reflux that is being medically managed. Others propose

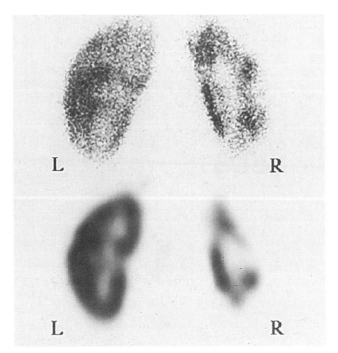

Figure 59-11. Dimercaptosuccinic acid (DMSA) renal scintigraphy. *Upper photographs,* Pinhole images showing normal left kidney and right kidney with multiple cortical defects. *Lower photographs,* Single-photon emission computed tomography (SPECT) study.

tailoring these studies to patients who have ultrasound abnormalities, high-grade reflux, or recurrent breakthrough infections (Merguerian et al, 1999).

Cystoscopy **has a limited role in the diagnosis of reflux by contemporary urologists.** There is little additional information to be gained in defining the anatomy of the ureters, urethra, and bladder neck that is not provided by VCUG and ultrasonography. The utility of cystoscopy was originally underscored by the study of Lyon et al, who described four orifice configurations of increasing abnormality: normal or cone, stadium, horseshoe, and golf-hole. These assumed progressively lateral positions and shorter intramural tunnel lengths and were increasingly likely to be associated with reflux (Lyon et al, 1969). Although these descriptive terms linger in the literature, their implications have assumed less importance with time. A few years later, measurements of submucosal tunnel length using calibrated ureteral catheters were also emphasized as having important prognostic implications for the outcome of reflux (King et al, 1974). In actuality, it is now well known that progressive bladder filling will give an orifice a more abnormal appearance. In addition, the muscular hiatus slides along the extravesical ureter as the bladder fills, in effect shortening the length of the submucosal tunnel. This phenomenon helps explain reflux that is seen only when the bladder is filled to extremes. **Orifice configuration was subsequently found to be of little value in predicting the presence of reflux or prognosticating the likelihood of its spontaneous resolution** (Duckett, 1983).

Other information that might be gained from cystoscopy, such as urethral calibration in female patients, has also lost importance, especially since actual urethral stenosis is exceedingly uncommon. Urethral dilatations of the "tight" sphincters associated with bladder dysfunction should be discouraged. If cystoscopy is performed, it is done in concert with a planned surgical repair. **The indications for cystoscopic evaluation immediately before surgery are shown** in Table 59–4. Although some surgeons routinely perform cystoscopy before reimplantation, deferring surgery on the basis of its findings is extremely uncommon, especially if a recent urine culture was negative.

Studies of urodynamics **are indicated for any child**

Table 59–4. RELATIVE INDICATIONS FOR CYSTOSCOPY

Nonvisualization of entire urethra on cystourethrography
Uncertainty in ureteral location or anomaly—duplication, ectopia, ureterocele
Inconclusive radiographic definition of lower or upper tract anatomy
Localization of paraureteral diverticulum
Suspected active infection

with a suspected secondary cause for reflux (e.g., valves, neurogenic bladder, non-neurogenic neurogenic bladder, voiding dysfunction) and help direct therapy (Koff et al, 1979b). This is becoming even more important with the realization that a significant number of patients with reflux have bladder instability, inadequate urethral relaxation during voiding, and voiding dysfunction (Yeung et al, 1998; Chandra and Maddix, 2000; Willemsen and Nijman, 2000). Complete evaluations include cystometrography, flow studies with electromyography, and video recordings. Valid urodynamic values can be difficult to obtain in the face of massive reflux. When this is the case, ureteral occlusion catheters can be placed to eliminate the dampening effect of deleterious pressures that reflux offers the severely neuropathic bladder (Woodard and Borden, 1982; Bomalaski and Bloom, 1997). Studies performed with the patient under general anesthesia are of equivocal value because the pharmacologic actions of the anesthetic can alter bladder dynamics.

REFLUX AND THE KIDNEY

Renal Scarring

The term *reflux nephropathy* encompasses a number of radiologic changes of the kidney associated with reflux. These include (1) focal thinning of renal parenchyma overlying a clubbed, distorted calyx; (2) generalized calyceal dilatation with parenchymal atrophy; and (3) impaired renal growth, associated with either focal scarring or global atrophy (Hodson and Edwards, 1960; Bailey, 1973). Parenchymal thinning without calyceal distortion that is more than 2.5 standard deviations of normal thickness should also be included and appears to represent scarring in evolution (Olbing et al, 1992), although this change is sometimes reversible. The sequelae of such findings, including proteinuria, hypertension, eclampsia in pregnancy, and renal failure, can be devastating, although the majority of scars never pose a health threat to the affected patient.

Hodson was the first to recognize the significance of renal scars in children with recurrent UTIs, 97% of whom had VUR in his initial report (Hodson, 1959). Reflux nephropathy was also noted in as many as 60% of kidneys associated with reflux in later series (Scott and Stansfeld, 1968; Dwoskin and Perlmutter, 1973; Filly et al, 1974; Smellie et al, 1975) and in 65% of patients entered in the IRSC. In addition, there is a direct relation between the grade of reflux and the incidence of nephropathy. In one retrospective review, for example, scars were distributed accordingly: grade I, 5%; grade II, 6%; grade III, 17%; grade IV, 25%; and grade V, 50% (Skoog et al,

1987). A variety of theories help explain the association of reflux and nephropathy, and a multifactorial etiology probably contributes in some patients.

Congenital Scars

Some scarring or renal dysmorphism presumably evolves on a congenital basis, although the pathophysiology undoubtedly differs from that of the more common acquired causes of pyelonephritis. Such an etiology is very likely in newborns with antenatally diagnosed disease. Despite being infection free, many (30% to 35%) of these infants have kidneys that are diminutive and/or dysmorphic and scarred, especially with higher grades of reflux (Najmaldin at al, 1990; Burge et al, 1992; Marra et al, 1994a) (Table 59–5, Fig. 59–12). Male infants are particularly prone because of their tendency to high grades of reflux (Hiraoka et al, 1997), and boys are much less likely to acquire scarring because they rarely have recurrent UTIs. One study reported primary (congenital) scarring in 86% of boys but in only 30% of girls, who were more likely to acquire scars from repeated infections (Wennerstrom et al, 2000). The histology differs between congenital and acquired lesions, although their radiologic appearance can be indistinguishable. In theory, the interplay between the ureteral bud and renal blastema during the first few weeks of gestation determines the development of the kidney as well as that of the UVJ. As Mackie and Stephens suggested, a ureteral bud that is laterally (cranially) positioned from a normal takeoff at the trigone offers an embryologic explanation for primary reflux, whereas those inferiorly (caudally) positioned are often obstructed (Mackie and Stephens, 1975) (Fig. 59–13). Variable degrees of renal dysplasia and caliectasis follow (Stecker et al, 1973; Sommer and Stephens, 1981; Stock et al, 1998). In addition to dysplasia, hypoplasia is commonly found in nephrectomy specimens of patients with reflux. Acquired cortical loss is often typically interspersed as a consequence of infection (Hinchliffe et al, 1992), although progressive renal scarring can be avoided if infections are prevented (Assael et al, 1998). Dysplasia has also been noted in patients with duplex collecting systems and upper ureteral ectopia (Mackie and Stephens, 1975), prune-belly syndrome (Manivel et al, 1989), or posterior urethral valves, where the effects of high-grade obstruction early in embryogenesis may also contribute to renal dysmorphism. In one series, as many as 50% of infants with urethral valves and reflux had clinically significant renal insufficiency at a time too early in infancy to be caused by infection (Hulbert et al, 1992).

Table 59–5. CONGENITAL RENAL SCARRING

Grade of Vesicoureteral Reflux	No. of Patients (Percentage)		
	Normal	*Slight Damage*	*Severe Damage*
I–III	13 (100%)	—	—
IV	8 (53%)	5 (34%)	2 (13%)
V	2 (15%)	5 (38%)	6 (46%)

Adapted from Marra G, Barbieri G, Dell'Agnola CA, et al: Congenital renal damage associated with primary vesicoureteric reflux. Arch Dis Child Fetal Neonatal Ed 1994;70:F147.

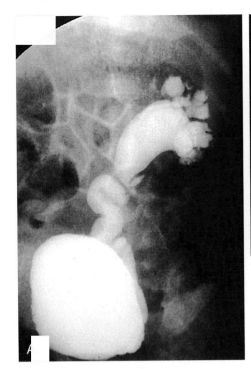

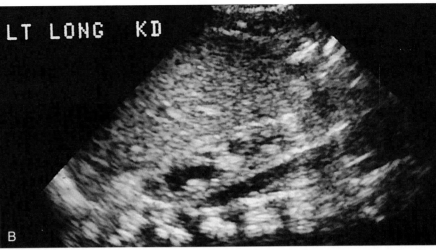

Figure 59–12. *A,* Massive reflux in a boy with antenatally diagnosed hydronephrosis. *B,* Ultrasound demonstrates kidney with poor internal differentiation. No function was seen on scan.

Scars and Sterile Reflux

The early work of Hodson and colleagues implicated sterile reflux and a high-pressure "water-hammer" effect as a significant cause of renal scarring (Hodson et al, 1975b). By surgically creating reflux and occluding the bladder outlet, reflux nephropathy could be induced in miniature pigs, even in the absence of infection. High intravesical pressures caused intrarenal reflux, usually in the polar

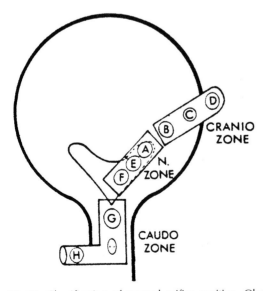

Figure 59–13. Classification of ureteral orifice position. Obstruction usually occurs in the caudo zone. Those ureters positioned in the cranio zone are likely to result in reflux. Ureters positioned in the normal (N) zone are associated with normal kidneys. Because of ureteral bud abnormality, renal dysplasia occurs with ureters projecting from both abnormal positions. (From Mackie GC, Stephens FD: Duplex kidneys: A correlation of renal dysplasia with position of the ureteral orifice. J Urol 1975;114:274.)

areas, and interstitial fibrosis whose radiologic appearance was similar to that seen in children with postinfectious reflux nephropathy. Other work also supported the concept of elevated bladder pressures causing reflux nephropathy (Mendoza and Roberts, 1992). The proximal projection of pressure causes a decrease in postglomerular blood flow to the medulla and cortex that results in ischemic damage (Roberts, 1992). This cause of nephropathy must be considered in the face of elevated bladder pressures and the high incidence of reflux associated with bladder dysfunction (Koff, 1992), urethral valves, or the high voiding pressures of newborns with antenatally diagnosed reflux (Elder, 1992). **However, more recent evidence in animal studies, obtained with newer imaging modalities, indicates that low-pressure sterile reflux into previously normal kidneys may lead to focal, chronic interstitial inflammation and fibrosis** (Paltiel et al, 2000).

Although abnormal bladder pressures might contribute to renal scarring in some children, the pathophysiology of most renal scarring was better defined by Ransley and Risdon (1981), who were unable to create scars in a model similar to Hodson's by keeping the bladder unobstructed and the urine sterile. Clinical verification of the importance of infection is documented by a number of reports that site new scars only in patients with reflux who have recurrent infections. In the combined series of Smellie and coauthors (1975) and Huland and Busch (1984), for example, new scars developed in only 17 (4%) of 446 patients, all of whom had interval UTIs. **The bulk of clinical and experimental studies underscore the importance of infection in the evolution of most renal scars.**

Postinfectious Scarring

An in-depth review of the pathophysiology of pyelonephritis is covered elsewhere, but several points deserve emphasis with regard to reflux. **Although pyelonephritis can commonly occur in the absence of VUR, reflux predisposes the kidney to ascending infections and may amplify the invasive effects of pathogens.** For example, acute pyelonephritis was documented twice as frequently in patients with high-grade reflux than in those with low-grade reflux in one series (Majd et al, 1991). In addition, most studies show a linear relation between grade of reflux and frequency of scarring (Winter et al, 1983; Weiss et al, 1992b). Primary renal dysgenesis could also contribute to the latter. Other factors determine the severity of renal injury in addition to grade, including include age of the patient, anatomic considerations, bacterial virulence factors, and host susceptibility and the inflammatory response to parenchymal infection.

PATIENT AGE

The development of scars is an age-related phenomenon. Just as the highest incidence of reflux is found in younger children, **the risk of scarring is greatest in children younger than 1 year of age** (Winberg, 1992). **Patients who experience their first febrile UTI before age 4 years have a much greater likelihood of developing a scar than children whose first episode of pyelonephritis occurs at a later age** (Smellie et al, 1985). **Reflux nephropathy occurs uncommonly after 5 years of age** (Rolleston et al, 1974). In the European arm of the IRSC, for example, new scars developed in approximately 24% of children who were younger than 2 years of age, 10% of those between age 2 and 4 years, and only 5% of those older than 5 years (Olbing et al, 1992). The clinical studies of Berg and Johansson also suggest that the infant kidney is more vulnerable to damage by infection during the first 3 years of life (Berg and Johansson, 1982). **The "big bang" theory of Ransley and Risdon (1978) underscored the susceptibility of young children with reflux to UTIs and proposed that the most severe degrees of renal parenchymal injury occur with the first infection.** Because all susceptible segments of the kidney are simultaneously affected, sequential scar formation is unusual, although "little bangs" do occur (Ransley and Risdon, 1981). The theory supports two clinical observations. **Most renal scarring in young children is as severe on initial imaging as is likely to develop in follow-up, unless severe episodes of pyelonephritis occur. In addition, the incidence of scarring is not significantly greater in children evaluated after their first infection than in those who present after multiple infections.** Age-based differences in treatment of pyelonephritis should not result from these observations, however, and **postinfectious scarring can develop in children of any age who are not properly treated** (Benador et al, 1997).

ANATOMIC CONSIDERATIONS

Papillary configuration also plays a role in protecting the renal parenchyma from urinary pathogens. **Compound or concave papillae, which are flattened and whose ducts open at right angles to the calyx, are more likely to allow intrarenal reflux than simple or convex papillae.** These project into the renal pelvis and have ducts that exit

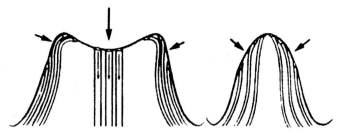

Figure 59–14. Papillary configuration in intrarenal reflux. Convex papilla *(right)* does not reflux—crescentic or slit-like openings of its collecting ducts open obliquely onto the papilla. In contrast, the concave *(left)* or flat papilla refluxes—collecting ducts open at right angles onto flat papilla. (From Ransley PG, Risdon RA: Reflux and renal scarring. Br J Radiol 1978;14[Suppl.]:1.)

obliquely into the calyx to provide a valvular action against the retrograde flow of urine into the collecting tubules of the renal medulla (Fig. 59–14). The configuration and action is very similar to the flap-valve created by the ureter itself. Compound papillae are located primarily in the polar regions of the kidney, where reflux nephropathy is much more likely to occur initially (Hodson et al, 1975b; Ransley and Risdon, 1978). Further deleterious distortion of normal papillae architecture can result from adjacent scarring, hydronephrosis, and high-pressure voiding to involve the entire collecting system. Early studies focused on intrarenal reflux (Fig. 59–15), which is observed in 5% to 15% of neonates and infants with reflux (Rose et al, 1975; Rolleston et al, 1974). When scarring occurred, it was always in the parenchyma overlying the segment with intrarenal reflux. Autopsy studies in newborns who died before 1 month of age demonstrated intrarenal reflux at pressures as low as 2 mm Hg. Later in development, greater amounts of pressure become necessary to produce the same effect (e.g., 20 mm Hg in a 1-year-old) (Funston and Cremin, 1978), and intrarenal reflux, like new scarring, is rarely seen radiographically after the age of 5 years. The crucial interplay of intrarenal reflux and UTI was also demonstrated by the seminal work by Ransley and Risdon (1975) in piglets, whose renal papillary morphology is similar to that of humans. **Scarring occurred only in areas**

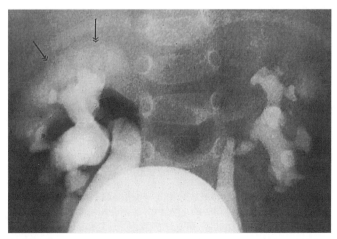

Figure 59–15. Intrarenal reflux *(arrows)* shown on voiding cystourethrogram.

exposed to both infected urine and intrarenal reflux. However, the presence of intrarenal reflux does not alter the likelihood of spontaneous resolution or management strategy if infections can be avoided.

BACTERIOLOGIC VIRULENCE

Bacteria causing UTIs express factors that facilitate colonization, enhance virulence, and increase the propensity to renal injury. The initial step in any infection is bacterial adhesion to uroepithelial cells. Adherence depends on the interaction between ligands or binding molecules that are located on the fimbriae of bacteria and host cell receptors. Serotyping of *Escherichia coli*, the most common uropathogen, has identified strains that are particularly pyelonephritogenic. O antigens are lipopolysaccharides that are part of the cell wall and are thought to be responsible for many of the systemic symptoms associated with infection. Of the 150 strains of *E. coli* identified by O antigens, 9 are present in most UTIs (Mannhardt et al, 1986). Another polysaccharide, the K antigen, is present within the capsules of virulent gram-negative organisms; it is thought to protect against phagocytosis and to inhibit host immune response. These organisms also commonly have fimbriae that show mannose-resistant hemagglutination and fail to react with mannose on the host cell surface. Some mannose-resistant bacteria also express P blood group ligands on their fimbriae, a property that further enhances bacterial adherence to the urothelium as well as renal epithelial cells (Vaisanen et al, 1981; Lichodziejewska et al, 1989). In one study, P pili bacteria were found in 91% of children with acute pyelonephritis (Kallenius et al, 1981), although their significance in severe reflux and nephropathy has been questioned (Lombard et al, 1983). Some have suggested that the adherence of bacteria to urothelial cells is independent of the P blood group antigen in the host (Lomberg et al, 1986), but others have noted that patients with the P1 blood group have a relative risk of pyelonephritis 11 times that of normal subjects (Roberts, 1995).

The ability of bacteria to adhere appears also to be affected by host epithelial cell surface receptors or soluble receptors in the urine. *E. coli* infections, for example, occur with greater frequency in children with Lewis (a−b−) phenotype, which is postulated to promote bacterial adherence (Jantausch et al, 1994). Tamm-Horsfall protein, which is secreted by the proximal renal tubules, binds to certain nonfimbrial adhesins and can prevent bacterial adherence to the mucus (glycoproteins or glycosaminoglycans) that normally coats the urothelium (Orskov et al, 1980). Differences in immunoglobulin A (Akerlund et al, 1979), blood group antigens (Blackwell et al, 1986), and the amount of mucopolysaccharide (Parsons et al, 1975) secreted by the bladder epithelium may also contribute to sexual and individual differences in the propensity to develop UTIs. However, no significant difference in genetic markers has been shown in children in the first year of life (Alberus et al, 1997).

Other virulence factors, including hemolysin, aerobactin, and bacterial iron-binding capacity, contribute to the host inflammatory response and degree of tissue destruction (Rushton, 1992). **Acute pyelonephritis that occurs when reflux is absent is usually caused by bacteria that express three or more virulence factors.** Less virulent bacteria can cause similar episodes in patients with reflux (Lomberg et al, 1984). In theory, once bacteria adhere to ureteral urothelium endotoxins cause a decrease in ureteral motility, ureteral dilatation, and an alteration in papillary configuration, thus allowing intrarenal reflux (Roberts, 1992).

HOST SUSCEPTIBILITY AND RESPONSE

The resiliency of most urinary tracts was shown 4 decades ago when the retrograde inoculation of more than 10^8 bacteria into the bladders of healthy volunteers did not result in clinical infections (Cox and Hinman, 1961). The defense against renal infections begins with the lower urinary tract, where a variety of host factors play a role. **The degree of preputial and vaginal bacterial colonization, which is determined by the host receptors discussed previously, influences periurethral colonization. Healthy girls have less bacterial colonization than those who are prone to UTIs** (Bollgren and Winberg, 1976), **and bacterial adherence to the prepuce probably explains why uncircumcised boys account for more than 90% of UTIs in infants younger than 6 months of age** (Rushton and Majd, 1992). More proximally, the composition of the urine can inhibit bacterial growth through its acidity and osmolality, and glycosaminoglycan secretion can trap and eradicate bacteria. But **the most important defense mechanism in any patient is effective bladder emptying on a regular basis.** Normal bladders empty almost to completion, leaving little if any culture medium for bacteria. In contrast, patients with bladder dysfunction commonly go for prolonged periods between voiding or emptying incompletely. The advantage provided an inoculum of bacteria is obvious.

After bacteria reach the kidney, the inflammatory response of the host contributes to the degree of scar development. Animal models demonstrate activation of complement followed by granulocytic aggregation and capillary obstruction. Renal ischemia and reperfusion injury result. In addition, the phagocytosis induced by endotoxins causes a respiratory burst that is accompanied by a release of oxygen free radicals and proteolytic enzymes that further amplifies cell death. The inflammatory response peaks at 24 hours (Roberts et al, 1990). Initial microabscess formation is followed by healing and scarring that results in the changes of chronic pyelonephritis. Allopurinol and superoxide dismutase, an antagonist of superoxide, have both been shown to retard this cascade and reduce renal injury (McCord and Fridovich, 1978; Roberts et al, 1986). Other means of tempering the immune response can alter the effects of pyelonephritis in animals, although a clinical applicability remains unclear. Oral corticosteroids reduced the incidence of scarring in kidneys with severe pyelonephritis in piglets, although antibiotics alone were equally effective with mild and moderate degrees of infections (Pohl et al, 1999). Bacterial immunization has been shown to have a mild protective effect on the development of reflux nephropathy in the piglet (Torres et al, 1984). In addition, the maternal immunization of monkeys can cause passive immunization in their offspring, with protective activity against experimental pyelonephritis (Kaack at al, 1988).

Clinically, early diagnosis and effective antibiotic treatment are instrumental to reducing the inflammatory response to acute pyelonephritis and decreasing the incidence and degree of renal scarring (see later discussion of clinical studies). Animal models also support this concept, though the optimal time for initiation of therapy remains undefined. Antibiotic treatment decreased reflux nephropathy in the pig (Ransley and Risdon, 1981), whereas studies in monkeys showed that renal damage could not be prevented if therapy was delayed for longer than 72 hours (Roberts et al, 1990). Studies in rodents have given mixed results, with protection provided by antibiotics if begun before 30 hours (Glauser et al, 1978), if begun within 24 hours (Slotki and Asscher, 1982), or even if delayed for up to 4 days (Miller and Phillips, 1981). Extrapolation of these data to humans must be done with care because of immunologic and anatomic differences. Nevertheless, prompt treatment is instrumental to minimizing the sequelae of chronic pyelonephritis in humans (Fig. 59–16). This principle is underscored by studies showing that delayed or improper treatment of acute pyelonephritis is responsible for reflux nephropathy in both infants and older children (Winberg at al, 1974: Winter et al, 1983; Smellie and Normand, 1985).

Hypertension

Reflux nephropathy is the most common cause of severe hypertension in children and young adults, although the actual incidence is unknown. Figures as high as 38% are cited in the literature (Wallace et al, 1978; Steinhardt, 1985; Wolfish et al, 1993), but methodologic flaws can be found in many study designs (Shannon and Feldman, 1990). **Arterial damage in the area of renal scarring presumably leads to segmental ischemia and renin-driven hypertension. Abnormalities of sodium-potassium adenosine triphosphatase activity have also been described** (Goonasekera and Dillon, 1998). Despite these limitations, renin profiles have been measured in children with a history of reflux, and many but not all were elevated (Eke et al, 1983; Savage et al, 1987). Elevated renins may be related to eventual hypertension for some patients, but others with high renins remain normotensive, while a small number revert to normal with extended follow-up

(Savage et al, 1978). In a 15-year follow-up of renin and blood pressure in a cohort of patients with reflux nephropathy, **plasma renin levels were found to be significantly higher than in control subjects but were not predictive of the development of hypertension** (Goonasekera et al, 1996b). **Most patients who develop hypertension have near-normal renal function, and the appearance of hypertension is uncommonly related to renal failure. Hypertension is related to the grade of reflux and the severity of scarring in most series, especially with bilateral involvement** (Torres et al, 1983; Winter et al, 1983; Hinchliffe et al, 1992). However, in the study by Wolfish and colleagues (1993), primary reflux was not associated with hypertension or with the severity of scarring unless there was preexisting dysplasia. The implications of scarring can be subtle. In one provocative study, normotensive children with renal scars demonstrated renal function and levels of renin and aldosterone similar to those of control subjects. They also demonstrated the same expected drops in nocturnal blood pressure but significantly faster heart rates, a possible risk factor for future cardiovascular morbidity (Pomeranz et al, 1998).

The elimination of reflux or its spontaneous resolution does not reverse the predisposition to hypertension once scarring is present. For example, Wallace and associates (1978) reported hypertension despite successful ureteral reimplantation in 18.5% of children with bilateral scarring and 11.3% of those with unilateral scarring after more than 10 years of follow-up. Hypertension did not develop without scars. This type of data emphasizes the need for periodic checks of blood pressure in any child with a history of reflux and scars. **Removing the offending renal parenchyma with partial or total nephrectomy can improve or correct hypertension in some patients** (Dillon and Smellie, 1984). Patients with one small, scarred, poorly functioning kidney may reasonably be considered candidates. Confirmation with selective renal vein renins (ratio greater than 1.5) is instrumental to selection but may still not ensure success with ablative surgery. Global changes in vascular resistance may contribute to hypertension that persists. Those patients with diffuse bilateral scarring are less than ideal candidates, because localization is difficult and sparing of renal parenchyma assumes primary importance.

Renal Growth

Factors that might contribute to the effects of reflux on renal growth include the congenital dysmorphism that often is associated with (30%) but is not caused by reflux; the number and types of UTIs and their resultant nephropathy; the quality of the contralateral kidney and its implications for compensatory hypertrophy; and the grade of reflux in the affected kidney. Studies that could be used to evaluate renal growth do so unreliably. In addition to the variability in interpretation that occurs with excretory urography or ultrasound (Redman et al, 1974; Hodson et al, 1975a), the response of the kidney to scarring, with its polar contracture and intermediate hypertrophy, makes interpretation of renal length alone unreliable. Other methods used to measure growth have included parenchymal thickness, renal area and length, and bipolar

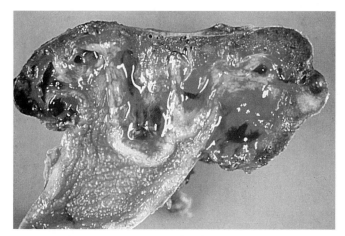

Figure 59–16. Gross specimen of a kidney severely affected by chronic pyelonephritis and reflux nephropathy from repeated urinary infections.

thickness (Lyon, 1973; Klare et al, 1980; Hannerz et al, 1989). Claesson and associates (1981) used planimetry to measure urograms and formulate a nomogram that allows determination of renal mass in relation to somatic size (Fig. 59–17).

With the exception of those kidneys that are developmentally arrested, most studies implicate infection as the cause for altered renal growth. Impaired growth was seen in kidneys with long-term reflux before the era of prophylactic antibiotics (Ibsen et al, 1977). It was subsequently shown that acceptable growth would occur if UTIs could be controlled. In their study of 111 kidneys with reflux managed medically, Smellie and coworkers (1981a) found slow growth in 11, 10 of whom had documented UTIs. **Successful antireflux surgery can accelerate renal growth but may not allow affected kidneys to return to normal size** (McRae et al, 1974; Willscher et al, 1976). In one study of 22 kidneys with reflux nephropathy, significant growth after reimplantation occurred in 15 (68%), 7 of which grew proportionally to their mates (Carson et al, 1982). The potential for renal growth was less optimistically portrayed by the studies of Hagberg and associates (1984) and Shimada and colleagues (1988), in which 75% of kidneys with significant nephropathy remained stunted despite reimplantation. In contrast, kidneys without radiographic evidence of scarring usually show rebound growth with the surgical correction of reflux or its spontaneous resolution. In addition, the results from the Birmingham Reflux Study Group (1987) and from the IRSC (Olbing et

al, 1992; Weiss et al, 1992b) showed no significant difference in rates of growth or parenchymal scarring whether managed medically or surgically.

Renal Failure and Function

Renal failure is an uncommon consequence of VUR as an isolated entity, with a risk estimated at less than 1% (Haycock, 1986; Sreenarasimhaiah and Hellerstein, 1998). Nevertheless, the implications of recurrent bouts of pyelonephritis cannot be ignored, especially at a young age. Severe scarring with renal failure probably does not occur after isolated episodes in adults. However, in a study by Jacobson and associates (1989), every adult who had their first infection during infancy had decreased renal function; hypertension was found in one third of these individuals, and end-stage renal disease occurred in 10%.

Chronic pyelonephritis was reported as the cause of end-stage renal disease in 15% to 25% of children and young adults in earlier studies (Scharer, 1971; Human Renal Transplant Registry, 1975; Smellie et al, 1985), although the presence of active reflux is probably less common, at an estimated 10% (Salvatierra and Tanagho, 1977). In many of these patients prior infection went unrecognized or became evident only with the diagnosis of end-stage renal disease. Increased awareness has had a positive effect on this complication. For example, chronic pyelonephritis accounted for less than 2.2% of end-stage renal disease in a more recent report from the North American Pediatric Renal Transplant Cooperative Study (1994). In addition, a better understanding and medical management of the renal nephropathy that accompanies scarring should further lessen the progressive nature of the disease. Glomerular lesions that resemble segmental glomerulosclerosis and may be caused by hyperfiltration have been identified (Hinchliffe et al, 1994), and preventive treatment may further retard the onset of disease. For example, the effects of therapy with an angiotensin-converting enzyme inhibitor (captopril) were studied in 16 patients with severe reflux nephropathy and microalbuminuria. After 2 years of follow-up, there was decreased proteinuria and stabilization of blood pressure and serum creatinine in each case (Lama et al, 1997).

Lesser degrees of renal impairment can also occur with reflux, in a progression that has been likened to that occurring with partial ureteral obstruction. The increased pressure of reflux presumably affects the distal nephron initially, though its effects are difficult to separate from those of associated infection. The defects in concentrating ability that result appear to be autonomous of infection and are inversely proportional to the grade of reflux; improvement often occurs with its cessation (Walker et al, 1973). Other parameters of tubular function can also be affected, including fractional excretion of magnesium and sodium (Walker, 1991). Renal tubular acidosis was identified in 9 (50%) of 18 children with primary reflux, 16 of whom had scars. Four of the affected children also had short stature (Guizar et al, 1996). **Glomerular function is usually unaffected unless global parenchymal damage has occurred.** Proteinuria accompanies significant renal insufficiency and scarring (Torres et al, 1983). Genetic mark-

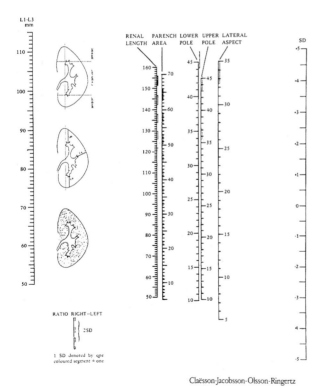

Claësson-Jacobsson-Olsson-Ringertz

Figure 59–17. Nomogram for measuring renal parenchymal thickness and area measured by planimetry allows comparison of observed and expected renal mass. (From Winberg J, Claesson I, Jacobsson B, et al: Renal growth after acute pyelonephritis in childhood: An epidemiological approach. In Hodson CJ, Kincaid-Smith P [eds]: Reflux Neuropathy. New York, Masson Publishing, 1979, pp 309–322.)

ers, including HLA-B12 in females, -B8 with -A9 or -BW15 in males, and -BW15 in both sexes have been found with end-stage reflux nephropathy and may represent a genetic link to a susceptibility to renal damage (Torres et al, 1980).

Somatic Growth

Children with VUR tend to be small for age (Dwoskin and Perlmutter, 1973; Polito et al, 1996), especially those with a history of recurrent UTIs. Eliminating infections with prophylactic antibiotics maintained normal somatic growth for 51 girls with known reflux (Smellie et al, 1983). Surgically correcting reflux was also shown to positively affect somatic growth (Merrell and Mowad, 1979; Polito et al, 1997). It remains unclear whether one form of treatment offers preferential benefit to this aspect of development, because a comparative study in a large series of children with extended follow-up is lacking (Sutton and Atwell, 1989).

ASSOCIATED ANOMALIES AND CONDITIONS

Ureteropelvic Junction Obstruction

The topic of ureteropelvic junction (UPJ) obstruction is covered in detail elsewhere in this textbook. **The incidence of VUR associated with UPJ obstruction ranges from 5% to 25%** (DeKlerk et al, 1979; Lebowitz and Blickman, 1983; Maizels et al, 1984; Hollowell et al, 1989). Most of the patients in these studies had reflux that was coincidentally discovered, was of low grade, and resolved spontaneously with time. Such patients typically exhibited a significant discrepancy in the minimal degree of ureteral dilatation seen below a dilated renal pelvis. **As contrast material enters an obstructed renal pelvis from below, the grade of reflux may be amplified. As a result, management decisions cannot be made on the basis of cystography alone.**

Conversely, the incidence of UPJ obstruction in patients with reflux ranges from 0.8% to 14% (Lebowitz and Blickman, 1983; Hollowell et al, 1989; Leighton and Mayne, 1989). Some cases of high-grade reflux result in kinking of the upper ureter and adjacent pelvic junction that causes obstruction. The chronic effects of reflux may also stretch the renal pelvis so that atonicity and an inability to propagate urine through the UPJ may occur (Whitaker, 1976). Inflammation and ureteritis can also contribute to transient or chronic obstruction. **In one series, high-grade reflux was five times more likely to be associated with UPJ obstruction than lower grades of reflux** (Bomalaski et al, 1997a). Impaired or absent filling of the pelvis by reflux that causes dilatation of the ureter below the UPJ is a sign suspicious of secondary kinking (Fig. 59–18). Postvoid films that demonstrate prompt drainage from the refluxing ureter but retention of contrast within the renal pelvis are also suggestive. Adequate drainage from the pelvis tends to rule out obstruction. Whether UPJ obstructions associated with reflux are similar to those that occur primarily is

unclear, but the dual nature of the problem poses the management dilemma of which anomaly, if any, to correct.

Therapy is directed at preserving renal function. If scintigraphy with catheter drainage documents obstruction, pyeloplasty rather than reimplantation should be performed. To correct the reflux initially risks amplifying the obstruction because of the distal ureteral edema that results. In addition, correcting reflux in the hope of alleviating kinking and the need for pyeloplasty is rarely successful (Bomalaski et al, 1997a). Improving urinary outflow is thought by some to increase the likelihood of cessation of reflux, although reimplantation is often necessary for patients whose reflux persists at a high grade after successful pyeloplasty. If, however, the pelvic dilatation associated with reflux is believed to be nonobstructive, ureteroneocystostomy becomes the procedure of choice. Three or four days of stent drainage is advisable during the early postoperative period to minimize any amplification of upper ureteral obstruction caused by distal ureteral edema.

Ureteral Duplication

VUR is the most common abnormality associated with complete ureteral duplications. The anatomy of patients with ureteral duplication typically follows the Weigert-Meyer rule (Weigert, 1877; Meyer, 1946), **wherein the upper pole ureter enters the bladder distally and medially and the lower pole ureter enters the bladder proximally and laterally. The incidence of reflux is increased in patients with complete ureteral duplication. Although urine may reflux into either ureter, it more commonly involves the ureter from the lower pole because of its lateral position and shorter submucosal tunnel** (Fig. 59–19). **Contrary to earlier teaching, the frequency of resolution of reflux appears to be the same in patients with either single or double ureters, although the duration until resolution may be somewhat increased.** One series of children with grades I to III reflux into the lower pole of a duplicated collecting system showed no significant difference in resolution of reflux or in the incidence of new scars, compared with control subjects with single ureters (Ben-Ami et al, 1989). Although management must be individualized, a more aggressive approach is probably not warranted in patients with reflux into duplicated systems (Husmann and Allen, 1991).

Bladder Diverticula

Bladder diverticula are mucosal herniations through areas of weakness in the muscular bladder wall. They were initially thought to occur only with bladder outlet obstruction and secondary detrusor hypertrophy and trabeculation. Hutch (1962) was the first to recognize that bladder diverticula were also congenital abnormalities that occurred primarily in smooth-walled normal bladders in children. Bladder diverticula also commonly occur with Ehlers-Danlos syndrome and Menkes' syndrome, causing an increased incidence of reflux in these conditions (Harcke et al, 1977; Levard et al, 1989). The most common location for diver-

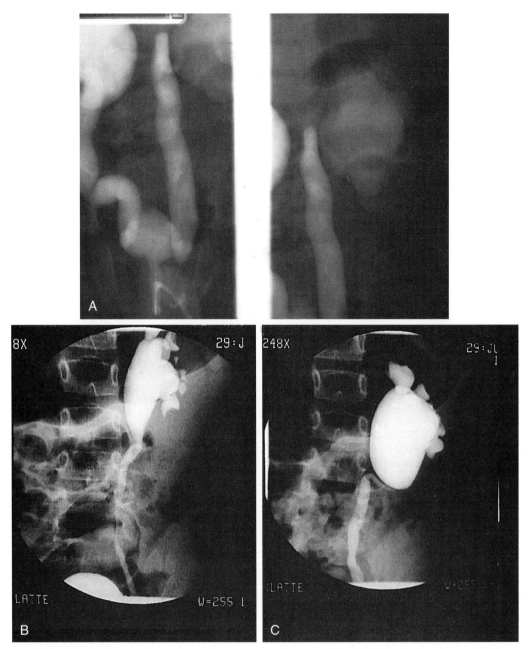

Figure 59–18. Reflux and ureteropelvic junction (UPJ) obstructions. *A,* Significant reflux fills the left ureter to the level of the UPJ. Minimal filling of the pelvis can be a sign of obstruction at that level. *B,* In a different patient, reflux is seen as the bladder fills. *C,* Significant kinking of the UPJ occurs with voiding.

ticula is lateral and cephalad to the ureteral orifice (Boechat and Lebowitz, 1978). These occasionally expand within Waldeyer's fascia to cause ureteral obstruction or project intraluminally to obstruct the bladder neck or urethra. Usually, however, they prolapse outside the bladder at the expense of paraureteral mucosa. This alters the anatomy of the UVJ and allows either transient or permanent reflux (Fig. 59–20). The management of reflux associated with diverticula differs from that of primary reflux depending on the degree of anatomic distortion that results. **Reflux associated with small diverticula resolves at rates similar to primary reflux and can be managed accord-**

ingly. In contrast, reflux found with paraureteral large diverticula is less likely to resolve and usually requires surgical correction. In any case, when the ureter enters the diverticulum, regardless of size, surgery is recommended (Atala et al, 1998; Pieretti and Pieretti-Vanmarcke, 1999).

Renal Anomalies

VCUG is indicated in any child with renal agenesis or multicystic dysplastic kidney. Reflux is a common

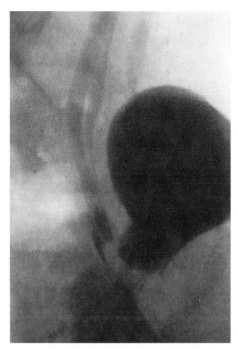

Figure 59–19. Reflux into both ureters of a complete duplication, as shown here, is less common than reflux into the lower pole ureter alone.

finding with renal agenesis and usually involves the contralateral ureter, although involvement of a blind-ending ipsilateral ureter also occurs. Incidences as high as 50% have been reported (Song et al, 1995; Cascio et al, 1999). The incidence of reflux is also increased with multicystic dys-

plastic kidneys, where the contralateral ureter is involved in 15% to 20% of cases (Gough et al, 1995; Selzman and Elder, 1995).

Megacystis-Megaureter Association

When massive bilateral reflux is present, incomplete emptying of the urinary tract results in marked dilatation of the ureters and bladder, the so-called megacystis-megaureter association. It is more frequently seen in males, and the differentiation from posterior urethral valves is an important one. A thin bladder wall and variable degrees of hydronephrosis are seen by ultrasound, while the absence of outlet obstruction is confirmed by VCUG (Mandell et al, 1992). Surgery is indicated once age permits. Effective bladder emptying occurs after reflux is corrected.

Other

Reflux is seen in children with the VACTERL association (*v*ertebral, *a*nal, *c*ardiac, *t*racheo*e*sophageal, *r*enal, and *l*imb anomalies) or the CHARGE syndrome (*c*oloboma, *h*eart disease, *a*tresia choanae, *r*etarded development, *g*enital hypoplasia, and *e*ar anomalies), both of which suggest a global insult in embryogenesis (Ragan et al, 1999; Kolon et al, 2000). Reflux is also a common finding with imperforate anus, whether neurogenic bladder dysfunction is present or not. A rectovesical or rectourethral fistula should be managed with a completely diverting colostomy to avoid problems with UTIs (Sheldon et al,

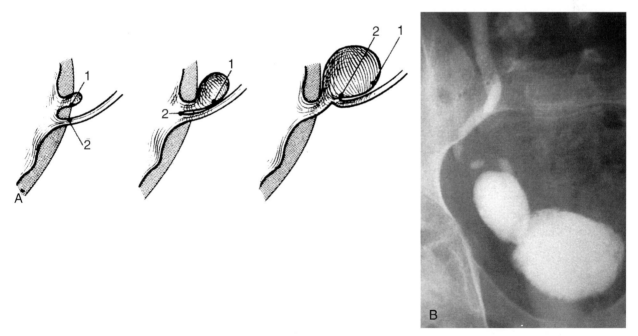

Figure 59–20. *A*, Schematic representation of bladder diverticulum. A small amount of mucosa initially herniates through a congenital defect in the bladder musculature. This enlarges with voiding. Finally, the ureteral orifice is incorporated into the diverticulum. (From Hernanz-Schulman M, Lebowitz RL: The elusiveness and importance of bladder diverticula in children. Pediatr Radiol 1995;15:399–402, copyright © 1995 by Springer-Verlag.) *B*, Reflux into right-sided paraureteral diverticulum and ureter seen on voiding cystography.

1991), and any patient with one of these conditions should have a VCUG as part of the evaluation of reflux.

PREGNANCY AND REFLUX

The morphology of the urinary tract is altered with the onset of pregnancy and increases throughout gestation (Beydoun, 1985). **Bladder tone decreases because of edema and hyperemia, changes that predispose the patient to bacteriuria. In addition, urine volume increases in the upper collecting system as the physiologic dilatation of pregnancy evolves.** The slower drainage that results can enhance the growth of organisms and increase the propensity to develop pyelonephritis. **It seems logical to assume that during pregnancy the presence of VUR in a system already prone to bacteriuria would lead to increased morbidity.** A number of studies have been conducted to examine this relationship.

The presence of active reflux appears to present a risk factor for the affected mother. In 1958, Hutch described a higher incidence of pyelonephritis during pregnancy in 23 women with a history of reflux and recurrent bacteriuria. Heidrick and associates (1967) evaluated 321 women with cystography either during the last trimester or within 30 hours after delivery. The incidence of pyelonephritis was 33% in women with reflux, compared to less than 5% in women without reflux. Finally, cystograms performed 4 to 6 months postpartum in 100 women with a history of asymptomatic bacteriuria during pregnancy showed reflux in 21%. Bacteriuria was easier to clear in patients without reflux (67%) than in those with reflux (33%) (Williams et al, 1968).

Maternal history also becomes a factor if past reflux, renal scarring, or a tendency to UTIs is included. Martinell and colleagues (1990) compared the outcome of pregnancy in matched controls with that in 41 women with and without renal scarring after childhood UTIs. They found that women with a history of prior infections had a high incidence of bacteriuria during pregnancy, whereas those with renal scarring and persistent reflux were more prone to develop acute pyelonephritis. In a similar study, the outcome of pregnancy was assessed in 88 women with previous bacteriuria. Women with known scars had a 3.3-fold increased incidence of hypertension, a 7.6-fold increased risk of preeclampsia, and a higher rate of obstetric interventions. Women with normal kidneys and reflux also had an increased risk of hypertension during the last trimester (McGladdery et al, 1992). Pregnant women with bilateral renal scars were also shown to have a higher incidence of preeclampsia than those with unilateral scarring (24% vs. 7%, respectively) (El-Khatib et al, 1994), and those with creatinine elevation are also at risk (Jungers et al, 1987). In a large study of 158 women with reflux nephropathy, pregnancy was uneventful in patients with normal blood pressure and renal function, whereas the risks of fetal demise and accelerated maternal renal disease were increased in women with impaired renal function (Jungers et al, 1996).

The implications of reimplantation surgery were studied by Austenfeld and Snow (1988), who found an increased risk of UTI and fetal loss in 31 women who had undergone ureteral reimplantation as children, despite correction of the anomaly. In a follow-up study comparing these patients with a new cohort of historical controls, women with UTIs and reflux who underwent reimplantation (suggesting an initially higher degree of reflux and increased renal scarring) were still at significant risk of UTI during pregnancy (Mansfield et al, 1995). However, they were not at a higher risk of miscarriage than the general population. In a larger study of 77 pregnancies in 41 women whose ureters had been reimplanted, Bukowski and coworkers (1998) reported that the incidence of pyelonephritis during pregnancy was slightly higher than in the general population but that the fetus and mother were at significant risk when renal scarring or hypertension was present.

In summary, the majority of studies examining the effects of VUR on pregnancy suggest that women with a history of reflux have increased morbidity during pregnancy because of infection-related complications, whether the reflux has been corrected or not. **Women with hypertension and an element of renal failure are particularly at risk.** Those with uncorrected reflux appear to be particularly at risk and should have their reflux corrected before pregnancy to minimize maternal and fetal morbidity. The morbidity during pregnancy of women with persistent reflux without renal scarring remains poorly defined, but the tendency to UTI seems to be increased. Because of the difficulty in predicting an outcome for this subset of patients, most clinicians recommend surgical correction for girls with reflux that persists beyond puberty, although there has been a trend toward discontinuation of prophylactic antibiotics in older girls with active reflux. Long-term follow-up studies of these patients through puberty are unavailable (see later discussion).

NATURAL HISTORY AND MANAGEMENT

Spontaneous Resolution

VUR spontaneously resolves in many children, although **the rate of resolution depends on the initial grade and age at presentation.** In theory, two mechanisms contribute to this phenomenon. The first is elongation of the submucosal tunnel that occurs with interval growth of the bladder and the longitudinal muscles of the ureter (Stephens and Lenaghan, 1962). The second, especially in neonates and infants, is a beneficial transition in bladder dynamics from a small-capacity, hyperreflexic voiding pattern to a more mature pattern having larger capacity and lessened intravesical pressures. In addition, experimental studies in puppies have implicated changes in the autonomic nervous system and an increase in adrenergic innervation as contributing in some way to the presence of reflux (Kiruluta et al, 1985). The clinical data in this regard are revealing.

Grade of Reflux

Most low grades (grades I or II) of reflux spontaneously resolve (King et al, 1974). Edwards and coauthors cited an 85% and Smellie and Normand an 80% rate of resolution in children with normal-caliber ureters (Edwards et al, 1977; Smellie and Normand, 1979). Similar results were reported by the Southwest Pediatric Nephrology study group, who noted resolution of 82% of grade I and 80% of grade II reflux after 5 years of medical management, and Duckett reported resolution in 63% of grade II cases (Duckett, 1983; Arant, 1992). Skoog and colleagues, using long-term medical management, noted resolution in 90% of grade I through grade III reflux after 5 years (Skoog et al, 1987). **Approximately 50% of intermediate-grade (grade III) reflux will resolve** (Duckett, 1983; Arant, 1992). A similar rate of resolution was reported after 5 years of medical management by McLorie and coworkers (1990).

Fewer high grades (grades III through V) of reflux spontaneously resolve. And it is with these higher grades, especially grades III and IV, that much of the debate over management exists. Historically, a more aggressive surgical stance has usually been taken with this severity of reflux, especially in the United States. The results of the IRSC, which commenced in 1980 to evaluate children with grades III and IV reflux, appear to support that bias. In the European arm of the study, 82 patients with bilateral grade III or IV reflux were monitored. Cessation of reflux occurred in only 7 (9%). Similarly, reflux resolved in only 4 (11%) of 31 children who had grade III or IV reflux on one side and low-grade (grades I through II) reflux on the other. Children with unilateral reflux alone had a more optimistic prognosis, with reflux abating in 23 (61%) of 38 cases. The results from the 41 patients entered in the American arm of the study were similarly discouraging, with reflux persisting in 75%, although the outcome of unilateral versus bilateral involvement was not reported (Weiss et al, 1992a; Tamminen-Mobius et al, 1992). Resolution rates of 41% with grades III to V reflux (Smellie and Normand, 1979); 30% for grade IV and 12% for grade V (McLorie et al, 1990); and as low as 9% for grade IV have been reported (Skoog et al, 1987). In addition, some studies have suggested no noticeable difference in resolution characteristics between grades III and IV (Tamminen-Mobius et al, 1992). Notably, the majority of patients in these studies were entered before the advent of antenatal diagnosis.

Age at Diagnosis

The age of the patient also assumes importance in any discussion of spontaneous resolution of reflux. Grade III reflux in a 3-year-old, for example, is probably different from that in a 3-month-old and, in fact, might have been grade V reflux if a diagnosis had been made at an earlier age. **Younger children are more likely to have reflux and also appear to be more likely to have spontaneous resolution of their reflux, regardless of grade. This is especially true of neonates** (Fig. 59–21) (Gordon et al, 1990; Zerin et al, 1993). In a study of perinatally diagnosed reflux, Burge and associates (1992) noted resolution in 54% of children with grade III or IV reflux within 3 years. The significance of the period of early development was also suggested by Skoog and colleagues (1987), who noted a significantly shorter duration until resolution in children diagnosed before 1 year of age (1.44 vs. 1.85 years). In contrast, McLorie and coworkers (1990) found

no difference in the degree of resolution of high-grade (grade III or IV) reflux between children younger than 1 year of age and those who were older.

Assuming that the theories of lower urinary tract development required to bring about the resolution of reflux are correct, intervals of significant growth and beneficial urodynamic change are most likely to re-enact change. This seems especially true of the newborn and infant (Belman, 1995). During childhood, gradual growth effects a more slowly cumulative, constant change, as suggested by the 15% to 20% overall yearly rate of resolution offered by Smellie and Normand (Smellie and Normand, 1979). **If resolution is to occur, it usually does so within the first few years after diagnosis.** Skoog and colleagues noted resolution rates of 30% to 35% per year in their study of low- and moderate-grade reflux. The various grades had similar disappearance curves, though higher grades took longer to cease (grade II, 1.56 years; grade III, 1.97 years) (Skoog et al, 1987). **The absence of improvement in degree of reflux on serial cystograms is a concerning sign that resolution may not occur with interval growth.** The duration of observation that should be allowed for the maturation of reflux remains undefined. However, in one series, 92% of grade III reflux that resolved did so within 4 years (McLorie et al, 1990). **Resolution of reflux sometimes occurs after 5 years but is especially uncommon if little improvement has occurred in the interim.** The onset of puberty does not initiate a period of accelerated resolution of reflux. Instead, **with the cessation of longitudinal growth the likelihood of having reflux resolve presumably ends,** though this has never been proven. In addition, the implications of reflux that persists into adulthood need to be more clearly defined.

DECISIONS IN MANAGEMENT

The surgeries designed to correct VUR have always set a high standard against which medical management is measured. Success rates of 99% are not uncommon (Duckett et al, 1992). Nevertheless, **it has become increasingly apparent that medical treatment is effective for many children with reflux.** Both modalities bring attendant risks and benefits that must be weighed in light of the natural history of the anomaly and its implications for the patient, as previously discussed. Walker summarized the premises that anchor the decision making in management of reflux as follows (Walker, 1994).

1. Spontaneous resolution of reflux occurs in many infants and children but is less likely to resolve with the onset of puberty.

2. More severe grades of reflux are less likely to spontaneously resolve.

3. Sterile reflux does not appear to cause significant nephropathy.

4. Extended prophylactic antibiotic therapy is well tolerated by children.

5. Antireflux surgeries are highly successful in capable hands.

An outline of rigid algorithms in management would be unfair to patients, whose treatment should be individual-

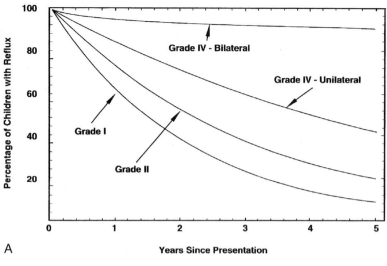

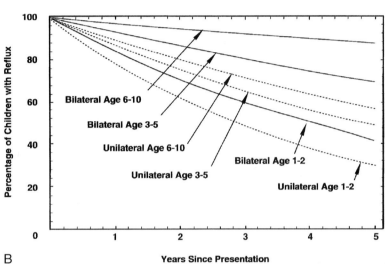

Figure 59–21. A, Percent chance of reflux persistence for grades I, II, and IV, for 1 to 5 years after presentation. B, Percent chance of reflux persistence by age at presentation, grade III, for 1 to 5 years after presentation. (From American Urological Association: Report on the Management of Vesicoureteral Reflux in Children. Baltimore, American Urological Association, Pediatric Vesicoureteral Reflux Clinical Guidelines Panel, 1997.)

ized, and to clinicians, who must gauge parental compliance with medical management and periodic radiologic follow-up, factor socioeconomic concerns, and also weigh their own personal experience with the anomaly. Nevertheless, some generalized recommendations can be made based on the likelihood of grade-related spontaneous resolution and the natural history of reflux previously discussed.

Medical management is initially recommended for prepubertal children with grade I to III reflux under the assumption that most cases will resolve. A period of observation and medical therapy also seems warranted for most grade IV reflux, especially in younger children and those with unilateral disease. Some trend toward improvement should become evident within 2 or 3 years. If not, surgery is recommended. Newborns with grade V reflux who can be maintained on prophylaxis should also be medically managed initially. Grade V reflux that persists or is discovered in older children is unlikely to spontaneously resolve. Surgery is recommended after infancy, although, again, a period of observation seems reasonable for perinatally diagnosed disease, especially because correction of megaureters in newborns can be challenging.

The onset of puberty and cessation of longitudinal growth alters the recommendations for adolescents whose reflux is being medically managed. Surgery is recommended for most girls with reflux that persists, in order to avoid the implications of active reflux for future pregnancies (see earlier discussion). This is especially true for patients who have nephropathy or have shown a tendency to UTIs in the past. Some clinicians discontinue antibiotics in adolescent girls as puberty approaches (Belman, 1995), in essence providing the child a "test." Those with normal kidneys or whose reflux is discovered serendipitously during sibling screening are particularly good candidates for this approach. Its risks must be fully understood by the family and treating physician, although episodes of pyelonephritis are uncommon and the appearance of new renal scars decreases with age. Surgery is reserved for those who develop significant infections. Because older boys are less prone to UTI, prophylaxis can be discontinued and most reflux observed, unless infection or other symptoms arise. In one study of 40 girls and 11 boys with persistent reflux who had been medically managed for an average of almost 5 years and whose medication was discontinued, surgery became necessary because of significant UTIs in 5 patients (9%) after an average follow-up period of 3.7 years. Reflux subsequently resolved in 10 others, and no scars developed in any patient. Longer follow-up is needed to more fully evaluate the efficacy of this approach, especially its implications for adults (Cooper et al, 2000). Reimplantation is recommended for adults who have presented with reflux and UTIs. It is noted, although rarely discussed, that reimplantation surgery in female patients is far more challenging after puberty. Maturation of the pelvic adnexa makes ureteral mobilization difficult and increases bleeding. Clinical guidelines for the management of primary VUR in children are summarized in Tables 59–6 and 59–7.

MEDICAL MANAGEMENT

There has been no clearcut demonstration of nephropathy developing in children with reflux whose urine is kept infection free. To achieve this end, medical management consists of continuous low-dosage prophylactic antibiotic therapy until the expected resolution of reflux occurs. A variety of different medications achieve high urinary concentrations and effectively control a broad spectrum of uropathogens, but preferences do exist. **Medications are usually given as suspensions once daily at one-half the standard therapeutic dose. Nighttime dosing in toilet-trained children is most effective because it precedes the longest period of urinary retention, when infection is most likely to develop.**

Amoxicillin or ampicillin is recommended for children up to 6 weeks of age. Although these medications favor the development of resistant fecal flora, they offer fewer side effects to the newborn. **After 6 weeks, the biliary system is mature enough to handle trimethoprim-sulfamethoxazole (Septra, Bactrim), which usually becomes the prophylactic drug of choice.** Side effects include gastrointestinal symptoms, allergies, Stevens-Johnson syndrome, and leukopenia, which resolves with discontinuance of the drug. A complete blood count should be obtained during the perioperative period from any child taking the medication, but periodic blood counts are probably unnecessary. **Nitrofurantoin (Macrodantin) is another acceptable option in prophylaxis, and it is the medication best suited to minimizing fecal resistance. Pulmonary fibrosis and interstitial pneumonia are rare but well-recognized complications of the medication.** Other side effects include nausea and vomiting, hemolytic anemia, peripheral neuropathies, and exfoliative dermatitis. Nitrofurantoin should not be given to children younger than 2 months old. Alternating Septra and Macrodantin every other day, or taking one drug in the morning and the other at night, has been an effective form of prophylaxis for children who develop infections with organisms that are resistant to single-agent therapy. Other options in prophylaxis for children who develop allergies include nalidixic acid, trimethoprim alone, and cephalosporins.

Guidelines for the nonoperative management of reflux are summarized in Tables 59–6 and 59–7. Improving toilet hygiene and bladder emptying by means of timed voids, double voiding, proper perineal wiping, and elimination of constipation also helps to achieve the goals of medical management. When present, bladder dysfunction should also be treated with anticholinergics. Periodic urine cultures are obtained every 3 months to evaluate for breakthrough infections. **Negative cultures are usually reliable, regardless of collection technique. When questions of culture validity arise, confirmation with catheterization becomes necessary.**

Yearly radiologic studies are also necessary, although some clinicians have gone to 18-month intervals. The latter method allows more time for interval growth, is cost-effective, and requires only two catheterizations for cystography during a 3-year period. A minor tradeoff is that 6 additional months of unnecessary medication might be given if reflux resolves during the first year of management. The combination of ultrasonography and nuclear cystography provides adequate follow-up of the urinary tract for directing the continuance or cessation of medical therapy. There is no need for serial DMSA scans unless recurrent bouts of pyelonephritis with scarring are suspected or have occurred. Standard VCUG provides better comparison of grade to monitor trends in resolution. Prophylaxis is discontinued once cystography has documented resolution of reflux. A repeat confirmatory cystogram is unnecessary in the asymptomatic child. However, families should be aware that these children sometimes remain prone to UTIs and be instructed to continue efforts at proper toilet hygiene. When infections do occur, they usually manifest with lower urinary tract symptoms. Complete reevaluations that include cystography are required for children who develop pyelonephritis.

The likelihood of resolution of reflux and expectations of medical management should be frankly discussed with the parents. The requirements of periodic radiologic follow-up and, in some cases, long-term prophylaxis cannot be fulfilled by certain families. In a study by Wan and colleagues (1996b), approximately one third of children treated nonsurgically for reflux were lost to follow-up, many after the first year. Intermittent treatment of infections is ineffective therapy. Data from patients treated only during symptomatic episodes demonstrate progressive nephropathy when compared with those who maintained chronic suppression. For example, Lenaghan and associates (1976) noted a 21% incidence of new renal scarring when intermittent antibiotics were given, in contrast to the 1% incidence noted with continuous antibiotics (Smellie et al, 1975). **When compliance is an issue, some children are best served by surgically correcting their reflux rather than embarking on a futile course of medical management or suboptimal follow-up.**

Clinical Studies

Since the early work of Smellie and Normand (1979), which involved a large group of children with reflux who were given continuous low-dose chemotherapy, a number of clinical studies have been done to assess the efficacy of medical management of reflux and better define certain aspects of its natural history.

The International Reflux Study in Children compared the medical and surgical management of high-grade (grade III or IV) reflux after randomization in children younger than 9 years of age in Europe and in the United States (see Table 59–7). **Surgery was more effective than medical**

Table 59–6. TREATMENT RECOMMENDATIONS FOR BOYS AND GIRLS WITH PRIMARY VESICOURETERAL REFLUX (VUR)*

Clinical Presentation		Initial (Antibiotic Prophylaxis or Open Surgical Repair)			Follow-up† (Continued Antibiotic Prophylaxis, Cystography, or Open Surgical Repair)		
VUR Grade and Laterality	*Age (Yr)*	*Guideline*	*Preferred Option*	*Reasonable Alternative*	*Guideline*	*Preferred Option*	*No Consensus‡*
For children without scarring at diagnosis	<1	Prophylaxis					Boys and girls
I–II, Unilateral or bilateral	1–5	Prophylaxis					Boys and girls
	6–10	Prophylaxis					Boys and girls
III–IV, unilateral or bilateral	<1	Prophylaxis			Bilateral: surgery if persistent§	Unilateral: surgery if persistent§	
	1–5	Unilateral: prophylaxis	Bilateral: prophylaxis			Surgery if persistent§	
	6–10		Unilateral: prophylaxis Bilateral: surgery	Bilateral: prophylaxis		Surgery if persistent§	
V, unilateral or bilateral	<1	Prophylaxis			Surgery if persistent§		
	1–5		Bilateral: prophylaxis Unilateral: prophylaxis	Bilateral: prophylaxis Unilateral: surgery	Surgery if persistent§		
	6–10	Surgery					
For children with scarring at diagnosis	<1	Prophylaxis					Boys and girls
I–II, unilateral or bilateral	1–5	Prophylaxis					Boys and girls
	6–10	Prophylaxis					Boys and girls
III–IV, unilateral	<1	Prophylaxis			Girls: surgery if persistent§	Boys: surgery if persistent§	
	1–5	Prophylaxis			Girls: surgery if persistent§	Boys: surgery if persistent§	
	6–10		Prophylaxis		Surgery if persistent§		
III–IV, bilateral	<1	Prophylaxis			Surgery if persistent§		
	1–5		Prophylaxis	Surgery	Surgery if persistent§		
	6–10	Surgery					
V, unilateral or bilateral	<1		Prophylaxis	Surgery	Surgery if persistent§		
	1–5	Bilateral: surgery	Unilateral: surgery			Surgery if persistent§	
	6–10	Surgery					

*Recommendations were derived from a survey of preferred treatment options from 36 clinical categories of children with reflux. The recommendations are classified as follows:
  Guidelines = Treatments selected by 8–9 of 9 panel members, given the strongest recommendation language
  Preferred Options = Treatments selected by 5–7 of 9 panel members
  Reasonable Alternatives = Treatments selected by 3–4 of 9 panel members
  No Consensus = Treatment selected by no more than 2 of 9 panel members
†For patients with persistent uncomplicated reflux after extended treatment with continuous antibiotic therapy.
‡No consensus was reached regarding the role of continued antibiotic prophylaxis, cystography, or surgery.
§See the text regarding the length of time that clinicians should wait before recommending surgery.
From American Urological Association: Report on the Management of Vesicoureteral Reflux in Children. Baltimore, American Urological Association, Pediatric Vesicoureteral Reflux Clinical Guidelines Panel, 1997.

Table 59–7. OUTCOMES OF MEDICAL AND SURGICAL THERAPY FOR CHILDREN WITH PRIMARY VESICOURETERAL REFLUX AND RENAL SCARRING

Registrant	No. of Patients	New Scars	Thinning
European			
Medical	155	19 (12%)	11 (7%)
Surgical	151	20 (13%)	15 (10%)
United States			
Medical	66	14 (20%)	9 (13%)
Surgical	64	16 (25%)	2 (3%)

International Reflux Study Committee: Medical versus surgical treatment of primary vesicoureteral reflux. Pediatrics 1981;67:392–400.

therapy in preventing pyelonephritis (10% vs. 21%), but the overall incidence of UTIs between the two groups was the same (38% to 39%). Both modalities were equally effective in preventing new renal scarring, although scars did develop regardless of therapy—further proof of the importance of host defense and bacterial virulence factors. In this regard, the European arm of the study considered the effects of dysfunctional voiding on reflux. When dysfunctional voiding was present (18%) and untreated, patients had more infections, greater variability in reflux grade during follow-up, and increased persistent reflux. Reflux nephropathy was not increased (Weiss et al, 1992a; Tamminen-Mobius et al, 1992; Van Gool et al, 1992). Cessation of reflux was seen in 34 (23%) of 151 patients who were medically managed in the European arm, although bilateral reflux was less likely to resolve (10%).

The Birmingham Reflux Study used a study design similar to that of the IRSC in treating 104 patients with severe reflux. Surgical and medical management were equally effective in preventing new renal scars. Between 50% and 80% of medically treated patients still had reflux after a 5-year period (Birmingham Reflux Study Group, 1987).

In *other studies,* the Southwest Pediatric Nephrology Group Study prospectively evaluated the medical management of low- and moderate-grade reflux (grades I to III) in 84 ureters of 59 patients. Grade-dependent resolution was seen in 67%. Despite strict medical therapy and close surveillance, breakthrough UTIs occurred in one third of the patients and grade-related renal scarring in 16%. No comparison with surgery was made (Arant, 1992). Another prospective randomized study by Scholtmeijer (1993) investigated 135 ureters in 93 children with varying grades of reflux. Spontaneous resolution occurred in 27 (57%) of 47 cases of grade III or IV reflux with 5 years of follow-up. Fifteen children (32%) required crossover to reimplantation because of breakthrough infections. New scars developed in 2 patients with grade II or III reflux who were being medically managed and in 6 who were surgically treated. Other prospective studies of reflux have been done, but not in a randomized fashion. Each emphasized the need to control breakthrough UTIs (Dunn et al, 1973; Edwards et al, 1977; King, 1977).

SURGICAL MANAGEMENT

The treatment of VUR is individualized. Before recommending surgery, consideration is given to the severity of

the reflux, possible underlying risk factors including bladder dysfunction, age at presentation and duration of the disorder, and the presence and quality of UTIs that may have occurred during medical management. Knowing that corrective surgery is usually successful does not allow for a broadening of its indications. Errors in selection set the stage for postoperative complications. Typical indications for antireflux surgery include

1. Breakthrough UTIs despite prophylactic antibiotics
2. Noncompliance with medical management
3. Severe grades of reflux (grade IV or V), especially with pyelonephritic changes
4. Failure of renal growth, new renal scars, or deterioration of renal function on serial ultrasounds or scans
5. Reflux that persists in girls as full linear growth is approached at puberty
6. Reflux associated with congenital abnormalities at the UVJ (e.g., bladder diverticula)

The expectations of surgery must be understood beforehand. Successful ureteral reimplantation should decrease but does not eliminate the incidence of pyelonephritis in children with reflux. A significant decrease (from 50% to 10%) was reported by Govan and Palmer (1969) after successful surgery. In the IRSC, the incidence of pyelonephritis in the surgical group (10%) was less than half that in the medically controlled group (21%) (Jodal et al, 1992). Nevertheless, UTIs still persist despite surgery. Bacteriuria is reported in as many as 40% of patients postoperatively, though most do not develop pyelonephritis (Willscher et al, 1976; Wacksman et al, 1978; Weiss et al, 1992b). Like medical management, surgery cannot completely protect the kidney. This is undoubtedly the consequence of host abnormalities such as dysfunctional voiding and bacterial virulence factors, especially because the incidence of bacteriuria is similar to that in children without reflux and in those whose reflux is being treated medically.

A variety of techniques have been described for the correction of VUR. These are anatomically categorized as *extravesical, intravesical, or combined,* depending on the approach to the ureter, and *suprahiatal or infrahiatal,* depending on the position of the new submucosal tunnel in relation to the original hiatus. Common to each method is the creation of a valvular mechanism that enables ureteral compression with bladder filling and contraction, re-enacting normal anatomy and function. A successful ureteroneocystostomy provides a submucosal tunnel for reimplantation having sufficient length and adequate muscular backing. A tunnel length of five times the ureteral diameter is cited as necessary for eliminating reflux (Paquin, 1959). Deviation from this basic principle is the most common cause of failed reimplantations and explains the lack of success seen with many earlier reimplantation techniques that are no longer employed (Winter, 1969). The technical details of the more widely used repairs follow.

Politano-Leadbetter Technique

The Politano-Leadbetter technique has been a reliable method for correction of VUR since it was described in

1958, although its popularity appears to be waning (Politano and Leadbetter, 1958). Any reluctance to use this suprahiatal, intravesical repair technique stems from the somewhat "blind" nature of its transfer of the ureter behind the bladder, especially when compared with the relatively simple cross-trigonal reimplantation method. This drawback can be overcome using the technique described here. Many surgeons still prefer the Politano-Leadbetter technique for unilateral reimplantations, avoiding possible disruption of the valvular mechanism of the contralateral ureter. Success rates between 97% and 99% are cited in the literature

(Brannon et al, 1973), although some authors noted a slightly higher complication rate with this technique when compared to the cross-trigonal method (Carpentier et al, 1982).

Method

The method for the Politano-Leadbetter technique is illustrated in Fig. 59–22.

1. A transverse skin incision is made along a skin crease

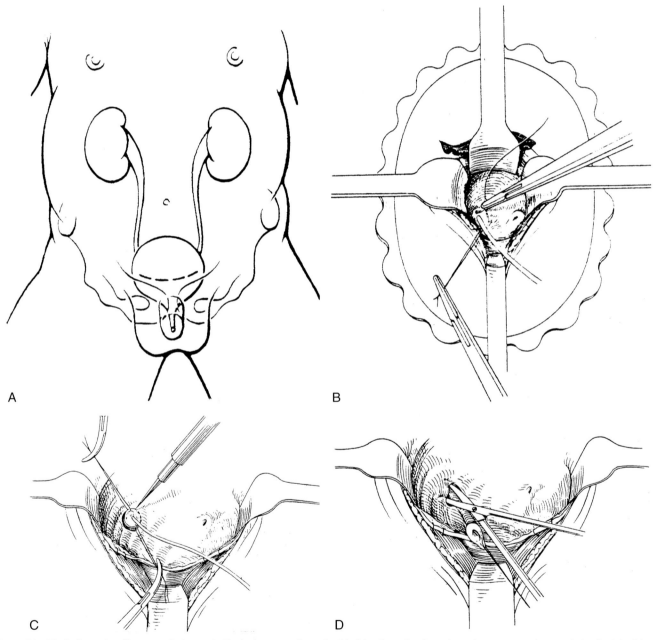

Figure 59–22. Politano-Leadbetter technique. *A,* Typical approach to the bladder for reimplantation. A transverse, lower abdominal incision is made along a skin crease one or two fingerbreadths above the symphysis pubis. *B,* Fine sutures are placed above and below the ureteral orifice for handling. A feeding tube in the ureter aids in the initial dissection. *C,* A needle-tip cautery outlines a circumferential incision around the orifice. *D,* Tenotomy scissors initially establish the plane of dissection inferiorly, where ureteral damage can be avoided. The plane is then carried around the ureter. (*A* through *D* from Retik AB, Colodny AH, Bauer SB: Pediatric urology. In Paulson DF [ed]: Genitourinary Surgery, vol 2. New York, Churchill Livingstone, 1984, pp 757–763.)

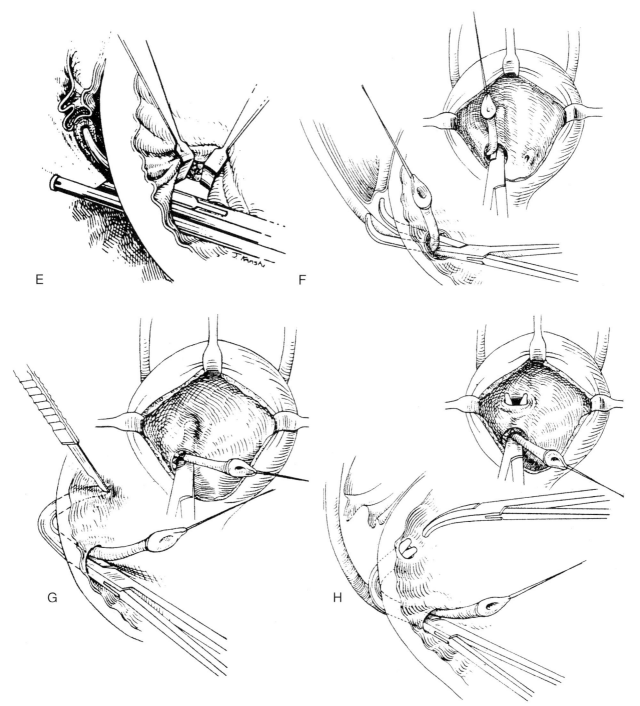

Figure 59–22 *Continued. E,* With the aid of a lighted suction tip and two Senn retractors, a fine gauze dissector is used to sweep the peritoneum from the posterior bladder wall. (From Keating MA, Retik AB: Management of failures of ureteroneocystostomy. In McDougal WS [ed]: Difficult Problems in Urologic Surgery. Chicago, Year Book, 1989, p 121.) *F,* After sweeping the peritoneum away, a blunt right-angle clamp indents the bladder from behind at a new hiatus approximately 2.5 cm superior and somewhat medial to the original hiatus. *G,* The clamp is incised upon from within and generously spread to make certain the new hiatus is wide enough. *H,* A second right-angle clamp follows the first from within the bladder to the original hiatus. *I,* The right-angle clamp grasps the stay suture and the ureter is pulled through the new hiatus.

Illustration continued on following page

two fingerbreadths above the symphysis pubis (Fig. 59–22A).

2. After the anterior rectus fascia is opened, flaps are developed superiorly and inferiorly above the muscles. The rectus and pyramidalis muscles are separated in the midline.

3. The transversalis fascia and peritoneum are swept from the dome of the bladder with the finger.

4. The bladder is opened in the midline with cautery to 2 cm above the bladder neck, and its inferior and lateral edges are sutured to the anterior rectus fascia. This elevates the bladder floor and aids in placement of the Denis

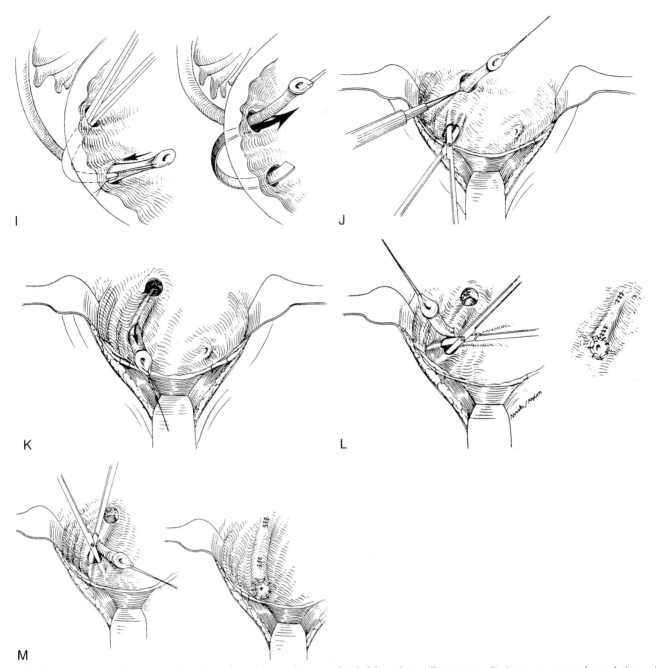

Figure 59–22 *Continued. J,* The inferior lip of muscle at the new hiatus is divided for a few millimeters to eliminate any ureteral angulation at its entrance to the submucosal tunnel that is created with scissors. *K,* The ureter is brought through the new tunnel to the original hiatus. *L,* The ureter is anastomosed to the original hiatus in the classic Politano-Leadbetter technique. Proximal mucosa can be closed over the ureter to give additional length to the tunnel. *M,* Ureteral advancement is also helpful, especially if the original hiatus is laterally positioned. A second submucosal tunnel can be created toward the bladder neck to place the new orifice in a more inferior position and gain additional length for the reimplant. *(F through M from Retik AB, Colodny AH, Bauer SB: Pediatric urology. In Paulson DF [ed]: Genitourinary Surgery, vol 2. New York, Churchill Livingstone, 1984, pp 757–763.)*

Browne retractor, whose lateral blades are positioned within the bladder.

5. Multiple moist 4 × 4 sponges are placed in the dome of the bladder behind the superior blade to further elevate the bladder floor. When the trigone is flattened and tense, the exposure is sufficient to proceed. Manipulation of the bladder with sponges, suction, or forceps is minimized to prevent edema and bleeding.

6. Ureteral dissection is performed with minimal tissue handling. A 5-0 chromic suture is placed above and below the orifice within the future perimeatal cuff. Placement of a fine (No. 3.5 or 5 Fr) feeding tube aids in the initial dissection of the ureter (Fig. 59–22B).

7. A generous mucosal cuff is outlined around the meatus using a needle-tip cautery. This facilitates later suturing of the ureter and helps avoid compromise of its lumen (Fig. 59–22C).

8. After the mucosa is incised and the superficial detru-

sor is taken down, the plane for ureteral dissection is found inferiorly by spreading a snap (Fig. 59–22D). Excessive dissection of the surrounding detrusor is unnecessary and causes annoying bleeding.

9. Sharp dissection parallel to the ureter with tenotomy scissors establishes the correct plane. It is important not to skeletonize the ureter and damage its adventitia. Hemostasis is accomplished with selective cautery using fine hemostats on the periureteral attachments. Kinks and angulations are straightened. If the distal ureter is narrow or unhealthy after being mobilized, it is excised back to healthy viable tissue and spatulated to avoid stenosis.

10. Visualization of the perivesical region and site for the neohiatus is aided by spreading the musculature of the old hiatus with a blunt right-angle clamp.

11. A fine gauze dissector is used to sweep the peritoneum from the posterior bladder wall with the aid of a lighted suction tip and two Senn retractors (Fig. 59–22E). The peritoneum must be completely swept from the proposed new hiatus to avoid placing the ureter through the peritoneum or viscera. In male patients, the vas is visualized and swept away as it crosses the peritoneum while perivesical vessels are fulgurated.

12. Adequate mobilization and length is mandatory. This usually occurs with 6 to 8 cm of dissection and leaves the ureter untethered on gentle traction. In some cases, it is necessary to elevate the peritoneum from the ureter to gain adequate length.

13. The right-angle clamp hugs the posterior wall and indents the proposed new hiatus from without. This location is superior, medial, and, in most instances, 2 to 2.5 cm from the old hiatus (Fig. 59–22F). Placement of the new hiatus must be carefully chosen. Excessive lateral placement can lead to ureteral obstruction as the bladder fills. Obstruction also can occur with excessively superior positions if the ureter has not been adequately mobilized.

14. The mucosa and muscle are then sharply incised and the right-angle clamp is spread generously on entering the bladder (Fig. 59–22G). Incomplete separation of the detrusor can cause obstruction at the new hiatus. Incising a few millimeters of its medial muscular lip helps avoid kinking, perhaps the technique's most common complication.

15. A second right-angle clamp is passed outside the bladder by the initial clamp and guides the ureter through the new hiatus into the bladder by grasping its stay sutures (Fig. 59–22H and I). Ureteral obstruction can result from twisting, and orientation must be maintained.

16. A fine infant feeding tube (No. 3.5 or 5 Fr) is passed intermittently to rule out obstruction. Inability to pass the tube warrants re-examination of the course of the ureter.

17. The mucosa surrounding the old hiatus is mobilized and its musculature is closed with interrupted polyglycolic acid sutures. Tenotomy scissors are used to develop a new submucosal tunnel that extends to the old hiatus and bladder neck (Fig. 59–22J). Wide mucosal mobilization is needed to avoid ureteral obstruction. When the bladder is scarred or trabeculated, it is sometimes easier to incise and raise mucosal flaps to form the ureteral bed.

18. A right-angle clamp delivers the ureter through the submucosal tunnel to its previous hiatus. After any necessary revisions, the distal ureter is sutured at the original

hiatus (classic Politano-Leadbetter technique) with interrupted 5-0 chromic suture (Fig. 59–22K and L). Ureteral spatulation is unnecessary. The most inferior three sutures include muscle as well as mucosa to anchor the repair. The remaining mucosa that has been mobilized is loosely reapproximated over the ureter, in effect increasing tunnel length.

19. Ureteral advancement can yield additional tunnel length and is especially helpful when the original orifice is laterally placed off the trigone. This is done by incising the mucosa inferiorly and advancing the ureter toward the bladder neck (Fig. 59–22M).

20. The bladder is closed with two layers of running polyglycolic acid sutures. In female patients, a multifenestrated No. 10 or 12 Fr soft red rubber catheter is placed transurethrally. Its position is secured to the abdominal wall by a 2-0 silk suture brought through the bladder with a Keith needle. The silk is tied over a button positioned just above the incision. In male patients, the bladder usually is drained with a Malecot (No. 12 or 14 Fr) catheter that exits a separate stab wound above the incision. Alternatively, a small-diameter Foley catheter may be left indwelling, making sure that the balloon is positioned distally. In infants and young children who are not toilet-trained, bladder drainage can be deferred. Perivesical drainage with Jackson-Pratt, Penrose, or other drains may also be used. However, an increasing number of surgeons are choosing not to use these types of drains, and morbidity has not increased (Chow et al, 1998).

Cohen Cross-Trigonal Technique

First described by Cohen in 1975, the versatile cross-trigonal reimplantation is probably the most popular technique in use today (Cohen, 1975). Achieving adequate submucosal length along the posterior aspect of the bladder is possible in virtually every patient with this intravesical, infrahiatal advancement; in addition, ease in performance and teaching is cited by its proponents. The cross-trigonal reimplantation is especially useful for correcting reflux in small bladders or neuropathic bladders that are significantly thickened, because a gentler ureteral curve is achieved than with the Politano-Leadbetter procedure (Glassberg et al, 1985). Cross-trigonal reimplantation is also the procedure of choice when bladder neck reconstructions are being performed so that the ureters can be superiorly positioned above the revision. Success rates of 96% to 99% have been reported (Burbige, 1991; Kennelly et al, 1995; McCool and Joseph, 1995). The technique's one drawback is the difficulty it presents to retrograde catheterization because of the lateral deviation of the ureters and their orifices. Fortunately, the introduction of flexible-tip retrograde catheters has obviated the combined approach of suprapubic cystostomy to deliver a catheter and cystoscopy to direct its position that originally was necessary to accomplish this feat (Lamesch, 1981).

Method

Figures 59–23 and 59–24 illustrate the Cohen cross-trigonal technique.

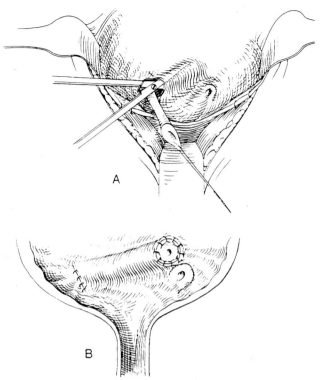

Figure 59–23. Cohen cross-trigonal technique, unilateral reimplantation. After the ureter is freed up *(A)*, a submucosal tunnel is made with the new mucosal hiatus just above the contralateral ureteral orifice *(B)*. (From Retik AB, Colodny AH, Bauer SB: Pediatric urology. In Paulson DF [ed]: Genitourinary Surgery, vol 2. New York, Churchill Livingstone, 1984, p 764.)

1. Initial exposure is obtained as in the Politano-Leadbetter procedure.

2. Mobilization of the ureter or ureters is similarly repeated. Less ureteral handling is necessary with this technique than with the Politano-Leadbetter method.

3. Excessive dissection of the trigone can usually be avoided when taking down the ureter. Hiatal closure is done if the opening is unusually patulous. After a medial groove is created in the detrusor to avoid a shelf at the ureteral entrance, the hiatus is reapproximated with interrupted 000 polyglycolic acid sutures. Inadequate closure can lead to diverticulum formation, the most common complication in early series (Ahmed and Tan, 1982). The hiatus should allow a Kelly clamp next to the ureter to avoid obstruction.

4. When one ureter is reimplanted, a submucosal tunnel is developed with tenotomy scissors to place the new mucosal hiatus just above the contralateral ureteral orifice (see Fig. 59–23). When both ureters are reimplanted, a submucosal tunnel for the superior-most ureter is made with a new mucosal hiatus located above the contralateral orifice. The other tunnel is then developed so that the new ureteral orifice is positioned at the inferior portion of the old contralateral hiatus (see Fig. 59–24). For some small bladders it helps to change the position of the ureteral entrance by incising the superolateral margin of the hiatus and mobilizing the peritoneum off the back of the bladder, giving the ureter a more lateral position and creating a longer tunnel.

5. Once the ureters have been brought across their new

tunnels, they are repositioned with polyglycolic acid and chromic sutures. Passage of a fine infant feeding tube ensures patency, and closure of the bladder and drainage are completed as described previously.

Glenn-Anderson Technique

The advantage of the Glenn-Anderson infrahiatal advancement is similar to that of the cross-trigonal method (Glenn and Anderson, 1967). Because the ureter remains in its original hiatus, obstruction or kinking is highly unusual. Success rates as high as 97% to 98% have been cited, although this technique is implicated in many referrals for persistent postreimplantation reflux (Gonzalez et al, 1972; Bellinger and Duckett, 1983). Again, selection is the key to success. The best candidates for this reimplantation technique are those whose ureters are laterally positioned and have enough distance to the bladder neck to allow for creation of a submucosal tunnel of adequate length. If the bladder is small or the ureters are medially positioned, a Mathisen-type (Mathisen, 1964) suprahiatal "cut-back" modification and more extensive transvesical dissection can be used to garner additional tunnel length (see later discussion).

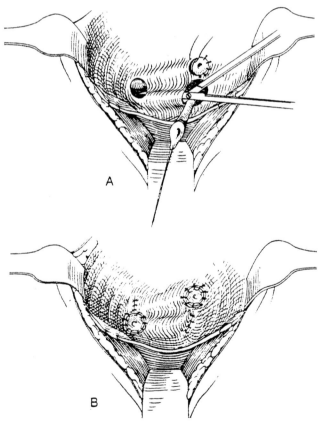

Figure 59–24. Cohen cross-trigonal technique, bilateral reimplant. *A,* The more superior ureter is tunneled transversely, with its new orifice just above the contralateral orifice. *B,* The other ureter is tunneled inferiorly, with its new orifice located at the inferiormost portion of the contralateral hiatus. (From Retik AB, Colodny AH, Bauer SB: Pediatric urology. In Paulson DF [ed]: Genitourinary Surgery, vol 2. New York, Churchill Livingstone, 1984, p 765.)

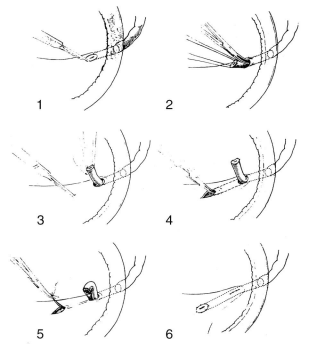

Figure 59–25. Glenn-Anderson technique. The ureter is mobilized and advanced beneath a new submucosal tunnel. (From Glenn JF, Anderson EE: Distal tunnel ureteral reimplantation. J Urol 1967;97: 623.)

Method

The method for the Glenn-Anderson technique is illustrated in Fig. 59–25.

1. Initial exposure is obtained as in the Politano-Leadbetter procedure.

2. The intravesical ureter is mobilized using similar techniques and should provide 2 to 3 cm of ureteral length.

3. A submucosal tunnel can be created with tenotomy scissors, although it is often simpler to sharply incise the mucosa to the bladder neck and raise flaps.

4. The widened hiatus is reapproximated with 000 polyglycolic acid sutures and the ureter is repositioned inferiorly near the bladder neck, where it is anchored with fine interrupted absorbable sutures.

5. When ureteral mobilization is inadequate, the muscular hiatus can be extended superolaterally by cutting the detrusor and mobilizing the peritoneum and other structures behind the bladder. This modification gains additional ureteral length and also provides extended backing when the muscle is ultimately closed beneath (Glenn and Anderson, 1978).

Gil-Vernet Technique

This simple infrahiatal advancement technique theoretically relies on the sphincteric action of intrinsic muscular fibers of the transmural ureter to prevent reflux, although the additional muscular backing and intramural length provided by the advancement also undoubtedly contribute to its effect (Gil-Vernet, 1984). High rates of success have been reported (94% with variable grades of reflux) (Solok

et al, 1988), but selection is crucial to meeting this standard. To be considered for the repair, the intravesical ureter must be freely mobile. Many ureters are not optional for this repair, especially ureters with higher grades of reflux and those of older children, whose periureteral attachments become more tenacious with age. The procedure has been recommended for the prevention of postoperative reflux in patients with unilateral reflux who have a pathologic appearance of a nonrefluxing contralateral ureteral meatus (Liard et al, 1999).

Method

The Gil-Vernet method is illustrated in Fig. 59–26.

1. Initial exposure is obtained as in the Politano-Leadbetter procedure.

2. Medially positioned traction sutures are placed near the ureteral orifices in the cuff to test ureteral mobility. If the ureters can be lifted from their beds to meet in the midline, they are good candidates for the technique.

3. A single transverse incision is made through the mucosa that joins both traction sutures.

4. Two 4-0 or 5-0 polydioxanone mattress sutures are placed through the intrinsic ureteral musculature and approximate the ureter to midline detrusor. Nonabsorbable

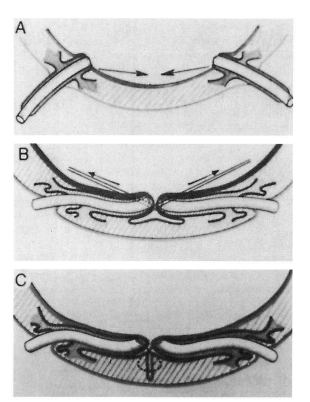

Figure 59–26. Gil-Vernet technique. *A,* The principle involves advancing the ureters across the trigone. *B,* Traction sutures are used to test mobility and demonstrate the desired result. *C,* On completion, the ureteral orifices are in close proximity near the midline and submucosal length has been increased, preserving intrinsic and extrinsic periureteral musculature. (From Gil-Vernet JM: A new technique for surgical correction of vesicoureteral reflux. J Urol 1984;131:456, copyright © 1984 by The Williams and Wilkins Company, Baltimore.)

sutures were used in the initial description, but they may migrate intravesically to become a nidus for stone.

5. Closing of the mucosa vertically with fine interrupted chromic sutures buries the absorbable stitch and completes the repair.

Extravesical Ureteral Reimplantation

The Lich-Gregoir extravesical reimplantation technique evolved concurrently in Europe (Gregoir and Van Regemorter, 1964) and in the United States (Lich et al, 1961), but it never achieved the widespread popularity in this country that it enjoyed overseas. Nevertheless, extended follow-up studies in large series have found the procedure to be as effective (90% to 98%) as any other (Gregoir and Schulman, 1977; Arap et al, 1981; Heimbach et al, 1995), and over the last decade its use has increased substantially in North America. Several modifications to the original procedure have been introduced by various centers over the years. This includes ending the paraureteral myotomy with an inverted Y, which facilitates detrusor muscle reapproximation (Lapointe et al, 1998; Barrieras et al, 1999); fixing the ureter to the detrusor with additional stitches (Vuckov et al, 1999); and multiple ureteral advancement procedures involving detrusorrhaphy. In a modification first introduced by Daines and Hodgson (1971), ureteral advancement sutures are used as an adjunct to extravesical reimplantation. Success rates of 93% to 99% have been reported (Zaontz et el, 1987; Wacksman et al, 1992; Mevorach et al, 1998).

Because the bladder is left intact, risks from urinary contamination are minimized. Bladder spasms and hematuria are also lessened. The Lich-Gregoir technique is also less invasive than most repairs, and hospitalization time is shortened. This method of implantation is particularly applicable to renal transplantation, although the placement of the donor ureter will differ.

Concerns about disrupting the nerves to the bladder cause some surgeons to defer the technique with bilateral reimplantations because of the risk of causing urinary retention, which has been reported in 4% to 36% of patients (Fung et al, 1995; Minevich et al, 1998a; Barrieras et al, 1999). Varying the techniques of repair does not seem to affect the incidence of urinary retention. Patients who had an inverted Y detrusorrhaphy had rates of urinary retention similar to those who had a ureteral advancement (Barrieras et al, 1999). Patients who had a ureteral advancement had the same incidence of urinary retention as those who had minimal detrusor dissection (Lipski et al, 1998). Children younger than 3 years of age, boys, patients with high-grade reflux, and children with a history of voiding dysfunction had higher incidences of urinary retention (Minevich et al, 1998a; Barrieras et al, 1999). Spontaneous resolution is seen after a maximum of 4 weeks of either Foley catheter drainage or intermittent catheterization (Houle et al, 1992; Minevich et al, 1998a). Long-term voiding efficacy is unaffected.

Because the bladder is not opened with the extravesical approach to ureteral reimplantation, associated pathology might be difficult to appreciate if cystoscopy were not done. In fact, periureteral diverticula are regarded as a contraindication to the Lich-Gregoir method by some surgeons (Linn et al, 1989), although they did not pose a technical problem for Jayanthi and associates (1995), who reported successful management in 22 of 23 patients with diverticula using this approach. The technique can also be used to reimplant duplicated ureters. Megaureters that require tailoring are also candidates if excisional tapering is not necessary (Wacksman et al, 1992).

Method

The Lich-Gregoir technique is illustrated in Fig. 59–27.

1. The bladder is moderately filled with a catheter. Initial exposure is obtained as in the Politano-Leadbetter procedure. The bladder is initially left intact and retracted medially to aid in extravesical identification of the ureter. The obliterated hypogastric artery is identified and ligated, and the ureter is isolated with a vessel loop above the bladder and then gently mobilized. The peritoneum is also cleared from the posterior aspect of the bladder intended for implantation. Major blood vessels are preserved during the perivesical dissection.

2. The serosal and muscular layers of the detrusor are opened along a straight course cephalad and lateral from the UVJ, freeing up the ureter during the dissection. A 4- or 5-cm length of detrusor is cleared along this route from the underlying mucosa to create the antirefluxing trough. Ureterotrigonal continuity is not disrupted. Any mucosal rents are closed with fine interrupted chromic sutures.

3. The ureter is placed in the trough, and the detrusor closed over it with interrupted 000 polyglycolic acid sutures. When present, most diverticula can simply be dunked into the bladder with the advanced ureter, closing the detrusor behind.

4. A Penrose drain is left in the perivesical space but bladder drainage is unnecessary.

Method Involving Detrusorrhaphy

See Fig. 59–27 for illustrations of this modification of the Lich-Gregoir method.

1. After exposing and mobilizing the ureter as in the Lich-Gregoir technique, additional ureteral dissection is performed circumferentially to the bladder mucosa so that the ureter is attached only at its juncture with the bladder mucosa.

2. The detrusor is incised proximally and distally to create a muscular defect, and the bladder mucosa is further freed in the region of the trigone to create submucosal flaps.

3. A pair of Vest-type sutures (4-0 polyglycolic acid) are placed that approximate, in succession, detrusor at the distal limit of the dissected trigone, proximal ureter, and detrusor (inside-out) to advance the ureter into the bladder and create a new, long submucosal ureter.

4. The detrusor defect is closed with interrupted sutures to recede the hiatus and buttress the submucosal ureter.

Special Surgical Considerations: Duplicated Ureters

Approximately 10% of children undergoing antireflux surgery have an element of ureteral duplication. The

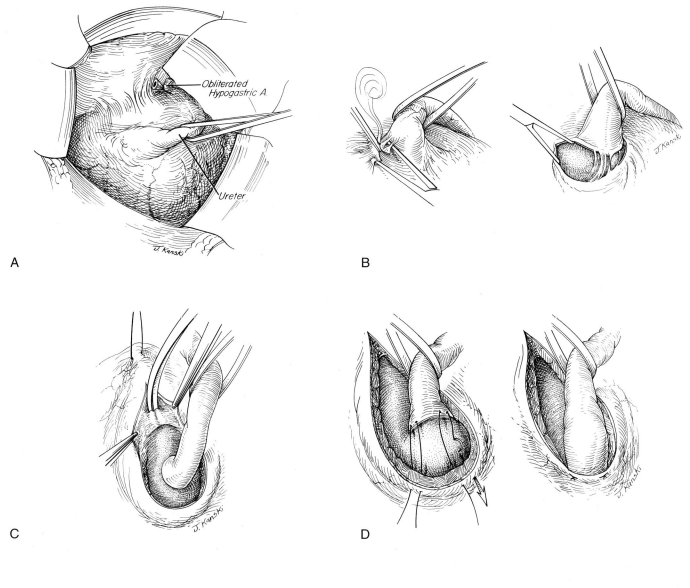

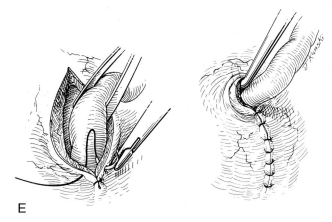

Figure 59–27. Modified Lich-Gregoir/detrusorrhaphy technique: *A,* The ureter is identified and gently grasped after ligation of the obliterated hypogastric artery. *B,* The ureter is circumferentially mobilized at its intersection with the bladder by incising the detrusor at the level of the ureteral hiatus. *C,* Serosal and muscular layers of the bladder (4 to 5 cm) are opened along a straight course cephalad and lateral from the ureterovesical junction to create the trough for reimplantation. Tacking suture aids in orientation. *D,* The bladder mucosa is elevated off muscle wall and Vest-type sutures are placed from the detrusor at the distal limit of dissection to the proximal ureteral adventitia and back again through same tissue planes. Tying of the Vest sutures advances and anchors the ureter onto the trigone. *E,* Reapproximation of the detrusor creates a long submucosal tunnel and completes the repair. (From Peters C, Retik AB: Ureteral reimplantation including megaureter repair. In Marshall FF [ed]: Textbook of Operative Urology. Philadelphia, WB Saunders, 1996, pp 868–870.)

most common configuration is a complete duplication that results in two separate orifices. This is best managed by preserving a cuff of bladder mucosa that encompasses both orifices. Because the pair typically share blood supply along their adjoining wall, mobilization as one unit with a "common sheath" preserves vascularity and minimizes trauma. Reimplantation then follows a sequence similar to that used in any of the techniques described earlier. In occasional instances, a "Y" or "V" ureteral configuration results in a single orifice that refluxes into both systems. If the common stem is long enough to be reimplanted alone, standard techniques can be used. Otherwise, to avoid obstruction at the union, the stem should be excised and the ureters converted to a complete duplication. A side-to-side reimplantation can then be completed. In rare instances, an unexpected ureteral duplication is encountered at surgery. These structures can be associated with functioning renal tissue or end blindly. Small ureteroceles that are unappreciated on preoperative studies have also been described. Common sheath reimplantation, rather than excision, is recommended (Bauer and Retik, 1978). Alternatively, ipsilateral ureteroureterostomy can be performed (Bieri et al, 1998). Although a duplicated system increases the risk associated with surgical management, it does not adversely affect surgical outcome (Ellsworth et al, 1996).

Postoperative Evaluation

Successful ureteroneocystostomy provides normal renal drainage and eliminates reflux. Ascending infections are usually controlled, although, for the reasons cited earlier, episodes of pyelonephritis sometimes reappear.

Several centers recommend limiting the postoperative imaging studies to those patients with abnormal preoperative ultrasound findings, voiding dysfunction, or high-grade reflux (Bomalaski et al, 1997b; Barrieras et al, 2000). However, most centers perform postoperative radiologic studies to assess initial and long-term surgical results and to monitor parameters of renal growth. A renal ultrasound study is obtained 6 weeks after surgery and should show minimal ureteral dilatation. A cystogram 3 to 6 months later checks the quality of the repair. If the imaging studies are satisfactory, further studies are unnecessary unless the patient develops upper tract changes or significant UTIs. The reappearance of hydronephrosis, new renal scars, retarded renal growth, or recurrent UTIs may warrant a complete radiographic re-evaluation. Periodic visits with blood pressure measurements are also recommended. Children with minimally symptomatic episodes of bacteriuria are evaluated for dysfunctional voiding and incomplete bladder emptying and treated accordingly.

Early Complications of Ureteral Reimplantation

Reflux

Postoperative reflux can occur in either the index ureter or a contralateral ureter that has been undisturbed. Presumably, these changes are secondary to trigonal edema from the operation. Exacerbations of bladder dysfunction during the perioperative period could also be implicated. Most postoperative reflux is of low grade and transient. In one study of 223 children who underwent antireflux surgery, the incidence of postoperative reflux in the reimplanted ureter was 3% at 4 months; in each case the reflux subsided within 1 year. **Reflux in the contralateral ureter occurs in 6% to 16% of patients, but seldom does it persist and require correction** (Willscher et al, 1976;

Burno et al, 1998; Minevich et al, 1998b). Correction of severe (grade V) reflux and reflux into duplex systems may place patients at risk for the development of contralateral reflux postoperatively (Diamond et al, 1996b). Parents should be reassured that conservative management is all that is required in most cases of postoperative reflux.

Obstruction

Early after surgery, various degrees of obstruction can be expected of the reimplanted ureter. Edema, subtrigonal bleeding, and bladder spasms all possibly contribute. Mucus plugs and blood clots are other causes. Most postoperative obstructions are mild and asymptomatic and resolve spontaneously. More significant obstructions are usually symptomatic. Affected children typically present 1 to 2 weeks after surgery with acute abdominal pain, nausea, and vomiting. Fever is less common. Renal scintigraphy usually shows marked delay in excretion, and severe hydroureteronephrosis is present on ultrasound. **The large majority of perioperative obstructions subside spontaneously, but placement of a nephrostomy tube or ureteral stent sometimes becomes necessary for symptoms that do not abate.** Treatment is otherwise supportive and includes parenteral antibiotics and hydration.

Late Complications of Ureteral Reimplantation

True failures of ureteroneocystostomy are rare, and success rates with reimplantation are high. For example, data from the IRSC indicate an overall success rate of greater than 97% in 394 ureters (Weiss et al, 1992a; Hjalmas et al, 1992). Strict attention to detail and adherence to the principles of the different operations discussed earlier are the best ways to minimize complications. **Before reoperation is considered, the cause of the complication should be fully defined so that any error of earlier surgery not be repeated. Standard radiologic studies (VCUG and excretory urography) and cystoscopy with retrograde ureterography provide anatomic detail, but additional diagnostic studies, including urodynamics and renal pressure perfusion studies, are sometimes helpful, especially when a functional cause is suspected.**

Reflux

VUR that persists after surgery usually results from failure to achieve sufficient submucosal length or failure to provide adequate muscular backing for the ureter within its tunnel. "Simplified" reimplantations consisting of minor submucosal advancements are common offenders. This approach to ureteroneocystostomy may be successful with mild degrees of ureteral dystopia, but for the most part it should be discouraged. **Another common error occurs when the dilated ureter is reimplanted. Reluctance to perform appropriate tailoring makes attainment of a proper diameter-to-tunnel ratio impossible. Less commonly, a ureter that is transmurally scarred**

from repeated infection is reimplanted but is unable to coapt because of fibrosis.

Other than technical errors, failure to identify and treat secondary causes of reflux is a common cause of its reappearance. Foremost among these are unrecognized neuropathic bladder and severe voiding dysfunction. Noe (1985) reported a 2% failure rate in 305 children after reimplantation. Of those with persistent reflux, 100% showed clinical signs of voiding dysfunction, and more than half of these cases resolved with behavior modification and anticholinergic medication alone. Performing ureteroneocystostomy in bladders that exhibit abnormal dynamics significantly lessens the likelihood of success. In severe cases, the early reappearance of hydroureteronephrosis followed by reflux is predictable when the recipient bladder incompletely empties or has high resting pressures with uninhibited contractions. Preoperative urodynamic studies are indicated in any child for whom a prior reimplantation has failed. Aggressive treatment of the underlying disorder with intermittent catheterization and anticholinergics will resolve some cases of recurrent reflux and must be effective to ensure the success of any secondary surgery that might be indicated. Enterocystoplasty or urinary diversion become necessary when medical measures do not improve bladder dynamics.

Obstruction

Significant postreimplantation ureteral obstruction varies in location and degree depending on its cause. **Complete obstructions usually occur as the result of ischemia.** Retrograde ureterography and catheterization at cystoscopy are often futile in their definition of the length of fibrosis and stricture, although the insult typically involves the implanted segment. **Other causes of partial or complete ureteral occlusion include angulation at the new hiatus, inadvertent passage through the peritoneum or viscera, and compromise at the hiatus or within an inadequately developed submucosal tunnel.** Intermittent obstructions are also encountered. Ureters reimplanted in abnormally lateral positions become increasingly angulated, with progressive bladder filling. Ureterectasis with "J" hooking of the distal ureter is seen by excretory urography. Voiding or catheterization results in alleviation of angulation with decompression. Revision is necessary if the obstruction becomes chronic.

Addressing the Failed Reimplant

After thoroughly defining a complication of ureteral reimplantation, the surgical approach to its correction is dictated by the type of failure, the degree of ureteral dilatation, and whether one or both ureters are affected.

Refluxing Ureter

An intravesical approach is used for ureters that reflux after ureteroneocystostomy. The technique of ureteral mobilization differs from that in standard reimplantation; the mucosa of the old submucosal tunnel is incised and scarred ureteral attachments are sharply removed. As much mobilization as possible is done within the bladder, but it is often necessary to move outside to gain adequate length for repair.

Obstructed Ureter

Intravesical mobilization is futile with the obstructed ureter, because it usually is irreparably damaged within the bladder wall. Instead, the bladder is opened to assess its interior and to plan the site for the new ureteral hiatus and tunnel. Attention is then turned extravesically. After the peritoneum is entered and the bowel packed away, virgin ureter is identified at the bifurcation of the iliac vessels. It is then freed as distally as possible and transected outside the bladder. The intramural segment remains untouched unless it hampers the planned repair. Possible exceptions to this approach include ureters obstructed from angulation and those suspected of having only meatal stenosis, which is rare. In both cases, attempts at intravesical mobilization might yield additional ureter length.

Surgical Options

With any type of ureter, mobilization is made to healthy tissue, and scarred or fibrotic tissue is excised. Any necessary tailoring of the dilated ureter is also completed. The surgical options are then dictated by the amount of viable ureter and the quality of the recipient bladder.

Refluxing ureters can be repaired in manner similar to that described for primary ureteroneocystostomy. Any standard method of reimplantation can be used to complete the repair intravesically, provided sufficient ureteral length is obtained from within. When the mobilization must be extended extravesically, selection of a neohiatus and reimplantation using a repair method similar to the Politano-Leadbetter technique is a good choice.

Obstructed ureters present the additional dilemma of obtaining adequate length for effective reimplantation. Careful proximal mobilization is the first maneuver used to obtain length. When this alone is inadequate, a psoas hitch can be used to bridge significant ureteral defects that remain. The bladder can be tacked to psoas tendon above the common iliac vessels and still maintain normal function despite this distortion. The technique provides lengths of as much as 8 to 10 cm and effective muscular backing along the bladder base, which is suitably immobile for creation of a new tunnel. In addition to bridging the defects of complications, the psoas hitch is also useful in primary cases to create longer submucosal tunnels when marginal reimplantations might result from use of standard techniques alone (Prout and Koontz, 1970).

Ureters with defects that cannot be bridged by a psoas hitch and those that continue to reflux despite repeated efforts at reimplantation are ideal candidates for transureteroureterostomy (TUU), in effect bypassing the problem. Historically, hesitation to use a TUU stemmed from its potential effect on the recipient ureter, which should be normal. This is not a problem if (1) the recipient ureter is minimally mobilized; (2) there is no angulation of the donor ureter under the sigmoid

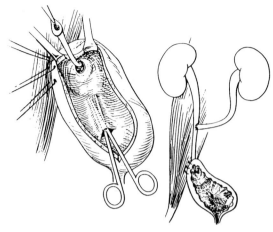

Figure 59–28. Psoas hitch can be used to effectively bridge significant ureteral defects. Its combination with transureteroureterostomy is ideal when both ureters are addressed in a reoperative setting. (From Keating MA, Retik AB: Management of failures of ureteroneocystostomy. In McDougal WS [ed]: Difficult Problems in Urologic Surgery. Chicago, Year Book, 1989, p 140.)

mesentery; and (3) a tension-free, widely spatulated anastomosis is created (Hendren and Hensle, 1980). The combination of psoas hitch and TUU is especially useful in cases of bilateral failures, where the feasibility of creating two adequately long tunnels would be limited by the anatomy of most bladders. Attempts at bilateral psoas hitches, which sacrifice one true hitch for two mediocre ones, should be discouraged. After both ureters are freed, the healthier and longer one can be reimplanted into a long submucosal tunnel using a psoas hitch. The second ureter is then joined to the reimplanted ureter as a TUU (Fig. 59–28) (Keating and Retik, 1989).

ENDOSCOPIC TREATMENT OF REFLUX

The concept of treating VUR endoscopically is valid. In theory, an object or injectable material is positioned behind the ureter to provide the backing necessary to enable its coaptation during bladder filling and contraction (Fig. 59–29). Surgically, such an approach, if successful, is particularly appealing because of its simplicity, lessened morbidity, and potential cost-effectiveness. However, endoscopic treatment is not as effective as open surgery. At best, cure rates of only about 70% may be obtained with a single injection. High-grade reflux, incorrect technique of injection, and voiding dysfunction may be some of the possible causes of an unsuccessful endoscopic treatment for reflux (Trsinar et al, 1999). Nonetheless, ease of treatment makes an endoscopic approach a viable option in selected patients. The decision making in the management of reflux often depends on balancing the uncertainty of spontaneous resolution against surgical morbidity. A significant reduction in the latter might very likely shift management decisions in the favor of endoscopic surgery in selected patients (Atala and Casale, 1990). In addition, there is a significant health care management cost savings. Calculated in 1996 health care dollars, the cost of an endoscopic injection per renal

unit was $1600, compared with $9144 for surgical reimplantation (Leonard et al, 1996).

Any endoscopic solution to treating reflux should have two major characteristics: *anatomic integrity,* or the ability of the material to be easily delivered and to conserve its volume, and *material safety,* meaning that the material is biocompatible, nonantigenic, and nonmigratory (Kershen and Atala, 1999). A number of different nonautologous and autologous options have been offered to meet these criteria.

General Endoscopic Technique

All patients are given a broad-spectrum preoperative antibiotic. The patient is placed in the dorsal lithotomy position. Routine cystoscopy is performed, and the ureters are visualized. A 20-gauge needle is advanced through the working channel. The needle tip is inserted under direct visualization at the 6 o'clock position into the subureteric space, approximately 4 to 6 mm distal to the ureteral orifice. Occasionally, proper placement of the needle may be facilitated by placing a No. 3 Fr catheter in the ureter. The needle is then advanced proximally. The bulking material is injected slowly until a bulge almost obliterates the ureteral orifice. A precise single injection should be made, because multiple puncture sites can allow extravasation of the material. The needle is kept in position for 2 to 3 minutes before being withdrawn, in order to minimize extravasation of the injected material through the needle track. **Clinical studies have shown that such methods can be performed in an outpatient setting, can be completed in less than 15 minutes, and have a low morbidity** (Geiss et al, 1990).

Nonautologous Materials

Teflon

The endoscopic treatment of VUR was given its origins by otolaryngologists who treated patients with vocal cord paralysis by injecting their cords with polytetrafluoroethy-

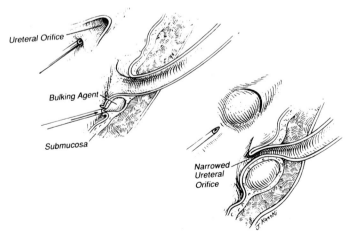

Figure 59–29. Principle of endoscopic treatment of reflux. Bulking agent is injected beneath the ureteral orifice with a needle. The buttress that is provided helps coapt the distal ureter.

lene (Teflon) paste (Arnold, 1962). Berg (1973) and Politano and colleagues (1974) realized the potential urologic applications of this bulking agent and applied the technology as a solution to urethral incontinence. The endoscopic treatment of reflux was first introduced by Matouschek (1981), who injected Teflon paste (polytef) into the subureteral region of a patient. O'Donnell and Puri (1984) later popularized the technique as the Sting procedure. Success rates vary from 66% to 92% depending on the grade of reflux and number of repeat treatments, which are required for as many as one third of patients (Bhatti et al, 1993; Dewan and Guiney, 1992; Puri and Granata, 1998).

Teflon has not fared well in the urinary tract, however. **Teflon particles are phagocytized into the reticuloendothelial system and are able to migrate locally and to distant sites.** This was first documented in a 76-year-old man who was successfully treated for urinary incontinence after a radical prostatectomy but was noted to have pulmonary Teflon granulomas at autopsy 4 years later (Mittleman and Marraccini, 1983). Malizia and colleagues (1984) subsequently demonstrated Teflon particle migration and granuloma formation in the lung, brain, and lymph nodes of dogs and monkeys after periurethral injection. Additional descriptions of Teflon migration in animals after periureteral injection followed these initial reports (Claes et al, 1989; Aaronson et al, 1993), although the particles were thought by some to be artifacts (Miyakita and Puri, 1994). Concerns regarding similar findings in children have prevented the widespread use of this substance for the treatment of reflux (Ferro et al, 1988; Rames and Aaronson, 1991; Aragona et al, 1997).

Collagen

Collagen has been used as an injectable soft tissue substitute for years, although its application as a cystoscopically delivered antireflux agent is a more recent development. Zyderm, Zyplast, and Contigen (Collagen Corporation, Palo Alto, California, and Bard Corporation, Atlanta, Georgia) are commercially available injectable cross-linked bovine corium collagen pastes composed almost solely of type I collagen (Frey et al, 1994). In vitro human and porcine cell culture studies demonstrate a stimulatory effect on fibroblasts by collagen causing ingrowth of the material. Success rates of 59% to 65% have been reported 3 months after one injection in children with variable grades of reflux (Leonard et al, 1991; Frey et al, 1995, 1997). Treatment with cross-linked collagen at a concentration of 65 mg/ml increased the success rate at 3 months to 88% (Frey et al, 1997). However, long-term results were not provided.

The major flaw of collagen is that its volume decreases with time. Biodegradation explains the reported high frequency of recurrent reflux and need for retreatment (Leonard et al, 1991; Frey et al, 1995). The results of some series suggest that repeat endoscopic collagen injections prolong the reflux-free period but remain ineffective in the long term (Haferkamp et al, 2000). Similar long-term failure rates have been reported with collagen used for the treatment of urinary incontinence (Monga et al, 1995). **As opposed to incontinence, reflux is largely a silent disease whose presence can be determined only through inva-** sive radiologic testing. **The major problem with any bulking agent that loses its volume is not knowing when reflux might reappear. "Successfully treated" patients may in fact redevelop recurrent reflux and its attendant health risks.** For these reasons, collagen has not been approved for the treatment of VUR by the U.S. Food and Drug Administration (FDA).

Silicone Microimplants

Textured silicone microparticles suspended in hydrogel have been used for the endoscopic treatment of urethral incontinence and VUR (Buckley et al, 1991; Henly et al, 1995; Ozyavuz et al, 1998). The substance is composed of fully vulcanized polydimethylsiloxane particles and water-soluble polyvinylpyrrolidone (PVP). The adverse publicity surrounding silicone gel–filled implants does not extend to these types of silicone elastomers. However, safety concerns do exist. In vivo experiments in animals have demonstrated particle migration to distant organs after their submucosal injection in the bladder (Buckley et al, 1991; Henly et al, 1995). Distant migration probably occurs more commonly when silicone particles smaller than 100 μm in diameter are included in the suspension. Nevertheless, these types of findings preclude the use of this material.

Deflux System

The Deflux system (Q-Med AB; Uppsala, Sweden) combines dextranomer microspheres with sodium hyaluronan, a common polysaccharide (Stenberg and Lackgren, 1995). The microspheres initially induce fibroblast and collagen deposition after their injection in the bladder. They disappear within 1 week, but endogenous tissue augmentation remains. Deflux was used to treat grades III and IV reflux in 101 ureters of 75 patients. Satisfactory results were achieved with 88% of grade III and 62% of grade IV cases, whereas treatment failed in 25 ureters. Follow-up was limited, and this detracts somewhat from these impressive results, especially because this material is biodegradable. Concerns about long-term efficacy, as with collagen, will determine the role of this agent in the treatment of reflux.

Detachable Membranes

A detachable, self-sealing silicone balloon has also been developed for the endoscopic treatment of VUR (Atala et al, 1992). The balloon is cystoscopically maneuvered into submucosa beneath the ureter and filled with a hydrogel through a catheter which is then withdrawn, leaving the membrane intact. Experiments in a pig model documented high rates of success. The system is currently being used in clinical trials approved by the FDA for the treatment of incontinence.

Autologous Injectable Materials

Alginate and Chondrocytes

Alginate, a biodegradable polymer, can be seeded with chondrocytes to serve as a synthetic substrate for the injectable delivery and maintenance of cartilage in vivo. Alginate-bovine chondrocyte cell allografts contained viable cartilage cells after implantation in athymic mice. The new cartilage that was formed retained the approximate shape and volume of the injected template (Atala et al, 1993a). Relying on these characteristics, Atala and colleagues (1994) used harvested chondrocytes effectively to eliminate reflux in a minipig model). Phase I FDA-approved clinical trials showed a success rate of 57% after one injection and 83% after two injections (Diamond and Caldamone, 1999). Combined phase II–III FDA clinical trials are currently ongoing.

Summary

The endoscopic treatment of VUR can be effective. The task remains to discover a material that is safe and provides long-term efficacy. The next several years will be instrumental to determining which autologous or nonautologous bulking agent is best for this innovative solution to reflux.

LAPAROSCOPIC MANAGEMENT OF REFLUX

Major advances have been made with laparoscopic surgery during the past decade. **The advantages of this approach over open surgery include smaller incisions, less discomfort, brief hospitalizations, and quicker convalescence.** The surge in laparoscopic urologic procedures and equipment in the 1990s led several investigators to explore so-called noninvasive alternatives to open ureteroneocystostomy. Successful laparoscopic correction of reflux in animals was reported in 1993 (Atala et al, 1993b). A laparoscopic modification of the Lich-Gregoir extravesical reimplantation, described later, was applied to minipigs (Lich et al, 1961; Gregoir and Van Regermorter, 1964). Laparoscopic correction of reflux was shown to be technically feasible in other animal models with varying techniques (Schimberg et al, 1994; McDougall et al, 1995; Cohen et al, 1999), as well as in humans (Atala, 1993; Ehrlich et al, 1994). **As with other laparoscopic procedures, a learning curve needs to be broached, and experience is essential to the success of this approach. Laparoscopic reimplantation requires a team with at least two surgeons. The repair is converted from an extraperitoneal to intraperitoneal approach. Many of the available instruments are less than ideal for use in children, operative time is greater than with open techniques, and cost is increased because of lengthier surgery and the expense of disposable equipment.** These considerations explain why, after an initial flurry of interest, laparoscopic reimplantation has not been widely used. It may be that improved instrumentation and more experience will allow better acceptance of the laparoscopic approach to reflux in the future.

Laparoscopic Technique

The laparoscopic technique is illustrated in Figure 59–30. A Veress needle is placed beneath the umbilicus, and pneumoperitoneum is obtained by insufflation of carbon dioxide (at a rate of 2 L/min) up to a pressure of 15 mm Hg. After adequate insufflation, two trocars are placed—one in the side opposite the refluxing ureter, at the midclavicular line 1 cm above the umbilicus (for various instruments), and one in the infraumbilical midline (for the camera). Two trocars are then positioned in the left and right midclavicular line, 2 cm above the level of the anterior superior iliac spine (for dissecting instruments and retractors). The table is then laterally rotated with the refluxing side up, allowing the bladder and viscera to fall away from the area of repair.

Ureteral mobilization is begun by identifying the obliterated umbilical artery along the pelvic sidewall. The bladder is then shifted away from the operative side by grasping and retracting its dome. This stretches the obliterated umbilical artery, which is traced deep into the pelvis until the ureter is seen passing beneath. After the artery is divided, periureteral adventitial tissue is gently grasped to retract the ureter away from the bladder. Blunt dissection is used to mobilize 4 cm of the ureter proximal to the UVJ to permit placement within a bladder trough. Small vessels are isolated and carefully fulgurated with cautery, and the UVJ is cleared of any bulky surrounding tissues. The bladder wall trough is created by incising the detrusor with electrocautery along a line from the UVJ superiorly for approximately 3 cm and inferiorly for 1 cm. Gentle spreading of the muscle fibers opens the trough until mucosa bulges outward. This level of dissection is developed for the entire length of the tunnel. Muscle fibers around the UVJ are also spread slightly, but no attempt is made to extensively dissect the UVJ free of the bladder wall.

The ureter is advanced by placing a pexing suture that approximates lateral muscle at the distal end of the trough, distal ureter, and medial bladder muscle tissue at the end of the trough. Once the advancement is complete, the detrusor is approximated over the ureter with an absorbable polydioxanone suture.

After the repair is complete, instruments and trocars are removed after checking for trocar site bleeding or visceral injury. The fascial defects and skin of each port are closed with absorbable sutures. A bladder catheter may be kept overnight.

MEGAURETERS

The spectrum of anomalies known as megaureters (MGUs) continues to challenge today's urologists. As with reflux, the surgical solutions to the anomaly are reliable. Where controversy arises is in differentiating nonobstructive from obstructive variants and better defining the indications for surgery. The debate that ensues is similar to that seen with different degrees of hydronephrosis caused by obstructions of the UPJ. **It is increasingly apparent that many urinary tract dilatations represent distortions of the collecting system that, although at times quite severe, do not represent an obstructive threat to their associated renal moiety.** Examples that have been recognized for some time include MGU found with prune-belly syndrome and the postobstructive upper tract dilatation associated with urethral valves (Glassberg et al, 1977).

Perinatal ultrasonography has altered the understanding

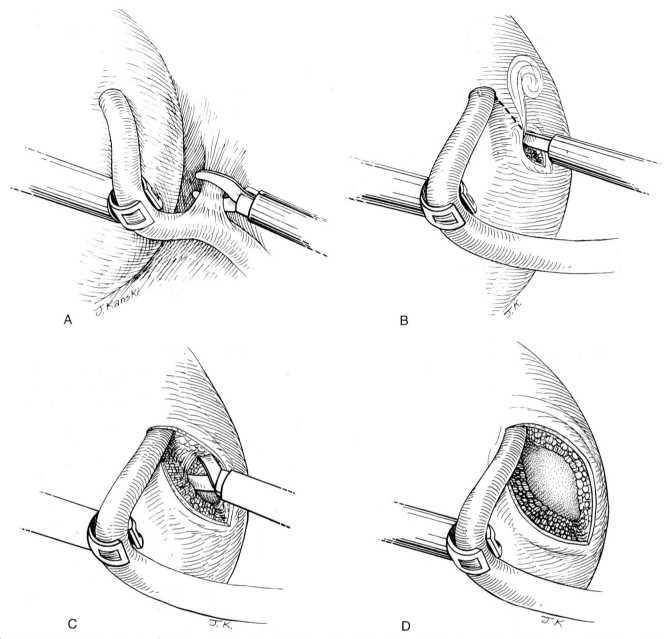

A

B

C

D

Figure 59–30. Laparoscopic reimplantation. *A,* Ureteral mobilization—the obliterated umbilical artery is identified and traced distally until the ureter is seen. *B,* The ureter is grasped gently, and the periureteral tissue is dissected bluntly toward the ureterovesical junction. *C* and *D,* Creation of bladder wall trough—the bladder wall is incised with electrocautery 3 cm proximal to the ureterovesical junction. Muscle fibers are gently cut and spread. Dissection is complete when mucosal tissue bulges outward.

and management of urologic anomalies and dilatations, with MGUs being no exception (Arger et al, 1986). In one series, MGU comprised 20% of antenatally diagnosed urologic anomalies, a percentage inordinately higher than that in historical series of urinary tract abnormalities, when most were discovered only after they became symptomatic (e.g., infection, calculi) (Preston and Lebowitz, 1989) and surgery was usually necessary. Today, through prenatal detection, the majority of children arrive with abnormalities that are totally asymptomatic. The denominator has increased, and its characteristics have changed. If left undetected, many MGUs might never become symptomatic—an observation that raises serious questions with regard to treatment. In the same manner, expectant treatment and serial ultrasonic follow-up studies have dramatically rede-

fined the natural history of multicystic dysplastic kidneys (Wacksman and Phipps, 1993), ureteroceles, and variants of UPJ obstructions (Homsy et al, 1986; Grignon et al, 1986, Johnson et al, 1987). The last are particularly significant, because mechanisms that affect the ureter at its junction with the renal pelvis and bring about the resolution of hydronephrosis may be similar to those that influence nonrefluxing MGUs.

Definitions

The normal ureteral diameter in children is rarely greater than 5 mm, and ureters wider than 7 mm can be considered MGUs (Hellstrom et al, 1985). The term *megaureter*

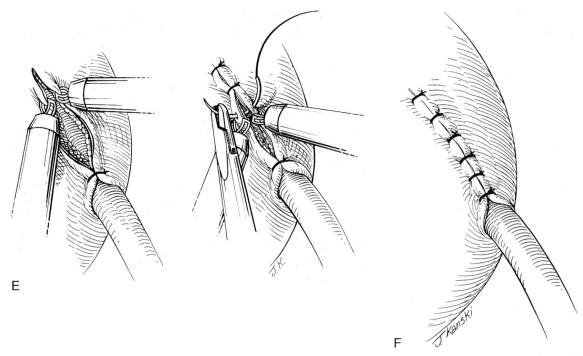

E

F

J.K.

J.Kanski

Figure 59–30 *Continued. E,* After the ureter is placed in the trough, grasping instruments wrap the superior aspect of the bladder wall around the ureter and a suture is placed proximally, immobilizing the ureter in the trough *(left).* Remaining sutures are placed throughout the length of the tunnel *(right). F,* Completed repair.

could be applied to any dilated or "big" (*mega*) ureter, but such use brings a generic connotation because it does not refer to any particular entity. This caused some confusion in the interpretation of earlier literature until an international classification system was derived (Smith, 1977); this system forms the basis of today's designations and serves as a useful guide for management when categorization is

possible (Fig. 59–31) (King, 1980). **The dilated ureter or MGU can be classified into one of four groups based on the cause of the dilatation: (1) refluxing, (2) obstructed, (3) both refluxing and obstructed, and (4) both nonrefluxing and nonobstructed.** Further subdivisions into primary or secondary causes assume additional importance for obvious reasons. A thorough evaluation of the entire uri-

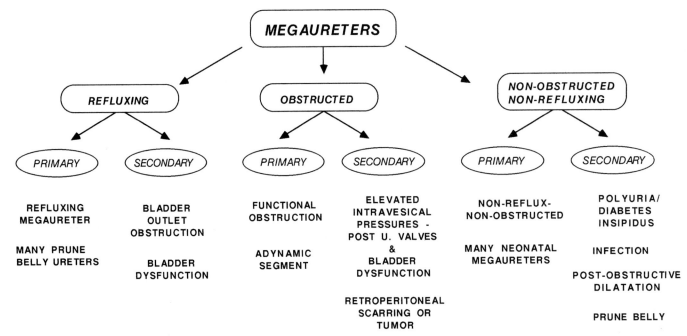

Figure 59–31. Three major classifications of megaureter based on primary and secondary etiologies. A combination of reflux and obstruction can also be seen with some megaureters.

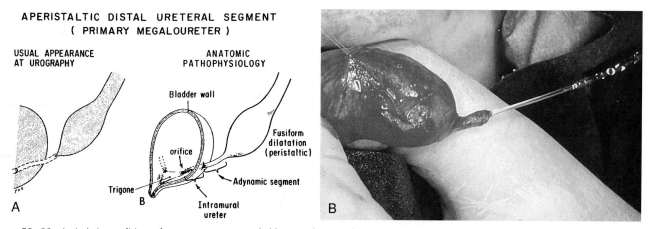

APERISTALTIC DISTAL URETERAL SEGMENT
(PRIMARY MEGALOURETER)

USUAL APPEARANCE
AT UROGRAPHY

ANATOMIC
PATHOPHYSIOLOGY

Bladder wall

Fusiform
dilatation
(peristaltic)

orifice

Trigone

Adynamic segment

Intramural
ureter

A   B   B

Figure 59–32. *A,* Artist's rendition of megaureter. Ureteral dilatation begins above the ureterovesical junction, usually a few millimeters or more above the bladder. (Courtesy of Dr. A.P. McLaughlin III). *B,* Typical appearance of distal portion of megaureter at exploration.

nary tract is required in every case, because therapeutic recommendations depend on proper categorization.

Pathophysiology

Primary and Secondary Refluxing Megaureter

The etiology of primary and secondary refluxing MGUs has already been discussed. **In addition, a small group of patients have an element of obstruction combined with reflux.** In one series of more than 400 refluxing ureters, obstruction was present in approximately 2% (Weiss and Lytton, 1974). A dysgenetic distal ureteral segment that not only fails to coapt within the intramural tunnel but also results in ineffective peristalsis is implicated. Identification is important, because management of obstruction, where expectant treatment is less likely to be successful, often differs from that of reflux alone.

Primary Obstructive Megaureter

It is generally agreed that the cause of primary obstructive MGU is an aperistaltic juxtavesical segment 3

to 4 cm long that is unable to propagate urine at acceptable rates of flow. The reason for this segmental aberrancy remains unclear (Fig. 59–32). True stenosis is rarely found, but a variety of histologic and ultrastructural abnormalities that alter function have been described. These include disorientation of muscle (Tanagho, 1973; MacKinnon, 1977), muscular hypoplasia, muscular hypertrophy, and mural fibrosis (McLaughlin et al, 1973) (Fig. 59–33). Excess collagen deposition is a common finding in light and electron microscopic studies (Gregoir and Debled, 1969; Hanna et al, 1976; Pagano and Passerini, 1977) (Figs. 59–34 and 59–35). In theory, increased matrix deposition alters cell-to-cell junctions and disrupts myoelectrical propagation and peristalsis. Ureteric profilometry shows irregular wave patterns within these segments, so-called "ureteroarrhythmias" (Shafik, 1998). Why the distal ureter is usually involved is unclear, but it may be related to arrested development in the musculature of this segment, which is the last portion of the ureter to develop (Tanagho, 1973).

Regardless of its origin, altered peristalsis prevents the free outflow of urine, and functional obstruction results. Retrograde regurgitation occurs as successive boluses of urine are unable to fully traverse the aberrant distal

Figure 59–33. *A,* Normal ureteral muscular orientation is sometimes seen with megaureters. *B,* Hypoplasia and atrophy of muscle is more common. (From McLaughlin AP III, Pfister RC, Leadbetter WF, et al: The pathophysiology of primary megaureter. J Urol 1973; 109:805–811, copyright © 1973 by The Williams and Wilkins Company, Baltimore.)

Normal   Hypoplasia

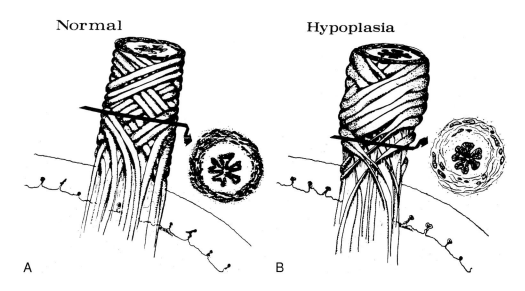

A   B

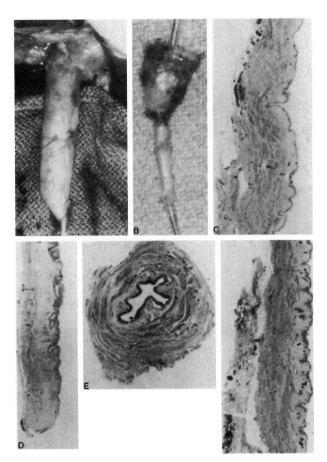

Figure 59–34. Primary obstructive megaureter. Light microscopic findings show various abnormalities. *A,* Operative exposure. *B,* Specimen. Obstructed segment admits probe. *C,* No abnormality seen on longitudinal section. *D,* Reduced muscle bulk seen in some megaureters. *E,* Preponderance of circular muscle. *F,* Thickened adventitia. (From Hanna MK, Jeffs RD, Sturgess JM, et al: Ureteral structure and ultrastructure: Part II. Congenital ureteropelvic junction obstruction and primary obstructive megaureter. J Urol 1978;116:728, copyright © 1973 by The Williams & Wilkins Company, Baltimore.)

segment. Pressure profiles of more proximal dilated ureter show arrhythmic patterns or virtually no rhythmic waves. The degree of ureteral dilatation that results depends on the amount of urine that is forced to coalesce proximally because of incomplete passage. This, in turn, is determined by the degree of distal obstruction and urinary output (Hutch and Tanagho, 1965). Disruption in ureteral dynamics has obvious implications for the renal parenchyma if the collecting system is unable to dampen the proximal pressures that can develop.

Other rare causes of primary obstructive MGU include congenital ureteral strictures (Allen, 1970) and ureteral valves (Albertson and Talner, 1972).

Secondary Obstructive Megaureter

This form of MGU most commonly occurs with neurogenic and non-neurogenic voiding dysfunction or infravesical obstructions such as posterior urethral valves. The ureter experiences increasing difficulty with propulsion of urine when an elevated pressure differential of greater than 40 cm H$_2$O exists across the UVJ. Progressive ureteral

dilatation, decompensation of the UVJ, reflux, and renal damage can be expected if such pressures continue unchecked. The dilatation that occurs with most of these variants largely resolves once the cause of the elevated intravesical pressures is addressed. In other cases, the ureter remains permanently dilated from what appears to be altered compliance or a permanent insult to the organ's peristaltic mechanisms, or both. Transmural scarring from chronic infection is implicated in some cases. Obstruction is not truly present within such ureters, but their abilities to buffer the kidney are lessened as elevated intravesical pressures are projected proximally as a noncompliant column (Jones et al, 1988). Other obstructive causes of ureteral dilatation, whose management is discussed in more detail elsewhere, include ureteroceles, ureteral ectopia, bladder diverticula, periureteral postreimplantation fibrosis, neurogenic bladder, and external compression by retroperitoneal tumors, masses, or aberrant vessels.

Secondary Nonobstructive, Nonrefluxing Megaureter

Nonobstructive, nonrefluxing MGUs are more common than once was recognized, and they often have an identifiable cause. **Significant ureteral dilatation can result from acute UTI accompanied by bacterial endotoxins that inhibit peristalsis.** Resolution is expected with appropriate antibiotic therapy (Retik et al, 1978). **Nephropathies and other medical conditions that cause significant increases in urinary output that overwhelm maximal peristalsis can also lead to progressive ureteral dilatation as collecting systems comply to handle the output from above. These include lithium toxicity, diabetes insipidus or mellitus, sickle cell nephropathy, and psychogenic polydipsia** (Keating, 1990). The most extreme examples of nonobstructed ureteral dilatations occur with the prunebelly syndrome. A spectrum exists, but many patients have markedly dilated and tortuous MGUs that belie the well preserved and normally functioning renal parenchyma above (Berdon et al, 1977; Keating and Duckett, 1993).

Primary Nonobstructive, Nonrefluxing Megaureter

Once reflux, obstruction, and secondary causes of dilatation have been ruled out, the designation of primary nonrefluxing, nonobstructive MGU is appropriate. Most newborn MGUs fall in this category (Keating et al, 1989; Rickwood et al, 1992; Baskin et al, 1994). In addition, many MGUs discovered in adults, where the distal ureteral spindle alone is dilated, are similarly categorized (Fig. 59–36). Explanations for the ureteral transformations that occur during development remain to be defined. However, a multifactorial etiology with a basis in transitional renal physiology and ureteral histoanatomy seems likely. The fetal kidney reportedly produces four to six times more urine before delivery than afterward, owing to differences in glomerular filtration, renal vascular resistance, and concentrating ability (Campbell et al, 1973). This relative deluge from above can "imprint" dilatation on the fetal ureter in a manner similar to that cited with the polyuric nephropa-

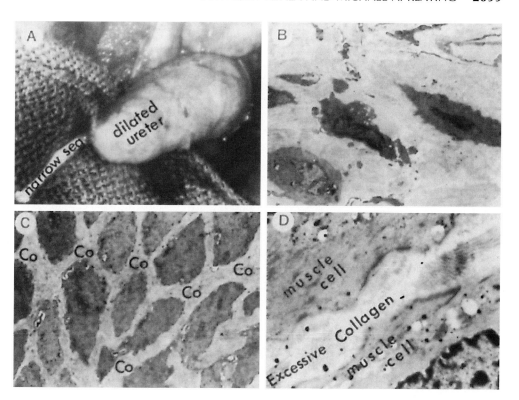

Figure 59–35. Primary obstructive megaureter: electron microscopic findings. *A,* Operative specimen. *B,* Muscle cell atrophy, absent nexus, and excessive ground substance and collagen in intracellular space from dilated ureter. *C,* Abnormal collagen fibers between muscle cells (×4000). *D,* Abnormality from narrow ureter (×17,000). (From Hanna MK, Jeffs RD, Sturgess JM, et al: Ureteral structure and ultrastructure: Part II. Congenital ureteropelvic junction obstruction and primary obstructive megaureter. J Urol 1978;116:728, copyright © 1973 by The Williams & Wilkins Company, Baltimore.)

thies, especially if a transient distal obstruction is present. Persistent fetal folds (Fig. 59–37) (Ostling, 1942), delays in the development of ureteral patency (Ruano-Gil et al, 1975), or immaturity of normal peristalsis are plausible causes of obstruction. The less compliant, hyperreflexic bladder of infancy (Baskin et al, 1994a) or a transient urethral obstruction that causes altered bladder compliance might also be implicated. Developmental alterations in ure-

teral compliance and changes in configuration could also result from differences in the deposition and orientation of elastin, collagen, and other matrices at different stages in development (Escala et al, 1989). **The newborn ureter is a more compliant conduit than that of the adult**—an impression borne out by the tortuous dilatations seen with distal obstruction in the infant, compared with the "pipe-stem" response that occurs at older ages. **As a result, the**

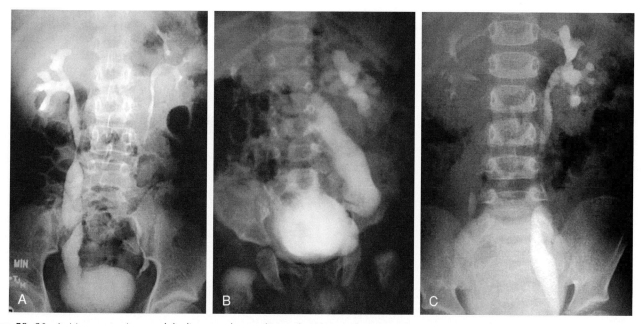

Figure 59–36. *A,* Megaureter in an adult discovered serendipitously. Most such cases are asymptomatic. The distal ureteral spindle typically is involved. *B,* Megaureter discovered antenatally and evaluated in the newborn period. It was thought to be a nonobstructive variant. *C,* Same child 2 years later. Continued maturation leaves the ureter with an appearance similar to that of adult.

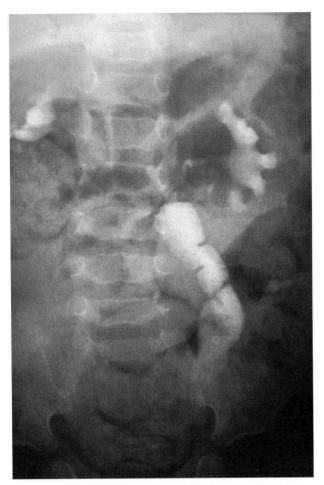

Figure 59–37. Ureteral folds perhaps implicated in early developmental obstructions. Lengthening with interval growth may bring about resolution.

kidneys of newborns are probably better buffered from the pressures of any partial or transient obstructions that might occur early in development than are kidneys obstructed at more proximal levels (UPJ) or at a later age.

Evaluation

Ultrasound is the initial study obtained in any child with a suspected urinary abnormality. It usually distinguishes MGU from UPJ obstruction as the most common cause of hydronephrosis; provides useful anatomic detail of the renal parenchyma, collecting system, and bladder; and offers a baseline standard for the degree of hydroureteronephrosis to use in serial follow-up studies (Fig. 59–38). Once ureteral dilatation is detected, a VCUG is obtained in most cases to rule out reflux and assess the quality of the bladder and urethra, where neurogenic dysfunction or outlet obstruction are common causes of secondary MGU. A study is also obtained to judge renal function and the degree of obstruction, if any. Excretory urography is rarely performed, because its functional data must be inferred. Substandard quality also presents a problem with neonates because of renal immaturity and bowel gas. The anatomic detail provided by an IVP is useful in cases where the level of obstruction cannot be defined, but this information can also be provided by retrograde pyelography at surgery. Instead, a diuretic renogram is preferred, because it offers objective, reproducible parameters of function and obstruction. ^{99m}Tc-DTPA and ^{99m}Tc-Mertiatide (MAG3) are the radionuclides most commonly used to provide parameters of function and clearance in the assessment of obstruction. However, the study has its shortcomings. Tracer dosing, timing in diuretic dosing, and patient hydration must be standardized to ensure valid comparison of test results. Subjective estimations must be made of the area of interest, which should include the lower ureter (Koff et al, 1984), and of the degree of filling of the affected system. These make timing of the administration of diuretic largely empirical, especially with MGUs. In addition, the immature glomeruli of the newborn kidney demonstrate a blunted response to diuretics. Whenever possible, it is preferable to defer the study for approximately 3 months to allow for glomerular maturation. Scans that evaluate drainage (half-life) alone routinely yield values indicative of obstruction because of the dilatation of the collecting system. As evaluators of function, however, these represent false-positive

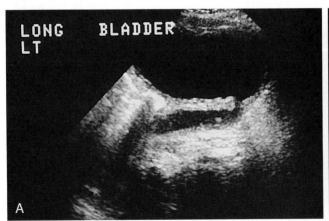
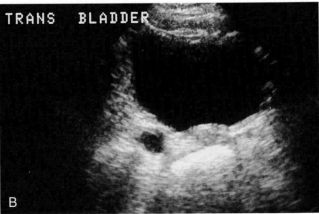

Figure 59–38. Urologic ultrasound study includes evaluation of the upper urinary tract as well as pelvis and bladder. A, Longitudinal study shows ureteral dilatation. B, Transverse study shows the same, behind the bladder on the right.

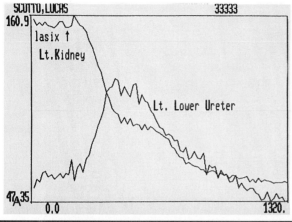

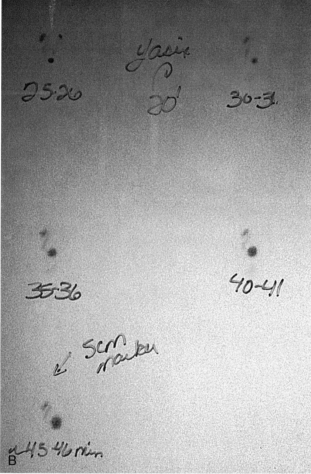

Figure 59-39. Diuretic renography (using diethylenetriamine penta-acetic acid, DTPA) of the megaureter shown in Fig. 59-38B. *A,* Washout curve from area of interest shows no evidence of obstruction, although delayed washout is commonly seen with such variants. *B,* Equal function was present on early sequences. Drainage is slightly impaired on the left.

studies. Useful information is provided when there is no evidence of obstruction (Fig. 59-39).

Radionuclide scans can also be used to estimate glomerular filtration rates and absolute renal function by measuring the uptake of radionuclide (DTPA) early after its systemic administration. Correlation with glomerular filtration is high (Heyman and Duckett, 1988). The percentage of the total dose, the so-called extraction factor, filtered by the kidneys can then be calculated and has been adopted by some institutions as a means of providing a more objective parameter for gauging significant obstruction. Fractional uptakes of radionuclide within the first few minutes should be approximately equal if significant function is not present. Ideally, these types of determinations offer functional correlates to hydroureteronephrosis by quantitating the effects of obstruction where it matters most, at the parenchymal level, rather than within the collecting system, where slow rates of washout are to be expected because of dilatation. Nevertheless, differentiating truly obstructive dilatations of the urinary tract from those that appear to represent no more than nonobstructive variants remains difficult. Particularly challenging can be bilateral MGUs, which do not provide a normal standard for comparison, and kidneys that may not function normally as a consequence of an earlier obstructive insult when actual obstruction no longer exists.

Whitaker's perfusion test (Whitaker, 1973) can also be used to evaluate obstruction, but its invasiveness is a drawback in children. In addition, the rate of flow at which intrapelvic pressures are measured (10 ml/min) is excessive for younger children and the parameters of obstruction empirically defined. The correlation of pressure perfusion with diuretic renography is good, but the study provides little additional data when compared with scintigraphy (Kass et al, 1983). Exceptions include renal moieties with extremely poor function and cases in which the diuretic renogram is equivocal or difficult to interpret because of a capacious collecting system. Cystoscopy is done in concert with surgery, if it becomes necessary. Retrograde imaging is rarely included in the initial evaluation of MGUs, whose anatomy can usually be defined by other means.

Recommendations

The therapeutic recommendations for MGUs that are truly obstructed and those that reflux are fairly well established. Where disagreement arises is in the differentiation of primary obstructed MGU from the nonrefluxing, nonobstructed variants, especially in the neonate. Given the constraints of the available diagnostic studies, classification is not always possible.

Primary Refluxing Megaureter

As discussed previously, the management of refluxing MGUs changed with the advent of antenatal detection. **Routinely recommending surgery in newborns and infants with grades IV or V reflux is no longer appropriate. Instead, medical management is appropriate during infancy and is continued if a trend to resolution is noted.** Otherwise, surgery remains the recommendation for persistent high-grade reflux in older children and adults. In the rare infant for whom medical management has failed but who is considered too small for reconstructive surgery, distal ureterostomy for unilateral reflux or vesicostomy for bilateral disease provides an ideal temporizing solution.

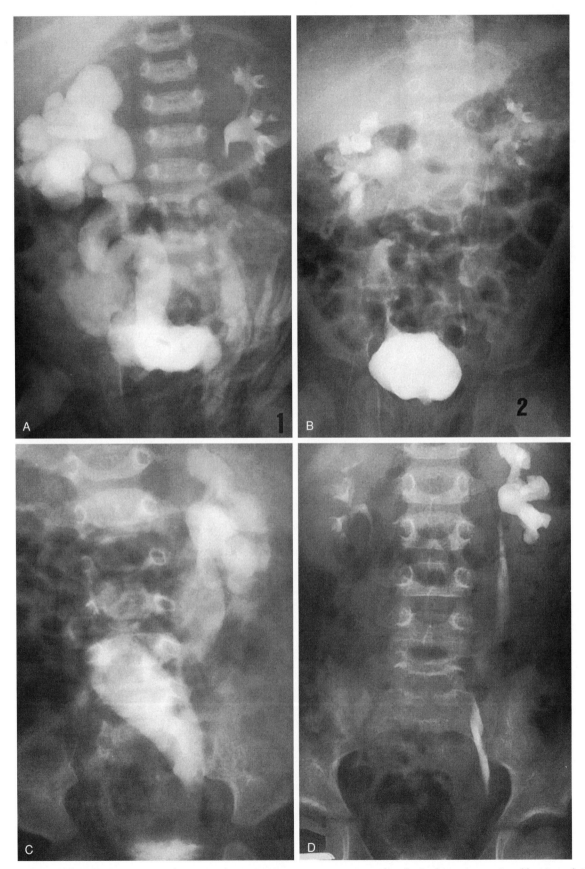

Figure 59–40. Neonatal megaureters managed expectantly. *A,* Excretory urogram at 3 weeks of age shows impressive dilatation of right ureter. The renal scan documented good function but delayed drainage. *B,* Excretory urogram in same patient 2 years later. *C,* Excretory urogram demonstrates impressively dilated left megaureter in a 6-week-old. *D,* Three years later, the appearance is almost normal.

Secondary Refluxing or Obstructive Megaureter

The management of secondary MGUs is directed at their cause. For example, impressive degrees of reflux and dilatation often improve with the ablation of urethral valves or medical management of neurogenic bladder. Other MGUs having secondary causes, including prune-belly syndrome, diabetes insipidus, or infection, require no more than observation alone. Chronic congenital distention, regardless of its source, imprints permanent dilatation on many collecting systems. As a result, some degree of nonobstructed hydroureteronephrosis usually persists, even after primary or secondary causes have been corrected. This dilation can be amplified with bladder filling, a finding that can pose a diagnostic dilemma because it mimics persistent or recurrent obstruction at the UVJ. Re-evaluation is often necessary.

Primary Nonobstructive, Nonrefluxing Megaureter

Deciding between surgery and expectant treatment sometimes becomes a function of clinical impression and experience. However, any haste in correcting MGUs in the newborn is tempered by the realization that their repair represents a technical challenge in smaller infants. Even in experienced hands, the complication rate of surgery is higher than in older children. For example, repeat surgeries were required for 5 (12%) of 42 infants operated on before 8 months of age in one series (Peters et al, 1989). **In light of such clinical observations, most clinicians now believe that as long as renal function is not significantly affected and UTIs do not become a problem, expectant management is preferred. Antibiotic suppression with close radiologic surveillance is appropriate in most cases.** Periodic checks of the urine and ultrasound scans every 3 to 6 months during the first year of life are appropriate. Renography is also sometimes repeated. The duration between studies is then extended if improvement in the degree of dilatation is seen. **When the hydroureteronephrosis is severe and shows no signs of improvement or the clinical status worsens, correction is undertaken when it is technically feasible, usually between the ages of 1 and 2 years.** For the occasional newborn who presents with massive ureteral dilatation or poor renal function (which is rare with MGUs) or develops recurrent infections, distal ureterostomy provides an effective panacea for poor drainage until the child is old enough to undergo reimplantation.

Clinical Correlates: Nonobstructive Megaureter

Past studies that have surgically addressed urinary tract obstructions and/or dilatations at both the UPJ and UVJ suffer from two weaknesses: (1) they lack a diagnostic modality that allows a uniform and reliable differentiation of nonobstructive from obstructive dilatations; and (2) they are unable to predict the degree of renal recoverability that

might occur after dilatations and/or obstructions have been corrected. In addition, data from surgical "corrections" of urinary tract dilatations in the neonate are skewed by a paradox peculiar to therapy at this age. That is, although truly obstructed kidneys are helped by surgery, operations also appear to benefit kidneys with preoperative dilatations that are not obstructed because of the increases in glomerular and tubular function expected of normal renal maturation. Obviously, the efficacy of surgery is difficult to judge in either instance (King et al, 1984; Peters et al, 1989; Koff and Campbell, 1992).

Antenatally diagnosed MGUs are different. Keating and coworkers (1989) evaluated 23 units in 17 newborns with observation alone. Renal scintigraphy (DTPA) and assessments of function rather than drainage defined the parameters of obstruction. Comparative IVP studies were also obtained in most patients. Notably, 20 (87%) of the 23 cases were deemed nonobstructive variants having no significant decrease in function and were followed up medically (Fig. 59–40). None showed a decrease in renal function after an average follow-up period of 7 years, and the improvement in dilatation that occurred in most was impressive (Baskin et al, 1994a). Others have since noted the same phenomenon, although functional deterioration or breakthrough UTI occurred in 13 (16%) of 82 neonatal MGUs in the combined series of Rickwood and associates (1992) and Liu and colleagues (1994). The rate of improvement seen with MGU is higher than the approximate 50% improvement seen in most series of UPJ obstructions (Homsy et al, 1986; Johnson et al, 1987). Expectant treatment of this type of MGU is not novel, however. Three decades ago, Williams and coworkers identified a subgroup of patients with obstructive ureters who had mild or negligible symptoms. Conservative management was recommended, although long-term follow-up results are unavailable (Williams and Hulme-Moir, 1970). Pitts and Muecke (1974) later observed a series of 80 patients with congenital MGU, 40% of whom required no therapy.

Primary MGUs coincidentally found in adults have radiographic appearances that usually remain stable over many years (Heal, 1973; Pfister and Hendren, 1978). Fusiform dilatations of the distal ureteral spindle comprise the most common variants although the entire ureter can be affected. Pyelocaliectasis is either absent or mild (Hanna and Wyatt, 1975). **It now appears that many perinatally diagnosed MGUs represent the anomaly at an earlier stage in its natural history and are precursors of the nonobstructive variants discovered serendipitously in adults in the past.**

Surgical Options

Once it has been determined that correction of a MGU is necessary, regardless of its etiology, the surgical objectives of ureteroneocystostomy are the same as for nondilated ureters. **Ureteral tailoring (excision or plication) is usually necessary to achieve the proper length-to-diameter ratio required of successful reimplantations. Narrowing of the ureter also theoretically enables its walls to coapt properly, leading to more effective peristalsis. Revising the distal segment intended for reimplantation**

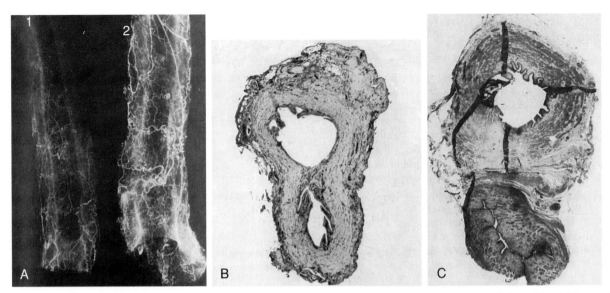

Figure 59–41. *A,* Comparison of microvasculature preservation in specimens obtained by excisional tapering *(left)* and by folding techniques *(right). B,* Histologic section of folded ureter 3 weeks postoperatively shows no obliteration of underfolded segment. *C,* Underfolded segment shows progressive obliteration at 3 months, although the lumen remains patent. (From Bakker HHR, Scholtameijer RJ, Klopper PJ: Comparison of 2 different tapering techniques in megaureters. J Urol 1988;140:1237.)

is all that is usually required. The proximal segments of most MGUs regain tone once they are unobstructed. Kinking is usually nonobstructive and will resolve. Children rarely have such massively dilated and tortuous ureters that straightening with removal of excess length and proximal revision becomes necessary (Hanna, 1979). Instead, extended stent drainage after tapering of such a ureter serves to decompress the system and allow for peristaltic recovery.

Two methods can be used to remodel MGUs. **Plication or infolding is useful for the moderately dilated ureter. Ureteral vascularity is preserved, and the revision can be taken down and redone if vascular compromise is suspected** (Bakker et al, 1988) (Fig. 59–41). **Bulk poses a problem with the extremely large ureter, however. Excisional tapering is preferred for the more severely dilated ureter or the ureter that is markedly thickened.** Plication of ureters greater than 1.75 cm in diameter experienced more complications in one series (Parrott et al, 1990). Remodeled MGUs have been generally reimplanted with standard cross-trigonal or Leadbetter-type techniques, but extravesical repairs can also be successfully done (Perovich, 1994). The success with reimplantation of remodeled MGUs, regardless of technique, is not as high as with nondilated ureters, yet the 90% to 95% approximated in most series is commendable (Hendren, 1969; Retik et al, 1978; Parrott et al, 1990).

Technique

The technique for repair of megaureter is shown in Figure 59–42.

1. The bladder is opened through a Pfannenstiel incision, and the ureter dissected from its intravesical and extravesical attachments as previously described. In some instances, it is possible to adequately mobilize the dilated ureter by staying within the bladder. When this is the case,

the maneuvers for reimplantation by either the Cohen or Politano-Leadbetter method are repeated after ureteral tailoring. However, when very large ureters are being tapered, it is advisable to go outside the bladder if there is any difficulty with mobilization to better define the blood supply.

2. If a method of reimplantation similar to the Politano-Leadbetter technique is chosen, it is wise to make the new hiatus before going extravesically. The hiatus is widened with a right-angle clamp, and the peritoneum swept from the base of the bladder, again using the lighted suction tip and Senn retractors. The clamp is incised upon and spread at an appropriate superior-medial location for the new hiatus. A red rubber catheter, which helps guide the ureter through its new hiatus, is engaged and carried extravesically and then back into the bladder, where it is snapped.

3. Dissection outside the bladder is begun by sweeping the lateral peritoneal attachments superiorly with a Kitner dissector. A right-angle clamp is used to pass the ureteral cuff stitch through the old hiatus to the perivesical space, and the ureter is brought extravesically.

4. The adventitia and blood supply to the lower ureter, which usually emanates medially, is carefully preserved. When working outside the bladder, it is helpful to divide the obliterated hypogastric artery to aid in the dissection and to eliminate it as a possible source of obstruction. Excessive mobilization and removal of proximal kinks is unnecessary.

5. After excision of any obstructive distal ureter or excessive length, ureteral tailoring is done over a No. 10 Fr red rubber catheter (No. 8 Fr in a baby). If the ureter is snug over the catheter, revisions are unnecessary. Otherwise, ureteral remodeling is recommended using one of the following methods:

Tapering (Fig. 59–43)—The technique used is similar to that originally described by Hendren (1969). Baby Allis clamps are placed laterally to define redundant

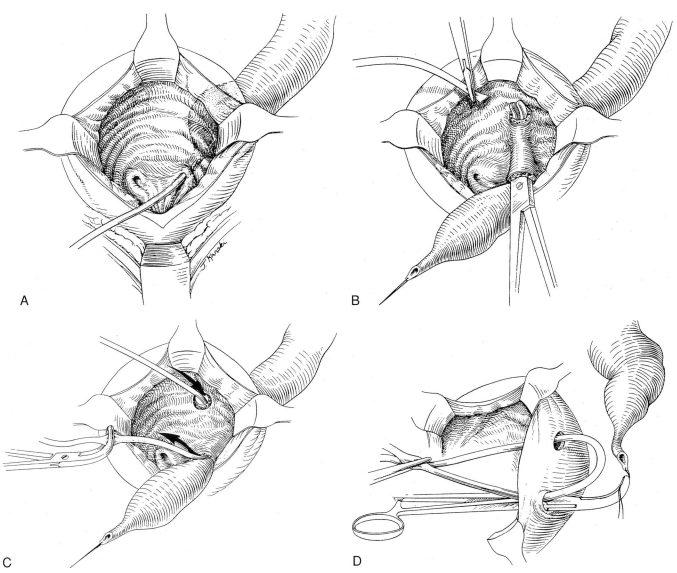

A

B

C

D

Figure 59–42. Technique for repair of megaureter. *A,* A No. 5 Fr feeding tube typically passes up a normal-caliber intravesical segment of primary obstructive megaureter. *B,* After the megaureter is freed from its intravesical and extravesical attachments, a blunt right-angle clamp is used to clear the peritoneum from the posterior and base of the bladder. If an extravesical dissection is necessary, it is advisable to make the new hiatus before moving outside the bladder. A right-angle clamp is incised upon and spread. *C,* A fine red rubber catheter marks the new hiatus by being pulled from within the bladder to the outside and then through the old hiatus. *D,* A right-angle clamp is guided from within the bladder to the perivesical space, where it is identified and incised upon. The ureter is brought extravesically by grasping the traction suture in the ureter.

ureter while preserving the medial vascular supply. Atraumatic clamps are applied around the catheter, and the excessive ureter is excised. Narrowing of the lumen should be avoided. A running, locking (to avoid reefing) 6-0 polydioxanone suture is used to reapproximate the proximal two thirds of the tapered ureter. Interrupted sutures complete the repair to allow for any shortening that might be necessary. The proximal portion of revised ureter should remain just outside the bladder after completion of the reimplantation with either tapering or plications.

Starr plication (Fig. 59–44)—Ureteral redundancy is again defined by briefly applying atraumatic clamps to mark the degree of necessary plication and preserve the best-vascularized portion of ureter. Starting proximally, the ureter is plicated anteriorly with interrupted

6-0 polydioxanone sutures placed in Lembert fashion along the clamp impressions (Starr, 1979).

Kalicinski plication (Fig. 59–45)—Two 6-0 polydioxanone sutures are placed along the clamp impressions, one at the proximal extent of the proposed revision and the other at the new meatus. The ureter is divided longitudinally by weaving one suture toward the other in running fashion, thus creating two lumens. The ureter is then reduced by folding its nonfunctional portion over the catheterized lumen (Kalicinski et al, 1977).

6. The reimplantation is completed using either the cross-trigonal or the Politano-Leadbetter technique. In the case of the latter, a right-angle clamp brings the revised ureter back into the bladder through the new hiatus, with the previously placed catheter used as a guide. It is often

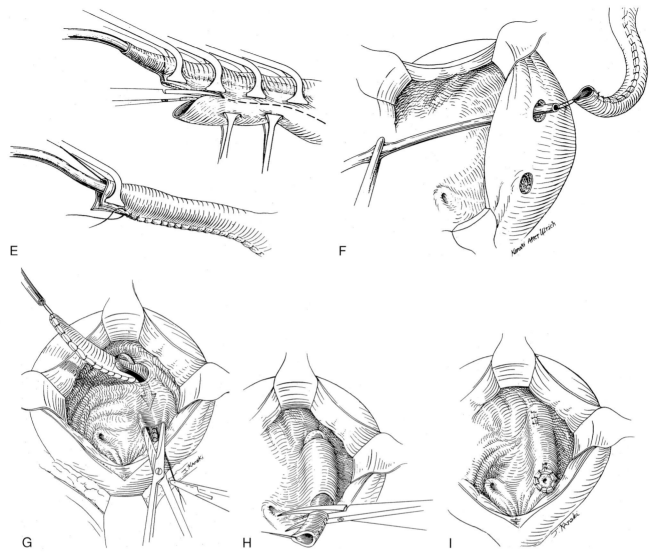

Figure 59-42 *Continued. E,* Ureteral tailoring is completed. Tapering is done over a No. 8 Fr red rubber catheter in infants or a No. 10 Fr in older children and adults. After vascularity is defined, special atraumatic clamps are placed over the catheter. Baby Allis clamps help retract the portion of ureter to be resected, which is usually lateral. It is important not to resect too much ureter. A running 5-0 polydioxanone or chromic suture is used to reapproximate the proximal two thirds of the ureter. Its distal third is closed with interrupted sutures to allow for shortening. *F,* The tailored ureter is brought back into the bladder through the new hiatus. *G,* After closing of the original hiatus, a new submucosal tunnel is made to the new hiatus. *H,* The distal portion of ureter is resected to match the length of the tunnel. *I,* The revised ureter is anastomosed to the bladder with fine interrupted sutures.

helpful to combine the repair with a psoas hitch, especially in smaller children.

7. Tapered ureters are stented for 5 to 7 days. Stentograms are unnecessary because leaks are rarely seen. Obstruction is also uncommon, although the stent itself often obstructs. Plicated ureters, in general, do not require stenting.

Results and Complications

The reimplantation of MGUs is associated with the same complications (i.e., persistent reflux and obstruction) as that of nondilated ureters, but at increased rates. Complications can occur regardless of whether excisional tapering or a folding technique is used. Perdzynski and Kalicinski (1996), for example, cited good results in 52 (93%) of 56

MGUs. Stenosis (2 cases) and reflux (2 cases) occurred in failures. Some authors have noted better results with obstructive MGU and higher rates of unresolved reflux after tailoring of refluxing variants (Johnston and Farkas, 1975). This has been attributed to a higher incidence of bladder dysfunction associated with the latter and to more dramatic abnormalities of their musculature.

The histologic study by Lee and colleagues (1992) demonstrated increased collagen deposition in refluxing MGUs and altered smooth muscle ratios that could severely affect function. In contrast, obstructive MGUs were not found to be statistically different from controls. In a subsequent study, the same investigators noted increased levels of type III collagen in refluxing MGUs. This less distensible subtype may cause an intrinsically stiffer ureter that lessens the surgical success in reimplantation of refluxing MGUs (Lee et al, 1998).

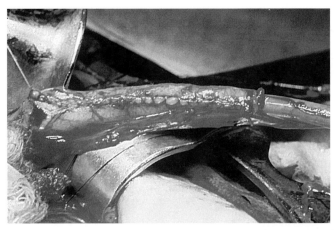

Figure 59–43. Megaureter shown in Figure 59–32*B* after excision of narrowed distal segment. Photography shows excisional tapering being completed.

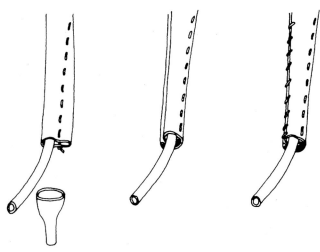

Figure 59–45. Ureteral folding technique. A running suture is longitudinally woven through the megaureter to create two lumens. This isolates the best-vascularized portion as functional ureter (catheter within) and excludes redundancy. The redundant portion is then folded, and the two are tacked together with interrupted sutures. (From Kalicinski ZH, Kansy J, Kotarbinska B, et al: Surgery of megaureters: Modification of Hendren's operation. J Pediatr Surg 1977;12:183.)

On rare occasions, reflux persists despite adequate ureteral tunnels in both tapered and normal-sized ureters. This may be a result of intrinsic ureteral dysfunction caused by transmural scarring after repeated infections or the insult of prior surgeries. The rigid distal ureter is incapable of normal peristalsis or appropriate coaptation during bladder contractions. TUU is ideal for unilateral disease. Bilateral cases can be treated by excising scarred distal ureter and creating exaggerated ureteral tunnels whose diameter-to-length ratio may exceed 10:1. In situ tailoring is another option for dilated ureters that continue to reflux after initial reimplantation. Vascularity is preserved and injury to the contralateral ureter avoided in unilateral cases (Diamond and Parulkar, 1998).

The Dilated Duplex Ureter

Duplications of the ureters are seen with anomalies commonly associated with reflux and/or obstruction that results in dilatation of one or both ureters. Examples include ureteroceles and ectopic ureters. With salvageable renal function, there are a number of surgical options, depending on the cause, the degree of dilatation, and whether one or both ureters are abnormal. Ureteroureterostomy provides an ideal solution when only one ureter of a duplex needs to be addressed. This can be done above the bladder through a lower-abdominal, extraperitoneal approach. Ureteropyelostomy is another option, but it leaves a segment of lower ureter unless a two-incision approach is used. When both ureters require correction, they can be mobilized within the bladder as a common sheath. One or both can then be tapered or plicated, depending on size. Tapering is performed on the side of the ureter (or ureters) away from the

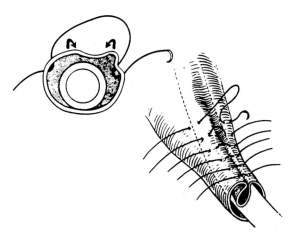

Figure 59–44. Ureteral plication is performed over the appropriate catheter with interrupted 5-0 polyglycolic sutures placed in Lembert fashion (after Starr). (From Keating MA, Retik AB: Management of failures of ureteroneocystostomy. In McDougal WS [ed]: Difficult Problems in Urologic Surgery. Chicago, Year Book, 1989, p 131.)

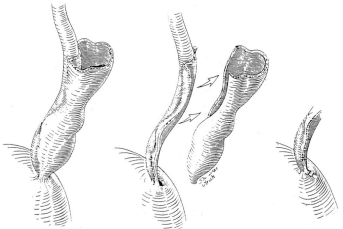

Figure 59–46. Excision of megaureter in a duplex system. Rather than separating its distal portion, the megaureter can be excised to this point. Distally, its inner wall is then excised to the bladder, leaving the common wall adjacent to the normal ureter intact. A suture is used to close its lumen at the bladder level. (From Retik AB, Colodny AH, Bauer SB: Pediatric urology. In Paulson DF (ed): Genitourinary Surgery, vol 2. New York, Churchill Livingstone, 1984, p 775.)

blood supply, which enters the adventitial septum between duplications (Weinstein et al, 1988). Reimplantation by a standard technique completes the repair. In cases where there is no function, excision of the MGU is done in concert with heminephrectomy. Because it is difficult to separate the distal segments of ureter, the common wall is left intact. After excision of lateral redundancy of the MGU, its lumen is closed distally at the bladder level (Fig. 59–46).

REFERENCES

Aaronson IA, Rames RA, Greene WB, et al: Endoscopic treatment of reflux: migration of Teflon to the lungs and brain. Eur Urol 1993;23:394–399.

Ahmed S, Tan H: Complications of transverse advancement ureteral reimplantation. J Urol 1982;127:970.

Akerlund A, Ahlstedt S, Hanson L, et al: Antibody responses in urine and serum against *Escherichia coli* O antigen in childhood urinary tract infection. Acta Pathol Microbiol 1979;87:29.

Albertson KW, Talner LB: Valves of the ureter. Radiology 1972;103:91.

Alberus MH, Salzano FM, Goldraich NP: Genetic markers and acute febrile urinary tract infection in the first year of life. Pediatr Nephrol 1997;11:691.

Allen TD: Congenital ureteral strictures. J Urol 1970;104:196.

Allen TD: Vesicoureteral reflux as a manifestation of dysfunctional voiding. In Hodson J, Kincaid-Smith P: Reflux Nephropathy. New York, Masson, 1979, pp 171–180.

Anderson NG, Abbott GD, Mogridge N, et al: Vesicoureteric reflux in the newborn: Relationship to fetal renal pelvic diameter. Pediatr Nephrol 1997;11:610.

Aragona F, D'Urso L, Scremin E, et al: Polytetrafluoroethylene giant granuloma and adenopathy: Long term complications following subureteral polytetrafluoroethylene injection for the treatment of vesicoureteral reflux in children. J Urol 1997;158:1539–1542.

Arant BS Jr: Medical management of mild and moderate vesicoureteral reflux: Follow-up studies of infants and young children. A preliminary report of the Southwest Pediatric Nephrology Group. J Urol 1992;148:1683.

Arap S, Abrao EG, Menezes de Goes G: Treatment and prevention of complications after extravesical antireflux technique. Eur Urol 1981;7:263.

Arger PH, Coleman BG, Mintz MC, et al: Routine fetal genitourinary tract screening. Radiology 1986;156:485.

Arnold GE: Vocal rehabilitation of paralytic dysphonia: Technique of intracordal injection. Arch Otolaryngol 1962;76:358.

Askari A, Belman AB: Vesicoureteral reflux in black girls. J Urol 1982;127:747.

Assael BM, Guez S, Marra G, et al: Congenital reflux nephropathy: A follow-up of 108 cases diagnosed perinatally. Br J Urol 1998;82:252.

Atala A: Laparoscopic technique for the extravesical correction of vesicoureteral reflux. Dialogues in Pediatric Urology 1993;16:12.

Atala A, Casale AJ: Management of primary vesicoureteral reflux. Inf Urol 1990;2:39–42.

Atala A, Cima LG, Kim W, et al: Injectable alginate seeded with chondrocytes as a potential treatment for vesicoureteral reflux. J Urol 1993a;150:745–747.

Atala A, Kavoussi LR, Goldstein DS, et al: Laparoscopic correction of vesicoureteral reflux. J Urol 1993b;150:748.

Atala A, Kim W, Paige KT, et al: Endoscopic treatment of vesicoureteral reflux with a chondrocyte-alginate suspension. J Urol 1994;152:641–643.

Atala A, Peters CA, Retik AB, Mandell J: Endoscopic treatment of vesico-ureteral reflux with a self-detachable balloon system. J Urol 1992;148:724.

Atala A, Ellsworth P, Share J, et al: Comparison of sonicated albumin enhanced sonography to fluoroscopic and radionuclide voiding cystography for detecting vesicoureteral reflux. J Urol 1998;160:1820.

Atala A, Wible, JH, Share JC, et al: Sonography with sonicated albumin in the detection of vesicoureteral reflux. J Urol 1993c;150:756–758.

Austenfeld MS, Snow BW: Complications of pregnancy in women after reimplantation for vesicoureteral reflux. J Urol 1988;140:1103–1106.

Bailey RR: The relationship of vesicoureteral reflux to urinary tract infection and chronic pyelonephritis-reflux nephropathy. Clin Nephrol 1973;1:132.

Baker R, Maxted W, Maylath J, et al: Relation of age, sex, and infection to reflux: Data indicating high spontaneous cure rate in pediatric patients. J Urol 1966;95:27.

Bakker HHR, Scholtameijer RJ, Klopper PJ: Comparison of 2 different tapering techniques in megaureters. J Urol 1988;140:1237.

Barrieras D, Lapointe S, Reddy PP, et al: Urinary retention after bilateral extravesical ureteral reimplantation: Does dissection distal to the ureteral orifice have a role? J Urol 1999;162:1197–1200.

Barrieras D, Lapointe S, Reddy PP, et al: Are postoperative studies justified after extravesical ureteral reimplantation? J Urol 2000;164:1064–1066.

Baskin LS, Meaney D, Landaman A, et al: Bovine bladder compliance increases with normal fetal development. J Urol 1994a;152:692.

Baskin LS, Zderic SA, Snyder HM, et al: Primary dilated megaureter: Long-term followup. J Urol 1994b;152:618.

Bauer SB, Retik AB: The non-obstructive ectopic ureterocele. J Urol 1978;119:804.

Bauer SB, Colodny AH, Retik AB: The management of vesicoureteral reflux in children with myelodysplasia. J Urol 1982;128:796.

Bellinger MF, Duckett JW: Vesicoureteral reflux: A comparison of non-surgical and surgical management. In Hodson J (ed): Reflux Nephropathy Update. Basel, S Karger, 1983, pp 81–93.

Bellinger MF, Duckett JW: Vesicoureteral reflux: A comparison of non-surgical and surgical management. Contrib Nephrol 1984;39:133.

Belman AB: A perspective on vesicoureteral reflux. Urol Clin North Am 1995;22:139.

Benador D, Benador N, Slosman D, et al: Are younger children at highest risk of renal sequelae after pyelonephritis? Lancet 1997;349:17.

Ben-Ami T, Gayer G, Hertz M, et al: The natural history of reflux in the lower pole of duplicated collecting systems: A controlled study. Pediatr Radiol 1989;19:308.

Berdon WE, Baker DH, Wigger HJ, Blanc WA: The radiologic and pathologic spectrum of prune belly syndrome. Urol Clin North Am 1977;15:83.

Berg S: Urethroplastie par injection de polytef. Arch Surg 1973;107:379.

Berg UB, Johansson SB: Age as a main determinant of renal function damage in urinary tract infection. Arch Dis Child 1982;58:963.

Beydoun SN: Morphologic changes in the renal tract in pregnancy. Clin Obstet Gynecol 1985;28:249.

Bhatti H, Khattak H, Boston V: Efficacy and causes of failure of endoscopic suburetric injection of Teflon in the treatment of primary vesicoureteric reflux. Br J Urol 1993;71:221.

Bieri M, Smith CK, Smith AY, Borden TA: Ipsilateral ureteroureterostomy for single ureteral reflux or obstruction in a duplicate system. J Urol 1998;159:1016–1018.

Birmingham Reflux Study Group: Prospective trial of operative versus non-operative treatment of severe vesicoureteric reflux in children: 5 Years observation. Br Med J (Clin Res Ed) 1987;295:237.

Bjorgvinsson E, Majd M, Eggli KD: Diagnosis of acute pyelonephritis in children: Comparison of sonography and 99mTc-DMSA scintigraphy. AJR Am J Roentgenol 1991;157:539.

Blackwell CC, May SJ, Brettle RP, et al: Host-parasite interactions underlying non-secretion of blood group antigens and susceptibility to recurrent urinary infections. In Lark D (ed): Protein Carbohydrate in Interactions in Biological Systems. London, Academic Press, 1986, p 229.

Blane CE, DiPietro MA, Zeim JM et al: Renal sonography is not a reliable screening examination for vesicoureteral reflux. J Urol 1993;150:752.

Blaufox MD, Gruskin A, Sandler P, et al: Radionuclide scintigraphy for detection of vesicoureteral reflux in children. J Pediatr 1971;79:239.

Blickman JG, Taylor GA, Lebowitz RL: Voiding cystourethrography as the initial radiologic study in the child with urinary tract infection. Radiology 1985;156:659–662.

Boechat MI, Lebowitz RL: Diverticula of the bladder in children. Pediatr Radiol 1978;7:22.

Bollgren I, Winberg J: The periurethral aerobic flora in girls highly susceptible to urinary tract infections. Acta Paediatr Scand 1976;65:81.

Bomalaski MD, Bloom DA: Urodynamics and massive vesicoureteral reflux. J Urol 1997;158:1236–1238.

Bomalaski MD, Hirschi RB, Bloom DA: Vesicoureteral reflux and ureteropelvic junction obstruction: Association, treatment options and outcome. J Urol 1997a;157:969.

Bomalaski MD, Ritcheny ML, Bloom DA: What imaging studies are necessary to determine outcome after ureteroneocystostomy? J Urol 1997b;158:1226–1228.

Bosio M: Cystosonography with echocontrast: A new imaging modality to detect vesicoureteric reflux in children. Pediatr Radiol 1998;28:250–255.

Boyarsky S, Labay P, Teague N: Aperistaltic ureter in upper urinary tract infection. Urology 1978;12:134–138.

Brannon W, Oschner MG, Rosencrantz DR, et al: Experiences with vesicoureteral reflux. J Urol 1973;109:46.

Bridge RAC, Roe CW: The grading of vesicoureteral reflux: A guide to therapy. J Urol 1969;101:821.

Brown T, Mandell J, Lebowitz RL: Neonatal hydronephrosis in the era of sonography. AJR Am J Roentgenol 1987;148:959–963.

Buckley JF, Scott R, Aitchison M, et al: Periurethral microparticulate silicone injection for stress incontinence and vesicoureteric reflux. Minin Invasive Ther 1991;1(Suppl. 1):72.

Bukowski TP, Betrus GG, Aquilina JW, et al: Urinary tract infections and pregnancy in women who underwent antireflux surgery in childhood. J Urol 1998;159:1286.

Buonomo C, Treves ST, Jones B, et al: Silent renal damage in symptom-free siblings of children with vesicoureteral reflux: Assessment with technetium Tc99m dimercaptosuccinic acid scintigraphy. J Pediatr 1993;122:721.

Burbige K: Ureteral reimplantation: A comparison of results with the cross-trigonal and Politano-Leadbetter techniques in 120 patients. J Urol 1991;146:1352.

Burbige KA, Lebowitz RL, Colodny AH, et al: Urinary tract infection in boys. J Urol 1984;132:541.

Burge D, Griffiths M, Malone P, et al: Fetal vesicoureteral reflux: Outcome following conservative postnatal management. J Urol 1992;148:1743.

Burger RH, Smith C: Hereditary and familial vesicoureteral reflux. J Urol 1971;106:845.

Burno DK, Glazier DB, Zaontz MR: Lessons learned about contralateral reflux after unilateral extravesical ureteral advancement in children. J Urol 1998;160:995–997.

Campbell S, Wladimiroff JW, Dewhurst CJ: The antenatal measurement of fetal urine production. J Obstet Gynaecol Br Common 1973;80:680.

Carpentier PJ, Bettink PJ, Hop WGJ, et al: A retrospective study of 100 ureteric implants by the Politano-Leadbetter method and 100 by the Cohen technique. Br J Urol 1982;54:230.

Carson CC III, Kelalis PP, Hoffman AD: Renal growth in small kidneys after ureteroneocystomy. J Urol 1982;127:1146.

Cascio S, Paran S, Puri P: Associated urological anomalies in children with unilateral renal agenesis. J Urol 1999;162:1081.

Chandra M, Maddix H: Urodynamic dysfunction in infants with vesicoureteral reflux. J Pediatr 2000;136:754–759.

Chandra M, Maddix H, McVicar M: Transient urodynamic dysfunction of infancy: Relationship to urinary infections and vesicoureteral reflux. J Urol 1996;155:673.

Choi KL, McNoe LA, French MC, et al: Absence of PAX2 gene mutation in patients with primary familial vesicoureteral reflux. J Med Genet 1998;35:338.

Chow SH, LaSalle MD, Stock JA, Hanna MK: Ureteroneocystostomy: To drain or not to drain. J Urol 1998;160:1001–1003.

Christie BA: Incidence and etiology of vesicoureteral reflux in apparently normal dogs. Invest Urol 1971;9:184.

Claes H, Stroobants D, Van Meerbeek J, et al: Pulmonary migration following periurethral polytetrafluoroethylene injection for urinary incontinence. J Urol 1989;142:821.

Claesson I, Jacobsson B, Olsson T, et al: Assessment of renal parenchymal thickness in normal children. Acta Radiol Diagn 1981;22:305.

Claesson I, Lindberg U: Asymptomatic bacteriuria in schoolgirls: VII. A follow-up study of the urinary tract in treated and untreated schoolgirls with asymptomatic bacteriuria. Radiology 1977;124:179.

Cohen RC, Moores D, Cooke-Yarborough C, Herrmann W: Laparoscopic bladder "wrap" technique for repair of vesicoureteric reflux in a porcine model. J Pediatr Surg 1999;34:1668–1671.

Cohen SH: Ureterozystoneostomie: Eine neue antirefluxtechnik. [A new technique for reflux prevention.] Aktuel Urol 1975;6:1.

Connolly LP, Treves ST, Connolly SA, et al: Vesicoureteral reflux in children: Incidence and severity in siblings. J Urol 1997;157:2287.

Connolly LP, Treves ST, Zurakowski D, et al: Natural history of vesicoureteral reflux in siblings. J Urol 1996;156:1805.

Conway JJ, Belman AB, King LR, Filmer RB: Direct and indirect radionuclide cystography. J Urol 1975;113:689.

Cooper CS, Chung BI, Kirsch AJ, et al: The outcome of stopping prophylactic antibiotics in older children with vesicoureteral reflux. J Urol 2000;163:269.

Cox CE, Hinman F: Experiments with induced bacteriuria, vesical emptying and bacterial growth in the mechanism of bladder defense to infection. J Urol 1961;117:472.

Crabbe DC, Thomas DF, Gordon AC, et al: Use of 99mtechnetium-dimercaptosuccinic acid to study patterns of renal damage associated with prenatally detected vesicoureteral reflux. J Urol 1992;148:1229–1231.

Craig JC, Knight JF, Sureshkumar P, et al: Vesicoureteric reflux and timing of micturating cystourethrography after urinary tract infection. Arch Dis Child 1997;76:275–277.

Daines SL, Hodgson NB: Management of reflux in total duplication anomalies. J Urol 1971;105:720.

Davey MS, Zerin JM, Reilly C, Ambrosius WT: Mild renal pelvic dilatation is not predictive of vesicoureteral reflux in children. Pediatr Radiol 1997;27:908–911.

Decter RM, Roth DR, Gonzalez ET: Vesicoureteral reflux in boys. J Urol 1988;40:1089.

DeKlerk DP, Reiner WG, Jeffs RD: Vesicoureteral reflux and ureteropelvic junction obstruction: Late occurrence of ureteropelvic obstruction after successful ureteroneocystotomy. J Urol 1979;121:816.

Dewan P, Guiney E: Endoscopic correction of primary vesicoureteral reflux in children. Urology 1992;39:162.

Dewan PA, Ehall H, Edwards GA: Ureteric tunnel incision in the fetal pig: A model for non-obstructive prenatal vesicoureteric reflux. Pediatr Surg Int 1999;15:350–352.

Diamond DA, Caldamone AA: Endoscopic correction of vesicoureteral reflux in children using autologous chondrocytes: Preliminary results. J Urol 1999;162:1185–1188.

Diamond DA, Parulkar BG: Ureteral tailoring in situ: A practical approach to persistent reflux in the dilated reimplanted ureter. J Urol 1998;160:998.

Diamond DA, Kleinman PK, Spevak M, et al: The tailored low dose fluoroscopic voiding cystogram for familial reflux screening. J Urol 1996a;155:681–682.

Diamond DA, Rabinowitz R, Hoenig D, Caldamone AA: The mechanism of new onset contralateral reflux following unilateral ureteroneocystostomy. J Urol 1996b;156:665–667.

Dillon MJ, Smellie JM: Peripheral renin activity, hypertension and renal scarring in children. Contrib Nephrol 1984;39:68.

Ditchfield MR, deCampo JF, Nolan TM, et al: Risk factors in the development of early renal cortical defects in children with urinary tract infection. Am J Radiol 1994;162:1393.

Ditchfield MR, Nadel HR: The DMSA scan in paediatric urinary tract infection. Australas Radiol 1998;42:318–320.

Dixon JS, Jen PY, Yeung CK, et al: The structure and autonomic innervation of the vesico-ureteric junction in cases of primary ureteric reflux. Br J Urol 1998;81:146.

Duckett JW: Vesicoureteral reflux: A "conservative" analysis. Am J Kidney Dis 1983;3:139.

Duckett JW, Walker RD, Weiss R: Surgical results: International reflux study in children—United States branch. J Urol 1992;148:1674.

Dunn M, Slade N, Gumpert JRW, et al: The management of vesicoureteral reflux in children. Br J Urol 1973;109:888.

Dwoskin JY, Perlmutter AD: Vesicoureteral reflux in children: A computerized review. J Urol 1973;109:888.

Dwoskin JY: Sibling uropathology. J Urol 1976;115:726.

Edwards D, Normand ICS, Prescod N, et al: Disappearance of vesicoureteral reflux during long-term prophylaxis of urinary tract infection in children. Br Med J 1977;2:228.

Ehrlich RM, Gershman A, Fuchs G: Laparoscopic vesicoureteroplasty in children: Initial case reports. Urology 1994;43:255.

Eke FU, Winterborn MH, Currie ABM, et al: Plasma renin activity in children after surgical relief of hydronephrosis. Int J Pediatr 1983;4:177.

Ekman H, Jacobsson B, Kock NG, et al: High diuresis: A factor in preventing vesicoureteral reflux. J Urol 1966;95:511.

Elder J: Commentary: Importance of antenatal diagnosis of vesicoureteral reflux. J Urol 1992;148:1750.

Elejalde BR, DeElejalde MM: Ureteral ejaculation of urine visualized by ultrasound. J Clin Ultrasound 1983;11:475–476.

El-Khatib M, Packham DK, Becker GJ, Kincaid-Smith P: Pregnancy-related complications in women with reflux nephropathy. Clin Nephrol 1994;41:50–55.

Ellsworth PI, Lim DJ, Walker RD, et al: Common sheath reimplantation yields excellent results in the treatment of vesicoureteral reflux in duplicated collecting system. J Urol 1996;155:1407–1409.

Escala JM, Keating MA, Boyd G, et al: Development of elastic fibers in the upper urinary tract. J Urol 1989;141:969.

Farnsworth JH, Rossleigh MA, Leighton DM, et al: Detection of reflux nephropathy in infants by 99m-technetium dimercaptosuccinic acid studies. J Urol 1991;145:542.

Ferro MA, Smith JH, Smith PJ: Periurethral granuloma: Unusual complications of Teflon periurethral injection. Urology 1988;31:422.

Filly RA, Friedland GW, Govan DE, et al: Urinary tract infections in children: Part II. Roentgenologic aspects. West J Med 1974;121:374.

Flood HD, Ritchey ML, Bloom DA, et al: Outcome of reflux in children with myelodysplasia managed by bladder pressure monitoring. J Urol 1994;152:1574.

Frey P, Gudinchet F, Jenny P: GAX65: New injectable cross-linked collagen for the endoscopic treatment of vesicoureteral reflux. A double-blind study evaluating its efficiency in children. J Urol 1997;158:1210–1212.

Frey P, Lutz N, Berger D, Herzog B: Histological behavior of glutaraldehyde cross-linked bovine collagen injected into the human bladder for the treatment of vesicoureteral reflux. J Urol 1994;152:632.

Frey P, Lutz N, Jenny P, Herzog B: Endoscopic subureteral collagen injection for the treatment of vesicoureteral reflux in infants and children. J Urol 1995;154:804.

Fung LCT, McLorie GA, Jain U, et al: Voiding efficacy after ureteral reimplantation: A comparison of extravesical and intravesical techniques. J Urol 1995;153:1972.

Funston MR, Cremin BJ: Intrarenal reflux: Papillary morphology and pressure relationships in children's necropsy kidneys. Br J Radiol 1978;51:665.

Geiss S, Alessandrini P, Allouch G, et al: Multicenter survey of endoscopic treatment of vesicoureteral reflux in children. Eur Urol 1990;17:328.

Gelfand MJ, Koch BL, Cordero GG, et al: Vesicoureteral reflux: Subpopulations of patients defined by clinical variables. Pediatr Radiol 2000;30:121.

Gil-Vernet JM: A new technique for surgical correction of vesicoureteral reflux. J Urol 1984;131:456.

Ginalski JM, Michaud A, Genton N: Renal growth retardation in children: Sign suggestive of vesicoureteral reflux? AJR Am J Roentgenol 1985;145:617.

Glassberg KI, Laungani G, Wasnick RJ, et al: Transverse ureteral advancement technique of ureteroneocystostomy (Cohen reimplant) and a modification for difficult cases (experience with 121 ureters). J Urol 1985;134:304.

Glassberg KI, Schneider M, Haller DO, et al: Observations on persistently dilated ureter after posterior urethral valve ablation. Urology 1977;9:1.

Glauser M, Lyons JM, Braude AI: Prevention of chronic pyelonephritis by suppression of acute suppuration. J Clin Invest 1978;61:403.

Glenn JF, Anderson EE: Distal tunnel ureteral reimplantation. J Urol 1967;97:623.

Glenn JF, Anderson EE: Technical considerations in distal tunnel ureteral reimplantation. J Urol 1978;119:194.

Gobet R, Cisek LJ, Chang B, et al: In a significant number of renal units experimental fetal vesicoureteral reflux induces renal tubular and glomerular damage, and is associated with persistent bladder instability. J Urol 1999;162:1090–1095.

Gobet R, Cisek LJ, Zotti P, Peters CA: Experimental vesicoureteral reflux in the fetus depends on bladder function and causes renal fibrosis. J Urol 1998;160:1058–1062; discussion, 1079.

Gonzalez ET, Glenn JF, Anderson EE: Results of distal tunnel ureteral reimplantation. J Urol 1972;107:572.

Goonasekera CD, Dillon MJ: Reflux nephropathy and hypertension: J Hum Hypertens 1998;12:497.

Goonasekera CD, Shah V, Dillon MJ: Tubular proteinuria in reflux nephropathy: Postureteric reimplantation. Pediatr Nephrol 1996a;10:559.

Goonasekera CD, Shah V, Wade AM, et al: 15-Year follow-up of renin and blood pressure in reflux nephropathy. Lancet 1996b;347:640.

Gordon AC, Thomas DF, Arthur RJ, et al: Prenatally diagnosed reflux: A follow-up study. Br J Urol 1990;65:407.

Gough DC, Postlewaite RJ, Lewis MA, et al: Multicystic renal dysplasia diagnosed in the antenatal period: A note of caution. Br J Urol 1995;76:244.

Govan DE, Palmer JM: Urinary tract infection in children: The influence of successful antireflux operations in morbidity from infection. Pediatrics 1969;44:677.

Gregoir W, Debled G: L'etiologie du reflux congenital et du mega-uretere primaire. Urol Int 1969;24:119.

Gregoir W, Schulman CC: Die extravesikale Antirefluxplastik. Urologe A 1977;16:124.

Gregoir W, Van Regemorter GV: Le reflux vesico-ureteral congenital. Urol Int 1964;18:122.

Grignon A, Filion R, Filiatrault D, et al: Urinary tract dilatation in utero: Classification and clinical applications. Radiology 1986;160:645.

Gruber GM: A comparative study of the intravesical ureter in man and experimental animals. J Urol 1929;21:567.

Gruss P, Walther C: PAX in development. Cell 1992;69:719.

Guizar JM, Kornhauser C, Malacara JM, et al: Renal tubular acidosis in children with vesicoureteral reflux. J Urol 1996;156:193.

Haberlik A: Detection of low-grade vesicoureteral reflux in children by color Doppler imaging mode. Pediatr Surg Int 1997;12:38–43.

Haferkamp A, Mohring K, Staehler G, Dorsam J: Pitfalls of repeat subureteral bovine collagen injections for the endoscopic treatment of vesicoureteral reflux. J Urol 2000;163:1919–1921.

Hagberg S, Hjalmas K, Jacobsson B, et al: Renal growth after antireflux surgery in infants. Z Kinderchir 1984;39:52.

Hanna MK: New surgical method for one-stage total remodeling of massively dilated and tortuous ureter: Tapering in situ method. Urology 1979;14:453.

Hanna MK, Jeffs RD, Sturgess JM, et al: Ureteral structure and ultrastructure: Part II. Congenital ureteropelvic junction obstruction and primary obstructive megaureter. J Urol 1976;116:725.

Hanna MK, Wyatt JK: Primary obstructive megaureter in adults. J Urol 1975;113:328.

Hannerz L, Wikstad I, Celsi G, et al: Influence of vesicoureteral reflux and urinary tract infection on renal growth in children with upper urinary tract duplication. Acta Radiol 1989;30:391.

Haraoka M, Senoh K, Ogata N, et al: Elevated interleukin-8 levels in the urine of children with renal scarring and/or vesicoureteral reflux. J Urol 1996;155:678.

Harcke HT, Capitanio MA, Grover WD, et al: Bladder diverticula and Menke's syndrome. Radiology 1977;124:459.

Harrison R: On the possibility and utility of washing out the pelvis of the kidney and ureters through the bladder. Lancet 1888;1:463.

Haycock GB: Investigation of urinary tract infection. Arch Dis Child 1986;61:1155.

Heal MR: Primary obstructive megaureter in adults. Br J Urol 1973;45:490.

Heidrick WP, Mattingly RF, Amberg JR: Vesicoureteral reflux in pregnancy. Obstet Gynecol 1967;29:571–578.

Heikel PE, Parkkulainen KV: Vesico-ureteric reflux in children: A classification and results of conservative treatment. Ann Radiol 1966;9:37.

Heimbach D, Bruhl P, Mallmann R: Lich-Gregoir anti-reflux procedure: Indications and results with 283 vesicoureteral units. Scand J Urol Nephrol 1995;29:311–316.

Hellstrom M, Hjalmas K, Jacobsson B, et al: Normal ureteral diameter in infancy and childhood. Acta Radiol 1985;26:433.

Hellstrom AL, Hjalmas K, Jodal U: Rehabilitation of the dysfunctional bladder in children: Method and 3-year followup. J Urol 1987a;138:847.

Hellstrom M, Judal U, Marild S, Wettergren B: Ureteral dilatation in children with febrile urinary tract infection or bacteriuria. AJR Am J Roentgenol 1987b;148:483.

Hendren WH: Operative repair of megaureter in children. J Urol 1969;101:491.

Hendren WH, Hensle TW: Transureteroureterostomy: Experience with 75 cases. J Urol 1980;123:826.

Henly DR, Barrett DM, Weiland TL, et al: Particulate silicone for use in periurethral injections: Local tissue effects and search for migration. J Urol 1995;153:2039–2043.

Henneberry MO, Stevens FD: Renal hypoplasia and dysplasia in infants with posterior urethral valves. J Urol 1980;123:912.

Herndon CD, McKenna PH, Kolon TF, et al: A multicenter outcomes analysis of patients with neonatal reflux presenting with prenatal hydronephrosis. J Urol 1999;162:1203–1208.

Heyman S, Duckett JW Jr: The extraction factor: An estimate of single kidney function in children during routine radionuclide renography with 99m technetium diethylenetriaminepentaacetic acid. J Urol 1988;140:780.

Hinchliffe SA, Chan YF, Jones H, et al: Renal hypoplasia and postnatally acquired cortical loss in children with vesicoureteral reflux. Pediatr Nephrol 1992;6:439.

Hinchliffe SA, Kreczy A, Ciftci AO, et al: Focal and segmental glomerulosclerosis in children with reflux nephropathy. Pediatr Pathol 1994;14:327.

Hinman F Jr: Nonneurogenic neurogenic bladder (the Hinman syndrome): 15 Years later. J Urol 1986;136:769.

Hinman FJ: Functional classification of conduits for continent urinary diversion. J Urol 1990;190:144.

Hinman F, Hutch JA: Atrophic pyelonephritis from ureteral reflux without obstructive signs (reflux pyelonephritis). J Urol 1962;87:230.

Hiraoka M, Hori C, Tsukahara H, et al: Congenitally small kidneys with reflux as a common cause of nephropathy in boys. Kidney Int 1997;52:811.

Hiraoka M, Hashimoto G, Hayashi S, et al: Ultrasonography for the detection of ureteric reflux in infants with urinary infection. Acta Paediatr Jpn 1996;38:248–251.

Hjalmas K, Lohr G, Tamminen-Mobius T, et al: Surgical results in the International Reflux Study in Children (Europe). J Urol 1992;148:1657.

Hodson CJ: The radiologic diagnosis of pyelonephritis. Proc R Soc Med 1959;52:669.

Hodson CJ, Davies Z, Prescod A: Renal parenchymal radiographic measurement in infants and children. Pediatr Radiol 1975a;3:16.

Hodson CJ, Edwards D: Chronic pyelonephritis and vesicoureteral reflux. Clin Radiol 1960;11:219.

Hodson J, Maling TMJ, McManamon PJ, et al: The pathogenesis of reflux nephropathy (chronic atrophic pyelonephritis). Br J Radiol Suppl 1975b;13:1.

Hollowell JG, Altman HG, Snyder H McC III, et al: Coexisting ureteropelvic junction obstruction and vesicoureteral reflux: Diagnostic and therapeutic implications. J Urol 1989;142:490.

Homsy YL, Nsouli I, Hamburger B, et al: Effects of oxybutynin on vesicoureteral reflux in children. J Urol 1985;134:1168.

Homsy YL, Williot P, Danais S: Transitional neonatal hydronephrosis: Fact or fantasy? J Urol 1986;136:339.

Horowitz M, Gershbein AB, Glassberg KI: Vesicoureteral reflux in infants with prenatal hydronephrosis confirmed at birth: Racial differences. J Urol 1999;161:248.

Houle AM, McLorie GA, Heritz DM, et al: Extravesical nondismembered ureteroplasty with detrusorrhaphy: A renewed technique to correct vesicoureteral reflux in children. J Urol 1992;148:704.

Howerton LW, Lich R Jr: The cause and correction of ureteral reflux. J Urol 1963;89:762.

Huland H, Busch R: Pyelonephritic scarring in patients with upper and lower urinary tract infections: Long-term follow-up in 213 patients. J Urol 1984;132:936.

Hulbert WC, Rosenberg HK, Cartwright PC, et al: The predictive value of ultrasonography in evaluation of infants with posterior urethral valves. J Urol 1992;148:122.

Human Renal Transplant Registry. The 12th report of the Human Renal Transplant Registry. JAMA 1975;233:787.

Husmann DA, Allen TD: Resolution of vesicoureteral reflux in completely duplicated systems: Fact or fiction? J Urol 1991;145:1022.

Hutch JA: Vesicoureteral reflux in the paraplegic: Cause and correction. J Urol 1952;68:457.

Hutch JA: The Ureterovesical Junction. Berkeley, University of California Press, 1958.

Hutch JA: Theory of maturation of the intravesical ureter. J Urol 1962;86:534.

Hutch JA: The mesodermal component: Its embryology, anatomy, physiology and role in prevention of vesicoureteral reflux. J Urol 1972;108:406.

Hutch JA, Tanagho EA: Etiology of nonocclusive ureteral dilatation. J Urol 1965;93:177.

Ibsen KK, Uldall P, Frokjaer O: The growth of kidney in children with vesicoureteral reflux. Acta Paediatr Scand 1977;66:741.

International Reflux Study Committee: Medical versus surgical treatment of primary vesicoureteral reflux. Pediatrics 1981;67:392–400.

Itoh K, Yamashita T, Tsukamoto E, et al: Qualitative and quantitative evaluation of renal parenchyma damage by 99mTc-DMSA planar and SPECT scintigraphy. Ann Nucl Med 1995;9:23.

Jacobson SH, Eklof O, Eriksson CG, et al: Development of hypertension and uraemia after pyelonephritis in childhood: 27 Year follow up. Br Med J 1989;299:703.

Jantausch BA, Criss VR, O'Donnell R, et al: Association of Lewis blood group phenotypes with urinary tract infection in children. J Pediatr 1994;124:863.

Jaswon MS, Dibble L, Puri S, et al: Prospective study of outcome on antenatally diagnosed renal pelvis dilatation. Arch Dis Child Fetal Neonatal Ed 1999;80:F135–F138.

Jayanthi VR, McLorie GA, Khang AE, Churchill BA: Extravesical detrusorrhaphy for refluxing ureters associated with paraureteral diverticula. Urology 1995;45:664.

Jeffs RD, Allen MS: The relationship between ureterovesical reflux and infection. J Urol 1962;88:691.

Jelakovic B, Benkovic J, Cikes N, et al: Antibodies to Tamm-Horsfall protein subunits prepared in vitro in patients with acute pyelonephritis. Eur J Clin Chem Clin Biochem 1996;34:315.

Jequier S, Jequier JC: Reliability of voiding cystourethrography to detect reflux. AJR Am J Roentgenol 1989;153:807.

Jequier S, Paltiel H, Lafortune M: Ureterovesical jets in infants and children: Duplex and color Doppler US studies. Pediatr Radiol 1990;175:349–353.

Jerkins GR, Noe HN: Familial vesico-ureteral reflux: A prospective study. J Urol 1982;128:774.

Jerkins GR, Noe HN, Hill D: Treatment of complications of cyclophosphamide cystitis. J Urol 1988;139:923.

Jodal U, Koskimies O, Hanson E, et al: Infection pattern in children with vesicoureteral reflux randomly allocated to operation or long-term antibacterial prophylaxis. The International Reflux Study in Children. J Urol 1992;148:1650.

Johnson CE, Shurin PA, Marchant CD, et al: Identification of children requiring radiologic evaluation for urinary infection. Pediatr Infect Dis 1985;4:656.

Johnson HW, Gleave M, Coleman GU, et al: Neonatal renomegaly. J Urol 1987;138:1023.

Johnson JH: Vesico-ureteral reflux: Its anatomical mechanism, causation, effects and treatment in the child. Ann R Coll Surg Engl 1962;30:324.

Johnston JH, Farkas A: The congenital refluxing megaureter: Experience with surgical reconstruction. Br J Urol 1975;47:153.

Jones DA, Holden D, George NJR: Mechanisms of upper tract dilatation in patients with thick-walled bladders, chronic retention of urine and associated hydroureteronephrosis. J Urol 1988;140:326.

Joseph DB, Young DW, Jordan SP: Renal cortical scintigraphy and single proton emission computerized tomography (SPECT) in the assessment of renal defects in children. J Urol 1990;144:595.

Jungers P, Houillier P, Chauveau D, et al: Pregnancy in women with reflux nephropathy. Kidney Int 1996;50:593.

Jungers T, Forget D, Houllier T, et al: Pregnancy in IgA nephropathy, reflux nephropathy, and focal glomerulosclerosis. Am J Kidney Dis 1987;9:334.

Kaack MB, Roberts JA, Baskin G: Maternal immunization with P fimbriae for the prevention of neonatal pyelonephritis. Infect Immun 1988;56:1.

Kaefer M, Curran M, Treves ST, et al: Sibling vesicoureteral reflux in multiple gestation births. Pediatrics 2000;105:800.

Kalicinski ZH, Kansy J, Kotarbinska B, et al: Surgery of megaureters: Modification of Hendren's operation. J Pediatr Surg 1977;12:183.

Kallenius G, Mollby R, Svenson SB, et al: Occurrence of P-fimbriated Escherichia coli in urinary tract infections. Lancet 1981;2:1369.

Kaplan GW: Postinfection reflux. Society for Pediatric Urology Newsletter 1980:April 9.

Kaplan WE, Firlit CF: Management of reflux in the myelodysplastic child. J Urol 1983;129:1195.

Kass EJ, Majd M, Belman AB: Comparison of the diuretic renogram and pressure-perfusion study in children. J Urol 1983;134:92.

Keating MA: A different perspective of the perinatal primary megaureter. In Kramer SA (ed): Problems in Urology. Philadelphia, JB Lippincott, 1990, p 583.

Keating MA, Duckett JW: Prune-belly syndrome. In Ashcraft KW, Holder TM (eds): Pediatric Surgery. Philadelphia, WB Saunders, 1993, p 721.

Keating MA, Escala J, Snyder HM, et al: Changing concepts in management of primary obstructive megaureter. J Urol 1989;142:636.

Keating MA, Retik AB: Management of failures of ureteroneocystostomy. In McDougal WS (ed): Difficult Problems in Urologic Surgery. Chicago, Year Book, 1989, pp 118–142.

Kennelly MJ, Bloom DA, Ritchey ML, Panzl AC: Outcome analysis of bilateral Cohen cross-trigonal ureteronecystostomy. Urology 1995;46:393–395.

Kershen RT, Atala A: New advances in injectable therapies for the treatment of incontinence and vesicoureteral reflux. Urol Clin North Am 1999;26:81–94.

King LR: Current management of vesicoureteral reflux. Journal of Continuing Education 1977.

King LR: Megaloureter: Definition, diagnosis and management. J Urol 1980;123:222.

King LR, Coughlin PWF, Bloch EC, et al: The case for immediate pyeloplasty in the neonate with ureteropelvic junction obstruction. J Urol 1984;132:725.

King LR, Kazmi SO, Belman AB: Natural history of vesicoureteral reflux: Outcome of a trial of nonoperative therapy. Urol Clin North Am 1974; 1:144.

Kiruluta HG, Fraser K, Owen L: The significance of the adrenergic nerves in the etiology of vesicoureteral reflux. J Urol 1985;136:232.

Klare B, Geiselhardt B, Wesch H, et al: Radiological kidney size in childhood. Pediatr Radiol 1980;9:153.

Koff SA: Relationship between dysfunctional voiding and reflux. J Urol 1992;148:1703.

Koff SA, Campbell K: Nonoperative management of unilateral neonatal hydronephrosis. J Urol 1992;148:525.

Koff SA, Fischer CP, Poznanski AK: The effect of reservoir height upon intravesical pressure. Pediatr Radiol 1979a;8:21.

Koff SA, Lapides J, Piazza DH: Association of urinary tract infection and reflux with uninhibited bladder contractions and voluntary sphincter obstruction. J Urol 1979b;122:373.

Koff SA, Murtaugh DS: The uninhibited bladder in children: Effect of treatment on recurrence of urinary infection and on vesicoureteral reflux resolution. J Urol 1983;130:1138.

Koff SA, Shore RM, Hayden LJ, et al: Diuretic radionuclide localization of upper urinary tract obstruction. J Urol 1984;132:513.

Koff SA, Wagner TT, Jayanthi VR: The relationship among dysfunctional elimination syndromes, primary vesicoureteral reflux and urinary tract infections in children. J Urol 1998;160:1019.

Kollerman VMW: Uberbewertung der pathogenetischen Bedeutung des vesiko-ureteralen Refluxes im Kindesalter. Z Urol 1974;67:573.

Kolon TF, Gray CL, Sutherland RW, et al: Upper urinary tract manifestations of the VACTERL association. J Urol 2000;163:1949.

Konda R, Sakai K, Ota S, et al: Urinary excretion of epidermal growth factor in children with reflux nephropathy. J Urol 1997;157:2282.

Kretschmer HL: Cystography: Its value and limitations in surgery of the bladder. Surg Gynecol Obstet 1916;23:709.

Kuhns LD, Hernandez R, Koff S, et al: Absence of vesicoureteral reflux in children with ureteral jets. Radiology 1977;124:185.

Kunin CM: Urinary tract infections in children. Hosp Pract 1976;11:91.

Lama G, Salsano ME, Pedulla M, et al: Angiotensin converting enzyme inhibitors and reflux nephropathy after 2-year follow-up. Pediatr Nephrol 1997;11:714.

Lamesch AJ: Retrograde catheterization of the ureter after antireflux plasty by the Cohen technique of transverse advancement. J Urol 1981; 125:73.

Lapides J, Diokno AC, Silber SJ, et al: Clean intermittent catheterization in the treatment of urinary tract disease. J Urol 1972;107:458.

Lapointe SP, Barrieras D, Leblanc B, Williot P: Modified Lich-Gregoir ureteral reimplantation: Experience of a Canadian center. J Urol 1998; 159:1662–1664.

Lattimer JK, Apperson JW, Gleason D, et al: The pressure at which reflux occurs: An important indicator of prognosis and treatment. J Urol 1963; 89:395.

Lebowitz RL: The detection and characterization of vesicoureteral reflux in the child. J Urol 1992;148:1640.

Lebowitz RL: Neonatal vesicoureteral reflux: What do we know? Radiology 1993;187:17.

Lebowitz RL, Avni F: Misleading appearances in pediatric uroradiology. Pediatr Radiol 1980;10:15–31.

Lebowitz RL, Blickman JG: The coexistence of ureteropelvic junction obstruction and reflux. AJR Am J Roentgenol 1983;140:231.

Lee BR, Partin AW, Epstein JI, et al: A quantitative histologic analysis of the dilated ureter of childhood. J Urol 1992;148:1482.

Lee BR, Silver RI, Parin AW, et al: A quantitative histologic analysis of collagen subtypes: The primary obstructed and refluxing megaureter of childhood. Urology 1998;51:820.

Leibovic SJ, Lebowitz RL: Reducing patient dose in voiding cystourethrography. Urol Radiol 1980;2:103–107.

Leighton DM, Mayne V: Obstruction in the refluxing urinary tract: A common phenomenon. Clin Radiol 1989;40:271.

Lenaghan D, Whitaker J, Jensen F, et al: The natural history of reflux and long term effects of reflux on the kidney. J Urol 1976;115:728.

Leonard MP, Canning DA, Peters CA, et al: Endoscopic injection of glutaraldehyde cross-linked bovine dermal collagen for correction of vesicoureteral reflux. J Urol 1991;145:115.

Leonard MP, Decter A, Mix LW, et al: Endoscopic treatment of vesicour-

eteral reflux with collagen: Preliminary report and cost analysis. J Urol 1996;155:1716–1720.

Levard G, Aigrain Y, Ferkadji L, et al: Urinary bladder diverticula and Ehlers-Danlos syndrome in children. J Pediatr Surg 1989;24:1184.

Liard A, Pfister C, Bachy B, Mitrofanoff P: Results of the Gil Vernet procedure in preventing contralateral reflux in unilateral ureteric reflux. BJU Int 1999;83:658–661.

Lich R, Howerton LL, Davis LA: Recurrent urosepsis in children. J Urol 1961;86:554.

Lichodziejewska M, Steadman R, Verrier Jones K: Variable expression of P-fimbriae in Escherichia coli urinary tract infection. Lancet 1989;1: 1414.

Linn R, Ginesin Y, Bolkier M, et al: Lich-Gregoir antireflux operation: A surgical experience and 5–20 years of follow-up in 149 ureters. Eur Urol 1989;16:200.

Lipski BA, Mitchelle ME, Burns MW: Voiding dysfunction after bilateral extravesical ureteral reimplantation. J Urol 1998;159:1019–1021.

Liu HYA, Dhillon HK, Yeung CK, et al: Clinical outcome and management of prenatally diagnosed primary megaureters. J Urol 1994;152: 614.

Loening-Baucke V: Urinary incontinence and urinary tract infection and their resolution with treatment of chronic constipation. Pediatrics 1997; 100:228.

Lombard H, Hanson LA, Jacobsson B, et al: Correlation of P blood group, vesicoureteral reflux and bacterial attachment in patients with recurrent pyelonephritis. N Engl J Med 1983;308:1189.

Lomberg H, Cedergren B, Leffler H, et al: Influence of blood group on the availability of receptors for attachment of uropathogenic Escherichia coli. Infect Immun 1986;51:919.

Lomberg H, Hellstrom M, Jodal U, et al: Virulence-associated traits in Escherichia coli causing first and recurrent episodes of urinary tract infections in children with and without reflux. J Infect Dis 1984;150: 561.

Lyon RP: Renal arrest. J Urol 1973;109:707.

Lyon RP, Marshall S, Tanagho EA: The ureteral orifice: Its configuration and competency. J Urol 1969;102:504.

Mackie GG, Stephens FD: Duplex kidneys: A correlation of renal dysplasia with position of the ureteral orifice. J Urol 1975;114:274.

MacKinnon KC: Primary megaureter. Birth Defects 1977;13:15.

Maizels M, Smith CK, Firlit CF: The management of children with vesicoureteral reflux and ureteropelvic junction obstruction. J Urol 1984;131:722.

Majd M, Rushton HG, Jantausch B, et al: Relationship among vesicoureteral reflux, P-fimbriated E. coli, and acute pyelonephritis in children with febrile urinary tract infection. J Pediatr 1991;119:578.

Malizia AA, Reiman HM, Myers RP, et al: Migration and granulomatous reaction after periurethral injection of polytef (Teflon). JAMA 1984; 251:3277.

Mandell J, Lebowitz RL, Peters CA, et al: Prenatal diagnosis of the megacystis-megaureter association. J Urol 1992;148:1487.

Manivel JC, Pettinata G, Reinberg Y, et al: Prune belly syndrome: Clinicopathologic study of 29 cases. Pediatr Pathol 1989;9:691.

Manley CB: Reflux in blond haired girls. Society for Pediatric Urology Newsletter 1981;October 14.

Mannhardt W, Schofer O, Schulte-Wiserman H: Pathogenic factors in recurrent urinary infection and renal scar formation in children. Eur J Pediatr 1986;145:330.

Mansfield JT, Snow BW, Cartwright PC, Wadsworth K: Complications of pregnancy in women after childhood reimplantation for vesicoureteral reflux: An update with 25 years of follow-up. J Urol 1995;154:787.

Marra G, Barbieri G, Dell'Agnola CA, et al: Congenital renal damage associated with primary vesicoureteral reflux detected prenatally in male infants. J Pediatr 1994a;124:726.

Marra G, Barbieri G, Moioli C, et al: Mild fetal hydronephrosis indicating vesicoureteric reflux. Arch Dis Child Fetal Neonatal Ed 1994b;70:F147.

Marshall JL, Johnson ND, DeCampo MP: Vesicoureteral reflux in children: Prediction with color Doppler imaging. Radiology 1990;175:355.

Martinell J, Jodal U, Lidin-Janson G: Pregnancies in women with and without renal scarring after urinary infections in childhood. Br Med J 1990;300:840.

Mathisen W: Vesicoureteral reflux and its surgical correction. Surg Gynecol Obstet 1964;118:965.

Matouschek E: Die Behandlung des vesikorenalen refluxes durch transuetherale (Einspritzung von polytetrafluoroethylenepaste). Urologe 1981;20:263.

Mayo ME, Burns MW: Urodynamic studies in children who wet. Br J Urol 1990;65:641.

Mazze RI, Schwartz FD, Slocum HC, et al: Renal function during anesthesia and surgery: 1. Effects of halothane anesthesia. Anesthesiology 1963;24:279.

McCool AC, Joseph BD: Postoperative hospitalization of children undergoing cross-trigonal ureteroneocystostomy. J Urol 1995;154:794–796.

McCord JM, Fridovich I: The biology and pathology of oxygen radicals. Ann Intern Med 1978;89:122.

McDonald A, Scranton M, Gillespie R, et al: Voiding cystourethrograms and urinary tract infections: How long to wait? Pediatrics 2000;105: E50.

McDougall EM, Urban DA, Kerbl K, et al: Laparoscopic repair of vesicoureteral reflux utilizing the Lich-Gregoir technique in the pig model. J Urol 1995;153:497.

McGladdery SL, Aparicio S, Verrier-Jones K, et al: Outcome of pregnancy in an Oxford-Cardiff cohort of women with previous bacteriuria. Q J Med 1992;83:533–539.

McLaughlin AP, Pfister RC, Leadbetter WF, et al: The pathophysiology of primary megaloureter. J Urol 1973;109:805.

McLorie GA, McKenna PH, Jumper BM, et al: High grade vesicoureteral reflux: Analysis of observational therapy. J Urol 1990;144:537.

McRae CU, Shannon FT, Utley WLF: Effect on renal growth of reimplantation of refluxing ureters. Lancet 1974;1:1310.

Melick WF, Brodeur AE, Karellos DN: A suggested classification of ureteral reflux and suggested treatment based on cineradiographic findings and simultaneous pressure recordings by means of the strain gauge. J Urol 1962;83:35.

Mendoza J, Roberts J: Effects of sterile high pressure vesicoureteral reflux on the monkey. J Urol 1992;148:1721.

Merguerian PA, Jamal MA, Agarwal SK, et al: Utility of SPECT DMSA renal scanning in the evaluation of children with primary vesicoureteral reflux. Urology 1999;53:1024–1028.

Merrell RW, Mowad JJ: Increased physical growth after successful antireflux operation. J Urol 1979;122:523.

Merrick M, Utley W, Wild S: The detection of pyelonephritic scarring in children by radioisotope imaging. Br J Radiol 1980;53:544.

Mevorach RA, Merguerian PA, Balcolm AH: Detrusorrhaphy for repair of unilateral vesicoureteral reflux: Report of 76 patients using a modified technique. J Urol 1998;51(5A Suppl):12–14.

Meyer R: Normal and abnormal development of the ureter in the human embryo: A mechanistic consideration. Anat Rec 1946;96:355.

Miller T, Phillips S: Pyelonephritis: The relationship between infection, renal scarring and antimicrobial therapy. Kidney Int 1981;19:654.

Minevich E, Aronoff D, Wacksman J, Sheldon CA: Voiding dysfunction after bilateral extravesical detrusorrhaphy. J Urol 1998a;160:1004–1006;1038.

Minevich E, Wacksman J, Lewis AG, Sheldon CA: Incidence of contralateral vesicoureteral reflux following unilateral extravesical detrusorrhaphy (ureteroneocystostomy). J Urol 1998b;159:2126–2128.

Mittleman RE, Marraccini JV: Pulmonary Teflon granulomas following periurethral polytetrafluoroethylene injection for urinary incontinence. Arch Pathol Lab Med 1983;107:611.

Miyakita H, Puri P: Particles found in lung and brain following subureteral injection of polytetrafluoroethylene paste are not Teflon particles. J Urol 1994;152:636.

Miyakita H, Puri P, Surana R, et al: Serum intercellular adhesion molecule (ICAM-1), a marker of scarring in infants with vesico-ureteric reflux. Br J Urol 1995;76:249.

Monga AK, Robinson D, Stanton SL: Periurethral collagen injections for genuine stress incontinence: A 2 year follow-up. Br J Urol 1995;76:156–160.

Najmaldin A, Burge DM, Atwell JD: Fetal vesicoureteral reflux. Br J Urol 1990;65:403.

Neal DE: Localization of urinary tract infections. AUA Update Series 1989;8:4.

Noe H: The role of dysfunctional voiding in the failure or complication of ureteral reimplantation for primary reflux. J Urol 1985;134:1172.

Noe HN: The relationship of sibling reflux to index patient dysfunctional voiding. J Urol 1988;140:119.

Noe HN: The long-term result of prospective sibling reflux screening. J Urol 1992;148:1739.

Noe HN, Wyatt RJ, Peeden JN Jr, et al: The transmission of vesicoureteral reflux from parent to child. J Urol 1992;148:1869.

North American Pediatric Renal Transplant Cooperative Study. Annual Report 1994. Hawthorn, NY, NAPRTCS Publications Committee, 1994.

O'Regan S, Yerbeck S, Schick E: Constipation, bladder instability, urinary tract infection syndrome. Clin Nephrol 1985;23:152.

O'Donnell B, Puri P: Treatment of vesicoureteric reflux by endoscopic injection of Teflon. Br Med J 1984;289:5–9.

Olbing H, Claesson I, Ebel K et al: Renal scars and parenchymal thinning in children with vesicoureteral reflux: The International Reflux Study in Children (European branch). J Urol 1992;148:1653.

Oliveira EA, Diniz JS, Silva JM, et al: Features of primary vesicoureteric reflux detected by investigation of foetal hydronephrosis. Int Urol Nephrol 1998;30:535–541.

Orskov I, Ferencz A, Orskov F: Tamm-Horsfall protein or uromucoid is the normal urinary slime that traps type I fimbriated *Escherichia coli*. Lancet 1980;1:887.

Ostling K: The genesis of hydronephrosis: Particularly with regard to the changes at the ureteropelvic junction. Acta Chir Scand Suppl 1942;86:72.

Ozyavuz R, Ozgur GK, Yuzuncu AK: Subureteric polydimethylsiloxane injection in the treatment of vesico-ureteric reflux. Int Urol Nephrol 1998;30:123–126.

Pagano P, Passerini G: Primary obstructed megaureter. Br J Urol 1977;49:469.

Paltiel JH, Rupich RC, Kiruluta HG: Enhanced detection of vesicoureteral reflux in infants and children with use of cyclic voiding cystourethrography. Radiology 1992;184:753.

Paltiel H, Mulkern RV, Perez-Atyde A, et al: Effect of chronic, low-pressure, sterile vesicoureteral reflux on renal growth and function in a porcine model: A radiological and pathological study. Radiology 2000;217:507.

Paquin AJ: Ureterovesical anastomosis: The description and evaluation of a technique. J Urol 1959;82:573.

Parrott TS, Woodard JR, Wolpert JJ: Ureteral tailoring: A comparison of wedge resection with infolding. J Urol 1990;144:328.

Parsons LC, Greenspan C, Mulholland GS: The primary antibacterial defense mechanism of the bladder. Invest Urol 1975;13:72.

Perdzynski W, Kalicinski ZH: Long-term results after megaureter folding in children. J Pediatr Surg 1996;31:1211.

Perovich S: Surgical treatment of megaureters using detrusor tunneling extravesical ureteroneocystostomy. J Urol 1994;152:618.

Persutte WH, Hussey M, Chyu J, Hobbins JC: Striking findings concerning the variability in the measurement of the fetal renal collecting system. Ultrasound Obstet Gynecol 2000;15:186–190.

Persutte WH, Koyle M, Lenke RR, et al: Mild pyelectasis ascertained with prenatal ultrasonography is pediatrically significant. Ultrasound Obstet Gynecol 1997;10:12–18.

Peters CA, Mandell J, Lebowitz RL, et al: Congenital obstructed megaureters in early infancy: Diagnosis and treatment. J Urol 1989;142:641.

Pfister RC, Hendren WH: Primary megaureters in children and adults: Clinical and pathophysiologic features in 150 ureters. Urology 1978;12:160.

Pieretti RV, Pieretti-Vanmarcke RV: Congenital bladder diverticula in children. J Pediatr Surg 1999;34:468–473.

Pitts WR, Muecke EC: Congenital megaureter: A review of 80 patients. J Urol 1974;111:468.

Pohl HG, Rushton HG, Park JS, et al: Adjunctive oral corticosteroids reduce renal scarring: The piglet model of reflux and acute experimental pyelonephritis. J Urol 1999;162:815.

Politano VA, Leadbetter WF: An operative technique for the correction of vesicoureteral reflux. J Urol 1958;79:932.

Politano VA, Small MP, Harper JM, Lynne CM: Teflon injection for urinary incontinence. J Urol 1974;111:180.

Polito C, La Manna A, Capacchione A, et al: Height and weight in children with vesicoureteral reflux and renal scarring. Pediatr Nephrol 1996;10:564.

Polito C, Marte A, Zamparelli M, et al: Catch-up growth in children with vesico-ureteral reflux. Pediatr Nephrol 1997;11:164.

Polito C, Moggio G, La Manna A, et al: Cyclic voiding cystourethrography in the diagnosis of occult vesicoureteric reflux. Pediatr Nephrol 2000;14:39–41.

Polk HC Jr: Notes on Galenic urology. Urol Surv 1965;15:25.

Pollet JE, Sharp PF, Smith RW, et al: Intravenous radionuclide cystography for the detection of vesicoureteral reflux. J Urol 1981;125:75.

Pomeranz A, Koretz Z, Regev A, et al: Is greater than normal nocturnal heart rate in children with reflux scars a predictor of reflux nephropathy? Blood Press Monit 1998;3:369.

Poznanski E, Poznanski AK: Psychogenic influences on voiding: Observations from voiding cystourethrography. Psychosomatics 1969;10:339.

Pozzi S: Ureteroverletzung bei Laparotomie. Zentrlbl Gynacol 1893;17:97.

Press SM, Badlani GH: Injection therapy for urinary incontinence. AUA Update Series 1995;14:14–20.

Preston A, Lebowitz RL: What's new in pediatric uroradiology? Urol Radiol 1989;11:217.

Prout GR Jr, Koontz WW Jr: Partial vesical immobilization: An important adjunct to ureteroneocystostomy. J Urol 1970;103:147.

Puri P, Cascio S, Lakshmandass G, et al: Urinary tract infection and renal damage in sibling vesicoureteral reflux. J Urol 1998;160:1028.

Puri P, Granata C: Multicenter survey of endoscopic treatment of vesicoureteral reflux using polytetrafluoroethylene. J Urol 1998;160:1007–1011;1038.

Ragan DC, Casale AJ, Rink RC, et al: Genitourinary anomalies with the CHARGE association. J Urol 1999;161:622.

Rames RA, Aaronson IA: Migration of polytef paste to the lung and brain following intravesical injection for the correction of reflux. Pediatr Surg Int 1991;6:239.

Ransley PG, Risdon RA: Reflux and renal scarring. Br J Radiol 1978;14(Suppl.):1.

Ransley PG, Risdon RA: Reflux nephropathy: Effects of antimicrobial therapy on the evolution of the early pyelonephritic scar. Kidney Int 1981;20:733.

Ransley PG, Risdon RA: Renal papillary morphology and intrarenal reflux in the young pig. Urol Res 1975;3:105.

Redman JF, Scriber LJ, Bissad NK: Apparent failure of renal growth secondary to vesicoureteral reflux. Urology 1974;3:704.

Retik AB, McElvoy JP, Bauer SB: Megaureters in children. Urology 1978;11:231.

Rickwood AMK, Jee LD, Williams MPL, et al: Natural history of obstructed and pseudo-obstructed megaureters detected by prenatal ultrasonography. Br J Urol 1992;70:322.

Ring E, Petritsch P, Riccabona M, et al: Primary vesicoureteral reflux in infants with a dilated fetal urinary tract. Eur J Pediatr 1993;152:523.

Roberts JA: Vesicoureteral reflux in the primate. Invest Urol 1974;12:88.

Roberts JA: Experimental pyelonephritis in the monkey: III. Pathophysiology of ureteral malfunction induced by bacteria. Invest Urol 1975;13:117.

Roberts J: Vesicoureteral reflux and pyelonephritis in the monkey: A review. J Urol 1992;148:1721.

Roberts JA: Mechanisms of renal damage in chronic pyelonephritis (reflux nephropathy). Curr Top Pathol 1995;88:265.

Roberts JA, Kaack MB, Baskin G: Treatment of experimental pyelonephritis in the monkey. J Urol 1990;143:150.

Roberts JA, Kaack MB, Fussell EF, et al: Immunology of pyelonephritis. VII. Effect of allopurinol. J Urol 1986;136:960.

Roberts JA, Kaack MB, Morvant AB: Vesicoureteral reflux in the primate, IV: Infection as a cause of prolonged high-grade reflux. Pediatrics 1988;82:91.

Roberts JA, Riopelle AJ: Vesicoureteral reflux in the primate: III. Effect of urinary tract infection on maturation of the ureterovesical junction. Pediatrics 1978;61:853.

Rolleston GL, Maling TMJ, Hodson CJ: Intrarenal reflux and the scarred kidney. Arch Dis Child 1974;49:531.

Rolleston GL, Shannon FT, Utley WLF: Follow-up of vesicoureteric reflux in the newborn. Kidney Int 1975;8:59.

Rose JS, Glassberg KI, Waterhouse K: Intrarenal reflux and its relationship to scarring. J Urol 1975;113:400.

Ruano-Gil D, Coca-Payeras A, Tejedo-Mateu A: Obstruction and normal recanalization of the ureter in the human embryo: Its relation to congenital ureteral obstruction. Eur Urol 1975;1:293.

Rushton HG: Genitourinary infections: Nonspecific infections. In Kelalis PP, King LR, Belman AB (eds): Clinical Pediatric Urology. Philadelphia, WB Saunders, 1992, pp 286–331.

Rushton HG, Majd M: Pyelonephritis in male infants: How important is the foreskin? J Urol 1992;148:733.

Rushton HG, Majd M, Chandra R, Yim D: Evaluation of 99m technetium-dimercapto-succinic acid renal scans in experimental acute pyelonephritis in piglets. J Urol 1988;140:1169.

Rushton HG, Majd M, Jantausch B, et al: Renal scarring following reflux and nonreflux pyelonephritis: Evaluation with ^{99m}technetium-dimercaptosuccinic acid scintigraphy. J Urol 1992;147:1327.

Salvatierra O Jr, Tanagho EA: Reflux as a cause of end stage kidney disease: Report of 32 cases. J Urol 1977;117:441.

Sampson JA: Ascending renal infections: With special reference to the reflux of urine from the bladder into the ureters as an etiological factor in its causation and maintenance. Johns Hopkins Hosp Bull 1903;14:334.

Sanyanusin P, Schimmenti LA, McNoe LA, et al: Mutation of the PAX2 gene in a family with optic nerve colobomas, renal anomalies and vesicoureteral reflux. Nat Genet 1995;9:358.

Sargent MA: What is the normal prevalence of vesicoureteral reflux? Pediatr Radiol 2000;9:587.

Savage JM, Koh CT, Shah V, et al: Renin and blood pressure in children with renal scarring and vesicoureteral reflux. Lancet 1978;8:441.

Savage JM, Koh CT, Shah V, et al: Five-year prospective study of plasma renin activity and blood pressure in patients with long-standing reflux nephropathy. Arch Dis Child 1987;62:678.

Scharer K: Incidence and causes of chronic renal failure in childhood. In Cameron D, Fries D, Ogg CS (eds): Dialysis and Renal Transplantation. Berlin, Pitman Medical, 1971, pp 211–217.

Schimberg W, Wacksman J, Rudd R, et al: Laparoscopic correction of vesicoureteral reflux in the pig. J Urol 1994;151:1664.

Scholtmeijer RJ: Treatment of vesicoureteric reflux: Results of a prospective study. Br J Urol 1993;71:346.

Scott JES, Stansfeld JM: Ureteric reflux and kidney scarring in children. Arch Dis Child 1968;43:468.

Scott JES, Lee REJ, Hunter EW, et al: Ultrasound screening of newborn urinary tract. Lancet 1991;338:1571.

Scott JES: Management of congenital posterior urethral valves. Br J Urol 1985;57:71.

Scott JES: Fetal ureteric reflux. Br J Urol 1987;59:291.

Selzman AA, Elder JS: Contralateral vesicoureteral reflux in children with a multicystic kidney. J Urol 1995;153:1252.

Semblinow VI: Zur pathologie der duech Bacterien bewinkten ambsteifenden Nephritis [1883 Dissertation]. Cited by Alksne J: Folia Urol 1907;1:338.

Seruca H: Vesicoureteral reflux and voiding dysfunction: A prospective study. J Urol 1989;142:494.

Shafik A: Ureterovesical junction inhibitory reflex and vesicoureteral junction excitatory reflex: Description of two reflexes and their role in the ureteric antireflux mechanism. Urol Res 1996;24:339.

Shafik A: Ureteric profilometry: A study of the ureteral pressure profile in normal and pathologic ureter. Scand J Urol Nephrol 1998;32:14.

Shannon A, Feldman W: Methodologic limitations in the literature on vesicoureteral reflux: A critical review. J Pediatr 1990;117:171.

Sheldon CA, Cormier M, Crone K, et al: Occult neurovesical dysfunction in children with imperforate anus. J Pediatr Surg 1991;26:49.

Shimada K, Matsui T, Ogino T, et al: Renal growth and progression of reflux nephropathy in children with reflux. J Urol 1988;140:1097.

Shopfner CE: Vesicoureteral reflux: Five year re-evaluation. Radiology 1970;95;637.

Sillen U: Vesicoureteral reflux in infants. Pediatr Nephrol 1999;13:355.

Sillen U, Bachelard M, Hansson S, et al: Video cystometric recording of dilating reflux in infancy. J Urol 1996;155:1711.

Skoog SJ, Belman AB: Primary vesicoureteral reflux in the black child. Pediatrics 1991;87:538.

Skoog SJ, Belman AB, Majd M: A nonsurgical approach to the management of primary vesicoureteral reflux. J Urol 1987;138:941.

Slotki IN, Asscher AW: Prevention of scarring in experimental pyelonephritis in the rat by early antibiotic therapy. Nephron 1982;30:262.

Smellie JM, Normand ICS: The clinical features and significance of urinary infection in childhood. Proc R Soc Lond 1966;59:415.

Smellie JM, Normand ICS: Experience of follow-up of children with urinary tract infection. In: O'Grady F, Brumditte W (eds): Urinary Tract Infection. London, Oxford University Press, 1968, p 123.

Smellie JM, Normand C: Reflux nephropathy in childhood. In Hodson CJ, Kincaid-Smith P (eds): Reflux Nephropathy. New York, Masson Publishing, 1979, pp 14–20.

Smellie JM, Normand ICS: Urinary tract infections in children 1985. Postgrad Med 1985;61:895.

Smellie JM, Edwards D, Hunter N, et al: Vesicoureteral reflux and renal scarring. Kidney Int 1975;8(Suppl 4):65.

Smellie JM, Edwards D, Normand ICS, et al: Effect of vesicoureteral reflux on renal growth in children with urinary tract infection. Arch Dis Child 1981a;56:593.

Smellie JM, Normand ICS, Katz G: Children with urinary infection: A comparison of those with and those without vesicoureteral reflux. Kidney Int 1981b;20:717.

Smellie JM, Preece MA, Paton AM: Normal somatic growth in children receiving low-dose prophylactic cotrimoxazole. Eur J Pediatr 1983;140:301.

Smellie JM, Ransley PG, Normand ICS, et al: Development of new renal scars: A collaborative study. Br Med J 1985;290:1957.

Smith ED: Report of working party to establish an international nomenclature for the large ureter. In Bergsman D, Duckett JW (eds): Birth Defects Original Articles Series 1977;13(5):3–8.

Solok V, Erozenci A, Kural A, et al: Correction of vesicoureteral reflux by the Gil-Vernet procedure. Eur Urol 1988;14:214.

Sommer JT, Stephens FD: Morphogenesis of nephropathy with partial ureteral obstruction and vesicoureteral reflux. J Urol 1981;125:67.

Song JT, Ritchie ML, Zerin JM, et al: Incidence of vesicoureteral reflux in children with unilateral renal agenesis. J Urol 1995;153:1249.

Sreenarasimhaiah S, Hellerstein S: Urinary tract infections per se do not cause end-stage kidney disease. Pediatr Nephrol 1998;12:210.

Starr A: Ureteral plication: A new concept in ureteral tapering for megaureter. Invest Urol 1979;17:153.

Stecker JF, Rose JG, Gillenwater JY: Dysplastic kidneys associated with vesicoureteral reflux. J Urol 1973;110:341.

Steinhardt GF: Reflux nephropathy. J Urol 1985;134:855.

Stenberg A, Lackgren G: A new bioimplant for the endoscopic treatment of vesicoureteral reflux: Experimental and short-term clinical results. J Urol 1995;154:800–803.

Stephens FD, Lenaghan D: The anatomical basis and dynamics of vesicoureteral reflux. J Urol 1962;87:669.

Stock JA, Wilson D, Hanna MK: Congenital reflux nephropathy and severe unilateral fetal reflux. J Urol 1998;160:1017.

Stockland E, Hellstrom M, Jacobsson B, et al: Early 99mTc dimercaptosuccinic acid (DMSA) scintigraphy in symptomatic first-time urinary tract infection. Acta Paediatr 1996;85:43–46.

Sutton R, Atwell JD: Physical growth velocity during conservative treatment and following subsequent surgical treatment for primary vesicoureteric reflux. Br J Urol 1989;63:245.

Tamminen-Mobius T, Brunier E, Ebel KD, et al: Cessation of vesicoureteral reflux for 5 years in infants and children allocated to medical treatment. The International Reflux Study in Children. J Urol 1992;148:1662.

Tanagho EA: Intrauterine fetal ureteral obstruction. J Urol 1973;109:196.

Tanagho EA, Hutch JA, Meyers FH, et al: Primary vesicoureteral reflux: Experimental studies of its etiology. J Urol 1965;93:165.

Tanagho EA, Meyers FH, Smith DR: The trigone: Anatomical and physiological considerations in relation to the ureterovesical junction. J Urol 1968;100:623.

Tarkington MA, Fildes RD, Levin K, et al: High resolution single photon emission computerized tomography (SPECT) 99m Technetium-dimercapto-succinic acid renal imaging: A state of the art technique. J Urol 1990;144:598.

Taylor A Jr: Quantitation of renal function with static imaging agents. Semin Nucl Med 1982;12:330.

Taylor CM, Corkery JJ, White RHR: Micturition symptoms and unstable bladder activity in girls with primary vesicoureteric reflux. Br J Urol 1982;54:494.

Torres M, Gomez-Pardo E, Dressler GR, et al: PAX-2 controls multiple steps of urogenital development. Development 1995;121:4057.

Torres VE, Kramer SA, Holley KE, et al: Effect of bacterial immunization on experimental reflux nephropathy. J Urol 1984;131:772.

Torres VE, Malek RS, Svensson JP: Vesicoureteral reflux in the adult: II. Nephropathy, hypertension and stones. J Urol 1983;130:41.

Torres VE, Moore SB, Kurtz SB, et al: In search of a marker for genetic susceptibility to reflux nephropathy. Clin Nephrol 1980;14:217.

Trsinar B, Cotic D, Oblak C: Possible causes of unsuccessful endoscopic collagen treatment of vesicoureteric reflux in children. Eur Urol 1999;36:635–639.

Urrutia EJ, Lebowitz TL: Re-reflux in blonde haired girls. Society for Pediatric Urology Newsletter 1983;October 14.

Vaisanen V, Tallgren L, Makela P, et al: Mannose-resistant hemagglutination and P-antigen recognition are characteristic of Escherichia coli causing primary pyelonephritis. Lancet 1981;2:1366.

Van den Abbeele AD, Treves ST, Lebowitz RL, et al: Vesicoureteral reflux in asymptomatic siblings of patients with known reflux: Radionuclide cystography. Pediatrics 1987;79:147.

Van Gool D, Hjalmas K, Tamminen-Mobius T, et al: Historical clues to the complex of dysfunctional voiding, urinary tract infection, and vesicoureteral reflux. The International Reflux Study in Children. J Urol 1992;148:1699.

Van Gool J, Tanagho EA: External sphincter activity and recurrent urinary tract infection in girls. Urology 1977;10:348.

Verber IG, Strudley MR, Meller ST: 99mTc dimercaptosuccinic acid (DMSA) scan as the first investigation of urinary tract infection. Arch Dis Child 1988;63:1320.

Vuckov S, Nikolic H, Kvesic A, Bukvic N: Our experience in the treatment of the vesico-ureteral reflux with Lich-Gregoir antireflux surgical procedure. Eur J Pediatr Surg 1999;9:33–36.

Wacksman J, Anderson EE, Glenn JF: Management of vesicoureteral reflux. J Urol 1978;119:814.

Wacksman J, Gilbert A, Sheldon CA: Results of the renewed extravesical reimplant for surgical correction of vesicoureteral reflux. J Urol 1992;148:359.

Wacksman J, Phipps L: Report of the multicystic kidney registry: Preliminary findings. J Urol 1993;150:1870.

Walker RD: Vesicoureteral reflux. In Gillenwater JY, Grayhack JT, Howards SS, et al (eds): Adult and Pediatric Urology, vol 2. Chicago, Year Book Medical Publishers, 1991, pp 1889–1920.

Walker RD: Vesicoureteral reflux update: Effect of prospective studies on current management. Urology 1994;43:279.

Walker RD, Duckett JW, Bartone F, et al: Screening school children for urologic disease. Pediatrics 1977;60:239.

Walker RD, Richard GA, Dobson D, et al: Maximum urinary concentration: Early means of identifying patients with reflux who may require surgery. Urology 1973;1:343.

Wallace DMA, Rothwell DL, Williams DI: The long term follow-up of surgically treated vesicoureteral reflux. Br J Urol 1978;50:479.

Walsh G, Dubbins PA: Antenatal renal pelvis dilatation: A predictor of vesicoureteral reflux? AJR Am J Roentgenol 1996;167:897.

Wan J, Greenfield SP, Ng M, et al: Sibling reflux: A dual center retrospective study. J Urol 1996a;156:677.

Wan J, Greenfield SP, Talley M, et al: An analysis of social and economic factors associated with follow-up of patients with vesicoureteral reflux. J Urol 1996b;156:668.

Weigert C: Ueber einige Bildunsfehler der Ureteren. Virchows Arch [Path Anat] 1877;70:490.

Weinberg B, Yeung N: Sonographic sign of intermittent dilatation of the renal collecting system in 10 patients with vesicoureteral reflux. J Clin Ultrasound 1998;26:65–68.

Weinstein AJ, Bauer SB, Retik AB et al: The surgical management of megaureters in duplex system: The efficacy of ureteral tapering and common sheath reimplantation. J Urol 1988;139:328.

Weiss R, Duckett J, Spitzer A, on behalf of the International Reflux Study in Children: Results of a randomized clinical trial of medical vs. surgical management of infants and children with grades III and IV primary vesicoureteral reflux (United States). J Urol 1992a;148:1667.

Weiss RM, Lytton B: Vesicoureteral reflux and distal ureteral obstruction. J Urol 1974;111:245.

Weiss R, Tamminen-Mobius T, Koskimies O, on behalf of the International Reflux Study in Children: Characteristics of entry in children with severe primary vesicoureteral reflux recruited for a multicenter international therapeutic trial comparing medical and surgical management. J Urol 1992b;148:1644.

Wennerstrom M, Hansson S, Jodal U, et al: Primary and acquired renal scarring in boys and girls with urinary tract infection. J Pediatr 2000;136:30.

Wettgren B, Jodal U, Jonasson G: Epidemiology of bacteriuria during the first year of life. Acta Paediatr Scand 1985;74:925.

Whitaker RH: Methods of assessing obstruction in dilated ureter. Br J Urol 1973;45:15.

Whitaker RH: Reflux induced pelvi-ureteric obstruction. Br J Urol 1976;48:555.

Willemsen J, Nijman RJ: Vesicoureteral reflux and videourodynamic studies: Results of a prospective study. Urology 2000;55:939–943.

Willi U, Treves S: Radionuclide voiding cystography. Urol Radiol 1983;5:161.

Williams GL, Davies DKL, Evans KT, Williams JE: Vesicoureteral reflux in patients with bacteriuria in pregnancy. Lancet 1968;2:1202.

Williams DI, Hulme-Moir I: Primary obstructive mega-ureter. Br J Urol 1970;42:140.

Willscher MK, Bauer SB, Zammuto PJ, et al: Renal growth and urinary infection following antireflux surgery in infants and children. J Urol 1976;115:722.

Wilson DB: Transcription factors: Regulators of gene expression in normal pathological states. Ann Med 1996;28:1.

Winberg J: Commentary: Progressive renal damage from infection with or without reflux. J Urol 1992;148:1733.

Winberg J, Andersen HJ, Bergstrom T, et al: Epidemiology of symptomatic urinary tract infection in childhood. Acta Pathol Scand Suppl 1974;252:1.

Winter AL, Hardy BE, Alton DJ, et al: Acquired renal scars in children. J Urol 1983;129:1190.

Winter CC: Vesicoureteral Reflux and Its Treatment. New York, Appleton-Century-Crofts, 1969.

Wiswell TE, Enzenauer RM, Holton ME, et al: Declining frequencies of circumcision: Implications for changes in the incidence of male to female sex ratio of upper tract infection in early infancy. Pediatrics 1987;79:338.

Wiswell TE, Roscelli JD: Corroborative evidence for the decreased incidence of urinary tract infections in circumcised male infants. Pediatrics 1986;78:96.

Wolfish NM, Delbrouck NF, Shanon A: Prevalence of hypertension in children with primary vesicoureteral reflux. J Pediatr 1993;123:559.

Woodard JR, Holden S: The prognostic significance of fever in childhood urinary infections: Observations in 350 consecutive patients. Clin Pediatr (Phila) 1976;15:1051.

Yen TC, Tzen KY, Lin WY, et al: Identification of new renal scarring in repeated episodes of acute pyelonephritis using Tc-99m DMSA renal SPECT. Clin Nucl Med 1998;23:828–831.

Yerkes EB, Adams MC, Pope JC, et al: Does every patient with prenatal hydronephrosis need voiding cystourethrography? J Urol 1999;162:1218.

Yeung CK, Godley ML, Dhillon HK, et al: The characteristics of primary vesico-ureteral reflux in male and female infants with pre-natal hydronephrosis. Br J Urol 1997;80:319.

Yeung CK, Godley ML, Dhillon HK, et al: Urodynamic patterns in infants with normal lower urinary tracts or primary vesico-ureteric reflux. Br J Urol 1998;81:461–467.

Young HH: Johns Hopkins Hosp Bull 1898;9:100.

Zaontz MR, Maizels M, Sugar EC, et al: Detrusorrhaphy: Extravesical ureteral advancement to correct vesicoureteral reflux in children. J Urol 1987;138:947.

Zerin JM, Ritchey ML, Chang AC: Incidental vesicoureteral reflux in neonates with antenatally detected hydronephrosis and other renal abnormalities. Radiology 1993;187:157.

60
PRUNE-BELLY SYNDROME

Edwin A. Smith, M.D.
John R. Woodard, M.D.

Prune-belly syndrome **is the most common term for the congenital absence, deficiency, or hypoplasia of the abdominal musculature accompanied by a large hypotonic bladder, dilated and tortuous ureters, and bilateral cryptorchidism** (Osler, 1901). Known since Frolich's description in 1839, it has been of interest to urologists since 1895, when Parker described the genitourinary involvement (Frolich, 1839; Parker, 1895). Because of the involvement of the abdominal musculature, urinary tract, and testicles, the term *triad syndrome* is commonly used. It is also referred to as the *Eagle-Barrett syndrome* (Eagle and Barrett, 1950). The reported incidence has ranged from 1 in 35,000 to 1 in 50,000 live births, with twins, blacks, and children born to younger mothers appearing to be at higher risk in at least one epidemiologic study (Garlinger and Ott, 1974; Druschel, 1995).

Historically, infants born with the full-blown syndrome have had a poor prognosis for long-term survival. A high percentage of such infants die from urinary sepsis, renal failure, or both (Lattimer, 1958; McGovern and Marshall, 1959; Burke et al, 1969; Barnhouse, 1972). Although the prognosis for these patients has improved, controversy exists between those who believe a more aggressive approach toward surgical reconstruction of the urinary tract might improve the survival and quality of life of these children (Hendren, 1972; Jeffs et al, 1977; Woodard and Parrott, 1978a; Randolph et al, 1981b; Fallat et al, 1989) and those who advocate limited or no surgical intervention (Woodhouse et al, 1979; Duckett, 1980).

In rare instances, a girl is affected by the abdominal wall defect of the abdominal muscles, but it is exceptional to find the characteristic urinary tract anomaly at the same time (Aaronson and Cremin, 1980). Virtually by definition, the fully developed syndrome occurs almost exclusively in boys. Infants with the prune-belly syndrome may be born of entirely normal pregnancies; however, oligohydramnios is more often the rule, and it is responsible for some of the associated and complicating conditions, especially the pulmonary and skeletal anomalies. With the increased use of diagnostic fetal ultrasound, it is no longer novel for a presumptive diagnosis of prune-belly syndrome to be made in utero. The clinical significance of such a fetal diagnosis is discussed later in this chapter. The appearance of the neonate is now so well known to neonatologists and pediatricians that it is unlikely to be missed (Fig. 60–1). The abdominal wall is thin and lax and, because of the sparsity of subcutaneous tissue, tends to be creased and wrinkled like a wizened prune. The liver edge, spleen, intestines, and distended bladder are often quite evident on viewing the abdominal wall externally.

The cause of prune-belly syndrome remains unknown. Some have suggested that both the abdominal wall defect and the intra-abdominal cryptorchidism are secondary to distention of the urinary tract during early fetal development. **Obstruction in the posterior urethra is a possible cause** of this distention and would explain the predominance of male patients (Pagon et al, 1979; Nakayama et al, 1984). This theory suggests that testicular de-

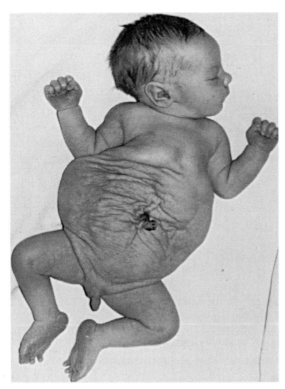

Figure 60–1. Newborn infant with the prune-belly syndrome, showing the characteristic appearance of the abdominal wall, the empty scrotum, and the talipes equinovarus.

scent is blocked by a distended bladder and that the abdominal wall defect occurs secondary to either urinary tract distention or fetal ascites. However, other types of severe obstruction in the posterior urethra (e.g., posterior urethral valves) do not result in either a similar abdominal wall defect or the same type of upper tract distortion. In addition, a similarly high incidence of cryptorchidism has not been observed in other obstructive uropathies.

Several investigators (Monie and Monie, 1979; Moerman et al, 1984) **have suggested that prostatic dysgenesis and fetal ascites are key factors in the causation of the syndrome, with fetal ascites producing the abdominal wall defect.** Although ascites is rarely present in patients with prune-belly syndrome (Smythe, 1981), it is speculated that ascites may be transient, with absorption toward the end of gestation. Another commonly quoted and at one time more popular theory is **that a primary mesodermal error might account for both the abdominal wall defect and the genitourinary abnormalities, because both arise from the paraxial intermediate and lateral plate mesoderm** (Smith, 1970). A genetic basis has been explored, but no clear inheritance pattern has emerged.

PATHOPHYSIOLOGY

Genitourinary Abnormalities

Kidney

Although the kidneys may be normal, **renal dysplasia and hydronephrosis are the two renal abnormalities typically associated with prune-belly syndrome.** Dysplasia may be present in more than 50% of cases, but involvement varies widely and is often asymmetric (Rogers and Ostrow, 1973). For example, a completely dysplastic multicystic kidney may be present on one side while the contralateral kidney demonstrates completely normal histology. This feature, which is an important determinant of prognosis, seems to be more severe in patients who have urethral stenosis, megalourethra, or imperforate anus (Potter, 1972).

Most patients with prune-belly syndrome display some degree of hydronephrosis, which similarly follows a spectrum of severity and does not appear to be related to the severity of abdominal wall deficiency. Dilation of the calyces may be random or global, and the renal pelvis may be of normal caliber or grossly dilated (Berdon et al, 1977). The severity of the hydronephrosis is often less than that anticipated from the degree of dilation of the ureter. It is also common to find that the renal parenchyma is thicker and of better quality than might be expected from the amount of distortion in the drainage system. Although these findings have prognostic importance, they also suggest that the mechanism for the hydronephrosis might differ from that characteristic of other obstructive uropathies.

Occasionally a patient also has ureteropelvic junction obstruction, and this possibility must not be overlooked in deciding on a plan of management. However, **recurrent infection, rather than obstruction, usually represents the greatest threat to renal parenchyma** that may already be compromised by an element of renal dysplasia.

Ureter

Ureteral abnormalities are detected at each level of pathologic observation. The gross features are tortuosity and segments of massive dilation alternating with segments of more normal caliber or even stenosis. **The proximal ureter usually displays a more normal appearance, an important feature when considering corrective surgery** (Fig. 60–2). Microscopically, the prune-belly ureter shows a reduced number of smooth muscle cells which are replaced by fibrous connective tissue (Palmer and Tesluk, 1974). Although involvement may be patchy, there is no greater fibrosis in regions of dilation or narrowing (Nunn and Stephens, 1961). However, the smooth muscle cell population is best represented proximally, where it may be arranged into normal layers. Gearhart and colleagues detected a more pronounced degree of fibrosis, reflected by an increased ratio of collagen to smooth muscle fibers, in refluxing ureters. Electron microscopy has demonstrated ultrastructural defects, with both thick and thin myofilaments reduced in number and less distinct than normal (Hanna et al, 1977).

The prune-belly ureter is disadvantaged mechanically by multiple factors. Severe ureteral dilation prohibits the luminal coaptation necessary for effective propulsion of urine. Also, the normal ureter allows a conduction wave to be propagated from smooth muscle cell to smooth muscle cell through intracellular junctions. In the prune-belly ureter, the excitatory wave reaches a smooth muscle cell population that is reduced in number, is separated by a collagen meshwork, and may be less capable of generating an

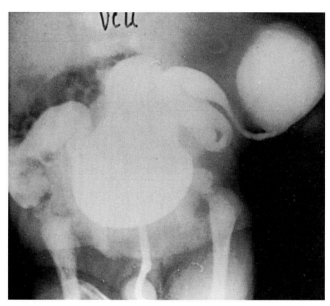

Figure 60–2. Cystogram showing massive bilateral vesicoureteral reflux. Note the marked difference in caliber of the left upper ureter compared with the lower ureter.

effective contraction owing to an abnormal myofilament content. Furthermore, the urine bolus that is moved forward reaches a progressively more severely affected segment of the ureter. Fluoroscopic observation confirms that these ureters can have markedly depressed peristaltic activity or may even be functionally inert (Nunn and Stephens, 1961; Williams and Berkholder, 1967). The resulting stasis within the upper tracts provides an opportunity for infection.

Bladder and Urachus

The ureters enter the bladder in a lateral and posterior position. The interureteric ridge, if discernible, is elongated

and often asymmetric (Barnhouse, 1972). Given the position and frequently patulous configuration of the ureteral orifices (see Fig. 60–2), the **high rate of vesicoureteral reflux, which may approach 85%,** is not surprising (Goulding and Garret, 1978). As with the ureteral architecture, there is replacement of the bladder smooth muscle with connective tissue. The bladder wall may be severely thickened by this process, yet the gross appearance of hypertrophied interlacing muscle bundles and trabeculation consistent with obstruction is absent. No abnormality in innervation has been detected. The large-capacity bladder is often elongated, with a wide urachal diverticulum that provides an hourglass configuration (Fig. 60–3). Patency of the urachus occurs most commonly when urethral atresia is present but may occur without definite urethral obstruction.

Usually, the **cystometrogram reveals excellent detrusor compliance; the end filling pressure assumes a normal value; and the bladder functions well as a reservoir.** However, bladder sensation during filling is shifted to the right with a delayed first sensation to void, and bladder capacity may be more than double the normal volume (Snyder et al, 1976). Less consistent and less favorable results are seen with the voiding profile. **The compressor capabilities of the detrusor are diminished by the frequent presence of vesicoureteral reflux and reduced detrusor contractility** (Kinahan et al, 1992). Despite these disadvantages, almost 50% of patients can void spontaneously, and a few display normal voiding pressures and generate normal flow rates with minimal postvoid residuals (Nunn and Stephens, 1961; Snyder et al, 1976; Kinahan et al, 1992). **Both spontaneous improvement and deterioration in the efficiency of voiding have been observed,** however, underscoring the importance of periodic urodynamic monitoring in those patients who can void spontaneously (Kinahan et al, 1992). In most cases in which a significant postvoid residual is present, there is no anatomic or urodynamic evidence of outflow obstruction and the voiding pressure is not elevated (Williams and Burkholder,

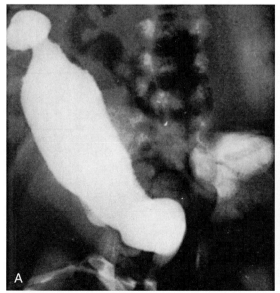

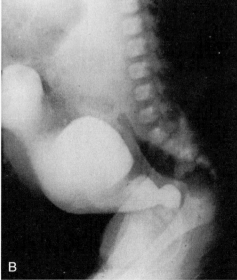

Figure 60–3. A and B, Voiding cystograms in two patients, showing the pseudodiverticulum configuration of the dome of the bladder. Note the wide, triangular prostatic urethra in both cystograms and the small utricular configuration in B.

1967; Snyder et al, 1976). The term *unbalanced voiding* has been used to describe the development of postvoid residuals as a consequence of the disproportion between detrusor contractility and the normal, although impeding, outflow resistance offered by the urethra. Internal urethrotomy has been employed to reduce urethral resistance and improve voiding efficiency (Snyder et al, 1976; Cukier, 1977).

Prostate and Accessory Sex Organs

The characteristically wide bladder neck merges with a grossly dilated prostatic urethra, so that the junction is almost imperceptible both radiographically and by gross inspection. The prostatic urethra does, however, taper to a relatively narrow membranous urethra at the urogenital diaphragm. This configuration produces an image on voiding cystourethrography that resembles that of posterior urethral valves. In fact, true anatomic obstruction of the posterior urethral by atresia, segmental stenosis, or posterior urethral valves is only rarely seen in surviving infants (Rogers and Ostrow, 1973; Welch and Kearney, 1974; Aaronson, 1983). Significant lesions have been more frequently reported in necropsy series of fetuses and neonates (Popek et al, 1991; Stephens and Gupta, 1994). Cystourethrography may also reveal reflux of contrast material into the ejaculatory ducts, and a utricular diverticulum is also often seen during the voiding phase (Kroovand et al, 1982).

Prostatic hypoplasia is responsible for the dilated radiographic appearance of the prostatic urethra. This is a uniform feature of the syndrome that is represented pathologically by a marked reduction in epithelial elements, reduced smooth muscle fibers, and increased connective tissue content (Deklerk and Scott, 1978; Popek et al, 1991). The configuration of severe prostatic sacculation combined with an obliquely implanted urethra has also been proposed as a mechanism of functional outflow obstruction (Monie and Monie, 1979). Involvement of other accessory sex organs has also been reported. In an autopsy series of affected fetuses and neonates, the seminal vesicles were in some cases rudimentary or absent, the vas deferens segmentally atretic, and the epididymal attachment to the testis tenuous (Stephens and Gupta, 1994).

Urethra

The anterior urethra and the penis are normal in most patients with prune-belly syndrome. However, hypospadias, penile torsion, ventral and dorsal chordee, and penile agenesis have been described (Kroovand et al, 1982; Kuga et al, 1998). **Congenital megalourethra, characterized by dilation of the anterior urethra without distal obstruction, occurs with increased frequency** in this syndrome. The scaphoid variety is represented by maldevelopment of the spongiosum, which produces urethral dilation with preservation of the corpora cavernosum and glans (Fig. 60–4). The more severe fusiform megalourethra involves maldevelopment of both the spongiosum and corpora, so that with voiding the entire phallus dilates in a fusiform fashion (Appel et al, 1986).

Urethral atresia also has a well-recognized association with prune-belly syndrome and most often portends a poor prognosis. In utero bladder decompression via a patent urachus may allow survival with variable impairment of renal and pulmonary function. Reinberg and colleagues (1993) identified a subset of patients with in utero spontaneous vesicocutaneous rupture and fistula formation which supported pulmonary and renal development. Urethral salvage by progressive dilation, the PADUA procedure, has been subsequently accomplished in this setting (Passerini-Glazel, 1988).

Testis

Bilateral cryptorchidism is a central feature of the prune-belly syndrome, and in most patients both testes are intra-abdominal, overlying the ureters at the pelvic brim near the sacroiliac level. Obstructed descent by the dilated urinary system (Silverman and Huang, 1950), gubernacular insufficiency as a consequence of its defective mesenchyme (Rajfer and Walsh, 1978), and an intrinsic abnormality of the testis have all been proposed as causes

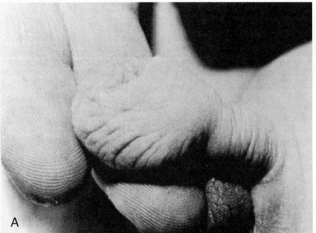
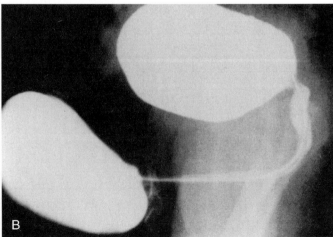

Figure 60–4. *A* and *B*, Elongated penis with ventral skin redundancy (*A*) accompanying a scaphoid megalourethra demonstrated by cystourethrography (*B*). (From Shrom SH, Cromie WJ, Duckett JW: Megalourethra. Urology 1981;17:152. Copyright © 1981 by Elsevier Science.)

of cryptorchidism in these patients. Nunn and Stephens (1961) noted that the histology of the testis in affected fetuses and neonates was equal to that in age-matched controls; others found decreased numbers of spermatogonia and Leydig cell hyperplasia (Orvis et al, 1988). In any case, the presence of spermatogonia in infant testes implies that early orchidopexy may preserve spermatogenesis for some patients. We recently observed viable sperm in the postejaculation urine of a postpubertal patient who had orchidopexy performed during early infancy (Woodard, 2000).

On a subcellular level, histochemical studies of infant testes have shown prominent placental alkaline phosphatase staining of the cell cytoplasmic membrane; atypical, enlarged nuclei; and prominent nuclei—features regarded as embryonic and common to normal fetal germ cells and intratubular testicular neoplasms (Massad et al, 1991). In fact, four cases of germ cell neoplasms in men with the prune-belly syndrome have now been reported (Woodhouse and Ransley, 1983; Duckett, 1986; Sayre et al, 1986).

Little information is available on sexual function in men with prune-belly syndrome. Preserved Leydig cell function usually allows for normal testosterone levels, although often in the presence of increased levels of luteinizing hormone. **Erection and orgasm are apparently normal, but no cases of paternity have been reported.** The potential for fertility in these patients is compromised not only by testicular abnormalities but also by multiple extratesticular factors. As mentioned, epididymal, vasal, and seminal vesical abnormalities may be present. The prostatic epithelium is hypoplastic, and the bladder neck is open. Therefore, retrograde ejaculation is common, and analysis of seminal fluid or postejaculation urine reveals azoospermia (Woodhouse and Snyder, 1985).

Extragenitourinary Abnormalities

Extragenitourinary abnormalities are frequently associated with prune-belly syndrome. Excluding the abdominal wall defect that is a consistent feature of the syndrome, as many as 75% of these patients may have other clinically significant problems (Geary et al, 1986). The range of possible abnormalities and their relative frequencies of occurrence are listed in Table 60–1.

Abdominal Wall Defect

Although most affected infants have a similar appearance, the abdominal wall defect varies in severity and is often asymmetric and patchy in distribution. **Characteristically, the abdominal muscles are absent in the lower and medial parts of the abdominal wall, although the upper rectus muscles and outer oblique muscles are developed.** Some practitioners (Welch and Kearney, 1974) have observed that the muscles are present but hypoplastic, whereas others (Afifi et al, 1972) have found that the deficiency ranges from slight hypoplasia to complete absence of muscles. In addition, although the muscle layers may be thin, their normal arrangement is preserved, or they may be fused to form a single fibrotic layer (Afifi et al, 1972). Innervation by the anterior spinal nerves is intact

Table 60–1. EXTRAGENITOURINARY ABNORMALITIES

Organ System	Frequency (%)	Observed Problems
Cardiac	10*	Patent ductus arteriosus
		Ventricular septal defect
		Atrial septal defect
		Tetralogy of Fallot
Pulmonary	55†	Lobar atelectasis
		Pulmonary hypoplasia
		Pneumothorax
		Pneumomediastinum
		Chronic bronchitis
		Recurrent pneumonia
Gastrointestinal	31‡	Intestinal malrotation
		Volvulus
		Intestinal atresias or stenosis
		Omphalocele
		Gastroschisis
		Hirschsprung's disease
		Imperforate anus
		Hepatobiliary anomalies
Orthopedic	40–63§	Chest wall deformity (pectus excavatum, pectus carinatum)
		Scoliosis
		Sacral agenesis (partial)
		Congenital hip subluxation or dislocation
		Genu valgum
		Talipes equinovarus
		Severe leg maldevelopment
Miscellaneous		Splenic torsion
		Adrenal cystic dysplasia

*Adebonojo, 1973.
†Geary et al, 1986.
‡Wright et al, 1986.
§Loder et al, 1992, and Brinker et al, 1995.

(Nunn and Stephens, 1961). A definite but nonspecific myopathology has been observed both histologically and ultrastructurally. Variation in muscle fiber diameter with haphazard arrangement of both atrophic and hypertrophic fibers, an increase in fibrous tissue surrounding the muscle fibers, and fatty infiltration are present. Disorganization persists at the ultrastructural level with disarray of myofibrils, mitochondrial proliferation, and clumping of glycogen granules (Afifi et al, 1972; Mininberg et al, 1973).

These features translate into a lax and redundant abdominal wall with bulging flanks and secondary flaring of the lower rib cage. **The poor support of the lower chest wall interferes with an effective cough mechanism and contributes to a greater vulnerability to respiratory infections.** These children also have difficulty in sitting up from the supine position. Although the wrinkled appearance is typical of the abdominal wall in the infant, it tends to take on a potbellied appearance in the older child (Fig. 60–5). Surprisingly, the defective abdominal wall causes little difficulty for the surgeon. Wound healing proceeds satisfactorily despite the absence of layers for suturing. Wound dehiscence and other wound complications are rare.

Pulmonary Aspects

The pulmonary status of the infant with prune-belly syndrome is particularly critical, and survival may be threatened by a variety of pulmonary complications. **Pulmonary**

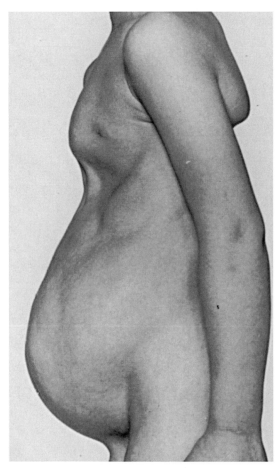

Figure 60–5. Older child with prune-belly syndrome, showing the absence of wrinkling, the "potbelly" appearance, and the consequent deformity of the lower ribs.

hypoplasia precipitated by oligohydramnios is particularly ominous. Moreover, pneumomediastinum or pneumothorax is a common occurrence in patients with hypoplastic lungs. Neonates in this category commonly die from respiratory failure. If the patient does survive the neonatal period, the lungs grow and eventually attain adequate capacity (Alford et al, 1978). As the patient becomes older, however, he still may have respiratory problems secondary to the deficiency of accessory muscles in the abdominal wall.

The other major category of pulmonary complications includes a tendency toward lobar atelectasis and pneumonia. Because the abdominal walls are important structures in powerful expiration, patients with prune-belly syndrome have a decreased ability to generate an effective cough. Consequently, they are more vulnerable to complications during periods of excess mucus production. A number of anesthetic complications have been reported (Hannington-Kiff, 1970; Karamanian et al, 1974). Sedatives and analgesics must be used judiciously to avoid respiratory depression. Apnea monitors play an important role in the neonatal surveillance of these patients.

Cardiac Anomalies

Ventricular septal defect, atrial septal defect, and tetralogy of Fallot occur with increased frequency in this patient population. **The incidence of cardiac abnormalities in patients with prune-belly syndrome is approximately 10%** (Adebonojo, 1973).

Gastrointestinal Anomalies

Most individuals with prune-belly syndrome have **intestinal malrotation secondary to a universal mesentery with an unattached cecum** (Silverman and Huang, 1950). Much less common is an imperforate anus, which is more likely to occur in association with urethral atresia and renal dysplasia. Gastroschisis and Hirschsprung's disease have also been reported in these patients (Willert et al, 1978; Cawthern et al, 1979). Constipation also appears to be a problem; it is secondary to deficiency of the abdominal musculature and may lead to acquired megacolon. Hepatobiliary anomalies including paucity of intralobar bile ducts (Aanpreung et al, 1993) and splenic torsion have also been reported (Heydenrych and Dutoit, 1978).

Orthopedic Deformities

In a literature review of 188 cases of prune-belly syndrome, Loder and associates noted **a 45% incidence of musculoskeletal involvement.** Although the most frequent and benign finding was a dimple on the outer aspect of the knee, club foot deformity occurred in 26%, hip dysplasia with dislocation in 5%, and spinal deformities in 5% of patients (Loder et al, 1992). Pectus carinatum and pectus excavatum deformities are also found relatively frequently. Fetal compression secondary to oligohydramnios is believed to be the cause of the various limb deformities. More severe malformations including lower extremity hypoplasias, and even amelias rarely occur. Because the lower extremities only are involved, compression of the iliac vessels by a distended bladder has been suggested as the pathogenic mechanism (Ralis and Forbes, 1971; Green et al, 1993).

CLINICAL PRESENTATION AND NATURAL HISTORY

Prenatal Diagnosis

Successful prenatal diagnosis of prune-belly syndrome by obstetric ultrasonography has been made as early as 14 weeks of gestation (Shimizu et al, 1992). However, the suggestive features of dilated ureters, bladder distention, and irregular dilatation of the abdominal circumference (Bovicelli et al, 1980; Christopher et al, 1982; Shih et al, 1982) are more readily imaged at 30 weeks (Okulski, 1977). **In clinical practice it has proved difficult to distinguish the fetus with prune-belly syndrome from one with primary vesicoureteral reflux or posterior urethral valves** (Kramer, 1983). Inaccuracies in diagnosis have resulted in application of in utero drainage procedures in at least 26 cases of prune-belly syndrome without evidence of definite benefit in regard to postnatal renal function (Elder et al, 1987; Sholder et al, 1988; Freedman et al, 1999). However, the rare observation of a patient with urethral atresia who survived in the presence of a patent urachus or spontaneous vesicocutaneous fistula or after placement of a

Table 60–2. SPECTRUM OF PRUNE-BELLY SYNDROME

Distinguishing Characteristics	Category Classification
Oligohydramnios, pulmonary hypoplasia, or pneumothorax. May have urethral obstruction or patent urachus.	I
Typical external features and uropathy of the full-blown syndrome but no immediate problem with survival. May have mild or unilateral renal dysplasia. May or may not develop urosepsis or gradual azotemia.	II
External feature may be mild or incomplete. Uropathy is less severe; renal function is stable.	III

vesicocutaneous shunt seems to suggest that in utero shunting might be useful in selected patients if it is delivered sufficiently early (Steinhardt et al, 1990; Reinberg et al, 1993). However, enthusiasm should be tempered by the realization that fetal renal damage seems to begin well before detection; that the ability of current interventional procedures to protect renal function in any fetal uropathy remains unproven; and that, for most patients with prune-belly syndrome, no obstruction can be found (Freedman et al, 1996).

Neonatal Period

Although all cases should be recognized by the pediatrician or neonatologist on routine postnatal examination, there is a considerable variability in the severity of the disorder and in the urgency with which urologic advice is sought. This is obviously a syndrome with a wide range of severity. Patients can be grouped according to severity. The classification shown in Table 60–2 is simple and clinically useful.

Category I includes neonates with severe pulmonary or marked renal dysplasia, either of which precludes survival beyond the first days of life. Some of these infants have a patent urachus and complete urethral obstruction. The more severely affected babies in this category may be stillborn. Because of severe oligohydramnios, others may have some of the features characteristic of renal agenesis, such as Potter's facies. The serum creatinine level is normal at birth but steadily rises thereafter. If these babies do not die quickly from pulmonary hypoplasia, they succumb only slightly later from renal failure. Drainage procedures result in a very scanty flow of dilute urine. In a few of these cases, in which there appears to be a chance for survival, a simple drainage procedure such as a vesicostomy may be justified.

Patients in category II have the potential to survive the neonatal period. They have the typical full-blown uropathy with diffuse dilatation of the urinary tract and hydronephrosis. Renal dysplasia may exist, but it is unilateral or less severe than that found in patients with category I disease. Most of these infants are able to void urine from the bladder and often do so with apparent ease. Others suffer a general failure to thrive with enormous abdominal distention. All such infants should be transferred to medical centers staffed by pediatric urologists, pediatric nephrolo-

gists, and other neonatal experts before any instrumentation is permitted.

Category III includes infants with definite but relatively mild or incomplete features of the syndrome. Some uropathy is present, but the renal parenchyma is apparently of high quality, renal function is normal, and urinary stasis is generally less marked. General agreement exists that patients in category III may require little if any urologic reconstructive surgery. However, they may later show signs of progressive upper tract deterioration, particularly if they are prone to urinary infection. They will also be candidates for treatment of cryptorchidism. All surviving patients require surveillance.

Infancy, Childhood, and Adolescence

The nadir creatinine during infancy has proven to be a useful predictor of long-term renal function. **If the nadir value is less than 0.7 mg/dl, renal function tends to be stable during childhood unless there is further renal compromise by pyelonephritis** (Geary et al, 1986; Reinberg et al, 1991; Noh et al, 1999). The importance of urinary tract monitoring by periodic cultures and prompt treatment of urinary tract infections cannot be overemphasized. Unfortunately, the risk of infection is constant in the setting of urinary tract dilation and stasis. **Circumcision is advisable, and prophylactic antibiotics should be provided, especially in patients with uncorrected reflux.** Despite these efforts, as many as 30% of patients, generally those with impaired renal function at initial evaluation, develop chronic renal failure during childhood or adolescence (Geary et al, 1986). Renal transplantation is necessary for these patients to ensure normal growth and development, and success with transplantation in prune-belly patients can be expected to equal that in other age-matched groups (Reinberg et al, 1989). Normal growth can be expected in most of the patients with normal renal function, although growth retardation in the absence of renal compromise was observed in one third of patients in one series (Geary et al, 1986). A normal pattern of secondary sexual development can be expected (Woodhouse and Snyder, 1985).

Adult Presentation

Although the diagnosis of prune-belly syndrome usually is made in the neonatal period or during early infancy, adult presentation still occasionally occurs. Symptoms of renal failure with associated hypertension most commonly bring these patients to medical attention (Lee, 1977; Wallner and Kramar, 1990; Kerbl and Pauer, 1993). In one case, a history of urinary tract infections was absent (Texter and Koontz, 1980). However, urinary stasis represents a persistent opportunity for infection, and patients have been reported who seem to do well for years with little treatment or no treatment only to succumb to urinary sepsis as adults (Culp and Flocks, 1954).

Female Syndrome

In the strictest sense, only a male patient may harbor the complete syndrome. Yet about 3% of reported cases occur in genetic females. The defect involves the abdominal wall, bladder, and upper urinary tract (Rabinowitz and Schillinger, 1977). Actually, fewer than 20 cases have been reported, and the principles of management are essentially the same as those for males. Many of the female patients have had incomplete forms of the syndrome with normal upper urinary tracts.

Incomplete Syndrome

Although it is exceptionally rare to encounter a normal urinary tract in association with the characteristic abdominal wall defect in a male, the converse is not unusual. Some patients (with "pseudo–prune-belly syndrome") have a normal or relatively normal abdominal wall but exhibit many or all of the internal urologic features. These features may include dysplastic or dysmorphic kidneys or dilated and tortuous ureters. **Bellah and coworkers (1996) described eight boys with relatively mild external features of the syndrome; five progressed to renal failure, evidence that these children remain vulnerable to renal deterioration.**

Genetic Aspects

The possibility of a genetic basis for prune-belly syndrome is suggested by the curious male-to-female ratio, the occasional occurrence of affected male siblings or cousins, and the rare patient with a karyotype abnormality. Mendelian inheritance patterns that have been considered include autosomal chromosome abnormalities, X chromosome abnormalities, and polygenic transmission (Garlinger and Ott, 1974; Adenyokunna et al, 1975; Riccardi and Grum, 1977; Lockhart et al, 1979). However, most cases are sporadic, and most patients have a normal karyotype. **One of the most powerful arguments against a genetic etiology rests with the observation of 100% discordance among all twins in whom monozygosity has been proven** (Ives, 1974). The reported associations with Turner's syndrome (Lubinsky et al, 1980; Adenyokunna and Familusi, 1982), monosomy 16 (Harley et al, 1972), trisomy 13 (Frydman et al, 1983), and trisomy 18 (Beckman et al, 1984) confound identification of a single gene locus.

MANAGEMENT

Initial Diagnostic Evaluation

Although the urologist is usually notified immediately, the affected neonate rarely represents a true urologic emergency. **The most urgent matters are actually those concerned with cardiopulmonary function.** Pulmonary complications including pulmonary hypoplasia, pneumomediastinum, pneumothorax, and cardiac abnormalities must be excluded. After stabilization, the urologic evaluation proceeds with physical examination and ultrasonography. Renal volume and the presence of dilated upper tracts may be palpated through the thin abdominal wall, and the infant is observed for voiding pattern and for the presence

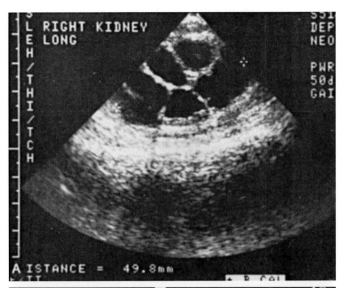

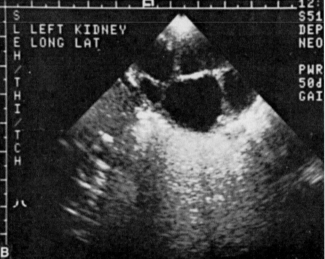

Figure 60–6. Right *(A)* and left *(B)* kidneys in a 1-day-old infant with typical prune-belly syndrome. The infant was seen at birth, prescribed antibiotics, and monitored closely with urine cultures, serum creatinine determinations, and renal ultrasound imaging. (From Woodard JR, Zucker I: Current management of the dilated urinary tract in prune-belly syndrome. Urol Clin North Am 1990;17:413.)

of a patent urachus. Further parenchymal assessment and definition of the collecting system, ureter, and bladder are provided by an ultrasound examination (Fig. 60–6). Serial electrolytes, serum creatinine, and routine urine culture complete an early urologic profile. An orthopedic examination should also be done initially. If spontaneous voiding is present and renal function is stable, other studies may be postponed. In particular, **imaging studies that require catheterization and the potential for introduction of bacteria should be avoided unless the results are needed for immediate clinical decision making.** Nevertheless, the occasional occurrence of obstructive urethral lesions argues for evaluation with a voiding cystourethrogram if voiding is impaired or if there is renal insufficiency. Attention to sterile technique is critical if invasive studies are performed. Once introduced, infection in a static system may be difficult to eradicate.

Category assignment becomes apparent during the neonatal period. There is general agreement that the fate of the category I patient is cannot be altered and that the category III patient is unlikely to require intervention beyond management of cryptorchidism. Within category II there is a gradient of severity that mandates an individualized approach. The stable infant may be observed with serial electrolytes, creatinine, urine cultures, and ultrasound studies. Evaluation of renal function and drainage is usually accomplished at 4 to 6 weeks of age to allow transitional parenchymal maturity. The technetium 99m (^{99m}Tc) dimercaptosuccinic acid (DMSA) renal scan evaluates renal parenchymal integrity, and clearance and drainage may be assessed by ^{99m}Tc-diethylene triamine pentaacetic acid (DTPA) or ^{99m}Tc-mercaptoacetyltriglycine (MAG3) scans. When diminished renal function or massive dilation compromises interpretation of radionuclide studies, a Whitaker test may prove useful. Early diversion procedures may be necessary in the setting of intractable infection or deterioration in renal function.

Controversies in Management of Category II Prune-Belly Syndrome

The motivation for aggressive surgical intervention was initially derived from observation of the poor prognosis for category II infants as a group. Because 20% were either stillborn or died in the neonatal period and an additional 30% died during the first 2 years of life, the outlook was dismal (Lattimer, 1958). Compilation of the cases reported in the literature between 1950 and 1970 by Waldbaum and Marshall (1970) revealed that 86% of the 56 accurately traceable patients had died, with or without surgical intervention. The obvious implication was that a more aggressive approach was necessary to improve the fate of the infant with prune-belly syndrome. With the recognition that infection and progressive renal insufficiency are the factors that most often pose the greatest threat to quality of life and survival, surgical reconstruction to normalize the anatomy and function of the genitourinary tract was advocated. Early retailoring of the urinary system to reduce stasis and eliminate reflux or obstruction has included ureteral shortening, tapering and vesicoureteral reimplantation, and reduction cystoplasty. Reconstruction is best delayed until the child is approximately 3 months of age to allow for pulmonary maturation. This approach has been successful in achieving anatomic and functional improvement evidenced by stable radiographic studies, stable creatinine values, and a reduced occurrence of infection (Waldbaum and Marshall, 1970; Jeffs et al, 1977; Woodard and Parrott, 1978a; Randolph et al, 1981b). In our experience with 17 category II patients observed from the neonatal period who underwent early reconstruction, 15 patients have maintained a normal creatinine level and only 2 have demonstrated moderate renal insufficiency, with follow-up ranging from 2 to 27 years.

An alternative approach of limited surgical intervention has also been applied. Proponents advocate close surveillance with medical management of bacteriuria and surgical intervention only in patients with proven obstruction or intractable infection. Opinions vary about the management of vesicoureteral reflux in the prune-belly population, although there is no reason to believe that reflux in this population is any less important, and correction of high-grade reflux seems prudent. Success with minimal surgical intervention has been reported (Woodhouse et al, 1979; Duckett, 1980; Tank and McCoy, 1983; McMullin et al, 1988). Woodhouse and his associates (1979) reviewed a series of patients with prune-belly syndrome managed conservatively. Nine of these 11 patients, who were monitored from infancy, remained well except for a few urinary tract infections for periods of up to 24 years. They were said to have normal voiding patterns and normal renal function. Certainly, patients in category III are candidates for this type of management (Fig. 60–7).

The paucity of long-term data for category II patients, the probable variation in assignment of disease severity in treatment groups, and the variable natural history of the disease make comparisons of these retrospective studies difficult. Spontaneous improvement in ureteral appearance and function may occur with normal growth and elongation of the ureters (Duckett, 1980). Also, some patients with gross abnormalities of the urinary collecting system have survived decades without medical attention (Asplund and Laska, 1975; Lee, 1977; Texter and Koontz, 1980). Yet, progressive uropathy is also well know to occur, and many patients with prune-belly syndrome ultimately require renal transplantation (Reinberg et al, 1989). Controversy will persist over category II patients until accurate application of a medical or surgical approach is possible based on distinct clinical features.

Nonoperative Management

When obstruction and vesicoureteral reflux have been excluded, a nonoperative stance may be taken toward patients with normal renal function despite gross dilation of the upper and lower tracts. This position demands close surveillance for the development of urinary tract infections, continuous monitoring of renal function, and routine radiographic imaging. Usually, antibiotic prophylaxis is provided, and a urinalysis is performed each month, with cultures performed as indicated. The upper tracts are monitored for increasing dilation and for evidence of obstruction by functional studies (radionuclide imaging). Suspicion of obstruction that cannot be fully defined with more routine studies should be further evaluated with a Whitaker test.

Surgical Management of Prune-Belly Syndrome

Surgical management of prune-belly syndrome uropathy is directed toward both correction of vesicoureteral dysfunction (vesicoureteral reflux, upper tract obstruction, and severe upper tract stasis) and correction of vesicourethral dysfunction including improvement of bladder emptying. As discussed, the timing of surgical intervention may be early in an attempt to protect a threatened system from further compromise, or it may be delayed until obstruction or infection mandates intervention.

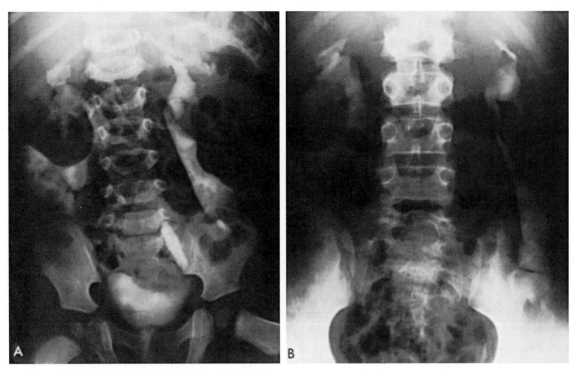

Figure 60–7. *A,* Intravenous urogram of a 2-year-old boy with prune-belly syndrome shows the classic appearance of tortuous, dilated ureters with relatively well preserved kidneys. *B,* Urogram in the same patient at age 19 years shows improvement in ureteric dilation without surgical treatment and no deterioration in renal function.

Orchiopexy is necessary in all patients. Abdominal reconstruction depends on the severity of the abdominal defect, but when indicated it should be performed early to allow the development of a normal physique as the child progresses through the formative years.

Vesicoureteral Dysfunction

TEMPORARY DIVERSION

Earlier efforts to improve the prognosis of the infant with prune-belly syndrome employed routine high supravesical urinary diversion followed by extensive reconstruction in infants with stable renal function (Carter et al, 1974; Burbige et al, 1987). Although enthusiasm for routine proximal diversion in the neonatal period has justifiably diminished, there remain situations in which urinary diversion is indicated. **In the presence of intractable infection or deterioration in renal function, a temporizing drainage procedure must be considered.** Cutaneous vesicostomy should be considered first in this situation. Vesicostomy is relatively simple to perform, is usually effective, and does compromise a more extensive reconstructive effort if such is indicated at a later date. The procedure is performed through a small transverse incision midway between the umbilicus and the symphysis pubis. A small ellipse of skin and rectus fascia is excised. The dome of the bladder is mobilized and delivered into the incision, at which point it is sutured to the rectus fascia and skin and a small bladder stoma is fashioned (Duckett, 1974). The urine is allowed to drain freely into a diaper, using no collection device or tubes. Vesicostomy is useful as a preliminary drainage procedure before a more extensive recon-

structive operation is undertaken at a later date. More proximal drainage, in the form of a cutaneous pyelostomy, remains useful in the unusual case of ureteropelvic junction or ureterovesical junction obstruction and in patients with unremitting infection. Although not as simple as a vesicostomy, it is still an expedient procedure and has the advantage of providing good proximal drainage to each kidney while permitting inspection and biopsy of the kidney at the time of operation. By allowing subsequent evaluation of differential kidney function, it may also aid in the planning of reconstructive operations. **Proximal ureterostomy should be avoided because it jeopardizes the segment of the ureter that is most useful in subsequent reconstruction efforts.**

URETERAL RECONSTRUCTION

The role of extensive surgical remodeling of the urinary tract in patients with prune-belly syndrome is understandably controversial, because some patients appear to do well without major reconstruction and others seem to have been harmed by unsuccessful surgical attempts. There is little question, however, that the urinary tract in patients with prune-belly syndrome is characterized by stasis and that this stasis predisposes to bacteriuria, which may lead to deterioration of renal function as well as troublesome clinical symptoms. Therefore, it is likely that many surgeons will continue their efforts to remodel these distorted urinary tracts. **Success in these surgical reconstructions depends to a great extent on the use of the upper few centimeters of ureter, which usually are less dilated, less tortuous, and morphologically better than the distal**

ureter. Meticulous surgical technique with adherence to established principles of ureteral tailoring and reimplantation surgery is required (Fig. 60–8E–G). Unfortunately, both the bladder and the ureter, by the very mature of this bizarre uropathy, are difficult structures with which to work. Elevation of the bladder mucosa during tunneling may be challenging, and it may be necessary to raise flaps to provide a trough of appropriate length, rather than tunneling beneath an intact mucosa. Despite these inherent difficulties, in experienced hands a reasonably high degree of success is possible with this extensive reconstructive surgery, both in the neonate as a primary procedure (Fig.

60–9) and in the older infant or child as a primary or staged procedure (Woodard and Parrott, 1978a; Woodard, 1990).

Vesicourethral Dysfunction

REDUCTION CYSTOPLASTY

Through reconfiguration of the bladder, the goal of reduction cystoplasty is to maximize the efforts of the poorly contractile detrusor. The most aggressive description of the procedure entailed not only removal of the wide urachal

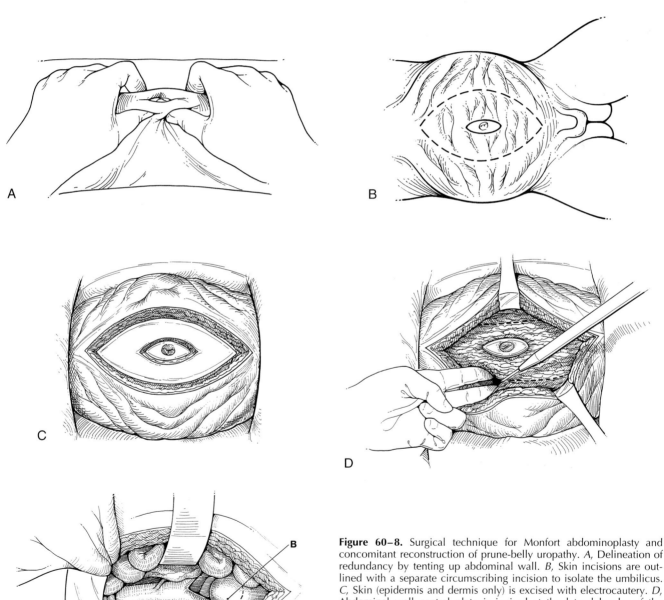

Figure 60–8. Surgical technique for Monfort abdominoplasty and concomitant reconstruction of prune-belly uropathy. *A,* Delineation of redundancy by tenting up abdominal wall. *B,* Skin incisions are outlined with a separate circumscribing incision to isolate the umbilicus. *C,* Skin (epidermis and dermis only) is excised with electrocautery. *D,* Abdominal wall central plate is incised at the lateral border of the rectus muscle on either side, from the superior epigastric to the inferior epigastric vessels, creating a central musculofascial plate. *E,* Adequate exposure is provided for concomitant transperitoneal genitourinary procedures.

Illustration continued on following page

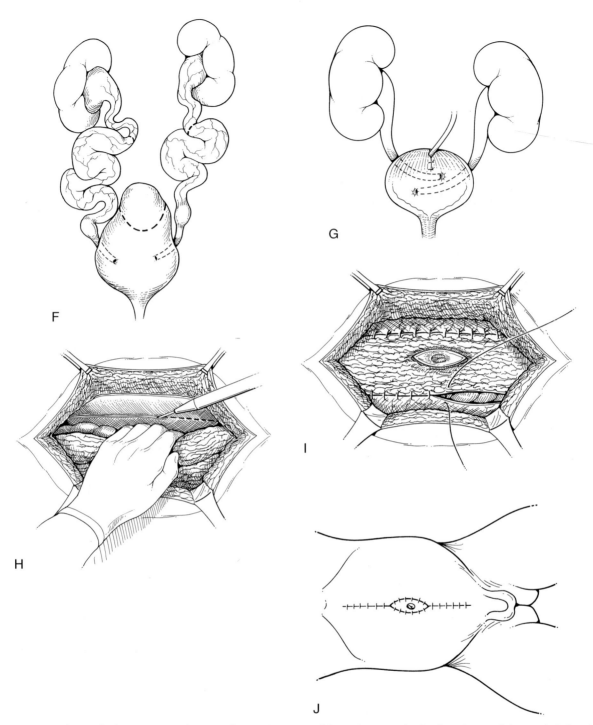

Figure 60–8 *Continued. F.* Only the more normal proximal ureter is preserved for vesicoureteral reimplantation, and the urachal diverticulum is excised. *G,* Transtrigonal ureteral reimplantation is performed with or without ureteral tapering as necessary. The bladder is closed in two layers, and ureteral stents (not shown) and a cystostomy tube are employed. *H,* Completion of abdominoplasty by scoring of the parietal peritoneum overlying the lateral abdominal wall musculature with electrocautery. *I,* The edges of the central plate are sutured to the lateral abdominal wall musculature along the scored line. *J,* Lateral flaps are brought together in the midline, with closed suction drains placed between the lateral flaps and the central plate. Skin is brought together in the midline, enveloping the previously isolated umbilicus. (From Woodard JR, Perez LM: Prune-belly syndrome. In Marshall FF [ed]: Operative Urology. Philadelphia, WB Saunders, 1996.)

diverticulum but also reshaping of the bladder into a more spherical form, either by further excision of the bladder dome or by overlapping the redundant detrusor muscle (Perlmutter, 1976). Benefit was believed to follow from removal of the tubelike dome, which often emptied poorly, and from alleviation of the acentric detrusor contraction caused by urachal tethering. The more spherical shape should also maximize the intravesical pressure generated by a detrusor contraction, as described by Laplace's law (Perlmutter, 1976). **Some initial improvement in voiding dy-**

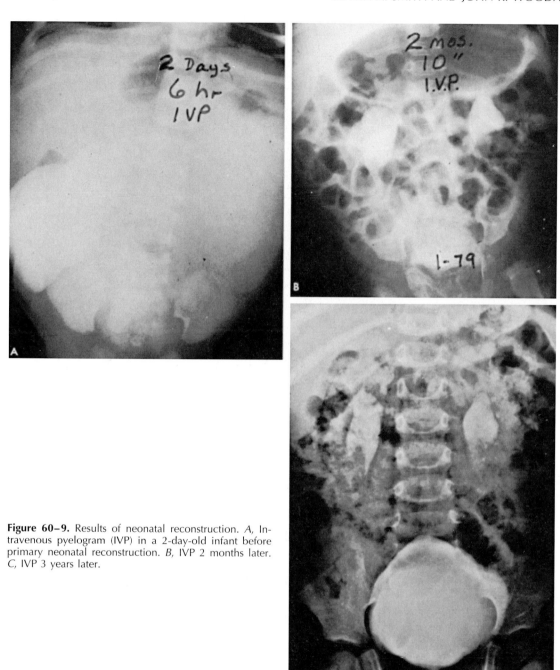

Figure 60–9. Results of neonatal reconstruction. *A,* Intravenous pyelogram (IVP) in a 2-day-old infant before primary neonatal reconstruction. *B,* IVP 2 months later. *C,* IVP 3 years later.

namics may be achieved by aggressive bladder remodeling. However, with long-term follow-up, there has been no evidence that this improvement is maintained, and excessive bladder volumes tend to recur with time (Bukowski and Perlmutter, 1994). Current use of reduction cystoplasty should be limited to simple excision of the large urachal diverticulum when it exists (see Fig. 60–8*F*).

INTERNAL URETHROTOMY

Internal urethrotomy is indicated in the rare patient with true anatomic urethral obstruction and in patients with urodynamic evidence of urethral obstruction by pressure flow studies. Application also has been extended to include those children who develop large postvoid residuals as a consequence of "unbalanced" vesicourethral function. Proponents suggest that improved flow rates and improved bladder emptying may be achieved by lowering urethral resistance (Snyder et al, 1976: Cukier, 1977). The procedure usually is considered in a child with increasing postvoid residuals, vesicoureteral reflux, or worsening ureteral dilation. Lower resting urethral pressures, improved flow rates, and a reduction in postvoid residuals with lowered infection rates have been reported (Snyder et al, 1976;

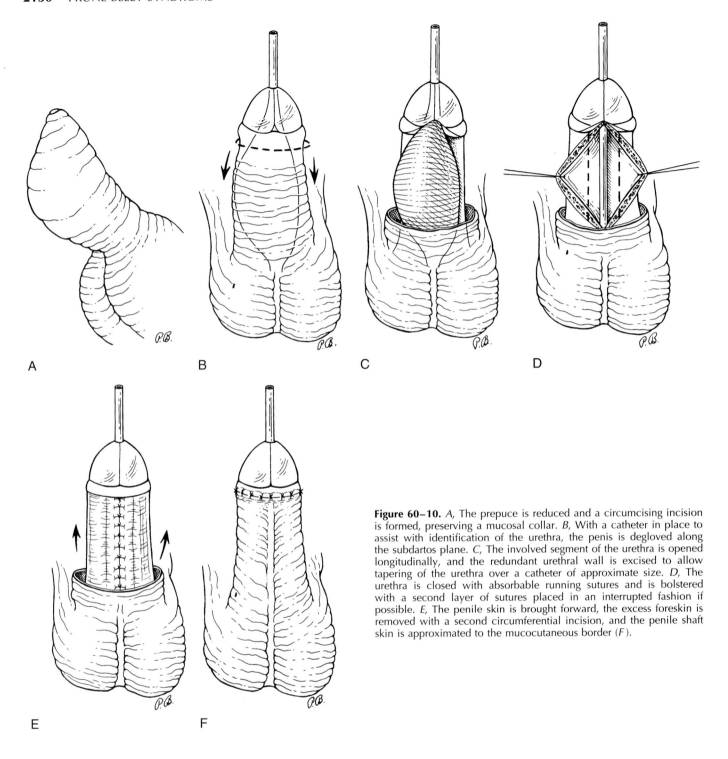

Figure 60–10. *A,* The prepuce is reduced and a circumcising incision is formed, preserving a mucosal collar. *B,* With a catheter in place to assist with identification of the urethra, the penis is degloved along the subdartos plane. *C,* The involved segment of the urethra is opened longitudinally, and the redundant urethral wall is excised to allow tapering of the urethra over a catheter of approximate size. *D,* The urethra is closed with absorbable running sutures and is bolstered with a second layer of sutures placed in an interrupted fashion if possible. *E,* The penile skin is brought forward, the excess foreskin is removed with a second circumferential incision, and the penile shaft skin is approximated to the mucocutaneous border (*F*).

Woodhouse et al, 1979). Even radiographic improvement of the upper tracts has been observed (Woodhouse et al, 1979). This approach certainly has some merit, although judicious use and correlation with urodynamic data are essential. Urethrotomy may be performed with the use of an Otis urethrotome or an endoscope. Williams (1979) advocated making one or two cuts anteriorly or anterolaterally to a size 24 or 30 Fr, followed by a period of catheter drainage. A visual urethrotomy seems preferable to the Otis procedure and should be made through the narrowed area in the urethra, which is typically at the end of the prostatic portion.

MEGALOURETHRA REPAIR

In the rare child in whom the anterior urethra is grossly dilated, surgery is required to reduce it to a normal caliber. Usually only the penile urethra is involved, and the meatus and the glanular portion are normal. In such a case, a circumferential incision around the coronal sulcus with degloving of the penile skin provides the best approach. The redundant wall of the urethra is excised, and the lumen is reconstructed over a catheter. The penile skin is then drawn forward and sutured (Fig. 60–10). In more severe cases, it may be necessary to cut back from the meatus

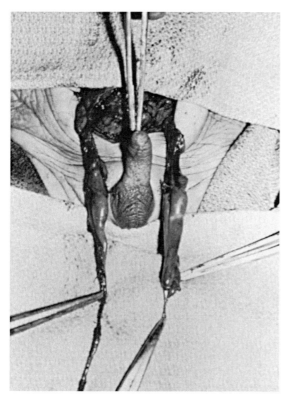

Figure 60–11. Operative photograph showing the ease with which the testes reach the scrotum after neonatal transabdominal mobilization of the spermatic cords.

both the redundant skin and the urethra, basing the reconstruction on the principles of hypospadias repair.

Management of Cryptorchidism

Orchidopexy in all patients is now usually performed during infancy in an effort to maintain the germ cell population and protect spermatogenesis. The potential for fertility in patients with prune-belly syndrome is clearly compromised. However, germ cells are known to be present in the testes of affected infants, mature sperm may develop after early orchidopexy, and testicular hormonal function will allow normal puberty. Therefore, orchidopexy is attempted in most patients. However, because the standard surgical techniques for orchidopexy are rarely successful, one of three alternatives is usually employed.

EARLY TRANSABDOMINAL ORCHIDOPEXY

In the neonate and in patients up to at least 6 months of age, transabdominal complete mobilization of the spermatic cord almost always allows the testis to be positioned in the dependent portion of the scrotum without dividing the vascular portion of the spermatic cord (Fig. 60–11) (Woodard and Parrott, 1978b). This procedure is particularly applicable to infants undergoing extensive ureteral reconstructive procedures during the neonatal period because it can be done simultaneously. In patients who do not require reconstructive surgery, the operation may be delayed 3 or 4 months to ensure stability of the upper urinary tract and the cardiopulmonary system.

FOWLER-STEPHENS (LONG LOOP VAS) TECHNIQUE

The Fowler-Stephens technique for performing orchidopexy in patients with intra-abdominal testes has become part of the standard urologic armamentarium (Fowler and Stephens, 1963). The operation relies on the presence of vascular anastomoses between the vessels of the vas deferens and the distal spermatic artery and on the redundancy of the looping vas deferens, which extends down beyond the testis and then returns superiorly to the epididymis. Preservation of the peritoneum over the vas deferens is important for protection of the collateral vessels. The spermatic vessel is divided above the level of the internal ring before its convergence with the vas. The vas and accompanying vasculature then allow placement of the testis in a scrotal position. In patients with prune-belly syndrome, the operation is done transperitoneally with a wider-than-usual exposure; the success rate has been reported as approximately 75% (Gibbons et al, 1979). This procedure represents a reasonable approach to the intra-abdominal testis in the patient with prune-belly syndrome and may allow greater flexibility in the timing of the procedure.

Enthusiasm has recently been generated for the so-called staged Fowler-Stephens operation, in which the spermatic vessels are ligated several months before the orchiopexy operation itself is performed. The rationale for this modification is to allow the development of increased collateral circulation between the vasal and distal testicular arteries, which may improve the success rate of the Fowler-Stephens procedure in these patients. The first stage may be accomplished by either open surgery or laparoscopy and is followed by either laparoscopic or open mobilization after an interval of 6 months (Docimo et al, 1995).

MICROVASCULAR AUTOTRANSPLANTATION

It is technically feasible to perform autotransplantation of the abdominal testis to the scrotum using microvascular anastomoses of the spermatic vessels to the inferior epigastric vessels. Although enthusiasm for this procedure is limited, the technique has been applied successfully in patients of various ages with prune-belly syndrome (McMahon et al, 1976; Wacksman et al, 1980). Despite the improbability of fertility in a patient with prune-belly syndrome, advances in the treatment of infertility may reduce the importance of extratesticular factors in these patients. Early orchiopexy may then assume even greater importance in preserving spermatogonia.

Abdominal Wall Reconstruction

Correction of the abdominal wall defect should be recognized as an important part of the management of patients with prune-belly syndrome. Not only does such a reconstruction produce a significant improvement in cosmesis and self image, but it also may improve bladder, bowel, and pulmonary function (Woodard et al, 1995; Smith et al, 1998). External support devices remain useful as a noninvasive means of managing abdominal wall. However, most parents and patients desire more definitive correction of the defect. Randolph and his colleagues carefully delineated

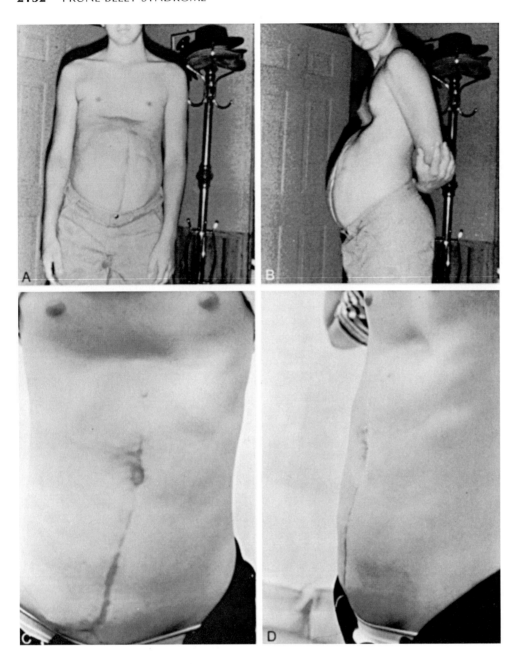

Figure 60–12. *A* and *B*, Anterior and lateral views of the abdomen of a 14-year-old boy who underwent major surgical remodeling of the urinary tract during early infancy with good results. Note typical abdominal configuration. *C* and *D*, Anterior and lateral views of the same boy 1 month after undergoing abdominoplasty with the technique described by Monfort.

the abdominal wall muscular defect by both electromyographic mapping and anatomic description. The lateral and upper parts of the abdominal wall are clearly the most normal, and the suprapubic region is the most affected (Randolph et al, 1981a; Fallat et al, 1989). This information forms the basis for each of the three procedures suggested for abdominal wall reconstruction.

RANDOLPH TECHNIQUE

The procedure developed by Randolph and colleagues (1981a) involves full-thickness removal of the abnormal region using a transverse incision extending from the tip of the 12th rib down to the symphysis pubis and back to the tip of the contralateral 12th rib. The redundant skin and deficient fascia are marked and excised, and the more healthy fascia is reapproximated to the anterior iliac spines, pubic tubercle, and fascia below. This procedure does suc-

ceed in reducing the protuberance of the abdomen, and the incision is carried out so that innervation to the anterior abdominal muscles is preserved. However, it does not improve abdominal wall thickness, and lateral bulging tends to remain uncorrected.

EHRLICH TECHNIQUE

Both the Ehrlich technique and the Monfort technique employ vertical overlapping of the abdominal fascia to eliminate redundancy, improve abdominal wall thickness, and generate a more normal physique (Fig. 60–12). Ehrlich's technique uses a midline incision followed by elevation of the skin and subcutaneous tissue from the attenuated muscular and fascial layers. A double-breasted overlapping advancement of each side toward the contralateral flank is then performed (Ehrlich et al, 1986). Preservation of the umbilicus requires mobilization on a vascular pedicle using the inferior epigastric vessels and appropriate repositioning during skin closure (Ehrlich and Lesavoy, 1993).

MONFORT TECHNIQUE

The Monfort abdominoplasty (see Fig. 60–8A through D and H through J) uses a vertically oriented elliptical incision to isolate the redundant skin, which is then elevated from the underlying fascia and excised. The umbilicus is circumscribed with a second incision and is left undisturbed. The abdominal cavity is then entered lateral to the rectus fascia, taking care to avoid interrupting the epigastric vessels at the superior and inferior aspects of the incision. Advancement of the lateral fascia over the central plate eliminates redundancy and provides increased thickness to the abdominal wall. Excellent results with a high degree of patient satisfaction have been reported with both the Ehrlich and Monfort techniques. Both procedures also provide adequate exposure for performance of concomitant genitourinary reconstruction (Ehrlich et al, 1986; Monfort et al, 1991).

OUTLOOK

The considerable improvements achieved in the medical, surgical, and urodynamic management of patients born with the prune-belly syndrome will certainly result in a prognosis far better than that previously reported, both for survival and for quality of life. The syndrome is clearly a disorder with a wide spectrum of severity. Some patients may benefit from major urologic reconstruction, but others require little if any such surgery. All patients need careful evaluation and individualized management, and, because urodynamics may change with age, long-term surveillance and periodic reappraisal are necessary.

REFERENCES

Aanpreung P, Bechwith B, Gelansky SH, et al: Association of paucity of interlobular bile ducts with prune belly syndrome. J Pediatr Gastroenterol Nutr 1993;16:81.

Aaronson IA: Posterior urethral valve masquerading as the prune belly syndrome. Br J Urol 1983;55:508.

Aaronson IA, Cremin BJ: Prune-belly syndrome in young females. Urol Radiol 1980;1:151.

Adebonojo FO: Dysplasia of the abdominal musculature with multiple congenital anomalies: Prune belly or triad syndrome. J Natl Med Assoc 1973;65:327.

Adenyokunna AA, Adenyu TM, Kolewole TM, et al: Prune-belly syndrome: A study of ten cases in Nigerian children with common and uncommon manifestations. East Afr Med J 1975;52:438.

Adenyokunna AA, Familusi JB: Prune belly syndrome in two siblings and a first cousin. Am J Dis Child 1982;136:23.

Affifi AK, Rebiez JM, Andonian SJ, et al: The myopathology of the prune belly syndrome. J Neurol Sci 1972;15:153.

Alford BA, Peoples WM, Resnick JS, et al: Pulmonary complications associated with the prune-belly syndrome. Pediatr Radiol 1978;129:401.

Appel RA, Kaplan GW, Brock WA, et al: Megalourethra. J Urol 1986;135:747.

Asplund J, Laska J: Prune belly syndrome at the age of 37. Scand J Urol Nephrol 1975;9:297.

Barnhouse DH: Prune belly syndrome. Br J Urol 1972;44:356.

Beckman H, Rehder H, Rauskolb R: Letter to the editor: Prune belly sequence associated with trisomy 13. Am J Med Genet 1984;19:603.

Bellah RD, States LJ, Duckett JW: Pseudoprune-belly syndrome: Imaging findings and clinical outcome. Am J Radiol 1996;167:1389.

Berdon WE, Baker DH, Wigger HJ, et al: The radiologic and pathologic spectrum of the prune belly syndrome: The importance of urethral obstruction in prognosis. Radiol Clin North Am 1977;15:83.

Bovicelli L, Rizzo N, Orsini LF, et al: Prenatal diagnosis of the prune belly syndrome. Clin Genet 1980;18:79.

Brinker M, Palutsis R, Sarwark J, et al: The orthopedic manifestations of prune-belly (Eagle-Barrett) syndrome. J Bone Joint Surg (Am) 1995;77:251.

Bukowski TP, Perlmutter AD: Reduction cystoplasty in the prune belly syndrome: A long term follow up. J Urol 1994;152:2113.

Burbige KA, Amodio J, Berdon WE, et al: Prune belly syndrome: 35 Years of experience. J Urol 1987;137:86.

Burke EC, Shin MH, Kelalis PP: Prune-belly syndrome. Am J Dis Child 1969;117:668.

Carter TC, Tomskey GC, Ozog LS: Prune-belly syndrome: Review of 10 cases. Urology 1974;3:279.

Cawthern TH, Bottene CA, Grant D: Prune-belly syndrome associated with Hirschsprung's disease. Am J Dis Child 1979;133:652.

Christopher CR, Spinelli A, Severt D: Ultrasonic diagnosis of prune-belly syndrome. Obstet Gynecol 1982;59:391.

Cukier J: Resection of the urethra in prune-belly syndrome. Birth Defects 1977;13:95.

Culp DA, Flocks RH: Congenital absence of abdominal musculature. J Iowa State Med Soc 1954;44:155.

Deklerk DP, Scott WW: Prostatic maldevelopment in the prune-belly syndrome: A defect in prostatic stromal-epithelial interaction. J Urol 1978;120:341.

Docimo SG, Moore RG, Kavoussi LR: Laparoscopic orchidopexy in the prune belly syndrome: A case report and review of the literature. Urology 1995;45:679.

Druschel CM: A descriptive study of prune belly in New York State, 1983 to 1989. Arch Pediatr Adolesc Med 1995;149:70.

Duckett JW Jr: Cutaneous vesicostomy in childhood: The Blocksom technique. Urol Clin North Am 1974;1:485.

Duckett JW Jr: The prune-belly syndrome. In Holder TM, Ashcroft KW (eds): The Surgery of Infants and Children. Philadelphia, WB Saunders, 1980, p 802.

Duckett JW: Prune-belly syndrome. In Welsh KJ, Randolph JG, Ravitch MM, et al (eds): Pediatric Surgery. Chicago, Year Book, 1986, pp 1193–1203.

Eagle JF, Barrett GS: Congenital deficiency of abdominal musculature with associated genitourinary anomalies: A syndrome. Reports of 9 cases. Pediatrics 1950;6:721.

Ehrlich RM, Lesavoy MA: Umbilicus preservation with total abdominal wall reconstruction in prune-belly syndrome. Urology 1993;43:3.

Ehrlich RM, Lesavoy MA, Fine RN: Total abdominal wall reconstruction in the prune-belly syndrome. J Urol 1986;136:282.

Elder JS, Duckett JW, Snyder HM: Intervention for fetal obstructive uropathy: Has it been effective? Lancet 1987;10:1007.

Fallat ME, Skoog SJ, Belman AB, et al: The prune-belly syndrome: A comprehensive approach to management. J Urol 1989;142:802.

Fowler R Jr, Stephens FD: The role of testicular vascular anatomy in the salvage of high undescended testes. In Stephens FD (ed): Congenital Malformations of the Rectum, Anus, and Genitourinary Tract. Baltimore, Williams & Wilkins, 1963.

Freedman AL, Bukowski TP, Smith CA, et al: Fetal therapy for obstructive uropathy: Specific outcomes diagnosis. J Urol 1996;156:720.

Freedman AL, Johnson MP, Smith CA, et al: Longterm outcome in children after antenatal intervention for obstructive uropathies. Lancet 1999;354:374.

Frolich F: Der mangei der muskeln, insbesondere der seitenbauchmuskeln [Dissertation]. Wurzberg, C.A. Zurn, 1939.

Frydman M, Magenis RE, Mohandas TK, et al: Chromosome abnormalities in infants with prune belly anomaly: Association with trisomy 18. Am J Med Genet 1983;15:145.

Garlinger P, Ott J: Prune-belly syndrome—possible genetic implications. Birth Defects 1974;10:173.

Geary DF, MacLusky IB, Churchill BM, et al: A broader spectrum of abnormalities in the prune belly syndrome. J Urol 1986;135:324.

Gibbons MD, Cromie WJ, Duckett JW: Management of the abdominal undescended testis. J Urol 1979;122:76.

Goulding FJ, Garrett RA: Twenty-five year experience with prune belly syndrome. Urology 1978;7:329.

Green NE, Lowery ER, Thomas R: Orthopaedic aspects of prune-belly syndrome. J Pediatr Orthop 1993;13:496.

Hanna MD, Jeffs RD, Sturgess JM, et al: Ureteral structure and ultrastructure: Part III. The congenitally dilated ureter (megaureter). J Urol 1977; 117:24.

Hannington-Kiff JG: Prune-belly syndrome and general anesthesia. Br J Anaesth 1970;42:649.

Harley LM, Chen Y, Rattner WH: Prune-belly syndrome. J Urol 1972; 108:174.

Hendren WH: Restoration of function in the severely decompensated ureter. In Johnston JH, Scholtmeijer RJ (eds): Problems in Paediatric Urology. Amsterdam, Excerpta Medica, 1972, pp 1–56.

Heydenrych J, Dutoit PE: Torsion of the spleen and associated prune-belly syndrome: Case report and review of the literature. S Afr Med J 1978;53:637.

Ives EJ: The abdominal muscle deficiency triad syndrome: Experience with ten cases. Birth Defects 1974;10:127.

Jeffs RD, Comisarow RH, Hanna MK: The early assessment for individualized treatment in the prune belly syndrome. Birth Defects 1977;13:97.

Karamanian A, Kravath R, Nagashima H, et al: Anesthetic management of the prune-belly syndrome in a 34 year old man. Int Urol Nephrol 1974;25:205.

Kerbl K, Pauer W: Renal failure and uraemia leading to the diagnosis of prune belly syndrome. Br J Anesthesiol 1993;46:897.

Kinahan TJ, Churchill BM, McLorie GA, et al: The efficiency of bladder emptying in the prune belly syndrome. J Urol 1992;148:600.

Kramer SA: Current status of fetal intervention for hydronephrosis. J Urol 1983;130:641.

Kroovand RL, Al-Ansari RM, Perlmutter AD: Urethral and genital malformations in prune-belly syndrome. J Urol 1982;127:94.

Kuga T, Esato K, Sase M, et al: Prune belly syndrome with penile and urethral agenesis: A report of a case. J Pediatr Surg 1998;33:1825.

Lattimer JK: Congenital deficiency of the abdominal wall musculature and associated genitourinary abnormalities: A report of 22 cases. J Urol 1958;79:343.

Lee ML: Prune-belly syndrome in a 54 year old man. JAMA 1977;237: 2216.

Lockhart JL, Reeve HR, Bredael JJ, et al: Siblings with prune belly syndrome and associated pulmonic stenosis, mental retardation, and deafness. Urology 1979;14:140.

Loder RT, Guiboux J, Bloom DA, et al: Musculoskeletal aspects of prune-belly syndrome. Am J Dis Child 1992;146:1224.

Lubinsky M, Koyle K, Trunca C: The association of prune-belly with Turner's syndrome. Am J Dis Child 1980;134:1171.

Massad CA, Cohen MB, Kogan BA, et al: Morphology and histochemistry of infant testes in the prune belly syndrome. J Urol 1991;146:1598.

McGovern JH, Marshall VF: Congenital deficiency of the abdominal musculature and obstructive uropathy. Surg Gynecol Obstet 1959;108:289.

McMahon RA, O'Brien MC, Cussen LJ: The use of microsurgery in the treatment of the undescended testis. J Pediatr Surg 1976;11:521.

McMullin ND, Hutson JM, Kelly JH: Minimal surgery in the prune belly syndrome. Pediatr Surg Int 1988;3:51.

Mininberg DT, Montoya F, Okada K, et al: Subcellular muscle studies in the prune belly syndrome. J Urol 1973;109:524.

Moerman P, Fryns JP, Goddeeris P, Lauweryns JM: Pathogenesis of the prune-belly syndrome: A functional urethral obstruction caused by prostatic hypoplasia. Pediatrics 1984;73:470.

Monfort G, Guys JM, Bocciardi A, et al: A novel technique for reconstruction of the abdominal wall in the prune belly syndrome. J Urol 1991;146:639.

Monie, IW, Monie BJ: Prune belly syndrome and fetal ascites. Teratology 1979;7:19.

Nakayama KD, Harrison MR, Chinn DH, de Lorimier AA: The pathogenesis of prune belly. Am J Dis Child 1984;138:834.

Noh PH, Cooper CS, Winkler AC, et al: Development of renal failure in children with the prune-belly syndrome. J Urol 1999;162:1399.

Nunn IN, Stephens FD: The triad system: A composite anomaly of the abdominal wall, urinary system and testes. J Urol 1961;86:782.

Okulski TA: The prenatal diagnosis of lower urinary tract obstruction using B scan ultrasound: A case report. J Clin Ultrasound 1977;5:268.

Orvis BR, Bottles K, Kogan BA: Testicular histology in fetuses with the prune belly syndrome and posterior urethral valves. J Urol 1988;139: 335.

Osler W: Congenital absence of the abdominal musculature, with distended and hypertrophied urinary bladder. Bull Johns Hopkins Hosp 1901;12:331.

Pagon RA, Smith DW, Shepard TH: Urethral obstruction malformation complex: A cause of abdominal muscle deficiency and the "prune belly." J Pediatr 1979;94:900.

Palmer JM, Tesluk J: Ureteral pathology in the prune belly syndrome. J Urol 1974;111:701.

Parker RW: Absence of abdominal muscles in an infant. Lancet 1895;1: 1252.

Passerini-Glazel G, Araguna F, Chiozza L, et al: The P.A.D.U.A. (progressive augmentation by dilating the urethra anterior). J Urol 1988; 140:1247.

Perlmutter AD: Reduction cystoplasty in prune belly syndrome. J Urol 1976;116:356.

Popek EJ, Tyson RW, Miller GJ, Caldwell SA: Prostate development in prune belly syndrome (PBS) and posterior urethral valves (PUV): Etiology of PBS—lower urinary tract obstruction or primary mesenchymal defect? Pediatr Pathol 1991;11:1.

Potter EL: Abnormal development of the kidney. In Potter EL (ed): Normal and Abnormal Development of the Kidney. Chicago, Year Book Medical Publishers, 1972, pp 154–220.

Rabinowitz R, Schillinger J: Prune belly syndrome in the female subject. J Urol 1977;118:454.

Rajfer J, Walsh PC: Testicular descent: Normal and abnormal. Urol Clin North Am 1978;5:223.

Ralis Z, Forbes M: Intrauterine atrophy and gangrene of the lower extremity of the fetus caused by megacystitis due to urethral atresia. J Pathol 1971;104:31.

Randolph J, Cavett C, Eng G: Abdominal wall reconstruction in the prune-belly syndrome. J Pediatr Surg 1981a;16:960.

Randolph J, Cavett C, Eng G: Surgical correction and rehabilitation for children with "prune-belly" syndrome. Ann Surg 1981b;6:757.

Reinberg Y, Manivel JC, Fryd D, et al: The outcome of renal transplantation in children with the prune-belly syndrome. J Urol 1989;142:1541.

Reinberg Y, Manivel JC, Pettinato G, et al: Development of renal failure in children with the prune belly syndrome. J Urol 1991;145:1017.

Reinberg Y, Chelimsky G, Gonzalez R: Urethral atresia and the prune belly syndrome: Report of six cases. Br J Urol 1993;72:112.

Riccardi VM, Grum CM: The prune-belly anomaly: Heterogeneity and superficial X-linkage mimicry. J Med Genet 1977;14:266.

Rogers LW, Ostrow PT: The prune belly syndrome: Report of 20 cases and description of a lethal variant. J Pediatr 1973;83:786.

Sayre R, Stephens R, Chonlo AM: Prune-belly syndrome and retroperitoneal germ cell tumor. Am J Med 1986;81:895.

Shih W, Greenbaum KD, Baro C: In utero sonogram in prune belly syndrome. Urology 1982;20:102.

Shimizu T, Ihara Y, Yomuro W, et al: Antenatal diagnosis of prune belly syndrome. Arch Gynecol Obstet 1992;251:211.

Sholder AJ, Maizels M, Depp R, et al: Caution in antenatal intervention. J Urol 1988;139:1026.

Silverman FM, Huang N: Congenital absence of the abdominal muscles associated with malformation of the genitourinary and alimentary tracts: Report of cases and review of literature. Am J Dis Child 1950;80:9.

Smith CA, Smith EA, Parrott TS, et al: Voiding function in patients with the prune-belly syndrome after Monfort abdominoplasty. J Urol 1998; 41:3.

Smith DW: Recognizable Patterns of Human Malformation. Philadelphia, WB Saunders, 1970, p 5.

Smythe AR: Ultrasound detection of fetal ascites and bladder dilation with resulting prune-belly. J Pediatr 1981;98:978.

Snyder HM, Harrison NW, Whitfield, HN, Williams DI: Urodynamics in the prune belly syndrome. Br J Urol 1976;48:663.

Stephens FD, Gupta D: Pathogenesis of the prune belly syndrome. J Urol 1994;152:2328.

Steinhardt G, Hogan W, Wood E, et al: Longterm survival in an infant with urethral atresia. J Urol 1990;143:336.

Tank ES, McCoy G: Limited surgical intervention in the prune belly syndrome. J Pediatr Surg 1983;18:688.

Texter JH, Koontz WW: Prune-belly syndrome seen in the adult. Soc Pediatr Urol Newsletter 1980; February 6.

Wacksman J, Dinner M, Staffon RA: Technique of testicular autotransplantation using a micro-vascular anastomosis. Surg Gynecol Obstet 1980;150:399.

Waldbaum RS, Marshall VF: The prune belly syndrome: A diagnostic therapeutic plan. J Urol 1970;103:668.

Wallner M, Kramar R: Detection of prune-belly syndrome in a 35 year old man: A rare cause of end-stage renal failure in the adult. Am J Nephrol 1990;10:413.

Welch KJ, Kearney GP: Abdominal musculature deficiency syndrome: Prune-belly. J Urol 1974;111:693.

Willert C, Cohen H, Yu YT, et al: Association of prune-belly syndrome and gastroschisis. Am J Dis Child 1978;132:526.

Williams DI: Prune-belly syndrome. In Harrison JH, Gittes RF, Perlmutter AD, et al (eds): Campbell's Urology, 4th ed. Philadelphia, WB Saunders, 1979, pp 1743–1755.

Williams DI, Burkholder GV: The prune-belly syndrome. J Urol 1967;98:244.

Woodard JR: The bladder in prune-belly syndrome. Dialog Pediatr Urol 1990;13:6.

Woodard JR: Prune-belly syndrome. State of the Art Podium Presentation. American Urological Association National Meeting, Atlanta, Georgia, May 2000.

Woodard JR, Parrott TS: Reconstruction of the urinary tract in prune-belly uropathy. J Urol 1978a;119:824.

Woodard JR, Parrott TS: Orchiopexy in the prune-belly syndrome. Br J Urol 1978b;50:348.

Woodard JR, Parrott TS, Broecker BH, et al: The Monfort abdominoplasty for patients with prune-belly syndrome. In Thuroff JW (ed): Societe Internationale d'Urologie Reports: Reconstructive Surgery of the Lower Urinary Tract in Children. Oxford, UK., Issis Medical Media, 1995.

Woodhouse RJ, Kellett MJ, Williams DI: Minimal surgical interference in the prune belly syndrome. Br J Urol 1979;51:474.

Woodhouse RJ, Ransley PG: Teratoma of the testis in the prune-belly syndrome. Br J Urol 1983;55:580.

Woodhouse RJ, Snyder HM: Testicular and sexual function in adults with prune belly syndrome. J Urol 1985;133:607.

Wright J, Barth R, Neff J, et al: Gastrointestinal malformations associated with prune-belly syndrome: Three cases and a review of the literature. Pediatr Pathol 1986;5:421.

61

EXSTROPHY, EPISPADIAS, AND OTHER BLADDER ANOMALIES

John P. Gearhart, MD

Types of Syndromes

Cloacal Exstrophy

Supra vesical Fissure

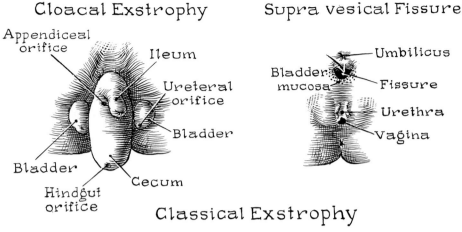

Classical Exstrophy

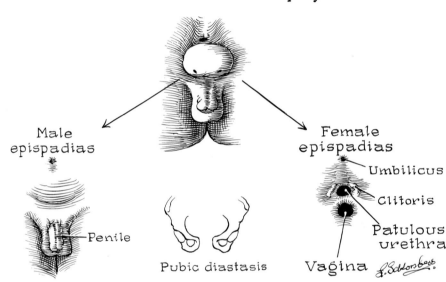

Figure 61–1. Various entities in the exstrophy-epispadias syndrome. (Drawings by Leon Schlossberg.)

The exstrophy-epispadias complex of genitourinary malformations can be as simple as a glandular epispadias or an overwhelming multisystem defect such as cloacal exstrophy (Fig. 61–1). This chapter deals mainly with the surgical management of bladder exstrophy, cloacal exstrophy, and epispadias. Other conditions involving the bladder are discussed, but a detailed approach to the modern management of the exstrophy-epispadias complex and the outcomes of such therapy are emphasized.

The primary objectives of the modern surgical management of classic bladder exstrophy are (1) a secure initial closure; (2) reconstruction of a functioning cosmetically acceptable penis in the male and external genitalia in the female; and (3) urinary continence with the preservation of renal function. Currently, these objectives can be achieved with newborn primary bladder and posterior urethral closure, early epispadias repair, and finally bladder neck reconstruction when the bladder reaches an appropriate volume for an outlet procedure and the child is ready to be dry. Occasionally, in highly selected patients, bladder closure and epispadias repair can be combined and then bladder neck repair performed when an adequate ca-

pacity is reached and again when the child is ready to be continent.

Formerly, surgical reconstruction of cloacal exstrophy, the most severe variant of the exstrophy complex, was considered futile. However, advances in pediatric anesthesia, neonatal care, and nutrition, along with the application of principles that have evolved in the treatment of classic bladder exstrophy, including the use of osteotomies in all patients, has markedly improved the outcome in this group of patients. Similarly, newer reconstructive techniques and better surgical repair have allowed a number of these patients to be raised in the male sex of rearing, obviating the need for gender conversion except in a few instances. In this chapter, the techniques for managing both bladder and cloacal exstrophy are discussed in a comprehensive manner and the surgical approach to these patients is presented. The long-term results presented here come from a database of 688 patients with the exstrophy complex treated at the author's institution since 1975.

The surgical management of epispadias, the least extensive anomaly of this complex, is straightforward and involves reconstruction of the external genitalia and restoration of urinary continence. In this chapter, techniques for managing the exstrophy-epispadias variants are discussed, a detailed description of our surgical approach to these anomalies is presented, and the results of surgical intervention are summarized. Also, management of exstrophy when initial or secondary closure has failed is discussed, along with bladders that fail to gain capacity, failed bladder neck reconstruction, and failed genitourethral reconstruction. Finally, techniques other than staged reconstruction are discussed in addition to malignancy, fertility, and the emotional impact of this birth defect on the child and family.

BLADDER EXSTROPHY

History

In older texts the first account of bladder exstrophy was ascribed to Assyro-Babylonian sources dating from the first and second millennium BC. At that time, birth anomalies in both humans and animals were carefully recorded on tablets for their importance as omens, based on their interpretation by divination experts. Feneley and Gearhart (2000) examined Assyro-Babylonian descriptions of congenital anomalies from cuneiform texts at the British Museum in London. Although references to anomalies involving the external genitalia were frequent (e.g., hermaphroditism, absence of external genitalia, unilateral and bilateral undescended testes), references to renal and bladder anomalies were few and difficult to interpret medically. Duplication and laterality of anomalies were described in detail owing to their distinct significance, but malformations in combination were not recorded. Based on these studies performed with a prominent Assyriologist, a definitive description of bladder or cloacal exstrophy was not corroborated. **The first recorded case of epispadias is attributed to the Byzantine Emperor Heraclius (AD 610 to 641) and the first description of bladder exstrophy to Schenck in 1595** (Feneley and Gearhart, 2000).

Incidence and Inheritance

The incidence of bladder exstrophy has been estimated as being between 1 in 10,000 and 1 in 50,000 (Lattimer and Smith, 1966) **live births. However, data from the International Clearinghouse for Birth Defects monitoring system estimated the incidence to be 3.3 cases in 100,000 live births** (Lancaster, 1987). **The male-to-female ratio of bladder exstrophy derived from multiple series is 2.3:1** (Shapiro et al, 1984). However, two series reported a 5:1 to 6:1 male-to-female ratio of exstrophy births (Ives et al, 1980; Lancaster, 1987).

The risk of recurrence of bladder exstrophy in a given family is approximately 1 in 100 (Ives et al, 1980). Shapiro and coworkers (1984) conducted a questionnaire of pediatric urologists and surgeons in North America and Europe and identified the recurrence of exstrophy and epispadias in only 9 of approximately 2500 indexed cases. Lattimer and Smith (1966) cited a set of identical twins with bladder exstrophy and another set of twins in whom only one child had exstrophy. Shapiro's series identified five sets of male and female nonidentical twins in whom

only one twin was affected with exstrophy; five sets of male identical twins in whom both twins were affected; one set of identical male twins in whom only one twin was affected; and three sets of female identical twins in whom only one twin had the exstrophy anomaly (Shapiro et al, 1985).

The inheritance pattern of bladder exstrophy in a literature review by Clemetson (1958) identified 45 women with bladder exstrophy who produced 49 offspring. None of their offspring demonstrated features of the exstrophy-epispadias complex. Bladder exstrophy or epispadias was not reported until the 1980s in the offspring of parents with the exstrophy-epispadias complex. Shapiro and colleagues (1984) described two women with complete epispadias who gave birth to sons with bladder exstrophy. They also reported that another woman with bladder exstrophy gave birth to a son with bladder exstrophy. The inheritance of these three cases of bladder exstrophy was identified in a total of 225 offspring (75 boys and 150 girls) produced by individuals with bladder exstrophy and epispadias. **Shapiro and colleagues determined that the risk of bladder exstrophy in the offspring of individuals with bladder exstrophy and epispadias is 1 in 70 live births, a 500-fold greater incidence than in the general population.** In a multinational review of exstrophy patients (Lancaster, 1987) two interesting trends were found: (1) bladder exstrophy tends to occur in infants of younger mothers, and (2) an increased risk at higher parity is observed for bladder exstrophy but not for epispadias.

Embryology

Bladder exstrophy, cloacal exstrophy, and epispadias are variants of the exstrophy-epispadias complex (see Fig. 61–1). The cause of this complex is thought to be the failure of the cloacal membrane to be reinforced by ingrowth of mesoderm (Muecke, 1964). The cloacal membrane is a bilaminar layer situated at the caudal end of the germinal disc that occupies the infraumbilical abdominal wall. Mesenchymal ingrowth between the ectodermal and endodermal layers of the cloacal membrane results in formation of the lower abdominal muscles and the pelvic bones. The cloacal membrane is subject to premature rupture, and, depending on the extent of the infraumbilical defect and the stage of development during which the rupture occurs, bladder exstrophy, cloacal exstrophy, or epispadias results (Ambrose and O'Brien, 1974).

After mesenchymal ingrowth occurs, the urorectal septum grows in a caudal direction and divides the cloaca into a bladder anteriorly and a rectum posteriorly (Fig. 61–2). Distally, the septum meets the posterior remnant of the bilaminar membrane, which eventually perforates and forms the urogenital and anal openings. The paired genital tubercles migrate medially and fuse in the midline, cephalad to the dorsal membrane before perforation.

The theory of embryonic maldevelopment in exstrophy held by Marshall and Muecke (1968) is that the basic defect is an abnormal overdevelopment of the cloacal membrane, which prevents medial migration of the mesenchymal tissue and proper lower abdominal wall development. The timing of the rupture of this defective cloacal membrane determines the variant of the exstro-

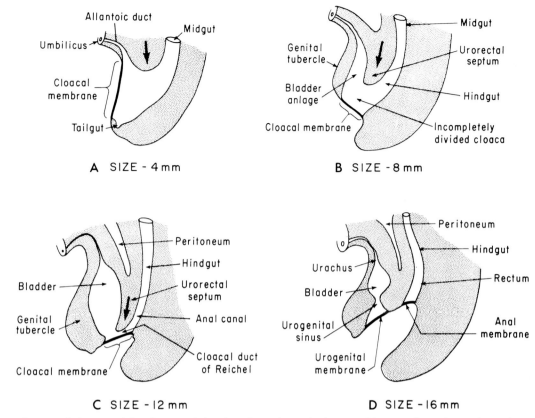

Figure 61–2. Developmental changes of the cloaca and the cloacal membrane in the 4- to 16-mm embryo. Arrow shows downward direction of growth of the urorectal septum. (Drawings not to scale.)

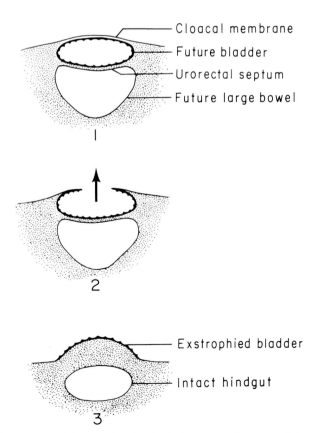

Figure 61–3. Diagram of embryological events and rupture of cloacal membrane leading to classic bladder exstrophy.

phy-epispadias complex that results (Figs. 61–3 and 61–4). This theory is supported by Muecke's work in the chick embryo and by the high incidence of expected central perforations, resulting in the preponderance of classic exstrophy variants. Classic exstrophy accounts for more than 50% of the patients born with this complex (Muecke, 1964; Marshall and Muecke, 1968).

However, other plausible theories concerning the cause of the exstrophy-epispadias complex exist. One group has postulated abnormal development of the genital hillocks caudal to the normal position, with fusion in the midline below rather than above the cloacal membrane. This view has been accepted by other investigators (Patten and Barry, 1952; Ambrose and O'Brien, 1974). Another interesting hypothesis that remains controversial describes an abnormal caudal insertion of the body stalk, which results in a failure of interposition of the mesenchymal tissue in the midline (Mildenberger et al, 1988). As a consequence of this failure, translocation of the cloaca into the depths of the abdominal cavity does not occur. A cloacal membrane that remains in a superficial infraumbilical position represents an unstable embryonic state with a strong tendency to disintegrate (Johnson and Kogan, 1974).

Anatomic Considerations

Exstrophy of the bladder is part of a spectrum of anomalies involving the urinary tract, the genital tract, the musculoskeletal system, and sometimes the intestinal tract. In classic bladder exstrophy, most anomalies are related to

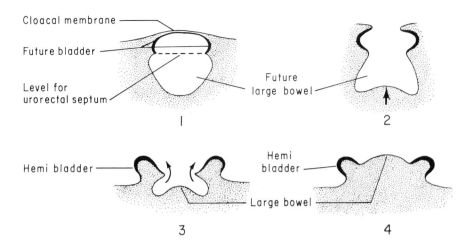

Figure 61–4. Diagram of premature rupture of cloacal membrane with eventration causing the formation of cloacal exstrophy.

defects of the abdominal wall, bladder, genitalia, pelvic bones, rectum, and anus (Fig. 61–5*A* and *B*). Because of the involved nature of this defect, the deficits are described here as they affect each system.

Skeletal Defects

Formerly, classic bladder exstrophy was thought only to show the characteristic widening of the pubic symphysis caused by malrotation of the innominate bones in relation to the sagittal plane of the body along both sacroiliac joints. In addition, there was an outward rotation or eversion of the pubic rami at their junction with the iliac bones. More recently, data by Sponseller and associates (1995) using CT of the pelvis with three-dimensional (3-D) reconstruction has further characterized the bony defect associated with both classic bladder exstrophy and cloacal exstrophy. **In reviewing a large group of patients with exstrophy of the bladder, using pelvic CT scans and age-matched controls, Sponseller and coworkers (1995) found that patients with classic bladder exstrophy have a mean external rotation of the posterior aspect of the pelvis of 12 degrees on each side, retroversion of the acetabulum, and a mean 18 degrees of external rotation of the anterior pelvis, along with 30% shortening of the pubic rami, in addition to the previously described diastasis of the symphysis pubis** (Fig. 61–6). In long-term follow-up there was a foot progression angle of 20 to 30 degrees of external rotation beyond the normal limits seen in early childhood, but this rotation improved with age. Likewise, patients with cloacal exstrophy not only had pelvic deformities to a greater degree, but also had asymmetry of the above-measured parameters between the right and left sides of the pelvis, malformation of the sacroiliac joints, and occasional dislocations of the hip (Sponseller et al, 1995).

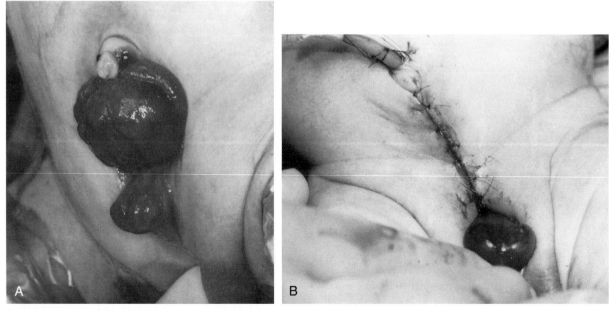

Figure 61–5. *A,* Newborn male with classic bladder exstrophy, excellent bladder template, but shortened urethral groove. *B,* Same patient at the end of surgical procedure after closure of bladder, posterior urethra, and abdominal wall. Note exit of suprapubic tube and ureteral stents from neoumbilicus.

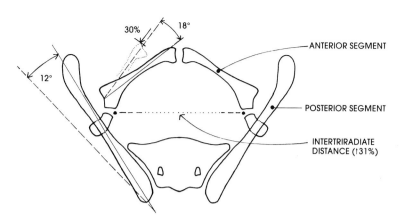

Figure 61–6. Abnormal anatomy seen in classic bladder exstrophy. The posterior bony segment is externally rotated a mean of 12 degrees on each side, but the length is not different. The anterior segment is externally rotated 18 degrees (6 degrees more than the posterior segment) and is shortened by a mean of 30%. There is a shortage of bone of 30%. The distance between the triradiate cartilage is increased by 31%.

New data from Stec and colleagues (Gearhart et al, 2002) using 3-D models from CT scans has gained further insight into the bony defect of children born with classic bladder exstrophy. Using age-matched controls, they found that the sacroiliac joint angle (before closure) was 10 degrees larger in the exstrophy pelvis, being 10 degrees more toward the coronal plane than sagittal. Also, the bony pelvis in exstrophy has 14.7 degrees more inferior rotation than in normal patients. Lastly, the sacrum in exstrophy patients has a 42.6% larger volume and 23.5% more surface area than in controls. These new findings will help with planning better osteotomies and better reduction of both the pubic diastasis and pubic long-term undergrowth in these patients.

These rotational deformities of the pelvic skeletal structures contribute to the short, pendular penis seen in bladder exstrophy. Outward rotation and lateral displacement of the innominate bones also accounts for the increased distance between the hips, waddling gait, and the outward rotation of the lower limbs in these children, which in itself causes little disability and usually corrects to some degree over time. However, new preliminary data from Sponseller and colleagues (2000b) shows an increased incidence of premature osteoarthritis of the hip in those adult patients who were closed without an osteotomy.

Pelvic Floor Defects

Gearhart, Stec, and colleagues (Gearhart et al, 2001), using 3-D models created from CT scans of children with classic bladder exstrophy and normal age-matched controls, found that the puborectal slings were supporting two times more body cavity area than normal. The levator ani group is positioned more posteriorly in exstrophy patients, with 68% located posterior to the rectum and 32% anterior (versus 52% posterior and 48% anterior in normal controls). The levators are also rotated outward 15.5 degrees and in the coronal aspect the levators are 31.7 degrees more flattened than normal. This deviation from normal makes the exstrophy puborectal sling more flattened than its normal conical shape. There was no significant difference in the length or thickness of these muscles between patients with exstrophy and normal controls. These new insights further elucidate the entire exstrophy defect, especially in regard to pelvic reconstruction.

Abdominal Wall Defects

The triangular defect caused by the premature rupture of the abnormal cloacal membrane is occupied by the exstrophy bladder and posterior urethra. The fascial defect is limited inferiorly by the intrasymphyseal band, which represents the divergent urogenital diaphragm. This band connects the bladder neck and posterior urethra to the pubic ramus on anatomic study. The anterior sheath of the rectus muscle has a fan-like extension behind the urethra and bladder neck that inserts into the intrasymphyseal band. **Complete dissection of this extension into the intrasymphyseal band and bladder neck area is required to achieve intrapelvic position of the bladder at the time of exstrophy closure.**

At the upper end of the triangular fascial defect is the umbilicus. In bladder exstrophy, the distance between the umbilicus and the anus is always foreshortened. Because the umbilicus is situated well below the horizontal line of the iliac crest, there is an unusual expanse of uninterrupted abdominal skin. Although an umbilical hernia is usually present, it is usually of insignificant size. The umbilical hernia is repaired at the time of the initial exstrophy closure. Omphaloceles, although rarely seen in conjunction with bladder exstrophy, are frequently associated with cloacal exstrophy. Omphaloceles associated with classic bladder exstrophy-epispadias complex are usually small and can be closed at the time of bladder closure.

The frequent occurrence of indirect inguinal hernias is attributed to a persistent processus vaginalis, large internal and external inguinal rings, and lack of obliquity of the inguinal canal. **Connelly and coauthors (1995), in a review of 181 children with bladder exstrophy, reported inguinal hernias in 81.8% of boys and 10.5% of girls.** At the time of closure of the bladder exstrophy, these hernias should be repaired by excision of the hernial sac and repair of the transversalis fascia and muscle defect to prevent recurrence or a direct inguinal hernia. The contralateral side should also be explored, because the incidence of synchronous or asynchronous bilaterality is very high.

Anorectal Defects

The perineum is short and broad and the anus is situated directly behind the urogenital diaphragm; it is

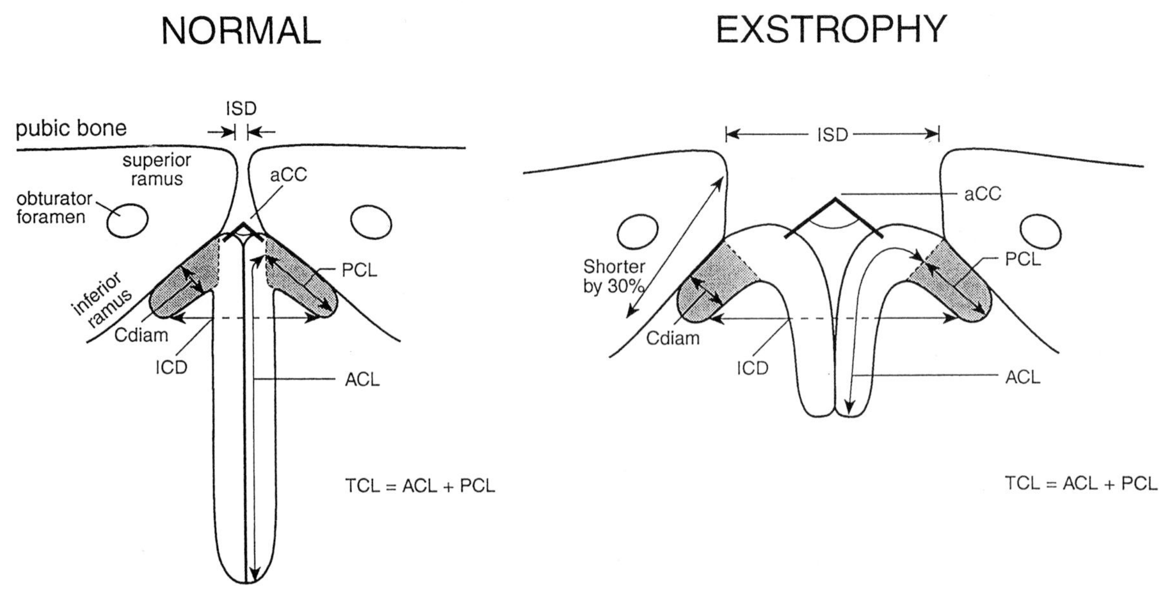

Figure 61–7. Penile and pelvic measurements in normal men and patients with classic exstrophy. ISD, intersymphyseal distance; aCC, corpora cavernosa sustended angle; Cdiam, corpus cavernosum diameter; PCL, posterior corporal length; ICD, intercorporal distance; ACL, anterior corporal length; TCL, total corporal length.

displaced anteriorly and corresponds to the posterior limit of the triangular fascial defect. The anal sphincter mechanism is also anteriorly displaced and should be preserved intact in case internal urinary diversion is required in future management.

The divergent levator ani and puborectalis muscles and the distorted anatomy of the external sphincter contribute to varying degrees of anal incontinence and rectal prolapse. Anal continence is usually imperfect at an early age. In rare patients, the rectal sphincter mechanism may never be adequate to control the liquid content of the bowel. Rectal prolapse frequently occurs in untreated exstrophy patients with a widely separated symphysis. It is usually transient and easily reduced. Prolapse virtually disappears after bladder closure or cystectomy and urinary diversion. The appearance of prolapse in an infant is an indication to proceed with definitive management of the exstrophied bladder. **If rectal prolapse occurs at any time after exstrophy closure, posterior urethral/bladder outlet obstruction should be suspected, and immediate evaluation of the outlet tract by cystoscopy should be performed** (Baker and Gearhart, 1998).

Male Genital Defect

The male genital defect is severe and is probably the most troublesome aspect of the surgical reconstruction, independent of the decision whether to treat with modern staged closure, combined closure, or some other form of urinary diversion. Formerly, it was thought that the individual corpora cavernosa were of normal caliber but appeared shorter because of the wide separation of the crural attachments, the prominent dorsal chordee, and the shortened urethral groove. **However, newer data by Silver and colleagues (1997b) described the genital defect in bladder exstrophy in much greater detail. They used magnetic resonance imaging (MRI) in adult men with bladder**

exstrophy and compared the results with those of age- and race-matched controls. They found that the anterior corporal length of male patients with bladder exstrophy was almost 50% shorter than that of normal controls (Fig. 61–7). However, although the posterior length of the corporal body was the same as in age-matched controls, the diameter of the posterior corporal segment was greater than in normal controls. It was also found on MRI that the diastasis of the symphysis pubis increased the intrasymphyseal and intercorporal distances but the angle between the corpora cavernosa was unchanged because the corporal bodies were separated in a parallel fashion. **Therefore, the penis appears short not only because of the diastasis of the pubic symphysis, as thought in the past, but also because of marked congenital deficiency of anterior corporal tissue** (Silver et al, 1997b).

A functional and cosmetically pleasing penis can be achieved when the dorsal chordee is released, the urethral groove lengthened, and the penis somewhat lengthened by mobilizing the crura in the midline. Patients with a very small or dystrophic penis should be considered for sex reassignment only after other opinions have been obtained and the parents have been counseled about the implications of this step.

In a study by Gearhart and associates (1993c), 13 adult men born with bladder exstrophy were evaluated with MRI of the pelvis to evaluate the size and configuration of the prostate and sex accessory organs. The volume, weight, and maximum cross-sectional area of the prostate appeared normal compared with published control values (Fig. 61–8). **However, in none of the patients did the prostate extend circumferentially around the urethra, and the urethra was anterior to the prostate in all patients.** Except for studies to document the presence of the prostate gland or its size, data do not exist concerning the function of the prostate gland in the

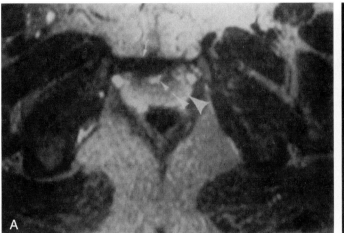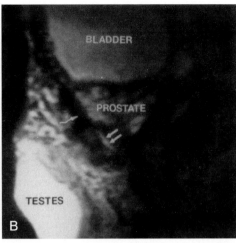

Figure 61–8. *A,* Axial T2-weighted image through mid-prostate gland in 20-year-old continent exstrophy patient. Lumen of urethra *(small arrowhead),* low-signal MRI central zone (including McNeal transitional zone, McNeal central zone, and periurethral stroma; *medium arrowhead),* and high signal MRI peripheral zone *(large arrowhead)* are shown. Note also fibrous band between diastatic symphysis, a structure of potential anterior support *(curved arrow). B,* Sagittal T2-weighted images through mid-prostate gland show anterior urethra *(double arrows)* and prostate gland posterior to it. Fibrous band anteriorly *(curved arrow)* extends along entire length of prostate gland.

patient with exstrophy. Silver and coworkers (1997a) reported free and total prostate-specific antigen levels for a group of adult men with bladder exstrophy. Although they were measurable, they were below the upper limits for established age-specific reference ranges for normal men. The vas deferens and ejaculatory ducts are normal in the exstrophy patient, provided they are not injured iatrogenically (Hanna and Williams, 1972). Also, the mean seminal vesicle length in men with exstrophy was normal compared with published controls. Additional evaluation of the puborectalis muscle group was undertaken, and these muscles were found to be widely separated and to provide only lateral support of the prostate in patients who were continent and had undergone prior iliac osteotomy.

Autonomic innervation of the corpus cavernosum is provided by the cavernous nerves. These autonomic nerves are displaced laterally in patients with exstrophy (Schlegel and Gearhart, 1989). **These nerves are preserved in almost all exstrophy patients as potency is preserved after surgery.** However, retrograde ejaculation may occur after bladder closure and later bladder neck reconstruction.

Testis function has not been studied in a large group of postpubertal exstrophy patients, but it is generally believed that fertility is not impaired by testicular dysfunction. The testes frequently appear undescended in their course from the widened separated pubic tubercles to the flat, wide scrotum. Most testes are retractile and have an adequate length of spermatic cord to reach the scrotum without the need for orchiopexy.

Female Genital Defects

Reconstruction of the female genitalia presents a less complex problem than in the male (Fig. 61–9*A* and *B*). **The vagina is shorter than normal, hardly greater than 6 cm in depth, but of normal caliber. The vaginal orifice is frequently stenotic and displaced anteriorly, the clitoris is bifid, and the labia, mons pubis, and clitoris are divergent. The uterus enters the vagina superiorly so that the cervix is in the anterior vaginal wall. The fallopian tubes and ovaries are normal.** The clitoral halves should be joined and the two ends of the labia minora joined to make a fourchette at the time of primary closure. Vaginal dilatation or episiotomy may be required to allow satisfactory intercourse in the mature female. The defective pelvic floor may predispose mature females to the development of uterine prolapse, making uterine suspension necessary. This usually occurs after childbirth but can occur in the nulliparous patient. Uterine prolapse does not appear to occur when osteotomy and closure of the anterior defect is performed early in life.

Urinary Defects

At birth, the bladder mucosa may appear normal; however, ectopic bowel mucosa, or an isolated bowel loop, or more commonly a hamartomatous polyp may be present on the bladder surface. If the bladder mucosa is not frequently irrigated with saline and protected from surface trauma by the interposition of some form of protective membrane before closure, cystic or metaplastic changes in the mucosal surface of the bladder may occur.

The size, distensibility, and neuromuscular function of the exstrophied bladder, as well as the size of the triangular fascial defect to which the bladder muscles attach, affects the decision to attempt repair. In the last several years, multiple basic science studies have been published that further delineate the exact nature of the exstrophied bladder in the newborn. **One of the first papers to characterize the neuromuscular function of the bladder was published by Shapiro and colleagues (1985). In this paper muscarinic cholinergic receptor density and binding affinity were measured in control subjects and in patients with classic bladder exstrophy. The density of the muscarinic cholinergic receptors in both the control and exstrophy groups were similar, as was the binding affinity of the muscarinic receptor.** Therefore, it was thought

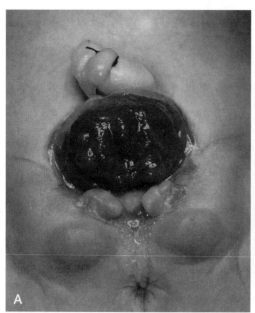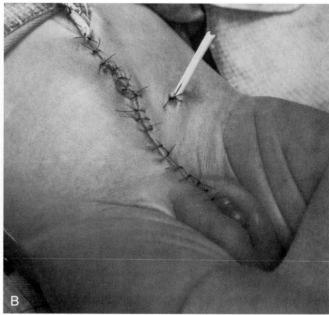

Figure 61–9. *A,* Newborn female with classic bladder exstrophy. Notice open urethral plate, bifid clitoral halves, and anterior displacement of the vaginal orifice. *B,* Same patient after closure and genitoplasty.

by the authors that the neurophysiologic composition of the exstrophied bladder is not grossly altered during its anomalous development. Studies have investigated both the neural innervation of the newborn exstrophy bladder and with its muscle and collagen content. **Lee and coworkers (1996), looked at bladder biopsies obtained from 12 newborns with bladder exstrophy, compared with age-matched controls, and found an increase in the ratio of collagen to smooth muscle in the newborns with bladder exstrophy. In addition, using anti-collagen antibodies, they evaluated various types of collagen in these bladders. Compared with normal control bladders, there was no statistical difference in the amount of type I collagen in the bladders of newborns with exstrophy at initial closure, but there was a threefold increase in type III collagen.** Peppas and associates (1999) found, in patients who gained adequate bladder capacities and were awaiting bladder neck reconstruction, that the ratio of collagen to smooth muscle decreased markedly after a successful closure and infection-free follow-up. Lais and coworkers (1996) reported similar findings, but they measured the ratio of smooth muscle to collagen and found it increased after a successful closure.

In an extension of the studies just cited, Mathews and coworkers (1999b) looked at the number of myelinated nerves per field in the newborn bladders of normal subjects and those with exstrophy. The average number of myelinated nerves per field was reduced in the exstrophy bladders compared with controls, and the difference was statistically significant. This reduction in nerve fibers appears to be the result of a lack of small fibers with preservation of larger nerve fibers. In light of the findings already mentioned, it is believed that bladder exstrophy in a newborn probably represents a maturational delay in overall bladder development.

In a large study by Rosch and colleagues (1997) from Germany, multiple immunocytochemical and histochemical markers were examined in patients with epispadias or classic bladder exstrophy. These studies involved indirect immunocytochemistry for vasoactive intestinal polypeptide (VIP), neuropeptide Y (NPY), substance P (SP), calcitonin gene-related product (CGRP), and protein gene product (PGP) 9.5, and nicotinamide adenine dinucleotide phosphate diaphorase (NADPHd). No evidence of bladder muscle dysinnervation was found morphologically in any cases of classic bladder exstrophy. Cases of bladder exstrophy after failed reconstruction had muscle innervation deficiencies that increased subepithelial and intraepithelial innervation. **Therefore, although a newborn with bladder exstrophy may have a maturational delay in bladder development, these bladders have the potential for normal development after a successful initial closure.**

However, when the bladder is small, fibrosed, inelastic, and covered with polyps, functional repair may be impossible (Fig. 61–10). The more normal bladder may be invaginated, or it may bulge through a small fascial defect, indicating the potential for satisfactory capacity after successful initial closure. **Also, not until examination under anesthesia can the true defect be adequately evaluated, because bladders that appear small in the nursery may have a good bit of bladder sequestered below the fascial defect. The depth of this extension often cannot be appreciated unless the infant is totally relaxed under anesthesia.**

Bladder function was assessed in a group of continent exstrophy patients with normal reflexive bladders. Normal cystometrograms were obtained in 70% to 90% of cases (Toguri et al, 1987). Diamond and associates (1999), looking at 30 patients with bladder exstrophy at various stages of reconstruction, found that 80% of patients had compliant

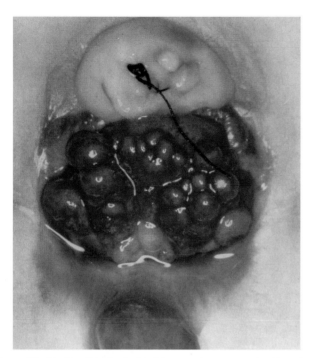

Figure 61-10. Small inelastic bladder template covered with polyps, unsuitable for primary closure.

and stable bladders before bladder neck reconstruction. After bladder neck reconstruction, approximately half of the patients maintained normal bladder compliance and a lesser number maintained normal stability. The authors believed that compliance and stability were impaired after bladder neck reconstruction and that 25% of patients with exstrophy may maintain normal detrusor function after reconstruction. In an earlier paper by Hollowell and colleagues (1993), 13 of 21 children revealed involuntary contractions and only four revealed stable bladders before bladder neck reconstruction. Also, 7 of 21 had increased pressures (greater than 10 cm H₂O), suggesting decreased compliance. The difference in findings between these two urodynamic studies is difficult to explain from an experimental perspective. However, standardized methods of bladder neck repair do not exist, and these differences may be reflected in the different urodynamic findings after bladder neck repair in these two groups of patients.

The urinary tract is usually normal, but anomalous development does occur. Horseshoe kidney, pelvic kidney, hypoplastic kidney, solitary kidney, and dysplasia with megaureter are all encountered in these patients. The ureters have an abnormal course in their termination. The peritoneal pouch of Douglas between the bladder and the rectum is enlarged and unusually deep, forcing the ureter down laterally in its course across the true pelvis. The distal segment of the ureter approaches the bladder from a point inferior and lateral to the orifice, and it enters the bladder with little or no obliquity. **Therefore, reflux in the closed exstrophy bladder occurs in 100% of cases, and subsequent surgery usually is required at the time of bladder neck reconstruction. If excessive outlet resistance is gained at the time of either initial closure or combined epispadias and bladder exstrophy closure, and recurrent infections are a problem even with sup-**

pressive antibiotics, then ureteral reimplantation is required before bladder neck reconstruction. Dilatation of the distal ureter frequently occurs on ultrasound and pyelogram studies and is a result of edema, infection, and fibrosis of the terminal ureter acquired after initial closure.

Exstrophy Complex and Variants

Because the entire exstrophy groups represents a spectrum of anomalies, it is not surprising that transitions between bladder exstrophy–epispadias–cloacal exstrophy have been reported. There is a close relationship among all forms of the exstrophy-epispadias complex, because the fault in its embryogenesis is common to all; therefore, all clinical manifestations are really variations on a theme. **The presence of a characteristic musculoskeletal defect of the exstrophy anomaly with no major defect in the urinary tract has been named "pseudoexstrophy"** (Marshall and Muecke, 1968). Predominant characteristics include an elongated, low-set umbilicus and divergent rectus muscles that attach to the separated pubic bones (Fig. 61-11). In this variant, the mesodermal migration has been interrupted in its superior aspect only, thus wedging apart the musculoskeletal elements of the lower abdominal wall without obstructing the formation of the genital tubercle.

In the superior vesical fistula variant of the exstrophy complex, the musculature and skeletal defects are exactly the same as those in classic exstrophy; however, the persistent cloacal membrane ruptures only at the uppermost portion, and a superior vesical fistula results which actually resembles a vesicostomy. Bladder extrusion is minimal and is present only over the normal umbilicus (Fig. 61-12).

Duplicate exstrophy occurs when a superior vesical fistula opens but there is later fusion of the abdominal wall and a portion of the bladder elements (mucosa) remains outside (Fig. 61-13). Three cases were reported by Arap and Geron (1986) in which the patients had classic musculoskeletal defects and two of the three were continent. Of the two male patients, one had an associated complete epispadias and the other had a completely normal penis. Therefore, the external genital manifestations in duplicate exstrophy can be quite variable.

In addition to pseudoexstrophy, superior vesical fistula, and duplicated exstrophy, isolated occurrences of a fourth entity, "covered exstrophy," have been reported (Cerniglia et al, 1989). This has also been referred to as split symphysis variant. A common factor in these patients is the presence of musculoskeletal defect associated with classic exstrophy but no significant defect of the urinary tract. Chandra and associates (1999) reported a covered exstrophy with incomplete duplication of the bladder. However, in most cases of covered exstrophy (Cerniglia et al, 1989; Narasimharao et al, 1985), there has been an isolated ectopic bowel segment present on the inferior abdominal wall near the genital area, which can either be colon or ileum with no connection with the underlying gastrointestinal tract and only epispadias in the male. A patient seen at our institution had the standard appearance of most split symphysis variants and one could actually see the bladder through a thin membrane of lower abdominal

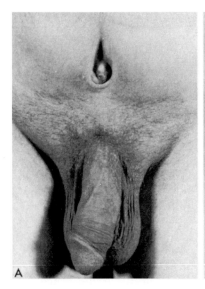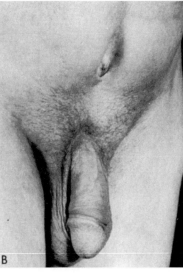

Figure 61–11. Pseudoexstrophy in an adult male patient. Musculoskeletal deformity characteristic of the exstrophy complex is present, but the urinary tract is intact.

skin. Although all of the classic musculoskeletal defects of exstrophy were present, there was no isolated ectopic bowel segment present on the lower abdominal wall (Fig. 61–14).

PRENATAL DIAGNOSIS AND MANAGEMENT

Currently, the prenatal diagnosis of bladder exstrophy is difficult to delineate. Many times the diagnosis of omphalocele or gastroschisis is made and the exstrophy condition is overlooked. Ultrasound evaluation of the fetus, by means of high-resolution real-time units, allows a thorough survey of the fetal anatomy, even during routine obstetric ultra-

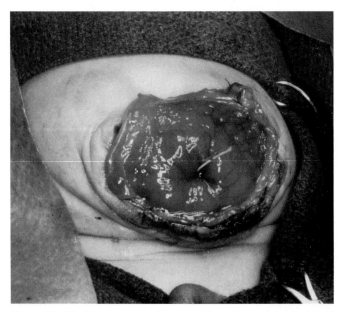

Figure 61–12. Superior vesical fissure. Note intact abdominal wall and normal penis.

sound examinations (Gearhart et al, 1995a). Several groups in the last few years have outlined important criteria for the diagnosis of classic bladder exstrophy prenatally. In these reviews, the absence of a normal fluid-filled bladder on repeat examinations suggested the diagnosis, as did a mass of echogenic tissue on the lower abdominal wall (Mirk et al, 1986; Verco et al, 1986). **In a review of 25 prenatal ultrasound examinations with the subsequent birth of a newborn with classic bladder exstrophy** (Gearhart et al, 1995), **several observations were made: (1) absence of bladder filling, (2) a low-set umbilicus, (3) widening pubis ramus, (4) diminutive genitalia, and (5) a lower abdominal mass that increases in size as the pregnancy progresses and as the intra-abdominal viscera increases in size** (Fig. 61–15). The main reason for the prenatal diagnosis of bladder exstrophy is so that the parents can be counseled regarding the risks and benefits and other aspects of the condition. After appropriate counseling, arrangements can be made for delivery of the baby in a specialized exstrophy center where immediate reconstruction of the exstrophy can occur. Presentations from various centers have shown that the sooner the bladder is closed, the more likely it is that the bladder will grow and will not require augmentation. **Delivery in a specialized exstrophy center allows the parents to be exposed to the expertise of multiple disciplines, including the all-important psychological support these young parents need when a child with a birth defect of this magnitude is delivered.**

MODERN SURGICAL RECONSTRUCTION

Sweetser and associates (1952) initially described a staged surgical approach for bladder exstrophy. Four to 6 days before bladder closure, bilateral iliac osteotomies were performed. Epispadias repair was performed as a separate procedure. The continence procedure was limited to freeing the fibers from the intrasymphyseal band and wrapping this

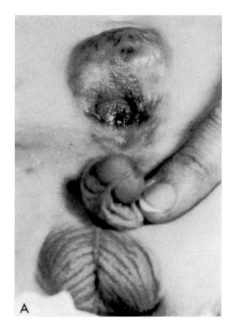
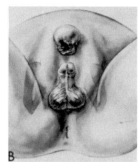
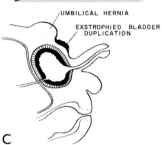

Figure 61–13. Duplicate exstrophy in a boy with an intact lower urinary tract.

band around the urethra at the time of closure to increase outlet resistance.

The modern staged approach to functional bladder closure included three separate stages: bladder, abdominal wall, and posterior urethral closure; bladder neck reconstruction and antireflux procedure; and later epispadias re-

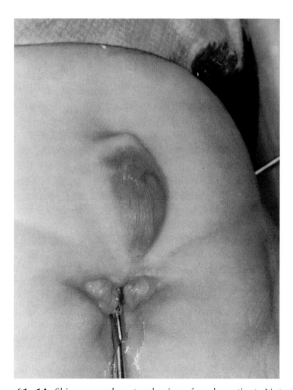

Figure 61–14. Skin-covered exstrophy in a female patient. Note urethral sound passing through the urethral meatus and its subcutaneous position on the abdominal wall. Notice there is no bowel sequestered on the lower abdominal wall as has been reported in the skin-covered exstrophy patients.

pair. This approach was recommended for most cases of exstrophy reconstruction beginning in the early 1970s (Cendron, 1971; Jeffs et al, 1972; Williams and Keaton, 1973; Gearhart and Jeffs, 1989b). **Although this procedure was successful, it has been significantly modified over the last 5 years to include bladder, posterior urethra, and abdominal wall closure in the newborn period with bilateral innominate and vertical iliac osteotomy, if indicated; epispadias repair at 6 months to 1 year of age; and bladder neck reconstruction along with antireflux procedure at age 4 to 5 years, when the child has achieved an adequate bladder capacity for bladder neck reconstruction and is motivated to participate in a postoperative voiding program** (Gearhart and Jeffs, 1998) (Table 61–1).

Other methods of treatment of the newborn with bladder exstrophy have been offered. Grady and Mitchell (1999) proposed combining bladder exstrophy closure with epispadias repair in the newborn period. Baka-Jakubiak (2000) recommended newborn exstrophy closure alone and combined bladder neck reconstruction and epispadias repair when the child reaches a satisfactory age for participation in a voiding program. Schrott and colleagues recommended bladder closure, ureteral reimplantation, epispadias repair, and bladder neck reconstruction in the newborn period. Lastly, Stein and coworkers (1999b) recommended ureterosigmoidostomy in the newborn period with abdominal wall and bladder closure. This chapter deals mainly with the author's preference of the modern approach to staged reconstruction with some emphasis on the use of the combined bladder closure and epispadias repair in highly selected patients.

Patient Selection

Successful treatment of exstrophy with functional closure demands that the potential for success in each child be

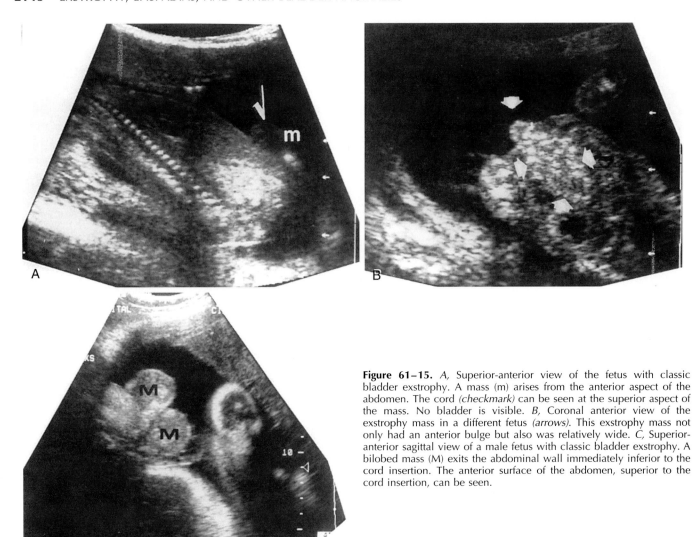

Figure 61–15. *A,* Superior-anterior view of the fetus with classic bladder exstrophy. A mass (m) arises from the anterior aspect of the abdomen. The cord *(checkmark)* can be seen at the superior aspect of the mass. No bladder is visible. *B,* Coronal anterior view of the exstrophy mass in a different fetus *(arrows).* This exstrophy mass not only had an anterior bulge but also was relatively wide. *C,* Superior-anterior sagittal view of a male fetus with classic bladder exstrophy. A bilobed mass (M) exits the abdominal wall immediately inferior to the cord insertion. The anterior surface of the abdomen, superior to the cord insertion, can be seen.

carefully considered at birth. The size and the functional capacity of the detrusor muscle are important considerations for the eventual success of functional closure. Correlation between apparent bladder size and the potential bladder capacity must not be confused. In minor grades of exstrophy that approach the condition of complete epispadias with incontinence, the bladder may be small yet may demonstrate acceptable capacity, either by bulging when the baby cries or by indenting easily when touched by a sterile gloved finger in the operating room with the child under anesthesia. **Sometimes a good bit of previously unappreciated bladder can be discovered behind the fascia under examination with anesthesia** (Gearhart and Jeffs, 1998) (Fig. 61–16). Once the bladder is relieved of surface irritation and repeated trauma, the small bladder can enlarge and increase in capacity with the absence of sphincter activity and with minimal outlet resistance. The exstrophied bladder that is estimated at the time of birth to have a capacity of 5 ml or more and demonstrates elasticity and contractility can be expected to develop useful size and capacity after successful bladder, posterior urethral, and abdominal wall closure with early epispadias repair (Gearhart and Jeffs, 1998).

Delivery Room and Nursery

At birth, although the bladder mucosa is usually smooth, pink, and intact, it is also sensitive and easily denuded. In the delivery room the umbilical cord should be tied with 2-0 silk close to the abdominal wall so that the umbilical clamp does not traumatize the delicate mucosa and cause excoriation of the bladder surface. The bladder can then be covered with a nonadherent film of plastic wrap (i.e., Saran Wrap) to prevent sticking of the bladder mucosa to clothing or diapers. In addition, each time the diaper is changed the plastic wrap should be removed, the bladder surface irrigated with sterile saline, and clean plastic wrap placed over the bladder surface area.

The distraught parents need reassurance at this stage. Counseling of the parents and decisions regarding eventual therapy should begin prenatally if the condition is diagnosed by prenatal ultrasound. The parents should be educated by a surgeon with a special interest and experience in managing cases of bladder or cloacal exstrophy. An exstrophy support team should be available and should include a pediatric orthopedic surgeon, pediatric anesthesiologist, social workers, nurses with special interest in bladder exstro-

Table 61-1. INITIAL PRESENTATION AND MANAGEMENT OF EXSTROPHY OF THE BLADDER

Age	Problem	Possible Solution
Initial Presentation		
0–72 hr	Classic exstrophy with reasonable capacity and moderate symphyseal separation; long urethral groove; mild dorsal chordee.	I: Midline closure of bladder, fascia, and symphysis to level of posterior urethra; no osteotomy. In *very* select cases combined bladder closure and epispadias repair.
0–72 hr	Above-mentioned findings with short urethra and severe dorsal chordee.	II: Close as in I, adding lengthening of dorsal urethral groove by paraexstrophy skin (cautiously).
0–72 hr	Above-mentioned findings with very wide separation of symphysis or late presentation of patient (beyond 72 hr up to 1–3 yr) for initial treatment.	Osteotomy (combined anterior and vertical iliac) and closure as in I or II.
0–2 wk	Male, penis duplex or extremely short.	Consider female sex of rearing and closure as in I or II (very rare).
0–2 wk	Very small, nondistensible bladder patch.	Prove by examination under anesthesia, then nonoperative expectant treatment awaiting internal or external diversion or delayed closure if bladder plate grows.
Incontinent period after initial closure		
1 mo–4 yr	Infection with residual resulting from outlet stenosis.	Urethral dilatation, occasional meatotomy or bladder neck revision.
	Infection, grade III reflux, with pliable outlet resistance.	Continuous antibiotic suppression with plan for early ureteroneocystostomy.
	Partial dehiscence at bladder neck or partial prolapse of bladder (both prevent bladder capacity increase).	Reclosure of bladder neck with osteotomy (with epispadias repair if older than 6 mo of life).
Epispadias repair continence		
6 mo–1 yr	Closed bladder with incontinence, normal ultrasound and good penile size and length of urethral groove.	Epispadias repair after preparation with testosterone.
	Epispadias penis, short with severe chordee, before bladder neck reconstruction.	Correction of chordee, lengthening of urethral groove, and epispadias repair, prepare with testosterone.
4–5 yr	Epispadias repair, capacity greater than 85 ml, child ready to be dry and be involved in voiding program.	Proceed to bladder neck plasty and ureteroneocystostomy.
4 yr or older	Completed repair of bladder, bladder neck, and epispadias with dry interval but wet pants.	Patience, biofeedback, oxybutynin chloride (Ditropan), imipramine, and time (up to 2 yr).
	Above-mentioned problems with marked stress incontinence and good bladder capacity.	Wait—may require bladder neck revision or endoscopic injection or possible artificial sphincter.
	Small-capacity bladder unchanged by time, epispadias repair, or attempted bladder neck reconstruction.	Consider augmentation cystoplasty and bladder neck transection/reconstruction; acceptance of intermittent catheterization with abdominal or urethral access may be necessary.
4–7 yr	Late presentation of untreated exstrophy, unsuitable for closure.	Consider temporary diversion by colon conduit with plan to undivert to bladder using bladder to form urethra and conduit for augmentation; in patients older than 5 yr, artificial sphincter or continent diversion can be considered.
4–7 yr	Small closed exstrophy unsuitable for bladder neck reconstruction or augmentation.	Consider permanent external or internal diversion; internal diversion direct by ureterosigmoidostomy or indirect by colocolostomy; evaluate day continence of anal sphincter and nighttime seepage before surgery or continent neobladder.
5–15 yr	Closed exstrophy with epispadias repaired with uncontrolled stress or dribbling incontinence.	Consider (1) revision of bladder neck reconstruction, (2) endoscopic injection, (3) augmentation and bladder neck revision, (4) artificial sphincter with omental wrap, and (5) continent diversion.
10–20 yr	Closed bladder with inadequate penis.	Consider penile lengthening, urethral reconstruction using free graft, pedicle grafts, and tissue transfer.
10–20 yr	Diverted exstrophy with inadequate penis.	As above-mentioned recommendations or penile lengthening without urethral reconstruction (prostatic fistula at base).

phy, and a child psychiatrist with expertise and experience in genital anomalies. The Association of Bladder Exstrophy Children is available and has a website for parents and family members to obtain further information about the bladder exstrophy condition. In addition, should the parents desire, websites are available in some major exstrophy centers for further information.

Although it is true that parents need to be educated as fully as possible about the exstrophy condition, this is especially true regarding the sex of rearing in males with bladder exstrophy. We have seen several families that were made even more distraught by being told that their child had ambiguous genitalia in addition to bladder exstrophy and that the child would need a change of gender. The

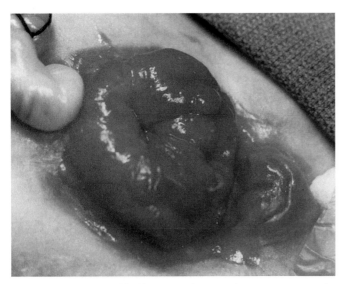

Figure 61–16. Classic bladder exstrophy in male patient. Notice the deep indentation of the bladder back into the pelvis indicating excellent potential both for excellent bladder growth and for successful closure. Note diminutive phallus.

need for changing the sex of rearing in classic bladder exstrophy is almost nonexistent in the male infant.

Early Management

Cardiopulmonary and general physical assessment measures can be carried out in the first few hours of life. Radionuclide scans and ultrasound studies can provide evidence of renal structure, function, and drainage, even in the first few hours of life before the patient undergoes closure of the exstrophy defect.

Circumstances may be less than ideal at birth. A thorough neonatal assessment may have to be deferred until transportation to a major children's medical center can be arranged. In these days of modern transportation, no child is ever more than a few hours away from a neonatal center with full diagnostic and consultative services. During travel the bladder should be protected by a plastic membrane, as in the nursery, to prevent damage to the delicate newborn bladder mucosa.

Small Bladder Unsuitable for Closure

A small, fibrotic bladder patch that is stretched between the edges of the small triangular fascial defect without elasticity or contractility cannot be selected for the usual closure procedure (Gearhart and Jeffs, 1998) (see Fig. 61–10). **Examination with the patient under anesthesia may at times be required to assess the bladder adequately, particularly if considerable edema, excoriation, and polyp formation has developed between birth and the time of assessment. Decisions regarding the suitability of bladder closure or the need for waiting should be made only by surgeons with a great deal of experience in the exstrophy condition** (Gearhart and Jeffs, 1998). Neonatal closure, even when the bladder is small, can al-

low for assessment of bladder potential, provides an initial step in genital reconstruction, and is helpful in reassuring the family. Some conditions preclude primary closure, including penoscrotal duplication, ectopic bowel within the extruded bladder (a relative contraindication), a hypoplastic bladder, and significant bilateral hydronephrosis.

In a review by Dodson and associates (2001) of cases at one institution, it was found on initial judgment that the bladder was too small for closure in 20 patients evaluated at birth. After a period of time when the bladder had grown sufficiently, closure was undertaken. Long-term follow-up revealed that 50% of these patients were dry after bladder neck reconstruction and 50% required other adjunctive procedures. **Ideally, waiting for the bladder template to grow for 4 to 6 months in the child with a small bladder is not as risky as submitting a small bladder template to closure in an inappropriate setting, resulting in dehiscence and allowing the fate of the bladder to be sealed at that point.** If the bladder does not grow to sufficient size after 4 to 6 months, other options include excision of the bladder and a nonrefluxing colon conduit or ureterosigmoidostomy. Another alternative involves urinary diversion with a colon conduit and placing the small bladder inside to be used later for the posterior urethra in an Arap-type procedure. Lastly, if the bladder is small and the presentation is for late primary closure, bladder augmentation, ureteral reimplantation, and an outlet procedure, in addition to a continent urinary stoma, can be considered.

Combined Bladder Closure and Epispadias Repair

The staged closure of bladder exstrophy has yielded consistently good cosmetic and functional results, and the utilization of osteotomy has improved the potential for successful initial closure and later continence. **In an effort to decrease costs, decrease the morbidity associated with multiple operative procedures, and possibly affect continence, there has been a recent interest in performing single-staged reconstruction or combining procedures in appropriately selected patients.** First described by Gearhart and Jeffs (1991a) for failed exstrophy closures and more recently by Grady and Mitchell for newborn patients (1999), results have now been reported in groups of boys undergoing single-stage reconstruction (bladder closure and epispadias repair) in infancy (Gearhart et al, 1998). In my opinion, this technique should be limited to boys of older age (older than 4 to 6 months) because of recent experimental evidence indicating that newborn bladders differ from bladders in older infants in the level of maturity of their muscle, connective tissue, and neural components (Gearhart et al, 1996).

These patients should be carefully selected, especially the newborns, because of the reasons just cited. Otherwise, boys presenting after failed initial closure or for primary closure at older than 4 to 6 months of age may be candidates for a combination of epispadias repair with bladder closure. **Children should be carefully selected based on phallic size and length, depth of the urethral groove, and size of the bladder template in those with delayed**

primary closures, as well as perivesical and urethral scarring in those who have undergone a prior failed closure (Gearhart and Jeffs, 1991; Gearhart et al, 1998). The operative description of this technique is presented later in this chapter.

SURGICAL PROCEDURE

Over the past two decades, modifications in the management of functional bladder closure have contributed to a dramatic increase in the success of the procedure. **The most significant changes in the management of bladder exstrophy have been (1) early bladder, posterior urethra, and abdominal wall closure, usually with osteotomy; (2) early epispadias repair; (3) reconstruction of a continent bladder neck and reimplantation of the ureters; and, most importantly, (4) definition of strict criteria for the selection of patients suitable for this approach.** The primary objective in functional closure is to convert the bladder exstrophy into a complete epispadias with incontinence with balanced posterior outlet resistance that preserves renal function, but stimulates bladder growth. Typically, epispadias repair is now performed between 6 months and 12 months of age, after testosterone stimulation. Bladder neck repair usually occurs when the child is 4 to 5 years of age, has an adequate bladder capacity, and, most important, is ready to participate in a postoperative voiding program.

Osteotomy

Pelvic osteotomy performed at the time of initial closure confers several advantages, including (1) easy approximation of the symphysis with diminished tension on the abdominal wall closure and elimination of the need for fascial flaps; (2) placement of the urethra deep within the pelvic ring, enhancing bladder outlet resistance; and (3) bringing of the large pelvic floor muscles near the midline, where they can support the bladder neck and aid in eventual urinary control (Fig. 61–17). After pubic approximation with osteotomy, some patients show the ability to stop and start the urinary stream, experience dry intervals, and in some cases become completely continent (Gearhart and Jeffs, 1991a). In a review of a large number of patients referred to our institution after failed exstrophy procedures, it was found that a majority of the patients who had partial or complete dehiscence of the bladder or major bladder prolapse had not undergone a prior osteotomy at the time of initial bladder closure (Gearhart et al, 1993b). **We recommend performing bilateral transverse innominate and vertical iliac osteotomy when bladder closure is performed after 72 hours of age** (Fig. 61–18). In addition, if the pelvis is not malleable or if the pubic bones are more than 4 cm apart at the time of initial examination under anesthesia, osteotomy should be performed, even if closure is done before 72 hours of age. A well coordinated surgery and anesthesia team can perform osteotomy and proceed to bladder closure without undue loss of blood or risk of prolonged anesthesia in the child. However, it must be realized that osteotomy together with

posterior urethral and bladder closure and abdominal wall closure, is a 5- to 7-hour procedure in these infants.

If the patient is less than 72 hours old and examination under anesthesia reveals that the pubic bones are malleable and able to be brought together easily in the midline by medial rotation of the greater trochanters, the patient can undergo closure without osteotomy. However, no chances should be taken with a decision of this magnitude. If there is any doubt, an osteotomy should be performed.

The most modern approach used for osteotomy today is the bilateral anterior innominate and vertical iliac osteotomy, popularized by Gearhart, Sponseller, and coworkers in 1996 (Gearhart et al, 1996b). This approach improves the ease of symphyseal approximation in the patient with exstrophy compared with posterior approaches, which require turning the patient. In my experience, this osteotomy is superior to the pubic mobilization seen with simple bilateral transverse anterior innominate osteotomy or even pubic ramotomy. With the ease of approximation obtained with this combined osteotomy, tension on the midline abdominal closure is lessened and the rate of bladder dehiscence and bladder prolapse are markedly decreased (Gearhart and Jeffs, 1998). In addition, pelvic closure allows approximation of the levator ani to strengthen the puborectalis sling, with positioning of the bladder neck and posterior urethra deep within the pelvic ring and improved continence rate. **Besides the ease of approximation, combined osteotomy was developed for three reasons: (1) osteotomy is performed with the patient in the supine position, as is the urologic repair, thereby avoiding the need to turn the patient; (2) the anterior approach to this osteotomy allows placement of an external fixator device and intrafragmentary pins under direct vision; and (3) the cosmetic appearance of this osteotomy is superior to that of the posterior iliac approach** (Gearhart et al, 1996b).

Although our experience with posterior iliac osteotomy is not associated with any failures after initial closure, the mobility of the pubis was disappointing, there was occasional malunion of the ileum, the blood loss was more than in the posterior approach, and, most importantly, the need to turn the patient intraoperatively from the prone to the supine position was always worrisome. Initially, the experience with osteotomy was in patients who had failed to benefit from initial exstrophy closure with or without iliac osteotomy or pubic ramotomy (Sponseller et al, 1991). The results of the new approach with combined horizontal transverse innominate osteotomy and vertical iliac osteotomy were so satisfactory that the approach is now being used in all primary closures of bladder exstrophy that require pelvic osteotomy (Gearhart et al, 1996b).

Combined osteotomy is performed by placing the patient in the supine position, preparing and draping the lower body below the costal margins, and placing soft absorbent gauze over the exposed bladder. The pelvis is exposed from the iliac wings inferiorly to the pectineal tubercle and posteriorly to the sacroiliac joints. The periosteum and sciatic notch are carefully elevated, and a Gigli saw is used to create a transverse innominate osteotomy exiting anteriorly at a point halfway between the anterior-superior and anterior-inferior spines (see Fig. 61–18). This osteotomy is

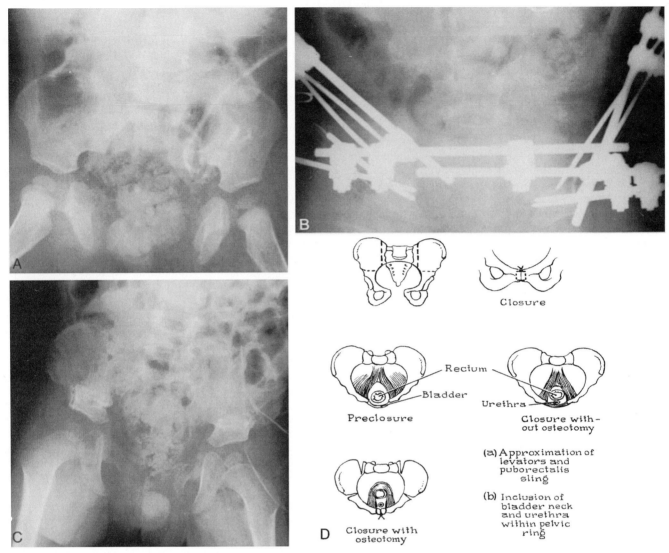

Figure 61–17. *A,* Eight-month-old patient with classic bladder exstrophy closed at birth without osteotomy with complete dehiscence, first seen at eight months of age. *B,* Patient after having undergone anterior innominate and vertical iliac osteotomy with placement of intrafragmentary pins and external fixator. *C,* The same patient four months after removal of external fixator and intrafragmentary pins. No dehiscence was observed with this closure. *D,* The technique of combined osteotomy showing the incision site and advantages of this approach. (Drawings by Leon Schlossberg.)

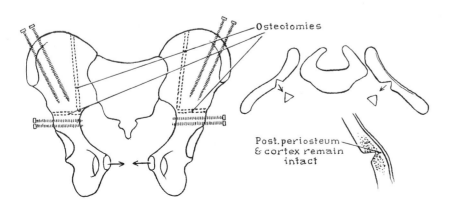

Figure 61–18. Depiction of the new combined transverse innominate and vertical iliac osteotomy showing intrafragmentary pin placement sites and pubic bone apposition. (Drawings by Leon Schlossberg.)

created at a slightly more cranial level than that described for a Salter osteotomy, in order to allow placement of external fixator pins in the distal segments. In addition to the transverse osteotomy, the posterior ileum may be incised from the anterior approach in an effort to correct the deformity more completely. This is important, because anatomic studies have shown that the posterior portion of the pelvis is also externally rotated in patients with exstrophy, and as patients age they lose elasticity of the sacroiliac ligaments. For this part of the osteotomy, an osteotome is used to create a closing wedge osteotomy vertically and just lateral to the sacroiliac joints. The proximal posterior iliac cortex is left intact and used as a hinge (see Fig. 61–18). This combination osteotomy easily corrects the abnormalities in both the anterior and posterior segments of the pelvis.

Two fixator pins are placed in inferior osteotomized segment, and two are placed in the wing of the ileum superiorly. Radiographs are obtained to confirm pin placement, soft tissues are closed, and the urologic procedure is performed (see Fig. 61–17). At the end of the procedure, the pelvis is closed with a suture between the two pubic rami. The external fixators are then applied between the pins to hold the pelvis in a correct position. In a newborn with less than optimal amounts of cancellous bone, only one pin is placed inferiorly and superiorly in the wing of the ileum, whereas older children have two pins in each bony wing.

Radiographs are taken 7 to 10 days after surgery to look for complete reduction of the symphyseal diastasis. If this diastasis has not been completely reduced, the right and left sides can be gradually approximated by means of the fixator bars over several days. Longitudinal skin traction is used to keep the legs still (Fig. 61–19). The patient remains supine in traction for approximately 4 weeks to prevent dislodgement of tubes and destabilization of the pelvis. The external fixator is kept on for approximately 6 weeks, until adequate callus is seen at the site of the osteotomy (see Fig. 61–17B and C). Postoperatively in newborns who undergo closure without osteotomy in the first 48 to 72 hours of life, the baby is immobilized in modified Bryant's traction in a position which the hips have 90 degrees of flexion. When modified Bryant's traction is used, the traction is employed for 4 weeks (Fig. 61–20). A horizontal mattress suture of No. 2 nylon is

placed between the fibrous cartilage of the pubic rami and tied anteriorly to the pubic closure at the time of bladder closure. **Evidence obtained by Sussman and associates (1997) from biomechanical testing in an intact piglet pelvic model revealed that all methods of pubic approximation were weak compared with the intact symphysis. However, the best technique with the strongest load-to-failure ratio was a No. 2 nylon horizontal mattress suture.** Should this suture work loose or cut through the tissues during healing, the anterior placement of a knot in the horizontal mattress suture ensures that it will not erode into the urethra and interfere with the bladder or urethral lumen.

Sponseller and colleagues (2000a) reported on a total of 82 combined bilateral anterior innominate and vertical iliac osteotomies performed in 88 children. Ten of these children had cloacal exstrophy, and 72 had bladder exstrophy with at least 2 years of clinical follow-up (mean 4.8 years). Complications included seven cases of transient left femoral nerve palsy which resolved fully by 12 weeks after surgery. There were no cases of right femoral nerve palsy, although the same surgeon performed the same technique on both sides. Patients with transient femoral nerve palsy were at bed rest for the first 6 to 8 weeks; a knee immobilizer was needed for the remaining 6 weeks until resolution. Other complications included three cases with delayed ileal union, one case of superficial infection of the ileal femoral incision that required irrigation and débridement, one case of transient right thigh abductor weakness, one infection of the ileum around a pin site requiring irrigation and débridement, and one case of transient right perineal palsy. Almost all patients had skin inflammation around the pins, particularly those in the proximal (iliac crest) segments. This was always controlled with the use of oral antibiotics. One child with classic exstrophy had bladder prolapse after primary bladder closure and combined osteotomies. Another child with classic exstrophy developed wound dehiscence after primary closure and pelvic osteotomy secondary to a respiratory virus and severe associated respiratory distress.

Whichever type of osteotomy is used, pelvic ring closure not only allows midline approximation of the abdominal wall structures but also allows the levator ani and puborectalis muscles to lend potential support to the bladder outlet,

Figure 61–19. A 15-month-old child with failed prior bladder exstrophy closure after reclosure of bladder exstrophy and application of external fixating device in modified Buck's traction.

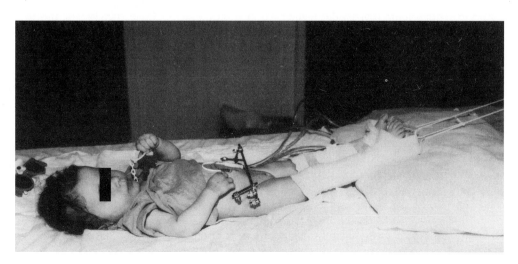

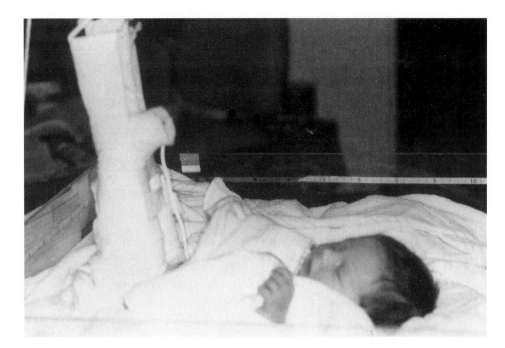

Figure 61–20. Newborn closure without osteotomy with patient placed in modified Bryant's traction.

thus increasing resistance to urinary outflow (see Fig. 61–17D) (Sponseller et al, 1991; Gearhart et al, 1993b, 1996b; Schmidt et al, 1993; McKenna et al, 1994). Furthermore, a continence procedure can be performed later on the bladder neck and urethra deep within the closed pelvic ring at a distance from the surface without independent movement of the two halves of the pubis. The urethra and bladder neck are set more deeply in the true pelvis, in a more normal relationship than when acutely angulated.

When good callus formation is seen on radiography, the fixating device and pins are removed with the patient under light sedation. The age of the patient plays a role in the amount of correction of the diastasis that is maintained over time. On review of the previously described types of osteotomy, both classic and cloacal exstrophy patients gained approximation, although the former group gained greater correction toward normal (Gearhart et al, 1996b). Greater postoperative diastasis as well as less optimal bone density in the newborn contributes to the greater difficulty in obtaining and maintaining closure of the pelvic bony deformity over time.

It is my impression that partial recurrence of diastasis in classic exstrophy occurs by two mechanisms. First, the pelvis may partially derotate owing to early loosening of pins before the time of osteotomy healing; this is seen mostly in infants. In the older child, increased bone density allows more rigid external fixation and thus better maintenance of the corrected position. Second, there is long-term undergrowth of the ischiopubic segment, which has been shown to be 33% smaller than normal in the adult with exstrophy, as the pelvis grows. Pubic diastasis increases with growth in the patient with uncorrected exstrophy. Therefore, even with some loss of approximation, significant correction remains in comparison to the unoperated state. We regard the main role of osteotomy to be relaxation of tension on the bladder, posterior urethra, and abdominal wall repair during healing. Therefore, we use osteotomy rarely in newborns and young infants, because

ligament laxity allows the pelvis to be closed without tension. However, it becomes essential in the older child with a failed exstrophy repair, in the patient with cloacal exstrophy, and in a newborn with a wide diastasis and excellent bladder template. **In patients undergoing combined exstrophy closure and epispadias repair, osteotomy allows the pubis to be joined, making it easier for the corpora to be brought over the closed proximal urethra** (Gearhart et al, 1998).

Bladder, Posterior Urethra, and Abdominal Wall Closure

Various steps in primary bladder closure illustrated in Fig. 61–21. A strip of mucosa 2 cm wide, extending from the distal trigone to below the verum montanum in the male and to the vaginal orifice in the female, is outlined for prostatic and posterior urethral reconstruction in the male and adequate urethral closure in the female. The male urethral groove may be adequate, in which case no transverse incision of the urethral plate need be performed for urethral lengthening (see Fig. 61–21A). We tend not to incise a urethral plate unless the length of the urethral groove from the veru montanum to the urethral glans is so short that it interferes with eventual penile length and reduces dorsal angulation. If so, then the urethral groove is lengthened after the manner of Johnston (1974) or Duckett (1977). The diagrams in Fig. 61–21B and C show marking of the incision with a blue marking pen just above the umbilicus, down the junction of the bladder and paraexstrophy skin, to the level of the urethral plate.

An appropriate plane is entered just above the umbilicus, and a plane is established between the rectus fascia and the bladder (Fig. 61–21E and F). The umbilical vessels are doubly ligated and incised and allowed to fall into the pelvis. The peritoneum is taken off the dome of the bladder at this point so that the bladder can be placed deep into

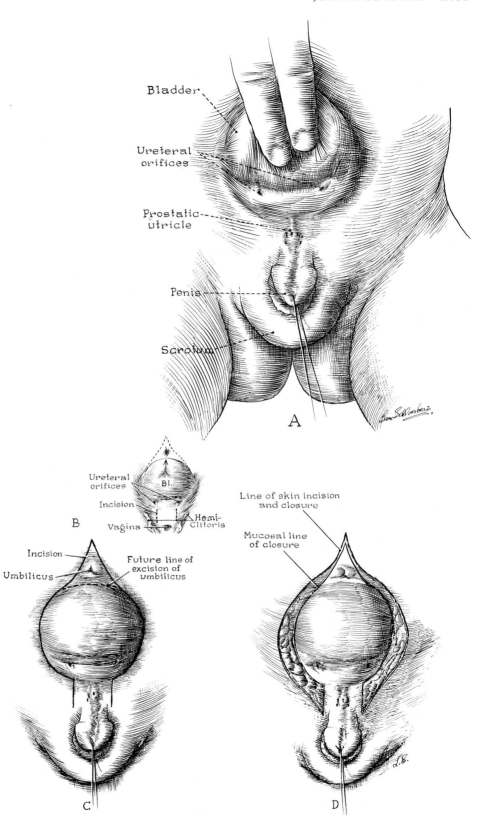

Figure 61–21. Steps in primary closure of the posterior urethra, bladder, and abdominal wall with or without osteotomy in the newborn patient. *A through D,* The incision line around the umbilicus and the bladder down to the urethral plate. If the urethral groove is adequate, no transverse incision is made in the urethral plate at the time of initial closure. Note in the female patient *(B)* that the inner aspect of the labia minora, and clitoral halves are denuded to allow for complete reconstruction of the external genitalia along with the bladder and urethral closure.

Illustration continued on following page

the pelvis at the time of closure. The plane is continued caudally down between the bladder and rectus fascia until the urogenital diaphragm fibers are encountered bilaterally. The pubis will be encountered at this junction, and a double-pronged skin hook can be inserted into the bone at this time and pulled laterally to accentuate the urogenital diaphragm fibers and help the surgeon radically incise these fibers between the bladder neck, posterior urethra, and pubic bone. Gentle traction on the glans at this point will show the insertion of the corporal body on the lateral

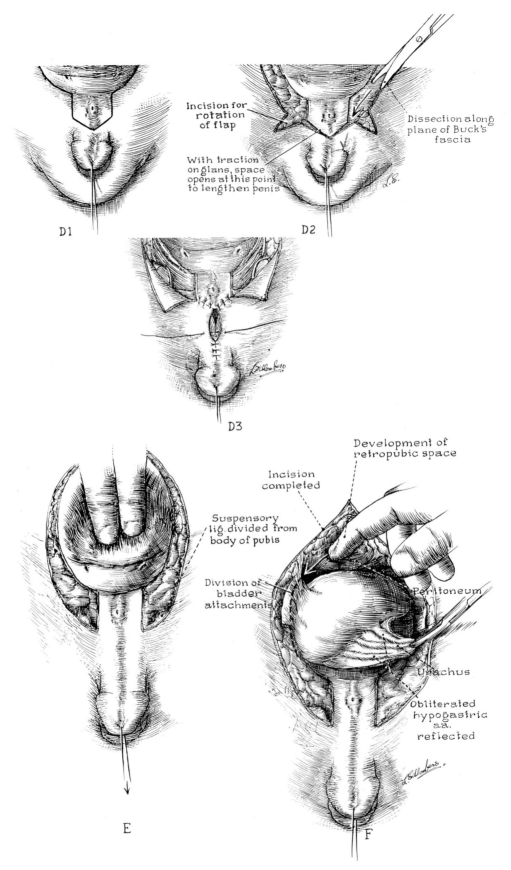

Figure 61–21 *Continued.* D1 *through* D3, Excision across the urethral plate using rotational flaps in the rare event that urethral lengthening must be done at the time of initial closure. E *and* F, Development of the retropubic space from below the area of the umbilical insertion to facilitate separation of the bladder from the rectus sheath and muscle.

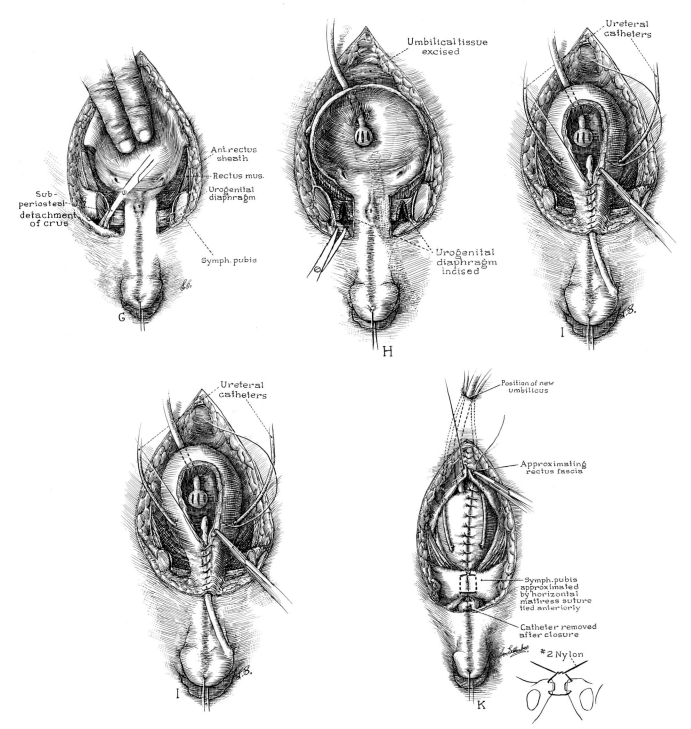

Figure 61–21 *Continued. G,* Medial extension of the rectus muscle attaching behind the prostate to the upper border of the urogenital diaphragm. The urogenital diaphragm and anterior corpus are freed from the pubis in a subperiosteal plane. *H,* Final incision deep into the remnant fibers of the urogenital diaphragm and placement of the suprapubic cystostomy tube. *I,* Exit of the ureteral stents from the lateral sidewall of the bladder and the first layer of the bladder wall closure. *J,* The second layer of the bladder wall closure is shown. *K,* Horizontal mattress sutures are tied on the external surface of the pubic symphysis as an assistant applies medial rotation of the greater trochanters. The suprapubic tube and ureteral stents are brought out cephalad to the bladder at the site of the neoumbilical opening. (Drawings by Leon Schlossberg.)

inferior aspect of the pubis. These urogenital diaphragm fibers are taken down sharply with electrocautery down to the pelvic floor in their entirety. If this maneuver is not performed adequately, the posterior urethra and bladder will not be placed deeply into the pelvis, and when the

pubic bones are brought together, the posterior vesical unit will be brought anteriorly into an unsatisfactory position for later reconstruction.

If the decision is made at this point that the urethral groove is to be transected, then the groove is cut distal to the veru montanum with continuity maintained between the thin, mucosal, non–hair-bearing skin adjacent to the posterior urethra and bladder neck and the skin and mucosa of the penile skin and glans. Flaps in the area of the thin skin are subsequently moved distally and rotated to reconstruct the urethral groove, resurfacing the penis dorsally (Fig. 61–21*D1* through *D3*). The corporal bodies are not brought together at this juncture, because later Cantwell-Ransley epispadias repair will require the urethral plate to be brought beneath the corporal bodies. If the urethral plate is left in continuity, it must be mobilized up to the level of the prostate in order to create as much additional urethral and penile length as possible. Further urethral lengthening can be performed at the time of epispadias repair.

Penile lengthening is achieved by exposing the corpora cavernosa bilaterally and freeing the corpora from their attachments to the suspensory ligaments on the anterior part of the inferior pubic rami. **However, since Silver and colleagues (1997b) showed that there is a 50% shortage of length of the corporal bodies in exstrophy versus normal controls, any penile length that is obtained is more correction of chordee and change in angulation of the penis rather than true penile lengthening.** The wide band of fibers and muscular tissue representing the urogenital diaphragm is detached subperiostally from the pubis bilaterally (see Fig. 61–21*G* and *H*). Reluctance to free the bladder neck and urethra well from the inferior ramus of the pubis moves the neobladder opening cephalad should any separation of the pubis occur during healing, thus increasing the chance of bladder prolapse. The mucosa and muscle of the bladder and posterior urethra are then closed well onto the penis in the midline anteriorly (see Fig. 61–21*I*). This will accommodate a No. 12 to 14 Fr sound comfortably. The size of the opening should allow enough resistance to aid in bladder adaptation and to prevent prolapse, but not enough outlet resistance to cause upper tract changes. The posterior urethra and bladder neck are buttressed with a second layer of local tissue if possible (see Fig. 61–21*J*). The bladder is drained by a suprapubic non-latex Malecot catheter for a period of 4 weeks. The urethra is not stented in order to avoid necrosis with accumulation of secretions in the neourethra. Stents provide drainage during the first 10 to 14 days after closure, and swelling caused by the pressure of closure of a small bladder can obstruct the ureters and give rise to obstruction and transient hypotension. If there are no problems with the stents during healing, we leave the stents in as long as 2 to 3 weeks.

When the bladder and urethra have been closed and the drainage tubes placed, pressure over the greater trochanters bilaterally allows the pubic bones to be approximated in the midline. Horizontal mattress sutures are placed in the pubis and tied with a knot away from the neourethra (Fig. 61–21*K*). Often, we are able to use another stitch of No. 2 nylon at the most caudal insertion of the rectus fascia onto the pubic bone. This maneuver adds to the security of the pubic closure. A V-shaped flap of abdominal skin at a point corresponding to the normal position of the umbilicus is tacked down to the abdominal fascia, and a drainage tube exits this orifice. The method described by Hanna (1986) is our most commonly performed procedure. Before and during the procedure, the patient is given broad-spec-

trum antibiotics in an attempt to convert a contaminated field into a clean surgical wound. Nonreactive sutures of polyglycolic acid (Dexon/Vicryl) and nylon are used to avoid an undesirable stitch reaction or stitch abscess.

Management after Primary Closure

The procedure just described converts a patient with exstrophy into one with complete epispadias and incontinence. **Before removal of the suprapubic tube, 4 weeks after surgery, the bladder outlet is calibrated by a urethral catheter or a urethral sound to ensure free drainage. A complete ultrasound examination is obtained to ascertain the status of the renal pelves and ureters, and appropriate urinary antibiotics are administered to treat any bladder contamination that might be present after removal of the suprapubic tube.** Residual urine is estimated by clamping the suprapubic tube, and specimens for culture are obtained before the patient leaves the hospital and at subsequent intervals to detect infection and ensure that the bladder is empty. If the initial ultrasound examination shows good drainage, upper tract imaging by ultrasound is repeated 3 months after discharge from the hospital and at intervals of 6 months to 1 year during the next 2 to 3 years to detect any upper tract changes caused by reflux, infection, or obstruction. Prophylactic antibiotics should be continuous, because all patients with bladder exstrophy, once closed, have vesicoureteral reflux. If a useful continence interval has resulted from the initial closure, a further operation for incontinence may not be required; however, this situation is quite unusual. In our experience with more than 85 primary closures, this has occurred in 3 patients, all of whom were girls. After the conversion from exstrophy to complete epispadias with incontinence, the bladder gradually increases in capacity as inflammatory changes in the mucosa resolve.

Cystoscopy and cystography at yearly intervals are used to detect bilateral reflux in almost 100% of patients and to provide an estimate of bladder capacity (Gearhart and Jeffs, 1998). Even in a completely incontinent patient, bladder capacity gradually increases to a point at which the bladder can be distended at cystography to its true capacity. **This must be done under anesthesia in young children, because the values obtained markedly differ from those obtained when trying to fill the bladder of a squirming infant on an x-ray table** (Gearhart and Jeffs, 1998). If the bladder has not achieved a capacity of at least 30 ml by 1 to 2 years, then concern must be voiced to the parents about the overall ability of the bladder to undergo a continence procedure. Currently, the only parameters available to predict overall success are the size of the bladder template at birth and a successful primary closure with absence of infections.

Should bladder outlet resistance be such that urine is retained within the bladder and reflux and ureteral dilatation develop with infected urine, it may be necessary to dilate the urethra or to begin intermittent catheterization (Baker et al, 1999). Sometimes the posterior urethral obstruction can be such that it requires a transurethral incision of the stricture to maintain an adequate posterior urethral outlet. **If bladder outlet resistance persists and**

infections continue, then an antireflux procedure may be required as early as 6 months to 1 year after initial closure (Mathews and Gearhart, 2001). If severe upper tract changes occur, surgical revision of the bladder outlet by advancing skin flaps into the orifice or even patching the stricture may be necessary to prevent scarring and further obstruction. As mentioned previously, transurethral incision of the urethral stricture to obtain a balanced outlet should be tried before surgical revision. Judgment is required to know when to avoid attempts at functional closure and to know when to return to urinary diversion as a means to preserve renal function. This change of plan is seldom necessary if an adequate outlet has been constructed at the initial closure and if careful attention has been paid to the details of follow-up of the bladder and posterior urethra. **An important caveat is that if there are recurrent urinary tract infections and if the bladder is distended on ultrasound, cystoscopy should be performed and the posterior urethra should be carefully examined anteriorly for erosion of the intrapubic stitch, which may be the cause of the recurrent infections** (Baker et al, 1999). If the intrapubic stitch is seen in the posterior urethra, a small suprapubic incision should be made and the stitch should be removed, or, if it can be grasped, it should be removed transurethrally.

Penile and Urethral Closure in Exstrophy

Epispadias Repair

Historically, bladder neck reconstruction was performed before penile and urethral reconstruction. However, an increase in bladder capacity in those patients with extremely small bladder capacities after epispadias repair prompted a change in the management program (Gearhart and Jeffs, 1989a) (Fig. 61–22). In a group of patients with a small bladder capacity after initial closure, there was a mean increase of 55 ml in males in only 22 months after epispadias repair. However, with the modern version of staged reconstruction, the epispadias repair is now performed at about 6 months of age in all patients. With this modification, possibly all patients can achieve an appropriate capacity at the time when they are ready physically and mentally to undergo bladder neck reconstruction. Because most boys with exstrophy have a somewhat small penis and a shortage of available penile skin, all patients undergo testosterone stimulation before urethroplasty and penile reconstruction (Gearhart and Jeffs, 1987).

Many techniques have been described for reconstruction of the penis and urethra in patients with classic bladder exstrophy. Current methods of epispadias repair in bladder exstrophy are the Cantwell-Ransley repair (1989), the modified Cantwell-Ransley repair (1992, 1995), and the penile disassembly technique described by Mitchell (1996) (Ransley et al, 1989; Gearhart et al, 1992, 1995c; Mitchell and Bagley, 1996).

Regardless of the surgical technique chosen for reconstruction of the penis in bladder exstrophy, four key concerns must be addressed to ensure a functional and cosmetically pleasing penis. These concerns include (1) correction of dorsal chordee, (2) urethral reconstruction, (3) glandular reconstruction, and (4) penile skin closure.

Although it is possible to achieve some penile lengthening with release of chordee at the time of initial closure, it is often necessary to perform formal penile elongation with release of chordee at the time of urethroplasty in exstrophy patients. Data by Silver and associates (1997b) clearly showed that this is more an apparent lengthening of the penis than a true lengthening, because the anterior corporal bodies in exstrophy patients have 50% less length than in those of age-matched controls in adult life. Certainly, all remnants of the suspensory ligaments and old scar tissue from the initial bladder closure must be excised. Also, further dissection of the corpora cavernosa from the inferior pubic ramus can be achieved. It is often surprising how little is accomplished in freeing the corporal bodies from the pubis at the time of initial exstrophy closure (Gearhart, 1991).

Lengthening of the urethral groove is also essential. Whether or not paraexstrophy skin flaps are used at the time of bladder closure, further lengthening will be needed. This can range from something as simple as Cantwell's original procedure to transection of the urethral plate and replacement of the genital tissue. However, in modern techniques of epispadias repair, replacement of the urethra is not typically performed. In the penile disassembly technique described by Mitchell and Bagley (1996), the urethral plate is dissected completely from the glans; in some patients it will not be long enough to reach the tip of the penis and as a result hypospadias will be present with further reconstruction needed at another setting. **I believe that because of the marked length disparity in male children with exstrophy compared with normal males, complete detachment of the urethra from the glans is an unnecessary step in light of the small amount of length that is obtained with this maneuver and the possibility of resulting hypospadias, which requires an additional surgical procedure.**

Chordee

Besides lengthening of the urethral groove, dorsal chordee must be addressed. To release dorsal chordee, one may lengthen the dorsomedial aspect of the corpora by incision and anastomosis of the corpora themselves (Ransley et al, 1992). Also, length can be gained by placement of a dermal graft to allow lengthening of the dorsal aspect of the corpora (Woodhouse, 1986). Another technique to improve dorsal chordee before urethroplasty is shortening or medial rotation of the ventral corpora (Koff and Eakins, 1984). However, most of these techniques, especially grafting, are reserved for patients who are seen in adolescent and adult years for epispadias surgery with the need for some increased penile length and correction of residual chordee.

Urethral Reconstruction

Urethral reconstruction is an important aspect of external genital reconstruction in exstrophy. This can be accomplished by many previously reported methods. Tubularization of the dorsal urethral groove as a modified Young

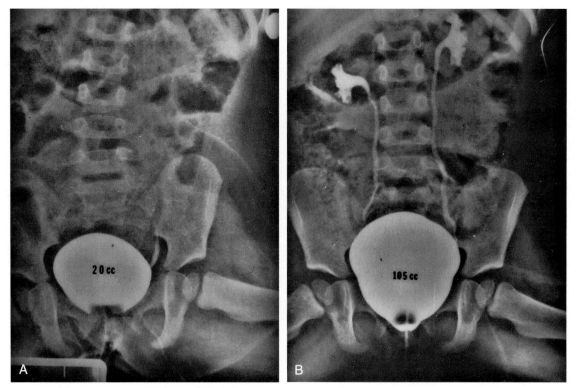

Figure 61–22. *A,* Initial cystogram under anesthesia showing small bladder capacity after exstrophy closure. *B,* Second film demonstrates much greater capacity after urethroplasty with volume of 105 cc under gravity cystogram under anesthesia. Interval is one year. (From Peters CA, Gearhart JP, Jeffs RD: Epispadias and incontinence: The child with a small bladder. J Urol 1988;140:1200, with permission.)

urethroplasty has been abandoned in our practice because of the high incidence of urethrocutaneous fistula and the less than optimal cosmetic appearance of the penis (Lepor et al, 1984). In the past, interposition of a free graft of genital or extragenital skin, or even bladder mucosa, has been used (Hendren, 1979). In addition, ventral transverse island flaps and double-faced island flaps have been used with some success for urethral reconstruction in exstrophy patients (Thomalla and Mitchell, 1984; Monfort et al, 1987). However, modern techniques of repair of epispadias repair associated with bladder exstrophy utilize tubularization of the urethral plate, moving the urethral plate under the corporal bodies after closure to lessen the incidence of urethrocutaneous fistula and also to give the penis a more downward deflection and more easily catheterizable urethral channel (Surer et al, 2000).

Penile Skin Closure

If skin closure continues to be a problem in genital reconstruction, owing to the paucity of skin associated with this condition, a Z-plasty incision and closure at the base of the penis prevents skin contraction and upward tethering of the penis. The ventral foreskin can be split in the midline and brought to the dorsum as lateral preputial flaps for coverage of the penile shaft. If the flaps are a bit asymmetrical, a staggered dorsal suture line results, with less upward tethering. Alternatively, a buttonhole can be created in the ventral foreskin and simply transposed to the dorsum for additional penile skin coverage.

Modified Cantwell-Ransley Repair

Our preference for urethroplasty and penile reconstruction, if the urethral groove has adequate length, is the modified Cantwell-Ransley repair (Gearhart et al, 1992, 1995c) (Fig. 61–23). Currently, in the modern applications of the staged reconstruction of bladder exstrophy, epispadias repair is performed when the child is 6 months to 1 year of age. The modified Cantwell-Ransley procedure is begun by placing an island stitch through the glans as a traction stitch. Incisions are made over two parallel lines marked previously on the dorsum of the penis that outline an 18-mm wide strip of urethral mucosa, extending from the prostatic urethral meatus to the tip of the penis (see Fig. 61–23A and B). For this procedure, a deep vertical incision (IPGAM) is made in the urethral plate distally. The incision is then closed with 6-0 polyglycolic sutures in a transverse fashion (see Fig. 61–23B and C). This procedure flattens the distal urethral plate and advances the urethra to the tip of the phallus so that it will be in excellent glandular position when the glandular wings are closed over the reconstructed urethra (see Fig. 61–23D). Glandular mucosal areas of the dorsal glans are excised adjacent to the urethral strip and thick glandar flaps are constructed bilaterally. Lateral skin flaps are mobilized and undermined. A Z-incision of the suprapubic area permits wide exposure and division of the suspensory ligaments and old scar tissue from initial exstrophy closure.

Ventral penile skin is taken down to the level of the scrotum (see Fig. 61–23E). Care is taken to preserve the mesentery to the urethral plate, which arises proximally

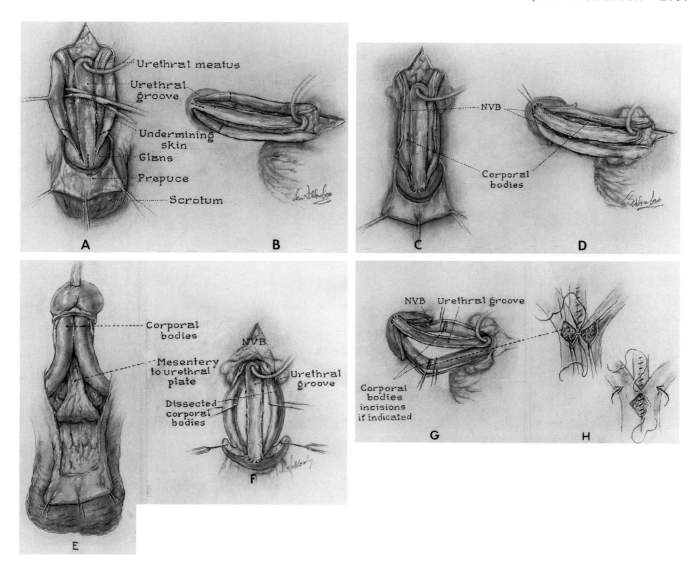

Figure 61–23. Modified Cantwell-Ransley procedure. *A* and *B,* Marking incision of the urethral groove and mobilization of the penile skin. *C* and *D,* Incision of the glans with the IPGAM maneuver exposure of the neurovascular bundles (NVB). *E* and *F,* Separation of the urethral plate from the corporal bodies with dissection initially started from below. Note that the entire urethral plate is separated from the corporal bodies, except for the last 1.5 cm of the plate, which is left attached to the corporal bodies and the glans distally. *G* and *H,* Mobilization of the neurovascular bundles from the corporal bodies and incision of the corporal bodies. Incisions in the corporal bodies are then closed with running sutures. This incision of the corporal bodies is used only if severe dorsal chordee cannot be corrected by radical mobilization of the urethral plate and simple rotation of the corpora.

Illustration continued on following page

and extends upward between the corporal blood supply to the urethral plate. Dissection of the corpora is begun ventrally with dissection on the surface of Buck's fascia covering the corporal bodies. The plan is followed closely until one exits on the dorsum of the penis between the corpus spongiosum and the corporal body, first on one side and then on the other (see Fig. 61–23*F*). The loops are placed around the corporal bodies and the dissection is extended proximally on the corpora to dissect the urethral plate free from the corporal bodies up to the level of the prostate (see Fig. 61–23*F*). Although one might expect difficulties when dissecting proximally where the paraexstrophy skin flaps had been sutured to the urethral plate, this has not been encountered in our experience, and dissection is kept just on the corporal bodies while proceeding proximally. The urethral plate is also dissected distally past the level of

the junction of the glans with the corporal bodies. In this manner, adequate mobilization is obtained, and it is not difficult to bring the corporal bodies over the urethra at the level of the corona. This almost separates the penis into three components, the two corpora and the urethral plate (see Fig. 61–23*F*). However, complete penile disassembly is not undertaken, and the distalmost 1-cm attachment of the mucosa plate to the glans is left intact (Surer et al, 2000).

The neurovascular bundles, situated between Buck's fascia and the corporal wall, are typically left intact in young patients if rotation of the corporal bodies over the urethra effectively straightens the penis. If not, then the neurovascular bundles are dissected free from the corporal bodies, with vessel loops being placed around these structures (see Fig. 61–23*G*) so that the neurovascular bundles will not be

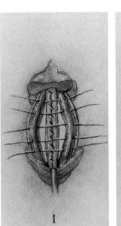
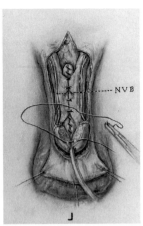
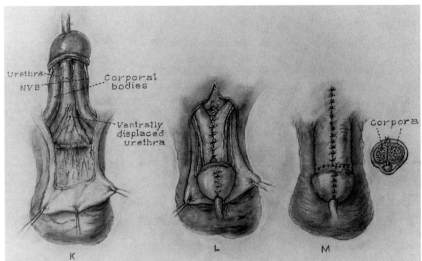

Figure 61–23 *Continued. I* and *J,* Closure and joining of the corporal bodies dorsally over the closed urethral plate. This is the typical situation in most repairs. Other sutures are used to bury the urethra under the corporal bodies. Distally the glans is coapted over the closed urethral plate. *K* through *M,* The urethra is shown under the corporal bodies and the mesentery coming from the ventral foreskin. The ventral foreskin is then split and sewn to the coronal margin and to itself in the midline. Oftentimes, a Z-plasty is used at the base of the penis. (Drawings by Leon Schlossberg.)

compromised when incisions are made in the corpora and the corpora is rotated medially over the neourethra (see Fig. 61–23*H*). After the corporal bodies are incised or rotated over the urethra, the urethral strip is closed in a linear manner from the prostatic opening to the glans over a No. 8 Fr silicone stent with 6-0 polyglycolic sutures. After this is accomplished, incisions are then made in the corporal bodies at the point of maximum curvature, opening a diamond-shaped effect in the erectile tissue (see Fig. 61–23*I*). The corpora are then closed over the neourethra with two running sutures of 5-0 polydiaxone, and the diamond-shaped defects in the adjacent area of the corpora are sutured to each other. This procedure effectively displaces the urethra ventrally in a normal position. This not only causes the downward deflection of the penis, but it also allows for some additional length by dorsal rotation and approximation of the corporal bodies over the neourethra. After the urethra has been transferred to the ventrum, further sutures of 4-0 polyglycolic acid are placed between the corporal bodies to bury the urethra further, especially at the level of the junction of the glans and the corporal bodies at the corona (see Fig. 61–23*J* and *K*).

The glans wings are then closed over the glandular urethra using subcuticular sutures of 5-0 polyglycolic acid, and the glans epithelium is closed with 6-0 polyglycolic acid sutures. The ventral skin is then brought up and sutured to the ventral edge of the corona, and the flaps are fashioned to provide adequate coverage and lengthening of the dorsum of the penis. The skin is reapproximated with interrupted 5-0 or 6-0 polyglycolic sutures (see Fig. 61–23*L* and *M*). A Z-plasty at the base of the penis is closed with interrupted 5-0 or 6-0 polyglycolic acid sutures. A silicone stent is left indwelling in the neourethra to provide drainage for 10 to 12 days.

Postoperative Problems

Postoperative pain and bladder spasms after extensive external genital reconstructive surgery require a combined effort of the pediatric anesthesia pain service and the surgical service. Controlling bladder spasms is paramount because they are associated with more urinary extravasation and fistula formation. All of our patients have a caudal epidural catheter placed at the time of surgery to help with postoperative pain control and bladder spasms. In addition, oxybutynin is started immediately after surgery to decrease the incidence of bladder spasms and enhance patient comfort. At the time of discharge, the plastic dressing on the penis is left intact and the child is discharged with narcotics, antispasmotics, and appropriate broad-spectrum antibiotic coverage.

Female Genitalia

We attempt to reconstruct the mons external genitalia at the time of initial exstrophy closure. Although this adds a bit of time to the operation, once the pubic bones are brought into apposition with osteotomy it is quite easy to reconstruct the female external genitalia.

The bifid clitoris is denuded medially and brought together in the midline at the time of closure along with labia minora reconstruction by creating a fourchette. A good closure with an attractive mons area and reconstruction of the female genitalia gives the parents a sense of well-being and markedly enhances the overall appearance of the female child born with bladder exstrophy (see Fig. 61–9).

Continence and Antireflux Procedure

Bladder capacity is measured with the child under anesthesia with a gravity cystogram at the 1-year anniversary of the initial closure (Gearhart and Jeffs, 1998). Formerly it was believed that if the bladder capacity was 60 ml or higher bladder neck reconstruction could

be planned (Gearhart and Jeffs, 1998). **However, Chan and colleagues (2001) found that, in selected exstrophy patients who underwent closure, epispadias repair, and bladder neck reconstruction at our institution, a median bladder capacity of 85 ml was more common in the group who were completely dry after bladder neck reconstruction. Most of these children were 4 to 5 years of age and were ready emotionally, maturationally, and intellectually to participate in a postoperative voiding program.** Continence and antireflux procedures performed at our institution are illustrated in Figure 61–24. The bladder is open through a transverse incision at the bladder neck with a vertical extension. The later midline closure of this incision is the width of the bladder neck and enlarges the vertical dimension of the bladder, which in exstrophy is often short. This illustration depicts a Cohen transtrigonal ureteral reimplantation or a cephalotrigonal reimplantation that moves the ureter across the bladder, above the trigone, or directs the ureter cephalad up onto the edge of the trigone (see Fig. 61–24B) (Canning et al, 1992). In addition, if the ureters are low on the trigone, there is a need to move the ureteral hiatus higher on the trigone. The hiatus is simply cut in a cephalad direction, and cross-trigonal reimplants are performed at the upper aspect of the trigone (see Fig. 61–24C).

The continence procedure is begun by selecting a posterior strip of mucosa 15 to 18 mm wide and 30 mm long which extends distally from the midtrigone to the prostate or posterior urethra (Fig. 61–24D). Bladder muscle lateral to the mucosal strip is denuded from the mucosa. It is often helpful at this juncture to use one or two epinephrine-soaked sponges to aid in the control of bleeding and the visualization of the denuded area. Tailoring of the denuded lateral muscle triangles is aided by multiple small incisions on the free edge bilaterally that allow the area of the reconstruction to assume a more cephalad position (see Fig. 61–24E). **These muscle flaps not only are smaller, but also are not incised transversely at their cephalad extent as described in the original Young-Dees procedure. We believe that, if these flaps are incised medially at the cephalad border where they join at the floor of the bladder, there is a significant risk of denervation and ischemia that will harm the bladder neck repair. The basic premise is to create a mucosal-lined tube inside a muscular funnel that narrows from its junction with the floor of the bladder that extends caudally.** The edges of the mucosa and underlying muscle are closed with interrupted sutures of 4-0 polyglycolic acid (see Fig. 61–24F). The adjacent denuded muscle flaps are overlapped and sutured firmly in place with a 3-0 polydiaxone suture to provide reinforcement of the bladder neck and urethral reconstruction (see Fig. 61–24G and H). A No. 8 Fr urethral stent may be used as a guide during urethral reconstruction, but it is removed after the bladder neck reconstruction is completed. After the bladder neck repair is completed, the repair is suspended to the rectus fascia (see Fig. 61–24I). **Very radical dissection of the bladder, bladder neck, and posterior urethra is required, not only within the pelvis but also from the posterior aspect of the pubic bar to provide enough mobility for the bladder neck reconstruction.** This maneuver allows for adequate bladder neck narrowing and tightening of the bladder neck repair

and subsequent anterior suspension of the newly created posterior urethra and bladder neck. If visualization of the posterior urethra is problematic, the intrasymphyseal bar can be cut, thus providing a widened field of exposure. The intrasymphyseal bar is approximated with 2-0 sutures of polydioxanone. If the intrasymphyseal bar is cut, mobility of the child should be restricted in the postoperative period to allow proper healing of the intrasymphyseal bar.

Postoperative Care

Ureteral stents are placed in the reimplanted ureters and brought out through the wall of the bladder, and the bladder is drained by suprapubic tube, which is left indwelling for a 3-week period. **At the end of 3 weeks the suprapubic tube is clamped and the patient is allowed to attempt to void. Initially, the tube should not be clamped for over 1 hour. If voiding does not occur, the child is given an anesthetic and a No. 8 Fr Foley catheter is placed.** This is left in place for 5 days, then removed, and another voiding trial is begun. This part of the postoperative period is most demanding on both the patient, family, and surgeon. Some children require several catheter placements before voiding is initiated. If the child can empty the bladder satisfactorily, the suprapubic tube is removed. Frequent bladder and renal ultrasound examinations are required in the first few months after bladder neck repair.

Combined Bladder Exstrophy and Epispadias Repair

Combined closure of exstrophy and epispadias repair is very similar at the beginning (Fig. 61–25A through J) **to closure of bladder exstrophy and the posterior urethra alone** (Gearhart et al, 1998). Evaluation of the bladder template is performed by inverting the bladder into the abdomen with a sterile gloved finger. This allows evaluation of the extent of the urethral plate, which may be larger than noted on visual inspection of the abdominal wall defect. Extent of bladder polyposis and scarring is also noted. In addition, the urethral plate is examined for its length and depth and the presence of scarring from any prior attempt at repair (see Fig. 61–25A). All patients receive preoperative testosterone to enhance penile size and testosterone cream to the urethral plate and bladder neck if prior surgery has led to scarring. The operative procedure begins and proceeds as with a standard closure of the bladder, posterior urethra, and abdominal wall, with only a few variations (see Fig. 61–25B and C). One major difference is that great care must be used to resect any remnants of the urogenital diaphragm fibers (see Fig. 61–25D and E). It is surprising how frequently these fibers are still intact in patients undergoing reclosure after failure of the initial operative procedures.

If adequate dissection has been performed, the entire posterior urethra/bladder unit can be moved posteriorly into the pelvis. Once the bladder and posterior urethra are adequately dissected, attention can be given to dissection of the penis, corporal bodies, and urethral plate. This part of the procedure (see Fig. 61–25F through O) progresses much as in a standard epispadias repair and exstrophy closure.

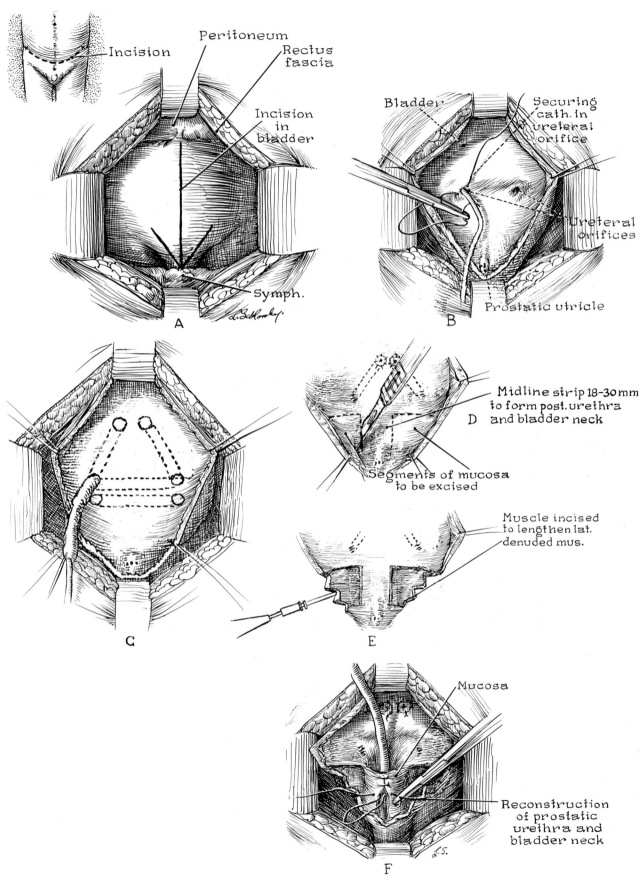

Figure 61–24. Modified Young-Dees-Leadbetter bladder neck repair. *A,* Vertical bladder incision with transverse incision distally where the bladder and posterior urethra go under the pubis. *B,* Ureteral mobilization with either transtrigonal or cephalotrigonal direction for ureteral reimplantation. *D* and *F,* A mucosal strip of trigone to form the bladder neck and prostatic urethra. Lateral denuded muscle triangles are lengthened by several incisions to allow tailoring and funneling of the bladder neck reconstruction area. Note: there is no transverse incision at the junction of the bladder neck repair with the bladder floor. A transverse incision in this area will create ischemic, poorly innervated flaps and will contribute to failure of the repair.

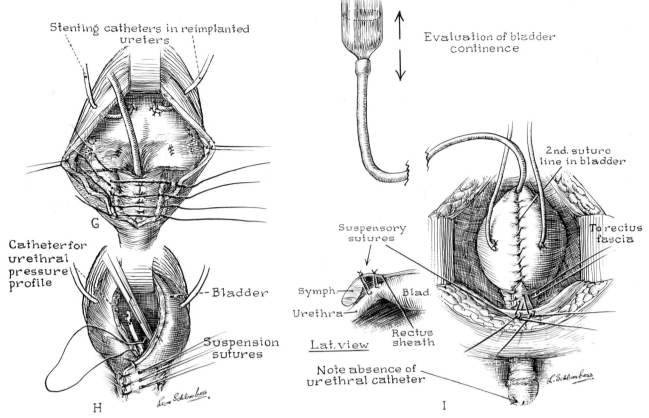

Figure 61–24 *Continued. G* and *H,* These illustrations depict the double-breasted nature and exact suture placement of the bladder neck reconstruction. A pressure profile catheter can be left and a urethral pressure profile can be obtained after closure of the bladder. *I,* suspension sutures are elevated mainly to estimate final outlet resistance. The bladder neck and urethra are unstented. Drainage is by ureteral catheter and suprapubic tube. Outlet resistance is estimated by water manometer. (Drawings by Leon Schlossberg.)

After dissection of the penis and corporal bodies, the urethral plate is then dissected off the corpora except for the distal 0.5 to 1 cm (see Fig. 61–25*P*). A No. 2 nylon suture is then placed in a horizontal mattress fashion in the pubis and used to bring the pelvis together (Fig. 61–25*Q* and *R*). In the child is older than 1 year of age and being managed with osteotomy, the fixator pins may be used to assist with rotation of the pelvis medially into place. In young children, the lack of ossified bones prohibits this maneuver. Approximation of the pubic tubercles allows the corpora to significantly rotate medially so that they can easily be brought over the closed urethral plate (see Fig. 61–25*R*).

Penile and glans reconstruction is completed with appropriate skin coverage using reverse Byars flaps or, in some cases, a Nesbitt turnover flap (see Fig. 61–25*S* through *U*). A Blake drain is placed next to the bladder closure, and the abdominal wall closure is completed. A No. 8 Fr Firlit stent is used to stent the urethra for 7 to 10 days. The external fixating device is then attached to the intrafragmentary pins and tightened.

External fixation of the pelvis is maintained for 4 weeks in children with primary closure and for 6 weeks in those undergoing reclosure of the bladder. **Follow-up is much the same as with standard exstrophy closure and includes monitoring of residual urines and upper tract imaging with ultrasound before removal of the suprapubic tube.** Although some of our patients have achieved long-term continence after these procedures, most require

bladder neck reconstruction when bladder capacity is deemed adequate and the child is able to participate in a postoperative voiding program (Gearhart et al, 1998).

MODERN STAGED FUNCTIONAL CLOSURE: OUTCOMES AND RESULTS

The use of functional bladder closure in bladder exstrophy has resulted in dramatic improvements in the success of reconstruction. Several series (Chisholm, 1979; Ansell, 1983; Mollard, 1980) have demonstrated the success and applicability of the staged functional closure approach to bladder exstrophy. Other series (Conner et al, 1988; Husmann et al, 1989a) have shown acceptable continence rates with preservation of renal function. More recent series (Perlmutter et al, 1991; Mollard et al, 1994; McMahon et al, 1996; Lotteman et al, 1998; Gearhart and Jeffs, 1998) have documented continued improvements in outcomes, acceptable urinary continence, and preservation of renal function in a majority of patients (Table 61–2).

Initial Closure

In a series by Chan and associates (2001), 90 patients with bladder exstrophy who were referred to our pediatric

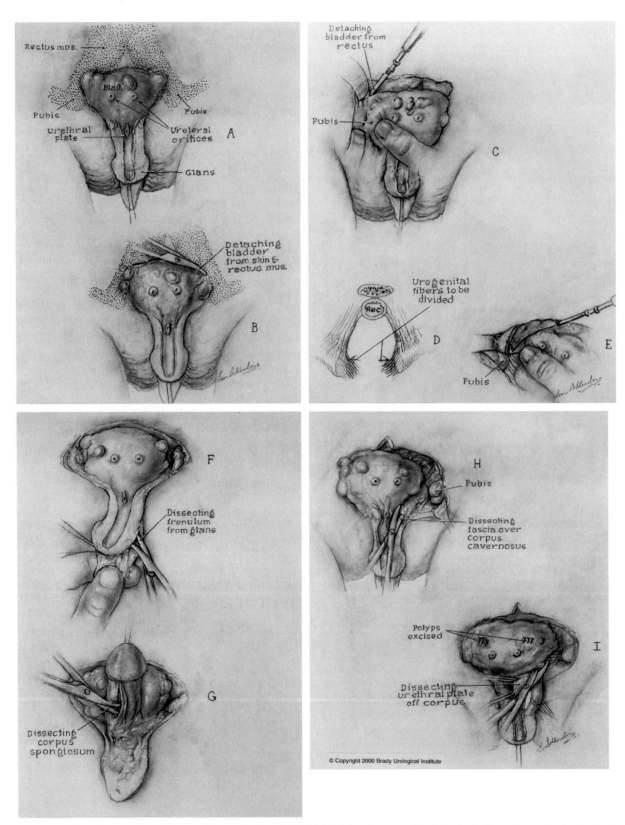

Figure 61–25. Combined exstrophy and epispadias repair. *A* and *B,* Initial incision between the abdominal skin and muscle developing the plane between the rectus fascia and the rectus muscle. *C,* Establishment of the retrovesical plane between the rectus muscle and the bladder. *D* and *E,* Urogenital diaphragm fibers with the bladder excluded in the initial area of incision of the urogenital diaphragm fibers to be divided from the base of the pubic bones to the posterior urethra and bladder neck area. *F* and *G,* Degloving of the penis as an initial approach to the urethral plate from below. *H* and *I,* Developing of the plane between the urethral plate and the corporal bodies and dissection of the urethral plate from the cephalad extent of the corporal bodies up under the bladder.

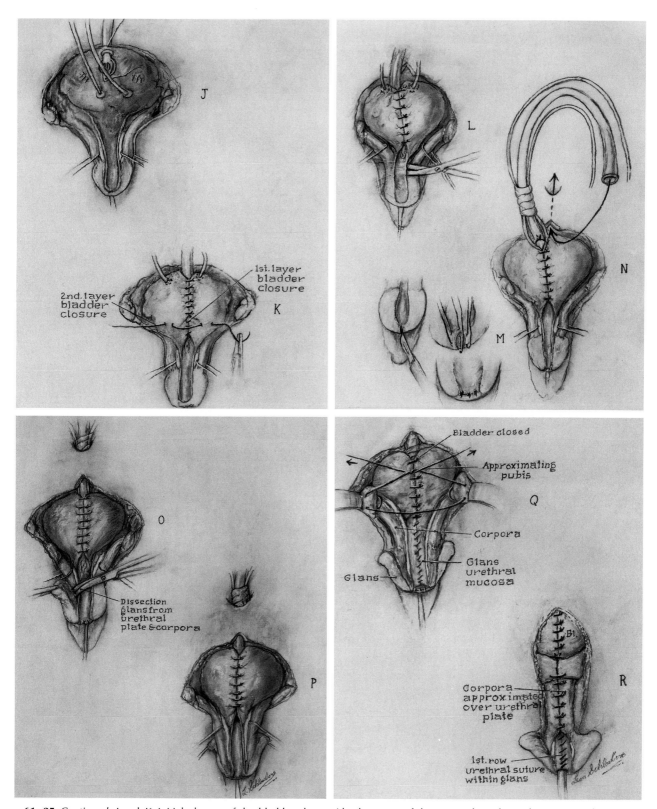

Figure 61–25 *Continued. J* and *K,* Initial closure of the bladder along with placement of the suprapubic tube and stents. *L* and *M,* Continuing dissection of the urethral plate from the dorsal aspect of the corporal bodies and bringing the suprapubic tube and stents out through the neoumbilicus. Insert shows the IPGAM maneuver to move the urethral plate to the distal tip of the glans. *O* and *P,* Dissection of the glanular tissue from the distal corporal bodies and the final dissection of the urethral plate from the entire corporal body except for the last 1.5 cm. *Q* and *R,* Closure of the pubic bones with horizontal mattress sutures before closure of the corporal bodies over the closed urethral plate.

Illustration continued on following page

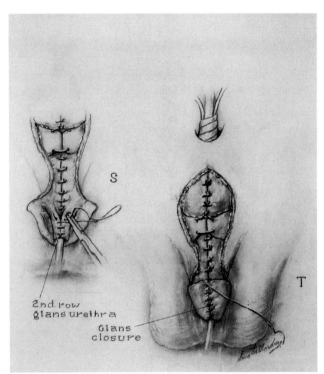
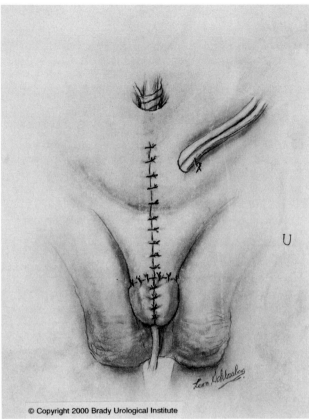

© Copyright 2000 Brady Urological Institute

Figure 61–25 *Continued. S* and *T,* Final closure of the glans over the closed urethral plate. *U,* completed closure with drains present. (Primary closure alone, no urethral stent is left indwelling. If secondary closure is performed, a urethral stent is left for 7 to 10 days.) (Drawings by Leon Schlossberg.)

urology service between 1975 and 1997 were evaluated. Complications from bladder closure, and additional surgical procedures required to correct these complications, are presented in Table 61–3. **The importance of a successful initial closure is emphasized by Oesterling and Jeffs (1987) and by Husmann and colleagues (1989a), who found that the onset of eventual continence was quicker and the continence rate higher in those who underwent a successful initial closure with or without osteotomy. In addition, Gearhart and associates (1996a) reported on 23 patients with bladder exstrophy who underwent more than two failed attempts at closure. If a patient underwent two closures, the chances of having an adequate bladder capacity for bladder neck reconstruction was 60%, and the chance of successful continence was 30%. Patients who had undergone three closures had only a 40% chance of obtaining an adequate bladder capacity and less than a 20% chance of being continent of urine.** In the evaluation of this group of selected exstrophy patients, it was found that at the time of initial closure

Table 61–2. URINARY CONTINENCE AFTER FUNCTIONAL BLADDER CLOSURE*

Series	Number of Closures Evaluated	Patients Who Became Continent
Perlmutter et al (1991)	15	77%
Mollard et al (1994)	73	69%
McMahon et al (1996)	33	70%
Lotteman et al (1998)	57	67%
Chan et al (2001)	90	90%†

*Includes only personal series (one or two surgeons only) repairing continence rates greater than 6%.
†74% dry day and night, 16% dry for >3 hr during day with some wet nights.

Table 61–3. COMPLICATIONS AND CORRECTIVE SURGICAL PROCEDURES IN 90 PRIMARY BLADDER CLOSURES*

Item	Number
Complication	
Bladder prolapse	3
Outlet obstruction	3
Bladder calculi	4
Renal calculi	2
Wound dehiscence	1
Stitch erosion	3
Procedure	
Repair prolapse/dehiscence	4
Cystolithopaxy	4
Urethrotomy	3
Nephrolithotomy	2
Removal of intrapubic stitch	3

*All closed primarily at the Johns Hopkins Hospital.
Chan DY, Jeffs RD, Gearhart JB: Determinates of continence in the bladder exstrophy population after bladder neck reconstruction. Urology 2001;165:1656.

19 of 23 patients had no form of osteotomy. Six of the patients had obtained bladder capacity suitable for bladder neck reconstruction; three were dry, and three were incontinent. Bladder size was inadequate in nine patients after being monitored for bladder growth. The chance of obtaining an adequate bladder capacity and eventual continence after more than one closure attempt is markedly diminished. These less than satisfactory results underline the paramount importance of a secure abdominal wall, posterior urethra, and bladder closure in these complex cases. Lastly, the importance of early initial closure was emphasized by data from Husmann and colleagues (1989a) showing than only 10% of those patients who undergo bladder closure before 1 year of age, but 40% of those who have the procedure at a later age, require eventual augmentation.

Epispadias Repair

Although urinary incontinence remains the most significant problem for patients with classic bladder exstrophy and epispadias, anxiety about inadequate and unattractive genitalia still poses the greatest concern to male patients. Formerly, the modified Young repair was the most commonly used technique at our institution to repair the epispadiac penis (Lepor et al, 1984). Because of the tortuosity of the urethra, high fistula rate, and significant dorsal chordee associated with this repair, a modification of the Cantwell-Ransley procedure was adopted as a new repair technique. We began using the modified Cantwell-Ransley repair in patients with classic exstrophy or epispadias in 1988 and have reported our early experience (Gearhart et al, 1992, Gearhart 1995c).

Since 1988 the modified Cantwell-Ransley repair has been performed for 93 male patients with either classic bladder exstrophy (79 patients) or epispadias (14 patients) (Surer et al, 1999). At the time of surgery, the patient age ranged from 1 to 18 years with an average age of 2.6 years. Over the last 2 years, however, the mean age at the time of epispadias repair decreased to 1.2 years. Of the 79 patients with bladder exstrophy, 31 had a short urethral groove requiring paraexstrophy skin flaps for penile lengthening at the time of initial bladder exstrophy closure. Of the 14 epispadiac patients, 11 had penopubic and 3 had penile epispadias at presentation.

This technique was used for primary urethroplasty in 65 patients with bladder exstrophy and 12 with epispadias. The modified Cantwell-Ransley repair was used as a secondary procedure after failed urethroplasty in 4 patients with exstrophy and 2 with epispadias and was combined with reclosure of bladder exstrophy in 10 patients. Early epispadias repair is performed when the patients were 6 months to 1 year of age. However, because of concerns about getting the urethra deeper under the corpora at the glandular level, beginning in 1994 we further modified the Cantwell-Ransley repair by detaching the mucosal plate from the corona except for the distal 0.5 to 1 cm of the plate. Intramuscular testosterone enanthate in oil was given to all children at a dose of 2 mg/kg at approximately 5 weeks and again at 2 weeks before surgery.

With mean follow-up of 68 months, 87 patients had a horizontal or downward-angled penis while standing. The

Table 61–4. OPERATIVE COMPLICATIONS AFTER URETHRAL RECONSTRUCTION

Complication*	Incidence	
	Number	*Percentage*
Fistula	21	23
Surgical closure	17	19
Spontaneous closure	4	4
Stricture	7	8
Superficial skin separation	5	5

*Classic exstrophy, 79 (primary 65), 31 closed with paraexstrophy skin flaps; epispadias, 14 (primary 12), 31 paraexstrophy flaps.

instance of urethrocutaneous fistula in the immediate postoperative period was 23%, and at 3 months it was 19% (Table 61–4). Seven patients developed a urethral stricture of the proximal anastomotic site, and five had minor skin separations of the dorsal skin closure. Cystoscopy with catheterization had been performed in 77 patients and had revealed an easily negotiable neourethral channel in all. With the patient standing, the penis dangled downward in 87 (93%) of patients; the remaining patients (5 with exstrophy and 1 with epispadias) needed further penile straightening surgery. The appearance of the penis was acceptable to both parents and children. Ten of the 12 patients who were older than 16 years of age had engaged in satisfactory intercourse and reported their penis to be acceptable, both functionally and cosmetically.

Modern penile reconstructive techniques should create a straight and functional penis with a glanular meatus, an easily catheterizable neourethral channel (if needed), and an acceptable cosmetic appearance. Many adolescents considered their odd-appearing genitalia with a short, widened penis to be a greater psychosocial problem than incontinence, and therefore every effort should be made to restore the penis to a normal condition. Historically, most repairs of the epispadiac penis came from Cantwell's original description in 1895. In 1989, Ransley and associates introduced a concept to release dorsal chordee by incision and anastomosis of the dorsomedial aspect of the corpora over the urethra and urethral meatotomy at the distal end of the glans, to move the meatus to a more normal position and secure good direction of the urinary stream. Ransley's group have reported their long-term experience with 95 patients in whom the modified Cantwell-Ransley repair was used: fistula occurred in only 4% of patients, and a urethral stricture in only 5% (Kajbafzadeh et al, 1995).

Dissection of the urethral strip to almost the tip of the glans provides a ventral position of the urethra and the glans and submerges the urethra well below the corpora at the glans level. This approximation of raw surface of glanular tissues dorsally over the urethra is clearly why the incidence of fistula in the area of the corona is very rare compared with the Young repair. Fistulas in our patients usually appear at the base of the penis, where the urethra comes up proximally between the corporal bodies. In modern exstrophy reconstructive techniques, most surgeons try to preserve the urethral plate at the time of exstrophy closure. Interestingly, we do not find a significant difference for fistula formation between those in whom paraexstrophy skin flaps were used at the time of initial closure and those in whom they were not.

Some authors have advised even more aggressive techniques than those proposed originally by Cantwell. Mitchell and Bagley (1996) described a complete penile disassembly technique in which the epispadiac phallus is completely disassembled into three components: the urethral plate and the right and left hemicorporal glandular bodies. A group of 10 patients with follow-up of 57 months were reported to be very happy with the horizontal direction of the penis. There were three fistulas after surgery, but these were in two patients who had undergone secondary repair. A multicenter report on the use of this repair in a total of 17 boys found that 3 of the 17 had a urethrocutaneous fistula, two of which closed spontaneously (Zaontz et al, 1998). One patient had a complete dehiscence, but all boys with intact repairs had straight erections, an orthotopic meatus, and a satisfactory appearance.

In my opinion, none of the current epispadias repairs offer any significant gain in penile length by removal of the entire urethral plate from the glans or even the use of a free graft. Data reported by Silver and colleagues (1997b) clearly showed that, although anterior corporal length is significantly less in patients with exstrophy, the posterior corporal length is normal. These findings suggest that penile lengthening procedures at the time of epispadias repair improve apparent penile length and straighten the penis but do not transfer additional tissue (i.e., length) to the corporal bodies. I have observed with increasing experience that the modified Cantwell-Ransley repair effectively corrects corporal chordee and adds some penile length. It can be hoped that dorsal penile curvature, which is often seen during the growth spurt at puberty, will be resisted. In those patients in whom corporal rotation is used without corporal incision and anastomosis, the neurovascular bundle is left intact and not dissected from its bed. However, if incision and anastomosis is needed, then mobilization of the neurovascular bundle is required. Typically in my experience, incision and rotation is used only for older patients with marked chordee. Although review of findings reveals that almost all penises are straight or deflected downward, many of these patients are still young children. The long-term assessment of penile and urethral reconstruction in exstrophy patients via the modified Cantwell-Ransley repair has shown that in patients with bladder exstrophy and epispadias there is some increase in penile length, and a relatively straight penis with an adequate urethral caliber, which is adequate to void and ejaculate through, can be achieved with minimal morbidity. These findings compare favorably with the series by Mesrobian and coworkers (1986) of 18 patients who underwent primary closure with a straight penis and downward angulation in 85% of patients. In a follow-up study of a group of postpubertal patients, those authors found that 86% of patients with a straight penis could achieve satisfactory intercourse when the penis was angulated downward (Mesrobian et al, 1986).

Bladder Neck Repair

Bladder neck reconstruction results in the exstrophy population have been reported by several groups. Some large experiences have come from the European groups in Lyon and Paris. Mollard and associates (1994) reported on 73 children with bladder exstrophy, 55 of which underwent the Mollard bladder neck repair along with an antireflux procedure. Follow-up ranged from 1 to 17 years. Sixty-nine percent of the patients had normal continence with volitional voiding, and the continence rate was higher in girls than in boys. Lotteman and colleagues (1998) presented a long-term follow-up study of Cendron's exstrophy patients who underwent complete reconstruction. With the Young-Dees repair they were able to achieve urinary continence in 71% of male patients and 53% of females. Overall continence was 65% with a mean follow-up of 12 years after bladder neck repair. Also, Jones and colleagues (1993), using their modification of the Young-Dees repair, reported 64% of patients dry and 18% partially dry in a group that included children with exstrophy, epispadias, and myelomeningocele. Series from North America using mainly the classic Young-Dees-Leadbetter repair reported continence rates ranging from 60% to 82% (Husmann et al, 1989a; Mergurian et al, 1991; Perlmutter et al, 1991; Franco et al, 1994; McMahon et al, 1996; Chan et al, 2001). **The most important long-term factor gleaned from a review of all these series is the fact that bladder capacity at the time of bladder neck reconstruction is a very important determinate of eventual success.**

Records of 90 patients who underwent all stages of bladder exstrophy reconstruction at our institution between 1975 and 1997 were reviewed by Chan and colleagues (2001). Sixty-two patients with bladder neck reconstruction were available for analysis after exclusion of 21 patients awaiting bladder neck reconstruction, 3 female patients who achieved continence without bladder neck repair, 3 patients with recent bladder neck repair, and 1 patient lost to follow-up. The current voiding status of each patient was obtained from parental or patient interview or direct observation by the nursing and physician staff. The patients were categorized as spontaneous voiding not on intermittent catheterization and were assigned a status of (1) completely dry day and night; (2) socially continent, being dry at least 3 hours during the day with occasional nighttime wetting; or (3) wet, being dry for less than 3 hours during the day and wet at night (Table 61–5).

Of the 62 patients who underwent bladder neck repair,

Table 61–5. URINARY CONTINENCE AFTER 62 INITIAL BLADDER NECK RECONSTRUCTIONS

Result*	Average Daytime Dry Interval (hr)	Patients	
		Number	Percentage
Continent (dry day and night)	3	46†	74
Social continence (dry >3 hr daytime, occasional nighttime wetness)	3	10	16
Wet	<3	4	10

*Two patients required diversion after bladder neck reconstruction for upper tract changes.
†Voiding per urethra without intermittent catheterization.

47 were male and 15 were female. The median age for primary closure was 9 days, and the mean was 4 months. The average age at bladder neck reconstruction was 4 years, and these patients had a median bladder capacity of 85 ml at the time of bladder neck repair. Of the 62 patients followed for over 1 year, 46 (74%) were continent and voiding urethrally without the need for augmentation or intermittent catheterization. Ten patients (16%) had social continence with only occasional nighttime accidents, two required diversion for continence after failed bladder neck repair, and four were wet. The renal units of all patients who underwent bladder neck reconstruction were evaluated by intravenous pyelography or ultrasound postoperatively on multiple occasions to assess the preservation of renal function after the continence procedure. One patient had reflux and hydronephrosis after bladder neck reconstruction and bilateral ureteral reimplantation and developed pyelonephritis on the left with mild scarring. A dimercaptosuccinic acid (DMSA) scan of this patient revealed nearly symmetrical renal function. Conservative management of vesicoureteral reflux over time led to the resolution of the reflux in this patient. No other patient developed significant upper tract pathology. There were no other major complications (e.g., ureteral obstruction). Bladder outlet obstruction required cystoscopy and placement of a urethral catheter in 18 patients and prolonged suprapubic drainage for voidings in 12 patients.

The findings in this series were that continence was more likely in those patients who underwent initial bladder closure before 72 hours of age or after 72 hours of age with an osteotomy. These results agree with those of Husmann and associates (1989a), who found that patients who underwent delayed closure without osteotomy showed a significantly lower rate of continence (10%). There was another revealing factor in this study. Although it was previously thought that a bladder capacity of 60 ml was adequate for successful bladder neck reconstruction, in this highly selected group of patients who underwent closure, epispadias repair, and bladder neck repair at our institution the continence rate was higher in those who had a median bladder capacity of 85 ml at the time of bladder neck repair. Therefore, bladder capacity determined under anesthesia before bladder neck reconstruction continues to be an important predictor of eventual urinary continence.

A continence procedure should be deferred until the bladder reaches a capacity of 85 ml and the child is motivated to be dry and to participate in a postoperative voiding program. In our particular series, the age at the time of bladder neck reconstruction was not as important as the capacity before bladder neck repair. The onset of continence is a very interesting phenomenon in this group of exstrophy patients. **The vast majority of patients achieve daytime continence in the first year after bladder neck reconstruction.** A few patients gain a longer daytime interval during the second year after bladder neck repair. However, patients who are not dry after 2 years are considered incontinent. **The onset of nighttime continence varies but often takes longer than the time needed to achieve daytime continence and can take 2 to 3 years.** Caione and coworkers (1999a) showed that use of desmopressin acetate (DDAVP) can increase the number of dry nights in these patients.

Combined Closure Results

In a recent series of 24 boys with classic bladder exstrophy who underwent combined closure and epispadias repair either as a secondary closure or as a delayed primary closure, there was a mean follow-up of 82 months (Gearhart and Mathews, 1998). Urethrocutaneous fistula was noted in three patients who underwent Cantwell-Ransley repair at the time of bladder closure, three who had a Young repair at the time of bladder closure, and one patient who had an island flap repair at the time of bladder closure. The urethrocutaneous fistula resolved spontaneously in four boys and required reoperative closure in three boys. A urethral stricture occurred in one boy who had a full thickness skin graft for initial reconstruction, necessitating a second repair with a skin graft.

At the time of evaluation, three boys were dry for longer than 3 hours after bladder closure and epispadias repair alone. Eleven boys had gone to modified Young-Dees-Leadbetter bladder neck reconstruction. Six of these 11 were totally dry day and night, and 3 were dry with 3-hour voiding intervals during the day and occasional wet nights; 2 patients required bladder augmentation with construction of a continent urinary stoma for continued incontinence. One boy had a bladder neck reconstruction combined with bladder augmentation and continent stoma construction. Twelve boys were awaiting the development of an adequate bladder capacity for bladder neck reconstruction, one was waiting for augmentation and continent stoma construction.

Grady and Mitchell (1999) reported that several patients in their series of 18 children with bladder exstrophy who underwent "complete primary closure" had "continent" intervals (i.e., dry for 2 hours during the day). However, 50% of the patients required reimplantation of the ureters during the first year of life because of uncontrolled upper urinary tract infections, even with the use of excellent suppressive antibiotics.

The combination of epispadias repair and bladder closure, as evidenced by these two studies, can be safely performed (Grady and Mitchell, 1999; Gearhart et al, 1991; Gearhart and Mathews, 2000). However, when complications do occur they can significantly affect the potential of the bladder. This approach, when successful, may have a positive influence on bladder capacity or even continence and may lead to a reduction in the number of procedures required for reconstruction. Data from the combined approach for exstrophy reconstruction are still young, and its use by the novice exstrophy surgeon should be discouraged. As experience is gained, these procedures may eventually take their place in the surgeon's armamentarium for exstrophy reconstruction.

EXSTROPHY RECONSTRUCTION FAILURES

Failed Closure

After primary closure, combined closure, or "complete repair," failures can manifest as complete bladder dehis-

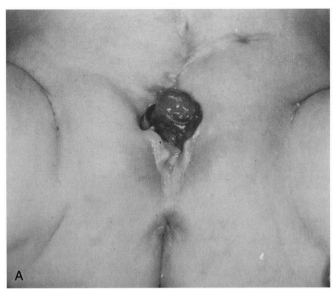
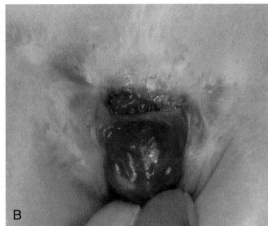

Figure 61–26. *A,* Complete dehiscence of bladder exstrophy repair in patient who underwent closure without osteotomy with greater than 4 cm pubic diastasis at birth. *B,* Prolapse of bladder after newborn closure without the use of osteotomy.

cence, bladder prolapse, or neourethral stricture and obstruction. It is prudent to consider referral of these complex management situations to a center where special expertise and experience in dealing with the exstrophy condition exists. **Dehiscence, which may be precipitated by incomplete mobilization of the pelvic diaphragm and inadequate pelvic immobilization postoperatively, wound infection, abdominal distention, or urinary tube malfunction, necessitates a 6-month recovery period before a second attempt at closure can be made** (Gearhart and Jeffs, 1991a; Gearhart et al, 1993) (Fig. 61–26*A*). Tension-free reclosure with osteotomy and immobilization are important factors in initial and subsequent closures. Unfortunately, the chance of obtaining adequate bladder capacity for bladder neck plasty and eventual continence after multiple closures is markedly diminished (Gearhart et al, 1996a). **Similarly, bladder prolapse is considered a failure and requires bladder reclosure/revision** (Fig. 61–26*B*). **In a patient with significant bladder prolapse or dehiscence, at the time of secondary closure we combine epispadias repair with bladder, posterior urethra, and abdominal wall closure** (McKenna et al, 1994). The patient is given testosterone enanthate intramuscularly 5 weeks and 2 weeks before surgical repair and undergoes an osteotomy with concomitant bladder, urethral, and abdominal wall closure. Although the results after reclosure are not as good as those obtained with a successful primary closure, the are respectable and may obviate the need for bladder augmentation. Neourethral stricture is often associated with paraexstrpohy skin flap use, pubic suture reaction, erosion, or the use of urethral stents. This may be somewhat subtle; however, warning signs consist of urinary tract infections, detectable increased bladder volumes on ultrasound, bladder stones, prolonged dry intervals, and unexplained rectal prolapse. In a review by Baker and colleagues (1999), posterior urethral obstruction was found in 41 patients. Most episodes occurred within 60 days after primary closure. If diversion was used for longer than 6 months, the ultimate fate of the bladder was augmentation.

If diversion was used for less than 6 months, most reconstructions were ultimately bowel free. Ultimately posterior urethral obstruction after exstrophy closure markedly decreased the success of staged repair. This complication presents a significant risk to the upper urinary tract and should be detected early.

Although all closed exstrophy bladders have vesicoureteral reflux, upper tract deterioration is the ultimate fate of significant outlet obstruction. At this point the management includes urethral dilation (incision), open urethroplasty, or upper tract diversion. If renal function is compromised, the choice must achieve unquestionable free drainage to allow the upper tracts and kidneys to fully recover. Further bladder neck or urethral reconstruction should not be performed until the posterior urethral stricture is clearly repaired and free drainage has been achieved.

Despite satisfactory closure, some bladders never achieve adequate capacity to act as functional bladders. It has become clear that multiple bladder closures, bladder prolapse, dehiscence, bladder calculi, recurrent infections, and vesicostomy have a negative impact on the potential of the exstrophy bladder (Silver et al, 1997b). We have used transurethral injection of collagen around the bladder neck to increase outlet resistance and stimulate the bladder to grow. However, in our hands this has not been as successful as was reported by Caione and colleagues (1993a, Caione 1993b) from Italy. If the bladder does not grow to a sufficient size for bladder neck reconstruction, bladder augmentation is recommended in this situation. If the bladder neck and/or urethra is problematic, a catheterizable continent stoma with or without bladder neck plasty or transection is performed, along with augmentation (Gearhart et al, 1995b).

Failed Bladder Neck Repair

If urinary continence, defined as a 3-hour dry interval, is not achieved within 2 years after bladder neck

reconstruction, failure to achieve dryness has resulted. Occasionally, the dry interval is nearly acceptable for daytime dryness (i.e., longer than 2 hours). In these situations, routine collagen injections into the bladder neck can move the dry interval up to 3 hours, but more than one injection may be required (Ben-Chaim et al, 1995a). **Some successes have been seen with repeat Young-Dees-Leadbetter repair if the bladder neck is patulous, the bladder capacity is adequate, and urodynamic evaluation reveals a stable bladder** (Gearhart et al, 1991). **A majority of bladder neck failures require eventual augmentation or continent diversion.** The artificial urinary sphincter has been used with some success in patients who have a good bladder capacity. However, in most of these failures the bladder capacity is small and augmentation will be required. At the time of reoperative surgery, either the bladder neck is transected proximal to the prostate with a Mitrofanoff substitution or a continence procedure is performed, such as an artificial sphincter or collagen injection, or both. In our extensive experience with failed bladder neck reconstructions, most of the patients have had several surgeries and need to be dry. In such cases, the most suitable alternative is bladder neck transection, augmentation, and a continent urinary stoma (Gearhart et al, 1995b; Hensle et al, 1995).

Delayed urinary continence has been reported at the onset of puberty in some males and has been attributed to prostatic growth. By MRI the prostate of exstrophy patients is clover-shaped and absent anteriorly, while its mean weight and maximal cross section and volume are normal (Hanna and Williams, 1969). Therefore, it is doubtful that growth of this abnormally configured prostate can have much impact on later urinary continence after failed bladder neck repair.

Failed Genitourethral Reconstruction

Common complications of modern epispadias repair include urethrocutaneous fistula formation. This has been reported in as few as 4% and as many as 19% of cases (Kajbafzadeh et al, 1995; Surer et al, 2000). Urethral tortuosity with difficult catheterization or strictures are uncommon with modern epispadias repair.

At an older age, unsightly penile scars and a short phallus may prompt further surgical intervention. Scar excision can be closed in a plastic fashion if enough penile skin is available. Otherwise, flaps or full-thickness skin grafts can be used. In severe cases tissue expanders can be placed under the penile skin and gradually inflated over 6 weeks to allow for more penile skin and obviate the need for grafting. Freeing all scar tissues and suspensory ligament tissue can maximize available penile length. A dorsal dermal corporal graft or ventral corporal plication or rotation may additionally help lengthen as well as correct any chordee. However, it must be recognized that the exstrophy penis, when compared with age- and race-matched controls, is congenitally deficient in anterior corporal tissue as assessed by MRI (Silver et al, 1997b). Therefore, overly aggressive attempts at penile lengthening may only result in corporal denervation and devascularization without additional lengthening.

Alternative Techniques of Reconstruction

Not all children with bladder exstrophy are candidates for staged functional closure or combined epispadias repair and bladder closure, because of a small bladder plate or significant hydronephrosis. Additional reasons for seeking other methods of treatment include failure of initial closure with a small remaining bladder and/or failure of continence surgery. Excluding those patients who fail initial treatment, this discussion deals with options available when modern staged functional closure or combined repair is not chosen by the surgeon or for other reasons has not been suitable.

Ureterosigmoidostomy

Whichever urinary diversion is chosen, the upper tracts and renal function initially are normal. This allows the reimplantation of normal-sized ureters in a reliable, nonrefluxing manner into the colon or other suitable reservoir. Historically, ureterosigmoidostomy was the first form of diversion to be popularized for patients with exstrophy. Although the initial series was associated with multiple metabolic problems, results improved markedly with newer techniques of reimplantation (Zarbo and Kay, 1986; Koo et al, 1996). Ureterosigmoidostomy is favored by some because of the lack of an abdominal stoma. **However, this form of diversion should not be offered until one is certain that anal continence is normal and after the family has been made aware of the potential serious complications, including pyelonephritis, hyperkalemic acidosis, rectal incontinence, ureteral obstruction, and delayed development of malignancy** (Spence et al, 1979; Duckett and Gazak, 1983). More recently, ureterosigmoidostomy has been proposed again as an initial treatment of bladder exstrophy with acceptable continence and renal preservation on follow-up of 10 years or longer. Stein and associates (1999a) treated a group of 128 patients with bladder exstrophy-epispadias with the Mainz technique for ureterosigmoidostomy. Continence was achieved in 95% of patients with a rectal reservoir. Their recommendation for treatment in a number of patients with severely impaired renal function was that a colonic conduit was the best method of choice for diversion. In those patients with a normal or slightly dilated upper tract and intact anal sphincters, a Mainz rectal reservoir was recommended. Although the group from Mainz reported no cancer in a long-term follow-up study of patients who underwent ureterosigmoidostomy, the risk for malignancy still exists and must be carefully considered in a young child. This is especially true in today's very mobile society, in which careful long-term follow-up may be difficult to guarantee.

Other Forms of Diversion

Alternative techniques of urinary diversion in bladder exstrophy have been described. Maydl described a method of trigonosigmoidostomy (Maydl, 1894). Boyce and Vest (1952) reported their results on long-term follow-up with these patients. Overall, renal function was normal in 91% and all children achieved daytime continence. A long-term report of Boyce's series by Kroovand and Boyce (1988) showed that most of the patients had stable upper tracts, minimal leakage, and no electrolyte imbalances or malignant changes in the vesical rectal reservoir.

Lastly, the procedure of Heinz-Boyer and Houvelaque (1912) included diverting the ureters into an isolated rectal segment and pulling the sigmoid colon through the anal sphincter just posterior to the rectum. Taccinoli and colleagues reviewed 21 patients with bladder exstrophy who had undergone this procedure with follow-up of 16 years. They reported 95% fecal and urinary continence, with no urinary calculi, electrolyte abnormalities, or postoperative mortality. Ureterorectal strictures developed in three patients and required surgical revision.

Continent Diversion in the Exstrophy Patient

In modern pediatric urology there is usually very little need for urinary diversion in the patient with bladder exstrophy. In a young child with a bladder that is too small to close, or in a failed closure where the bladder template is too small to reclose, I recommend a nonrefluxing colon conduit. This protects the kidneys from vesicoureteral reflux, and undiversion can be performed when clinically indicated at an older age.

An innovative approach by Rink and Retik (1987) was the creation of a nonrefluxing ileocecal segment that could be rejoined to the sigmoid colon. In this procedure, the terminal limb is intussuscepted to the ileocecal valve and stabilized against the cecal wall to prevent desusception. A nipple then serves as an antirefluxing mechanism. The cecum is anastomosed to the lower sigmoid colon and the ureters to the ileal tail "proximal to the intussusception." Results from the patient's point of view were the same as after intact ureterosigmoidostomy, with urine passed with the feces, and again urinary control depends on an intact anal sphincter. However, because the transitional epithelium of the ureter is in a sterile environment above the antireflux nipple, an increased risk of later malignancy is theoretically decreased. Gearhart and coworkers (1995b) reported on a series of continent diversion cases; the continence rate was greater than 90%, and the complication rate was acceptable in a large series of patients with failed exstrophy repairs. Multiple reports of the use of urinary diversion in patients with failed exstrophy repair or nonreconstructable conditions have been published (Bassiouny, 1992; Ulman et al, 1998).

SEXUAL FUNCTION AND FERTILITY IN THE EXSTROPHY PATIENT

The Male Patient

Reconstruction of the male genitalia and preservation of fertility were not primary objectives in early surgical management of bladder exstrophy. **Sporadic instances of pregnancy or the initiation of pregnancy by males with bladder exstrophy have been reported.** In two large exstrophy series, male fertility was documented. Only 3 of 68 men in one study (Bennett, 1973) and 4 of 72 in another (Woodhouse et al, 1983) had successfully fathered chil-

dren. In a large series of 25 patients exstrophy and epispadias (Shapiro et al, 1984), there were 38 males who had fathered children.

Hanna and Williams (1972) compared semen analyses in men who had undergone primary closure and ureterosigmoidostomy. A normal sperm count was found in only one of eight men after functional closure and in four of eight men with diversion. The difference in observed fertility potential is probably attributable to iatrogenic injury to the verumontanum during functional closure or bladder neck reconstruction. Retrograde ejaculation may also account for low sperm counts after functional bladder closure. **In a long-term study from our institution, Ben-Chaim and associates (1996) found that 10 of 16 men reported they ejaculated a few cubic centimeters of volume, 3 ejaculated only a few drops, and 3 had no ejaculation. Semen analysis was obtained in 4 patients: 3 had azoospermia and 1 had oligospermia. The average ejaculated volume of these patients who had sperm counts was 0.4 ml.** In another large series by Stein and colleagues (1994) from Germany, the authors found that none of the patients who had reconstruction of the external genitalia could ejaculate normally, nor had they fathered children. Five patients who did not undergo reconstruction had normal ejaculation, and two had fathered children. The conclusion was that male patients with genital reconstruction and closure of the urethra demonstrated high risk of infertility.

Assisted reproductive techniques have been applied to the exstrophy population. **Bastuba and coworkers (1993) reported pregnancies achieved with the use of assisted reproductive techniques. Regardless of the method of reconstruction of the external genitalia and bladder neck, newer techniques such as gamete intrafallopian transfer (GIFT) or intracytoplasmic sperm injection (ICSI) can be used to assist these patients in their goal of pregnancy achievement.**

Sexual function and libido in exstrophy patients are normal (Woodhouse, 1998). The erectile mechanism in patients who have undergone epispadias repair appears to be intact, because 87% of boys and young men in the Hopkins series experienced erections after repair of epispadias (Surer et al, 2000). Poor or absent ejaculation may occur after genital reconstruction. Complete absence of ejaculation is rare, but the emission that does occur may be slow and may occur for several hours. Milking the urethra in an antegrade fashion from proximal to distal has provided pregnancy in some cases (Woodhouse, 1999). **In papers from both Woodhouse (1998) and Ben-Chaim and colleagues (1996), most patients reported satisfactory orgasm; half of the men and all of the women described intimate relationships as serious and long-term.** In the series by Ben-Chaim, the only patients who had no ejaculation were two patients who had undergone cystectomy. Overall, it seems from the experience in England, Germany, and the United States that most men with exstrophy achieve erection and have a reasonable sex life.

The Female Patient

Further reconstruction of the female genitalia, if needed, can occur during adolescent years. In our experience, the external genitalia are fully reconstructed at the time of initial exstrophy closure, because with the use of osteotomy a nice mons pubis can be created and the bifid clitoris and labia can easily be brought together in the midline. **Occasionally, vulvoplasty is performed in patients before they become sexually active. However, in Woodhouse's experience (1999), most patients required vaginoplasty before intercourse could take place.** Woodhouse reported successful intercourse in all of his patients, but three found it painful. Stein and associates (1995) from Germany reviewed a large series of patients with exstrophy and found that a cut-back vaginoplasty was required before intercourse in 23 patients. We have seen several patients who have not had vulvoplasty, have two clitoral halves, have a normal sex life and normal orgasm, and desire no surgical repair of this condition.

Mons plasty is very important, either in infancy or adolescence, because hair-bearing skin and fat needs to cover the midline defect. As mentioned earlier, we perform this procedure at the time of initial closure. It certainly can be done in adolescence with the use of rhomboid flaps, as popularized by Kramer and colleagues (1986).

Obstetric Implications

Review of the literature reveals 45 women with bladder exstrophy who successfully delivered 49 normal offspring. The main complication after pregnancy was cervical and uterine prolapse, which occurred frequently (Krisiloff et al, 1978). Burbage and coworkers (1986) described 40 women ranging from 19 to 36 years of age who were treated in infancy for bladder exstrophy; 14 pregnancies in 11 of these women resulted in 9 normal deliveries, 3 spontaneous abortions, and 2 elective abortions. Uterine prolapse occurred in 7 of the 11 patients during pregnancy. All had undergone prior permanent urinary diversions. Spontaneous vaginal deliveries were performed in those women, and cesarean sections were performed in women with functional bladder closures to eliminate stress on the pelvic floor and to avoid traumatic injury to the urinary sphincter mechanism (Krisiloff et al, 1978). With modern reconstructive techniques, successful pregnancies have been reported in female patients who have undergone continent urinary diversion (Kennedy et al, 1993).

Woodhouse and associates (1999) reported prolapse in a number of patients, and it was said to be a considerable problem to correct. Seven patients had total prolapse, one of whom had never had intercourse or a pregnancy. Woodhouse believes that prolapse may occur in up to half of patients after pregnancy. Stein and colleagues (1995), in a large exstrophy series from Germany, found that uterine fixation was required to correct prolapse in 13 patients with long-term follow-up of more than 25 years. The reason for uterine prolapse is that the cervix is close to the introitus and the weak pelvic floor and poor uterine support make prolapse common. I believe that widespread application of pelvic osteotomy and better closure of the pelvic floor will markedly decrease the incidence of uterine prolapse in years to come.

Regardless of the method of repair, the uterus must be anchored in such a way that it is fixated in the pelvis and less prone to prolapse. Some authors have advocated fixation of the uterus to the anterior abdominal wall in child-hood; this, they say, prevents prolapse but still allows normal pregnancy. Woodhouse (1999) believed that, although prophylactic surgery may be helpful, once prolapse occurs, anterior fixation is insufficient to correct uterine prolapse in the exstrophy patient.

LONG-TERM ADJUSTMENT ISSUES

Interest has increased in long-term adjustment issues in patients with bladder exstrophy. Children with exstrophy undergo multiple reconstructive surgeries and have potential problems with respect to urinary incontinence and sexual dysfunction. However, the ultimate outcome would be better measured by how these children adjust overall in society. The severe nature of the exstrophy disorder could predict that this birth defect could have substantial psychological implications. Parental reaction to the child's medical condition may change the way the parents interact with the child. Incontinence may have a negative impact on social function and self-esteem. Multiple hospitalizations may interfere with the ability to be like other children. Concerning the potential medical and psychological implications of this anomaly, children born with exstrophy may be at increased risk for difficulties.

However, there has been a limited amount of information in the literature concerning this condition and its treatment, and whether or not it has a deleterious effect on children and their families. Montagnino and coworkers (1998) evaluated younger children who performed more poorly and had disturbed behavior, specifically in skills related to function in school. Children who achieved continence after the age of 5 years were more likely to have problems with acting-out behavior. There were no differences in adjustment based on male or female sex, bladder versus cloacal exstrophy, type of continence strategy, or gender reassignment versus no reassignment. **The conclusions of this long-term study were that children with exstrophy do not have clinical psychopathology** (Montagnino et al, 1998). There was acting-out behavior rather than depression or anxiety, suggesting that improved outcomes may be achieved through a focus on normal adaptation rather than potential psychological stress.

Reiner (1999) studied 42 children with exstrophy and presented preliminary results suggesting that these patients tend to have more severe behavioral and developmental problems than children with other anomalies, significant body distortion, and self-esteem problems. Although these problems were not severe, Reiner recommended intervention with the exstrophy patient and family to continue with long-term psychiatric support into adult life. In a study from Europe, Feitz and associates (1994) found a more positive picture when they evaluated 11 women and 11 men with exstrophy, of whom 91 (82%) did not endorse any clinical levels of psychological stress. The authors concluded that these adults had a positive attitude toward life.

Being born with exstrophy does not result in childhood psychopathology. **Children with exstrophy exhibit some tendency toward increased problems with acting out or lack of attainment of age-appropriate adaptive behavior** (Montagnino et al, 1998; Reiner, 1999). Therefore, all experts in childhood psychology tend to agree that counseling should come from the nursing and medical staff early on in the exstrophy condition. Likewise, the patient and parents should be served by an experienced exstrophy support team, and psychological support and counseling should be extended into adult life.

CLOACAL EXSTROPHY

Cloacal exstrophy represents one of the most severe congenital anomalies compatible with intrauterine viability. It is exceedingly rare, occurring 1 in 200,000 to 400,000 live births (Hurwitz et al, 1987). Most recent reports indicate a male-female sex ratio of 2:1 (Gearhart and Jeffs, 1998). Inheritance of cloacal exstrophy is unknown, because offspring have never been produced by patients with this disorder.

Prenatal Diagnosis

Since its initial description in the early 1980s, further refinements in the prenatal diagnosis of cloacal exstrophy have occurred (Meizner and Bar-Ziv, 1985). Chitrit and colleagues (1993) reported the diagnosis of monozygotic twins with cloacal exstrophy detected during antenatal ultrasound screening. Since their report, there have only been occasional case reports of prenatal diagnosis of cloacal exstrophy, and only 15% of patients with this anomaly have been diagnosed by prenatal ultrasonography, according to the literature. With the marked improvements in survival in the last 20 years and the common application of fetal ultrasound, early diagnosis may expedite the care of patients with cloacal exstrophy.

In 1998, Austin and colleagues reviewed 20 patients with this abnormality and proposed major and minor criteria for the prenatal diagnosis of cloacal exstrophy, based on the frequency of occurrence rather than the severity. A criterion was considered major if it was present in more than 50% of cases. The gestational age for diagnosis of cloacal exstrophy ranged between 15 and 32 weeks (mean, 22 weeks). Major diagnostic criteria included nonvisualization of the bladder in 91%, a large midline infraumbilical anterior wall defect or a cystic anterior wall structure in 82%, an omphalocele in 77%, and a myelomeningocele in 68%. Minor criteria included lower-extremity defects in 23%, renal anomalies in 23%, ascites in 41%, widened pubic arches in 18%, narrow thorax in 9%, hydrocephalus in 9%, and a single umbilical artery in 9%. Hamada and coauthors (1999) reported a single case in which ultrasound revealed a wavy cord-like segment of soft tissue protruding from the anterior abdominal wall of the fetus below the umbilicus. This was found to be prolapsed terminal ileum, which resembled the trunk of an elephant. The authors suggested that this sonographic image be added to the criteria described by Austin and associates (1998) for making a prenatal diagnosis of cloacal exstrophy.

Embryology and Anatomy

Typically, after 4 weeks of life, the urorectal septum divides the cloaca into an anterior urogenital sinus and a posteroanorectal canal. Simultaneously, the cloacal membrane is invaded by lateral mesodermal folds at approximately 4 weeks of gestation. It is postulated that if a mesodermal invasion does not occur, the infraumbilical cloacal membrane persists, with subsequently poor abdominal wall development. Because of its inherent instability, the cloacal membrane eventually ruptures. If it does so before the urorectal septum descends at 6 to 8 weeks of gestation, then cloacal exstrophy results. However, in the developing embryo, a stage similar in appearance to cloacal exstrophy does not exist. Therefore, the anomaly must not represent an arrest in development, but more likely some form of embryogenetic defect. **According to Muecke (1964), an abnormally extensive cloacal membrane produces a wedge effect, serving as a mechanical barrier to mesodermal migration, which results in impaired development of the abdominal wall, failure of fusion of the paired genital tubercles, and diastasis pubis. Exstrophy of the cloaca results when the wedge effect occurs before the formation of a urorectal septum at 6 weeks.**

Animal models similar to cloacal exstrophy have been created in chick embryos by placing a plastic wedge in the area of the cloacal membrane, thus preventing migration of the mesoderm into the membrane, or by using a carbon dioxide laser to open the cloacal membrane before fusion of the urorectal septum with the cloacal membrane (Thomalla et al, 1985). All the experimental evidence in the present theory of embryogenesis relies on occurrence of the inciting event in the first 6 to 8 weeks of embryonic development. However, ultrasound evidence of later cloacal membrane rupture, between 18 and 24 weeks of gestation, coupled with previous reports of cloacal membrane rupture occurring between 22 and 26 weeks, cast doubt on these theories. **Langer (1992) and Bruch (1996) and their colleagues reported the prenatal diagnosis of cloacal exstrophy with an intact cloacal membrane after 18 to 24 weeks of gestation.** Vermeij-Keers and coworkers (1996) postulated that the embryologic maldevelopment of cloacal exstrophy is caused by poorly orchestrated cellular proliferation and apoptosis, with resultant poor mesodermal formation from the umbilical ectodermal placode. Rather than debate about the exact timing of the disintegration of the cloacal membrane (8 versus 22 weeks), they described the urorectal septum, abdominal wall, and cloacal membrane as related with a similar origin (i.e., ectodermal placodes) and timing of the rupture as representing the balance between cellular proliferation and apoptotic cell death.

Anatomically there is exstrophy of the foreshortened hindgut or cecum, which displays its bulging mucosa between the exstrophied hemibladders (Fig. 61–27). The orifice of the terminal ileum, rudimentary tailgut, and a single appendix are apparent on the surface of the everted cecum. The tailgut is blind-ending and is of various lengths. The ileum may be prolapsed, the pubic symphysis widely separated, the hips externally rotated and abducted, and the phallus separated into right and left halves with an adjacent labial or scrotal half (Fig. 61–28). Sponseller and associates (1995) described the anatomy of the bony pelvis in the patient with cloacal exstrophy with the use of 3-D CT scans. Marked external rotation deformities were reported, of both the anterior and posterior pelvis. Unlike bladder exstrophy, where there is a 30% shortage of bone in the pubis, in patients with cloacal exstrophy there were marked

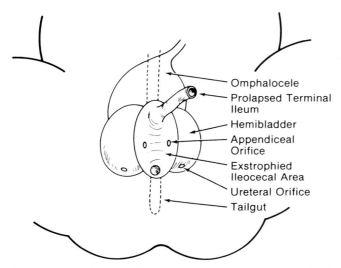

Figure 61–27. Schematic drawing showing gastrointestinal and urinary defects in children of either sex born with cloacal exstrophy. (Courtesy of Dr. Richard Hurwitz.)

asymmetries in the pubis, sacroiliac joint malformations, and occasional hip malformations.

Schlegel and Gearhart (1989) defined the neuroanatomy of the pelvis in the child with cloacal exstrophy (Fig. 61–29). **The innervation of the hemibladders and corporal bodies arises from a pelvic plexus on the anterior surface of the rectum. The nerves to the hemibladders travel the midline along the posteroinferior surface of the rectum and extend laterally to the hemibladders. Innervation to the duplicated corporal bodies arises from the sacral plexus, travels in the midline, perforates the interior portion of the pelvic floor, and courses medially to the hemibladders.**

Manzoni and associates (Hurwitz et al, 1987) have suggested a gridlike schema to describe cloacal exstrophy and to better delineate its variants. The grid in Fig. 61–30 shows type I classic cloacal exstrophy. In this type, the hemibladders may be confluent cranial to the bowel patch, lateral to the bowel (most common), and confluent caudal to the bowel. Type IIA grids show variations of the bladder (covered bladder or hemibladder); type IIB grids show variations of distal exstrophied bowel segments (duplications); and type IIC grids depict the situation in which both bowel and bladder variations occur. The grid also describes the penis (divided or united) and the status of the clitoris and vagina (duplications). We have modified the grid concept to describe the status of the hindgut remnant (Gearhart and Jeffs, 1992).

In a large review by Diamond (1990), associated anomalies were seen in multiple organ systems. In this large series, the incidence of spina bifida varied from 29% to 75%, including patients with both meningoceles and lipomeningoceles. When spina bifida patients were stratified according to neural involvement, myelomeningocele was noted in 17% to 52% of cases. In this report, 72% of myelomeningocele defects were found to be lumbar, 14% sacral, and 14% thoracic.

Upper urinary tract anomalies occurred in 41% to 60% of patients in Diamond's review. The most common anomalies were pelvic kidney and renal agenesis, both occurring in up to one third of patients. Hydronephrosis and

hydroureter were common, occurring in one third of patients. Multicystic dysplastic kidneys and fusion anomalies were seen less frequently. Ectopic ureters draining to the vasa in the male and into the uterus, vagina, or fallopian tubes in the female were also reported (Diamond, 1990).

Müllerian anomalies were reported in several patients. Duplication of the uterus and vagina were reported in a number of patients. **The most commonly reported müllerian anomaly was uterine duplication, seen in 95% of patients** (Diamond, 1990). The vast majority of these patients had partial uterine duplication, predominantly a bicornate uterus. Vaginal duplication occurred in 65% of cases, and vaginal agenesis was seen in 25% to 50% of patients. In a report by Hurwitz and colleagues (1987), cases of complete duplication of the uterus and fallopian tubes associated with both vaginal duplication and vaginal agenesis were noted. Gearhart and Jeffs (1991b) recommended preservation of all mullerian duplication anomalies that could be used in reconstructing the lower urinary tract.

Skeletal and limb anomalies were reported by Diamond (1990) in 12% to 65% of cases. The vast majority were club foot deformities, although absent of feet, severe tibial or fibular deformities, and congenital hip dislocations were commonly noted in this group of patients.

Gastrointestinal tract anomalies occur in virtually all patients with cloacal exstrophy. **In Diamond's series (1990), the incidence of omphalocele was 88%, and a majority of all series reported an incidence of 95% or greater.** Omphaloceles do vary in size and usually contain small bowel or liver, or both. Immediate closure of the omphalocele defect in the newborn period is advised to prevent subsequent rupture. **In addition, Hurwitz and colleagues (1987), in a large review of cloacal exstrophy patients, reported a 46% incidence of associated gastrointestinal**

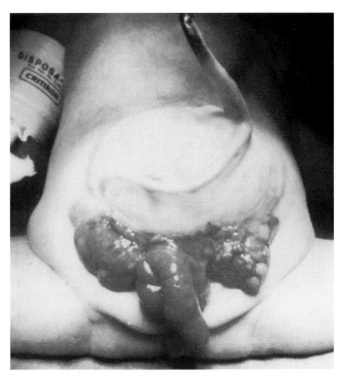

Figure 61–28. Cloacal exstrophy. Newborn female showing omphalocele, prolapsed ileocecal valve, and symmetric bladder halves.

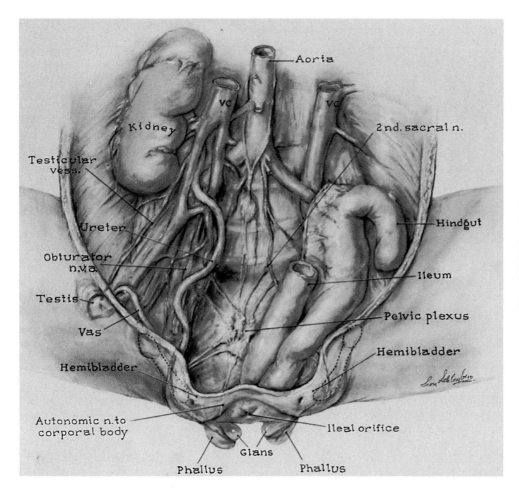

Figure 61–29. Internal view of patient with cloacal exstrophy. Pudendal vessels, nerves, as well as other vessels and autonomic innervation of the corporal bodies, are demonstrated. Internal structures of the pelvis along with duplication of the vena cava in the dissected specimen is also shown. (Drawing by Leon Schlossberg.)

tract anomalies, with malrotation, duplication anomalies, and anatomically short bowel occurring with equal frequency. Hurwitz noted a 23% incidence of short gut syndrome, which is compatible with 25% incidence reported by Diamond (Hurwitz et al, 1987; Diamond, 1990). It now seems well accepted that short gut syndrome may occur in the presence of normal small bowel length, suggesting absorptive dysfunction and emphasizing the absolute need to preserve as much large bowel as possible.

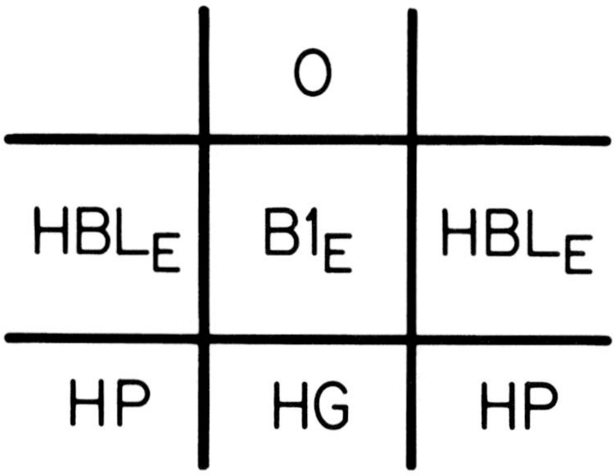

Life-threatening cardiovascular and pulmonary anomalies are rarely seen in cloacal exstrophy. Reported cases included two patients with cyanotic heart disease and one with aortic duplication. A bilobed lung was reported in two patients, and an atretic right upper lung in one. Also, Schlegel and Gearhart (1989) reported caval duplication in their anatomic dissection of a patient with cloacal exstrophy.

Initial Management

Immediate management is directed to the medical stabilization of the infant. Evaluation and appropriate management of associated malformations should be undertaken. For infants who have few other associated malformations and are medically stable, staged closure can be considered (Table 61–6). The bowel should be moistened with saline and covered with protective plastic dressing. Evaluation of the genitalia and gender assignment should be made by a gender assignment team, including a pediatric urologist, pediatric surgeon, pediatrician, and pediatric endocrinologist. Consultations from social work, pediatric orthopedic surgery, and other disciplines should be obtained. In a large medical center with experience in dealing with these patients, these multiple consultations should be done in a

Figure 61–30. Coding grid used to describe classic cloacal exstrophy and its variants. O, omphalocele; HBL$_E$, hemi-bladder; B1$_E$, everted bowel; HP, hemi-phallus; HG, hindgut. (Modified from Hurwitz RS, Manzoni GA, Ransley PG, Stephen FD: Cloacal exstrophy: A report of 34 cases. J Urol 1987;138:1060.)

Table 61–6. MODERN STAGED FUNCTIONAL RECONSTRUCTION OF CLOACAL EXSTROPHY

Immediate neonatal assessment
  Evaluate associated anomalies
  Decide whether to proceed with reparative surgery
Functional bladder closure (soon after neonatal assessment)
  One-stage repair (few associated anomalies)
    Excision of omphalocele
    Separation of cecal plate from bladder halves
    Joining and closure of bladder halves and urethroplasty
    Bilateral anterior innominate and vertical iliac osteotomy
    Gonadectomy in males with unreconstructible phallus
    Terminal ileostomy/colostomy
    Genital revision if needed
  Two-stage repair
    First stage (newborn period)
      Excision of omphalocele
      Separation of cecal plate from bladder halves
      Joining of bladder halves
      Gonadectomy in male with unreconstructible phallus
      Terminal ileostomy/colostomy
    Second stage
      Closure of joined bladder halves and urethroplasty
      Bilateral anterior innominate and vertical iliac osteotomy
      Genital revision if needed
Anti-incontinence/reflux procedure (age 4–5 yr)
  Bladder capacity ≥85 ml (small select group of patients):
    Young-Dees-Leadbetter bladder neck reconstruction
    Bilateral Cohen ureteral reimplantations
    Bowel and/or stomach segment used to augment bladder
           or
  Continent diversion with abdominal/perineal stoma
Vaginal reconstruction
  Vagina constructed or augmented using colon, ileum, or full-thickness skin graft

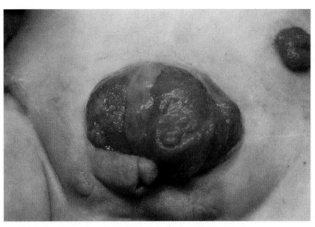

Figure 61–31. 46,XY cloacal male exstrophy with a dominant right hemi-phallus prior to bladder closure and epispadias repair with the male sex of rearing.

short period of time. If there is a medical concern, delayed closure after initial intestinal diversion is appropriate (Mathews et al, 1998).

Gender Assignment

Gender assignment is limited to the genetic male patient with cloacal exstrophy. Male gender assignment is appropriate for males with adequate bilateral or unilateral phallic structures (Fig. 61–31). A difficult situation arises when a male neonate with minimal phallic structures presents for closure. Although modern techniques of genital reconstruction allow better closure and better genital reconstruction, some of these patients may be more appropriately raised as females with excision of gonads (Husmann et al, 1989b). This decision cannot be made unilaterally, and it should be made in conjunction with parental counseling and input from multiple disciplines, including pediatric endocrinology and a trained pediatric psychiatrist or psychologist who is familiar with treating patients with genital anomalies. This consultant should be an integral part of the exstrophy management team to help the parents, and later the developing child, deal with questions of sexuality and body image. Initial data from one pilot study seemed to indicate a high frequency of psychosexual dysfunction, but this may be improved to some degree after appropriate hormonal manipulation (Reiner et al, 2002). Improvements in phallic reconstruction may eventually allow most genetic males to be assigned a male gender. If long-term psychological out-

comes prove to be poor in those 46,XY patients who are raised as females, then complete phallic reconstruction will need to be performed at an appropriate age.

Surgical Reconstruction

Surgical reconstruction may be considered in the infant who is medically stable. This would include closure of the omphalocele, closure of the bladder and urethra, bony pelvis closure, and repair of the external genitalia. Cloacal exstrophy patients should undergo carefully planned and individualized reconstructions (Ricketts et al, 1991; Lund and Hendren, 1993; Mathews et al, 1998). For infants with spinal dysraphism and myelocystocele, neurosurgical consultation should be obtained and closure undertaken as soon as the infant is medically stable. After closure of the myelocystocele, long-term follow-up is mandatory to evaluate for subtle changes in the neurologic evaluation that could herald cord tethering.

Once the infant has recovered from closure of the myelocystocele repair, reconstruction should focus on management of the gastrointestinal tract. Omphalocele closure is combined with gastrointestinal diversion or reconstruction. Formerly, initial attempts focused on ileostomy with resection of the hindgut remnant. **Since the recognition of the metabolic changes that occur in patients with ileostomy, an attempt is always made to use the hindgut remnant to provide additional length of bowel for fluid absorption** (Mathews et al, 1998). Enlargement of the hindgut remnant and increased water absorption have been noted in children who have had the segment incorporated into construction of a fecal colostomy. The hindgut segment may be anastomosed in an isoperistaltic or retroperistaltic fashion to increase motility and generate formed stool. Children who have anal stenosis and nonimperforate anus may have the capability for later continence and may be treated with a pull-through procedure. If the hindgut remnant is not used for bowel reconstruction, it should be left as a mucus fistula to be used for later bladder augmentation and/or vaginal reconstruction (Lund and Hendren, 1993; Mathews et al, 1998). If gastrointestinal reconstruction is combined with bladder closure, approximation of the pubis, usually with osteotomies, is beneficial in reconstruction of the pelvic ring and increases the potential for successful bladder and abdominal wall closure (Mathews et al, 1998).

Role of Osteotomy

Infants who are medically stable may be considered for urinary tract reconstruction in the immediate postnatal period. **Osteotomy is indicated in all children with cloacal exstrophy at the time of bladder closure, because of the wide diastasis that is invariably present** (Mathews et al, 1998). Osteotomy allows the pelvic ring, bladder, and abdominal wall to be closed without undue tension on the closure. Reduction in dehiscence and postoperative ventral hernias has been noted in patients treated with osteotomy. **In a large series reported by Ben-Chaim and associates (1995c), significant complications occurred in 89% of patients who underwent closure of the cloacal exstrophy without osteotomy but in only 17% of patients who underwent osteotomy at the time of initial cloacal exstrophy closure.** Interestingly, the patients who underwent osteotomy and those who did not were similar in terms of size of the omphalocele, presence of myelomeningocele, and time of primary closure. However, it is not surprising that osteotomy had no affect on eventual continence of patients with cloacal exstrophy.

Currently, combined anterior innominate and vertical iliac osteotomies are routinely used at our institution (Silver et al, 1999). This approach does not require the patient to be repositioned on the operating table before commencing bladder and abdominal wall closure. In addition, this method obviates the use of a posterior approach and any complication of the procedure related to the spinal or back closure. **In a series of five patients with extreme pubic diastasis greater than 10 cm, Silver and colleagues (1999) described initial pelvic osteotomy and gradual pelvic closure of the fixator for 1 to 2 weeks, followed by abdominal wall closure and bladder closure.** Closure was successful in all patients without technical problems or complications. This technique of staged pelvic closure may provide reliable initial secondary repair in patients with cloacal exstrophy in whom one-stage pelvic closure is infeasible, even with pelvic osteotomy.

Pelvic and Phallic Reconstruction

The urinary tract reconstruction may be performed at the time of omphalocele closure. The medial edges of the bladder halves are initially closed to generate a bladder exstrophy that can be closed and placed into the pelvis if complete repair is feasible in the newborn period. Inguinal hernias may be repaired if identified. In genetic females and in genotypic male subjects undergoing gender reassignment, reconstruction should be performed to improve the appearance of the genitalia.

Reconstruction of the external genitalia in the immediate postnatal period is performed to make the infant appear more congruent with the gender assigned. The psychiatric studies of children who have had gender assignment has fueled interest in male gender assignment if adequate unilateral or bilateral corporal tissue is present (Reiner et al, 2002). Histologic studies indicate normal histology in the testes of male subjects who have had gender reassignment despite the presence of cryptorchidism (Mathews et al, 1999a). Results of phallic reconstruction in male patients with minimal or no penile tissue in the past have been disappointing. For male-to-female reassignment, initial female genital reconstruction should bring the phallic halves together in the midline as a clitoris.

However, in instances with adequate corporal tissue, either unilaterally or bilaterally, epispadias repair can be performed at the time of initial closure or later, depending on the situation. Vaginal reconstruction can be performed early in the genetic female patient. In gender-converted male patients who require reconstruction of a neovagina, delayed reconstruction is appropriate. Reconstruction may be performed by using a preserved hindgut segment or expanded perineal skin. Long-term dilatation of the neovagina may be required.

Improvements in preoperative and postoperative care of the pediatric patient and modern surgical techniques have led to a reduction in mortality and improved functional and cosmetic results. A good pelvic osteotomy at the time of closure helps to get the genitalia together in the midline and improve the "mons" appearance of the lower part of the closure.

Techniques to Create Urinary Continence

Urinary continence is possible in most children but usually requires bladder augmentation and the use of intermittent catheterization. Multiple series by Gearhart and Jeffs (1991b), Mitchell and associates (1990), and Hendren (1992) have shown the applicability of modern techniques for lower tract reconstruction to help these patients achieve urinary continence. Enhancement of bladder capacity may be performed using a hindgut segment, if available; ileum; or stomach. Continence appears to be more difficult to achieve in male patients who undergo gender reassignment, and a continent stoma may be most applicable in this special group of patients (Mathews, 1998). In genetic female patients, successful continence has been achieved after Young-Dees-Leadbetter bladder neck reconstruction, but the vast majority of patients have required intermittent catheterization (Husmann et al, 1999). similar findings were reported in a series by Mitchell and associates (1990). **Husmann and colleagues (1999) reported that the success rate of Young-Dees-Leadbetter bladder neck reconstruction in the cloacal exstrophy population was closely related to the presence of coexisting neurologic abnormalities.**

Urinary continence can be achieved in these individuals in many ways. An orthotopic urethra can be constructed from local tissue, vagina, ileum, stomach, or ureter. A catheterizable stoma can be constructed from ileum when enough bowel is present and fluid loss is not a problem. The bladder may be augmented with unused hindgut, ileum, or stomach. However, surgery to provide a continent urinary reservoir should be delayed until a method of evacuation can be taught and the child is old enough to participate in self-care. The choice between a catheterizable urethra and an abdominal stoma depends on the adequacy of the urethra and bladder outlet, interest and dexterity of the child, and orthopedic status regarding the spine, hip joints, braces, and ambulation. In a series by Gearhart and Jeffs (1991b) and in another series by Mitchell and associates (1990), multiple techniques were used to produce continence in patients with cloacal exstrophy. An innovative approach is required to find a suitable solution for each individual patient according to the patient's bladder size and function and mental, neurologic, and orthopedic status. With the advent of modern pediatric anesthesia and intensive care, the newborn survival rate is high. Improving survivorship makes reconstructive techniques applicable in a large percentage of patients born with this condition.

Long-Term Concerns

Spinal cord untethering may be required years after closure for the myelocystocele. In a series reported by McLaughlin and coworkers (1995), changes in urinary continence represented the initial evidence of a tethered cord. Early evaluation with MRI allows rapid treatment and prevention of further loss of function. In their series of patients with long-term follow-up (McLaughlin et al, 1995), 12 patients were fully evaluated with myelography, CT, and/or MRI of the lumbosacral spinal cord. Spinal exploration and repair of tethered cord was performed in 11 patients, 2 of whom subsequently underwent reoperation for retethering of the cord. These authors reported an incidence of spinal cord or vertebral anomalies in 100% of their patients, which is higher than formerly reported in the urologic literature. They recommended MRI of the spinal cord as part of the initial evaluation of all newborns with cloacal exstrophy and recommended lifelong attention to the risk of spinal cord tethering, which can affect the neurologic outcome of these individuals.

Gastrointestinal Function

Preservation of all bowel and performance of colostomy has led to improvement in the gastrointestinal management of cloacal exstrophy. The life-threatening complications of a terminal ileostomy can be obviated with this approach if hindgut is available to be used. Usually, intestinal absorption problems are resolved by 3 to 4 years of age and gastrointestinal reconstruction can then be considered. **In a minority of children, pull-through procedures may be successful** (Ricketts et al, 1991; Mathews, 1998). However, most children still require a bowel stoma. Involvement of a pediatric gastroenterologist who is interested in the complex care of these patients is mandatory.

Long-Term Psychological and Psychosexual Issues

Sixteen patients evaluated at our institution with a genotype of 46,XY and diminutive genitalia had gender reas-

signment; four children with adequate unilateral or bilateral corpora were raised as boys (Mathews et al, 1998). **Reiner and coauthors (2002) evaluated six children between 9 and 14 years of age who had had sex reassignment, and developmental difficulties were noted in all.** None of these children had received any exogenous female hormones, and most expressed typical male behavior. Two children spontaneously declared themselves boys at age 9.5 and 12 years, respectively; neither child had prior knowledge of their genetic sex. Initial sex reassignment in all patients was performed in conjunction with extensive family counseling as well as continued counseling of the parents and children. Nonetheless, this is a worrisome finding which will require long-term psychological studies in a larger subset of patients with cloacal exstrophy.

Summary

The management of cloacal exstrophy has advanced to provide improvement in quality of life for these children. Reconstruction by means of a complete closure, if the neonate's condition allows, or by the modern staged approach, seems applicable in most children. Neurologic and gastrointestinal management takes precedence over urologic and genital reconstruction. Improvements in diagnosis in surgical management have served to reduce life-threatening complications and progression of the neurologic deficit. Urinary continence is now possible in most children. Further advances in reconstructive surgery may some day enable congruent rearing for all male patients with cloacal exstrophy.

EPISPADIAS

Epispadias varies from a mild glanular defect in a covered penis, to the penopubic variety with complete incontinence in males or females, to the complete variety associated with exstrophy of the bladder.

Male Epispadias

Male epispadias is a rare anomaly, with a reported incidence of 1 in 117,000 males. Most male epispadias patients (about 70%) have complete epispadias with incontinence (Gearhart and Jeffs, 1998). Epispadias is explained by a defective migration of the primordium of the genital tubercles, which migrates toward the midline superior to the cloacal membrane to form the genital tubercle at about the 5th week of gestation. The resulting malformation consists of a defect in the dorsal wall of the urethra. The normal urethra is replaced by a broad, mucosal strip lining the dorsum of the penis toward the bladder, with incompetence of the sphincter mechanism. The displaced meatus is free of penile deformity, and occurrence of urinary incontinence is related to the degree of the dorsally displaced urethral meatus (Gearhart and Jeffs, 1998). The displaced meatus may be found on the glans, penile shaft, or penopubic region. All types of epispadias are associated with varying degrees of dorsal chordee. In penopubic or

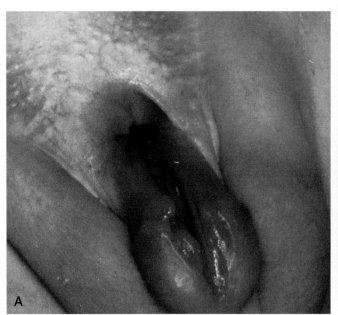 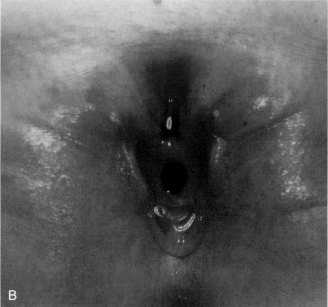

Figure 61–32. *A,* Three-month-old male with complete epispadias. *B,* Six-month-old female with complete epispadias. Note bifid clitoris, bifid labia minora, and large urethral cleft.

subsymphyseal epispadias, the entire penile urethra is opened and the bladder outlet may be large enough to admit the examining finger, indicating obvious gross incontinence (Fig. 61–32*A* and *B*). To a lesser extent than those with classic bladder exstrophy, patients with epispadias have a characteristic widening of the symphysis pubis caused by outward rotation of the innominate bones. This separation of the pubis causes divergent penopubic attachments that contribute to the short, pendular penis with dorsal chordee. **Therefore, the penile deformity is virtually identical to that observed in bladder exstrophy. The reported male-to-female ratio of epispadias varies between 3:1** (Dees, 1949) **and 5:1** (Kramer and Kelalis, 1982a).

Kramer and Kelalis (1982a) reviewed their surgical experience with 82 male patients with epispadias. Penopubic epispadias occurred in 49 cases, penile epispadias in 21, and glandular epispadias in 12. Urinary incontinence was observed in 46 of 49 patients with penopubic epispadias, in 15 of 21 patients with penile epispadias, and in no patient with glandular epispadias. The goals of the treatment of complete male epispadias include creation of a normal urinary control and establishment of a straight, cosmetically acceptable penis of adequate length that is functional for normal sexual intercourse. It has been postulated that complete male epispadias is similar to classic bladder exstrophy, except that in complete epispadias the bladder is closed and bladder closure procedures are not required.

Associated Anomalies

Anomalies associated with complete epispadias are usually confined to deformities of the external genitalia, diastasis of the pubic symphysis, and deficiency of the urinary continence mechanism. The only real anomaly observed in 11 cases of epispadias was agenesis of the left kidney

(Campbell, 1952). In a review by Arap and associates (1988), 1 case of renal agenesis and 1 ectopic kidney occurred among 38 patients.

The ureterovesical junction is inherently deficient in complete epispadias, and the incidence of reflux has been reported in a number of series to be between 30% and 40% (Kramer and Kelalis, 1982a; Arap et al, 1988). In a review by Ben-Chaim and colleagues (1995b) of a series of 15 patients with complete male epispadias treated at our institution, there was a significantly lower rate of vesicoureteral reflux, compared with male patients with classic bladder exstrophy (100% versus 82%, respectively); the rate of inguinal hernias (33%) was also significantly lower. A possible explanation for the lower incidence of reflux in complete male epispadias is that the pouch of Douglas is not as enlarged and deep. Therefore, the distal ureter enters the bladder in a more oblique fashion than in classic exstrophy (Gearhart and Jeffs, 1998).

Surgical Management

The objectives of repair of penopubic epispadias include achievement of urinary continence with preservation of the upper urinary tracts and the reconstruction of cosmetically acceptable genitalia. The surgical management of incontinence in penopubic epispadias is virtually identical to that in closed bladder exstrophy.

Young (1922) reported the first cure of incontinence in a male patient with complete epispadias. Since Young reported his approach to obtain continence, results have progressively improved (Burkholder and Williams, 1965; Kramer and Kelalis, 1982a; Arap et al, 1988; Peters et al, 1988; Mollard et al, 1998).

In patients with complete epispadias and good bladder capacity, epispadias and bladder neck reconstruction can be performed in a single-stage operation. Urethroplasty for-

Table 61–7. URINARY CONTINENCE AFTER BLADDER NECK RECONSTRUCTION (BNR) IN PATIENTS WITH COMPLETE EPISPADIAS

Item	Ben-Chaim et al (1995b)	Gearhart et al (1993a)	Kramer and Kelalis (1982a)	Arap et al (1988)	Burkholder and Williams (1965)
No. patients	15	11	53	38	27
Males					
No. treated with BNR	11	—	32*	21	17
No. with surgically corrected incontinence	9	—	22	15	8
Percentage with surgically corrected incontinence	82	—	69	71	47
Females					
No. treated with BNR	0	9	8	9	10
No. with surgically corrected incontinence	0	8	8	7	7
Percentage with surgically corrected incontinence	0	87	88	77	70

*All complete female epispadias cases.

merly was performed after bladder neck reconstruction (Kramer and Kelalis, 1982a; Arap et al, 1988). However, results with the small bladder associated with exstrophy (Gearhart and Jeffs, 1989a) and the small bladder associated with epispadias (Peters et al, 1988) have led us to perform urethroplasty and penile elongation before bladder neck reconstruction. A small, incontinent bladder with reflux is hardly an ideal situation for bladder neck reconstruction and ureteral reimplantation. Before bladder neck reconstruction there was an average increase in bladder capacity of 95 ml within 18 months in those patients with a small bladder capacity initially associated with epispadias and a continence rate of 87% after the continence procedure (Peters et al, 1988). **In a recent series by Ben-Chaim and colleagues (1995b) composed exclusively of patients with complete male epispadias, bladder capacity increased by an average of 42 ml within 18 months after urethroplasty.** Nine (82%) of 11 patients were dry day and night after an average of 9 months.

In the epispadias group, much as in the exstrophy group, bladder capacity is the most predominant indicator of eventual continence (Richey et al, 1988). **In a series by Arap and coworkers (1988), there was a much higher continence rate in those patients who had an adequate bladder capacity before bladder neck reconstruction than in those with an inadequate capacity (71% versus 20%, respectively).** In addition, in Arap's group of patients with complete epispadias patients, most obtained continence within 2 years, similar to results in patients with classic bladder exstrophy.

A firm intrasymphyseal band bridges the divergent symphysis, and an osteotomy is not usually performed. The Young-Dees-Leadbetter bladder neck plasty, Marshall-Marchetti-Krantz suspension, and ureteral reimplantation are performed when the bladder capacity reaches approximately 80 to 85 ml, which usually occurs between 4 and 5 years of age. Genital reconstruction procedures in epispadias and exstrophy are similar. The following reconstructive maneuvers must take place: release of dorsal chordee and division of the suspensory ligaments; dissection of the corpora from their attachments to the inferior pubic ramus; lengthening of the urethral groove; and lengthening of the corpora, if needed, by incision and anastomosis or grafting, or by medial rotation of the ventral corpora in a more downward direction.

Urethral reconstruction in complete epispadias has been performed in many ways. A transverse island flap was used by Monfort (1987). The urethra, once reconstructed, can be positioned between and below the corpora (Cantwell, 1895; Ransley et al, 1989; Gearhart et al, 1992; Gearhart et al, 1995c). Mitchell and Bagley reported their experience with a complete penile disassembly technique (1996), and a multicenter experience with the technique was later reported in a total of 17 patients from four institutions (Zaontz et al, 1998). Chordee was reliably corrected, erectile function was preserved, the urethra was eventually situated in a cosmetic fashion, and satisfactory cosmesis was achieved. In a larger series by Ransley and by Surer and their associates, excellent results were obtained with the modified Cantwell-Ransley procedure, saving cavernocavernostomy for those patients with very severe chordee and especially those in the older age group (Kajbafzadeh et al, 1995; Surer et al, 2000). For surgical reconstruction, see the previous discussion of bladder exstrophy.

Achievement of urinary continence after epispadias repair in patients with epispadias is summarized in Table 61–7. A majority of these patients underwent reconstruction by means of a Young-Dees-Leadbetter bladder neck plasty. Urinary continence was obtained in 82% of male patients (Ben-Chaim et al, 1995b). As in the exstrophy population, repair of the epispadiac deformity results in an increase of outlet resistance and possible increase in bladder capacity before bladder neck reconstruction. Although both complete epispadias and bladder exstrophy patients achieve somewhat better bladder capacity after epispadias repair, the mean increase in overall capacity is higher in those with complete epispadias. This increase in bladder capacity may account for increased continence in this group, compared with the classic bladder exstrophy population. **Clinically, these bladders are more supple, easier to mobilize, and more amenable to bladder neck reconstruction.**

Ben-Chaim and colleagues (1995b) reported that the mean time to initial continence was 90 days in those patients with complete male epispadias, compared with 110 days in those with bladder exstrophy. These results suggest that, for patients with complete epispadias, bladder capacity before reconstruction and the rate of achieving continence afterward are better than for patients with bladder exstrophy. The reason might be that the bladder is not exposed in utero and does not undergo primary closure; therefore, its potential for expansion is higher. It was formerly thought that the effect of urethral lengthening and prostatic enlargement might be significant in complete epispadias by increasing outlet resistance if continence was not perfect as the child became older. Earlier in a series by Arap and associates (1988), the establishment of continence had no relation to puberty and usually occurred within 2 years; usually preceded puberty by several years. In the series reported by Ben-Chaim and coworkers (1995b), as stated previously, all patients obtained daytime continence at a mean of 9 months after bladder neck reconstruction, and 9 (82%) of 11 patients attained total day and night continence. All patients voided spontaneously. After a mean follow-up of 7 years, all patients maintained normal upper tracts and kidney function. All of them had cosmetically pleasing genitalia, as judged by parents, patients, and physicians, and experienced normal erections. A 36-year-old patient was married and had fathered three children. Many of the patients were younger than 16 years of age and had not yet become sexually active.

Results of urethroplasty in epispadias have been reported in a number of publications (Mesrobian et al, 1986; Ransley et al, 1989; Kajbafzadeh et al, 1995; Zaontz et al, 1998). In a modern series of modified Cantwell-Ransley repairs reported by Surer and colleagues (2000), the incidence of postoperative fistula in the 3-month period after surgery was 19%, and the incidence of urethral stricture formation was less than 10%. Catheterization and cystoscopy could easily negotiate the neourethral channel in all patients who underwent a modified Cantwell-Ransley epispadias repair. In another modern series reported by Mollard and coworkers (1998), the continence rate was 84% and the fistula rate was less than 10%. In Mollard's series there was good long-term follow-up. Patients had normal erections; the vast majority had regular sexual intercourse, and most had normal ejaculation or had fathered children. Most of Surer's patients were quite young, and assessment of genital reconstruction must be deferred until these patients are sexually mature and active (2000). Although many methods of epispadias repair exist, meticulous follow-up of the urethra, patient selection, and surgical experience remain the milestone of success. Lastly, Ransley and colleagues (Kajbafzadeh et al, 1995) obtained very good results using a modified Cantwell-Ransley repair in a large number of patients with epispadias. The fistula rate was 4%, and the urethral stricture rate was 5.3%.

In a different approach to the treatment of epispadias reported by Duffy and Ransley (1998), 12 boys age 3 to 7 years underwent endoscopic submucosal injection of plastic microspheres. All patients had undergone a modified Cantwell-Ransley epispadias repair before injection. The procedure was performed 24 times, with a total volume of 83 ml of material injected into 59 sites in the posterior urethra. Mean follow-up was 10.8 months. Three patients (25%) were rendered completely dry, the degree of incontinence was improved in six, and there was no change in three. The authors offered this as an alternative to bladder neck reconstruction in patients with primary epispadias. Ben-Chaim and coworkers (1995a) reported that submucosal injection of collagen in the bladder neck area can have a

role in improving stress incontinence when the patient with complete epispadias has incomplete urinary control or as an adjunct after bladder neck reconstruction.

Kramer and associates (Mesrobian et al, 1986) reported the success of genital reconstruction in epispadias, with good long-term follow-up ending with a straight penis angled downward in almost 70% of patients, with normal erectile function. Of this group, 80% had satisfactory sexual intercourse, and of 29 married patients, 19 had fathered children. These results were mirrored in the long-term follow-up study of Mollard and associates (1998).

A carefully constructed and well-planned approach to the management of urinary incontinence in genital deformities associated with complete epispadias should provide a satisfactory cosmetic appearance, normal genital function, and preservation of fertility potential in most patients.

Female Epispadias

Female epispadias is a rare congenital anomaly; it occurs in 1 of every 484,000 female patients (Gearhart and Jeffs, 1998). We use the classification of Davis (1928), which describes three degrees of epispadias in female patients. In the least degree of epispadias, the urethral orifice simply appears patulous. In intermediate epispadias, the urethra is dorsally split along most of the urethra. In the most severe degree of epispadias, the urethral cleft involves the entire length of the urethra and sphincteric mechanism and the patient is rendered incontinent (see Fig. 61–32). The genital defect is characterized by a bifid clitoris. The mons is depressed in shape and coated by a smooth, glabrous area of skin. Beneath this area, there may be a moderate amount of subcutaneous tissue and fat, or the skin may be closely applied to the anterior and inferior surface of the symphysis pubis. The labia minora are usually poorly developed and terminate anteriorly at the corresponding half of the bifid clitoris, where there may be a rudiment of a preputial fold. These external appearances are most characteristic: on minimal separation of the labia, one sees the urethra, which may vary considerably, as mentioned previously. The symphysis pubis is usually closed but may be represented by a narrow fibrous band. The vagina and internal genitalia are usually normal.

Associated Anomalies

The ureterovesical junction is inherently deficient in cases of epispadias, and the ureters are often laterally placed in the bladder with a straight course so that reflux occurs. The incidence of reflux is reported to be 30% to 75% (Kramer and Kelalis, 1982b; Gearhart et al, 1993). Because there is no outlet resistance, the bladder is small and the wall is thin. However, after urethral reconstruction, the mild urethral resistance created allows the bladder to develop an acceptable capacity so that in the future the child can undergo bladder neck reconstruction.

Surgical Objectives

Objectives for repair of female epispadias parallel those devised for male patients: (1) achievement of uri-

nary continence, (2) preservation of the upper urinary tracts, and (3) reconstruction of a functional and cosmetically acceptable external genitalia.

Operative Techniques

With the patient in the lithotomy position, the defect of the female epispadias with incontinence is apparent (Fig. 61–33A). The two halves of the clitoris are widely apart, and the roof of the urethra is cleft between the 9 o'clock to 3 o'clock position. The smooth mucosa of the urethra tends to blend cephalad with the thin, hairless skin over the mons. The urethral incision is begun at the cephalad extent of the vertical incision at the base of the mons and is brought inferiorly through the full thickness of the urethral wall at the 9 o'clock and 3 o'clock positions (see Fig. 61–33B and C). Sutures can be placed in the urethra at this juncture and used to retract the cephalad extent of the urethra downward so that the roof of the urethra is excised to a level near the bladder neck. Often, one finds the dissection under the symphysis at this juncture (see Fig. 61–33D). An inverting closure of the urethra is then performed over a No. 12 or 10 Fr Foley catheter. Suturing is begun near the bladder neck and progresses downward until narrowing of the new urethra is accomplished (Fig. 61–33E and F). Attention is then given to denuding the medial half of the bifid clitoris and the labia minora so that proper genital coaptation can be obtained. After this is done, fat from the mons and subcutaneous tissue can be used to cover the suture line and obliterate the space in front of the pubic symphysis (see Fig. 61–33G). The two halves of the clitoris and labia minora are brought together using interrupted sutures of 6-0 polyglycolic acid. The corpora may be partially detached from the anterior ramus of the pubis to aid in the urethral closure. Also, bringing these tissues together may contribute by adding resistance to the urethra. Mons closure is further aided by mobilizing subcutaneous tissue laterally and bringing it medially to fill any prior depression that remains (see Fig. 61–33H). The subcutaneous layer is closed with 4-0 polyglactin in an interrupted fashion (see Fig. 61–33J). The skin is closed with interrupted sutures of 6-0 polypropylene (see Fig. 61–33J through L). A No. 10 Fr catheter is left indwelling for 5 to 7 days. Should the patient undergo simultaneous bladder neck reconstruction, a Foley catheter is not left in the urethra and the patient is placed in the supine position for the abdominal part of the procedure.

Achievement of a satisfactory cosmetic appearance of the external genitalia and of satisfactory urinary continence in the female child with epispadias represents a surgical challenge. Many operations have been reported to control continence in the epispadias group, but the results are disappointing. These procedures include transvaginal plication of the urethra and bladder neck, muscle transplantations, urethra twisting, cauterization of the urethra, bladder flap, and Marshall-Marchetti vesicourethral suspension (Stiles, 1911; Davis, 1926; Marshall et al, 1949; Gross and Kresson, 1952). These procedures may increase urethral resistance, but they do not correct incontinence or the malformed anatomy of the urethra, bladder neck, and genitalia. The challenge of the small bladder in the female epispadias patient is comparable to a situation often seen in patients with closed bladder exstrophy. The small, incontinent bladder, with or without reflux, is hardly an ideal setting for a successful bladder neck reconstruction and ureteral reimplantation. A third of all incontinent epispadias patients have a small bladder capacity of less than 60 ml, in our experience and that of Kramer and Kelalis (1982b). Bladder augmentation, injection of polytetrafluoroethylene (Teflon) in the bladder neck area, and/or simultaneous bladder neck reconstruction and bladder neck augmentation have been offered as a solution to this challenge. However, primary closure of the epispadiac urethra in children with closed exstrophy was found to increase bladder capacity without causing hydronephrosis, and this approach has been applied to male and female patients with epispadias (Peters et al, 1988; Gearhart and Jeffs, 1989a; Ben-Chaim et al, 1995b). Although we typically perform urethral and genital reconstruction at about 1 year of age, we advocate delaying bladder neck reconstruction until the child is 4 to 5 years old. Not only does this delay allow the bladder to increase in capacity, but it also allows the child to accept essential instructions for toilet training, which is critical to achieving satisfactory continence in the postoperative state.

Surgical Results

The continence rate of 87.5% in our female patients is comparable to that of Hanna and Williams (1972), who found a 67% continence rate in female patients with a good bladder capacity, and that of Kramer and Kelalis (1982b), who reported an 83% continence rate in patients with an adequate bladder capacity. All of the author's patients seen for primary treatment have achieved a capacity in excess of 80 ml.

Hendren (1981) and Kramer and Kelalis (1982b) showed that genitourethral reconstruction can be accomplished with satisfactory results. At our institution, patients who underwent prior urethral and genital reconstruction had a mean bladder capacity at bladder neck reconstruction of 121 ml, making the bladder suitable for the reconstruction and eventual continence without the use of augmentation cystoplasty or need for intermittent catheterization.

The time interval to achieve continence in our patients was a mean of 18 months for those who underwent genitourethral and bladder neck reconstruction in one procedure and 23 months for those who underwent preliminary urethroplasty and genital reconstruction after bladder neck reconstruction. In a series by Klauber and Williams (1974), the mean interval to acceptable continence was 2.25 years. Also, in a series by Kramer and Kelalis (1982b), some patients became continent within a short period, whereas complete continence was delayed for several years in others. The time delay for achieving continence may represent increased pelvic muscular development, as suggested by Kramer and Kelalis (1982b). In regard to the interval to continence, no advantage appears to be gained by preliminary urethroplasty. However, I believe that the advantage gained by increased bladder capacity at the time of bladder neck reconstruction outweighs any advantage gained by a combined approach.

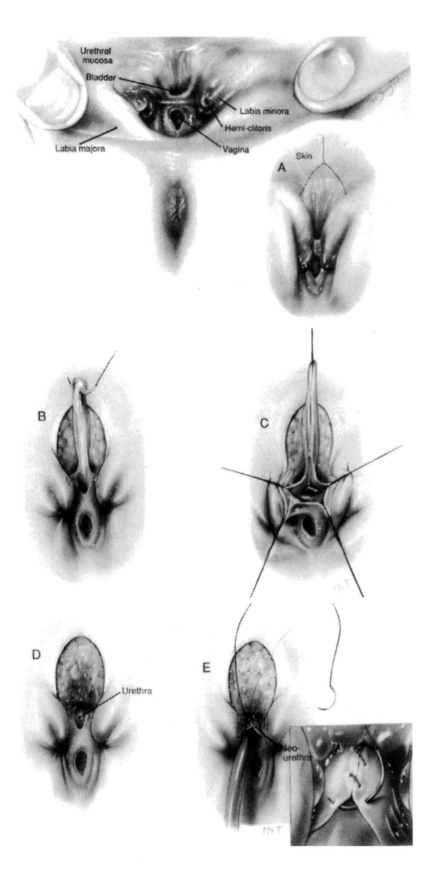

Figure 61–33. *A,* Typical appearance of female epispadias. Insert shows initial incision for surgical repair. *B* and *C,* Excision of glabrous skin of the mons and parallel urethral incisions taken cephalad toward the bladder neck. *D* and *E,* Urethral reconstruction begun over a catheter with running sutures of 5-0 polyglycolic acid.

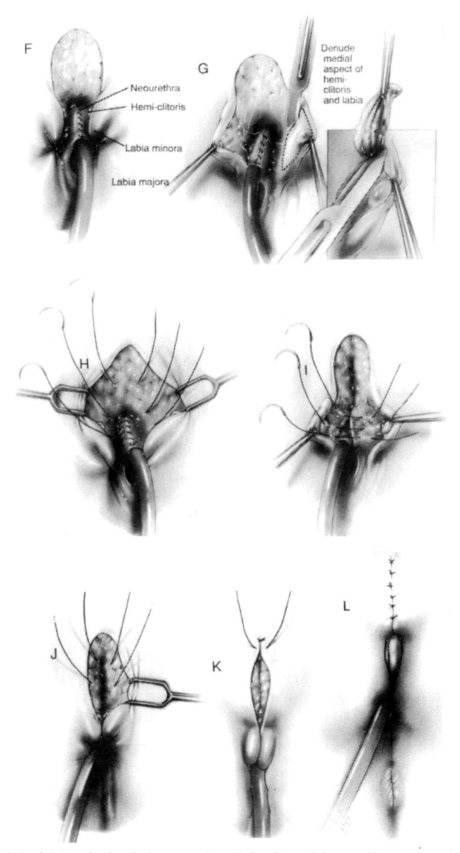

Figure 61–33 *Continued. F* and *G,* Completed urethral reconstruction with denuding medial aspect of labia minora and clitoris. *H* and *I,* Closure of periurethral tissues over neourethra with coaptation of labial and clitoral halves. *J* and *K,* Closure of subcutaneous area to build up mons area and skin closure. *L,* Completed urethral and genital reconstruction. (Drawings by M. Yung Toi.)

OTHER BLADDER ANOMALIES

Agenesis and Hypoplasia

Agenesis of the bladder is an extremely rare congenital anomaly, with only 44 cases reported in the English literature up to 1988. Vakili (1973) reported seven cases, all in female patients. Glenn (1959) found only 1 case among 600,000 cases seen at Duke University Hospital over 20 years. Agenesis of the bladder is seldom compatible with life, and only 15 live births have been reported, all except one being female (Adkes et al, 1988; Aragona et al, 1988; Krull et al, 1988). The cause of agenesis of the bladder is uncertain. Because the hindgut is normal in these infants, it may be assumed that embryonic division of the cloaca into urogenital sinus and anorectum has proceeded normally. Bladder agenesis may be the result of secondary atrophy of the anterior division of the cloaca, and perhaps a lack of distention with urine caused by failure of incorporation of the mesonephric ducts and ureters into the trigone, thus preventing urine from accumulating in the bladder (Krull et al, 1988).

The results of this anomaly depend on the sex of the fetus. In the female with normally developed müllerian structures, the ureteral orifices may end in the uterus, anterior vaginal wall, or vestibule. In these cases with ectopic ureteral openings, there is usually some preservation of renal function (Krull et al, 1988). In the male, the only means to achieve adequate outlet drainage would be cloacal persistence, with the ureters draining into the rectum or by way of a patent urachus. Considering the severity of this defect, it is not surprising that bladder agenesis is most often associated with neurologic, orthopedic, or other urogenital anomalies, such as solitary kidney, renal agenesis, renal dysplasia, or absence of prostate, vagina, seminal vesicles, or penis (Aragona et al, 1988). In most reported cases, surviving infants underwent urinary diversion by either ureterosigmoidostomy or external stoma (Glenn, 1959).

The small bladder may be dysplastic or hypoplastic. Dysplasia is observed in conditions such as duplicate exstrophy or hemibladder exstrophy, in which the rudiment is small, fibrotic, and nondistensible. Hypoplastic bladders have little capacity when an adequate amount of urine is stored in the bladder during fetal life (epispadias with incontinence, urogenital sinus abnormalities in females, bilateral renal agenesis, or renal dysplasia) or when the bladder is bypassed altogether (e.g., bilateral ureteral ectopia with distal urethra or vaginal orifices in a female). Hypoplastic bladders have the potential to enlarge, but more commonly they require augmentation.

Duplication

Complete duplication of the bladder and urethra is rare, with only 45 cases reported in the literature (Kapoor and Saha, 1987). Complete duplication of the bladder involves two bladder halves, each with a full-thickness muscular wall, and each with its own ipsilateral ureter and urethra (Fig. 61–34). Anomalies are observed more commonly in males than females. Associated congenital anomalies of

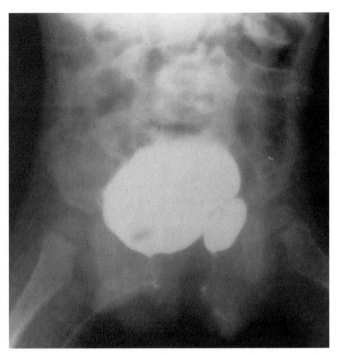

Figure 61–34. Complete bladder and urethral duplication in a 6-month-old child.

other systems are present in the majority of cases of complete duplication of the bladder and urethra. In 40 cases reviewed by Kossow and Morales (1973), 90% had some type of duplication of the external genitalia, and 42% had duplication of the lower gastrointestinal tract. Spinal duplication and fistulas in the rectum, vagina, and urethra were other associated abnormalities. In incomplete duplication, the bladder is divided by a full-thickness septum, either sagittally or coronally. This also involves two full-thickness bladder halves, each with its own ureter. However, in contrast to complete bladder duplication, the two halves communicate and drain into a common urethra. Unlike the complete bladder duplication anomaly, genital and other anomalies (e.g., anorectal) are not usually associated with this incomplete form of bladder duplication. This condition usually is not associated with serious sequelae.

Congenital Bladder Diverticulum

Congenital bladder diverticulum not associated with posterior urethral valves or a neurogenic bladder is unusual (Johnson, 1960; Barrett et al, 1976). This entity almost always occurs in male patients. Congenital bladder diverticula usually occur in a smooth-walled bladder; they are most often solitary and occur without evidence of outflow obstruction. In children, the most common location for a bladder diverticulum is lateral and cephalad to the ureteral orifice. The cause of these diverticula is an inherent weakness in the bladder musculature and herniations of bladder mucosa between fibers of the detrusor muscle. As the diverticulum enlarges, it may incorporate the ureteral tunnel, and the ureter may drain into the diverticulum with resultant reflux. These congenital diverticula are often larger than those associated with neurogenic bladder or lower tract obstructive anomalies. These structures may also cause outlet obstruction at the bladder neck or at the urethral location (Taylor et al, 1979) or ureteral obstruction (Lelione and Gonzales, 1985). These bladder diverticula are uncommon but not rare. Blane and colleagues (1994) reported that of 5084 children, bladder diverticula were found in 1.7%. These diverticula are not difficult to diagnose on voiding cystourethrography, especially with postvoiding images. Upper tract imaging, although important, is not believed to be the best method to diagnose a bladder diverticulum initially. Only 2 of the 24 patients in the series by Atwell and Allah (1980) had bladder diverticula seen on intravenous urography.

Acquired bladder diverticula are usually multiple and associated with bladder outlet obstruction. They are usually secondary to bladder outlet obstruction, infection, or iatrogenic causes. Bladder neck or urethral obstruction with posterior urethral valves, anterior urethral diverticulum, urethral stricture, neuropathic bladder dysfunction, or external sphincter dyssynergia are all known causes of bladder diverticula. Also, bladder diverticula may be acquired iatrogenically, such as after antireflux surgery in which defects of the ureteral hiatus are not repaired adequately with a resulting bladder diverticulum.

It is now well recognized that a majority of bladder diverticula in young children are solitary and occur in a small bladder. The etiologic factor is believed to be an inherent weakness in the detrusor musculature, in particular deficiencies of the fascial sheath. Congenital bladder diverticula have been described in children with Ehlers-Danlos syndrome and Menkes' syndrome (Harcke et al, 1977; Burrows et al, 1998). Menkes' syndrome, a neurodegenerative and connective tissue disorder, involves characteristic increases in tissue copper content and metallothionein. Eleven cases of congenital bladder diverticula have been described in children with Ehlers-Danlos syndrome. This is a congenital connective tissue disorder characterized by abnormalities of collagen structure and function. However, the link between the connective tissue disorder and the bladder diverticulum have yet to be proven. The reported cases of congenital bladder diverticulum associated with Ehlers-Danlos syndrome have occurred in male patients (Levard et al, 1989). Lastly, bladder diverticula have been seen in Williams' syndrome, a disorder characterized by growth, mental retardation, facial anomalies, and aortic stenosis, and in prune-belly syndrome. In addition to the above-mentioned obstruction of the ureters or posterior urethra, it has also been noted that children with bladder diverticula have abnormal voiding patterns on urodynamic evaluation, including detrusor sphincter dyssynergia, hyperreflexia, or hypertonia. These findings, in addition to stasis of urine associated with diverticula, predispose children with bladder diverticulum to recurrent lower tract infections in the absence of reflux.

Surgical intervention for congenital bladder diverticulum may be required when recurring infections, persistent vesicoureteral reflux, bladder outlet obstruction, or significant ureteral obstruction is present. The surgical approach to bladder diverticulum depends on anatomic considerations such as the relationship of the diverticulum to the bladder neck, whether there is associated reflux or obstruction, the need for ureteral reimplantation, and so on.

Congenital Megacystis

Congenital megacystis is an entity in which the bladder is associated with massively refluxing megaureters. It was first described by Williams (1957). The physiologic result of massive reflux is constant cycling of urine with massively dilated reflux in megaureters and the bladder. Bladder contractibility is normal, although a majority of each vessel contraction empties into the upper tracts. This constant recycling of urine results in a progressive increase in urine and bladder capacity. The trigone is wide and fully developed with lateral gaping, incontinent orifices. The diagnosis can be made prenatally, and the patient should be prescribed prophylactic antibiotics.

The rarity of this condition in present urologic practice suggests an acquired origin. *Escherichia coli* infection and reflux in a normal system may cause bladder and ureteral atony with subsequent dilatation. The dilated bladder in neonates may be difficult to determine. Prenatal temporary obstruction, metabolic abnormalities, and cerebral anoxia have been implicated. Congenital megacystis can also be associated with microcolon intestinal hyperperistalsis syndrome or Ehlers-Danlos syndrome, or it may occur secondary to an outlet obstruction phenomenon. The treatment of patients with primary congenital megacystis is primarily directed at the massive vesicoureteral reflux, and a reduction in bladder size often is not needed. Care must be taken to reimplant the ureters, because the bladder wall is often thin, and it can be difficult to construct a plane between the bladder mucosa and bladder muscle.

Urachal Abnormalities

Anatomy and Histology

The urachus lies between the peritoneum and transversalis fascia, adjacent to the umbilical ligaments and the remnants of the umbilical arteries; it extends from the anterior dome of the bladder toward the umbilicus (Fig. 61–35). The urachus varies from 3 to 10 cm in length and from 8 to 10 mm in diameter. The urachus is encased between two layers of umbilicovesical fascia, which tends to contain the spread of urachal disease. The urachus is adjacent to the umbilical arteries. It is present as a muscular tube, and three distinct tissue layers are recognized: (1) an epithelial canal with cuboidal or transitional epithelium, (2) a submucosal connective tissue layer, and (3) an outer layer of smooth muscle that is thickest near the bladder. The central lumen is regular and beaded and is filled with desquamated epithelial debris and epithelial islands. If the urachus becomes a fibrous cord, there are generally no recognizable urachal elements (Baig, 1927; Hammond et al, 1941; Hector, 1961; Steck and Helwig, 1965).

Embryology

The allantois is an extraembryonic cavity located within the body stalk that projects onto the anterior surface of the

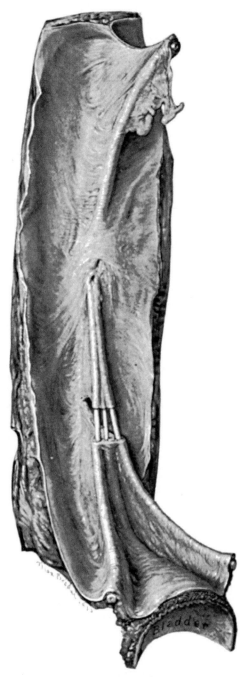

Figure 61–35. Posterior view of the umbilical region of the anterior abdominal wall showing the relation of the urachus to the umbilical ligaments, peritoneum, and bladder dome. The urachus does not extend fully to the umbilicus. Ligamentum teres is seen superior to the umbilicus. (From Cullen TS: Embryology, Anatomy and Diseases of the Umbilicus. Philadelphia, WB Saunders, 1916.)

cloaca, the future bladder. Descent of the bladder into the pelvis is associated with elongation of the urachus, a tubular structure that extends from the fibrotic allantoic duct to the anterior bladder. During the 4th and 5th months of gestation, the urachus narrows into a small-caliber epithelial tube (Nix et al, 1958). During fetal development, as the bladder descends into the pelvis, its proportion narrows progressively into a fibromuscular strand of urachus, which maintains continuity with the allantoic duct. As the fetus

develops, the urachus loses its attachment to the umbilicus. Hammond and coworkers (1941) observed that the continuity of the urachus with the posterior surface of the umbilicus and apex of the bladder persisted only in 50% of fetal specimens. Shortly after the embryonic stage of development the tract apparently obliterates, because patency was observed in only 2% of adult specimens.

Obliteration of the urachus results in different patterns of urination. In type I, the urachus fails to retain its attachment to the dome of the bladder separate from each umbilical artery. In type II variants, the urachus fuses with one of the umbilical arteries and continues as a single fibrous cord to the umbilicus. In type III variants, the urachus fuses with both the umbilical arteries and continues as a single structure with the umbilicus. Lastly, a type IV variant occurs when the urachus forms and terminates before fusing with the umbilical arteries, ending within the fascia or blending into a band of fibrous tissue (Hammond et al, 1941; Nex et al, 1958; Blichert-Toft and Nielson, 1971a, 1971b). Between the 4th and 5th months of gestation, the potential communication between the apex of the bladder and the urachal canal is segmentally obstructed by desquamated epithelium.

Patent Urachus

Congenital patent urachus is a lesion that is usually recognized in the neonate as a rare anomaly occurring in only 3 of more than 1,000,000 admissions to a large pediatric center (Nix et al, 1958). **Two forms of congenital patent urachus exist: (1) persistent patent urachus with a partially distended bladder and (2) a vesicoumbilical fistula representing failure of the bladder to descend** (Fig. 61–36). When the bladder forms, the bladder apex never forms a true urachal tract. The more common form of a patent urachus results when there is failure of obliteration of the urachal remnant. Persistence of the urachus has been attributed to intrauterine obstruction; however, only 14% of neonates born with a patent urachus have evidence of urinary obstruction. It is unlikely that urinary obstruction is directly related to the development of a patent urachus, because even the most severe cases of posterior urethral valves are not associated with this anomaly. Furthermore, urethral tubularization occurs after obliteration of the urachal remnant, suggesting that urinary obstruction is not the major factor in the production of patent urachus (Schreck and Campbell, 1972).

In a large series of urachal anomalies, Cilento et al (1998b) found a patent urachus to be present in only 15% of patients. The patent urachus is rarely diagnosed when there is a free discharge of urine through the umbilicus. The patent urachus should be suspected when a local cord is enlarged and edematous or when its normal slough is delayed. On occasion, the fistula is tiny and the discharge of urine is minimal or intermittent. The diagnosis of a patent urachus and patients with these symptoms should be differentiated from that of omphalitis, granulation of a healing umbilical stump, patent omphalomesenteric duct, infected umbilical vessel, or external urachal sinus. Analysis of the periumbilical fluid for creatinine and urea is useful in differentiating a patent urachus from these other conditions, and a fistulogram with radiopaque contrast is

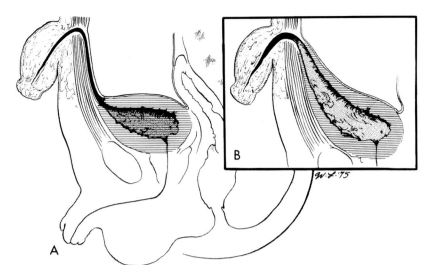

Figure 61–36. Forms of patent urachus. Note high hydrops of the umbilical cord. *A*, Typical patent urachus. *B*, Vesicoumbilical fistula.

often diagnostic. Voiding cystourethrography is helpful in fully evaluating the lesion and any associated bladder outlet obstruction. This distinguishes the condition from a patent mesenteric duct. The presence of both urinary and enteric fistulas at the umbilicus is exceedingly rare (Davis and Nilhaus, 1926; Herbst, 1937; Steck and Helwig, 1965; Mendoza et al, 1968; Keningsburg, 1975). Antenatal diagnosis of patent urachus was reported by Persuit and coworkers (1988) and by Cilento and associates (1994a). Not only is prenatal diagnosis helpful, but postnatal confirmation of these anomalies can be readily accomplished with high-resolution ultrasound imaging (Cilento et al, 1998b). In the management of patent urachus, observation may be indicated for young infants with symptoms, because closure of the urachus is not completed at birth and spontaneous closure can occur within the first few months of life.

Urachal Cyst

A cyst may form in the isolated urachal canal if the lumen is enlarged with epithelial desquamation and degeneration. Connection frequently persists between the tract and the bladder and potential bacterial infection which becomes loculated (Fig. 61–37A). Infected cysts occur more commonly in adults (Sterling and Goldsmith, 1953; Blichert-Toft and Nielson, 1971b) but have been reported in infants (Geist, 1952; Hinman, 1961). The cyst manifests

because infection has developed. The organism most commonly cultured in the cyst fluid is *Staphylococcus aureus* (Tauber and Bloom, 1951; McMillan et al, 1973). The cyst may drain into the bladder or through the umbilicus, or it may drain intermittently, resulting in alternating sinus (Sterling and Goldsmith, 1953; Hinman, 1961; Blichert-Toft and Nielson, 1971b). **These lesions are far more common than was originally thought. In a series of 45 urachal anomalies, Cilento and coworkers (1998b) found this anomaly in 16 patients (36%). The urachal cyst develops most commonly in the distal one third of the urachus, but it also can occur in the proximal third, depending on the type of urachal termination variant that it occurs in.** These cysts rarely manifest in the newborn period but may become symptomatic during late childhood or early adult life. Serious complications of an infected urachal cyst include rupture of the preperitoneal tissues, rupture into the peritoneal cavity causing significant peritonitis, and, rarely, inflammatory involvement of the adjacent bowel and formation of an enteric fistula (Nunn, 1952; Berman et al, 1988).

Symptoms and signs of a loculated and infected urachal cyst are lower abdominal pain, fever, voiding symptoms, midline hypogastric tenderness, and, often, a palpable mass and evidence of urinary infection. A urachal cyst should be suspected when localized suprapubic pain and tenderness are present with disturbed micturition, even when the urine

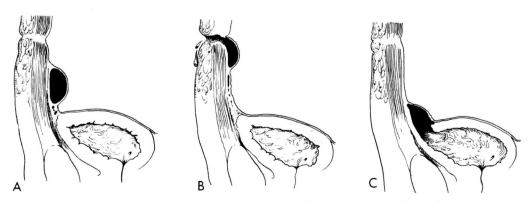

Figure 61–37. *A*, Urachal cyst. *B*, External urachal sinus. *C*, Urachal diverticulum.

remains clear. A diagnosis of urachal cyst is most often made by ultrasound, delineating the location of the cyst relative to the bladder and peritoneum and the limited extension. CT studies may be occasionally useful in further delineating the extent of the cyst and involvement of adjacent structures, such as bowel. Other useful diagnostic studies include excretory urography and cystoscopy.

Treatment of the urachal cyst depends on the symptoms. In children who have only a small, asymptomatic mass, watchful waiting may be appropriate. However, in the setting of an infected urachal cyst, the primary treatment includes excision and drainage of the cyst, marsupialization, or percutaneous catheter drainage. Definitive treatment with surgical excision should be performed once the inflammation subsides. The staged approach to treating an infected urachal cyst helps to limit the amount of bladder wall resected and reduces the risk of injury to the adjacent intraperitoneal structures.

External Urachal Sinus

Persistence of the urachal apex alone results in a blind external site that opens at the umbilicus (Fig. 61–37*B*). This may become symptomatic at any age with infected discharge. In adults umbilical disease can mimic an external sinus (Steck and Helwig, 1965). In a series reported by Cilento and associates (1998b), this anomaly occurred in 22 (49%) of patients with urachal anomalies. Because the differential diagnosis also includes the lesions listed in the previous section, proper radiologic evaluation should be undertaken before surgery. The sinus extends inferiorly, unlike an omphalic mesenteric duct remnant, which usually extends inward toward the peritoneal cavity. As mentioned earlier, an alternating sinus may be formed when a small urachal cyst becomes chronically infected and drains into the umbilicus or the bladder. In the presence of a draining sinus at the umbilicus, a sinogram with radiopaque contrast is diagnostic. As soon as the associated infection is controlled, complete excision of the sinus tract along with resection of the omphalic mesenteric duct remnant should

be performed. At the time of resection care should be taken to avoid damaging the peritoneal structures that may be densely inherent to the posterior aspect of the inflammatory mass.

Urachal Diverticulum

A diverticulum of the bladder apex (see Fig. 61–37*C*) is a blind internal sinus, an incidental finding in radiographic studies that does not require treatment. However, lesions of massive proportions reported in adults have required percutaneous drainage and eventual surgery (Berman et al, 1988). A large urachal diverticulum, as frequently seen in prune-belly syndrome (Lattimer, 1958) and occasionally associated with severe urethral obstruction, may require resection. These diverticula may be poorly contracted or may even expand during voiding. Urachal diverticula occasionally contain calculi (Ney and Freedenburg, 1968). Although they occasionally contain calculi, most diverticula are non-obstructive, drain well, and therefore do not predispose to stagnation of urine or infection. However, urachal carcinoma has been known to develop within these anomalies.

Treatment

Therapy for a patent urachus requires excision of all anomalous tissue in the bladder. Some workers advocate conservative treatment initially, reserving radical surgical excision of the urachus for persistent cases or recurrences. Simple drainage of a urachal cyst is associated with recurrent infections in 30% of cases, and late occurrence of adenocarcinoma has been reported (Nix et al, 1958; Blichert-Toft and Nielson, 1971a). In a more modern series, Cilento and coworkers (1998b) recommended routine excision of both the anomaly and a cuff of bladder.

In the treatment of a benign urachal lesion in children, it is rarely necessary to remove the umbilicus; whenever possible, cosmetic consideration should prevail. In infants, a small, curved subumbilical incision is usually ample, because at this age the bladder dome is still high and readily

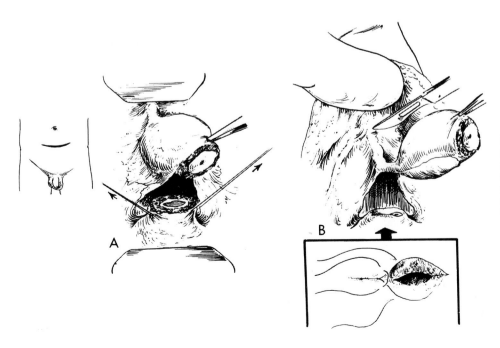

Figure 61–38. Surgical removal of a urachal cyst. Transverse midhypogastric incision. *A,* Lesion removed with a cuff of the bladder apex. *B,* Urachal stalk detached from the posterior umbilicus. A cuff of adherent peritoneum is excised with the specimen.

accessible to exposure. A transverse, midhypogastric incision is adequate in older children and adults and allows for both superior and inferior dissection. Surgical management of umbilical anomalies is depicted in Figure 61–38. The urachal stump or fibrous urachal remnant should be detached from the dermis posterior to the umbilicus. A buttonhole in the umbilical area is of no consequence. Application of a small gauze pledget under the dressing obliterates dead space, maintains the umbilical configuration, and allows the skin to close secondarily.

When peritoneal and umbilical ligaments are adherent to the inflammatory mass, these structures should be excised with the lesion. A vertical midline incision is the best method of removal. Elliptical incision of the umbilicus may be necessary if it is involved in the inflammatory process, especially with an external urachal sinus or alternating sinus. A separate infection within a cyst or external sinus may require initial excision and drainage with treatment as for an abscess. After healing is complete, an internal excision of all urachal tissue should be performed.

Acknowledgment

This chapter is dedicated to Leon Schlossberg, B.S., M.S., M.D. (Hon.), for his contributions to the discipline of Medical Illustration. His accurate and life-like illustrations have permitted complex surgical procedures to be understood by all students of surgery.

REFERENCES

Adkes A, Iseric C, Ozgurs S, Kirhilaz Z: Bladder agenesis. Int J Urol Nephrol 1988;20:261.
Ambrose SS, O'Brien DP: Surgical embryology of the exstrophy-epispadias complex. Surg Clin North Am 1974;54: 1379.
Ansell JE: Exstrophy and epispadias. In Glenn JF (ed): Urologic Surgery. Philadelphia, JB Lippincott, 1983, p 647.
Aragona F, Passerini G, Carembella P, et al: Agenesis of the bladder: A case report and review of the literature. Urol Radiol 1988;10:207.
Arap S, Nahas WC, Giron AM, et al: Continent epispadias: Surgical treatment of 38 cases. J Urol 1988;140:577.
Arap S, Giron AN: Duplicated exstrophy: Report of three cases. Eur Urol 1986;12:451.
Atwell JD, Allah NH: The inter-relationship between periureteric diverticula, vesicoureteric reflux and duplication of the pelvic calyceal collecting system: a family study. BJU Int 1980;52:269.
Austin P, Holmsy YL, Gearhart JP, et al: Prenatal diagnosis of cloacal exstrophy. J Urol 1998;160:1179.
Baig RC: The urachus umbilical fistula. J Anat 1927;64:170.
Baka-Jakubiak M: Combined bladder neck, urethral and penile reconstruction in boys with exstrophy-epispadias complex. Br J Urol Int 2000;86: 513.
Baker LA, Gearhart JP: Staged approach to bladder exstrophy and the role of osteotomy. World J Urol 1998;16:205.
Baker LA, Jeffs RD, Gearhart JP: Urethral obstruction after primary exstrophy closure: What is the fate of the genitourinary tract? J Urol 1999;161:618.
Barrett DM, Maleck RS, Kelalis DP: Observations of vesical diverticulum in children. J Urol 1976;116:234.
Bassiouny IE: Continent urinary reservoir in exstrophy/epispadias complex. Br J Urol 1992;70:558.
Bastuba MD, Alper MM, Oats RD: Fertility and the use of assisted reproductive techniques in the adult male exstrophy patient. Fertil Steril 1993;60:733.
Ben-Chaim J, Jeffs RD, Peppas DS, et al: Submucosal bladder neck injections of glutaraldehyde cross linked bovine collagen for the treatment of urinary incontinence in patients with the exstrophy-epispadias complex. J Urol 1995a;154:862.

Ben-Chaim J, Jeffs RD, Reiner WG, et al: The outcome of patients with classic bladder exstrophy in adult life. J Urol 1996;155:1251.
Ben-Chaim J, Peppas DS, Jeffs RD, Gearhart JP: Complete male epispadias: Genital reconstruction achieving continence. J Urol 1995b;153: 1665.
Ben-Chaim J, Peppas DS, Sponseller PD, et al: Application of osteotomy in the cloacal exstrophy patient. J Urol 1995c;154:865.
Bennett AH: Exstrophy of the bladder treated by ureterosigmoidostomies. Urology 1973;2:165.
Berman SM, Tolia BM, Laor E, et al: Urachal remnants in adults. Urology 1988;131:17.
Blane CE, Zeron JM, Bloom DA: Bladder diverticula in children. Radiology 1994;190:695.
Blichert-Toft M, Nielson OV: Congenital patent urachus and acquired variants. Acta Chir Scand 1971a;137:807.
Blichert-Toft M, Nielson OV: Diseases of the urachus simulating intraabdominal disorders. Am J Surg 1971b;122:123.
Boyce WH, Vest SA: A new concept concerning treatment of exstrophy of the bladder. J Urol 1952;677:503.
Bruch SW, Isaac NS, Goldstein RB: Etiology and embryogenesis of cloacal exstrophy. J Pediatr Surg 1996;31:768.
Burbage KA, Hensle TW, Chambers WJ, et al: Pregnancy and sexual function in bladder exstrophy. Urology 1986;28:12.
Burkholder GV, Williams DI: Epispadias and incontinence: Surgical treatment in 27 children. J Urol 1965;94:674.
Burrows MP, Monk BE, Harrison JB, et al: Giant bladder diverticulum in Ehlers-Danlos syndrome type I causing outflow obstruction. Clin Exp Dermatol 1998;23:109.
Caione P, Kapoza N, Lais A, et al: Female genito-urethroplasty and submucosal periurethral collagen injections as adjunctive procedures for continence in the exstrophy-epispadias complex. Br J Urol 1993a;71: 350.
Caione P, Lais A, Dejenaro N, et al: Glutaraldehyde cross linked bovine collagen in the exstrophy-epispadias complex. J Urol 1993b;150:631.
Caione P, Napo S, DeCastro R: Low dose desmopressin in the treatment of nocturnal urinary incontinence in exstrophy-epispadias complex. BJU Int 1999;84:329.
Campbell M: Epispadias: A report of 15 cases. J Urol 1952;67:988.
Canning DA, Gearhart JP, Peppas DS, Jeffs RD: The cephalotrigonal reimplant in bladder neck reconstruction for patients with exstrophy or epispadias. J Urol 1992;150:156.
Cantwell FV: Operative technique of epispadias by transplantation of the urethra. Ann Surg 1895;22:689, 1895.
Cendron J: La reconstruction vesicale. Ann Chir Infant 1971;12:371.
Cerniglia F, Roth DA, Gonzalez ET: Covered exstrophy and visceral sequestration in a male newborn. J Urol 1989;141:903.
Chan DY, Jeffs RD, Gearhart JP: Determinates of continence in the bladder exstrophy population after bladder neck reconstruction. Urology 2001;165:1656.
Chandra S, Sharma A, Bharga S: Covered exstrophy with incomplete duplication of the bladder. Pediatr Surg Int 1999;15:422.
Chisholm TC: Exstrophy of the urinary bladder. In Kiesewetter WB: Pediatric Surgical Symposium: Long-term Follow-up in Congenital Anomalies, vol 6, Pittsburgh, Pittsburgh Children's Hospital, 1979, p 31.
Chitrit Y, Zorn B, Filidori M et al: Cloacal exstrophy in monozygotic twins detected through antenatal ultrasound scanning. J Clin Ultrasound 1993;21:339.
Cilento BG Jr, Bauer SB, Retik AB, et al: Urachal anomalies: Defining the best diagnostic modality. Urology 1998a;52:120.
Cilento BG, Retik AB, Peters CA, et al: Urachal abnormalities: Defining the best diagnostic modality. Urology 1998;52:120.
Clemetson CAB: Ectopia vesicae and split pelvis. J Obstet Gynaecol Br Commonwealth 1958;65:973.
Connely JA, Peppas DS, Jeffs RD, Gearhart JP: Prevalence in repair of inguinal hernia in children with bladder exstrophy. J Urol 1995;154: 1900.
Conner JP, Lattimer JK, Hensle TW, Burbige KA: Primary bladder closure of bladder exstrophy: Long-term functional results in 137 patients. J Pediatr Surg 1988;23:1102.
Davis DM: Epispadias in females and the surgical treatment. Surg Gynecol Obstet 1928;47:600.
Davis NH, Nilhaus FW: Persistent omphalomesenteric duct and urachus in the same case. JAMA 1926;86:685.
Dees JE: Congenital epispadias with incontinence. J Urol 1949;62:513.
Diamond DA: Management of cloacal exstrophy. Dial Pediatr Urol 1990; 13:2.

Diamond DA, Bauer SB, Dinlenc C, et al: Normal urodynamics in patients with bladder exstrophy are they achievable? J Urol 1999;162:841.

Dodson J, Jeffs RD, Gearhart JP: The small exstrophy bladder unsuitable for closure. J Urol 2001;165:1656.

Duckett JW: Use of paraexstrophy skin pedicle grafts for correction of exstrophy and epispadias repair. Birth Defects 1977;13:171.

Duckett JW, Gazak JM: Complications of ureterosigmoidostomy. Urol Clin North Am 1983;10:473.

Duffy PG, Ransley PG: Endoscopic treatment of urinary incontinence in children with primary epispadias. Br J Urol 1998;81:309–311.

Feitz WF, Vangrunsven VJ, Froeling FM: Outcome analysis of the psychosexual and socioeconomic development of adults born with bladder exstrophy. J Urol 1994;152:1417.

Feneley M, Gearhart JP: A history of bladder and cloacal exstrophy. (Abstract.) American Urological Association Annual Meeting, May 1, 2000, Anaheim, California.

Franco I, Culligan M, Reed EF, et al: The importance of catheter size in achievement of urinary continence in patients undergoing a Young-Dees-Leadbetter procedure. J Urol 1994;152:710.

Gearhart JP: Failed bladder exstrophy closure: Evaluation and management. Urol Clin North Am 1991;18:687.

Gearhart JP, Ben-Chaim J, Jeffs RD, et al: Criteria for the prenatal diagnosis of classic bladder exstrophy. Obstet Gynecol 1995a;85:961.

Gearhart JP, Ben-Chaim J, Scortino C: The multiple reoperative bladder exstrophy closure: What affects the potential of the bladder. Urology 1996a;47:240.

Gearhart JP, Canning DA, Jeffs RD: Failed bladder neck reconstruction: Options for management. J Urol 1991;146:1082.

Gearhart JP, Forschner DC, Jeffs RD, et al: A combined vertical and horizontal pelvic osteotomy approach for primary and secondary repair of bladder exstrophy. J Urol 1996b;155:689.

Gearhart JP, Jeffs RD: The use of parenteral testosterone therapy in genital reconstructive surgery. J Urol 1987;138:1077.

Gearhart JP, Jeffs RD: Bladder exstrophy: Increase in capacity following epispadias repair. J Urol 1989a;142:525, 1989b.

Gearhart JP, Jeffs RD: State of the art reconstructive surgery for bladder exstrophy at the Johns Hopkins Hospital. Am J Dis Child 1989b;143: 1475, 1989a.

Gearhart JP, Jeffs RD: Management of the failed exstrophy closure. J Urol 1991a;146:610.

Gearhart JP, Jeffs RD: Techniques to create urinary continence in cloacal exstrophy patients. J Urol 1991b;146:616.

Gearhart JP, Jeffs RD: The bladder exstrophy-epispadias complex. In Walsh PC, et al (eds): Campbell's Urology, 7th ed. Philadelphia, WB Saunders, 1998, p 1939.

Gearhart JP, Leonard MP, Burgers JK: Cantwell-Ransley technique for repair of epispadias. J Urol 1992;148:851.

Gearhart JP, Mathews RI, Taylor S, et al: Combined bladder closure in epispadias repair and the reconstruction of bladder exstrophy. J Urol 1998;160:1182.

Gearhart JP, Peppas DS, Jeffs RD: Complete genitourinary reconstruction of female epispadias. J Urol 1993a;149:1010.

Gearhart JP, Peppas DS, Jeffs RD: Failed exstrophy closure: Strategy for management. Br J Urol 1993b;71:217.

Gearhart JP, Peppas DS, Jeffs RD: The application of continent urinary stomas to bladder augmentation replacement in the failed exstrophy reconstruction. Br J Urol 1995b;75:87.

Gearhart JP, Scortino C, Ben-Chaim J: The Cantwell-Ransley repair in exstrophy and epispadias: Lessons learned. Urology 1995c;46:92.

Gearhart JP, Stec A, et al: Pelvic floor anatomy in classic bladder exstrophy: First insights. J Urol 2001;166:1444..

Gearhart JP, Stec A, et al: Evaluation of the bony pelvis in classic bladder exstrophy: Further insights. Urology (accepted for publication, 2002).

Gearhart JP, Yang A, Leonard MP, et al: Prostate size and configuration in adult patients with bladder exstrophy. J Urol 1993c;149:308.

Geist D: Patent urachus. Am J Surg 1952;84:118.

Glenn JR: Agenesis of the bladder. JAMA 1959;169:2016.

Grady R, Mitchell ME: Complete repair of exstrophy. J Urol 1999;162: 1415.

Gross RE, Kresson SL: Exstrophy of the bladder: Observations from 80 cases. JAMA 1952;149:1640.

Hamada H, Pakano K, Shinah H, et al: New ultrasonographic criterion for the prenatal diagnosis of cloacal exstrophy: Elephant trunk-like image. J Urol 1999;162:2123.

Hammond G, Yglesis L, David JE: The urachus, its anatomy and associated fascia. Anat Rec 1941;80:271.

Hanna MN: Reconstruction of the umbilicus during functional closure of bladder exstrophy. Urology 1986;27:340.

Hanna MK, Williams DI: Genital function in males with vesical exstrophy and epispadias. BJU Int 1969;44:1972.

Hanna MK, Williams DI: Genital function in males with exstrophy and epispadias. Br J Urol 1972;44:1969.

Harcke HT, Capitano MA, Grover WD, et al: Bladder diverticula and Menkes' syndrome. Radiology 1977;124:459.

Hector A: Les vestiges de l'ouraque et leur pathologie. J Surg (Paris) 1961;81:499.

Heitz-Boyer M, Hovelaque A: Creation d'une nouvelle vessie et d'une nouvelle uretre. J Urol 1912;1:237.

Hendren WH: Penile lengthening after previous repair of epispadias. J Urol 1979;12:527.

Hendren WH: Congenital female epispadias with incontinence. J Urol 1981;125:58.

Hendren WH: Ileal nipple for continence in cloacal exstrophy. J Urol 1992;148:372.

Hensle TW, Hirsch AJ, Kennedy WA, et al: Bladder neck closure associated with continent urinary diversion. J Urol 1995;154:883.

Herbst WP: Patent urachus. South Med J 1937;30:711.

Hinman F Jr: Surgical disorders of the bladder and umbilicus of urachal origin. Surg Gynecol Obstet 1961;113:605.

Hollowell JG, Hill PD, Duffy PG, et al: Evaluation and treatment of incontinence after bladder neck reconstruction in exstrophy and epispadias. Br J Urol 1993;140:743.

Hurwitz RS, Manzoni GA, Ransley PG, Stephen FD: Cloacal exstrophy: A report of 34 cases. J Urol 1987;138:1060.

Husmann DA, McLorie GA, Churchill BM: Closure of the exstrophic bladder: An evaluation of the factors leading to its success and its importance on urinary continence. J Urol 1989a;142:522.

Husmann DA, McLorie Ga, Churchill BM: Phallic reconstruction in cloacal exstrophy. J Urol 1989b;142:563.

Husmann DA, Vanderstein VR, McLorie GA, et al: Urinary continence after staged bladder reconstruction in cloacal exstrophy: The affect of co-existing neurological abnormalities on urinary continence. J Urol 1999;161:1598.

Ives E, Coffey R, Carter CO: A family study of bladder exstrophy. J Med Genet 1980;17:139.

Jeffs RD, Charrios R, Mnay M, Juransz AR: Primary closure of the exstrophied bladder. In Scott R (ed): Current Controversies in Urologic Management. Philadelphia, WB Saunders, 1972, p 235.

Johnson JH: Vesical diverticula without urinary obstruction in childhood. J Urol 1960;84:535.

Johnson JH, Kogan SJ: The exstrophic anomalies and their surgical reconstruction. Curr Probl Surg 1974;46:1–39.

Johnston JH: Lengthening of the congenital or acquired short penis. Br J Urol 1974;46:685.

Jones JA, Mitchell ME, Rink RC: Results using the modification of the Young-Dees-Leadbetter bladder neck repair. Br J Urol 1993;71:555.

Kajbafzadeh AN, Duffy PG, Ransley PG: The evolution of penile reconstruction and epispadias repair: A report of 180 cases. J Urol 1995;154: 858.

Kapoor R, Saha MM: Complete duplication of the bladder, common urethra, and external genitalia in the neonate: A case report. J Urol 1987;137:1243.

Keningsberg K: Infection of umbilical artery simulating patent urachus. Pediatrics 1975;86:151.

Kennedy WA, Hensle TW, Riley EA: Pregnancy after orthotopic continent urinary diversion. Surg Obstet Gynecol 1993;177:405.

Klauber G, Williams DI: Epispadias with incontinence. J Urol 1974;111: 110.

Koff SA, Eakins M: The treatment of penile chordee using corporeal rotation. J Urol 1984;131:931.

Koo HP, Avolio L, Duckett JW Jr: Long-term results of ureterosigmoidostomy in children with bladder exstrophy. J Urol 1996;156:2037.

Kossow JH, Morales PA: Duplication of the bladder and urethra and associated anomalies. Urology 1973;1:71.

Kramer SA, Jackson IT: Bilateral rhomboid flaps for reconstruction of the external genitalia in epispadias—exstrophy. Plast Reconstr Surg 1986; 77:621.

Kramer SA, Kelalis P: Assessment of urinary continence in epispadias: Review of 94 patients. J Urol 1982a;128:290.

Kramer SA, Kelalis PP: Surgical correction of female epispadias. Eur Urol 1982b;8:321.

Krisiloff M, Puchner PJ, Tretter W, et al: Pregnancy in women with bladder exstrophy. J Urol 1978;119:478.

Kroovand RL, Boyce WH: Isolated vesicorectal internal urinary diversion: A 37-year-review of the Boyce-Vest procedure. J Urol 1988;140:572.

Krull CL, Hanes CF, DeKlerk DP: Agenesis of the bladder and urethra: A case report. J Urol 1988;140:793.

Lais A, Paolocci N, Ferro N, et al: Morphometric analysis of smooth muscle in the exstrophy-epispadias complex. J Urol 1996;156:819.

Lancaster PAL: Epidemiology of bladder exstrophy: A communication from the International Clearinghouse for Birth Defects monitoring systems. Teratology 1987;36:221.

Langer JC, Brennan B, Lappalainen RE: Cloacal exstrophy: Prenatal diagnosis before rupture of the cloacal membrane. J Pediatr Surg 1992;27;1352.

Lattimer JK: Congenital deficiency of the abdominal musculature and associated genitourinary anomalies: A report of 22 cases. J Urol 1958;79;343.

Lattimer JK, Smith MJK: Exstrophy closure: A follow up on 70 cases. J Urol 1966;95:356.

Lee BR, Perlman EJ, Partin AW, et al: Evaluation of smooth muscle and collagen subtypes in normal newborns and those with bladder exstrophy. J Urol 1996;156:203.

Lelione PM, Gonzales ET: Congenital bladder diverticula causing ureteral obstruction. Urology 1985;25:273.

Lepor H, Shapiro E, Jeffs RD: Urethral reconstruction in males with classical bladder exstrophy. J Urol 1984;131:512.

Levard G, Aigran Y, Farkaji L, et al: Urinary bladder diverticula in Ehlers-Danlos syndrome in children. J Pediatr Surg 1989;24:1184.

Lotteman H, Melon Y, Lombrail P, et al: Reconstruction of bladder exstrophy: Retrospective study of 57 patients with evaluation of factors in favor of acquisition of continence. Ann Urol 1998;32:233.

Lund DT, Hendren WH: Cloacal exstrophy: Experience with 20 cases. J Pediatr Surg 1993;28:1360.

Marshall VF, Marchetti AA, Krantz KE: The correction of stress incontinence by simple vesicourethral suspension. Surg Gynecol Obstet 1949;88:509.

Marshall VF, Muecke C: Congenital abnormalities of the bladder. In Handbuch de Urologie. New York, Springer-Verlag, 1968, p 165.

Mathews RI, Gearhart JP: Ureteral reimplantation before bladder neck repair: Indications and outcome. J Urol (submitted for publication, 2001).

Mathews R, Jeffs RD, Reiner WG, et al: Cloacal exstrophy: Improving the quality of life–The Johns Hopkins experience. J Urol 1998;160:2552.

Mathews RI, Perlman E, Gearhart JP: Gonadal morphology in cloacal exstrophy: Implications in gender assignment. BJU Int 1999a;83:484.

Mathews RI, Wills M, Perlman E, et al: Neural innervation of the newborn exstrophy bladder: An immunohistological study. J Urol 1999b;162:506.

Maydl K: Uer die Radical therapie der ectopia vesical urinarie. Wien Med Wochenschr 1894;25:1113, 1894.

McKenna PH, Khouri AE, McLorie GA, et al: Iliac osteotomy: A model to compare the options in bladder and cloacal exstrophy reconstruction. J Urol 1994;151:182.

McLaughlin KT, Rink RC, Kalsbeck GE et al: Cloacal exstrophy: The neurological implications. J Urol 1995;154:782.

McMahon DR, Kane MP, Husmann DA, et al: Vesical neck reconstruction in patients with the exstrophy-epispadias complex. J Urol 1996;155:1411.

McMillan RW, Schulinger JN, Santucci VT: Pyourachus: An unusual surgical problem. J Pediatr Surg 1973;8:87.

Meizner I, Bar-Ziv J: In utero prenatal ultrasonic diagnosis of a rare case of cloacal exstrophy. J Clin Ultrasound 1985;13:500.

Mendoza CB, Cuerto J, Payan H, Gerwig WH Jr: Complete urachal tract associated with Meckel's diverticulum. Arch Surg 1968;96:438.

Mergurian PA, McLorie GA, McMullin ND, et al: Continence in bladder exstrophy: Determinates of success. J Urol 1991;145:350.

Mesrobian H, Kelalis P, Kramer SA: Follow up of cosmetic appearance and genital function in boys with exstrophy: Review of 53 patients. J Urol 1986;136:256.

Mildenberger H, Lkuth D, Dziuba M: Embryology of bladder exstrophy. J Pediatr Surg 1988;23:116.

Mirk M, Calisti A, Feleni A: Prenatal sonographic diagnosis of bladder exstrophy. J Ultrasound Med 1986;5:291.

Mitchell MI, Bagley DJ: Complete penile disassembly for epispadias repair: The Mitchell technique. J Urol 1996;155:300.

Mitchell ME, Brito CG, Rink RC: Cloacal exstrophy reconstruction for urinary continence. J Urol 1990;144:554.

Mollard P: Bladder reconstruction in exstrophy. J Urol 1980;124:523.

Mollard P, Bassett T, Mure PY: Male epispadias: Experience with 45 cases. J Urol 1998;160:55–59.

Mollard P, Mouriquand PE, Buttin X: Urinary continence after reconstruction of classic bladder exstrophy (73 cases). Br J Urol 1994;73:298.

Monfort G, Morisson-Lacombe GM, Guys JM, Coguel M: Transverse island flap and double flap procedure in the treatment of congenital epispadias in 32 patients. J Urol 1987;138;1069.

Montagnino B, Czyzewski DI, Runyon RD, et al: Adjustment issues in patients with exstrophy. J Urol 1998;160:1471.

Muecke EC: The role of the cloacal membrane in exstrophy: The first successful experimental study. J Urol 1964;92:659.

Narasimharao KI, Chana RS, Mitra SR, Pathak IC: Covered exstrophy and visceral sequestration: A rare exstrophy variant. J Urol 1985;133:274.

Ney C, Freidenberg RM: Radiographic findings in the anomalies of the urachus. J Urol 1968;99:288.

Nix JT, Menville JG, Albert M, Wendt DL: Congenital patent urachus. J Urol 1958;79:264.

Nunn LL: Urachal cysts and their complications. Am J Surg 1952;84:252.

Oesterling JE, Jeffs RD: The importance of a successful initial bladder closure in the surgical management of classical bladder exstrophy: Analysis of 144 patients treated at the Johns Hopkins Hospital between 1975 and 1985. J Urol 1987;137:258.

Patton BR, Barry A: The genesis of exstrophy of the bladder and epispadias. Am J Anat 1952;90:35.

Peppas DS, et al: A quantitative histology of the bladder in various stages of reconstruction utilizing color morphometry. In: Gearhart JP, Mathews RI (eds): Exstrophy-Epispadias Complex: Research Concepts and Clinical Applications. New York, Plenum Publishers, 1999, p 41.

Perlmutter AD, Weinstein MD, Rademan C: Vesical neck reconstruction in patients with the exstrophy-epispadias complex. J Urol 1991;146:613.

Persuit WH, Lenke RR, Kropp K, Chareb C: Antenatal diagnosis of fetal patent urachus. J Ultrasound Med 1988;7:399.

Peters CA, Gearhart JP, Jeffs RD: Epispadias and incontinence: The child with a small bladder. J Urol 1988;140:1199.

Ransley PG, Duffy PG, Wollin M: Bladder exstrophy closure and epispadias repair. In Operative Surgery: Paediatric Surgery, 4th ed. Edinburgh, Butterworths, 1989, p 620.

Reiner WG: Psychosocial concerns in bladder and cloacal exstrophy patients. Dial Pediatr Urol 1999;22:8.

Reiner WG, Bahlberg H, Gearhart JP: Long-term psychosexual dysfunction in the cloacal exstrophy patient. J Urol (submitted for publication).

Ricketts R, Woodard JR, Zwiren GT: Modern treatment of cloacal exstrophy. J Pediatr Surg 1991;26:444.

Rink RC, Retik AB: Ureteroileocecalsigmoidostomy and avoidance of carcinoma of the colon. In King LR, Stone AS (eds): Bladder Reconstruction and Continent Urinary Diversion. Chicago, Year Book Medical Publishers, 1987, p 172.

Ritchey ML, Kramer SA, Kelalis PP: Vesical neck reconstruction in patients with epispadias and exstrophy. J Urol 1998;139:1278.

Rosch W, Christela, Strauss B: Comparison of preoperative innervation pattern and post reconstructive urodynamics in the exstrophy-epispadias complex. Urol Int 1997;59:6.

Schlegel PN, Gearhart JP: Neuroanatomy of the pelvis in an infant with cloacal exstrophy: A detailed microdissection with histology. J Urol 1989;141:583.

Schmidt AH, Teenan TL, Tank ES: Pelvic osteotomy for bladder exstrophy. J Pediatr Orthop 1993;13:214.

Schrenck WR, Campbell WA: The relationship of bladder outlet obstruction to urinary umbilical fistula. J Urol 1972;108:641.

Schrott KM, Siegel A, Schrott G: Fruhzeitige total reconstruktion der blasenexstrophie. In Rodeck R (ed): Verh ber Dtsch ges Urol, 35. Tagung. Berlin, Springer, 1984, pp 383–386.

Shapiro E, Jeffs RD, Gearhart JP, Lepor H: Muscarinic cholinergic receptors in bladder exstrophy: Insights into surgical management. J Urol 1985;134:309.

Shapiro E, Lepor H, Jeffs RD: The inheritance of classical bladder exstrophy. J Urol 1984;132:308.

Silver RI, Partin AW, Epstein JI, et al: Prostate specific antigen in men born with bladder exstrophy. Urology 1997a;49:253.

Silver RI, Sponseller PG, Gearhart JP: Staged closure of the pelvis in cloacal exstrophy: First description of a new approach. J Urol 1999;161:263.

Silver RI, Yang A, Ben-Chaim J et al: Penile length in adulthood after exstrophy reconstruction. J Urol 1997b;158:999.

Spence HM, Hoffman WW, Fosmire PP: Tumors of the colon as a later complication of ureterosigmoidostomy of exstrophy of the bladder. Br J Urol 1979;51:466.

Sponseller PD, Bisson, L, Jani L, et al: Anterior innominate osteotomy in repair of bladder exstrophy. J Bone Joint Surg (Am) (submitted for publication, 2001).

Sponseller P, et al: Premature osteoarthritis of the hip in the older exstrophy patient: A cause for concern (submitted for publication, 2001).

Sponseller PD, Bisson LJ, Gearhart JP, et al: The anatomy of the pelvis in the exstrophy complex. J Bone Joint Surg (Am) 1995;77:177.

Sponseller PD, Gearhart JP, Jeffs RD: Anterior innominate osteotomies for failure or late closure bladder exstrophy. J Urol 1991;146:137.

Steck WD, Helwig E: Umbilical granulomas: Pilonidal disease and the urachus. Surg Gynecol Obstet 1965;120:1043.

Stein R, Fisch M, Bauer H, et al: Operative reconstruction in external and internal genitalia in female patients with bladder exstrophy and epispadias. J Urol 1995;154:1002.

Stein R, Fisch M, Black P: Strategies for reconstruction after unsuccessful or unsatisfactory primary treatment of patients with bladder exstrophy and incontinent epispadias. J Urol 1999a;161:1934.

Stein R, Fisch M, Black P, Hohenfellner R: Strategies for reconstruction after unsuccessful or unsatisfactory primary treatment of patients with bladder exstrophy or incontinent epispadias. J Urol 1999b;161:1934.

Stein R, Stuckel M, Fisch M, et al: Fate of the adult exstrophy patient. J Urol 1994;152:1413.

Sterling JH, Goldsmith R: Lesions of the urachus which appear in the adult. Ann Surg 1953;137:120.

Stiles HJ: Epispadias in the female: Surgical treatment. Surg Gynecol Obstet 1911;13:127.

Surer I, Baker LA, Jeffs RD, Gearhart JP: The modified Cantwell-Ransley repair in exstrophy and epispadias: 10 year experience. J Urol 2001; 164:1040.

Sussman J, Sponseller PD, Gearhart JP, et al: A comparison of methods of repairing the symphysis pubis in bladder exstrophy by tensile testing. BJU Int 1997;79:979.

Sweetser TH, Chisolm TC, Thompson WH: Exstrophy of the urinary bladder: Discussion of anatomic principles applicable to repair with a preliminary report of a case. Minn Med 1952;35:654.

Taccinoli M, Laurenti C, Racheli T: Sixteen years experience with the Heitz-Boyer–Hovelacque procedure for exstrophy of the bladder. Br J Urol 1977;49:385.

Tauber J, Bloom B: Infected urachal cyst. J Urol 1951;66:692.

Taylor WN, Alton D, Taguri A, et al: Bladder diverticulum causing posterior urethral obstruction in children. J Urol 1979;122:415.

Thomalla J, Mitchell ME: Ventral preputial island flap technique for the repair of epispadias with or without exstrophy. J Urol 1984;132:985.

Thomalla J, Rudolph RA, Rink RC, et al: Induction of cloacal exstrophy in the chick embryo with a CO_2 laser. J Urol 1985;134:991.

Toguri AG, Churchill BM, Schillinger JF, Jeffs RD: Continence in cases of bladder exstrophy. J Urol 1987;119:538.

Ulman I, Erguno E, Avanoglua A, et al: The place of Mitrofanoff neo-urethra in repair of exstrophy-epispadias complex. Eur J Pediatr Surg 1998;8:353.

Vakili BF: Agenesis of the bladder. J Urol 1973;104:510.

Verco PW, Khor BH, Barbary J, Enthoven C: Ectopic vesicae in utero. Australas Radiol 1986;30;117.

Vermeij-Keers C, Hartwig N, van der Werff J, et al: Embryonic development of the ventral body and its congenital malformations. Semin Pediatr Surg 1996;5:82.

Williams DI: Congenital bladder neck obstruction in megaureter. BJU Int 1957;29:389.

Williams DI, Keaton J: Vesical exstrophy: Twenty years' experience. Br J Surg 1973;60:203.

Woodhouse CRJ: The management of erectile deformity in adults with exstrophy and epispadias. J Urol 1986;135:932.

Woodhouse CRJ: Sexual function in boys with exstrophy, myelomeningocele, and micropenis. Urology 1998;52:3.

Woodhouse CRJ: The gynecology of exstrophy. BJU Int 1999;83:34.

Woodhouse CRJ, Ransley PC, Williams DI: The exstrophy patient in adult life. Br J Urol 1983;55:632.

Young HH: An operation for the cure of incontinence associated with exstrophy. J Urol 1922;7:1.

Zaontz M, Steckler RE, Shortliffe LM, et al: Multicenter experience with the Mitchell technique for epispadias repair. J Urol 1998;160:1972.

Zarbo A, Kay R: Uterosigmoidostomy in bladder exstrophy: A long-term follow-up. J Urol 1986;136:396.

62
SURGICAL TECHNIQUE FOR ONE-STAGE RECONSTRUCTION OF THE EXSTROPHY-EPISPADIAS COMPLEX

Richard W. Grady, MD
Michael E. Mitchell, MD

Background

Disassembly Technique with Complete Primary Exstrophy Repair—Considerations

Preoperative Care

Postoperative Care

Operative Considerations

Complete Primary Exstrophy Repair Surgical Technique—Bladder Exstrophy
Initial Dissection
Penile-Urethral Dissection

Complete Penile Disassembly
Proximal Dissection
Primary Closure

Complete Primary Exstrophy Repair—Cloacal Exstrophy

Results

Complications

Conclusions

In the effort to effectively treat patients with the exstrophy-epispadias complex, surgeons have come up with a large array of operative procedures. These operations for exstrophy fall largely into **two approaches**. The **first approach** includes operations designed to remove the exstrophic bladder and replace it with a form of urinary diversion. **The second approach includes anatomically oriented procedures designed to reconstruct the bladder either in multiple stages or in a single stage.** Surgeon preference, patient anatomy, previous surgical procedures, availability of tertiary care facilities, and access to medical care all play a role in which operative procedure is chosen for a particular patient. No standard of care exists for this patient population. However, because of the complexity of care involved, specialists with an interest in the exstrophy-epispadias complex usually manage these patients most effectively.

In the late 1980s, one of us (MM) devised an anatomic approach to exstrophy repair that could be performed in one stage. This operation evolved out of a technique developed (by MM) for the treatment of epispadias: the complete penile disassembly technique. This approach allowed the tissue deformation in exstrophy to return most closely to an anatomically oriented position. We have used this approach—the disassembly technique with complete primary exstrophy repair (CPER) or Mitchell technique—exclusively for the surgical treatment of newborns with exstrophy since 1990. We also frequently employ this technique or its principles in reoperative or delayed repairs for exstrophy.

BACKGROUND

The thing that hath been, it is that which shall be; and that which is done is that which shall be done: and there is no new thing under the sun.

ECCLESIASTES 1:9

Anatomic and single-stage operations to repair exstrophy are not new. Trendelenberg attempted to reconstruct an exstrophic bladder to achieve urinary continence at the beginning of the 20th century (Trendelenberg, 1906). This was the first time in recorded history that a surgeon had attempted such a reconstruction, and Trendelenberg did it by reconfiguring the bladder in as anatomically normal a position as could be achieved. **Trendelenberg (1906) used sacroiliac disarticulation and emphasized the importance of pubic reapproximation in front of the reconstructed bladder to achieve continence and prevent dehiscence.** The patient ultimately did not gain continence despite initial urinary control after the operation. These discouraging results led to the abandonment of functional reconstruction of exstrophy by most surgeons for cystectomy and urinary diversion. Ureterosigmoidostomy became the preferred approach to the treatment of exstrophy. Ureterosigmoidostomy remains the first treatment choice in some areas of the world and offers a reliable means to achieve urinary continence for patients who may not have reliable access to health care facilities or who have not achieved urinary continence despite attempts at functional reconstruction (Stein et al, 1999).

Some surgeons still attempted functional reconstruction for children with exstrophy despite the common use of urinary diversion in the early 20th century. Successful results with anatomic reconstruction were sporadic. H. H. Young reported a successful primary bladder closure in 1942 when urinary continence was achieved in a young girl after reconstruction of her exstrophic bladder (Young, 1942). Later, other investigators intermittently achieved satisfactory results with one-stage reconstructive efforts to repair exstrophied bladders. Ansell, an early advocate for primary reconstruction in the newborn with exstrophy, reported a successful outcome with a one-stage closure in a newborn female in 1971. He eventually reported 28 cases closed in this fashion (Ansell, 1971, 1979). Montagnani also described a one-stage functional bladder reconstruction in two female babies aged 8 and 13 months. His bladder reconstruction procedure included innominate osteotomy, bladder closure, an antireflux procedure, and narrowing of the bladder outlet followed by pubic reapproximation. Continence was achieved in one of the two patients. The second patient required further bladder neck reconstruction to achieve continence (Montagnani, 1982). Fuchs achieved urinary continence in 8 of 15 patients who underwent a single-stage repair (Fuchs et al, 1996). Other large series of patients who underwent single-stage reconstruction in the 1960s and 1970s resulted in lower continence rates of only 10% to 30%. Specifically, continence rates ranged from 0 to 45%, with an average of 17% for single-stage reconstructions in these older series (Ezell and Carlson, 1970; Marshall and Muecke, 1970; Cendron, 1971; King and Wendel, 1972; Engel, 1973; Megalli and Lattimer, 1973; Williams and Keeton, 1973; Johnston and Kogan, 1974). Renal damage was as high as 90% in these patients, generally because of bladder outlet obstruction (King and Wendel, 1972).

Because of these complications and the low rate of urinary continence, reconstructive surgical efforts were subsequently directed toward staged bladder reconstruction, an approach pioneered and advocated by Dr. Robert Jeffs and others from the 1970s to the 1990s (Jeffs, 1977; Saltzman et al, 1985). More recently, new techniques of single-stage reconstruction for exstrophy have been advocated by Mitchell, Fuchs, Kelly, and others that appear to be safer than the techniques used in the past. Continence rates in their series approach or equal those reported with a staged surgical reconstruction approach (Fuchs et al, 1996; Grady and Mitchell, 1999). **The single-stage anatomic approach offers many advantages. It offers the possibility to correct the penile abnormalities, bladder abnormalities, and bladder neck abnormalities in one setting. These new techniques also have a lower complication rate than reported in older series of single-stage reconstruction efforts. Finally, urinary continence can be achieved for many of these patients without the need for further bladder neck reconstruction.**

DISASSEMBLY TECHNIQUE WITH COMPLETE PRIMARY EXSTROPHY REPAIR—CONSIDERATIONS

CPER, or Mitchell technique, is optimally performed in the newborn period (Fig. 62–1). Primary reconstruction in the newborn period is technically easier than when performed in a delayed fashion. It also offers theoretical advantages that are now being observed with normal bladder development that may improve the potential for urinary continence. The bony pelvis also remains pliable in the newborn period so that osteotomies may be avoided in some cases—usually if closure occurs within the first 72 hours of life. Neonatal closure by this technique optimizes the chance for early bladder cycling, which may maximize potential for bladder development.

CPER effectively moves the bladder, bladder neck, and urethra posteriorly, thus positioning the proximal urethra within the pelvic diaphragm in an anatomically normal position. This takes advantage of the pelvic muscles and support structures in securing urinary continence. Posterior positioning of the bladder neck and urethra also helps to

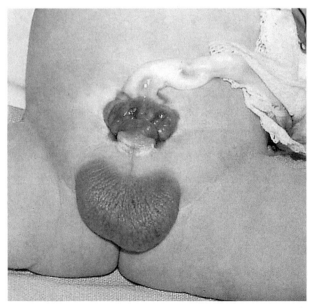

Figure 62–1. Newborn male with classic bladder exstrophy.

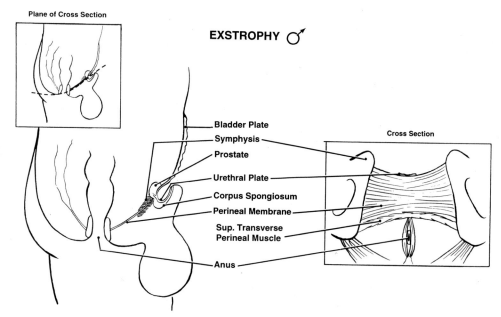

EXSTROPHY ♂

Plane of Cross Section

Cross Section

- Bladder Plate
- Symphysis
- Prostate
- Urethral Plate
- Corpus Spongiosum
- Perineal Membrane
- Sup. Transverse Perineal Muscle
- Anus

Figure 62–2. Schematic cross-sectional drawing of a male infant demonstrating the anterior placement of the urethral wedge in relation to the urethral diaphragm and intersymphyseal ligaments.

reapproximate the pubic symphysis and to create a more anatomically normal muscular pelvic diaphragm.

CPER reduces anterior tension on the urethra and abdominal wall because the urethra is separated from its attachments to the underlying corporal bodies and pelvic diaphragm. Left attached, the urethra will be anteriorly tethered; this prevents posterior placement of the proximal urethra and bladder neck in the pelvis. Tension reduction increases the success of initial primary bladder closure. It also reduces the tension on the corporal bodies that contributes to dorsal chordee and deflection in male children with exstrophy-epispadias. Combining the epispadias repair with primary closure allows for the most important aspect of primary closure—division of the intersymphyseal ligament or band (anterior portion of the pelvic diaphragm)

located **posterior** to the urethra in these patients (Figs. 62–2 and 62–3). This allows for posterior positioning of the bladder, bladder neck, and urethra in a more anatomically normal position. **The goal of the complete primary repair approach is to combine the stages of staged anatomic reconstruction in a single operation (i.e., bladder closure, epispadias repair, and achievement of urinary continence).**

PREOPERATIVE CARE

After delivery, the umbilical cord should be ligated with silk suture rather than a plastic or metal clamp to prevent trauma to the exposed bladder plate. We believe it is im-

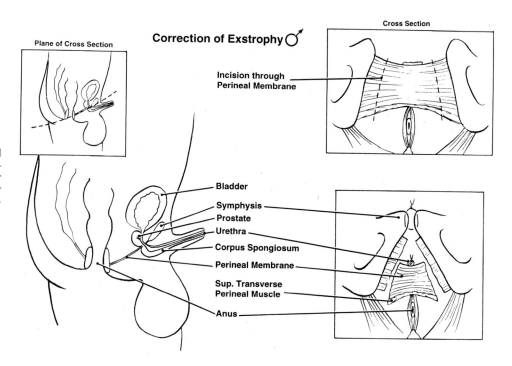

Plane of Cross Section

Cross Section

Correction of Exstrophy ♂

- Incision through Perineal Membrane

- Bladder
- Symphysis
- Prostate
- Urethra
- Corpus Spongiosum
- Perineal Membrane
- Sup. Transverse Perineal Muscle
- Anus

Figure 62–3. Schematic cross-sectional drawing demonstrating the approximation to anatomically normal posterior positioning of the bladder, bladder neck, and urethra achieved after complete disassembly has been performed.

portant to protect the exstrophic bladder against the elements by whatever means are available. We advocate hydrated gel dressings such as Vigilon (Bard Inc., Murray Hill, NJ). This type of dressing is easy to use, keeps the bladder plate from desiccating, and stays in place to allow handling of the infant with minimal risk of trauma to the bladder. The exposed bladder may be covered with plastic wrap as an acceptable alternative. Dressings should be replaced daily, and the bladder should be irrigated with normal saline with each diaper change. Other authors have advocated the use of a humidified air incubator to minimize bladder trauma (Churchill et al, 1997).

We also recommend the routine use of the following measures:

1. Intravenous antibiotic therapy in the preoperative and postoperative period to decrease the chance for infection

2. Preoperative ultrasonography to assess the kidneys preoperatively and to establish a baseline examination for later ultrasonographic studies

3. Preoperative spinal sonographic examination if sacral dimpling or other signs of spina bifida occulta are noted on physical examination

POSTOPERATIVE CARE

The patient must be immobilized to decrease lateral stresses on the closure after any primary reconstructive procedure for exstrophy. A number of options exist for this purpose. We prefer to use a spica cast for immobilization. Spica casting for 3 weeks to prevent external hip rotation and optimize pubic apposition can facilitate early discharge and home care (Fig. 62–4). Modified Buck's traction has been used by many groups for a period of 3 to 4 weeks. A posterior lightweight splint can be used in newborns when the child is out of traction to facilitate home care and early removal of traction. We have stopped using Buck's traction because spica casts are easier for the families to care for at home. External fixation devices have also been advocated by several centers. Fixator pins for

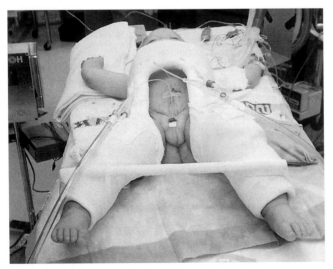

Figure 62–4. The use of the spica cast to maintain immobilization in the postoperative period after complete primary exstrophy repair.

these devices should be cleaned several times a day to reduce the chance for infection. Internal fixation may be necessary in older patients. "Mummy wrapping" should *not* be used to immobilize the pelvis, because it is unreliable (Gearhart, 1999).

Because of the high incidence of vesicoureteral reflux (VUR), we prescribe low-dose suppressive antibiotic therapy for all newborns after bladder closure. This is continued until the VUR is corrected or resolves spontaneously. Postoperative factors that appear to directly affect the success of initial closure include the following (Lowe and Jeffs, 1983; Husmann et al, 1989):

1. Postoperative immobilization
2. Use of postoperative antibiotics
3. Ureteral stenting catheters
4. Adequate postoperative pain management
5. Avoidance of abdominal distention
6. Adequate nutritional support
7. Secure fixation of urinary drainage catheters

OPERATIVE CONSIDERATIONS

In the newborn period, we perform primary exstrophy closure using general inhalation anesthesia. We advise against the use of nitrous oxide during primary closure because it can cause bowel distention, which decreases surgical exposure during the operation and increases the risk of wound dehiscence. Some advocate the use of nasogastric tube drainage to decrease abdominal distention in the postoperative period (Gearhart, 1999). We do not use nasogastric suction in most patients but do routinely use a one-time caudal block to reduce the inhaled anesthetic requirement during the operation.

For patients older than 3 days, and for newborns with a wide pubic diastasis, we perform anterior iliac osteotomies. Osteotomies assist closure and enhance anterior pelvic floor support, which may improve later urinary continence (Aadalen et al, 1980; Ben-Chaim et al, 1995).

Factors that are important in the operative period include the following (Lowe and Jeffs, 1983; Husmann et al, 1989):

1. Use of osteotomies in selected cases and for newborn closures more than 24 to 48 hours after birth
2. Ureteral stenting catheters placed intraoperatively for use in the postoperative period to divert urine
3. Avoidance of abdominal distention
4. Use of intraoperative antibiotics

COMPLETE PRIMARY EXSTROPHY REPAIR SURGICAL TECHNIQUE— BLADDER EXSTROPHY

Initial Dissection

After standard preparation of the surgical field, we place No. 3.5 Fr umbilical artery catheters into both ureters and suture them in place with 5-0 chromic suture (Fig. 62–5). Initial dissection begins superiorly and proceeds inferiorly

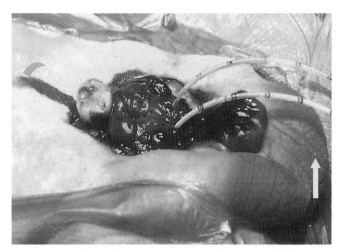

Figure 62–5. The purple markings indicate lines of initial dissection. The curved arrow indicates where the incision is carried above the vessels of the cord so that the umbilicus can be constructed superiorly. Arrow demonstrates stay sutures in hemiglans of the penis.

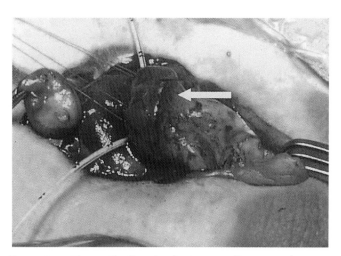

Figure 62–6. The penile dissection begins ventrally. A ventral incision is made at the base of the glans penis (circumcising incision).

to separate the bladder plate from the adjacent skin and fascia. We use fine-tip electrocautery (**Colorado tip** [Stryker Leibinger, Kalamazoo, MI]) during this dissection. The umbilical vessels are ligated, but we leave the inferior aspect of the umbilicus in place and use it as the location to bring out the suprapubic catheter at the end of the operation.

Penile-Urethral Dissection

To aid in dissection, traction sutures are placed into each hemiglans of the penis. These sutures are placed at the beginning of the operation and are initially oriented **transversely** in the hemiglans. The sutures rotate to a parallel vertical orientation as the corporal bodies rotate medially after dissection of the corporal bodies and the urethral wedge (urethral plate plus underlying corpora spongiosa) from each other.

We begin the penile dissection along the **ventral aspect** of the penis as a circumcising incision (Fig. 62–6). This should precede dissection of the urethral wedge from the corporal bodies because it is easier to identify Buck's fascia ventrally. We develop the initial plane of dissection just above Buck's fascia. Buck's fascia stops at the corpora spongiosum during the dissection; therefore, as the dissection progresses medially, the plane shifts subtly from above Buck's fascia to just above the tunica albuginea. Dorsally, methylene blue or brilliant green helps differentiate urothelium from squamous epithelium. Injection of the surrounding tissues with 0.25% lidocaine and 1:200,000 units/ml epinephrine also improves hemostasis, which assists the dissection. The margins of the dorsal urethra are usually obvious. The surgeon must take care not to narrow the urethral wedge, which will be tubularized later. Urethral wedge dissection is carried proximally to the bladder neck. Careful lateral dissection of the penile shaft skin and dartos fascia from the corporal bodies is paramount, because the neurovascular bundles are located laterally on the corpora of the epispadic penis. The lateral dissection of the penis is

always superficial to Buck's fascia because the neurovascular bundles are located laterally in the epispadic penis. Medially, under the urethral wedge, the dissection plane is on the tunica albuginea of the corpora cavernosa.

Complete Penile Disassembly

As described by Mitchell and Bagli (1996), the penis is disassembled into three components—the right and left corporal bodies with their respective hemiglans and the urethral wedge (urothelium with underlying corpora spongiosa). This is done primarily to provide exposure to the intersymphyseal band and to allow adequate proximal dissection. It is easiest to initiate the dissection proximally and ventrally. The plane of dissection should be carried out at the level of the tunica albuginea on the corpora (Fig. 62–7). After a plane is established between the urethral wedge and the corporal bodies, this dissection is carried distally to separate the three components from each other.

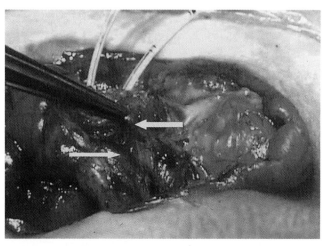

Figure 62–7. White arrows indicate the corpora cavernosa (*inferior arrow*) and the urethral wedge (*superior arrow*). During the dissection of the corpora from the urethra, it is important to keep the corpora spongiosa with the urethra to preserve its blood supply.

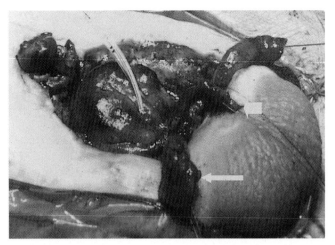

Figure 62–8. Separation of the corporal bodies from each other and the urethral wedge. This dissection is then carried proximally to separate the proximal corpora from the bulbar urethra.

This maximizes the degree of freedom for the best repair. The corporal bodies may be completely separated from each other since they exist on a separate blood supply (Fig. 62–8). It is important to keep the underlying corpora spongiosa with the urethral plate; the blood supply to the urethral plate is based on this corporal tissue, which should appear wedge-shaped after its dissection from the adjacent corpora cavernosa. The urethral/corporal spongiosal component will later be tubularized and placed ventral to the corporal bodies. Paraexstrophy skin flaps *cannot* be used with this technique, because this maneuver will devascularize the distal urethra. Fortunately, because **the bladder and urethra are moved posteriorly in the pelvis as a unit,** division of the urethral wedge is not required. How-

ever, in some cases, a male patient is left with a hypospadias that will require later surgical reconstruction.

Proximal Dissection

Proximal dissection of the urethral wedge from the corporal bodies is critical to the posterior placement of the bladder neck and proximal urethra. Deep incision of the intersymphyseal ligaments posterior and lateral to each side of the urethral wedge is absolutely necessary to allow the bladder to achieve a posterior position in the pelvis (Fig. 62–9). This dissection should be carried until the pelvic floor musculature becomes visible. CT of the pelvis demonstrates that these ligaments lie posterior to the bladder neck and urethra. **Failure to adequately dissect the bladder and urethral wedge from these surrounding structures will create anterior tension along the urethral plate and prevent posterior movement of the bladder in the pelvis.**

Primary Closure

Once the bladder and urethral wedge are adequately dissected from the surrounding tissues, the majority of the procedure is done and the closure is straightforward and anatomic. Before the bladder is reapproximated, a suprapubic tube is placed and brought out through the umbilicus. We then perform a primary closure of the bladder using a three-layer closure with monofilament absorbable suture (i.e., Monocryl and Vicryl [Ethicon, New Brunswick, NJ]). The urethra is tubularized using a two-layer running closure with monofilament and Vicryl suture as well (Figs. 62–10 and 62–11). The tubularized urethra

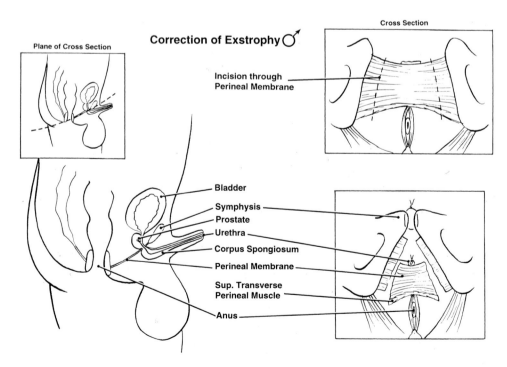

Figure 62–9. Schematic cross-sectional diagram demonstrating incision of the intersymphyseal ligaments to allow posterior positioning of the bladder neck and urethra.

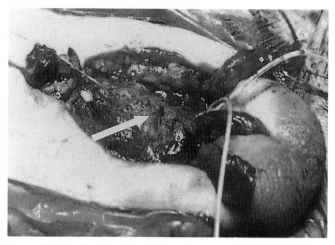

Figure 62–10. The bladder and urethra are reapproximated using running absorbable suture material. The white arrow identifies the reapproximated bladder.

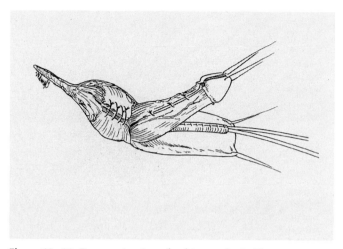

Figure 62–12. Reapproximation of pubis symphysis. The corpora cavernosa are still separated at this point. Knots remain anterior to decrease the risk of suture erosion.

is then placed ventral to the corpora in an anatomically normal position.

We then reapproximate the pubic symphysis using 0-0 polydioxanone interrupted sutures. Knots are left anterior to prevent suture erosion into the bladder neck (Fig. 62–12). Rectus fascia is reapproximated using a running 2-0 polydioxanone suture. Penile shaft skin is reconfigured using either a primary dorsal closure or reversed Byars flaps if needed to provide dorsal skin coverage. Skin covering the abdominal wall is reapproximated using a two-layer running closure of absorbable monofilament suture.

The corporal bodies tend to rotate medially with closure when the lateral margins of Buck's fascia of the corpora cavernosa are approximated. This rotation assists in correcting the dorsal deflection and can be readily appreciated by observing the vertical lie of the previously horizontally placed glans traction sutures. Occasionally, significant discrepancies in the dorsal and ventral lengths of the corpora necessitate dermal graft insertion. However, this is **rarely** needed in the **newborn closure.** The corpora are reapprox-

imated with fine interrupted sutures along their dorsal aspect.

The urethra can then be brought up to each hemiglans ventrally to create an orthotopic meatus (Fig. 62–13). The glans is reconfigured using interrupted mattress sutures of polydioxanone suture (i.e., PDS [Ethicon, New Brunswick, NJ]), followed by horizontal mattress sutures of 7-0 monofilament suture (i.e., Maxxon) to reapproximate the glans epithelium. The neourethra is matured with 7-0 braided polyglactin suture (i.e., Vicryl), similar to our standard hypospadias repair. We also perform glans tissue reduction to create a conical-appearing glans. In roughly half of our

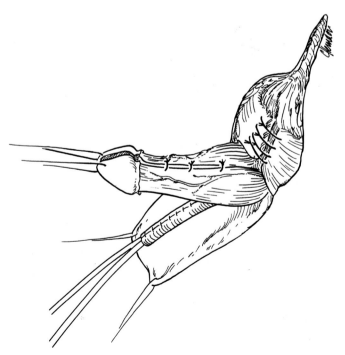

Figure 62–13. Schematic drawing of ventral positioning of the urethra. This allows the bladder and urethra to be positioned posteriorly in an anatomically more normal location.

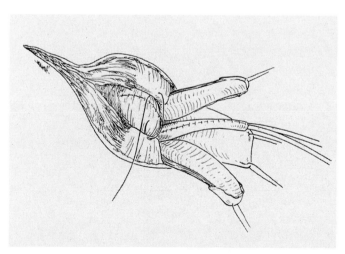

Figure 62–11. Schematic drawing of bladder and urethral closure. The urethra and bladder are closed in continuity.

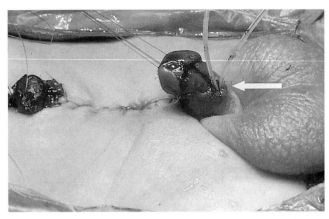

Figure 62–14. White arrow indicates midshaft hypospadias that can occur during closure for the complete primary exstrophy repair (CPER). Hypospadias occurs in this situation because the urethra is too short after the bladder has been positioned posteriorly in the pelvis.

cases, the urethra lacks enough length to reach the glans. In this situation the urethra may be matured along the ventral aspect of the penis to create a hypospadias (Fig. 62–14). This can be corrected at a later date as a second-stage procedure. We often leave redundant shaft skin ventrally in these patients to assist in later penile reconstructive procedures.

COMPLETE PRIMARY EXSTROPHY REPAIR—CLOACAL EXSTROPHY

When possible we perform a one-stage closure for patients with cloacal exstrophy using components of the CPER technique described previously. **The decision to proceed with one-stage closure versus staged reconstruction must be weighed carefully.** The importance of including surgeons experienced in the care of these patients cannot be overemphasized. Factors that affect a decision to proceed with a single-stage reconstruction include the size of the omphalocele, the extent of the pubic diastasis, and coexisting medical conditions. A large omphalocele, in particular, will make single-stage closure hazardous.

When it is not possible to perform a single-stage reconstruction, we prefer to remove the hindgut in its entirety from the exstrophic bladder and then reapproximate the bladder plates (Figs. 62–15 and 62–16). This essentially recreates the anatomy of classic bladder exstrophy. Once the baby has recovered sufficiently to tolerate another surgical procedure, we proceed with functional reconstruction of the bladder, bladder neck, and genitalia using the CPER technique (Plaire and Mitchell, 2000).

Because of the wide pubic diastasis in cloacal exstrophy, pubic reapproximation often requires iliac osteotomies even if the closure is performed within the first 48 hours of life. We determine the need for osteotomies by assessing the lower extremities and external genitalia for ischemia during pubic reapproximation before osteotomies are performed. We have used osteotomies to assist in the reconstruction of the majority of these patients. Other authors prefer to avoid the use of osteotomies because they believe that they make

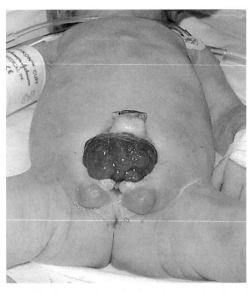

Figure 62–15. Newborn male with cloacal exstrophy. The size of the anatomic defect precludes the use of complete primary exstrophy repair (CPER) as the primary procedure in this patient.

the abdominal closure more difficult (Husmann and Vandersteen, 1999). This has not been our experience.

RESULTS

The important thing is to make the lesson of each case tell on your education.

—Sir William Osler

At our institution, between 1989 to 1999, 24 children with bladder exstrophy (16 boys and 8 girls) and 7 with

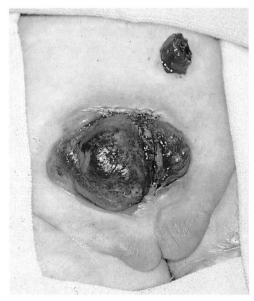

Figure 62–16. The hindgut has been removed and kept in continuity with the remaining intestines. The bladder plates have undergone anastomosis in the midline. The remaining exstrophic bladder defect will be closed later using the complete primary exstrophy repair (CPER) technique.

cloacal exstrophy (5 boys and 2 girls) underwent the disassembly technique with complete primary repair as a primary procedure. Twenty-three patients underwent this procedure during the first day of life.

Initial assessment of the bladder plate preoperatively indicated a very small plate in one patient; the rest were considered satisfactory in size. Operative time ranged from 2.4 to 5.1 hours (median, 4.1 hours). Median operative time in girls was 3.2 hours; in boys, it was 4.7 hours. Estimated blood loss associated with this operation ranged from 10 to 100 ml (median, 45 ml). We performed osteotomies for one patient with bladder exstrophy repaired at 9 months of age, for one patient who was born weighing more than 5 kg, and for three patients with cloacal exstrophy who underwent closure after 72 hours of life.

We reported previously on a series of patients who underwent CPER (Grady and Mitchell, 1999). Follow-up in this group of patients now ranges from 4 months to 10 years (median, 60 months); approximately half of the patients in this series have reached toilet training age. We define urinary continence by the ability to void volitionally in combination with dry intervals of 2 hours or longer. All eighteen patients with bladder exstrophy in this series now have documented dry intervals after primary repair. Overall, urinary continence in this group approaches 80% after toilet training, including 8 of the 10 patients—4 girls and 4 boys—with bladder exstrophy who have reached an appropriate age for toilet training (Grady and Mitchell, 1999).

Of the patients with cloacal exstrophy, two have achieved urinary continence. Both are boys; one of these patients had inclusion of the hindgut in his bladder at primary closure and so effectively has an augmentation cystoplasty. One girl has dry intervals between urinations but is not continent, and one boy is not continent and does not have dry intervals. One of the girls with cloacal exstrophy required bladder neck reconstruction to achieve dry intervals (Grady and Mitchell, 1999; Plaire and Mitchell, 2000).

We monitor all patients with serial ultrasonography. Growth by serial ultrasonographic examinations has been used as a surrogate for serum studies when serum studies were not available. In our series, 12 of 18 patients with bladder exstrophy now have a normal ultrasonographic examination of the kidneys. Six patients demonstrated mild to moderate hydronephrosis in one or both kidneys at their most recent follow-up examination; all of these patients have had less than 2 years of follow-up since CPER. Mild hydronephrosis was also noted in four of the other patients but resolved on serial examination. Of the patients with cloacal exstrophy, three have normal kidneys by ultrasound examination; three patients have mild hydronephrosis. Based on serial ultrasound examinations and serum studies, 98% of the renal units show no evidence of renal deterioration.

As with any other form of anatomic reconstruction, VUR is common after bladder closure using a complete primary repair technique. VUR is seen in the majority of patients in our series. All patients with VUR are maintained on suppressive antibiotic therapy. However, febrile urinary tract infections despite suppressive antibiotic therapy have necessitated neoureterocystostomy in many of our patients with VUR.

Other centers have reported on their experience using the CPER (Mitchell) technique to reconstruct bladder exstrophy. Long-term data are not yet available, but short-term results suggest favorable cosmesis and a low rate of postoperative complications (Hafez et al, 2000).

COMPLICATIONS

Inadequate application of an effective therapy is not a reason to abandon it.

−RUPERT TURNBULL, JR., MD

As is the case with any operation, operative complications can occur after CPER. These include urethrocutaneous fistula formation. In our experience, these fistulas often close spontaneously with proper urinary diversion. Dehiscence of the primary closure can also occur. **After CPER, if the bladder and urethra have been adequately dissected, fascial dehiscence should not jeopardize the bladder and urethral closure.** This is in marked contrast to the devastating consequences of wound dehiscence after a staged primary closure

After CPER, some patients develop bladder and kidney infections. They should be appropriately evaluated to ensure that they have no evidence of outlet obstruction. We routinely maintain our patients on suppressive antibiotic therapy if they have VUR.

Other complications that have been reported after CPER include atrophy of the corpora cavernosa and urethra. These complications can occur if the blood supply to the corporal bodies or urethral wedge is damaged during dissection. These complications have been described after the initial stage of a staged reconstruction as well (Gearhart, 2000). In experienced hands, these complications are unusual. They do underscore the importance of involving surgeons who are experienced in the surgical management of these patients in their care.

CONCLUSIONS

The CPER technique represents a logical extension of previous efforts at anatomic exstrophy reconstruction beginning with Trendelenberg's attempts at the turn of the century. The CPER technique also incorporates principles of the modified Cantwell-Ransley repair and orthopedic reconstruction. The key features of this single-stage technique largely involve the extended dissection that can be effectively performed only by separating the corporal bodies from each other. This extended dissection occurs along anatomic planes and allows the bladder and urethra to move posteriorly into a more normal anatomic position. Bladder reconstruction of the exstrophic patient remains a challenge. The CPER technique will not replace the skills and experience needed to effectively care for these patients. It does, however, offer the promise of improving their care by streamlining the operations these children require and by hastening their time to continence.

REFERENCES

Aadalen RJ, O'Phelan EH, Chisholm TC, et al: Exstrophy of the bladder: Long-term results of bilateral posterior iliac osteotomies and two-stage anatomic repair. Clin Orthop 1980;151:193–200.

Ansell JS: Primary closure of exstrophy in the newborn: A preliminary report. Northwest Medicine 1971;70:842–844.

Ansell JS: Surgical treatment of exstrophy of the bladder with emphasis on neonatal primary closure: Personal experience with 28 consecutive cases treated at the University of Washington hospitals from 1962 to 1977. Techniques and results. J Urol 1979;121:650–653.

Ben-Chaim J, Peppas DS, Sponseller PD, et al: Applications of osteotomy in the cloacal exstrophy patient. J Urol 1995;154:865–867.

Cendron J: Bladder reconstruction: Method derived from that of Trendelenberg. Ann Chir Infant 1971;12:371–381.

Churchill B, Merguerian PA, Khoury AE, et al: Bladder exstrophy and epispadias. In O'Donnell S (ed): Pediatric Urology, 3rd ed. Oxford, England, Reed Elsevier, 1997, pp 495–508.

Engel RM: Bladder exstrophy: Vesicoplasty or urinary diversion? Urology 1973;2:20–24.

Ezell WW, Carlson HE: A realistic look at exstrophy of the bladder. Br J Urol 1970;42:197–202.

Fuchs J, Gluer S, Mildenberger H: One-stage reconstruction of bladder exstrophy. Eur J Pediatr Surg 1996;6:212–215.

Gearhart J: Bladder and cloacal exstrophy. In Gonzales ET, Bauer S (eds): Pediatric Urology Practice. Philadelphia, Lippincott Williams & Wilkins, 1999, pp 339–363.

Gearhart J: Complete repair of bladder exstrophy in the newborn: Complications and management. (Abstract 150.) BJU Int 2000;85(suppl. 4):74.

Grady RW, Mitchell ME: Complete primary repair of exstrophy (see comments). J Urol 1999;162:1415–1420.

Hafez A, Elsherbiny MT, Ghoneim MA: Complete repair of exstrophy: Preliminary experience in neonates and in children with failed initial closure. BJU Int 2000;85(Suppl. 4):72–73.

Husmann DA, McLorie GA, Churchill BM: Closure of the exstrophic bladder: An evaluation of the factors leading to its success and its importance on urinary continence. J Urol 1989;142:522–524; discussion, 542–543.

Husmann D, Vandersteen DR: Anatomy of cloacal exstrophy: The surgical implications. In Gearhart J, Matthews RJ (eds): The Exstrophy-Epispadias Complex: Research Concepts and Clinical Applications. New York, Kluwer Academic/Plenum Publishers, 1999, pp 199–206.

Jeffs RD: Functional closure of bladder exstrophy. Birth Defects Orig Artic Ser 1977;13:171–173.

Johnston JH, Kogan SJ: The exstrophic anomalies and their surgical reconstruction. Curr Probl Surg 1974;1:1–39.

King L, Wendel E: Primary cystectomy and permanent urinary diversion in the treatment of exstrophy of the urinary bladder. In Scott R Jr, Gordon H, Carlton C, Beach P (eds): Current Controversies in Urologic Management. Philadelphia, WB Saunders, 1972, pp 242–250.

Lowe FC, Jeffs RD: Wound dehiscence in bladder exstrophy: An examination of the etiologies and factors for initial failure and subsequent success. J Urol 1983;130:312–315.

Marshall VF, Muecke EC: Functional closure of typical exstrophy of the bladder. J Urol 1970;104:205–212.

Megalli M, Lattimer JK: Review of the management of 140 cases of exstrophy of the bladder. J Urol 1973;109:246–248.

Mitchell ME, Bagli DJ: Complete penile disassembly for epispadias repair: The Mitchell technique. J Urol 1996;155:300–304.

Montagnani CA: One stage functional reconstruction of exstrophied bladder: Report of two cases with six-year follow-up. Z Kinderchir 1982;37:23–27.

Plaire J, Mitchell ME: Single-stage reconstruction of cloacal exstrophy, In Weiner J (ed): New Concepts in the Management of Cloacal Exstrophy. New York, WJ Miller Publishing, 2000, pp 4–5.

Saltzman B, Mininberg DT, Muecke EC: Exstrophy of bladder: Evolution of management. Urology 1985;26:383–388.

Stein R, Fisch M, Black P, et al: Strategies for reconstruction after unsuccessful or unsatisfactory primary treatment of patients with bladder exstrophy or incontinent epispadias. J Urol 1999;161:1934–1941.

Trendelenberg F: The treatment of ectopia vesicae. Ann Surg 1906;44:981–989.

Williams DI, Keeton JE: Further progress with reconstruction of the exstrophied bladder. Br J Surg 1973;60:203–207.

Young H: Exstrophy of the bladder: The first case in which a normal bladder and urinary control have been obtained by plastic operations. Surg Gynecol Obstet 1942;74:729–737.

63
POSTERIOR URETHRAL VALVES AND OTHER URETHRAL ANOMALIES

Edmund T. Gonzales, Jr., MD

Posterior Urethral Valves
　Clinical Presentation
　Pathophysiology
　Management
　Prenatal Considerations
　Prognosis

Anterior Urethral Obstruction

Megalourethra

Urethral Duplication

Prostatic Urethral Polyps

Posterior urethral valves and other congenital obstructions of the urethra are particularly important clinical disorders because severe urethral obstruction results in widespread damage and dysfunction of the entire urinary tract, affecting glomerular filtration, ureteral and bladder smooth muscle function, and urinary continence. Posterior urethral valves remains the single most common urologic cause for renal failure and need for renal transplantation in children. These anomalies are unique to male children. Occasionally girls with bladder outlet obstruction secondary to ureteroceles or neoplasm may present with a similar clinical picture; however, there are no parallel urethral anomalies in girls similar to those described here in boys.

The embryology of the male urethra is complex and is not completely understood. **Development of the urethra can be considered in two separate phases: differentiation of the urogenital sinus portion, commonly known as the posterior urethra, and tubularization of the urethral plate, the anterior urethra.** The mature male urethra is divided into four segments: (1) the prostatic urethra—from the bladder neck to the proximal margin of the urogenital diaphragm; (2) the membranous urethra—the segment that traverses the urogenital diaphragm (the striated sphincter); (3) the bulbous urethra—the portion from the distal margin of the membranous urethra to the penoscrotal angle; and (4) the penile urethra—that segment which traverses the length of the penile shaft, including the glans.

The prostatic and membranous portions of the urethra are not entirely androgen dependent, because these segments of the urethra also develop in the female. However, it is obvious that androgen action on the tissues of the

prostate gland and the mesonephric ducts (the embryologic anlage of the male genital ducts) has a significant impact on final differentiation of these segments of the male urethra.

The bulbous and penile portions of the urethra are uniquely male and are entirely dependent on androgen action for differentiation. The presence of inadequate androgenization in peripheral tissues, as a result of abnormal androgen receptor number or function, 5α-reductase deficiency, or inadequate androgenic steroid production by the testes, results in incomplete tubularization of the anterior segments of the male urethra. These multiple disorders represent the various syndromes of incomplete virilization that can be seen in genotypic (XY) males, spanning the anatomic spectrum from mild degrees of hypospadias to complete phenotypic females (testicular feminization syndrome) (Griffin and Wilson, 1989).

This chapter, however, is concerned with anomalies of the male urethra not known or believed to result from androgen deficiency and includes the following topics:

1. Posterior urethral valves
2. Anterior urethral valves
3. Syringoceles
4. Megalourethra
5. Urethral duplications
6. Prostatic urethral polyps

Normal urethral embryology is described elsewhere. This chapter emphasizes the abnormal embryology, as it is generally understood, to explain the individual anomalies discussed here.

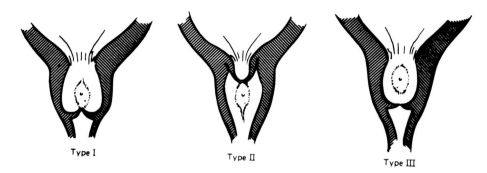

Figure 63–1. The original classification and diagrammatic depiction of urethral valves as presented by Young and coworkers. (Adapted from Young HH, Frontz WA, Baldwin JC: Congenital obstruction of the posterior urethra. J Urol 1919;3:289, with permission.)

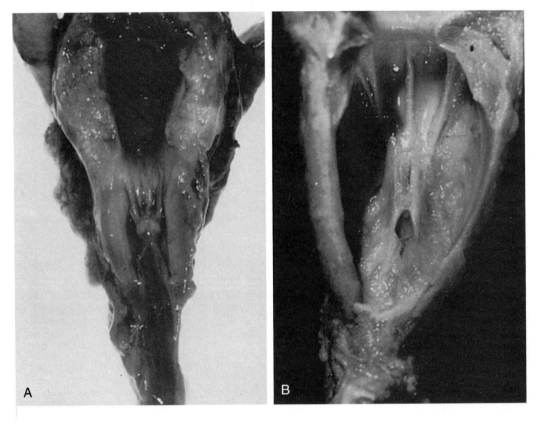

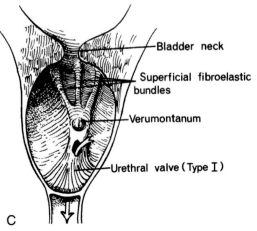

Figure 63–2. *A,* A posterior urethral valve specimen unfolded after an anterior urethra midline incision gives the impression of two folds coapting in the midline. *B,* Another specimen opened by unroofing rather than incision of the anterior urethral wall shows the folds to be an oblique diaphragm fused anteriorly. Note also the proximal folds, which could be confused with type II valves. *C,* Drawing of typical appearance of type I urethral valve. (*B* from Robertson WB, Hayes JA: Br J Urol 1969;41:592, with permission.)

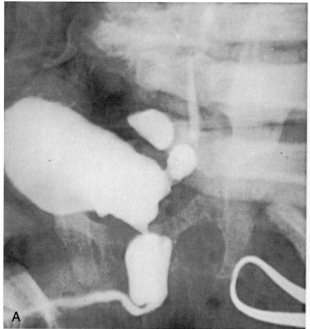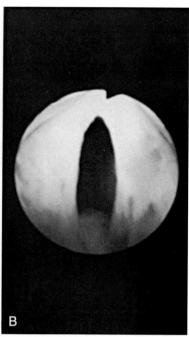

Figure 63–3. *A,* Radiologic appearance of type I urethral valve. Note the bulging anterior membrane, the posteriorly positioned perforation in the valve, the dilated prostatic urethra, and the narrowed and thickened bladder neck. These findings are typical of type I valves when the urethra is viewed in an oblique position. *B,* Cystoscopic picture of type I valve. The verumontanum is the small nodule at the 6 o'clock position.

POSTERIOR URETHRAL VALVES

Dr. H. Hampton Young is generally given credit for the first clear description and classification of posterior urethral valves (Young et al, 1919). He recognized three distinct varieties of congenital proximal urethral obstructions and classified these as types I, II, and III urethral valves (Fig. 63–1).

A type I urethral valve is an obstructing membrane that arises from the posterior and inferior edge of the verumontanum and radiates distally toward the membranous urethra, inserting anteriorly near the proximal margin of the membranous urethra. Although type I valves are usually represented in line sketches as two coapting folds, they actually are a single membranous structure with the opening in the membrane positioned posteriorly near the verumontanum (Robertson and Hayes, 1969) (Fig. 63–2). During voiding, the fused anterior portion of the membrane bulges into the membranous urethra and possibly into the bulbous urethra, leaving only a narrow opening that is compressed along the posterior wall of the urethra. This predictable anatomy gives type I urethral valves a characteristic radiologic appearance (Fig. 63–3). Retrograde passage of a urethral catheter is usually possible without resistance because the catheter slides along the outer surface of the valve and is directed posteriorly to the small opening.

The embryology of type I valves is not completely understood, but it is generally believed that they represent the end result of anomalous insertion of the mesonephric ducts into the primitive fetal cloaca. Normally, the mesonephric ducts insert laterally on the cloaca. As the cloaca folds inward in its midportion to separate the anorectal canal from the urogenital sinus, the ostium of each mesonephric duct migrates posteromedially and cranially to assume a final position at the verumontanum. In the normal male urethra, this pathway of migration persists as the plicae colliculi—delicate mucosal folds that emanate from

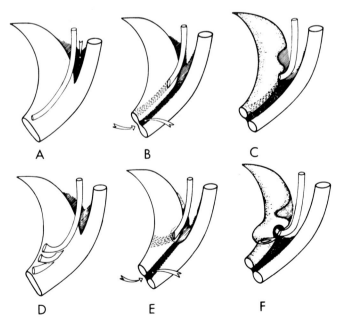

Figure 63–4. Development of type I valves. *A–C,* Development of the normal urethral crest. Migration of the orifice of the wolffian duct from its anterolateral position in the cloaca to the site of the Müller tubercle on the posterior wall of the anorectal septum occurs synchronously with cloacal division (*dots* denote pathway of migration). This wolffian remnant is more lateral and posterior and remains as the normal inferior crest and the plicae colliculi. *D,* Abnormal anterior positions of the wolffian duct orifices. *E,* Abnormal migration of the terminal ends of the ducts. *F,* Circumferential obliquely oriented ridges that compose the valve. (From Kelalis PP, King LR [eds]: Clinical Pediatric Urology. Philadelphia, WB Saunders, 1976, with permission.)

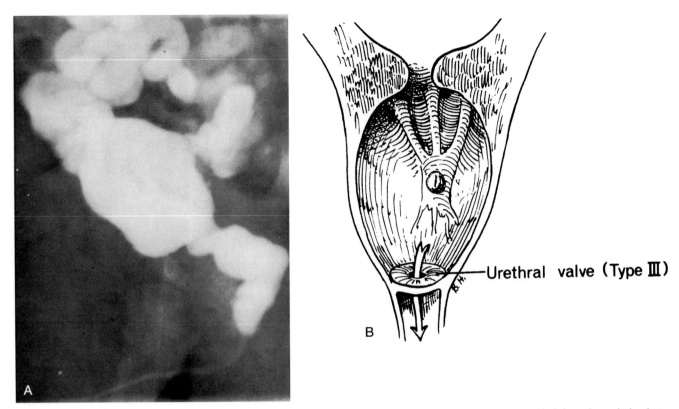

Urethral valve (Type Ⅲ)

Figure 63–5. *A,* Congenital urethral membrane (Young's type III urethral valve) causing severe obstruction with bilateral renal dysplasia; a retrograde catheter could not be passed. *B,* Drawing of typical appearance of type III urethral valve.

the verumontanum in a distal and slightly lateral direction along the posterior (dorsal) floor of the urethra. Type I posterior urethral valves are thought to develop when the mesonephric ducts enter the cloaca more anteriorly than normal. During infolding and separation of the cloaca, their migration is impeded and they may fuse in the midline anteriorly (Stephens, 1983). Children with classic type I valves do not have plicae colliculi (Fig. 63–4). Although the specific mechanisms for development of urethral valves are not clear, genetic factors undoubtedly play a role, because valves have been described in twins (Livne, 1983) and in successive generations (Hanlon-Lundberg, 1994).

Type II urethral valves were initially described as folds radiating in a cranial direction from the verumontanum to the posterolateral aspect of the bladder neck. It is now generally accepted that these folds are not obstructive but rather represent hypertrophy of the thin superficial muscle that runs from the ureteral orifice to the opening of the ejaculatory duct on the verumontanum (muscle derived from the tissue of the mesonephric ducts as the ureter and the vas deferens separate). When there is resistance to urine flow through the urethra, these muscle bands hypertrophy. This is found when true mechanical obstruction is present, but it may also be seen in cases of functional obstruction (neuropathic bladder, detrusor-sphincter dyssynergy).

Type III valves are believed to represent incomplete dissolution of the urogenital membrane. The obstructing membranes are situated distal to the verumontanum at the level of the membranous urethra (Fig. 63–5). Classically described as a discrete, ringlike membrane with a

central aperture, these lesions can assume the most bizarre configurations, depending on the elasticity of the membrane and the location of the perforation in it (Fig. 63–6). Long, willowy folds may prolapse well down into the urethra during voiding and suggest more of a bulbar urethral obstruction—the classic windsock valve described by Field and Stephens (1974) (Fig. 63–7).

Although it is generally accepted that type II valves do not exist, the traditional classification scheme is so ingrained in the urologic vernacular that the usual congenital obstructions of the proximal urethra continue to be described as type I and type III. This accepted classification will be continued for this chapter.

Overall, type I urethral valves make up more than 95% of the lesions in large series; type III valves make up the remainder. However, despite their different embryology, there is no clear difference in the clinical presentation, pathophysiology, or management of children with either type, and the following discussion applies to both anomalies. Although the number of children with type III valves is small, as a group they seem to have a worse prognosis than children with type I valves (Rosenfeld et al, 1994).

The incidence of congenital valvular obstruction is not clearly known, in part because the presentation is variable and different series include patients of many different ages and degrees of obstruction. The incidence is generally accepted to be somewhere between 1 in 5000 and 1 in 8000 male births. However, large screening studies of fetuses with hydronephrosis place the likely incidence slightly higher; in one study (Gunn et al, 1995), the incidence was 1 case of urethral valves in every 1250 fetal ultrasounds.

Figure 63-6. Development of congenital urethral membranes (type III valves). *A–D,* Normal canalization of the urogenital membrane. *D* shows normal slight constriction at the level of the perineal membrane. *E,* Stricture formation. *F,* Canalization by central downgrowth and circumferential ingrowth resulting in bulging membrane with a central stenotic orifice. *G* and *H,* Side openings creating valvular windsock membranes. (Drawings and descriptions supplied through the courtesy of Dr. F.D. Stephens. From Kelalis PP, Kin LR [eds]: Clinical Pediatric Urology. Philadelphia, WB Saunders, 1976, with permission.)

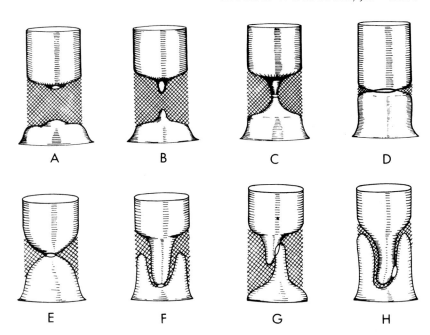

Stephens (1983) suggested the existence of an additional type of proximal urethral obstruction, which he termed a type IV valve. Seen most often in the prune-belly syndrome, these obstructions occur when a flabby, poorly supported prostate folds on itself and causes relative outlet obstruction. This phenomenon is not discussed in this chapter.

Clinical Presentation

Children with congenital posterior urethral obstruction present in a variety of ways, depending primarily on the degree of obstruction. Classically, presenting symptoms are age dependent. In the newborn, palpable abdominal masses (distended bladder, hydronephrosis), ascites, or respiratory distress from pulmonary hypoplasia suggests the possibility of severe bladder outlet obstruction. Other features may include an obstetric history of oligohydramnios (the bulk of the amniotic fluid is fetal urine) and findings in the neonate consistent with Potter's syndrome (dysmorphic facial features, fetal growth retardation, positional limb deformations, pulmonary hypoplasia). The neonate with severely obstructing valves has a very thick-walled bladder that is often easily palpable through the flaccid abdomen of this age group—even when the bladder empties completely. The dilated renal pelves and large, tortuous, tense ureters are often readily felt on abdominal examination.

Neonatal ascites results from many diverse causes, but almost 40% of patients with ascites have urinary ascites secondary to obstructive uropathy, most often infravesical in location (Adzick et al, 1985) (Fig. 63–8) The ascites is thought to represent transudation of retroperitoneal urine across the thin and permeable peritoneum

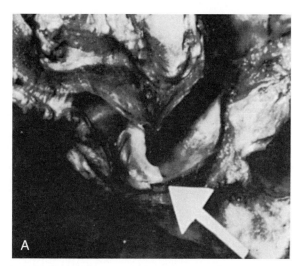

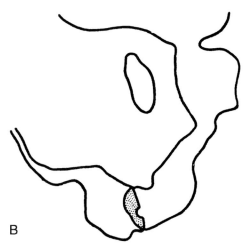

Figure 63-7. Windsock membrane. *A,* Obstructing membrane *(arrow)* attached in membranous urethra and ballooned like a windsock into expanded bulbous urethra (autopsy specimen). *B,* Diagram of the anatomic findings. (From Field PL, Stephens FD: Congenital urethral membranes causing urethral obstruction. J Urol 1974;111:250.)

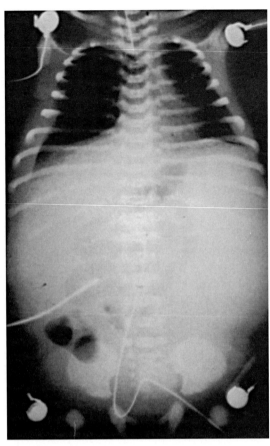

Figure 63–8. Typical radiographic findings with urinary ascites in a neonate, showing the centrally positioned bowel loops, ground-glass appearance of the abdomen, and bulging flanks.

of the neonate. Extravasation may develop at any number of sites, but most often it is seen at the renal fornix (Fig. 63–9). **Although newborns with urinary ascites may develop severe electrolyte abnormalities and life-threatening abnormal fluid shifts shortly after birth, the presence of ascites actually bodes a somewhat more favorable prognosis regarding ultimate renal function than for a similar group of children without ascites** (Rittenberg et al, 1988).

Pulmonary hypoplasia is frequently associated with severe obstructive uropathy, especially when oligohydramnios is present also. Although several theories have been proposed to explain the origin of pulmonary hypoplasia, the most accepted one proposes that oligohydramnios cramps the fetus and prevents normal chest mobility and lung expansion in utero (Landers and Hanson, 1990). These infants have reduced branching of the bronchial tree as well as reduced numbers and size of alveoli.

At birth, these infants are cyanotic and have low Apgar scores. They require immediate pulmonary resuscitation with endotracheal intubation and positive-pressure ventilation, and they may develop pneumothorax or pneumomediastinum, which necessitates placement of chest tubes. Some centers are employing the technique of extracorporeal membrane oxygenation (ECMO) to assist the severely affected infant during the early postpartum period (Dieter and Gibbons, 1990; Gibbons et al, 1993). **Today, most neonates who die as a result of posterior urethral valves**

die from respiratory causes, not from renal or infectious causes. Indeed, newborns with urethral valves and significant pulmonary hypoplasia still have a mortality rate as high as 50% (Nakayama et al, 1986).

Severely affected neonates who are not recognized at birth most commonly present within a few weeks with urosepsis, dehydration, and electrolyte abnormalities. Some infants have only failure to thrive because they develop renal insufficiency. Less commonly, a dribbling urinary stream may call attention to the problem.

Patients presenting during the toddler years are likely to have somewhat better renal function and usually present because of urinary infection or voiding dysfunction. School-age boys—the least common age for presentation—more often have voiding dysfunction, which is usually manifested as urinary incontinence, as their primary complaint (Pieretti, 1993). Not all children presenting late do well, however. In one series, 35% of patients who presented at more than 5 years of age had renal insufficiency, and 10% ultimately developed end-stage renal failure (Bomalaski et al, 1999).

Today, the majority of infants with bladder outlet obstruction are recognized on prenatal ultrasound (Fig. 63–10). **In one series, posterior urethral valves was the cause of fetal hydronephrosis in 10% of all cases of congenital obstructive uropathy recognized by fetal ultrasound evaluation** (Thomas and Gorddon, 1989). Currently, it is estimated that two thirds of patients with poste-

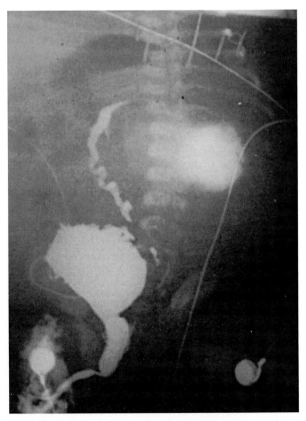

Figure 63–9. Voiding cystourethrogram in the patient with ascites shown in Figure 63–8. In this study, reflux occurred on the left, demonstrating the site of urinary extravasation to be at the renal fornix.

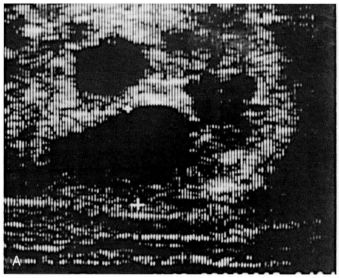

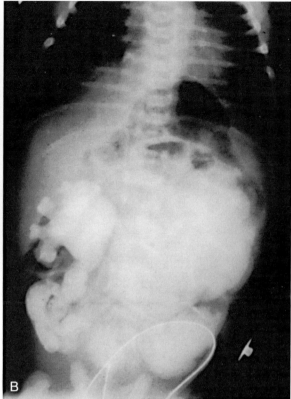

Figure 63–10. *A,* Typical findings with a urethral valve on prenatal ultrasound (bilateral hydronephrosis; distended, thickened bladder). *B,* Postnatal intravenous pyelogram of same patient.

rior urethral valves are identified prenatally (Greenfield, 1997). However, if the ultrasound is performed before the fetus is 24 weeks of age, almost half of infants with urethral valves may be missed (Dinneen et al, 1993; Hutton et al, 1994). Today these infants are evaluated and treated promptly after birth with immediate relief of obstruction and prevention of infection. Our current ability to diagnose this problem before birth also raises the possibility that intervention before birth (percutaneous placement of vesicoamniotic shunts or primary fetal surgery) may better preserve renal and pulmonary function in some babies than if we electively wait to initiate treatment at birth. A more detailed discussion of prenatal diagnosis and the issues surrounding fetal intervention is presented later.

Pathophysiology

Congenital urethral obstruction causes a broad array of abnormalities in the urinary tract, including damage to the renal parenchyma as well as to the smooth muscle function of the ureter and bladder. **These changes may persist despite successful relief of the primary obstruction.** Because urethral valves are present during the earliest phase of fetal development, primitive tissues mature in an abnormal environment of high intraluminal pressures and organ distention. Increasingly, studies are demonstrating that this situation results in permanent maldevelopment and long-lasting functional abnormalities (McConnell, 1989; Keating, 1994). The pathophysiology of the urinary tract associated with congenital urethral obstruction is discussed under five categories: reduced glomerular filtration, abnormal renal tu-

bular function, hydronephrosis (luminal dilatation), vesicoureteral reflux, and detrusor dysfunction.

Glomerular Filtration

The ultimate goal of management of posterior urethral valves is to maximize and preserve glomerular filtration. Although this issue has always been the area of primary concern, it is especially important now because of our ability to suspect the diagnosis of urethral valves with reasonable accuracy in the fetus. Today, decisions regarding management for the unborn, both timing and technique, may have significant impact on ultimate renal function. The data relative to patient survival as well as the anticipated levels of renal function are gradually being revised.

In the early 1980s, 25% of children with urethral valves died within the first year of life, 25% died later in childhood, and the remaining half survived into the young adult years with varying degrees of renal insufficiency (Churchill et al, 1983). Today, a neonatal death from renal insufficiency or sepsis is rare. Dialysis and, ultimately, renal transplantation are available to the youngest babies. Neonatologic and nephrologic support are universally available, and the overall outlook is greatly improved. Children who die within the neonatal period usually die from pulmonary hypoplasia (Churchill et al, 1990). Nonetheless, children with posterior urethral valves may have severe renal insufficiency at birth and may demonstrate gradual loss of renal function over time, the cause of which often remains elusive (Burbige and Hensle, 1987). Deteriorating renal function may result from renal parenchymal dysplasia, incomplete relief of obstruction, parenchymal injury from infection or hypertension and, perhaps, progressive glomerulosclerosis from hyperfiltration.

Renal parenchymal dysplasia is commonly associated with urethral valves. The renal dysplasia tends to be microcystic in nature and develops most severely in the peripheral cortical zone. It has long been suspected that this dysplasia is a result of maturation of the primitive metanephric blastema in the presence of high intraluminal pressures. Experimental data suggest that this probably does play a role. Beck (1971) first reported that cystic, dysplastic changes developed in the kidneys of sheep that underwent ureteral obstruction created in the midtrimester. Subsequent experimental studies by Glick and coworkers (1984) and by Gonzalez and associates (1990) in lambs also demonstrated the development of dysplastic changes in fetal kidneys after creation of fetal ureteral or urethral obstruction.

Henneberry and Stephens (1980), however, argued that the dysplasia seen with urethral valves may also be a primary embryologic abnormality resulting from abnormal positioning of the primitive ureteral bud along the mesonephric duct. In a careful anatomic dissection of the trigone in 11 cases of urethral valves (22 renal units), they noted that, in 11 instances, the ureters were very laterally ectopic (D position) and that these kidneys were more dysplastic than those associated with more normally positioned ureters. Hoover and Duckett (1982) observed that a relationship exists between nonfunction of a kidney (severe dysplasia) and the presence of ipsilateral massive vesicoureteral reflux in patients with urethral valves. Commonly known as the VURD syndrome (*v*alves, *u*nilateral *r*eflux, *d*ysplasia), this finding is thought to be another clinical manifestation of abnormal ureteral budding in this anomaly.

Regardless of the mechanism that initiates abnormal parenchymal histology, it is clear that the development of dysplasia is an early embryologic event. The severity of the renal dysplasia is the single most significant abnormality that will determine ultimate renal function, and it is perhaps the only aspect of this congenital disorder over which the clinician has no impact.

On the other hand, satisfactory relief of the high intravesical and intraureteral pressures associated with urethral obstruction should prevent progressive renal parenchymal damage from the obstruction. Therefore, prompt relief of obstruction is mandatory as soon as the diagnosis is confirmed. What is not clearly known is which therapeutic approach for managing valves (e.g., primary ablation, temporary diversion) is most likely to prevent further damage and allow for maximal recovery of renal function. In the newborn and very young infant, in particular, data have suggested that satisfactory relief of obstruction allows an absolute increase in glomerular filtration (Mayor et al, 1975). It is assumed that this "recovery" of glomerular filtration rate in the very young indicates that hyperplasia has occurred, providing growth of new renal tissue (Hayslett, 1983). This item is discussed in greater detail under specifics of management (see later), but controversy exists regarding the optimal approach to therapy in relation to ultimate renal function.

Other causes for progressive renal failure are recurring urinary tract infection and, perhaps, glomerulo- sclerosis associated with hyperfiltration. Although these children are at risk for recurring urinary tract infection because of the presence of vesicoureteral reflux, ureteral stasis, or incomplete bladder emptying, careful selected surgical intervention and the use of long-term chemoprophylaxis, where necessary, should prevent significant, progressive damage from infection. The significance of hyperfiltration has been very controversial (Brenner et al, 1982). When experimental animals with a significant reduction in renal mass are fed diets that result in a high renal solute load, thereby requiring significant renal work to excrete the metabolic by-products, progressive deterioration of renal function occurs much faster than in a similar group fed a diet with a low renal solute load. Whether this phenomenon might play a role in the child who has had posterior urethral valves and who now has moderate renal insufficiency remains unclear. Of the major food groups, proteins provide a higher renal solute load by weight than either fats or carbohydrates. Experimentally, diets high in protein are most often associated with progressive renal functional deterioration. At this time, however, it is not entirely clear what effect severely limited protein intake in children would have on somatic and central nervous system growth, and there is not yet great enthusiasm for embracing a protein-restricted diet in an infant with significant renal insufficiency (Klahr, 1989).

Several anatomic conditions seen in association with urethral valves appear to be associated with generally improved renal function, presumably by allowing lower intraluminal pressures during fetal development (Conner et al, 1988; Rittenberg et al, 1988). **These conditions include the following: (1) massive unilateral vesicoureteral reflux, (2) large bladder diverticula, and (3) urinary ascites.** In each situation, there is a "pop-off valve," which potentially absorbs high intraluminal pressures and thereby allows the fetal renal parenchyma to develop in a more normal environment. However, one study of 12 boys with valves and massive unilateral vesicoureteral reflux (VURD syndrome) did not support an improved outcome for this group. Sixty-seven percent of the boys had a normal creatinine concentration at 2 years of age, but only 30% were within the normal range at 8 years of age (Cuckow et al, 1997).

Renal Tubular Function

Because high ureteral pressures always affect the most distal aspect of the nephron first, almost half of the patients with posterior urethral valves will have significant impairment of urinary concentrating ability (Dinneen, 1995). In fact, significant urinary concentration defects may be present when the glomerular filtration rate is normal (Parkhouse and Woodhouse, 1990). This abnormality is an acquired form of nephrogenic diabetes insipidus and results in persistently high urinary flow rates regardless of fluid intake or state of hydration. This phenomenon has two significant consequences.

The newborn or infant with a fixed high urinary flow rate is particularly prone to development of severe episodes of dehydration and electrolyte imbalance whenever there is increased fluid loss elsewhere, such as excessive gastrointestinal losses (vomiting, diarrhea), high fever, or third-space fluid sequestration. As long as adequate fluid and electrolytes can be taken orally, the high urinary output is of limited significance. If the infant is unable to maintain adequate oral intake, he or she may rapidly dehydrate because of the persistently high urinary output despite significant total body water depletion.

The second major consequence of high urinary flow involves ureteral and vesical dysfunction. Significantly high ureteral flow rates may cause persistent ureteral dilation that would otherwise seem less significant with a lower urinary flow rate. In addition, high urinary flow rates rapidly fill the bladder. In situations in which poor bladder compliance is present, this means that higher resting bladder pressures are achieved much more quickly. High urinary flow rates can be controlled to some extent with the use of diets that provide a low renal solute load. Hormonal therapy with antidiuretic hormone (ADH) is usually not successful because this renal diabetes insipidus results from damage to the collecting ducts, and these ducts no longer respond to ADH.

Hydronephrosis

In the presence of significant urethral obstruction, ureteral dilatation of varying, but usually considerable, degree is expected. After satisfactory relief of the obstruction, either by endoscopic destruction of the valve or by vesicostomy, gradual but substantial reduction in the degree of hydronephrosis usually occurs (Fig. 63–11) When this does not happen, several specific diagnostic possibilities must be investigated to elucidate the cause of the problem. Is the persisting dilatation a result of true ureterovesical junction (UVJ) obstruction? Is the ureteral musculature faulty and unable to generate effective peristalsis (Gearhart et al, 1995)? In this situation, the dilatation of the ureters may be a permanent facet of the child's disorder. Could these changes be the result of high intravesical pressures, or could they be secondary to high urinary flow rates? Each of these factors may play a role in an individual case.

Johnston and Kulatilake (1971) demonstrated many years ago that it may take years after primary valve ablation for final improvement in ureteral caliber to occur. They suggested that the responsible physician should not be anxious to proceed with further surgical therapy on the ureter in young infants as long as renal function is stable and urinary infection is controlled. When it is evident that substantial recovery is not going to occur, then it becomes necessary to address the role of each of the issues noted previously (Fig. 63–12).

Properly performed vesical urodynamic studies are essential. If the child has a noncompliant bladder associated with high intravesical pressures, this condition must be corrected before any attempt at surgical remodeling of the ureter is considered. Addressing the bladder dysfunction may be sufficient to allow the hydronephrosis to resolve. An accurate assessment of a timed urinary volume is also an important factor in this evaluation. As noted previously, many children who have had urethral valves have significant hyposthenuria and excrete very large urinary volumes. As in children with primary diabetes insipidus, this excessive, high-flow state may also contribute to persistent ureteral dilatation.

The most controversial issue has been the evaluation and assessment of the presence of true UVJ obstruction. For many years it was thought that the lower ureter and UVJ were abnormal (and thus obstructing) in children with urethral valves, or that the thickened detrusor impaired effective ureteral emptying. Hence, reduction ureteroplasty and ureteral reimplantation were encouraged. In 1973, Whitaker introduced the concept of percutaneous antegrade pressure/perfusion studies to more objectively assess whether obstruction was truly present. In a series of 70 patients with persisting hydronephrosis after valve destruction, he demonstrated that true UVJ obstruction was rare. Subsequent series by Tietjen (1997), Glassberg (1982), and Smith (1996) and their colleagues confirmed Whitaker's initial observations. Therefore, it would seem that surgical reconstruction of the distal ureter and UVJ is rarely indicated and should be considered only after thorough investigation of all possible causes for the persisting hydronephrosis has been completed.

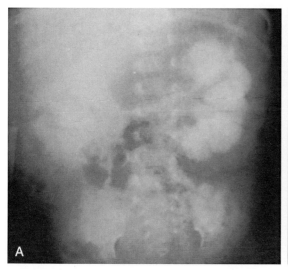
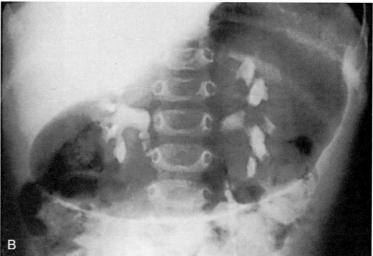

Figure 63–11. *A,* Initial intravenous pyelogram (IVP) at the time of diagnosis of posterior urethral valves. *B,* IVP 3 months after valve ablation alone, showing marked reduction in the degree of hydronephrosis.

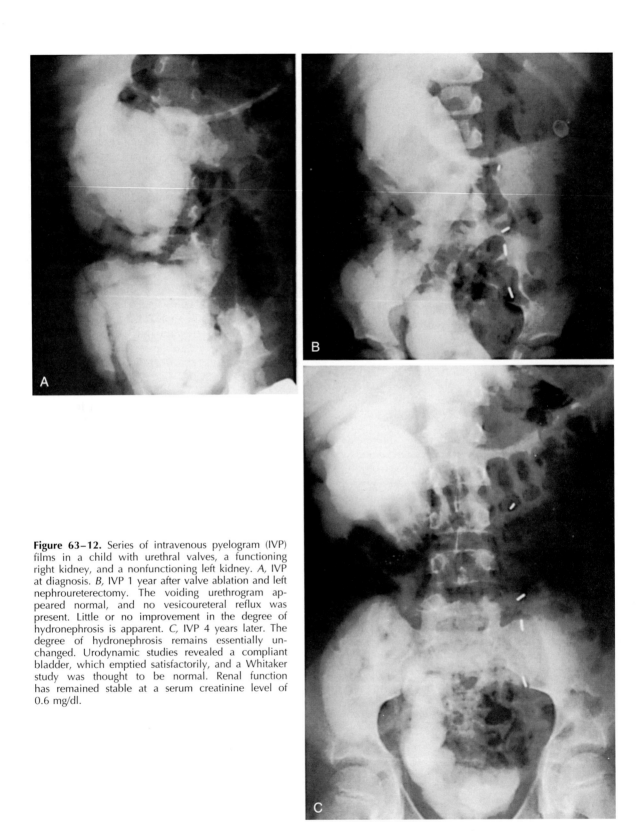

Figure 63–12. Series of intravenous pyelogram (IVP) films in a child with urethral valves, a functioning right kidney, and a nonfunctioning left kidney. *A,* IVP at diagnosis. *B,* IVP 1 year after valve ablation and left nephroureterectomy. The voiding urethrogram appeared normal, and no vesicoureteral reflux was present. Little or no improvement in the degree of hydronephrosis is apparent. *C,* IVP 4 years later. The degree of hydronephrosis remains essentially unchanged. Urodynamic studies revealed a compliant bladder, which emptied satisfactorily, and a Whitaker study was thought to be normal. Renal function has remained stable at a serum creatinine level of 0.6 mg/dl.

Vesicoureteral Reflux

Vesicoureteral reflux (VUR) is commonly found in association with posterior urethral valves. Between one third and one half of these children have reflux at the time of initial diagnosis. Most often, this represents secondary VUR resulting from high intravesical pressures, development of paraureteral diverticula, and loss of ureterovesical valvular competence. In some instances, however, the reflux is primary and may be caused by a ureteral bud anomaly. As noted previously, Henneberry and Stephens (1980), in their study of fetuses and newborn infants with severe posterior urethral valves, reported a significant incidence of lateral ectopia of the ureteral orifice.

The presence of VUR has long been associated with a poorer prognosis in patients with urethral valves. As early as 1979, Johnston reported on a series of patients in which those with bilateral reflux had a much higher mortality rate (57%) than those without reflux (9%). Those with unilateral VUR fell in between, at 17%. Parkhouse and coworkers (1988) confirmed this observation a decade later with a second series of patients who were observed for up to 20 years. The specific mechanisms relating VUR to increased renal parenchymal damage remain unknown.

The presence of VUR should not in itself influence the initial management of children with posterior urethral valves (Johnston, 1979). **In about one third of cases, the reflux resolves spontaneously after obstruction is eliminated.** In another one third of the cases, the reflux persists but is no problem as long as chemoprophylaxis is maintained. Decisions regarding reimplantation then should be made after a period of observation following initial valve ablation, as long as urinary infection is able to be controlled with maintenance chemoprophylaxis. Even if reflux persists, dilated ureters usually decrease in caliber over time. If reimplantation is ultimately necessary, this surgery probably can be accomplished without extensive tailoring or remodeling of the ureter. About one third of the patients have problems associated with their reflux during follow-up and are best managed by earlier reimplantation.

Vesical Dysfunction

For many years, it has been recognized that most children treated for urethral valves have varying degrees of abnormal bladder function. Most often, this abnormality presents as urinary incontinence, with half of the boys still damp during the day well into late childhood (Parkhouse et al, 1988; Churchill et al, 1990). In the past, investigators assumed that this incontinence was primarily a result of incompetent sphincter function caused by either primary maldevelopment of the membranous urethra and bladder neck (because of the anatomic location of the valve at the level of the voluntary sphincter, causing distention and dilatation of that region of the urethra during embryogenesis) or by direct injury to the sphincter at the time of endoscopic valve ablation. However, with the application of modern urodynamics to pediatric urology, it has become increasingly obvious that primary vesical dysfunction is commonly present in association with urethral valves, that this vesical dysfunction does not necessarily abate after relief of the obstruction, and that, ultimately, this abnormal bladder function has a significant impact on prognosis.

Tanagho (1974) and Lome and associates (1972) first brought attention to the difficulties encountered in establishing adequate bladder volume after a period of bladder defunctionalization in some children with urethral valves (usually after high loop urinary diversion). Review of these data from the 1960s and 1970s shows that many children included in these series had also had had previous bladder surgery or placement of indwelling suprapubic tubes for initial management of the urethral valves. How much impact this previous bladder surgery had on final bladder function was not clearly defined. Subsequently, several groups of investigators, including Glassberg (1982), Bauer (1979), Campaiola (1985), and Peters (1990) and their coworkers, reported several abnormalities of detrusor function, including primary myogenic failure, uninhibited bladder activity, and findings consistent with poor compliance of the detrusor muscle in children with urethral valves. **In a more recent study, Holmdahl and associates (1995) demonstrated that urodynamic patterns can change when bladder function is evaluated over time in infants with urethral valves.** In this study of 16 infants, all patients had urodynamic testing before valve ablation and were monitored with serial urodynamic studies postoperatively. In all boys preoperatively, the bladder was small in capacity and hypercontractile. After destruction of the valves, the bladder capacity increased, although the bladder continued to show some instability and some boys demonstrated incomplete emptying. Holmdahl and colleagues (1996) subsequently reported on a second series of boys with follow-up into late adolescence. They observed that the pattern of bladder abnormality changed as the children got older, progressing from instability during infancy to findings more consistent with myogenic failure in older boys.

The cause for the detrusor dysfunction remains unclear, although experimental evidence suggests that fetal urethral obstruction results in irreversible changes in the organization and function of the smooth muscle cells of the bladder (Karim, 1992, 1993) and may also result in deposition of abnormal quantity and type of intercellular collagen (Keating, 1994; Peters, 1994).

Ultimately boys with incontinence do achieve dryness in the majority of cases (Parkhouse et al, 1988; Smith, 1996), **but the primary bladder dysfunction may also be a factor causing renal function to deteriorate.** Parkhouse and associates (1988) monitored their series of children with urethral valves into adolescence. They observed that those who were incontinent during childhood ultimately developed more severe degrees of renal insufficiency during adolescence than did the children who had demonstrated normal urinary control. They proposed that boys who were incontinent had more severe bladder dysfunction than boys who had normal urinary control. Presumably, at puberty, the persisting detrusor abnormality, along with the development of the prostate, which increases outlet resistance, improves continence but raises intravesical pressures, resulting in unfavorable effects on renal function. Unfortunately, routine urodynamic studies were not consistently performed in all of these children to unquestionably support these observations and conclusions.

Depending on the extent and nature of bladder dysfunction and the ability of the bladder to empty, management may consist of anticholinergic therapy to reduce uninhibited detrusor contractions; clean, inter-

mittent catheterization to afford satisfactory bladder emptying; or bladder augmentation to improve bladder volume and compliance (Glassberg, 1985). In older, cooperative boys, a program of planned, timed voidings might keep bladder volumes sufficiently low that intravesical pressures remain acceptable.

Management

Management of posterior urethral valves depends on the degree of renal insufficiency as well as the age of the child. Older children who present with voiding dysfunction or urinary tract infection but satisfactory renal function are easily and effectively treated initially by endoscopic destruction of the urethral valve alone. Decisions concerning selective surgery for persisting VUR, lingering UVJ obstruction (uncommon), or detrusor dysfunction are made on an individual basis.

The main controversies related to treatment of urethral valves involve the very young infant. In these situations, it is believed that there is a potential for recovering some renal function. In addition, the increasing recognition of urethral valves in the fetus raises ongoing questions about timing for intervention and offers the responsible physician an opportunity to perform procedures that will decompress the urinary tract and allow for maximal recoverability of renal function during a period when growth of new renal tissue is ongoing.

In the past, most infants with urethral valves presented because of urosepsis or failure to thrive. At presentation these infants were often dehydrated and had renal insufficiency, severe acidosis, and electrolyte abnormalities. In any case, management usually began with placement of a small transurethral catheter to provide unobstructed vesical drainage and the initiation of appropriate antibiotics and parenteral fluid rehydration. A small feeding tube was preferred rather than a Foley catheter because of concerns that the retention balloon might increase detrusor irritability and spasm and impair urethral drainage. Initiation of these measures allowed for immediate improvement of renal function in most cases. In general, 5 to 7 days of catheter drainage allowed for adequate assessment of the existing level of glomerular filtration. In this situation, much of the improvement in renal function probably reflected improved hydration and renal parenchymal perfusion rather than relief of obstruction alone.

Currently, more patients with posterior urethral valves are being recognized by observation of hydronephrosis on prenatal ultrasound than by one of the more traditional histories just described. At birth, these children have renal function parameters equivalent to maternal renal function. **The placement of a urethral catheter and initiation of prophylactic antibiotic management allow for assessment of the baseline level of renal function during the first few days after birth. In each of these situations, further management is dictated by the level of renal function.**

In the presence of normal or satisfactory renal function (most often described as a serum creatinine concentration of less than 1.0 mg/dl in the newborn after several days of catheter drainage, although a healthy neonate at 4 weeks of age may have a concentration of 0.2 to 0.4 mg/dl), endoscopic destruction of the valves would be preferred in all cases. Today, endoscopes with excellent optics are available in sufficiently small caliber for even the tiniest newborn. Most systems accept small operating cautery electrodes sufficient for destruction of the valve. For the child whose urethra is too small to accept the available endoscopes, antegrade destruction of the valve by percutaneous access to the bladder was described by Zaontz and Firlit (1985). McAninch (personal communication) suggested that this technique is made easier by use of the rigid ureteroscope. The longer instrument allows the endoscopist increased maneuverability—one of the limiting factors in this technique when the short pediatric cystoscope is used. Other techniques employed for primary destruction of urethral valves include use of the neodymium: yttrium-aluminum-garnet laser (Ehrlich and Shanberg, 1988; Biewald and Schier, 1992) and the potassium titanyl phosphate (KTP)-532 laser (Gholdoian et al, 1998); the cautery hook as originally described by Williams and improved by Deane and coworkers (1988); the antegrade extraction of a balloon catheter (Kolicinski, 1988); and the valvulotome (Cromie et al, 1994).

Valve ablation must be done carefully. Only a single wire (not a loop) or a small electrode should be used. The current on the electrosurgical unit should be set at a level just sufficient to incise the valve but not so high as to diffuse thermal injury to surrounding urethral tissues. I prefer to incise the valve at the 4 o'clock, 8 o'clock and 12 o'clock positions but I believe that the 12 o'clock incision is most important, because it is the one that separates the anteriorly fused membrane. The cautery wire or electrode is advanced in a retrograde fashion from the proximal margin of the membranous urethra into the dilated prostatic urethra (Fig. 63–13). If the bladder is distended during the valvulotomy, the increased luminal pressure balloons the valve, making retrograde incision easy and safe. A Credé cystogram on the operating table can confirm that the obstruction has been adequately relieved. This approach significantly minimizes the risk of injury to the urethral sphinc-

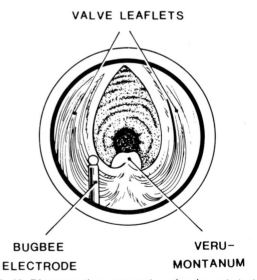

VALVE LEAFLETS

BUGBEE ELECTRODE

VERUMONTANUM

Figure 63–13. Diagrammatic representation of endoscopic incision of type I posterior urethral valve. Note that the electrode is positioned distal to the valve and will be advanced toward the prostatic urethra. (From Kaplan GW, Scherz HC: Infravesical obstruction. In Kelalis PP, King LR, Belman AB [eds]: Clinical Pediatric Urology, 3rd ed. Philadelphia, WB Saunders, 1992, p 846, with permission.)

ter, which might occur if the valve is pulled down in an antegrade fashion by the resectoscope wire. A small transurethral catheter may be left in place for 1 or 2 days but usually is not needed.

After satisfactory destruction of the valve is accomplished, the child should be observed expectantly with regular estimates of renal function as well as imaging studies to assess whether improvement occurs in the degree of hydronephrosis or VUR. A follow-up voiding cystourethrogram is usually done 2 months after the valve ablation to be sure that the obstruction was satisfactorily relieved. If renal function remains stable and infection is avoided (chemoprophylaxis is generally recommended), improvement in the anatomy of the urinary tract and continued stabilization of renal function can be expected. The improvement in ureteral dilation may be gradual and may take months, or occasionally years.

Careful endoscopic destruction of valves, even in the newborn, has not been associated with a significant incidence of urethral stricture. Nijman and Scholtmeyer (1991) reported an incidence of only 5% urethral injury in a group of 85 boys undergoing electroincision of urethral valves. **In the unusual situation in which the newborn urethra seems too small to accommodate the available endoscopes, an elective vesicostomy is appropriate and safe.** Indeed, Walker preferred a vesicostomy rather than endoscopic ablation in the neonate, believing that this technique is safer and reduces the incidence of urethral strictures (Walker and Padron, 1990). However, a review of this approach did not suggest any benefit in overall improvement of renal function, compared with endoscopic management of valves only (Walker and Padron, 1990). Performing a vesicostomy does not appear to harm ultimate bladder function (Kim et al, 1996).

The major area of continuing controversy involves the most appropriate approach to treating the infant who has significant renal insufficiency that persists after a satisfactory period of transurethral drainage. The options for managing this group of children include endoscopic destruction of the urethral valves only, elective vesicostomy, or a supravesical temporizing ureteral diversion. The issue of concern is which therapeutic approach maximizes recoverability of renal function and brings the urodynamics of the upper urinary tract most nearly to normal (Gonzales, 1990).

During the 1960s, high-loop ureterostomy was a commonly performed approach for the initial management of infants with urethral valves (Johnston, 1963). After ureterostomy, renal function usually improved initially and then remained stable, ureteral diameter decreased, and the infant often exhibited surprisingly good health. Reconstruction of the ureters and valve ablation was then done electively within 1 to 2 years in a larger, more robust child.

During the same period, a few investigators experimented with various techniques to destroy valves transurethrally. Johnston (1966) demonstrated that many infants treated in this manner also showed stabilization or improved renal function and gradual, but progressive, reduction in the degree of hydronephrosis. When better endoscopes became available in the 1970s, most pediatric urologists switched to primary endoscopic destruction as their preferred form of management.

Krueger and associates, in 1980, published a provocative article that compared two series of children with posterior

urethral valves: one group treated by high-loop ureterostomy and a second group treated by endoscopic ablation only. Their data suggested that children who presented with renal insufficiency and who were managed by high-loop cutaneous ureterostomy ultimately showed improved glomerular filtration rate and somatic growth potential when compared with similar children managed by endoscopic destruction of valves only. They proposed that high-loop diversion is probably better at lowering ureteral luminal pressures and thereby allows the renal parenchyma to recover in a more nearly normal environment, compared with valve ablation only. This report was challenged by Duckett and Norris (1989) and Reinberg (1992) on the basis that it was not a controlled study and that similar data of their own did not support this conclusion, with comparable groups treated by valve ablation or temporizing diversion showing no difference in outcome. This area remains controversial, although fewer temporizing diversions are being done now than in the recent past, because no one has proven that temporary diversion of any type truly improves ultimate renal function in the long term. In addition, Close and associates (1997) have suggested that preservation of bladder cycling in the newborn by doing valve ablation initially may be very important in preserving more normal bladder function.

The decision to proceed with a high-loop ureterostomy is a significant one, because it commits the child to a major reconstructive procedure later, with its attendant complications. Severe urosepsis that does not respond to appropriate chemotherapy would be one indication, but similar results today can usually be achieved by placing percutaneous nephrostomy tubes—a less morbid procedure that sometimes can be done even without general anesthesia. More often, the decision to perform a temporizing urinary diversion depends on whether this procedure is likely to offer the child overall improved renal function. The study by Krueger and associates (1980) does have certain experimental design flaws, especially when one considers that two separate groups collected at different times and managed arbitrarily by two different techniques were compared without a true control group. Considering all these variables, as well as the observation that within the first few months after birth the kidney may continue to grow new cells (as evidenced by increased DNA content) (Hayslett, 1983), I believe there is still a place for occasional use of temporizing diversion in these infants. My own criterion is a nadir serum creatinine concentration of 2.0 mg/dl or greater after several days of transurethral catheter drainage. However, in this situation, careful discussion with the parents is essential, because no clear, objective data exist to know how the procedure will affect the ultimate outcome.

It is important to remember that the "valve bladder" may be very irritable, and placement of an indwelling catheter can induce severe detrusor spasm with secondary ureteral obstruction. Noe and Jerkins (1983) observed an infant who was anuric during the period of transurethral catheterization but had normal renal function after loop ureterostomy. A similar observation was reported by Jordan and Hoover (1985). The infant who has a high nadir creatinine concentration on catheter drainage that falls to near-normal levels immediately after ureterostomy probably represents the same phenomenon. The purpose of considering a temporizing diversion is long-term, gradual improvement in renal function through maximization of renal growth potential, not immediate improvement in renal function. It is prudent during the period of catheter drainage, if renal function does not improve to satisfactory levels, to consider anticholinergic therapy to reduce detrusor spasm.

If the decision is made to proceed with a diversion, I recommend a vesicostomy if bilateral VUR is present, a ureterostomy if reflux is not present on at least one side. Several techniques have been described to perform loop ureterostomies (Fig. 63–14). I prefer a single-loop procedure (Novak and Gonzales, 1978). The more complex procedures require more operative time and incur a greater risk of immediate surgical complications (Sober, 1972; Williams and Cromie, 1975). These procedures are being done in the sickest infants, and I recognize no significant benefit from making the procedure more complex, although the latter two techniques do allow some urine to reach the bladder and maintain bladder cycling.

Vesicostomy is technically easy to perform and to close, and it has not been shown to decrease ultimate bladder capacity. Care must be taken to place the stoma high on the bladder (beyond the urachus) to minimize the risk of vesical prolapse. The Blocksom vesicostomy is simple and effective in the infant because the bladder is an abdominal organ and skin flaps or detrusor flaps are not necessary to reach the anterior abdominal wall without tension (Fig. 63–15). Stomal stenosis may occur, but usually it is easily managed either by simple dilatation and initiation of intermittent catheterization of the stoma or by revision of the cicatricial band.

Several years ago, there was enthusiasm by some surgeons to proceed in short order with total reconstruction of the urinary tract when significant decompression of the upper tracts did not occur quickly after endoscopic destruction of the valve (Hendren, 1971). This included reduction ureteroplasty and ureteral reimplantation in very young infants with thick-walled, dysfunctional bladders. It was believed that this procedure was indicated to relieve possible obstruction at the UVJ, reduce urinary stasis, improve the effectiveness of ureteral peristalsis, and minimize the risk of urinary infection. Although this approach to management has been shown to be safe in skilled hands, enthusiasm for early major reconstruction has waned because there is no convincing evidence that it provides better results than the more selective approach described previously. Over the two past decades, it has come to be recognized that true UVJ obstruction is uncommon in children with urethral valves. **In addition, improved understanding of the dysfunctional aspects of the valve bladder has focused more attention on the bladder as a major lingering cause for progressive renal deterioration in children with urethral valves.**

Prenatal Considerations

Today, many, probably most, patients with urethral valves are recognized on prenatal ultrasound. If one accepts that some of the renal parenchymal damage associated with urethral valves is progressive, then it is reasonable to ask

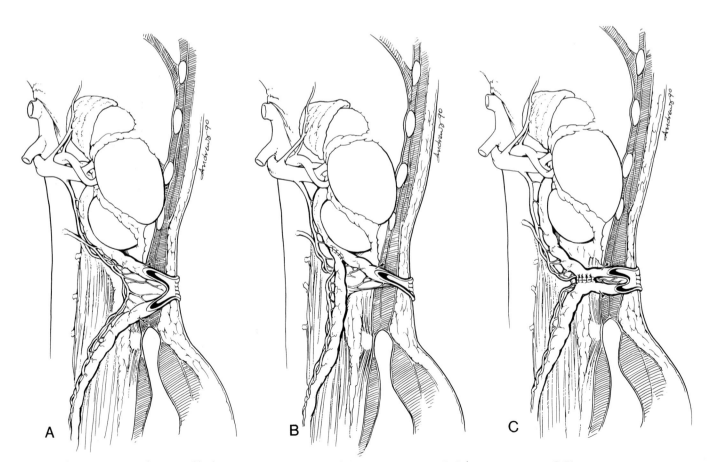

Figure 63–14. Techniques of high cutaneous ureterostomy. A, Loop ureterostomy. B, Sober ureterostomy. C, Ring ureterostomy.

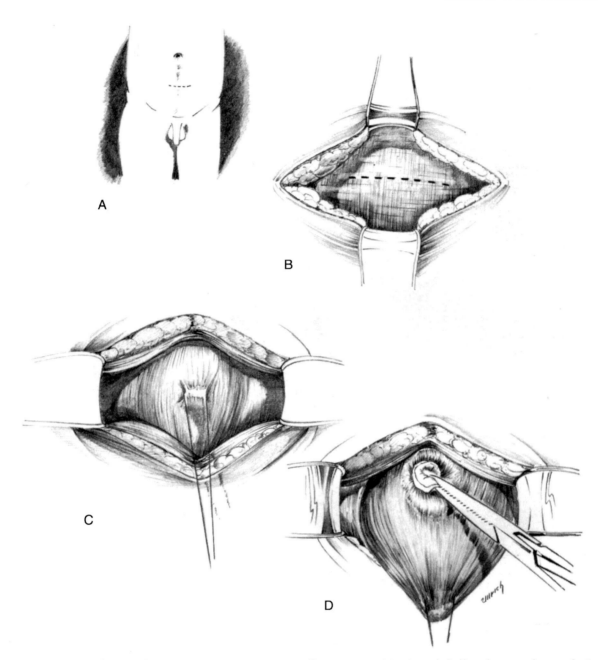

Figure 63–15. Blocksom technique of cutaneous vesicostomy. *A,* A small transverse incision is made halfway between the symphysis pubis and umbilicus. *B,* The rectus fascia is incised transversely, and the rectus muscles are divided in the midline, exposing the bladder. *C* and *D,* The bladder is mobilized superiorly with the aid of traction sutures and the peritoneum peeled off the dome, which is mobilized into the incision.

Illustration continued on following page

how soon after recognition should appropriate relief of obstruction be accomplished. Initial enthusiasm for prenatal intervention waned after it became evident that certain inherent problems existed: (1) inability to make the diagnosis of urethral valves with absolute certainty on prenatal ultrasound; (2) difficulty in ensuring placement and patency of vesicoamniotic shunt catheters; (3) fetal and maternal risks directly related to the procedure (e.g., hemorrhage, infection, initiation of early labor); (4) the lack of objective data indicating any benefit of prenatal intervention greater than what would have occurred had the infant been treated promptly and appropriately at birth.

Modern ultrasound technology offers greatly improved imaging, and the diagnostic accuracy of prenatal ultrasound is substantially improved over what it was a decade ago. **The characteristic findings in a fetus with posterior urethral valves are bilateral hydronephrosis, a distended and *thickened* bladder, a dilated prostatic urethra (seen occasionally), and varying degrees of amniotic fluid abnormality. The renal parenchyma can often be described as normal or echodense (the latter suggesting dysplasia).** However, similar findings can be described for the prune-belly syndrome, a disorder not generally thought to be primarily obstructive in nature. An infant with massive bilateral VUR might have marked hydronephrosis and a distended (although usually not thickened) bladder. Either of these two latter problems might be mistaken for urethral valves on prenatal evaluation, yet prenatal drainage would

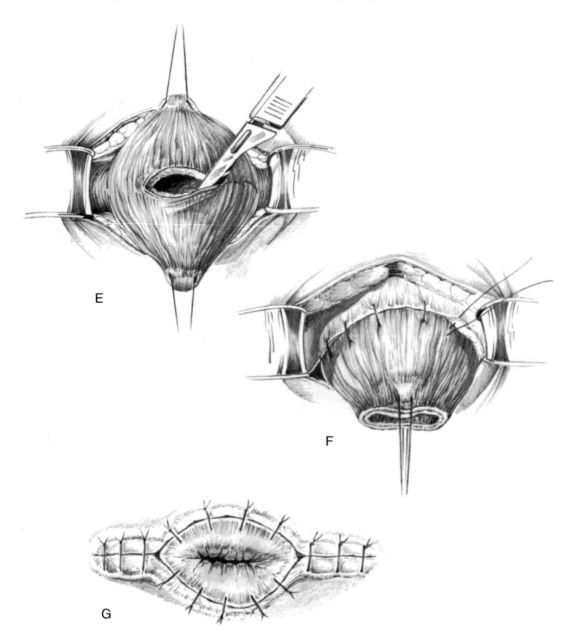

Figure 63–15 *Continued. E,* An incision is made in the dome of the bladder. *F,* The bladder wall is sutured to the fascia with interrupted chromic catgut. *G,* The edges of the bladder are sutured to the skin with interrupted chromic catgut or Dexon.

not be indicated. Diagnostic inaccuracies are still present in the technique (Skolder et al, 1988; Abbott et al, 1998). An exciting addition to fetal diagnosis is fetal cystoscopy, which has been done successfully and permits antegrade destruction of urethral valves in a fetus (Quintero et al, 1995). However, this technique is new, has yet to accumulate a significant number of successes, and cannot be recommended for routine use at this time.

Any technically oriented procedure incurs certain risks, which should gradually lessen as individuals become more familiar with the procedure and its technology. The most serious complications are those that risk both mother and fetus and include severe hemorrhage, infection, and induction of premature labor. In the selected cases done to date, these risks have been thought to be acceptable. However, the incidence is directly related to the experience of the

center and the personnel involved. It is still prudent that these prenatal procedures be done in a limited number of medical centers that have the most experience. There is little doubt that technology and techniques will improve, and this area of fetal medicine deserves careful monitoring.

The greatest deterrent to more frequent use of prenatal intervention has been the lack of any objective data to measure whether prenatal intervention is beneficial in terms of ultimate renal function (Freedman et al, 1999). It is generally believed that dysplasia is an early gestational event and that it occurs before the fetus is large enough to even be considered for prenatal manipulation. Absolutely no data are available indicating that dysplasia improves after relief of obstruction. In addition, the spectrum of severity of obstruction from urethral valves is very wide, and the level of glomerular filtration does not correlate directly with the severity of ureteral dilation. Because of this, some children would undergo diversion who do not really require urgent drainage, increasing the risks associated with prenatal intervention.

Certain parameters can be used to suggest the degree of renal functional compromise. First, as noted previously, dysplastic renal parenchyma is echodense when compared with normal renal parenchyma. Second, the majority of the amniotic fluid is made from urine. Severe oligohydramnios suggests poor renal function, but a normal volume of amniotic fluid does not mean normal renal function. Lastly, Glick and associates (1985) have developed a technique of percutaneous urine sampling with measurement of certain urinary parameters (Table 63–1). Fetal urine is normally low in sodium and is dilute relative to serum. High sodium losses and isosthenuria suggest poor overall renal function. A fetus with unfavorable urine parameters probably would not benefit from prenatal drainage.

None of these observations, however, directly relates to whether prenatal intervention or early postnatal management makes any difference in regard to long-term renal outlook. Therefore, decisions regarding prenatal intervention should be highly selective and should be made with full knowledge of the potential risks involved. **Perhaps the most objective finding today that suggests that prenatal intervention should be considered is when a fetus with ultrasound findings of infravesical obstruction initially is judged to have normal amounts of amniotic fluid but then is noted on follow-up ultrasound examinations to have developed oligohydramnios.**

Additional considerations that influence decisions regarding fetal intervention involve the possible benefits of protecting the fetus from developing pulmonary hypoplasia. Just as the degree of urinary obstruction associated with urethral valves varies widely, the pathophysiology of the pulmonary hypoplasia that may develop is also variable. The presence of oligohydramnios is associated with an increased risk of pulmonary hypoplasia, but some infants with severe oligohydramnios have good pulmonary function, and some with normal amniotic fluid volume have pulmonary insufficiency. The development of pulmonary

hypoplasia may be multifaceted, and factors other than amniotic fluid volume alone undoubtedly play a role (Landers and Hanson, 1990). However, clinical and experimental evidence has suggested that increasing the amniotic fluid volume, after it was initially reduced, lowers the overall risk of severe pulmonary insufficiency (Harrison et al, 1982). Within the broad picture of offering the parents of a newborn with severe renal insufficiency the option of continuous peritoneal dialysis and eventual transplantation, the prevention of pulmonary hyperplasia is another possible indication for considering prenatal intervention in selected cases.

As experience with prenatal evaluation increases, more is being learned about the pathophysiology of posterior urethral valves. The first observation is that children with significant urethral obstruction may not be recognized on prenatal ultrasonograms obtained before 24 weeks of gestational age. In one series, 90% of infants who presented acutely after birth with urethral valves had no recognized urologic pathology on an earlier fetal ultrasonogram (Dinneen et al, 1993). Also, despite enthusiasm for prenatal diagnosis and prompt postpartum management, the early available data do not suggest a significant improvement in ultimate outlook for renal function, compared with postpartum treatment of infants without a prenatal diagnosis (Reinberg, 1992; Jee, 1993). In another study, patients recognized early in gestation (less than 24 weeks) fared much worse in regard to renal function than those fetuses first recognized later in pregnancy or at birth after earlier normal fetal ultrasound studies (Hutton et al, 1994).

Prognosis

The prognosis for children with urethral valves is improving, and current management is gradually rewriting the historical data. In most modern large series neonatal deaths make up only 2% to 3% of the series (Churchill et al, 1990). Early (prenatal) recognition, control of infection, appropriate and selective surgery, recognition of harmful urodynamic abnormalities, modern nephrologic management, and eventual dialysis and transplantation all combine to increase survival now to an extent unheard of in the past. The original series reported total mortality rates as high as 50% by the end of the adolescent period (Johnston and Kulatilake, 1972). Certainly, those statistics no longer hold true today. **In all series, prognosis relates closely to nadir serum creatinine. Warshaw and associates (1985) noted that infants with a serum creatinine concentration of less than 1.0 mg/dl at 1 year of age generally fared well, although this level does not ensure long-term satisfactory renal function.** The fact remains that many children with urethral valves have significant degrees of parenchymal dysplasia and demonstrate gradual but progressive loss of renal function during their lifetime (Burbige and Hensle, 1987; Parkhouse et al, 1988; Tejani et al, 1986; Reinberg, 1992). **It is important that parents be aware that the diagnosis of urethral valves means a long-term commitment to surveillance and care and that even today the eventual outcome is unclear in many instances.**

One bright spot in management of patients with posterior urethral valves has been the success of renal transplantation (Indudhara et al, 1998; Crowe et al, 1998).

Table 63–1. PROGNOSTIC VARIABLES FOR THE FETUS WITH POSTERIOR URETHRAL VALVES

Variable	Predicted Renal Function Postpartum	
	Good	*Poor*
Amniotic fluid volume	Normal to moderately decreased	Moderate to severely decreased
Sonographic appearance of renal parenchyma	Normal to slightly increased echogenicity	Definitely increased echogenicity to frankly cystic
Fetal urinary chemistries		
Sodium (mEq/L)	<100	>100
Chloride (mEq/L)	<90	>90
Osmolarity (mOsm)	<210	>210
Urinary output (mL/hr)	>2	<2

From Glick PL, Harrison MR, Golbus MS, et al: Management of the fetus with congenital hydronephrosis: II. Prognostic criteria and selection for treatment. J Pediatr Surg 1985;20:376.

Despite the recognized bladder dysfunction in many patients, overall graft survival approaches that in patients who require renal transplants but have no uropathy whatsoever (Groene-wegen et al, 1993; Bryant et al, 1991). Careful urodynamic evaluation and selective vesical reconstruction (including enterocystoplasty and clean intermittent catheterization) provides these patients the best chance for successful management of their renal failure (Zaragoza et al, 1993; Koo et al, 1999; Salomon et al, 2000). Even when the patient has a supravesical diversion, transplantation into the native bladder has

usually been successful (Ross, 1994). One study showed an increased risk of urinary infection after transplantation in boys who had urethral valves compared with a similar matched group who had normal bladders, although the long-term significance of this observation in regard to graft survival remains unknown (Mochon, 1992).

As the outlook for boys with urethral valves improves, it is increasingly evident that a significant number of these patients will have problems with fertility. The cause is not always clear and may be multifaceted. Injury to the ejacu-

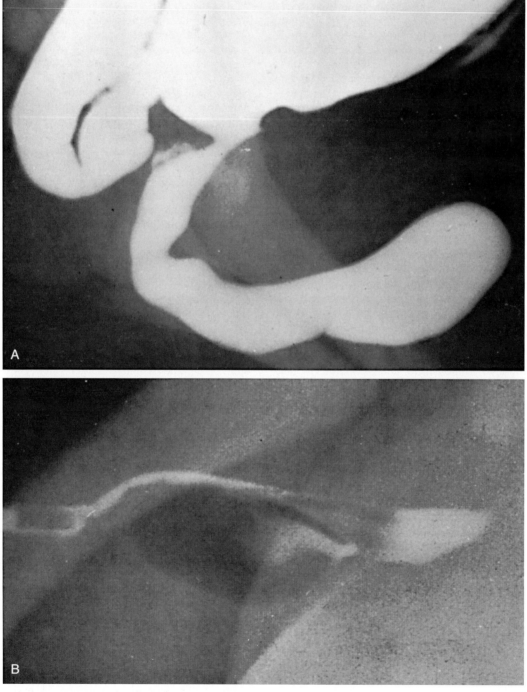

Figure 63–16. *A,* Anterior urethral diverticulum (valve). This voiding cystourethrogram in a newborn boy shows severe obstruction associated with reflux into a dysplastic left kidney and compromised right renal function. *B,* Demonstration of anterior diverticulum, using air injected retrograde with compression of urethra in perineum, followed by contrast injection, showing neck of diverticulum and mechanism of obstruction.

latory ducts at the time of valve ablation and retrograde ejaculation are two possible sequelae from the treatment itself (Parkhouse and Woodhouse, 1990). About 10% of boys with valves also have cryptorchidism (Krueger, 1980a). Again, the reasons are unclear, but this observation suggests there may be a primary mesonephric anomaly responsible for both the valve and the cryptorchidism. However, overall, the majority of men with urethral valves demonstrate normal erectile function and ejaculation, and many, if not all, are able to father children (Parkhouse and Woodhouse, 1990).

ANTERIOR URETHRAL OBSTRUCTION

Congenital obstruction of the more distal urethra is much less common than obstruction of the proximal urethra. Congenital obstruction of the anterior urethra is varied and can include anterior urethral valves (congenital diverticulum of the urethra), valvular obstruction of the fossa navicularis, and cystic dilation of the ducts of Cowper's glands (syringoceles). Of these, the most common abnormality is anterior urethral valves.

An anterior urethral valve in almost all cases is actually a congenital urethral diverticulum (Tank, 1987) (Fig. 63–16). **During voiding, the diverticulum expands, ballooning ventrally and distally beneath the thinned corpus spongiosum. The flaplike dorsal margin of the diverticulum then extends into the urethral lumen, occluding urinary flow (an obstructing valve).** Anterior urethral valves have been described in every portion of the anterior urethra with almost equal incidence. They may be small, minimally obstructive, and of limited clinical concern (Fig. 63–17). Often, though, they are severely obstructing and result in all the findings seen with posterior urethral valves.

The diagnosis of anterior urethral valves is confirmed on voiding cystourethrography. At times, difficulty with catheterization may be encountered because the catheter preferentially slips into the diverticulum. However, this occurs less often than one might expect because the proximal wall of the diverticulum is often not hollowed out nearly as extensively as the distal wall. Because the diverticula almost always are placed in the midline ventrally, a dorsally oriented coudé-tipped catheter can usually be negotiated with less difficulty into the more proximal urethra. To establish the diagnosis, the entire penile urethra must be included in the voiding phase of the cystourethrogram, or more distally located lesions will be missed.

The etiology of these anomalies is not entirely clear, but they seem to represent incomplete fusion of a segment of the urethral plate. Another possible cause might be a focally incomplete development of the corpus spongiosum with ballooning of the urethral mucosa due to inadequate support. Small, nonobstructing diverticula often appear stable for many years and do not show continuous enlargement and progressively worsening obstruction.

Initial management of a congenital anterior urethral valve parallels that for the more commonly seen posterior urethral valve. Initial imaging studies assess the extent of hydronephrosis, the thickness and quality of the renal parenchyma (echogenicity on renal ultrasound, uptake on renal scan), and the presence or absence of VUR. Infants presenting with urosepsis and/or severe renal insufficiency require a period of transurethral or suprapubic (by percutaneous route) catheter drainage for stabilization, antibiotics, electrolyte management, and assessment of renal functional improvement. As with infants with posterior urethral valves, a temporizing, tubeless diversion (vesicostomy, loop ureterostomy) might be chosen on an individual basis (Rushton et al, 1987).

Management of the urethral anomaly may be endoscopic or open. A hooked, single-wire, electrocautery "knife" can engage the distal margin of the diverticulum and incise it in the midline. When performing this procedure, the surgeon must be very careful not to place the tip of the wire too close to the floor of the diverticulum. At this location, the wall of the urethra can be very thin, and thermal injury might result in the development of a urethrocutaneous fistula. Even after satisfactory destruction of the leaflet, postoperative urethrography is often disappointing, because the appearance of the diverticulum may be unchanged. One must carefully assess the quality of flow (flow rate if the child is old enough) and the extent of filling of the urethra distal to the anomaly to evaluate the results of the procedure.

Some surgeons have advocated open resection and reconstruction of the diverticulum (Tank, 1987). This technique allows one to completely excise the distal lip and provide a more homogeneous caliber to the urethra. In most cases, a patch graft urethroplasty is the preferred procedure. If the diverticulum is on the penile shaft, a sleeve dissection of the penile shaft skin from the corona to the penoscrotal angle allows the urethroplasty to be completed without overlapping suture lines.

Some anterior urethral valves may not be associated with

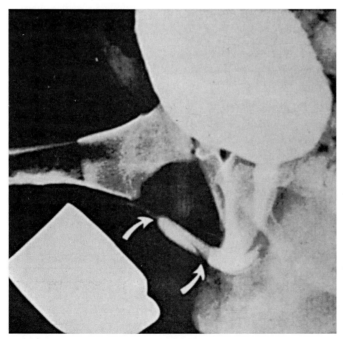

Figure 63–17. Anterior urethral diverticulum (valve) demonstrated by voiding cystourethrogram in a 4-year-old boy with symptoms of straining to void and a fine stream.

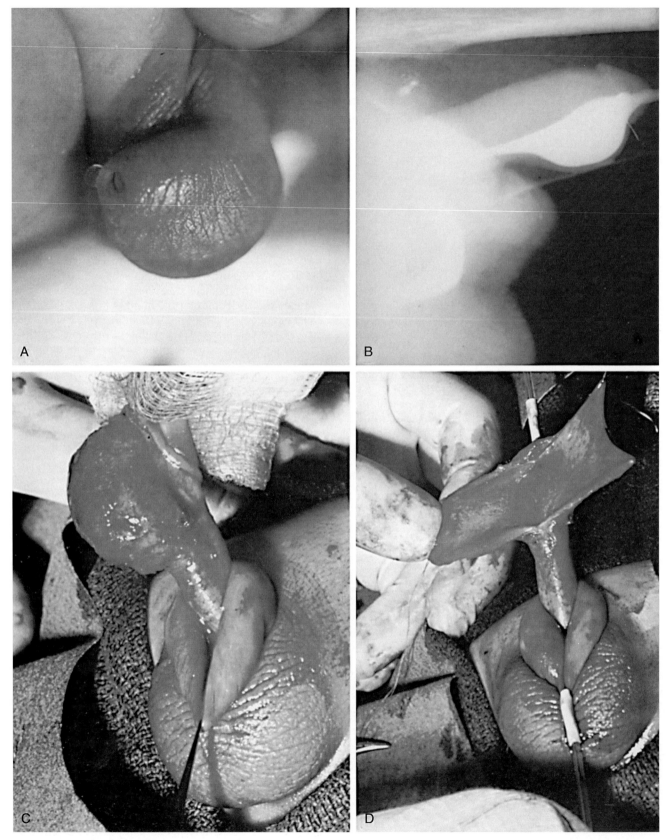

Figure 63–18. *A,* Photograph showing megalourethra in a newborn boy. This photograph was taken during the act of micturition. *B,* Voiding urethrogram of same patient. *C,* Appearance of the urethra after degloving of the penis. *D,* The dilated segment of the urethra has been opened. Excess urethral tissue is excised, leaving just enough to reconstruct a urethra of normal caliber.

a urethral diverticulum. DeCastro and colleagues (1987) described three children who had anterior urethral membranes without the associated diverticulum. Scherz and associates (1987) described valvular obstruction in the region of the fossa navicularis in three children. Whether these isolated variations represent a portion of the spectrum described earlier is not known.

Syringoceles are cystic dilations of the duct of Cowper's gland within the bulbous urethra (Maizels et al, 1983). They are usually small, inconsequential lesions; but, rarely, they can be of sufficient size to cause varying degrees of outlet obstruction. Management, when necessary, is usually by endoscopic unroofing. After unroofing, a diverticulum-like defect may result on the posterolateral wall of the bulbous urethra. However, these defects are rarely obstructing and do not need further management.

MEGALOURETHRA

Nonobstructive urethral dilation (megalourethra) is a rare entity that is associated with abnormal development of the corpus spongiosum and, occasionally, with abnormal development of the corpora cavernosum. Traditionally, megalourethra has been divided into two varieties: scaphoid megalourethra and fusiform megalourethra. In the scaphoid variety, the corpus spongiosum is thought to be the only abnormal segment, whereas the fusiform variety is associated with defects of the corpora cavernosa also. However, this distinction is arbitrary and is not based on any recognized embryologic difference between the two varieties (Appel et al, 1986). Although megalourethra may be an isolated event, it is often associated with upper tract abnormalities. Appropriate imaging of the urinary tract is indicated in every case. **Megalourethra is especially common in association with the prune-belly syndrome and may represent a defect in development of the mesoderm, one of the proposed causes for the prune-belly anomaly** (Mortensen et al, 1985).

Management of the megalourethra itself is primarily cosmetic if the upper tracts are satisfactorily normal (Fig. 63–18). The large bulbous urethra can be trimmed and tailored for a more homogeneous and normal urethral caliber. When the corpora cavernosa are severely deficient, concern regarding sexual function is often raised. In the past, one might have considered a change in the gender of rearing. Considering the current controversy regarding the appropriateness of deciding on a gender of rearing for children with intersex states or dysmorphic genital development, I would be reluctant to recommend such a change today. These anomalies are not known to result from any deficiency of testosterone action. Therefore, testosterone imprinting on the brain is likely to be normal.

A subset of boys with distal megalourethra are often classified as having a variant of hypospadias. These anomalies were described by Duckett and Keating (1989) as the "megameatus, intact prepuce." The patients present with a coronally positioned, wide-mouthed meatus and a fully formed foreskin. The urethra for 1 cm or so is often very large, and the corpus spongiosum is very thin. Ventral chordee is not present. This anomaly contrasts with the more usual variety of hypospadias, thought to represent a fetal androgen deficiency, in which the meatus is often small, the distal urethra is narrowed and inelastic, the foreskin is unfused ventrally, and ventral chordee is expected.

URETHRAL DUPLICATION

Duplication of the urethra is an uncommon anomaly. Urethral duplications are complex anomalies, and different embryologic abnormalities are thought to be responsible for the many variations seen. A universally accepted classification has not yet been described (Ortolano and Nasaralloh, 1986). **Urethral duplications are conveniently divided into dorsal and ventral duplications. Most duplications occur in the same sagittal plane; that is, they occur one on top of the other** (Fig. 63–19). Less commonly, duplex urethras lie side by side. This is the usual finding in children with a completely duplicated phallus, but occasionally it can occur when the phallus is fused but widened. This anatomic appearance is also more common when the bladder is completely duplicated.

In the dorsal variety, where an accessory meatus is positioned above a glandular meatus, the normal urethra is the ventrally positioned channel that usually

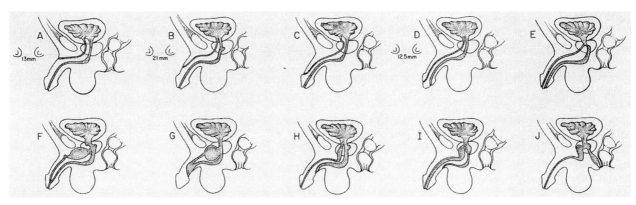

Figure 63–19. Variations in presentation of urethral duplication in the sagittal plane. Note in each of these drawings that the ventrally positioned channel is depicted in the central region of the prostate, indicating that it is the more "normal" urethra. (From Colodny A: Urethral lesions in infants and children. In Gillinwater JY, Grayhack JT, Howards SS, Duckett JW [eds]: Adult and Pediatric Urology, 2nd ed. St. Louis, Mosby–Year Book, 1991, p 2013.)

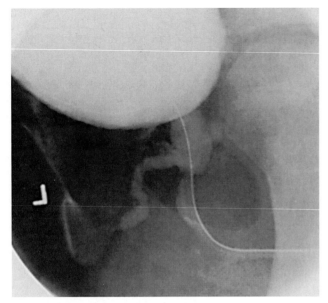

Figure 63–20. Voiding cystourethrogram in a 17-year-old male patient with ventral urethral duplication, with one meatus at the anus. The catheter is passed up the perineal opening. The penile urethra was very atretic.

ends in a normal meatus on the glans. The accessory (abnormal) channel opens on the shaft in an epispadiac position anywhere from the glans to the base of the penis. Often, dorsal penile chordee is present, and the foreskin may be unfused dorsally. The abnormal dorsal segment extends proximally beneath the symphysis pubis for a varying length. Many end blindly before reaching the bladder. If these abnormal urethras do reach the bladder, the patient usually is incontinent. Widening of the symphysis pubis may also be found. These findings suggest a relationship between this anomaly and the exstrophy-epispadias complex (Campbell et al, 1987; Sharma et al, 1987). Cases have been described in which this accessory channel never entered the bladder but continued along the ventral surface of the bladder and joined with the urachus, suggesting that it might represent more of an abortive duplication of the bladder rather than of the urethra. Because the normally positioned urethra has a normal bladder neck and sphincter mechanism, excision of the abnormal epispadiac urethra usually cures any incontinence affecting the patient. Significant penile chordee may also have to be repaired.

Ventral duplications of the urethra are less clearly understood embryologically. They may be complete, with two separate urethras coming off the bladder. Other cases are incomplete, with the urethra bifurcating somewhere distal to the bladder neck. Patients may have a hypospadiac meatus on the penile shaft. However, the most serious variation occurs when the ventral meatus is present at the anterior anal margin. The dorsal penile urethra is often narrowed and inelastic (Fig. 63–20). **Urinary flow is preferentially through the perianal urethral opening, and the ventral urethra is usually considered the more normal urethra, because it traverses the sphincter mechanism** (Salle et al, 2000).

Urethral duplication may not always require surgical management, and some cases are noted incidentally during voiding cystourethrography (Hoekstra and Jones, 1985). Management of the more severe perianal duplication has usually involved advancement of the ventral channel to the perineum as the initial procedure, followed by a formal urethroplasty. Usually, this has been accomplished by excising the existing dorsal urethra and then performing a standard urethroplasty. The more normally positioned dorsal channel is often very narrowed, with focal areas of atresia, and usually has not been used in the reconstruction (Holst and Peterson, 1988). However, Passerini-Glazel and coworkers (1988) demonstrated that if the dorsal urethra can be catheterized—even if the lumen is very tiny—gentle, gradual, prolonged dilation in situ may allow for eventual use of this urethral channel.

PROSTATIC URETHRAL POLYPS

Urethral polyps are rare abnormalities of male children that usually manifest with hematuria or obstructive symptoms (Raviv et al, 1993). If the lesion is large enough and on a long stalk, strangury may occur. The diagnosis is best confirmed by voiding cystourethrography but may be detected by ultrasonography. The polyps are almost always in the prostatic fossa, although anterior urethral polyps have been reported (Coleman and Nensle, 1991).

Urethral polyps have been speculated to represent a developmental error in the invagination process of the submucous glandular material of the inner zone of the prostate (Walsh et al, 1993). They are benign lesions (not to be confused with the polypoid masses of a sarcoma botryoides), and transurethral excision of the polyps is curative (Gleason and Kramer, 1994).

REFERENCES

Abbott JF, Levine D, Wapner R: Posterior urethral valves: Inaccuracy of prenatal diagnosis. Fetal Diagn Ther 1998;13:179.

Adzick NS, Harrison MR, Flake AW, de Lorimier AA: Urinary extravasation in the fetus with obstructive uropathy. J Pediatr Surg 1985;20:608.

Appel RA, Kaplan GW, Brock WA, Streit D: Megalourethra. J Urol 1986;135:747.

Bauer SB, Dieppa RA, Labib K, et al: The bladder in boys with posterior urethral valves: A urodynamic assessment. J Urol 1979;121:769.

Beck AD: The effect of intra-uterine urinary obstruction upon the development of the fetal kidney. J Urol 1971;105:784.

Biewald W, Schier F: Laser treatment of posterior urethral valves in neonates. Br J Urol 1992;69:425.

Bomalaski MD, Arema JG, Coplen DE, et al: Delayed presentation of posterior urethral valves: A not so benign condition. J Urol 1999;162:2130.

Brenner BM, Meyer TW, Hostetler TH: Dietary protein intake and the progressive nature of kidney disease. N Engl J Med 1982;307:652.

Bryant JE, Joseph DB, Kohaut EC, Diethelm AG: Renal transplantation in children with posterior urethral valves. J Urol 1991;146:1585.

Burbige KA, Hensle TW: Posterior urethral valves in a newborn: Treatment and functional results. J Pediatr Surg 1987;22:165.

Campaiola JM, Perlmutter AP, Steinhardt GF: Noncompliant bladder resulting from posterior urethral valves. J Urol 1985;134:708.

Campbell J, Beasley S, McMullin N, Hutson JM: Congenital prepubic sinus: Possible variant of dorsal urethral duplication. J Urol 1987;137:505.

Churchill BM, Krueger RP, Fleisher MH, et al: Complications of posterior urethral valve surgery. Urol Clin North Am 1983;10:519.

Churchill BM, McLorie GA, Khoury AE, et al: Emergency treatment and long-term follow-up of posterior urethral valves. Urol Clin North Am 1990;17:343.

Close CE, Carr MC, Burns MW, Mitchell ME: Lower urinary tract changes after early valve ablation in neonates and infants: Is early diversion warranted? J Urol 1997;157:984.

Coleman NH, Nensle TW: Anterior urethral polyp associated with hematuria in six year old child. Urology 1991;38:143.

Colodny A: Urethral lesions in infants and children. In Gillenwater JY, Grayhack JT, Howards SS, Duckett JW (eds): Adult and Pediatric Urology, 2nd ed. St. Louis, Mosby–Year Book, 1991, p 2013.

Conner JP, Hensle TW, Berdon W, Burbige KA: Contained neonatal urinoma: Management and functional results. J Urol 1988;140:1319.

Cromie WJ, Cain MP, Bellinger MF, et al: Urethral valve incision using a modified venous valvulotome. J Urol 1994;151:1053.

Crowe A, Cairns HS, Wood S, et al: Renal transplantation following renal failure due to urological disorders. Nephrol Dial Transplant 1998;13:2065.

Cuckow PM, Dinneen MD, Risdon RA, et al: Long-term renal function in the posterior urethral valves, unilateral reflux and renal dysplasia syndrome. J Urol 1997;158:1004.

Deane AM, Whitaker RH, Sherwood T: Diathermy hook ablation of posterior urethral valves in neonates and infants. Br J Urol 1988;62:593.

DeCastro R, Battaglino F, Casolari E, et al: Valves of the anterior urethra without diverticulum: Description of three cases. Pediatr Med Chir 1987;9:211.

Djeter S, Gibbons D: The newborn value. In Gonzales ET, Roth DR (eds): Common Problems in Pediatric Urology. Houston, Mosby–Year Book, 1990, p 76.

Dinneen MD, Duffy PG, Barratt TM, Ransley PG: Persistent polyuria after posterior urethral valves. Br J Urol 1995;75:236.

Dinneen MD, Phillon HK, Ward HC, et al: Antenatal diagnosis of posterior urethral valves. Br J Urol 1993;72:364.

Duckett JW, Keating MA: Technical challenge of the megameatus intact prepuce hypospadias variant: The pyramid procedure. J Urol 1989;141:1407.

Duckett JW, Norris M: The management of neonatal valves with advanced hydronephrosis and azotemia. In Carlton CE (ed): Controversies in Urology. Chicago, Year Book, 1989, p 2.

Ehrlich RM, Shanberg A: Neodymium-YAG laser ablation of posterior urethral valves. Dialogues Pediatr Urol 1988;11:29.

Field PL, Stephens FD: Congenital urethral membranes causing urethral obstruction. J Urol 1974;111:250.

Freedman AL, Johnson MP, Smith CA, et al: Long-term outcome in children after antenatal intervention for obstructive uropathies. Lancet 1999;354:374.

Gearhart JP, Lee BR, Partin AW, et al: A quantitative histological evaluation of the dilated ureter of childhood: II. Ectopia, posterior urethral valves, and the prune belly syndrome. J Urol 1995;153:172.

Gholdoian CG, Thayer K, Hald D, et al: Applications of the KTP laser in the treatment of posterior urethral valves, ureteroceles, and urethral strictures in the pediatric patient. J Clin Laser Med Surg 1998;16:39.

Gibbons MD, Horan JJ, Dejter SW, Keszler M: Extracorporeal membrane oxygenation: An adjunct in the management of the neonate with severe respiratory distress and congenital urinary tract anomalies. J Urol 1993;150:434.

Glassberg KI: Current issues regarding posterior urethral valves. Urol Clin North Am 1985;12:175.

Glassberg KL, Schneider M, Haller JO, et al: Observations on persistently dilated ureter after posterior urethral valve ablation. Urology 1982;20:20.

Gleason PE, Kramer SA: Genitourinary polyps in children. Urology 1994;44:106.

Glick PL, Harrison MR, Adzick NS, et al: Correction of congenital hydronephrosis in utero IV: In utero decompression prevents renal dysplasia. J Pediatr Surg 1984;19:649.

Glick PL, Harrison MR, Golbus MS, et al: Management of the fetus with congenital hydronephrosis: II. Prognostic criteria and selection for treatment. J Pediatr Surg 1985;20:376.

Gonzales ET: Alternatives in the management of posterior urethral valves. Urol Clin North Am 1990;17:335.

Gonzalez R, Reinberg, Y, Burke, B, et al: Early bladder outlet obstruction in fetal lambs induces renal dysplasia and the prune-belly syndrome. J Pediatr Surg 1990;25:342.

Greenfield SP: Posterior urethral valves: New concepts (Editorial.) J Urol 1997;157:996.

Griffin JE, Wilson JD: The androgen resistance syndromes: 5α-reductase deficiency, testicular feminization, and related syndromes. In Scriner CR, Beaudet AL, Sly WS, Valle D (eds): The Metabolic Basis of Inherited Disease. New York, McGraw-Hill, 1989, pp 1919–1944.

Groenewegen AA, Sukhai RN, Nanta J, et al: Results of renal transplantation in boys treated for posterior urethral valves. J Urol 1993;149:1517.

Gunn TR, Mora JD, Pease P: Antenatal diagnosis of urinary tract abnormalities by ultrasonography after 28 weeks gestation: Incidence and outcome. Am J Obstet Gynecol 1995;172:479.

Hanlon-Lundberg KM, Verp MS, Loy G: Posterior urethral valves in successive generations. Am J Perinatol 1994;11:37.

Harrison MR, Nakayamo DK, Rooll R: Correction of congenital hydronephrosis in utero: II. Decompression versus the effects of obstruction on the fetal lung and urinary tract. J Pediatr Surg 1982;17:965.

Hayslett JP: Effect of age on compensatory renal growth. Kidney Int 1983;23:599.

Hendren WH: Posterior urethral valves in boys. A broad clinical spectrum. J Urol 1971;106:298.

Henneberry MO, Stephens FA: Renal hypoplasia and dysplasia in infants with posterior urethral valves. J Urol 1980;123:912.

Hoekstra I, Jones B: Duplication of the male urethra: Report of three cases. Clin Radiology 1985;36:529.

Holmdahl G, Sillen U, Bachelard M, et al: The changing urodynamic pattern in valve bladders during infancy. J Urol 1995;153:463.

Holmdahl G, Sillen U, Hanson E, et al: Bladder dysfunction in boys with posterior urethral valves before and after puberty. J Urol 1996;155:694.

Holst S, Peterson NE: Fulguration-ablation of atypical accessory urethra. J Urol 1988;140:347.

Hoover DL, Duckett JW: Posterior urethral valves, unilateral reflux, and renal dysplasia: A syndrome. J Urol 1982;128:994.

Hutton KAR, Thomas DFM, Arthur RF, et al: Prenatally detected posterior urethral valves: Is gestational age at detection a predictor of outcome? J Urol 1994;152:698.

Indudhara R, Joseph DB, Perez LM, Diethelm AG: Renal transplantation in children with posterior urethral valve revisited: A 10-year followup. J Urol 1998;160:1201.

Jee LD, Rickwood AM, Turnock RR: Posterior urethral valves: Does prenatal diagnosis influence prognosis. Br J Urol 1993;72:830.

Johnston JH: Temporary cutaneous ureterostomy in the management of advanced congenital urinary obstruction. Arch Dis Child 1963;38:161.

Johnston JH: Vesicoureteric reflux with urethral valves. Br J Urol 1979;51:100.

Johnston JH: Posterior urethral valves: An operative technique using an electric auriscope. J Pediatr Surg 1996;1:583.

Johnston JH, Kulatilake AE: The sequelae of posterior urethral valves. Br J Urol 1971;43:743.

Johnston JH, Kulatilake AE: Posterior urethral valves: Results and sequelae. In Johnston JH, Scholtmeyer RY (eds): Problems in Pediatric Urology. Amsterdam, Excerpta Medica, 1972, p 161.

Jordan GH, Hoover DL: Inadequate decompression of the upper tracts using a Foley catheter in the valve bladder. J Urol 1985;134:137.

Kaplan GW, Scherz HC: Infravesical obstruction. In Kelalis PP, King LR, Belman AB (eds): Clinical Pediatric Urology, 3rd ed. Philadelphia, WB Saunders, 1992, p 846.

Karim OM, Cendron M, Mostwin JL, Gearhart JP: Developmental alterations in the fetal lamb bladder subjected to partial urethral obstruction in utero. J Urol 1993;150:1060.

Karim OM, Seki N, Pienta KJ, Mastwin JL: The effect of age on the response of the detrusor to intracellular mechanical stimulus: DNA replication and the cell actin matrix. J Cell Biochem 1992;48:373.

Keating MA: The noncompliant bladder: Principles in pathogenesis and pathophysiology. Prob Urol 1994;8:348.

Kim YH, Horwitz M, Combs A: Comparative urodynamic findings after primary valve ablation, vesicostomy, or proximal diversion. J Urol 1996;156:673.

Klahr S: The modification of diet in renal disease study. N Engl J Med 1989;320:864.

Kolicinski ZH: Foley balloon procedure in posterior urethral valves. Dialogues Pediatr Urol 1988;11:7.

Koo HP, Bunchman TE, Flynn JT, et al: Renal transplantation in children with severe lower urinary tract dysfunction. J Urol 1999;161:240.

Krueger RP, Hardy BE, Churchill BM: Cryptorchidism in boys with posterior urethral valves. J Urol 1980a;124:101.

Krueger RP, Hardy BE, Churchill BM: Growth in boys with posterior urethral valves. Urol Clin North Am 1980b;7:265.

Landers S, Hanson TN: Pulmonary problems associated with congenital renal malformations. In Gonzales ET, Roth DR (eds): Common Problems in Pediatric Urology. Houston, Mosby–Year Book, 1990, p 85.

Livne PM, Delaune J, Gonzales ET: Genetic etiology of posterior urethral valves. J Urol 1983;130:781.

Lome LG, Howat JM, Williams DI: The temporarily defunctionalized bladder in children. J Urol 1972;107:469.

Maizels M, Stephens FD, King LR, Firlit CF: Cowper's syringocele: A classification of dilatations of Cowper's duct based upon clinical characteristics of 8 boys. J Urol 1983;129:111.

Mayor G, Genton R, Torrado A, Geirgnard J: Renal function in obstructive nephropathy: Long-term effects of reconstructive surgery. Pediatrics 1975;58:740.

McConnell JD: Detrusor smooth muscle development. Dialogues Pediatr Urol 1989;12.

McVary KT, Maizels M: Urinary obstruction reduces glomerulogenesis in the developing kidney: A model in the rabbit. J Urol 1989;142:646.

Mochon M, Kaiser BA, Dunn S, et al: Urinary tract infection in children with posterior urethral valves after kidney transplantation. J Urol 1992; 148:1874.

Mortensen PH, Johnson HW, Coleman GU, et al: Megalourethra. J Urol 1985;134:358.

Nakayama DK, Harrison MR, de Lorimier AA: Prognosis of posterior urethral valves presenting at birth. J Pediatr Surg 1986;21:43.

Nijman RJ, Scholtmeyer RJ: Complications of transurethral electro-incision of posterior urethral valves. Br J Urol 1991;67:324.

Noe HN, Jerkins GR: Oliguria and renal failure following decompression of the bladder in children with posterior urethral valves. J Urol 1983; 129:595.

Novak ME, Gonzales ET: Single stage reconstruction of urinary tract after loop cutaneous ureterostomy. Urology 1978;11:134.

Ortolano V, Nasaralloh PF: Urethral duplication. J Urol 1986;136:909.

Parkhouse HF, Barratt TM, Dillon MJ, et al: Long-term outcome of boys with posterior urethral valves. Br J Urol 1988;62:59.

Parkhouse HF, Woodhouse CR: Long-term status of patients with posterior urethral valves. Urol Clin North Am 1990;17:373.

Passerini-Glazel G, Araguna F, Chiozza L, et al: The P.A.D.U.A. (Progressive Augmentation by Dilating the Urethra Anterior) procedure for the treatment of severe urethral hypoplasia. J Urol 1988;140:1247.

Peters CA: Congenital bladder obstruction. Probl Urol 1994;8:333.

Peters CA, Bolkier M, Bauer SB, et al: The urodynamic consequences of posterior urethral valves. J Urol 1990;144:122.

Pieretti RV: The mild end of the clinical spectrum of posterior urethral valves. J Pediatr Surg 1993;28:701.

Quintero RA, Hume R, Smith C, et al: Percutaneous fetal cystoscopy and endoscopic fulguration of posterior urethral valves. Am J Obstet Gynecol 1995;172:206.

Raviv G, Leibovitch I, Hanani J, et al: Hematuria and voiding disorders in children caused by congenital urethral polyps: Principles of diagnosis and management. Eur Urol 1993;23:382.

Reinberg Y, deCastano I, Gonzalez R: Influence of initial therapy on progression of renal failure and body growth in children with posterior urethral valves. J Urol 1992a;148:532.

Reinberg Y, deCastano I, Gonzalez R: Prognosis for patients with prenatally diagnosed posterior urethral valves. J Urol 1992b;148:125.

Rittenberg MH, Hulbert WC, Snyder HM, Duckett JW: Protective factors in posterior urethral valves. J Urol 1988;140:993.

Robertson WB, Hayes JA: Congenital diaphragmatic obstruction of the male posterior urethra. Br J Urol 1969;41:592.

Rosenfeld B, Greenfield SP, Springate JE, Feld LG: Type III posterior urethral valves: Presentation and management. J Pediatr Surg 1994;29: 81, 1994.

Ross JH, Kay R, Novick AC, et al: Long-term results of renal transplantation into the valve bladder. J Urol 1994;151:1500.

Rushton HG, Parrott TS, Woodard JR, Walther M: The role of vesicostomy in the management of anterior urethral valves in neonates and infants. J Urol 1987;138:107.

Salle JL, Sibai H, Rosenstein D, et al: Urethral duplication in the male: Review of 16 cases. J Urol 2000;163:1936.

Salomon L, Fontaine E, Guest G, et al: Role of the bladder in delayed failure of kidney transplants in boys with posterior urethral valves. J Urol 2000;163:1282.

Scherz HC, Kaplan GW, Packer MG: Anterior urethral valves in the fossa navicularis in children. J Urol 1987;138:1211.

Sharma SK, Kapoor R, Kumar A, Mandal AK: Incomplete epispadiac urethral duplication with dorsal penile curvature. J Urol 1987;138:585.

Skolder AJ, Maizels M, Depp R, et al: Caution in antenatal intervention. J Urol 1988;139:1026.

Smith GHH, Duckett JW: Urethral lesions in infants and children. In Gillenwater JY, Grayhack JT, Howards SS, Duckett JW (eds): Adult and Pediatric Urology, 3rd ed. St. Louis, Mosby–Year Book, 1996, p 2411.

Smith GHH, Canning DA, Schulmon SL, et al: The long-term outcome of posterior urethral valves treated with primary valve ablation and observation. J Urol 1996;155:1730.

Sober I: Pelvioureterostomy-en-Y. Urology 1972;107:473.

Stephens FD: Congenital Malformations of the Urinary Tract. New York, Praeger, 1983, pp 96, 103.

Tanagho EA: Congenitally obstructed bladders: Fate after prolonged defunctionalization. J Urol 1974;111:102.

Tank ES: Anterior urethral valves resulting from congenital urethral diverticula. Urology 1987;30:467.

Tejani A, Butt K, Glassberg K, et al: Predictors of eventual end stage renal disease in children with posterior urethral valves. J Urol 1986; 136:857.

Thomas DFM, Gorddon AC: Management of prenatally diagnosed uropathies. Arch Dis Child 1989;64:58.

Tietjen DN, Gloor JM, Husmann DA: Proximal urinary diversion in the management of posterior urethral valves: Is it necessary? J Urol 1997; 158:1008.

Walker RD, Padron M: Management of posterior urethral valves by initial vesicostomy and delayed valve ablation. J Urol 1990;144:1212.

Walsh IK, Keane PF, Herron B: Benign urethral polyps. Br J Urol 1993; 72:937.

Warshaw BL, Hymes LC, Trulock TS, et al: Prognostic features in infants with obstructive uropathy due to posterior urethral valves. J Urol 1985; 133:240.

Whitaker RH: The ureter in posterior urethral valves. Br J Urol 1973;45: 395.

Williams PI, Cromie WJ: Ring ureterostomy. Br J Urol 1975;47:789.

Woodbury PW: Constant pressure perfusion: A method to determine obstruction in the upper urinary tract. J Urol 1989;142:632.

Young HH, Frontz WA, Baldwin JC: Congenital obstruction of the posterior urethra. J Urol 1919;3:289.

Zaontz MR, Firlit CF: Percutaneous antegrade ablation of posterior urethral valves in premature or underweight term neonates: An alternative to primary vesicostomy. J Urol 1985;134:139.

Zaragoza MR, Ritchey ML, Bloom DA, McGuire EJ: Enterocystoplasty in renal transplantation candidates: Urodynamic evaluation and outcome. J Urol 1993;150:1463.

64
VOIDING DYSFUNCTION IN CHILDREN: NEUROGENIC AND NON-NEUROGENIC

Stuart B. Bauer, MD
Stephen A. Koff, MD
Venkata R. Jayanthi, MD

SECTION A: NEUROPATHIC DYSFUNCTION OF THE LOWER URINARY TRACT

Stuart B. Bauer, MD

INTRODUCTION

At least 25% of the clinical problems seen in pediatric urology are the result of neurologic lesions that affect lower urinary tract function. As pediatric urology developed in the latter half of the 20th century, urinary diversion initially was the mainstay of treatment for these children with either intractable incontinence or normal or abnormal upper urinary tracts (Smith, 1972). **The advent of clean intermittent catheterization (CIC) in the early 1970s by Lapides** (Lapides et al, 1972), **refinements in techniques of urodynamic studies in children** (Gierup and Ericsson, 1970; Blaivas et al, 1977; Blaivas, 1979), **and the development of surgical modalities to manage**

incontinence dramatically changed the way this group of children was traditionally managed. Along with this change came a greater understanding of the pathophysiology of the many diseases that affect children primarily. With the increased reliability of data collection, the applicability of urodynamic testing expanded, and most pediatric urologic centers now believe that functional assessment of the lower urinary tract is an essential element in the evaluation process and as important as radiographic visualization in characterizing and managing these abnormal conditions (McGuire et al, 1981; Bauer et al, 1984). **The natural outcome of early functional investigation has been the advocacy of proactive or early aggressive management in these children, who are now considered to be at risk**

for urinary tract deterioration based on specific hostile urodynamic parameters (Perez et al, 1992; Edelstein et al, 1995; Kaufman et al, 1996). **This has resulted in (1) a statistically significant decrease in upper urinary tract deterioration, compared with those children followed expectantly in the past, and (2) a dramatic reduction in the need for augmentation cystoplasty** (Wu et al, 1997; Kaefer et al, 1999; Bauer, 2000). Furthermore, there is now evidence that molecular changes occur intracellularly when prophylactic treatment is begun as early as possible (Park et al, 1999; Ohnishi et al, 2000). Because urodynamic testing has become such an integral part of any discussion of the subject, this chapter first defines the testing process as it applies to children, outlines its pitfalls and advantages, and then elaborates on the various neurologic abnormalities that are prevalent in children.

URODYNAMIC EVALUATION

Before a urodynamic study is performed, it is important for the child and the family to have full knowledge of the procedure. Therefore, an explanation of the test and a questionnaire are sent to each family before the appointment. A booklet is provided so that parents will know what to expect and can explain the test to their child, or the child can read about it if he or she is old enough. Attempts are made to minimize anxiety in children who are able to understand what will happen by providing reasons for specific portions of the test and explaining exactly what the child will experience. The questionnaire tries to elicit information about the mother's pregnancy history, the child's birth and development, his or her current bladder and bowel habits, and any other information that might be pertinent at the time of the procedure.

Rarely is any premedication given either orally or intramuscularly, but the child is conscientiously attended to in order to minimize his or her fears. Since 1993, EMLA cream, a topical anesthetic, has been applied to the perineum about 45 minutes before the electromyography (EMG) needle is inserted to record sphincter activity. If possible, the child is instructed to come to the urodynamic suite with a full bladder to obtain an initial representative uroflow. The time of the child's previous urination is noted to calculate an average rate of urine production per unit of time. In addition, this information allows the nurse to record a reliable residual urine volume when catheterizing the child after voiding. The flowmeter is located in a private bathroom that contains a one-way mirror so that voiding can be viewed unobtrusively. This allows the investigator to see whether a Credé or a Valsalva maneuver is employed by the child to help empty the bladder.

Next, the nurse reviews the test and shows the child all the equipment in an attempt to make the patient feel as comfortable as possible. The child is catheterized with either a No. 7 Fr or a No. 11 Fr triple-lumen urodynamic catheter (Cook Urological Inc, Spencer, IN)—the smaller, the better—after a small amount of liquid Xylocaine (1%) has been injected into the urethra and held in place for a moment or two. First, the intravesicular pressure is recorded. Then the bladder is drained and the residual urine is carefully measured, yielding a pressure at residual volume (Kaefer et al, 1997a). Sometimes it is necessary to

aspirate the catheter to get accurate information on the volume of residual urine, especially if the bladder is hypotonic (particularly if the child is taking anticholinergic medication) or has been previously augmented and secretes mucus (because it may not drain completely after insertion of a catheter).

A small balloon catheter is passed into the rectum at this time to measure intra-abdominal pressure during the cystometrogram to identify artifacts of motion and monitor increases in abdominal pressure during the filling and emptying phases of the study (Bates et al, 1970; Bauer, 1979). Uninhibited contractions and straining to empty can be clearly differentiated by this maneuver.

Before the bladder is filled, a urethral pressure profile is sometimes obtained by infusing saline through the side-hole channel at a rate of 2 ml/min as the catheter is withdrawn at a rate of 2 mm/sec (Yalla et al, 1980). Another way of determining maximal urethral closure pressure is by measuring the leak point pressure at various stages of bladder filling as well as with a bladder contraction or Valsalva maneuver (Ghoniem et al, 1990; Homma et al, 1999). When the maximum resistance is known, the catheter is positioned so that the urethral pressure port is located at that or any other point of interest. This area can then be monitored throughout the urodynamic study.

Urethral pressure profilometry (UPP) measures the passive resistance of a particular point within the urethra to stretch (Gleason et al, 1974). Many factors contribute to this resistance, including the elastic properties of the tissues surrounding the lumen and the tension generated by the smooth and skeletal muscles of the urethra, which are constantly changing during the micturition cycle (Fig. 64–1) (Abrams, 1979; Evans et al, 1979). Therefore, the static urethral pressure profile is a measure of resistance in a specific set of circumstances (Yalla et al, 1979). It is difficult to extrapolate data obtained when the bladder is empty and apply it to periods when the bladder is full, is responding to increases in abdominal pressure, or is in the process of emptying (Fig. 64–2). Failure to recognize this fact leads to false assumptions and improper treatment.

External urethral sphincter EMG is performed using a 24-gauge concentric needle electrode (Diokno et al, 1974; Blaivas et al, 1977b) inserted perineally in boys or paraurethrally in girls and advanced into the skeletal muscle component of the sphincter until individual motor unit action potentials are seen or heard on a standard EMG recorder. Alternatively, perineal electrodes (Maizels and Firlit, 1979) or abdominal patch electrodes (Koff and Kass, 1982) have been used to record the bioelectric activity in the sphincter muscle. Disagreements exist concerning the accuracy of these surface electrode measurements, compared with those obtained with needle electrodes, particularly during voiding. The intactness of sacral cord function is easily measured with needle electrodes by (1) looking at the characteristic wave form of individual motor unit action potentials when the patient is relaxed and the bladder is empty, (2) performing and recording the responses to bulbocavernosus and anal stimulation and to Credé and Valsalva maneuvers, (3) asking the patient to voluntarily contract and relax the external sphincter, and (4) seeing the reaction of the sphincter to filling and emptying of the bladder (Fig. 64–3) (Blaivas et al, 1977a; Blaivas, 1979b).

The rate of bladder filling per minute usually is selected

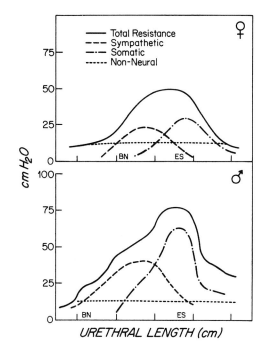

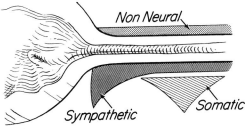

Figure 64–1. Components of urethral wall tension according to their geographic distribution and effect along the urethra in males and females. BN, bladder neck; ES, external sphincter. (From Bauer SB: Urodynamic evaluation and neuromuscular dysfunction. In Kelalis PP, Kin LR, Belman AB [eds]: Clinical Pediatric Urology, 2nd ed, vol 1. Philadelphia, WB Saunders, 1985, pp 283–310.)

by first calculating the child's predicted capacity and then dividing the result by 10 in order to fill the bladder slowly. The average capacity in milliliters for a child older than 2 years of age is determined by adding 6 to half of the child's age in years and multiplying the result by 30; for younger children, it is determined by adding 2 to twice the child's age and multiplying the result by 30 (Kaefer et al, 1997b). In children with myelodysplasia, the average bladder capacity fits the following formula: $24.5 \times$ age in years + 62 (Palmer et al, 1997). It has been shown that more rapid filling rates may yield falsely low levels of detrusor compliance and may minimize uninhibited contractions (Turner-Warwick 1975; Joseph, 1992). In an attempt to avoid this problem, the bladder is filled slowly with saline warmed to 37°C. When it is important to determine very mild degrees of hypertonicity, even slower rates of filling are used to measure its true incidence (Kerr et al, 1994; Yeung et al, 1995; Zermann et al, 1997). Some investigators have recorded pressure at residual volume to measure natural filling pressure as the most accurate means of denoting hypertonicity (Kaefer et al, 1997a; Walter et al, 1998). During filling, it is helpful to try to divert the child's attention by asking unrelated questions, reading a

story aloud, or showing a movie or cartoon. If the examiner wishes to elicit uninhibited contractions, the child is asked to cough (Mayo, 1978); alternatively, a cold solution may be instilled at a rapid rate.

The study is not considered complete until the child urinates and voiding pressures are measured. The small size of the urodynamic catheter does not seem to affect micturition pressures adversely, even in very young children. The normal voiding pressure varies from 55 to 80 cm H_2O in boys and from 30 to 65 cm H_2O in girls (Blaivas et al, 1977b; Blaivas, 1979a; Gierup et al, 1979). Infants tend to have higher voiding pressures than older children. Sometimes it is difficult to get the child to void; patience and time are needed in this situation. Placing a bedpan under the buttocks of the child who is supine or dripping tepid water on the genital area often stimulates the child sufficiently to begin urinating. Having the child listen to the audio channel of the EMG amplifier machine while he or she tightens and/or relaxes the sphincter provides a means of biofeedback training to get the child to void. Once the child has voided, it is important to do the following:

1. Analyze the pressure curve to determine whether the contraction is sustained until voiding is complete
2. Determine whether abdominal pressure has been used to facilitate the emptying process
3. Listen to changes in EMG activity of the sphincter to determine whether it remained quiet throughout the voiding process
4. Note whether the flow rate curve was bell-shaped or intermittent
5. Measure the voided volume
6. Calculate whether the patient voided to completion
7. Observe whether an after-contraction occurred

Video urodynamics has gained popularity since its introduction in 1970 (Bates et al, 1970). Visualization of the bladder and bladder neck during filling and of the urethra during voiding has added a dimension for more accurately integrating all aspects of lower urinary tract function and characterizing an abnormality (Glazier et al, 1997). Incompetency of the bladder neck or pelvic floor or the location of any posterior urethral obstruction can be correlated with pressure measurements recorded simultaneously. Sometimes, aberrations noted on pressure monitoring of sphincter EMG tracings can be confirmed, enhancing these findings (Passerini-Glazel et al, 1992; Weerasinghe and Malone, 1993). Ambulatory urodynamics has become available and feasible in children with the development of microtransducers mounted on small catheters positioned in the bladder (Kulseng-Hanssen and Klevmark, 1996; McInerney et al, 1991). Data can be stored up to 24 hours at a time and analyzed later. When combined with techniques to monitor wetness, it can be a very effective way to determine the cause of incontinence (Webb et al, 1991). There are many difficulties and artifacts inherent with this technique (Heslington and Hilton, 1996), but over time it may provide the most accurate way to evaluate lower urinary tract function in a natural setting (Bristow and Neal, 1996).

Often, because it is appropriate to see the effects of drug administration, studies are repeated under similar circumstances several weeks to months later. This is especially true when one is trying to treat detrusor hypertonicity or

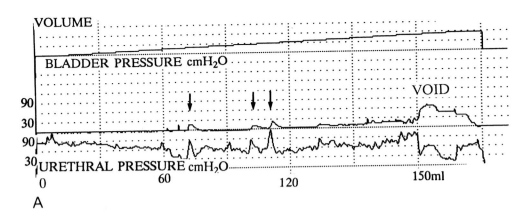

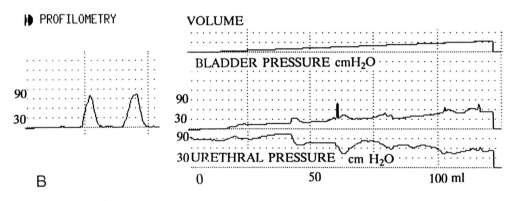

Figure 64–2. *A,* Urodynamic study in an 8-year-old boy with enuresis with the urethral pressure profilometry (UPP) port of the multichannel urodynamic catheter positioned in the midurethra. Note that urethral resistance is adequate at the start of filling, but it decreases just before and then increases with each uninhibited contraction *(arrows).* At capacity, the resistance is very high, but then it equals bladder pressure during voiding. *B,* A 7-year-old girl with myelomeningocele has a very good level of resistance when a urethral pressure profile is performed initially. During bladder filling, with the catheter positioned in the midurethra, urethral resistance drops from 90 to 58 cm H_2O at capacity.

hyperreflexia medically. To determine the maximum effect, the usual dose of most drugs is taken 2 to 3 hours before the test is performed a second time. The most commonly used drugs that affect lower urinary tract function are listed in Table 64–1, along with their appropriate dose ranges.

NEUROSPINAL DYSRAPHISMS

Myelodysplasia

The most common cause of neurogenic bladder dysfunction in children is abnormal development of the spinal canal and internecine spinal cord. Formation of the spinal cord and vertebral column begins at about the 18th day of gestation. Closure of the canal proceeds in a caudal direction from the cephalad end and is complete by 35 days. The exact mechanism that results in closure and what produces a dysraphic state are yet to be elucidated, but numerous factors have been implicated. **The incidence was reported as 1 per 1000 births in the United States** (Stein et al, 1982), **but there has been a definite decrease in this rate in the last 20 years** (Laurence, 1989; Lary and Edmonds, 1996). With the advent of prenatal screening, many affected fetuses are being identified and the pregnancies terminated before 16 weeks of gestation, thereby lowering the number of children born with this disease (Palomaki et al, 1999). **If spina bifida is already present in one member of a family, there is a 2% to 5% chance that a second sibling will be conceived with the same condition** (Scarff and Fronczak, 1981). The incidence doubles when more than one family member has a

neurospinal dysraphism (Table 64–2). Therefore, when the disease is already present in a family, the **Medical Research Council Vitamin Study Group recommends that women of childbearing age take 400 μg (0.4 mg) of folic acid per day beginning at least 1 month before the time they plan on becoming pregnant** (Committee on Genetics, American Academy of Pediatrics, 1999). There is strong evidence that folate deficiency can lead to a myelodysplastic abnormality de novo, and maternal ingestion of 400 μg of folate per day in all women of child-bearing age can reduce the incidence of spina bifida by 50% (Laurence et al, 1981; MRC Vitamin Study Research Group, 1991; Czeizel and Dudas, 1992).

Pathogenesis

Myelodysplasia is an all-inclusive term used to describe the various abnormal conditions of the vertebral column that affect spinal cord function. More specific labels for each abnormality include the following: a *meningocele* occurs when just the meninges but no neural elements extend beyond the confines of the vertebral canal; in a *myelomeningocele,* neural tissue, either nerve roots or portions of the spinal cord, has evaginated with the meningocele (Fig. 64–4); the term *lipomyelomeningocele* denotes that fatty tissue has developed with the cord structures and both are extending with the protruding sac. **Myelomeningocele accounts for more than 90% of all open spinal dysraphic states** (Stark, 1977). **Most spinal defects occur at the level of the lumbar vertebrae, with the sacral, thoracic, and cervical areas, in decreasing order of frequency, less affected** (Bauer et al, 1977) (Table 64–3). An over-

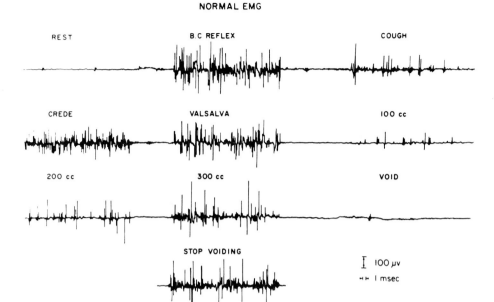

Figure 64–3. Normal reaction of the external urethral sphincter on electromyogram to all the sacral reflexes and to bladder filling and emptying. (From Bauer SB: Urodynamic evaluation and neuromuscular dysfunction. In Kelalis PP, King LR, Belman AB [eds]: Clinical Pediatric Urology, 2nd ed, vol 1. Philadelphia, WB Saunders, 1985, pp 283–310.)

whelming number of meningoceles are directed posteriorly, but on rare occasions they may protrude anteriorly, particularly in the sacral area. Usually the meningocele is made up of a flimsy covering of transparent tissue, but it may be open and leaking cerebrospinal fluid. For this reason urgent repair is necessary, with sterile precautions being followed in the interval between birth and closure. **In 85% of affected children, there is an associated Arnold-Chiari malformation, in which the cerebellar tonsils have herniated down through the foramen magnum, obstructing the fourth ventricle and preventing the cerebrospinal fluid from entering the subarachnoid space surrounding the brain and spinal cord.**

Table 64–1. DRUGS THAT AFFECT LOWER URINARY TRACT FUNCTION

Type	Dosage	
	Minimum	*Maximum*
Cholinergic		
Bethanechol (Urecholine)	0.7 mg/kg tid	0.8 mg/kg qid
Anticholinergic		
Propantheline (Pro-Banthine)	0.5 mg/kg bid	0.5 mg/kg qid
Oxybutynin (Ditropan)	0.2 mg/kg bid	0.2 mg/kg qid
Glycopyrrolate (Robinul)	0.01 mg/kg bid	0.03 mg/kg tid
Hyoscyamine (Levsin)	0.03 mg/kg bid	0.1 mg/kg tid
Tolterodine (Detrol)	0.01 mg/kg bid	0.04 mg/kg bid
Sympathomimetic		
Phenylpropanolamine (alpha)	2.5 mg/kg tid	2.5 mg/kg qid
Ephedrine (alpha)	0.5 mg/kg tid	1.0 mg/kg tid
Pseudoephedrine (alpha)	0.4 mg/kg bid	0.9 mg/kg tid
Sympatholytic		
Prazosin (alpha) (Minipress)	0.05 mg/kg bid	0.1 mg/kg tid
Phenoxybenzamine (alpha)	0.3 mg/kg bid	0.5 mg/kg tid
Propranolol (beta)	0.25 mg/kg bid	0.5 mg/kg bid
Smooth muscle relaxant		
Flavoxate (Urispas)	3.0 mg/kg bid	3.0 mg/kg tid
Dicyclomine (Bentyl)	0.1 mg/kg bid	0.3 mg/kg tid
Other		
Imipramine (Tofranil)	0.7 mg/kg bid	1.2 mg/kg tid

In the past 2 years, several centers in the United States have begun closing the defect in fetuses between 25 and 29 weeks of gestation in an attempt to improve the neurologic defect in these children (Adzick et al, 1998; Holzbeierlein et al, 2000; Bruner et al, 1999). Thus far this procedure has not altered the incidence of abnormal findings on urodynamic assessment in the postnatal period, but, surprisingly, aqueduct obstruction and hydrocephalus have not occurred at birth. **It is possible that leakage of cerebrospinal fluid accounts for the herniation of the posterior brain stem down the foramen magnum, leading to the development of hydrocephalus.**

The neurologic lesion produced by this condition can be variable, depending on what neural elements, if any, have everted with the meningocele sac. The bony vertebral level often provides little or no clue to the exact neurologic level or lesion produced. The height of the bony level may differ from the highest extent of the neurologic lesion from one to three vertebrae in either direction (Bauer et al, 1977). Furthermore, there may be differences in function from one side of the body to the other at the same neurologic level and from one neurologic level to the next owing to asymmetry of the affected neural elements. **It is important to remember that no two children have the same neurourologic defect.** In addition, in 20% of

Table 64–2. FAMILIAL RISK OF MYELODYSPLASIA IN THE UNITED STATES PER 1000 LIVE BIRTHS

Relationship	Incidence
General population	0.7–1.0
Mother with one affected child	20–50
Mother with two affected children	100
Patient with myelodysplasia	40
Mother older than 35 years	30
Sister of mother with affected child	10
Sister of father with affected child	3
Nephew who is affected	2

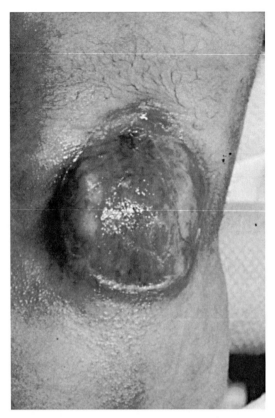

Figure 64–4. Typical appearance of a newborn with an open myelomeningocele.

Table 64–3. SPINAL LEVEL OF MYELOMENINGOCELE

Location	Incidence (%)
Cervical–high thoracic	2
Low thoracic	5
Lumbar	26
Lumbosacral	47
Sacral	20

area may not provide sufficient information to make a concrete inference. As a result, urodynamic evaluation in the neonatal period is now recommended at most pediatric centers in the United States, because it not only provides a clear picture of the function of the sacral spinal cord and lower urinary tract but also has predictive value in babies at risk for future urinary tract deterioration and progressive neurologic change (McGuire et al, 1981; Van Gool et al, 1982; Bauer, 1984b; Sidi et al, 1986). The advent of hostility scores and the reliability of urodynamic risk factors has led many clinicians to initiate prophylactic therapy in those newborns considered to be at risk for urinary tract deterioration (Perez et al, 1992).

Newborn Assessment

Ideally, it would be best to perform urodynamic testing immediately after the baby is born, but the risk of spinal infection and the exigency for closure have not made this a viable option. It was accomplished in one study, however, and the results showed that fewer than 5% of children experienced a change in neurologic status as a result of the spinal canal closure (Kroovand et al, 1990). Therefore, **renal ultrasonography and measurement of residual urine are performed as early as possible after birth,** either before or immediately after the spinal defect is closed; **urodynamic studies are delayed until it is safe to transport the child to the urodynamic suite** and place him or her on back or side for the test. **If the infant cannot empty the bladder after a spontaneous void or with a Credé maneuver, CIC is begun** even before urodynamic studies are conducted. If the Credé maneuver is effective in emptying the bladder, it is performed on a regular basis instead of using CIC until the lower urinary tract can be evaluated. The normal bladder capacity in the newborn period is 10 to 15 ml; therefore, a residual urine of less than 5 ml is acceptable. **Other tests that should be performed in the neonatal period include a urine analysis and culture, serum creatinine, and a careful neurologic examination of the lower extremities.**

Once the spinal closure has healed sufficiently, a renal ultrasonogram or excretory urogram and renal scan are performed to reassess upper urinary tract architecture and function. Next, a voiding cystourethrogram (VCUG) and urodynamic study are conducted. **These studies meet several objectives: they provide baseline information** about the radiologic appearance of the upper and lower urinary tracts as well as the condition of the sacral spinal cord and the central nervous system (CNS); **they provide results that can be compared with findings on subsequent assessments,** so that early signs of deterioration of urinary tract function and drainage, or of progressive neurologic

affected children a vertebral bony or intraspinal abnormality occurs more cephalad than the vertebral defect and meningocele, and this can affect function in those portions of the cord. **Children with thoracic or upper lumbar meningoceles often have complete reconstitution of the spine in the sacral area, and these individuals frequently have intact sacral reflex arc function involving the sacral spinal roots (in our series of patients with high-level lesions, 74% of newborns and 54% of older children were affected thusly)** (Pontari et al, 1995). In fact, it is more likely that children with upper thoracic or cervical lesions will have just a meningocele and no myelomeningocele. **Children with neurologic deficits at S1 or lower may also manifest a variety of findings on urodynamic testing,** ranging from normal function to upper and/or lower motor neuron lesions involving either the bladder or the external urethral sphincter (Dator et al, 1992). Finally, **the differing growth rates of the vertebral bodies and the elongating spinal cord add a dynamic factor in the developing fetus that further complicates the picture** (Lais et al, 1993). Superimposed on all this is the Arnold-Chiari malformation, which can have a profound effect on the brain stem and pontine center, areas that are involved in control of lower urinary tract function.

Therefore, **the neurologic lesion produced by this condition influences lower urinary tract function in a variety of ways and cannot be predicted just by looking at the spinal abnormality or the neurologic function of the lower extremities.** Even careful assessment of the sacral

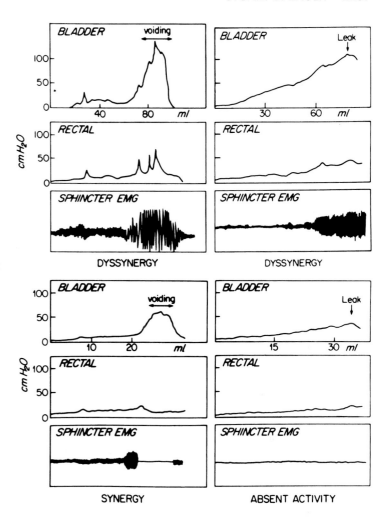

Figure 64–5. Various patterns of urodynamic findings on electromyography (EMG) in newborns with myelodysplasia. Note that a hypertonic detrusor with a nonrelaxing sphincter is also labeled dyssynergy. (From Bauer SB: Early evaluation and management of children with spina bifida. In King LR [ed]: Urologic Surgery in Neonates and Young Infants. Philadelphia, WB Saunders, 1988, pp 252–264.)

denervation, can be detected; **they help to identify babies at risk for urinary tract deterioration** as a result of detrusor hypertonicity or outflow obstruction from detrusor-sphincter dyssynergia (DSD), which allows initiation of prophylactic measures before the changes actually take place; and **they help the physician to counsel parents** about the child's future bladder and sexual function (McGuire et al, 1981; Bauer et al, 1984; Bauer, 1984a; Sidi et al, 1986; Lais et al, 1993).

Findings

Ten to fifteen percent of newborns have an abnormal urinary tract on radiologic examination when first evaluated (Bauer, 1985); 3% have hydroureteronephrosis secondary to spinal shock, probably from the closure procedure (Chiaramonte et al, 1986), and 10% have abnormalities that developed in utero as a result of abnormal lower urinary tract function in the form of outlet obstruction.

Urodynamic studies in the newborn period have shown that 57% of infants have bladder contractions. This is also true in children with upper lumbar or thoracic lesions in whom the sacral spinal cord is spared, 50% of whom have detrusor contractions (Pontari et al, 1995). **Forty-three percent have an areflexic bladder** with compliance during filling that is either good (25%) or poor (18%) in this subgroup (Bauer et al, 1984). **EMG assess-**

ment of the external urethral sphincter demonstrates an intact sacral reflex arc with no evidence of lower motor neuron denervation in 40% of newborns; partial denervation is seen in 24%, and complete loss of sacral cord function is noted in 36%** (Lais et al, 1993).

A combination of bladder contractility and external sphincter activity results in **three categories of lower urinary tract dynamics: synergic (19%), dyssynergic with and without detrusor hypertonicity (45%), and complete denervation (36%)** (Fig. 64–5) (Bauer et al, 1984; Sidi et al, 1986). DSD occurs when the external sphincter fails to decrease or actually increases its activity during a detrusor contraction or a sustained increase in intravesical pressure as the bladder is filled to capacity (Blaivas et al, 1986). Frequently, a poorly compliant bladder with a high intravesical pressure occurs in conjunction with a dyssynergic sphincter, resulting in a bladder that empties only at high intravesical pressures (Van Gool et al, 1982; Sidi et al, 1986). Synergy is characterized by complete silencing of the sphincter during a detrusor contraction or when capacity is reached at the end of filling. Voiding pressures are usually within the normal range. Complete denervation is noted when no bioelectric potentials are detectable in the region of the external sphincter at any time during the micturition cycle or in response to sacral stimulation or a Credé maneuver.

The **categorization** of lower urinary tract function in

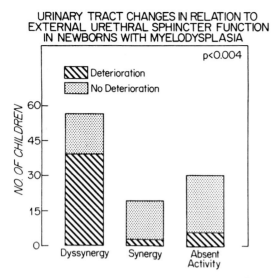

Figure 64–6. Urinary tract deterioration is related to outflow obstruction and is most often associated with dyssynergy. Children with synergy converted to dyssynergy, and patients with complete denervation developed fibrosis with a fixed high outlet resistance in the external sphincter, before any changes occurred in the urinary tract. (From Bauer SB: Early evaluation and management of children with spina bifida. In King LR [ed]: Urologic Surgery in Neonates and Young Infants. Philadelphia, WB Saunders, 1988, pp 252–264.)

this way has been extremely useful because it **reveals which children are at risk for urinary tract changes, which ones should be treated prophylactically, which need close surveillance, and which can be monitored at greater intervals. Within the first 3 years of life, 71% of newborns with DSD had urinary tract deterioration on initial assessment or subsequent studies, whereas only 17% of synergic children and 23% of completely denervated individuals developed similar changes** (Fig. 64–6). The infants in the synergic group who showed deterioration did so only after they converted to a dyssynergic pattern of sphincter function. Among the infants with complete denervation, the ones who showed deterioration were those who had increased levels of urethral resistance, presumably caused by fibrosis of the skeletal muscle component of the external sphincter. Therefore, it appears that **outlet obstruction is a major contributor to the development of urinary tract deterioration in these children** (Fig. 64–7). **Bladder tonicity plays an important role in this regard, especially when outlet resistance exceeds 40 cm H_2O** (McGuire et al, 1981; Tanaka et al, 1999). Detrusor compliance seems to be worse in children with high levels of outlet resistance (Ghoniem et al, 1989). Bloom and colleagues (1990) noted an improvement in compliance when outlet resistance was reduced after gentle urethral dilation in these children; however, the reasons for this change are unclear, and the long-term effect of the maneuver remains uncertain.

It may be that bladder filling pressures need to be looked at in a more critical way to determine whether they are an important factor in upper urinary tract deterioration. **Landau and colleagues (1994) developed the concept of low detrusor filling pressure (less than 30 cm H_2O) at specific volumes adjusted for age and not at maximum capacity. Applying this idea, they noted significantly im-**proved sensitivity in predicting upper urinary tract deterioration. The ability to predict accurately which newborns are at risk for urinary tract deterioration prompted the initiation of prophylactic therapy with CIC and anticholinergic drugs** (Geranoitis et al, 1988; Kasabian et al, 1992). **Long-term success has been achieved in preventing reflux and hydronephrosis and in reducing the need for augmentation cystoplasty, from between 27% and 41% to between 11% and 17%** (Edelstein et al, 1995; Wu et al, 1997; Kaefer et al, 1999). Others believe that aggressive observation and prompt intervention yields similar long-term results with less morbidity from catheterization (Teichman et al, 1994), but only time will delineate which avenue of treatment is most efficacious (Tanaka et al, 1999).

Recommendations

Because expectant treatment has revealed that infants with outlet obstruction in the form of DSD are at considerable risk for urinary tract deterioration, the idea of treating these children prophylactically has emerged as an important alternative. When CIC is begun in the newborn period, it is easy for parents to master, even in uncircumcised boys, and for children to accept as they grow older (Joseph et al, 1989). Complications such as meatitis, epididymitis, and urethral injury are rarely encountered, and urinary infections occur in fewer than 30% (Kasabian et al, 1992).

CIC alone or in combination with anticholinergic agents, when detrusor filling pressures exceed 40 cm H_2O and voiding pressures are higher than 80 to 100 cm H_2O, **resulted in an incidence of urinary tract deterioration of only 8% to 10%** (Geranoitis et al, 1988; Kasabian et al, 1992; Edelstein et al, 1995). This represents a significant drop in the occurrence of detrimental changes compared with children observed expectantly (McGuire et al, 1981; Bauer et al, 1984; Sidi et al, 1986; Teichman et al, 1994). Oxybutynin hydrochloride is administered in a dose of 1.0 mg per year of age every 12 hours to help lower detrusor filling pressures. In neonates and children younger than 1 year of age, the dose is lowered to less than 1.0 mg in relation to the child's age at the time and increased proportionately as the age approaches 1 year. Side effects have not been manifest when oxybutynin is administered according to this schedule (Joseph et al, 1989; Kasabian et al, 1992). On rare occasions when a hyperreflexive or hypertonic bladder fails to respond to these measures, a cutaneous vesicostomy may have to be performed (Fig. 64–8) (Duckett, 1974; Mandell et al, 1981).

Neurologic Findings and Recommendations

It has been documented that **the neurologic lesion in myelodysplasia is a dynamic disease process in which changes take place throughout childhood** (Epstein, 1982; Reigel, 1983; Venes and Stevens, 1983; Oi et al, 1990), **especially in early infancy** (Spindel et al, 1987) **and later at puberty** (Begger et al, 1986), **when the linear growth rate accelerates again.** When a change is noted on neurologic, orthopedic, or urodynamic assessment, radiologic investigation of the CNS often reveals (1) tethering of the

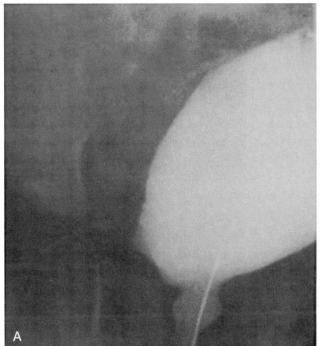

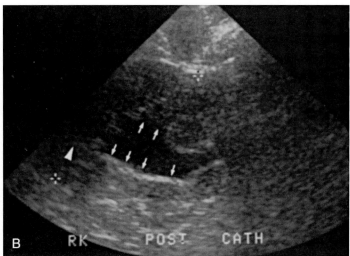

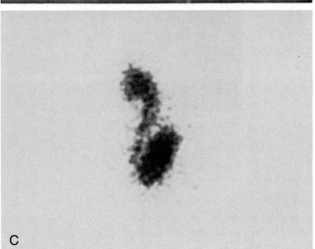

Figure 64–7. *A,* A voiding cystourethrogram in a newborn girl with dyssynergy and elevated voiding pressures demonstrates no reflux and a smooth-walled bladder. Her initial renal echogram was normal. She was started on clean intermittent catheterization and oxybutynin chloride (Ditropan) but did not respond. Within 1 year, she developed right hydronephrosis *(B, white arrows)* and severe reflux on a radionuclide cystogram *(C).*

spinal cord (Fig. 64–9), (2) a syrinx or hydromyelia of the cord, (3) increased intracranial pressure due to a shunt malfunction, or (4) partial herniation of the brain stem and cerebellum. Children with completely intact or only partially denervated sacral cord function are particularly vulnerable to progressive changes. Today, **MRI is the test of choice because it reveals anatomic details of the spinal column and CNS** (Just et al, 1990). **However, it is not a functional study, and when used alone it cannot provide exact information about a changing neurologic lesion.**

Sequential urodynamic testing on a yearly basis beginning in the newborn period and continuing until the child is 5 years old provides a means of carefully monitoring these children to detect signs of change, thus offering the hope that early detection and neurosurgical intervention may help to arrest or even reverse a progressive pathologic process. **Changes occurring in a group of newborns monitored in this manner involved both the sacral reflex arc and the pontine–sacral reflex interac-**

tion (Fig. 64–10) (Lais et al, 1993). Most children who undergo such changes tend to do so in the first 3 years of life (Fig. 64–11). Twenty-two of 28 children in whom the neurologic picture became worse underwent a second neurosurgical procedure; 11 of them had a beneficial effect from the surgery and showed improvement in urethral sphincter function (Lais et al, 1993). Babies with only sacral level deficits have a 47% risk of deterioration (Dator et al, 1992). Even children with normal neurourologic function at birth have a 32% risk, mostly DSD or upper motor findings, of developing a tethered spinal cord (Tarcan et al, 2001).

As a result of these developments, **it is recommended that all babies with myelodysplasia be monitored according to the guidelines set forth in Table 64–4.** It is not enough to look at just the radiologic appearance of the urinary tract; scrutiny of the functional status of the lower urinary tract is important as well. In addition to the reasons cited previously, it may be necessary to repeat a urody-

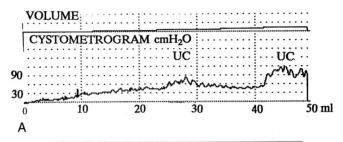

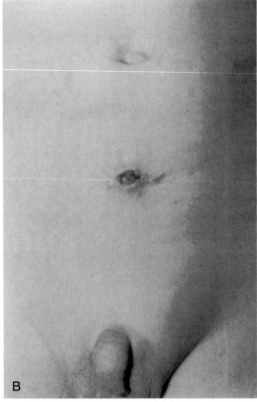

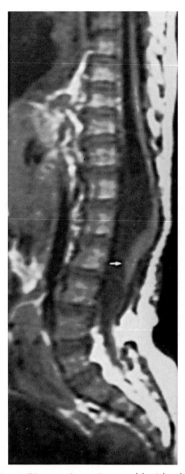

Figure 64–9. An MRI scan in a 9-year-old girl who developed a tethered cord after myelomeningocele repair reveals the conus opposite the L3–4 vertebrae *(arrow)*.

Figure 64–8. *A,* A 6-month-old boy with a myelomeningocele and detrusor sphincter dyssynergy fails to lower bladder filling and detrusor contractile pressures on oxybutynin. UC, uninhibited contraction. *B,* Because the lower ureters showed increasing dilation on ultrasonography, in addition to this poor response to medication in lowering intravesical pressure, a vesicostomy was performed.

namic study if the upper urinary tract dilates secondary to impaired drainage from a hypertonic detrusor.

Management of Reflux

Vesicoureteral reflux occurs in 3% to 5% of newborns with myelodysplasia, usually in association with detrusor hypertonicity or DSD (Flood et al, 1994). **It is rare to find reflux in any neonate without DSD or poor compliance** (Bauer, 1984b; Geranoitis et al, 1988; Edelstein et al, 1995). **If left untreated, the incidence of reflux in these infants at risk increases with time until 30% to 40% are afflicted by 5 years of age** (Bauer, 1984a). **Prophylactic treatment that lowers detrusor filling and voiding pressures with oxybutynin and empties the bladder by means of CIC significantly reduces this rising incidence of reflux** (Edelstein et al, 1995).

In children with reflux grades 1 to 3 (International Classification) who void spontaneously or have complete lesions with little or no outlet resistance and empty their bladder completely, **management consists solely of prophylaxis with antibiotics to prevent recurrent infection. In children with high-grade reflux (grade 4 or 5), CIC is begun to ensure complete emptying. Children who cannot empty their bladder spontaneously, regardless of the grade of reflux, are treated with CIC to empty the bladder efficiently. Children with detrusor hypertonicity with or without hydroureteronephrosis are also started on oxybutynin to lower intravesical pressure** and ensure adequate upper urinary tract decompression (Flood et al, 1994). **When reflux is managed in this manner there has been a dramatic response, with reflux resolving in 30% to 55% of individuals** (Kass et al, 1981; Bauer, 1984b; Joseph et al, 1989; Flood et al, 1994). **Bacteriuria is seen in as many as 56% of children on CIC** but usually it is not harmful except in the presence of high-grade reflux, because symptomatic urinary infection and renal scarring rarely occur with lesser grades of reflux (Kass et al, 1981; Cohen et al, 1990).

Credé voiding should be avoided in children with reflux, especially those with a reactive external sphincter. In this circumstance, the Credé maneuver results in a reflex response in the external sphincter that increases urethral resistance and raises the pressure needed to expel urine from the bladder (Barbalais et al, 1983) (Fig. 64–

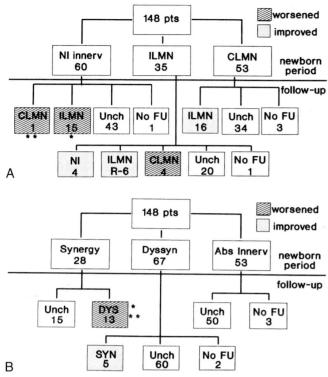

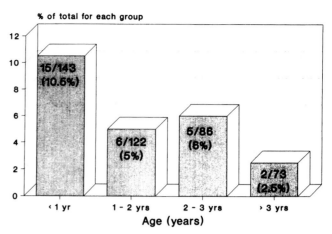

Figure 64–11. The propensity for a change in ureteral sphincter innervation is greatest in the first year of life. (From Lais A, Kasabian NG, Dyro FM, et al: Neurosurgical implications of continuous neuro-urological surveillance of children with myelodysplasia. J Urol 1993; 150:1879–1883.)

Figure 64–10. The changes in innervation of the purely sacral *(A)* and pontine-sacral *(B)* reflex arc pathways that occurred in a group of children with myelodysplasia who were monitored with sequential urodynamic studies beginning in the newborn period. ILMN, incomplete lower motor neuron lesion; CLMN, complete lower motor neuron lesion; NL, normal innervation; Unch, unchanged; FU, follow-up; DYS, dyssynergy; Syn, synergy. In *A*, the double asterisk indicates 1 patient changed from synergy to dyssynergy, and the single asterisk indicates 4 of 15 patients so changed. In *B*, the single asterisk indicates 1 patient changed from normal to partial and then complete denervation, and the double asterisk indicates 4 patients changed from normal to partial denervation. (From Lais A, Kasabian NG, Dyro FM, et al: Neurosurgical implications of continuous neuro-urological surveillance of children with myelodysplasia. J Urol 1993;150:1879–1883.)

Jeffs and colleagues (1976) were the first to show that **antireflux surgery can be very effective in children with neurogenic bladder dysfunction as long as it is combined with measures to ensure complete bladder emptying.** Before this observation was made, the results of ureteral reimplantation were so dismal that most physicians treating these children advocated urinary diversion as a means of managing reflux (Smith, 1972; Cass, 1976). Since the advent of CIC, success rates for antireflux surgery have approached 95% (Kass et al, 1981; Woodard et al, 1981; Bauer et al, 1982; Kaplan and Firlit, 1983). Bilateral surgery for unilateral disease need not be done, because contralateral reflux does not occur postoperatively (Bauer, 1984a).

Continence

Urinary continence is becoming an increasingly important issue that demands attention at an early age as parents try to mainstream their handicapped children. **Initial attempts at achieving continence include CIC and drug**

12). This has the effect of aggravating the degree of reflux and accentuating its water-hammer effect on the kidneys. Vesicostomy drainage (Duckett, 1974; Mandell et al, 1981) is rarely required today but is reserved for those infants who have such severe reflux that CIC and anticholinergic medication fail to improve upper urinary tract drainage or whose parents cannot adapt to the catheterization program.

The indications for antireflux surgery are not very different from those applicable to children with normal bladder function. They include recurrent symptomatic urinary infection while receiving adequate antibiotic therapy and appropriate catheterization techniques; persistent hydroureteronephrosis despite effective emptying of the bladder and lowering of intravesical pressure; severe reflux with an anatomic abnormality at the ureterovesical junction; reflux that persists into puberty; and the presence of reflux in any child undergoing surgery to increase bladder outlet resistance. Although some clinicians do not advocate reimplanting ureters in patients with low-grade reflux who are undergoing augmentation cystoplasty to lower intravesical pressure, this concept is not universally accepted (Nasrallah and Aliabadi, 1991).

Table 64–4. SURVEILLANCE IN INFANTS WITH MYELODYSPLASIA*

Sphincter Activity	Recommended Tests	Frequency
Intact–synergic	Postvoid residual volume	q 4 mo
	IVP or renal echo	q 12 mo
	UDS	q 12 mo
Intact–dyssynergic†	IVP or renal echo	q 12 mo
	UDS	q 12 mo
	VCUG or RNC‡	q 12 mo
Partial denervation	Postvoid residual volume	q 4 mo
	IVP or renal echo	q 12 mo
	UDS§	q 12 mo
	VCUG or RNC‡	q 12 mo
Complete denervation	Postvoid residual volume	q 6 mo
	Renal echo	q 12 mo

IVP, intravenous pyelogram; echo, sonogram; UDS, urodynamic study; VCUG, voiding cystourethrogram; RNC, radionuclide cystogram.
*Until age 5 years.
†Patients receiving intermittent catheterization and anticholinergic agents.
‡If detrusor hypertonicity or reflux is already present.
§Depending on degree of denervation.

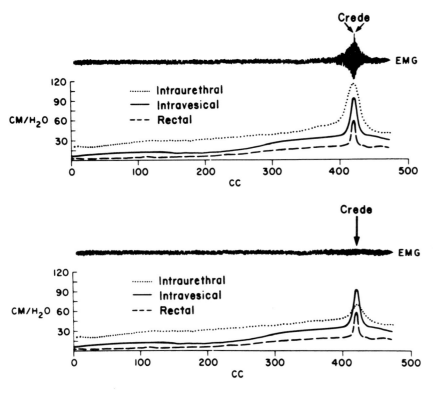

Figure 64–12. When the external sphincter is reactive *(top graph),* a Credé maneuver produces a reflex increase in electromyographic (EMG) activity of the sphincter and a concomitant rise in urethral resistance, resulting in high "voiding" pressure. A child whose sphincter is denervated and nonreactive *(bottom graph)* will not have a corresponding rise in EMG activity, urethral resistance, or voiding pressure. A Credé maneuver here will not be detrimental. (From Bauer SB: Early evaluation and management of children with spina bifida. In King LR [ed]: Urologic Surgery in Neonates and Young Infants. Philadelphia, WB Saunders, 1988, pp 252–264.)

therapy designed to maintain low intravesical pressures and a reasonable level of urethral resistance (Figs. 64–13 and 64–14). Although these measures can be initiated on a trial-and-error basis, it is more efficient to use exact treatment protocols based on specific urodynamic findings. As a result, urodynamic testing is performed if initial attempts with CIC and oxybutynin fail to achieve continence.

Without urodynamic studies it is hard to know whether (1) a single drug is effective, (2) the dose should be increased, or (3) a second drug should be added to the regimen.

At this point, **if detrusor hypertonicity or uninhibited contractions have not been dealt with effectively, another anticholinergic agent may be combined with or given instead of oxybutynin** (see Table 64–1). Glycopyr-

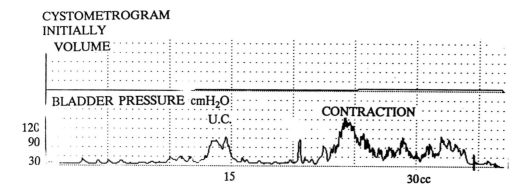

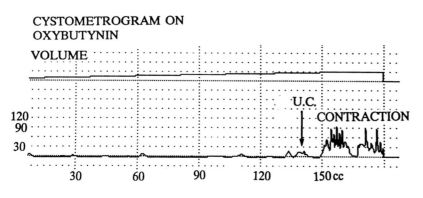

Figure 64–13. Oxybutynin is a potent anticholinergic agent that dramatically delays detrusor contractions and lowers contraction pressure, as demonstrated on these two graphs. U.C., uninhibited contraction.

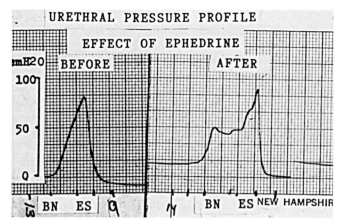

Figure 64–14. α-Sympathomimetic agents potentially have their greatest effect in the bladder neck region, where the highest concentration of α-receptor sites exists. They can raise outlet resistance and improve continence in many individuals. BN, bladder neck; ES, external sphincter.

rolate is the most potent oral anticholinergic drug available today, but it may have the typical belladonna-like side effects common to all these drugs. Tolterodine, a newly approved anticholinergic drug, is equally effective as oxybutynin in reducing hyperreflexia and improving compliance but with fewer side effects, especially constipation (Goessl et al, 2000). Hyoscyamine produces fewer side effects still, but its potency is less. Intravesical instillation of oxybutynin has been proven to be successful in lowering detrusor pressures and has fewer side effects compared with oral administration; serum concentrations may reach similar levels regardless of the route of intake (Greenfield and Fera, 1991; Massad et al, 1992). Inconvenience of administration, however, seems to preclude its long-term use (Kasabian et al, 1994).

If urodynamic testing reveals that urethral resistance is inadequate to maintain continence because either the sphincter fails to react to increases in abdominal pressures or resistance drops with bladder filling (see Fig. 64–2B), **α-sympathomimetic agents are added to the regimen** (see Table 64–1); phenylpropanolamine is the most effective drug in this regard.

Surgery becomes a viable option when this program of drug therapy fails to achieve continence. In general, surgical intervention is not considered until the child is about 5 years of age and ready to start school. Persistent hypertonicity or hyperreflexia may be treated with either enterocystoplasty (Mitchell and Piser, 1987; Sidi et al, 1987; Hernandez et al, 1994), autoaugmentation (Cartwright and Snow, 1989a, 1989b), or a combination thereof (Duel et al, 1998). **Sigmoid, cecum, and small intestine, in that order, have been used to enlarge the bladder. Although the ileocecal segment is a favored source for bladder replacement in adults, it is avoided in children with myelodysplasia** because removing it might aggravate the bowel dysfunction that is so often a factor in these children. **Detubularization of the bowel is needed to minimize the intrinsic contractions of the intestinal segment** and prevent it from causing intractable incontinence once it has been added to the bladder (Goldwasser et al, 1987; Hinman, 1988). **In the last 15 years, gastrocysto-**

plasty has been advocated when bowel augmentation is considered because it has fewer intrinsic contractions; the diamond-shaped patch does not have to be reconfigured, so there are fewer suture lines; the spherical reservoir created by the patch is the most efficient way to store fluid; it provides an acid milieu; and it is free of mucus secretions, which can lead to repeated urinary infections (Adams et al, 1988; Atala et al, 1993).

Concerns have been expressed about gastric segments because they can cause hyponatremic hypochloremic metabolic alkalosis (Gosalbez et al, 1993) **or an abnormality called the hematuria dysuria syndrome** (Nguyen et al, 1996). As a result, some surgeons have advocated peeling the detrusor muscle off the dome of the bladder, leaving the mucosa intact, and augmenting this bladder with demucosalized intestine (Gonzalez et al, 1994) or stomach (Nguyen et al, 1996). However, this too has not yielded a uniform long-term success rate in providing a bladder of adequate capacity and good compliance (Carr et al, 1999).

If bladder neck or urethral resistance is insufficient to allow adequate storage capacity, several operations are available to improve this continence mechanism. Bladder neck reconstruction can be undertaken in a variety of ways, including the Young-Dees or Leadbetter procedures (Young, 1919; Dees, 1949; Leadbetter, 1964) or the more recently described operation by Kropp (Kropp and Angwafo, 1986), which was modified by Salle to make catheterization easier (Salle et al, 1994). A fascial sling procedure that suspends the bladder neck and buttresses it against the undersurface of the pubis has been advocated enthusiastically by several clinicians (McGuire et al, 1986; Raz et al, 1988; Peters et al, 1989). Its effectiveness does not seem to diminish over time (Elder, 1990). Each of these operations, however, necessitates the use of CIC to empty the bladder postoperatively. The artificial sphincter (Barrett and Furlow, 1982; Light and Scott, 1983; Light et al, 1983) also increases bladder outlet resistance, and its mechanism of action allows emptying at low urethral pressures. Any patient who can empty his or her bladder before the device is implanted should be able to do so afterward without the need for CIC. Poor detrusor compliance can develop postoperatively if the preoperative cystometrogram is not carefully scrutinized for signs of hypertonicity (Woodside and McGuire, 1982; Bauer et al, 1986), and this may lead to progressive renal failure if not treated in a timely fashion with medications or augmentation cystoplasty (Bauer et al, 1993). Long-term results with the artificial sphincter have shown that it is a viable option in children with neurogenic bladder dysfunction (Bosco et al, 1991; Levesque et al, 1996; Kryger et al, 1999).

In an attempt to avoid many of the complications associated with these invasive procedures, glutaraldehyde crosslinked bovine collagen has been injected endoscopically around the bladder neck to increase urethral resistance (Ben-Chaim et al, 1995). Although early reports were encouraging, longer-term assessment has been discouraging, with many patients requiring repeated injections to stay dry (Perez et al, 1996; Silveri et al, 1998). More recently, Atala and associates developed a self-sealing, detachable membrane balloon that can be placed submucosally at the bladder neck to improve outlet resistance (Yoo et al, 1997).

Initial results revealed improvement in continence (Diamond et al, 1999), but no long-term data are available.

Urinary diversion, once considered a panacea for children with myelodysplasia, has turned out to be a Pandora's box of new clinical problems (Schwarz and Jeffs, 1975; Shapiro et al, 1975). **Pyelonephritis and renal scarring, calculi, ureterointestinal obstruction, strictures of the conduit, and stomal stenosis are often encountered** in children who are monitored on a long-term basis. Although antirefluxing colon conduits seem to have fewer complications, they are still not ideal. In the last 15 years very successful attempts have been made to reverse urinary tract diversions in children who probably would not be diverted today (Hendren, 1973, 1990). Few if any children undergo urinary diversion now; if they do, it is in the form of a continent stoma.

Continent urinary diversion with closure of the bladder neck has been used to provide a better quality of life for those with intractable urethral incompetence despite bladder outlet surgery, or to make it easier to catheterize those individuals who cannot easily catheterize themselves.

Several operations have been devised, but the ones that achieved the most publicity initially were the Kock pouch in adults (Kock, 1971; Skinner et al, 1987) and the Indiana reservoir in children (Rowland et al, 1987). **Mitrofanoff (1980) created a continence mechanism by tunneling one end of the vermiform appendix into the bladder, as if reimplanting the ureter to prevent reflux, with the other end being brought out through the skin as a catheterizable stoma. This principle has been extended to the ureter.** After the ureter is transected at the pelvic brim, a proximal transureteroureterostomy is performed, and the cut end of the distal segment is brought to the skin as a stoma (Duckett and Snyder, 1986); the continence mechanism is provided by the intramural detrusor tunnel of the ureter. Other narrow structures (e.g., fallopian tube, a rolled strip of stomach, a tapered ileal segment) have been implanted either into the native bladder or along the tinea of a detubularized portion of sigmoid or cecum acting as a urinary reservoir (Woodhouse et al, 1989; Reidmiller et al, 1990; Bihrie et al, 1991). **The success rate for achieving continence has been excellent, approaching 85%, primarily owing to the flap valve effect of the intramural tunnel** (Hinman, 1990; Watson et al, 1995; Kaefer et al, 1997). For this reason, it is now the preferred method for continent urinary diversion.

Sexuality

Sexuality in this population is becoming an increasingly important issue as more individuals reach adulthood and want to marry or to have meaningful long-term relationships with the opposite sex (Cromer et al, 1990). Investigators are looking into the concerns, fears, self-imagery, and desires of teenagers and young adults, and at the ability of males to procreate and females to bear children (Bomalaski et al, 1995). However, few studies are available that look critically at sexual function in these patients. It is important to remember that **sexual development depends on socialization and the ability of the child to make** friends and discuss shared experiences and thoughts. **Mental handicaps, poor manual dexterity, lack of education, and overprotective parents often prevent independent behavior and, as a result, lead to poor understanding of sexual issues** (Joyner et al, 1998).

In several studies researchers interviewed groups of teenagers and reported that **28% to 40% of them had had one or more sexual encounters, and almost all of them had a desire to marry and ultimately to bear children** (Cromer et al, 1990; Palmer et al, 1999). **In one study, 72% of male subjects claimed they were able to have an erection, and two thirds of these were able to ejaculate** (Decter et al, 1997). **Other studies revealed that 70% to 80% of myelodysplastic women were able to become pregnant and to have an uneventful pregnancy and delivery, although urinary incontinence in the latter stages of gestation was common in many, as was delivery by cesarean section** (Laurence and Beresford, 1975; Cass et al, 1986; Bomalaski et al, 1995). In the same studies, **17% to 39% of male subjects claimed that they were able to father children,** and another 25% had a good prognosis for siring them (Laurence and Beresford, 1975; Bomalaski et al, 1995; Decter et al, 1997). **It is more likely that men will have problems with erectile and ejaculatory function because the sacral spinal cord is frequently involved, whereas reproductive function in women, which is under hormonal control, is not affected. Men with neurologic lesions at S1 or lower are likely to have normal or adequate reproductive sexual function, but only 50% of those with lesions above that level have adequate function** (Woodhouse, 1994).

Sexuality or the ability to interact with the opposite sex in a meaningful and lasting way is just as important as knowledge of one's precise sexual function. **The degree of sexuality is inversely proportional to the level of neurologic dysfunction** (Joyner et al, 1998; Palmer et al, 1999). Until recently, however, this **subject has been taboo** (Decter et al, 1997). Sexual identity, education, and social mores have been taken out of the realm of secrecy and are now openly discussed and taught to handicapped people. **Boys reach puberty at an age similar to the age for normal males, whereas breast development and menarche tend to start as much as 2 years earlier than usual in myelodysplastic girls.** The cause of this early hormonal surge is uncertain, but it may be related to changes in pituitary function in girls secondary to hydrocephalus (Hayden, 1985).

Bowel Function

There is no unanimity regarding the ideal bowel management program for myelodysplastic children. The external anal sphincter is innervated by the same (or similar) nerves that modulate the external urethral sphincter, whereas the internal anal sphincter is influenced by more proximal nerves from the sympathetic nervous system. As a result, the internal anal muscle reflexively relaxes in response to anal distention. Consequently, **bowel incontinence is frequently unpredictable;** it is often related to the consistency of fecal material and how rapidly the anal area refills after an evacuation, the degree of intactness of sacral cord sensation and motor function, and reflex reactivity of the external anal sphincter muscle (Younoszai, 1992).

A majority of pediatricians believe that a regular and efficient bowel emptying regimen is mandatory. Most programs begin at about 1 year of age, but the best method of attaining these objectives is still controversial. **Usually the children are placed on diets** that are intended to create formed but not severely constipated stool. Roughage in the form of fruits and bran and stool softeners (in older children) is given to achieve this goal. **Suppositories that help evacuate the rectum are used on a regular basis to help train the lower bowel to fill and empty.** Some physicians believe that enemas are more effective in evacuating a greater portion of the lower bowel, but one problem with them is the difficulty of retaining the fluid when the anal sphincter muscle is lax. **Biofeedback training programs to strengthen the external anal sphincter are no more effective than a good bowel management program in attaining fecal continence** (Loening-Baucke et al, 1988). **Electrostimulation of the bowel has resulted in variable improvement** in fecal continence from 0 to 36% (Marshall and Boston, 1997; Palmer et al, 1997). **When a carefully constructed bowel regimen is adhered to, most children with myelomeningocele can achieve some degree of fecal continence** (Myers, 1984), but the uncertainty of accidents always makes this a tenuous situation. **Often the urinary incontinence is effectively managed with CIC, drugs, and/or surgery but episodes of fecal soiling remain a problem,** particularly in socially minded adolescents (Hayden, 1985). When diet, medications, and manual evacuation fail to achieve predictable bowel emptying without soiling, **a continent cutaneous pathway from the lower abdominal wall to the cecum may be created using the vermiform appendix; this is called the ACE procedure, for *a*ntegrade *c*ontinence *e*nema** (Griffiths and Malone, 1995). Enemas are instilled daily or every other day to evacuate the colon. Cleansing the colon in this manner has resulted in complete continence in 89% of children in whom it has been tried (Squire et al, 1993).

Lipomeningocele and Other Spinal Dysraphisms

Diagnosis

There is a group of congenital defects that affect the formation of the spinal column but do not result in an **open vertebral canal** (James and Lassman, 1972) (Table 64–5). **They occur once in 4000 live births** (Bruce and Schut, 1979). These lesions can be very subtle and have no obvious outward signs, but **in more than 90% of children there is a cutaneous abnormality overlying the lower spine** (Anderson, 1975; Pierre-Kahn et al, 1997). This varies from a small dimple or skin tag to a tuft of hair, a dermal vascular malformation, or a very noticeable subcutaneous lipoma (Fig. 64–15). In addition, **on careful inspection of the legs, one may note a high arched foot or feet; alterations in the configuration of the toes with hammer or claw digits; a discrepancy in muscle size,**

Table 64–5. TYPES OF OCCULT SPINAL DYSRAPHISMS

Lipomeningocele
Intradural lipoma
Diastematomyelia
Tight filum terminale
Dermoid cyst/sinus
Aberrant nerve roots
Anterior sacral meningocele
Cauda equina tumor

shortness, and decreased strength in one leg compared to the other, typically at the ankle; and/or a gait abnormality, especially in older children (Dubrowitz et al, 1965; Weissert et al, 1989). **Absent perineal sensation and back pain are common symptoms** in older children and young adults (Linder et al, 1982; Yip et al, 1985; Weissert et al, 1989). **Lower urinary tract function is abnormal in 40% to 90% of affected older individuals, with the incidence of an abnormality increasing proportionately with age** (Mandell et al, 1980; Koyangi et al, 1997; Pierre-Kahn et al, 1997). **The child may experience difficulty with toilet training, urinary incontinence after an initial period of dryness once they are toilet trained (especially during the pubertal growth spurt), recurrent urinary infections, and/or fecal soiling.** Occasionally, some patients without an obvious back lesion escape detection until they develop urinary (66%) or lower extremity (19%) symptoms or back pain (14%) after puberty caused by delayed traction on the spinal cord (Satar et al, 1995).

Findings

When these children are evaluated in the newborn period or early infancy, **the majority have a perfectly normal neurologic examination** (Atala et al, 1992). **Urodynamic testing, however, reveals abnormal lower urinary tract function in about one third of babies younger than 18 months of age** (Keating et al, 1988) (Fig. 64–16). Such studies may provide the only evidence of a neurologic injury involving the lower spinal cord (Keating et al, 1988; Foster et al, 1990; Atala et al, 1992, Satar et al, 1997). **When present, the most likely abnormality is an upper motor neuron lesion** characterized by detrusor hyperreflexia and/or hyperactive sacral reflexes (Fone et al, 1997; Pierre-Kahn et al, 1997); mild forms of DSD are rarely noted. **Lower motor neuron signs with denervation potentials in the sphincter or detrusor areflexia occur in only 10% of young children.**

In contrast, practically all individuals older than 3 years of age who have not been operated on or in whom an occult dysraphism has been belatedly diagnosed have either an upper or lower motor neuron lesion or a combination thereof, on urodynamic testing (92%) (see Fig. 65–16) or neurologic signs of lower extremity dysfunction (Yip et al, 1985; Kondo et al, 1986; Keating et al, 1988; Atala et al, 1992; Satar et al, 1997). **When such children were observed expectantly from infancy after the diagnosis was made, 58% deteriorated within 2 years** (Andar et al, 1997; Cornette et al, 1998). There does not seem to be a preponderance of one type of

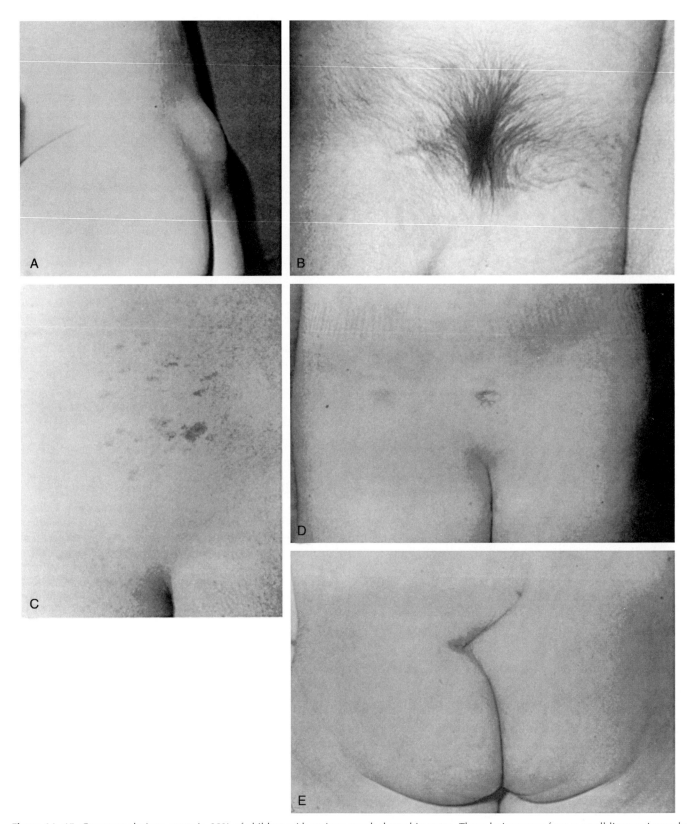

Figure 64–15. Cutaneous lesions occur in 90% of children with various occult dysraphic states. These lesions vary from a small lipomeningocele (*A*) to a hair patch (*B*), a dermal vascular malformation (*C*), a dimple (*D*), or an abnormal luteal cleft (*E*).

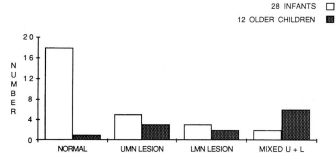

Figure 64–16. Most newborns with a covered spinal dysraphism have normal lower urinary tract function, whereas older children tend to have both upper motor neuron (UMN) and lower motor neuron (LMN) lesions.

lesion over the other (i.e., upper versus lower motor neuron); each occurs with almost equal frequency, and often the child shows signs of both (Hellstrom et al, 1986; Kondo et al, 1986). In one study of children older than 3 years of age, 43% had denervation in the sphincter and 52% detrusor areflexia, with a total of 81% having an abnormality (Satar et al, 1995).

Pathogenesis

Various occult spinal dysraphic lesions produce different neurourologic findings. When they do cause an abnormality, lipomas of the cauda equina invariably cause an upper motor neuron lesion (70%), alone or in combination with a lower motor neuron deficit (30%) (Satar et al, 1997). The split cord syndrome results in an isolated upper or lower motor neuron lesion in 25% each or a combined lesion in 50% (Proctor et al, 2000).

The reason for this difference in neurologic findings may be related to (1) compression on the cauda equina or sacral nerve roots by an expanding lipoma or lipomeningocele (Yamada et al, 1983), **(2) tension on the cord from tethering secondary to differential growth rates in the bony vertebrae and neural elements while the lower end of the cord is held in place by the lipoma or by a thickened filum terminale** (Dubrowitz et al, 1965), **or (3) fixation of the split lumbosacral cord by an intravertebral bony spicule or fibrous band** (Pang et al, 1992; Pang, 1992; Andar et al, 1997). **Under normal circumstances, the conus medullaris ends just below the L2 vertebra at birth and recedes upward to T12 by adulthood** (Barson, 1970). **When the cord does not "rise" because of one of these lesions, ischemic injury may ensue** (Yamada et al, 1981). **Correction of the lesion in infancy has resulted not only in stabilization but also in improvement in the neurologic picture in many instances** (Koyangi et al, 1997, Cornette et al, 1998; Proctor et al, 2000) (Fig. 64–17). **Sixty percent of babies with abnormal urodynamic findings preoperatively revert to normal postoperatively,** with improvement noted in 30%; 10% become worse with time. **In older children there is a less dramatic change after surgery, with only 27% becoming normal**, 27% improving, 27% stabilizing, but 19% actually becoming worse with time (see Fig. 64–17) (Keating et al, 1988; Satar et al, 1997). Older children with hyperreflexia tend to improve, whereas those with areflexic

bladders do not (Hellstrom et al, 1986; Kondo et al, 1986; Flanigan et al, 1989). **Finally, 5% to 27% of children operated on in early childhood develop secondary tethering when observed for several years**, suggesting that early surgery has both beneficial and sustaining effects in patients with this condition (Pierre-Kahn et al, 1997; Satar et al, 1997; Proctor et al, 2000).

As a result of these findings, it is apparent that urodynamic testing may be the only way to document that an occult spinal dysraphism is actually affecting lower spinal cord function (Keating et al, 1988; Khoury et al, 1990; Pierre-Khan et al, 1997). Some investigators have shown that posterior tibial somatosensory evoked potentials are an even more sensitive indicator of tethering and should be an integral part of the urodynamic evaluation (Roy et al, 1986). The implication of this finding lies in the fact that early detection and early intervention can both reverse the progress of the lesion, which does not happen in the older child (Yamada et al, 1983; Tami et al, 1987; Kaplan et al, 1988), and offer a degree of protection from subsequent tethering (Pierre-Kahn et al, 1997; Satar et al, 1997; Proctor et al, 2000), which seems to be a frequent occurrence when the lesion is not dealt with expeditiously in infancy (Chapman, 1982; Seeds and Jones, 1986).

Recommendations

Consequently, in addition to MRI studies (Tracey and Hanigan, 1990), **urodynamic testing** including EMG of the external urethral sphincter **should be performed in every child who has a questionable cutaneous or bony abnormality of the lower spine** (Packer et al, 1986; Hall

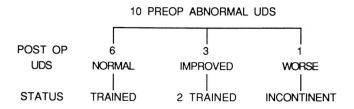

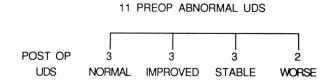

Figure 64–17. The potential for recoverable function is greatest in infants (6 of 10, 60%) and less so in older children (3 of 11, 27%). The risk of damage to neural tissue at the time of exploration to those with normal function is small (2 of 19, 11%). UDS, urodynamic study.

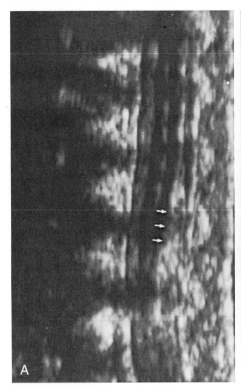

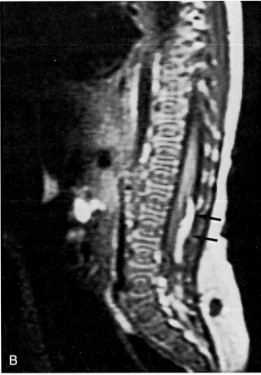

Figure 64–18. *A,* During the first few months of life, ultrasound can clearly demonstrate intravertebral anatomy because the posterior arches have not completely ossified. Note that the spinal cord along with its central canal is displaced anteriorly *(white arrows)* beginning at L3 because of an intradural lipoma. *B,* The MRI is juxtaposed to confirm the ultrasound findings. The longitudinal white intraspinal mass *(black arrows)* is the lipoma; the longitudinal gray mass is the spinal cord.

et al, 1988; Campobasso et al, 1988). This test provides the most accurate measure of sacral spinal cord function at diagnosis and provides a basis for comparison with subsequent studies when the children are either operated on or carefully observed. **If the child is younger than 4 to 6 months of age, ultrasound may be useful in visualizing the spinal canal before the vertebral bones have had a chance to ossify** (Fig. 64–18) (Raghavendra et al, 1983; Scheible et al, 1983). In the past, these conditions were usually treated only by removal of the superficial skin lesions, without delving further into the spinal canal to remove or repair the entire abnormality. Today, most neurosurgeons advocate laminectomy and removal of the intraspinal process as completely as possible without injuring the nerve roots or cord, in order to release the tether and prevent further injury with subsequent growth (Linder et al, 1982; Kondo et al, 1986; Kaplan et al, 1988; Foster et al, 1990; Atala et al, 1992; Pierre-Kahn et al, 1997; Proctor et al, 2000).

Sacral Agenesis

Sacral agenesis has been defined as the absence of part or all of two or more lower vertebral bodies. The cause of this condition is still uncertain, but teratogenic factors may play a role, because **insulin-dependent mothers have a 1% chance of giving birth to a child with this disorder. Conversely, 16% or more of children with sacral agenesis have an affected mother** (Passarge and Lenz, 1966; Guzman et al, 1983; Wilmshurst et al, 1999). Often the mothers have only gestational insulin-dependent diabetes. The disease has been reproduced in chicks by exposing embryos to insulin (Landauer, 1945; White and

Klauber, 1976). Maternal insulin-antibody complexes have been noted to cross the placenta, and their concentration in the fetal circulation is directly correlated with macrosomia (Menon et al, 1990). It is possible that a similar cause-and-effect phenomenon occurs in sacral agenesis. There is evidence that **a deletion of the seventh chromosome (7q36) leading to the absence of a transcription factor may be responsible for this anomaly** (Papapetrou et al, 1999).

Diagnosis

The presentation is bimodal, with more than three quarters of the children being detected in early infancy and the remainder discovered between 4 and 5 years of age (Wilmshurst et al, 1999). **The diagnosis is often delayed until failed attempts at toilet training bring the child to the attention of a physician. Sensation, including that in the perianal dermatomes, is usually intact, and lower extremity function is normal** (Koff and De-Ridder, 1977; Jakobson et al, 1985). Because these children have normal sensation and little or no orthopedic deformity in the lower extremities (although high arched feet or claw or hammer toes may be present), the underlying lesion is often overlooked. In fact, 20% escape detection until the age of 3 or 4 years (Guzman et al, 1983). **The only clue, besides a high index of suspicion, is flattened buttocks and a low, short gluteal cleft** (Bauer, 1990) (Fig. 64–19). Palpation of the coccyx is used to detect the absent vertebrae (White and Klauber, 1976). **The diagnosis is most easily confirmed with a lateral film of the lower spine, because this area is often obscured by the overlying gas pattern on an anteroposterior projection** (White and Klauber, 1976; Guzman et al, 1983) (Fig. 64–20). Recently, MRI has been used to visualize the spinal cord in these cases; **MRI reveals a sharp cut-off of the conus at T12 as a consistent finding** (Pang, 1993) (Fig. 64–21).

Findings

On urodynamic evaluation, an almost equal number of individuals manifest either an upper or a lower motor neuron lesion (35% versus 40%, respectively); 25% have no sign of denervation at all (Guzman et al, 1983; Boemers et al, 1994). Upper motor neuron lesions are characterized by detrusor hyperreflexia, exaggerated sacral reflexes, absence of voluntary control over sphincter function, DSD, and no EMG evidence of denervation potentials in the sphincter (White and Klauber, 1976; Koff and De-Ridder, 1977; Guzman et al, 1983). A lower motor neuron lesion is noted when detrusor areflexia and partial or complete denervation of the external urethral sphincter with diminished or absent sacral reflexes are seen. **The presence or absence of the bulbocavernosus reflex is an indicator (but not a foolproof one) of an upper or a lower motor neuron lesion, respectively** (Schlussel et al, 1994). **The number of affected vertebrae does not seem to correlate with the type of motor neuron lesion present** (Boemers et al, 1994) (Fig. 64–22). **The injury appears to be stable and rarely shows signs of progressive denervation** as the child grows. Sacral sensation is relatively spared, even in the presence of extensive sacral motor deficits (Boemers et al, 1994; Schlussel et al, 1994). **Urinary tract infection (UTI) may be detected in 75% of children**

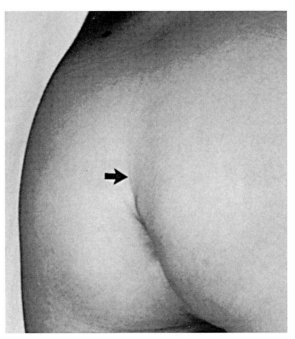

Figure 64–19. Characteristically, the gluteal crease is short and is seen only inferiorly *(below arrow)* because of the flattened buttocks in sacral agenesis.

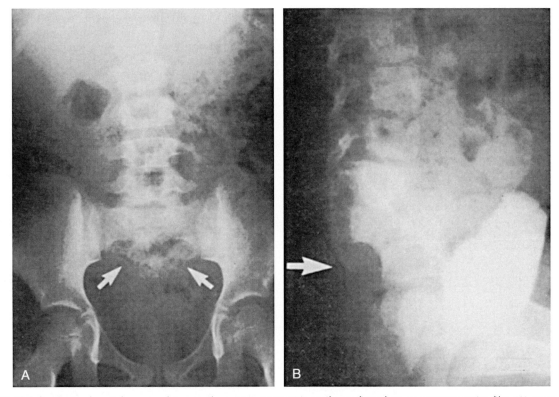

Figure 64–20. The diagnosis of partial or complete sacral agenesis *(arrows)* is easily confirmed on an anteroposterior film *(A)*, or on a lateral film *(B)* of the spine if bowel gas obscures the sacral area. (From Bauer SB: Urodynamic evaluation and neuromuscular dysfunction. In Kelalis PP, King LR, Belman AB [eds]: Clinical Pediatric Urology, 2nd ed, vol 1. Philadelphia, WB Saunders, 1985, pp 283–310.)

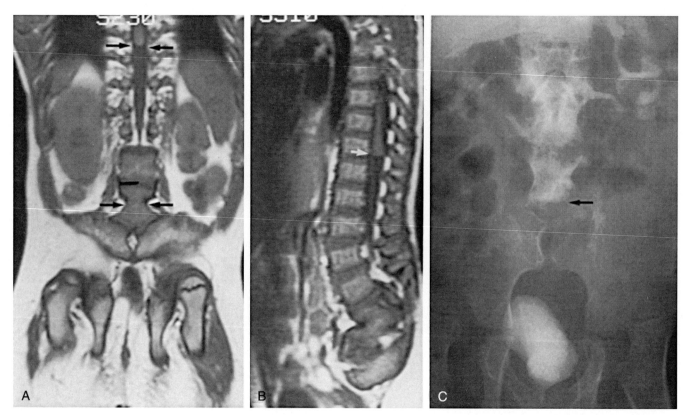

Figure 64–21. Coronal *(A)* and sagittal *(B)* magnetic resonance images in a 10-year-old boy with sacral agenesis beginning at L5. Note the squared lower limit of the cord adjacent to T11 *(A, upper arrows; B, white arrow)* and the two sacroiliac joints *(A, lower arrows)*, which are in the midline because of absence of the sacrum. *C,* An anteroposterior radiograph from an excretory urogram shows no vertebral bodies below L4 *(arrow)*.

over time, with vesicoureteral reflux diagnosed in 37%. Reflux is most likely in those with an upper (75%) versus a lower (40%) motor neuron lesion (Schlussel et al, 1994).

Recommendations

Because most children who are diagnosed with this condition have a neurologic deficit, **urodynamic testing is**

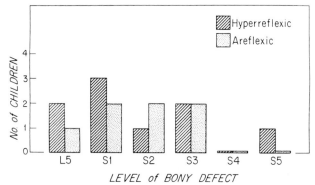

COMPARISON OF TYPE OF BLADDER FUNCTION
TO HEIGHT OF ABSENT VERTEBRAE

Figure 64–22. Bladder contractility is unrelated to the number of absent vertebrae. (From Bauer SB: Urodynamic evaluation and neuromuscular dysfunction. In Kelalis PP, King LR, Belman AB [eds]: Clinical Pediatric Urology, 2nd ed, vol 1. Philadelphia, WB Saunders, 1985, pp 283–310.)

mandatory at the time of diagnosis. Renal ultrasonography and nuclear or conventional cystography should be included as part of the evaluation process, especially if the child has a history of urinary infection. Additional imaging studies may be required based on the child's history and findings from baseline studies.

Management depends on the specific type of neurourologic dysfunction seen on urodynamic testing. Anticholinergic agents should be given to children with upper motor neuron findings of uninhibited contractions, whereas CIC and α-sympathomimetic medications may have to be given to individuals with lower motor neuron deficits who cannot empty their bladders or stay dry between catheterizations. The bowels manifest a similar picture of dysfunction and need as much characterization and treatment as the lower urinary tract. It is important to identify these individuals as early as possible so that they can become continent and out of diapers at an appropriate age, thus avoiding the social stigma of fecal or urinary incontinence.

Associated Conditions—Imperforate Anus

Imperforate anus is a condition that can occur alone or as part of a constellation of anomalies that have been called the VATER or VACTERL syndrome (Barry and Auldist, 1974). **This mnemonic denotes all the organs that can possibly be affected (V, vertebral; A,**

Table 64-6. WINGSPREAD CLASSIFICATION OF ANORECTAL MALFORMATIONS

Female	Male
High	High
Anorectal agenesis	Anorectal agenesis
With rectovaginal fistula	With rectourethral (prostatic)
Without fistula	fistula
Rectal atresia	Without fistula
Intermediate	Rectal atresia
Rectovestibular fistula	Intermediate
Rectovaginal fistula	Rectovestibular urethral fistula
Anal agenesis without fistula	Anal agenesis without fistula
Low	Low
Anovestibular fistula	Anocutaneous fistula
Anocutaneous fistula	Anal stenosis
Anal stenosis	Rare malformation
Cloacal malformation	
Rare malformation	

anal; C, cardiac; TE, tracheo-esophageal fistula; R, renal; L, limb). The incidence of anorectal malformations varies between 1 in 4000 and 1 in 5000 live births (Templeton and O'Neill, 1986). **There is a male predominance of 1.5:1. The majority of female patients have low lesions, whereas males tend to have high ones** (Santulli et al, 1971). Several classification systems have been devised, but the most commonly used one is the Wingspread Workshop on Anorectal Malformations (Table 64-6) (Shaul and Harrison, 1997). **This format attempts to divide the lesions into high, intermediate, or low, depending on whether the rectum ends above, at, or below the levator ani muscle, respectively. The relative incidence for the various levels of the defect is 36% high, 14% intermediate, 47% low, and 1% a cloacal lesion.**

Associated Findings

A fistulous communication with the lower urinary tract is a common occurrence, related in part to the sex of the child and the extent of the lesion: 87% of male and 79% of female babies with a high or intermediate lesion have a connection, whereas 7% of male and 10% of female children with a low lesion have such a communication (Templeton and O'Neill, 1986; Holschneider et al, 1994). **Urinary tract abnormalities have been noted in 26% to 52% of affected children, with renal agenesis (primarily left-sided) and vesicoureteral reflux the most common associated findings** (Parrott, 1985). Again, **the highest incidence of an abnormality is in those children with a high versus a low lesion** (Shaul and Harrison, 1997), **with boys more prone than girls to having an anomaly** (50% versus 29%) (Metts et al, 1997). **Spinal bony abnormalities range in incidence from 30% to 44%,** but patients with a high lesion are more likely to be affected (48% to 54%) than those with a low lesion (15% to 27%) (Carson et al, 1984; Tsakayannis and Shamberger, 1995; Long et al, 1996). **Spinal cord abnormalities including a tethered cord, thickened or fatty filum terminale, and a lipoma have been noted in 18% to 50% of patients, with the incidence varying proportionally in relation to the height of the rectal lesion** (Shaul and Harrison, 1997).

Not all patients with a spinal cord abnormality have a bony defect, so intraspinal imaging is mandatory to ensure the presence of a normal spinal cord (Rivosecchi et al, 1995). Often, this can be found in patients even without one of the commonly associated other anomalies. **Neurogenic bladder dysfunction is a frequent finding** (Kakizaki et al, 1994) and usually manifests as incontinence, **but its occurrence is rare when no spinal cord malformation exists** (Fig. 64-23). It often manifests when the child is older and the parents have difficulty with toilet training. It is not certain whether the dysfunction is caused by a spinal cord defect or by trauma to the nerves supplying the lower urinary tract or the pelvic floor musculature occasioned during surgery to repair the spinal cord or rectal defect (Parrott and Woodard, 1979). With the advent of the Peña posterior sagittal midline approach, the latter etiology is less likely (Peña, 1986; Boemers et al, 1994).

Evaluation

Initial evaluation in the newborn period should include a careful inspection of the perineum looking for a fistulous site from the bowel, an examination of the upper and lower extremities, and an assessment of the bony spine and spinal cord (Carson et al, 1984). A prone cross-table lateral image with the child held in that position for 3 minutes and a radio-opaque marker placed on the perineum will help delineate the distance from the end of the rectum to the skin in order to classify the extent of the rectal defect. Gas, meconium, or a gram-negative infection in the urine strongly suggests a rectal-urinary tract fistula, which then necessitates a divided colostomy very early in the postnatal period. **Once the child is stable clinically, radiologic investigation of the urinary tract is begun, first with renal ultrasonography and then with a VCUG, to define the presence of an abnormality and discover any clues for possible neurogenic bladder dysfunction.** Other imaging modalities include ultrasonography of the spine within the first 3 months of life, before the vertebral bodies have ossified, and, if necessary, a spinal MRI to rule out any intraspinal process (see Fig. 64-23) (Barnes et al, 1986; Tunell et al, 1987; Karrer et al, 1988). **Urodynamic studies are reserved for those children with either a bony abnormality of the spine, a spinal cord defect, or the telltale signs of dysfunction on a VCUG or renal ultrasonography.** These studies should be conducted early in infancy before the child has had any definitive surgery for the imperforate anus, and again after a pull-through operation has been performed on the rectum, to determine, respectively, the true incidence of neurogenic bladder dysfunction and any changes that might have occurred as a result of the surgery. The presence of an abnormality on urodynamic testing in early infancy may warrant either intervention at that time to correct a spinal cord defect or watchful waiting to determine whether the lesion is progressive.

The most common finding on urodynamic testing is an upper motor neuron lesion with uninhibited contractions and/or bladder-urethral sphincter dyssynergy (Boemers et al, 1994), but a lower motor neuron lesion with detrusor areflexia and a denervated sphincter may be seen as well (see Fig. 64-23) (Greenfield and Fera, 1991).

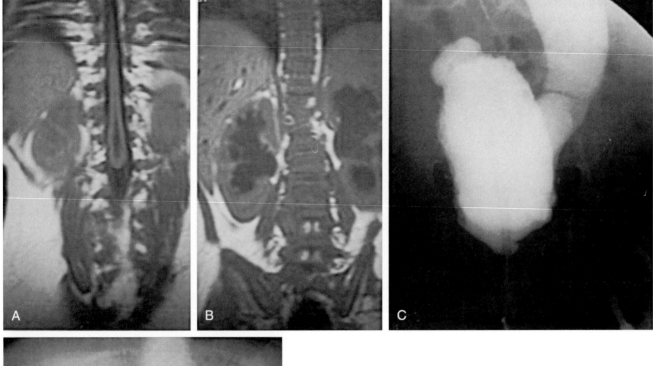

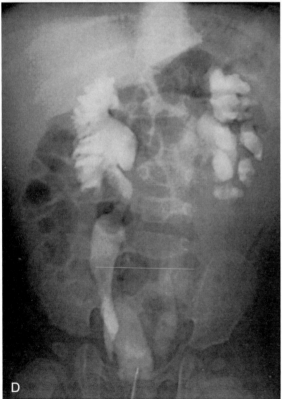

Figure 64–23. *A* and *B,* A 1-year-old girl with an imperforate anus and bony vertebral abnormalities has a tethered cord and bilateral hydronephrosis on MRI. *C,* Voiding cystourethrogram reveals significant trabeculation and reflux on the left. *D,* Excretory urogram demonstrates bilateral hydronephrosis secondary to the reflux on the left and a ureterovesical junction obstruction on the right. Subsequent urodynamic study revealed detrusor hypertonicity and dyssynergy.

EMG assessment of the perianal musculature at this time helps determine the exact location of the future anus. In addition, it can provide precise information about the innervation to the levator ani muscle and its competence to function as a sphincter. The posterior midline approach espoused by Peña (1986) minimizes the chances of injuring the pelvic nerves that innervate the pelvic floor muscles and therefore reduces the risk of an iatrogenic cause for neurogenic bladder dysfunction.

CENTRAL NERVOUS SYSTEM INSULTS

Cerebral Palsy

Etiology

Cerebral palsy is a nonprogressive injury of the brain occurring in the perinatal period that produces a neuromuscular disability or a specific symptom complex or cerebral dysfunction (Kuban and Leviton, 1994). **Its incidence is approximately 1.5 per 1000 births, but the incidence is increasing as smaller and younger premature infants survive in intensive care units** (Kuban and Leviton, 1994). **The condition is usually caused by a perinatal infection (e.g., sepsis, meningoencephalitis) or by a period of anoxia (or hypoxia) that affects the CNS** (Nelson and Ellenberg, 1986; Naeye et al, 1989). It most commonly appears in babies who were premature, weighed less than 2 kg at birth, had intraventricular hemorrhage, and received mechanical ventilation for a prolonged time in the postnatal period, and in premature infants weighing more than 2 kg who experienced a neonatal seizure (Kim et al, 1999). Maternal urinary infection in the later stages of pregnancy increases the risk of having an affected child by four to five times (Polivka et al, 1997).

Diagnosis

Affected children have delayed gross motor development, abnormal fine motor performance, altered muscle tone, abnormal stress gait, and exaggerated deep tendon reflexes. These findings can vary substantially, from obvious to very subtle when no discernible lesion is present, unless a careful neurologic examination is performed. These abnormalities may not manifest in the postnatal period, but they do become evident over time, because myelination of axons and maturation of neurons in the basal ganglia are required before spasticity, dystonia, and athetosis become apparent (Kyllerman et al, 1982). The lesions are classified according to which extremities are involved (monoplegia, hemiplegia, diplegia, and quadriplegia) and what kind of neurologic dysfunction is present (spastic, hypotonic, dystonic, athetotic, or a combination thereof). Among the more overtly affected individuals, spastic diplegia is the most common of the five types of dysfunction that characterize this disease, accounting for almost two thirds of the cases (Kuban and Leviton, 1994).

Findings

Most children with cerebral palsy develop total urinary control. Incontinence is a feature in some, but the exact incidence has never been truly determined (McNeal et al, 1983; Decter et al, 1987). **The presence of incontinence is related to the extent of the physical impairment, often because the handicap prevents the child from getting to the bathroom on time, causing an episode of wetting** (Murphy et al, 1995). A number of chil-

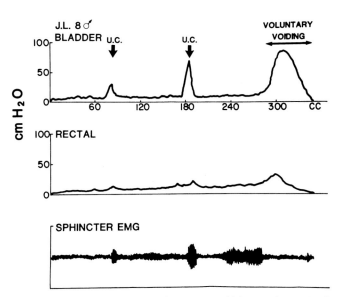

Figure 64–24. Electromyogram of an 8-year-old boy with spastic diplegia shows a typical partial upper motor neuron type bladder with uninhibited contractions (U.C.) associated with increased sphincter activity but normal voiding dynamics at capacity. Wetting is caused by these contractions when they are unaccompanied by the heightened sphincter activity.

dren have such a severe degree of mental retardation that they are not trainable, but the majority have sufficient intelligence to learn basic societal protocols with patient and persistent handling. **Often continence is achieved at a later than expected age. Therefore, urodynamic evaluation is reserved for children who appear to be trainable and do not seem to be hampered too much by their physical impairment but have not achieved continence by late childhood or early puberty.**

In one review (Decter et al, 1987), urodynamic studies were performed in 57 children with cerebral palsy (Table 64–7). **Forty-nine (86%) had the expected picture of a partial upper motor neuron type of dysfunction,** with exaggerated sacral reflexes, detrusor hyperreflexia, and/or DSD (Fig. 64–24), even though they manifested voluntary control over voiding. **Six (11%) of the 57 had evidence of both upper and lower motor neuron denervation** with detrusor areflexia or abnormal motor unit potentials on sphincter EMG assessment (Table 64–8). **Most of the children who exhibited these latter findings were found to have an episode of cyanosis in the perinatal period** when their records were analyzed on a retrospective basis (Table 64–9). **Therefore, a lower motor neuron lesion may be seen in addition to the expected upper motor neuron dysfunction.** Similar findings have been noted more recently (Mayo, 1992; Reid and Borzyskowski, 1993). Upper urinary tract imaging is usually normal even in children with upper motor neuron lesions (Brodak et al, 1994).

Recommendations

Treatment usually centers on abolishing the uninhibited contractions with the use of anticholinergic medications, but residual urine must be monitored closely to ensure complete evacuation with each void. CIC may be

Table 64–7. LOWER URINARY TRACT FUNCTION IN CEREBRAL PALSY

Type	Number	%
Upper motor neuron lesion	49	86
Mixed upper + lower motor neuron lesion	5	9.5
Incomplete lower motor neuron lesion	1	1.5
No urodynamic lesion	2	3

Adapted from Decter RM, Bauer SB, Khoshbin SJ, et al: Urodynamic assessment of children with cerebral palsy. J Urol 1987; 138:1110.

Table 64–8. URODYNAMIC FINDINGS IN CEREBRAL PALSY*

Type of Lesion	No. of Patients
Upper motor neuron	
Uninhibited contractions	35
Detrusor sphincter dyssynergy	7
Hyperactive sacral reflexes	6
No voluntary control	3
Small-capacity bladder	2
Hypertonia	2
Lower motor neuron	
Excessive polyphasia	5
↑ Amplitude + ↑ duration potentials	4

*Some patients had more than one finding.
Adapted from Decter RM, Bauer SB, Khoshbin S, et al: Urodynamic assessment of children with cerebral palsy. J Urol 1987; 138:1110.

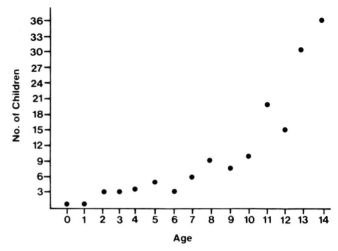

Figure 64–25. Increasing frequency of spinal injury with age. (From Anderson JM, Schutt AH: Spinal injury in children: A review of 156 cases seen from 1958 through 1980. Mayo Clin Proc 1980;55:499–504, with permission.)

required for those who cannot empty their bladder. Selective dorsal rhizotomy has improved bladder capacity, reduced the number of uninhibited contractions, and increased compliance, thus rendering the patient more continent, in a selected group of children who failed to respond to less invasive measures (Houle et al, 1998). The risk of neurourologic deterioration from this procedure is extremely low (Steinbok and Schrag, 1998). Upper and lower urinary tract imaging is not recommended unless UTI has occurred (Reid and Borzyskowski, 1993).

Traumatic Injuries to the Spine

Diagnosis

Despite exposure to and the potential for traumatic spinal cord injuries, **such injuries are rarely encountered in children. Their incidence tends to increase geometrically with age** (Anderson and Schutt, 1980) (Fig. 64–25). When an injury does occur, **it is more likely to happen in a male than a female child, and it is usually the result of a motor vehicle or bicycle accident, a fall from a high place, a gunshot wound, or a diving or sports incident**

Table 64–9. PERINATAL RISK FACTORS IN CEREBRAL PALSY

Factor	UMN (No. of Patients)	LMN (No. of Patients)
Prematurity	10	1
Respiratory distress/arrest/apnea	9	2
Neonatal seizures	5	—
Infection	5	—
Traumatic birth	5	—
Congenital hydrocephalus	3	—
Placenta previa/abruption	2	2
Hypoglycemia ± seizures	2	—
Intracranial hemorrhage	2	—
Cyanosis at birth	1	3
No specific factor noted	15	—

UMN, upper motor neuron lesion; LMN, lower motor neuron lesion.
Adapted from Decter RM, Bauer SB, Khoshbin S, et al: Urodynamic assessment of children with cerebral palsy. J Urol 1987; 138:1110.

(Cass et al, 1984; Hadley et al, 1988; Decter and Bauer, 1993). **It may also occur iatrogenically after surgery to correct scoliosis, kyphosis, other intraspinal processes, congenital aortic anomalies, or patent ductus arteriosus** (Cass et al, 1984; Batista et al, 1995). **Newborns are particularly prone to hyperextension injuries during high forceps delivery** (Adams et al, 1988; Lanska et al, 1990). Among younger children, girls are affected as often as boys (Ruge et al, 1988).

Pathogenesis

Spinal cord injuries in children are intrinsically different from those in adults owing to a variety of factors, including the mechanism of injury and the difference in configuration of the cord in children compared with adults. In addition, the horizontal versus vertical orientation of the facet joints in vertebral bodies that predisposes to anteroposterior subluxation in children, the delayed supportive effect of the paraspinous musculature and ligaments, and the relative heaviness of the head, which causes a fulcrum of maximal flexion of the upper cervical region in infants and young children, all contribute to a high degree of hypermobility that predisposes the child's spinal cord to ischemic necrosis (Decter and Bauer, 1993).

Findings

The lower urinary tract dysfunction that ensues is not likely to be an isolated event but is usually associated with loss of sensation and paralysis of the lower limbs. Radiologic investigation of the spine may not reveal any bony abnormality, although momentary subluxation of osseous structures resulting from the elasticity of the vertebral ligaments can result in a neurologic injury (Pollack et al, 1988). This condition has been seen only in children (usually younger than 8 years old) and has been labeled SCIWORA (*s*pinal *c*ord *i*njury *w*ithout *r*adiologic *a*bnormality) (Pang and Wilberger, 1982; Pang and Pollack, 1989). Myelography and CT show swelling of the cord below the level of the lesion (Adams et al, 1988; Lanska et al, 1990). **Often, what appears to be a permanent lesion initially turns out to be a transient phenomenon with time. Although sensation and motor function in the lower extremities may be restored relatively quickly, the dysfunction involving the bladder and rectum may persist considerably longer.**

During the acute phase of the injury, the bladder is often areflexic and the urethral sphincter nonreactive, although normal-appearing bioelectric potentials can be recorded on sphincter EMG (spinal shock). Over an undefined period of time, detrusor contractility and sphincter reactivity return as spinal cord edema subsides. With this return of function, detrusor hyperreflexia and bladder-sphincter dyssynergy develop. When the lesion affects the cauda equina, there is probably little to no return of bladder or sphincter function. Sacral sensation and peripheral reflexes are not good indicators of ultimate lower urinary tract function (Shenot et al, 1998). Over time, the predominant urodynamic pattern in patients with a thoracic-level lesion is a hyperreflexive detrusor with DSD, high voiding pressures, eventual hydronephrosis, and vesicoureteral reflux. Often children exhibit a good compliant bladder for a portion of bladder filling but then have C fiber–mediated, small, ineffective rhythmic contractions of the detrusor with simultaneous waxing and waning of external urethral sphincter activity. Some urinary leakage may occur with these contractions, but in general the bladder does not empty with them. Patients with an upper thoracic or cervical lesion are likely to exhibit autonomic dysreflexia with a spontaneous discharge of α_1-stimulants during bladder filling and with contractions of the detrusor. Monitoring of blood pressure and availability of α-antagonists are mandatory during urodynamic studies (Vaidyanathan et al, 1998b; Perkash, 1997).

Management

If urinary retention occurs immediately after the injury, an indwelling Foley catheter is passed into the bladder and left in place for as short a time as possible, until the patient is stable and aseptic intermittent catheterization can be started safely on a regular basis (Guttmann and Frankel, 1966; Barkin et al, 1983). **There is no difference in the incidence of urinary infection or in the development of stones in patients using sterile versus clean catheterization techniques** to empty the bladder (Prieto-Fingerhut et al, 1997; VanHala et al, 1997). **Rates of infection are as high as 60% to 80%** (Biering-Sorensen et al, 1999), **and stone formation occurs in 1.5% to 3% within the first 5 years after the trauma** (McKinley et al, 1999; Donnellan and Bolton, 1999). When the child starts to void again, the timing of catheterization can be regulated so that it is used as a means of measuring the residual urine after a spontaneous void. Residual urine volumes of 25 ml or less are considered safe enough to allow reducing the frequency or even stopping the catheterization program (Barkin et al, 1983). After 4 to 6 weeks, if there is no improvement in lower urinary tract function, urodynamic studies are conducted to determine whether the condition is the result of spinal shock or actual nerve root or spinal cord injury. Detrusor areflexia is not uncommon

under these circumstances (Iwatsubo et al, 1985). On the other hand, EMG recording of the sphincter often reveals normal motor units without fibrillation potentials but absent sacral reflexes and a nonrelaxing sphincter with bladder filling, a sign that transient spinal shock has occurred (Iwatsubo et al, 1985). The outcome of this situation is guarded but good, because most cases resolve completely as edema of the cord in response to the injury subsides, leaving no permanent damage (Iwatsubo et al, 1985; Fanciullacci et al, 1988).

If and when bladder function returns and emptying is incomplete, it has been shown in the rat (Xiaa et al, 1999) that peripheral L7 dermatome stimulation initiates a micturition reflex without DSD; whether this becomes a reliable treatment in humans remains to be seen. Incomplete emptying may be enhanced by the judicious use of phenoxybenzamine (Al-Ali et al, 1999). **The goal is balanced voiding at pressures lower than 40 cm H_2O, which reduces the 30% risk for urinary tract deterioration seen in poorly managed patients** (Giannantoni et al, 1998; Kim et al, 1998). If this cannot be achieved, then CIC is continued. **Anticholinergics, oxybutynin either orally or intravesically** (Vaidyanathan et al, 1998a; Wein, 1998), **or capsaicin** (an inhibitor of C-fiber stimulation [Wiart et al, 1998]) **have been added and are effective in reducing detrusor hyperreflexia,** but at the cost of significant side effects. Alternative pathways that have been effective to ensure complete emptying at low pressure include external urethral sphincterotomy (Kim et al, 1998), a urethral stent (Chancellor et al, 1999) or injection of botulinum A toxin (Botox) (Schurch et al, 1997). **In some cases, a continent catheterizable abdominal urinary stoma may be created** to facilitate self-catheterization in patients with low cervical or upper thoracic lesions, or to minimize the embarrassment of periodic genital organ exposure when care providers need to repeatedly catheterize the bladder (Sylora et al, 1997).

Recommendations

Most permanent traumatic injuries involving the spinal cord produce an upper motor neuron type lesion with detrusor hyperreflexia and DSD. The potential danger from this outflow obstruction is obvious (Donnelly et al, 1972). **Substantial residual urine volumes, high-pressure reflux, urinary infections, and their sequelae are the leading causes of long-term morbidity and mortality in patients with spinal cord injury** (Giannantoni et al, 1998). Even patients who involuntarily but spontaneously void to completion are not immune to urinary tract changes (Decter and Bauer, 1993). Urodynamic studies are imperative to identify which patients are at risk (Barkin et al, 1983). **These studies should be performed within 2 to 3 months after the injury, again 6 to 9 months later, and possibly at 2 years after the trauma to determine the stability of lower urinary tract function, the need for continued CIC, and whether adjuvant drug or surgical therapy should be added to achieve good long-term success.** When these measures are employed judiciously, effective management can be achieved (Pannek et al, 1997). Renal ultrasonography early in the course, and a VCUG if signs of bladder outlet obstruction are present on urodynamic testing or if recurrent urinary infection ensues, are also recommended. **Radionuclide cystography is indicated if the patient has repeated urinary infections or develops hydronephrosis** (Phillips et al, 1997). **Because stone formation can be insidious, periodic imaging of the kidneys and bladder is necessary.** Early identification and proper management may prevent the signs and effects of outlet obstruction before they become apparent on radiographic examination of the urinary tract (Pearman, 1976; Ogawa et al, 1988).

REFERENCES

Introduction

Bauer SB: The effects and challenges of bladder outlet obstruction. (Editorial.) J Urol 2000;163:3.

Bauer SB, Hallet M, Khoshbin S, et al: The predictive value of urodynamic evaluation in the newborn with myelodysplasia. JAMA 1984; 152:650.

Blaivas JG: A critical appraisal of specific diagnostic techniques. In Krane RJ, Siroky MB (eds): Clinical Neurourology. Boston, Little, Brown, 1979, pp 69–110.

Blaivas JG, Labib KB, Bauer SB, Retik AB: Changing concepts in the urodynamic evaluation of children. J Urol 1977;117:777.

Edelstein RA, Bauer SB, Kelly MD, et al: The long-term urologic response of neonates with myelodysplasia treated proactively with intermittent catheterization and anticholinergic therapy. J Urol 1995;154: 1500.

Gierup J, Ericsson NO: Micturition studies in infants and children: Intravesical pressure, urinary flow and urethral resistance in boys with intravesical obstruction. Scand J Urol Nephrol 1970;4:217.

Kaefer M, Pabby A, Kelly M, et al: Improved bladder function after prophylactic treatment of the high risk neurogenic bladder in newborns with myelo-meningocele. J Urol 1999;162:1068–1071.

Kaufman AM, Ritchey ML, Roberts AC, et al: Decreased bladder compliance in patients with myelomeningocele treated with radiologic observation. J Urol 1996;156:2031–2033.

Lapides J, Diokno AC, Silber SJ, Lowe BS: Clean intermittent self-catheterization in the treatment of urinary tract disease. J Urol 1972; 107:458.

McGuire EJ, Woodside JR, Borden TA, Weiss RM: The prognostic value of urodynamic testing in myelodysplastic patients. J Urol 1981;126:205.

Ohnishi N, Horan P, Levin SS, Levin RM: Intermittent catheterization limits rabbit bladder dysfunction in response to partial outlet obstruction. J Urol 2000;163:292–295.

Park JM, Bauer SB, Freeman MR, Peters CA: Oxybutynin chloride inhibits proliferation and suppresses gene expression in bladder smooth muscle cells. J Urol 1999;162:1110–1114.

Perez LM, Khoury J, Webster D: The value of urodynamic studies in infants less than one year old with congenital spinal dysraphism. J Urol 1992;148:584.

Smith ED: Urinary prognosis in spina bifida. J Urol 1972;108:115.

Wu HY, Baskin LS, Kogan BA: Neurogenic bladder dysfunction due to myelomeningocele: Neonatal versus childhood treatment. J Urol 1997; 157:2295–2297.

Urodynamic Evaluation

Abrams PH: Perfusion urethral profilometry. Urol Clin North Am 1979;6: 103.

Bates CP, Whiteside CG, Turner-Warwick RT: Synchronous cine/pressure/flow/cysto-urethrography with special reference to stress and urge incontinence. Br J Urol 1970;42:714.

Bauer SB: Pediatric neurourology. In Krane RJ, Siroky MB (eds): Clinical Neurourology. Boston, Little, Brown, 1979, pp 275–294.

Blaivas JG: A critical appraisal of specific diagnostic techniques. In Krane RJ, Siroky MB (eds): Clinical Neurourology. Boston, Little, Brown, 1979a, pp 69–110.

Blaivas JG: EMG: Other uses. In Barrett DM, Wein AJ (eds): Controversies in Neuro-urology. New York, Churchill Livingstone, 1979b, pp 103–116.

Blaivas JG, Labib KB, Bauer SB, Retik AB: A new approach to electromyography of the external urethral sphincter. J Urol 1977a;117:773.

Blaivas JG, Labib KB, Bauer SB, Retik AB: Changing concepts in the urodynamic evaluation of children. J Urol 1977b;117:777.

Bristow SE, Neal DE: Ambulatory urodynamics. Br J Urol 1996;77:333.

Diokno AC, Koff SA, Bender LF: Periurethral striated muscle activity in neurogenic bladder dysfunction. J Urol 1974;112:743.

Evans AT, Felker JR, Shank RA, Sugarman SR: Pitfalls of urodynamics. J Urol 1979;122:220.

Ghoniem GM, Roach MB, Lewis VH, et al: The value of leak point pressure and bladder compliance in the urodynamic evaluation of myelomeningocele patients. J Urol 1990;144:1440.

Gierup J, Ericsson NO, Okmain L: Micturition studies in infants and children. Scand J Urol Nephrol 1979;3:1.

Glazier DB, Murphy DP, Fleisher MH, et al: Evaluation of the utility of video-urodynamics in children with urinary tract infection and voiding dysfunction. Br J Urol 1997;80:806–808.

Gleason DM, Reilly RJ, Botacini MR, Pierce MJ: The urethral continence zone and its relation to stress incontinence. J Urol 1974;112:81.

Heslington K, Hilton P: Ambulatory urodynamic monitoring. Br J Obstet Gynecol 1996;103:393.

Homma Y, Batista JE, Bauer SB, et al: Urodynamics. In Abrams P, Khoury S, Wein A (eds): Incontinence. Plymouth, UK, Plymbridge Distributors Ltd., 1999, pp 353–399.

Joseph DB: The effect of medium-fill and slow-fill cystometry on bladder pressure in infants and children with myelodysplasia. J Urol 1992;147: 444.

Kaefer M, Rosen A, Darbey M, et al: Pressure at residual volume: A useful adjunct to standard fill cystometry. J Urol 1997a;158:1268–1271.

Kaefer M, Zurakowski D, Bauer SB, et al: Estimating normal bladder capacity in children. J Urol 1997b;158:2261–2264.

Kerr LA, Bauer SB, Staskin DR: Abnormal detrusor function precipitating hydronephrosis identified by extended voiding cystometry. J Urol 1994; 152:89.

Koff SA, Kass EJ: Abdominal wall electromyography: A noninvasive technique to improve pediatric urodynamic accuracy. J Urol 1982;127: 736.

Kulseng-Hanssen S, Klevmark B: Ambulatory urodynamic monitoring in women. Scand J Urol Nephrol Suppl 1996;30:27.

Maizels M, Firlit CF: Pediatric urodynamics: Clinical comparison of surface vs. needle pelvic floor/external sphincter electromyography. J Urol 1979;122:518.

Mayo ME: Detrusor hyperreflexia: The effect of posture and pelvic floor activity. J Urol 1978;119:635.

McInerney PD, Harris SA, Pritchard A, Stephenson TP: Night studies for primary diurnal and nocturnal diuresis and preliminary results of "clam" ileocystoplasty. Br J Urol 1991;67:42.

Palmer LS, Richards I, Kaplan WE: Age related bladder capacity and bladder capacity growth in children with myelomeningocele. J Urol 1997;158:1261–1264.

Passerini-Glazel G, Cisternino A, Camuffo MC, et al: Video-urodynamic studies of minor voiding dysfunction in children: An overview of 13 years' experience. Scand J Urol Nephrol Suppl 1992;141:70.

Turner-Warwick RT: Some clinical aspects of detrusor dysfunction. J Urol 1975;113:539.

Walter JS, Wheeler JS Jr, Markley J, et al: Home monitoring of bladder pressure and volume in individuals with spinal cord injury and multiple sclerosis. J Spinal Cord Med 1998;21:7–14.

Webb RJ, Ramsden PD, Neal DE: Ambulatory monitoring and electronic measurement of urinary leakage in the diagnosis of detrusor instability and incontinence. Br J Urol 1991;68:148.

Weerasinghe N, Malone PS: The value of video-urodynamics in the investigation of neurologically normal children who wet. Br J Urol 1993; 71:539.

Yalla SV, Rossier AB, Fam B: Vesico-urethral pressure recordings in the assessment of neurogenic bladder functions in spinal cord injury patients. Urol Int 1979;32:161.

Yalla SV, Sharma GURK, Barsamian EM: Micturitional static urethral pressure profile method of recording urethral pressure profiles during voiding and implications. J Urol 1980;124:649.

Yeung CK, Godley ML, Duffy PG, Ransley PG: Natural filling cystometry in infants and children. Br J Urol 1995;76:531.

Zermann DH, Lindner H, Huschke T, Schubert J: Diagnostic value of natural fill cystometry in neurogenic bladder in children. Eur Urol 1997;32:223–228.

Myelodysplasia

Adams MC, Mitchell ME, Rink RC: Gastrocystoplasty: An alternative solution to the problem of urological reconstruction in the severely compromised patient. J Urol 1988;140:1152.

Adzick NS, Sutton LN, Crombleholme TM, Flake AW: Successful fetal surgery for spina bifida. Lancet 1998;352:1675–1676.

Atala A, Bauer SB, Hendren WH, Retik AB: Effect of gastric augmentation on bladder function. J Urol 1993;149:1099–1102.

Barbalais GA, Klauber GT, Blaivas JG: Critical evaluation of the Credé maneuver: A urodynamic study of 207 patients. J Urol 1983;130:720.

Barrett DM, Furlow WL: The management of severe urinary incontinence in patients with myelodysplasia by implantation of the AS791/792 urinary sphincter device. J Urol 1982;128:44.

Bauer SB: Vesico-ureteral reflux in children with neurogenic bladder dysfunction. In Johnston JH (ed): International Perspectives in Urology, vol 10. Baltimore, Williams & Wilkins, 1984a, pp 159–177.

Bauer SB: Myelodysplasia: Newborn evaluation and management. In McLaurin RL (ed): Spina Bifida: A Multidisciplinary Approach. New York, Praeger, 1984b, pp 262–267.

Bauer SB: The management of spina bifida from birth onwards. In Whitaker RH, Woodard JR (eds): Paediatric Urology. London, Butterworths, 1985, pp 87–112.

Bauer SB: Early evaluation and management of children with spina bifida. In King LR (ed): Urologic Surgery in Neonates and Young Infants. Philadelphia, WB Saunders, 1988, pp 252–264.

Bauer SB: Bladder neck reconstruction. In Glenn JF, Graham SD (eds): Urologic Surgery. Philadelphia, JB Lippincott, 1990, pp 509–522.

Bauer SB, Colodny AH, Retik AB: The management of vesico-ureteral reflux in children with myelodysplasia. J Urol 1982;128:102.

Bauer SB, Hallet M, Khoshbin S, et al: The predictive value of urodynamic evaluation in the newborn with myelodysplasia. JAMA 1984;152:650.

Bauer SB, Kelly MD, Darbe M, Atala A: Late onset detrusor instability in patients with the artificial urinary sphincter. (Abstract 597.) Presented at the Annual Meeting of the American Urologic Association, San Antonio, May 18, 1993.

Bauer SB, Labib KB, Dieppa RA, et al: Urodynamic evaluation in a boy with myelodysplasia and incontinence. Urology 1977;10:354.

Bauer SB, Reda EF, Colodny AH, Retik AB: Detrusor instability: A delayed complication in association with the artificial sphincter. J Urol 1986;135:1212.

Begger JH, Meihuizen de Regt MJ, Hogen Esch I, et al: Progressive neurologic deficit in children with spina bifida aperta. Z Kinderchir 1986;41(suppl. 1):13.

Ben-Chaim J, Jeffs RD, Peppas DS, Gearhart JP: Submucosal bladder neck injections of glutaraldehyde cross-linked bovine collagen for treatment of urinary incontinence in patients with exstrophy/epispadias complex. U Urol 1995;154:862–864.

Bihrie R, Klee LW, Adams MC, et al: Transverse colon-gastric tube composite reservoir. Urology 1991;37:36–40.

Blaivas JG, Sinka HP, Zayed AH, et al: Detrusor-sphincter dyssynergia: A detailed electromyographic study. J Urol 1986;125:545.

Bloom DA, Knechtel JM, McGuire EJ: Urethral dilation improves bladder compliance in children with myelomeningocele and high leak point pressures. J Urol 1990;144:430.

Bomalaski MD, Teague JL, Brooks B: The long-term impact of urologic management on the quality of life in children with spina bifida. J Urol 1995;156:778.

Bosco PJ, Bauer SB, Colodny AH, et al: The long-term follow-up of artificial urinary sphincters in children. J Urol 1991;146:396.

Bruner JP, Tulipan N, Paschall RL, et al: Fetal surgery for myelomeningocele and the incidence of shunt dependent hydrocephalus. JAMA 1999;282:1819–1825.

Carr MC, Docima SG, Mitchell ME: Bladder augmentation with urothelial preservation. J Urol 1999;162:1133–1137.

Cartwright PC, Snow BW: Bladder autoaugmentation: Early clinical experience. J Urol 1989a;142:505.

Cartwright PC, Snow BW: Bladder autoaugmentation: Partial detrusor excision to augment bladder without use of bowel. J Urol 1989b;142:1050.

Cass AS: Urinary tract complications of myelomeningocele patients. J Urol 1976;115:102.

Cass AS, Bloom BA, Luxenberg M: Sexual function in adults with myelomeningocele. J Urol 1986;136:425.

Chiaramonte RM, Horowitz EM, Kaplan GA, et al: Implications of hydronephrosis in newborns with myelodysplasia. J Urol 1986;136:427.

Cohen RA, Rushton HG, Belman AB, et al: Renal scarring and vesicoureteral reflux in children with myelodysplasia. J Urol 1990;144:541.

Committee on Genetics, American Academy of Pediatrics, Desposito F (Chairperson): Folic acid for the prevention of neural tube defects. Pediatrics 1999;104:325–327.

Cromer BA, Enrile B, McCoy K, et al: Knowledge, attitudes and behavior related to sexuality in adolescents with chronic disability. Dev Med Child Neurol 1990;32:602.

Czeizel AE, Dudas I: Prevention of the first occurrence of neural-tube defects by preconceptual vitamin supplementation. N Engl J Med 1992;321:1832.

Dator DP, Hatchett L, Dyro EM, et al: Urodynamic dysfunction in walking myelodysplastic children. J Urol 1992;148:362–365.

Decter RM, Furness PD, Nguyen TA, et al: Reproductive understanding, sexual functioning and testosterone levels in men with spina bifida. J Urol 1997;157:1466–1468.

Dees JE: Congenital epispadias with incontinence. J Urol 1949;62:513.

Diamond DA, Atala A, Bauer SB: Initial experience with the transurethral self-detachable balloon system for urinary incontinence. (Abstract 92). Presented at the Annual Meeting of the Section on Urology of the American Academy of Pediatrics, Washington, DC, October 11, 1999.

Duckett JW: Cutaneous vesicostomy in childhood. Urol Clin North Am 1974;1:485.

Duckett JW, Snyder HM III: Continent urinary diversion: Variations of the Mitrofanoff principle. J Urol 1986;136:58.

Duel B, Gonzalez R, Barthold JS: Alternative techniques for augmentation cystoplasty. J Urol 1998;159:998–1005.

Edelstein RA, Bauer SB, Kelly MD, et al: The long-term urologic response of neonates with myelodysplasia treated proactively with intermittent catheterization and anticholinergic therapy. J Urol 1995;154:1500.

Elder JS: Periurethral and pubovaginal sling repair for incontinence in patients with myelodysplasia. J Urol 1990;144:434.

Epstein F: Meningocele: Pitfalls in early and late management. Clin Neurosurg 1982;30:366.

Flood HD, Ritchey ML, Bloom DA, et al: Outcome of reflux in children with myelodysplasia managed by bladder pressure monitoring. J Urol 1994;152:1574.

Geranoitis E, Koff SA, Enrile B: Prophylactic use of clean intermittent catheterization in treatment of infants and young children with myelomeningocele and neurogenic bladder dysfunction. J Urol 1988;139:85.

Ghoniem GM, Bloom DA, McGuire EJ, Stewart KL: Bladder compliance in meningocele children. J Urol 1989;141:1404.

Goessl C, Sauter T, Michael T, et al: Efficacy and tolerability of tolterodine in children with hyperreflexia. Urology 2000;55:414–418.

Goldwasser B, Barrett DM, Webster GD, Kramer SA: Cystometric properties of ileum and right colon after bladder augmentation, substitution and replacement. J Urol 1987;138:1007.

Gonzalez R, Reid C, Remberg Y, Buson H: Seromuscular enterocystoplasty lined with urothelium (SEIU): Experience with 12 patients. J Urol 1994;151:235.

Gosalbez R Jr, Woodard JR, Broecker BH, Warshaw B: Metabolic complications of the use of stomach for urinary reconstruction. J Urol 1993;150:710.

Greenfield SP, Fera M: The use of intravesical oxybutynin chloride in children with neurogenic bladder. J Urol 1991;146:532.

Griffiths DM, Malone PS: The Malone antegrade continence enema. J Pediatr Surg 1995;30:68–71.

Hayden P: Adolescents with meningomyelocele. Pediatr Rev 1985;6:245.

Hendren WH: Reconstruction of the previously diverted urinary tracts in children. J Pediatr Surg 1973;8:135.

Hendren WH: Urinary tract refunctionalization after long-term diversion. Am Surg 1990;212:478.

Hernandez RD, Hurwitz RS, Foote JE, et al: Nonsurgical management of threatened upper urinary tracts and incontinence in children with myelomeningocele. J Urol 1994;152:1582.

Hinman F Jr: Selection of intestinal segments for bladder substitution: Physical and physiological characteristics. J Urol 1988;139:519.

Hinman F Jr: Functional classification of conduits for continent diversion. J Urol 1990;144:27.

Holzbeierlein J, Pope JC, Adams MC, et al: The urodynamic profile of myelodysplasia in childhood with spinal canal closure during gestation. J Urol 2000;164:1336.

Jeffs RD, Jones P, Schillinger JF: Surgical correction of vesico-ureteral reflux in children with neurogenic bladder. J Urol 1976;115:449.

Joseph DB, Bauer SB, Colodny AH, et al: Clean intermittent catheterization in infants with neurogenic bladder. Pediatrics 1989;84:78.

Joyner BD, McLorie GA, Khoury AE: Sexuality and reproductive issues in children with myelomeningocele. Eur J Pediatr Surg 1998;8:29–34.

Just M, Schwarz M, Ludwig B, et al: Cerebral and spinal MR findings in patients with post repair myelomeningocele. Pediatr Radiol 1990;20:262.

Kaefer M, Pabby A, Kelly M, et al: Improved bladder function after prophylactic treatment of the high risk neurogenic bladder in newborns with myelomeningocele. J Urol 1999;162:1068–1071.

Kaefer M, Tobin M, Hendren WH, et al: Continent urinary diversion: The Children's Hospital experience. J Urol 1997;157:1394–1399.

Kaplan WE, Firlit CF: Management of reflux in myelodysplastic children. J Urol 1983;129:1195.

Kasabian NG, Bauer SB, Dyro FM, et al: The prophylactic value of clean intermittent catheterization and anticholinergic medication in newborns and infants with myelodysplasia at risk of developing urinary tract deterioration. Am J Dis Child 1992;146:840.

Kasabian NG, Vlachiotis JD, Lais A, et al: The use of intravesical oxybutynin chloride in patients with detrusor hypertonicity and detrusor hyperreflexia. J Urol 1994;151:944.

Kass EJ, Koff SA, Lapides J: Fate of vesico-ureteral reflux in children with neuropathic bladders managed by intermittent catheterization. J Urol 1981;125:63.

Khoury AE, Hendrick EB, McLorie GA, et al: Occult spinal dysraphism: Clinical and urodynamic outcome after division of the filum terminale. J Urol 1990;144:426.

Kock NG: Ileostomy without external appliances: A survey of 25 patients provided with intra-abdominal intestinal reservoir. Ann Surg 1971;173:545.

Kroovand RL, Bell W, Hart LJ, Benfeld KY: The effect of back closure on detrusor function in neonates with myelodysplasia. J Urol 1990;144:423.

Kropp KA, Angwafo FF: Urethral lengthening and reimplantation for neurogenic incontinence in children. J Urol 1986;135:533.

Kryger JV, Spencer Barthold J, Fleming P: The outcome of artificial urinary sphincter placement after a mean of 15 years' follow-up in a paediatric population. Br J Urol 1999;83:1026–1031.

Lais A, Kasabian NG, Dyro FM, et al: Neurosurgical implications of continuous neuro-urological surveillance of children with myelodysplasia. J Urol 1993;150:1879–1883.

Landau EH, Churchill BM, Jayanthi VR, et al: The sensitivity of pressure specific bladder volume versus total bladder capacity as a measure of bladder storage dysfunction. J Urol 1994;152:1578.

Lary JM, Edmonds LD: Prevalence of spina bifida at birth—United States, 1983–1990: A comparison of two surveillance systems. MMWR Morb Mortal Wkly Rep 1996;45:15–26.

Laurence KM: A declining incidence of neural tube defects in UK. Z Kinderchir 1989;44(suppl. 1):51.

Laurence KM, Beresford A: Continence, friends, marriage and children in 51 adults with spina bifida. Dev Med Child Neurol 1975;17(suppl. 35):128.

Laurence KM, James M, Miller MH, et al: Double-blind randomized controlled trial of folate treatment before conception to prevent recurrence of neural tube defects. Br Med J 1981;282:1509.

Leadbetter GW Jr: Surgical correction for total urinary incontinence. J Urol 1964;91:261.

Levesque PE, Bauer SB, Atala A, et al: Ten-year experience with artificial urinary sphincter in children. J Urol 1996;156:625.

Light JK, Hawila M, Scott FB: Treatment of urinary incontinence in children: The artificial sphincter vs. other methods. J Urol 1983;130:518.

Light JK, Scott FB: Use of the artificial urinary sphincter in spinal cord injury patients. J Urol 1983;130:1127.

Loening-Baucke V, Deach L, Wolraich M: Biofeedback training for patients with myelomeningocele and fecal incontinence. Dev Med Child Neurol 1988;30:781.

Mandell J, Bauer SB, Colodny AH, Retik AB: Cutaneous vesicostomy in infancy. J Urol 1981;126:92.

Marshall DF, Boston VE: Altered bladder and bowel function following cutaneous electrical field stimulation in children with spina bifida: Interim results of a randomized double-blind placebo-controlled trial. Eur J Pediatr Surg 1997;7:41–43.

Massad CA, Kogan BA, Trigo-Rocha FE: The pharmacokinetics of intravesical and oral oxybutynin chloride. J Urol 1992;148:548.

McGuire EJ, Wang CC, Usitalo H, Savastano J: Modified pubovaginal sling in girls with myelodysplasia. J Urol 1986;135:94.

McGuire EJ, Woodside JR, Borden TA, Weiss RM: The prognostic value of urodynamic testing in myelodysplastic patients. J Urol 1981;126:205.

Mitchell ME, Piser JA: Intestinocystoplasty and total bladder replacement in children and young adults: Follow-up of 129 cases. J Urol 1987;138:1140.

Mitrofanoff P: Cystometric continente trans-appendiculaire dans le traitement de vessies neurologiques. Chir Pediatr 1980;21:297.

MRC Vitamin Study Research Group: Prevention of neural tube defects: Results of the Medical Research Council Vitamin Study. Lancet 1991;338:131.

Myers GJ: Myelomeningocele: The medical aspect. Pediatr Clin North Am 1984;31:165.

Nasrallah PF, Aliabadi HA: Bladder augmentation in patients with neurogenic bladder and vesicoureteral reflux. J Urol 1991;146:563.

Nguyen DH, Mitchell ME, Horowitz M, et al: Demucosalized augmentation gastrocystoplasty with bladder autoaugmentation in pediatric patients. J Urol 1996;156:206–209.

Oi S, Yamada H, Matsumoto S: Tethered cord syndrome versus low-placed conus medullaris in an over-distended cord following initial repair for myelodysplasia. Childs Nerv Syst 1990;6:264.

Palmer JS, Kaplan WE, Firlit CF: Sexuality of the spina bifida male and female: Anonymous questionnaires. (Abstract 13.) Presented at the Annual Meeting of the Section on Urology of the American Academy of Pediatrics, Washington, DC, October 9, 1999.

Palmer LS, Richards I, Kaplan WE: Transrectal electrostimulation therapy for neuropathic bowel dysfunction in children with myelomeningocele. J Urol 1997;157:1449–1452.

Palomaki GE, Williams JR, Haddow JE: Prenatal screening for open neural-tube defects in Maine. N Engl J Med 1999;340:1049–1050.

Perez LM, Khoury J, Webster GD: The value of urodynamic studies in infants less than one year old with congenital spinal dysraphism. J Urol 1992;148:584.

Perez LM, Smith EA, Parrott TS, et al: Submucosal bladder neck injection of bovine dermal collagen for stress urinary incontinence in the pediatric population. J Urol 1996;156:633–636.

Peters CA, Bauer SB, Colodny AH, et al: The use of rectus fascia to manage urinary incontinence. J Urol 1989;142:516.

Pontari MA, Keating M, Kelly MD, et al: Retained sacral function in children with high level myelodysplasia. J Urol 1995;154:775.

Raz S, Ehrlich RM, Ziedman EJ, et al: Surgical treatment of the incontinent female patient with myelomeningocele. J Urol 1988;139:524.

Riedmiller H, Burger R, Muller S, et al: Continent appendix stoma: A modification of the Mainz pouch technique. J Urol 1990;143:1115.

Reigel DH: Tethered spinal cord. Concepts Pediatr Neurosurg 1983;4:142.

Rowland RG, Mitchell ME, Birhle R, et al: Indiana continent urinary reservoir. J Urol 1987;137:1136.

Salle JLP, Amarante FA, Silveira ML, et al: Urethral lengthening with anterior bladder wall flap for urinary incontinence: A new approach. J Urol 1994;152:803.

Scarff TB, Fronczak S: Myelomeningocele: A review and update. Rehab Lit 1981;42:143.

Schwarz GR, Jeffs RD: Ileal conduit urinary diversion in children: Computer analysis of follow-up from 2 to 16 years. J Urol 1975;114:285.

Shapiro SR, Lebowitz RL, Colodny AH: Fate of 90 children with ileal conduit urinary diversion a decade later: Analysis of complications, pyeloplasty, renal function and bacteriology. J Urol 1975;114:289.

Sidi AA, Aliabadi H, Gonzalez R: Enterocystoplasty in the management and reconstruction of the pediatric neurogenic bladder. J Pediatr Surg 1987;22:153.

Sidi AA, Dykstra DD, Gonzalez R: The value of urodynamic testing in the management of neonates with myelodysplasia: A prospective study. J Urol 1986;135:90.

Silveri M, Capitanucci ML, Mosiello G, et al: Endoscopic treatment for urinary incontinence in children with a congenital neuropathic bladder. Br J Urol 1998;82:694–697.

Skinner DG, Lieskovsky G, Boyd SD: Construction of a continent ileal reservoir (Kock pouch) as an alternative to cutaneous urinary diversion: An update after 250 cases. J Urol 1987;137:1140.

Smith ED: Urinary prognosis in spina bifida. J Urol 1972;108:115.

Spindel MR, Bauer SB, Dyro FM, et al: The changing neuro-urologic lesion in myelodysplasia. JAMA 1987;258:1630.

Squire R, Kiely EM, Carr B, et al: The clinical application of the Malone antegrade colonic enema. J Pediatr Surg 1993;28:1012–1015.

Stark GD: Spina Bifida: Problems and Management. Oxford, Blackwell Scientific Publications, 1977.

Stein SC, Feldman JG, Freidlander M, et al: Is myelomeningocele a disappearing disease? Pediatrics 1982;69:511.

Tanaka H, Kakizaki H, Kobayashi S, et al: The relevance of urethral resistance in children with myelodysplasia: Its impact on upper urinary tract deterioration and the outcome of conservative management. J Urol 1999;161:929–932.

Tarcan T, Bauer S, Olmedo E, et al: Long-term follow-up of newborns with myelodysplasia and normal urodynamic findings: Is it necessary? J Urol 2001;165:564–567.

Teichman JMH, Scherz HC, Kim KD, et al: An alternative approach to myelodysplasia management: Aggressive observation and prompt intervention. J Urol 1994;152:807.

Van Gool JD, Juijten RH, Donckerwolcke RA, Kramer PP: Detrusor-sphincter dyssynergia in children with myelomeningocele: A prospective study. Z Kinderchir 1982;37:148.

Venes JL, Stevens SA: Surgical pathology in tethered cord secondary to meningomyelocele repair. Concepts Pediatr Neurosurg 1983;4:165.

Watson HS, Bauer SB, Peers CA, et al: Comparative urodynamics of appendiceal and ureteral Mitrofanoff conduits in children. J Urol 1995;154:878.

Woodard JR, Anderson AM, Parrott TS: Ureteral reimplantation in myelodysplastic children. J Urol 1981;126:387.

Woodhouse CRJ: The sexual and reproductive consequences of congenital genitourinary anomalies. J Urol 1994;152:645.

Woodhouse CRJ, Malone PR, Cumming J, Reilly TM: The Mitrofanoff principle for continent urinary diversion. Br J Urol 1989;63:53.

Woodside JR, McGuire EJ: Techniques for detection of detrusor hypertonia in the presence of urethral sphincter incompetence. J Urol 1982;127:740.

Wu H-Y, Baskin LS, Kogan BA: Neurogenic bladder dysfunction due to myelomeningocele: Neonatal versus childhood treatment. J Urol 1997;157:2295–2297.

Yoo JJ, Magliochetti M, Atala A: Detachable self-sealing membrane system for the endoscopic treatment of incontinence. J Urol 1997;158:1045–1048.

Young HH: An operation for the cure of incontinence of urine. Surg Gynecol Obstet 1919;28:84.

Younoszai MK: Stooling problems in patients with myelomeningocele. South Med J 1992;85:718.

Lipomeningocele and Other Spinal Dysraphisms

Andar UB, Harkness WF, Hayward RD: Split cord malformations of the lumbar region: A model for the neurosurgical management of all types of "occult" spinal dysraphism? Pediatr Neurosurg 1997;26:17–24.

Anderson FM: Occult spinal dysraphism: A series of 73 cases. Pediatrics 1975;55:826.

Atala A, Bauer SB, Dyro FM, et al: Bladder functional changes resulting from a lipomeningocele repair. J Urol 1992;148:592.

Barson AJ: The vertebral level of termination of the spinal cord during normal and abnormal development. J Anat 1970;106:489.

Bruce DA, Schut L: Spinal lipomas in infancy and childhood. Brain 1979;5:92.

Campobasso P, Galiani E, Verzerio A, et al: A rare cause of occult neuropathic bladder in children: The tethered cord syndrome. Pediatr Med Chir 1988;10:641.

Chapman PH: Congenital intraspinal lipomas: Anatomic considerations and surgical treatment. Childs Brain 1982;9:37.

Cornette L, Verpooten C, Lagae L, et al: Tethered spinal cord in occult spinal dysraphism: Timing and outcome of surgical release. Neurology 1998;50:1761–1765.

Dubrowitz V, Lorber J, Zachary RB: Lipoma of the cauda equina. Arch Dis Child 1965;40:207.

Flanigan RF, Russell DP, Walsh JW: Urologic aspects of tethered cord. Urology 1989;33:80.

Fone PD, Vapnek JM, Litwiller SE, et al: Urodynamic findings in the tethered spinal cord syndrome: Does surgical release improve bladder function? J Urol 1997;157:604–609.

Foster LS, Kogan BA, Cogan PH, Edwards MSB: Bladder function in patients with lipomyelomeningocele. J Urol 1990;143:984.

Hall WA, Albright AL, Brunberg JA: Diagnosis of tethered cord by magnetic resonance imaging. Surg Neurol 1988;30(suppl. 1):60.

Hellstrom WJ, Edwards MS, Kogan BA: Urologic aspects of the tethered cord syndrome. J Urol 1986;135:317.

James CM, Lassman LP: Spinal Dysraphism: Spina Bifida Occulta. New York, Appleton-Century-Crofts, 1972.

Kaplan WE, McLone DG, Richards I: The urologic manifestations of the tethered spinal cord. J Urol 1988;140:1285.

Keating MA, Rink RC, Bauer SB, et al: Neuro-urologic implications of changing approach in management of occult spinal lesions. J Urol 1988;140:1299.

Khoury AE, Hendrick EB, McLorie GA, et al: Occult spinal dysraphism: Clinical and urodynamic outcome after diversion of the filum terminale. J Urol 1990;144:426.

Kondo A, Kato K, Kanae S, Sakakibara T: Bladder dysfunction secondary to tethered cord syndrome in adults: Is it curable? J Urol 1986;135:313.

Koyangi I, Iwasaki Y, Hida K, et al: Surgical treatment supposed natural history of the tethered cord with occult spinal dysraphism. Childs Nerv Syst 1997;13:268–274.

Linder M, Rosenstein J, Sklar FH: Functional improvement after spinal surgery for the dysraphic malformations. Neurosurgery 1982;11:622.

Mandell J, Bauer SB, Hallett M, et al: Occult spinal dysraphism: A rare but detectable cause of voiding dysfunction. Urol Clin North Am 1980;7:349.

Packer RJ, Zimmerman RA, Sutton LN, et al: Magnetic resonance imaging of spinal cord diseases of childhood. Pediatrics 1986;78:251.

Pang D: Split cord malformation. II. Clinical syndrome. Neurosurgery 1992;31:481–500.

Pang D, Dias M, Ahab-Barmada M: Split cord malformation. I. A unified theory of embryogenesis for double spinal cord malformations. Neurosurgery 1992;31:451–481.

Pierre-Kahn A, Zeral M, Renier D, et al: Congenital lumbosacral lipomas. Childs Nerv Syst 1997;13:298–334.

Proctor M, Bauer SB, Scott MR: The effect of surgery for the split spinal cord malformation on neurologic and urologic function. Pediatr Neurosurg 2000;32:13–19.

Raghavendra BN, Epstein FJ, Pinto RS, et al: The tethered spinal cord: Diagnosis by high-resolution real-time ultrasound. Radiology 1983;149:123.

Roy MW, Gilmore R, Walsh JW: Evaluation of children and young adults with tethered spinal cord syndrome: Utility of spinal and scalp recorded somatosensory evoked potentials. Surg Neurol 1986;26:241.

Satar N, Bauer SB, Scott RM, et al: Late effects of early surgery on lipoma and lipomeningocele in children less than two years old. J Urol 1997;157:1434–1437.

Satar N, Bauer SB, Shefner J, et al: The effects of delayed diagnosis and treatment in patients with an occult spinal dysraphism. J Urol 1995;154:754.

Scheible W, James HE, Leopold GR, Hilton SW: Occult spinal dysraphism in infants: Screening with high-resolution real-time ultrasound. Radiology 1983;146:743.

Seeds JW, Jones FD: Lipomyelomeningocele: Prenatal diagnosis and management. Obstet Gynecol 1986;67(suppl.):34.

Tami S, Yamada S, Knighton RS: Extensibility of the lumbar and sacral cord: Pathophysiology of the tethered cord in cats. J Neurosurg 1987;66:116.

Tracey PT, Hanigan WC: Spinal dysraphism: Use of magnetic resonance imaging in evaluation. Clin Pediatr 1990;29:228.

Weissert M, Gysler R, Sorensen N: The clinical problem of the tethered cord syndrome: A report of three personal cases. Z Kinderchir 1989;44:275.

Yamada S, Knierim D, Yonekura M, et al: Tethered cord syndrome. J Am Paraplegic Soc 1983;6(suppl. 3):58.

Yamada S, Zincke DE, Sanders D: Pathophysiology of "tethered cord syndrome." J Neurosurg 1981;54:494.

Yip CM, Leach GE, Rosenfeld DS, et al: Delayed diagnosis of voiding dysfunction: Occult spinal dysraphism. J Urol 1985;124:694.

Sacral Agenesis

Bauer SB: Urodynamics in children. In Ashcraft KW (ed): Pediatric Urology. Orlando, FL, Grune & Stratton, 1990, pp 49–76.

Boemers TM, Van Gool JD, deJong TPVM, Bax KMA: Urodynamic evaluation of children with caudal regression syndrome (caudal dysplasia sequence). J Urol 1994;151:1038.

Guzman L, Bauer SB, Hallet M, et al: The evaluation and management of children with sacral agenesis. Urology 1983;23:506.

Jakobson H, Holm-Bentzen M, Hald T: Neurogenic bladder dysfunction in sacral agenesis and dysgenesis. Neurourol Urodyn 1985;4:99.

Koff SA, DeRidder PA: Patterns of neurogenic bladder dysfunction in sacral agenesis. J Urol 1977;118:87.

Landauer W: Rumplessness of chicken embryos produced by the injection of insulin and other chemicals. Exp Zool 1945;98:65.

Menon RK, Cohen RM, Sperling MA, et al: Transplacental passage of insulin in pregnant women with insulin-dependent diabetes mellitus. N Engl J Med 1990;323:309.

Pang D: Sacral agenesis and caudal spinal cord malformations. Neurosurgery 1993;32:755.

Papapetrou C, Drummond F, Reardon W, et al: A genetic study of the human T gene and its exclusion as a major candidate gene for sacral agenesis with anorectal atresia. J Med Genet 1999;36:208–213.

Passarge E, Lenz K: Syndrome of caudal regression in infants of diabetic mothers: Observations of further cases. Pediatrics 1966;37:672.

Schlussel RN, Bauer SB, Kelly MD, et al: The clinical and urodynamic findings in 35 patients with sacral agenesis. (Abstract 412.) Presented at the Annual Meeting of the American Urological Association, San Francisco, May 16, 1994.

White RI, Klauber GT: Sacral agenesis: Analysis of twenty-two cases. Urology 1976;8:521.

Wilmshurst JM, Kelly R, Borzyskowski M: Presentation and outcome of sacral agenesis: 20 years' experience. Dev Med Child Neurol 1999;41:806–812.

Imperforate Anus

Barnes PD, Lester PD, Yamanashi WS, Prince JR: MRI in infants and children with spinal dysraphism. Am J Radiol 1986;147:339.

Barry JE, Auldist AW: The Vater syndrome. Am J Dis Child 1974;128:769.

Boemers TM, Van Gool JD, deJong TPVM, Bax KMA: Urodynamic evaluation of children with the caudal regression syndrome (caudal dysplasia sequence). J Urol 1994;151:1038.

Carson JA, Barnes PD, Tunell WP, et al: Imperforate anus: The neurologic implication of sacral abnormalities. J Pediatr Surg 1984;19:838.

Greenfield SP, Fera M: Urodynamic evaluation of the patient with imperforate anus: A prospective study. J Urol 1991;146:539.

Holschneider AM, Pfrommer W, Gerresheim B: Results in the treatment of anorectal malformations with special regard to the histology of the rectal pouch. Eur J Pediatr Surg 1994;4:303–309.

Kakizaki H, Nonomura K, Asano Y, et al: Preexisting neurogenic voiding dysfunction in children with imperforate anus: Problems in management. J Urol 1994;151:1041.

Karrer FM, Flannery AM, Nelson MD Jr, et al: Anal rectal malformations: Evaluation of associated spinal dysraphic syndromes. J Pediatr Surg 1988;23:45.

Long FL, Hunter JV, Mahboubi S, et al: Tethered cord and associated vertebral anomalies in children and infants with imperforate anus: Evaluation with MR imaging and plain radiography. Radiology 1996;200:377–382.

Metts JC, Kotkin L, Kasper S, et al: Genital malformations and coexistent urinary tract or spinal anomalies in patients with imperforate anus. J Urol 1997;158:1298–1300.

Parrott TS: Urologic implications of anorectal malformations. Urol Clin North Am 1985;12:13–21.

Parrott T, Woodard J: Importance of cystourethrography in neonates with imperforate anus. Urology 1979;13:607.

Peña A: Posterior sagittal approach for the correction of anal rectal malformations. Adv Surg 1986;19:69.

Rivosecchi M, Lucchetti MC, Zaccara A, et al: Spinal dysraphism detected by magnetic resonance imaging in patients with anorectal anomalies: Incidence and clinical significance. J Pediatr Surg 1995;30:488.

Santulli TV, Schullinger JN, Kiesewetter WB, et al: Imperforate anus: A survey from the members of the Surgical Section of the American Academy of Pediatrics. J Pediatr Surg 1971;6:484–487.

Shaul DB, Harrison EA: Classification of anorectal malformation: Initial approach, diagnostic test, and colostomy. Semin Pediatr Surg 1997;6:187–195.

Templeton JM, O'Neill JA Jr: Anorectal malformations. In Welch KJ, Randolph JG, Ravitch MM, et al (eds): Pediatric Surgery. Chicago, Year Book Medical Publishers, 1986, pp 1022–1037.

Tsakayannis DE, Shamberger RC: Association of imperforate anus with occult spinal dysraphism. J Pediatr Surg 1995;30:1010–1012.

Tunell WP, Austin JC, Barnes TP, Reynolds A: Neuroradiologic evaluation of sacral abnormalities in imperforate anus complex. J Pediatr Surg 1987;22:58.

Cerebral Palsy

Brodak PP, Sherz HC, Packer M, Kaplan GW: Is urinary screening necessary for patients with cerebral palsy? J Urol 1994;152:1586.

Decter RM, Bauer SB, Khoshbin S, et al: Urodynamic assessment of children with cerebral palsy. J Urol 1987;138:1110.

Houle AM, Vernot O, Jednak R, et al: Bladder function before and after sacral rhizotomy in children with cerebral palsy. J Urol 1998;160:1088–1091.

Kim JN, Namburg R, Chang W, et al: Prospective evaluation of perinatal risk factors for cerebral palsy and delayed development in high risk infants. Yonsei Med J 1999;40:363–370.

Kuban KCK, Leviton A: Cerebral palsy. N Engl J Med 1994;330:188.

Kyllerman M, Bogen B, Bensch J, et al: Dyskinetic cerebral palsy: I. Clinical categories, associated neurological abnormalities and incidences. Acta Paediatr Scand 1982;71:543.

Mayo ME: Lower urinary tract dysfunction in cerebral palsy. J Urol 1992;147:419.

McNeal DM, Hawtrey CE, Wolraich ML, Mapel JR: Symptomatic neurogenic bladder in a cerebral-palsied population. Dev Med Child Neurol 1983;25:612.

Murphy KP, Molnar GE, Lankasky K: Medical and functional status of adults with cerebral palsy. Dev Med Child Neurol 1995;37:1075–1084.

Naeye RL, Peters EC, Bartholomew M, Landis R: Origins of cerebral palsy. Am J Dis Child 1989;143:1154.

Nelson KB, Ellenberg JH: Antecedents of cerebral palsy. N Engl J Med 1986;315:81.

Polivka BJ, Nickel JT, Wilkins JR III: Urinary tract infection during pregnancy: A risk factor for cerebral palsy? J Obstet Gynecol Neonatal Nurs 1997;26:405–413.

Reid CJD, Borzyskowski M: Lower urinary tract dysfunction in cerebral palsy. Arch Dis Child 1993;68:739.

Steinbok P, Schrag C: Complications after selective sacral rhizotomy for spasticity in children with cerebral palsy. Pediatr Neurosurg 1998;28:300–313.

Traumatic Injuries to the Spine

Adams C, Babyn PS, Logan WJ: Spinal cord birth injury: Value of computed tomographic myelography. Pediatr Neurol 1988;4:109.

Al-Ali M, Salman G, Rasheed A, et al: Phenoxybenzamine in the management of neuropathic bladder following spinal cord injury. Aust N Z J Surg 1999;69:660–663.

Anderson JM, Schutt AH: Spinal injury in children: A review of 156 cases seen from 1950 through 1978. Mayo Clin Proc 1980;55:499.

Barkin M, Dolfin D, Herschorn S, et al: The urologic care of the spinal cord injury patient. J Urol 1983;129:335.

Batista JE, Bauer SB, Shefner JM, et al: Urodynamic findings in children with spinal cord ischemia. J Urol 1995;154:1183.

Biering-Sorensen F, Nielans HM, Dorflinger T, Sorensen B: Urological situation five years after spinal cord injury. Scand J Urol Nephrol 1999;33:157–161.

Cass AS, Luxenberg M, Johnson CF, Gleich P: Management of the neurogenic bladder in 413 children. J Urol 1984;132:521.

Chancellor MB, Bennett C, Simoneau AR, et al: Sphincteric stents versus external sphincterotomy in spinal cord injured men: Prospective randomized multicenter trial. J Urol 1999;161:1893–1898.

Decter RM, Bauer SB: Urologic management of spinal cord injury in children. Urol Clin North Am 1993;20:475.

Donnellan SM, Bolton DM: The impact of contemporary bladder management techniques on struvite calculi associated with spinal cord injury. BJU Int 1999;84:280–285.

Donnelly J, Hackler RH, Bunts RC: Present urologic status of the World War II paraplegic: 25-year follow-up comparison with status of the 20-year Korean War paraplegic and 5-year Vietnam paraplegic. J Urol 1972;108:558.

Fanciullacci F, Zanollo A, Sandri S, Cantanzaro F: The neuropathic bladder in children with spinal cord injury. Paraplegia 1988;26:83.

Giannantoni A, Scivoletto G, DiStasi SM, et al: Clean intermittent catheterization and prevention of renal disease in spinal cord injured patients. Spinal Cord 1998;36:29–32.

Guttmann L, Frankel H: The value of intermittent catheterization in the early management of traumatic paraplegia and tetraplegia. Paraplegia 1966;4:63.

Hadley MN, Zabramski JM, Browner CM, et al: Pediatric spinal trauma: Review of 122 cases of spinal cord and vertebral column injuries. J Neurosurg 1988;68:18.

Iwatsubo E, Iwakawa A, Koga H, et al: Functional recovery of the bladder in patients with spinal cord injury: Prognosticating programs of an aseptic intermittent catheterization. Acta Urol Japan 1985;31:775.

Kim YH, Kattan NW, Boon TB: Bladder leak point pressure: The measure for sphincterotomy success in spinal cord injured patients with external detrusor sphincter dyssynergia. J Urol 1998;159:493–496.

Lanska MJ, Roessmann U, Wiznitzer M: magnetic resonance imaging in cervical cord birth injury. Pediatrics 1990;85:760.

McKinley WO, Jackson AB, Cardenas DD, DeVivo JM: Long-term medical complications after traumatic spinal cord injury: A regional model systems analysis. Arch Phys Med Rehabil 1999;80:1402–1410.

Ogawa T, Yoshida T, Fujinaga T: Bladder deformity in traumatic spinal cord injury patients. Acta Urol Japan 1988;34:1173.

Pang D, Pollack IF: Spinal cord injury without radiographic abnormalities in children: The SCIWORA syndrome. J Trauma 1989;29:654.

Pang D, Wilberger JE Jr: Spinal cord injury without radiographic abnormalities in children. J Neurosurg 1982;57:114.

Pannek J, Diederichs W, Botel U: Urodynamically controlled management of spinal cord injury in children. Neurourol Urodyn 1997;16:285–292.

Pearman JW: Urologic follow-up of 99 spinal cord injury patients initially managed by intermittent catheterization. Br J Urol 1976;48:297.

Perkash I: Autonomic dysreflexia and detrusor-sphincter dyssynergia in spinal cord injury patients. J Spinal Cord Med 1997;20:365–370.

Phillips JR, Jadvar H, Sullivan G, et al: Effect of radionuclide renograms on treatment of patients with spinal cord injuries. AJR Am J Roentgenol 1997;169:1045–1047.

Pollack IF, Pang D, Sclabassi R: Recurrent spinal cord injury without radiographic abnormalities in children. J Neurosurg 1988;69:177.

Prieto-Fingerhut T, Banovac K, Lynne CM: A study comparing sterile and non-sterile urethral catheterization in patients with spinal cord injury. Rehabilitation Nursing 1997;22:299–302.

Ruge JR, Sinson GP, McLone DG, et al: Pediatric spinal injury: The very young. J Neurosurg 1988;68:25.

Schurch B, Hodler J, Rodic B: Botulism A toxin as a treatment of detrusor-sphincter dyssynergia in patients with spinal cord injury: MRI controlled transperineal injections. J Neurol Neurosurg Psychiatry 1997;63:474–476.

Shenot PJ, Rivas DA, Watanabe T, Chancellor MB: Early predictors of bladder recovery and urodynamics after spinal cord injury. Neurourol Urodyn 1998;17:25–29.

Sylora JA, Gonzalez R, Vaughn M, Reinberg Y: Intermittent self-catheterization by quadriplegic patients via a catheterizable Mitrofanoff channel. J Urol 1997;151:48–50.

Vaidyanathan S, Soni BM, Brown E, et al: Effect of intermittent urethral catheterization and oxybutynin bladder instillation on urinary continence status and quality of life in a select group of spinal cord injury patients with neuropathic bladder dysfunction. Spinal Cord 1998a;36:409–414.

Vaidyanathan S, Soni BM, Sett P, et al: Pathophysiology of autonomic dysreflexia: Long-term treatment with terazosin in adult and pediatric spinal cord injury patients manifesting recurrent dysreflexic episodes. Spinal Cord 1998b;36:761–770.

VanHala S, Nelson VS, Hurvitz EA, et al: Bladder management in patients with pediatric onset neurogenic bladders. J Spinal Cord Med 1997;20:410–415.

Wein AJ: Pharmacologic options for the overactive bladder. Urology 1998;51(2A suppl.):43–47.

Wiart L, Joseph PA, Petit H, et al: The effects of capsaicin on the neurogenic hyper-reflexic detrusor: A double blind placebo controlled study in patients with spinal cord disease. Preliminary results. Spinal Cord 1998;36:95–99.

Xiaa CG, deGroat WC, Godec CJ, et al: "Skin-CNS-Bladder" reflex pathway for micturition after spinal cord injury and its underlying mechanisms. J Urol 1999;162:936–942.

SECTION B: NON-NEUROGENIC LOWER URINARY TRACT DYSFUNCTION

Stephen A. Koff, MD
Venkata R. Jayanthi, MD

Developmental Biology of Urinary Control

Dysfunctional Elimination Syndromes of Childhood
  Guidelines for Evaluation and Management
  The Non-Neurogenic Neurogenic Bladder
  The Unstable Bladder

Infrequent Voiding Syndrome
Functional Bowel Disturbances
Postvoid Dribbling
Daytime Urinary Frequency Syndrome
Nocturnal Enuresis
Worrisome Signs and Symptoms

This new chapter in *Campbell's Urology* reflects a new stage in the evolution of pediatric urology, in which certain non-neurogenic or functional lower urinary tract disorders have become recognized as causes for urinary infection, obstruction, and vesicoureteral reflux. It is no doubt because these disorders lack an anatomic or neurogenic etiology and represent subtle and often difficult to diagnose alterations in urinary control that their potential for urinary tract injury has remained obscure for so long. The development and use of specialized pediatric radiographic and urodynamic techniques have made it possible to observe and define the maturation of urinary tract function. This has permitted characterization of these functional disturbances to provide a more rational basis for therapy. Physicians who care for children with urinary tract problems must be aware of these functional disorders and able to diagnose and manage them effectively.

DEVELOPMENTAL BIOLOGY OF URINARY CONTROL

Historically, bladder function in the infant was believed to be characterized by instability, with bladder contraction occurring frequently as a result of a simple unsupervised spinal cord reflex (Hjalmas, 1988; Yeung et al, 1995). The detrusor contracts whenever sufficient urine volume distends the bladder to stimulate the afferent limb of this reflex arc. The periurethral striated muscles that make up the voluntary (external) urinary sphincter are fully integrated into this reflex, even in infants. As the bladder fills, the urinary sphincter constricts progressively to prevent incontinence. This sphincter relaxes synchronously with detrusor contraction to permit complete, low-pressure bladder emptying.

Actual studies of the voiding habits and urodynamic functions of normal infants and children refuted many historical beliefs and revealed that bladder function in the young child is not simply a miniaturized version of bladder function in older children or adults. Healthy preterm and term infants void regularly, usually hourly, but with great variability, and their voids are typically stimulated by feeding. Because infants sleep almost 16 hours each day, it is not surprising that about two thirds of voids occur during sleep. However, more than half of the time, bladder emptying is neither complete nor coordinated; it often takes two to three small voids to completely empty the bladder, and residual urine volumes of up to 30% capacity are typical. Urodynamic studies in normal control infants have confirmed this discoordinated pattern of voiding, have indicated that bladder instability is very uncommon in normal infants and children (5% to 18% of infants, decreasing to 5% to 8% of those older than 8 years of age), and have demonstrated that young children, especially boys, void at very high pressures (up to 100 cm H_2O is normal) compared with adults (Holmdahl et al, 1996; Yeung et al, 1995, 1998; Wen and Tong, 1998; Bachelard et al, 1999; Sillen et al, 2000).

As a child matures, successful toilet training involves achieving an adult pattern of urinary control and depends on the outcome of at least three separate events in the development of bladder form and function (Nash, 1949). **First, bladder capacity must increase to serve as an adequate reservoir.** Capacity begins to change soon after infancy. Voiding frequency progressively decreases as bladder capacity enlarges, so that by 2 years of age voiding occurs only about 11 times per day (Goellner et al, 1981). Subsequently, during the childhood years, voided volumes and bladder capacity increase parallel with one another. With the capacity of the newborn bladder at about 30 to 60 ml and bladder capacity increasing by about 30 ml/yr each year almost until puberty, bladder capacity in childhood

may be reasonably well estimated by a simple formula (capacity in ounces = age in years + 2) (Koff, 1983), although a number of other formulas have been proposed (Berger et al, 1983; Hjalmas, 1988; Kaefer et al, 1997).

Second, voluntary control over the periurethral striated muscle sphincter must occur to allow for decisive initiation and termination of voiding. As with other acquired striated muscle skills, sphincter control fits into an orderly scheme of developmental landmarks and usually occurs by the age of 3 years.

Third, direct volitional control over the spinal reflex that controls the detrusor smooth muscle must develop for the child to be able to voluntarily initiate or inhibit detrusor contraction. This third phase in the development of urinary control is the most complex, but once it is accomplished the ability to void or inhibit voiding voluntarily at any degree of bladder filling sets humans apart from almost all other mammals. Although the ability to have voluntary control over detrusor smooth muscle seems perplexing even to physiologists, the nature and accuracy of this phenomenon have been documented (Lapides et al, 1957).

By the age of 4 years, many if not most children have matured their urinary tract function and developed an adult pattern of urinary control. They are generally dry during the day and the night. **The adult pattern is characterized during bladder filling by an absence of unstable or uninhibited (involuntary) detrusor contractions. Urodynamic studies have confirmed that even at bladder capacity and when the desire to void is strong, detrusor contraction will not occur unless it is voluntarily initiated** (Diokno et al, 1974). During bladder filling, the striated sphincter muscles are activated reflexively, and constriction becomes maximal at bladder capacity. This is a guarding reflex that prevents urinary incontinence. When detrusor contraction is initiated voluntarily, simultaneous reflex relaxation of the sphincter permits low-pressure bladder emptying.

DYSFUNCTIONAL ELIMINATION SYNDROMES OF CHILDHOOD

Guidelines for Evaluation and Management

In the absence of anatomic urinary tract obstruction or neurologic disease, there exists in otherwise normal children a group of functional disorders that may cause urinary obstruction and produce significant uropathology. They usually reach clinical awareness because of voiding symptoms and urinary incontinence or urinary infection and are thought to be caused by behavioral factors that affect toilet training and prevent successful transition from the infantile to the adult pattern of urinary control. These syndromes of dysfunctional elimination differ greatly in manifestation, prognosis, and pathophysiology and comprise a clinical spectrum that varies widely (Table 64–10).

At the severe end of the spectrum are a small group of patients with **Hinman's syndrome, also termed the non-neurogenic neurogenic bladder, dysfunctional voiding,**

Table 64–10. DYSFUNCTIONAL ELIMINATION SYNDROMES

Non-neurogenic neurogenic bladder
Unstable bladder
   Urgency incontinence syndrome
   Small-capacity hypertonic bladder
   Continent bladder instability
Infrequent voiding syndrome
Functional bowel disturbances
   Constipation or fecal retention
Giggle incontinence
Postvoid dribbling
Daytime urinary frequency syndrome
Nocturnal enuresis

or occult neuropathic bladder (Datta et al, 1970; Hinman, 1974; Williams et al, 1974; Allen, 1977). They demonstrate a functional obstruction which occurs during voiding to produce severe clinical manifestations that are as prominent as those observed in patients with true neurogenic bladder (NGB) disease. Despite having no neurologic defect or anatomic obstruction, these children characteristically display urinary retention, altered bladder anatomy, and upper urinary tract dilatation and scarring.

Less severe uropathology is observed in the large group of children who present with refractory and often severe symptoms that reflect incomplete toilet training with diminished urinary control. Their **obstruction is caused by an incoordination between bladder and sphincter that occurs only during bladder filling in the presence of unstable bladder contractions** and is, therefore, of less potential risk to the urinary tract. Although these children have also come to be called "dysfunctional voiders," that term was coined almost 3 decades ago to describe the rather specific syndrome (Hinman's syndrome), as noted earlier (Hinman and Baumann, 1973). The term has evolved to become nonspecific and is now used to refer to almost any child who presents with voiding symptoms or urinary incontinence, many of whom have no functional obstruction at all. The term is still useful, if only because it lumps these diverse clinical entities together. Because **the term "dysfunctional voiding" causes the practitioner to focus on the urinary tract abnormalities and to overlook functional gastrointestinal disturbances that in many cases may be their underlying cause, the term and concept of dysfunctional elimination syndromes (DES) has been proposed** to provide an inclusive categorization of all functional bladder, sphincter, and gastrointestinal disorders that pathologically affect the pediatric urinary tract (Koff et al, 1998). **In addition to Hinman's syndrome, these disorders include the unstable bladder, the infrequent voiding syndrome, and constipation and fecal retention.**

Lastly, there exists a group of children with identifiable symptom complexes that include **giggle incontinence, postvoid dribbling, the daytime urinary frequency syndrome, and nocturnal enuresis (NE).** They are considered separately because they do not present with uropathology and because the principles of their evaluation and management are different than for children with DES.

In making the transition from an infantile to an adult pattern of urinary control, many children transiently display voiding disturbances or episodes of urinary incontinence that suggest bladder and sphincter dysfunction. Provided these are neither sustained nor repetitive, they do not appear to be of any long-term significance. Consequently, because of the great variability in the timing and manner with which young children develop urinary control, one must be extremely cautious about overinterpreting complaints and misdiagnosing innocuous symptoms; transient symptoms are best ignored, and intermittent ones can usually be safely observed. However, when functional disturbances persist after toilet training and produce characteristic symptoms that imply pathologic potential, investigations must be instituted to exclude anatomic, neurologic, and functional causes.

In evaluating and treating urinary control symptoms in children, the primary goal is to differentiate benign disturbances from those that are potentially harmful and capable of producing uropathology. Initial examination should include a complete history and physical examination (including examination of the lumbosacral spine) and a urinalysis (with specific gravity determination) and culture. This is usually sufficient for children who do not display potentially pathologic signs and symptoms such as combined day and night symptoms, overt anatomic or neurologic abnormalities, or an acute UTI or history of one. Their urinary tracts are usually normal, and they do not require radiologic investigation, endoscopy, or urodynamic study. However, those children with worsening or worrisome signs or symptoms require at least a screening ultrasonogram of the kidneys and bladder, and some may need additional diagnostic studies such as VCUG and urodynamic investigation. The ultrasonogram should include measurement of bladder wall thickness; the empirical criterion for bladder wall thickening is a measurement greater than 0.30 cm with full bladder or 0.50 cm empty. If the ultrasonographic study of the kidneys, ureters, and bladder is normal and without evidence of hydroureteronephrosis, bladder wall thickening, or postvoiding residue, it virtually excludes significant uropathology and indicates that the current symptoms are not being caused by a significant anatomic or neurologic disorder (Fig. 64–26). An awareness of the natural history and clinical features of these conditions allows the practitioner to distinguish benign voiding disturbances from more ominous conditions and greatly facilitates patient management.

The Non-Neurogenic Neurogenic Bladder

Clinical Features

Although occasionally recognized in the newborn period or in early infancy (Jayanthi et al, 1997), patients typically present after toilet training and before puberty with a symptom complex that combines nocturnal and diurnal urinary incontinence with variable patterns of dribbling, overflow, and urgency incontinence. Bowel dysfunction characteristically coexists in the form of encopresis, constipation, and fecal impaction. Recurrent UTI is almost invariably noted (Hinman and Baumann, 1973; Allen, 1977; Hinman,

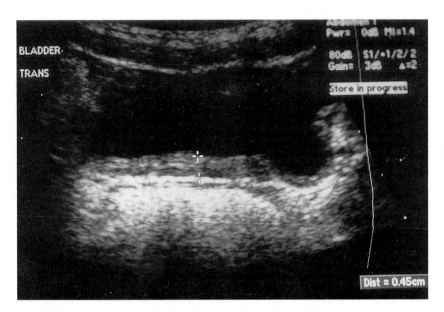

Figure 64–26. Screening urinary tract ultrasound examination demonstrates bladder wall thickness of full bladder to be 0.45 cm, which is thickened and requires further evaluation.

1986). Some children have been noted to have a stressful family environment.

Physical and neurologic examination is typically normal except for a palpably enlarged bladder. Rectal examination discloses normal sphincter tone and may reveal fecal impaction; impaction may be recognizable during urinary tract ultrasonography as dilatation of the rectum (Asselman et al, 2000).

The clinical and radiographic characteristics result from

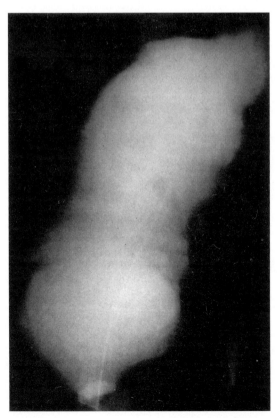

Figure 64–27. Hinman's syndrome, showing the large, thick-walled, dumbbell-shaped bladder.

voiding against a closed sphincter. Radiographic studies of the spine are normal and do not show spinal dysraphism, although spina bifida occulta may be observed. However, radiographic studies of the urinary tract are characteristically abnormal. The bladder often appears neuropathic, with a pear or dumbbell shape, and has a thick wall with saccules and diverticula (Fig. 64–27); a decompensated, smooth-walled bladder of large capacity can sometimes be seen. VCUG usually displays a large postvoid residual and a bladder neck and urethra that are nonobstructed (Fig. 64–28). At times the VCUG appearance is striking and indistinguishable from that of posterior urethral valves, with a dilated prostatic urethra and an abrupt narrowing in caliber distal to the veru montanum (Fig. 64–29). However, no obstruction is noted when endoscopic inspection of the bladder and urethra are performed, although secondary bladder neck hypertrophy may exist. The cause of this radiographic misdiagnosis may be obvious on video urodynamic study: DSD with dilatation of the prostatic urethra during voiding (Fig. 64–30). Renal imaging demonstrates various degrees of upper urinary tract dilatation and damage with vesicoureteric reflux present in about 50% of cases.

Urodynamic Diagnosis

The child with suspected non-neurogenic neurogenic bladder (NNGNGB) should undergo urodynamic studies. However, DSD is not always identifiable because of bladder decompensation that may interfere with voiding, cause the child to void by straining, and produce urodynamic misinterpretation. Although more than 75% of cases display bladder instability, this is not diagnostic; however, **when bladder instability is combined with signs of impaired or obstructed bladder emptying** (low or intermittent flow rate, increased residual urine volume, and/or high intravesical pressures) **in the absence of anatomic or neurologic disease, the diagnosis of NNGNGB is strongly suggested** (Hinman and Baumann, 1973; Hinman, 1974; Allen, 1977; Mix, 1977; Bauer et al, 1980).

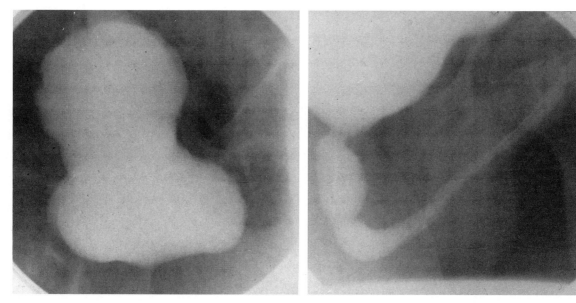

Figure 64–28. Hinman's syndrome. Voiding cystourethrogram demonstrates dumbbell-shaped bladder and nonobstructed urethra.

Etiology

Historically, the etiology of this syndrome was debated by those who viewed it as a neuropathy of occult and obscure pathology (Dorfman et al, 1969; Datta et al, 1970; Williams et al, 1974; Bucy and Carlin, 1975) and by those who suggested it was a manifestation of acquired voiding dysfunction (Hinman and Baumann, 1973; Hinman, 1974; Allen 1977; Bauer et al, 1980; Hinman, 1986). The terms "non-neurogenic neurogenic bladder," "dysfunctional voiding," and, more recently, "the Hinman syndrome" (Hinman, 1986) have been used to describe a condition currently believed to be **caused by voluntary dyssynergia between the detrusor and the striated muscle sphincter during voiding** (Allen and Bright, 1978). It is thought to represent persistence of a pattern of voiding that is transitional between the infant and adult types and that develops from overlearned responses to bladder instability (Allen, 1977). For unknown reasons, the child who has learned to constrict the striated muscle sphincter in order to stay dry during an unstable bladder contraction applies voluntary constriction of the sphincter inappropriately during normal voiding to create a functional obstruction. Depending on the frequency, duration, and severity of obstruction, the clinical spectrum ranges from mild to severe symptoms that are virtually indistinguishable from those in patients with urethral valves or a true NGB.

Diagnostic overlap between the NNGNGB and occult neuropathy exists and can present diagnostic difficulty because of the lack of neurologic and urodynamic tests that are able to distinguish these conditions (see discussion in the earlier part of this chapter). To add confusion, there exists an inherited pattern of voiding dysfunction (Ochoa syndrome), recently identified in Colombian children, that combines features of neuropathy and NNGNGB. These children display dysfunctional voiding features (incontinence, constipation, reflux, hydronephrosis, and bladder instability) but also demonstrate a peculiar painful-appearing facial expression during laughter (similar to a sixth nerve palsy), all of which are inherited in an autosomal recessive pattern (Ochoa and Gorlin, 1987). Resolution of voiding dysfunction may occur at the same time as resolution of the facial distortions, suggesting a functional etiology.

Treatment

A variety of programs have been employed successfully to treat the NNGNGB; no one therapy works for all patients, and each must receive individualized care. Because of the similarity to NGB disease, the methods of management generally follow the lines of treatment for NGB.

After the urine is sterilized and maintained infection free, bladder function must be restored to normal. In children without significant upper urinary tract involvement, this may be accomplished by instituting a comprehensive **bladder retraining program.** Retraining requires strong psychological support, suggestion therapy (including hypnosis in some cases), and the motivation and help of the parents (Baumann and Hinman, 1974) and others (Hanson et al, 1987). **Biofeedback techniques supplement these methods.** By making visible pelvic floor EMG and uroflow data, biofeedback aims to make the child aware that the elements of voiding are under voluntary control and to teach the child to relax the urinary sphincter and pelvic floor striated muscles during bladder emptying. Results have been excellent in controlling symptoms, but disassociation can be noted between subjective symptom relief and objective improvement in clinical and urodynamic parameters (Wennergren and Oberg, 1995; Combs et al, 1998; McKenna et al, 1999; Van Gool et al, 2000).

In addition to bladder retraining, **bowel function needs to be normalized** by adjusting the diet and using laxatives to eliminate fecal accumulation and its potentially obstructive effects on the urinary tract. **Pharmacologic therapy** aimed at the patient's own specifically identified urodynamic disturbance is required in many cases. This may

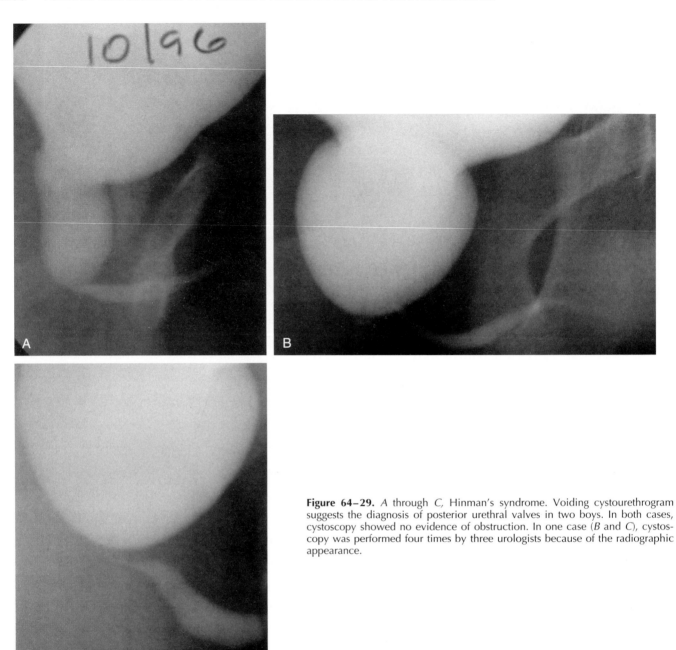

Figure 64–29. *A* through *C*, Hinman's syndrome. Voiding cystourethrogram suggests the diagnosis of posterior urethral valves in two boys. In both cases, cystoscopy showed no evidence of obstruction. In one case (*B* and *C*), cystoscopy was performed four times by three urologists because of the radiographic appearance.

include anticholinergic drugs to eliminate unstable bladder contractions, or sympatholytic agents and diazepam to reduce outflow resistance in the region of the bladder neck and urethral sphincter, respectively. Because of the significant psychological overlay observed in certain patients, appropriate **psychological counseling** should be employed as needed. Parental re-education is also required.

Children who present with more severe degrees of bladder decompensation and upper urinary tract dilatation and damage may require additional therapy with **clean intermittent catheterization** (Fig. 64–31). CIC affords complete low-pressure bladder emptying, and once it is working well and the patient begins voiding more normally, the catheterization frequency may be reduced to monitor postvoiding residual urine volumes. This may provide a very early alert that residual volumes are increasing and voiding dysfunction has recurred.

The secondary effects of altered bladder function in NNGNGB, namely vesicoureteric reflux and hydroureteronephrosis, can at times seem to be a primary disease process requiring surgical intervention. In the past the correct diagnosis of NNGNGB was often made too late, only after operative failure. It cannot be emphasized too strongly that unless the bladder and sphincter functions are treated first, the results of surgery will be attended by unacceptably high complication and failure rates. Of equal significance is

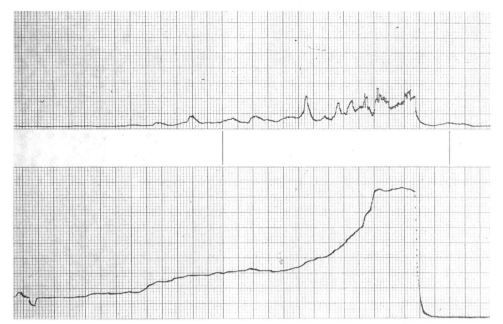

Figure 64–30. Hinman's syndrome. Combined cystometrogram *(bottom)* and periurethral striated muscle integrated electromyogram *(top)* reveals detrusor sphincter dyssynergia during voiding.

the fact that, after function is restored to normal, the sequelae often improve spontaneously and make operative treatment unnecessary (Hinman and Baumann, 1976; Noe, 1985; Koff et al, 1998).

The Unstable Bladder

Etiology

Unstable bladder, the most common pattern of urinary dysfunction in childhood, occurs in up to 57% of *symptomatic* children aged 3 to 14 years (Ruarte and Quesada, 1987). It is characterized by bladder hyperactivity occurring before true detrusor contraction and has been termed the infantile, uninhibited, or overactive bladder. It usually does not represent a neuropathy. These uncontrolled contractions have been viewed as the normal mechanism for infant voiding, and their persistence into childhood reflects a functional or organic delay in CNS maturation that prevents some children from gaining voluntary control over the micturition reflex (Nash, 1949; Lapides and Diokno, 1969; Bauer et al, 1980; Koff et al, 1980). However, this view is not compatible with recent observations (noted previously) regarding bladder function in *asymptomatic* infants and young children, in whom a very low incidence of bladder instability (5% to 18%) has been observed (Yeung, 1995; Wen and Tong, 1998). This inconsistency suggests that either asymptomatic bladder instability, when present in infancy, persists and becomes symptomatic instability in older children or that symptomatic bladder instability is an acquired condition that develops de novo (in response to transient obstruction) during toilet training mishaps or in association with other forms of dysfunctional elimination.

Pathophysiology

If the unstable bladder is considered simply as **bladder hyperactivity occurring during bladder filling**, its patho-

physiology will never appear to be more of a problem than day or night incontinence. Significance depends on how the toilet-trained child responds. Because unstable contractions are involuntary and often insuppressible, a child attempting to maintain continence during them tries to constrict the urinary sphincter to stay dry. This results in a simultaneous and unphysiologic contraction (dyssynergia) of bladder and sphincter. Even though the child is not actually attempting to void, an obstruction to bladder emptying occurs and high intravesical pressures develop that persist until the bladder either relaxes or empties. If the child decides to void during the unstable contraction, voiding will be normal and at low pressure, because the urinary sphincter will relax appropriately during bladder contraction. With regard to urodynamic detection, the only difference between normal children and those with this condition is the latter's inability to suppress the unstable bladder contraction. Consequently, cystometric diagnosis of DSD associated with bladder instability depends on instructing the patient to keep from wetting during an unstable contraction. If the patient is permitted to void during the unstable contraction, then no urodynamic abnormality will be identified.

Clinical and Urodynamic Features

Voluntary constriction of the urinary sphincter during unstable bladder contractions produces urinary obstruction with high intravesical pressures (Koff et al, 1979; Van Gool 1979; Bauer et al, 1980). The clinical spectrum depends on the frequency and forcefulness of bladder contraction and on the effectiveness of sphincteric constriction. It ranges from the harmless urgency-incontinence syndrome to the severely affected child with UTI and reflux.

The clinical features of bladder hyperactivity—urgency, frequency, and precipitate voiding—occur in about 60% to 70% of affected patients (Koff et al, 1979; Bauer et al, 1980). These symptoms characterize the commonly occurring **urgency-incontinence syndrome** in children whose

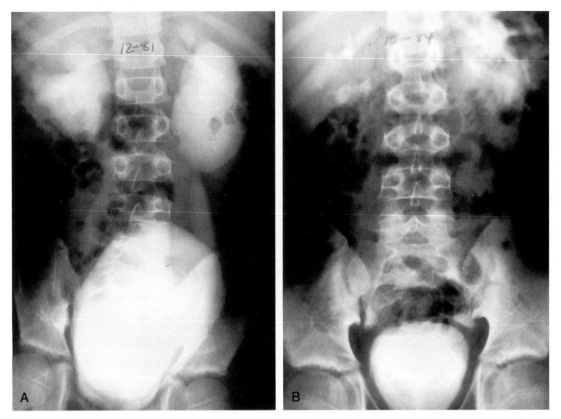

Figure 64–31. Hinman's syndrome requiring clean intermittent catheterization (CIC). *A,* Pretreatment intravenous pyelogram demonstrates bilateral hydroureteronephrosis and distended bladder. *B,* After 1 year with retraining, voiding had returned to normal and CIC was stopped. Twenty-two months later, upper tracts remain decompressed and stable with the child on a bowel and bladder program.

bladder instability elicits a weak or absent sphincteric response. Incontinence may vary in severity. **Urodynamic study is not required in most cases for diagnosis;** it may be safely reserved for children who fail an empiric trial of anticholinergic drug therapy. When performed, it confirms bladder instability with minimal evidence of dyssynergia or obstruction. Consequently, UTI is not a major feature of this subcategory. Ultrasonography of the urinary tract is characteristically normal except for bladder wall thickening, and VCUG, if performed to evaluate for UTI, typically demonstrates a smooth-walled bladder with capacity nearly appropriate for age. Children with bladder instability void normally to completion without residue, so the occurrence of a large residual urine volume should make the diagnosis suspect. One sign that is almost pathognomonic is Vincent's curtsey, so named because the child squats with the heel of one foot compressing the perineum and urethra to prevent urinary leakage (Vincent, 1966) (Fig. 64–32).

The **small-capacity, hypertonic bladder** subcategory is characterized clinically by more prominent symptoms and urodynamically by more obvious bladder-sphincter dyssynergia causing functional obstruction. UTIs commonly occur and are associated with prominent urgency and incontinence that characteristically persist after eradication of the infection. Typically, functional bladder capacity is observed to be reduced during urodynamic study or cystography. This appears to be the result of chronic repetitive functional obstruction during unstable contractions, which is reflected in radiographic studies that may show bladder wall thickening, saccules, and diverticula.

Paradoxically, **up to one third of children with bladder instability have no incontinence** (Koff et al, 1979; Koff and Murtagh, 1983). This is apparently the result of their ability to overcome even forceful bladder contractions by extremely tight sphincter constriction. Unfortunately, this occurs at the expense of raised intravesical pressure. These patients are prone to develop recurrent UTI because of the repeated high intravesical pressures that interfere with bladder wall blood supply and promote bacterial colonization (Chandra, 1995; Chandra et al, 1996; Koff et al, 1979, 1998). In addition to infection, this repetitive functional obstruction produces a spectrum of intravesical anatomic distortions that includes trabeculation, saccules, diverticula, and abnormalities of the ureteric orifices. These secondary changes are responsible for the occurrence and persistence of vesicoureteric reflux in up to 50% of children with unstable bladders (Koff et al, 1979); once acquired, these sequelae tend to persist long after the symptoms of bladder dysfunction resolve or are eliminated (Johnston et al, 1978). **Diagnosis of bladder instability can be difficult in this continent subgroup of patients because the pathologic sequelae of DSD are often considered to be primary (e.g., reflux). A high level of suspicion of bladder dysfunction and urodynamic studies are required to correctly establish the diagnosis.**

Most children have primary bladder instability and

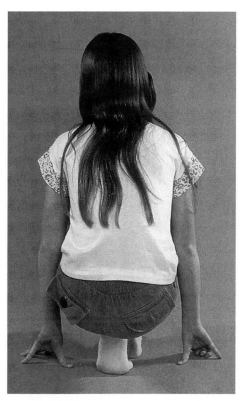

Figure 64–32. Vincent's curtsey. This girl is squatting to keep from leaking urine during an insuppressible bladder (instability) contraction. Note position of heel, which is used to compress the vulva to produce tight mechanical compression of the urethra.

are described as never having been toilet trained completely; however, those with secondary bladder instability were perfectly toilet trained for years before developing symptoms. Although this secondary pattern usually reflects successful sphincter control of occult bladder instability that becomes symptomatic only after the bladder wall thickens and bladder contraction power increases, **the possibility of spinal cord tethering must be considered, especially in the older child who suddenly develops significant urgency and urge incontinence.**

Treatment

Treatment of unstable bladder in childhood is influenced by the observation that with maturation **contractions cease in most children as they develop adult patterns of urinary control.** Until this occurs, the goal of therapy is elimination of the unstable contractions without interfering with normal voiding. **Anticholinergic medication is the mainstay of treatment** (Lapides and Costello, 1969; Koff et al, 1979; Bauer et al, 1980; Homsy et al, 1983, 1985; Koff, 1983; Koff and Murtagh, 1983; Seruca, 1989; Scholtjmeier and van Mastrigt, 1991; Curran et al, 2000). **They appear to work by decreasing detrusor hyperactivity and by shifting the cystometric curve to the right to increase the threshold volume at which unstable contractions occur and thereby enlarge the functional capacity of the bladder.** Bladder instability can be induced or exacerbated by fecal retention or constipation, and these

in turn can be caused by anticholinergic medication. Consequently, an awareness of gastrointestinal functional status is required before anticholinergic therapy is initiated, because a diet/laxative program may be needed during anticholinergic treatment. **Besides medication, fluid restriction, elimination of caffeine, and frequent voidings are essential therapeutic adjuncts to keep bladder volumes below the new threshold for unstable bladder contractions.** Consequently, except in the presence of an acute UTI, **the practice of forcing fluids to children with bladder instability is inappropriate therapy; it causes the bladder to rapidly overfill to exceed threshold volumes.** Therapy is effective in eliminating symptoms in more than 80% of children; however, mean time to complete resolution may exceed 2.5 years in problematic children with day and night symptoms (Curran et al, 2000). In addition to symptom relief, successful therapy may eliminate recurrent infection and hasten the resolution of reflux.

Infrequent Voiding Syndrome

Clinical Features

This syndrome is more common in girls and includes a spectrum of disorders that range from simply voiding infrequently to bladder decompensation. It includes children with urinary incontinence, those with large-capacity bladders who develop UTI, and patients who develop urinary retention without neuropathy or obstruction. Children who present at the minor end of the spectrum were thought to have a "lazy bladder" in the past; however, use of this term should be discouraged because it inappropriately blames the child as being lazy. History is the mainstay of diagnosis. Because voiding infrequency is a relative term, a precise definition of infrequent voiding is more difficult than is recognition and clinical diagnosis. Characteristically, these children are dry at night and do not void in the morning on awakening. Fecal retention from infrequent defecation may also coexist. Unless reminded by a parent to do so, they may not void for 8 to 12 hours or longer while at school or other activities. A single cause does not explain this condition. In some cases the bladder was large in utero (megacystis); in others there may be a behavioral or even a psychogenic cause; and a large-capacity bladder may represent an end stage for children who continue to hold their urine after bladder instability has resolved.

Urologic investigation of these patients with radiographic and urodynamic tests is required if symptoms are significant, to exclude underlying neuropathy or obstruction. In their absence, diagnostic studies are usually normal. The bladder is not thickened on ultrasound study, and hydronephrosis is absent. Urodynamic study is characteristically normal also, except for a larger than normal bladder capacity for age, unless the condition has progressed to bladder decompensation. There is usually no DSD. In the absence of obstruction or neuropathy, bladder retraining with a frequent voiding program is usually successful even for children with partial urinary retention, in whom residual urine volume disappears. Urinary incontinence improves as well.

Psychogenic urinary retention, an extreme variation of

infrequent voiding, is rare in children (Khan, 1971; Stams et al, 1982; Baldew and van Gelderen, 1983). The diagnosis is one of exclusion and requires a complete investigation. The mechanism of the retention is unknown, but it may involve overactive contraction of the external sphincter. Barrett (1978) reported on urodynamic findings in 12 patients. All had a delayed sensation of bladder fullness, and none had evidence of neuropathy. Psychological stressors were found in some but not all of the patients.

Management

Treatment of infrequent voiding involves patient education and bladder retraining using a timed voiding schedule. Use of an elimination (urinary and bowel) diary may be helpful to document voiding frequency; discover coexisting constipation, which may make management difficult; and demonstrate improvement. Correction of occult fecal retention is necessary so that the child can better perceive the sensation of bladder fullness. A successful program permits bladder capacity to decrease with time. In children with severe infrequent voiding, bladder decompensation, and urinary retention, CIC may be required. After bladder recompensation and return of voiding, a modified CIC program can be used as needed to monitor postvoiding residual urine volumes to prevent a recurrence of urinary retention.

Functional Bowel Disturbances

A long, historical relationship exists in children among bladder dysfunction, UTI, and functional gastrointestinal tract disorders, specifically constipation and fecal retention. Schopfner (1968) noted that fecal retention was associated with reflux, hydronephrosis, enuresis, and UTI. Radiographically, alteration of the shape of the bladder neck and urethra by the fecal mass and abnormal voiding patterns with a hesitant and interrupted stream were observed. In some cases this resulted in urinary retention (Gallo, 1970). Neumann and associates (1973) confirmed the association between constipation and UTI and noted that, when constipation was successfully treated, recurrent UTI decreased to 20%, compared with 88% among those untreated. In studying children with constipation/fecal retention, UTI, and bladder instability, O'Regan and colleagues (O'Regan and Yazbeck, 1985; O'Regan et al, 1986) observed that, after treatment for constipation, bladder instability completely disappeared and wetting symptoms and UTI markedly improved. They concluded that bladder instability could be produced by constipation and that the combination induced UTI. Interestingly, the diagnosis of constipation was surprisingly elusive; children had no prior gastrointestinal history, and more than 50% of mothers were unaware of retentive behavior. More recently, Loening-Baucke (1997) observed that constipated children constricted rather than relaxed their pelvic floor during emptying attempts, a pattern similar to DSD, which explains how successful treatment of constipation helped improve dysfunctional voiding symptoms and wetting in 89% and eliminated UTI in all 234 constipated children. The direct relationship between constipation and UTI is supported by other studies

(Blethyn et al, 1995; Chandra, 1995; Wan et al, 1995), especially that of Dohil and colleagues (1994), who found that 66% of constipated children had significant residual volume before treatment of constipation, which decreased to 21% after treatment, compared with only 5% of normal controls. More recently, fecal retention and dysfunctional voiding have been causally related to recurrent UTI and also to vesicoureteral reflux (Koff et al, 1998).

Diagnosis and Therapy

From a pediatric urologic perspective, constipation and fecal retention are very common and usually are not caused by any structural, biochemical, or endocrine disease. The diagnosis of constipation in children is similar to that in adults and requires the presence of hard stools occurring less often than two to three times per week. In contrast, fecal retention, the most common cause of constipation and fecal soiling (encopresis) in children, is thought to result from repetitive attempts to avoid defecation because of fear or temporary pain. A fecal mass accumulates in the rectum or higher in the colon. Infrequent, large stools characterize this condition (Rasquin-Weber et al, 1999).

After toilet training many parents (and physicians) are largely unaware of the frequency and character of bowel movements unless symptoms or signs such as painful fissures or bleeding occur. Diagnosis requires a combination of history, physical examination of the abdomen and rectum, and an abdominal film. A negative physical and rectal examination does not exclude fecal retention, but in about 75% of children the diagnosis can be made on plain abdominal film. In some cases, severe compression of the bladder and bladder neck can be observed. When necessary, standardized criteria have been described for quantifying fecal retention and for assessing follow-up (Rockney et al, 1995) (Fig. 64–33).

Treatment of functional bowel disease in children can and should be initiated by the pediatric urologist when the genitourinary signs and symptoms appear to be secondary to gastrointestinal dysfunction. The principles of management include an initial clean-out with laxatives and enemas, followed by a maintenance program that combines oral laxatives and/or stool softeners with dietary manipulation (fiber, fruits, and vegetables) to generate bowel movements on an almost daily basis. Unfortunately, only about 50% of patients are cured for the long term (Loening-Baucke, 1997). Consultation with a pediatric gastroenterologist is recommended to help select specific therapeutic agents and to establish guidelines for successful therapy and follow-up. It is therefore important that both parents and patient recognize the genitourinary signs of recurrent gastrointestinal dysfunction and be prepared to restart or modify therapy.

Often multiple syndromes of elimination dysfunction coexist, and although it may be difficult to determine which one is primary, this determination is important. The fact that large fecal accumulations can induce bladder dysfunction by producing bladder instability has important treatment implications, because anticholinergic drug therapy is central to the treatment of bladder instability yet these same medications produce constipation and fecal retention. Caution must be exercised in using anticholinergic drugs in

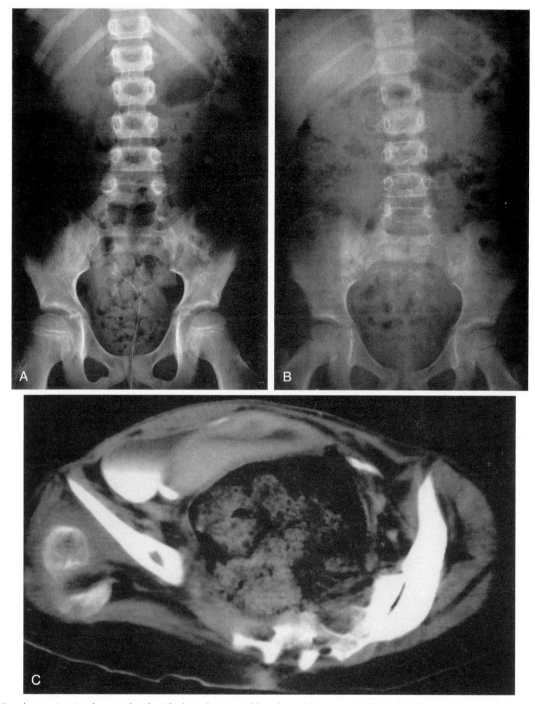

Figure 64–33. Fecal retention is often easily identified on the scout film of a voiding cystourethrogram *(A)*, on a routine abdominal film *(B)*, or, in some cases, by severe compression of the bladder by the fecal mass *(C)*.

susceptible children, because fecal accumulation may result and lead to an increase rather than a decrease in bladder hyperactivity.

Association between Dysfunctional Elimination Syndromes, Reflux, and Urinary Tract Infections

Although UTI and reflux can clearly be caused by anatomic and neurogenic obstruction, their relation to DES was not well considered until 1974, when Hinman described the anatomic consequences of functional urinary obstruction in NNNGNGB. Since then, multiple studies have confirmed the pathophysiologic consequences of other functional causes of urinary tract obstruction. These include the unstable bladder, the infrequent voiding syndrome, and constipation and fecal retention.

Considering the bladder function–altering effects of constipation noted previously, the causal relationship between dysfunctional voiding syndromes and reflux should not be surprising. It is analogous to—although less severe than—the dysfunction that occurs in NGB. Hutch (1952) originally noted paraureteric diverticula and reflux in paraplegic patients with DSD in whom anatomic outflow obstruction was absent. Their urodynamic abnormalities were almost identical to those seen in children with instability and DSD, except that sphincter incoordination in these neurologically normal children occurs voluntarily during bladder filling and does not lead to large residual urine volumes.

Several studies have closely examined the relationship between bladder instability, UTI, and vesicoureteral reflux (Homsy et al, 1983, 1985; Koff and Murtagh, 1983, 1998; Seruca, 1989; Scholtjmeier and van Mastrigt, 1991; Van Gool et al, 1992; Homsy 1994; Chandra, 1995; Chandra et al, 1996). Successful treatment of bladder instability produces a twofold to threefold increase in the rate of reflux resolution and a reduced rate of recurrent UTI compared with controls. Although obstruction during instability-induced DSD is pathophysiologic, video urodynamic cystography shows that reflux does not necessarily occur at the peak or even during an uninhibited contraction; it occurs unpredictably throughout bladder filling. Reflux does not appear to be caused simply by a high intravesical pressure spike (Conway, 1984; Godley et al, 1990). Rather, the culprit is the repeated high pressures that gradually produce alterations to bladder anatomy (wall thickening, trabeculation, saccules, and diverticula). These deform the ureterovesical junction and interfere with its antireflux function (Koff et al, 1998), but because voiding occurs normally the deleterious effects are blunted compared with Hinman's syndrome.

Studies in newborns have demonstrated that high-grade reflux occurs mainly in male infants, is usually bilateral, and is associated with bladder dysfunction characterized by high voiding pressure, low capacity, and hypercontractility (instability) (Yeung et al, 1997; Sillen, 1999). The rate of spontaneous resolution of high-grade reflux is much higher in infants (44% in 15 months) than in older children. Coincidental with reflux resolution is normalization of bladder function. This strongly incriminates bladder dysfunction occurring in utero as a cause for reflux in this population and suggests that the management of high-grade reflux in neonates should be different than in older children.

In addition to bladder instability, other DES that affect the bladder during filling have been shown to influence the behavior of the ureterovesical junction and the inheritance (Noe, 1988) and natural history of reflux (Koff et al, 1998). These include infrequent voiding and constipation or fecal retention. In the presence of DES, reflux resolves more slowly: with DES, grade 2 reflux takes 1.6 years longer to resolve than grade 3 reflux does in children without DES. DES also appear to increase the risk of complications accompanying antireflux surgery (Savage, 1973; Noe, 1985, 1998). Failure of surgery to completely eliminate reflux, recurrence of reflux after surgery, and occurrence of contralateral reflux after unilateral reimplantation are all more likely in patients with DES. Furthermore, with DES breakthrough UTI is three times more likely, as is recurrence of UTI after reflux resolution. Voiding dysfunction is also a risk factor for renal damage in children with UTI and reflux. The significance of this risk

was defined by the observation that more than 75% of children who develop new renal scars while taking antibiotic prophylaxis for reflux have voiding dysfunction (Naseer and Steinhardt, 1997).

Giggle Incontinence

MacKeith coined the term "giggle incontinence" in 1959 (MacKeith, 1964). The term itself is not widely known, although the condition is surprisingly common in girls. In one study, almost 25% of student nurses experienced giggle incontinence at some time, and in 10% it persisted past the age of 20 years (Christmas et al, 1991). There is some evidence that the condition may be inherited.

Urodynamic studies are often normal but may show detrusor hyperreflexia or tetanic detrusor contractions during laughter, confirming the relationship (Rogers et al, 1982). The cause is unknown, but it has similarities to other disorders that display strong emotion-induced muscle hypotonia. This suggests that giggle incontinence may be a centrally mediated disorder (Sher, 1994). For example, cataplexy, a part of the narcoleptic syndrome complex, displays sudden hypotonia or paralysis of the muscles of the face, neck, or trunk lasting from seconds to minutes. Laughter is the most common precipitating event.

History is all that is needed to establish a diagnosis of giggle incontinence. These patients typically have completely normal voiding habits aside from incontinence. Unless there is a prior history of UTIs, imaging studies are unnecessary, as are studies such as VCUG or urodynamics.

Simple measures should be tried first, such as frequent voiding, especially before events or situations that may lead to wetting. Although occasional improvement has been noted with anticholinergic medications or Kegel exercises, these usually are not helpful.

CNS stimulants that are useful in narcolepsy have been tried in giggle incontinence. Methylphenidate, used either on a daily basis or as needed before precipitating situations, is reported to be effective (Sher, 1994; Sher and Reinberg, 1996).

Postvoid Dribbling

Postvoid dribbling occurs almost exclusively in normal girls after toilet training. Voiding is normal, and there is no urgency or urge incontinence. Dry nights are typical. The **condition results from vaginal reflux,** a harmless and transient event that is asymptomatic in most girls and often can be observed radiographically during VCUG. However, in some girls, the urine is temporarily trapped in the vagina because of prepubertal narrowing and compression. When they stand up after voiding, the urine leaks out slowly until the vagina is empty. The problem usually improves with age and growth but may be treated by two simple maneuvers designed to open the introitus or tilt the vaginal canal: (1) the child voids by facing the back of the commode, which allows the thighs to spread apart laterally or (2) after voiding and while sitting on the commode, the child leans forward to touch her toes with her hands, to allow urine to evacuate.

Daytime Urinary Frequency Syndrome

The daytime urinary frequency syndrome is relatively common (Crowther et al, 1988; Zoubek, 1990). It is characterized by the development of sudden, severe, and often dramatic daytime urinary frequency without incontinence in healthy young children (mean age, 4.5 years) without any identifiable antecedent illness or injury and with no history of UTI. Voiding occurs as often as every 10 to 20 minutes. Characteristically, symptoms stop as soon as the child falls asleep, although NE may precede or coexist. The natural history is of spontaneous resolution after several months. Recurrence is low (3%), except when NE is present (40%).

The cause is unknown. Seasonal variation has been observed (Koff and Byard, 1988) but not confirmed. Viral cultures are generally negative (Robson and Leung, 1993). Some series have suggested that psychosocial stresses may be a trigger, but no cause and effect relation has been established (Zoubek, 1990; Bass, 1991; Watemberg and Shalev, 1994). Hypercalciuria has also been noted in almost 30% of these children.

The diagnosis remains one of exclusion and is suggested by a characteristic history. The presence of significant urinary incontinence should suggest bladder instability instead. Physical examination is required to exclude occult neuropathy; the bladder should not be palpable. Although the meatus always looks small in young boys, meatal stenosis does not cause this syndrome and meatotomy is not curative. Renal ultrasound excludes urologic pathology and, if the results are normal, VCUG and urodynamic studies are not indicated.

There is no known therapy for this condition until it resolves spontaneously. Parents should be advised that the child is not willfully producing symptoms and reassured that with time it will stop. Anticholinergic medications usually are ineffective.

Nocturnal Enuresis

Enuresis is defined as involuntary voiding; when it occurs at night it is termed *nocturnal* enuresis, and daytime incontinence is termed *diurnal* enuresis. Because urinary incontinence occurs normally in infants and young children, its significance depends on the age of the patient, parental expectations, and social and cultural factors. **Approximately 15% of children still wet at night at age 5 years.** Although NE persisting after this age or until the child enters school generally causes concern, it is not until age 7 years that most parents, peers, and physicians begin to expect dryness, because the NE interferes with socialization (Moffatt, 1994). In contrast, diurnal enuresis that persists or recurs after toilet training may be a problem. More girls than boys are dry both day and night by the age of 2 years, and NE is 50% more common in boys than in girls. NE has a spontaneous resolution rate of 15% per year, so that by age of 15 years it persists in only 1% of the population (Table 64–11). More than 80% of enuretics wet only at night and have no other abnormalities in their urologic history; they are classified as having monosymptomatic NE (MNE). This subgroup of patients with MNE

Table 64–11. ENURESIS LAWS OF 15
15% of 5-year-old children wet
5% of 10-year-old children wet
1% of 15-year-old adolescents wet
15% of enuretics have encopresis
15% of enuretics become dry each year
15% of enuretics have daytime symptoms
15% of enuretics have an initial dry period
15% of nonenuretics have nocturnal polyuria
15% of nonenuretics have nocturnal awakenings

After Glassberg K: Personal communication.

have such unified features that they must be clearly distinguished from patients who have both nighttime incontinence and daytime symptoms (urgency, frequency, or incontinence).

Most nocturnal enuretics have never been dry; their incontinence is termed *primary enuresis.* Unfortunately, the development of urinary control is not always final. Approximately 25% of children who attain initial nighttime dryness by 12 years of age relapse and wet for a period averaging 2.5 years. These children have *secondary enuresis*.

Etiology

MNE is a symptom rather than a disease. A number of theories have been proposed to explain why children with MNE fail to recognize or respond to their full or contracting bladder during sleep. Although these theories, which include behavioral, genetic, developmental, neurologic, psychological, urodynamic, and organic causes, are diverse and may be able to explain selected cases, there is no single explanation for this symptom, and in each individual multiple factors may be operative. Clearly, the vast majority of children with MNE do not suffer from psychiatric, neurologic, or urologic disturbances, and investigation and treatment along these lines is both inappropriate and unrewarding.

URODYNAMIC FINDINGS

The single most important urodynamic observation in MNE is a reduced bladder capacity (Starfield, 1967). This reduction was shown to be functional, not anatomic, by measurements of bladder capacity under anesthesia (Troup and Hodgson, 1971). It is not the cause for the enuresis, although it often increases coincidently with cure. A number of nocturnal enuretics have diurnal symptoms of frequency and urgency, or even incontinence, which suggests bladder instability (Wu et al, 1988). However, although more than 50% of children with night wetting have unstable bladder contractions observed during awake cystometry, in those with pure MNE the incidence is low (15% to 20%) and is similar to that in normal subjects (Hjalmas, 1976; Norgaard et al, 1985, 1989b, 1997).

Most enuretics are not incontinent because of bladder instability. During sleep urodynamic studies, an enuretic event appears to be almost identical to voluntary daytime voiding, rather than involving unstable contractions with a single bladder contraction leading to emptying. Unstable contractions can occur at some time in half of sleep cystometric studies, but these contractions do not necessarily lead to incontinence; about 45% of the time the children awaken to void. Provocative urodynamic studies with fast filling of the bladder (30 ml/min) during sleep provide further insight into the relation between instability and enuresis. Bladder contraction occurs in almost all patients, but the patient is equally likely to awaken to void as to wet (Norgaard et al, 1989b). It therefore appears that it is the child's neurologic response to the uninhibited contraction that determines whether sleep wetting or awakening to void will occur, and this can be assessed by EMG monitoring of the pelvic floor muscles. If muscle activity occurs, it signals an arousal response and leads to awakening, whereas a silent pelvic floor during bladder contraction reflects a nonresponsiveness that is associated with sleep wetting (Norgaard et al, 1989a).

In summary, bladder instability does not occur in children with MNE at a higher rate than in normal subjects, and in most enuretics unstable contractions are not the cause for sleep wetting. Consequently, therapy aimed at eliminating uninhibited contractions is generally ineffective (Kosar et al, 1999).

SLEEP FACTORS

The fact that wetting occurs during sleep has led to the hypothesis that enuretics have a disturbance of sleep which allows them to sleep too deeply or prevents them from awakening. Sophisticated nighttime encephalography (EEG) and monitoring of eye movements, urodynamic parameters, pulse, blood pressure, and so on indicate that sleep is not simply a progressive and passive slowing of body and brain processes. The relationships between sleep, arousal, and sleep wetting are neither simple nor intuitive, and **the sleep disturbance hypothesis is false.**

Sleep occurs in stages and begins with so-called non–rapid eye movement (NREM) sleep, which is divisible into four progressively deeper stages of sleep (stages 1 through 4), each characterized by specific EEG changes. In addition, a particularly light stage of sleep is recognized that is characterized by bursts of conjugate rapid eye movements (REM sleep). REM sleep is associated with increased autonomic activity, generalized muscle atonia, and dreaming. Normal sleep structure is composed of cycles of NREM sleep, REM sleep, and occasional awakenings. In older children and adults, these cycles last about 1 to 1.5 hours, and the percentage of time spent in REM sleep increases as the cycles progress through the night (Rechtschaffen and Kales, 1968).

Enuretics often appear to be very deep sleepers, and enuresis was originally considered to be the result of sleeping too soundly or awakening with difficulty (Broughton, 1968). Early sleep studies demonstrated that enuresis often occurred during deep sleep and that older enuretics were often very deep sleepers whose wetting could sometimes be improved with the administration of amphetamines that lightened sleep (Strom-Olsen, 1950). Clearly, when children are aroused from deep sleep, they are often hard to

awaken, appear to be confused and disoriented, and stumble when they are walked to the toilet. The observation that enuretics are especially deep sleepers is a misconception, because parents usually do not attempt to awaken their nonenuretic children. When they do so, they are usually surprised to find them sleeping equally soundly (Boyd, 1960; Graham, 1973). However, some enuretic boys are truly more difficult to arouse than age-matched controls. Because sleep arousal thresholds decrease with age, this elevated arousal threshold may reflect a developmental delay (Wolfish, 1999).

Controlled sleep studies have shown that children with enuresis sleep no more soundly than normal children and that a number of enuretics actually wet during very light sleep or while temporarily awake, as do many infants. They have also proven that neither hypothesis—deep sleep or an arousal disorder—is accurate in describing enuretic sleep or is a cause for sleep wetting. Enuretic episodes occur throughout the night on a random basis, and wetting occurs in each sleep stage in proportion to the time actually spent in that stage (Mikkelsen et al, 1980; Norgaard et al, 1989a; Reimao et al, 1993).

Nocturnal sleep and bladder monitoring studies by Robert and others (1993) have been able to distinguish three types of enuretic episodes:

1. Gradually undulating elevations in bladder pressure culminate in wetting; these are associated with prominent somatic and visceral reactions, including tachycardia, body movements, increasing respirations, and progressive awakening. The awakening reaction is strong, and the child struggles to keep from wetting.

2. A very quick micturition is associated with minimal body movement and visceral signs. The awakening reaction is very brief, and the struggle to keep from wetting is very limited.

3. Complete parasomnia, a total lack of CNS reaction and response to bladder contraction, occurs; neither bladder filling nor bladder contraction registers on the EEG, and involuntary voiding occurs without any modification of sleep.

These three patterns appear to reflect the various stages in the normal development of nocturnal urinary control and suggest that wetting during sleep is to a great extent determined by CNS maturation.

Watanabe and Azuma (1989) further defined three discrete types of enuresis based on cystometric and EEG observations (Table 64–12). Follow-up analysis of patients with these three patterns indicated that 20% of patients with type IIb enuresis will change to type IIa and 60% to type I, whereas 78% of patients with type IIa will change to type I (Watanabe et al, 1994). The evolution of these distinct patterns of EEG and urodynamic responses suggests that with time maturational changes take place that include increasing CNS recognition of bladder fullness and contraction along with increasing CNS control over the micturition reflex. **These findings suggest that the sleep patterns of enuretics are not different from those of normal children, and that most enuretics neither have a disorder of arousal nor wet as a consequence of sleeping too deeply. Instead, they lend support to the con-**

Table 64–12. TYPES OF ENURESIS BASED ON CYSTOMETRIC AND ELECTROENCEPHALOGRAPHIC (EEG) OBSERVATIONS

Type I:	A stable bladder with an EEG response during an enuretic episode
Type IIa:	A stable bladder with no EEG response during an enuretic episode
Type IIb:	An unstable bladder with no EEG response during an enuretic episode

From Watanabe H, Azuma Y: A proposal for a classification system of enuresis based on overnight simultaneous monitoring of electroencephalography and cystometry. Sleep 1989;12:257–264.

cept that enuresis is related to a delay in CNS development or, more accurately, a dual delay in the development of the perception and inhibition of bladder filling and contraction by the CNS (Koff, 1995).

ALTERATIONS IN VASOPRESSIN SECRETION AND NOCTURNAL URINE PRODUCTION

About 50% less urine is normally excreted during the night than during the day. George and colleagues (1975) demonstrated that **a circadian rhythm of plasma arginine vasopressin (AVP), which increased at night, is responsible for this fact. Many children with enuresis have similar levels of AVP during both the day and the night. This causes them to produce larger amounts of dilute urine at night,** so that their nocturnal urine production can equal or exceed diurnal output and in some cases may exceed functional bladder capacity (Norgaard et al, 1989c, 1997; Rittig et al, 1989). Although this relationship between nocturnal polyuria caused by decreased excretion of AVP and enuresis has led some to suggest that AVP deficiency is the cause for NE, other opinions have been contradictory. **In some studies, no difference in day and night urine output was observed;** others found that only a small proportion of children with NE had a significant decrease in nocturnal AVP levels compared with controls (Vulliamy, 1956; Steffens et al, 1993). Likewise, **in large population studies, Kawauchi and Watanabe (1993) found no significant difference in nocturnal urine osmolality between enuretic and nonenuretic children at any age.** Although failure of AVP to increase during the night and nocturnal polyuria may occur in some children with enuresis, the frequency, mechanism, and pathophysiologic significance of altered AVP excretion in enuresis requires further clarification.

AVP is stored in the posterior pituitary and is released into the blood stream in response to action potentials in nerve fibers that synthesize the hormone. In addition to well recognized factors such as changes in serum osmotic pressure and extracellular fluid volume, a variety of other stimuli can alter vasopressin secretion, including pain, emotion, exercise, and medication. Moreover, established patterns of AVP secretion can be modified by sleep and by light. Sleep is known to affect pituitary hormone secretion, and its effect can be seen in individuals who nap after lunch and have increases in AVP secretion. Alterations in sleep also produce changes in established AVP circadian

rhythms, a phenomenon that is well recognized in night-shift workers who display a reversal of their AVP circadian rhythm (Aschoff, 1965; Moore-Ede, 1986).

Evidence suggests that **AVP secretion may also be influenced by bladder fullness.** In clinical studies, Kawauchi and associates (1993) observed that (1) after supravesical urinary diversion, the normal difference between day and night levels of AVP disappeared, and (2) during cystometry, AVP levels were higher when the bladder was full than when it was empty. Experimental studies by Ohne (1995) examined the effect of urinary retention on AVP production and found that within 2 hours after urethral obstruction there occurred increased activity in hypothalamic cells that produce AVP. It was hypothesized that bladder wall fullness and wall stretching induced by urinary retention affects, via neuronal stimulation, the regulation of AVP secretion from the hypothalamus. **These observations suggest that bedwetting, by emptying the bladder during the night, may actually be the cause of low levels of nocturnal AVP secretion in enuretics, because the empty bladder removes a stimulus for AVP secretion.**

Evidence also suggests that the absence of an AVP circadian rhythm may represent a normal delay in development rather than a true pathophysiologic process (Koff, 1995). Measurement of urinary osmolality in first morning urine specimens from enuretic and nonenuretic children demonstrated that children younger than 4 years of age had significantly lower osmolality than children older than 5 years, yet there was no difference in osmolality between enuretic and nonenuretic children (Kawauchi and Watanabe, 1993; Vande Walle et al, 1998). This immaturity in nighttime urine concentration does not appear to be a result of renal concentrating ability, which reaches adult levels by 18 months of age; nor does it appear to be caused by serum AVP levels, which reach adult levels by 12 months of age (Rascher et al, 1986). It suggests that the **circadian rhythmicity of AVP matures over time** and indicates that **enuresis associated with AVP-induced nocturnal polyuria may simply represent another manifestation of developmental delay.** Observations by Knudsen and coworkers (1991), who noted that 25% of enuretics who initially lacked AVP rhythmicity ultimately developed a circadian rhythm of AVP, support this concept and show how this delay improves with time. Interestingly, even after increasing their nocturnal AVP secretion, these patients improved but did not cure their enuresis.

DEVELOPMENTAL DELAY

The aforementioned, seemingly unrelated alterations in urodynamic function, sleep, AVP secretion, and urinary osmolality that characterize older children with MNE all occur normally in infants and young children and actually represent varied expressions of neurophysiologic immaturity. **In most children MNE represents a delay in development, and each of these physiologic alterations tends to improve with time and to resolve spontaneously.**

The theory that NE reflects a degree of developmental delay is well supported clinically. Population control studies have shown that associated developmental delays, such as fine and gross motor clumsiness, perceptual dysfunction, and speech delays, do not occur in nonwetting control subjects (Mimouni et al, 1985; Jarvelin, 1989). In addition, a significant number of children with enuresis were small for gestational age at birth, display retardation in skeletal maturation (bone age), and exhibit a generalized delay in attaining developmental landmarks and in achieving functional maturation of the CNS (Bakwin, 1961). Delayed development of both day and nighttime urinary control and the high rate of spontaneous resolution (15% per year) in MNE support this theory, as does the tendency for encopresis to occur more commonly in enuretics (10% to 25%).

However, it appears that a single delay in development cannot explain fully the enuretic event, because for wetting to occur during sleep there must be not only a failure of inhibition of the bladder contraction but a failure to awaken in response to the bladder contraction. Sleep wetting must therefore reflect a dual developmental delay involving both afferent and efferent CNS limbs: failure to inhibit bladder contraction (efferent limb) and failure to perceive bladder fullness or awaken to the contraction (afferent limb) (Koff, 1995). It is noteworthy that, although NE requires both CNS limbs to be dysfunctional, cure of enuresis can be achieved by eliminating only one dysfunction. This may explain why therapies for enuresis that focus on only one of these two CNS limbs generally have lower efficacy.

These findings suggest that achieving urinary control at night is an integral part of a child's general development, which can be delayed or retarded by a variety of factors. In most cases, NE represents a delay in development that to the casual observer may appear to be an isolated physiologic disturbance. However, careful study has shown that this developmental delay is not isolated, that it is associated with other lags in development, and that in almost all cases maturation will occur with time and enuresis will cease spontaneously.

HEREDITARY FACTORS

Enuresis is inherited: the likelihood for child bedwetting is 77% if it occurred in both parents, 43% if one parent wet, and 15% if neither wet (Bakwin, 1973). Bladder control is delayed on average 1.5 years if two first-degree relatives had enuresis. In twin studies, enuresis is more common in monozygotic than in dizygotic boys (70% vs. 31%) or girls (65% vs. 44%) (Norgaard et al, 1997; Hublin et al, 1998). NE is inherited as an autosomal dominant tendency with variable penetrance that may be influenced by environmental and other genetic factors. Already characterized is the ENUR1 gene located on chromosome 13; it has two markers, 13q13 and 13q14.2, that are associated with the clinical phenotype (Norgaard et al, 1997), but inheritance patterns suggest linkage to chromosome 22 and the possibility of another gene on chromosome 12 (Arnell et al, 1997; Von Gontard et al, 1999). Response to desmopressin (DDAVP) also appears to have a genetic predisposition; Hogg and Husmann (1993) noted that, whereas an overall response rate to DDAVP could be achieved in 75% of patients, the response by patients with a positive history of enuresis was 91%.

Enuresis appears to be influenced by hereditary factors. It occurs in boys more commonly than in girls. A significant number of parents and siblings of an enuretic child had or have enuresis, and if both parents were enuretic there is an overwhelming likelihood that their child will also wet.

ORGANIC URINARY TRACT DISEASE

Most children with MNE do not have an organic urinary tract cause for their wetting; the incidence is less than 0.4% (Kawauchi et al, 1996). In the past, many children underwent surgical procedures on the urethra and bladder neck in a misguided attempt to treat conditions that nowadays are not considered pathologic (Mahony, 1971; Arnold and Ginsberg, 1973). **Obstructive urethral lesions such as meatal stenosis and urethral stricture do not cause nighttime wetting without daytime symptoms.** Consequently, meatotomy or urethral dilatation should not be used to treat MNE. In contrast to those with MNE, children with lower urinary tract obstruction may display coexisting day and night symptoms and pollakiuria (Cutler et al, 1978; Kawauchi et al, 1996). **The need to distinguish MNE from NE associated with diurnal symptoms cannot be overemphasized. If daytime symptoms are present, children, especially boys, should undergo urinary tract imaging at least with an ultrasonogram to search for signs of possible obstruction: bladder wall thickening, hydronephrosis, or incomplete bladder emptying. A normal examination provides reassuring confirmation that a significant obstruction is absent.**

MISCELLANEOUS FACTORS

Enuresis is not typically caused by a psychological disturbance. If it were the somatic expression of an emotional disorder, then from a psychodynamic viewpoint its elimination might produce worsening of the psychopathology or cause substitute symptoms to develop. In fact, the opposite occurs after enuresis cure. Treatment of enuresis does not produce any negative effect on adolescent health, growth, or development; it is beneficial (Fergusson et al, 1986; Moffatt, 1989; Norgaard et al, 1997). **In general, if psychological disturbance is present, enuresis may be a cause rather than a consequence.**

Children with attention deficit hyperactivity disorder (ADHD) appear to have an increased incidence of nocturnal and diurnal enuresis. Recognition of these patients is useful because their treatment outcome has generally been disappointing (Husmann, 1996; Robson et al, 1997).

There is no objective evidence relating allergy to enuresis for most patients. In selected cases, an association may exist and be treatable. Egger and colleagues (1992) and Zaleski and associates (1972) showed that food allergy may cause bladder hyperactivity and a reduced functional bladder capacity, which can improve after elimination of the dietary allergen. However, in those patients whose wetting appeared to be caused by food allergy, no difference could be observed in the level of immunoglobulin E, which is often elevated with allergenic phenomena (Kaplan, 1973).

Sudden-onset enuresis and urinary frequency in young girls may be caused by *Enterobius vermicularis* (pinworm)

Table 64–13. CHARACTERISTICS OF A NEGATIVE SCREENING EVALUATION FOR ENURESIS

Age prepubertal
Enuresis has been lifelong
Wetting occurs only at night
No daytime symptoms of wetting, urgency, or polyuria
No history of urinary infection
Negative urinalysis and culture
Normal physical examination, including lumbosacral spine

infestation even in the absence of perineal itching. Diagnosis is made by recovery of characteristic eggs in feces, from perianal skin, or from under fingernails. Dramatic relief of symptoms follows appropriate antihelmintic therapy (Sachdev and Howards, 1975).

Evaluation

A carefully obtained history, physical examination, and urinalysis are sufficient for most children with primary MNE. The goal of evaluation is to identify those children who require further study. Clues such as a history of urinary infection, diurnal incontinence, or obstructive symptoms or subtle signs of neuropathy must be pursued. In their absence, there is generally no indication for radiographic studies or cystoscopy because the incidence of associated uropathology is so low (Table 64–13). As noted previously, ultrasonography of the kidneys and bladder is a reasonable, initial noninvasive method of excluding obstructive uropathy in the child with NE who requires additional study. A cystometrogram is not useful in the routine evaluation of children with MNE.

Treatment

A number of treatment modalities have been used for NE, but their effectiveness, even in controlled studies, has been difficult to assess because of the high spontaneous annual remission rate (15%) and the extremely high placebo improvement effect, which can exceed 65% (Mishra et al, 1980). **Proven, reproducible, and effective therapy has evolved along two lines: drug therapy and behavioral modification.**

Before beginning therapy, the physician must recognize that **many families do not actually seek treatment but simply come to the urologist to exclude an organic cause for the wetting.** Parents have very different attitudes and expectations about bedwetting and its cure than do physicians. About 60% of surveyed parents believe that bedwetting is a significant problem, severe enough for 35% to warrant punishment of the child. Although most parents believe that their child should be dry at a much younger age than their physician does, **only 63% of parents believe that enuresis should actually be treated, compared with almost 90% of physicians.** Likewise, the vast majority of parents (93%) believe that medication is not a good form of treatment for bedwetting (Haque et al, 1981). The ideal age to start treatment is likewise not well defined. In most families, nocturnal wetting is not perceived to be a problem before the child is 5 years old, and at that age about 15% of the population still wet. **We generally dis-** courage treatment before 7 years of age and have not witnessed many treatment successes before that age. This is the age when children, peers, and parents generally begin to expect dryness and when bedwetting starts to interfere with social activities such as sleepovers (Moffatt, 1994).

PHARMACOLOGIC THERAPY

Effective pharmacologic therapy exists for MNE but does not include sedatives, stimulants, or sympathomimetic agents. Anticholinergic therapy has likewise been relatively disappointing, with an effectiveness ranging from only 5% to 40% (Person-Junemann et al, 1993; Kosar et al, 1999). Although anticholinergic agents have been shown to increase the functional capacity of the bladder, improvement in enuresis after therapy to expand the bladder occurs in fewer than half of these cases (Johnstone et al, 1977). However, anticholinergic agents are extremely effective for certain subgroups of enuretics; they are very effective (87.5%) in treating patients with combined day and nighttime wetting and those with proven bladder instability (Kass et al, 1979).

Imipramine, typical of a class of tricyclic antidepressants, has been effective in a large number of well-controlled clinical studies. It can cure enuresis in about 40% to 50% of cases and results in improvement in another 10% to 20%. However, discontinuation of medication causes relapse in up to 60% of patients. Clinical response has been shown to correlate with plasma levels (Jorgensen et al, 1980; De Gatta et al, 1984). However, routine measurement of imipramine or its metabolites is not clinically useful (Devane et al, 1984), because normal or even high plasma levels do not ensure a response. The usual recommended dose of imipramine is 25 mg for children between 5 and 8 years of age and 50 mg for older children (0.8 to 1.6 mg/kg/day), given as a single dose shortly before bedtime. This produces a therapeutic plasma concentration in only 30% of patients. Care must be exercised when prescribing higher doses because of potential toxicity.

Imipramine drug therapy has two potentially problematic consequences. The first is drug toxicity. Although side effects are usually infrequent, personality changes, adverse effects on sleep and appetite, gastrointestinal symptoms, and nervousness have been reported (Kardash et al, 1968; Shaffer et al, 1968). Because of the low ratio between beneficial effect and toxic effect, overdose is a potential hazard. At greatest risk are the younger siblings of enuretics who unwarily ingest the medication in large amounts. Poisoning is characterized by severe myocardial depression and electrocardiographic changes that are not observed at therapeutic doses (Rohner and Sanford, 1975). Should a toxic reaction occur, specific therapeutic protocols exist to effect a reversal (Green and Cromie, 1981).

The second potentially problematic effect of imipramine is its ability to improve wetting symptoms not only in cases of enuresis but also when incontinence is caused by an organic abnormality, such as neuropathy (Epstein and DeQuevedo, 1964; Cole and Fried, 1972). As a result, the use of imipramine as a therapeutic test to distinguish organic from nonorganic incontinence is not advisable.

Desmopressin (DDAVP). Reduction of urine output at

Table 64–14. DDAVP CURE RATE IN NOCTURNAL ENURESIS

| Author | Number of Patients | Mean Wet Nights | | Percentage Totally Dry |
		Placebo	DDAVP	
Aladjem et al, 1982	32	8.8	3	35
Birkasova et al, 1978	22	11	4.2	23
Dimson, 1977	17	9.9	6.9	12
Ferrie, 1984	22	8.8	7.9	N/S
Fjellestad-Paulsen, 1987	30	9.0	5.6	10
Janknegt and Smans, 1990	22	10.6	6.8	N/S
Pedersen et al, 1985	37	7.7	5.0	16
Post et al, 1983	52	10	7.8	12
Ramsden et al, 1982	24	8	4.3	38
Rittig, 1989b	28	6.7	1.8	86
Sukhai et al, 1989	28	5.8	3.8	58
Terho, 1991	52	9.4	5.0	29
Tuvemo, 1978	18	8.0	3.2	44
Wille, 1986	50	9.8	13.8	N/S
Number Totally Dry/Total Number Subjects = 24.5%				

DDAVP, desmopressin; N/S, Not stated.
From Moffatt MEK, Harlos S, Kirshen AJ, Burd L: Desmopressin acetate and nocturnal enuresis: How much do we know? Pediatrics 1993;92:420–425. Reproduced by permission of Pediatrics, vol. 92, pp 420–425, copyright 1993.

night is theoretically attractive for treating bedwetting. However, simply limiting fluids or using diuretics during the daytime to produce relative dehydration at night has not been effective (Scott and Morrison, 1980). In contrast, manipulation of antidiuretic hormone (ADH) levels has proved to be useful because some enuretics demonstrate reduced nocturnal vasopressin concentrations and have nocturnal polyuria (Norgaard et al, 1989c). DDAVP, an analogue of vasopressin and free from its dangerous and unpleasant side effects, has been shown to have a significant, albeit temporary, antienuretic effect because it produces a state of nocturnal antidiuresis. It can be given intranasally or orally, it has no pressor or smooth muscle activity in the therapeutic dose range, and its effect lasts 7 to 12 hours. In double-blind studies, DDAVP was more effective than placebo in treating enuresis. The usual clinical dose ranges between 20 and 40 μg per night for the nasal spray and between 200 and 400 μg per night for the tablet; response may be dose dependent. Efficacy is similar in oral and nasal formulations (Fjellestad-Paulsen et al, 1987; Matthiesen et al, 1994; Skoog et al, 1997).

In Moffatt's review of randomized clinical studies using DDAVP therapy (Moffatt et al, 1993), **all but one study demonstrated a statistically significant reduction in wet nights, yet only 25% of patients actually became dry for 14 or more consecutive days on therapy** (Table 64–14). With long-term therapy, the cure rate may even be lower, 19% (Tullus et al, 1999). DDAVP therefore appears to be much more effective in reducing the number of wet nights than in curing bedwetting, an observation that has been confirmed by others (Klauber, 1989; Rew and Rundle, 1989; Bloom, 1993). The response to DDAVP has been found to correlate with the presence of nocturnal polyuria and with a large functional bladder capacity (Norgaard et al, 1997; Rittig et al, 1997; Eller et al, 1998). Although spot urine osmolality is not useful in predicting DDAVP response, home recordings of nocturnal volume may help identify potential responders and guide therapy. Enuretic children without polyuria and with a normal circadian rhythm of ADH do not respond to DDAVP, nor do those with a small bladder capacity (Eller et al, 1997; Rushton et al, 1996).

The therapeutic effect of DDAVP is temporary, and once treatment is stopped 50% to 90% of children relapse and resume their original pattern of wetting (Kahan et al, 1998). **In those who were studied after being cured, a much higher proportion (75%) became dry by developing nocturia, compared with controls (5%)** (Lackgren et al, 1998). **When DDAVP is used for periods longer than 1 year there appear to be no adverse changes in vasopressin secretion, diurnal urinary output, and urine osmolality after the medication is stopped** (Knudsen et al, 1991).

Desmopressin is capable of producing side effects. Nonserious side effects are infrequent, the most common being nasal irritation associated with the nasal spray. Serious side effects can occur in the form of water intoxication leading to hyponatremic seizures. At least 40 separate cases have been reported (Beach et al, 1992; Hjalmas and Bengtsson, 1993; Donoghue et al, 1998). **The mechanism for this serious side effect is related to a large fluid intake at night while taking DDAVP. To minimize this risk, it has been recommended that children limit fluids to no more than 8 ounces (240 ml) on any night that DDAVP is administered** (Beach et al, 1992; Robson et al, 1996).

In summary, although DDAVP is very effective at decreasing the number of wet nights per week, it is very ineffective at eliminating sleep wetting. Complete cure while taking DDAVP occurs in less than one third of patients, and relapse is common. Because DDAVP is relatively expensive, is less effective than the urinary alarm worn on the body, and may be associated with serious side effects, it should not be used as a first-line therapy in treating NE.

BEHAVIOR MODIFICATION

Modification of behavior to control enuresis has met with varied success. Although generalized supportive measures designed to improve self-confidence and provide encouragement are unpredictably effective, certain specific behavioral approaches produce the most effective and reproducible rate of sustained cure and **should be considered the first-line approach to the management of enuresis.**

Techniques that have been used include bladder training, responsibility reinforcement, and classic conditioning therapy with a urinary alarm. Often, a successful treatment program combines several of these techniques, which may also be used in conjunction with drug therapy.

Bladder training, specifically retention control training (Kimmel and Kimmel, 1970), was developed to reverse the reduced functional bladder capacity that characterizes many enuretics. Because an increase in bladder functional capacity is associated with reduced bedwetting, the rationale for this treatment appears well founded. The goal is to progressively increase the time interval between voidings so that the functional bladder capacity is enlarged. Parents typically encourage their child to hold the urine for as long as possible after first feeling an urge to void. With retention control therapy, mean bladder capacity can be increased sizably in enuretic subjects compared with controls (approximately 35%). Unfortunately, this increase does not generally translate into an improvement in bedwetting for most children (Doleys, 1977; Harris and Purohit, 1977). However, when retention control is combined with conditioning therapy using the urinary alarm (see later discussion), results can be highly successful (Scott and Morrison, 1980; Geffken et al, 1986).

Behavior modification techniques using ***responsibility reinforcement*** are successful in treating enuresis, but they require a motivated child, conscientious parents, and close rapport between the physician and family. The program aims to motivate the child to assume both the responsibility for wetting and the credit for dryness. The child keeps a progress record or "gold star" chart. Progressively longer dry intervals and dry nights are rewarded. The consequence of these stepwise rewards for changes in behavior is often progressive attainment of continence. For selected, highly motivated children, improvement may be more rapid and the relapse rate lower than with other types of programs (Marshall et al, 1973). Responsibility reinforcement is particularly useful as part of a multicomponent behavioral program (Scott et al, 1992).

Randomized controlled trials and clinical studies have both shown that ***conditioning therapy using the urinary alarm*** is the most effective means of eliminating bedwetting (Werry and Cohrsen, 1965; McKendry et al, 1975; Moffatt et al, 1987; Butler et al, 1990; Van Londen et al, 1993). Conditioning therapy using a body-worn urinary alarm has evolved from the bell and pad popularized in 1938 (Mowrer and Mowrer, 1938). The success of the urinary alarm method has been explained by classic conditioning theory. It consists of a battery-operated detector that is activated by urine. Ideally, the child must awaken or be awakened by the bell to get up and complete voiding into the toilet. Ultimately, those factors that are present and associated with micturition during sleep, such as the sensation of a full or contracting bladder, are conditioned to produce the same inhibition to voiding as does the alarm and to awaken the child before wetting occurs (Doleys, 1977). Alarm therapy is associated with a significant in-

crease in nocturnal bladder capacity in those children who become dry. This allows them to sleep through the night after becoming dry, instead of developing nocturia, as occurs with DDAVP therapy (Oredsson and Jorgenson, 1998). **Conditioning therapy using a urinary alarm appears to be the most effective approach available for NE.**

The single most important cause for failure is a lack of child and parental understanding and commitment. This problem can be minimized by proper instruction and supervision as well as recognition that the period of therapy can be lengthy, perhaps 3 to 4 months. Once enuresis has been cured completely (for at least 14 days) or converted to nocturia, relapse can be prevented by the use of overlearning techniques (Young and Morgan, 1973). These involve forcing fluids before bedtime to promote bladder overdistention and provide a stronger conditioning stimulus.

In controlled studies, the urinary alarm is superior to drug therapy, either imipramine or DDAVP, with a cure rate of 60% to 100% (80% in our experience) after discontinuation. When compared directly to DDAVP, the alarm cure rate is significantly better, and after therapy the relapse rate with DDAVP is ten times greater (Wagner et al, 1982; Wille, 1986). Although as many as 25% of patients relapse, this is often preventable with the use of overlearning techniques. In addition, retreatment produces a secondary cure in a significant proportion of patients (Forsythe and Butler, 1989; Scott et al, 1992). Conditioning therapy is effective under a variety of circumstances; age and intelligence are not factors in achieving dryness, nor is the degree or frequency of wetting. Even deep sleepers can be treated successfully by having their parents awaken them at the sound of the bell. Conditioning therapy using the urinary alarm may be combined with pharmacotherapy or behavior modification to create individually tailored treatment. About 80% of children so treated are cured (i.e., dry for 14 consecutive days), and only 24% relapse (Houts et al, 1986; Ellsworth et al, 1995).

Summary

The physician who cares for patients with enuresis must develop an orderly, practical, and effective approach to evaluating and treating the large number of children who present with this complaint:

1. Identify medically serious conditions such as urinary infection, neuropathy, and obstruction; for children with MNE a history, physical examination, and urinalysis is sufficient.

2. Reassure the parents and the child that bedwetting is medically harmless, is not the child's fault, may have been inherited from the parents, is subject to a high (15% per year) spontaneous cure rate, and usually disappears by puberty.

3. Recognize that not all parents want and not all children are ready for a treatment program.

4. Determine whether the child is sufficiently old, mature, and motivated (usually by 7 years of age) and the family is supportive enough to begin a treatment program that might be lengthy and might not be successful initially.

5. Recommend the body-worn urinary alarm as the initial treatment, because it is statistically the most effective

Table 64–15. WORRISOME SIGNS AND SYMPTOMS

Signs
    Lumbosacral spine abnormalities
        Hairy patches
        Lipomas
        Cutaneous dimples or tracts
        Bony irregularities
    Reduced anal sphincter tone
    Fixed low urinary specific gravity
    Palpable bladder
Symptoms
    Day and night frequency and wetting
    Painful urination
    Rectal pain
    Penile pain or discharge
    Vaginal pain or discharge
    Straining to urinate

means of achieving complete dryness and has no known side effects.

6. Avoid pharmacologic therapy initially, because most children do not achieve complete dryness during or after drug therapy, and side effects can occur and be significant.

7. Reassure the family that relapses after successful therapy may occur, are often transient, and respond well to retreatment.

Worrisome Signs and Symptoms

When certain signs and symptoms are noted in children with voiding dysfunction, diagnostic testing is required to exclude occult neurologic or urologic disease (Table 64–15). However, sometimes pain is atypical, the site of discomfort is vaguely suggested, or penile or vaginal discharge is described or noted. Because these symptoms do not necessarily fit a specific pattern or syndrome, they should not be dismissed as innocuous. The possibility of sexual abuse must be considered; telltale signs must be sought, if necessary with the help of appropriate investigative and counseling teams.

REFERENCES

Allen TD: The non-neurogenic neurogenic bladder. J Urol 1977;117:232.

Allen TD, Bright TC: Urodynamic patterns in children with dysfunctional voiding problems. J Urol 1978;119:247.

Arnell H, Hjalmas K, Jagervall M, et al: The genetics of primary enuresis: Inheritance and suggestion of a second major gene on chromosome 12q. J Med Genet 1997;34:360–365.

Arnold SJ, Ginsberg A: Enuresis, incidence and pertinence of genitourinary disease in healthy enuretic children. Urology 1973;2:437.

Aschoff J: Circadian rhythms in man: A self-sustained oscillator with an inherent frequency underlies 24-hour periodicity. Science 1965;148:1427–1432.

Asselman M, Dik P, Vijverberg MAW, de Jong T: The diameter of the rectum on ultrasonography of the bladder as a diagnostic tool for fecal constipation in children with dysfunctional voiding. Presented at AAP-ESPU Joint Meeting, Tours, France, 2000.

Bachelard M, Sillen U, Hansson S, et al: Urodynamic patterns in asymptomatic infants: Siblings of children with vesicoureteral reflux. J Urol 1999;162:1733–1738.

Bakwin H: Enuresis in children. J Pediatr 1961;58:806–819.

Bakwin H: The genetics of enuresis. Clin Dev Med 1973;48/49:73–77.

Baldew IM, van Gelderen HH: Urinary retention without organic cause in children. Br J Urol 1983;55:200–202.

Barrett DM: Evaluation of psychogenic urinary retention. J Urol 1978;120:191–192.

Bass LW: Pollakiuria, extraordinary daytime urinary frequency: Experience in a pediatric practice. Pediatrics 1991;87:735–737.

Bauer SB, Retik AB, Colodny AH, et al: The unstable bladder of childhood. Urol Clin North Am 1980;7:321.

Baumann FW, Hinman F: Treatment of incontinent boys with non-obstructive disease. J Urol 1974;111:114.

Beach PS, Beach RE, Smith LR: Hyponatremic seizures in a child treated with desmopressin to control enuresis. Clin Pediatr 1992;31:566–569.

Berger RM, Maizels M, Moran GC, et al: Bladder capacity (ounces) equals age (years) plus 2 predicts normal bladder capacity and aids in diagnosis of abnormal voiding patterns. J Urol 1983;129:347–349.

Blethyn AJ, Jenkins HR, Roberts R, Verrier Jones K: Radiological evidence of constipation in urinary tract infection. Arch Dis Child 1995;73:534–535.

Bloom D: The American experience with desmopressin. Clin Pediatr 1993;Special No:28–31.

Boyd MM: The depth of sleep in enuretic school children and nonenuretic controls. J Psychosom Res 1960;4:274.

Broughton RJ: Sleep disorders: Disorders of arousal? Science 1968;159:1070.

Bucy JG, Carlin MR: The silent neurogenic bladder. J Urol 1975;114:296.

Butler RJ, Forsythe WI, Robertson J: The body worn alarm in the treatment of childhood enuresis. Br J Clin Pract 1990;44:237.

Chandra M: Reflux nephropathy, urinary tract infection, and voiding disorders. Curr Opin Pediatr 1995;7:164–170.

Chandra M, Maddix H, McVicar M: Transient urodynamic dysfunction of infancy: Relationship to urinary tract infections and vesicoureteral reflux. J Urol 1996;155:673–677.

Christmas TJ, Noble JG, Watson GM, Turner-Warwick RT: Use of biofeedback in treatment of psychogenic voiding dysfunction. Urology 1991;37:43–45.

Cole AT, Fried FA: Favorable experiences with imipramine in the treatment of neurogenic bladder. J Urol 1972;107:44.

Combs AJ, Glassberg KI, Gerges D, Horowitz M: Biofeedback therapy for children with dysfunctional voiding. Urology 1998;52:312–315.

Conway JJ: Radionuclide cystography. Contrib Nephrol 1984;39:1–19.

Crowther P, Pead PJ, Pead L, Maskell R: Daytime urinary frequency in children. Br Med J 1988;297:855.

Curran MJ, Kaefer M, Peters C, et al: The overactive bladder in childhood: Long-term results with conservative management. J Urol 2000;163:574–577.

Cutler C, Middleton AW, Nixon GW: Radiographic findings in children surveyed for enuresis. Urology 1978;11:480.

Datta NS, Martin D, Schweitz B: The occult neurological bladder: Detection by electromyography of the anal sphincter. Surg Forum 1970;21:545.

De Gatta MF, Garcia MJ, Acosta A: Monitoring of serum levels of imipramine and desipramine and individualization of dose in enuretic children. J Ther Drug Monit 1984;6:438–443.

De Paepe H, Hoebeke P, Renson C, et al: Pelvic-floor therapy in girls with recurrent urinary tract infections and dysfunctional voiding. Br J Urol 1998;81:109–113.

Devane R, Walker RD, Sawyer WP, et al: Concentrations of imipramine and its metabolites during enuresis therapy. Pediatr Pharmacol 1984;4:245–251.

Diokno AC, Koff SA, Bender L: Periurethral striated muscle activity in neurogenic bladder dysfunction. J Urol 1974;112:743.

Dohil R, Roberts E, Verrier Jones K, Jenkins HR: Constipation and reversible urinary tract abnormalities. Arch Dis Child 1994;70:56–57.

Doleys DM: Behavioral treatments for nocturnal enuresis in children: A review of the recent literature. Psychol Bull 1977;1:30.

Donoghue MB, Latimer E, Pillsbury HL, Herzog JH: Hyponatremic seizure in a child using desmopressin for nocturnal enuresis. Arch Pediatr Adolesc Med 1998;152:290–292.

Dorfman LE, Bailey J, Smith JP: Subclinical neurogenic bladder in children. J Urol 1969;101:48.

Egger J, Carter CH, Soothill JF, Wilson J: Effect of diet treatment on enuresis in children with migraine or hyperkinetic behavior. Clin Pediatr 1992;31:302–307.

Eller DA, Austin PF, Tanguay S, Homsy YL: Daytime functional bladder capacity as a predictor of response to desmopressin in monosymptomatic nocturnal enuresis. Eur Urol 1998;33(suppl. 3):25–29.

Eller DA, Homsy YL, Austin PF, et al: Spot urine osmolality, age and bladder capacity as predictors of response to desmopressin in nocturnal enuresis. Scand J Urol Nephrol 1997;31(suppl. 183):41–45.

Ellsworth PI, Merguerian PA, Copening ME: Sexual abuse: Another causative factor in dysfunctional voiding. J Urol 1995;153:773–776.

Epstein SJ, DeQuevedo A: The control of enuresis with imipramine in the presence of organic bladder disease. Am J Psychiatry 1964;120:908.

Fergusson DM, Horwood LJ, Shannon FT: Factors related to the age of attainment of nocturnal bladder control: An eight-year longitudinal study. Pediatrics 1986;78:884–890.

Fjellestad-Paulsen A, Wille S, Harris AS: Comparison of intranasal and oral desmopressin for nocturnal enuresis. Arch Dis Child 1987;62:674–677.

Forsythe WI, Butler RJ: Fifty years of enuretic alarms. Arch Dis Child 1989;64:879–885.

Gallo D: Urinary retention due to fecal impaction in children. Pediatrics 1970;45:292–294.

Geffken G, Johnson SB, Walker D: Behavioral interventions for childhood nocturnal enuresis: The differential effect of bladder capacity on treatment, progress and outcome. Health Psychol 1986;5:261–272.

George CPL, Messeril FH, Gennest J, et al: Diurnal variation of plasma vasopressin in man. J Endocrinol Metab 1975;41:332.

Godley ML, Ransley PG, Parkhouse HF, Gordon I: Quantitation of vesicoureteral reflux by radionuclide cystography and urodynamics. Pediatr Nephrol 1990;4:485–490.

Goellner MH, Ziegler EE, Fomon SJ: Urination during the first three years of life. Nephron 1981;28:174–178.

Graham P: Depth of sleep and enuresis: A critical review. In Kolvin I, MacKeith RC, Meadow SR (eds): Bladder Control and Enuresis. London, W. Heinemann Medical Books Ltd., 1973, pp 78–83.

Green AS, Cromie WJ: Treatment of imipramine overdose in children. Urology 1981;18:314.

Hanson E, Hellstrom AL, Hjalmas K: Non-neurogenic discoordinated voiding in children: The long-term effect of bladder retraining. Z Kinderchir 1987;42:109–111.

Haque M, Ellerstein NS, Gundy JH, et al: Parental perceptions in enuresis: A collaborative study. Am J Dis Child 1981;135:809.

Harris LS, Purohit AP: Bladder training and enuresis: A controlled trial. Behav Res Ther 1977;15:485.

Hinman F: Urinary tract damage in children who wet. Pediatrics 1974;54:142.

Hinman F: Non-neurogenic neurogenic bladder (the Hinman syndrome): 15 years later. J Urol 1986;136:769.

Hinman F, Baumann FW: Vesical and ureteral damage from voiding dysfunction in boys without neurologic or obstructive disease. J Urol 1973;109:727.

Hinman F, Baumann FW: Complications of vesicoureteral operations from incoordination of micturition. J Urol 1976;116:638.

Hjalmas K: Micturition in infants and children with normal lower urinary tract. Scand J Urol Nephrol Suppl 1976;37:1–150.

Hjalmas K: Urodynamics in normal infants and children. Scand J Urol Nephrol 1988;114:20–27.

Hjalmas K: Urinary incontinence in children: Suggestions for definitions and terminology. Scand J Urol Nephrol Suppl 1992;141:1–6.

Hjalmas K, Bengtsson B: Efficacy, safety, and dosing of desmopressin for nocturnal enuresis in Europe. Clin Pediatr 1993;Special No:19–24.

Hoebeke P, Walle JV, Theunis M, et al: Outpatient pelvic-floor therapy in girls with daytime incontinence and dysfunctional voiding. Urol 1996;48:923–927.

Hogg RJ, Husmann D: The role of family history in predicting response to desmopressin in nocturnal enuresis. J Urol 1993;150:444–445.

Holmdahl G, Hanson E, Hanson M, et al: Four-hour voiding observation in healthy infants. J Urol 1996;156:1809–1812.

Homsy YL: Dysfunctional voiding syndromes and vesicoureteral reflux. Pediatr Nephrol 1994;8:116–121.

Homsy YL, Nsouli I, Hamburder B, et al: Effects of oxybutynin on vesicoureteral reflux in children. J Urol 1985;134:1168.

Homsy YL, Van Gool J, Koff SA, et al: Vesicoureteral reflux: The urodynamic dimension. Dial Pediatr Urol 1983;6:1–8.

Houts AC, Peterson JK, Whelan JP: Prevention of relapse in full-spectrum home training for primary enuresis: A component analysis. Behav Ther 1986;17:462–469.

Hublin C, Kaprio J, Partinen M, Koskenvuo M: Nocturnal enuresis in a nationwide twin cohort. Sleep 1998;21:579–585.

Husmann DA: Enuresis. Urology 1996;48:184–193.

Hutch JA: Vesicoureteral reflux in the paraplegic: Cause and correction. J Urol 1952;68:457.

Jarvelin MR: Developmental history and neurological findings in enuretic children. Dev Med Child Neurol 1989;31:728–736.

Jayanthi VR, Khoury AE, McLorie GA, Agarwal SK: The nonneurogenic bladder of early infancy. J Urol 1997;158:181–185.

Johnston JH, Koff SA, Glassberg KI: The pseudo-obstructed bladder in enuretic children. Br J Urol 1978;50:505.

Johnstone JMS, Ardvan GM, Ramsden PD: A preliminary assessment of bladder distension in the treatment of enuretic children. Br J Urol 1977;49:43–49.

Jorgensen OS, Lober M, Christiansen J, Gram LF: Plasma concentration and clinical effect in imipramine treatment of childhood enuresis. Clin Pharmacokinet 1980;5:386–393.

Kaefer M, Zurakowski D, Bauer SB, et al: Estimating normal bladder capacity in children. J Urol 1997;158:2261–2264.

Kahan E, Morel D, Amir J, Zelcer C: A controlled trial of desmopressin and behavioral therapy for nocturnal enuresis. Medicine (Baltimore) 1998;77:384–388.

Kahmi B, Horowitz MI, Kovetz A: Isolated neurogenic dysfunction of the bladder in children with urinary tract infection. J Urol 1971;106:151.

Kaplan G: Serum IgE and allergy in enuresis. Presented at Section on Urology, American Academy of Pediatrics, Chicago, October 22, 1973.

Kardash S, Hillman ES, Werry J: Efficacy of imipramine in childhood enuresis: A double blind control study with placebo. Can Med Assoc J 1968;99:263.

Kass EJ, Diokno AC, Montealegre A: Enuresis: Principles of management and result of treatment. J Urol 1979;121:794–796.

Kawauchi A, Kitamori T, Imada N, et al: Urological abnormalities in 1328 patients with nocturnal enuresis. Eur Urol 1996;29:231–234.

Kawauchi A, Watanabe H: Development of bladder capacity, nocturnal urinary volume and urinary behavior in non-enuretic and enuretic children. Nippon Hinyokika Gakkai Zasshi 1993;84:1811–1820.

Kawauchi A, Watanabe H, Kitamori T, et al: The possibility of centripetal stimulation from the urinary bladder for vasopressin excretion. J Kyoto Pref Univ Med 1993;102:747–752.

Khan AU: Psychogenic urinary retention in a boy. J Urol 1971;106:432–434.

Kimmel HD, Kimmel EC: An instrumental conditioning method for the treatment of enuresis. J Behav Ther Exp Psychiatry 1970;1:121.

Klauber GT: Clinical efficacy and safety of desmopressin in the treatment of nocturnal enuresis. J Pediatr 1989;114:719–722.

Knudsen UB, Rittig S, Norgaard JP, et al: Long term treatment of nocturnal enuresis with desmopressin. Urol Res 1991;19:237–240.

Koff SA: Estimating bladder capacity in children. Urology 1983;21:248.

Koff SA: Why is desmopressin sometimes ineffective at curing bedwetting? Scand J Urol Nephrol 1995;29(suppl. 173):103–108.

Koff SA, Byard MA: The daytime urinary frequency syndrome of childhood. J Urol 1988;140:1280–1281.

Koff SA, Lapides J, Piazza DH: Association of urinary tract infection and reflux with uninhibited bladder contractions and voluntary sphincteric obstruction. J Urol 1979;122:373.

Koff SA, Murtagh DS: The uninhibited bladder in children: Effect of treatment on vesicoureteral reflux resolution. J Urol 1983;130:1138–1141.

Koff SA, Solomon MH, Lane GA, Lieding KC: Urodynamic studies in anesthetized children. J Urol 1980;123:61.

Koff SA, Wagner TT, Jayanthi VR: The relationship among dysfunctional elimination syndromes, primary vesicoureteral reflux and urinary tract infections in children. J Urol 1998;160:1019–1022.

Kosar A, Arikan N, Dincel C: Effectiveness of oxybutynin hydrochloride in the treatment of enuresis nocturna. Scand J Urol Nephrol 1999;33:115–118.

Lackgren G, Lilia B, Neveus T, Stenberg A: Desmopressin in the treatment of severe nocturnal enuresis in adolescents: A 7 year study. Br J Urol 1998;81(suppl. 3):17–23.

Lapides J, Costello RT: Uninhibited neurogenic bladder: A common cause for recurrent urinary infection in normal women. J Urol 1969;101:539.

Lapides J, Diokno AC: Persistence of the infant bladder as a cause for urinary infection in girls. Trans Am Assoc Genitourin Surg 1969;61:51.

Lapides J, Sweet RB, Lewis LW: Role of striated muscle in urination. J Urol 1957;77:247.

Loening-Baucke V: Urinary incontinence and urinary tract infection and their resolution with treatment of chronic constipation. Pediatrics 1997;100:228–232.

MacKeith RC: Micturition induced by giggling. Guy's Hospital Reports 1964;113:250–260.

Mahony DT: Studies of enuresis: I. Incidence of obstructive lesions and pathophysiology of enuresis. J Urol 1971;106:951.

Marshall S, Marshal HH, Lyon RP: Enuresis: An analysis of various therapeutic approaches. Pediatrics 1973;52:813.

Matthiesen TB, Rittig S, Djurhuus JC, Norgaard JP: A dose titration, and an open 6-week efficacy and safety study of desmopressin tablets in the management of nocturnal enuresis. J Urol 1994;151:460–463.

McKendry JBJ, Stewart DA, Kahnna F, Netley C: Primary enuresis: Relative success of three methods of treatment. Can Med Assoc J 1975; 113:953–955.

McKenna PH, Herndon CD, Connery S, Ferrer FA: Pelvic floor muscle retraining for pediatric voiding dysfunction using interactive computer games. J Urol 1999;162:1056–1062; discussion, 1062–1063.

Mikkelsen EJ, Rapoport JL, Nee L, et al: Childhood enuresis: I. Sleep patterns and psychopathology. Arch Gen Psychiatry 1980;37:1139.

Mimouni M, Schuper A, Mimouni F, et al: Retarded skeletal maturation in children with primary enuresis. J Pediatr 1985;144:234–235.

Mishra PC, Agarwal VK, Rahman H: Therapeutic trial of amitriptyline in the treatment of nocturnal enuresis: A controlled study. Indian Pediatr 1980;17:279–285.

Mix L: Occult neuropathic bladder. Urology 1977;10:1.

Moffatt MEK: Nocturnal enuresis: Psychologic implications of treatment and nontreatment. J Pediatr 1989;114:697–704.

Moffatt MEK: Nocturnal enuresis: Is there a rationale for treatment? Scand J Urol Nephrol Suppl 1994;163:55–67.

Moffatt MEK, Harlos S, Kirshen AJ, Burd L: Desmopressin acetate and nocturnal enuresis: How much do we know? Pediatrics 1993;92:420–425.

Moffatt MEK, Kato C, Pless IB: Improvements in self-concept after treatment of nocturnal enuresis: Randomized controlled trial. J Pediatr 1987;110:647–652.

Moore-Ede MC: Physiology of the circadian timing systems: Predictive vs reactive homeostasis. Am J Physiol 1986;250:737–752.

Mowrer OH, Mowrer WM: Enuresis: A method for its study and treatment. Am J Orthopsychiatry 1938;8:436.

Naseer SR, Steinhardt GF: New renal scars in children with urinary tract infections, vesicoureteral reflux and voiding dysfunction. J Urol 1997; 158:566–568.

Nash DFE: The development of micturition control with special reference to enuresis. Ann R Coll Surg Engl 1949;5:318.

Neumann PZ, deDomenico IJ, Nogrady MB: Constipation and urinary tract infection. Pediatrics 1973;52:241–245.

Noe HN: The role of dysfunctional voiding in failure or complication of ureteral reimplantation for primary reflux. J Urol 1985;134:1172.

Noe HN: The relationship of sibling reflux to index patient dysfunctional voiding. J Urol 1988;140:119–120.

Noe HN: The risk and risk factors of contralateral reflux following repair of simple unilateral primary reflux. J Urol 1998;160:849–850.

Norgaard JP, Djurhuus JC, Watanabe H, et al: Experience and current status of research into pathophysiology of nocturnal enuresis. Br J Urol 1997;79:825–835.

Norgaard JP, Hansen JH, Nielsen JB, et al: Simultaneous registration of sleep stages and bladder activity in enuresis. Urology 1985;26:316–319.

Norgaard JP, Hansen JH, Nielsen JB, et al: Sleep patterns in enuretics: A polygraphic study of EEG and bladder activity. Scand J Urol Nephrol 1989a;125:73–78.

Norgaard JP, Hansen JH, Wildschiotz G: Cystometries in children with nocturnal enuresis. J Urol 1989b;141:1156.

Norgaard JP, Rittigs J, Djurhuus JC: Nocturnal enuresis: An approach to treatment based on pathogenesis. J Pediatr 1989c;114:705–710.

Ochoa B, Gorlin RJ: Urofacial (Ochoa) syndrome. Am J Med Genet 1987;27:661.

Ohne T: The increase in c-Fos expression in vasopressin- and oxytocin-immunoreactive neurons in paraventricular and supraoptic nucleus of the hypothalamus following urinary retention. J Kyoto Pref Univ Med 1995;104:393–403.

Oredsson AF, Jorgenson TM: Changes in nocturnal bladder capacity during treatment with the bell and pad for monosymptomatic nocturnal enuresis. J Urol 1998;160:166–169.

O'Regan S, Schick E, Hamburger B, Yazbeck S: Constipation associated with vesicoureteral reflux. Urology 1986;28:394–396.

O'Regan S, Yazbeck S: Constipation: A cause of enuresis, urinary tract infections and vesicoureteral reflux in children. Med Hypotheses 1985; 17:409–413.

Person-Junemann C, Seemann O, Kohrmann KU, et al: Comparison of urodynamic findings and response to oxybutynin in nocturnal enuresis. Eur Urol 1993;24:92–96.

Rascher W, Rauh W, Brandeis WE, et al: Determinants of plasma arginine-vasopressin in children. Acta Paediatr Scand 1986;75:111–117.

Rasquin-Weber A, Hyman PE, Cucchiara S, et al: Childhood functional gastrointestinal disorders. Gut 1999;45:1160–1168.

Rechtschaffen A, Kales A (eds): A Manual of Standardized Terminology, Techniques and Scoring System for Sleep Stages of Human Subjects. Los Angeles, Brain Information Service/Brain Research Institute, UCLA, 1968, pp 1–12.

Reimao R, Pachelli LC, Carneiro R, Faiwichow G: Primary sleep enuresis in childhood: Polysomnographic evidences of sleep stage and time modulation. Arq Neuropsiquiatr 1993;51:41–45.

Rew DA, Rundle JSH: Assessment of the safety of regular DDAVP therapy in primary nocturnal enuresis. Br J Urol 1989;63:352–353.

Rittig S, Knudsen UB, Norgaard JP, et al: Abnormal diurnal rhythm of plasma vasopressin and urinary output in patients with enuresis. Am J Physiol 1989;256:664.

Rittig S, Schaumburg H, Schmidt F, et al: Long-term home studies of water balance in patients with nocturnal enuresis. Scand J Urol Nephrol 1997;31(suppl. 183):25–27.

Robert M, Averous M, Besset A, et al: Sleep polygraphic studies using sleep cystomanometry in twenty patients with enuresis. Eur Urol 1993; 24:97–102.

Robson WL, Jackson HP, Blackhurst D: Enuresis in children with attention-deficit hyperactivity disorder. South Med J 1997;90:503–505.

Robson WL, Leung AK: Extraordinary urinary frequency syndrome. Urology 1993;42:321–324.

Robson WL, Norgaard JP, Leung AKC: Hyponatremia in patients with nocturnal enuresis treated with DDAVP. Eur J Pediatr 1996;155:959–962.

Rockney RM, McQuade WH, Days AL: The plain abdominal roentgenogram in the management of encopresis. Arch Pediatr Adolesc Med 1995;149:623–627.

Rogers MP, Gittes RF, Dawson DM, Reich P: Giggle incontinence. JAMA 1982;247:1446–1448.

Rohner TJ, Sanford EJ: Imipramine toxicity. J Urol 1975;114:402.

Ruarte AC, Quesada EM: Urodynamic evaluation in children. Int Perspect Urol 1987;14:114.

Rushton HG, Belman AB, Zaontz M, et al: The influence of small bladder capacity and other predictors on the response to desmopressin in the management of monosymptomatic nocturnal enuresis. J Urol 1996;156: 651–655.

Sachdev YV, Howards SS: *Enterobius vermicularis* infestation and secondary enuresis. J Urol 1975;113:143.

Savage JP: The deleterious effect of constipation upon the reimplanted ureter. J Urol 1973;109:501.

Scholtjmeier RJ, van Mastrigt R: The effect of oxyphenonium bromide and oxybutynin chloride on detrusor contractility and reflux in children with vesicoureteral reflux and bladder instability. J Urol 1991;146:660.

Schopfner CE: Urinary tract pathology associated with constipation. Radiology 1968;90:865–877.

Scott MA, Barclay DR, Houts AC: Childhood enuresis: Etiology, assessment, and current behavioral treatment. Prog Behav Modif 1992;28:83–117.

Scott R, Morrison LH: Diuretic treatment of enuresis: Preliminary communication. J R Coll Surg Edinb 1980;25:470.

Seruca H: Vesicoureteral reflux and voiding dysfunction: A prospective study. J Urol 1989;68:457.

Shaffer D, Costell AJ, Hill ID: Control of enuresis with imipramine. Arch Dis Child 1968;43:665.

Sher PK: Successful treatment of giggle incontinence with methylphenidate. Pediatr Neurol 1994;10:81.

Sher PK, Reinberg Y: Successful treatment of giggle incontinence with methylphenidate. J Urol 1996;156:656–658.

Sillen U: Vesicoureteral reflux in infants. Pediatr Nephrol 1999;13:355–361.

Sillen U, Solsnes E, Hellstrom AL, Sandberg K: The voiding pattern of healthy preterm infants. J Urol 2000;163:278–281.

Skoog SJ, Stokes A, Turner KL: Oral desmopressin: A randomized double-blind placebo controlled study of effectiveness in children with primary nocturnal enuresis. J Urol 1997;158:1035–1040.

Stams UK, Martin CH, Tan TG: Psychogenic urinary retention in eight-year-old boy. Urology 1982;20:83–85.

Starfield B: Functional bladder capacity in enuretic and non-enuretic children. J Pediatr 1967;70:777–781.

Steffens J, Netzer M, Isenberg E, et al: Vasopressin deficiency in primary nocturnal enuresis: Results of a controlled prospective study. Eur Urol 1993;24:366–370.

Strom-Olsen R: Enuresis in adults and abnormality of sleep. Lancet 1950; 2:133.

Troup CW, Hodgson NB: Nocturnal functional bladder capacity in enuretic children. Wis Med J 1971;70:171–173.

Tullus K, Bergstrom R, Fosdal I, et al: Efficacy and safety during long-term treatment of primary monosymptomatic nocturnal enuresis with desmopressin. Acta Paediatr 1999;88:1274–1278.

Van Gool JD: Bladder infection and pressure. In Hodson J, Kincaid-Smith P (eds): Reflux Nephropathy. New York, Masson, 1979, Chapter 19.

Van Gool JD, De Heij R, Nijman R, et al: A prospective study of treatment plans in children with non-neuropathic bladder-sphincter dysfunction. Presented at AAP-ESPU Joint Meeting, Tours, France, June, 2000.

Van Gool JD, Hjalmas K, Tamminen-Mobius T, et al: Historical clues to the complex of dysfunctional voiding, urinary tract infection and vesicoureteral reflux. J Urol 1992;148:1699–1702.

Van Londen A, Van Londen-Barensten MWM, Van Son MJM, Mulder GALA: Arousal training for children suffering from nocturnal enuresis: A 2 1/2-year follow-up. Behav Res Ther 1993;31:613–615.

Vande Walle J, Hoebeke P, Van Laecke E, et al: Persistent enuresis caused by nocturnal polyuria is a maturation defect of the nyctohemeral rhythm of diuresis. Br J Urol 1998;81(suppl. 3):40–45.

Vincent SA: Postural control of urinary incontinence: The curtsey sign. Lancet 1966:2:631.

Von Gontard A, Eiberg H, Hollman H, et al: Molecular genetics of nocturnal enuresis: Linkage to locus on chromosome 22. Scand J Urol Nephrol 1999;202(suppl.):76–80.

Vulliamy D: The day and night output of urine in enuresis. Arch Dis Child 1956;31:439–443.

Wagner W, Johnsson SS, Walker D, et al: A controlled comparison of two treatments for nocturnal enuresis. J Pediatr 1982;101:302–307.

Wan J, Kaplinsky R, Greenfield S: Toilet habits of children evaluated for urinary tract infections. J Urol 1995;154:797–799.

Watanabe H, Azuma Y: A proposal for a classification system of enuresis based on overnight simultaneous monitoring of electroencephalography and cystometry. Sleep 1989;12:257–264.

Watanabe H, Kawauchi A, Kitamori T, Azuma Y: Treatment system for nocturnal enuresis according to an original classification system. Eur J Urol 1994;25:43–50.

Watemberg N, Shalev H: Daytime urinary frequency in children. Clin Pediatr 1994;33:50–53.

Wen JG, Tong EC: Cystometry in infants and children with no apparent voiding symptoms. Br J Urol 1998;81:468–473.

Wennergren H, Oberg B: Pelvic floor exercises for children: A method of treating dysfunctional voiding. Br J Urol 1995;76:9–15.

Werry JS, Cohrsen J: Enuresis: An etiologic and therapeutic study. J Pediatr 1965;67:423–431.

Wille S: Comparison of desmopressin and enuresis alarm for nocturnal enuresis. Arch Dis Child 1986;61:30–33.

Williams DI, Hirst G, Doyle D: The occult neuropathic bladder. J Pediatr Surg 1974;9:35.

Wolfish N: Sleep arousal function in enuretic males. Scand J Urol Nephrol 1999;202:24–26.

Wu HHH, Chen MT, Lee YH: Urodynamics studies and primary nocturnal enuresis. Chin Med J (Taipei) 1988;41:227–232.

Yeung CK: The normal infant bladder. Scand J Urol Nephrol 1995;173:19–23.

Yeung CK, Godley ML, Dhillon HK, et al: The characteristics of primary vesico-ureteric reflux in male and female infants with pre-natal hydronephrosis. Br J Urol 1997;80:319–327.

Yeung CK, Godley ML, Dhillon HK, et al: Urodynamic patterns in infants with normal lower tracts or primary vesico-ureteric reflux. Br J Urol 1998;81:461–467.

Yeung CK, Godley ML, Duffy PG, Ransley PG: Natural filling cystometry in infants and children. Br J Urol 1995;73:531–537.

Young GC, Morgan RTT: Conditioning technics and enuresis. Med J Aust 1973;2:329.

Zaleski A, Shokeir MK, Gerrad JW: Enuresis: Familial incidence and relationship to allergic disorders. Can Med Assoc J 1972;106:30.

Zoubek J: Extraordinary urinary frequency. Pediatrics 1990;85:1112–1114.

65
HYPOSPADIAS

Alan B. Retik, MD
Joseph G. Borer, MD

TRIBUTE TO DR. JOHN W. DUCKETT, JR.

The current authors of this chapter and the pediatric urology community as a whole are deeply indebted to Dr. John W. Duckett, Jr., for his significant contributions to the field he named *hypospadiology* and defined as "the in-depth study of the art and science of the surgical correction of hypospadias" (Duckett, 1981, 1995). His major influence is evident in three decades of peer-reviewed publications, numerous mentored disciples, and multiple chapters regarding all aspects of hypospadias, including this chapter in several previous editions of *Campbell's Urology*. Perhaps Dr. Duckett's most poignant remarks regarding this "currently flourishing" field are summarized in what he referred to as two of his favorite quotes: "Skepticism blossoms on the compost of experience" and "Opinions abound where truths are hard to prove" (Duckett, 1995).

INTRODUCTION

Definition

Hypospadias, in boys, may be defined classically as an association of three anatomic and developmental anomalies of the penis: (1) an abnormal ventral opening of the urethral meatus, which may be located anywhere from the ventral aspect of the glans penis to the perineum; (2) an abnormal ventral curvature of the penis (chordee); and (3) an abnormal distribution of foreskin, with a "hood" present dorsally and deficient foreskin

ventrally (Mouriquand et al, 1995) (Fig. 65–1). The second and third of these typical characteristics are not present in all cases (Fig. 65–2).

Diagnosis

The diagnosis of hypospadias, in boys, is usually evident on newborn physical examination. However, this is not always the case for boys with milder forms of hypospadias or for those with the megameatus intact prepuce (MIP) variant (Duckett and Keating, 1989; Hatch et al, 1989). These particular boys may escape diagnosis until such time as the foreskin is fully retracted or the newborn circumcision is complete (see Fig. 65–2). **It must be kept in mind that apparent simple, isolated hypospadias may be the only visible indication of a significant underlying abnormality** (Aarskog, 1971).

Classification Schemes

Many different classification systems with varying utility have been proposed through history, as reviewed by Sorensen (1953) and summarized more recently by Sheldon and Duckett (1987). **Culp, in 1959, was perhaps the first to classify the level of hypospadias after any necessary treatment of penile curvature (orthoplasty) and to realize the importance of this method. In 1973, Barcat more formally proposed designating the location of the hypospadiac meatus, and thus the true extent of the**

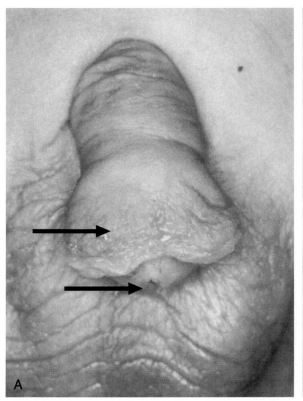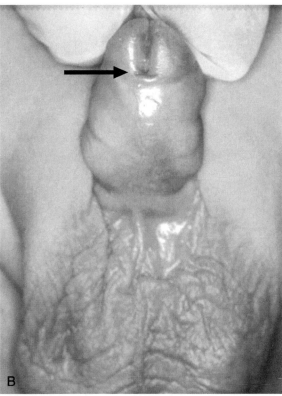

Figure 65–1. Typical appearance of hypospadias. *A,* Dorsal "hood" foreskin *(upper arrow)* and distal glanular groove *(lower arrow). B,* Ventral view of same patient showing paucity of foreskin and proximally placed meatus *(arrow).*

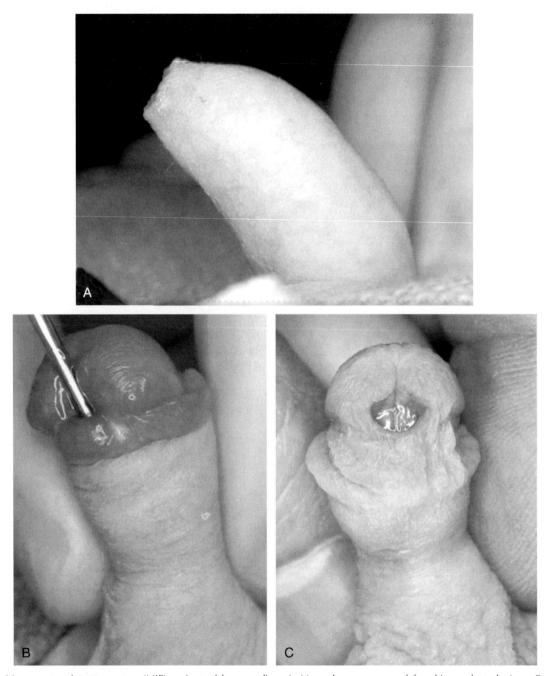

Figure 65–2. Megameatus, intact prepuce (MIP) variant of hypospadias. *A,* Normal appearance of foreskin on lateral view. *B,* Sound passed within gaping hypospadiac meatus. *C,* Typical appearance of meatus following newborn circumcision in a patient with the MIP variant.

urethral defect requiring repair, after orthoplasty. Most would agree with this important concept of classification. However, although categoric designations of anterior (distal), middle, and posterior (proximal) hypospadias are helpful, the use of more specific, anatomically descriptive terms for designating the level of the hypospadiac meatus is preferred (Fig. 65–3).

In all commonly used classification systems, glanular, coronal, and subcoronal (anterior) defects constitute the great majority (approximately 50% to 70%) of hypospadias cases (Sheldon and Duckett, 1987; Sauvage et al, 1993; Borer et al, 2001). Duckett (1998) reported overall

rates of approximately 50%, 30%, and 20% for anterior, middle, and posterior hypospadias, respectively.

DEVELOPMENT

Embryology

Glenister (1954) performed serial sectioning of 37 human fetuses (21 male, 12 female, and 4 in the indifferent stage) in order to evaluate embryologic development of the urethral plate and urethra. **Based on a thorough review of**

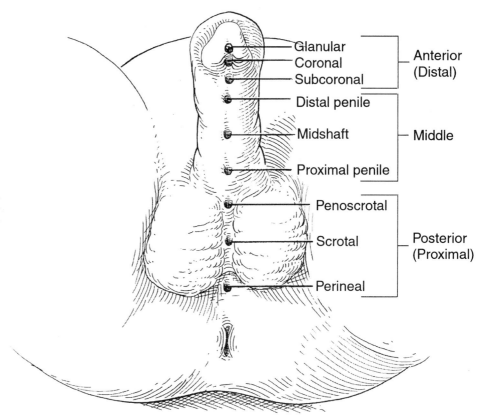

Figure 65–3. Anatomically descriptive levels of hypospadias within the three major categories, based on the level of the meatus following orthoplasty.

Labels in figure:
- Glanular
- Coronal
- Subcoronal
- Anterior (Distal)
- Distal penile
- Midshaft
- Proximal penile
- Middle
- Penoscrotal
- Scrotal
- Posterior (Proximal)
- Perineal

the subject, with comparison and contrast to his findings, Glenister believed the origin of the urethral plate to be an outgrowth from the walls of the cloaca and urogenital sinus. According to Glenister, development of the urethra begins at the 10 mm stage (approximately 4th week of development) (Stephens et al, 1996), when the urethral plate is recognizable as a thickening of the anterior wall of the endodermal cloaca. **A *urethral groove* is established by the development of the urethral folds on the ventrum of the phallic portion of the urogenital sinus on either side of the urethral plate.** These folds are covered by surface epithelium, and it is suggested that the groove between them be called the *primary* urethral groove (Glenister, 1954). A *secondary* urethral groove develops at the 35 mm stage (approximately 8th week) (Stephens et al, 1996) as a result of disintegration of the roof of the primary groove. Continuation of this process eventually establishes the *definitive* urethral groove.

In the male fetus, at the 50 mm stage (approximately 11th week of development) (Stephens et al, 1996), when the interstitial (Leydig) cells of the testis increase in number, size, and function, the urethral folds begin to fuse ventrally in the midline to form the urethra (Glenister, 1954). Via a similar process, the proximal portion of the glanular urethra forms shortly thereafter and is thus derived from the urethral plate (endodermal origin). **The distal portion of the glanular urethra is formed by lamellar ingrowth of the surface epithelium (ectodermal origin), which grows toward the distal extent of the urethral plate, becoming stratified squamous epithelium at the completion of development.** This classic "ecto-

dermal ingrowth theory" for development of the distal glanular urethra has recently been challenged by the "endodermal differentiation theory" (Fig. 65–4) (Kurzrock et al, 1999).

The ***endodermal differentiation theory* described by Kurzrock and colleagues (1999)** is based on the results of immunohistochemical staining for different cytokeratins in 36 serially sectioned human fetal phallic specimens of gestational ages 5 to 22 weeks. **According to these investigators the urethral plate extends to the tip of the phallus and maintains patency and continuity throughout urethral development; therefore, the epithelium of the entire urethra originates from the urogenital sinus (endoderm).** Sections of the distal glanular urethra showed no evidence of ectodermal tissue ingrowth. **Kurzrock and colleagues (1999) provided further support for the endodermal differentiation theory using tissue recombinant grafting techniques, suggesting that under the correct cellular signaling conditions endodermally derived epithelium (urethral plate) differentiates into the stratified squamous epithelial phenotype present in the fully developed distal glanular urethra.**

Interestingly, significant ventral curvature exists in the phallus of both the male and female fetus early in development (Glenister, 1954). Further discussion of this finding and its implications are addressed subsequently in the section regarding the etiology of penile curvature. **With regard to preputial development, Hunter (1935) noted that at the 40 mm stage preputial tissue did not uniformly surround the phallus in the form of a circle; rather, it was present in an oblique orientation, radiat-**

Ectodermal Ingrowth Theory

Endodermal Differentiation Theory

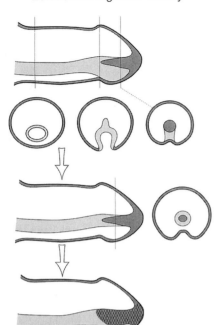

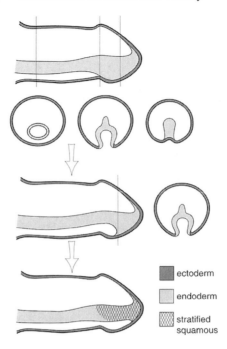

Figure 65–4. Classical (ectodermal ingrowth) and recently purported (endodermal differentiation) theories of distal glanular urethral development. (From Kurzrock EA, Baskin LS, Cunha GR: Ontogeny of the male urethra: Theory of endodermal differentiation. Differentiation 1999;64:115–122, with permission.)

■ ectoderm

☐ endoderm

▨ stratified squamous

ing out on either side of the phallus from the point of the urethral opening, with the urethral opening placed "well back" on the ventral surface of the phallus at this stage of development. According to Hunter, at this early stage of development the preputial tissue appears as a "hood" dorsally and gradually becomes less well marked ventrally as it approaches the urethral meatus. Complete preputial covering of the glans occurs at approximately the 130 mm stage (20th week) of development (Stephens et al, 1996).

Neurovascular Anatomy

Using immunohistochemical localization and three-dimensional computer reconstructive techniques, Baskin and colleagues (1998) studied neural and vascular anatomic features of 10 normal and 1 hypospadiac fetal penis. They showed that **the nerves that innervate the penis originate proximally as two well-defined bundles under the pubic rami superior and slightly lateral to the urethra. This was similar for both the hypospadiac and normal fetal penises compared. As the two crural bodies converge into the corpora cavernosa, the nerves diverge, spreading around the corpora cavernosa to the junction with the urethral spongiosum. Nervous tissue fans out in this manner from the 11 and 1 o'clock positions all along the penis and does not remain confined to two well-defined bundles.** The absence of neuronal structures at the 12 o'clock position along the entire shaft of the penis was also noted (Baskin et al, 1998).

On further comparison of normal and hypospadiac fetal penile anatomy with the use of immunostaining techniques, Baskin and colleagues (1998) noted that the most striking difference detected was that of relative vascularity. **There was extensive vascularity of the distal urethral spongiosum and glans in the hypospadiac compared with the normal penises examined. Baskin and colleagues (1998) proposed implications for hypospadias repair in that incision of these sites (i.e., distal urethral spongiosum and glans), which are rich in large endothelial-lined sinuses, results in release of epithelial growth factors that encourage tissue repair without significant scar or stricture formation.** The authors stressed the importance of knowledge of normal and hypospadiac penile anatomy, particularly the neural and vascular aspects, for safe and efficacious penile reconstructive procedures.

ETIOLOGY

Hypospadias

In simple terms, hypospadias is thought to be caused by incomplete closure of tissue on the undersurface of the penis, known as the urethral folds, which form the urethra (Winslow and Devine, 1996). **A fascinating, detailed report by Sorensen (1953) and more recent reviews by Sweet and colleagues (1974) and by Baskin (2000) suggest a multifactorial etiology of hypospadias, fitting a polygenic model. In this vein, responsible etiologic factors may include one or more of the following: an environmental or other endocrine disruptor; a native endocrinologic, enzymatic, or local tissue abnormality; and a manifestation of arrested development.**

More specifically, the defects of the hypospadias anomaly may result from (1) abnormal androgen production by the fetal testis, (2) limited androgen sensitivity in the target tissues of the developing external genitalia, and/or (3) premature cessation of androgenic stimulation secondary to

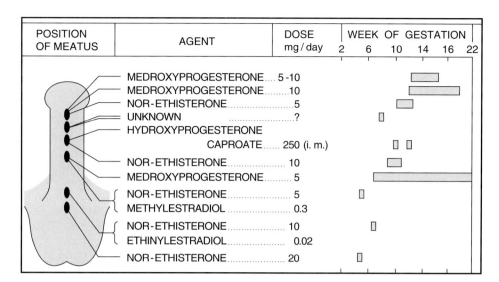

POSITION OF MEATUS	AGENT	DOSE mg / day	WEEK OF GESTATION
	MEDROXYPROGESTERONE	5-10	
	MEDROXYPROGESTERONE	10	
	NOR-ETHISTERONE	5	
	UNKNOWN	?	
	HYDROXYPROGESTERONE CAPROATE	250 (i. m.)	
	NOR-ETHISTERONE	10	
	MEDROXYPROGESTERONE	5	
	NOR-ETHISTERONE	5	
	METHYLESTRADIOL	0.3	
	NOR-ETHISTERONE	10	
	ETHINYLESTRADIOL	0.02	
	NOR-ETHISTERONE	20	

Figure 65–5. Hypospadias associated with maternal (gestational) treatment with progestins. (From Aarskog D: Maternal progestins as a possible cause of hypospadias. N Engl J Med 1979;300: 75–78, with permission.)

premature involution of Leydig cells of the fetal testis (Devine and Horton, 1977). **Other possible etiologic factors include insufficient synthesis of testosterone or dihydrotestosterone or both (presumably from defective or deficient 5α-reductase enzyme activity) and/or defects in androgen receptor quality or quantity or both. Several entities in the spectrum of androgen resistance (androgen insensitivity syndromes) have been elucidated at the clinical and molecular level** (Griffin and Wilson, 1987; Griffin, 1992).

Several endocrinopathic/enzymatic factors have been identified in humans and in animal models of hypospadias. **It has been observed that genotypic male infants born with a severe deficiency of 3β-hydroxysteroid dehydrogenase enzyme (a microsomal enzyme essential in biosynthesis of almost every biologically active steroid hormone) have incomplete masculine development and hypospadias** (Goldman and Bongiovanni, 1967). Additional evidence, in humans, of an endocrinopathic etiology was provided in several detailed reports (Allen and Griffin, 1984; Aaronson et al, 1997; Albers et al, 1997), including monozygotic twin studies (Roberts and Lloyd, 1973; Fredell et al, 1998).

Allen and Griffin (1984) evaluated 15 boys younger than 4 years of age with "advanced degrees" of hypospadias for an endocrinopathy. Six different endocrine-related abnormalities were identified in 11 boys. One child each had been exposed to progesterone given to the mother during the first trimester of pregnancy, had an abnormal karyotype, and had a unilateral nonpalpable gonad. One patient with a family history of Reifenstein's syndrome (partial androgen resistance) had low receptor numbers, and three patients with normal receptor levels exhibited a poor genital response to exogenous testosterone (perhaps because of abnormal receptor function or dihydrotestosterone production). **According to Allen and Griffin (1984), the most striking finding was the poor testosterone response to injections of human chorionic gonadotropin (hCG), observed in seven patients. In several instances this improved or normalized with time, suggesting that hypospadias is a local manifestation of an endocrinopathy rather than a local dysmorphic problem, and that one**

major cause may be a delay in maturation of the hypothalamic-pituitary-testicular axis.

Experimentally, the importance of steroid hormone synthesis in normal genitalia development has been reinforced. Genotypic male rats experience peak activity of 3β-hydroxysteroid dehydrogenase enzyme in the testis at the time of urethral fold fusion (Goldman and Bongiovanni, 1967). Greene and colleagues (1938) showed that administration of estrogens antenatally reproducibly causes feminization in male rats. The same **investigators produced profound congenital adrenal hyperplasia experimentally with the use of a 3β-hydroxysteroid dehydrogenase enzyme inhibitor. The experimental gonadal males had severe hypospadias. The critical period for production of hypospadias by the inhibitor corresponded to the beginning of activity of the enzyme in the rat testis and was time dependent** (Goldman and Bongiovanni, 1967).

With regard to endocrine disruptors, Aarskog (1979) retrospectively studied a personal series of 130 hypospadiac patients with special reference to pathogenetic mechanisms that might have interfered with fetal testicular differentiation and/or function. In 11 patients there was a history of maternal progestin intake early in pregnancy, either for treatment of threatened abortion or in combination with estrogen for pregnancy testing. **When the position of the urethral meatus was compared with the week of gestation at which progestin therapy was begun, a positive correlation was noted for more proximal hypospadias in mothers treated during the first month of pregnancy** (Fig. 65–5).

The implication of a role for maternal progestin exposure in the development of hypospadias has been both supported (Goldman and Bongiovanni, 1967) and discounted (Mau, 1981). Alternatively, Paulozzi suggested that the real risk factor for hypospadias in these patients is related to that responsible for threatening the loss of pregnancy rather than the progestin itself (Paulozzi, 2000). However, this would not explain hypospadias development in offspring of those exposed to a combination of progestin and estrogen during pregnancy testing. **Further support of an endocrine disruptor etiology for hypospadias may be provided by markedly increased rates of hypospadias in** male offspring conceived by in vitro fertilization (i.e., when progesterone is given early for pregnancy support) (Macnab and Zouves, 1991; Silver et al, 1999). Although a possible causative role for environmental factors and endocrine disruptors in hypospadias is of significant concern, it is not yet established (Myers, 2000; Paulozzi, 2000).

The hypothesis of an "arrest of development," as noted by Mettauer (1842) and Van Hook (1896) would seem the most plausible explanation for hypospadias. Although this theory does not identify a possible specific cause of the arrested development, it would account for the concomitant occurrence of all three typical characteristics of hypospadias—penile curvature, hypospadiac meatus, and deficient foreskin. Complete straightening of the phallus does not occur until approximately the same time as the completion of urethral closure and just before completion of preputial formation. In addition, the dorsal "hood" of the prepuce described by Hunter (1935) in the early stages of development is an exact description of the observed appearance of the preputial defect typically associated with hypospadias. This "hood" appearance is present at a time during development when the meatus is still hypospadiac in location. Slight variations in timing of the developmental arrest may account for hypospadias variants such as the MIP.

Baskin (2000) proposed that future areas of study, such as endocrine disruptors, mesenchymal-epithelial interactions, and mechanisms of penile growth, may hold the key to explaining the etiology of hypospadias. Baskin's group has shown that disruption of the fibroblast growth factor 10 (FGF-10) gene results in hypospadias (Baskin et al, 2000). FGF-10 is known to be important in growth, development, and wound healing.

Penile Curvature (Chordee)

According to E.D. Smith (1997), Galen (130–199 AD) was the first to use the term "hypospadias" and the first to emphasize the major significance of penile curvature. Although there were references to penile curvature in the 1500s (Ambrose Paré) and in the 1700s (Pierre Dionis), there was apparently no understanding of its cause until the attempt by Mettauer in 1842. Mettauer (1842) described "contracted structures" situated in the "subcutaneous cellular texture" which from some cause had lost the ability to elongate with the contiguous structures and may produce curvature. The exact location of this culpable tissue was not stated by Mettauer, but, according to E.D. Smith (1997), **Mettauer implicated subcutaneous structures proximal to the meatus and described a "skin tethering" etiology for penile curvature. This concept was ignored for more than 100 years until championed by D.R. Smith in 1955.**

In a critical review of the subject and his own experience, D.R. Smith (1955) discussed what he believed was a common misunderstanding about the true anatomic aspects of hypospadias, particularly the component of curvature. He stated that, "with few exceptions, the corpus spongiosum is perfectly normal." He believed that the major cause of curvature was skin and that correction of curvature depended on freeing attachments of the ventral skin and corpora cavernosa distal to the urethral meatus (Smith, 1955). **Creevy, in 1958,** acknowledged D.R. Smith's thoughts regarding the significance of skin and **proposed his own hypothesis regarding the etiology of penile curvature, implicating the tissue now commonly referred to as the urethral plate by stating that the "urethra distal to the urinary meatus appears as a modified strip of mucosa covering a band of dense fibrous tissue composed of abortive corpus spongiosum"** (Creevy, 1958). Creevy went on to state that this tissue (urethral plate) is shorter than the corresponding segment of penis, and "so produces the characteristic ventral bowing."

More recently, **study of penile development via examination of fetal specimens has led to the understanding that penile curvature is a part of the early stages of normal penile development** (Glenister, 1954; Kaplan and Lamm, 1975). It follows that interruption of development or other detrimental effect on fetal development during these stages could result in fixation of penile development at a time when curvature is present and therefore the condition would be observed in the newborn carried to term. These observations support the "arrest of development" hypothesis for etiology of hypospadias as proposed by Mettauer (1842) and Van Hook (1896). **Currently, three major theories are proposed for the cause of penile curvature: (1) abnormal development of the urethral plate; (2) abnormal, fibrotic mesenchymal tissue at the urethral meatus; and (3) corporal disproportion or differential growth of normal dorsal corpora cavernosal tissue and abnormal corporal tissue ventrally** (Kaplan and Lamm, 1975; Bellinger, 1981; Duckett et al, 1996).

Perhaps the most enlightening information regarding the etiology of hypospadias comes from microscopic evaluation of the urethral plate distal to the hypospadiac meatus. **This report by Snodgrass and colleagues (2000) challenges most of the historical tenets that typically vilified the urethral plate as the sole source or contributing factor in chordee or penile curvature. Using light microscopy and routine staining techniques, these investigators showed that subepithelial biopsy of the urethral plate in 17 boys with hypospadias, including 5 with curvature and 4 with penoscrotal defects, revealed well-vascularized smooth muscle and collagen without fibrous bands or dysplastic tissue.** These results were consistent with histologic findings at autopsy in a boy with proximal hypospadias (Marshall et al, 1978) and in a fetus with distal hypospadias (Baskin et al, 1998).

Penile Curvature without Hypospadias

Although commonly associated with hypospadias, congenital penile curvature (chordee) may also occur with an orthotopically positioned urethral meatus. Devine and Horton (1973) described three classes of chordee or penile curvature without hypospadias. In class I, the most severe defect, there is a very thin "mucous membrane" urethra and deficiency of corpus spongiosum from the site at which curvature begins and continuing to the level of the glans. According to these authors, the presence of dense fibrous tissue lying beneath the urethra is the cause of curvature in these cases. In class II, the urethra is surrounded by normal corpus spongiosum with abnormal Buck's and dartos fascia present. In class III, only the dartos fascia is abnormal.

Several authors have described this entity in similar terms of classification and treatment (Cendron and Melin, 1981; Hurwitz, 1986; Devine et al, 1991; Caldamone and Diamond, 1999). A report from **Donnahoo and colleagues (1998) evenly divided the etiology of congenital penile curvature without hypospadias in a series of 87 patients into three categories: (1) skin tethering, (2) fibrotic dartos and Buck's fasciae, and (3) corporal disproportion. According to these authors, a congenitally short urethra was a rare cause of isolated curvature.**

Dorsal or lateral curvatures of the penis, both with and without hypospadias, have also been described (Udall, 1980; Redman, 1983; Spiro et al, 1992; Adams et al, 1999). **Various methods used for treatment of congenital penile curvature without hypospadias are identical to those used for curvature with hypospadias** and are discussed later in this chapter.

EPIDEMIOLOGY

Prevalence: General Population

In a comprehensive review, Sorensen (1953) credited Rennes in 1831 with reporting a prevalence for hypospadias in 1 in 300 "recruits" and also reported the same figure for live male births in Denmark. In 1896, Van Hook quoted Orth's figure for hypospadias prevalence of 1 in 300 live births, and in a postmortem series of 12,280 children, Campbell in 1947 reported a prevalence of 1 in 1100 boys. **In the frequently quoted Rochester, Minnesota, community-wide case-control study of hypospadias, Sweet and colleagues (1974) reported their 30-year experience and reviewed the epidemiology of hypospadias. During the period 1940 to 1970, inclusive, 113 cases of hypospadias were noted in 13,776 live male births (1 of every 122). Of note, 87% of defects were coronal or glanular. In their review of the literature from five different countries, Sweden had the lowest reported prevalence, 1 in 1250 live male births.**

In 1997, two independent and well-established surveillance systems in the United States, the Metropolitan Atlanta Congenital Defects Program (MACDP) and the nationwide Birth Defects Monitoring Program (BDMP), reported near-doubling of hypospadias rates in the most recent compared with the immediately preceding decades (Paulozzi et al, 1997). As measured by the BDMP, hypospadias rates increased from 2.02 per 1000 male births in 1970 to 3.97 per 1000 in 1993. In other words, approximately 1 in every 250 live male births was a boy with hypospadias. **The rate of severe hypospadias increased threefold to fivefold, from 0.11 per 1000 male births in 1968 to between 0.27 and 0.55 per 1000 male births per year from 1990 to 1993, as recorded by the MACDP**

(Paulozzi et al, 1997). The rising trend may simply reflect more frequent or earlier diagnosis of mild forms of hypospadias over time or an increasing tendency to report to registries of congenital anomalies. However, the results suggest that the ratio of minor to severe cases is decreasing, not increasing, as would be expected if the change in hypospadias rates were secondary to more frequent reporting of minor forms (Dolk, 1998).

Prevalence: Other

Pertinent familial aspects include the finding of hypospadias in approximately 6% to 8% of fathers of affected boys and 14% of male siblings of the index case of hypospadias (Sweet et al, 1974; Bauer et al, 1979, 1981; Sorber et al, 1997). **Roberts and Lloyd (1973) noted an 8.5-fold higher rate of hypospadias in one of monozygotic male twins, compared with singleton live male births. They suggested that this strong association of monozygotic twinning and hypospadias may be the result of an inability of a single placenta and reduced hCG levels to meet the requirements of two developing male fetuses.** In an evaluation of monozygotic male twins discordant for hypospadias, Fredell and colleagues (1998) found that 16 boys with hypospadias, from 18 such pairs, had a statistically significant lower birth weight than their unaffected twin, as well as a more pronounced difference in birth weight than that found in unaffected monozygotic twin males. This would seem to further support an endocrinopathic etiology, namely mismatch in the "supply and demand" of hCG (of placenta and fetus, respectively), as suggested by Roberts and Lloyd (1973).

ASSOCIATED FINDINGS

Genetic Associations

Aarskog (1970) was one of the first to perform cytogenetic analyses in patients with hypospadias. He found a normal karyotype in all cases of glanular hypospadias and noted that abnormal karyotypes tended to occur among patients with the most severe degrees of hypospadias, especially among those with associated cryptorchidism. Yamaguchi and colleagues (1991) studied 110 consecutive patients who had cryptorchidism and/or hypospadias. Seven (6.4%) of these patients were found to have chromosomal anomalies. **The incidence of chromosomal anomalies in patients with cryptorchidism only was 4.8% (4/83), in patients with hypospadias only it was 5.6% (1/18), and in concomitant cases the incidence was 22.2% (2/9).**

Cryptorchidism and Inguinal Hernia

Associated abnormalities include cryptorchidism (8% to 9%) and inguinal hernia and/or hydrocele (9% to 16%) (Sweet et al, 1974; Khuri et al, 1981; Sorber et al, 1997). **These overall rates for males with hypospadias**

increase significantly in those with more proximal defects. The concomitant occurrence of hypospadias and cryptorchidism even in the setting of nonambiguous genitalia should alert the urologist to evaluate for the possible presence of an intersex state, as discussed in detail later.

Syndromes and Diagnoses

According to the authoritative, encyclopedic reference, *Smith's Recognizable Patterns of Human Malformation,* there are approximately 49 recognized syndromes in which hypospadias is either a "frequent" (15) or an "occasional" (34) associated finding (Jones, 1997) (Table 65–1). **Of these 49 syndromes in which hypospadias is an associated finding, 38 (78%) also have associated micropenis, cryptorchidism, and/or a scrotal abnormality. This would seem to further support an endocrinopathic etiology for hypospadias.** The issue of intersexuality is not specifically discussed in this reference (Jones, 1997).

Intersex States

Based on his experiments in the rabbit fetus, Jost regarded all hypospadias as a form of male pseudohermaphroditism (Aarskog, 1971). **A high index of suspicion for an intersex state should accompany presumed males with any degree of hypospadias and cryptorchidism** (Rajfer and Walsh, 1976; Borer et al, 1995; Albers et al, 1997; Smith and Wacksman, 1997; Kaefer et al, 1999). In 1976, Rajfer and Walsh reported the incidence of intersexuality in children with cryptorchidism, hypospadias, and otherwise nonambiguous genitalia to be 27%.

In a detailed evaluation of hypospadias level and exact status of concomitant cryptorchidism, **Kaefer and colleagues (1999) evaluated 79 presumed males presenting with one or both undescended testes and hypospadias.** Intersex conditions were identified with almost equal frequency in the 44 cases (30%) of unilateral and 35 (32%) of bilateral cryptorchidism. **In the group with unilateral cryptorchid testis, patients with a nonpalpable testis were at least threefold more likely to have an intersex condition than those with a palpable undescended testis (50% versus 15%). In the bilateral cryptorchid group, patients with one or more nonpalpable testes were also almost three times as likely to have an intersex condition compared with those who had bilateral palpable undescended gonads (47% versus 16%).** Meatal position was graded as anterior in 33% of cases, middle in 25%, and posterior in 41%, with the more posterior location conferring a significantly greater likelihood of intersexuality (anterior, 2 of 26 cases; middle, 1 of 20; posterior, 21 of 33) (Kaefer et al, 1999).

SPECIAL CONSIDERATIONS: PREOPERATIVE

Indications

According to Cecil (1932), the only reason for operating on any hypospadiac patient is to correct deformities that interfere with the function of urination and procreation. There is no question that more severe degrees of hypospadias require repair in order to provide the ability to micturate in a standing position, achieve sexual intercourse, and effectively inseminate. However, questions regarding the need for repair of anterior hypospadias are noted throughout history. **Early on, unsatisfactory results of anterior hypospadias repair were responsible for the sentiment that the balanitic type of hypospadias is best treated by "masterly neglect"** (Cabot, 1936). **This sentiment has changed because of both superior results with current techniques and caregiver concern regarding cosmesis.** As Backus and De Felice (1960) stated, "The cosmetic considerations are definitely secondary and usually of more concern to the parents than the patient. However, this does not constitute a valid excuse to dismiss them entirely."

Few have studied the natural history of untreated distal hypospadias. One such report by Fichtner and colleagues (1995) examined the meatal location in 500 adult men admitted for transurethral treatment of either prostatic or bladder disease. A meatus located in the distal one third of the glans was considered to be in the "normal" position and was noted in only 55% of the 500 men examined. Sixty-five (13%) of the men had either glanular (49), coronal (15), or subcoronal (1) hypospadias. **Of the 16 men with a coronal or subcoronal defect, only 6 were aware of the abnormality, all reported no difficulties with sexual intercourse or voiding in a standing position without downward deflection of the stream, and all 15 heterosexuals had fathered children** (Fichtner et al, 1995). This data led Fichtner and colleagues to narrow their indications for repair of anterior hypospadias.

Intersex Evaluation

Although it is not indicated for isolated anterior or middle hypospadias, the necessity for an intersex evaluation in the setting of concomitant hypospadias and cryptorchidism has been discussed. **The idea that evaluation for an endocrine abnormality and/or intersex state should be undertaken in those with posterior hypospadias, regardless of gonadal position or palpability, is controversial but is supported in the literature, because significant, identifiable, and treatable abnormalities are common** (Allen and Griffin, 1984; Aaronson et al, 1997; Albers et al, 1997). It has been suggested that for patients with severe, apparently isolated hypospadias, a standardized set of diagnostic evaluations including ultrasonographic, genitographic, chromosomal, gonadal (histologic), biochemical, and molecular studies should be performed as a minimum (Rajfer and Walsh, 1976; Albers et al, 1997). Detailed discussion regarding evaluation for specific intersex states is available in Chapter 68.

Radiologic Evaluation

In general, the literature does not support routine imaging of the urinary tract with either ultrasonogra-

Table 65–1. SYNDROMES IN WHICH HYPOSPADIAS IS A FEATURE

Syndrome (s.)	Relative or Approximate % of Cases with Hypospadias	Other Notable Findings of the Genitalia
Aniridia–Wilms tumor association	Frequent	Cryptorchidism
Deletion 4p s.	Frequent	Cryptorchidism
Deletion 11q s.	50%	Cryptorchidism
Deletion 13q s.	Frequent	Cryptorchidism
Fetal trimethadione s. (Tridione s.)	Frequent	Ambiguous genitalia
Fraser s. (cryptophthalmos s.)	Frequent	Cryptorchidism
Fryns s.	86%	Cryptorchidism, bifid scrotum
Opitz s. (hypertelorism-hypospadias s., Opitz-Frias s., Opitz oculo-genito-laryngeal s.)	Frequent	Cryptorchidism, bifid scrotum
Rapp-Hodgkin ectodermal dysplasia s. (hypohidrotic ectodermal dysplasia, autosomal dominant type)	Frequent	—
Rieger s.	Frequent	—
Schinzel-Giedion s.	100%	Micropenis, hypoplastic scrotum
Smith-Lemli-Opitz s.	70%	Micropenis, hypoplastic/bifid scrotum
Triploidy s. and diploid/triploid mixoploidy s.	Frequent	Micropenis, cryptorchidism
X-linked α-thalassemia/mental retardation (ATR-X) s.	Frequent	Micropenis, hypoplastic scrotum
Brachmann-de Lange s. (Cornelia de Lange s., de Lange s.)	33%	Cryptorchidism (73%)
Beckwith-Wiedemann s. (exomphalos-macroglossia-gigantism s.)	Occasional	Cryptorchidism
Craniofrontonasal dysplasia	Occasional	—
Dubowitz s.	Occasional	—
Duplication 4p s. (trisomy for the short arm of chromosome 4, trisomy 4p s.)	Occasional	Micropenis, cryptorchidism
Duplication 9p s. (trisomy 9p s.)	Occasional	Micropenis, cryptorchidism
Escobar s.	Occasional	Cryptorchidism
Duplication 10q s.	Occasional	Cryptorchidism, streak gonads
Fanconi pancytopenia s.	20%	Micropenis, cryptorchidism
Fetal hydantoin s. (fetal dilantin s.)	Occasional	Cryptorchidism, micropenis, ambiguous genitalia
Fetal rubella effects (fetal rubella s.)	Occasional	Cryptorchidism
Fetal valproate s.	Occasional	—
FG s.	Occasional	Cryptorchidism (36%)
Hay-Wells s. of ectodermal dysplasia (ankyloblepharon-ectodermal dysplasia-clefting s., AEC s.)	Occasional	Micropenis
Hydrolethalus s.	Occasional	—
Johanson-Blizzard s.	Occasional	Micropenis, cryptorchidism
Killian/Teschler-Nicola s. (Pallister mosaic s., tetrasomy 12p)	Occasional	—
Lenz-Majewski hyperostosis s.	Occasional	Cryptorchidism
Peters'-Plus s.	Occasional	Cryptorchidism
Levy-Hollister s. (lacrimo-auriculo-dento-digital s., LADD s.)	Occasional (coronal)	—
Marden-Walker s.	Occasional	Micropenis, cryptorchidism
Multiple lentigines s. (leopard s.)	Occasional	Cryptorchidism, hypogonadism
Oto-palato-digital s., type II	Occasional	Cryptorchidism
Restrictive dermopathy	Occasional	—
Roberts-SC phocomelia (pseudothalidomide s., hypomelia-hypotrichosis-facial hemangioma s.)	Occasional	Cryptorchidism
Russell-Silver s. (Silver s.)	Occasional	Seminoma
Shprintzen s. (velo-cardio-facial s.)	Occasional	Cryptorchidism
Simpson-Golabi-Behmel s.	Occasional	Cryptorchidism
Townes-Brocks s.	Occasional	—
Trisomy 13 s. (D1 trisomy s.)	<50%	Cryptorchidism (>50%)
Trisomy 18 s.	<10%	Cryptorchidism (≥50%), bifid scrotum (<10%)
XXY s., Klinefelter s.	Occasional	Micropenis, cryptorchidism
XXXY s. and XXXXY s.	Occasional	Micropenis (80%), cryptorchidism (28%)
XYY s.	Occasional	Micropenis, cryptorchidism
Zellweger s. (cerebro-hepato-renal s.)	Occasional	Cryptorchidism

Adapted from Jones KL: Smith's Recognizable Patterns of Human Malformation, 5th ed. Philadelphia, WB Saunders, 1997, p 835, with permission.

phy (Cerasaro et al, 1986; Davenport and MacKinnon, 1988) **or intravenous urography** (McArdle and Lebowitz, 1975; Cerasaro et al, 1986) **for evaluation of children with isolated hypospadias,** particularly when the hypospadiac meatus is middle or anterior in location. Retrograde injection of radiographic contrast material into the presumed urethral meatus (genitogram) is an essential component of the intersex evaluation when such an evaluation is deemed appropriate. **Preoperative evaluation is more extensive in patients with posterior hypospadias and at**

Table 65–2. EARLY CONTRIBUTIONS TO HYPOSPADIOLOGY

Contributor	Date	Reference	Contribution
Heliodor and Antyl	1st, 2nd, 3rd centuries AD	Hauben, 1984	First description of hypospadias and hypospadias repair
Galen	130–199 AD	Smith, 1997	First to use the term "hypospadias" and to emphasize significance of penile curvature
Ambrose Paré	1510–1590	Hauben, 1984; Smith, 1997	Extensive discussions of hypospadias and penile curvature and their treatment
Pierre Dionis	1658–1718	Hauben, 1984; Smith, 1997	Described methods for treating hyposadias, "chordea," and hermaphroditism; wrote a complete treatise on the surgery of hypospadias
Dieffenbach	1836	Murphy, 1972	Attempted urethroplasty via tubularization of ventral local tissue
Mettauer	1842	Mettauer, 1842	"Arrest of development" theory for hypospadias etiology; "skin tethering" theory for curvature etiology
Bouisson	1860	Mayo, 1901; Murphy, 1972; Smith, 1997	Incorporated scrotal skin into hypospadias repair (see Rosenberger, 1891 and Landerer, 1891 in Van Hook, 1896 and Bucknall, 1907); ventral orthoplasty with interposition skin graft (see Hagner, 1932)
Thiersch	1869	Thiersch, 1869	Local tissue tubularized urethroplasty for epispadias repair (see Duplay, 1880)
Wood	1875	Mayo, 1901; Murphy, 1972	"Buttonhole," transfer of intact preputial skin and use of scrotal skin as onlay
Duplay	1880	Duplay, 1880	Acknowledged Thiersch; described tubularized urethroplasty for hypospadias repair, following first-stage ventral orthoplasty
Rosenberger	1891	Van Hook, 1896	Use of scrotal skin flaps for repair of hypospadias
Landerer	1891	Van Hook, 1896	First-stage scrotal fixation and second-stage release with scrotal skin incorporation into urethroplasty
Van Hook	1896	Van Hook, 1896	First description of "pedunculate flap" tubularized urethroplasty (see Asopa et al, 1971; Duckett, 1980; Hodgson, 1970; Wehrbein, 1943)
Beck	1898	Beck, 1898	Distal circumferential urethral dissection and advancement via glans tunnel
Nové-Josserand	1897, 1914	Nové-Josserand, 1897, 1914	First description (1897) of tubularized free skin graft urethroplasty (see Devine and Horton, 1961; Humby, 1941; McIndoe, 1937)
Russell	1900	Russell, 1900	"Clergyman's stole" strip of prepuce in continuity with longitudinal, ventral penile skin strips for proximal hypospadias (see Des Prez et al, 1961; Koyanagi et al, 1994) or distal (see Aronoff, 1963)
Mayo	1901	Mayo, 1901	Acknowledged Van Hook; described pedicled prepuce and dorsal penile skin tubularized urethroplasty (see Broadbent et al, 1961; Davis, 1940)
Bucknall	1907	Bucknall, 1907	First-stage scrotal fixation and second-stage release with scrotal skin incorporation into urethroplasty
Edmunds	1913, 1926	Edmunds, 1913, 1926	Three-stage ventrally repositioned prepuce via buttonholed pedicle followed by tubularized urethroplasty (see Browne, 1936; Byars, 1951; Nesbit, 1941; Retik et al, 1994; Smith, 1973)
Bevan	1917	Bevan, 1917	Proximal "perimeatal" ventral penile skin tubularized and advanced via glans channel (see Mustarde, 1965)
Hagner	1932	Hagner, 1932	Ventral corpora cavernosa interposition (full-thickness) skin graft orthoplasty
Ombredanne	1932	Ombredanne, 1932	Buttonhole ventral shaft skin coverage with "intact" prepuce
Mathieu	1932	Mathieu, 1932	Proximal "perimeatal" ventral penile skin "flip-flap" (onlay) urethroplasty
Blair	1933	Blair et al., 1933	Three-stage ventral transposition of prepuce, tubularized urethroplasty, and scrotal skin coverage
D. Browne	1936	Browne, 1936	Acknowledged Edmunds; described "transplantation of prepuce" to dorsum of penile shaft followed by lateral, longitudinal perimeatal based flap urethroplasty
McIndoe	1937	McIndoe, 1937	Free skin graft urethroplasty
Davis	1940, 1951	Davis, 1940, 1951	Ventrally transposed pedicled prepuce and dorsal penile skin tubularized urethroplasty
Nesbit	1941	Nesbit, 1941	Two-stage ventrally repositioned intact prepuce via buttonholed pedicle followed by tubularized urethroplasty
Humby	1941	Humby, 1941	Tubularized free skin graft urethroplasty; inner upper arm, thigh, "mucous membrane from the lower lip" donor sites descrbed (see Bürger et al., 1992; Dessanti et al., 1992, regarding buccal mucosa free graft urethroplasty)
Cecil	1946	Cecil, 1946	Popularized staged scrotal skin incorporation into urethroplasty

Table 65–2. EARLY CONTRIBUTIONS TO HYPOSPADIOLOGY *Continued*

Contributor	Date	Reference	Contribution
Memmelaar	1947	Memmelaar, 1947	First description of bladder mucosa use for one-stage urethroplasty (see Hendren and Reda, 1986; Marshall and Spellman, 1955)
D. Browne	1949, 1953	Browne, 1949	"Buried" urethral plate strip urethroplasty
Byars	1951	Byars, 1951	"Split" ventral preputial transposition with second-stage tubularized urethroplasty
Byars	1955	Byars, 1955	"Byars' flaps"; ventrally repositioned "split" prepuce for ventral skin coverage
Marshall and Spellman	1955	Marshall and Spellman, 1955	Two-stage tubularized bladder mucosa urethroplasty
DesPrez	1961	Des Prez et al., 1961	Described "island pedicle flap" that circumscribes the meatus and extends along the inner aspect of the prepuce
Devine and Horton	1961	Devine and Horton, 1961	Popularized one-stage free skin graft urethroplasty
Broadbent	1961	Broadbent et al., 1961	One-stage urethroplasty with dorsolateral penile skin
Aronoff	1963	Aronoff, 1963	Described "bi-pedicle (bucket handle) transposition flap" use of prepuce for distal hypospadias repair

our institution includes voiding cystourethrography (VCUG) in those with a scrotal or perineal defect to evaluate the frequent presence and extent of a prostatic utricle (Retik, 1996).

Hormonal Manipulation

There is considerable controversy surrounding the use of hormonal stimulation or supplementation for the purpose of penile enlargement before hypospadias repair. Topics of debate include whether to administer any adjunctive gonadotropins or hormones and, if so, which agent, route, dose, dosing schedule, and timing of treatment is to be employed.

Androgen Stimulation (hCG)

Koff and Jayanthi (1999) recently presented evidence that supports the use of hCG before repair of proximal hypospadias. An increase in penile size and length was noted in 12 boys aged 8 to 14 months who received a 5-week course of hCG preoperatively. The significant increase in penile length occurred primarily proximal to the urethral meatus, advancing the meatus distally anywhere from 6 to 19 mm. Observations included decreased hypospadias and chordee severity in all patients, increased vascularity and thickness of proximal corpus spongiosum, and allowance for more simple repairs in 3 of the 12 boys receiving hCG preoperatively. Shima and colleagues (1986) noted impaired gonadotropin and testosterone response to luteinizing hormone-releasing hormone and hCG stimulation in prepubertal boys with hypospadias. These authors did not discuss the penile or meatal response to stimulation.

Androgen Supplementation or Replacement

Various preparations, including testosterone ointment, applied to the glans penis for 2 weeks before surgery, have been used to stimulate penile growth (Perovic and Vukadi-

novic, 1994). Citing variable absorption and inconsistent results with the use of topical testosterone, **Gearhart and Jeffs (1987) administered testosterone enanthate intramuscularly (2 mg/kg body weight), 5 and 2 weeks before reconstructive penile surgery. They noted a 50% increase in penile size and an increase in available skin and local vascularity in all patients. A near-doubling (from 3 to 5 cm) of the mean transverse length of the inner prepuce was also noted in some.** In addition, they reported minimal side effects and return of plasma testosterone levels to within the normal range for age within 6 months after therapy. Others have employed variations in the total dose and schedule of testosterone enanthate administration, using 25 mg intramuscularly once weekly for a total of either two (Belman, 1997) or three injections (Stock et al, 1995).

Monfort and Lucas (1982) used a 4-week period of local penile stimulation with **daily application of dihydrotestosterone (DHT) cream before repair of hypospadias or epispadias. They reported a mean increase in penile circumference and length by 50% of pretreatment measurements, without any lasting side effects or gonadotropin level perturbation, and without any effects in the pubertal or postpubertal period.**

Timing of Hormonal Manipulation

Hormonal manipulation at any age is not without risk. Caution must be exercised with regard to neonatal administration of hCG, in that evidence obtained from an experimental rat micropenis model supports delaying hormonal therapy until the pubertal period (McMahon et al, 1995). However, in their study of boys with congenital hypogonadotropic hypogonadism and micropenis, **Bin-Abbas and colleagues (1999) concluded that one or two short courses of testosterone therapy in infancy and childhood (puberty) augmented adult penile size into the normal range.** These results refute the theoretical concern and experimental evidence that testosterone treatment in infancy or childhood impairs penile growth in adolescence and compromises adult penile length. **The conclusion that prepubertal exogenous testosterone administration does** *not* adversely affect ultimate penile growth has been supported by the study of men with true precocious puberty or congenital adrenal hyperplasia (Sutherland et al, 1996) and by the study of growth and androgen receptor status of testosterone-stimulated human fetal penile tissue in vitro (Baskin et al, 1997).

HISTORICAL ASPECTS OF HYPOSPADIAS REPAIR

Hauben (1984) credited Heliodor and Antyl (first, second, and third centuries AD) as the first to describe hypospadias and its surgical correction. Perhaps no surgical concern in history has inspired such widespread and varied opinion with regard to management as has hypospadias. From the earliest recorded description of hypospadias to the present, several hundred surgical approaches and/or variations on a theme have been described. Early contributors to the field of hypospadiology and a brief description of their contributions are listed in Table 65–2. In addition, several comprehensive accounts of historical aspects (Murphy, 1972; Hauben, 1984; Smith, 1997; Hodgson, 1999) and early technical reviews (Cecil, 1932; Young and Benjamin, 1948; Creevy, 1958; Backus and De Felice, 1960) regarding hypospadias are available.

GENERAL PRINCIPLES OF HYPOSPADIAS REPAIR

Regardless of the technique employed for repair of hypospadias and its associated defects, attention to penile curvature and its correction (orthoplasty), urethroplasty, meatoplasty and glanuloplasty, and finally skin coverage, are universal concerns.

Orthoplasty

Assessment of Penile Curvature

Preoperatively, the degree of penile curvature may be assessed in the infant or young boy who has an erection at the time of examination. A photograph taken at home during an erection in the adolescent or adult may also be very helpful in assessing penile curvature with or without hypospadias. Alternatively or adjunctively, **intraoperative assessment of penile curvature by either artificial or pharmacologic methods is a critical step in hypospadias repair and is typically performed after degloving of the penile shaft skin. A subjective impression or an objective (protractor) measurement** (Bologna et al, 1999) **of the observed curvature helps guide management.**

ARTIFICIAL ERECTION

Gittes and McLaughlin were the first to describe artificial erection as an aid to the evaluation of penile curvature (Gittes and McLaughlin, 1974). This technique has gained wide acceptance (Horton and Devine, 1977) and is depicted in Fig. 65–6*A*. **Injection of normal saline with a "butterfly" needle into the corpora** directly is performed

by insertion of the needle through the lateral aspect of one or the other corpora cavernosa. Alternatively, **the needle may be passed through the glans in order to decrease or eliminate the possibility of hematoma formation beneath Buck's fascia. It is important to note that the degree of curvature may vary with the force of injection or the method used to impede saline outflow.**

PHARMACOLOGIC ERECTION

Intracorporal injection of the arterial vasodilator prostaglandin E_1 (PGE_1) has been used for pharmacologic induction of erection during hypospadias repair (Perovic et al, 1997; Kogan, 2000). **Proponents of a pharmacologically induced erection argue that the physiologic erection allows for a more accurate and continued assessment of penile curvature before, during, and after its correction.** It would seem wise to defer use of the pharmacologic method if underlying neurologic pathology or injury is either known or suspected. Many options have been described for those requiring a penile straightening (orthoplasty) procedure.

Management of Penile Curvature with or without Hypospadias

Aside from simple release of skin tethering for correction of mild curvature, **penile curvature may be addressed with procedures that are carried out on either the dorsal, ventral, or lateral aspect of the penis. The site for orthoplasty and the specific technique employed are dictated by the direction and severity of curvature, by penile size, or both.** Except where indicated in the technique description, orthoplasty techniques may be performed on any surface of the penis. **Occasionally, repair of severe ventral curvature without hypospadias may require concomitant (interposition) urethroplasty to achieve lasting success.**

SKIN RELEASE AND TRANSFER

Penile skin may be the sole source or only a contributor to penile curvature (Smith, 1955) **or torsion** (Culp, 1966). In 1968, Allen and Spence observed this association with distal hypospadias, when on making a circumcising incision proximal to a coronal hypospadiac meatus they noted that freeing of penile shaft skin from the underlying urethra permitted penile straightening. As part of the repair, preputial skin was transposed ventrally. **King (1970) recognized the utility of this concept and incorporated it into tubularized urethroplasty and later summarized the concept of "cutaneous chordee"** (King, 1981). As summarized by Smith (1955), others have employed ventrally transposed, pedicled preputial skin as an aid to correction of penile curvature in two-stage correction of severe hypospadias. A similar technique has been described for correction of minor penile curvature without hypospadias (Allen and Roehrborn, 1993).

PLICATING AND HEINEKE-MIKULICZ TECHNIQUES

Nesbit (1965) described removing "vertical elliptical segments" of tunica albuginea (transversely oriented)

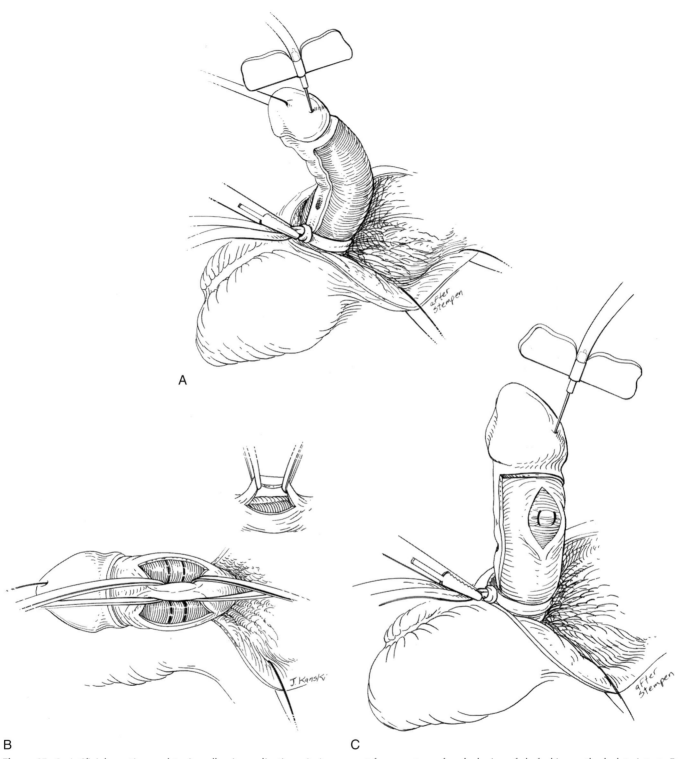

A

B

C

Figure 65–6. Artificial erection and tunica albuginea plication. *A,* Assessment for curvature after degloving of shaft skin, urethral plate intact. *B,* Neurovascular bundles isolated and elevated. Proposed parallel lines of incision bilaterally are opposite point of maximal curvature. *C,* Outer edges of incisions have been approximated, and both the intervening strip of tunica albuginea and the knots are buried. (Modified from Baskin LS, Duckett JW: Dorsal tunica albuginea plication (TAP) for hypospadias curvature. J Urol 1994;151:1668, with permission.)

from the disproportionately longer, convex aspect of the penis in order to correct curvature. Another method for correcting the disparity in tunica albuginea length consists of lengthening the shorter concave surface by using the Heineke-Mikulicz principle (Udall, 1980). Several transverse incisions in the tunica are closed longitudinally

to achieve lengthening of the concave aspect of the penis (Saalfeld et al, 1973). The Nesbit and Heineke-Mikulicz techniques can be used simultaneously on opposing aspects of the curvature (Udall, 1980). Either the Nesbit technique or simple dorsal plicating sutures may be used to repair the "glans tilt" deformity. Cross-hatched incisions of the corpora cavernosa followed by simple plicating sutures has been described as a successful orthoplasty technique (Perovic et al, 1998). **Multiple parallel plicating sutures placed opposite the site of maximal curvature is a more recently reported technique that has become the preferred method for the treatment of penile curvature by the reporting authors** (Baskin and Lue, 1998). Interestingly, Nesbit had repaired one patient with plicating sutures only, and on recurrence of curvature at 6 months developed the technique for which he has become famous (Nesbit, 1965).

TUNICA ALBUGINEA PLICATION

Initially described by Baskin and colleagues (Baskin and Duckett, 1994), **the tunica albuginea plication has become a popular technique for correction of penile curvature** (Klevmark et al, 1994). **After degloving the penile shaft of its skin, the neurovascular bundles are dissected free from the surface of the corpora cavernosa bilaterally** (see Fig. 65–6). Vessel loops are placed around the neurovascular bundles to elevate them away from the corpora during plication. **Parallel lines of incision approximately 1 cm in length and 0.5 to 1 cm apart are marked bilaterally on the anterolateral surface of the tunica albuginea, directly opposite the point of maximal penile curvature.** The tunica albuginea is incised at these sites with a fine knife. A tourniquet placed at the base of the penis decreases blood loss and optimizes visualization during this procedure. **After incision, the outer edges of the parallel incisions are approximated with 4-0 polydioxanone suture with simple interrupted technique and inverting of the knot. This technique buries the intervening strip of tunica albuginea and shortens the disproportionately long corporal surface, thus correcting the opposing penile curvature.**

CORPORAL ROTATION

Corporal rotation, achieved via a ventral, midline longitudinal incision alone, was described by Koff and Eakins (1984) for correction of ventral penile curvature in a hypospadiac patient. **Medial rotation and suture fixation of the dorsal aspect of both corpora cavernosa has been described for management of severe curvature. This may be performed with** (Snow, 1989) **or without** (Kass, 1993) **simultaneous longitudinal incision of the corporal septum in the ventral midline.** Decter (1999) described a similar technique for correction of ventral curvature in severe hypospadias in which, after urethral plate division, the septum between the corpora cavernosa is partially split with a ventral midline incision. This incision and freeing of the neurovascular bundles on the dorsal aspect of the corpora cavernosa facilitate medial rotation of the dorsal aspect of the corpora. Nonabsorbable sutures are placed in the area of maximal convex curvature from the dorsolateral aspect of one corpus cavernosum across the midline to the other side, so that the corpora are rotated toward the dorsal midline. **The corporal rotation technique allows one-stage reconstruction while achieving or maintaining maximal penile length.**

DERMAL GRAFT

The dermal graft has been used extensively for repair of significant penile curvature (Devine and Horton, 1975; Hendren and Keating, 1988; Hendren and Caesar, 1992; Horton et al, 1993; Pope et al, 1996; Lindgren et al, 1998). **This orthoplasty technique is ideal for the short phallus with severe penile curvature, for which the Nesbit wedge or tunica albuginea plications may be inadequate to correct the curvature or may further shorten the phallus to an unacceptable degree.** After assessing the degree of curvature, the dermal graft is harvested from a nonhair-bearing donor site, typically in the groin (Fig. 65–7). The donor site is marked in an elliptical shape at a length slightly longer than the ventral defect to be created by transverse linear corporotomy. The donor site is then injected with saline below the dermis to ease dissection after incision of the skin. Silk stay sutures placed in both corners of the graft facilitate its sharp dissection. The graft is then defatted and placed in saline. **A transverse incision is made at the site of maximal curvature (concavity) and the dermal graft is anastomosed to the edges of the corporal defect** with a running simple suture of 6-0 polyglactin.

TUNICA VAGINALIS GRAFT

Use of a tunica vaginalis free graft as a ventral corporal patch orthoplasty technique was reported by Perlmutter and colleagues (1985) for repair of severe curvature in 11 boys with chordee and hypospadias. Only one patient had "some degree" of ventral angulation on follow-up ranging from 2 to 37 months. Others have reported a 91% success rate at 33 months mean follow-up for correction of curvature with a tunica vaginalis patch graft as the first stage (orthoplasty) of a two-stage repair of severe hypospadias (Stewart et al, 1995).

TOTAL PENILE DISASSEMBLY

A radical approach of penile disassembly and corporoplasty was described by Perovic and colleagues (1998). According to these authors, the total penile disassembly technique is ideal for correction of (1) glans tilt, (2) ventral curvature without hypospadias (neourethral tube interposed as needed), and (3) curvature with hypospadias. They also reported that the total penile disassembly technique corrects curvature without the need for placement of an interposition corporal graft, thus minimizing the work of straightening the penis and lengthening the urethra in those patients with associated hypospadias (Perovic et al, 1998).

Urethroplasty

Neourethral Formation

Several basic principles and techniques govern successful urethroplasty during hypospadias repair. Among these is the term *tissue transfer,* **which implies the movement of tissues for the purpose of reconstruction. Techniques for urethroplasty typically use immediately**

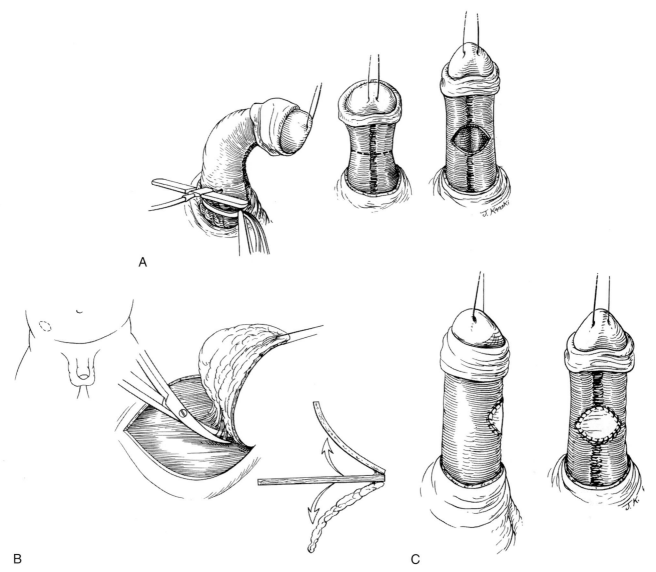

Figure 65–7. Dermal graft. *A,* Degree of curvature is noted with artificial erection and a transverse incision has been made at the site of maximal curvature. *B,* Isolation of elliptical dermal graft from nonhair-bearing donor site. Graft is then defatted. *C,* Dermal graft sutured to the edges of the defect. (From Retik AB: Proximal hypospadias. In Marshall FF [ed]: Textbook of Operative Urology. Philadelphia, WB Saunders, 1996, with permission.)

adjacent tissue, local tissue flaps, free grafts of genital or extragenital tissue, or some combination of these.

IMMEDIATELY ADJACENT TISSUE

The neourethra may be formed via reconfiguration of tissue immediately juxtaposed to the hypospadiac meatus and/or along the path of proposed urethroplasty. This may be the least risky and least technically challenging of all forms of urethroplasty. An example would be simple tubularization of the urethral plate.

LOCAL TISSUE FLAPS

Although immediately adjacent tissue is moved to some degree when it is incorporated into urethroplasty, in other techniques specific local penile or other genital tissue may be transferred to the penile ventrum to be used in the

urethroplasty or another component of hypospadias repair. **The term *flap* implies that the tissue used is excised and transferred with its vasculature preserved or surgically reestablished at the recipient site** (Jordan, 1999a, 1999b). Tissue flaps may be classified by their vascularity. A *random* flap does not have a defined cutaneous vascular territory. **The term *axial* flap implies the presence of specific, defined vasculature in the base of the flap.** With regard to elevation technique, another means of flap classification, the vascular and cutaneous continuity of the flap remains intact in a *peninsula* flap, whereas **the term *island* flap implies maintenance of vascular and division of cutaneous continuity** (Jordan, 1999b).

Local tissue flaps used for urethral reconstruction must be thin, nonhirsute, and reliably tailored. These flaps are properly termed *fasciocutaneous* flaps, and the extended fascial system is called the dartos fascia (Jordan, 1999b). **The vessels of the fasciocutaneous flap are**

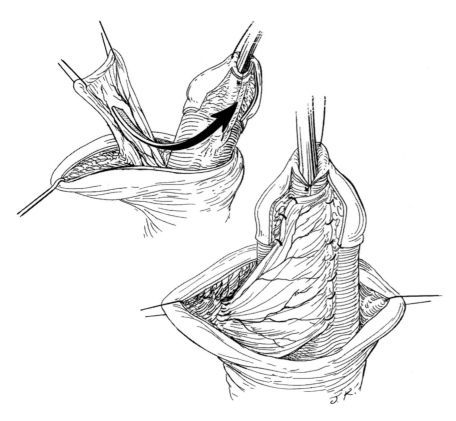

Figure 65–8. Second layer coverage of neourethra with subcutaneous (dartos) tissue flap harvested from lateral or dorsal penile shaft and repositioned ventrally over the neourethra. (From Retik AB, Borer JG: Primary and reoperative hypospadias repair with the Snodgrass technique. World J Urol 1998;16:186, with permission.)

preserved within the fascia, which provides a conduit for smaller arteries and veins. Axial blood supply and drainage are typically provided by branches of the deep and superficial external pudendal vessels, which are medial branches of the femoral vessels (Hinman, 1991; Jordan, 1999b; Standoli, 1988).

LOCAL OR EXTRAGENITAL FREE GRAFTS

The term *graft* implies that tissue has been excised from one location and transferred to a graft host bed, where a new blood supply develops by a process called "take" (Jordan, 1999b). As with all free grafts, a well-vascularized recipient site is crucial for optimal graft survival. The initial phase of take, called *imbibition*, relies on diffusion of nutrient material from the adjacent graft host bed into the graft and requires approximately 48 hours. This is followed by the second phase of take, *inosculation*, which is the formation of new and permanent vascularization of the graft and also requires approximately 48 hours (Jordan, 1999b).

Neourethral Coverage (Second Layer)

SUBCUTANEOUS (DARTOS) FLAP

Second-layer coverage of the neourethra with the use of various vascularized flaps has significantly decreased urethrocutaneous fistula as a complication of hypospadias repair (Smith, 1973; Churchill et al, 1996; Belman, 1988; Retik et al, 1988). As previously described by Retik and colleagues (Retik et al, 1988, Retik et al, 1994), the dorsal prepuce is unfolded and the underlying dartos layer

is sharply dissected to the base of the penis and then incised longitudinally in the midline (Fig. 65–8). One side of the flap or, alternatively, a dartos flap raised from the lateral penile shaft skin is then brought around to the ventral aspect of the penis and secured over the neourethra with simple interrupted fine absorbable suture. **Glans wings must be incised deeply to accommodate this additional tissue cover of the neourethra.**

TUNICA VAGINALIS

Tunica vaginalis tissue may be used as an alternative for second-layer coverage of the neourethra (Kirkali, 1990; Snow, 1986, Snow et al, 1995) (Fig. 65–9). Before tunica vaginalis coverage, the inferolateral border of the neourethral mesentery may be advanced over the edges of the neourethra as a buttress. The testis to be used as the donor of tunica vaginalis is delivered into the operative field and isolated from its scrotal attachments. The tunica vaginalis is incised, and an appropriate width of flap is isolated from the testis and widely mobilized on its own vascular pedicle. (Tunica vaginalis is harvested similarly for corporal patch graft orthoplasty.) The tunica vaginalis flap is then secured over the neourethra by placement of simple interrupted sutures, and the testicle is replaced in the scrotum.

CORPUS SPONGIOSUM

Paraurethral (spongiosal) tissue approximation in the midline as a second cover of the initial suture line was initially described by van Horn and Kass (1995) as an

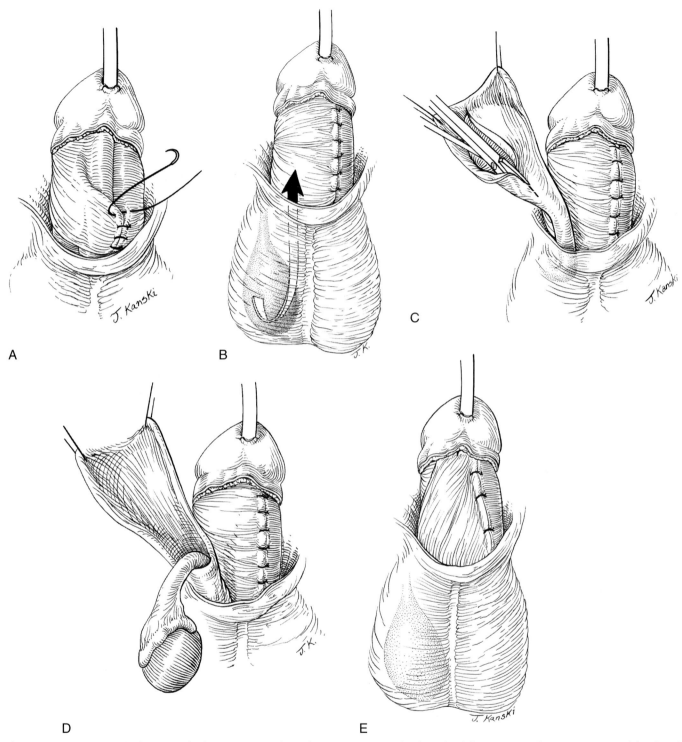

A

B

C

D

E

Figure 65–9. Tunica vaginalis neourethral coverage. (Performed over mesentery of onlay island flap repair in this case.) *A*, Lateral border of onlay or tube pedicle may be advanced as a second layer of neourethral coverage. *B*, Testis to be delivered for harvest of tunica vaginalis as supplemental or sole source for second layer coverage. *C*, Harvest of tunica vaginalis. *D*, Isolation of flap from testis and distal spermatic cord. *E*, Tunica vaginalis has been secured over the neourethra. (From Retik AB: Proximal hypospadias. In Marshall FF [ed]: Textbook of Operative Urology. Philadelphia, WB Saunders, 1996, with permission.)

adjunct to distal hypospadias repair. In a recent cohort repaired with this technique, the complication rate was 1.7% for distal and 7.7% for midshaft hypospadias repair (Kass and Chung, 2000). Similarly, Yerkes and colleagues (2000) described mobilizing distal spongiosum lateral to

the open urethra along with the urethral plate away from the corpora cavernosa, subsequently wrapping it around various types of urethroplasty for distal hypospadias in order to prevent fistula formation. In 25 patients with follow-up of longer than 1 year, there were no urethrocutaneous fistulas. **The distal wrap of corpus spongiosum appears to avoid fistula formation without causing residual or recurrent curvature.**

Meatoplasty and Glanuloplasty

These two components of hypospadias repair are discussed together because, for the most part, successful completion of one is intimately dependent on the other. Although nuances of glanuloplasty and meatoplasty are typically discussed in relation to specific hypospadias repair techniques, some principles may have more broad application. In 1977, Devine and Horton described the "V-flap" glanuloplasty as an adjunct to tubularized skin graft urethroplasty. This technique involves extensive dissection of the glans penis with development of a midline, anteriorly based flap of glans epithelium. Underlying subepithelial tissue is removed from the glans flap, and the flap is fixed to the tunica of the corpora cavernosa, consistently fashioning a widely patent, complication-free meatus. Others have incorporated a glanular "W-shaped" flap meatoplasty with urethroplasty (Sensöz et al, 1997).

Penile Shaft Skin Coverage

Various techniques have been employed for the purpose of completing hypospadias with adequate skin coverage of the penis. These techniques have included **ventral transfer of preputial skin either with a buttonhole through the skin for through passage of the glans penis** (Ombredanne, 1932; Nesbit, 1941) **or a midline longitudinal split of the prepuce or dorsal penile skin followed by lateral transfer of the skin on either side of the penis for ventral coverage** (Thiersch, 1869; Byars, 1951; Mustarde, 1965).

SPECIAL CONSIDERATIONS: PERIOPERATIVE

Timing (Age at Repair)

In 1975, an ad hoc committee of the American Academy of Pediatrics, composed of urologists and pediatricians, concluded that the optimal time for surgery, from a psychological perspective, was during the fourth or fifth year of life (Kelalis et al, 1975). Then, in 1979, Lepore and Kesler reported a prospective study of boys undergoing hypospadias repair between 2 and 6 years of age. They noted a distinctive pattern of postoperative behavior characterized by anger, aggression, and negative interactions, compared with children undergoing other types of surgery. This and other studies that followed (Manley and Epstein, 1981; Schultz et al, 1983) prompted **a more recent review of the subject by the American Academy of Pediatrics** (Kass et al, 1996). **In this report, as a result of a combination of factors including an improved understanding of the psychological implications of genital surgery in children, improvement in the technical aspects of surgery for hypospadias, and advances in pediatric anesthesia, it was suggested that "the best time for surgery**

for hypospadias is between 6 and 12 months of age." Hypospadias repair before 1 year of age is the current standard. Results of a recent report by Hensle and colleagues (2001) suggest a significantly higher complication rate for hypospadias repair in older patients, further supporting the benefit of repair at a younger age.

Anesthesia
General

General anesthesia, typically with endotracheal intubation, has been the mainstay of anesthetic technique for hypospadias repair. General anesthesia provides uninterrupted performance of the repair without concern for patient movement or sensation of pain. Adjunctive analgesia in the form of long-acting injectable agents, delivered via a caudal route or as a penile block, has proved safe and efficacious.

Local and Regional

A popular agent for adjunctive analgesia is bupivacaine hydrochloride (0.25%), administered as a caudal or penile block. Bupivacaine given in this manner at the beginning of hypospadias repair allows time for onset of action during the planning and preliminary stages of the repair. Newer concepts regarding perioperative analgesia administration have been reported by Chhibber and colleagues (1997). Patients undergoing outpatient hypospadias repair were randomly assigned to receive a penile block with the same total dose of bupivacaine at the completion of surgery, before the incision, or both before and at the completion of surgery. **A statistically significant improvement in postoperative pain control was noted for those patients who received a penile block both at the beginning and at completion of hypospadias repair, compared with the other groups** (Chhibber et al, 1997).

Antibiotics

In general, perioperative antibiotics are not indicated for routine outpatient hypospadias repair. However, **one intravenous dose of a broad-spectrum antibiotic may be indicated for those in whom the urethra is catheterized intraoperatively.** We prefer administration of a prophylactic antibiotic during use and for several days beyond removal of an indwelling urethral catheter. Preferential use of perioperative antibiotics has been described by others (Winslow and Devine, 1996).

Hemostasis

Based on the hypothesis that some complications (e.g., urethrocutaneous fistula, repair breakdown) are in part a result of ischemic tissue necrosis, use of electrocautery should be limited during hypospadias repair, if it is used at all (Zaontz, 1990). **The current of monopolar cautery is dispersed to the remote grounding site, usually along the vessels, and in this way may irrepara-**

bly damage tissue microvasculature (Jordan, 1999). Others employing electrocautery prefer the bipolar variant and the use of fine-point neurologic forceps (Winslow and Devine, 1996). **We favor injection of a vasoconstrictive agent (epinephrine diluted 1:200,000 with lidocaine [Xylocaine]) deep to proposed glanular incisions, as well as intermittent use of a tourniquet** at the base of the penis during urethroplasty. Other options **for effective temporary hemostasis without permanent tissue devitalization** include intermittent compression with gauze soaked in iced saline or epinephrine solution or both.

Optical Magnification

Wacksman (1987) reported that a new microscope (mouth-controlled operating room microscope) compared favorably to loupe magnification and allowed use of small sutures with great accuracy. Shapiro (1989) compared the results of hypospadias repair using 3.5× magnification (loupes) and using the Zeiss reconstruction microscope. There was no significant difference in outcome, and Shapiro's prediction that the microscope would be used more often in the repair of hypospadias in the future does not appear to have come to fruition.

Sutures and Suture Technique

Stay sutures are used whenever possible to limit tissue handling. Delicate forceps with fine teeth may limit crushing of tissues when handling is necessary. Typically, a subcuticular technique is employed during longitudinal closure of the neourethra when performing a tubularization technique. **Perhaps the most important aspect of closure of the neourethra is the exact placement of each suture such that the edge of the epithelial surface is inverted and the raw surfaces of the subepithelial tissue are approximated.** Healing then provides a "watertight" anastomotic suture line that, at least theoretically, decreases the risk of urethrocutaneous fistula formation. However, Hakim and coworkers (1996) reported that the technique, either subcuticular or full thickness, did not affect results provided the suture used was of polyglactin composition. In contrast, Ulman and colleagues documented a statistically significant lower fistula rate (4.9% versus 16.6%) for subcuticular compared with full-thickness technique (Ulman et al, 1997). **DiSandro and Palmer (1996) reported a fourfold increase in urethral stricture rate after hypospadias repair with polydioxanone suture compared with chromic or polyglycolic acid suture.**

Laser Techniques

Although its use in hypospadias repair is not popular as yet, Scherr and Poppas (1998) have published an exhaustive review of current laser technology. **Kirsch and colleagues (1997) updated their experience with the use of laser-tissue welding for urethral surgery,** either as an adjunct to suturing in 25 patients or as the primary means of tissue approximation in 11. Preoperative diagnoses included hypospadias, urethral stricture, urethral diverticulum,

and urethral fistulas. With follow-up ranging from 3 months to 3 years, no strictures or diverticula developed. Overall, five patients developed fistulas between 2 weeks and 6 months postoperatively. Among those patients with hypospadias, the meatus was scrotal or penoscrotal in four. Two urethrocutaneous fistulas developed after sutureless, reoperative urethroplasty, including one after traumatic catheterization for urinary retention. **In the initial experience (Kirsch et al, 1996), the overall complication rate using laser soldering was 19%, with one half of the complications occurring in reoperative repairs. More recently, the fistula rate was 14% overall and 6% for primary cases** (Kirsch et al, 1996). The application of protein solders, temperature control, and chromophore control have improved the safety and efficacy of the laser-tissue welding process, and report of a randomized, prospective study is expected.

Neourethral Intubation

Another source of controversy in hypospadias repair is the use or omission of postoperative urethral catheterization. Stressing the importance of a watertight urethroplasty, Rabinowitz (1987) performed Mathieu hypospadias repair without urethral catheter drainage or urinary diversion in 59 boys, achieving excellent cosmetic and functional results with few complications. **In a multicenter report combining the experience of four institutions** (Hakim et al, 1996), **excellent results were obtained in 96.7% of 336 patients repaired with the Mathieu technique** as modified by Rabinowitz (1987). Complications occurred in 11 patients and consisted of urethrocutaneous fistula in 9, meatal retraction in 1, and meatal stenosis in 1. **Results were not affected by urethral catheterization status.** In a prospective, randomized study, McCormack and colleagues (1993) found no difference in outcome when comparing 19 boys with urinary diversion and indwelling urethral catheter versus 16 boys without, all of whom underwent Mathieu hypospadias repair. Further experience with limited use of a urethral catheter in more than 200 patients undergoing Mathieu hypospadias repair was reported by Retik and colleagues (1994), who noted a complication rate of 0.98% and no urethrocutaneous fistulas.

Others report rates of urethrocutaneous fistula formation and meatal stenosis twofold greater in patients with a urethral catheter compared with those diverted suprapubicly after hypospadias repair (Demirbilek and Atayurt, 1997). **Based on these results and those for the more extensively studied Mathieu repair, there does not appear to be an advantage to or necessity for use of a urethral catheter after some hypospadias repairs.** This may be true for some of the more recently described techniques as well (Steckler and Zaontz, 1997).

Dressing

An ideal penile dressing should be nonadherent, slightly absorbent and compressive, and yet somewhat elastic and soft to allow for slight swelling. In order to achieve these goals, several different dressing techniques have been described (Cromie and Bellinger, 1981). In

1982, De Sy and Oosterlinck (1982) described a soft, pliable foam dressing, the "silicone foam elastomer," as a significant improvement in postoperative penile dressing. Elastomer and catalyst are mixed, and the sterile foam is molded around the penis. This dressing appears to be well tolerated and is easily removed in 4 to 6 days. This silicone foam elastomer has been used in conjunction with a pantaloon spica cast for postoperative immobilization after free graft hypospadias repair (Cilento et al, 1997). Although the urethrocutaneous fistula rate was similar to previous experience, this method of postoperative care significantly reduced the hospitalization time and cost.

In two prospective randomized trials, it was shown that there is little or no advantage to the application of a dressing to the operated hypospadias (McLorie et al, 1999; Van Savage et al, 2000). Patients were randomly assigned to receive either transparent film dressing, elastic wrap dressing, or no dressing. Antibiotic ointment was used to coat the penis in those receiving "no dressing." **The method of postoperative care (dressing versus no dressing) did not affect surgical success rate or wound healing. In general, a regimen of no dressing appears to result in increased patient comfort and decreased burden for the caregiver.**

Postoperative Penile Erection and Bladder Spasm

Stock and Kaplan (1995) reported use of ketoconazole as a reliable method for preventing postoperative penile erections after penile surgery in eight patients ranging in age from 14 to 42 years. **Ketoconazole reduces adrenal and testicular androgen production through the inhibition of 17,20-desmolase, thereby preventing the conversion of cholesterol to testosterone. Hepatotoxicity is a recognized side effect of ketoconazole.** The authors recommended obtaining liver function tests before starting therapy, on day 3 of therapy, and after completion of therapy. **Amyl nitrite has also been used to prevent penile erections** (Horton and Horton, 1988). Judicious use of anticholinergic medication has been described for postoperative bladder spasm in stented patients (Horton and Horton, 1988; Minevich et al, 1999). Follow-up schedule and length of follow-up are specific to surgeon preference but in general should be at least 6 to 12 months for successful repairs (Caldamone and Diamond, 1999).

INTRAOPERATIVE ALGORITHM

At surgery, the decision-making process for determining an appropriate repair for a given defect begins with a general assessment of native meatal location, penile size and curvature, and characteristics of ventral, proximal shaft skin (Fig. 65–10). Occasionally, it may be necessary to longitudinally incise ventral, deficient skin and urethral tissue proximal to the hypospadiac meatus in order to incorporate healthy, well-developed tissue at the proximal extent of the repair (Fig. 65–11).

The penile shaft is degloved of its skin with care taken to preserve the urethral plate in all but the most severe (scrotal and perineal) defects. **Assessment and manage-**

ment of penile curvature (as previously discussed) follows and is perhaps the most important aspect of any hypospadias repair. In general, both the level of the hypospadiac meatus and the severity of penile curvature dictate appropriate repair options. Usually, anterior, middle, and some proximal hypospadias are amenable to repair by preservation of the urethral plate, dorsal orthoplasty procedure as needed, and then one of several appropriate urethroplasty techniques discussed in detail later in this chapter.

The use of well-vascularized local tissue is preferred for urethroplasty. The most distal defects are typically repaired with one of several advancement techniques. However, in instances where simple advancement is not sufficient or appropriate, defects may be managed with various tubularization or flap techniques. Defects with a deep glanular groove and a phallus (including urethral plate) with sufficient width are perhaps amenable to a simple tubularization technique. However, if the glanular groove is shallow or the urethral plate is narrow, or both, a midline, longitudinal incision of the urethral plate may allow neourethral tubularization free of tension.

Various perimeatal-based flap techniques using ventral, proximal shaft skin may also be employed in the setting of a shallow glanular groove and narrow urethral plate, provided the proximal extent of the flap does not include hair-bearing skin. However, perimeatal-based flaps may not be favored secondary to inferior meatal cosmesis and flap vascularity relative to other repairs. In the setting of a small phallus that is inadequate in width for tubularization alone or with an adjunctive midline, longitudinal incision of the urethral plate, and in the specific case of a conical (convex ventral) glans with a shallow groove, an onlay technique may be preferred. **Thus far, preferable technical options assume either absent, mild, or moderate penile curvature (amenable to dorsal orthoplasty techniques) and allow preservation of the urethral plate and its incorporation into the neourethra.**

For more proximal defects, with mild to moderate curvature, dorsal orthoplasty techniques may be sufficient, allowing preservation of the urethral plate and performance of one of several tubularization or flap urethroplasty techniques. **In some proximal hypospadias cases, the associated curvature is severe and the urethral plate may have a tethering effect on the penis, being at least in part responsible for the observed curvature. In this setting, with or without a relatively small penis, it may be necessary to divide the urethral plate (i.e., incise it transversely at the distal extent) and then to dissect the urethral plate proximally off the ventral aspect of the corpora cavernosa to the level of the meatus. Curvature, if persistent, may then be corrected with placement of a ventral interposition graft (ventral orthoplasty technique) before urethroplasty** performed via tubularization of either pedicled local skin, a free graft of local or extragenital tissue, or, alternatively, a two-stage repair.

PRIMARY HYPOSPADIAS REPAIR

There is no single, universally applicable technique for hypospadias repair. Several well established tech-

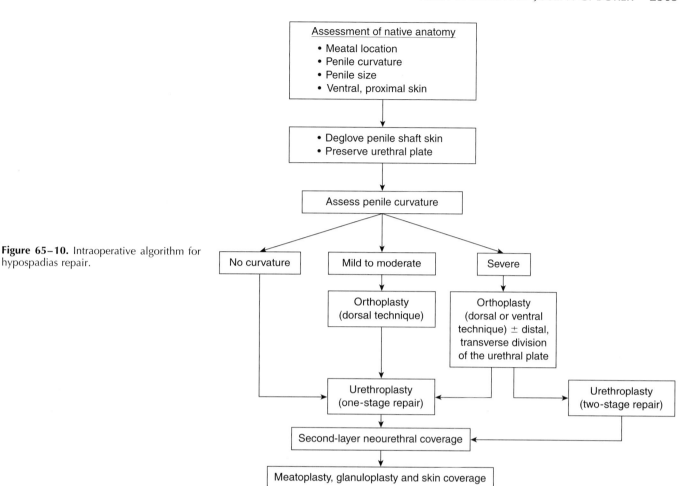

Figure 65–10. Intraoperative algorithm for hypospadias repair.

niques exist for the repair of all hypospadias defects with which the surgeon is presented. A discussion of various currently popular techniques for hypospadias level follows. Techniques listed and discussed are intended to be neither exhaustive nor exclusive for the level of hypospadias described. Generalizations are presented with the expectation of overlap and/or exclusion of technique applicability for a given defect based on surgeon preference and case-specific anatomy. Included in the discussion are specifics of technique, from our experience, for several of the most commonly performed repairs.

Anterior Hypospadias Procedures

Advancement Techniques

Glanular and some coronal hypospadias defects are amenable to the meatoplasty and glanuloplasty (MAGPI) technique (Fig. 65–12), with excellent functional and cosmetic results provided there is adequate urethral mobility and no penile curvature (Duckett, 1981; Duckett and Snyder, 1992; Park et al, 1995). The MAGPI technique is performed by first making a circumferential incision 5 to 7 mm proximal and parallel to the corona of the glans and proximal to the hypospadiac meatus. If present, the typical transverse glanular tissue "bridge" in the urethral plate that separates the hypospadiac meatus and distal glanular groove is incised longitudinally.

The incised tissue edges are then approximated transversely in Heineke-Mikulicz fashion. This single step obliterates the tissue bridge and advances the meatus slightly. The ventral edge of meatus is pulled distally with the aid of a stay suture placed in the midline, and the medial edges of the glans are then trimmed before midline approximation in two layers. Approximation of the glans and skin with simple interrupted fine absorbable suture completes the repair.

Another successful technique for the repair of glanular and coronal defects is a modification of the MAGPI **technique described by Arap** and colleagues (1984). According to these authors, incorporation of urethroplasty (distal tubularization) with meatal advancement and glanuloplasty enables treatment of the more severe cases of distal hypospadias. Proponents of other modifications on the theme of **distal urethral advancement and glanuloplasty** have reported long-term success rates of 95% or greater and low reoperation rates of 2% (Harrison and Grobbelaar, 1997) and 5% (Caione et al, 1997).

Distal urethral **circumferential dissection and advancement** was first described by Beck in 1898 for repair of distal hypospadias. Taken to the extreme, the principle of urethral advancement may gain 2 to 2.5 cm of urethral length in children, with mobilization of the urethra to the bulbar level using the **bulbar elongation anastomotic meatoplasty (BEAM)** procedure for hypospadiac urethroplasty (Turner-Warwick et al, 1997). According to Turner-Warwick and colleagues, this degree of mobilization is necessary to prevent the formation of penile curvature.

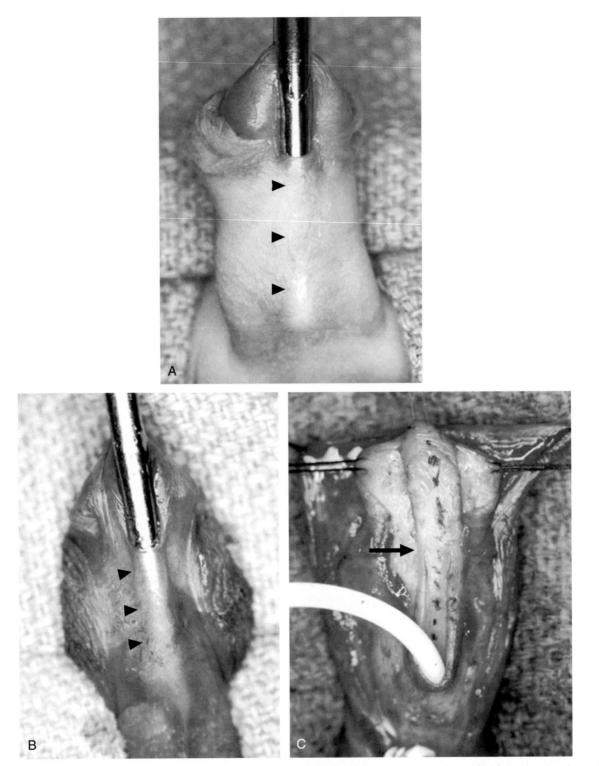

Figure 65–11. Ventral skin proximal to the hypospadiac meatus is evaluated for thickness/integrity prior to deciding on reparative technique. Note urethral sound passed into meatus. *A,* Thick, healthy skin overlying urethra *(arrowheads)* proximal to hypospadiac meatus. *B,* Thin, near transparent skin and urethra *(arrowheads)* proximal to meatus prior to midline incision. *C,* Same patient as in *B* following midline incision proximally from site of the native meatus *(arrow)* to the point of encountering healthy tissue in preparation for urethroplasty. Note catheter within neomeatus. The urethral plate has been outlined with incisions and marked in the midline with a longitudinal dotted line (see *Fig. 65–13C–G*).

Tubularization Techniques

Thiersch (1869) and Duplay (1880) were the initial descriptors of the simple urethral plate tubularization technique that has come to be known as the Thiersch-

Duplay urethroplasty. Several techniques, including that **described by King** (1970, 1981), employ tubularization of the urethral plate for repair of distal hypospadias. The **glans approximation procedure (GAP)** described by Zaontz (1989), is an ideal repair for glanular and coronal

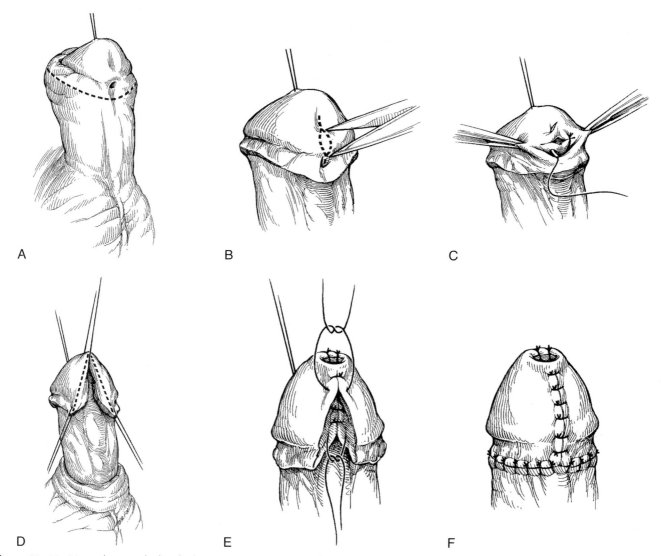

A   B   C

D   E   F

Figure 65–12. Meatoplasty and glanuloplasty (MAGPI). *A,* Circumferential subcoronal incision is marked. *B,* Longitudinal incision, and *C,* transverse approximation (Heineke-Mikulicz procedure) of transverse glanular "bridge" in urethral plate. *D,* Ventral edge of meatus is pulled distally and medial glans "trimming" incisions are marked. *E,* Deep suture approximation of the glans. *F,* Superficial approximation of the glans and skin. (From Duckett JW: Hypospadias. In Walsh PC, Retik AB, Vaughan ED Jr, Wein AJ [eds]: Campbell's Urology, 7th ed, vol 2. Philadelphia, WB Saunders, 1998, pp 2093–2119, with permission.)

defects with a deep glanular groove. This technique has excellent functional and cosmetic results. **A study involving more than 500 repairs with the combined use of the Heineke-Mikulicz meatoplasty and the GAP reported a complication and reoperation rate of only 2.1% for the entire group** (Stock and Hanna, 1997). **Glanuloplasty and in situ tubularization** of the urethral plate has been touted as an excellent technique for distal and midshaft hypospadias (van Horn and Kass, 1995). In a recent cohort of patients repaired with this technique, the complication rate decreased to 1.7% for distal and 7.7% for midshaft hypospadias repair (Kass and Chung, 2000).

A modification of the Thiersch-Duplay technique was described by Snodgrass (1994). The tubularized incised plate (TIP) urethroplasty, combines modifications of the previously described techniques of urethral plate incision (Rich et al, 1989) **and tubularization** (Thiersch, 1869; Duplay, 1880). **The concept of a urethral plate "relaxing incision" as an adjunct to hypospadias repair**

that allows tension-free neourethral tubularization was also described simultaneously by Perovic and Vukadinovic (1994). Since that initial description for use in distal hypospadias repair, additional experience using the TIP urethroplasty technique for distal and more proximal defects has been reported by several centers (Snodgrass et al, 1996; Snodgrass et al, 1998; Ross and Kay, 1997; Steckler and Zaontz, 1997; Retik and Borer, 1998; Decter and Franzoni, 1999). Excellent results have also been reported for TIP urethroplasty in reoperative and complex hypospadias repairs (Snodgrass et al, 1996; Retik and Borer, 1998; Borer et al, 2001). **Complication rates of approximately 2% to 5% have been reported for primary hypospadias repair with the TIP urethroplasty technique.**

Modifications to the TIP urethroplasty technique have been previously described (Retik and Borer, 1998; Borer and Retik, 1999) and are summarized here (Fig. 65–13). After stay suture placement in the glans, the urethral plate is outlined at a width of approximately 7 to 9 mm, depend-

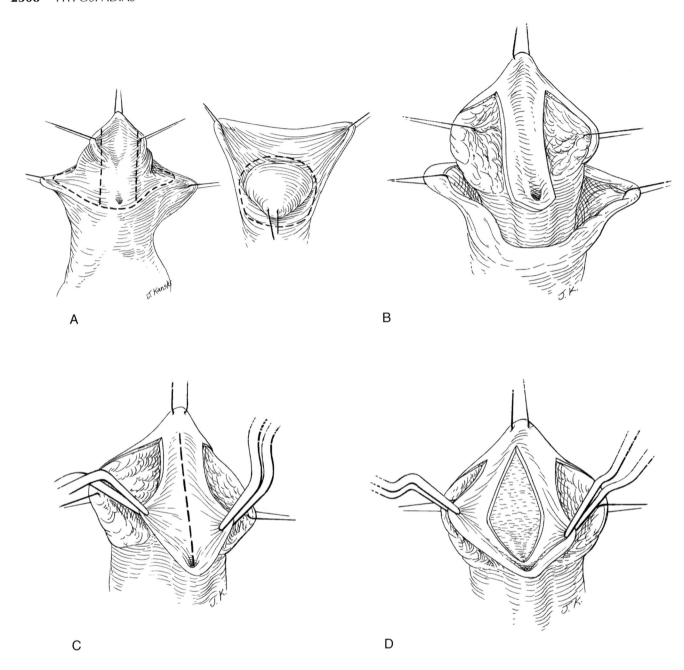

Figure 65–13. Tubularized incised plate (TIP) urethroplasty in distal, primary hypospadias repair. *A,* Stay sutures are placed, and proposed urethral plate demarcating and circumferential incisions are marked. *B,* Parallel longitudinal and circumferential incisions have been made. *C,* Proposed longitudinal line of incision in the midline of the urethral plate. *D,* Urethral plate has been incised.

ing on the size of the phallus. Dilute epinephrine is injected deep to the proposed sites of incision, and parallel longitudinal incisions demarcating the urethral plate are made from the tip of the glans to the hypospadiac meatus. A transverse incision across the skin overlying the urethra completes the U-shaped incision outlining the urethral plate. A circumferential incision 5 to 7 mm proximal to the coronal margin is extended from each longitudinal incision, followed by degloving of the penile shaft skin. Orthoplasty is performed as needed, with paired dorsal tunica albuginea plications.

The *first* critical point in the TIP urethroplasty in-

volves a longitudinal midline incision of the urethral plate from the tip of the penis to, as necessary, the level of the hypospadiac meatus. The depth of the urethral plate incision depends primarily on the configuration of the glans and the glanular groove. With the aid of a tourniquet, the urethral plate is then tubularized over a No. 6 Fr Silastic catheter with a running subcuticular fine polyglactin suture. The *second* critical point involves the fashioning of a wide meatus. Second-layer coverage of the neourethra with a well-vascularized subcutaneous (dartos) tissue flap, harvested from the dorsal preputial and shaft skin, is the *third* critical aspect of the TIP

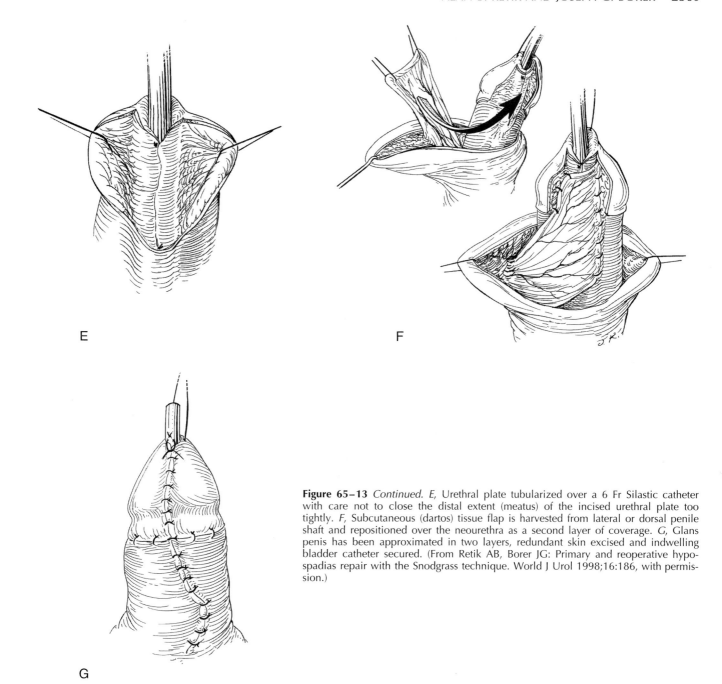

E

F

G

Figure 65–13 *Continued. E,* Urethral plate tubularized over a 6 Fr Silastic catheter with care not to close the distal extent (meatus) of the incised urethral plate too tightly. *F,* Subcutaneous (dartos) tissue flap is harvested from lateral or dorsal penile shaft and repositioned over the neourethra as a second layer of coverage. *G,* Glans penis has been approximated in two layers, redundant skin excised and indwelling bladder catheter secured. (From Retik AB, Borer JG: Primary and reoperative hypospadias repair with the Snodgrass technique. World J Urol 1998;16:186, with permission.)

urethroplasty. **For more proximal repairs, a tunica vaginalis flap may be used for this purpose.** The glans wings are then approximated without tension in two layers, the indwelling Silastic urethral catheter is secured to the glans penis, and skin coverage completes the repair. The TIP urethroplasty technique is performed similarly for previously circumcised boys and for more proximal defects (see Fig. 65–11C), and it results in a normal appearing penis with a "slit-like," vertically oriented meatus.

Flap Techniques

Among the more commonly used local tissue flap techniques for coronal and subcoronal defects is the **Mathieu, perimeatal-based flap technique** (Mathieu, 1932). **In**

1994, Retik and colleagues reported a series of 204 perimeatal-based repairs performed with the addition of dorsal dartos flap coverage of the neourethra and a complication rate of 0.98% (Retik et al, 1994b). **In a multicenter report combining the experience of four institutions, an excellent functional and cosmetic result was obtained in 96.7% of 336 patients repaired with a modified Mathieu technique** (Hakim et al, 1996). **Urethrocutaneous fistula, the most common complication, occurred in only nine patients.**

The *Mathieu* hypospadias repair (Fig. 65–14) **is begun by measuring the length of the defect from the urethral meatus to the glans tip. An equal distance from the meatus is measured on the proximal penile shaft skin.** With the aid of calipers, the urethral plate and

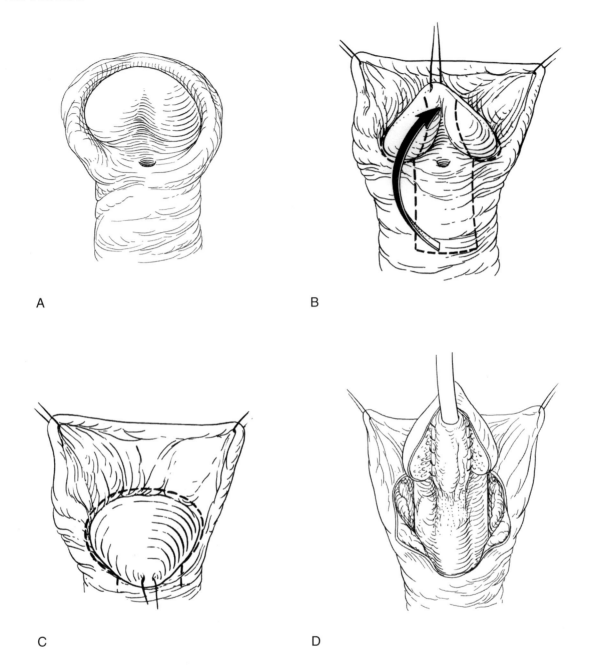

Figure 65–14. Mathieu hypospadias repair. *A,* Subcoronal hypospadias. *B,* Appropriate flap size is outlined proximal to urethral meatus. *C,* Proposed circumferential incision. *D,* Proximal flap has been elevated from penile ventrum and sutured to the urethral plate with running subcuticular technique.

perimeatal-based flap are then marked at appropriate widths. Typically, a width of 7.5 mm is measured for the proximal flap. This width is tapered to 5.5 mm at the distal extent of the glans, and longitudinal lines outlining the urethral plate are then drawn. A line is marked beginning at either lateral margin of the previously marked urethral plate and carried around the dorsal aspect of the penis, approximately 5 to 7 mm proximal to the corona of the glans. Injection of dilute epinephrine is followed by skin and glanular incisions. **The glans wings are incised deeply, the penile shaft skin is degloved, and the penis is evaluated for curvature.**

After a straight penis is either appreciated or achieved with an orthoplasty technique, the premeasured segment of penile skin proximal to the meatus is mobilized off the urethra in a proximal-to-distal direction with the aid of skin hooks, fine stay sutures, and tenotomy scissors. This tissue is folded over at the meatus (perimeatal-based flap), and bilateral, longitudinal, running subcuticular sutures approximate this flap to the lateral aspects of the urethral plate, thereby creating the neourethra. Tubularization is performed over a No. 6 Fr Silastic catheter using fine polyglactin suture. The meatus is matured at the glans tip with simple interrupted fine absorbable suture,

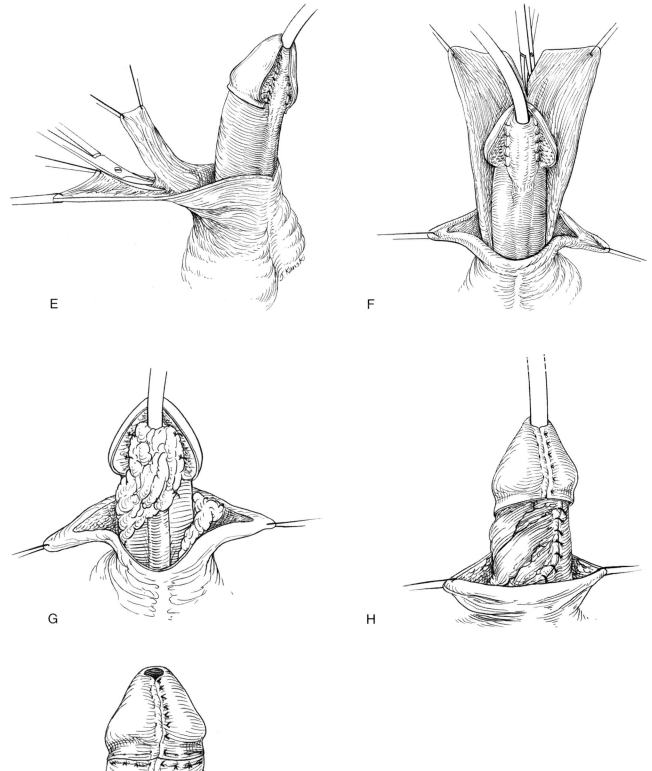

E

F

G

H

I

Figure 65–14 *Continued. E,* Dorsal subcutaneous pedicled flap is harvested, and *F,* divided in the midline. *G,* One-half of subcutaneous flap has been secured over neourethra. *H,* Glans closure with subcutaneous simple suture and skin with mattress technique. *I,* Skin coverage of shaft and repair have been completed. (From Atala A, Retik AB: Hypospadias. In Libertino JA [ed]: Reconstructive Urologic Surgery, 3rd ed. St. Louis, Mosby–Year Book, 1998, p 467, with permission.)

and **second-layer neourethral coverage is performed with dorsal dartos tissue.** The glans wings are then approximated without tension in two layers, and skin coverage is completed.

The **Barcat balanic groove** technique is similar to the Mathieu repair but includes dissection of the urethral plate distal to the meatus and advancement of the approximated (now tubularized) flaps to the tip of the glans (Barcat, 1973; Redman, 1987; Koff et al, 1994; Barthold et al, 1996). **Perimeatal-based flap repairs such as the Mathieu technique and the initial and modified Barcat balanic groove procedures incorporate the use of tissue flaps with blood supply that may be compromised** (Keating and Duckett, 1995). **In addition, these repairs require ventral penile shaft skin of sufficient length without incorporation of proximal hair-bearing skin.** Often, this results in a skin defect that requires complex rotational skin flaps for coverage and a horizontally oriented, abnormal-appearing urethral meatus. A **technique described initially by Bevan** (Bevan, 1917) **and later by Mustarde** (Mustarde, 1965) **represents a combination of a** perimeatal-based, ventral skin flap which is then tubularized and passed through a glans channel to achieve a meatus at the penile tip.

Other Techniques

The megameatus intact prepuce (MIP) technique (see Fig. 65–2), **a variant of distal hypospadias so named by Duckett and Keating (1989), was simultaneously described by Hatch and colleagues (1989).** A repair specific to this hypospadias variant, the "pyramid" procedure was also described by Duckett and Keating (Duckett and Keating, 1989). Other techniques, including the MAGPI, Thiersch-Duplay urethroplasty, and Mathieu techniques, have been used to successfully repair this particular defect (Hatch et al, 1989; Hill et al, 1993; Nonomura et al, 1998). The split prepuce in situ onlay technique (Rushton and Belman, 1998) has been reported for use in distal and middle hypospadias and is discussed in detail in the next section.

Middle Hypospadias Procedures

Numerous successful procedures with acceptable complication rates have been described for the repair of middle hypospadias with mild-to-moderate penile curvature. Popular techniques include the **TIP urethroplasty** (Snodgrass et al, 1996; Retik and Borer, 1998; Borer et al, 2001) and the **Mathieu, perimeatal-based flap** (Mathieu, 1932), both of which have been described for repair of distal hypospadias. Although its primary utility may be in repair of coronal and subcoronal (anterior) defects, the Mathieu technique may also be employed for repair of distal penile shaft defects, with usefulness in more proximal hypospadias limited.

Onlay Techniques

Among the most commonly used techniques for repair of middle hypospadias is the onlay island flap (onlay, or OIF) technique (Elder et al, 1987). **Since its in-**troduction for the repair of subcoronal and midshaft hypospadias, use of the OIF technique has expanded both in frequency and indication to include more proximal defects as well. In 1994, Baskin and colleagues reported use of the OIF in 33% of their total hypospadias repairs during a 5-year period. Complications requiring reoperation occurred in 32 (8.6%) of 374 patients. Twenty-three (6%) of the patients developed a urethrocutaneous fistula.

The *onlay island flap* hypospadias repair (Fig. 65–15) **is begun by placing a traction suture in the glans penis and fine stay sutures at the corners of the prepuce. The urethral plate is measured to a width of approximately 6 mm, and proposed parallel longitudinal incisions outlining the urethral plate are marked from the hypospadiac meatus to the glans tip.** A near-circumferential incision that preserves the urethral plate is also marked on the distal penile shaft. Dilute epinephrine solution is injected to facilitate hemostasis, and the skin incisions are then made with a fine knife. **After evaluation for and correction of penile curvature, as necessary, the length of the defect from the urethral meatus to the glans tip is measured. This is the length required of the rectangular preputial onlay to be harvested for repair. We typically use a width of 9 to 10 mm for the onlay flap when used for repair in infants.** The preputial skin is marked, incised, and then dissected with its pedicle from the outer preputial layer and dorsal penile shaft skin. Dissection of the pedicle to the base of the penis minimizes torque on the penis and tension on the repair.

The rectangular preputial OIF is held with a fine stay suture in each corner and is passed around the penis to the ventrum. Care is taken to ensure that the flap reaches the site of anastomosis without tension on its pedicle. Tubularization is performed over a No. 6 Fr Silastic catheter and is begun with a full-thickness running 6-0 or 7-0 polyglactin suture that approximates the previous proximal edge of the onlay flap (now oriented longitudinally), with the edge of urethral plate ipsilateral to the side of flap transfer. A full-thickness running suture is also used for the transverse proximal anastomosis, and the remainder of the tubularization is performed with a running subcuticular technique. **The inferolateral border of the pedicle is advanced over the lines of anastomosis as a buttress, and a tunica vaginalis flap may be employed for second-layer neourethral coverage.** Maturation of the urethral meatus, securing of the Silastic catheter, glans approximation, and skin closure are then performed.

Rushton and Belman (1998) reported excellent results with the **split prepuce in situ onlay** (Fig. 65–16) modification of the OIF technique. In this modification, **preservation of the whole blood supply to one half of the prepuce (onlay segment harvested in longitudinal orientation and transferred ventrally) used for coronal to midshaft hypospadias repair is responsible, they believe, for the low 4% urethrocutaneous fistula and 5% reoperative rates.** In further contrast to the standard OIF repair (onlay segment harvested in transverse orientation) (Elder et al, 1987), **the split prepuce island onlay does not require separate mobilization of both inner preputial and skin vascular supplies. The outer epithelial layer is simply excised, simplifying the repair and optimizing blood supply to the onlay flap.** The authors sug-

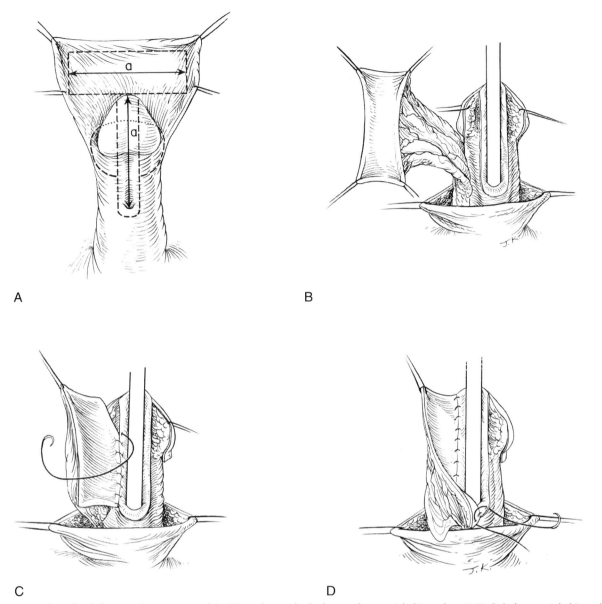

A

B

C

D

Figure 65–15. Onlay island flap repair. *A,* Proposed incisions for urethral plate and preputial skin onlay. *B,* Pedicled preputial skin onlay with stay sutures. *C,* Initial full-thickness suture approximation of onlay flap and urethral plate. *D,* Approximation at proximal extent.

Illustration continued on following page

gested that this technique would be applicable for more proximal repairs as well (Rushton and Belman, 1998). Yerkes and colleagues (2000) also reported excellent preliminary results with this technique. Another variation of the onlay, the **double onlay preputial flap,** as described by Gonzalez and colleagues primarily for the repair of posterior hypospadias, has also been employed for repair of midshaft hypospadias (Gonzalez et al, 1996; Barroso et al, 2000).

Tubularization Techniques

Other popular and successful techniques include the tubularization **technique described by King** (1970), whose initial description of the technique involved a patient with midshaft hypospadias, and the **TIP urethroplasty.** As stated in the discussion of anterior hypospadias repair, the TIP urethroplasty has become a popular technique for pri-

mary and reoperative repair of middle as well as anterior hypospadias (Snodgrass et al, 1996; Retik and Borer, 1998; Borer et al, 2001).

Posterior Hypospadias Procedures

Posterior hypospadias defects represent the most challenging and complex manifestations of this entity and may be successfully treated with one of several one- or two-stage repair procedures.

One-Stage Repairs

ONLAY TECHNIQUES

The *onlay island flap,* **initially described for distal and midshaft repairs** (Elder et al, 1987)**, has been increas-**

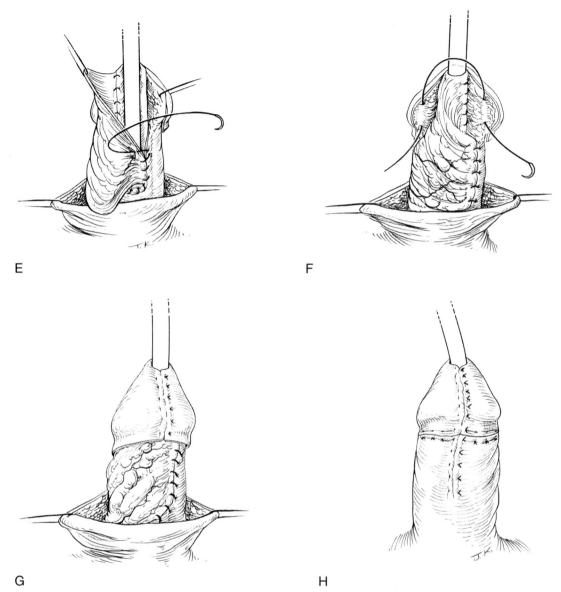

E

F

G

H

Figure 65–15 *Continued. E,* Completion of anastomosis with running subcuticular technique. *F,* Inferolateral border of onlay pedicle has been advanced as a second layer coverage of proximal and longitudinal suture lines. *G,* Approximated glans. *H,* Completed repair. (From Atala A, Retik AB: Hypospadias. In Libertino JA [ed]: Reconstructive Urologic Surgery, 3rd ed. St. Louis, Mosby–Year Book, 1998, p 467, with permission.)

ingly employed for repair of more severe hypospadias (Hollowell et al, 1990; Dewan et al, 1991; Mollard et al, 1991; Gearhart and Borland, 1992; Baskin et al, 1994; Perovic and Vukadinovic, 1994). Baskin and colleagues (1994) reported the repair of penoscrotal and perineal hypospadias defects in 33 and 5 patients, respectively, with excellent results.

The *onlay-tube-onlay urethroplasty* technique, a variation of the onlay principle that comprises a central tubularized and distal and proximal onlay components, has been described. This repair, based on the same strip of penile shaft and preputial skin (harvested in longitudinal orientation) (Perovic and Vukadinovic, 1994) or preputial skin alone (harvested transversely) (Flack and Walker, 1995), has been described in four patients each with "severe" and perineal hypospadias. Other modifications of this onlay-tube combination have been reported (Kocvara and Dvoracek, 1997).

The **double-onlay preputial flap,** as described by Gonzalez and colleagues (1996), combines the principles of the OIF and the double-face preputial flap. The preputial onlay segment is harvested transversely and transposed ventrally with a "buttonhole" in the vascular pedicle. **This repair preserves the urethral plate, as do other onlay techniques, but obviates the need for separation of the inner and outer preputial layers and the need for separate skin coverage of the onlay segment used for urethroplasty.** Use in proximal hypospadias included 11 patients with a penoscrotal and 1 with a perineal meatus. According to the authors, there were no problems with vascular supply to the flaps or ventral bulkiness. Complications requiring reoperation occurred in four patients with penoscrotal hypospadias (Gonzalez et al, 1996). Barroso and colleagues (2000) have recently updated their experience with this technique. They have now performed the double-onlay preputial flap in a total of 47 patients. Complications requiring

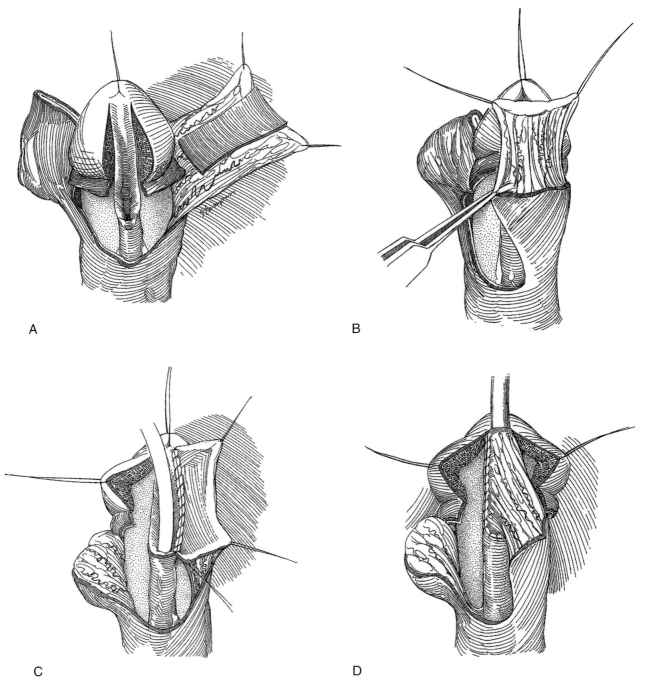

A

B

C

D

Figure 65–16. Split prepuce in situ onlay technique. *A*, Penile shaft skin is degloved, prepuce is split in the dorsal midline and the urethral plate is outlined. The one half of split prepuce used for the island flap is isolated by de-epithelializing adjacent inner prepuce. *B*, Outer skin of preputial onlay is de-epithelialized. *C*, The onlay flap is sutured to the urethral plate beginning with a running 7-0 polyglactin suture, and *D*, completed with subcuticular technique.

Illustration continued on following page

reoperation occurred in 12 patients (25%). In eight boys (17%), a fistula developed; six of them had perineal and two had penoscrotal hypospadias. Successful closure was achieved with one procedure in six patients, required an additional fistula repair in one, and remained to be determined in another. Diverticula, meatal recession, and persistent penile curvature requiring repeat dorsal plication occurred in 4 (9%), 2 (4%), and 2 (4%) patients, respectively. Revision for a bulky ventral skin strip was required in one boy (2%) (Barroso et al, 2000).

TUBULARIZATION TECHNIQUES

Credit for the first description of preputial skin use for a tubularized, pedicled flap neourethra goes to Weller Van Hook, who in 1896 described use of a pedicled preputial flap for creation of a tubularized neourethra in a patient with proximal hypospadias. Several others have described similar techniques (Wehrbein, 1943; Hodgson, 1970; Toksu, 1970; Duckett, 1980; Harris, 1984).

In 1969, Hamilton described urethroplasty with a **longi-**

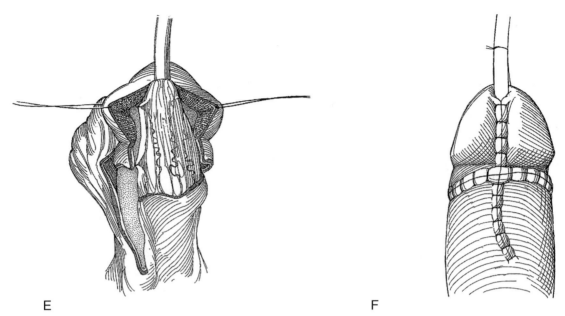

E   F

Figure 65-16 *Continued. E,* Edges of the vascular pedicle are secured lateral to neourethral suture lines as second layer coverage, and *F,* the repair is completed with skin coverage and securing of an 8 Fr intravesical stent to the glans. (From Rushton HG, Belman AB: The split prepuce in situ onlay hypospadias repair. J Urol 160:1134–1136, with permission.)

tudinally oriented preputial island flap. A similar technique was described by Chen and colleagues in 1993. In 1971, **Asopa and colleagues** described use of preputial skin for formation of a tubularized neourethra transferred to the ventrum for hypospadias repair as a single unit, with the inner prepuce as the tubularized neourethra and the attached outer prepuce for skin cover. A similar technique for repair of midshaft or proximal hypospadias in 26 patients with a success rate of 92.3% was reported by Yavuzer and colleagues (1998).

The transverse preputial island flap (TPIF) employs preputial skin for formation of a tubularized neourethra transferred to the ventrum for hypospadias repair as separate components of the repair: inner prepuce with its vascular pedicle for the neourethra, separated from and followed by transfer of the longitudinally split outer prepuce as skin cover. The TPIF described, named, and popularized by Duckett (1980) is often referred to as the "Duckett tube," and it is perhaps the most frequently performed one-stage tubularized repair for proximal hypospadias.

The TPIF technique (Fig. 65–17) begins with placement of fine traction sutures in the glans and prepuce. A ventral midline longitudinal incision is marked from the urethral meatus to the distal circumcising incision. The urethral meatus is marked circumferentially for planned incision as well. The skin is incised, the penile shaft is degloved, and the penis is assessed for curvature. **Curvature that persists after release of skin and tethering subcutaneous tissues may require division of the urethral plate. Curvature is then reassessed and, if necessary, corrected with a ventral orthoplasty technique. After orthoplasty, a transversely oriented rectangle of preputial skin is marked at a length equal to the distance from the urethral meatus to the glans tip and approximately 15 mm in width.** Once dissected from the outer layer of prepuce and dorsal penile skin, the pedicled inner prepuce is tubu-

larized over a No. 6 Fr Silastic catheter to form the neourethra. The anastomosis is performed in a running, subcuticular first-layer closure with fine polyglactin suture and a second layer with inverting Lembert technique using the same material. The last 0.5 to 1.0 cm of the anastomosis is closed with a simple interrupted technique to allow future tailoring of the distal neourethral length.

The neourethra is transferred to the penile ventrum on a tension-free pedicle and oriented so that the sutured line of anastomosis is facing the ventral surface of the corpora cavernosa after anastomosis. The dorsal aspect of the native meatus, before anastomosis with the neourethra, is fixed with simple interrupted sutures to the ventrum of the corpora cavernosa so as to stabilize the anastomosis. Additionally, a small circular incision is marked in the glans penis at the proposed site for the neomeatus. **A wide channel is fashioned, initially with tenotomy scissors and finally to a No. 16 to 18 urethral sound caliber, in order to accommodate passage of the distal neourethra. A core of glans tissue is excised to achieve sufficient channel caliber. Alternatively, the glans may be deeply incised in the midline to allow advancement of the neourethra and proper placement of the meatus.** The proximal anastomosis is performed first with two separate sutures and a running, locking full-thickness technique. The distal extent of the neourethra is then passed through the glans channel and the meatus is trimmed, if necessary, to appropriate length and fixed to the glans with fine polyglactin simple interrupted suture. **The inferolateral border of the pedicle is advanced over the neourethra and then covered by a tunica vaginalis flap.** Securing of the Silastic catheter and skin closure complete the repair.

In a comparison of techniques for the repair of proximal hypospadias, Wiener and colleagues (1997) reported similar results in overall complication rate (31% versus 36%) and fistula rate (14% versus 17%) for the OIF when compared

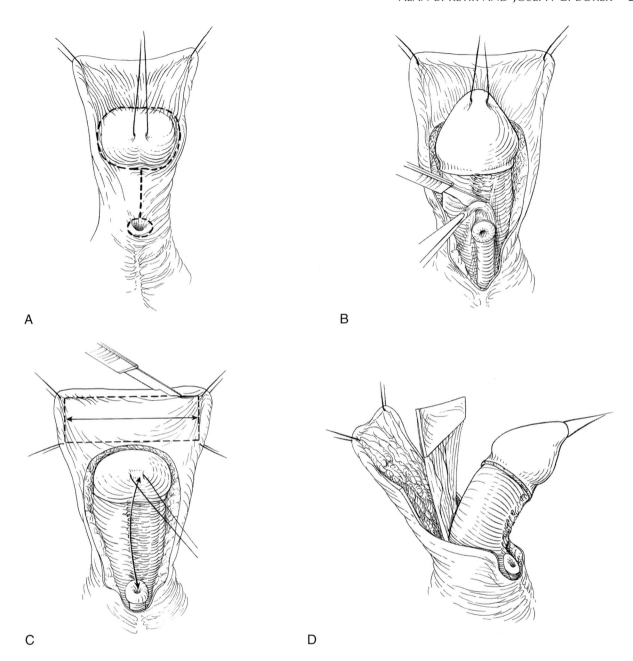

A

B

C

D

Figure 65–17. Transverse preputial island flap repair. *A*, Proposed initial incisions for proximal shaft/penoscrotal hypospadias. *B*, Release of tethering urethral plate and "dropping" of meatus proximally. *C*, Incision of preputial skin of appropriate dimensions for length of defect and width for desired luminal diameter. *D*, Harvested transverse preputial island flap.

Illustration continued on following page

with the TPIF. Baskin and colleagues (1994) reported similar fistula rates for the OIF and TPIF, 10% versus 15%, respectively, and postulated that the lower fistula rate for the OIF may be a result of improved healing of the repair with preservation of the spongiosal supported urethral plate.

OTHER TECHNIQUES

A modification of the TPIF incorporates tubularization of proximal nonhirsute interscrotal tissue as an adjunct to the TPIF (Glassberg, 1987). Tubularization of the nonhirsute interscrotal tissue was described previously

as an adjunct to distal skin graft urethroplasty (Devine and Horton, 1977). In some cases, where anatomy necessitates division of the urethral plate, we have performed **a similar modification with incorporation of a longitudinal, midline incision and tubularization of the urethral plate, proximally, with repair of the remaining distal defect using the TPIF technique. These modifications, in effect, decrease the length of defect requiring repair with the TPIF technique.**

A one-stage urethroplasty with the **parameatal foreskin flap** technique described for repair of proximal hypospadias with or without penoscrotal transposition has been promoted as having universal applicability (Koyanagi et al,

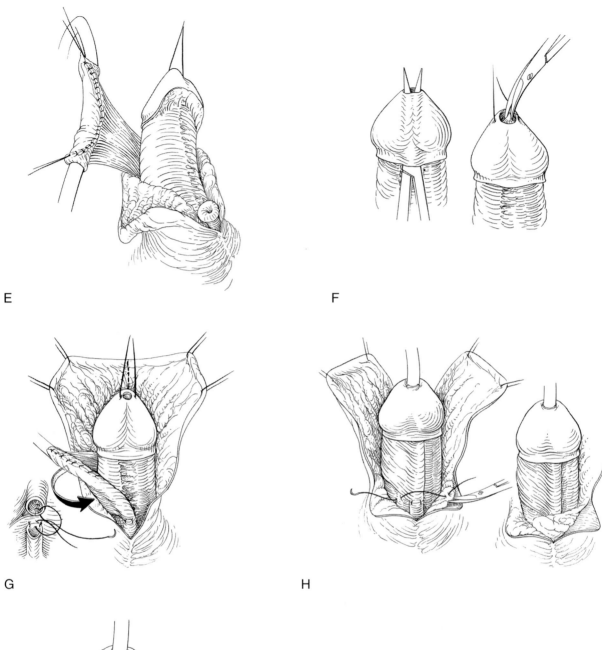

E

F

G

H

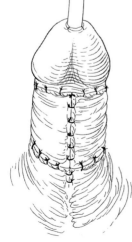

I

Figure 65–17 *Continued. E,* Running subcuticular suture tubularization has been performed over a Silastic catheter to be followed by a second layer running Lembert suture. *F,* Generous glans channel is fashioned for neourethral passage. A core of glans tissue is excised in order to achieve sufficient caliber. *G,* Native urethral meatus is fixed to corpora cavernosa prior to performing proximal anastomosis with the neourethra. *H,* Subcutaneous (dartos) tissue coverage of anastomosis. *I,* Maturation of neourethral meatus and penile shaft skin coverage have been completed. (From Atala A, Retik AB: Hypospadias. In Libertino JA [ed]: Reconstructive Urologic Surgery, 3rd ed. St. Louis, Mosby–Year Book, 1998, p 467, with permission.)

1994). This technique has also been referred to as the meatal based "manta-wing flap," and it has similarities to the "clergyman's stole" (strip of prepuce in continuity with longitudinal, ventral penile skin strips) technique described by Russell in 1900. Complication rates continue to approach 50% for this procedure (Koyanagi et al, 1994; Glassberg et al, 1998). **Radical bulbar dissection** has been described as a rapid adjunctive technique that is applicable to all proximal hypospadias (Baker et al, 2000). According to the authors, benefits realized by this technique include release of proximal tethering of the scrotum and subcutaneous fibrous bands, resulting in correction of curvature in some and at times decreased severity of the hypospadias defect requiring repair.

Two-Stage Repairs

Because the majority of hypospadias can be repaired with a one-stage procedure, the use of two-stage techniques for repair of posterior hypospadias is controversial. In the setting of scrotal or perineal hypospadias, severe curvature, and a small penis, we prefer to perform a two-stage repair as described by Retik and colleagues (Retik et al, 1994a; Retik, 1996). In a series of 58 repairs performed with this two-stage technique, a urethrocutaneous fistula developed in 3 patients (5.2%) postoperatively (Retik et al, 1994a).

At the *first stage*, orthoplasty is performed and the prepuce is repositioned ventrally (Fig. 65–18). Depending on the severity of penile curvature, resection of ventral tethering tissue and division of the urethral plate, with dropping of the urethral meatus proximally, may not be sufficient for correction. **Orthoplasty may be performed with one of several techniques. We prefer to use an interposition dermal graft inlay after transverse incision of the corpora cavernosa directly at the apex of maximal concave curvature.** When flat, the glans penis is deeply incised in the ventral midline distally to the point of the eventual neomeatus. For those with a deep glanular groove, longitudinal incisions may be placed lateral to the groove, bilaterally. Another option would be to leave the glans intact, cover the ventral shaft with approximation of prepuce to the subcoronal circumcising incision, and perform TIP urethroplasty for the distal aspect of the neourethra at the second stage of the repair.

A midline longitudinal incision is made in the preputial and dorsal distal penile shaft skin. Each half is brought around its respective lateral aspect of the penis and anastomosed with fine interrupted absorbable sutures to the penile ventrum, beginning at the distal apex of the glans incision. Identical sutures are placed with simple interrupted full-thickness technique to approximate the transferred skin in the ventral midline. Simple interrupted sutures approximate transferred skin and native meatus proximally. **In some cases, it may take all of the preputial skin to cover the ventral aspect of the liberated and straightened shaft. This step prepares well-vascularized tissue to be used for neourethral formation (tubularization) at the second stage.**

The *second stage* is performed 6 months or longer after completion of the first stage. The primary goal of the second stage of the procedure is to create a neour-

ethra that bridges the defect between the hypospadiac meatus and the tip of the penis. Tubularization of local skin in Thiersch-Duplay fashion is the preferred technique. Tissue to be used for neourethral construction is marked on the ventral aspect of the penis **at a width of approximately 15 mm, centered on the midline.** Once incised, the lateral edges of this tissue are dissected only minimally toward the midline, so as preserve the vascular supply to the neourethra. **Second-layer neourethral coverage is either with local subcutaneous tissues or with a tunica vaginalis flap.** Subcutaneous tissues and penile skin are approximated in the ventral midline with "pullout" running sutures of 4-0 nylon. Urinary diversion is achieved with a urethral and/or suprapubic catheter for approximately 7 to 10 days postoperatively.

Free Graft for Neourethral Formation

Various techniques incorporating the use of free skin, bladder, or buccal mucosa graft alone or in combination have also been described for the repair of posterior hypospadias. These include graft of nonhair-bearing skin (genital or extragenital) (Hendren and Horton, 1988; Hendren and Keating, 1988), bladder mucosa (Hendren and Reda, 1986; Baskin and Duckett, 1994), and buccal mucosa (Bürger et al, 1992; Dessanti et al, 1992; Baskin and Duckett, 1994, 1995), which may be used alone or in combination (Ransley et al, 1987; Retik, 1996).

The use of skin for urethroplasty was first described by Nové-Josserand in 1897 (Nové-Josserand, 1897, Nové-Josserand, 1914). **In 1941, Humby used tubularized skin as a free graft for primary hypospadias repair in 12 patients, and Devine and Horton popularized use of the tubularized skin graft with their description of a preputial, free graft tubularized neourethra in 1961.** Bracka (1995a, 1995b) has continued to be a proponent of the skin graft tube as the second stage of a universally applicable two-stage technique for hypospadias repair.

The use of bladder mucosa was first reported by Memmelaar in 1947, and later by others (Marshall and Spellman, 1955; Hendren and Reda, 1986), **for primary repair of severe hypospadias in cases with a paucity of local tissue.** However, protruding mucosa at the neomeatus resulted in a significant reoperation rate for revision at that site. **Unlike bladder mucosa, which tends to shrink and requires a greater size of tissue at harvest in relation to the defect to be repaired, buccal mucosa may be harvested in a one-to-one ratio** (Bürger et al, 1992; Dessanti et al, 1992; Baskin and Duckett, 1994, 1995). **This characteristic of buccal mucosa results from a lamina propria rich with vascularity. As with all free grafts, a well-vascularized graft host bed is a necessity for successful take via the processes of imbibition and inosculation.**

Bladder mucosa is harvested by distending the bladder with saline and dissecting the detrusor muscle, anteriorly, off the underlying mucosa (Fig. 65–19). A rectangular donor site is marked to a size 10% greater than the size of the defect to be repaired. **As part of a composite repair, tubularized skin or buccal mucosa may be added to the distal extent of the tubularized bladder mucosa graft to decrease the risk of meatal complica-**

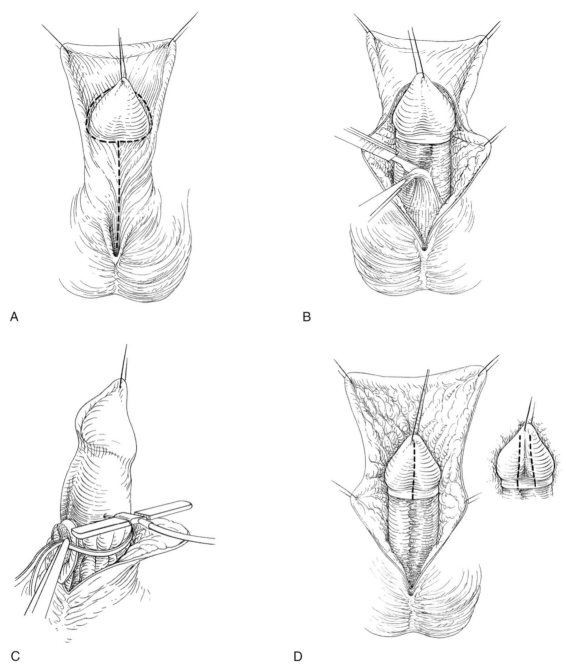

A

B

C

D

Figure 65–18. Two-stage hypospadias repair. *A, First stage:* proposed initial incisions for penoscrotal/scrotal hypospadias. *B,* Release of tethering urethral plate and "dropping" of meatus proximally. *C,* Artificial erection assessment for curvature. *D,* Midline incision or alternatively, longitudinal incisions on either side of a deep glanular groove, is/are placed in the glans.

tions. **The length of bladder mucosa graft harvested should equal that of the defect when used in a composite repair.** The two grafts are approximated with two running sutures of 6-0 or 7-0 polyglactin. The composite graft is then tubularized over a Silastic catheter using a running, locking technique. The proximal anastomosis is performed with two running, locking sutures of fine polyglactin, and the neomeatus is matured with simple interrupted fine absorbable suture. **A second layer of neourethral coverage is provided by either a dorsal subcutaneous flap or tunica vaginalis.** The bladder is drained with a suprapubic

catheter, and the repair is stented for 7 to 10 days postoperatively with a Silastic catheter. **Immobilization of the patient in the early postoperative period is crucial to graft survival.**

The technique for use of *buccal mucosa* in hypospadias repair begins with induction of general anesthesia and *nasotracheal* intubation. A self-retaining retractor is then placed in the oral cavity, and **with care taken to avoid Stensen's duct, a graft of appropriate size is marked on the mucosa of the cheek and/or lip** (see Fig. 65–19). **Epinephrine (diluted 1:200,000 in 0.5% lido-**

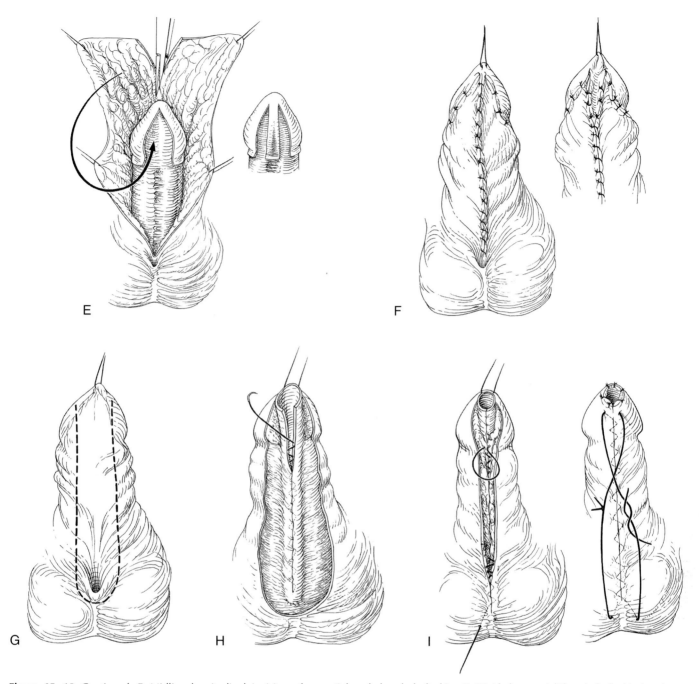

Figure 65–18 *Continued. E,* Midline longitudinal incision of preputial and dorsal shaft skin. *F,* Divided preputial/dorsal shaft skin has been transferred to the penile ventrum. *G, Second stage:* Line of incision for Thiersch-Duplay tubularization. *H,* Running subcuticular closure of neourethra. *I,* The meatus is secured to the glans, the subcutaneous tissues approximated and the skin closed with nylon suture, the ends of which are tied to each other. (From Retik AB: Proximal hypospadias. In Marshall FF [ed]: Textbook of Operative Urology. Philadelphia, WB Saunders, 1996, with permission.)

caine) is injected submucosally, fine stay sutures are placed in the corners of the graft, and the graft is harvested with sharp dissection superficial to the buccinator muscle. Buccal mucosal edges at the harvest site are approximated with 5-0 chromic catgut suture in a running simple fashion. The graft is defatted on a sterile cardboard scaffold and then tubularized in a manner similar to that for bladder mucosa. Proximal and meatal anastomoses and second-layer neourethral and skin coverage and closure are performed similarly as well. The repair is stented for 7

to 10 days postoperatively. Improved results are noted when buccal mucosa is used in an onlay fashion compared with a tubularized technique (Ahmed and Gough, 1997; Duckett et al, 1995).

COMPLICATIONS

Complications of hypospadias repair include bleeding/hematoma, meatal stenosis, urethrocutaneous fistula, ure-

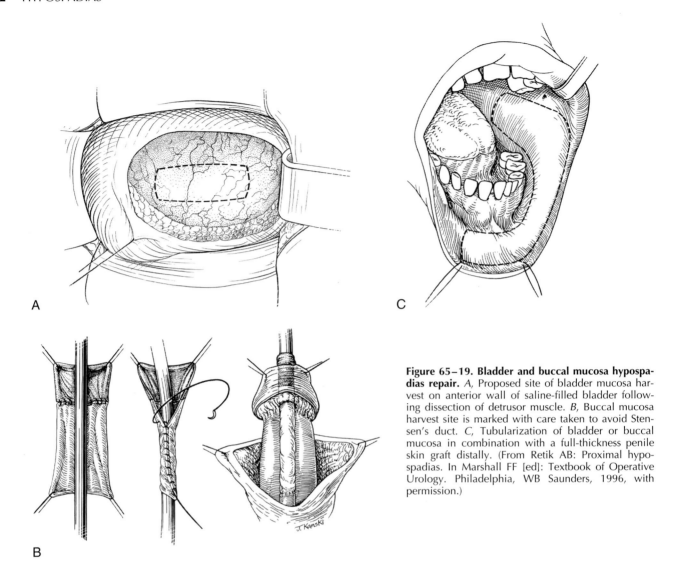

Figure 65–19. Bladder and buccal mucosa hypospadias repair. *A,* Proposed site of bladder mucosa harvest on anterior wall of saline-filled bladder following dissection of detrusor muscle. *B,* Buccal mucosa harvest site is marked with care taken to avoid Stensen's duct. *C,* Tubularization of bladder or buccal mucosa in combination with a full-thickness penile skin graft distally. (From Retik AB: Proximal hypospadias. In Marshall FF [ed]: Textbook of Operative Urology. Philadelphia, WB Saunders, 1996, with permission.)

thral stricture, urethral diverticulum, wound infection, impaired healing, and breakdown of the repair (Duckett et al, 1980; Horton and Horton, 1988; Retik et al, 1988; Keating and Duckett, 1995). When reoperation is indicated, complications such as meatal stenosis, urethrocutaneous fistula, and urethral stricture can be repaired expeditiously, with appropriate timing. However, more serious complications involving either partial or complete breakdown of the hypospadias repair may require a major reconstructive effort. At times, this involves the task of performing a complete repair in the face of less than optimal tissues and conditions. **In general, unless immediate re-exploration is indicated for bleeding, infection or débridement, reoperation for complications should not be performed less than 6 months after previous repair.**

Bleeding and Hematoma

Bleeding has been noted as the most common complication of hypospadias repair. This may require addition of a compressive dressing due to persistent oozing. At **other times, significant postoperative bleeding may require immediate exploration to identify and treat the source.** Hematoma may form as a result of persistent bleeding; if large in size, it may require wound exploration and hematoma evacuation. Consequences of hematoma formation range from simple temporary cosmetic issues to wound or repair breakdown (Elbakry et al, 1998). **Patients with excessive bleeding and/or hematoma formation, particularly those requiring reoperation, should undergo evaluation for bleeding diathesis/dyscrasias** (Horton and Horton, 1988).

Meatal Stenosis

The complication of meatal stenosis is perhaps most commonly caused by technical issues at the time of repair, such as fashioning of the urethral meatus with too narrow a lumen or performance of glanuloplasty too tightly. Urethral (meatal) dilation or meatotomy may be sufficient for the mildest forms of meatal stenosis. However, a more complex distal urethral stricture also involving the meatus may require a more extensive flap procedure (De Sy, 1984).

Urethrocutaneous Fistula

The suspicion of a **urethrocutaneous fistula is often reported by a parent or caregiver. This can be confirmed on physical examination with or without voiding, or with retrograde injection of dye such as methylene blue, either alone or with glycerin** (Horton and Horton, 1988; Retik et al, 1988). Fistula may result from, or be associated with, distal stricture or meatal stenosis. Other risk factors include failure to invert all epithelial edges at urethroplasty, devitalization of tissue, and failure to add appropriate second-layer urethroplasty coverage. **Second-layer coverage of the neourethra has been shown to significantly reduce the fistula rate as reported by several authors** (Smith, 1973; Belman, 1988; Retik et al, 1988; Churchill et al, 1996). **Repair of urethrocutaneous fistula is optimized by the same principle** (Davis, 1940; Cecil, 1946; Goldstein and Hensle, 1981; Retik et al, 1988). **At times, larger or multiple fistulas may require incision of the intact skin bridges and delayed repeat hypospadias repair.**

Infection

Infection is an uncommon complication of hypospadias repair. When infection is suspected, culture, incision and drainage, and débridement, when indicated, are incorporated with appropriate empirical and definitive antibiotic therapy. Severe infection may lead to breakdown of the entire repair.

Urethral Diverticula

Although infrequent, urethral diverticulum formation may occur after hypospadias repair. **Similar to urethrocutaneous fistula, urethral diverticulum may be associated with distal stricture or meatal stenosis.** Zaontz and colleagues (1989) described repair of this entity with circumferential skin incision, penile shaft skin degloving, diverticular excision and urethral closure, followed by "pants over vest" subcutaneous tissue coverage of the repair, with excellent results. For more extensive lesions, Aigen and colleagues (1987) described repair similar to that for megalourethra.

Balanitis Xerotica Obliterans

Balanitis xerotica obliterans (BXO) is a chronic inflammatory process of unknown cause. BXO can arise spontaneously or occur after minor trauma or penile surgery such as circumcision or hypospadias repair. Kumar and Harris (1999) reported on eight patients with histologically proven BXO. Seven of these patients presented with difficult micturition and meatal stenosis or neourethral

stricture, at varying periods from 1 to 8 years after primary hypospadias repair. **These authors recommended use of bladder or buccal mucosal free grafts for repair of such cases, in order to improve on an alarming 50% complication rate with the use of skin grafts for urethroplasty.**

Recurrent Penile Curvature

Late-onset, recurrent curvature has been described by several authors as a complication of orthoplasty performed alone or in conjunction with hypospadias repair. Farkas (1967) reported that a second operation (and sometimes more) was required in approximately 50% of cases of hypospadias and initial severe curvature. In a more contemporary report, **late-onset curvature in 22 patients with initial proximal penile or penoscrotal hypospadias and successful orthoplasty was thought to be caused equally by extensive fibrosis of the reconstructed urethra, corporeal disproportion, or both** (Vandersteen and Husmann, 1998).

Urethral Stricture

Urethral stricture other than meatal stenosis may be a complication of proximal hypospadias repair. The proximal anastomotic site of a tubularized repair such as the TPIF appears to be particularly at risk. **This type of stricture may be successfully treated with less invasive means, such as endoscopic cold knife urethrotomy** (Scherz et al, 1988). **However, a more extensive stricture may warrant patch with free graft or, preferably, pedicled flap urethroplasty; either of these two techniques achieves greater success when used as an onlay rather than a tubularized segment.** In a thorough review of anterior urethral stricture repair techniques, Wessells and McAninch (1998) reported near-identical overall success rates of approximately 85% for both free graft and pedicled skin flap methods. However, these authors noted that many of the reports reviewed did not specifically state the site of repair.

Others have discussed the usefulness of mucosal grafts for treatment of urethral stricture disease (Baskin and Duckett, 1994; Ahmed and Gough, 1997). In 1989, Schreiter described a two-stage mesh-graft urethroplasty using split-thickness skin, for application in the absence of available pedicled flap tissue or an appropriate graft bed (Schreiter and Noll, 1989; Wessells and McAninch, 1998). The mesh-graft technique would be useful in those instances when all other options have failed.

Repair Breakdown

Repair breakdown may occur secondary to devascularization of local tissues or flaps used in urethroplasty or other components of hypospadias repair. **Breakdown may also result from urethroplasty and/or approximation of the glans (glanuloplasty) under tension, or from devitalized tissue resulting from excessive use of electrocautery, unidentified vascular pedicle injury during repair,** or hematoma formation (Elbakry et al, 1998). **Regardless of the cause, repair breakdown may require débridement of devascularized, necrotic tissue before repair** (Horton and Horton, 1988).

Hypospadias Cripples

Horton and Devine (1970) used the term "hypospadias cripple" to describe the patient who has undergone multiple, unsuccessful hypospadias repair attempts, with significant resultant penile deformity. These patients represent perhaps the most perplexing of hypospadias repair complications in that they require extensive repair amidst scarred and devitalized tissue. Options for treatment of the hypospadias cripple are discussed in the next section.

REOPERATIVE HYPOSPADIAS REPAIR

General Principles

In general, attempts at reoperative hypospadias surgery should not be undertaken before 6 months after the previous failure. Certainly, no attempt at repair should be entertained until all edema, infection, and inflammation have resolved and healing is complete. Radiographic imaging with retrograde urethrogram or VCUG, or both, for complete urethral visualization may be necessary in complex reoperative hypospadias cases as an important aspect of preparation for definitive repair. **Inspection of available tissue, to determine whether adequate local tissue exists or there is need for an extragenital tissue graft, significantly affects and dictates repair options.** This decision-making process is critical to achieving a successful result.

Specific Techniques

Immediately Adjacent or Local Tissue Flap

When possible, the use of immediately adjacent or local pedicled, well-vascularized tissue is preferred for reoperative hypospadias surgery. This may be in the form of a simple tubularization procedure or a modification such as the tubularized, incised plate urethroplasty. The TIP urethroplasty technique is performed similarly for previously operated patients as for primary repair (see Fig. 65–13). The applicability and advantages of TIP urethroplasty use in reoperative hypospadias repair were initially described by Snodgrass and colleagues (1996) in their report of a multicenter experience. **Based, in part, on a 95% success rate for primary hypospadias repair, we have employed TIP urethroplasty for reoperative hypospadias. Results are similar to those for primary repair when all components of the TIP technique, as described for primary repair, are incorporated** (Borer et al, 2001).

For reoperative hypospadias repair, advantages of the TIP urethroplasty include use of local, usually supple tissue with well-established vascularity for urethroplasty and skin coverage, as well as a cosmetically superior result. The TIP urethroplasty technique is ideal for repair after failed Mathieu, OIF, and tubularization procedures because, theoretically, the native vascularity of the urethral plate has not been altered. **The absence of preputial skin in reoperative cases makes TIP urethroplasty an ideal option because additional skin flaps are not necessary for urethroplasty or for skin coverage, since mobilized ventral penile shaft skin is usually sufficient for the latter.**

Based on issues of tissue availability, it has been our experience that the OIF is rarely a feasible option in reoperative hypospadias repair. However, this impression is not universal. **In a report of reoperative repair using Mathieu and OIF techniques, secondary complications occurred in 24% and 14% of reoperative surgeries performed with these techniques, respectively** (Simmons et al, 1999). With similar concerns regarding skin coverage and a complication rate of 30% in reoperative cases (Koff et al, 1994), we would not recommend the modified Barcat technique as a viable alternative in such cases. Johanssen (1953) described a useful two-stage technique for repair of severe urethral stricture after hypospadias repair.

Joseph and Perez (1999) reported use of the **tunica vaginalis flap** as an onlay salvage procedure after multiple previously failed hypospadias repairs in 10 boys and 1 adult man. **This option for reoperative hypospadias has fallen into disfavor because of a complication rate of 60% for both meatal stenosis and urethral stricture.** A tubularized technique with tunica vaginalis tissue was previously described in several patients (Snow and Cartwright, 1992).

Ehrlich and Alter (1996) described the use of split-thickness skin graft and tunica vaginalis flaps for reoperative hypospadias. Using a two-stage procedure, 10 patients with one or more failed hypospadias repairs were treated by a varied combination of split-thickness mesh-graft urethroplasty and tunica vaginalis flap. A bed for the mesh graft in three patients was provided by a tunica vaginalis flap. Tunica vaginalis flaps were also used as an intermediate layer during stage two of the repair. No strictures or fistulas occurred in eight patients. Two patients were awaiting the second stage of repair after successful placement of the mesh graft. **The combination of split-thickness mesh-graft urethroplasty and a tunica vaginalis flap appears to achieve success in the difficult patient with complex hypospadias subsequent to multiple failed repairs.**

Free Graft with Local or Extragenital Tissue

Horton and Devine (1970) described the use of a tubularized free skin graft urethroplasty in patients with multiple, previously failed hypospadias repairs. This nonhirsute skin graft may be from a genital or extragenital source. **Similarly, and perhaps for use in more severe reoperative cases, free graft bladder mucosa** (Baskin and Duckett, 1994), **buccal mucosa ("dry" or "wet," onlay or tubularized)** (Baskin and Duckett, 1994; Duckett et al,

1995; Ahmed and Gough, 1997; Caldamone et al, 1998), **or a combination of these sources may be used** (Ransley et al, 1987; Retik, 1996).

Free graft of bladder mucosa has been used for successful repair in the most complex reoperative cases (Mollard et al, 1989). Buccal mucosa is used as a "dry" onlay (first stage of a planned two-stage repair), followed by tubularization at the second-stage repair for the hypospadias cripple. **Split-thickness mesh skin graft as first stage, followed by tubularization at second stage, may be a last resort for the hypospadias cripple in whom multiple previous attempts at repair have failed** (Schreiter and Noll, 1989).

LONG-TERM FOLLOW-UP

Gender Identity Issues

Sandberg and colleagues studied gender-role behavior of middle childhood boys (175 boys aged 6 to 10 years of age) with hypospadias (Sandberg et al, 1995). Parents completed standardized questionnaires regarding their son's behavior. Both questionnaires, the *Child Behavior and Attitude Questionnaire* and the *Child Game Participation Questionnaire*, may help to differentiate between gender-typical boys and boys with gender-identity disorders. **Hypospadias subjects did not show consistent differences from a community control group, and the severity of hypospadias was unrelated to gender-role behavior.** A greater number of hospitalizations was associated with increased gender-atypical behavior, but overall **it was concluded that hypospadias and possible associated "hypoandrogenization" did not interfere with development of gender-typical masculine behavior.**

Eberle and colleagues (1993) reported "satisfactory" results in two thirds of the 42 patients who were available for long-term follow-up after childhood posterior hypospadias repair. However, there were 13 patients who at follow-up still presented with complex sexual ambiguity. In six of these patients, androgen receptor defects were detected by means of biochemical as well as molecular-biologic investigations. **These authors emphasized the importance of androgen metabolism for male sexual development and underlined the necessity of careful evaluation in children with posterior hypospadias.**

Patient Satisfaction

Cosmesis

Mureau and colleagues studied children and adolescents (1995a) and men with previous hypospadias repair (1995b). **Although many of the children and adolescents (39%) desired functional and/or cosmetic penile improvement, they were reluctant to seek advice for these and other issues; therefore, such patients should be monitored through adolescence** (Mureau et al, 1995a). Similarly, adult hypospadias patients reported a more negative genital appraisal than comparison subjects, and 37% desired functional or cosmetic penile improvement (Mureau et al, 1995b).

Psychosexual Issues

Mureau and colleagues (1995a) studied psychosexual adjustment of children and adolescents. In relation to "comparison" subjects, 116 boys aged 9 to 18 years had a more negative genital appraisal and anticipated more ridicule by a partner because of penile appearance than comparison subjects, but sexual adjustment did not differ. The surgical procedures, the number of operations, and the age at final surgery did not significantly affect outcome. Mureau and colleagues (1995b, 1997) also evaluated psychosexual adjustment, sexual functioning, and genital appraisal in adult hypospadias patients 18 years of age or older. A total of 73 hypospadias patients and 50 comparison subjects received a semistructured interview. **More hypospadias patients (32.8%) than comparison subjects (12.8%) had been inhibited in seeking sexual contacts. The severity of hypospadias negatively affected genital appraisal. Patient age at final operation positively correlated with sociosexual development. The majority of hypospadias patients experienced a normal adult sex life but were reluctant to seek advice for problems.** This subject has been reviewed by others (Bracka, 1999; Woodhouse, 1994).

Functional Issues

Uroflow

Several authors have evaluated uroflowmetry parameters in normal boys (Szabo and Fegyverneki, 1995; Gutierrez Segura, 1997) and in boys after hypospadias repair (Svensson and Berg, 1983; Garibay et al, 1995; Jayanthi et al, 1995; Malyon et al, 1997). **At some centers, this noninvasive study is part of a postoperative evaluation routine and has been of value in identifying asymptomatic urethral stricture in some patients** (Garibay et al, 1995). Jayanthi and colleagues (1995) reviewed uroflowmetry data obtained after TPIF repair and after stricture and/or fistula repair and concluded that the neourethra was functionally equivalent to a normal urethra in most boys.

Sexual Function and Fertility

Several authors have reported relatively normal adult sexual function and fertility after hypospadias repair (Berg et al, 1981; Bracka, 1999; Mureau et al, 1995b; Svensson and Berg, 1983; Woodhouse, 1994). Selection bias may influence these results, because those with a less than optimal outcome or outlook may not wish to divulge such information and therefore may not be represented in these reports.

CURRENT TRENDS

It is clear that preservation of the urethral plate, if at all possible, has become a priority in current hy[.]pa-

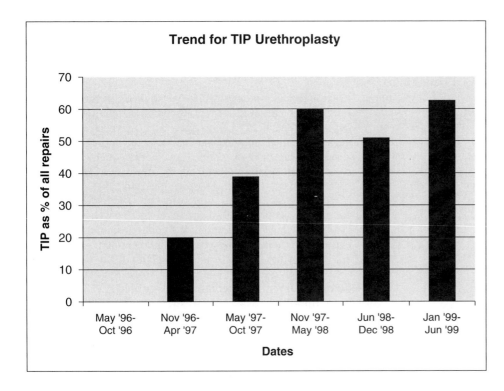

Figure 65–20. Bar graph representation of trend for frequency of TIP urethroplasty use during the consecutive 32 month period (November 1996 through June 1999) following incorporation of the technique. Experience is divided into intervals of approximately 6 months. Note that no TIP urethroplasty procedures were performed prior to November 1996.

dias repair. This, in part, explains the popularity and increasing indications for use of several tubularization and onlay techniques. For a relatively wide range of hypospadias, the tubularized, incised plate urethroplasty has gained popularity; it has become the technique of choice for both primary and reoperative middle and anterior hypospadias repair at our institution (Fig. 65–20) (Borer et al, 2001) and is touted as the ideal repair for distal hypospadias by others (Decter and Franzoni, 1999). **As the use of TIP urethroplasty for reoperative repair increases, perhaps the need for extragenital tissue use in this setting will decrease.**

Many, including its originators, have favored the OIF technique for a wide and increasing range of hypospadias (Baskin et al, 1994). In 1994, Baskin and colleagues reported use of the OIF in 374 or 33% of the total hypospadias repairs performed during a 5-year period. This represented an increase from 10% of total repairs in the immediately preceding 5-year period. The decreased fistula rate relative to the TPIF was thought to be a result of improved healing of the repair with preservation of the spongiosal supported urethral plate. **The current preference for onlay versus tubularized techniques, whenever possible, was predicted by Hodgson (1993).**

A variation of the OIF, the split prepuce in situ onlay technique described by Rushton and Belman (1998), has achieved excellent early results and has become the preferred technique for anterior hypospadias repair at some institutions (Yerkes et al, 2000). The OIF and several modifications are gaining popularity for repair of more proximal defects, complementing proven success over an already wide range of hypospadias. **This trend is supported by a comparison of results for proximal hypospadias repair using free grafts as an onlay versus a tube, with significantly higher proximal stricture rates**

for the latter (Powell et al, 2000). **Transition away from the use of free grafts and toward increased use of pedicled, vascularized flaps has also been reported** (Winslow and Devine, 1996).

FUTURE CONCEPTS

To this point, detailed principles and techniques for treatment of hypospadias have been discussed. With regard to hypospadias repair, tissue used for urethroplasty is typically obtained from either genital skin, extragenital skin, or mucosal grafts of bladder or buccal origin. **Although it is at times the only viable option for repair, the use of extragenital donor tissue may increase the morbidity of the procedure and/or the length of hospital stay for the patient. Ideally, a readily available and biocompatible alternative source of tissue would be helpful in this setting.**

Atala and colleagues (1999) have explored the use of a human cadaveric, bladder submucosal, collagen-based inert matrix as a potential substitute for use in hypospadias repair. In their preliminary report, four patients with one or more failed previous repairs underwent urethroplasty with the collagen-based inert matrix material in an onlay fashion. Length of tissue used ranged from 5 to 15 cm, and all repairs were covered with a tunica vaginalis flap. One patient developed a urethrocutaneous fistula, which was repaired by standard techniques. Postoperative urethrography and endoscopy showed a normal-appearing urethra in all patients. **Although this was a preliminary report, the *human cadaveric, bladder submucosal, collagen-based inert matrix* material may have a specific role for use in more complex reoperative cases with insufficient local tissue** (Atala et al, 1999). **Ideally, this type of urethral** tissue substitute would obviate the need for use of extragenital skin in the future.

CONCLUSIONS

Innovative concepts and techniques continue to emerge in the field of hypospadiology and with time may herald improvements to even the most basic of principles necessary for successful hypospadias repair. Hypospadiologists must be cognizant of the general principles of repair, be well versed in several appropriate techniques for all levels of hypospadias, and, most importantly, be dedicated to meticulous and uncompromising surgical technique and patient care as they strive for perfection in this *ever* flourishing field.

REFERENCES

Introduction

Aarskog D: Intersex conditions masquerading as simple hypospadias. Birth Defects Original Article Series 1971;7:122–130.

Barcat J: Current Concepts of Treatment. Boston: Little, Brown, 1973.

Borer JG, Bauer SB, Peters CA, et al: Tubularized, incised plate urethroplasty: Expanded use in primary and repeat surgery for hypospadias. J Urol 2001;165:581–585.

Culp OS: Experiences with 200 hypospadiacs: Evolution of a therapeutic plan. Surg Clin North Am 1959;39:1007–1023.

Duckett JW: Foreword: Symposium on hypospadias. Urol Clin North Am 1981;8:371–373.

Duckett JW: The current hype in hypospadiology. Br J Urol 1995;76(suppl. 3):1–7.

Duckett JW: Hypospadias. In Walsh PC, Retik AB, Vaughan ED Jr, Wein AJ (eds): Campbell's Urology, vol 2. Philadelphia, WB Saunders, 1998, pp 2093–2119.

Duckett JW, Keating MA: Technical challenge of the megameatus intact prepuce hypospadias variant: The pyramid procedure. J Urol 1989;141:1407–1409.

Hatch DA, Maizels M, Zaontz MR, et al: Hypospadias hidden by a complete prepuce. Surg Gynecol Obstet 1989;169:233–234.

Mouriquand PD, Persad R, Sharma S: Hypospadias repair: Current principles and procedures. Br J Urol 1995;76(suppl. 3):9–22.

Sauvage P, Becmeur F, Geiss S, et al: Transverse mucosal preputial flap for repair of severe hypospadias and isolated chordee without hypospadias: A 350-case experience. J Pediatr Surg 1993;28:435–438.

Sheldon CA, Duckett JW: Hypospadias. Pediatr Clin North Am 1987;34:1259–1272.

Sorensen HR: Hypospadias with special reference to aetiology. Copenhagen, Ejnar Munksgaard, 1953.

Development

Baskin LS, Erol A, Li YW, et al: Anatomical studies of hypospadias. J Urol 1998;160:1108–1115; discussion, 1137.

Glenister JW: The origin and fate of the urethral plate in man. J Anat 1954;288:413–418.

Hunter RH: Notes on the development of the prepuce. J Anat 1935;70:68–75.

Kurzrock EA, Baskin LS, Cunha GR: Ontogeny of the male urethra: Theory of endodermal differentiation. Differentiation 1999;64:115–122.

Stephens FD, Smith ED, Hutson JM: Embryogenesis of hypospadias. In Stephens FD (ed): Congenital Anomalies of the Urinary and Genital Tracts. Oxford, UK: Isis Medical Media Ltd, 1996, pp 80–90.

Etiology

Aaronson IA, Cakmak MA, Key LL: Defects of the testosterone biosynthetic pathway in boys with hypospadias. J Urol 1997;157:1884–1888.

Aarskog D: Maternal progestins as a possible cause of hypospadias. N Engl J Med 1979;300:75–78.

Adams MC, Chalian VS, Rink RC: Congenital dorsal penile curvature: A potential problem of the long phallus [see comments]. J Urol 1999;161:1304–1307.

Albers N, Ulrichs C, Gluer S, et al: Etiologic classification of severe hypospadias: Implications for prognosis and management [see comments]. J Pediatr 1997;131:386–392.

Allen TD, Griffin JE: Endocrine studies in patients with advanced hypospadias. J Urol 1984;131:310–314.

Baskin LS: Hypospadias and urethral development. J Urol 2000;163:951–956.

Baskin LS, Erol A, Li YW, et al: Anatomical studies of hypospadias. J Urol 1998;160:1108–1115; discussion, 1137.

Baskin LS, Liu W, Li Y, et al: FGF-10 gene disruption results in hypospadias. In Section on Urology Program for Scientific Sessions (Poster 31). Presented at 2000 Annual Meeting of the American Academy of Pediatrics, October 28, 2000. Chicago, American Academy of Pediatrics, 2000.

Bellinger MF: Embryology of the male external genitalia. Urol Clin North Am 1981;8:375–382.

Caldamone AA, Diamond DA: Contemporary hypospadiology. Contemp Urol 1999;11:61–77.

Cendron J, Melin Y: Congenital curvature of the penis without hypospadias. Urol Clin North Am 1981;8:389–395.

Creevy CD: The correction of hypospadias: A review. Urol Surv 1958;8:2–47.

Devine CJ Jr, Blackley SK, Horton CE, et al: The surgical treatment of chordee without hypospadias in men. J Urol 1991;146:325–329.

Devine CJ Jr, Horton CE: Chordee without hypospadias. J Urol 1973;110:264–271.

Devine CJ Jr, Horton CE: Hypospadias repair. J Urol 1977;118:188–193.

Donnahoo KK, Cain MP, Pope JC, et al: Etiology, management and surgical complications of congenital chordee without hypospadias. J Urol 1998;160:1120–1122.

Duckett JW, Devine CJ Jr, Mitchell ME, et al: Controversies in hypospadias surgery. Dial Pediatr Urol 1996;19:8.

Fredell L, Lichtenstein P, Pedersen NL, et al: Hypospadias is related to birth weight in discordant monozygotic twins. J Urol 1998;160:2197–2199.

Glenister JW: The origin and fate of the urethral plate in man. J Anat 1954;288:413–418.

Goldman AS, Bongiovanni AM: Induced genital anomalies. Ann N Y Acad Sci 1967;142:755–767.

Greene RR, Burrill MW, Ivy AC: Experimental intersexuality: The production of feminized male rats by antenatal treatment with estrogens. Science 1938;88:130–131.

Griffin JE: Androgen resistance: The clinical and molecular spectrum. N Engl J Med 1992;326:611–618.

Griffin JE, Wilson JD: Syndromes of androgen resistance. Hosp Pract (Off Ed) 1987;22:159–164.

Hunter RH: Notes on the development of the prepuce. J Anat 1935;70:68–75.

Hurwitz RS: Chordee without hypospadias. Dial Pediatr Urol 1986;9:1–8.

Kaplan GW, Lamm DL: Embryogenesis of chordee. J Urol 1975;114:769–772.

Macnab AJ, Zouves C: Hypospadias after assisted reproduction incorporating in vitro fertilization and gamete intrafallopian transfer. Fertil Steril 1991;56:918–922.

Marshall M Jr, Beh WP, Johnson SH, et al: Etiologic considerations in penoscrotal hypospadias repair. J Urol 1978;120:229–231.

Mau G: Progestins during pregnancy and hypospadias. Teratology 1981;24:285–287.

Mettauer JP: Practical observations in those malformations of the male urethra and penis, termed hypospadias and epispadias, with an anomalous case. Am J Med Sci 1842;4:43–58.

Myers JP: Endocrine disruption: Emerging science vitally important for pediatric urologists. (Special issue: The impact of the environment and endocrine disruptors on pediatric urology.) Dial Pediatr Urol 2000;23:8.

Paulozzi LJ: Is hypospadias an "environmental" birth defect. (Special issue: The impact of the environment and endocrine disruptors on pediatric urology.) Dial Pediatr Urol 2000;23:8.

Redman JF: Dorsal curvature of penis. Urology 1983;21:479–481.

Roberts CJ, Lloyd S: Observations on the epidemiology of simple hypospadias. BMJ 1973;1:768–770.

Silver RI, Rodriguez R, Chang TS, et al: In vitro fertilization is associated with an increased risk of hypospadias. J Urol 1999;161:1954–1957.

Smith DR: Hypospadias: Its anatomic and therapeutic considerations. J Int Coll Surg 1955;24:64.

Smith ED: The history of hypospadias. Pediatr Surg Int 1997;12:81–85.

Snodgrass W, Patterson K, Plaire JC, et al: Histology of the urethral plate: Implications for hypospadias repair. J Urol 2000;164:988–990.

Sorensen HR: Hypospadias with special reference to aetiology. Copenhagen, Ejnar Munksgaard, 1953.

Spiro SA, Seitzinger JW, Hanna MK: Hypospadias with dorsal chordee. Urology 1992;39:389–392.

Sweet RA, Schrott HG, Kurland R, et al: Study of the incidence of hypospadias in Rochester, Minnesota, 1940–1970, and a case-control comparison of possible etiologic factors. Mayo Clin Proc 1974;49:52–58.

Udall DA: Correction of 3 types of congenital curvatures of the penis, including the first reported case of dorsal curvature. J Urol 1980;124:50–52.

Van Hook W: A new operation for hypospadias. Ann Surg 1896;23:378–393.

Winslow BH, Devine CJ Jr: Principles in repair of hypospadias. Semin Pediatr Surg 1996;5:41–48.

Epidemiology

Bauer SB, Bull MJ, Retik AB: Hypospadias: A familial study. J Urol 1979;121:474–477.

Bauer SB, Retik AB, Colodny AH: Genetic aspects of hypospadias. Urol Clin North Am 1981;8:559–564.

Campbell MF: Hypospadias: When to operate. Am J Surg 1947;74:795–796.

Dolk H: Rise in prevalence of hypospadias. Lancet 1998;351:770.

Fredell L, Lichtenstein P, Pedersen NL, et al: Hypospadias is related to birth weight in discordant monozygotic twins. J Urol 1998;160:2197–2199.

Paulozzi LJ, Erickson JD, Jackson RJ: Hypospadias trends in two US surveillance systems. Pediatrics 1997;100:831–834.

Roberts CJ, Lloyd S: Observations on the epidemiology of simple hypospadias. Br Med J 1973;1:768–770.

Sorber M, Feitz WF, de Vries JD: Short- and mid-term outcome of different types of one-stage hypospadias corrections. Eur Urol 1997;32:475–479.

Sorensen HR: Hypospadias with special reference to aetiology. Copenhagen, Ejnar Munksgaard, 1953.

Sweet RA, Schrott HG, Kurland R, et al: Study of the incidence of hypospadias in Rochester, Minnesota, 1940–1970, and a case-control comparison of possible etiologic factors. Mayo Clin Proc 1974;49:52–58.

Van Hook W: A new operation for hypospadias. Ann Surg 1896;23:378–393.

Associated Findings

Aarskog D: Clinical and cytogenetic studies in hypospadias. Acta Paediatr Scand Suppl 1970;203:1–61.

Aarskog D: Intersex conditions masquerading as simple hypospadias. Birth Defects Original Article Series 1971;7:122–130.

Albers N, Ulrichs C, Gluer S, et al: Etiologic classification of severe hypospadias: Implications for prognosis and management [see comments]. J Pediatr 1997;131:386–392.

Borer JG, Nitti VW, Glassberg KI: Mixed gonadal dysgenesis and dysgenetic male pseudohermaphroditism. J Urol 1995;153:1267–1273.

Jones KL: Smith's Recognizable Patterns of Human Malformation, 5th ed, vol 1. Philadelphia, WB Saunders, 1997.

Kaefer M, Diamond DA, Hendren WH, et al: The incidence of intersexuality in children with cryptorchidism and hypospadias: Stratification based on gonadal palpability and meatal position. J Urol 1999;162:1003–1006; discussion, 1006–1007.

Khuri FJ, Hardy BE, Churchill BM: Urologic anomalies associated with hypospadias. Urol Clin North Am 1981;8:565–571.

Rajfer J, Walsh PC: The incidence of intersexuality in patients with hypospadias and cryptorchidism. J Urol 1976;116:769–770.

Smith EP, Wacksman J: Evaluation of severe hypospadias [see comments]. (Editorial; comment.) J Pediatr 1997;131:344–346.

Sorber M, Feitz WF, de Vries JD: Short- and mid-term outcome of different types of one-stage hypospadias corrections. Eur Urol 1997;32:475–479.

Sweet RA, Schrott HG, Kurland R, et al: Study of the incidence of hypospadias in Rochester, Minnesota, 1940–1970, and a case-control comparison of possible etiologic factors. Mayo Clin Proc 1974;49:52–58.

Yamaguchi T, Kitada S, Osada Y: Chromosomal anomalies in cryptorchidism and hypospadias. Urol Int 1991;47:60–63.

Special Considerations: Preoperative

Aaronson IA, Cakmak MA, Key LL: Defects of the testosterone biosynthetic pathway in boys with hypospadias. J Urol 1997;157:1884–1888.

Albers N, Ulrichs C, Gluer S, et al: Etiologic classification of severe hypospadias: Implications for prognosis and management [see comments]. J Pediatr 1997;131:386–392.

Allen TD, Griffin JE: Endocrine studies in patients with advanced hypospadias. J Urol 1984;131:310–314.

Backus LH, De Felice CA: Hypospadias: Then and now. Plast Reconstr Surg 1960;25:146.

Baskin LS, Sutherland RS, DiSandro MJ, et al: The effect of testosterone on androgen receptors and human penile growth. J Urol 1997;158:1113–1118.

Belman AB: Hypospadias update. Urology 1997;49:166–172.

Bin-Abbas B, Conte FA, Grumbach MM, et al: Congenital hypogonadotropic hypogonadism and micropenis: Effect of testosterone treatment on adult penile size: why sex reversal is not indicated. J Pediatr 1999;134:579–583.

Cabot H: The treatment of hypospadias in theory and practice. N Engl J Med 1936;214:871–875.

Cecil AB: Surgery of hypospadias and epispadias in the male. J Urol 1932;27:507–537.

Cerasaro TS, Brock WA, Kaplan GW: Upper urinary tract anomalies associated with congenital hypospadias: Is screening necessary? J Urol 1986;135:537–538.

Davenport M, MacKinnon AE: The value of ultrasound screening of the upper urinary tract in hypospadias. Br J Urol 1988;62:595–596.

Fichtner J, Filipas D, Mottrie AM, et al: Analysis of meatal location in 500 men: Wide variation questions need for meatal advancement in all pediatric anterior hypospadias cases. J Urol 1995;154:833–834.

Gearhart JP, Jeffs RD: The use of parenteral testosterone therapy in genital reconstructive surgery. J Urol 1987;138:1077–1078.

Koff SA, Jayanthi VR: Preoperative treatment with human chorionic gonadotropin in infancy decreases the severity of proximal hypospadias and chordee [see comments]. J Urol 1999;162:1435–1439.

McArdle F, Lebowitz R: Uncomplicated hypospadias and anomalies of upper urinary tract: Need for screening? Urology 1975;5:712–716.

McMahon DR, Kramer SA, Husmann DA: Micropenis: Does early treatment with testosterone do more harm than good? J Urol 1995;154:825–829.

Monfort G, Lucas C: Dihydrotestosterone penile stimulation in hypospadias surgery. Eur Urol 1982;8:201–203.

Perovic S, Vukadinovic V: Onlay island flap urethroplasty for severe hypospadias: A variant of the technique. J Urol 1994;151:711–714.

Rajfer J, Walsh PC: The incidence of intersexuality in patients with hypospadias and cryptorchidism. J Urol 1976;116:769–770.

Retik AB: Proximal hypospadias. In Marshall FF (ed): Textbook of Operative Urology. Philadelphia, WB Saunders, 1996, pp 977–984.

Shima H, Ikoma F, Yabumoto H, et al: Gonadotropin and testosterone response in prepubertal boys with hypospadias. J Urol 1986;135:539–542.

Stock JA, Scherz HC, Kaplan GW: Distal hypospadias. Urol Clin North Am 1995;22:131–138.

Sutherland RS, Kogan BA, Baskin LS, et al: The effect of prepubertal androgen exposure on adult penile length. J Urol 1996;156:783–787; discussion, 787.

Historical Aspects of Hypospadias Repair

Aronoff M: A one-stage operative technique for the treatment of subglandular hypospadias in children. Br J Plastic Surgery 1963;16:59–62.

Asopa HS, Elhence IP, Atri SP, et al: One stage correction of penile hypospadias using a foreskin tube: A preliminary report. Int Surg 1971;55:435–440.

Backus LH, De Felice CA: Hypospadias: Then and now. Plast Reconstr Surg 1960;25:146–160.

Beck C: A new operation for balanic hypospadias. N Y Med J 1898;67: 147.

Bevan AD: A new operation for hypospadias. JAMA 1917;68:1032–1033.

Blair VP, Brown JB, Hamm WG: The correction of scrotal hypospadias and of epispadias. Surg Gynecol Obstet 1933;57:646–653.

Broadbent TR, Woolf RM, Toksu E: Hypospadias: One-stage repair. Plast Reconstr Surg 1961;27:154–157.

Browne D: An operation for hypospadias. Lancet 1936;1:141.

Browne D: An operation for hypospadias. Proc R Soc Med 1949;42:466–468.

Bucknall TH: A new operation for penile hypospadias. Lancet 1907;2: 887–890.

Bürger RA, Muller SC, el-Damanhoury H, et al: The buccal mucosal graft for urethral reconstruction: A preliminary report. J Urol 1992;147:662–664.

Byars LT: Functional restoration of hypospadias deformities: With a report of 60 completed cases. Surg Gynecol Obstet 1951;92:149–154.

Byars LT: Technique of consistently satisfactory repair of hypospadias. Surg Gynecol Obstet 1955;100:184–190.

Cecil AB: Surgery of hypospadias and epispadias in the male. J Urol 1932;27:507–537.

Cecil AB: Repair of hypospadias and urethral fistula. J Urol 1946;56:237–242.

Creevy CD: The correction of hypospadias: a review. Urol Surv 1958;8: 2–47.

Davis DM: The pedicle tube-graft in the surgical treatment of hypospadias in the male: With new method of closing small urethral fistulas. Surg Gynecol Obstet 1940;71:790–796.

Davis DM: Surgical treatment of hypospadias, especially scrotal and perineal. J Urol 1951;65:595–602.

Des Prez JD, Persky L, Kiehn CL: A one-stage repair of hypospadias by island flap technique. Plast Reconstr Surg 1961;28:405–410.

Dessanti A, Rigamonti W, Merulla V, et al: Autologous buccal mucosa graft for hypospadias repair: An initial report. J Urol 1992;147:1081–1083; discussion, 1083–1084.

Devine CJ Jr, Horton CE: A one stage hypospadias repair. J Urol 1961; 85:166–172.

Duckett JW: Transverse preputial island flap technique for repair of severe hypospadias. Urol Clin North Am 1980;7:423–430.

Duplay LS: Sur le traitement chirurgical de l'hypospadias et de l'epispadias. Arch Gen Med 1880;5:257–276.

Edmunds A: An operation for hypospadias. Lancet 1913;1:447–449.

Edmunds A: Pseudo-hermaphroditism and hypospadias: Their surgical treatment. Lancet 1926;1:323–327.

Hagner FR: A new method for straightening the penis in hypospadias. JAMA 1932;99:116.

Hauben DJ: The history of hypospadias. Acta Chir Plast 1984;26:196–199.

Hendren WH, Reda EF: Bladder mucosa graft for construction of male urethra. J Pediatr Surg 1986;21:189–192.

Hodgson NB: A one-stage hypospadias repair. J Urol 1970;104:281–283.

Hodgson NB: History of hypospadias. In Ehrlich RM, Alter GJ (eds): Reconstructive and Plastic Surgery of the External Genitalia: Adult and Pediatric. Philadelphia, WB Saunders, 1999, pp 13–17.

Humby G: A one-stage operation for hypospadias. Br J Surg 1941;29:84–92.

Koyanagi T, Nonomura K, Yamashita T, et al: One-stage repair of hypospadias: Is there no simple method universally applicable to all types of hypospadias? [see comments]. J Urol 1994;152:1232–1237.

Marshall VF, Spellman RM: Construction of urethra in hypospadias using vesical mucosal grafts. J Urol 1955;73:335.

Mathieu P: Traitement en un temps de l'hypospadias balanique ou juxtabalanique. Journal de Chirurgie 1932;39:481–486.

Mayo CH: Hypospadias. JAMA 1901;36:1157–1162.

McIndoe AH: The treatment of hypospadias. Am J Surg 1937;38:176–185.

Memmelaar J: Use of bladder mucosa in a one-stage repair of hypospadias. J Urol 1947;58:68.

Mettauer JP: Practical observations in those malformations of the male urethra and penis, termed hypospadias and epispadias, with an anomalous case. Am J Med Sci 1842;4:43–58.

Murphy LJT: The urethra. In Murphy LJT (ed): The History of Urology. Springfield, Charles C Thomas, 1972, pp 453–481.

Mustarde JC: One-stage correction of distal hypospadias: And other people's fistulae. Br J Plast Surg 1965;18:413–422.

Nesbit RM: Plastic procedure for correction of hypospadias. J Urol 1941; 45:699–702.

Nové-Josserand G: Traitement de l'hypospadias; nouvelle methode. Lyon Med 1897;85:198–200.

Nové-Josserand G: Resultats eloignes de l'uretroplastie par la tunnellisation et la greffe dermo-epidermique dans les formes graves de l'hypospadias et de l'epispadias. J d'Urologie 1914;5:393–406.

Ombredanne L: Clinique et Operation de Chirurgie Infantile. Paris, Masson, 1932.

Retik AB, Bauer SB, Mandell J, et al: Management of severe hypospadias with a 2-stage repair. J Urol 1994;152:749–751.

Russell RH: Operation for severe hypospadias. BMJ 1900;2:1432–1435.

Smith D: A de-epithelialised overlap flap technique in the repair of hypospadias. Br J Plast Surg 1973;26:106–114.

Smith ED: The history of hypospadias. Pediatr Surg Int 1997;12:81–85.

Thiersch C: Ueber die entstehungsweise und operative behandlung der epispadie. Arch Heilkunde 1869;10:20–35.

Van Hook W: A new operation for hypospadias. Ann Surg 1896;23:378–393.

Wehrbein HL: Hypospadias. J Urol 1943;50:335–340.

Young F, Benjamin JA: Repair of hypospadias with free inlay skin graft. Surg Gynecol Obstet 1948;86:439–451.

General Principles of Hypospadias Repair

Allen TD, Roehrborn CG: Pedicled preputial patch in repair of minor penile chordee with or without hypospadias. Urology 1993;42:63–65.

Allen TD, Spence HM: The surgical treatment of coronal hypospadias and related problems. J Urol 1968;100:504–508.

Baskin LS, Duckett JW: Dorsal tunica albuginea plication for hypospadias curvature. J Urol 1994;151:1668–1671.

Baskin LS, Lue TF: The correction of congenital penile curvature in young men. Br J Urol 1998;81:895–899.

Belman AB: De-epithelialized skin flap coverage in hypospadias repair. J Urol 1988;140:1273–1276.

Bologna RA, Noah TA, Nasrallah PF, et al: Chordee: Varied opinions and treatments as documented in a survey of the American Academy of Pediatrics, Section of Urology. Urology 1999;53:608–612.

Byars LT: Functional restoration of hypospadias deformities: With a report of 60 completed cases. Surg Gynecol Obstet 1951;92:149–154.

Churchill BM, van Savage JG, Khoury AE, et al: The dartos flap as an adjunct in preventing urethrocutaneous fistulas in repeat hypospadias surgery. J Urol 1996;156:2047–2049.

Culp OS: Struggles and triumphs with hypospadias and associated anomalies: Review of 400 cases. J Urol 1966;96:339–351.

Decter RM: Chordee correction by corporal rotation: The split and roll technique. J Urol 1999;162:1152–1154; discussion, 1155.

Devine CJ Jr, Horton CE: Use of dermal graft to correct chordee. J Urol 1975;113:56–58.

Devine CJ Jr, Horton CE: Hypospadias repair. J Urol 1977;118:188–193.

Gittes RF, McLaughlin AP: Injection technique to induce penile erection. Urology 1974;4:473–474.

Hendren WH, Caesar RE: Chordee without hypospadias: Experience with 33 cases. J Urol 1992;147:107–109.

Hendren WH, Keating MA: Use of dermal graft and free urethral graft in penile reconstruction. J Urol 1988;140:1265–1269.

Hinman F Jr: The blood supply to preputial island flaps. J Urol 1991;145: 1232–1235.

Horton CE, Devine CJ Jr: Simulated erection of the penis with saline injection, a diagnostic maneuver. Plast Reconstr Surg 1977;59:138–139.

Horton CE Jr, Gearhart JP, Jeffs RD: Dermal grafts for correction of severe chordee associated with hypospadias. J Urol 1993;150:452–455.

Jordan GH: Penile reconstruction, phallic construction, and urethral reconstruction. Urol Clin North Am 1999a;26:1–13, vii.

Jordan GH: Techniques of tissue handling and transfer. J Urol 1999b;162: 1213–1217.

Kass EJ: Dorsal corporeal rotation: An alternative technique for the management of severe chordee. J Urol 1993;150:635–636.

Kass EJ, Chung AK: Glanuloplasty and in situ tubularization of the urethral plate: Long-term followup. J Urol 2000;164:991–993.

King LR: Hypospadias—A one-stage repair without skin graft based on a new principle: Chordee is sometimes produced by the skin alone. J Urol 1970;103:660–662.

King LR: Cutaneous chordee and its implications in hypospadias repair. Urol Clin North Am 1981;8:397–402.

Kirkali Z: Tunica vaginalis: An aid in hypospadias surgery. Br J Urol 1990;65:530–532.

Klevmark B, Andersen M, Schultz A, et al: Congenital and acquired curvature of the penis treated surgically by plication of the tunica albuginea. Br J Urol 1994;74:501–506.

Koff SA, Eakins M: The treatment of penile chordee using corporeal rotation. J Urol 1984;131:931–932.

Kogan BA: Intraoperative pharmacological erection as an aid to pediatric hypospadias repair. J Urol 2000;164:2058–2061.

Lindgren BW, Reda EF, Levitt SB, et al: Single and multiple dermal grafts for the management of severe penile curvature. J Urol 1998;160:1128–1130.

Mustarde JC: One-stage correction of distal hypospadias: And other people's fistulae. Br J Plast Surg 1965;18:413–422.

Nesbit RM: Plastic procedure for correction of hypospadias. J Urol 1941;45:699–702.

Nesbit R: Congenital curvature of the phallus: Report of three cases with description of corrective operation. J Urol 1965;93:230–232.

Ombredanne L: Clinique et Operation de Chirurgie Infantile. Paris, Masson, 1932.

Perlmutter AD, Montgomery BT, Steinhardt GF: Tunica vaginalis free graft for the correction of chordee. J Urol 1985;134:311–313.

Perovic S, Djordjevic M, Djakovic N: Natural erection induced by prostaglandin-E1 in the diagnosis and treatment of congenital penile anomalies. Br J Urol 1997;79:43–46.

Perovic SV, Djordjevic ML, Djakovic NG: A new approach to the treatment of penile curvature. J Urol 1998;160:1123–1127.

Pope JC, Kropp BP, McLaughlin KP, et al: Penile orthoplasty using dermal grafts in the outpatient setting. Urology 1996;48:124–127.

Retik AB, Keating M, Mandell J: Complications of hypospadias repair. Urol Clin North Am 1988;15:223–236.

Retik AB, Mandell J, Bauer SB, et al: Meatal based hypospadias repair with the use of a dorsal subcutaneous flap to prevent urethrocutaneous fistula. J Urol 1994;152:1229–1231.

Saalfeld J, Ehrlich RM, Gross JM, et al: Congenital curvature of the penis. Successful results with variations in corporoplasty. J Urol 1973;109:64–65.

Sensöz Ö, Celebioglu S, Baran CN, et al: A new technique for distal hypospadias repair: Advancement of a distally deepithelialized urethrocutaneous flap. Plast Reconstr Surg 1997;99:93–98; discussion, 99.

Smith DR: Hypospadias: Its anatomic and therapeutic considerations. J Int Coll Surg 1955;24:64.

Smith D: A de-epithelialised overlap flap technique in the repair of hypospadias. Br J Plast Surg 1973;26:106–114.

Snow BW: Use of tunica vaginalis to prevent fistulas in hypospadias surgery. J Urol 1986;136:861–863.

Snow BW: Transverse corporeal plication for persistent chordee. Urology 1989;34:360–361.

Snow BW, Cartwright PC, Unger K: Tunica vaginalis blanket wrap to prevent urethrocutaneous fistula: An 8-year experience. J Urol 1995;153:472–473.

Standoli L: Vascularized urethroplasty flaps: The use of vascularized flaps of preputial and penopreputial skin for urethral reconstruction in hypospadias. Clin Plast Surg 1988;15:355–370.

Stewart TS, Bartkowski DP, Perlmutter AD: Tunica vaginalis patch graft for treatment of severe chordee. J Urol 1995;153(suppl.):340A.

Thiersch C: Ueber die entstehungsweise und operative behandlung der epispadie. Arch Heilkunde 1869;10:20–35.

Udall DA: Correction of 3 types of congenital curvatures of the penis, including the first reported case of dorsal curvature. J Urol 1980;124:50–52.

van Horn AC, Kass EJ: Glanuloplasty and in situ tubularization of the urethral plate: A simple reliable technique for the majority of boys with hypospadias. J Urol 1995;154:1505–1507.

Yerkes EB, Adams MC, Miller DA, et al: Y-to-I wrap: Use of the distal spongiosum for hypospadias repair. J Urol 2000;163:1536–1538; discussion, 1538–1539.

Special Considerations: Perioperative

Caldamone AA, Diamond DA: Contemporary hypospadiology. Contemp Urol 1999;11:61–77.

Chhibber AK, Perkins FM, Rabinowitz R, et al: Penile block timing for postoperative analgesia of hypospadias repair in children. J Urol 1997;158:1156–1159.

Cilento BG Jr, Stock JA, Kaplan GW: Pantaloon spica cast: An effective method for postoperative immobilization after free graft hypospadias repair. J Urol 1997;157:1882–1883.

Cromie WJ, Bellinger MF: Hypospadias dressings and diversions. Urol Clin North Am 1981;8:545–558.

De Sy WA, Oosterlinck W: Silicone foam elastomer: A significant improvement in postoperative penile dressing. J Urol 1982;128:39–40.

Demirbilek S, Atayurt HF: One-stage hypospadias repair with stent or suprapubic diversion: Which is better? J Pediatr Surg 1997;32:1711–1712.

DiSandro M, Palmer JM: Stricture incidence related to suture material in hypospadias surgery. J Pediatr Surg 1996;31:881–884.

Hakim S, Merguerian PA, Rabinowitz R, et al: Outcome analysis of the modified Mathieu hypospadias repair: Comparison of stented and unstented repairs. J Urol 1996;156:836–838.

Hensle T, Tennenbaum S, Reiley E, et al: Hypospadias repair in the adult population: Adventures and misadventures. J Urol 2001;165:77–79.

Horton CE Jr, Horton CE: Complications of hypospadias surgery. Clin Plast Surg 1988;15:371–379.

Jordan GH: Techniques of tissue handling and transfer. J Urol 1999;162:1213–1217.

Kass E, Kogan SJ, Manley C: Timing of elective surgery on the genitalia of male children with particular reference to the risks, benefits, and psychological effects of surgery and anesthesia. Pediatrics 1996;97:590–594.

Kelalis P, Bunge R, Barkin M: The timing of elective surgery on the genitalia of male children with particular reference to undescended testes and hypospadias. Pediatrics 1975;56:479–483.

Kirsch AJ, Canning DA, Zderic SA, et al: Laser soldering technique for sutureless urethral surgery. Tech Urol 1997;3:108–113.

Kirsch AJ, de Vries GM, Chang DT, et al: Hypospadias repair by laser tissue soldering: Intraoperative results and follow-up in 30 children. Urology 1996;48:616–623.

Lepore AG, Kesler RW: Behavior of children undergoing hypospadias repair. J Urol 1979;122:68–70.

Manley CB, Epstein ES: Early hypospadias repair. J Urol 1981;125:698–700.

McCormack M, Homsy Y, Laberge Y: "No stent, no diversion": Mathieu hypospadias repair. Can J Surg 1993;36:152–154.

McLorie GA, Joyner BD, Bagli DJ, et al: A prospective randomized clinical trial to evaluate methods of postoperative care in hypospadias. Pediatrics 1999;104(suppl):813A.

Minevich E, Pecha BR, Wacksman J, et al: Mathieu hypospadias repair: Experience in 202 patients. J Urol 1999;162:2141–2142; discussion, 2142–2143.

Rabinowitz R: Outpatient catheterless modified Mathieu hypospadias repair. J Urol 1987;138:1074–1076.

Retik AB, Mandell J, Bauer SB, et al: Meatal based hypospadias repair with the use of a dorsal subcutaneous flap to prevent urethrocutaneous fistula. J Urol 1994;152:1229–1231.

Scherr DS, Poppas DP: Laser tissue welding. Urol Clin North Am 1998;25:123–135.

Schultz JR, Klykylo WM, Wacksman J: Timing of elective hypospadias repair in children. Pediatrics 1983;71:342–351.

Shapiro SR: Hypospadias repair: Optical magnification versus Zeiss reconstruction microscope. Urology 1989;33:43–46.

Steckler RE, Zaontz MR: Stent-free Thiersch-Duplay hypospadias repair with the Snodgrass modification. J Urol 1997;158:1178–1180.

Stock JA, Kaplan GW: Ketoconazole for prevention of postoperative penile erection. Urology 1995;45:308–309.

Ulman I, Erikci V, Avanoglu A, et al: The effect of suturing technique and material on complication rate following hypospadias repair. Eur J Pediatr Surg 1997;7:156–157.

Van Savage JG, Palanca LG, Slaughenhoupt BL: A prospective randomized trial of dressings versus no dressings for hypospadias repair. J Urol 2000;164:981–983.

Wacksman J: Repair of hypospadias using new mouth-controlled microscope. Urology 1987;29:276–278.

Winslow BH, Devine CJ Jr: Principles in repair of hypospadias. Semin Pediatr Surg 1996;5:41–48.

Zaontz MR: Nuances of hypospadias. Probl Urol 1990;4:705–721.

Primary Hypospadias Repair

Ahmed S, Gough DC: Buccal mucosal graft for secondary hypospadias repair and urethral replacement. Br J Urol 1997;80:328–330.

Arap S, Mitre AI, De Goes GM: Modified meatal advancement and glanuloplasty repair of distal hypospadias. J Urol 1984;131:1140–1141.

Asopa HS, Elhence IP, Atri SP, et al: One stage correction of penile hypospadias using a foreskin tube: A preliminary report. Int Surg 1971; 55:435–440.

Baker LA, Mathews RI, Docimo SG: Radical bulbar dissection to correct severe chordee and proximal hypospadias. J Urol 2000;164:1347–1349.

Barcat J: Current Concepts of Treatment. Boston, Little, Brown, 1973.

Barroso UJ, Jednak R, Spencer Barthold J, et al: Further experience with the double onlay preputial flap for hypospadias repair. J Urol 2000;164: 998–1001.

Barthold JS, Teer TL, Redman JF: Modified Barcat balanic groove technique for hypospadias repair: Experience with 295 cases. J Urol 1996; 155:1735–1737.

Baskin LS, Duckett JW: Mucosal grafts in hypospadias and stricture management. AUA Update Series 1994;13:270–275.

Baskin LS, Duckett JW: Buccal mucosa grafts in hypospadias surgery. Br J Urol 1995;76(suppl. 3):23–30.

Baskin LS, Duckett JW, Ueoka K, et al: Changing concepts of hypospadias curvature lead to more onlay island flap procedures. J Urol 1994; 151:191–196.

Beck C: A new operation for balanic hypospadias. N Y Med J 1898;67: 147.

Bevan AD: A new operation for hypospadias. JAMA 1917;68:1032–1033.

Borer JG, Bauer SB, Peters CA, et al: Tubularized, incised plate urethroplasty: Expanded use in primary and repeat surgery for hypospadias. J Urol 2001;165:581–585.

Borer JG, Retik AB: Current trends in hypospadias repair. Urol Clin North Am 1999;26:15–37, vii.

Bracka A: Hypospadias repair: The two-stage alternative [see comments]. Br J Urol 1995a;76(suppl. 3):31–41.

Bracka A: A versatile two-stage hypospadias repair. Br J Plast Surg 1995b;48:345–352.

Bürger RA, Muller SC, el-Damanhoury H, et al: The buccal mucosal graft for urethral reconstruction: A preliminary report. J Urol 1992;147:662–664.

Caione P, Capozza N, Lais A, et al: Long-term results of distal urethral advancement glanuloplasty for distal hypospadias. J Urol 1997;158: 1168–1170; discussion, 1170–1171.

Chen S, Wang G, Wang M: Modified longitudinal preputial island flap urethroplasty for repair of hypospadias: Results in 60 patients. J Urol 1993;149:814–816.

Decter RM, Franzoni DF: Distal hypospadias repair by the modified Thiersch-Duplay technique with or without hinging the urethral plate: A near ideal way to correct distal hypospadias. J Urol 1999;162:1156–1158.

Dessanti A, Rigamonti W, Merulla V, et al: Autologous buccal mucosa graft for hypospadias repair: An initial report. J Urol 1992;147:1081–1083; discussion, 1083–1084.

Devine CJ Jr, Horton CE: A one stage hypospadias repair. J Urol 1961; 85:166–172.

Devine CJ Jr, Horton CE: Hypospadias repair. J Urol 1977;118:188–193.

Dewan PA, Dinneen MD, Duffy PG, et al: Pedicle patch urethroplasty. Br J Urol 1991;67:420–423.

Duckett JW: Transverse preputial island flap technique for repair of severe hypospadias. Urol Clin North Am 1980;7:423–430.

Duckett JW: MAGPI (meatoplasty and glanuloplasty): A procedure for subcoronal hypospadias. Urol Clin North Am 1981;8:513–519.

Duckett JW, Coplen D, Ewalt D, et al: Buccal mucosal urethral replacement [see comments]. J Urol 1995;153:1660–1663.

Duckett JW, Keating MA: Technical challenge of the megameatus intact prepuce hypospadias variant: The pyramid procedure. J Urol 1989;141: 1407–1409.

Duckett JW, Snyder HM: Meatal advancement and glanuloplasty hypospadias repair after 1,000 cases: Avoidance of meatal stenosis and regression. J Urol 1992;147:665–669.

Duplay LS: Sur le traitement chirurgical de l'hypospadias et de l'epispadias. Arch Gen Med 1880;5:257–276.

Elder JS, Duckett JW, Snyder HM: Onlay island flap in the repair of mid and distal penile hypospadias without chordee. J Urol 1987;138:376–379.

Flack CE, Walker RD 3rd: Onlay-tube-onlay urethroplasty technique in primary perineal hypospadias surgery. J Urol 1995;154:837–839.

Gearhart JP, Borland RN: Onlay island flap urethroplasty: Variation on a theme. J Urol 1992;148:1507–1509.

Glassberg KI: Augmented Duckett repair for severe hypospadias. J Urol 1987;138:380–381.

Glassberg KI, Hansbrough F, Horowitz M: The Koyanagi-Nonomura 1-stage bucket repair of severe hypospadias with and without penoscrotal transposition. J Urol 1998;160:1104–1107; discussion, 1137.

Gonzalez R, Smith C, Denes ED: Double onlay preputial flap for proximal hypospadias repair. J Urol 1996;156:832–834; discussion, 834–835.

Hakim S, Merguerian PA, Rabinowitz R, et al: Outcome analysis of the modified Mathieu hypospadias repair: Comparison of stented and unstented repairs. J Urol 1996;156:836–838.

Hamilton JM: Island flap repair of hypospadias. South Med J 1969;62: 881–882.

Harris DL: Splitting the prepuce to provide two independently vascularised flaps: A one-stage repair of hypospadias and congenital short urethra. Br J Plast Surg 1984;37:108–116.

Harrison DH, Grobbelaar AO: Urethral advancement and glanuloplasty (UGPI): A modification of the MAGPI procedure for distal hypospadias. Br J Plast Surg 1997;50:206–211.

Hatch DA, Maizels M, Zaontz MR, et al: Hypospadias hidden by a complete prepuce. Surg Gynecol Obstet 1989;169:233–234.

Hendren WH, Horton CE Jr: Experience with 1-stage repair of hypospadias and chordee using free graft of prepuce. J Urol 1988;140:1259–1264.

Hendren WH, Keating MA: Use of dermal graft and free urethral graft in penile reconstruction. J Urol 1988;140:1265–1269.

Hendren WH, Reda EF: Bladder mucosa graft for construction of male urethra. J Pediatr Surg 1986;21:189–192.

Hill GA, Wacksman J, Lewis AG, et al: The modified pyramid hypospadias procedure: Repair of megameatus and deep glanular groove variants. J Urol 1993;150:1208–1211.

Hodgson NB: A one-stage hypospadias repair. J Urol 1970;104:281–283.

Hollowell JG, Keating MA, Snyder HM, et al: Preservation of the urethral plate in hypospadias repair: Extended applications and further experience with the onlay island flap urethroplasty. J Urol 1990;143:98–100; discussion, 100–101.

Humby G: A one-stage operation for hypospadias. Br J Surg 1941;29:84–92.

Kass EJ, Chung AK: Glanuloplasty and in situ tubularization of the urethral plate: Long-term followup. J Urol 2000;164:991–993.

Keating MA, Duckett JW: Failed hypospadias repair. In Cohen MS, Resnick MI (eds): Reoperative Urology. Boston, Little, Brown, 1995, pp 187–204.

King LR: Hypospadias—A one-stage repair without skin graft based on a new principle: Chordee is sometimes produced by the skin alone. J Urol 1970;103:660–662.

King LR: Cutaneous chordee and its implications in hypospadias repair. Urol Clin North Am 1981;8:397–402.

Kocvara R, Dvoracek J: Inlay-onlay flap urethroplasty for hypospadias and urethral stricture repair. J Urol 1997;158:2142–2145.

Koff SA, Brinkman J, Ulrich J, et al: Extensive mobilization of the urethral plate and urethra for repair of hypospadias: The modified Barcat technique. J Urol 1994;151:466–469.

Koyanagi T, Nonomura K, Yamashita T, et al: One-stage repair of hypospadias: Is there no simple method universally applicable to all types of hypospadias? [see comments]. J Urol 1994;152:1232–1237.

Marshall VF, Spellman RM: Construction of urethra in hypospadias using vesical mucosal grafts. J Urol 1955;73:335.

Mathieu P: Traitement en un temps de l'hypospadias balanique ou juxtabalanique. J Chir 1932;39:481–486.

Memmelaar J: Use of bladder mucosa in a one-stage repair of hypospadias. J Urol 1947;58:68.

Mollard P, Mouriquand P, Felfela T: Application of the onlay island flap urethroplasty to penile hypospadias with severe chordee. Br J Urol 1991;68:317–319.

Mustarde JC: One-stage correction of distal hypospadias: And other people's fistulae. Br J Plast Surg 1965;18:413–422.

Nonomura K, Kakizaki H, Shimoda N, et al: Surgical repair of anterior hypospadias with fish-mouth meatus and intact prepuce based on anatomical characteristics. Eur Urol 1998;34:368–371.

Nové-Josserand G: Traitement de l'hypospadias; nouvelle methode. Lyon Med 1897;85:198–200.

Nové-Josserand G: Resultats eloignes de l'uretroplastie par la tunnellisation et la greffe dermo-epidermique dans les formes graves de l'hypospadias et de l'epispadias. J d'Urologie 1914;5:393–406.

Park JM, Faerber GJ, Bloom DA: Long-term outcome evaluation of patients undergoing the meatal advancement and glanuloplasty procedure [see comments]. J Urol 1995;153:1655–1656.

Perovic S, Vukadinovic V: Onlay island flap urethroplasty for severe hypospadias: A variant of the technique. J Urol 1994;151:711–714.

Ransley PG, Duffy PG, Oesch IL, et al: Autologous bladder mucosa graft for urethral substitution. Br J Urol 1987;59:331–333.

Redman JF: The Barcat balanic groove technique for the repair of distal hypospadias. J Urol 1987;137:83–85.

Retik AB: Proximal hypospadias. In Marshall FF (ed): Textbook of Operative Urology. Philadelphia, WB Saunders, 1996, pp 977–984.

Retik AB, Bauer SB, Mandell J, et al: Management of severe hypospadias with a 2-stage repair. J Urol 1994a;152:749–751.

Retik AB, Borer JG: Primary and reoperative hypospadias repair with the Snodgrass technique. J Urol 1998;16:186–191.

Retik AB, Mandell J, Bauer SB, et al: Meatal based hypospadias repair with the use of a dorsal subcutaneous flap to prevent urethrocutaneous fistula. J Urol 1994b; 152:1229–1231.

Rich MA, Keating MA, Snyder HM, et al: Hinging the urethral plate in hypospadias meatoplasty. J Urol 1989;142:1551–1553.

Ross JH, Kay R: Use of a de-epithelialized local skin flap in hypospadias repairs accomplished by tubularization of the incised urethral plate. Urology 1997;50:110–112.

Rushton HG, Belman AB: The split prepuce in situ onlay hypospadias repair. J Urol 1998;160:1134–1136; discussion, 1137.

Russell RH: Operation for severe hypospadias. BMJ 1900;2:1432–1435.

Snodgrass W: Tubularized, incised plate urethroplasty for distal hypospadias. J Urol 1994;151:464–465.

Snodgrass W, Koyle M, Manzoni G, et al: Tubularized incised plate hypospadias repair: Results of a multicenter experience. J Urol 1996; 156:839–841.

Snodgrass W, Koyle M, Manzoni G, et al: Tubularized incised plate hypospadias repair for proximal hypospadias [see comments]. J Urol 1998;159:2129–2131.

Steckler RE, Zaontz MR: Stent-free Thiersch-Duplay hypospadias repair with the Snodgrass modification. J Urol 1997;158:1178–1180.

Stock JA, Hanna MK: Distal urethroplasty and glanuloplasty procedure: Results of 512 repairs. Urology 1997;49:449–451.

Thiersch C: Ueber die entstehungsweise und operative behandlung der epispadie. Arch Heilkunde 1869;10:20–35.

Toksu E: Hypospadias: One-stage repair. Plast Reconstr Surg 1970;45: 365–369.

Turner-Warwick R, Parkhouse H, Chapple CR: Bulbar elongation anastomotic meatoplasty (BEAM) for subterminal and hypospadiac urethroplasty. J Urol 1997;158:1160–1167.

Van Hook W: A new operation for hypospadias. Ann Surg 1896;23:378–393.

van Horn AC, Kass EJ: Glanuloplasty and in situ tubularization of the urethral plate: A simple reliable technique for the majority of boys with hypospadias. J Urol 1995;154:1505–1507.

Wehrbein HL: Hypospadias. J Urol 1943;50:335–340.

Wiener JS, Sutherland RW, Roth DR, et al: Comparison of onlay and tubularized island flaps of inner preputial skin for the repair of proximal hypospadias. J Urol 1997;158:1172–1174.

Yavuzer R, Baran C, Latifoglu O, et al: Vascularized double-sided preputial island flap with W flap glanuloplasty for hypospadias repair. Plast Reconstr Surg 1998;101:751–755.

Yerkes EB, Cain MP, Casale AJ, et al: Experience with split-prepuce in situ island onlay for anterior hypospadias. J Urol 2000;163(suppl.):138.

Zaontz MR: The GAP (glans approximation procedure) for glanular/coronal hypospadias. J Urol 1989;141:359–361.

Complications

Ahmed S, Gough DC: Buccal mucosal graft for secondary hypospadias repair and urethral replacement. Br J Urol 1997;80:328–330.

Aigen AB, Khawand N, Skoog SJ, et al: Acquired megalourethra: An uncommon complication of the transverse preputial island flap urethroplasty. J Urol 1987;137:712–713.

Baskin LS, Duckett JW: Mucosal grafts in hypospadias and stricture management. AUA Update Series 1994;13:270–275.

Belman AB: De-epithelialized skin flap coverage in hypospadias repair. J Urol 1988;140:1273–1276.

Cecil AB: Repair of hypospadias and urethral fistula. J Urol 1946;56:237–242.

Churchill BM, van Savage JG, Khoury AE, et al: The dartos flap as an adjunct in preventing urethrocutaneous fistulas in repeat hypospadias surgery. J Urol 1996;156:2047–2049.

Davis DM: The pedicle tube-graft in the surgical treatment of hypospadias in the male: With new method of closing small urethral fistulas. Surg Gynecol Obstet 1940;71:790–796.

De Sy WA: Aesthetic repair of meatal stricture. J Urol 1984;132:678–679.

Duckett JW, Kaplan GW, Woodard JR, et al: Panel: Complications of hypospadias repair. Urol Clin North Am 1980;7:443–454.

Elbakry A, Shamaa M, Al-Atrash G: An axially vascularized meatal-based flap for the repair of hypospadias [see comments]. Br J Urol 1998;82:698–703.

Farkas LG: Hypospadias: Some causes of recurrence of ventral curvature of the penis following the straightening procedure. Br J Plast Surg 1967;20:199–203.

Goldstein HR, Hensle TW: Simplified closure of hypospadias fistulas. Urology 1981;18:504–505.

Horton CE, Devine CJ Jr: A one-stage repair for hypospadias cripples. Plast Reconstr Surg 1970;45:425–430.

Horton CE Jr, Horton CE: Complications of hypospadias surgery. Clin Plast Surg 1988;15:371–379.

Keating MA, Duckett JW: Failed hypospadias repair. In Cohen MS, Resnick MI (eds): Reoperative Urology. Boston, Little, Brown, 1995, pp 187–204.

Kumar MV, Harris DL: Balanitis xerotica obliterans complicating hypospadias repair. Br J Plast Surg 1999;52:69–71.

Retik AB, Keating M, Mandell J: Complications of hypospadias repair. Urol Clin North Am 1988;15:223–236.

Scherz HC, Kaplan GW, Packer MG, et al: Post-hypospadias repair urethral strictures: A review of 30 cases. J Urol 1988;140:1253–1255.

Schreiter F, Noll F: Mesh graft urethroplasty using split thickness skin graft or foreskin. J Urol 1989;142:1223–1226.

Smith D: A de-epithelialised overlap flap technique in the repair of hypospadias. Br J Plast Surg 1973;26:106–114.

Vandersteen DR, Husmann DA: Late onset recurrent penile chordee after successful correction at hypospadias repair. J Urol 1998;160:1131–1133; discussion, 1137.

Wessells H, McAninch JW: Current controversies in anterior urethral stricture repair: Free-graft versus pedicled skin-flap reconstruction. World J Urol 1998;16:175–180.

Zaontz MR, Kaplan WE, Maizels M: Surgical correction of anterior urethral diverticula after hypospadias repair in children. Urology 1989;33:40–42.

Reoperative Hypospadias Repair

Ahmed S, Gough DC: Buccal mucosal graft for secondary hypospadias repair and urethral replacement. Br J Urol 1997;80:328–330.

Baskin LS, Duckett JW: Mucosal grafts in hypospadias and stricture management. AUA Update Series 1994;13:270–275.

Borer JG, Bauer SB, Peters CA, et al: Tubularized, incised plate urethroplasty: Expanded use in primary and repeat surgery for hypospadias. J Urol 2001;165:581–585.

Caldamone AA, Edstrom LE, Koyle MA, et al: Buccal mucosal grafts for urethral reconstruction. Urology 1998;51:15–19.

Duckett JW, Coplen D, Ewalt D, et al: Buccal mucosal urethral replacement [see comments]. J Urol 1995;153:1660–1663.

Ehrlich RM, Alter G: Split-thickness skin graft urethroplasty and tunica vaginalis flaps for failed hypospadias repairs. J Urol 1996;155:131–134.

Horton CE, Devine CJ Jr: A one-stage repair for hypospadias cripples. Plast Reconstr Surg 1970;45:425–430.

Johanssen B: Reconstruction of the male urethra in strictures: Application of the buried intact epithelium tube. Acta Chir Scand Suppl 1953; 176:1.

Joseph DB, Perez LM: Tunica vaginalis onlay urethroplasty as a salvage repair. J Urol 1999;162:1146–1147.

Koff SA, Brinkman J, Ulrich J, et al: Extensive mobilization of the urethral plate and urethra for repair of hypospadias: The modified Barcat technique. J Urol 1994;151:466–469.

Mollard P, Mouriquand P, Bringeon G, et al: Repair of hypospadias using a bladder mucosal graft in 76 cases. J Urol 1989;142:1548–1550.

Ransley PG, Duffy PG, Oesch IL, et al: Autologous bladder mucosa graft for urethral substitution. Br J Urol 1987;59:331–333.

Retik AB: Proximal hypospadias. In Marshall FF (ed): Textbook of Operative Urology. Philadelphia, WB Saunders, 1996, pp 977–984.

Schreiter F, Noll F: Mesh graft urethroplasty using split thickness skin graft or foreskin. J Urol 1989;142:1223–1226.

Simmons GR, Cain MP, Casale AJ, et al: Repair of hypospadias complications using the previously utilized urethral plate. Urology 1999;54: 724–726.

Snodgrass W, Koyle M, Manzoni G, et al: Tubularized incised plate hypospadias repair: Results of a multicenter experience. J Urol 1996; 156:839–841.

Snow BW, Cartwright PC: Tunica vaginalis urethroplasty. Urology 1992; 40:442–445.

Long-Term Follow-Up

Berg R, Svensson J, Astrom G: Social and sexual adjustment of men operated for hypospadias during childhood: A controlled study. J Urol 1981;125:313–317.

Bracka A: Sexuality after hypospadias repair. BJU Int 1999;83(suppl. 3): 29–33.

Eberle J, Uberreiter S, Radmayr C, et al: Posterior hypospadias: Long-term followup after reconstructive surgery in the male direction. J Urol 1993;150:1474–1477.

Garibay JT, Reid C, Gonzalez R: Functional evaluation of the results of hypospadias surgery with uroflowmetry. J Urol 1995;154:835–836.

Gutierrez Segura C: Urine flow in childhood: a study of flow chart parameters based on 1,361 uroflowmetry tests. J Urol 1997;157:1426–1428.

Jayanthi VR, McLorie GA, Khoury AE, et al: Functional characteristics of the reconstructed neourethra after island flap urethroplasty [see comments]. J Urol 1995;153:1657–1659.

Malyon AD, Boorman JG, Bowley N: Urinary flow rates in hypospadias. Br J Plast Surg 1997;50:530–535.

Mureau MA, Slijper FM, Nijman RJ, et al: Psychosexual adjustment of children and adolescents after different types of hypospadias surgery: A norm-related study. J Urol 1995a;154:1902–1907.

Mureau MA, Slijper FM, Slob AK, et al: Psychosocial functioning of children, adolescents, and adults following hypospadias surgery: A comparative study. J Pediatr Psychol 1997;22:371–387.

Mureau MA, Slijper FM, van der Meulen JC, et al: Psychosexual adjustment of men who underwent hypospadias repair: A norm-related study. J Urol 1995b;154:1351–1355.

Sandberg DE, Meyer-Bahlburg HF, Yager TJ, et al: Gender development in boys born with hypospadias. Psychoneuroendocrinology 1995;20: 693–709.

Svensson J, Berg R: Micturition studies and sexual function in operated hypospadiacs. Br J Urol 1983;55:422–426.

Szabo L, Fegyverneki S: Maximum and average urine flow rates in normal children: The Miskolc nomograms. Br J Urol 1995;76:16–20.

Woodhouse CR: The sexual and reproductive consequences of congenital genitourinary anomalies. J Urol 1994;152:645–651.

Current Trends and Future Concepts

Atala A, Guzman L, Retik AB: A novel inert collagen matrix for hypospadias repair. J Urol 1999;162:1148–1151.

Baskin LS, Duckett JW, Ueoka K, et al: Changing concepts of hypospadias curvature lead to more onlay island flap procedures. J Urol 1994; 151:191–196.

Borer JG, Bauer SB, Peters CA, et al: Tubularized, incised plate urethroplasty: Expanded use in primary and repeat surgery for hypospadias. J Urol 2001;165:581–585.

Decter RM, Franzoni DF: Distal hypospadias repair by the modified Thiersch-Duplay technique with or without hinging the urethral plate: A near ideal way to correct distal hypospadias. J Urol 1999;162:1156–1158.

Hodgson NB: Editorial comment. J Urol 1993;149:816.

Powell CR, McAleer I, Alagiri M, et al: Comparison of flaps versus grafts in proximal hypospadias surgery. J Urol 2000;163:1286–1288; discussion, 1288–1289.

Rushton HG, Belman AB: The split prepuce in situ onlay hypospadias repair. J Urol 1998;160:1134–1136; discussion, 1137.

Winslow BH, Devine CJ Jr: Principles in repair of hypospadias. Semin Pediatr Surg 1996;5:41–48.

Yerkes EB, Cain MP, Casale AJ, et al: Experience with split-prepuce in situ island onlay for anterior hypospadias. J Urol 2000;163(suppl.):138.

66

ABNORMALITIES OF THE GENITALIA IN BOYS AND THEIR SURGICAL MANAGEMENT

Jack S. Elder, MD

Normal Genitalia and Association with Other Abnormalities

Male Genital Anomalies
Penile Anomalies

Scrotal Anomalies
Vascular Lesions of the Genitalia
Miscellaneous Genital Anomalies

Neonatal genital anomalies are common and may result from a disorder of sexual differentiation, genital differentiation, or genital growth. Many genital anomalies are associated with developmental abnormalities of other organ systems. **Although most genital deformities are recognized at birth, occasionally they may be detected in utero** (Shapiro, 1999). For example, Cheikhelard and colleagues (2000) reported that in 43 cases in which a genital abnormality was identified by sonography at a mean gestational age of 29 weeks, the diagnosis was accurate in 34 (79%).

Recognition of normal embryology is essential to understanding the pathogenesis of genital anomalies. **In the male embryo, differentiation of the external genitalia occurs between weeks 9 and 13 of gestation and requires production of testosterone by the testes as well as conversion of testosterone into dihydrotestosterone (DHT) under the enzymatic influence of 5α-reductase in the genital anlagen. Under the influence of DHT, the genital tubercle differentiates into the glans penis, the genital folds become the shaft of the penis, and the genital swellings migrate inferomedially, fusing in the midline to become the scrotum. In the female, because of the absence of testosterone and DHT, the genital tubercle develops passively into the clitoris, the genital folds become the labia minora, and the genital swellings become the labia majora.** The same changes may also occur in males with an abnormality in fetal testosterone production, a 5α-reductase deficiency, or an androgen receptor defect.

NORMAL GENITALIA AND ASSOCIATION WITH OTHER ABNORMALITIES

In a normal, full-term male neonate, the penis is 3.5 ± 0.7 cm in stretched length and 1.1 ± 0.2 cm in diameter (Table 66–1). At birth, the inhibitory effect of maternal estrogens on the fetal pituitary is no longer present; this change in the hormonal milieu causes a rebound surge in gonadotropins that results in an **early, transient surge in testosterone production by the Leydig cells that stimulates penile growth during the first 3 months of life.** During the remainder of childhood, the penis grows much more slowly. Normally, the penis has a fully developed foreskin and a median raphe on the shaft. However, **in 10% of males, the raphe deviates, usually to the left side** (Ben-Ari et al, 1985). Although deviation of the raphe may be associated with penile torsion or chordee without hypospadias, it is usually an insignificant finding. However, in the newborn male with deviation of the raphe, careful inspection of the glans is important. Congenital ventral or lateral curvature of the penis affects approximately 0.6% of male neonates (Yachia et al, 1993). A urethral deformity such as hypospadias or epispadias occurs in approximately 1 of every 250 males.

Congenital anomalies of the genitalia are often associated with abnormalities of other organ systems or are part of recognized syndromes (Table 66–2). **As many as 50% of children with congenital anorectal malformations**

Table 66–1. STRETCHED PENILE LENGTH (CENTIMETERS) IN NORMAL MALE SUBJECTS

Age	Mean ± SD	Mean − 2.5 SD
Newborn, 30 wk gestation	2.5 ± 0.4	1.5
Newborn, 34 wk gestation	3.0 ± 0.4	2.0
0–5 mo	3.9 ± 0.8	1.9
6–12 mo	4.3 ± 0.8	2.3
1–2 yr	4.7 ± 0.8	2.6
2–3 yr	5.1 ± 0.9	2.9
3–4 yr	5.5 ± 0.9	3.3
4–5 yr	5.7 ± 0.9	3.5
5–6 yr	6.0 ± 0.9	3.8
6–7 yr	6.1 ± 0.9	3.9
7–8 yr	6.2 ± 1.0	3.7
8–9 yr	6.3 ± 1.0	3.8
9–10 yr	6.3 ± 1.0	3.8
10–11 yr	6.4 ± 1.1	3.7
Adult	13.3 ± 1.6	9.3

Data from Feldman KW, Smith DW: Fetal phallic growth and penile standards for newborn male infants. J Pediatr 1975;86:895; Schonfeld WA, Beebe GW: Normal growth and variation in the male genitalia from birth to maturity. J Urol 1987;30:554; Tuladhar R, Davis PG, Batch J, Doyle LW: Establishment of a normal range of penile length in preterm infants. J Paediatr Child Health 1998; 34:471.

also have an associated urologic malformation (Hoekstra et al, 1983), and frequently the external genitalia are involved. For example, **in a series of boys with high imperforate anus, 29% had an abnormality of the external genitalia, including hypospadias, penile duplication, micropenis, or scrotal deformity, whereas hypospadias was the primary genital abnormality in those with low imperforate anus** (Hoekstra et al, 1983). Among boys with esophageal atresia or tracheoesophageal fistula, genital anomalies also are common, including hypospadias (6%), penile agenesis, penoscrotal transposition, scrotal malformation, and scrotal agenesis (1.5% each) (Berkhoff et al, 1989). Consequently, involvement of the urologist in the initial evaluation and long-term management of these patients is important. A guide to the early diagnosis and management of genital anomalies has been published by the American Academy of Pediatrics (AAP) Committee on Genetics and Sections on Endocrinology and Urology (2000).

MALE GENITAL ANOMALIES

Penile Anomalies

Phimosis

At birth, there is a physiologic phimosis or inability to retract the foreskin in the majority of neonates because natural adhesions exist between the prepuce and the glans. During the first 3 to 4 years of life, as the penis grows, epithelial debris (smegma) accumulates under the prepuce, gradually separating the foreskin from the glans. Intermittent penile erections cause the foreskin to become completely retractable. **By 3 years of age, 90% of foreskins can be retracted, and fewer than 1% of males have phimosis by 17 years of age** (Oster, 1968).

Early forceful retraction of the foreskin generally is not recommended, because recurrent adhesions between the de-epithelialized glans and foreskin may occur, and a cicatrix may form at the tip of the foreskin, causing secondary phimosis. However, **in boys older than 4 or 5 years of age and in those who develop balanitis or balanoposthitis, application of a topical corticosteroid cream (e.g., 0.1% dexamethasone) to the foreskin three to four times daily for 6 weeks loosens the phimotic ring in two thirds of the cases and usually allows the foreskin to be retracted manually** (Monsour et al, 1999). Topical corticosteroids are beneficial even if the foreskin is involved with balanitis xerotica obliterans. Formal lysis of adhesions is rarely indicated. In uncircumcised boys older than 7 or 8 years of age with phimosis that is resistant to topical corticosteroids and in boys with phimosis that causes ballooning of the foreskin or recurrent balanitis, strong consideration should be given to performing a circumcision or dorsal slit.

Table 66–2. MALE GENITAL ANOMALIES THAT COMMONLY OCCUR IN VARIOUS SYNDROMES (MICROPHALLUS, HYPOSPADIAS, AMBIGUOUS GENITALIA, AND BIFID SCROTUM)

Anencephaly
Aniridia-Wilms' tumor association (WAGR syndrome)
Bladder exstrophy
Borjeson-Forssman-Lehman syndrome (microcephaly, mental retardation, large ears)
Carpenter's syndrome (acrocephaly, polydactyly and syndactyly of feet, congenital heart disease)
CHARGE association (*c*oloboma, *h*eart malformation, *a*tresia choanae, *r*etarded growth and development, *g*enital anomalies, *e*ar anomalies and/or deafness)
Cloacal syndrome
Fraser's syndrome (cryptophthalmos, mental retardation, ear anomalies)
Johanson-Blizzard syndrome (hypoplastic alae nasi, hypothyroidism, mental retardation, pancreatic insufficiency, deafness)
Meckel-Gruber syndrome (occipital encephalomeningocele, micrognathia, polydactyly, cystic renal dysplasia)
Noonan syndrome (webbed neck, pectus excavatum, pulmonic stenosis, short stature)
Opitz syndrome (hypertelorism, hypospadias, mild to moderate mental retardation)
Pallister-Hall syndrome (hypothalamic hamartoblastoma, hypopituitarism, imperforate anus)
Popliteal pterygium syndrome (popliteal web, cleft palate, lower lip pits)
Prader-Willi syndrome (hypotonia, obesity, small hands and feet, mild to moderate mental retardation)
Rapp-Hodgkin ectodermal dysplasia syndrome (hypohidrosis, oral clefts, dysplastic nails)
Rieger syndrome (iris dysplasia, hypodontia)
Robinow syndrome ("fetal face syndrome"; flat facial profile, hypertelorism, short forearms, thoracic hemivertebrae)
Schinzel-Giedian syndrome (growth deficiency, mental retardation, widely patent fontanelles, short forearms and legs, renal anomalies)
Smith-Lemli-Opitz syndrome (ptosis of eyelids, syndactyly of second and third toes, microcephaly, failure to thrive with short stature, mental retardation)
Triploidy syndrome
Trisomy 4p, 9p, 18, 20p, 21, 22, 9p, 10q, 11p, or 15q deficiency
XXY, XXXXY

From Jones KL: Smith's Recognizable Patterns of Human Malformation, 5th ed. Philadelphia, WB Saunders, 1997.

Circumcision

In pediatrics, few topics generate as much controversy as whether the newborn male should undergo a circumcision, perhaps because it is the most common surgical procedure in the United States and because it is usually performed for cosmetic reasons. In 1975, the AAP declared, "There is no absolute medical indication for routine circumcision of the newborn" (Thompson et al, 1975). This stance was supported by the American College of Obstetricians and Gynecologists.

Reasons given in support of circumcision include prevention of penile cancer, urinary tract infection (UTI), sexually transmitted disease (STD), and phimosis, as well as lessening of the risk of balanitis.

Carcinoma of the penis develops almost exclusively in men who were not circumcised at birth. Schoen and coworkers (2000b) reported that, of 89 men in a large health maintenance organization with invasive penile cancer, only 2 (2%) had been circumcised at birth. Furthermore, of 116 men with penile carcinoma in situ, 16 (14%) had had a neonatal circumcision. On the other hand, although carcinoma of the penis develops primarily in uncircumcised men, in Scandinavian countries, where few men are circumcised and genital hygiene is excellent, the incidence of penile cancer is quite low.

Uncircumcised newborns and infants are predisposed to UTI. For example, in a study of 100 neonates with UTI, Ginsburg and McCracken (1982) found that only 3 (5%) of the 62 males who developed a UTI were circumcised. Subsequently, Wiswell and colleagues (1985) studied more than 2500 male infants and found that 41 had symptomatic UTIs; of these, 88% were uncircumcised. In that study, uncircumcised males were almost 20 times more likely than circumcised neonates to develop a UTI. Other studies of larger groups of infants have confirmed these reports (Wiswell, 1992, 2000) and have demonstrated that neonatal circumcision is less costly than treating UTIs in uncircumcised boys (Schoen et al, 2000a). **The increased risk seems to affect boys at least through 5 years of age** (Craig et al, 1996) and the incidence of epididymitis is reduced (Bennett et al, 1998). **The increased risk of UTIs is attributed to colonization of the prepuce by urinary pathogens** (Wiswell et al, 1988).

Whether circumcision reduces the risk of STDs has been controversial. An increased risk has been attributed to minor frenular injuries acquired during intercourse and to the larger surface area of the penis in uncircumcised men. In some studies, however, an increased incidence of STDs in uncircumcised men has been attributed to demographic factors. Nevertheless, Lavreys and associates (1999) studied 746 men who were seronegative for HIV-1 infection and **found that uncircumcised men were four times more likely to become HIV-1 positive and 2.5 times more likely to develop genital ulcers, compared with circumcised men. However, there was not an increased incidence of genital warts in uncircumcised men.** There have been other studies with similar findings (Schoen et al, 2000c).

In 1989, the AAP reviewed its policy and concluded, **"Newborn circumcision has potential medical benefits and advantages as well as disadvantages and risks. When circumcision is being considered, the benefits and** risks should be explained to the parents and informed consent obtained" (AAP Task Force on Circumcision, 1989). More recently, the AAP again updated its policy statement (AAP Task Force on Circumcision, 1999, 2000). Its position was essentially unchanged, with the exception that it emphasized the importance of local anesthesia for the procedure. The AAP does not endorse routine circumcision. There has been an ongoing dialogue on this topic, with some arguing against circumcision at all (Anonymous, 1999) and others believing that neonatal circumcision confers sufficient benefits to warrant its routine practice (Schoen et al, 2000c).

When neonatal circumcision is performed, local anesthesia is recommended. Available options include topical application of a cream containing eutectic mixture of local anesthetic (EMLA; lidocaine and prilocaine), dorsal penile nerve block, and a penile ring block (Hardwick-Smith et al, 1998). Randomized controlled trials have demonstrated that a dorsal penile nerve block is more effective than EMLA cream (Howard et al, 1999; Taddio et al, 2000). In addition, the **prilocaine in EMLA cream poses a risk for methemoglobinemia** (Cooper, 2000), although the risk is quite low. Consequently, **a dorsal penile nerve block or ring block at the base of the penis with 1% lidocaine is preferred.** Circumcision can be performed under local anesthesia even in older boys. For example, Jayanthi and colleagues (1999) reported a series of 287 infants aged 3 days to 9 months (20% older than 3 months) who underwent office circumcision with the use of local anesthesia. The mean cost (excluding professional fees) was $196, compared with $1805 for circumcision under general anesthesia.

Circumcision should not be performed in neonates with hypospadias, chordee without hypospadias, a dorsal hood deformity, a webbed penis, or a small penis. In addition, many neonates with a large hydrocele or hernia are more likely to develop secondary phimosis and a buried penis if circumcision is performed. In a report by Williams and associates (2000), 8% of boys referred for initial circumcision had an "inconspicuous penis" (see later discussion), as did 63% of boys referred for circumcision revision.

Some newborn boys are not circumcised owing to illness (e.g., prematurity, sepsis, congenital heart disease) or parental choice, and when the child is older the family requests that a circumcision be performed under general anesthesia. The most common indications for "delayed" circumcision include balanoposthitis (23% to 36%), social reasons (23% to 39%), improved hygiene (13%), UTI (7%), coincident with other surgical procedure (27%), and phimosis (3%) (Larsen and Williams, 1990). An alternative to circumcision for phimosis is "preputial plasty," which is essentially a minimal dorsal slit through the phimotic ring (Cuckow et al, 1994).

CIRCUMCISION COMPLICATIONS

The complication rate for newborn circumcision is 0.2% to 3% (Ross, 1996; Christakis et al, 2000). **Minor complications include early problems such as bleeding, wound infection, penile adhesions, removal of too much or too little skin, secondary phimosis with a trapped or hidden penis** (see later discussion), **and injury to the**

glans, urethra, or penile shaft by inadvertent excision or by a thermal injury (Baskin et al, 1996). The main late complication is meatal stenosis.

Bleeding usually results from oozing from the frenulum or occasionally from a large arterial or venous vessel on the penile shaft. Bleeding usually can be controlled with compression, but occasionally cautery with a silver nitrate stick or ophthalmic cautery is necessary, and in some cases hemorrhage must be controlled with a suture. If cautery is used, ventrally one must be careful not to injure the urethra. Wound infection is rare and usually is prevented by applying antibiotic ointment to the circumcision wound. Another potential complication is severe penile vasoconstriction secondary to inadvertent injection of concentrated epinephrine instead of lidocaine. Treatment of this unusual problem is either local infiltration with 0.4 mg of phentolamine or insertion of a caudal catheter to induce a sympathetic block (Adams et al, 2000).

Many of the other problems with healing can be managed in the office if the baby is seen 2 or 3 weeks after the circumcision. **Filmy penile adhesions are common and have been reported to be present in 71% of infants, 30% of 1- to 5-year-olds, and 2% of those older than 9 years of age** (Van Howe, 1997; Ponsky et al, 2000). These adhesions usually cause no problems and come apart on their own over time. Occasionally epithelial debris accumulates and helps to separate the adhesion. In some cases dense skin bridges form between the penile shaft and glans—these never come apart and need to be excised. This procedure often can be performed in the office under local anesthesia, but, if the adhesions are extensive, excision under general anesthesia is necessary. **If too much penile shaft skin is removed, application of an antibiotic ointment and adherent gauze to the open wound usually yields a satisfactory result. Typically, most of the skin grows back and bridges the defect. Immediate skin grafting rarely is necessary** and may result in a disfigured penis and graft site. In addition, suturing the skin edges together to bridge the gap is not recommended, because the penile shaft may end up with insufficient skin. If too much skin is left, then revision of circumcision may need to be considered. In some babies, the penis retracts into the suprapubic fat pad or scrotum. This situation is most common if the baby had a large hydrocele or hernia or was born with a webbed penis. A cicatricial scar may result, producing a trapped penis, which can cause urinary retention and/or UTI in the most severe cases. If this situation is recognized early, the cicatrix may be opened bluntly in the office. Alternatively, application of a topical corticosteroid cream may loosen the scar tissue. If the problem is not corrected satisfactorily, then correction of hidden penis under anesthesia is necessary when the child is older.

The most serious circumcision complications are urethral injury and removal of part of the glans or part or all of the penile shaft. **Partial glans removal has been reported to occur with a Mogen clamp; in these cases, the excised tissue should be preserved and immediately sutured back to the penis** (Sherman et al, 1996). **A microscopic repair is unnecessary. When repair is performed within 8 hours after the injury, the penis heals nicely in the vast majority of cases.**

In extremely rare cases, penile necrosis can result from thermal injury. One way a thermal injury can occur is if a metal clamp is applied to the foreskin and the cautery is used to excise the foreskin; if the cautery comes into contact with the metal clamp, then an electrical/thermal injury to the shaft can result. Thermal injury to the penis also can result from inappropriate use of the yttrium-aluminum-garnet (YAG) contact laser in performing a circumcision. **When an ablative penile injury occurs, the optimal therapy is unresolved at this time. One option is to reassign the baby to a female gender and perform bilateral orchiectomy** (Bradley et al, 1998). **Unfortunately, these children may grow up with a male identity, presumably from androgen imprinting in utero and shortly after birth** (Reiner, 1996; Diamond and Sigmundson, 1997; Diamond, 1999). **On the other hand, current efforts for penile reconstruction in such cases have suboptimal cosmetic and functional results. These patients should be referred immediately to a tertiary center with a team approach that includes specialists from pediatric urology, endocrinology, plastic surgery, child psychiatry, and ethics for definitive management.**

MEATAL STENOSIS

Meatal stenosis is a condition that almost always is acquired after neonatal circumcision. One theory is that, after disruption of the normal adhesions between the prepuce and glans and removal of the foreskin, a significant inflammatory reaction occurs, causing severe meatal inflammation and cicatrix formation, which results in a narrow meatus, a membranous web across the ventral aspect of the meatus, or an eccentric healing process that produces a prominent lip of ventral meatal tissue. Symptoms of meatal stenosis vary with the appearance. Another theory is that the abnormality results from meatal devascularization caused by cutting of the frenular artery during circumcision (Persad et al, 1995).

In most cases, meatal stenosis does not become apparent until after the child is toilet trained. If the meatus is pinpoint, the boy voids with a forceful, fine stream that has a great casting distance. Some boys have a dorsally deflected stream or a prolonged voiding time. Dysuria, frequency, terminal hematuria, and incontinence are symptoms that may lead to discovery of meatal stenosis but generally are not attributable to this abnormality. In other boys with meatal stenosis, deflection of the urinary stream is the only sign. These concepts of meatal stenosis reflect the philosophy espoused by the Section on Urology of the AAP (AAP Committee from the Urology Section, 1978).

In a boy with suspected meatal stenosis, the meatus should be calibrated with a bougie (Table 66–3) or assessed with infant sounds. Not infrequently, an asymptomatic boy with suspected meatal stenosis actually has a compliant meatus of normal caliber. If the meatus is diminished in size or if the child has abnormal voiding symptoms, a renal and bladder ultrasound examination is indicated. If the child has a history of UTIs, a voiding cystourethrogram (VCUG) should be done also. However, **meatal stenosis rarely causes obstructive changes in the urinary tract.** In boys with UTIs, it is often uncertain whether the infection is the result of meatal stenosis. In a series of 280 children with meatal stenosis, 5% of the patients had surgically significant lesions on VCUG, and

Table 66–3. NORMAL SIZE OF URETHRAL MEATUS IN BOYS

Age	Size (Fr)	Number (%)	Size (Fr)	Number (%)
6 wk–3 yr	< 8	62/425 (15%)	10	363/425 (85%)
4–10 yr	tight 8	41/508 (8%)	12	384/508 (76%)
11–12 yr	< 10	4/85 (5%)	14	64/85 (75%)

Adapted from Litvak AS, Morris JA Jr, McRoberts JW: Normal size of the urethral meatus in boys. J Urol 1976;115:736; and Morton HG: Meatus size in 1,000 circumcised children from two weeks to sixteen years of age. J Fla Med Assoc 1986;50:137.

only 1% had upper tract abnormalities (Noe and Dale, 1975). All of the patients with radiologic findings had experienced UTIs.

In many cases, meatoplasty can be accomplished in the physician's office using EMLA cream for local anesthesia (Cartwright and Snow, 1996). In addition, 1% lidocaine with 1:100,000 epinephrine may be infiltrated in the ventral web with a 26-gauge needle for local anesthesia and vasoconstriction. A ventral incision is made toward the frenulum and long enough to provide a meatus of normal caliber, which can be checked with the bougie. The urethral mucosa is sutured to the glans with fine chromic catgut sutures. If the procedure is performed under general anesthesia, the bladder may be filled with saline and compressed manually to be certain that the stream is straight. **Cystoscopy is unnecessary unless the child has obstructive symptoms and has not had a VCUG.**

When meatal stenosis is congenital, it occurs primarily in neonates with coronal or subcoronal hypospadias. Obstruction in these cases is unusual, but occasionally UTI occurs or catheterization is necessary during hospitalization, and urgent meatoplasty may need to be performed.

In rare cases, a boy with suspected meatal stenosis and obstructive symptoms has an anterior urethral valve in the fossa navicularis (Scherz et al, 1987). Another form of meatal stenosis that can result in urinary retention is balanitis xerotica obliterans. In these cases, topical application of corticosteroid cream may be effective in reducing the risk of recurrent meatal stenosis.

Penile Cysts

The most common cystic lesion of the penis is accumulation of epithelial debris, or smegma, under the unretractable foreskin. In young boys, the foreskin should not be retracted unless infection or inflammation is associated, because eventually it will retract by itself.

Congenital epidermal cysts occasionally form along the median penile raphe on the penile shaft or on the glans (Fig. 66–1). Epidermal inclusion cysts may form after circumcision, hypospadias repair, or other forms of penile surgery, and result when islands of epithelium are left behind in the subcutaneous tissue. These cystic lesions should be treated with simple excision.

Inconspicuous Penis

The term *inconspicuous penis* refers to a penis that appears to be small (Bergeson et al, 1993). **Several entities are included in this term, including webbed penis, concealed penis, and trapped penis, in which the penis is normal in size, and micropenis, in which the penis is abnormally small.** When an infant is found to have an inconspicuous penis, prompt evaluation is necessary for proper treatment, and the family must be informed as to whether the penis is or is not normal. **The stretched penile length should be measured from the pubic symphysis to the top of the glans. In addition, the diameter of the penile shaft may be measured by palpation.**

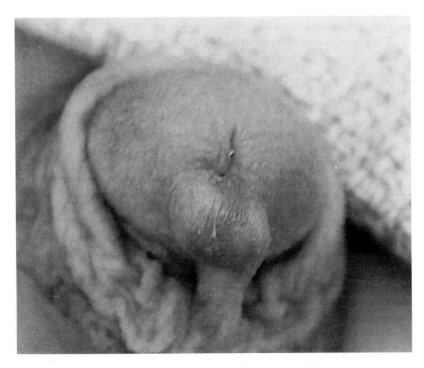

Figure 66–1. Epithelial inclusion cyst of glans.

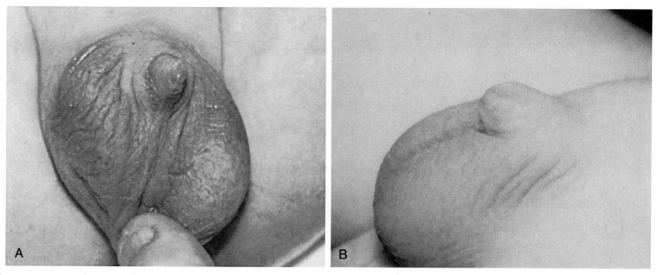

Figure 66-2. *A* and *B,* Examples of webbed penis. The penile shaft is normal in length. In *A,* there is also scrotal engulfment of the penile shaft.

WEBBED PENIS

Webbed penis is a condition in which the scrotal skin extends onto the ventrum of the penis (Fig. 66-2). When this condition is congenital, the penis, the urethra, and the remainder of the scrotum typically are normal and **the deformity represents an abnormality of the attachment between the penis and the scrotum.** This condition also may be iatrogenic after circumcision or other penile surgery, in which case it results from excessive removal of ventral penile skin.

Although the webbed penis is usually asymptomatic, the cosmetic appearance often is unacceptable. Occasionally this condition may be corrected by incising the web transversely, separating the penis from the scrotum, and closing the skin vertically. In other cases a circumferential incision is made 1.5 cm proximal to the coronal sulcus, Byars' preputial skin flaps are transferred to the ventral surface of the penis, and the redundant foreskin is excised. The scrotum may be anchored to the base of the penis to prevent recurrence of the webbed appearance. **In rare cases, the distal urethra is hypoplastic, necessitating urethral reconstruction.**

CONCEALED (BURIED OR HIDDEN) PENIS

A concealed penis is a normally developed penis that is camouflaged by the suprapubic fat pad; this anomaly may be congenital, or it may occur iatrogenically after circumcision (Fig. 66-3). In infants and young children, the congenital condition has been thought to result from the inelasticity of the dartos fascia (which normally allows the penile skin to slide freely on the deep layers of the shaft); extension of the penis is restricted because the penile skin is not anchored to the deep fascia. In older children and obese adolescents, the abundant fat on the abdominal wall may hide the penile shaft.

On inspection, the contour of the penile shaft and the glans cannot be seen. However, careful palpation allows one to determine that the penile shaft actually is concealed and normal in size and is not a microphallus or a penis

that has undergone circumcision injury. It is important to determine whether the glans can be exposed simply by retracting the skin covering the glans. If so, it remains the surgeon's judgment whether correction is warranted.

Numerous techniques have been described to correct the concealed penis (Donahoe and Keating, 1986; Maizels et al, 1986; Shapiro, 1987; Cromie et al, 1998; Alter and Ehrlich, 1999; Casale et al, 1999; Smuelders et al, 2000). The indications for this type of surgery and the timing of reconstruction are controversial. In moderately severe cases, the dysgenic bands of tissue, which are located primarily on the dorsal surface of the shaft of the penis, must be removed. The prepuce should be unfurled and used for ventral skin coverage. In addition, the subcutaneous tissue on the dorsal aspect of the penis should be fixed to the pubic fascia, and the subcutaneous tissue of the scrotum should be fixed to the ventral aspect of the base of the penile shaft with nonabsorbable suture. In addition, penoscrotal Z-plasty and lateral penile shaft Z-plasty often are necessary. In the most severe cases, the suspensory ligament of the penis must be divided, suprapubic fat excised, and the spermatic cords protected. Liposuction has been reported to be helpful in severe cases (Maizels et al, 1986; Shenoy et al, 2000). However, this technique should be reserved for adolescent boys, because prepubertal boys may

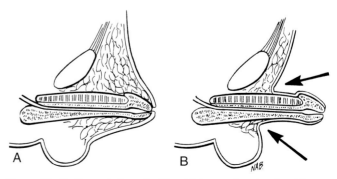

Figure 66-3. Concealed penis *(A),* which may be visualized by retracting skin lateral to penile shaft *(B).*

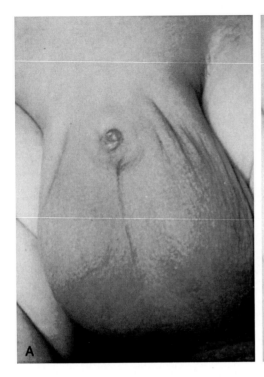 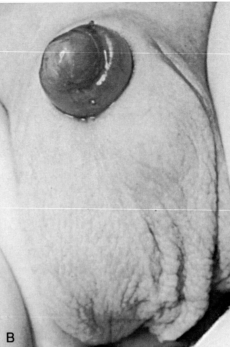

Figure 66–4. *A,* Trapped (concealed) penis resulting from circumcision. *B,* Same patient after revision of circumcision.

lose their fat pad with somatic growth. In some cases, an island pedicle of ventral preputial skin may be used to cover the penis and aid in reconstruction.

TRAPPED PENIS

Trapped penis is an acquired form of inconspicuous penis; the term refers to a phallus that has become embedded in the suprapubic fat pad after circumcision. This deformity may occur after neonatal circumcision in a baby who has significant scrotal swelling due to a hydrocele or hernia or after routine circumcision in a baby with a webbed penis. In some neonates the penile shaft seems to retract naturally into the scrotum, and if circumcision is performed in this situation the skin at the base of the penis may form a cicatrix over the retracted phallus (Fig. 66–4). **In its most severe form, this complication can predispose the child to UTIs and may cause urinary retention.** If the condition is recognized in a newborn, the cicatrix may be opened in the office. Alternatively, correction under general anesthesia may be considered, although the anesthetic risk is higher in the first few months of life. Elective repair of the trapped penis at 6 months is preferred. The surgical technique is similar to that for concealed penis.

Micropenis

Micropenis is defined as a normally formed penis that is at least 2.5 standard deviations (SD) below the mean in size (Aaronson, 1994) (Fig. 66–5*A*). **Typically, the ratio of the length of the penile shaft to its circumference is normal.** In a few cases, the corpora cavernosa are severely hypoplastic. The scrotum usually is fused but often is diminutive. The testes usually are small and frequently are undescended.

Assessment of length is made by measuring the penis from its attachment to the pubic symphysis to the tip of the glans (see Fig. 66–5*B*). In an obese infant or child, one must be careful to depress the suprapubic fat pad completely to obtain an accurate measurement. Stretched penile length is used because it correlates more closely with erectile length than does the relaxed length of the penis. The measurements should be compared with standards for penile length (see Table 66–1). **In general, the penis of a full-term newborn should be at least 1.9 cm long. A webbed or concealed penis often resembles micropenis, but examination shows a normal penile shaft.**

Knowledge of the endocrinologic regulation of penile development allows an understanding of how micropenis occurs. Differentiation of the male external genitalia is complete by the 12th week of gestation and requires a normal testis producing testosterone, stimulated by maternal human chorionic gonadotropin (hCG). During the second and third trimesters, growth of the penis occurs under the direction of fetal androgen, which is controlled by the secretion of fetal luteinizing hormone (LH). An abnormality in the production or use of testosterone results not only in a small penis but usually in hypospadias also, whereas a true micropenis often seems to be a consequence of a deficiency of gonadotropic hormones. **Therefore, micropenis results from a hormonal abnormality that occurs after 14 weeks of gestation.**

There are numerous causes of micropenis (Table 66–4), including isolated gonadotropin defects without involvement of other organ systems and generalized endocrinopathies that may be associated with central nervous system defects. **The most common causes of micropenis are (1) hypogonadotropic hypogonadism, (2) hypergonadotropic hypogonadism (primary testicular failure), and (3) idiopathic** (Lee et al, 1980b; Gonzales, 1983). **In addition, micropenis is often associated with major chromosomal**

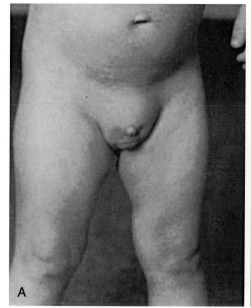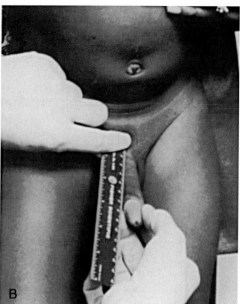

Figure 66–5. *A,* Microphallus. *B,* Technique of measuring stretched penile length.

A

B

defects, including Klinefelter's syndrome (47,XXY), other X polysomy syndromes, and translocations, deletions, and trisomy involving chromosomes 8, 13, and 18 (Aaronson, 1994).

The most common cause of micropenis is failure of the hypothalamus to produce an adequate amount of gonadotropin-releasing hormone (GnRH). This condi-

Table 66–4. ETIOLOGY OF MICROPENIS

I. Deficient testosterone secretion
  A. Hypogonadotropic hypogonadism
    1. Isolated, including Kallmann's syndrome
    2. Associated with other pituitary hormone deficiencies (e.g., CHARGE association)
    3. Prader-Willi syndrome
    4. Laurence-Moon syndrome
    5. Bardet-Biedl syndrome
    6. Rud's syndrome
  B. Primary hypogonadism
    1. Anorchia
    2. Klinefelter's syndrome and poly X syndrome
    3. Gonadal dysgenesis (incomplete)
    4. Luteinizing hormone receptor defects (incomplete)
    5. Genetic defects in testosterone steroidogenesis (incomplete)
    6. Noonan's syndrome
    7. Down syndrome
    8. Robinow's syndrome
    9. Bardet-Biedl syndrome
    10. Laurence-Moon syndrome
II. Defects in testosterone action
  A. Growth hormone/insulin-like growth factor-I deficiency
  B. Androgen receptor defects (incomplete)
  C. 5α-reductase deficiency (incomplete)
  D. Fetal hydantoin syndrome
III. Development anomalies
  A. Aphallia
  B. Cloacal exstrophy
IV. Idiopathic
V. Associated with other congenital malformations

Adapted from Bin-Abbas B, Conte FA, Grumbach MM, Kaplan SL: Congenital hypogonadotropic hypogonadism and micropenis: Effect of testosterone treatment on adult penile size—Why sex reversal is not indicated. J Pediatr 1999; 134:579.

tion, termed hypogonadotropic hypogonadism, may result from hypothalamic dysfunction, as in Kallmann's syndrome (genito-olfactory dysplasia), Prader-Willi syndrome, Laurence-Moon-Biedl syndrome (Walsh et al, 1978; Danish et al, 1980), **and the CHARGE association** (Ragan et al, 1999). In other cases, there is an associated growth hormone deficiency (Burstein et al, 1979) or neonatal hypoglycemia secondary to congenital hypopituitarism (Lovinger et al, 1975). Other major causes include congenital pituitary aplasia and midline brain defects such as agenesis of the corpus callosum and occipital encephalocele.

Another cause of micropenis is primary testicular failure. Micropenis secondary to hypergonadotropic hypogonadism may result from gonadal dysgenesis or rudimentary testes syndrome, and it also occurs in Robinow's syndrome (Lee et al, 1980b). Failure of serum testosterone to rise appropriately after stimulation by hCG has been the test most frequently used to identify this subgroup. However, in patients with Kallmann's syndrome and undescended testes, the serum testosterone level may not increase after hCG administration. Rarely, a patient with partial androgen insensitivity syndrome has micropenis; more commonly, the patient has sexual ambiguity.

Some patients have an idiopathic form of micropenis and a normal hypothalamic-pituitary-testicular axis as demonstrated by endocrine studies. In these cases, micropenis may result from improper timing or delayed onset of gonadotropin stimulation in the fetus (Lee et al, 1980a).

A karyotype analysis should be performed for all patients with micropenis. Consultation usually is obtained from the pediatric endocrinology service to help determine the cause of the micropenis and to assess whether other abnormalities are also present. **Several issues need to be addressed, the most important of which is the growth potential of the penis. In addition, the endocrine abnormality needs to be defined. Testicular function may be assessed by measuring serum testosterone levels before and after hCG stimulation.** Primary testicular failure produces an absent response and elevated basal concentrations of LH and follicle-stimulating hormone (FSH). In some cases, a GnRH stimulation test is done also. Anterior pituitary screening tests include serial measurements of serum glucose, sodium and potassium concentrations, serum cortisol levels, and thyroid function tests. The endocrine evaluation of patients with micropenis is not standardized. **MRI of the head should be done to determine the anatomic integrity of the hypothalamus and the anterior pituitary gland as well as the midline structures of the midbrain.**

Before extensive evaluation of the hypothalamic-pituitary-testicular axis, **androgen therapy should be administered to determine the end-organ response. In general, intramuscular testosterone enanthate, 25 mg per month for 3 months, is given. Although prolonged treatment might advance skeletal maturation, short courses of treatment do not affect height** (Burstein et al, 1979). Transdermal testosterone also has been used in these patients (Choi et al, 1993). Levy and Husmann (1996) proposed the use of growth hormone alone to stimulate penile development in boys with micropenis and isolated growth hormone deficiency; in a series of eight patients, seven had an adult stretched penile length in the normal range, but the average was 1.73 SD below the mean. In contrast, using a combination of growth hormone and testosterone in five boys with multiple pituitary hormone deficiencies, Bin-Abbas and coworkers (1999) reported that the mean stretched adult penile length was only 0.56 SD below the mean.

If androgen treatment in a neonate with a micropenis is used to increase the size of the penis so that it falls within the normal range, what will happen at puberty? The answer is not known with certainty. In a mouse model of hypogonadotropic hypogonadal micropenis, there was evidence that significant prepubertal exposure of the penis to androgens reduced the ultimate growth response to androgens (Husmann and Cain, 1994; McMahon et al, 1995). However, more recently Bin-Abbas and coworkers (1999) reported on **eight boys with micropenis who were treated with androgens both at birth and at puberty. The final penile stretched length averaged 10.3 cm and was in the normal range in all cases.** Until more long-term studies are available, exogenous stimulation at birth and at puberty with testosterone enanthate seems most reasonable (Baskin et al, 1997; Tietjen et al, 1998a, 1998b).

If the penis does not respond to testosterone, the question of whether to recommend gender reassignment is controversial. In the past gender reassignment was recommended, but more recently this position has come under criticism, in large part because of the lack of long-term data regarding the risks and benefits of reassigning these patients to a female gender (Calikoglu, 1999; Diamond, 1999).

In an important long-term retrospective study, Reilly and Woodhouse (1989) reported on 20 patients with a primary diagnosis of micropenis in infancy. Of these, 8 patients were prepubertal and 12 were postpubertal; almost all had received androgen therapy during childhood. Only one child in the prepubertal group had a stretched penile length above the 10th percentile; none of the adults had a penis in the satisfactory range. All parents of patients in the prepubertal group considered their children to be normal boys

and thought that the penile appearance was satisfactory but expressed concern about the size of the penis and wondered whether sexual function in adulthood would be a problem. All of the boys stood to urinate. Nine of the 12 patients in the adult group had a normal male appearance; 3 appeared eunuchoid despite regular testosterone therapy. All had a strong male identity, although half had experienced teasing because of their genital appearance. Nine of the 12 patients were sexually active. This study demonstrated that, **although their ultimate penile size may not fall within what is considered a normal range, the majority of these patients can still have satisfactory sexual function.**

Penile Torsion

Penile torsion is a rotational defect of the penile shaft (Fig. 66–6). **Almost always the shaft is rotated in a counterclockwise direction (i.e., to the left side).** In most cases, penile size is normal and the condition is unrecognized until circumcision is performed or until the foreskin is retracted. Penile torsion may also be associated with hypospadias or a dorsal hood deformity without a urethral abnormality. In most cases of penile torsion, the median raphe spirals obliquely around the shaft. In general, the defect has primarily cosmetic significance, and **correction is unnecessary if the rotation is less than 60 to 90 degrees from the midline.**

Although the glans may be directed more than 90 degrees from the midline, the orientation of the corporal bodies and the corpus spongiosum at the base of the penis is normal. In the milder forms of penile torsion, the penile skin may be degloved and simply reoriented so that the median raphe is restored to its normal position. However, in boys with penile torsion of 90 degrees or more, simply rearranging the skin on the shaft of the penis is not sufficient. In these more severe forms of the disorder, the base of the penis must be mobilized so that dysgenic bands of tissue can be identified and incised. If the penis still remains rotated, correction may be accomplished by placing a nonabsorbable suture through the lateral aspect of the base of the corpora cavernosa on the side opposite the direction of the abnormal rotation (i.e., on the right corporal body) and fixing it to the pubic symphysis dorsal to the penile shaft (Elder, 2002).

Lateral or Dorsal Curvature of the Penis

Lateral penile curvature usually is caused by overgrowth or hypoplasia of one corporal body (Fitzpatrick, 1976). Lateral penile curvature usually is congenital; however, it is often unrecognized until later in childhood because the penis is normal when flaccid and the disparity in corporal size becomes apparent only during an erection. Surgical repair of this lesion involves degloving the penis and performing a modified Nesbit procedure, in which ellipses of tunica albuginea are excised from the site of maximum curvature to allow straightening of the penis.

Another deformity is **congenital dorsal penile curvature. These boys have been observed to have a slender phallus more than 2 SD above the mean (unstretched**

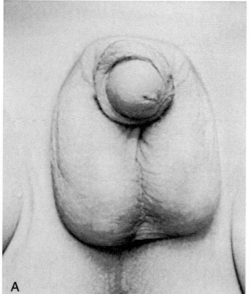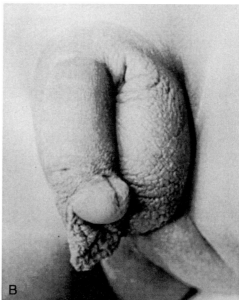

Figure 66–6. Penile torsion in a 1-year-old infant *(A)* and in a 9-year-old boy *(B)*.

length) (Adams et al, 1999). **As many as half have hypospadias.** Repair is performed by excising ellipses from the ventral corporal bodies.

The intraoperative technique of artificial erection using a normal saline solution is critical to the procedure's success. An alternative is to inject alprostadil, 14 μg, into the corpora intraoperatively while manually compressing the corporal base (Kogan, 2000). This technique allows tumescence throughout the penile repair. Detumescence is induced by infiltrating the corporal bodies with phenylephrine, 40 μg. During correction, one must be careful to avoid injury to the neurovascular bundles (Baskin and Lue, 1998; Baskin et al, 2000).

Genital Lymphedema

Lymphedema of the genitalia is a disfiguring disorder characterized by impaired lymphatic drainage that causes progressive penile and/or scrotal swelling. Lymphedema usually is caused by a congenital abnormality of the lymphatics that may appear at various ages. *Milroy's disease* refers to congenital lymphedema, whereas *Meige's disease* occurs later in childhood. The disorder may occur at or just before puberty and is termed *lymphedema praecox* (Hilliard et al, 1990). The lymphedema may involve the penis, scrotum, or both (Fig. 66–7).

Initial management involves observation. If lymphedema remains significant or progresses, then surgical therapy is necessary. The goal of surgical treatment is to remove all involved tissue. On the penile shaft, the penis is degloved and all tissue between Buck's fascia and the skin must be excised, as well as redundant penile skin. If the scrotum is involved, all scrotal tissue, with the exception of the skin, testes, and spermatic cords, must be removed. Usually most of the scrotal skin must be excised, with the exception of the posterior skin (Ross et al, 1998). **The penis may be covered with local skin flaps, and the scrotal contents may be covered with uninvolved posterior skin flaps** (Bolt et al, 1998; Ross et al, 1998). **If inadequate healthy skin is available, the penis and/or scrotum must be covered with split-thickness skin flaps** (Morey et al, 1997). After definitive surgical therapy, recurrence in adjacent areas may occur.

Megaprepuce

Megaprepuce refers to a severely redundant inner foreskin covering a normal glans penis. The foreskin cannot be retracted. Typically, during voiding there is tremendous penoscrotal swelling; significant discomfort or even UTI may be present, and the urine trapped in the foreskin is often malodorous. Manual decompression of the swelling typically relieves the discomfort. Correction of this problem involves degloving of the penis and excision of the redundant skin (Shenoy and Rance, 1999; Summerton et al, 2000). Ideally the penile shaft should be covered with the dorsal penile skin, which should be anchored to Buck's fascia in each quadrant.

Aphallia

Penile agenesis results from failure of development of the genital tubercle. The disorder is rare and has an estimated incidence of 1 in 10,000,000 births; approximately 80 cases have been reported. In these cases, **the karyotype almost always is 46,XY and the usual appearance is that of a well-developed scrotum with descended testes and an absent penile shaft** (Fig. 66–8). The anus usually is displaced anteriorly. The urethra often opens at the anal verge adjacent to a small skin tag; in other cases, it opens into the rectum.

Associated malformations are common and include cryptorchidism, vesicoureteral reflux, horseshoe kidney, renal agenesis, imperforate anus, and musculoskeletal and cardiopulmonary abnormalities (Skoog and Belman, 1989; Evans et al, 1999). **The connection between the genitourinary and gastrointestinal tract is variable.** Skoog and Belman (1989) reviewed 60 reports of aphallia

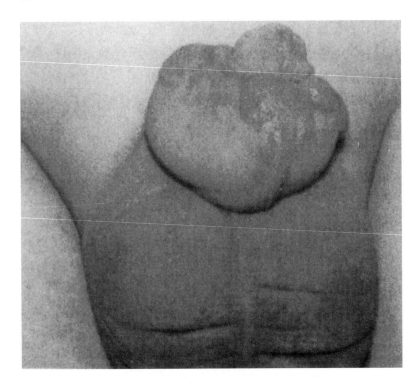

Figure 66–7. Lymphedema of penile shaft in a 1-year-old boy (From Ross JH, Kay R, Yetman RJ, Angermeier K: Primary lymphedema of the genitalia in children and adolescents. J Urol 1998;160:1485, with permission.)

and found that the more proximal the urethral meatus, the higher the incidence of other anomalies and the greater the likelihood of neonatal death. At least 60% of patients had a postsphincteric meatus located on a peculiar appendage at the anal verge (see Fig. 66–8*B*). There were an average of 1.2 associated anomalies, and the mortality rate was 13%. Among the 28% of patients who had a presphincteric urethral communication (prostatorectal fistula), the mortality rate was 36%. In the 12% with a vesicorectal fistula and urethral atresia, there were an average of four anomalies per patient, and mortality rate was 100%.

Children with this lesion should be evaluated immediately with a karyotype and other appropriate studies to determine whether there are associated malformations of the urinary tract or other organ systems. **Gender reassignment was recommended for affected newborns in the past. However, with more recent revelations that some of these patients have a male gender identity despite reconstruction as a female (Diamond, 1999), the recommendation to perform gender reassignment should be made very carefully, and only after full evaluation by an ambiguous genitalia assessment team that includes a pediatric urologist, endocrinologist, and psychiatrist.** As a male, the patient would potentially be fertile, but currently there is an inability to construct a cosmetically acceptable phallus that would allow normal urinary, sexual,

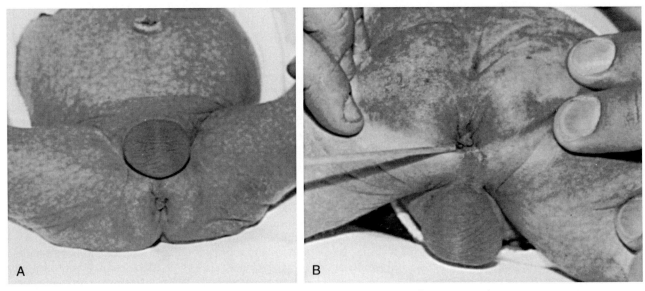

Figure 66–8. *A,* Neonate with aphallia. *B,* Urethral meatus at skin tag on anal verge.

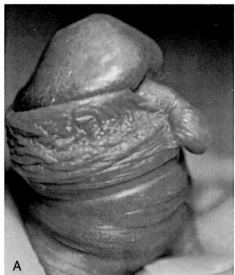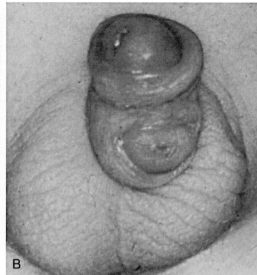

Figure 66–9. *A,* Diphallia. Urethra is in diminutive phallic structure. *B,* Second example of diphallia. (*A,* Courtesy of Richard Hurwitz, MD.)

and reproductive function. The issues are similar to those under consideration in many genetic males born with cloacal exstrophy. Gender reassignment involves orchiectomy and feminizing genitoplasty in the newborn period. At a later age, construction of a neovagina is necessary. Urinary tract reconstruction with simultaneous construction of an intestinal neovagina through a posterior sagittal and abdominal approach in patients with penile agenesis has been described (Stolar et al, 1987; Hendren, 1997).

Diphallia

Duplication of the penis is a rare anomaly and has a range of appearances from a small accessory penis (Fig. 66–9) **to complete duplication** (Hollowell et al, 1977). In some cases each phallus has only one corporal body and urethra, whereas others seem to be a variant of twinning, with each phallus having two corpora cavernosa and a urethra. The penes usually are unequal in size and lie side by side. Associated anomalies are common, including hypospadias, bifid scrotum, duplication of the bladder, renal agenesis or ectopia, and diastasis of the pubic symphysis (Kapoor and Saha, 1987; Maruyama et al, 1999). Anal and cardiac anomalies also are common. Evaluation should include imaging of the entire urinary tract. Sonography has been reported to aid in assessment of the extent of phallic development (Marti-Bonmati et al, 1989). MRI can also be used to assess penile development. Treatment must be individualized to attain a satisfactory functional and cosmetic result.

Congenital Urethral Fistula

A rare anomaly is the congenital urethral fistula, in which **the urethra and meatus are normal and a urethrocutaneous fistula is present, typically coronal or subcoronal** (Fig. 66–10). This abnormality **usually is an isolated deformity, but it may be associated with imperforate anus or ventral chordee** (Ritchey et al, 1994). In a series of 14 boys with a congenital fistula, 4 had distal hypospadias and 2 had chordee (Caldamone et al, 1999). In

the patient portrayed in Fig. 66–10, at birth there was a small ventral penile cyst, resembling an epithelial inclusion cyst; it ruptured at 1 to 2 weeks of age and became a small fistula. The cause of congenital urethral fistula is unknown but probably involves a focal defect in the urethral plate that prevents fusion of the urethral folds. Some reported patients have undergone circumcision before diagnosis (Caldamone et al, 1999), raising the possibility that in some of these cases the fistula may have been iatrogenic rather than congenital. Treatment usually consists of one of two techniques: (1) the fistula can be circumscribed and

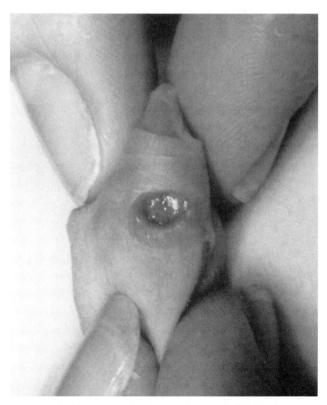

Figure 66–10. Infant with subcoronal congenital urethral fistula.

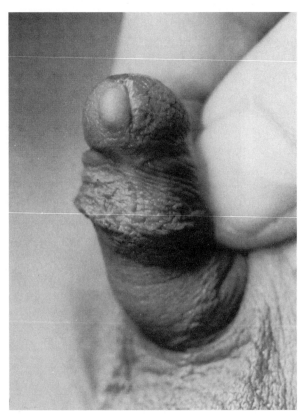

Figure 66–11. Example of parameatal urethral cyst.

Parameatal Urethral Cysts

The parameatal urethral cyst is another rare anomaly (Fig. 66–11). Shiraki (1975) suggested that these cysts may result from occlusion of paraurethral ducts, or in other cases from faulty preputial separation from the glans along the coronal sulcus. The cyst wall has been reported to consist of transitional and squamous as well as columnar epithelium (Hill and Ashken, 1977). Treatment consists of simple excision under anesthesia, with care taken not to cause meatal stenosis.

Scrotal Anomalies

Penoscrotal Transposition (Scrotal Engulfment)

Penoscrotal transposition may be partial or complete (Figs. 66–12 and 66–13). **Its less severe forms have been termed bifid scrotum, doughnut scrotum, prepenile scrotum, and shawl scrotum. Frequently, the condition occurs in conjunction with perineal, scrotal, or penoscrotal hypospadias with chordee.** It also has been associated with caudal regression (Lage et al, 1987; MacKenzie et al, 1994), Aarskog syndrome (Shinkawa et al, 1983), and sex chromosome abnormalities (Yamaguchi et al, 1989). **When there is complete penoscrotal transposition and a normal scrotum, as many as 75% of patients have a significant urinary tract abnormality** (MacKenzie et al, 1994), **and a renal sonogram and VCUG should be performed.** Presumably, this anomaly results from incomplete or failed inferomedial migration of the labioscrotal swellings.

When scrotal engulfment is associated with severe hypospadias, hypospadias repair usually is accomplished with the use of a transverse preputial island flap in conjunction

then closed in multiple layers, similar to a urethrocutaneous fistula after hypospadias repair, or (2) if the glans bridge is thin, the ventral glans can be opened through the distal urethra, the distal urethra then being closed by a Thiersch-Duplay technique.

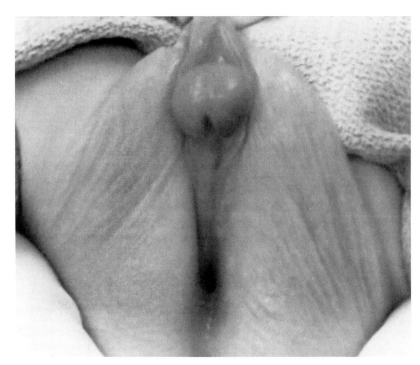

Figure 66–12. Scrotal engulfment in a child with scrotal hypospadias and chordee.

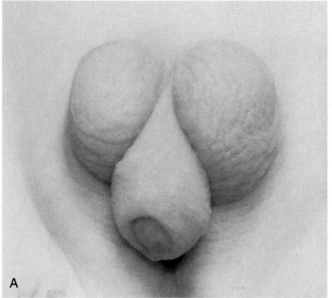

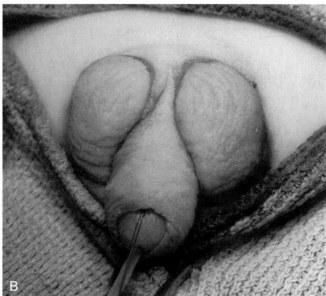

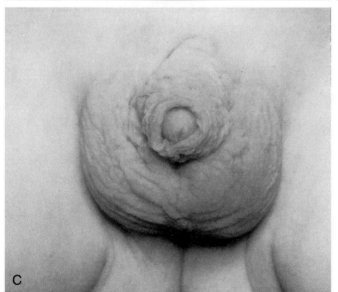

Figure 66–13. *A,* Complete penoscrotal transposition. The urethral meatus is at the tip of the glans, but the urethra is short. *B,* Skin flaps for scrotoplasty. *C,* Completed two-stage repair: first stage, scrotoplasty; second stage, urethroplasty.

with Thiersch-Duplay tubularization of the proximal urethra. To minimize the possibility of devascularizing the preputial flap, correction of the scrotal engulfment usually is done as a second-stage procedure 6 months later (Elder and Duckett, 1990; Germiyanoglu et al, 1994). If the penis is normal, scrotoplasty can be accomplished when the child is 6 to 12 months of age.

Scrotoplasty is begun by circumscribing the superior aspects of each half of the vertical aspect of the scrotum and extending these incisions laterally to include at least half of the scrotum (Fig. 66–14). The medial aspects of the incision are joined on the ventral aspect of the penis, and the incision is carried down the midline along the median raphe for 4 or 5 cm. Before making the incision, it is helpful to infiltrate the skin with 1% lidocaine with 1:100,000 epinephrine to diminish bleeding. Traction sutures are placed on the superior aspect of the scrotal flaps, and these are dissected out in the areolar layer. Deeper dissection may result in cutting of the tunica vaginalis and may injure the spermatic cord. The scrotal wings are rotated medially

under the penis and are sutured together in the midline in an everted manner. During this dissection, moderate oozing from the areolar tissue frequently occurs, and it may be necessary to leave a small dependent Penrose drain in place for 24 to 48 hours. In many cases, the bare area on either side of the penis can be closed. However, in more severe cases of penoscrotal transposition, dorsal interposition flaps may be necessary, allowing caudal advancement of the skin of the abdominal wall (Dresner, 1982). Usually, scrotoplasty can be accomplished as an outpatient procedure.

An alternative technique is to identify the correct position for the penis and create a buttonhole by excising a plug of epidermis, dermis, and suprapubic fat. The penis is then degloved and the penile shaft is brought through the buttonhole. The penile shaft skin remains behind and is split down the ventrum and mobilized superiorly to the penile shaft. A window of the dartos pedicle is created, and the penile shaft is brought through this window. The degloved penis is then resurfaced with shaft skin. In a

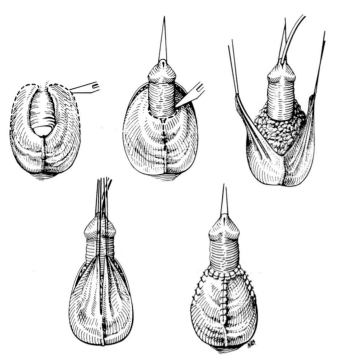

Figure 66–14. Repair of penoscrotal transposition (see discussion in text).

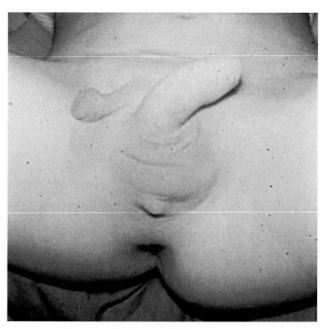

Figure 66–15. Child with ectopic scrotum.

report of 15 patients who underwent this technique, all had an excellent cosmetic result (Kolligian et al, 2000).

Ectopic Scrotum

Ectopic scrotum, the anomalous position of one hemiscrotum along the inguinal canal, is a rare condition. Most commonly, it is suprainguinal (Fig. 66–15), although it may also be infrainguinal or perineal (Elder and Jeffs, 1982). This anomaly has been associated with cryptorchidism, inguinal hernia, and exstrophy as well as the popliteal pterygium syndrome (Cunningham et al, 1989). In one review, 70% of boys with a suprainguinal ectopic scrotum exhibited ipsilateral upper urinary tract anomalies, including renal agenesis, renal dysplasia, and ectopic ureter (Elder and Jeffs, 1982). Another study indicated that an associated perineal lipoma was found in 83% of these children; 68% of those with a lipoma had no associated anomalies, where 100% of those without a lipoma had associated genital or renal malformations (Sule et al, 1994). Consequently, children with this anomaly should undergo upper urinary tract imaging. Because the embryology of the gubernaculum and that of the scrotum are intimately related chronologically and anatomically, it seems likely that the ectopic scrotum results from a defect in gubernacular formation that prevents migration of the labioscrotal swellings (Hoar et al, 1998). Scrotoplasty and orchiopexy may be performed at 6 to 12 months of age, or earlier if other surgical procedures are necessary.

Bifid Scrotum

The term *bifid scrotum* refers to the deformity in which the labioscrotal folds are completely separated. Almost al-

ways this anomaly is associated with proximal hypospadias (Fig. 66–16).

Scrotal Hypoplasia

Scrotal hypoplasia is the underdevelopment of one or both sides of the scrotum. This anomaly **occurs most com-**

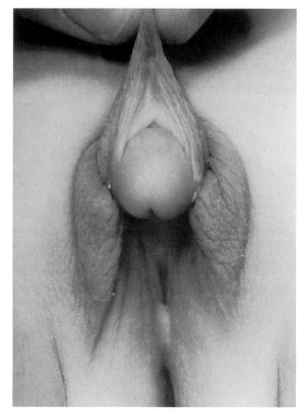

Figure 66–16. Child with bifid scrotum and perineal hypospadias.

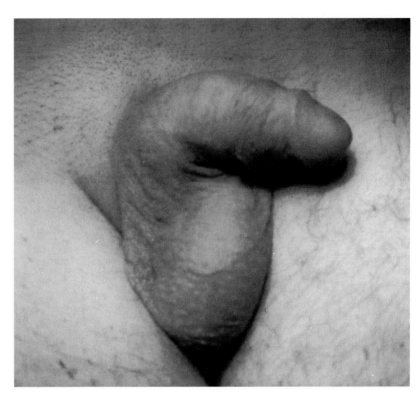

Figure 66–17. Boy with hypoplastic right hemiscrotum and right undescended testis.

monly in boys with an undescended testis (Fig. 66–17) and frequently is noted in infants with genital ambiguity. The deformity probably results from lack of gubernacular swelling of the labioscrotal folds.

Vascular Lesions of the Genitalia

Vascular lesions of the genitalia are uncommon, and there is disagreement regarding their classification, etiology, and treatment. These deformities **include hemangiomas and vascular malformations. A hemangioma is on the skin and often is present at birth. It may show significant growth in the postnatal period followed by slow involution. Vascular malformations, on the other hand, are present at birth in the subcutaneous tissues, and tend to persist or enlarge. They may expand secondary to trauma, sepsis, or hormonal changes** (Ramos et al, 1999). Vascular malformations can be subdivided into either slow-flow (capillary, lymphatic, venous) or fast-flow (arterial, arteriovenous) types.

Congenital hemangiomas are common and affect the genitalia in approximately 1% of cases (Alter et al, 1993). **Strawberry hemangiomas, the most common type, result from proliferation of immature capillary vessels.** These are also categorized as cutaneous hemangiomas because they occur on the skin. Although the lesions may undergo a period of rapid growth lasting 3 to 6 months, gradual involution is common, and **most lesions require no treatment** (Casale and Menashe, 1989). If ulceration develops, intervention is necessary to prevent complications from bleeding. The most popular form of therapy is short-term oral steroid therapy. In some cases, surgical excision is necessary.

In 1990, Smith reported using an argon laser to treat a bladder hemangioma because the pigments melanin and hemoglobin absorb the argon laser, which emits a wavelength of 488 to 524 nm. Then, because of limited tissue penetration, he abandoned the argon laser in favor of the neodymium:YAG laser. However, the high degree of scatter with resultant tissue injury and the twofold increase in depth of penetration makes use of this laser potentially dangerous in the treatment of cutaneous hemangiomas of the genitalia in the pediatric population. The potassium thiophosphate (KTP) laser is a frequency-doubled neodymium:YAG laser. The 1060-nm wave length of the neodymium:YAG laser is passed through a KTP crystal, producing a wave length of 532 nm, which is highly absorbed in hemoglobin and produces less tissue scatter. Preliminary work with the KTP laser in children with cutaneous and urethral hemangiomas has been encouraging (Kennedy et al, 1993).

Subcutaneous hemangiomas, also referred to as cavernous hemangiomas, are much less common than the cutaneous variety (Sule et al, 1993; Ferrer and McKenna, 1995) and are probably more appropriately classified as a vascular malformation. They may be detected at birth or later in life. In contrast to cutaneous hemangiomas, which tend to involute, cavernous hemangiomas **tend to enlarge gradually. Physical examination reveals a "bag of worms" sensation** similar to that of a varicocele, although the lesions tend to be firm and do not decompress when the patient is recumbent. Because examination does not disclose the extent of the lesion, ultrasound with color Doppler, CT scan, or MRI is advised to delineate the size of the hemangioma. **Definitive treatment by en bloc resection is advised,** and preoperative angioembolization may be helpful to reduce the size of the mass and the risk of bleeding.

Vascular malformations may also affect the penis. Although these lesions are congenital, they usually are not diagnosed until the teenage years or young adulthood and are characterized as a faint blue patch or a soft blue mass. If the lesion affects the glans penis, the neodymium:YAG laser may yield a better result than surgical excision (Ramos et al, 1999).

Miscellaneous Genital Anomalies

Cysts of the median raphe can occur on the perineum, scrotum, or shaft of the penis (Little et al, 1992). The lesions probably result from epithelial rests that become buried during the urethral infolding process. Excision is recommended unless the cysts are small and asymptomatic.

Juvenile xanthogranulomas appear as one or more lesions of rapid onset; they measure 2 to 20 mm in diameter and are orange, gold, or brown in color. These lesions can affect the penis (Hautmann and Bachor, 1993) or scrotum (Goulding and Traylor, 1983). As many as 20% are present at birth. The lesion often is self-limited, and a period of 1 year of expectant waiting is advised to avoid potentially unnecessary ablative genital surgery.

Meconium peritonitis causes genital manifestations on occasion, among them meconium hydrocele (Ring et al, 1989) **and congenital rupture of the scrotum, termed** *scrotoschisis* (Pippi Salle et al, 1992; Chun and St-Vil, 1997). When an unusual inflammatory condition of the scrotum is detected, the clinician should suspect meconium peritonitis and proceed with the appropriate evaluation.

REFERENCES

Aaronson IA: Micropenis: Medical and surgical implications. J Urol 1994; 152:4.

Adams MC, Chalian VS, Rink RC: Congenital dorsal penile curvature: A potential problem of the long phallus. J Urol 1999;161:1304.

Adams MC, McLaughlin KP, Rink RC: Inadvertent concentrated epinephrine injection at newborn circumcision: Effect and treatment. J Urol 2000;163:592.

Alter GJ, Ehrlich RM: A new technique for correction of the hidden penis in children and adults. J Urol 1999;161:455.

Alter GJ, Trengove-Jones G, Horton CE Jr: Hemangioma of penis and scrotum. Urology 1993;42:205.

American Academy of Pediatrics, Committee from the Urology Section: Urethral meatal stenosis in males. Pediatrics 1978;61:778.

American Academy of Pediatrics, Committee on Genetics, Section on Endocrinology, Section on Urology: Evaluation of the newborn with developmental anomalies of the external genitalia. Pediatrics 2000;106: 138.

American Academy of Pediatrics, Task Force on Circumcision: Report of the Task Force on Circumcision. Pediatrics 1989;84:388.

American Academy of Pediatrics, Task Force on Circumcision: Circumcision policy statement. Pediatrics 1999;103:686.

American Academy of Pediatrics, Task Force on Circumcision. 1999–2000: Circumcision debate. Pediatrics 2000;106:641.

Anonymous: Circumcision. BJU Int 1999;83(Suppl 1):1.

Baskin LS, Canning DA, Snyder HM, Duckett JW: Treating complications of circumcision. Pediatr Emerg Care 1996;12:62.

Baskin LS, Erol A, Li YW, Liu WH: Anatomy of the neurovascular bundle: Is safe mobilization possible? J Urol 2000;164:2122.

Baskin LS, Sutherland RS, DiSandro MJ, et al: The effect of testosterone on androgen receptors and human penile growth. J Urol 1997;158:1113.

Baskin LS, Lue TF: The correction of congenital penile curvature in young men. Br J Urol 1998;81:895.

Ben-Ari J, Merlob P, Minouni F, Reisner SH: Characteristics of the male genitalia in the newborn: Penis. J Urol 1985;134:521.

Bennett RT, Gill B, Kogan SJ: Epididymitis in children: The circumcision factor? J Urol 1998;160:1842.

Bergeson PS, Hopkin RJ, Bailey RB Jr, et al: The inconspicuous penis. Pediatrics 1993;92:794.

Berkhoff WBC, Scholtmeyer RJ, Tibboel D, Molenaar JC: Urogenital tract abnormalities associated with esophageal atresia and tracheoesophageal fistula. J Urol 1989;141:362.

Bin-Abbas B, Conte FA, Grumbach MM, Kaplan SL: Congenital hypogonadotropic hypogonadism and micropenis: Effect of testosterone treatment on adult penile size—Why sex reversal is not indicated. J Pediatr 1999;134:579.

Bolt RJ, Peelen W, Nikkels PG, de Jong TP: Congenital lymphoedema of the genitalia. Eur J Pediatr 1998;157:943.

Bradley SJ, Oliver GD, Chernick AB, Zucker KJ: Experiment of nurture: Ablatio penis at 2 months, sex reassignment at 7 months, and a psychosexual follow-up in young adulthood. Pediatrics 1998;102:E9.

Burstein S, Grumbach MM, Kaplan SL: Early determination of androgen-responsiveness is important in the management of microphallus. Lancet 1979;2:193.

Caldamone AA, Chen S-C, Elder JS, et al: Congenital anterior urethrocutaneous fistula. J Urol 1999;162:1430.

Calikoglu AS: Should boys with micropenis be reared as girls? J Pediatr 1999;134:537.

Cartwright PC, Snow BW, McNees DC: Urethral meatotomy in the office using topical EMLA cream for anesthesia. J Urol 1996;156:857.

Casale AJ, Beck SD, Cain MP, et al: Concealed penis in childhood: A spectrum of etiology and treatment. J Urol 1999;162:1165.

Casale AJ, Menashe DS: Massive strawberry hemangioma of the male genitalia. J Urol 1989;141:593.

Cheikhelard A, Luton D, Philippe-Chomette P, et al: How accurate is the prenatal diagnosis of abnormal genitalia? J Urol 2000;164:984.

Choi SK, Han SW, Kim DH, de Lignieres B: Transdermal dihydrohydrotestosterone therapy and its effects on patients with microphallus. J Urol 1993;150:657.

Christakis DA, Harvey E, Zerr DM, et al: A trade-off analysis of routine newborn circumcision. Pediatrics 2000;105:246.

Chun K, St-Vil D: Scrotoschisis associated with contralateral meconium periorchitis. J Pediatr Surg 1997;32:864.

Cooper RT: Methaemoglobinaemia secondary to topical lignocaine/prilocaine in a circumcised neonate. J Paediatr Child Health 2000;36:406.

Craig JC, Knight JF, Suresh Kumar P, et al: Effect of circumcision on incidence of urinary tract infection in preschool boys. J Pediatr 1996; 128:23.

Cromie WJ, Ritchey ML, Smith RC, Zagaja GP: Anatomical alignment for the correction of buried penis. J Urol 1998;160:1482.

Cuckow JC, Rix G, Mouriquand PDE: Preputia plasty: A good alternative to circumcision. J Pediatr Surg 1994;29:561.

Cunningham LN, Keating MA, Snyder HM, Duckett JW: Urological manifestations of the popliteal pterygium syndrome. J Urol 1989;141:910.

Danish RK, Lee PA, Mazur T, et al: Micropenis: II. Hypogonadotropic hypogonadism. Johns Hopkins Med J 1980;146:177.

Diamond M: Pediatric management of ambiguous and traumatized genitalia. J Urol 1999;162:1021.

Diamond M, Sigmundson HK: Sex reassignment at birth: Long term review and clinical implications. Arch Pediatr Adolesc Med 1997;151: 298.

Donahoe PJ, Keating MA: Preputial unfurling to correct the buried penis. J Pediatr Surg 1986;21:1055.

Dresner ML: Surgical revision of scrotal engulfment. Urol Clin North Am 1982;9:305.

Elder JS: Penile torsion. In Frank JD, Snyder HM III (eds): Operative Paediatric Urology, 2nd ed. London, Churchill Livingstone, 2002.

Elder JS, Duckett JW: Complications of hypospadias surgery. In Smith RB, Ehrlich RM (eds): Complications of Urologic Surgery. Philadelphia, WB Saunders, 1990, p 549.

Elder JS, Jeffs RD: Suprainguinal ectopic scrotum and associated anomalies. J Urol 1982;127:336.

Evans JA, Erdile LB, Greenberg CR, Chudley AE: Agenesis of the penis: Patterns of associated malformations. Am J Med Genet 1999;84:47.

Feldman KW, Smith DW: Fetal phallic growth and penile standards for newborn male infants. J Pediatr 1975;86:395.

Ferrer FA, McKenna PH: Cavernous hemangioma of the scrotum: A rare benign genital tumor of childhood J Urol 1995;153:1262.

Fitzpatrick TJ: Hemihypertrophy of the human corpus cavernosum. J Urol 1976;115:560.

Germiyanoglu C, Ozkardes H, Altug U, Erol D: Reconstruction of peno-scrotal transposition. Br J Urol 1994;73:200.

Ginsburg CM, McCracken GH Jr: Urinary tract infections in young infants. Pediatrics 1982;69:409.

Gonzales JR: Micropenis. AUA Update Series 1983;2(39):1.

Goulding FJ, Traylor RA: Juvenile xanthogranuloma of the scrotum. J Urol 1983;129:841.

Hardwick-Smith S, Mastrobattista JM, Wallace PA, Ritchey ML: Ring block for neonatal circumcision. Obstet Gynecol 1998;91:930.

Hautmann RE, Bachor R: Juvenile xanthogranuloma of the penis. J Urol 1993;150:456.

Hendren WH: The genetic male with absent penis and urethrorectal communication: Experience with 5 patients. J Urol 1997;157:1469.

Hill JT, Ashken MH: Parameatal urethral cysts: A review of 6 cases. Br J Urol 1977;49:323.

Hilliard RI, McKendry JBJ, Phillips MJ: Congenital abnormalities of the lymphatic system: A new clinical classification. Pediatrics 1990;86:988.

Hoar RM, Calvano CJ, Reddy PP, et al: Unilateral suprainguinal ectopic scrotum: The role of the gubernaculum in the formation of an ectopic scrotum. Teratology 1998;57:64.

Hoekstra WJ, Scholtmeijer RJ, Molenaar JC, et al: Urogenital tract abnormalities associated with congenital anorectal anomalies. J Urol 1983;130:962.

Hollowell JG Jr, Witherington R, Ballagas AJ, Burt JN: Embryologic considerations of diphallus and associated anomalies. J Urol 1977;117:728.

Howard CR, Howard FM, Fortune K, et al: A randomized, controlled trial of a eutectic mixture of local anesthetic cream (lidocaine and prilocaine) versus penile nerve block for pain relief during circumcision. Am J Obstet Gynecol 1999;181:1506.

Husmann DA, Cain MP: Microphallus: Eventual phallic size is dependent on the timing of androgen administration. J Urol 1994;152:734.

Jayanthi VR, Burns JE, Koff SA: Postneonatal circumcision with local anesthesia: A cost-effective alternative. J Urol 1999;161:1301.

Kapoor R, Saha MM: Complete duplication of the bladder, urethra, and external genitalia in a neonate: A case report. J Urol 1987;137:1243.

Kennedy WA II, Hensle TW, Giella J, et al: Potassium thiophosphate laser treatment of genitourinary hemangioma in the pediatric population. J Urol 1993;150:950.

Kogan BA: Intraoperative pharmacological erection as an aid to pediatric hypospadias repair. J Urol 2000;164:2058.

Kolligian ME, Franco I, Reda EF: Correction of penoscrotal transposition: A novel approach. J Urol 2000;164:994.

Lage JM, Driscoll SG, Bieber FR, et al: Transposition of the external genitalia associated with caudal regression. J Urol 1987;138:387.

Larsen GL, Williams SD: Postneonatal circumcision: Population profile. Pediatrics 1990;85:808.

Lavreys L, Rakwar JP, Thompson ML, et al: Effect of circumcision on incidence of human immunodeficiency virus type 1 and other sexually transmitted diseases: A prospective cohort study of trucking company employees in Kenya. J Infect Dis 1999;180:330.

Lee PA, Danish RK, Major T, Migeon CJ: Micropenis: III. Primary hypogonadism, partial androgen insensitivity syndrome, and idiopathic disorders. Johns Hopkins Med J 1980a;147:175.

Lee PA, Mazur T, Danish R, et al: Micropenis: I. Criteria, etiologies and classification. Johns Hopkins Med J 1980b;146:156.

Levy JB, Husmann DA: Micropenis secondary to growth hormone deficiency: Does treatment with growth hormone alone result in adequate penile growth? J Urol 1996;156:214.

Little LS Jr, Keating MA, Rink RC: Median raphe cysts of the genitalia. J Urol 1992;148:1872.

Litvak AS, Morris JA Jr, McRoberts JW: Normal size of the urethral meatus in boys. J Urol 1976;115:736.

Lovinger RD, Kaplan SL, Grumbach MM: Congenital hypopituitarism associated with neonatal hypoglycemia and microphallus: Four cases secondary to hypothalamic hormone deficiencies. J Pediatr 1975;87:1171.

MacKenzie J, Chitayat D, McLorie G, et al: Penoscrotal transposition: A case report and review. Am J Med Genet 1994;49:103.

Maizels M, Zaontz M, Donovan J, et al: Surgical correction of the buried penis: Description of a classification system and a technique to correct the disorder. J Urol 1986;136:268.

Mandell J, Bromley B, Peters CA, Benacerraf BR: Prenatal sonographic detection of genital malformations. J Urol 1995;153:1994.

Marti-Bonmati L, Menor F, Gomez J, et al: Value of sonography in true complete diphallia. J Urol 1989;142:356.

Maruyama K, Takahashi A, Kobayashi T, et al: Diphallia and the VATER association. J Urol 1999;162:2144.

McMahon DR, Kramer SA, Husmann DA: Micropenis: Does early treatment with testosterone do more harm than good? J Urol 1995;154:825.

Monsour MA, Rabinovitch HH, Dean GE: Medical management of phimosis in children: Our experience with topical steroids. J Urol 1999;162:1162.

Morey AF, Meng MV, McAninch JW: Skin graft reconstruction of chronic genital lymphedema. Urology 1997;50:423.

Morton HG: Meatus size in 1,000 circumcised children from two weeks to sixteen years of age. J Fla Med Assoc 1986;50:137.

Noe HN, Dale GA: Evaluation of children with meatal stenosis. J Urol 1975;114:455.

Oster J: Further fate of the foreskin: Incidence of preputial adhesions, phimosis, and smegma among Danish schoolboys. Arch Dis Child 1968;43:200.

Persad R, Sharma S, McTavish J, et al: Clinical presentation and pathophysiology of meatal stenosis following circumcision. Br J Urol 1995;75:91.

Pippi Salle JL, de Fraga JCS, Wojciechowski M, Antunes CRH: Congenital rupture of the scrotum: An unusual complication of meconium peritonitis. J Urol 1992;148:1292.

Ponsky LE, Ross JH, Knipper N, Kay R: Penile adhesions after neonatal circumcision. J Urol 2000;164:495.

Ragan DC, Casale AJ, Rink RC, et al: Genitourinary anomalies in the CHARGE association. J Urol 1999;161:622.

Ramos LM, Pavon EM, Barrilero AE: Venous malformation of the glans penis: Efficacy of treatment with neodymium:yttrium-aluminum-garnet laser. Urology 1999;53:779.

Reilly JM, Woodhouse CRJ: Small penis and the male sexual role. J Urol 1989;142:569.

Reiner WG: Case study: Sex reassignment in a teenage girl. J Am Acad Child Adolesc Psychiatr 1996;35:799.

Ring KS, Axelrod SL, Burbige KA, Hensle TW: Meconium hydrocele: An unusual etiology of a scrotal mass in the newborn. J Urol 1989;141:1172.

Ritchey ML, Sinha A, Argueso L: Congenital fistula of the penile urethra. J Urol 1994;151:1061.

Ross JH: Circumcision: Pro and con. In Elder JS (ed): Pediatric Urology for the General Urologist. New York, Igaku-Shoin, 1996, p 49.

Ross JH, Kay R, Yetman RJ, Angermeier K: Primary lymphedema of the genitalia in children and adolescents. J Urol 1998;160:1485.

Scherz HC, Kaplan GW, Packer MG: Anterior urethral valves in the fossa navicularis in children. J Urol 1987;138:1211.

Schoen EJ, Colby CJ, Ray GT: Newborn circumcision decreases incidence and costs of urinary tract infections during the first year of life. Pediatrics 2000a;105:789.

Schoen EJ, Oehrli M, Colby CJ, Machin G: The highly protective effect of newborn circumcision against invasive penile cancer. Pediatrics 2000b;105:E36.

Schoen EJ, Wiswell TE, Moses S: New policy on circumcision: Cause for concern. Pediatrics 2000c;105:620.

Shapiro E: The sonographic appearance of normal and abnormal fetal genitalia. J Urol 1999;162:530.

Shapiro SR: Surgical treatment of the "buried" penis. Urology 1987;30:554.

Shenoy MU, Rance CH: Surgical correction of congenital megaprepuce. Pediatr Surg Int 1999;15:593.

Shenoy MU, Srinivasan J, Sully L, Rance CH: Buried penis: Surgical correction using liposuction and realignment of skin. BJU Int 2000;86:527.

Sherman J, Borer JG, Horowitz M, Glassberg KI: Circumcision: Successful glanular reconstruction and survival following traumatic amputation. J Urol 1996;156:842.

Shinkawa T, Yamauchi Y, Osada Y, Ishisawa N: Aarskog syndrome. Urology 1983;22:624.

Shiraki IW: Parameatal cysts of the glans penis: A report of 9 cases. J Urol 1975;114:544.

Skoog SJ, Belman AB: Aphallia: Its classification and management. J Urol 1989;141:589.

Smith JA Jr: Laser treatment of bladder hemangioma. J Urol 1990;143:282.

Smuelders N, Wilcox DT, Cuckow PM: The buried penis: An anatomical approach. BJU Int 2000;86:523.

Stolar CJH, Wiener ES, Hensle TW, et al: Reconstruction of penile agenesis by a posterior sagittal approach. J Pediatr Surg 1987;22:1076.

Sule JS, Lemmers MJ, Barry JM: Scrotal arteriovenous malformation: Case report and literature review. J Urol 1993;150:1917.

Sule JD, Skoog SJ, Tank ES: Perineal lipoma and the accessory labioscrotal fold: An etiological relationship. J Urol 1994;151:475.

Summerton DJ, McNally J, Denny AJ, Malone PSJ: Congenital megaprepuce: An emerging condition—How to recognize and treat it. BJU Int 2000;86:519.

Taddio A, Pollock N, Gilbert-MacLeod C, et al: Combined analgesia and local anesthesia to minimize pain during erection. Arch Pediatr Adolesc Med 2000;154:620.

Thompson HC, King LR, Knox E, Keanes SB: Report of the ad hoc task force on circumcision. Pediatrics 1975;56:610.

Tietjen DN, Uramoto GY, Tindall DJ, Husmann DA: Characterization of penile androgen receptor expression in micropenis due to hypogonadotropic hypogonadism. J Urol 1998a;160:1075.

Tietjen DN, Uramoto GY, Tindall DJ, Husmann DA: Micropenis in hypogonadotropic hypogonadism: Response of the penile androgen receptor to testosterone treatment. J Urol 1998b;160:1054.

Tuladhar R, Davis PG, Batch J, Doyle LW: Establishment of a normal range of penile length in preterm infants. J Paediatr Child Health 1998; 34:471.

Van Howe RS: Variability in penile appearance and penile findings: A prospective study. Br J Urol 1997;80:776.

Walsh PC, Wilson JD, Allen TD, et al: Clinical and endocrinological evaluation of patients with congenital microphallus. J Urol 1978;120: 90.

Williams CP, Richardson BG, Bukowski TP: Importance of identifying the inconspicuous penis: Prevention of circumcision complications. Urology 2000;56:140.

Wiswell TE: Prepuce presence portends prevalence of potentially perilous periurethral pathogens. J Urol 1992;148:739.

Wiswell TE: The prepuce, urinary tract infections, and the consequences. Pediatrics 2000;106:860.

Wiswell TE, Miller GM, Gelston HM Jr, et al: Effect of circumcision status on periurethral bacterial flora during the first year of life. J Pediatr 1988;113:442.

Wiswell TE, Smith FR, Bass JW: Decreased incidence of urinary tract infections in circumcised male infants. Pediatrics 1985;75:901.

Yachia D, Beyar M, Aridogan IA, Dascalu S: The incidence of congenital penile curvature. J Urol 1993;150:1478.

Yamaguchi T, Hamasuna R, Hasui Y, et al: 47,XXY/48,XXY, +21 chromosomal mosaicism presenting as hypospadias with scrotal transposition. J Urol 1989;142:797.

67
ABNORMALITIES OF THE TESTES AND SCROTUM AND THEIR SURGICAL MANAGEMENT

Francis X. Schneck, MD
Mark F. Bellinger, MD

NORMAL GONADAL AND EXTERNAL GENITAL DEVELOPMENT AND DIFFERENTIATION IN THE MALE

Male Sex Determination and Differentiation

Genital development is a complex process of genetic interactions, the critical components of which occur during embryogenesis. Development of the male phenotype is determined by the presence or absence of the Y chromosome and can be divided into two distinct stages: sex determination and sexual differentiation. **Sex determination is the process of gonadal development resulting in either ovary or testis formation, whereas sexual differentiation is the subsequent process of gonad formation that ultimately results in either the female or the male phenotype.** The genetics of male sex determination and gonadal development are incompletely understood, although critical components of this process have been elucidated.

2353

Because the Y chromosome confers the male sex, it was postulated that the genes responsible for testis determination were present on the Y chromosome. Through the investigation of sex-reversed XX male patients, portions of translocated Y chromosomal material important in male sexual differentiation were localized (Guellaen et al, 1984; Muller et al, 1986). Analysis of these patients led to the identification of the ZFY (zinc finger Y) gene within a 140-kilobase (kb) region just proximal to the pseudoautosomal region of the short arm of the Y chromosome (Page et al, 1987). Localization of this conserved gene helped to isolate another gene, the testicular differentiation gene, to a 35-kb region on the short arm of the Y chromosome by characterizing sex-reversed patients with testicular differentiation and no identifiable Y chromosomal material containing ZFY (Sinclair et al, 1990). A conserved Y chromosome–specific sequence within this region was later identified and named SRY for sex-determining region–Y chromosome. The SRY gene encodes a DNA-binding motif, referred to as the high mobility group (HMG) box, which is associated with genes encoding proteins that preferentially bind to specific DNA sequences and are expressed in a tissue-specific or developmentally regulated fashion (Parker et al, 1999).

The importance of the SRY gene in sex determination has been substantiated in experiments with transgenic mice and in mutational analysis of the 46,XY sex reversal cluster within the HMG box of the SRY gene (Haqq et al, 1994). Almost all SRY mutations responsible for sex reversal occur within the highly conserved HMG box. Other subsets of HMG box proteins have been isolated because of their homology to SRY and are termed SOX genes. Mutations in SOX9 have also been shown to result in sex reversal. In particular, camptomelic dysplasia, an autosomal dominant skeletal malformation syndrome mapped to chromosome 17q24.3-q25.1, is characterized by cardiac, skeletal, and renal abnormalities, as well as impaired testicular development resulting in 46,XY sex reversal (Foster et al, 1994; Waner et al, 1994; Cameron and Sinclair, 1997).

Although the SRY gene appears to be primarily responsible for male sexual differentiation through complex interactions involving both activation and repression of other male-specific genes, little is known about its mode of action or about downstream target genes that convert the bipotential gonad into the testis. Evidence exists to suggest that the SRY product may not activate a developmental cascade positively; instead, it may repress a negative regulator that inhibits male sex determination (McElreavey et al, 1993). This would explain other types of sex reversal in mammals, in particular XY females containing SRY.

Coordinated expression of multiple genes, both sex-linked and autosomal, is responsible for gonadogenesis. Other non-Y genes that have been implicated in sex determination prior to sexual differentiation include WT1, DAX1, and SF1, and there is increasing evidence that there is a close functional relationship among the protein products of these genes (Nachtigal et al, 1998).

During male sexual differentiation, hormones produced by the fetal testes initiate and sustain normal male development, whereas absence of testicular hormones result in the female sexual differentiation. Normal male sexual differentiation involves gonadal development, stabilization of the wolffian (mesonephric) ducts with simultaneous regression of müllerian (paramesonephric) duct structures, and testicular descent into the scrotum. **The hormones that control embryonic male sexual differentiation include the testicular androgens, produced by the Leydig cells, and müllerian inhibiting substance (MIS), produced by the Sertoli cells. Androgens (testosterone, dihydroxytestosterone [DHT]) mediate the differentiation of the paired wolffian ducts into the seminal vesicles, epididymis, vas deferens, and ejaculatory ducts.** Masculinization of the external genitalia is under similar influence of the testicular androgens.

Gonadal development involves the differentiation of cells from four bipotential cell lineages: germ cells, supporting cells, steroidogenic cells, and connective tissue cells. Germ cells migrate to the gonadal ridge from the hindgut. Supporting cells differentiate into Sertoli cells and organize into testicular cords following expression of SRY. SRY is expressed in the pre-Sertoli cells within the fetal testis (Rossi et al, 1993). The protein product of the SRY gene is also present in both adult Sertoli cells and germ cells, and although the role of SRY in germ cell development is unclear at this time, it may play an important role in germ cell development or maintenance (Salas-Cortes et al, 1999). The steroidogenic cells differentiate into Leydig cells within the interstitium around the cords containing the Sertoli cells and primordial germ cells. By 10 weeks of gestation, the fetal testis is histologically distinguishable from the ovary.

Embryology

The embryologic origin of testicular development begins early in fetal life. Although chromosomal sex is determined at the time of fusion of the gametes by the presence or absence of the Y chromosome, male sexual differentiation does not begin until **testicular differentiation is initiated in the 7th week** of gestation by the SRY gene. At 4 to 6 weeks' gestation, the genital ridges organize. This is followed by migration of primordial germ cells (Wylie, 1993). Primordial germ cells, located along the caudal wall of the embryonic yolk sac near the allantoic stalk, begin migration by amoeboid movement to the genital ridges via the dorsal mesentery. At this stage, the gonadal primordium is indifferent and arises from a thickening of the coelomic epithelium between the root of the mesentery and the mesonephros. The segmented mesonephros extends along the posterior abdominal wall as a ridge from the lower cervical to the lumbar region. The coelomic epithelium develops epithelial cords (germinal cords) into the underlying mesenchyme to form the genital ridges. Chemotactic factors are produced by the thickened coelomic epithelium and attract the primordial germ cells.

Cells other than germ cells, including Sertoli cells, are derived from cells that migrated from the mesonephros. **By 7 weeks, primitive Sertoli cells have developed. Germ cells differentiate into gonocytes upon entering the testicular cords to become fetal spermatogonia by 15 weeks of gestation.** Gonocytes and Sertoli cells form testicular cords within the testis and canalize to form seminiferous tubules; however, a lumen will not be present within the tubule until puberty. **By the 8th week of gestation, Leydig cells have differentiated** around the testicular cords in the gonadal mesenchyme between the seminiferous tubules (Huhtaniemi et al, 1994). The testicular cords are separated from the coelomic epithelium by a well-vascularized connective tissue layer that later becomes the tunica albuginea. The rete testis forms at the ends of the testicular cords and converges at the hilus of the testis to connect to the efferent ductules that differentiate from the mesonephric tubules. The gonadal ridge rounds off into an oval organ.

During the 8th week, the fetal testis begins to secrete testosterone and MIS independent of pituitary hormonal regulation. This signals the stabilization and differentiation of the wolffian ducts and external genitalia. Fetal Leydig cells secrete testosterone, a paracrine hormone, which is converted by intercellular 5α-reductase in target tissues to DHT. DHT is responsible for inducing differentiation of the wolffian duct into the epididymis and vas deferens. Testosterone synthesis and secretion is regulated by maternal human chorionic gonadotropin (hCG) and peaks at 12 to 14 weeks of gestation. **MIS is secreted by the Sertoli cells and causes degeneration of the müllerian structures after the 8th week of gestation** (Lee and Donahue, 1993). MIS expression is detectable by week 7 and is limited to Sertoli cells only. MIS induces degeneration of basement membrane integrity of the epithelial and mesenchymal müllerian cells within the genital ridge (Catlin et al, 1993). The gene for MIS maps to chromosome 19p13.3 (Cohen-Haguenauer et al, 1987).

The gubernaculum appears at the 7th week of embryologic development as a condensation of mesenchymal tissue within the subserous fascia on either side of the vertebral column that extends from the gonad to the fascia between the developing external and internal oblique muscles. The cranial aspect of the gubernaculum envelops the cauda epididymis and lower pole tunica albuginea of the testis and extends caudally into the inguinal canal, where it maintains a firm attachment. This distal attachment has been shown experimentally to be important in the normal development of the processus vaginalis (Clarnette et al, 1996). Mechanical disruption of the gubernaculum resulted in lack of development of the processus vaginalis, but proximal gubernaculectomy had no effect on development of the processus vaginalis when the testis descended into the scrotum. Heyns (1987) demonstrated in dissections of fetuses of less than 23 weeks' gestation, before descent of the testis, that the gubernaculum does not extend beyond the external inguinal ring (Heyns, 1987). Controversy as to the caudal extent of gubernaculum attachment during development is especially relevant when considering the theoretical mechanisms of gubernacular function during testicular descent. **Many investigators have observed that the gubernaculum itself does not extend into the scrotum during fetal development** (Heyns, 1987). The gubernaculum is not firmly attached to the scrotum but is in continuum with the scrotum by mesenchymatous tissue that fills the scrotum.

Before descent, the testis lies atop the gubernaculum, which resembles a cylindrical, Wharton's jelly–like structure covered by peritoneum on all sides except posteriorly along the mesorchium, which is retroperitoneal. Histologically, the gubernaculum is composed of undifferentiated spindle-shaped cells with a large amount of extracellular material containing glycosaminoglycans (GAG). Just before testicular descent, the gubernaculum undergoes a significant increase in length as well as a rapid enlargement in gubernacular mass due to increased water uptake. The GAG fraction within the gubernaculum is probably responsible for the increase in water in the extracellular matrix (Heyns et al, 1990). Backhouse (1964) suggested that this may serve to dilate the inguinal canal to facilitate testicular passage. Gubernacular swelling coincides with lengthening of the testicular vasculature and vas deferens. The bulbous lower end of the gubernaculum loses its firm attachments to the inguinal canal after the testis descends through the canal. Therefore, it has been observed that **the gubernaculum has an important role in fixation of the testis to the inguinal canal before descent, but its role in descent of the testis through the canal and into the scrotum is less obvious and requires further analysis.**

As the cranial portion of the mesonephros involutes, a mesenchymatous ridge persists between the gonad and the diaphragm, which becomes part of the cranial gonadal mesentery (Backhouse, 1982a). Backhouse (1982a) considered this embryologic structure, the cranial suspensory ligament (CSL), to have an insignificant role in the mechanism of testicular descent, an observation that has been clinically correlated. The testes, like the ovaries, are initially located near the developing kidney positioned between the CSL and gubernaculum. The CSL in the male regresses while the gubernaculum proliferates during the transabdominal and transinguinal phases of descent. Evidence suggests that androgens mediate the regression of the CSL and possibly the transinguinal phase of descent, although the normal positioning of the ovaries in 46,XX individuals with prenatal androgen exposure demonstrates that regression of the CSL alone is insufficient to cause gonadal descent (Scott, 1987).

This is also the stage when the inguinal canal develops. Its role is to convey the testes to the developing scrotum. The developing trilaminar anterior abdominal wall musculature is present at 6 weeks' gestation. During the 8th week, the inguinal canal begins development as a caudal evagination of the abdominal wall that forms in conjunction with caudal elongation of the processus vaginalis. The processus vaginalis develops as a herniation of peritoneum at the deep inguinal ring and lies on the anterior aspect of the gubernaculum. The processus encounters the three layers of the abdominal wall via the large hiatus of the transversus abdominis muscle. The first layer is the transversalis fascia, which lies just deep to the transversus abdominis muscle at the deep inguinal ring. This eventration embryologically becomes the internal spermatic fascia of the spermatic cord. The next layer encountered, the internal oblique muscle, becomes the cremasteric muscle of the spermatic cord, although there is debate as to the origin of this layer (Backhouse, 1964). The cremasteric muscle extends along the developing processus vaginalis. The last layer is the external oblique muscle, which becomes the external spermatic fascia. The anatomic boundaries of the inguinal canal are the deep (internal) inguinal ring superiorly and the superficial (external) inguinal ring inferomedially. The canal itself is filled by mesenchyme, through which the genital branch of the genitofemoral nerve and ilioinguinal nerve pass (Backhouse, 1982a).

The external genitalia develop between the 8th and 16th weeks of gestation. Differentiation is induced by DHT, the active androgen converted from testosterone by 5α-reductase. The genital swellings contain undifferentiated mesenchyme and differentiate under androgenic stimulation into the scrotum. The testes at this time are intra-abdominal and develop never more than 1.3 mm from the internal ring (Hutson, 1986). **The testes lie dormant within the abdomen until about the 23rd week** of gestation, during which time the processus vaginalis continues its elongation into the scrotum. The testis, epididymis, and gubernaculum have been observed to descend en mass through the inguinal canal posterior to the patent processus vaginalis. Transinguinal transit of the testes is a rapid process that probably occurs within a period of several days (Scorer and Farrington, 1971; Backhouse, 1982b; Heyns, 1987; Sampaio and Favorito, 1998). Heyns (1987) found that 75% of testes passed through the inguinal canal between 24 and 28 weeks of gestation and only 2.6% of testes were present within the inguinal canal during the period of descent. His postmortem dissections of spontaneously aborted human fetuses showed that testicular descent had occurred in 10% at 24 weeks' gestation, in 50% at 27 weeks, in 75% at 28 weeks, and in 80% at 34 weeks to birth. This coincides with a 72% descent rate reported in fetuses weighing less than 1200 g or having a crown-rump length greater than 270 mm (Heyns, 1987). **Sampaio and Favorito (1998) observed, similarly, that before 23 weeks of gestation the majority of testes remained intra-abdominal, yet by 30 weeks all testes were descended into the scrotum.** Complete descent from the external ring to the bottom of the scrotum may take more than 3 to 4 weeks (Curling, 1843; Scorer and Farrington, 1971). Sampaio and Favorito (1998) reported that transinguinal migration occurred between 21 and 25 weeks after conception. In addition, testes remained undescended in fetuses weighing less than 990 g or having a crown-rump length of 245 mm or less, whereas all testes were descended in fetuses weighing more than 1220 g or having a crown-rump length greater than 275 mm. **These data support epidemiologic findings in newborn boys with cryptorchidism and suggest that fetal and birth weights are a significant determinant of descent in males after 30 weeks' gestation.**

THE UNDESCENDED TESTIS

Definition

The cause of cryptorchidism is multifactorial. The undescended testis can be located anywhere between the abdominal cavity and just outside the anatomic scrotum. Less commonly, the testis can also migrate to ectopic positions outside of the scrotum, not along the normal path of descent. *Cryptorchidism* is a term that has been used interchangeably with the term *undescended testis*. Both terms refer to an abnormally positioned testis, but cryptorchidism literally means "hidden testis." Therefore, undescended testis may be a more appropriate term, because most testes

that are not within the scrotum at birth are detectable by palpation. In order to fully appreciate the diversity of this congenital disorder, one must concede that this is not a single disease process with a common pathogenesis but a group of commonly recognized clinical abnormalities with multiple etiologies. Evidence for this is that cryptorchid testes exhibit a wide variation in phenotypic expression. Differences in the resting anatomic position of the testis, unilateral versus bilateral maldescent, paratesticular structural anomalies, intrinsic structural and hormonal abnormalities of the testis, and association with other congenital conditions (e.g., hypospadias) represent common variations of cryptorchidism. Clinical debate also exists concerning categorization of testes that are retractile, ectopic, or absent or have ascended to an abnormal location late in childhood, with respect to the comparative developmental and pathophysiologic origins of cryptorchidism. A large body of research and clinical observation has begun to answer important etiologic questions, but to date the exact mechanism of what is perhaps the most common congenital abnormality at birth in male children is unknown.

Incidence

Isolated cryptorchidism is one of the most common congenital anomalies at birth, affecting upward of 3% of full-term male newborns (Scorer and Farrington, 1971; John Radcliffe Hospital, 1992; Berkowitz et al, 1993; Thong et al, 1998). Unilateral cryptorchidism is more common than bilateral cryptorchidism, which occurs in 1.6% to 1.9% of boys. Testicular descent into the scrotum is usually complete by the second trimester; however, a significantly higher rate of cryptorchidism in premature boys suggests that the process of descent may not be complete until close to term. Scorer and Farrington (1971) reported a 30.3% incidence of undescended testes in premature infants. Many other studies have confirmed similar results in preterm male infants with less than 37 weeks of gestation and weighing less than 2500 g. Several large series have identified groups of newborns at risk for cryptorchidism to characterize the natural history and factors that affect postnatal descent. **These studies found that undescended testes are significantly more prevalent among preterm, small-for-gestational-age, low-birth-weight, and twin neonates.** The Cryptorchidism Study Group prospectively examined more than 7400 consecutive normal boys at birth and showed that the rate of cryptorchidism was 7.7%, 2.5%, and 1.41% at 3 months of age for babies weighing, respectively, less than 2000 g, between 2000 and 2499 g, and 2500 g or more (John Radcliffe Hospital, 1992).

Berkowitz and colleagues (1993) reported that the rate of cryptorchidism in 6935 newborn boys declined from 3.7% at birth to 1.0% by 3 months of age and remained essentially constant by 1 year of age. **Approximately 70% to 77% of cryptorchid testes will spontaneously descend, usually by 3 months of age.** Factors that predict complete spontaneous descent by 3 months of age include low birth weight, bilateral cryptorchidism, normal scrotal anatomy, and testis that are positioned lower along the normal path of descent; boys with a small or poorly rugated scrotum and those with hypospadias are more likely to be cryptorchid at 3 months (John Radcliffe Hospital, 1992). Other factors that may help determine late testicular descent include black or Hispanic ethnicity, a family history of cryptorchidism, low birth weight and preterm birth delivery, and cola consumption during pregnancy (Berkowitz and Lapinski, 1996). **By 1 year of age, the incidence of cryptorchidism declines to about 1% and remains constant throughout adulthood.**

Epidemiology

Establishing epidemiologic factors that affect the risk of undescended testes is made more difficult by the complex interactions among anatomy, heredity, hormonal milieu, and socioeconomic and environmental conditions. Nevertheless, the risk factors for the presence of an undescended testis at birth and by 1 year of age need to be considered. As described earlier, cryptorchidism is more common in premature and low-birth-weight male newborns. This includes boys born prematurely due to maternal, fetal, and unknown causes, intrauterine growth retardation, and twin gestation. **However, more accurate analysis of data leads to the conclusion that birth weight alone is the principal determinant of cryptorchidism at birth and at 1 year of life, independent of the length of gestation** (Hjertkvist et al, 1989; Mayr et al, 1999). Jones and associates (1998) found that gestational age was not an independent risk factor after adjusting for birth weight, as did Weidner and coworkers (1999), who found that the risk of cryptorchidism and hypospadias both increased with decreasing birth weight, independent of gestational age.

A study of 1002 Malaysian male newborns found that premature infants with an undescended testis were more likely than term newborns to demonstrate complete testicular descent (Thong et al, 1998). This implicates factors that result in low birth weight, such as intrauterine growth retardation and poor placental function, to be a more important risk factor for testicular maldescent. Neonates with congenital malformations, who often have low birth weight, are at increased risk for cryptorchidism. Other studies examining maternal causes of cryptorchidism have discovered a number of possible risk factors. Important factors common to all reports include pre-eclampsia, breech presentation of the fetus, delivery by cesarean section or complicated delivery, and a family history of cryptorchidism (Hjertkvist et al, 1989; Mori et al, 1992; Berkowitz and Lapinski, 1996; Jones et al, 1998; Akre et al, 1999; Mayr et al, 1999). This again implicates factors that may disrupt uteroplacental function, affecting fetal viability and development. Few studies have examined ethnicity; however, Asian descent may be a relative risk factor for the development of cryptorchidism (Berkowitz and Lapinski, 1996). Investigators have postulated a possible common genetic, hormonal, or environmental cause for cryptorchidism and hypospadias. Simultaneous presence of hypospadias and cryptorchidism has been shown to occur more commonly than would be predicted (Weidner et al, 1999). Czeizel and associates (1981) reported that the occurrence of undescended testes in families was 1.5% to 4.0% among

the fathers and 6.2% among the brothers of index patients with cryptorchidism, supporting a multifactorial pattern of inheritance. However, to date the molecular mechanism underlying cryptorchidism in humans remains unknown.

Classification

By definition, cryptorchidism is a developmental defect in which there is failure of the testis to descend into the scrotum. Although this is a useful general definition, there is considerable anatomic variation among cryptorchid testes. In addition, classification by anatomic position alone no doubt underestimates the variable anatomy, physiology, etiology, and natural history of the undescended testis and skews many published studies. Anatomic variation in testicular size and consistency, epididymal and vasal anomalies, and associated patent processus vaginalis or inguinal hernia should be taken into account. These factors reflect the dimorphic nature of male sexual differentiation and suggest that multiple etiologies may be responsible for the variations in phenotypic expression. Consideration of the normal embryologic sequence of testicular descent helps in understanding the possible ectopic positions the testis may attain when it fails to descend to an orthotopic intrascrotal position.

It is sometimes difficult to accurately classify the position, integrity, and presence of the undescended testis. Body habitus, testicular position, and compliance of the child during the examination can significantly complicate the clinical evaluation and account for diagnostic error. Classification systems can be useful in determining management and predicting outcome. Although there are a number of classification systems, Kaplan (1993) proposed the most popular system, which categorizes cryptorchid testes as either *palpable* or *nonpalpable*. The subjective nature of the physical examination confounds the accurate classification of testicular position; a more accurate assessment of occurs at the time of surgery. **Cryptorchid testicular position is most simply described as intra-abdominal, intracanalicular, extracanalicular (suprapubic or infrapubic), or ectopic.**

The *intra-abdominal testis* is usually located just inside the internal ring, commonly within a few centimeters, although intra-abdominal testes have been observed anywhere along a line between the lower pole of the kidney and the internal ring. Testes may also lie at a high annular position at the internal ring. These testes have been referred to as "peeping," because they can move between the abdominal cavity and inguinal canal. Rarely, a testis is found in ectopic intra-abdominal positions such as in the perihepatic and perisplenic regions. The *intracanalicular testis* is occasionally difficult to palpate and by definition lies within the inguinal canal, between the internal and external ring. The emergent or *suprapubic testis* lies just beyond the external ring, above the level of pubic symphysis, and the *infrapubic testis* lies just below the pubic symphysis, often just outside the anatomic scrotum in the retroscrotal space. The testis may also be located in an ectopic position. The *ectopic testis* completes normal transinguinal migration but is misdirected outside the normal path of descent below the external ring. **The most common ectopic location is within a superficial pouch between external oblique fascia and Scarpa's fascia, which has been termed the Denis-Browne pouch. Other abnormal locations include transverse scrotal, femoral, perineal, and prepenile ectopia.** Theories of descent do not include adequate data, either observational or experimental, to explain testicular ectopia, and presently the mechanism of pathologic descent is unknown. Studies of human fetuses by both Backhouse in 1981 and Heyns in 1987 did not support the finding of multiple distal attachments of the gubernaculum, originally credited to Lockwood in 1888 to account for testicular ectopia (Heyns, 1987).

The terms "nonpalpable testis" and "retractile testis" are ubiquitous. These terms deserve further definition and incorporation into this discussion because they may confound the accurate classification of cryptorchidism. **The term "nonpalpable testis" implies that the testis cannot be detected on physical examination and therefore is either intra-abdominal, absent (vanishing), atrophic, or missed on physical examination.** A vanishing or absent testis is usually encountered during exploration for a nonpalpable testis. The anatomic hallmark of the vanishing testis is blind-ending spermatic vessels that are found just proximal to the internal inguinal ring. An atrophic testis is a smaller than normal testis that may be cryptorchid. These testes can be encountered anywhere along the course of normal descent from within the abdomen to the scrotum.

The "retractile testis" is withdrawn out of the scrotum by an active cremasteric reflex but can easily be brought down into an orthotopic position within the scrotum and remains there after traction has been released. The retractile testis can be found anywhere along the course of descent, but it is usually palpable in the groin. Retractile testes most commonly present clinically between the ages of 3 and 7 years of age. The retractability of the testes is caused by an overactive cremasteric reflex. A cremasteric reflex, initiated by stroking the skin of the inner aspect of the thigh, is present in about 50% of boys younger than 30 months and in most boys older than 30 months of age (Caesar and Kaplan, 1994). If a testis can be milked down to the bottom of the scrotum, it is probably retractile and does not require therapy (Wyllie, 1984). However, there is debate as to whether retractile testes are a subtle variant of their undescended counterpart. The retractile testis is truly not cryptorchid, although an uncommon phenomenon of delayed spontaneous testicular ascent has been perhaps falsely ascribed to the retractile testis. In cases of ascent, boys previously documented to have normally descended testes are found later in childhood to be cryptorchid. Ascent likely represents an undescended testis that is almost completely descended. Rabinowitz and Hulbert (1997) observed that the etiology of this condition is a missed diagnosis at a younger age. The testis usually is located in a superficial inguinal pouch and declares itself undescended with somatic growth. Therefore, children with retractile testes should be monitored regularly at least until puberty, until the testes are no longer retractile and remain intrascrotal. This phenomenon was noted by Scorer and Farrington (1971) and other investigators, who reported a higher incidence of cryptorchidism in 5-year-old boys than

in younger children. Although Puri and Nixon (1977) reported that children with retractile testes have normal testicular volume and a normal fertility rate in adulthood, testicular development has been reported to be abnormal in both retractile testes and ascending testes, with histology similar to that of undescended testes (Ito et al, 1986; Saito and Kumamoto, 1989; Han et al, 1999).

Testicular Maldescent

Theories of Descent and Maldescent

The past two centuries have resulted in theories of testicular descent and maldescent that remain controversial, because they are mired in myth, misconceptions, and misinterpretation of previous data. As yet, there is no unified (universally agreed upon) theory of descent, but important pieces of the puzzle have been postulated based on careful anatomic and embryologic observations. Testicular descent and maldescent are now being explored on a molecular level, but most of our current understanding is based on observation. John Hunter, an English anatomist, published the first important and highly accurate description of testicular descent in 1762. He is credited with describing and naming the gubernaculum, which is derived from the Latin word meaning *helm* or *rudder*. Hunter also recognized the importance of this structure with regard to testicular descent but was cautious in postulating its function (Backhouse, 1982a). Since that time, many theories have been proposed involving the effect of intra-abdominal pressure, gravity, cremasteric muscle contraction, endocrine factors, and structures unique to the male fetus—however, none more important than the gubernaculum. The popular theories of descent are presented in this section to underscore the diversity and complexity of this condition.

In order for normal spermatogenesis to occur, it is necessary for the testes to descend into the scrotum, a specialized, low-temperature environment that maintains a temperature 2° to 3°F lower than core body temperature. Under normal embryologic conditions in humans, the fetal testis begins its multistaged descent into the scrotum from the position of origin, the abdominal cavity. Gier and Marion (1969) proposed three phases of testicular descent in the human fetus: (1) nephric displacement by degeneration of the mesonephros at 7 to 8 weeks' gestation, (2) transabdominal passage of the testis from the metanephros to the inguinal ring by 21 weeks, and (3) inguinal transit of the testis from the peritoneal cavity to along the processus vaginalis at 28 weeks. **Conceptually, testicular descent is best illustrated in three phases: (1) transabdominal, (2) transinguinal, and (3) extracanalicular migration (descent from the external ring to the scrotum).**

To briefly review, transabdominal descent of the testis toward the internal ring results from differential growth of the lumbar vertebral column and pelvis. The testis is adjacent to the kidney by the 8th week of gestation, and further migration does not begin until about the 23rd week. The intra-abdominal position of the testis before transinguinal descent is just inside the internal ring. The rapid transinguinal phase of descent requires the testis to travel through the inguinal canal alongside and posterior to the processus vaginalis into the scrotum. The final phase of descent, from the external ring to the scrotum, occurs after 28 weeks; in most cases testicular descent is complete between the 30th and 32nd week. Many investigators agree with this basic outline and time course, but controversy exists as to the mechanism of descent after 23 weeks of gestation until the testis is intrascrotal, because most theories are extrapolated from static observation of fetal human dissections. Animal models have not provided a satisfactory comparison to human testicular descent. Most theories of testicular descent are concentrated on development of the gubernaculum, processus vaginalis, inguinal canal, spermatic vessels, and scrotum because the analogous structures in the female fetus are substantially different, and the gubernaculum truly has no analog in the female (Heyns and Hutson, 1995).

Endocrine Factors

A normal hypothalamic-pituitary-gonadal axis is usually a necessary prerequisite for testicular descent to occur (Toppari and Kaleva, 1999). Defects may occur in gonadotropin production, androgen biosynthesis, or androgen action. The primary hormones that regulate the testes are luteinizing hormone (LH) and follicle-stimulating hormone (FSH). Both hormones are secreted by the basophilic cells in the anterior pituitary. The primary site of action of FSH is on the epithelium of the seminiferous tubule. Gonadotropin regulation is under the control of luteinizing hormone–releasing hormone (LHRH) stimulation from the hypothalamus, which interacts with high-affinity cell surface receptor sites on the plasma membrane of pituitary gonadotrophs. Plasma FSH levels are often elevated in patients with testicular pathology, including patients with cryptorchidism. FSH stimulates Sertoli cells and therefore has an important role in spermatogenesis. Plasma FSH levels usually correlate inversely with spermatogenesis, and therefore FSH is considered the most clinically useful endocrine marker in the evaluation of infertile men. However, in children, circulating FSH, LH, and testosterone levels may not accurately reflect testicular development or the presence of testicular pathology.

ANDROGENS

The androgens testosterone and DHT are necessary for testicular descent to occur. They may act either directly or indirectly, such as in the neuroendocrine modulation of the genitofemoral nerve and release of calcitonin gene-related peptide (CGRP), as proposed by Hutson and associates in 1994. Clinical examples supporting this theory include patients with androgen insensitivity syndrome (AIS) and hypogonadotropic hypogonadism who have bilateral cryptorchidism. In the majority of humans with AIS, the testes are located in close proximity to the inguinal canal, indicating that transabdominal descent has not been effected (Ahmed et al, 2000). The testes were palpable in the labioscrotal folds or the inguinal region in 77% and 41% of cases of complete AIS and partial AIS, respectively. In addition,

transabdominal descent occurs normally in mice with androgen insensitivity (Hutson, 1986). Prenatal exposure to an anti-androgen, flutamide, did not interfere with transabdominal descent in rats (Shono et al, 1994).

From these data it can be surmised that androgens do not mediate the first phase of testicular descent. However, androgens appear to be important for the inguinal-scrotal phase of testicular descent. Failure of gubernacular involution has been observed in humans with AIS (Hutson, 1986). In animal models, delayed gubernacular migration and regression are described in gonadotropin deficiency associated with low testosterone concentrations and in AIS. Additional support for androgen action is the presence of androgen binding by the gubernaculum in rodent models. Evidence indicating that androgens mediate CSL regression includes (1) persistence of CSL in humans with AIS and (2) persistence of CSL in animal models with prenatal anti-androgen exposure (Hutson, 1986; Shono et al, 1994). **Therefore, impaired androgen biosynthesis or action can impede the second phase of testicular descent.**

Analysis of the androgen receptor in DNA samples obtained from 21 boys with isolated unilateral or bilateral cryptorchidism identified no abnormalities (Wiener et al, 1998). However, exon 1 was not evaluated, and it contains a polymorphic CAG trinucleotide repeat expansion. Longer repeats are associated with decreased androgen action, manifested as an increased incidence of oligozoospermia or azoospermia in otherwise normal men (Tut et al, 1997, Dowsing et al, 1999). Undervirilized 46,XY patients have been found to have longer CAG repeats, suggesting that this locus functions as a modifier locus (Lim et al, 2000). Therefore, variations in the trinucleotide repeat in exon 1 of the androgen receptor may have a role in cryptorchidism.

In utero testosterone deficiency can be caused by decreased LH, by impaired function of the gonadotropin-releasing hormone (GnRH) or LH receptors, or by loss of function mutations in the proteins involved in testosterone biosynthesis. Complete loss of function mutations are associated with sex reversal in 46,XY fetuses and with variable testicular location. The spectrum of testicular location includes intra-abdominal position to labia majora. Experimental evidence links gonadotropin deficiency and cryptorchidism. Although a small penis is a common clinical finding in boys with gonadotropin deficiency, cryptorchidism does occur (Van Dop et al, 1987). Hypogonadotropic hypogonadism due to mutations in KAL, DAX1, and the GnRH receptor genes are monogenic disorders associated with gonadotropin deficiency in which cryptorchidism has been described as one of the clinical features (Habiby et al, 1996; Pralong et al, 1999). Because anosmia occurs infrequently in the majority of patients with cryptorchidism, KAL mutations are probably an extremely rare cause of isolated cryptorchidism. Deletion of the GnRH gene in GnRH[hpg] mice often results in intra-abdominal testes (Mason et al, 1986). Mutations in the GnRH receptor (GNRHR) gene are associated with autosomal recessive hypogonadotropic hypogonadism (de Roux et al, 1997; Layman et al, 1998). Abnormalities of the LH receptor show a theoretical possibility of affecting testicular descent. Two variants of the LHβ gene have been described that show an increased clearance rate from serum, although the relationship to cryptorchidism has not been evaluated (Furui et al, 1994; Suganuma et al, 1996). A mutation in the LHβ gene has been shown to impair the ability of LH to bind to its receptor and is associated with impaired steroidogenesis and infertility in heterozygotic carriers that results in delayed puberty, oligospermia, and Leydig cell hypoplasia (Weiss et al, 1992). Cryptorchidism has been described in association with Leydig cell hypoplasia, an autosomal recessive disorder characterized by impaired Leydig cell differentiation secondary to loss of function mutations in the LH receptor gene (LHR) (Martinez-Mora et al, 1991; Kremer et al, 1995; Wu et al, 1998).

Errors in testosterone biosynthesis have also been associated with cryptorchidism. The specific enzyme genes include 17α-hydroxylase/17,20-lyase (CYP17), 3β-hydroxysteroid dehydrogenase type 2 (HSD3B2), and 17β-hydroxysteroid dehydrogenase type 3 (HSD17B3). Children with complete **CYP17 deficiency** are usually assigned to female gender at birth and present in adolescence with delayed puberty. Affected 46,XY individuals can have intra-abdominal testes or genital ambiguity with undescended testes (Biason et al, 1991; Lin et al, 1991; Geller et al, 1997). **β-Hydroxysteroid dehydrogenase type 2 deficiency** is a rare cause of congenital adrenal hyperplasia in which the affected 46,XY fetus is undervirilized due to mutations in HSD3B2 (Kenny et al, 1971; Rheaume et al, 1992). Whereas hypospadias is typical, testicular position is variable (Rheaume et al, 1994). Affected 46,XY individuals with **17β-hydroxysteroid dehydrogenase type 3 deficiency** demonstrate a female phenotype or ambiguous genitalia at birth, with undescended testes (Gross et al, 1986). Testicular conversion of androstenedione to testosterone is affected, and these individuals often present in adolescence with virilization and primary amenorrhea (Geissler et al, 1994; Andersson et al, 1996; Park et al, 1996). The clinical spectrum of **5α-reductase type 2 (SRD5A2) deficiency** ranges from female phenotype to hypospadias. Testicular position is variable and ranges from intra-abdominal to labial-scrotal (Imperato-McGinley et al, 1991; Nordenskjold and Ivarsson, 1998).

MÜLLERIAN INHIBITING SUBSTANCE

MIS is secreted by the fetal Sertoli cells and is responsible for regression of the müllerian ducts. MIS has also been implicated in effecting testicular descent. MIS levels normally surge in the first year of life, peak at 4 to 12 months, and subsequently decline with age. **Yamanaka and colleagues (1991) reported that patients with cryptorchidism do not demonstrate a surge in the first year of life, and mean MIS serum concentrations in cryptorchid boys are significantly lower than in controls.** There was also a significant reduction of the mean MIS level in children with bilateral cryptorchidism compared with those with unilateral undescended testis. However, the authors concede that the difference in MIS levels may have resulted from secondary intrinsic Sertoli cell dysfunction, rather than being a consequence of cryptorchidism.

MIS has been further investigated as a factor mediating testicular descent, because cryptorchidism is a common presenting feature of persistent müllerian duct syndrome (PMDS) (Hutson and Donahoe, 1986). PMDS is characterized by normal male differentiation with failure of regression of müllerian duct derivatives secondary to mutations in the MIS or MIS II receptor gene (Knebelmann et al, 1991; Josso et al, 1993; Imbeaud et al, 1996). However, it is more likely that anatomic obstruction is the cause of cryptorchidism associated with PMDS, because the testes are tethered to the intra-abdominal müllerian duct derivatives. Therefore, the weight of evidence suggests that MIS does not play a significant role in the regulation of testicular descent, based on the following: (1) normal testicular descent occurs in MIS-deficient knock-out mice (Behringer et al, 1994); (2) normal testicular descent occurs in fetal rabbits immunized against bovine MIS (Tran et al, 1986); (3) ovarian descent is not observed in transgenic female mice overexpressing MIS (Behringer et al, 1994); and (4) the majority of patients with intra-abdominal testes do not have retained müllerian derivatives.

ESTROGEN

Estrogens have been postulated to impair testicular descent. Prenatal treatment with diethylstilbesterol (DES), a nonsteroidal synthetic estrogen, is associated with urogenital abnormalities of both male and female fetuses. Undescended testes is one of the abnormalities observed in 46,XY fetuses (Stillman, 1982). Animal studies on mice confirmed that prenatal estrogen exposure disrupts the transabdominal phase of testicular descent (McLachlan et al, 1975; Shono et al, 1994). Estrogens are thought to impair gubernacular development and to cause persistence of müllerian duct derivatives. Testicular position was noted to be similar in Insl3 knock-out animals and in DES-exposed normal animals. To determine the relationship between prenatal estrogen exposure and Insl3 expression, experimental evidence determined that prenatal DES exposure was associated with decreased testicular Insl3 expression in mice. However, no change in SF1 expression was noted in DES-treated animals (Emmen et al, 2000). In a different animal model, testicular expression of SF1 was decreased by prenatal DES exposure (Majdic et al, 1997). Prenatal testosterone treatment does not correct cryptorchidism induced by prenatal estrogen exposure, indicating independent mechanisms of action (Hutson and Watts, 1990).

Skakkebaek and colleagues maintained that the frequency of cryptorchidism and poor semen quality is increasing and speculated that this was occurring because of greater exposure to endocrine disruptors in the environment (Toppari and Shakkebaek, 1998). Evidence cited against their hypothesis included the absence of differences in maternal estrogen concentrations during pregnancy between woman who had sons with cryptorchidism and controls (Key et al, 1996). However, because the maternal circulation is far removed from local fetal hormone concentrations, maternal estrogen concentrations may not be valid measures of fetal estrogen exposure.

DESCENDIN

Conflicting views on the role of androgen stimulation and gubernacular development resulted in the concept of an androgen-independent factor, descendin, a gubernacular specific growth factor. Hosie and associates (1999) demonstrated a direct androgen stimulation of the human gubernaculum testis via specific intranuclear hormone receptor binding, implicating its role in gubernacular swelling through an increase in glycosaminoglycans. Quality and quantity of androgen receptors would therefore theoretically influence the extent of transinguinal testicular descent. However, evidence suggests that gubernacular development is not completely androgen dependent. In dogs, fetal orchiectomy prevented gubernacular swelling and regression but was not completely resuscitated by testosterone supplementation (Baumans et al, 1982, 1983). Gubernacular regression was not completely prevented by fetal supplementation of testosterone, and some descent of the remaining epididymis occurred. On the other hand, dogs orchidectomized neonatally and supplemented with an autotransplant of testicular tissue demonstrated normal gubernacular development and epididymal descent. Cryptorchidism induced by the antiandrogen flutamide was also shown to specifically inhibit only gubernacular regression (McMahon et al, 1995). Furthermore, normal gubernacular development was observed to occur in the presence of complete testicular feminization (Hutson and Donahoe, 1986). Indirect evidence that growth of the gubernaculum during descent is not the result of androgen stimulation supports the existence of an androgen-independent factor (Hens and Pape, 1991). Testicular descent was examined in a fetal porcine model, and it was demonstrated that, during the first phase of testicular descent, a bioactive, low-molecular-weight factor is present that stimulates gubernacular cell growth (Fentener van Vlissingen et al, 1988). This paracrine factor, descendin, is believed to be secreted from the testis in an androgen-independent fashion and to be responsible for changes in the first phase of gubernaculum development, which is characterized by rapid cell proliferation (outgrowth) and concomitant synthesis of sulfated glycosaminoglycans, hyaluronic acid, and collagen (Fentener van Vlissingen, 1989).

Gubernaculum

The singular importance of the gubernaculum in testicular descent cannot be underestimated; however, its exact physiologic mechanism is of considerable debate and study. There are many theories as to the function of the gubernaculum. These include the gubernaculum as a guide into the scrotum, the gubernaculum as a wedge that swells and dilates the inguinal passage of the testis, and various theories espousing gubernacular contraction, involution, traction, and stationary fixation in combination with differential somatic growth. Heyns (1987) defined the primary differences between the countervailing theories of gubernaculum-mediated testicular descent in relation to three points: (1) the cranial and caudal attachments, (2) the type of cell forming its "active" constituent, and (3) gubernacular morphogenesis relative to inguinal-scrotal development during testicular descent. All evidence implicates the gubernaculum as the major factor responsible for testicular descent.

Research from many species has simultaneously advanced and muddled our understanding of testicular descent; nonetheless, several key mechanistic properties of the gubernaculum have been established. The earliest theo-

ries were based on preconceived notions of testicular descent and suggested that the testis was pulled into the scrotum by the gubernaculum. However, there is substantial evidence indicating that there is no firm scrotal attachment of the gubernaculum to the scrotum (Wensing, 1968, 1988; Scorer and Farrington, 1971; Heyns, 1987; Hutson et al, 1997). **Consequently, the testis cannot be pulled *into* the scrotum.** The gubernaculum is anchored near the future inguinal canal and stabilizes the testis near the groin while the kidney migrates to a cranial position. The processus vaginalis allows the previously intra-abdominal testis to migrate from the abdominal cavity (Heyns, 1995). Once the testis has passed through the inguinal canal and descent is complete, the bulb of the gubernaculum is resorbed (Backhouse, 1966). Clinical and experimental data indicate that hormones, transcription factors, and possibly neural factors influence development. At present, it appears that testicular descent is a complex event mediated by both hormonal and mechanical factors.

Genitofemoral Nerve and Calcitonin Gene-Related Peptide

Hutson first presented data suggesting that the genitofemoral nerve (GFN) induces testicular descent and gubernacular differentiation. Transection of the GFN in rats resulted in the testes' remaining in the abdomen and prevented gubernacular migration (Beasley and Hutson, 1987; Fallat et al, 1992). This concept is based on evidence that androgens increase the number of GFN cell bodies and promote gubernacular migration, which is mediated by calcitonin gene-related peptide (CGRP) (Hutson and Beasley, 1987). CGRP has been identified as a neurotransmitter in the GFN and its nerve branches (Larkins et al, 1991). Gubernacula in vivo showed rhythmic contractility and demonstrated a high degree of motility during testicular descent (Park and Hutson, 1991). This theory is supported by evidence that the androgen receptor is present in the lumbar spinal cord near the cremaster nucleus before the onset of maximal androgenic action (Cain et al, 1994).

GFN morphology has been shown to be altered by reduction of motoneuron number and neural diameter in association with flutamide-induced cryptorchidism (Husmann et al, 1994). Prenatal androgen blockade with flutamide has been shown to inhibit masculinization of the GFN, with significant reduction of its CGRP content (Goh et al, 1994). These findings support the hypothesis that androgens directly regulate the development and morphology of the sexually dimorphic GFN during testicular descent and that CGRP acts as a second messenger. However, a number of studies present evidence to the contrary of this hypothesis, including the observation that CGRP release is increased by androgen withdrawal and that the cremaster nucleus may not be androgen dependent (Popper and Micevych, 1989; Barthold et al, 1994, 1996). CGRP also fails to induce murine testicular descent (Houle and Gagne, 1995). Additionally, CGRP is a neuromuscular transmitter that has been demonstrated to act on the muscular component of the rodent's developing gubernaculum, which is primarily cremasteric muscle (Husmann and Levy, 1995). The human gubernaculum lacks a muscular component;

this fact most likely excludes CGRP from playing a significant role in human testicular descent (Heyns, 1987).

Epididymis

The theoretical association uniting normal testicular descent to epididymal function is based on the observation that epididymal abnormalities often accompany cryptorchidism. The difficulty arises in that it is unknown whether epididymal anomalies are the cause or the result of the undescended testis. The concept that normal testicular descent depends on the epididymis is challenged by the demonstration that either elimination of the epididymis or epididymal agenesis does not impede testicular descent (Frey and Rajfer, 1982; Baikie and Hutson, 1990). Many of the theories related to epididymal anomalies link the causative theories of cryptorchidism, and it stands to reason that the same factors are responsible for both cryptorchidism and fusion anomalies of the epididymis (Merksz, 1998). Most theories suggest that fetal androgen deficiency plays an important role in this association.

Embryologically, the epididymis is in direct contact with the gubernaculum and precedes the testis into the scrotum. It has been suggested that abnormal embryologic attachment of the cranial gubernaculum may account for abnormalities evidenced in the mode of descent of adjacent paratesticular structures (Abe et al, 1996). Epididymal anomalies are encountered in undescended testes (including ectopic testes), hernias, and hydroceles. Epididymal abnormalities were found to be more common in undescended testes (41%) than in the ectopic testes (25.9%) (Kucukaydin et al, 1998). One large series of 652 cases of cryptorchidism reported that epididymal and vasal anomalies occurred with an overall frequency of 36% (Mollaeian et al, 1994). **Koff reported similar findings but found a much higher incidence of complex epididymal abnormalities in cryptorchidism, approaching 90%** (Koff and Scaletscky, 1990). Thirty-nine percent of ectopic testes displayed more severe epididymal abnormalities, whereas 33% showed only an elongated epididymis and 29% were normal. The higher the arrest of testicular descent, the more grossly abnormal the associated ductal system (Gill et al, 1989). Epididymal anomalies associated with cryptorchidism also include a significantly higher incidence of patent processus vaginalis. Barthold and Redman (1996) found that epididymal anomalies were more frequent in association with undescended rather than descended testes (72% versus 34%, respectively), with a greater frequency depending on the extent of patency of the processus vaginalis. A closed, partially closed, or open processus vaginalis was associated with an abnormal epididymis in 14%, 36%, and 69% of cases, respectively.

Elder (1992a) concluded that most epididymal abnormalities probably do not contribute to testicular maldescent by comparing epididymal abnormalities in descended testes. Excluding intra-abdominal testes, 50% of boys with a hydrocele or hernia had an epididymal abnormality if the processus was patent and communicated with the testis, compared with only 10% if no communication was present. Among those children with an undescended testis, 71% had an epididymal abnormality if there was a patent processus, versus 16% without a patent processus.

Epididymal abnormalities range from minor structural findings, such as elongation, to more complex anatomic aberrations of fusion, to complete disjunction, to an absent structure altogether. **Perhaps the most salient point concerning this association as it relates to future fertility is that, despite early surgical treatment of children with cryptorchidism to preserve normal germ cell development, fusion anomalies commonly exist that ultimately must affect sperm maturation and transport** (Mollaeian et al, 1994). **In addition, biopsy of the testes with severe anomalies of ductal fusion showed preservation of germ cells in 69% and diminished germ cells in 31%** (Gill et al, 1989). **Therefore, prognostic indicators of future fertility should consider the epididymal anomalies detected at the time of surgery, because such anomalies might coexist with excellent testis histology.**

Intra-abdominal Pressure

Conditions that result in cryptorchidism hypothetically associated with decreased intra-abdominal pressure include prune-belly syndrome, cloacal exstrophy, omphalocele, gastroschisis, and a number of syndromes that include both cryptorchidism and congenital abdominal wall muscular defects or agenesis (Levard and Laberge, 1997; Koivusalo et al, 1998). Abdominal pressure probably has an ancillary role in migration of the testis from the abdominal cavity to the inguinal canal, but thereafter it plays a more significant role in transinguinal descent into the scrotum (Quinlan et al, 1988; Attah and Hutson, 1993; Hutson et al, 1997). The patent processus vaginalis probably works in conjunction with intra-abdominal pressure, which is transmitted to the testis during transinguinal migration. Androgens may also play a role in combination with abdominal pressure at this stage of development to deliver the testis into the scrotum (Frey et al, 1983; Frey and Rajfer, 1984; Hadziselimovic et al, 1987a). Frey demonstrated experimentally that in the presence of androgen a silicone prosthesis will descend from the abdominal cavity into the scrotum, but this occurs less frequently when androgen is removed (Frey et al, 1983; Frey and Rajfer, 1984).

Histopathology

Normal germ cell development during childhood is a continuous process that is completed at puberty (Hadziselimovic et al, 1987b). The concept that a testis was more likely to be histologically abnormal the longer it remains cryptorchid was proposed by Cooper in 1929. Undescended testes demonstrate more pronounced impairment of germ cell development the higher the testes are located, although newborns with intra-abdominal testes have a normal number of germ cells (Hadziselimovic et al, 1987b). **The histopathologic hallmarks associated with cryptorchidism are evident between 1 and 2 years of age and include decreased numbers of Leydig cells, degeneration of Sertoli cells, delayed disappearance of gonocytes, delayed appearance of adult dark (Ad) spermatogonia, failure of primary spermatocytes to develop, and reduced total germ cell counts** (Huff et al, 1987, 1993; Rune et al, 1992). **A decrease in cryptorchid testis volume by 6**

months of age has been reported (Cendron et al, 1993). **The earliest postnatal histologic abnormality in cryptorchid testes was hypoplasia of the Leydig cells, which was observed from the first month of life** (Huff et al, 1991). Minenberg and colleagues (1982) reported peritubular fibrosis by 1 year of age in undescended testes. Huff and associates (1989) documented significantly defective maturation of gonocytes in bilateral testicular biopsies of unilaterally cryptorchid boys aged 1 to 13 years, as well as decreased numbers of germ cells from the first year of life. Specifically, transformation of gonocytes to Ad spermatogonia, which normally is complete at age 6 months, and transformation of Ad spermatogonia to primary spermatocytes, which normally initiates at age 3 years, were delayed or defective or both. Total germ cell count was similar to normal controls until the seventh month of age, when secondary degeneration of untransformed gonocytes led to a decrease in the total germ cell count (Huff et al, 1991). Numbers of Leydig cells were also abnormally decreased. Similar pathology was observed in the contralateral descended testis, although to a lesser extent, which supports the theory of hypogonadotropic hypogonadism as the possible cause of the increased incidence of infertility seen in males with unilateral cryptorchidism (Huff et al, 1989, 1993). McAleer and coworkers (1995) reported similar abnormalities in the undescended and descended testes of boys with unilateral cryptorchidism; no significant differences were seen in fertility index in children before 1 year of age, but there were significant differences in all other age groups. Hadziselimovic and colleagues (1987c) showed a positive correlation between the number of germ cells in prepubertal testes and sperm count after puberty. A continuous process of Sertoli cell degeneration is also evident from 1 year of age in undescended testis; it is not related to age but depends on testicular position (Rune et al, 1992). Sertoli cell degeneration may help account for the reduction in germ cell number.

These reports all demonstrate early histopathologic evidence of abnormal spermatogenesis in boys well before 2 years of age that is probably related, in part, to deficient hormonal stimulation. Other parameters that provide evidence of testicular injury include the physical examination and the appearance of the testis at the time of orchiopexy. Circulating concentrations of gonadotropins and gonadal hormones correlate with testicular dysfunction in adults; however, because of the relative quiescence of the pituitary during infancy and early childhood, these hormones do not provide an accurate indirect measurement of testicular maturation and pathology in young boys.

Consequences of Cryptorchidism

Infertility

Impairment of germ cell maturation is a well-recognized consequence of cryptorchidism. A tenet of treatment is that early surgical repositioning of the testis into the scrotum before the onset of histopathologic changes reduces the risk of subfertility. However, there is increasing evidence to suggest that orchiopexy does not significantly reduce this risk. Initial reports focused on histologic changes that were seen in undescended testes after 1 year of age as a rationale for early surgical treatment to preserve spermatogenic function. McAleer and coworkers (1995) reported that no significant difference in the fertility index was seen in patients 1 year old or younger when comparing undescended to descended testes, but fertility index differences were significantly abnormal in all other age groups. However, fertility index measurements were significantly decreased from normal expected values in all age groups with unilateral cryptorchidism, which suggests that potential fertility may be significantly impaired regardless of patient age at the time of surgery. One study conducted after orchiopexy noted severe changes in histomorphologic characteristics of the testicular tissue if surgery was performed after 5 years of age (Tzvetkova and Tavetkov, 1996).

Grasso and associates (1991) assessed the fertility of 91 patients with unilateral cryptorchidism who underwent postpubertal orchiopexy and found that 83.5% of patients were azoospermic or oligospermic, with or without asthenospermia. Another study concluded that in postpubertal males presenting with unilateral cryptorchidism, the undescended testis should be removed because of the risk of future malignancy, because the majority of testes cannot contribute to fertility (only 1 of 52 orchiectomy specimens showed normal spermatogenesis), and because of the risk of torsion (Rogers et al, 1998). Two patients (4%) had carcinoma in situ of the testicle. Fifteen percent of men treated for unilateral cryptorchidism between 4 and 14 years of age were found to be azoospermic, and an additional 30% were oligospermic (sperm count less than 20×10^6/mL). Untreated men with unilateral cryptorchidism had very similar spermiograms. No untreated, bilaterally cryptorchid patient had normal fertility, whereas a quarter of those who were treated achieved normal fertility (Chilvers et al, 1986). Experimental evidence has demonstrated that early orchiopexy can reverse the histologic changes in cryptorchid testes (Lugg et al, 1996). These data provide support to the value of orchiopexy in the treatment of cryptorchidism.

Lee (1993) postulated that paternity would be a better index for verification than sperm count, since it is known that men with subnormal sperm counts can have normal paternity rates. **Compared with a control group, paternity was significantly compromised in men with previous bilateral, but not unilateral, cryptorchidism (53% versus 75%, respectively)** (Lee et al, 1995). It was also demonstrated that paternity was not correlated with age at orchiopexy. In another study, 87% of men with unilateral undescended testes demonstrated paternity, whereas only 33% of men with bilateral undescended testes fathered children (Cendron et al, 1989). Higher FSH levels and lower sperm counts were shown to correlate inversely, both in formerly unilaterally cryptorchid men compared with controls and in the subset of men who reported unsuccessful attempts at paternity compared with those reporting paternity; LH, testosterone, and other results of semen analysis did not differ (Lee et al, 1998). Therefore, increased FSH and low sperm count may be weighed as risks for infertility in formerly cryptorchid men. Other risk factors include the placement of a parenchymal testicular suture at the time of orchiopexy (Bellinger et al, 1989; Coughlin et al, 1998).

Neoplasia

It is a well-established fact that children born with undescended testes are at increased risk for testicular malignancy. Testis tumors usually develop during puberty and thereafter, although there are reports of tumor development before 10 years of age. Approximately 10% of testicular tumors arise from an undescended testis (Whitaker, 1970; Abratt et al, 1992). **The incidence of a testicular tumor in the general population is 1 in 100,000, and the incidence of a germ cell tumor in men formally cryptorchid is 1 in 2550; therefore, the relative risk is approximately 40 times greater** (Farrer et al, 1985). It is controversial whether orchiopexy affects the natural history of development of a testicular tumor, although there is emerging evidence to support the claim that prepubescent orchiopexy may lessen the risk. An indication for orchiopexy is to allow for a more thorough examination of the testis that would theoretically allow for earlier detection of malignant degeneration.

Uncorrected cryptorchidism is now rarely seen in the West, but 14% of adult patients from New Delhi, India, with primary germ cell tumors of testis were found to have cryptorchidism (Raina et al, 1995). The United Kingdom Testicular Cancer Study Group (1994a, 1994b) found a significant association of testicular cancer with undescended testis and inguinal hernia. However, the risk associated with undescended testis was eliminated in men who had had an orchiopexy before 10 years of age and therefore it was concluded that the trend to perform orchiopexy at younger ages may reduce the associated risk of testicular malignancy. The study also found that the increased risk of tumor formation was associated with early age at puberty and low amounts of exercise. These findings may be related to effects of exposure to endogenous hormones and may partly contribute to the increasing rates of testicular cancer observed in the past few decades (United Kingdom Testicular Cancer Study Group, 1994a).

Moller and associates (1996) reported on a large cohort of men in Denmark and observed the relative risk (RR) of testicular cancer in men with treated or persisting cryptorchidism to be 3.6 (95% confidence interval [CI], 1.8 to 6.9), but no increase in risk was observed in men who reported a history of undescended testes that demonstrated spontaneous descent. This study also provided evidence that the relative risk for cancer in men who were treated for cryptorchidism increased with age at treatment. Testicular atrophy was associated with both testicular cancer and cryptorchidism. Contrary to the previous study, inguinal hernia was not associated with testicular cancer in the absence of cryptorchidism or testicular atrophy. Another study demonstrated that the incidence of undescended testes was statistically significantly higher in both black and mixed-race patients compared with white patients presenting with testis tumors (Abratt et al, 1992). However, a study bias probably accounts for this finding, because the orchiopexy rate was 71% among mixed-race patients, 87% among whites, and zero among blacks. In addition, the mean age at presentation was 40 years for black patients, 32 years for those of mixed race, and 33 years for whites. Black patients also presented with abdominal or inguinal tumors rather than scrotal tumors.

These studies provide evidence to support the contention that orchiopexy may protect against the development of malignancy. Although the study by Prener and coworkers (1996) found the risk for testicular cancer to be increased in men with a history of cryptorchidism (RR, 5.2; 95% CI, 2.1% to 13.0%), there was no observed decrease in risk associated with treatment in early childhood.

Location of the undescended testis also affects the relative risk of developing a tumor. The higher the position of the undescended testis, the greater the risk of developing a malignancy (Martin and Menck, 1975; Martin, 1982). Almost half of the tumors that develop from undescended testes are in testes located abdominally, sixfold higher than for inguinal testes (Campbell, 1942). **The most common tumor that develops from a cryptorchid testis is seminoma** (Martin, 1979, 1982; Batata et al, 1980; Abratt et al, 1992). Of 125 patients treated with a history of cryptorchidism and testicular germ cell tumor, 54 were found to have pure seminoma, embryonal carcinoma was found in 35, teratocarcinoma in 33, and pure choriocarcinoma in 3 (Batata et al, 1980).

The cause of the increased risk for malignant degeneration of the undescended testis is at this time theoretical. Theories have included exposure of the testis to increased temperature, but most compelling is the idea of an intrinsic pathologic process affecting both testes. This theory is supported by evidence of increased risk of tumor formation in normally descended contralateral testes (Johnson et al, 1968; Batata et al, 1980; Martin, 1982). One study found that the relative risk of testicular cancer in the contralateral, normally descended testis in unilaterally cryptorchid men was increased to 3.6 (Prener et al, 1996). The risk of developing a testis tumor is 15% for the contralateral testis in men with bilaterally undescended testes when the other testis is already involved with tumor (Gilbert and Hamilton, 1970).

In 1972, Skakkebaek reported finding carcinoma in situ in the testis of an infertile man with an undescended testis who developed a germ cell tumor 16 months later. Since that time, it has been estimated that **the prevalence of carcinoma in situ is 1.7% in patients with cryptorchidism.** Carcinoma in situ is more commonly detected in abdominal testes than in testes that have undergone further descent (Ford et al, 1985). These findings bring into question the extent to which testicular biopsies taken during childhood orchiopexy can exclude the development of a tumor in adult life. Premalignant changes could not be demonstrated in biopsies of cryptorchid testis before adulthood (Muffly et al, 1984). In addition, no evidence of histologic premalignant changes occurring before the onset of puberty was observed in men who later developed testicular malignancies (Parkinson et al, 1994). **Therefore, routine testicular biopsy during childhood orchiopexy appears to have no predictive value for the development of later malignant degeneration.**

Hernia

A patent processus vaginalis is found in more than 90% of patients with an undescended testis (Scorer and Farrington, 1971; Grosfeld, 1989; Elder, 1992a). The processus normally closes between the period after complete testicular descent and the first month after birth. A higher incidence of epididymal anomalies is associated with a patent processus vaginalis, supporting the theory that androgenic stimulation may be required for closure of the processus (Barthold and Redman, 1996). The clinical significance of a patent processus vaginalis is that it has been shown to affect the efficacy of hormonal treatment of cryptorchidism. This was investigated in children with cryptorchidism who received hCG and later underwent inguinal herniorrhaphy. The incidence of testicular descent was 49.5% in patients with a nonpatent (normal) processus vaginalis and zero in the testes associated with a patent vaginal process (Varela Cives et al, 1996). Adamsen and colleagues (1989) unexpectedly found a hernia or hydrocele at surgery in 77% of cases after failed hCG treatment for cryptorchidism.

Testicular Torsion

The increased susceptibility of the testis to undergo torsion is the result of a developmental anatomic abnormality between the testis and its mesentery. The mechanism is believed to be related to a greater relative broadness of the testicle compared with its mesentery (Scorer and Farrington, 1971). This may explain the phenomenon of torsion of an undescended testis associated with a testicular tumor. Riegler (1972) found that 64% of adults with torsion in an undescended testis had an associated germ cell tumor. Intravaginal spermatic cord torsion and testicular infarction were reported in an infant with bilateral cryptorchidism who was receiving hCG treatment (Sawchuk et al, 1993). Although torsion of an undescended testis is rare, it should be considered in any child who presents with abdominal or groin pain and an empty ipsilateral hemiscrotum.

Work-up

When a child is referred for an undescended testis, the testis is palpable in approximately 80% and the remainder are nonpalpable. Most nonpalpable testes are intra-abdominal. However, a nonpalpable testis does not exclude an intracanalicular or absent testis. Approximately 20% of nonpalpable testes are absent, and 30% are atrophic. Determination as to whether the testis is present on physical examination is critically important, because it guides further work-up and treatment. Many times children are found to have retractile testes; often these require only follow-up examination to document a normally palpable state without retraction of the testis. Furthermore, up to 25% of children with cryptorchidism present with bilaterally undescended testes. The work-up begins with a thorough history that includes the following:

1. Preterm and maternal history, including the use of gestational steroids
2. Perinatal history, including documentation of a scrotal examination at birth
3. The child's medical and previous surgical history
4. Family history of cryptorchidism or syndromes (Table 67–1)

The physical examination ideally requires a relaxed child observed first in the supine position. Examination of the child in general should include any other birth defects that might suggest a syndromic association. The genital examination includes inspection for any penile malformations, including hypospadias, micropenis, or ambiguous genitalia. It should be noted whether there is asymmetry or underdevelopment of the scrotum. The examination also includes inspection of the inguinal canal and common sites of testicular ectopia for any masses. If only one testis is descended, this gonad should be carefully examined for size, turgor, any palpable paratesticular anomalies, and the presence of a hernia or hydrocele. In cases of a unilaterally nonpalpable testis, contralateral testicular hypertrophy of the normally descended testis has been suggested to represent ipsilateral testicular absence. Huff (1992) found that the mean volume of the contralateral descended testis of boys with an absent testis was greater than that of boys with an intra-abdominal testis at all ages, but this was not a reliable criterion for differentiating the two conditions. It has also been suggested, based on spermiograms, that compensatory hypertrophy of one testis does not prevent testicular insufficiency in adulthood (Laron et al, 1980). The child may be placed in one of several positions in order to assist in locating the undescended testis, including a sitting or squatting position. The examination for the undescended testis is best performed with warm hands and soapy water on the fingertips to reduce skin friction. The examiner's fingers are swept down from just above the internal ring along the inguinal canal into the scrotum. The clinician should feel either a testis moving back under the fingertips against the direction of palpation or a "pop" as the testis springs back into its cryptorchid position. Ectopic areas of testicular descent should also be carefully examined.

The overall accuracy of radiologic testing for the undescended testis is 44% (Hrebinko and Bellinger, 1993). The purpose of testing is usually to determine the location or presence of the undescended testis. But because surgical exploration is necessary in either case, imaging becomes a fruitless and expensive endeavor that in most situations does not influence the decision to operate, the surgical approach, or the viability or salvageability of the cryptorchid testis. Many modalities have been employed including ultrasound, CT scanning, MRI, testicular angiography and venography, pneumoperitoneography, and herniography. Many of these techniques are either invasive, require anesthesia, are technically difficult to perform, or are associated with a significant rate of false-negative results.

The work-up for bilateral nonpalpable testes merits special consideration, because this may represent a life-threatening situation if it is associated with either hypospadias or ambiguous genitalia. The diagnosis of bilateral anorchia should be considered if a male karyotype is confirmed. Endocrinologic evaluation is necessary and may help to determine whether one or both testes are present. Childhood is a quiescent phase in testicular activity, and the hCG stimulation test is widely used to evaluate testicular function. The hCG stimulation test can be administered to induce testosterone production and would confirm the presence of at least one testis. However, there may be a false-negative response if the Leydig cells are unresponsive to exogenous hCG. **If basal gonadotropin levels, FSH in particular, are increased in a prepubescent boy, then**

Table 67–1. SYNDROMIC ASSOCIATIONS WITH CRYPTORCHIDISM

Syndrome/ Associations	Major Characteristics	Genitourinary Characteristics Including Cryptorchidism	Gene/Chromosome	Inheritance
Aarskog	Hypertelorism, unusual facies, brachy-dactyly	Shawl scrotum, hernia	FGDY1 at Xp11.21	X-linked recessive
Acrodysostosis	Short hands with peripheral dysotosis, low nasal bridge, vertebral defects, MR	Hypogonadism		AD
Beckwith-Wiedemann	Aniridia, hemihypertrophy, macroglossia, macrosomia, omphalocele, adrenocortical cytomegaly, MR	Wilms' tumor, renal hyperplasia and dysplasia, interstitial	WT1, 11p13	Sporadic
Borjeson-Forssman-Lehmann	Large ears, MR	Hypogonadotropic hypogonadism, delayed second-degree sexual characteristics	—	X-linked recessive
Carpenter	Acrocephaly, polydactyly and syndactyly of feet, lateral displacement of inner canthi, limb abnormalities, MR	Hypogonadism	—	AR
Cloacal exstrophy sequence	Common cloaca with exstrophy, short gut, omphalocele, vertebral anomalies, failure of fusion of genital tubercle and pubic rami	Pelvic kidneys, other renal anomalies including renal duplication, agenesis, cystic dysplasia	—	—
Congenital microgastria–limb reduction complex	Microgastria, limb defects, splenic abnormalities	Renal anomalies	—	—
Deletion 4p	Hypertelorism, broad-beaked nose, microcephaly, low-set ears, MR, GR	Hypospadias	4p16.3 (cr)	—
Deletion 5p (cridu chat)	Cat-like cry, microcephaly, downward slant of palpedral fissures, hypertelorism, GR, MR	Renal agenesis, inguinal hernia	5p15.3 (cr)	—
Deletion 9p	Craniostenosis with trigonocephaly, up-slanting palpebral fissures, hypoplastic supraorbital ridges, limb and cardiac anomalies	Micropenis	9p24 (bp)	—
Deletion 11q	Trigonencephaly, large, carp-like mouth, hypertelorism, cardiac defects, MR	Hypospadias; occasional inguinal hernia, renal malformations	11q24.1 (cr)	—
Deletion 13q	Microcephaly, high nasal bridge, other facial anomalies, eye defects, thumb hypoplasia, cardiac defects, MR, GR	Hypospadias, focal lumbar agenesis	—	—
Deletion 18q	Midfacial hypoplasia, prominent antihelix of ears, whirl digital pattern	Hypogonadism; occasional horseshoe kidney	18q21.3 or q22.2 to qter	—
Distal arthrogryposis	Distal limb contractures, clenched hands at birth	—	—	AD with variable expressivity
Duplication 3q	Severe postnatal GR, MR, broad nasal root, hypertrichosis, high arched palate	Renal anomalies	3q21–qter	—
Duplication 4p	Characteristic facial anomalies, MR, GR	Micropenis, hypospadias	4p15.2–16.1	—
Duplication 10q	Microcephaly, ptosis, camptodactyly, short palpebral fissures, MR, IUGR	Renal malformations	10q24–qter	—
Duplication 15q	Sloping forehead, prominent nose with broad nasal bridge, micrognathia, camptodactyly, cardiac defects, MR, GR	—	15q21, 15q23 (bp's)	—
Early urethral obstruction sequence	Oligohydramnios deformation sequence, abdominal muscle deficiency, colon malrotation, persistent urachus, lower limb deficiency	Urethral obstruction (urethral valve, atresia), hydronephrosis, megacystis, renal dysplasia	—	—
Escobar	Multiple pterygia, camptodactyly, syndactyly, small stature, multiple facial anomalies	Hypospadias	—	AR
Fanconi's pancytopenia	Pancytopenia, short stature, hyperpigmentation, radial hypoplasia (thumb deformity), microcephaly, MR	Small testes, hypergonadotropic hypogonadism, renal malformations (ranging from duplication and ectopia, to agenesis)	At least two loci: distal 20q and 9q22.3	AR

Table 67–1. SYNDROMIC ASSOCIATIONS WITH CRYPTORCHIDISM *Continued*

Syndrome/ Associations	Major Characteristics	Genitourinary Characteristics Including Cryptorchidism	Gene/Chromosome	Inheritance
FG	Imporforate anus, hypotonia, prominent forehead, MR	—	—	X-linked recessive
Fraser	Cryptophthalmos, auricle defect, MR, cutaneous syndactyly	Incomplete development, hypospadias; renal hypoplasia or agenesis	—	AR
Freeman-Sheldon	"Whistling" and mask-like facies, hypoplastic alae nasi, ulnar deviation of hands, postnatal GR	Inguinal hernia	—	AD (AR reported)
Frontometaphyseal dysplasia	Craniofacial anomalies including prominent supraorbital ridges, joint contractures, splayed metaphyses	Obstructive uropathy	—	X-linked
Fryns	Coarse facies, abnormal ear shape, cleft palate, microretrognathia, diaphragmatic abnormalities, distal digital hypoplasia, CNS abnormalities (50%)	Hypospadias, scrotalization of phallus, bifid scrotum, cystic kidney disease	—	AR
Johanson-Blizzard	Hypoplastic alae nasi, hypothyroidism, anorectal malformations, deafness, MR	Hydronephrosis, micropenis, hypospadias	—	AR
Kallmann 1	Anosmia, hypogonadotropic hypogonadism, mirror hand movements, ataxia; GnRH deficiency	Micropenis, unilateral renal agenesis, testicular atrophy	KAL1, Xp22.3	X-linked
Kallmann 2	Hypogonadotropic hypogonadism, anosmia, MR, choanal atresia, heart defects, short stature, NS hearing loss	—	KAL2	AD
Lenz's dysplasia	Microphthalmia or anophthalmos, limb/digit abnormalities, MR, GR, microcephaly, cleft lip/palate, webbed neck, heart defects, imperforate anus	Hypospadias, renal hypoplasia, hydronephrosis	—	X-linked
Lethal multiple pterygium	IUGR, epicanthal folds, hypertelorism, cleft palate, pterygia, flexion contractures	—	—	AR; X-linked recessive reported
Lenz-Majewski hyperostosis	FTT, MR, proximal symphalangism, short-absent middle phalanges, diffuse cortical sclerosis and thickening of bone, hypotrophic skin	Inguinal hernia	—	Unknown, sporadic cases
Lowe	Hypotonia, cataract, MR	Renal tubular dysfunction	—	X-linked
McDonough	MR, unusual facies, short stature, diastasis recti, heart defects, kyphoscoliosis	—	—	AR
Meckel-Gruber	CNS anomalies including encephalocele, microcephaly; facial anomalies including, microphthalmia, cleft palate, polydactyly	Cystic dysplasia of kidneys, incomplete development of external/internal genitalia	17q21–q24	AR
MHS1	Hyperthermia, myopathy, rhabdomyolysis, hypertonicity, metabolic abnormalities, second-degree general anesthesia	—	19q13.1–q13.2	AD
Miller-Dieker	Incomplete brain development, microcephaly	Pelvic kidney, cystic dysplasia of kidneys	17p13.3	—
Multiple lentigines	Multiple lentigines, cardiac anomalies, deafness	Unilateral renal and/or gonadal agenesis/hypoplasia, hypogonadism	—	AD
Noonan	Short stature, FTT (infancy), webbed neck, pectus excavatum, pulmonic stenosis, bleeding diathesis including von Willebrand's disease and abnormal intrinsic pathway deficiencies, thrombocytopenia, vertebral abnormalities	Occasional hypogonadism	12q22–qter (AD)	Genetic heterogeneity; AD
Opitz	Hypertelorism, swallowing difficulties, MR	Hypospadias, bifid scrotum, inguinal hernia, occasional renal anomalies	22q11.2–Xp22	AD, X-linked
Oto-palato-digital, type II	Craniofacial anomalies including hypertelorism and cleft palate; conductive hearing loss, multiple distal limb abnormalities	Hypospadias, absent adrenal	—	X-linked
Pena-Shokeir phenotype	Rigid facies, hypertelorism, multiple ankylosis, pulmonary hypoplasia	—	—	AR (?)

Table continued on following page

Table 67–1. SYNDROMIC ASSOCIATIONS WITH CRYPTORCHIDISM *Continued*

Syndrome/ Associations	Major Characteristics	Genitourinary Characteristics Including Cryptorchidism	Gene/Chromosome	Inheritance
Perlman	Fetal ascites without hydrops, fetal gigantism, macrosomia, anteverted upper lip, depressed nasal bridge, micrognathia, open mouth, hyperinsulinism, abdominal muscular hypoplasia, visceromegaly, cardiac defects	Wilms' tumor, renal hamartomas, nephroblastomatosis	Similar deletions at 11p as Wilms' tumor	AR
Peter-plus	MR, short limb dwarfism, hypertelorism, Peter's anomaly of the eyes, cardiac defects	Hydronephrosis, renal duplication anomalies	—	AR
Popliteal pterygium	Mouth anomalies include lower lip pits, cleft palate, popliteal web	Bifid scrotum, and other scrotal abnormalities; occasional ambiguous genitalia, ectopic testes, penile anomalies, hernia	—	AD
Prader-Willi	FTT, rapid weight gain >1yr, obesity, short stature, small hands and feet, MR, hypotonia,	Hypogonadotropic hypogonadism	Deletion 15q11.2–q12	
Ptosis of eyelids with diastasis recti and hip dysplasia	Blepharoptosis, partial abdominal muscle agenesis, hip dislocation	—	—	AR
Roberts-SC phocomelia	MR, microcephaly, profound growth deficiency, cleft lip/palate, midfacial defect (hemangioma), hypomalia	—	—	AR
Robinow	Hypertelorism, flat facial profile, short forearms, vertebral anomalies, short stature	Hypogonadism, renal anomalies	—	AD, AR
Rubinstein-Taybi	Broad thumbs and toes, slanted palpebral fissures, hypoplastic maxilla, MR	—	16p13.3	Sporadic
Seckel	Microcephaly, severe short stature, prominent nose	Hypoplastic external genitalia	—	AR
Senter-KID	Keratitis, ichythyosis, deafness	—	—	AD; AR described
Simpson-Golabi-Behmel	Somatic overgrowth, macrocephaly, hypertelorism, vertebral defects	Inguinal hernias, occasional renal anomalies, hypospadias	Xq26 (GPC3)	X-linked recessive
Smith-Lemli-Opitz	Anteverted nostrils ± ptosis of eyelids, syndactyly second and third toes, simian crease, short stature, MR, microcephaly	Hypospadias	—	AR
TKCR	Torticollis/keloids/cryptorchidism/renal dysplasia	Oligospermia	Xq28	X-linked with incomplete dominance
Triploidy	Large placenta with hydatidiform changes, GR, syndactyly, craniofacial anomalies	Hypospadias, micropenis, Leydig cell hyperplasia, renal anomalies including cystic dysplasia and hydronephrosis, adrenal hypoplasia	—	Complete extra set of chromosomes, usually paternally derived
Trisomy 9 mosaic	Joint contractures, cardiac anomalies, low-set malformed ears, prenatal GR, MR	Hypoplastic external genitalia, cystic dilatation of renal tubules, bladder diverticula, hydronephrosis	—	—
Trisomy 13	Midface defects, eye and forebrain abnormalities, MR, polydactyly, skin defects	Abnormal scrotum	—	—
Trisomy 18	Clenched hand, short sternum, low arch dermal ridge pattern of fingertips	Inguinal hernia, small pelvis; renal anomalies including horseshoe kidney, ectopic kidney, hydronephrosis, PCKD	—	—
Varadi-Papp	Growth retardation, cleft lip/palate, oral frenula, digital asymmetry, reduplicated big toes, hexadactyly, absent olfactory bulbs and tracts, heart defects	Adult PCKD; occasional hypogonadotropic hypogonadism	—	AR

Table 67–1. SYNDROMIC ASSOCIATIONS WITH CRYPTORCHIDISM *Continued*

Syndrome/ Associations	Major Characteristics	Genitourinary Characteristics Including Cryptorchidism	Gene/Chromosome	Inheritance
Weaver	Macrosomia, accelerated skeletal maturation, camptodactyly, unusual facies, macrocephaly, MR	Inguinal hernia	—	—
X-Linked α-thalassemia/MR (ATR-16)	Severe MR, microcephaly, unusual facies	Testicular dysgenesis, shawl/hypoplastic scrotum, small penis, hypospadias; occasional renal agenesis, hydronephrosis	16p13.3	—
XXXY/XXXXY	Decreased pronation at elbow, low dermal ridge pattern on fingertips; greater degree of aneuploidy, more severe the GR	Hypogenitalism: small penis, small testes with hypoplastic tubules and diminished Leydig cells, hypoplastic scrotum; occasional hypospadias	—	—

AD, autosomal dominant; AR, autosomal recessive; bp, break point; CNS, central nervous system; cr, critical region; FGDY, fasciogenital dysplasia; FTT, failure to thrive; GnRH, gonadotropin-releasing hormone; GR, growth hormone; IUGR, in utero growth retardation; MR, mental retardation; NS, nonsignificant; PCKD, polycystic kidney disease; WT, Wilms' tumor.

further endocrine work-up is unnecessary, because this probably represents bilateral anorchia (Jarow et al, 1986). If gonadotropin levels are normal in a boy with bilateral nonpalpable testes, then an hCG stimulation test can be performed to further establish the diagnosis. However, all boys with nonpalpable testes and normal serum gonadotropins must undergo surgical exploration regardless of the results of the hCG stimulation test. MIS and inhibin B are also specific testicular markers, and their measurement may be of benefit in determining whether testicular tissue is present. Inhibin B, a testicular peptide regulating FSH secretion, is a marker of Sertoli cell function and spermatogenesis in adults (Byrd et al, 1998) and probably regulates FSH secretion in early childhood. In contrast to the other hormones of the hypothalamic-pituitary-gonadal axis, it is secreted in detectable amounts during childhood and may predict prepubertal testicular function (Raivio and Dunkel, 1999; Kubini et al, 2000).

Management of Cryptorchidism

Tenets of Treatment

The important tenets for the treatment of a child who presents with an undescended testis include the following:

1. Proper identification of the anatomy, position, and viability of the undescended testis
2. Identification of any potential coexisting syndromic abnormalities
3. Placement of the testis within the scrotum in a timely fashion to prevent further testicular impairment of either fertility potential or endocrinologic function
4. Attainment of permanent fixation of the testis with a normal scrotal position that allow for easy palpation
5. No further testicular damage resulting from the treatment

Definitive treatment of the undescended testis should occur before 1 year of age. Because spontaneous descent occurs in most boys by 3 months of age and uncommonly thereafter, consideration for earlier intervention should be made to theoretically prevent complications of cryptorchidism that may be manifested before 1 year of age. Approach and timing should be predicated on the anatomic position and whether both testes are undescended. For instance, there may be a theoretical advantage to bringing down a solitary undescended testis before 1 year of age if the contralateral testis is absent or intra-abdominal. Every effort should be made to preserve any testicular tissue at an early age, especially in children with unilateral or bilateral intra-abdominal testes. This is based on the poor paternity rates in men with a history of bilateral cryptorchidism. Orchiectomy is typically reserved for postpubescent males with a contralateral normally descended testis when the cryptorchid testis is either anatomically or morphologically abnormal or too far from the scrotum to allow for tension-free placement without compromising the vascular integrity to the testis. Extraordinary means are occasionally necessary to preserve a solitary testis or bilateral intra-abdominal testes, especially when the clinical presentation is late.

Hormonal Therapy

There are two types of medical treatment for the undescended testis: exogenous hCG and exogenous GnRH or LHRH. The mechanism of action in both cases increases serum testosterone production by stimulation at different levels of the hypothalamic-pituitary-gonadal cascade. This therapy is based on experimental observations that descent is androgen mediated, involving testicular synthesis of the active metabolite in high local concentrations (Rajfer and Walsh, 1977). hCG stimulates Leydig cells directly to produce testosterone, whereas GnRH stimulates the pituitary to release LH and thereby promote testicular production of testosterone. Serum testosterone levels during therapy for cryptorchidism in prepubertal boys are much higher with hCG than with GnRH (Rajfer et al, 1986).

Patient selection has been found to be critical in achieving good results. Successful results are more commonly reported in older groups of children and in testes that were retractile or below the external inguinal ring—that is, **the lower the pretreatment position, the better the success rate** (Rajfer et al, 1986; De Muinck Keizer-Schrama et al, 1987; Pyorala et al, 1995; Fedder and Boesen, 1998). A retrospective evaluation of boys treated with LHRH revealed a previous scrotal position of the testes in 43% of those with successful treatment but in only 17% of those with failed treatment (De Muinck Keizer-Schrama et al, 1987). Similar results were reported by Fedder and Boesen (1998), who found a 56% success rate in boys whose testes were documented to both be descended by 1 week after birth. These findings certainly help explain the earlier studies that reported high success rates with hormonal therapy. In most of these cases, surgical exploration revealed an anatomic anomaly that most likely caused testicular ascent. Regular reexamination of children treated with hormonal therapy is indicated, because reascent has been reported in up to 25% of patients. Hormonal treatment is not indicated in patients with previously operated testes or surgery that would result in inguinal scar tissue formation, in those with ectopic testes, or in those with an inguinal hernia. Presently, only hCG is available for patient use in the United States.

Use of hCG in the treatment of cryptorchidism has been both widespread and debated since the 1930s. hCG is structurally analogous to LH and is a potent stimulator of Leydig cells. Reported therapeutic success rates have varied considerably, from 14% to 59% (Erlich et al, 1969; Job et al, 1982; Adamsen et al, 1989). Treatment regimens have also varied greatly, and the most effective treatment was demonstrated to be a total dose of at least 10,000 IU to achieve maximal stimulation of the Leydig cells and avoid the complications of doses exceeding 15,000 IU (Job et al, 1982). A typical treatment schedule is 1500 IU/m² given by intramuscular injection twice a week for 4 weeks. A downside of hCG treatment is that it must be given parenterally on a frequent basis. FSH appears to influence the spontaneous descent of the testis and to induce LH receptors; however, efficacy studies of combination treatment with hCG have shown mixed results and cannot be recommended at this time (Saggese et al, 1989; Hoorweg-Nijman et al, 1994).

Side effects of hormonal treatment include increased rugation and pigmentation of the scrotum. Rarely, there is an increase in the size of the penis and development of pubic hair, which regresses after cessation of therapy. Significant increase in weight increment velocity was seen in 7- to 9-year-olds treated with a dose of 10,000 IU (Adamsen et al, 1989). A number of studies have evaluated the controversial issue of adverse histologic effects on the testis after hCG treatment. Although hCG induced a significant increase in the volume density of both interstitial tissue and blood vessels in normally descended and undescended testes, there appeared to be no permanent damage (Kaleva et al, 1996). However, hCG withdrawal was implicated as the mechanism of increased germ cell apoptosis in the hor-

monal treatment of cryptorchidism (Heiskanen et al, 1996). hCG should also be avoided in immunosuppressed patients because of a transient decrease in the absolute number of total peripheral blood lymphocytes, total T cells, T helper-inducer cells, and of CD8⁺ subsets during therapy. In addition, the percentage of CD8⁺ cells and lymphocyte response to the mitogen concanavalin A decreased significantly with hCG treatment and returned to normal after hCG withdrawal (Mahnie et al, 1991).

Exogenous GnRH was developed as a therapy for cryptorchidism because of the less than ideal results of exogenous hCG. It has the advantage of nasal spray administration, and an effective dose for stimulating LH is 1.2 mg/day for 4 weeks (Rajfer et al, 1986). Results of previous trials may have been falsely optimistic owing to the inclusion of patients with retractile testes; the reported success rates ranged from 32% to 65% (Illi et al, 1977; Hadziselimovic, 1982; Witjes et al, 1990). Rajfer and associates (1986) found that testicular descent into the scrotum occurred in 19% of patients treated with GnRH and in 6% of those treated with hCG. In addition, there appears to be a difference in success rate between unilateral and bilateral cryptorchidism. One multicenter study demonstrated the effect of LHRH in cryptorchid boys and found a therapeutic gain in 8.1% of those with bilaterally undescended testes and no effect in those with unilateral undescended testis (Olsen et al, 1992). A success rate of 9% for LHRH nasal spray and 8% for placebo was reported in 252 prepubertal boys with 301 undescended testes (De Muinck Keizer-Schrama et al, 1987). Hormonal evaluation revealed no abnormalities in cryptorchid boys compared with control subjects. These results confirmed similar findings reported by Pyolala and coworkers (1995), who performed a meta-analysis of 33 studies from 1958 to 1990 that assessed the results of LHRH and hCG in the treatment of 3282 boys with cryptorchidism. Analysis of randomized, controlled trials showed that LHRH was not significantly more effective than hCG (21% versus 19%). The low success rate with GnRH has been demonstrated not to be caused by defective LH secretion by the hypothalamus or testosterone secretion by the testes (Rajfer et al, 1986).

In summary, the overall efficacy of hormonal treatment is less than 20% for cryptorchid testes and is significantly dependent on testicular pretreatment location. Therefore, surgery remains the gold standard in the management of the undescended testis.

Surgical Treatment

It is very useful to examine the child after the induction of general and regional anesthesia to reaffirm testicular position, or to attempt to establish testicular position in the case of a previously nonpalpable testis. With anesthesia, the anterior abdominal musculature relaxes, offering the surgeon the opportunity to perform a more thorough physical examination in the occasional case in which the initial examination was complicated by body habitus, uncooperative behavior, or guarding. In general, success rates for orchiopexy are directly related to anatomic position of the testis. The 1995 analysis of surgical therapy for undescended testes by Docimo revealed an orchiopexy success rate of 92% for testes below the external

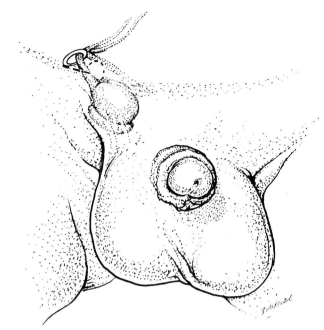

Figure 67–1. A transverse skin incision is made in an inguinal skin crease.

ring, 89% for inguinal testes, 84% for microvascular orchiopexies, 81% for standard abdominal orchiopexies, 77% for staged Fowler-Stephens orchiopexies, and 67% for standard Fowler-Stephens orchiopexies.

STANDARD ORCHIOPEXY

The key steps of this procedure are (1) complete mobilization of the testis and spermatic cord, (2) repair of the patent processus vaginalis by high ligation of the hernia sac, (3) skeletonization of the spermatic cord without sacrificing vascular integrity in order to achieve tension-free placement of the testis within the dependent position of the scrotum, and (4) creation of a superficial pouch within the hemiscrotum to receive the testis.

A transverse inguinal skin incision is made in the midinguinal canal, usually in a skin crease in children younger than 1 year of age (Fig. 67–1). The dermis is opened with electrocautery, and subcutaneous tissue and Scarpa's fascia are opened sharply. The skin and subcutaneous tissues are quite elastic in younger children and allow for a tremendous degree of mobility by retractor positioning in order to view the entire length of the inguinal canal. Therefore, a large incision is usually unnecessary. Be careful to observe that the testis is in the superficial inguinal pouch and that it lies between Scarpa's fascia and the external oblique fascia. Sharp dissection cleans the surface of the external oblique fascia of prefascial fat, and gentle spreading over Poupart's ligament defines the full lateral extent of the external oblique fascia. This maneuver is helpful to maintain anatomic orientation in defining the area directly over the inguinal canal.

The testis will be lying within its tunics either in the inguinal canal or just outside it in most cases. If the testis is intracanalicular, the external oblique fascia is opened with a small superficial incision that is carried through the

external ring, with care taken to preserve the ilioinguinal nerve (Fig. 67–2A). The tunics overlying the testis are grasped, and the distal gubernacular attachments are sharply dissected; this frees the testis up into the wound. Cremasteric muscular fibers and any anomalous fibrous attachments from the superficial peripheral fascia are then dissected sharply away from the testis and spermatic cord (Fig. 67–2B). Once the spermatic cord is freely mobilized to the internal ring from cremasteric attachments in the inguinal canal, the tunica vaginalis is opened over the testis. This is a good time to carefully inspect the anatomy and integrity of the paratesticular structures and measure the testis.

Complete mobilization of the spermatic cord is essential to achieve adequate cord length for tension-free placement of the testis into the scrotum. This should not be done at the risk of devitalizing the vascular supply to the testis or damaging paratesticular structures, including the vas deferens. The key steps in this part of the operation include (1) complete transsection of the fused fibers between the cremasteric muscle and the internal oblique muscle; (2) complete separation of the patent processus vaginalis from the elements of the spermatic cord (Fig. 67–3), with mobilization of the hernia sac/peritoneum to at least just inside the internal ring (Fig. 67–4); and (3) dissection of internal spermatic fascia from the cord structures (Fig. 67–5). In most cases, division of the processus vaginalis and cremasteric muscle attachments provides adequate cord length to allow for placement of the testis in the scrotum. It is also helpful to separate the vas deferens from the vascular elements from the level of the internal ring, because these structures diverge at this level. If additional cord length is needed at this point, retroperitoneal dissection is necessary. A Ragnell retractor placed within the internal ring allows for adequate visualization of the spermatic vessels cephalad for gentle blunt mobilization with either a Q-Tip, sponge, or kipner. The external oblique should be opened above the level of the internal ring, and the internal oblique muscle can be divided 1 to 2 cm from the superior lateral margin of the internal ring.

Experimental evidence has documented that transparenchymal suture fixation causes testicular damage by inducing an inflammatory reaction regardless of suture size and material. **In comparison, dartos-fixed testes demonstrated complete circumferential adherence with only 5% of the animals in the dartos pouch group demonstrating an inflammatory response and normal spermatogenesis in 94%** (Bellinger et al, 1989; Dixon et al, 1993). Based on these studies, transparenchymal suture should be avoided. There are only two exceptional circumstances: for a tethered testis when its position is tenuous after complete mobilization of the spermatic cord and short-term external fixation to a nylon button is required, and for testicular fixation of the ipsilateral and contralateral testes due to clinical torsion of the spermatic cord. A significant variation of the technique, however, is to completely avoid deep transparenchymal placement of the sutures by superficial placement of the sutures just under the tunica albuginea. The sutures used in these cases are fine, permanent monofilament suture, such as 5-0 or 6-0 Prolene, on a noncutting needle. **It is important to be familiar with the intragonadal vascular anatomy in such cases, especially**

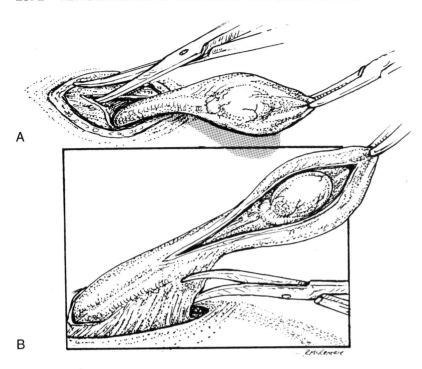

A

B

Figure 67–2. *A,* The external ring is opened. *B,* Cremasteric fibers are dissected from the cord.

when ligation of the spermatic vessels is contemplated. The collateral arterial circulation through the deferential artery, which communicates with the internal spermatic arterial system both in the spermatic cord and at the lower pole of the testis, was found to be compromised in all testes with placement of a traction suture (Jarow, 1991).

The testis can be adequately and permanently secured in the scrotum by placement of the testis within a superficial dartos pouch. The dartos pouch has a long and proven record of success. Placement of the testis within the dartos pouch results in complete circumferential adherence of the tunica albuginea to the scrotal skin. A transverse midscrotal superficial skin incision is made within a rugal skin fold, and a mosquito hemostat is then used to develop a tissue plane just under the scrotal skin of the ipsilateral hemiscrotum (Fig. 67–6). The scrotal pocket should be developed from the median raphe and the lateral scrotal margin, with creation of the space inferiorly to encourage preferential fixation of the testis as dependently in the scrotum as possible. After the testis and cord are completely mobilized and the tunica vaginalis is opened and everted over the testis, a hemostat is passed just over the pubic symphysis

from the inguinal incision through the tough dartos fascia into the scrotum (Fig. 67–7A). It is important to pass the hemostat into the medial aspect of the scrotum to avoid lateral placement or migration of the testis. The most direct path to the scrotum allows for the most dependent placement of the testis. A second hemostat is back-passed from the scrotum into the inguinal incision; the most dependent tunica vaginalis or remnant of gubernaculum is grasped, and the testis is passed into the scrotum, with care taken to avoid torsion of the spermatic cord (Fig. 67–7B,C).

The dartos fascial window is closed with a fine absorbable suture, with the option of placing this suture through the redundant tunica vaginalis well above the level of the testis in order to indirectly secure the cord at this position. The testis is then placed within the dartos pouch, and the scrotal skin closed with fine interrupted absorbable sutures such as 4-0 chromic vertical mattress sutures. The external oblique fascia is closed with running or interrupted absorbable suture with re-creation of the external ring, although not to such a degree as to impinge on the spermatic cord or redirect the cord from keeping the most direct path to the scrotum. Subcutaneous tissues and skin are closed in the usual fashion. We prefer interrupted subcuticular clo-

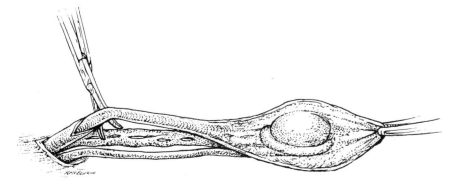

Figure 67–3. Dissection to separate the processus vaginalis from the cord structures.

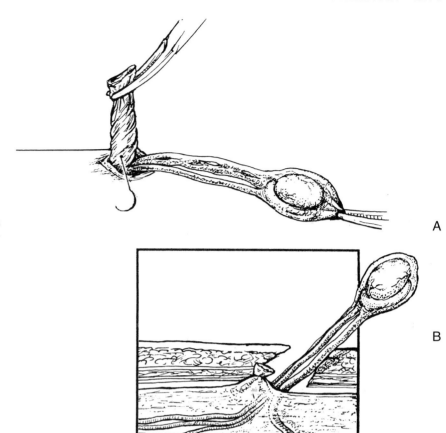

Figure 67–4. *A,* High ligation of the processus vaginalis at the internal inguinal ring. *B,* The ligated processus and the cord structures.

sure of the skin with fine absorbable suture and collodion placed as a dressing.

ANCILLARY TECHNIQUES FOR THE HIGH UNDESCENDED TESTIS

Occasionally, greater mobilization of the proximal spermatic cord structures does not provide adequate length to allow for tension-free placement of the testis within the scrotum. Greater cord length can be obtained by mobilizing the spermatic vessels medially. The spermatic vessels are usually the limiting factor in these circumstances. The Prentiss maneuver was described in 1960 and occasionally is helpful in adding length to the spermatic vessels by positioning the spermatic vessels medially and thereby choosing the hypotenuse of the triangle, or most direct course to the scrotum, created by the natural course of the vessels laterally through the internal ring (Prentiss et al, 1960). It is performed by incising the floor of the inguinal canal through the external ring and dividing the inferior epigastric vessels. The internal ring and transversalis fascia are then closed lateral to the cord. In addition, a thorough retroperitoneal dissection, especially of the lateral attachments, is carried out in conjunction with this procedure.

If adequate length is not achieved, a staged orchiopexy can be performed, as described by Persky and Albert in 1971. The testis is anchored to the external ring or pubic symphysis after maximal mobilization in the first stage, and a second procedure is performed 6 to 12 months later.

Wrapping of the cord and testis in a Silastic sheath may reduce adhesion formation and render the second-stage procedure less difficult (Corkery, 1975; Steinhardt et al, 1985).

REOPERATIVE ORCHIOPEXY

Reoperative orchiopexy is performed in cases of secondary cryptorchism after orchiopexy or inguinal hernia repair. Testes that are at risk for iatrogenic ascent after a hernia repair many times appear to be normally descended when in fact they are retractile or represent a subtle variant of a cryptorchid testis. In this case, the testis may be ectopic, in a low-lying position within a superficial pouch. In many cases, the testis is also in a retroscrotal plane just outside the confines of the anatomic scrotum. The testis is usually located near the pubic tubercle, but, depending on age and the delay to treatment, it may be as high as just outside the external ring. The skin incision and initial exposure should be in a previously nonoperated area in order to identify landmarks and approach the testis from normal tissue to scarred.

The initial dissection should be toward the lower pole of the testis. The inguinal ligament should also be identified early in the procedure. After the testis is freed, care is taken to mobilize the spermatic cord, which probably has been previously skeletonized. Dense scarring may be found between the anterior aspect of the cord and the undersurface of the external oblique fascia. To lessen the risk of injury to the spermatic vessels, dissection lateral and me-

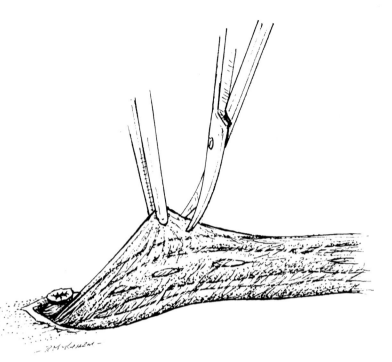

Figure 67–5. Separation of the internal spermatic fascia from the cord structures after ligation of the processus vaginalis.

dial to the cord in more normal tissues is performed, and in some cases it is beneficial to leave a strip of fascia overlying the cord during the initial mobilization. It may also be necessary to mobilize the cord proximally above the internal ring in order to gain length in a now relatively inelastic cord. The usual surgical principles of a standard orchiopexy can then be applied, including positioning the cord more medially.

Management of Intra-abdominal Testis

LAPAROSCOPY

Laparoscopy is a safe and effective method of assessing the nonpalpable testis. The accuracy of transperitoneal laparoscopy in locating a nonpalpable testis approaches 100% and subsequently defines the management options. Once the presence or absence of the testis is verified by diagnostic laparoscopy, an orchiopexy or orchiectomy may be performed with laparoscopic assistance. The initial purpose of diagnostic laparoscopy is to plan the subsequent surgical approach or to avoid an open exploration. **The three likely findings at diagnostic laparoscopy for a nonpalpable testis are (1) blind-ending vessels above the internal ring, (2) cord structures entering the internal ring, and (3) an intra-abdominal testis.** When blind-ending spermatic vessels are found, no further surgical investigation is necessary. The testis is considered "vanished," most likely as the result of a prenatal vascular accident. **When spermatic vessels, even hypoplastic ones, are visualized entering the internal ring, inguinal exploration is mandatory.** Vessels entering the inguinal canal signify a possible intracanalicular testis, especially if the processus vaginalis is patent. Inguinal exploration also examines the distal structures, and the remnant nubbin of testicular tissue is removed if present. Rozanski and colleagues (1996)

characterized the histologic features of remnant testicular tissue distal to the internal inguinal ring and found evidence of ischemia and necrosis (scar, calcification, hemosiderin, and hyalinization) that were suggestive of a vascular accident. Most importantly, a 10% incidence of viable germ cells was identified, which warrants excision of all nubbin remnants.

The intra-abdominal testis can be managed by either an "open" surgical or laparoscopic orchiopexy procedure or by orchiectomy. The orchiopexy can either be staged or per-

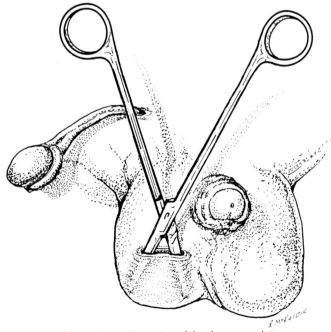

Figure 67–6. Formation of the dartos pouch.

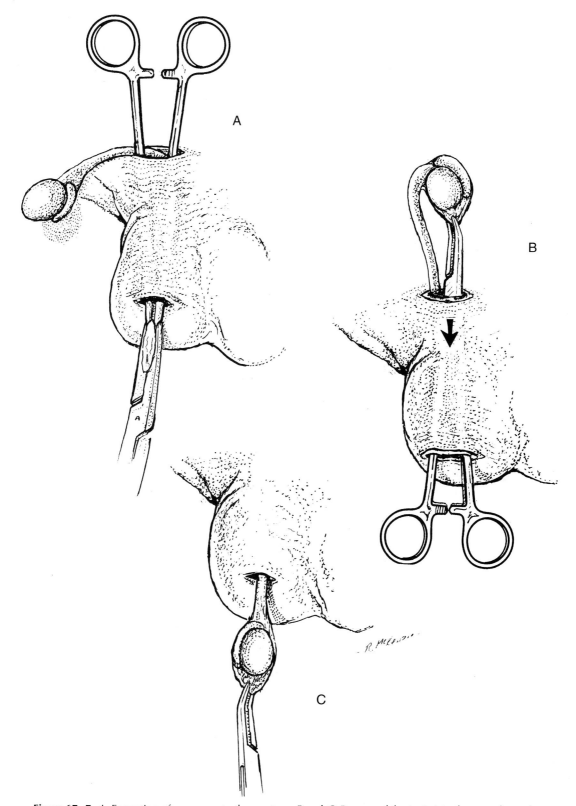

Figure 67–7. *A,* Formation of a passage to the scrotum. *B* and *C,* Passage of the testis into the scrotal pouch.

formed with complete mobilization of the testis into the scrotum in one procedure. The choice of repair technique depends on the viability of the testis, the anatomy of the paratesticular structures, the distance of the testis from the scrotum, the status of the contralateral testis, and, most importantly, the surgeon's experience and ability. A microsurgical autotransplantation of the intra-abdominal testis is an extreme measure with few indications.

Laparoscopic techniques, advantages, and contraindications are discussed elsewhere in this text, but a natural extension of the diagnostic laparoscopy is first-stage clip ligation of the spermatic vessels for a true intra-abdominal testis. Endoscopic clip ligation of the proximal spermatic vessels with delayed second-stage open or laparoscopic vasal pedicle orchiopexy 6 months later offers comparable results (Bloom, 1991; Rozanski and Bloom, 1995). Bloom (1991) and Jordan and Winslow (1994) reported their initial experience in the management of the intra-abdominal testis by laparoscopic techniques by one- and two-stage procedures. The low intra-abdominal testis can be delivered to the scrotum without dividing the spermatic vessels. The Prentiss maneuver is applied by diverting the exit of the testis medial to the inferior epigastric vessels. High intra-abdominal testes are best managed by a two-stage procedure. Proponents of laparoscopic techniques point to these advantages over standard open surgical techniques: (1) more complete and proximal dissection of the spermatic vessels to their origin, (2) magnified view of the main and collateral vasculature, and (3) less morbidity.

FOWLER-STEPHENS ORCHIOPEXY

Ligation of the testicular vessels occasionally becomes a necessary consideration, especially in the management of the high inguinal or intra-abdominal testis. The testicular artery and veins often limit the distal mobility of these testes. The surgical complexity of this condition was recognized well before the 20th century. Bevan's 1899 attempt at remedying this conundrum resulted in a procedure that included testicular artery division. The results of this technique were poor and produced testicular atrophy. It was not until 1959 that Fowler and Stephens studied the vascular anatomy of the testis and devised a means to repair the high undescended testis and preserve its blood supply via collateral circulation. The testis has three sources of arterial blood supply: the testicular artery (primary), the deferential artery of the vas deferens, and the cremasteric arteries (Fowler and Stephens, 1959). **When the spermatic vessels are divided, blood supply to the testis is dependent on collateral circulation from the deferential artery, a branch of the inferior vesical artery, and the cremasteric system, a branch of the inferior epigastric artery.**

The technique described by Fowler and Stephens was originally a one-stage procedure, but it may also be performed in two stages. If a one-stage repair is to be performed, it is critical early in the dissection that a wide pedicle of peritoneum be preserved with the vas deferens in order to maintain collateral blood flow. It is also important to remember that the testis is technically a retroperitoneal organ, as is its blood supply and the vas deferens. A high transverse inguinal incision is made that can be extended laterally in a cranial direction. The external oblique fascia is opened in the direction of its fibers, and the contents of the inguinal canal are examined. If a hernia sac is present, it is carefully dissected up to the level of the internal ring and opened. More commonly, there is no canal or sac, and therefore anterior abdominal muscles are opened to expose the peritoneum which is opened.

After the testis is identified, it is gently mobilized up into the incision without transecting any structures proximal to the testis. Careful inspection is then required to identify the primary and collateral vessels to the testis, as well as the course of the vas deferens. Anatomic variations of the vascular supply to the testis are especially common in associated cases of a long-looping vas. It has been reported that this most important requirement for successful Fowler-Stephens orchiopexy is present in less than one third of boys with true intra-abdominal testes (Bloom et al, 1994). Children with a long-looping vas that extends down the inguinal canal are the ideal candidates for a one-stage repair. True intra-abdominal testes lie at least 1 cm from internal ring and have shortened spermatic vessels. If a long-looping vas is present, it is carefully mobilized and protected up from the inguinal canal. Once it has been determined that the testis will not traverse the distance to the scrotum, the spermatic vessels are divided.

The Fowler-Stephens test is a method of testing the collateral blood supply to the testis. It is performed by temporarily occluding the testicular artery with a vascular clamp for 5 minutes and inspecting the testis for color as well as making a small incision in the tunica albuginea of the testis to document arterial bleeding. Care must be taken to distinguish the tunical blood supply, which tends to be preserved despite testicular arterial occlusion, from the true blood supply to the testicular parenchyma. If the blood supply is at this point considered tenuous, then a two-stage repair should be performed to allow for development of the collateral circulation.

If the testis appears viable, then the testicular artery is tied and divided high above the testis. The testis is then mobilized on a wide swath of peritoneum with the vas deferens. An incision is made in the lateral peritoneal reflection, and the peritoneum medial to the testis is left undisturbed. Care is taken not to injure the ureter during dissection of the deep vasal pedicle. If a long-looping vas is present, the loop is straightened by dividing the peritoneum in the center, the loop to extend the length of the pedicle. The course of the vasal pedicle should be as medial as possible in order to choose the shortest distance to the scrotum. This may require a direct placement of the testis and pedicle through a neohiatus in the abdominal wall over the symphysis pubis, or medial to the inferior epigastric vessels using the Prentiss maneuver. From this point forward the procedure is carried out as a standard orchiopexy with creation of a dartos pouch.

The anticipated advantage of a two-stage orchiopexy with spermatic vessel ligation is twofold: (1) to allow for development of the collateral blood supply to compensate for division of the main blood supply to the testis, and (2) to allow for greater mobility of the testis in order to place it within the scrotum (Elder, 1989, 1992b). The two-stage orchiopexy is typically performed by ligating the spermatic vessels in situ as close to the origin as possible, and then returning after 6 months or longer to complete the vasal-peritoneal pedicle mobilization using the standard Fowler-Stephens technique. Koff and Sethi (1996) reported excellent results with a technique of low spermatic vessel ligation and demonstrated that high ligation of the spermatic vessels does not need to be performed to preserve testicular viability.

MICROVASCULAR AUTOTRANSPLANTATION

The indications to perform autotransplantation of the intra-abdominal testis must be weighed in light of the circumstances of the clinical presentation; the indications are similar to those for a Fowler-Stephens orchiopexy. **An important consideration that weighs in favor of this procedure is the variability of collateral blood supply in patients with a high undescended testis that may potentially compromise the Fowler-Stephens procedure.** The results of testicular autotransplantation have been demonstrated to be superior to the predicted results reported with division of the spermatic vessels for the high intra-abdominal testis. The success of this technique is heavily dependent on microvascular expertise, which may not be universally available and most likely accounts for why this approach has not been more widely adopted.

Silber and Kelly (1976) first reported using a microvascular anastomosis to bring extra blood supply to the testicle after mobilization of a high intra-abdominal testicle in a child with prune-belly syndrome. Initial series were limited to older boys whose internal spermatic artery was large enough to be anastomosed to the inferior epigastric artery, but the technique was demonstrated to be successful in boys younger than 2 years of age (Harrison et al, 1990). Overall success rates are in excess of 80% (Wacksman et al, 1982; Bianchi, 1984; Harrison et al, 1990; Bukowski et al, 1995a, 1995b). Bukowski and associates (1995a) reported a 96% success rate for testicular autotransplantation over a 17-year period. Diagnostic laparoscopy is used in conjunction with autotransplantation to locate and assess the viability of the testis. Laparoscopically assisted testicular autotransplantation was reported to be successful in five children, with a median operative time of 5 hours (Wacksman et al, 1996). Therefore, microvascular testicular autotransplantation may be the procedure of choice for the solitary, high intra-abdominal testis, compared with an open or two-stage Fowler-Stephens approach.

Before surgery, hCG or testosterone can be given to increase vascular caliber. The procedure is performed through a Gibson incision that offers high intraperitoneal exposure. Donor vessel preparation requires 1 to 3 cm of the vessel to be dissected free of surrounding tissue for the anastomosis of the spermatic vessels to the ipsilateral inferior epigastric artery and vein. The spermatic vessels are mobilized proximally and are divided near their origin after the vas and its collateral vessels have been preserved and mobilized on a wide patch of peritoneum. Vascular spasm can be relieved with 1% lidocaine, and systemic anticoagulation with heparin may be used. Further preparation of the vessels and anastomoses are based on microvascular techniques. Fixation of the testis in the scrotum is performed by the dartos pouch method. Doppler ultrasound or radioactive isotope perfusion scanning can be used postoperatively to determine the patency of the anastomosis.

COMPLICATIONS OF ORCHIOPEXY

Complications of orchiopexy include testicular retraction, hematoma formation, ilioinguinal nerve injury, postoperative torsion (either iatrogenic or spontaneous), damage to the vas deferens, and testicular atrophy. Atrophy of the testis is the most devastating complication, but it is seldom seen with standard orchiopexies. Devascularization with atrophy of the testis can result from skeletonization of the cord, from overzealous electrocautery, from inadvertent torsion of the spermatic vessels during passage of the testis into the scrotum, or as a result of ligation and division of the spermatic vessels during a Fowler-Stephens orchiopexy. Devascularization may also be caused by excessive axial tension on the spermatic vessels, particularly if the collaterals are poor. Some degree of postoperative hematoma is common, but a large hematoma increases the risk of infection and abscess formation. Although retraction is usually caused by inadequate retroperitoneal dissection, insufficient cord length precludes successful orchiopexy no matter how much dissection is performed. If the patent processus vaginalis is ligated within the canal and not above the internal ring, the peritoneum remains adherent to the spermatic vessels, and complete retroperitoneal mobilization of vessels is not feasible.

HERNIAS AND HYDROCELES

The differential diagnosis of acute and chronic swelling of the inguinal and scrotal area is of daily concern to the urologist who deals with children. Although there has been a trend toward imaging of the groin in some circles, physical examination and a history of the clinical findings remain the hallmarks of physical diagnosis.

Hydrocele

As the testis descends into the scrotum from its abdominal position, it carries with it a tongue of peritoneum (the processus vaginalis). Normally, the processus is obliterated from the internal inguinal ring to the upper scrotum, leaving a small potential space in the scrotum that partially surrounds the testis. During the normal embryologic processes that involve descent of the testis and closure and obliteration of the processus vaginalis, a number of embryologic misadventures may occur that can result in commonly seen inguinal or scrotal pathology (hydrocele, hydrocele of the cord, and communicating hydrocele).

A simple (scrotal) hydrocele is an accumulation of fluid within the tunica vaginalis. All hydroceles in infants and children result from persistence of or delayed closure of the processus vaginalis. Simple hydroceles, in which the processus appears to be obliterated and fluid trapped within the tunica vaginalis of the scrotum persists, are commonly seen at birth, are frequently bilateral, and may be quite large. They transilluminate and may seem quite tense but are not painful. No fluid is evident in the groin in most cases, but occasionally a large, simple hydrocele extends toward the internal inguinal ring. Most simple scrotal hydroceles found at birth deserve long-term observation, and most resolve during the first 2 years of life. Aspiration of infant hydroceles is contraindicated because of the risk of infection, which, in the case of a patent processus, would extend into the peritoneal cavity. If surgical repair of an infant hydrocele is elected, an inguinal approach should be used in case a patent processus is encountered.

Communicating Hydrocele and Inguinal Hernia

Persistence of the processus vaginalis allows peritoneal fluid to freely communicate with the scrotal limits of the processus, and a communicating hydrocele results. **The classic description of a communicating hydrocele is that of a hydrocele that vacillates in size, usually related to activity.** Most communicating hydroceles are smaller in the morning and become more prominent as the day progresses, enlarging in response to the upright position, activities that increase intra-abdominal pressure, and, in many cases, fever. The scrotal swelling may be soft or tense, and it may change in consistency. In infants, the hydrocele sac may be thick or thin. Thin sacs frequently present a bluish hue through thin scrotal skin. Hydroceles easily transilluminate. Tense hydroceles may prohibit adequate palpation of the testis. Because most undescended testes are found at exploration to have an accompanying patent processus, it is important that a cryptorchid testis not be missed when assessing a child with a communicating hydrocele. Inguinal hernias represent the same anatomic defect that is seen in cases of communicating hydrocele. Small intestine, omentum, bladder, or genital contents may be found in the sac.

Communicating hydroceles may be diagnosed by history or by physical examination. If a scrotal hydrocele can be compressed and the fluid within the scrotum evacuated into the abdomen, a patent processus must be present. In many cases, however, the processus is small and it is not possible to express fluid out of the scrotum. In these cases, one must rely on the observations of the child's caretakers to determine whether a communication exists. In most cases, observation permits differentiation of simple from communicating hydroceles. On occasion, however, a hydrocele is explored because of the assumption that it communicates and is found to have an obliterated processus vaginalis.

Communicating hydroceles are by definition congenital in origin. However, it is not uncommon for a communicating hydrocele to manifest clinically for the first time in an older child or adolescent. In our experience, many of these late-onset communicating hydroceles are found to be omental hernias, in which descent of a plug of omentum through the internal inguinal ring has caused a sudden increase in the amount of fluid in the scrotum. In some of these cases, a palpable thickening in the inguinal canal may suggest the presence of entrapped omentum.

All communicating hydroceles should be explored through an inguinal incision. A small incision, 1 cm or less in length, placed in an inguinal skin crease, should be used. The subcutaneous tissue and Scarpa's fascia are incised. The cord structures may be isolated outside of the external inguinal ring in infants because of the very short oblique course of the inguinal canal; however, in most cases a short incision through the aponeurosis of the external oblique or through the external ring provides adequate access to the cord just below the internal inguinal ring. Once the cord structures have been isolated, the cremasteric fibers are spread to identify the shiny sac, which

should be located on the anteromedial aspect of the cord. The sac may be isolated from the cord structures or opened on its anterior wall, allowing the back wall to be dissected off the cord under direct vision. This technique is particularly appealing and offers safety to the cord structures when a very large sac is present. It is imperative that the sac is opened when the anatomy is confusing or when the sac is very thickened. Failure to do so may result in disastrous consequences if bowel, bladder, or ovary is contained in the sac and is not recognized.

Once the sac has been isolated from the cord structures, it should be divided distal to the internal ring. High ligation of the stump of the sac is then performed at the internal ring after the sac is twisted to strengthen it for suture ligation. If the internal ring is patulous, it may be tightened with one or two sutures, with care taken not to close it too tightly around the remaining cord structures. If the cord was pulled into the wound during the procedure, the testis should now be pulled back into the scrotum. The distal sac does not need to be completely removed. If fluid remains in the distal sac, the proximal portion of the distal hydrocele can be unroofed through the inguinal incision, or a small needle can be passed through the scrotum to aspirate the remaining fluid. If there is concern that the testis is not completely in the scrotum, a scrotal incision and orchidopexy are indicated. The external oblique, subcutaneous tissue, and dermis are then closed with absorbable sutures.

The quandary of whether to explore the asymptomatic contralateral inguinal canal in cases of inguinal hernia or communicating hydrocele in children has been a controversial topic since the 1950s. Several areas of concern are raised when this question is discussed, including the incidence of a contralateral patent processus vaginalis, the incidence of clinically apparent hernia or communicating hydrocele that develops after unilateral inguinal herniorrhaphy, and the potential for injury to the vas or testicular blood supply that is inherent in repair of an inguinal hernia. The incidence of patent processus vaginalis has been confirmed at exploration to be between 48% and 63% and varies with the age of the child (Rowe et al, 1969; Holder and Ashcraft, 1980). Rowe reviewed 1965 infants and children with a clinically unilateral hernia who underwent contralateral exploration, finding a patent processus in 46%, with an incidence of 63% in those younger than 2 months of age and 41% in those aged 2 to 16 years. These data must be considered in light of the much smaller incidence of contralateral clinical hernia and communicating hydrocele developing after unilateral inguinal herniorrhaphy. Sparkman (1962) analyzed data from seven studies and found the average incidence to be 15.8%, similar to the finding of 14.9% in the study by Bock and Sobye (1970) and 22% in the study by McGregor and colleagues (1980). In practice, the incidence of contralateral exploration has varied according to patient age from institution to institution. Wiener and coworkers (1996) surveyed the Surgery Section of the American Academy of Pediatrics in 1996 and found that open contralateral exploration was carried out in 65% of boys up to 2 years of age and in 84% of girls up to 4 years of age.

A concern was raised by Sparkman about the morbidity of contralateral inguinal exploration, which causes pathologically proven vas injury in 1.6% of patients. He postulated that the true incidence of vas injury might be much higher. With the advent of small laparoscopic instrumentation, evaluation of the contralateral internal inguinal ring can be performed endoscopically, a trend that has grown significantly over the past several years (DuBois et al, 1997; Gardner et al, 1998; Yerkes et al, 1998; Van Glabeke et al, 1999; Owings and Georgeson, 2000). This technique would seem to obviate any concerns about injury to the vas and vessels.

No consensus has been reached about either which technique to use or the age below which evaluation of the contralateral inguinal canal should be strongly considered in cases of clinically unilateral inguinal hernia or communicating hydrocele. However, it is important that the question of contralateral disease be addressed completely by both history and examination at the time of initial consultation. Any past or present history of contralateral inguinal or scrotal pathology should be considered an indication for contralateral evaluation at the time of herniorrhaphy. In addition, any child with ventriculoperitoneal shunt or other source of increased intraperitoneal fluid (e.g., peritoneal dialysis) should undergo bilateral exploration.

Hydrocele of the Cord

One of the vagaries of closure of the processus vaginalis that may occur is segmental closure of the processus, which leaves a loculated hydrocele of the cord that may or may not communicate with the peritoneal cavity (communicating hydrocele of the cord). Hydrocele of the cord usually presents as a painless groin mass contiguous with the cord structures and located at any position from just above the testis to the inguinal canal. The mass is mobile and transilluminates. The mass may vacillate in size when communication with the peritoneal cavity is present. Differential diagnosis of inguinal masses also includes sarcomas of the cord and paratesticular tissues and inguinal hernia (especially with impacted omentum). Inguinal exploration of hydrocele of the cord in most cases delineates a circumscribed, cystic mass connected to an obliterated or patent processus vaginalis. High ligation of a patent processus at the internal ring and excision or unroofing of the encysted hydrocele are curative.

Abdominoscrotal Hydrocele

Abdominoscrotal hydrocele is a rare clinical entity in which a large, bilobed hydrocele spans the internal inguinal ring, consisting of a large inguinoscrotal component and a large intra-abdominal component. It is thought that the abdominal component results from a large inguinoscrotal hydrocele that is separated from the peritoneal cavity by only a short obliterated segment at the internal ring. As fluid continues to accumulate, the hydrocele expands into the relatively low pressure of the abdominal cavity, forming the abdominal component (Gentile et al, 1998). Diagnosis is usually made on physical examination when a child with a large hydrocele presents with a palpable abdominal mass. Pressure on the abdominal mass usually results in an in-

Table 67–2. DIFFERENTIAL DIAGNOSIS OF THE ACUTE/SUBACUTE SCROTUM

Torsion of the spermatic cord
Torsion of the appendix testis
Torsion of the appendix epididymis
Epididymitis
Epididymo-orchitis
Inguinal hernia
Communicating hydrocele
Hydrocele
Hydrocele of the cord
Trauma/insect bite
Dermatologic lesions
Inflammatory vasculitis (Henoch-Schönlein purpura)
Idiopathic scrotal edema
Tumor
Spermatocele
Varicocele
Nonurogenital pathology (e.g., adductor tendinitis)

crease in size of the scrotal hydrocele. Ultrasound examination is definitive. At inguinal exploration, it is important to remove all of the abdominal component, which is advanced into the wound as the proximal end of the sac is dissected. Failure to recognize the abdominal component is a cause for recurrence.

ACUTE SCROTUM

The presentation of a child or adolescent with acute scrotal pain, tenderness, or swelling should be looked upon as an emergency situation requiring prompt evaluation, differential diagnosis, and potentially immediate surgical exploration. Adolescent males do not always understand the potential significance of acute scrotal conditions, and presentation in many cases is delayed. As a result, the presentation of a subacute or even chronic scrotal condition may in certain situations merit prompt evaluation and intervention.

Differential Diagnosis

The list of differential diagnoses for the acute scrotum is extensive. In all instances, it is imperative to rule out torsion of the spermatic cord, the clinical diagnosis requiring emergency surgical intervention (Table 67–2).

Torsion of the Spermatic Cord (Intravaginal)

Torsion of the spermatic cord is a true surgical emergency of the highest order. Irreversible ischemic injury to the testicular parenchyma may begin as soon as 4 hours after occlusion of the cord. Bartsch and colleagues (1980) demonstrated that, although testes operated on less than 8 hours after the onset of symptoms of torsion retained normal testis size and showed only slight changes in testicular morphology, only 50% of men whose testes were

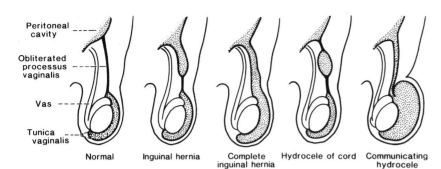

Peritoneal cavity

Obliterated processus vaginalis

Vas

Tunica vaginalis

Normal   Inguinal hernia   Complete inguinal hernia   Hydrocele of cord   Communicating hydrocele

Figure 67–8. Anomalies of the inguinal canal and scrotum that may result from anomalous closure of the processus vaginalis. (From Welch KA, Randolph JG, et al (eds): Pediatric Surgery, 4th ed, vol 2. St. Louis, Year Book Medical, 1986, p 780, with permission.)

detorsed less than 4 hours after symptoms began had normal semen analyses. It appears that the degree of torsion that occurs may have a significant influence on the potential for viability of the testis over time. The significance of this situation is magnified by the findings of Barada and coworkers (1989), who reported that patients younger than 18 years of age were more prone to testicular loss after acute torsion because of a median delay in presentation for medical attention of 20 hours after the onset of scrotal pain, an indication of the need for improved awareness of the significance of scrotal pain in adolescents.

Intravaginal torsion, or torsion of the cord within the space of the tunica vaginalis, may result from lack of normal fixation of an appropriate portion of the testis and epididymis to the fascial and muscular coverings that surround the cord within the scrotum. In effect, the normally segmental area of the free space between the parietal and visceral layers of the tunica vaginalis is expanded to surround the testis and epididymis and extends proximally up the cord for a variable distance. This creates an abnormally mobile testis that hangs freely within the tunical space (a "bell-clapper deformity") (Fig. 67–8).

Although torsion of the cord does occur in prepubertal males, it appears that the added weight of the testis after puberty adds a physical dimension that may be more likely to allow the testis to twist on its vascular stalk. Torsion can occur in relation to trauma or athletic activity, but in most cases spontaneous torsion of the cord is reported; in many cases the adolescent is awakened from sleep. It is thought that sudden contraction of the cremasteric muscle, which inserts onto the cord in a spiral configuration, is the inciting event in most cases, initiating a rotational effect on the testis as it is pulled upward. The cord may twist as many as several complete (360-degree) rotations.

The classic presentation of acute torsion of the spermatic cord is that of an acute onset of scrotal pain, but in some instances the onset appears to be more gradual, and in some boys the degree of pain is minimized. A large number of boys who present with acute scrotal pain give a history of prior episodes of severe, self-limited scrotal pain and swelling. It is likely that these represent prior episodes of intermittent torsion of the cord with spontaneous detorsion. Nausea and vomiting may accompany acute torsion, and some boys present with pain referred to the ipsilateral lower quadrant of the abdomen. Dysuria and other bladder symptoms are usually absent.

History is an important factor in the differential diagnosis of acute scrotum, but the physical examination may be perhaps even more crucial in determining whether the diagnosis is torsion of the cord or otherwise (i.e., whether the patient does or does not require immediate surgical exploration). Inspection of the genitalia may prove helpful if the affected testis is high-riding in the scrotum, perhaps indicating foreshortening of the spermatic cord as the result of twisting of the cord. In some cases, the affected testis has an abnormally transverse orientation, but in many cases, in particular when several hours have passed since onset, an acute hydrocele or massive scrotal edema obliterates all landmarks. **The absence of a cremasteric reflex is a good indicator of torsion of the cord.** Rabinowitz (1984) found 100% correlation between absence of a cremasteric reflex and the presence of torsion in 245 boys over a 7-year period. In some cases, the assessment of this physical finding is difficult. When the patient is cooperative enough to allow examination of the affected hemiscrotum, an effort should be made to assess anatomic landmarks, looking primarily for an appreciation of normal structures in an effort to identify a swollen and tender epididymis or a torsed appendix of the testis or epididymis. If torsion of the cord seems likely, manual detorsion should be attempted as a part of the initial examination, because the patient may be uncooperative to an extended examination because of discomfort. Classically, torsion of the cord occurs such that the anterior surface of each testis turns toward the midline as viewed from the patient's perspective (Sparks, 1971). To detorse the cord, a rotational effort should be made in the opposite direction. Kieslinger and associates (1984) described detorsion through two planes, with rotation in a caudal-to-cranial direction and simultaneous medial-to-lateral rotation. In actuality, the examiner should try to twist or "unscrew" the testis in one direction (usually outward, toward the thigh) and then in the opposite direction if the first attempt is unsuccessful. When detorsion is successful, the testis "flips" into a different rotation and pain relief may be almost instantaneous, with the cord appearing to lengthen and the testis dropping into the scrotum. **Manual detorsion may not totally correct the rotation that has occurred, and prompt exploration usually is still indicated.** However, when the patient becomes almost immediately comfortable, it can be assumed that blood flow to the testis has been restored, at least to a significant degree.

When the diagnosis of torsion of the cord is suspected, prompt surgical exploration is warranted. Although adjunctive tests are commonly used to aid in differential diagnosis of the acute scrotum, these are most appropriately used when their purpose is to confirm the absence of torsion of the cord in cases where surgical intervention is believed to be unnecessary.

Doppler examination of the cord and testis to determine whether blood flow is present was once touted as a helpful diagnostic test, but false-positive and false-negative results have led most examiners to abandon this technique. Color Doppler ultrasound examination has become the adjunctive investigation of choice in many institutions for the evaluation of both acute and chronic scrotal conditions. Color Doppler studies allow an assessment of anatomy (e.g., presence of a hydrocele, swollen epididymis) while determining the presence or absence of blood flow to the testis. Baker and associates (2000) showed that, in patients with acute scrotal swelling and an uncertain diagnosis, color Doppler examination had a diagnostic sensitivity of 88.9% and a specificity of 98.8%, with a 1% rate of false-positive results. Allen and Elder (1995), however, reported five cases in which color Doppler interpretations were inconsistent with findings at surgery. It is clear that, as in most clinical situations, ultrasound imaging is inherently operator dependent.

Radionuclide imaging, originally the study of choice for assessment of the acute scrotum, is more limited because it allows only an assessment of testicular blood flow (Kogan et al, 1979). Although Levy and associates (1983) found the study to have a positive predictive value of 75%, a sensitivity of 90%, and a specificity of 89%, false impression of blood flow may result from hyperemia of the scrotal wall. In addition, children with small scrotal sacs and testes that are not dependent may be difficult to image with radionuclide imaging techniques. In spite of these shortcomings, Paltiel and colleagues (1998) found the efficacy of color Doppler imaging and radionuclide imaging in the diagnosis of torsion of the spermatic cord in boys who presented with indeterminate clinical diagnoses to be equivocal. In most institutions, clinicians learn to place most trust in the imaging technique and in the radiographers with the most interest, experience, and reliability in differential diagnosis of the acute scrotum.

When surgical exploration is elected, it should be performed promptly. A median raphe scrotal incision may be used to explore both sides, or a transverse incision following the skin creases may be placed in each hemiscrotum. The separate incisions are more appropriate for dartos pouch placement of the testes. The affected side should be examined first. After the skin has been incised, a dartos pouch may be created into which the testis can later be placed; then the tunica vaginalis is entered and the testis is examined. The cord should be detorsed to re-establish blood flow to the testis. Testes with marginal viability should be placed in warm sponges and re-examined after several minutes. A necrotic testis should be removed by dividing the cord into two or three segments and doubly ligating each segment with silk suture. Testes with marginal viability may be preserved, although there has been some concern about "sympathetic orchiopathy" to the contralateral testis secondary to circulating antibodies released from the injured testis (Cosentino et al, 1985; Nagler and White, 1982). The validity of comparing animal studies with the human situation, however, has been called into question, and most urologists choose to preserve testes that seem marginally viable.

If the testis is to be preserved, it should be placed into the dartos pouch without suture fixation, as in most standard orchidopexy procedures. It has been shown experimentally that placing sutures through the tunica albuginea of the testis can produce local injury to the testis, and that suture fixation may be suboptimal when compared with the fixation offered by the dartos pouch placement (Bellinger et al, 1989). If suture fixation is elected, fine, nonreactive, nonabsorbable sutures should be used, and they should be placed so as to avoid superficial blood vessels on the surface of the testis. **When torsion of the spermatic cord is found, exploration of the contralateral hemiscrotum must be carried out. In almost all cases, a bell-clapper deformity is found. The contralateral testis must be fixed to prevent subsequent torsion.**

Intermittent Torsion of the Spermatic Cord

A significant percentage of adolescents who present with acute torsion of the spermatic cord give a history of prior episodes of acute, self-limited scrotal pain that appear clinically to have been episodes of intermittent torsion with spontaneous detorsion (Stillwell and Kramer, 1986). It is not uncommon to be asked to evaluate an adolescent for one or more episodes of acute scrotal pain that resolved spontaneously, was severe in nature, and in many cases was associated with vomiting or even a visit to the emergency room. At the time of evaluation a normal physical examination will be found. **If the suspicion is strong that episodes of intermittent torsion and spontaneous detorsion have occurred, our experience has been that the finding of a bell-clapper deformity at exploration can be expected. Elective scrotal exploration should be performed, and scrotal fixation of both testes should be performed when bell-clapper deformities are found.** The purpose of prophylactic fixation of the testes is to prevent an episode of torsion that might lead to testicular atrophy.

Torsion of the Testicular and Epididymal Appendages

The appendix testis, a müllerian duct remnant, and the appendix epididymis, a wolffian remnant, are prone to torsion in adolescence, presumably as a result of hormonal stimulation that increases their mass and makes them more likely to twist on the small vascular pedicle upon which they are based.

The presentation of torsion of an appendage is extremely variable, from an insidious onset of scrotal discomfort to an acute presentation identical to that seen with torsion of the cord. In this sense, torsion of an appendage and epididymitis might be difficult to distinguish clinically. When seen at an early stage, an adolescent with torsion of an appendage may present with localized tenderness of the upper pole of the testis or epididymis, where a tender nodule may be palpated. In some instances, the infarcted appendage is visible through the skin as a "blue dot sign" (Dresner, 1973). In cases in which inflammatory changes are more severe, scrotal wall edema and erythema may be severe. The cremasteric reflex should be present, and the testis should be mobile. Radionuclide scans or color Doppler studies may show normal or increased flow, and ultrasound imaging may delineate the swollen appendage.

When the diagnosis of a torsed appendage is confirmed clinically or by imaging, nonoperative management allows most cases to resolve spontaneously. Limitation of activity, administration of nonsteroidal anti-inflammatory agents, and observation allow most symptoms to subside as the acute changes of ischemic necrosis resolve. In an occasional clinical situation, acute exploration is performed because of suspicion of torsion of the cord, or delayed exploration is performed because of failure of spontaneous resolution of the inflammatory changes and discomfort. Simple excision of the torsed appendage in these cases is therapeutic.

Epididymitis

Inflammation or infection of the epididymis is an important part of the differential diagnosis of the acute scrotum. Epididymitis is reported to be a rare clinical diagnosis in the pediatric age group. Siegel and associates (1987) reported fewer than five cases per year at a major pediatric hospital, most documented at the time of scrotal exploration. Likitnukul and colleagues (1987) reported 35 cases in a 20-year retrospective review. The most common clinical symptoms at presentation are scrotal swelling, erythema, and pain; these symptoms are found equally in boys found subsequently to have anatomic anomalies of the urogenital system and in boys with normal anatomy. In fact, it appears that in many cases the diagnosis of epididymitis is a "wastebasket" diagnosis for patients without torsion of the spermatic cord who have swollen, painful scrotal contents. It is possible that some cases of appendage torsion, for example, are misdiagnosed as epididymitis. This results, in part, from the varied severity of presentation of the symptoms of epididymitis, from localized epididymal tenderness, to tenderness and swelling of the entire epididymis, to a massively inflamed hemiscrotum with absence of definable landmarks and increased blood flow on scrotal scintigraphy or color Doppler study.

The clinical presentation of epididymitis is classically described as an indolent process, in contrast to the rather acute onset of torsion of the spermatic cord. Adolescents, however, frequently present with a less easily categorized clinical distinction between the two entities. The presence of dysuria and fever is more common in the epididymitis group, although many boys with clinical epididymitis present have neither. A past history of urinary tract infections, urethritis, urethral discharge, sexual activity, urethral catheterization, or urinary tract surgery may indicate a higher likelihood of epididymitis. Epididymitis has also been associated with Henoch-Schönlein purpura, presumably on a systemic inflammatory basis, and has been noted in boys treated with the antiarrhythmic agent amiodarone (Hutcheson et al, 1998). Physical examination may reveal localized epididymal tenderness, a swollen and tender epididymis, or a massively swollen hemiscrotum with absence of landmarks. **The cremasteric reflex should be present in epididymitis, and its absence is highly suggestive of torsion of the spermatic cord;** however, it may be difficult to demonstrate in the acutely swollen scrotum of epididymitis (Rabinowitz, 1984).

The presence of pyuria, bacteriuria, or a positive urine culture is important evidence that epididymitis should be high on the list of differential diagnoses, although urine cultures may be sterile in 40% to 90% of patients. A normal urinalysis does not rule out epididymitis. Gram-negative bacteria is the most common finding in this age group (Likitnukul et al, 1987; Siegel et al, 1987). Our experience, in fact, would demonstrate that most boys with a clinical diagnosis of epididymitis have sterile urine (Gislason et al, 1980; Likitnukul et al, 1987; Siegel et al, 1987). Conversely, there is a low incidence of clinical epididymitis in patients who require nonsterile intermittent catheterization. Thirumavalavan and Ransley (1992) found the incidence in this group to be only about one episode of epididymitis per 10 patient-years. Bennett and colleagues (1998) documented a relationship between epididymitis in boys with infected urine and the presence of an uncircumcised penis.

Scrotal imaging may be an important part of making the diagnosis of epididymitis, and thus avoiding unnecessary surgery, especially in the patient with a massively swollen scrotum. Color flow Doppler and radionuclide imaging reveal increased blood flow; ultrasound may reveal a swollen testis or testis and epididymis, frequently with the presence of a hydrocele, which may contain echogenic debris when bacterial infection is present. In current practice, the trend toward imaging of the acute scrotum has made the finding of epididymitis at scrotal exploration less common.

Radiographic imaging of the urinary tract is commonly performed during follow-up of boys diagnosed with epididymitis. Likitnukul and coworkers (1987) found radiographic abnormalities in four of five such boys with positive urine cultures. These included urethral stricture, ureteral ectopia into the seminal vesicle, and reflux of contrast into the seminal vesicles in two patients. In Siegel's series, 47% of prepubertal boys with epididymitis were found to have radiographic abnormalities, including ectopia of the vasa or ureter and urethral anomalies, all having the common end result of predisposing the genital duct system to reflux of urine (Siegel et al, 1987). The younger the child with epididymitis, the more likely it is that a urinary tract infection, radiographic anomaly, or both will be found (Merlini et al, 1998). **Because the majority of boys with epididymitis have sterile urine and apparently radiographically normal urinary tracts, it would seem most appropriate to screen all boys with renal and bladder ultrasonography and to perform both ultrasound evaluation and voiding cystourethrography in prepubertal boys and those with positive urine cultures.** When epididymitis is diagnosed on color Doppler study, it is expeditious to proceed with imaging of the bladder and the upper urinary tract at the same sitting.

Epididymitis in adolescents should be treated aggressively, whether in an early or advanced stage. Because all boys with acute scrotal swelling of any cause will clinically worsen when allowed to resume normal activities, limitation of activity, especially that of a strenuous nature, should be enforced. In many cases, bed rest for 1 to 3 days results in a less protracted clinical course of pain and scrotal swelling. Following this period with a more extended course of relative restriction (sports, gymnastics) continues to promote resolution of scrotal swelling and discomfort. Scrotal elevation, the use of an athletic supporter, and the application of cold or warmth to the area may prove beneficial in reducing discomfort. Prompt and aggressive parenteral antibiotic therapy should be instituted when urinary tract infection is documented or suspected. Urethral instrumentation should be avoided if at all possible. After the acute episode has subsided, prophylactic antibiotic therapy should be continued until the voiding cystourethrogram is performed. In boys with sterile urine, the same limitations of physical activity should be imposed. Oral nonsteroidal anti-inflammatory agents may promote the resolution of inflammation.

Miscellaneous Causes of Acute Scrotal Swelling

Scrotal swelling, erythema, or pain may be initiated by lesions primary to the scrotal contents, the scrotal wall or skin, or the inguinal canal. On occasion, pain thought to originate in the scrotum is found to have an extrascrotal origin.

Acute idiopathic scrotal edema is a self-limited process of unknown cause that usually is not associated with scrotal erythema (Qvist, 1956). Fever is not present, and scrotal tenderness is usually minimal, but pruritus may be significant. Although the process is considered to be idiopathic, allergic or chemical dermatitis, insect bites, trauma, and other known potential causes of scrotal inflammation may be responsible but undiagnosed. Examination should include a complete assessment of the perineum and perianal region to rule out scrotal edema secondary to a contiguous process (e.g., perirectal abscess). In most cases, the scrotal wall is thickened but the testes can be palpated. When doubt about the cause of scrotal edema exists, ultrasound evaluation with color flow Doppler should be performed. No therapy is indicated.

Henoch-Schönlein purpura is a systemic vasculitis that can cause scrotal swelling secondary to involvement of the testis, epididymis, or both (Clark and Kramer, 1986). The cause of vasculitis is unknown. The purpura is a nonthrombocytopenic process that may manifest with abdominal and joint pain, nephritis and hematuria, and skin lesions. Scrotal involvement is merely a part of the systemic presentation; it is seen in up to 35% of patients. Scrotal findings are generally diffuse, with swelling, erythema, and tenderness. Urinalysis may demonstrate hematuria and proteinuria. Color Doppler study or scintigraphy shows increased blood flow. Observation of the scrotal findings is a part of managing the systemic symptom complex, which is usually a self-limited process.

Perinatal Torsion of the Spermatic Cord

Torsion of the spermatic cord may occur prenatally (months, weeks, or days before birth or during the process of labor) or in the immediate postnatal period. **Although the term *perinatal torsion* has been used to group both prenatal and postnatal torsion into a single clinical diagnosis, they in fact may represent distinctly different pathophysiologic processes that should be approached very differently.** The major points of contention that arise when perinatal torsion is discussed are the utility of prompt surgical exploration and the need for contralateral scrotal exploration.

Prenatal (in utero) torsion is typified by the finding at delivery of a hard, nontender testis fixed to the overlying scrotal skin. The skin is commonly discolored by the underlying hemorrhagic necrosis. This clinical scenario is pathognomonic of a resolving infarction process, the acute phase of which occurred before delivery. Pathologic examination of testes that have undergone prenatal torsion reveals that, in most cases, extravaginal torsion (torsion of the cord and its tunics) has occurred. Duckett (1991) argued that the incidence of prenatal torsion is probably much higher than is usually quoted. He postulated that the blind-ending spermatic cord ("vanishing testis") discovered on exploration for a nonpalpable testis is in many cases the result of antenatal torsion. This thought is corroborated by the common finding of hemosiderin in the pathologic examination of the distal sections of blind-ending spermatic cords removed surgically. Prenatal torsion may merely be a late gestational representation of the same process that, if it had occurred earlier, would have produced a blind-ending spermatic cord (Duckett, 1991).

Classic teaching has held that testes found to be hard, nontender, and fixed to the skin at birth do not merit surgical exploration because of the delayed nature of the pathologic process at the time of presentation. In fact, the reported salvage rates of testes presumed torsed before birth is negligible. Despite prompt exploration, Brandt found no salvageable testes in 25 explorations, a finding confirmed by others (Brandt et al, 1992; Stone et al, 1995). However, controversy has arisen regarding the need for prompt exploration of the contralateral testis.

Contralateral scrotal exploration traditionally has not been recommended in cases of prenatal torsion because extravaginal torsion is not associated with the testicular fixation defect (bell-clapper deformity) that is recognized as the cause of intravaginal torsion. However, reports of asynchronous perinatal torsion have made the practice of avoiding prompt surgical exploration of the contralateral testis controversial (Olguner et al, 2000).

The postnatal presentation of acute scrotal swelling may present a problem for the urologist who is unsure of whether the process is truly a prenatal or a postnatal event. Postnatal torsion is usually associated with swelling and tenderness of the scrotum. Fixation of the skin usually is not present. Burge (1987) described 30 infants with acute scrotal swelling, 18 of whom underwent prompt surgical exploration. Ten were found to have extravaginal torsion, 3 had intravaginal torsion, 2 had torsion of an appendix testis, 1 had torsion of an undescended testis, and 1 had a normal testis. Pinto and coworkers (1987) described salvage of 2 of 10 testes explored within 6 hours of discovery. Diagnosis may be aided by color flow Doppler examination, even in small neonates (Stone et al, 1995).

Prompt exploration of suspected postnatal torsion of the spermatic cord is indicated (in conjunction with exploration of the contralateral testis) when the patient's general condition and anesthetic considerations

allow for a safe procedure. The 17% incidence of bell-clapper deformity and the 20% incidence of salvage of a solitary contralateral testis (prevention of anorchia) must be weighed against the risk of general anesthesia for neonates. Tiret and associates (1988) reported the incidence of major anesthetic-related complications in children older than 1 year of age to be 0.5 in 1000, and in those younger than 1 year it was 0.7 in 1000. Mortality occurred in 1 of 40,000 anethesias. Others showed that the incidence of intraoperative and postoperative complications was greatest in infants younger than 1 month of age (Cohen et al, 1990). Clearly, the decision to subject a neonate with suspected torsion of the spermatic cord to surgery should be carefully considered, weighing the clinical assessment of the acuity of the torsion episode, the risk to the contralateral testis, and the risk of general anesthesia. The decision may be even more difficult when the neonate is located at a distance from a tertiary referral center that can offer skilled pediatric anesthesia, because both the risk of neonatal transport and the time lost in transport may be critical if acute postnatal torsion is to be salvaged. **Clearly, if the cause of scrotal swelling appears to be related to an acute postnatal event, all efforts should be made to pursue prompt surgical intervention.**

Exploration, when elected, should be carried out through an inguinal incision to allow for the most efficacious treatment of other potential or unexpected causes of scrotal swelling. **If torsion is confirmed, contralateral scrotal exploration with testicular fixation should be carried out** (Bellinger, 1985). The most effective and safest form of testicular fixation involves dartos pouch placement (Bellinger et al, 1989).

VARICOCELE

Dilated and tortuous veins of the pampiniform plexus of the spermatic cord are found in approximately 15% of male adolescents, with a marked left-sided predominance (Steeno et al, 1976). It was documented in the 1880s that varicoceles predominated on the left side, were rarely observed before puberty, and were in some cases associated with ipsilateral testicular volume loss that appeared to be reversible in some instances after varicocele ligation (Barwell, 1885). In fact, Bennett in 1889 described improved seminal fluid after varicocele ablation. **Varicoceles rarely become clinically evident before early adolescence. Once present, they are not thought to regress. Because varicoceles rarely have been reported to arise in older men, it seems that the population of boys with varicoceles probably represents the population of adults who will have varicoceles.** The prevalence of varicocele in adolescence, the association of varicocele with male infertility, and the improvement in semen quality that may be seen in infertile men after varicocele ligation have brought increased interest to the study of the adolescent varicocele and its associated spermatogenic dysfunction.

Anatomy

Approximately 90% of varicoceles are left-sided. **Because retrograde flow of blood in the internal spermatic vein is responsible for venous dilation and tortuosity, differences in the configuration of the right and left internal spermatic veins and their embryologic origins are thought to contribute to this marked left-sided predominance.** The left spermatic vein enters the left renal vein at a right angle, rather than entering obliquely into the vena cava as the right internal spermatic vein does. The insertion of the left renal vein into the vena cava is 8 to 10 cm more craniad than the insertion of the right internal spermatic vein. As a result, the left internal spermatic vein has an 8- to 10-cm greater head of pressure, and its effluent faces a relatively slower flow of blood.

Etiology

Varicocele formation has been attributed to one of three primary factors: increased venous pressure in the left renal vein, collateral venous anastomoses, and incompetent valves of the internal spermatic vein. Increased venous pressure may be attributed to one of several factors, including a proximal "nutcracker" phenomenon (caused by compression of the left renal vein between the aorta and the superior mesenteric artery); a distal "nutcracker" effect described by Coolsaet (compression of the left common iliac vein by the common iliac artery, which results in retrograde flow via the deferential and external spermatic veins); and anomalies of the left renal vein (Coolsaet et al, 1980). Collateral venous channels have been demonstrated by venography in patients undergoing sclerotherapy. These are thought in most cases to represent persistent intercardinal anastomoses, which are a result of disordered involution of the embryonic venous channels that normally regress to form the inferior vena cava (Braedel et al, 1994). **Absence or incompetence of valves in the proximal internal spermatic vein are probably responsible for varicocele formation in the majority of cases, with left-sided predominance in part caused by the higher venous pressures in the left internal spermatic venous system.**

Pathophysiology

Although varicoceles are commonly discovered for the first time in adolescence, the pathophysiology of varix formation remains the subject of conjecture. Oster (1971) surveyed 1072 schoolboys and found the incidence of varicocele to be 0% in those younger than 10 years of age and 16.2% in those aged 10 to 19 years. Other studies have estimated the incidence between 10 and 17 years of age to be between 9% and 25.8%, with an incidence in adulthood of approximately 15% (Skoog et al, 1997). However, because most adolescent varicoceles are asymptomatic and many are discovered on routine physical examination, the true incidence of adolescent varicocele is likely to be much higher than expected, especially in later adolescence. The pathophysiology of adolescent varicocele may be multifactorial, but some consider that normal physiologic changes that occur during puberty and result in increased testicular blood flow might expose underlying venous anomalies to overperfusion and cause venous ectasia to become clinically evident.

Pathology of Testicular Dysfunction

The presence of a varicocele is known to be associated with an adverse effect on spermatogenesis in a subset of men. The pathophysiology of this testicular dysfunction has been attributed to one or a combination of several mechanisms, including reflux of adrenal metabolites, hyperthermia, hypoxia, local testicular hormonal imbalance, and intratesticular hyperperfusion injury. Concrete evidence remains elusive in both clinical and laboratory investigations. Harrison created varicoceles in monkeys and in a subset of animals performed simultaneous ipsilateral adrenalectomy. No differences in testicular histology were noted in either group, suggesting absence of a role for adrenal metabolites in testicular dysfunction (Harrison et al, 1969). Similarly, it was shown that serum levels of testosterone in both peripheral and internal spermatic venous blood of patients with varicoceles and in normal controls are not significantly different (Ando et al, 1985). The possible role of testicular hypoxia in spermatogenic dysfunction was investigated independently by Donohue and Brown (1969) and by Netto and colleagues (1977), with both studies failing to find evidence to support a causal relationship.

Normal arterial and venous flow to and from the testis is such that the veins exiting from the tunica albuginea disperse into an intercommunicating mesh of veins (the pampiniform plexus), which encircles the arteries and supplies the testes as they pass through the inguinal canal into the scrotum. It is thought that this normal anatomic arrangement produces an effective countercurrent heat-exchange mechanism that permits arterial blood to be cooled from intra-abdominal temperature to the cooler temperature found in the scrotum. The presence of varicosities impedes this countercurrent exchange mechanism, and this is perhaps a critical alteration in normal homeostasis, because it is considered that elevated scrotal temperature associated with varicocele formation can inhibit spermatogenesis. Zorgnotti and MacLeod (1973) compared scrotal temperatures in oligospermic men with varicocele with those in controls and found lower intrascrotal temperature in the control group, as well as in a group of infertile men without varicocele. Agger (1971) subsequently found a correlation between improved scrotal temperature and improved sperm count after varicocele ablation. Green and Turner (1984) independently studied laboratory preparations of varicocele in animals and concluded that increased intratesticular microvascular blood flow induced by varicocele induction was associated with histologic changes and elevated intratesticular temperatures that mimicked the changes seen in idiopathic human varicocele. It has been postulated that abnormal elevation of microvascular blood flow and intratesticular temperature produces increases phosphorylase activity and metabolism, which acts to deplete intracellular glycogen stores and thereby induces testicular parenchymal injury (Gorelick and Goldstein, 1992). In addition, germ cell enzymes involved in DNA recombination and polymerase activity function optimally at 33° to 34°C and are inhibited at higher temperatures (Fujisawa and Yoshida, 1988).

Toxic effect of varicocele may manifest as testicular growth failure, semen abnormalities, Leydig cell dysfunction, and histologic changes (tubular thickening, interstitial fibrosis, decreased spermatogenesis, maturation arrest). Lyon and Marshall (1982) found ipsilateral volume loss in 77% of testes associated with a varicocele; this was confirmed by Steeno (1991), who documented diminished ipsilateral volume loss in 34.4% of boys with a grade 2 varicocele and in 81.2% of boys with a grade 3 varicocele. Because testis volume increases rapidly during adolescence, it should not be surprising that differences in testis size are most easily appreciated in teenagers. This ipsilateral growth failure is reversible in some cases after varicocele ablation.

Because the rapid increase in testis volume in adolescence is in part caused by an increase in seminiferous tubule diameter and an increase in germ cell number, it is not surprising that testicular growth failure secondary to varicocele may be associated with a decrease in sperm count. **Semen analysis is rarely performed in adolescents, and the utility of this most important measure of varicocele effect is limited when the effect of varicocele on the adolescent testis is analyzed. As a result, testis volume, a much less precise and more end-stage manifestation of orchiopathy, is used to guide therapy.**

Leydig cell dysfunction in patients with varicocele may be in part caused by diminished intratesticular testosterone levels, but serum levels of FSH, LH, and testosterone are not predictably abnormal, and normal peripheral blood levels of these hormones cannot exclude the possibility that Leydig cell dysfunction exists (Su and Goldstein, 1995). Castro-Magana and colleagues (1990) found exaggerated LH and FSH levels in adolescents with unilateral varicocele after stimulation with GnRH and testosterone and concluded that normalization of gonadotropin and testosterone responses to GnRH stimulation occurred after varicocele ablation in boys whose testis biopsies demonstrated no histologic abnormalities. Kass, however, measured the gonadotropin response pattern in 53 adolescents and found that an abnormal response paralleled a finding of ipsilateral testicular volume loss, concluding that increased serum FSH and LH levels after gonadotropin stimulation may indicate an irreversible testicular parenchymal injury to both Leydig cells and germinal epithelium (Kass et al, 1993). Hudson and Perez-Marrero (1985) confirmed these findings, showing that exaggerated gonadotropin response to GnRH stimulation correlated with abnormal sperm density.

Histologic evaluation of the testes in men with unilateral varicocele and infertility may show bilateral findings that include decreased spermatogenesis, maturation arrest, and tubular thickening. In addition, Leydig cell abnormalities may be found, ranging from atrophy to hyperplasia. These findings are present in both testes and are more pronounced on the side ipsilateral to the varicocele. Hadziselimovic (1986) studied bilateral testis biopsies in adolescents with unilateral varicocele. Histologic findings in the seminiferous tubules included impaired spermatogenesis and varying degrees of degenerative changes in the Sertoli cells. When changes in the Sertoli cells were not irreversible, Leydig cell atrophy was present. However, when Leydig cell hyperplasia was found, irreversible Sertoli cell damage was seen. Hadziselimovic concluded that normal testicular histology was seen in all boys younger than 13 years of age. Abnormal histologic findings, when present, were found in both testes but were more pronounced ipsilateral to the varicocele. Leydig cell atrophy was invariably present, with Leydig cell hyperplasia uncommon.

Clinical Presentation

Because adolescent varicocele is usually asymptomatic, many are discovered on routine physical examinations performed for school entry, driver's license examinations, or preseason sports participation. In large part because of dissemination of information regarding self-examination for the detection of testicular cancer, an increasing number of adolescents have sought medical evaluation because of self-discovered scrotal masses. Many scrotal masses of unknown origin referred from primary care physicians are found to be varicoceles. Inguinal hernia, communicating hydrocele, omental hernia, hydrocele of the cord, epididymal cyst (spermatocele), and scrotal hydrocele are common differential diagnoses for such generally painless scrotal masses in adolescents. Rarely, an adolescent seeks evaluation for a painful varicocele, usually one that is symptomatic with inguinal or scrotal aching discomfort that in many cases is relieved by assuming the supine position.

Physical examination should be carried out in a warm room with the patient in both the supine and standing positions and with and without a Valsalva maneuver. Failure to use the standing position or Valsalva may result in missing some cases of varicocele. A varicocele presents as a painless, compressible mass above and in some cases surrounding the testis. The classic description of the varices is the consistency of a "bag of worms" that decompresses when the patient is in the supine position. Varicoceles have been graded based on physical characteristics: grade III (large, visible through the scrotal skin); grade II (moderate-sized, easily palpable without Valsalva); and grade I (small, palpable only with Valsalva). Bilateral varicoceles are palpable in fewer than 2% of males.

A crucial part of the physical examination of all boys with varicocele is an accurate assessment of testicular volume and consistency. Although the assessment of testicular consistency (firmness) is extremely subjective, measurement of testis volume can be accurately and reproducibly assessed by the use of either a Prader or disk orchidometer (Nagu and Takahira, 1979). In standard practice, the volume of the left testis is compared with that of the right. Behre and Nashan (1991) showed that the measurement of testis volume by ultrasound offers little practical advantage and significant expense when compared with orchidometer measurement.

Adjunctive Assessment

The assessment of subclinical varicocele by Doppler examination does not have a role in adolescent varicocele evaluation, primarily because the significance of subclinical varicocele in adolescents is unknown. Although Kass (1990) found an exaggerated response to GnRH stimulation in 43% of adolescents with grade II or III varicocele independent of testicular volume differential, the relation between GnRH stimulation testing and future fertility issues in adolescents remains unclear. Carillo and coauthors (1996) studied nine boys and found four with an exaggerated response to GnRH stimulation. They also measured levels of inhibin B but failed to find a correlation with varicocele size or laterality or with asymmetry in testicular volume. It appears that few pediatric urologists rely on hormonal stimulation as a basis for determination of which patients should undergo varicocele ablation.

Varicocele Ablation: Treatment Considerations

Few studies are available regarding the effect of varicocele on semen analysis in adolescents. Paduch and Niedzielski (1996) compared 36 boys without varicocele to 38 boys with varicocele and found statistically significant differences in sperm motility and viability and total sperm count between the two groups, indicating that varicocele does have a noxious effect on semen parameters in adolescents. Because semen analysis in adolescent boys is not usually considered practical from a psychological and ethical point of view, and because of the lack of widespread acceptance of hormonal stimulation testing, testis volume measurements have become the mainstay of assessment of whether surgical indication is appropriate. Volume determinations may be aided by the use of a Prader orchidometer or a disk orchidometer, as described by Nagu and Takahira (1979). Although volume measurements, even when aided with the use of an orchidometer, are somewhat subjective, they appear to be reproducible in the hands of an experienced examiner. **In adults and adolescents, testis size (volume) should be approximately equal bilaterally, with the differential normally not greater than 2 ml or 20% of volume** (Kass, 1990). When the testis ipsilateral to a varicocele varies by more than this differential, many examiners believe that varicocele ablation is indicated, in a large part because catch-up growth has been reported after varicocele ablation in adolescents.

Ipsilateral testis catch-up growth after varicocele ablation has been evaluated by several observers. Kass and Belman (1987) studied 20 adolescents with grade II or III varicocele and ipsilateral testicular volume loss averaging 70%. At an average interval of 3.3 years after varicocele ligation, a statistically significant increase in testis volume (50% to 104%; average, 91%) was found in 16 of the 20 patients. The remaining 4 patients had an ipsilateral testis volume increase that was not statistically significant. Gershbein and associates (1999) retrospectively studied 42 patients (average age, 14.7 years) with palpable varicoceles at least 6 months after ligation (average follow-up, 22.6 months). Preoperatively, 54.8% had a small ipsilateral testis. Postoperatively, 38% developed left testicular hypertrophy (testis volume at least 10% greater than that of the contralateral side). Although not statistically significant, the hypertrophy was found to be more common in the younger boys and in those with smaller varicoceles. Further data, perhaps from a prospective multicenter study, is needed to sort out the specifics of patient age, varicocele size, and the potential for reversibility of testicular volume loss as related to GnRH stimulation and future semen parameters. Until such data are available, **it appears that an ipsilateral testis volume loss greater than 2 ml is a reasonable criterion to use as an indicator for adolescent varicocele ablation, offering expected improvement in testis volume to a majority of those undergoing ablation.**

Treatment Alternatives

When varicocele ablation is determined to be appropriate, several therapeutic options must be considered. Because most of the available techniques for varicocele ablation have proved to have very nearly the same efficacy, it is imperative that the relative advantages and disadvantages of each technique be reviewed with particular attention to the unique circumstances posed by adolescents. Currently, it appears that multiple different techniques are applied clinically, with the choice of technique guided by the experience of the surgeon and taking into account the age, body habitus, and peculiarities of the patient and varicocele in question.

Retroperitoneal and Laparoscopic Ligation

Retroperitoneal ligation of the internal spermatic vein, described by Palomo in 1949, remains a commonly used technique for varicocele ablation in adolescents, in part because of a relatively short operative time and quick recovery. The procedure is commonly performed with the adolescent under general anesthesia in an outpatient setting. A small (1.5-inch) muscle-splitting incision is made at the level of the anterior superior iliac spine, and the retroperitoneal space is entered, with the peritoneal envelope swept medially to identify the internal spermatic vessels. At this level, the testicular artery and a single vein or a small number of veins may be present. Ligation is performed, the wound is closed with running absorbable sutures, a local anesthetic is infiltrated, and the patient is discharged soon after the procedure. Retroperitoneal ligation may be performed with mass ligation of the spermatic vessels or by an artery-sparing technique. Preservation of the artery can be difficult to accomplish in adolescents even with the assistance of optical magnification, owing to both the small size of the testicular artery and the small size and rather deep dissection that is encountered during this technique. Kass and Marcol (1992) found no recurrences when the mass ligation technique was used but an 11% incidence of persistent varicocele when testicular artery sparing was attempted.

Laparoscopic varicocele ligation is a technique that is easily mastered by surgeons familiar with laparoscopic technique and is in many ways similar to open retroperitoneal ligation of the internal spermatic vein. Mandressi compared open versus laparoscopic techniques in adults and concluded that laparoscopic varix ligation was much more costly than open techniques because of the added equipment and operating room time, although hospitalization was briefer. The conclusion was that there was little indication to use laparoscopy (Mandressi et al, 1996). Ogura and colleagues (1994) found a similar diminution in recovery time in adults. Ulker and associates (1997) found the laparoscopic technique to be superior for preservation of the testicular artery.

Inguinal Ligation and Subinguinal Ligation

Inguinal ligation (opening of the external oblique aponeurosis) is performed through a small incision over the inguinal canal that follows the skin lines. The inguinal canal is opened through the external inguinal ring along the direction of the fascial fibers to gain access to the cord just below the internal ring. The cord is isolated over a Penrose drain, excluding the ilioinguinal nerve, and is delivered into the wound. With optical magnification and the help of Doppler ultrasound, the testicular artery should be located and preserved. The veins of the cord, except those associated with the vas, are doubly ligated with 4-0 silk and divided. Attention should be paid to lymphatic vessels, which should be preserved when possible. The inguinal approach is best avoided when a prior inguinal surgical procedure has been performed.

The subinguinal approach involves a transverse skin fold incision below the inguinal ring at about the level of the pubic tubercle, with isolation and delivery of the testis as in the inguinal approach. The inguinal canal is not opened. At this level, a larger number of veins will be encountered and the testicular artery may be more difficult to identify. Dissection of the cord should follow the technique described for dissection within the inguinal canal. When either the inguinal or the subinguinal approach is used, a cord block or caudal block may provide adequate postoperative analgesia (Ogura et al, 1994).

When using the inguinal or subinguinal approach for varicocele ablation, several adjunctive techniques may be considered that have been reported to improve results in several series. Doppler identification of the testicular artery is an important adjunct. Goldstein and coworkers (1992) reported that delivery of the testis out of the wound allows improved access for ligation of external spermatic and gubernacular vessels, thought to be avenues of persistent venous drainage in some cases of persistent or recurrent varicocele. Lemack and colleagues (1998), in addition to delivering the testis for ligation of the cremasteric and gubernacular vessels, performed microsurgical ligation of the spermatic veins, a technique that has become standard in the practice of many adult fertility specialists and that seems to minimize the potential for recurrence. Intraoperative spermatic venography has been reported to improve the success of varicocele ablation in adolescents (Levitt et al, 1987; Hart et al, 1992).

Transvenous Occlusion

Interventional radiographic techniques typically involve transfemoral access to the spermatic vein for venography and embolization, with the use of detachable balloons or steel coils to accomplish venous occlusion. Although trans-

Table 67–3. OUTCOME OF VARICOCELE ABLATION PROCEDURES

Technique	Hydrocele	Recurrence or Failure
Open inguinal/subinguinal	3%–9%	15% average
Microscopic inguinal/subinguinal	<1%	1%–3%
Retroperitoneal mass ligation	7.2%	2%
Retroperitoneal artery sparing	<7.2%	11%
Laparoscopic	Similar to open	Similar to open
Embolization	None	10%–25%

venous embolization in adults can often be carried out under local anesthesia, adolescents usually require general anesthesia and the procedures may take several hours to complete. In addition, the relatively small caliber of the adolescent venous system makes the potential for vascular complications higher in this age group.

Comparison of Techniques and Complication Rates

The potential complications of varicocelectomy of primary concern are hydrocele formation, varicocele recurrence (failure to decompress the varicocele), and testicular infarction (atrophy). Hydrocele formation is related to failure to preserve spermatic vessels associated with the spermatic cord and its vessels. Hydrocele formation seems most common after retroperitoneal ligation, especially when a mass ligation technique is used, and it is least likely to occur after transvenous embolization. Failure to decompress a varicocele or recurrence appears to be minimized by microsurgical ligation. Table 67–3 compares the success and complication rates of the various varicocele ablation procedures.

Conclusion

Adolescent varicocele presents the urologist with many dilemmas, including questions about the necessity of intervention, the timing of intervention, and the method of intervention. It is hoped that further studies will clarify some of the answers to these uncertainties.

CONGENITAL ANOMALIES OF THE VAS DEFERENS, SEMINAL VESICLES, AND EPIDIDYMIS

The closely parallel development of the müllerian and wolffian ducts and the structures that derive from them invites the formation of a wide spectrum of congenital anomalies of the lower genital and urinary tracts. Congenital anomalies of the vas deferens, seminal vesicles, epididymis, and lower urinary tract are encountered with regularity in both adult and pediatric urologic practices. It is not feasible to catalog every known congenital anomaly of the genital ducts because of the infinite number of variations that may present clinically. However, an appreciation of

the broad categorization of the potential embryologic misadventures involved in various clinical scenarios will promote optimal evaluation and management of each case.

Agenesis of the Vas Deferens

Agenesis of the vas deferens may occur unilaterally or bilaterally. Bilateral agenesis has been closely associated with cystic fibrosis, occurring in 65% to 95% of men with the disease (Vohra and Morgentaler, 1997). The relationship between cystic fibrosis and vasal anomalies appears to be related to the cystic fibrosis transmembrane conductance regulator (CFTR) gene, mutations of which may result in cystic fibrosis, unilateral absence of the vas, bilateral absence of the vas, unilateral or bilateral absence of the ejaculatory duct, or unilateral or bilateral epididymal obstruction (Stuhrmann and Dork, 2000). In fact, it has been suggested that all men with idiopathic obstructive azoospermia deserve genetic counseling and molecular genetic analysis of the CFTR gene. Bilateral agenesis of the vas results in infertility, whereas unilateral agenesis may be clinically inconsequential.

Agenesis of the vas deferens may be associated with unilateral or bilateral hypoplasia or absence of other portions of the wolffian duct derivatives. In the presence of unilateral agenesis of the vas, 75% of patients have only the caput of the epididymis present, 20% have no ipsilateral epididymis; 86% have ipsilateral agenesis of the seminal vesicle, and 20% have bilateral seminal vesicle agenesis. In bilateral vas agenesis, 68% have absence of a portion of the epididymis bilaterally, and approximately 45% have seminal vesical absence (Schlegel et al, 1996). **Men with vasal agenesis should be screened with renal ultrasonography.** In men with bilateral vas agenesis, the incidence of renal anomalies is 14% to 21%, and in men with unilateral agenesis, it is 26% to 79%. The most common renal anomaly found is unilateral renal agenesis.

Persisting Mesonephric Duct

The term *persisting mesonephric duct* was first used by Schwarz and Stephens (1978) to describe junction of the vas and ureter. In reality, this anomaly probably represents failure of incorporation of the distal mesonephric duct into the urogenital sinus and subsequent separation of the ureteral bud from the mesonephric (wolffian) duct. In most cases the ipsilateral kidney is poorly functioning, and in many cases renal dysplasia is found. Boys with persisting mesonephric duct may present with urinary tract infection or epididymitis. Persisting mesonephric duct syndrome has been associated with imperforate anus (Vordermark, 1983). The focus of surgical intervention depends primarily on the function in the unilateral kidney.

Epididymal Attachment Anomalies

Anomalies of attachment of the epididymis to the testis are commonly described at orchiopexy. Gill and associates (1989) described two classes of anomaly: fusion anomalies that cause the caput epididymis to be detached from the testis, and suspension anomalies in which other segments of the epididymis are poorly attached to the body of the testis. Elder (1992a) reported similar anomalies in 31% of boys after exploration for repair of an inguinal hernia or communicating hydrocele. Although some of these anomalies have implications regarding fertility, some are clinically insignificant and might in many cases be merely normal variants. It has been postulated that epididymal anomalies seen in association with cryptorchidism may indicate a role for the epididymis in testicular descent (Elder, 1992a).

Epididymal Cyst (Spermatocele)

Epididymal cysts are usually asymptomatic, and in adolescents they are often found on routine physical examination, in many cases a preparticipation sports-related examination. Increased awareness of the importance of testicular self-examination in adolescents has made self-discovery an important contribution to the diagnosis of spermatocele. Patients with von-Hippel-Lindau disease have an increased incidence of epididymal cysts, as do the offspring of women treated with DES (Vohra and Morgentaler, 1997).

Epididymal cysts are smooth, spherical, and in many cases located at the head of the epididymis. Although most cysts are small, on occasion a large cyst or one that has gradually enlarged is identified. The cysts transilluminate. Usually, physical examination is sufficient to differentiate an epididymal cyst from other scrotal pathology. Scrotal ultrasound has proved successful in the differential diagnosis of scrotal masses in children and adolescents (Finkelstein et al, 1986). Surgical excision of epididymal cysts may be performed if continued enlargement of the cysts or pain occurs. However, long-term observation has shown that in most cases intervention is unnecessary.

REFERENCES

Abe T, Aoyama K, Gotoh T, et al: Cranial attachment of the gubernaculum associated with undescended testes. J Pediatr Surg 1996;31:652–655.

Abratt RP, Reddi VB, Sarembock LA: Testicular cancer and cryptorchidism. Br J Urol 1992;70:656–659.

Adamsen S, Aronson S, Borjesson B: Prospective evaluation of human chorionic gonadotropin in the treatment of cryptorchidism. Acta Chir Scand 1989;155:509–514.

Agger P: Scrotal and testicular temperature: its relation to sperm count before and after operation for varicocele. Fertil Steril 1971;22:286–297.

Ahmed SF, Cheng A, Dovey L, et al: Phenotypic features, androgen receptor binding, and mutational analysis in 278 clinical cases reported as androgen insensitivity syndrome. J Clin Endocrinol Metab 2000;85:658–665.

Akre O, Lipworth L, Cnattingius S, et al: Risk factor patterns for cryptorchidism and hypospadias (see comments). Epidemiology 1999;10:364–369.

Allen TD, Elder JS: Shortcomings of color Doppler sonography in the diagnosis of testicular torsion. J Urol 1995;154:1508–1510.

Andersson S, Geissler WM, Wu L, et al: Molecular genetics and pathophysiology of 17 beta-hydroxysteroid dehydrogenase 3 deficiency. J Clin Endocrinol Metab 1996;81:130–136.

Ando S, Giacchetto C, Beraldi E, et al: Progesterone, 17-OH-progesterone, androstenedione and testosterone plasma levels in spermatic venous blood of normal men and varicocele patients. Horm Metab Res 1985;17:99–103.

Attah AA, Hutson JM: The role of intra-abdominal pressure in cryptorchidism. J Urol 1993;150:994–996.

Backhouse KM: The gubernaculum testis Hunteri: testicular descent and maldescent. Ann R Coll Surg Engl 1964;35:15–33.

Backhouse KM: The natural history of testicular descent and maldescent. Proc R Soc Med 1966;59:357–360.

Backhouse KM: Embryology of testicular descent and maldescent. Urol Clin North Am 1982a;9:315–325.

Backhouse KM: Development and descent of the testis. Eur J Pediatr 1982b;139:249–252.

Baikie G, Hutson JM: Wolffian duct and epididymal agenesis fails to prevent testicular descent. Pediatr Surg Int 1990;5:458–462.

Baker LA, Sigman D, Matthews RI, et al: An analysis of clinical outcomes using color Doppler testicular ultrasound for testicular torsion. Pediatrics 2000;105:604–607.

Barada JH, Weingarten JL, Cromie WJ: Testicular salvage and age related delay in the presentation of testicular torsion. J Urol 1989;142:746–748.

Barthold JS, Mahler HR, Newton BW: Lack of feminization of the cremaster nucleus in cryptorchid androgen insensitive rats. J Urol 1994;152:2280–2286.

Barthold JS, Mahler HR, Sziszak TJ, Newton BW: Lack of feminization of the cremaster nucleus by prenatal flutamide administration in the rat and pig. J Urol 1996;156:767–771.

Barthold JS, Redman JF: Association of epididymal anomalies with patent processus vaginalis in hernia, hydrocele and cryptorchidism. J Urol 1996;156:2054–2056.

Bartsch G, Frank S, Marberger H, Mikuz G: Testicular torsion: late results with special regard to fertility and endocrine function. J Urol 1980;124:375–378.

Barwell R: One hundred cases of varicocele treated by subcutaneous wire loop. Lancet 1885;1:978.

Batata MA, Whitmore WF Jr, Chu FC, et al: Cryptorchidism and testicular cancer. J Urol 1980;124:382–387.

Baumans V, Dijkstra G, Wensing CJ: The effect of orchidectomy on gubernacular outgrowth and regression in the dog. Int J Androl 1982;5:387–400.

Baumans V, Dijkstra G, Wensing CJ: The role of a non-androgenic testicular factor in the process of testicular descent in the dog. Int J Androl 1983;6:541–552.

Beasley SW, Hutson JM: Effect of division of genitofemoral nerve on testicular descent in the rat. Aust N Z J Surg 1987;57:49–51.

Behre HM, Nashan D: Objective measurement of testicular volume by ultrasonography. Int J Androl 1991;12:395.

Behringer RR, Finegold MJ, Cate RL: Müllerian-inhibiting substance function during mammalian sexual development. Cell 1994;79:415–425.

Bellinger M: The blind-ending vas: the fate of the contralateral testis. J Urol 1985;133:644–645.

Bellinger MF, Abromowitz H, Brantley S, Marshall G: Orchiopexy: an experimental study of the effect of surgical technique on testicular histology. J Urol 1989;142:553–555; discussion, 572.

Bennett R, Gill B, Kogan S: Epididymitis in children: the circumcision factor? J Urol 1998;160:1842–1844.

Bennett WH: Varicocele, particularly with reference to its radical cure. Lancet 1889;1:261–268.

Berkowitz GS, Lapinski RH: Risk factors for cryptorchidism: a nested case-control study. Paediatr Perinat Epidemiol 1996;10:39–51.

Berkowitz GS, Lapinski RH, Dolgin SE, et al: Prevalence and natural history of cryptorchidism. Pediatrics 1993;92:44–49.

Bevan AD: Operation for undescended testicle and congenital inguinal hernia. JAMA 1899;33:733.

Bianchi A: Microvascular orchiopexy for high undescended testes. Br J Urol 1984;56:521–524.

Biason A, Mantero F, Scaroni C, et al: Deletion within the CYP17 gene together with insertion of foreign DNA is the cause of combined complete 17 alpha-hydroxylase/17,20-lyase deficiency in an Italian patient. Mol Endocrinol 1991;5:2037–2045.

Bloom DA: Two-step orchiopexy with pelviscopic clip ligation of the spermatic vessels. J Urol 1991;145:1030–1033.

Bloom DA, Ritchey ML, Manzoni G: Laparoscopy for the nonpalpable testis. In Holcomb GWI (ed): Pediatric Endoscopic Surgery. Norwalk, CT, Appleton and Lange, 1994.

Bock JE, Sobye JV: Frequency of contralateral inguinal hernia in children. Acta Chir Scand 1970;136:707.

Braedel HU, Steffens J, Ziegler M, et al: A possible ontogenic etiology for idiopathic left varicocele. J Urol 1994;151:62–66.

Brandt MT, Sheldon CA, Wacksman J, Matthews P: Prenatal testicular torsion: principles of management. J Urol 1992;147:670–672.

Bukowski TP, Wacksman J, Billmire DA, et al: Testicular autotransplantation: a 17-year review of an effective approach to the management of the intra-abdominal testis (see comments). J Urol 1995a;154:558–561.

Bukowski TP, Wacksman J, Billmire DA, Sheldon CA: Testicular autotransplantation for the intra-abdominal testis. Microsurgery 1995b;16:290–295.

Burge DM: Neonatal testicular torsion and infarction: aetiology and management. Br J Urol 1987;59:70–73.

Byrd W, Bennett MJ, Carr BR, et al: Regulation of biologically active dimeric inhibin A and B from infancy to adulthood in the male. J Clin Endocrinol Metab 1998;83:2849–2854.

Caesar RE, Kaplan GW: The incidence of the cremasteric reflex in normal boys. J Urol 1994;152:779–780.

Cain MP, Kramer SA, Tindall DJ, Husmann DA: Expression of androgen receptor protein within the lumbar spinal cord during ontologic development and following antiandrogen induced cryptorchidism. J Urol 1994;152:766–769.

Cameron FJ, Sinclair AH: Mutations in SRY and SOX9: testis-determining genes. Hum Mutat 1997;9:388–395.

Campbell HE: Incidence of malignant growth of the undescended testicle: a critical and statistical study. Arch Surg 1942;44:353.

Carrillo A, Gershbein A, Glassberg KI, Danon M: Serum inhibin B levels and the response to gonadotropin stimulation test in pubertal boys with varicocele. J Urol 1999;162:875–877.

Castro-Magana M, Angulo M, Canas A, Uy J: Leydig cell function in adolescent boys with varicoceles. Arch Androl 1990;24:73–79.

Catlin EA, MacLaughlin DT, Donahoe PK: Müllerian inhibiting substance: new perspectives and future directions. Microsc Res Tech 1993;25:121–133.

Cendron M, Huff DS, Keating MA, et al: Anatomical, morphological and volumetric analysis: a review of 759 cases of testicular maldescent. J Urol 1993;149:570–573.

Cendron M, Keating MA, Huff DS, et al: Cryptorchidism, orchiopexy and infertility: a critical long-term retrospective analysis. J Urol 1989;142:559–562; discussion, 572.

Chilvers C, Dudley NE, Gough MH, et al: Undescended testis: the effect of treatment on subsequent risk of subfertility and malignancy. J Pediatr Surg 1986;21:691–696.

Clarnette TD, Hutson JM, Beasley SW: Factors affecting the development of the processus vaginalis in the rat. J Urol 1996;156:1463–1466.

Clark W, Kramer S: Henoch-Schönlein purpura and the acute scrotum. J Pediatr Surg 1986;21:991–992.

Cohen M, Cameron C, Duncan PG: Pediatric anesthesia morbidity and mortality in the perioperative period. Anesth Analg 1990;70:160–167.

Cohen-Haguenauer O, Picard JY, Mattei MG, et al: Mapping of the gene for anti-mullerian hormone to the short arm of human chromosome 19. Cytogenet Cell Genet 1987;44:2–6.

Coolsaet BLRA: The varicocele syndrome: venography determining the optimal level for surgical management. J Urol 1980;124:833–839.

Cooper ER: The histology of the retained testis in the human subject at different ages and its comparison with the testis. J Anat 1929;64:5–10.

Corkery JJ: Staged orchiopexy: a new technique. J Pediatr Surg 1975;10:515–518.

Cosentino J, Nishida M, Rabinowitz R, Cockett ATK: Histological changes occurring in the contralateral testes of prepubertal rats subjected to various durations of unilateral spermatic cord torsion. J Urol 1985;133:906–911.

Coughlin MT, Bellinger MF, LaPorte RE, Lee PA: Testicular suture: a significant risk factor for infertility among formerly cryptorchid men. J Pediatr Surg 1998;33:1790–1793.

Curling JB: A Practical Treatise on the Diseases of the Testis, and of the Spermatic Cord and Scrotum. London, Samuel Highley, 1843.

Czeizel A, Erodi E, Toth J: Genetics of undescended testis. J Urol 1981;126:528–529.

De Muinck Keizer-Schrama SM, Hazebroek FW, Drop SL, et al: LH-RH nasal spray treatment for cryptorchidism: a double-blind, placebo-controlled study. Eur J Pediatr 1987;146(Suppl. 2):S35–S37.

de Roux N, Young J, Misrahi M, et al: A family with hypogonadotropic hypogonadism and mutations in the gonadotropin-releasing hormone receptor. N Engl J Med 1997;337:1597–1602.

Dixon TK, Ritchey ML, Boykin W, et al: Transparenchymal suture fixation and testicular histology in a prepubertal rat model. J Urol 1993;149:1116–1118.

Docimo SG: The results of surgical therapy for cryptorchidism: a literature review and analysis. J Urol 1995;154:1148–1152.

Donohue RE, Brown JS: Blood gases and pH determination in the internal spermatic veins of subfertile men with varicocele. Fertil Steril 1969;20:365–369.

Dowsing AT, Yong EL, Clark M, et al: Linkage between male infertility and trinucleotide repeat expansion in the androgen-receptor gene (see comments). Lancet 1999;354:640–643.

Dresner M: Torsed appendage: blue dot sign. Urology 1973;1:63–66.

DuBois JJ, Jenkins JR, Egan JC: Transinguinal laparoscopic examination of the contralateral groin in pediatric herniorrhaphy. Surg Laparosc Endosc 1997;7:384–387.

Duckett J: Routine contralateral exploration and fixation is unjustified. Dial Pediatr Urol 1991;14:7–8.

Ehrlich RM, Dougherty LJ, Tomashefsky P, Lattimer JK: Effect of gonadotropin in cryptorchism. J Urol 1969;102:793–795.

Elder JS: Laparoscopy and Fowler-Stephens orchiopexy in the management of the impalpable testis. Urol Clin North Am 1989;16:399–411.

Elder JS: Epididymal anomalies associated with hydrocele/hernia and cryptorchidism: implications regarding testicular descent. J Urol 1992a;148:624–626.

Elder JS: Two-stage Fowler-Stephens orchiopexy in the management of intra-abdominal testes. J Urol 1992b;148:1239–1241.

Emmen JM, McLuskey A, Adham IM, et al: Involvement of insulin-like factor 3 (Insl3) in diethylstilbestrol-induced cryptorchidism. Endocrinology 2000;141:846–849.

Fallat ME, Williams MPL, Farmer PJ, Hutson JM: Histologic evaluation of inguinoscrotal migration of the gubernaculum in rodents during testicular descent and its relationship to the genitofemoral nerve. Pediatr Surg Int 1992;7:265–270.

Farrer JH, Walker AH, Rajfer J: Management of the postpubertal cryptorchid testis: a statistical review. J Urol 1985;134:1071–1076.

Fedder J, Boesen M: Effect of a combined GnRH/hCG therapy in boys with undescended testicles: evaluated in relation to testicular localization within the first week after birth. Arch Androl 1998;40:181–186.

Fentener van Vlissingen JM, van Zoelen EJ, Ursem PJ, Wensing CJ: In vitro model of the first phase of testicular descent: identification of a low molecular weight factor from fetal testis involved in proliferation of gubernaculum testis cells and distinct from specified polypeptide growth factors and fetal gonadal hormones. Endocrinology 1988;123:2868–2877.

Fentener van Vlissingen JM, Koch CA, Delpech B, Wensing CJ: Growth and differentiation of the gubernaculum testis during testicular descent in the pig: changes in the extracellular matrix, DNA content, and hyaluronidase, beta-glucuronidase, and beta-N-acetylglucosaminidase activities. J Urol 1989;142:837–845.

Finkelstein MS, Rosenberg HK, Snyder HMd, Duckett JW: Ultrasound evaluation of scrotum in pediatrics. Urology 1986;27:1–9.

Ford TF, Parkinson MC, Pryor JP: The undescended testis in adult life. Br J Urol 1985;57:181–184.

Foster JW, Dominguez-Steglich MA, Guioli S, et al: Campomelic dysplasia and autosomal sex reversal caused by mutations in an SRY-related gene. Nature 1994;372:525–530.

Fowler R, Stephens FD: The role of testicular vascular anatomy and the salvage of high undescended testes. Aust N Z Surg 1959;29:92.

Frey HL, Peng S, Rajfer J: Synergy of abdominal pressure and androgens in testicular descent. Biol Reprod 1983;29:1233–1239.

Frey HL, Rajfer J: Epididymis does not play an important role in the process of testicular descent. Surg Forum 1982;33:617–621.

Frey HL, Rajfer J: Role of the gubernaculum and intraabdominal pressure in the process of testicular descent. J Urol 1984;131:574–579.

Fujisawa M, Yoshida S: Deoxyribonucleic acid polymerase activity in the testes of infertile men with varicocele. Fertil Steril 1988;50:795–800.

Furui K, Suganuma N, Tsukahara S, et al: Identification of two point mutations in the gene coding luteinizing hormone (LH) beta-subunit, associated with immunologically anomalous LH variants. J Clin Endocrinol Metab 1994;78:107–113.

Gardner TA, Ostad M, Mininberg DT: Diagnostic flexible peritoneoscopy: assessment of the contralateral internal inguinal ring during unilateral herniorrhaphy. J Pediatr Surg 1998;33:1486–1489.

Geissler WM, Davis DL, Wu L, et al: Male pseudohermaphroditism caused by mutations of testicular 17 beta-hydroxysteroid dehydrogenase 3 (see comments). Nat Genet 1994;7:34–39.

Geller DH, Auchus RJ, Mendonca BB, Miller WL: The genetic and functional basis of isolated 17,20-lyase deficiency. Nat Genet 1997;17:201–205.

Gentile DP, Rabinowitz R, Hulbert WC: Abdominoscrotal hydrocele in infancy. Urology 1998;51(Suppl.):20–22.

Gershbein AB, Horowitz M, Glassberg KI: The adolescent varicocele: I. Left testicular hypertrophy following varicocelectomy. J Urol 1999;162: 1447–1449.

Gier HT, Marion GB: Development of mammalian testes and genital ducts. Biol Reprod 1969;1(Suppl. 1):1–23.

Gilbert JB, Hamilton JB: Incidence and nature of tumors in ectopic testes. Surg Gynecol Obstet 1970;71:731.

Gill B, Kogan S, Starr S, et al: Significance of epididymal and ductal anomalies associated with testicular maldescent. J Urol 1989;142:556–558; discussion, 572.

Gislason T, Norohna R, Gregory J: Acute epididymitis in boys: a 5 year retrospective study. J Urol 1980;124:533–537.

Goh DW, Middlesworth W, Farmer PJ, Hutson JM: Prenatal androgen blockade with flutamide inhibits masculinization of the genitofemoral nerve and testicular descent. J Pediatr Surg 1994;29:836–838.

Goldstein M, Gilbert BR, Dicker AP, et al: Microsurgical inguinal varicocelectomy with delivery of the testis: an artery and lymphatic sparing technique. J Urol 1992;148:1808–1811.

Gorelick JI, Goldstein M: Loss of fertility in men with a varicocele. Fertil Steril 1992;57:174.

Grasso M, Buonaguidi A, Lania C, et al: Postpubertal cryptorchidism: review and evaluation of the fertility. Eur Urol 1991;20:126–128.

Green KF, Turner TT: Varicocele, reversal of testicular blood flow and temperature effect by varicocele repair. J Urol 1984;131:1208.

Grosfeld JL: Current concepts in inguinal hernia in infants and children. World J Surg 1989;13:506–515.

Gross DJ, Landau H, Kohn G, et al: Male pseudohermaphroditism due to 17 beta-hydroxysteroid dehydrogenase deficiency: gender reassignment in early infancy. Acta Endocrinol (Copenh) 1986;112:238–246.

Guellaen G, Casanova M, Bishop C, et al: Human XX males with Y single-copy DNA fragments. Nature 1984;307:172–173.

Habiby RL, Boepple P, Nachtigall L, et al: Adrenal hypoplasia congenita with hypogonadotropic hypogonadism: evidence that DAX-1 mutations lead to combined hypothalamic and pituitary defects in gonadotropin production (see comments). J Clin Invest 1996;98:1055–1062.

Hadziselimovic F: Treatment of cryptorchidism with GnRH. Urol Clin North Am 1982;9:413–420.

Hadziselimovic F: The value of testicular biopsy in patients with varicocele. J Urol 1986;135:707.

Hadziselimovic F, Duckett JW, Snyder HMd, et al: Omphalocele, cryptorchidism, and brain malformations. J Pediatr Surg 1987a;22:854–856.

Hadziselimovic F, Herzog B, Buser M: Development of cryptorchid testes. Eur J Pediatr 1987b;146(Suppl. 2):S8–S12.

Hadziselimovic F, Herzog B, Hocht B, et al: Screening for cryptorchid boys risking sterility and results of long-term buserelin treatment after successful orchiopexy. Eur J Pediatr 1987c;146(Suppl. 2):S59–S62.

Han SW, Lee T, Kim JH, et al: Pathological difference between retractile and cryptorchid testes. J Urol 1999;162:878–880.

Haqq CM, King CY, Ukiyama E, et al: Molecular basis of mammalian sexual determination: activation of müllerian inhibiting substance gene expression by SRY (published erratum appears in Science 1995;267: 317). Science 1994;266:1494–1500.

Harrison CB, Kaplan GW, Scherz HC, et al: Microvascular autotransplantation of the intra-abdominal testis. J Urol 1990;144:506–507; discussion, 512–503.

Harrison RM, Lewis RW, Roberts JA: Pathophysiology of varicocele in non-human primates: long-term seminal and testicular changes. Fertil Steril 1969;20:365–369.

Hart RR, Rushton HG, Belman AB: Intraoperative spermatic venography during varicocele surgery in adolescents. J Urol 1992;148:1514–1516.

Heiskanen P, Billig H, Toppari J, et al: Apoptotic cell death in the normal and cryptorchid human testis: the effect of human chorionic gonadotropin on testicular cell survival. Pediatr Res 1996;40:351–356.

Heyns CF: The gubernaculum during testicular descent in the human fetus. J Anat 1987;153:93–112.

Heyns CF, Human HJ, Werely CJ, De Klerk DP: The glycosaminoglycans of the gubernaculum during testicular descent in the fetus. J Urol 1990; 143:612–617.

Heyns CF, Hutson JM: Historical review of theories on testicular descent. J Urol 1995;153:754–767.

Heyns CF, Pape VC: Presence of a low capacity androgen receptor in the gubernaculum of the pig fetus. J Urol 1991;145:161–167.

Hjertkvist M, Damber JE, Bergh A: Cryptorchidism: a registry based study in Sweden on some factors of possible aetiological importance. J Epidemiol Community Health 1989;43:324–329.

Holder TM, Ashcraft KW: Groin hernias and hydroceles. In Textbook of Pediatric Surgery. Philadelphia, WB Saunders, 1980, p 594.

Hoorweg-Nijman JJ, Havers HM, Delemarre-van de Waal HA: Effect of human chorionic gonadotrophin (hCG)/follicle-stimulating hormone treatment versus hCG treatment alone on testicular descent: a double-blind placebo-controlled study. Eur J Endocrinol 1994;130:60–64.

Hosie S, Wessel L, Waag KL: Could testicular descent in humans be promoted by direct androgen stimulation of the gubernaculum testis? Eur J Pediatr Surg 1999;9:37–41.

Houle AM, Gagne D: Human chorionic gonadotropin but not the calcitonin gene-related peptide induces postnatal testicular descent in mice. Int J Androl 1995;16:143–147.

Hrebinko RL, Bellinger MF: The limited role of imaging techniques in managing children with undescended testes. J Urol 1993;150:458–460.

Hudson RW, Perez-Marrero R, Crawford VA, McKay DE: Hormonal parameters of men with varicocele before and after varicocelectomy. Fertil Steril 1985;43:905–910.

Huff DS, Hadziselimovic F, Duckett JW, et al: Germ cell counts in semithin sections of biopsies of 115 unilaterally cryptorchid testes: the experience from the Children's Hospital of Philadelphia. Eur J Pediatr 1987;146(Suppl. 2):S25–S27.

Huff DS, Hadziselimovic F, Snyder HM, et al: Postnatal testicular maldevelopment in unilateral cryptorchidism. J Urol 1989;142:546–548; discussion, 572.

Huff DS, Hadziselimovic F, Snyder HM, et al: Early postnatal testicular maldevelopment in cryptorchidism. J Urol 1991;146:624–626.

Huff DS, Hadziselimovic F, Snyder HM, et al: Histologic maldevelopment of unilaterally cryptorchid testes and their descended partners. Eur J Pediatr 1993;152(Suppl. 2):S11–S14.

Huff DS, Snyder HM, Hadziselimovic F, et al: An absent testis is associated with contralateral testicular hypertrophy. J Urol 1992;148:627–628.

Huhtaniemi I: Fetal testis: a very special endocrine organ. Eur J Endocrinol 1994;130:25–31.

Hunter J: Observations on the state of the testis in the foetus and on the hernia congenita. In London HW (ed): Medical Commentaries, vol 1. London, A. Hamilton, 1762.

Husmann DA, Boone TB, McPhaul MJ: Flutamide-induced testicular undescent in the rat is associated with alterations in genitofemoral nerve morphology. J Urol 1994;151:509–513.

Husmann DA, Levy JB: Current concepts in the pathophysiology of testicular undescent. Urology 1995;46:267–276.

Hutcheson J, Peters C, Diamond D: Amiodarone induced epididymitis in children. J Urol 1998;160:515–517.

Hutson JM: Testicular feminization: a model for testicular descent in mice and men. J Pediatr Surg 1986;21:195–198.

Hutson JM, Baker M, Terada M, et al: Hormonal control of testicular descent and the cause of cryptorchidism. Reprod Fertil Dev 1994;6: 151–156.

Hutson JM, Beasley SW: The mechanisms of testicular descent. Aust Paediatr J 1987;23:215–216.

Hutson JM, Donahoe PK: The hormonal control of testicular descent. Endocr Rev 1986;7:270–283.

Hutson JM, Hasthorpe S, Heyns CF: Anatomical and functional aspects of testicular descent and cryptorchidism. Endocr Rev 1997;18:259–280.

Hutson JM, Watts LM: Both gonadotropin and testosterone fail to reverse estrogen-induced cryptorchidism in fetal mice: further evidence for non-androgenic control of testicular descent in the fetus. Pediatr Surg Int 1990;5:13–18.

Illig R, Exner GU, Kollmann F, et al: Treatment of cryptorchidism by intranasal synthetic luteinising-hormone releasing hormone: results of a collaborative double-blind study. Lancet 1977;2:518–520.

Imbeaud S, Belville C, Messika-Zeitoun L, et al: A 27 base-pair deletion of the anti-müllerian type II receptor gene is the most common cause of the persistent müllerian duct syndrome. Hum Mol Genet 1996;5: 1269–1277.

Imperato-McGinley J, Miller M, Wilson JD, et al: A cluster of male pseudohermaphrodites with 5 alpha-reductase deficiency in Papua New Guinea. Clin Endocrinol (Oxf) 1991;34:293–298.

Ito H, Kataumi Z, Yanagi S, et al: Changes in the volume and histology of retractile testes in prepubertal boys. Int J Androl 1986;9:161–169.

Jarow JP: Clinical significance of intratesticular arterial anatomy. J Urol 1991;145:777–779.

Jarow JP, Berkovitz GD, Migeon CJ, et al: Elevation of serum gonadotropins establishes the diagnosis of anorchism in prepubertal boys with bilateral cryptorchidism. J Urol 1986;136:277–279.

John Radcliffe Hospital Cryptorchidism Study Group. Cryptorchidism: a prospective study of 7500 consecutive male births, 1984–1988. Arch Dis Child 1992;67:892–899.

Job JC, Canlorbe P, Garagorri JM, Toublanc JE: Hormonal therapy of cryptorchidism with human chorionic gonadotropin(HCG). Urol Clin North Am 1982;9:405–411.

Johnson DE, Woodhead DM, Pohl DR, Robison JR: Cryptorchism and testicular tumorigenesis. Surgery 1968;63:919–922.

Jones ME, Swerdlow AJ, Griffith M, Goldacre MJ: Prenatal risk factors for cryptorchidism: a record linkage study. Paediatr Perinat Epidemiol 1998;12:383–396.

Jordan GH, Winslow BH: Laparoscopic single stage and staged orchiopexy. J Urol 1994;152:1249–1252.

Josso N, Picard JY, Imbeaud S, et al: The persistent müllerian duct syndrome: a rare cause of cryptorchidism. Eur J Pediatr 1993; 152(Suppl. 2):S76–S78.

Kaleva M, Arsalo A, Louhimo I, et al: Treatment with human chorionic gonadotropin for cryptorchidism: clinical and histological effects. Int J Androl 1996;19:293–298.

Kaplan GW: Nomenclature of cryptorchidism. Eur J Pediatr 1993; 152(Suppl. 2):S17–S19.

Kass EJ: The evaluation and management of the adolescent with a varicocele. AUA Update Series 1990;12:90–95.

Kass EJ, Belman AB: Reversal of testicular growth failure by varicocele ligation. J Urol 1987;137:475–476.

Kass EJ, Freitas JE, Salisz JA, Steinert BW: Pituitary gonadal dysfunction in adolescents with varicocele (see comments). Urology 1993;42:179–181.

Kass EJ, Marcol B: Results of varicocele surgery in adolescents: a comparison of techniques. J Urol 1992;148:694–696.

Kenny FM, Reynolds JW, Green OC: Partial 3-hydroxysteroid dehydrogenase (3-HSD) deficiency in a family with congenital adrenal hyperplasia: evidence for increasing 3-HSD activity with age. Pediatrics 1971;48:756–765.

Key TJ, Bull D, Ansell P, et al: A case-control study of cryptorchidism and maternal hormone concentrations in early pregnancy. Br J Cancer 1996;73:698–701.

Kieslinger VJ, Schroeder DE, Pauljev P, Hull J: Spermatic cord block and manual reduction: primary treatment for spermatic cord torsion. J Urol 1984;132:921–923.

Knebelmann B, Boussin L, Guerrier D, et al: Anti-Müllerian hormone Bruxelles: a nonsense mutation associated with the persistent Müllerian duct syndrome. Proc Natl Acad Sci U S A 1991;88:3767–3771.

Koff WJ, Scaletscky R: Malformations of the epididymis in undescended testis. J Urol 1990;143:340–343.

Koff SA, Sethi PS: Treatment of high undescended testes by low spermatic vessel ligation: an alternative to the Fowler-Stephens technique. J Urol 1996;156:799–803; discussion, 803.

Kogan SJ, Lutzker LG, Perez LA, et al: The value of the negative radionuclide scrotal scan in the management of the acutely inflamed scrotum in children. J Urol 1979;122:223–225.

Koivusalo A, Taskinen S, Rintala RJ: Cryptorchidism in boys with congenital abdominal wall defects. Pediatr Surg Int 1998;13:143–145.

Kremer H, Kraaij R, Toledo SP, et al: Male pseudohermaphroditism due to a homozygous missense mutation of the luteinizing hormone receptor gene. Nat Genet 1995;9:160–164.

Kubini K, Zachmann M, Albers N, et al: Basal inhibin B and the testosterone response to human chorionic gonadotropin correlate in prepubertal boys. J Clin Endocrinol Metab 2000;85:134–138.

Kucukaydin M, Ozokutan BH, Turan C, et al: Malformation of the epididymis in undescended testis. Pediatr Surg Int 1998;14:189–191.

Larkins SL, Hutson JM, Williams MPL: Localization of calcitonin gene-related peptide immunoreactivity within the spinal nucleus of the genitofemoral nerve. Pediatr Surg Int 1991;6:176–179.

Laron Z, Dickerman Z, Ritterman I, Kaufman H: Follow-up of boys with unilateral compensatory testicular hypertrophy. Fertil Steril 1980;33:297–301.

Layman LC, Cohen DP, Jin M, et al: Mutations in gonadotropin-releasing hormone receptor gene cause hypogonadotropic hypogonadism. (Letter.) Nat Genet 1998;18:14–15.

Lee MM, Donahue PK: Müllerian inhibiting substance: a gonadal hormone with multiple functions. Endocr Rev 1993;14:152–164.

Lee PA: Fertility in cryptorchidism: does treatment make a difference? Endocrinol Metab Clin North Am 1993;22:479–490.

Lee PA, Bellinger MF, Coughlin MT: Correlations among hormone levels, sperm parameters and paternity in formerly unilaterally cryptorchid men. J Urol 1998;160:1155–1157; discussion, 1178.

Lee PA, O'Leary LA, Songer NJ, et al: Paternity after cryptorchidism: lack of correlation with age at orchidopexy. Br J Urol 1995;75:704–707.

Lemack GE, Uzzo RG, Schlegel PN, Goldstein M: Microsurgical repair of the adolescent varicocele. J Urol 1998;160:179–181.

Levard G, Laberge JM: The fate of undescended testes in patients with gastroschisis. Eur J Pediatr Surg 1997;7:163–165.

Levitt S, Gill B, Katlowitz N, et al: Routine intraoperative post-ligation venography in the treatment of the pediatric varicocele. J Urol 1987; 137:716–718.

Levy OM, Gittleman MC, Strashun AM: Diagnosis of acute testicular torsion using radionuclide scanning. J Urol 1983;129:975–977.

Likitnukul S, McCracken G, Nelson J, Votteler T: Epididymitis in children and adolescents. Am J Dis Child 1987;141:41–44.

Lim HN, Chen H, McBride S, et al: Longer polyglutamine tracts in the androgen receptor are associated with moderate to severe undermasculinized genitalia in XY males. Hum Mol Genet 2000;9:829–834.

Lin D, Harikrishna JA, Moore CC, et al: Missense mutation serine 106-proline causes 17 alpha-hydroxylase deficiency. J Biol Chem 1991;266:15992–15998.

Lugg JA, Penson DF, Sadeghi F, et al: Prevention of seminiferous tubular atrophy in a naturally cryptorchid rat model by early surgical intervention. J Androl 1996;17:726–732.

Lyon RP, Marshall S, Scott MP: Varicocele in childhood and adolescence: implication in adult fertility. Urology 1982;19:641–644.

Maghnie M, Valtorta A, Moretta A, et al: Effects of short-term administration of human chorionic gonadotropin on immune functions in cryptorchid children. Eur J Pediatr 1991;150:238–241.

Majdic G, Sharpe RM, Saunders PT: Maternal oestrogen/xenoestrogen exposure alters expression of steroidogenic factor-1 (SF-1/Ad4BP) in the fetal rat testis. Mol Cell Endocrinol 1997;127:91–98.

Mandressi A, Buizza C, Antonelli D, Chisena S: Is laparoscopy a worthy method to treat varicocele? Comparison between 160 cases of two-port laparoscopic and 120 cases of open inguinal spermatic vein ligation. J Endourol 1996;10:435–441.

Martin DC: Germinal cell tumors of the testis after orchiopexy. J Urol 1979;121:422–424.

Martin DC: Malignancy in the cryptorchid testis. Urol Clin North Am 1982;9:371–376.

Martin DC, Menck HR: The undescended testis: management after puberty. J Urol 1975;114:77–79.

Martinez-Mora J, Saez JM, Toran N, et al: Male pseudohermaphroditism due to Leydig cell agenesis and absence of testicular LH receptors (see comments). Clin Endocrinol (Oxf) 1991;34:485–491.

Mason AJ, Hayflick JS, Zoeller RT, et al: A deletion truncating the gonadotropin-releasing hormone gene is responsible for hypogonadism in the hpg mouse. Science 1986;234:1366–1371.

Mayr JM, Lawrenz K, Berghold A: Undescended testicles: an epidemiological review. Acta Paediatr 1999;88:1089–1093.

McAleer IM, Packer MG, Kaplan GW, et al: Fertility index analysis in cryptorchidism. J Urol 1995;153:1255–1258.

McElreavey K, Vilain E, Abbas N, et al: A regulatory cascade hypothesis for mammalian sex determination: SRY represses a negative regulator of male development. Proc Natl Acad Sci U S A 1993;90:3368–3372.

McGregor DB, Halverson K, McVay CB: The unilateral pediatric inguinal hernia: Should the contralateral side be explored? J Pediar Surg 1980; 15:313.

McLachlan JA, Newbold RR, Bullock B: Reproductive tract lesions in male mice exposed prenatally to diethylstilbestrol. Science 1975;190:991–992.

McMahon DR, Kramer SA, Husmann DA: Antiandrogen induced cryptorchidism in the pig is associated with failed gubernacular regression and epididymal malformations. J Urol 1995;154:553–557.

Merksz M: Fusional anomalies of the testis and epididymis. Acta Chir Hung 1998;37:153–170.

Merlini E, Rotundi F, Seymandi PL, Canning DA: Acute epididymitis and urinary tract anomalies in children. Scand J Urol Nephrol 1998;32:273–275.

Mininberg DT, Rodger JC, Bedford JM: Ultrastructural evidence of the onset of testicular pathological conditions in the cryptorchid human testis within the first year of life. J Urol 1982;128:782–784.

Mollaeian M, Mehrabi V, Elahi B: Significance of epididymal and ductal anomalies associated with undescended testis: study in 652 cases. Urology 1994;43:857–860.

Moller H, Prener A, Skakkebaek NE: Testicular cancer, cryptorchidism, inguinal hernia, testicular atrophy, and genital malformations: case-control studies in Denmark. Cancer Causes Control 1996;7:264–274.

Mori M, Davies TW, Tsukamoto T, et al: Maternal and other factors of cryptorchidism: a case-control study in Japan. Kurume Med J 1992;39:53–60.

Muffly KE, McWhorter CA, Bartone FF, Gardner PJ: The absence of premalignant changes in the cryptorchid testis before adulthood. J Urol 1984;131:523–525.

Muller U, Donlon T, Schmid M, et al: Deletion mapping of the testis determining locus with DNA probes in 46,XX males and in 46,XY and 46,X,dic(Y) females. Nucleic Acids Res 1986;14:6489–6505.

Nachtigal MW, Hirokawa Y, Enyeart-VanHouten DL, et al: Wilms' tumor 1 and Dax-1 modulate the orphan nuclear receptor SF-1 in sex-specific gene expression. Cell 1998;93:445–454.

Nagler H, White R: The effect of testicular torsion on the contralateral testis. J Urol 1982;128:1343–1347.

Nagu T, Takahira H: A new apparatus for the measurement of testicular volume. Jpn J Fertil Steril 1979;24:12.

Netto NR, Lemos GC, De Goes GM: Varicocele, relation between anoxia and hypospermatogenesis. Int J Fertil 1977;22:174–178.

Nordenskjold A, Ivarsson SA: Molecular characterization of 5 alpha-reductase type 2 deficiency and fertility in a Swedish family. J Clin Endocrinol Metab 1998;83:3236–3238.

Ogura K, Matsuda T, Terachi T, et al: Laparoscopic varicocelectomy: invasiveness and effectiveness compared with conventional open retroperitoneal high ligation. Int J Urol 1994;1:62–66.

Olguner M, Akgur FM, Aktug T, Derebek E: Bilateral asynchronous perinatal testicular torsion: a case report. J Pediatr Surg 2000;35:1348–1349.

Olsen LH, Genster HG, Mosegaard A, et al: Management of the non-descended testis: doubtful value of luteinizing-hormone-releasing-hormone (LHRH). A double-blind, placebo-controlled multicentre study. Int J Androl 1992;15:135–143.

Oster J: Varicocele in children and adolescents. Scand J Urol Nephrol 1971;5:27.

Owings EP, Georgeson KE: A new technique for laparoscopic exploration to find contralateral patent processus vaginalis. Surg Endosc 2000;14:114–116.

Paduch DA, Niedzielski J: Semen analysis in young men with varicocele: preliminary study. J Urol 1996;156:788–790.

Page DC, Mosher R, Simpson EM, et al: The sex-determining region of the human Y chromosome encodes a finger protein. Cell 1987;51:1091–1104.

Palomo AR: Radical cure of varicocele by a new technique: preliminary report. J Urol 1949;61:604–607.

Paltiel HJ, Connolly LP, Atala A, et al: Acute scrotal symptoms in boys with an indeterminate clinical presentation: comparison of color Doppler sonography and scintigraphy. Radiology 1998;207:223–231.

Park D, Lee PA, Witchel SF: Progressive virilization of a pubertal phenotypic female: 17 beta-hydroxysteroid dehydrogenase deficiency. J Pediatr Adolesc Gynecol 1996;9:9–11.

Park WH, Hutson JM: The gubernaculum shows rhythmic contractility and active movement during testicular descent. J Pediatr Surg 1991;26:615–617.

Parker KL, Schedl A, Schimmer BP: Gene interactions in gonadal development. Annu Rev Physiol 1999;61:417–433.

Parkinson MC, Swerdlow AJ, Pike MC: Carcinoma in situ in boys with cryptorchidism: when can it be detected? Br J Urol 1994;73:431–435.

Persky L, Albert DJ: Staged orchiopexy. Surg Gynecol Obstet 1971;132:43–45.

Pinto K, Noe H, GR: Management of neonatal testicular torsion. J Urol 1987;158:1196–1197.

Popper P, Micevych PE: The effect of castration on calcitonin gene-related peptide in spinal motor neurons. Neuroendocrinology 1989;50:338–343.

Pralong FP, Gomez F, Castillo E, et al: Complete hypogonadotropic hypogonadism associated with a novel inactivating mutation of the gonadotropin-releasing hormone receptor. J Clin Endocrinol Metab 1999;84:3811–3816.

Prener A, Engholm G, Jensen OM: Genital anomalies and risk for testicular cancer in Danish men. Epidemiology 1996;7:14–19.

Prentiss RJ, Weickgenant CJ, Moses JJ, Frazier DB: Undescended testis: surgical anatomy of spermatic vessels, spermatic surgical triangles, and lateral spermatic ligament. J Urol 1960;83:686.

Puri P, Nixon HH: Bilateral retractile testes: subsequent effects on fertility. J Pediatr Surg 1977;12:563–566.

Pyorala S, Huttunen NP, Uhari M: A review and meta-analysis of hormonal treatment of cryptorchidism. J Clin Endocrinol Metab 1995;80:2795–2799.

Quinlan DM, Gearhart JP, Jeffs RD: Abdominal wall defects and cryptorchidism: an animal model. J Urol 1988;140:1141–1144.

Qvist O: Swelling of the scrotum in infants and children and non-specific epididymitis: a study of 158 cases. Acta Chir Scand 1956;110:417–419.

Rabinowitz R: The importance of the cremasteric reflex in acute scrotal swelling in children. J Urol 1984;132:89–90.

Rabinowitz R, Hulbert WC Jr: Late presentation of cryptorchidism: the etiology of testicular re-ascent. J Urol 1997;157:1892–1894.

Raina V, Shukla NK, Gupta NP, et al: Germ cell tumours in uncorrected cryptorchid testis at Institute Rotary Cancer Hospital, New Delhi. Br J Cancer 1995;71:380–382.

Raivio T, Dunkel L: Inverse relationship between serum inhibin B and FSH levels in prepubertal boys with cryptorchidism. Pediatr Res 1999;46:496–500.

Rajfer J, Handelsman DJ, Swerdloff RS, et al: Hormonal therapy of cryptorchidism: a randomized, double-blind study comparing human chorionic gonadotropin and gonadotropin-releasing hormone. N Engl J Med 1986;314:466–470.

Rajfer J, Walsh PC: Hormonal regulation of testicular descent: experimental and clinical observations. J Urol 1977;118:985–990.

Rheaume E, Simard J, Morel Y, et al: Congenital adrenal hyperplasia due to point mutations in the type II 3 beta-hydroxysteroid dehydrogenase gene. Nat Genet 1992;1:239–245.

Rheaume E, Sanchez R, Simard J, et al: Molecular basis of congenital adrenal hyperplasia in two siblings with classical nonsalt-losing 3 beta-hydroxysteroid dehydrogenase deficiency. J Clin Endocrinol Metab 1994;79:1012–1018.

Riegler HC: Torsion of intra-abdominal testis: an unusual problem in diagnosis of the acute surgical abdomen. Surg Clin North Am 1972;52:371–374.

Rogers E, Teahan S, Gallagher H, et al: The role of orchiectomy in the management of postpubertal cryptorchidism. J Urol 1998;159:851–854.

Rossi P, Dolci S, Albanesi C, et al: Direct evidence that the mouse sex-determining gene Sry is expressed in the somatic cells of male fetal gonads and in the germ cell line in the adult testis. Mol Reprod Dev 1993;34:369–373.

Rowe MI, Copelson LW, Clatworthy HW: The patent processus vaginalis and the inguinal hernia. J Pediatr Surg 1969;4:102.

Rozanski TA, Bloom DA: The undescended testis: theory and management. Urol Clin North Am 1995;22:107–118.

Rozanski TA, Wojno KJ, Bloom DA: The remnant orchiectomy. J Urol 1996;155:712–713; discussion, 714.

Rune GM, Mayr J, Neugebauer H, et al: Pattern of Sertoli cell degeneration in cryptorchid prepubertal testes. Int J Androl 1992;15:19–31.

Saggese G, Ghirri P, Gabrielli S, Cosenza GC: Hormonal therapy for cryptorchidism with a combination of human chorionic gonadotropin and follicle-stimulating hormone: success and relapse rate. Am J Dis Child 1989;143:980–982.

Saito S, Kumamoto Y: The number of spermatogonia in various congenital testicular disorders. J Urol 1989;141:1166–1168.

Salas-Cortes L, Jaubert F, Barbaux S, et al: The human SRY protein is present in fetal and adult Sertoli cells and germ cells. Int J Dev Biol 1999;43:135–140.

Sampaio FJ, Favorito LA: Analysis of testicular migration during the fetal period in humans. J Urol 1998;159:540–542.

Sawchuk T, Costabile RA, Howards SS, Rodgers BM: Spermatic cord torsion in an infant receiving human chorionic gonadotropin. J Urol 1993;150:1212–1213.

Schlegel PN, SHIN D, Goldstein M: Urogenital anomalies in men with congenital absence of the vas deferens. J Urol 1996;155:1644.

Schwarz R, Stephens F: The persisting mesonephric duct syndrome: high junction of the vas and ureter. J Urol 1978;120:592–596.

Scorer CG, Farrington GH: Congenital Deformities of the Testis and Epididymis. New York, Appleton-Century-Crofts, 1971.

Scott JE: The Hutson hypothesis: a clinical study. Br J Urol 1987;60:74–76.

Shono T, Ramm-Anderson S, Goh DW, Hutson JM: The effect of flutamide on testicular descent in rats examined by scanning electron microscopy. J Pediatr Surg 1994;29:839–844.

Siegel A, Snyder H, Duckett JW: Epididymitis in infants and boys: underlying urogenital anomalies and efficacy of imaging modalities. J Urol 1987;138:1100–1103.

Silber SJ, Kelly J: Successful autotransplantation of an intra-abdominal testis to the scrotum by microvascular technique. J Urol 1976;115:452–454.

Sinclair AH, Berta P, Palmer MS, et al: A gene from the human sex-determining region encodes a protein with homology to a conserved DNA-binding motif (see comments). Nature 1990;346:240–244.

Skoog SJ, Roberts KP, Goldstein M, Pryor JL: The adolescent varicocele: what's new with an old problem in young patients? Pediatrics 1997; 100:112–121.

Sparkman RS: Bilateral exploration in inguinal hernia in juvenile patients. Surgery 1962;51:393.

Sparks JP: Torsion of the testis. Ann R Coll Surg Engl 1971;49:77.

Steeno OP: Varicocele in the adolescent. Adv Exp Med Biol 1991;286: 295–321.

Steeno O, Knops J, Declerck L: Prevention of fertility disorders by detection and treatment of varicocele at school and college age. Andrologia 1976;8:47–53.

Steinhardt GF, Kroovand RL, Perlmutter AD: Orchiopexy: planned 2-stage technique. J Urol 1985;133:434–435.

Stillman RJ: In utero exposure to diethylstilbestrol: adverse effects on the reproductive tract and reproductive performance and male and female offspring. Am J Obstet Gynecol 1982;142:905–921.

Stillwell T, Kramer S: Intermittent testicular torsion. Pediatrics 1986;77: 908–911.

Stone KT, Kass EJ, Cacciarelli AA, Gibson DP: Management of suspected antenatal torsion: what is the best strategy? J Urol 1995;153: 782–784.

Stuhrmann M, Dork T: CFTR gene mutations and male infertility. Andrologia 2000;32:71–83.

SU 293. Su L, Goldstein M: The effect of varicocelectomy on serum testosterone levels in infertile men with varicoceles. J Urol 1995;154: 1752.

Suganuma N, Furui K, Kikkawa F, et al: Effects of the mutations (Trp8 Arg and Ile15 Thr) in human luteinizing hormone (LH) beta-subunit on LH bioactivity in vitro and in vivo. Endocrinology 1996;137:831–838.

Thirumavalan V, Ransley P: Epididymitis in children and adolescents on clean intermittent catheterization. Eur Urol 1992;22:53–56.

Thong M, Lim C, Fatimah H: Undescended testes: incidence in 1,002 consecutive male infants and outcome at 1 year of age (see comments). Pediatr Surg Int 1998;13:37–41.

Tiret L, Desmonts J, Vourc'h G: Complications related to anesthesia in infants and children: a prospective survey of 40,240 anesthetics. Br J Anaesth 1988;61:263–269.

Toppari J, Kaleva M: Maldescendus testis. Horm Res 1999;51:261–269.

Toppari J, Skakkebaek NE: Sexual differentiation and environmental endocrine disrupters. Baillieres Clin Endocrinol Metab 1998;12:143–156.

Tran D, Picard JY, Vigier B, et al: Persistence of müllerian ducts in male rabbits passively immunized against bovine anti-müllerian hormone during fetal life. Dev Biol 1986;116:160–167.

Tut TG, Ghadessy FJ, Trifiro MA, et al: Long polyglutamine tracts in the androgen receptor are associated with reduced trans-activation, impaired sperm production, and male infertility. J Clin Endocrinol Metab 1997; 82:3777–3782.

Tzvetkova P, Tzvetkov D: Etiopathogenesis of cryptorchidism and male infertility. Arch Androl 1996;37:117–125.

Ulker V, Garibyan H, Kurth KH: Comparison of inguinal and laparoscopic approaches in the treatment of varicocele. Int Urol Nephrol 1997;29:71–77.

United Kingdom Testicular Cancer Study Group. Aetiology of testicular cancer: association with congenital abnormalities, age at puberty, infertility, and exercise (see comments). BMJ 1994a;308:1393–1399.

United Kingdom Testicular Cancer Study Group. Social, behavioural and medical factors in the aetiology of testicular cancer: results from the UK study. Br J Cancer 1994b;70:513–520.

Van Dop C, Burstein S, Conte FA, Grumbach MM: Isolated gonadotropin deficiency in boys: clinical characteristics and growth. J Pediatr 1987; 111:684–692.

Van Glabeke E, Khairouni A, Gall O, et al: Laparoscopic diagnosis of contralateral patent processus vaginalis in children under 1 year of age with unilateral inguinal hernia: comparison with herniography. J Pediatr Surg 1999;34:1213–1215.

Varela Cives R, Bautista Casasnovas A, et al: The influence of patency of the vaginal process on the efficacy of hormonal treatment of cryptorchidism. Eur J Pediatr 1996;155:932–936.

Vohra S, Morgentaler A: Congenital anomalies of the vas deferens, epididymitis, and seminal vesicles. Urology 1997;49:313–321.

Vordermark J: The persisting mesonephric duct syndrome: the description of a new syndrome. J Urol 1983;130:958–960.

Wacksman J, Billmire DA, Lewis AG, Sheldon CA: Laparoscopically assisted testicular autotransplantation for management of the intraabdominal undescended testis. J Urol 1996;156:772–774.

Wacksman J, Dinner M, Handler M: Results of testicular autotransplantation using the microvascular technique: experience with 8 intra-abdominal testes. J Urol 1982;128:1319–1321.

Wagner T, Wirth J, Meyer J, et al: Autosomal sex reversal and camptomelic dysplasia are caused by mutations in and around the SRY-related gene SOX9. Cell 1994;79:1111–1120.

Weidner IS, Moller H, Jensen TK, Skakkebaek NE: Risk factors for cryptorchidism and hypospadias. J Urol 1999;161:1606–1609.

Weiss J, Axelrod L, Whitcomb RW, et al: Hypogonadism caused by a single amino acid substitution in the beta subunit of luteinizing hormone (see comments). N Engl J Med 1992;326:179–183.

Wensing CJG: Testicular descent in some domestic mammals: I. Anatomical aspect of testicular descent. Proc Kon Ned Akad Wetensch 1968; 71(Series C):423–434.

Wensing CJ: The embryology of testicular descent. Horm Res 1988;30: 144–152.

Whitaker RH: Management of the undescended testis. Br J Hosp Med 1970;4:25.

Wiener ES, Touloukian RJ, Rodgers BM, et al: Hernia survey of the Section on Surgery of the American Academy of Pediatrics. J Pediatr Surg 1996;31:1166–1169.

Wiener JS, Marcelli M, Gonzales ET Jr, et al: Androgen receptor gene alterations are not associated with isolated cryptorchidism. J Urol 1998; 160:863–865.

Witjes JA, de Vries JD, Lock MT, Debruyne FM: Use of luteinizing-hormone-releasing hormone nasal spray in the treatment of cryptorchidism: is there still an indication? A clinical study in 78 boys with 103 undescended testicles. Eur Urol 1990;17:226–228.

Wu SM, Hallermeier KM, Laue L, et al: Inactivation of the luteinizing hormone/chorionic gonadotropin receptor by an insertional mutation in Leydig cell hypoplasia. Mol Endocrinol 1998;12:1651–1660.

Wylie CC: The biology of primordial germ cells. Eur Urol 1993;23:62–66.

Wyllie GG: The retractile testis. Med J Aust 1984;140:403–405.

Yamanaka J, Baker M, Metcalfe S, Hutson JM: Serum levels of müllerian inhibiting substance in boys with cryptorchidism. J Pediatr Surg 1991; 26:621–623.

Yerkes EB, Brock JW III, Holcomb GW III, Morgan WM III: Laparoscopic evaluation for a contralateral patent processus vaginalis: part III. Urology 1998;51:480–483.

Zorgniotti AW, MacLeod J: Studies in temperature: human semen quality and varicocele. Fertil Steril 1973;24:854–863.

68
SEXUAL DIFFERENTIATION: NORMAL AND ABNORMAL

David A. Diamond, MD

Disorders of sexual differentiation are among the most fascinating and complex disease processes encountered by the urologist. Indeed, since antiquity physicians have been fascinated by sexual differentiation. In the 2nd century AD, Galen suggested that sperm from the right testis was "male," that from the left testis was "female," and a hermaphrodite resulted when sperm from both testes joined in fertilization. Considerable progress has been made since then. In particular, over the past decade, remarkable advances in molecular biology and genetic research have provided new insight into the precise mechanisms responsible for sexual differentiation and for specific intersex disorders.

NORMAL SEXUAL DIFFERENTIATION

Under normal circumstances, sexual differentiation is a dynamic and sequential process. **According to the Jost paradigm, three steps must occur: establishment of chromosomal sex at fertilization, which determines development of the undifferentiated gonads into testes or ovaries, and subsequent differentiation of the internal ducts and external genitalia as a result of endocrine functions associated with the type of gonad present** (Jost et al, 1973). Therefore, development of the sexual phenotype represents the result of complex interactions of genetic and hormonal signals. Interference with this highly ordered process at any step can result in a disorder of sexual differentiation.

Chromosomal Sex

In 1921, Painter demonstrated cytologically that humans have X and Y chromosomes. Based on chromosomal studies of *Drosophila,* it was assumed that sex was determined by the X chromosomes possessed by the individual (Bridges, 1921). The Y chromosome was thought to impart no genetic information until karyotyping of mammalian chromosomes, developed in the 1950s, demonstrated that the Y chromosome specified development of the testis. Specifically, reports in the late 1950s describing the karyotype 47,XXY as male with Klinefelter's syndrome and 45,XO as female with Turner's syndrome demonstrated that the presence of a Y chromosome, independent of the number of X chromosomes, resulted in the development of a male embryo, whereas in the absence of a Y chromosome the embryo developed as a female (Ford et al, 1959; Jacobs and Strong, 1959). Therefore, the Y chromosome appeared to possess a gene or genes that determined the destiny of the bipotential gonad as a testis or ovary. **In the human, the hypothetical Y-chromosomal gene was termed TDF (testis-determining factor).**

During the following years, the search for TDF was the focus of intense research. The observation that antibodies raised in inbred female mice transplanted with male skin grafts resulted in graft rejection whereas female-to-male skin grafts were accepted in the same strain of mice led to the proposal that the histocompatibility Y or H-Y antigen was the product of TDF (Eichwald and Silmser, 1955).

2395

Assays for quantifying H-Y antigen were developed. With the use of these assays, it was discovered that the presence of a testis resulted in serologically detectable levels of H-Y antigen. This was confirmed in normal and intersex patients as well as in males of other species. **Therefore, it was believed that the H-Y gene was the TDF** (Wachtel, 1977). **This theory was considered valid for more than 10 years.**

Problems with the H-Y antigen theory developed, however. A number of women with 45,X gonadal dysgenesis were found to be H-Y antigen positive. In addition, a mouse model for the male sex reversal syndrome (XX male) was studied in which mice have two X chromosomes and testes because a fragment of Y is translocated onto one of the X chromosomes (McLaren et al, 1984). These mice were H-Y antigen negative and azoospermic. **As a result of these findings, the hypothesis that the H-Y antigen was the product of TDF was excluded.**

Further study of the Y chromosome suggested that the genetic information responsible for maleness was on the short arm of the chromosome near the centromere. This theory was supported by experiments of nature in which the short arm of the Y chromosome was lost and only the long arm remained, the result being a female phenotype.

Further progress was made by studying 46,XX males, paradoxical individuals who develop as phenotypic males in the presence of a normal female 46,XX karyotype (Magenis et al, 1982). The simplest explanation for their sex reversal would be the presence of Y chromosomal material (including TDF) owing to mosaicism or in submicroscopic cellular quantities. The application of molecular techniques to evaluate Y chromosomal sequences present in XX males, as well as deletions of the Y chromosome in XY females, led to the cloning of TDF (Lukusa et al, 1992). **Deletion maps based on the genomes of these individu-** **als were constructed by a number of laboratories, and TDF was mapped to the most distal aspect of the Y-unique region of the short arm of the Y chromosome, adjacent to the pseudoautosomal boundary** (Fig. 68–1).

ZFY

Page and coworkers (1987) constructed a more detailed genomic map and defined a 140-kilobase (kb) interval thought to contain the TDF by aligning the Y-specific DNA present in an XX male with a Y chromosome deletion of the same region in an XY female. These investigators identified a gene encoding a protein with multiple "zinc finger" domains, characteristic of a class of proteins that bind DNA in a sequence-specific manner and regulate transcription. In addition, these sequences demonstrated evolutionary conservation. **Based on its position and structural similarity to regulatory genes, ZFY (zinc finger gene on Y chromosome) was proposed as a candidate for the TDF.**

However, in subsequent years, data were accumulated that excluded *ZFY* as the TDF. This included the discovery that in marsupials *ZFY* was located not on the sex chromosomes but on autosomes (Sinclair et al, 1988). **ZFY was excluded with certainty as a candidate for TDF when four individuals with testicular development were found to have inherited a fragment of the Y chromosome that did not include ZFY** (Palmer et al, 1989).

The renewed search for TDF led to the discovery of Y-specific sequences in XX males lacking ZFY and imposing new limits on the location of TDF to a 35-kb region adjacent to the pseudoautosomal boundary (Fig. 68–2). **Using probes from this region, Sinclair and colleagues (1990) discovered a single-copy male-specific sequence that was evolutionarily conserved. This gene was**

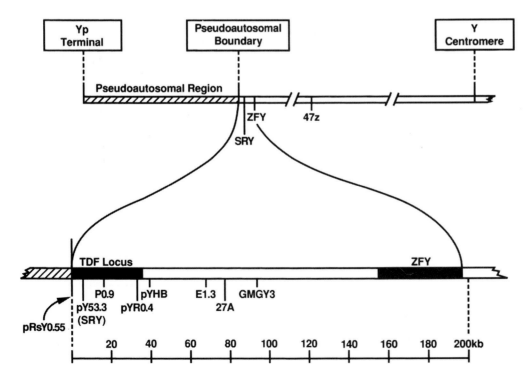

Figure 68–1. Genetic map of the short arm of the human Y chromosome. The top of the diagram shows the pseudoautosomal region of the short arm of the Y chromosome and the locus of the *SRY* and *ZFY* genes near the pseudoautosomal boundary. The lower part of the diagram represents an enlargement of the Y chromosome near the pseudoautosomal boundary and the location of the *SRY* and *ZFY* genes. (From Migeon CJ, Berkovitz GD, Brown TR: Sexual differentiation and ambiguity. In Kappy MS, Blizzard RN, Migeon CJ (eds): Wilkins, The Diagnosis and Treatment of Endocrine Disorders in Childhood and Adolescence. Springfield, Ill, Charles C Thomas, 1994, p 588, with permission.)

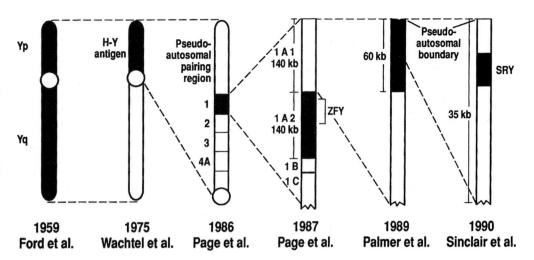

Figure 68–2. Diagrammatic representation of the historical search for the testis-determining factor (TDF). The shaded area on the Y chromosome is the region to which this factor has been localized. (From Grumbach MM, Conte FH: Disorders of sex differentiation. In Wilson JD, Foster DW (eds): Williams Textbook of Endocrinology. Philadelphia, WB Saunders, 1998, p 1315, with permission.)

termed *SRY* (sex-determining region Y gene) in humans and *Sry* in mice. Analysis of the *SRY* gene demonstrated there to be a highly conserved region with homology to a DNA-binding motif referred to as high-mobility group (HMG) box (Fig. 68–3). When the HMG box was used as a probe, a subfamily of closely related genes was identified. Members of this family, defined as those encoding a region with 60% or greater amino acid similarity to the *SRY* HMG-box motif, were called *SOX* (SRY-box-related) genes (Goodfellow and Lovell-Badge, 1993).

Considerable evidence has accumulated that *SRY* is the TDF. In the mouse, expression of *Sry* correlates with testicular determination in the gonadal ridge (Koopman et al, 1990). *SRY* is an evolutionarily conserved gene on the Y chromosome of mammals. Chromosomal fragments related to *SRY* (i.e., the *SOX* genes) are very much conserved evolutionarily, being demonstrated in various vertebrates and marsupials. ***SRY* is localized to the smallest region of the Y chromosome capable of inducing testicular differentiation in humans and in mice** (Gubbay et al, 1992). In fact, Koopman and coworkers (1991) introduced into XX mouse embryos a 14-kb mouse genomic DNA fragment containing *Sry* and no other Y-linked gene sequences and demonstrated that it was capable of giving rise to normal testicular development in the transgenic mice.

SRY appears to be capable of recognizing specific sites on DNA, and, by binding and producing bending of the DNA, it is able to activate downstream gene expression (Fig. 68–4).

An expectation for TDF was that mutations in its protein sequence would result in sex reversal. Examination of the *SRY* sequence in XY females has identified more than 20 mutations in the protein coding sequences. All but one of these point mutations and microdeletions lie within the DNA-binding domain. Another prediction for TDF is that its presence can cause XX male sex reversal. All but one XX male with Y-specific sequences have been found to contain *SRY* (Goodfellow and Lovell-Badge, 1993). This suggests a causative role of *SRY* in these cases of XX sex reversal. **Therefore, genetic and molecular data have established that *SRY* can be equated to the TDF.** Biochemical data have provided insight into how the gene may function, but the identities of genes that interact directly with *SRY*, both upstream and downstream, are currently unknown (Bogan and Page, 1994). However, the initial step—establishment of gonadal sex in the previously undifferentiated urogenital ridge—provides a model of a genetic switch in organogenesis. Identification of *SRY* as the testis-determining factor may potentially lead to biochemical characterization of this switch.

Figure 68–3. Diagram of the *SRY* (sex-determining region Y gene) locus, with the so-called high-mobility group (HMG)-related box in the center. The HMG box encodes the DNA binding region of the SRY protein. Various arrows represent the location of the mutations which have been identified in patients with 46,XY complete gonadal dysgenesis. (From Migeon CJ, Berkovitz GD, Brown TR: Sexual differentiation and ambiguity. In Kappy MS, Blizzard RN, Migeon CJ (eds): Wilkins, The Diagnosis and Treatment of Endocrine Disorders in Childhood and Adolescence. Springfield, Ill, Charles C Thomas, 1994, p 620, with permission.)

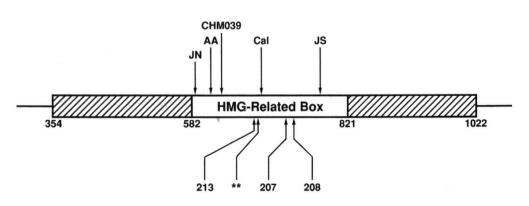

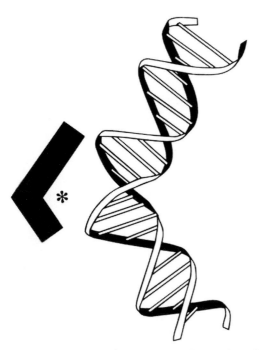

Figure 68–4. Schematic model of the L-shaped HMG box *(left)* and bent DNA site *(right)*. (From Peters R, King CY, Ukiyama E, et al: An SRY mutation causing human sex reversal resolves a general mechanism of structure-specific DNA recognition: Application to the four-way DNA junction. Biochemistry 34(14):4569–4576, 1995.

Other Genes Involved in Sex Determination

Genes other than *SRY* that have been found to be involved in sex determination include *WT-1, SF-1, SOX-9,* and *DSS* (Fig. 68–5).

WT-1

The *WT-1* gene was originally isolated in cloning experiments that identified an oncogene on human chro- mosome **11 as being involved in the etiology of Wilms' tumor** (Call et al, 1990). This gene, originally localized by examining chromosomal deletions in children with WAGR syndrome (Wilms' tumor, aniridia, genitourinary abnormalities, gonadoblastoma, and mental retardation), was found to be expressed primarily in the kidney and gonads of the developing human embryo (Kreidberg et al, 1993). The first reported mutations in the Denys-Drash syndrome, which includes Wilms' tumor, renal failure, and gonadal and genital abnormalities, were found to involve the WT-1 protein (Pelletier et al, 1991a, 1991b). Indeed, mutations involving *WT-1* have been found in the majority of patients with Denys-Drash syndrome who were tested. **Research on *Wt-1* in the mouse suggests that it exerts its effects upstream of *Sry* and is likely to be necessary for commitment and maintenance of gonadal tissue** (Lim and Hawkins, 1998).

SF-1

Experiments in the mouse have demonstrated the nuclear receptor, SF-1, to be expressed in all steroidogenic tissue, including adrenal cortex, testis (Leydig cells), ovarian theca, granulosa cells, and corpus luteum. SF-1 appears to be a key regulator of enzymes involved in steroid production, including the sex hormones. In addition, it may well play a role in early gonadal differentiation. **SF-1 appears to be a regulator of müllerian inhibiting substance** (MIS) (Shen et al, 1994; Imbeaud et al, 1995).

SOX-9

The *SOX-9* gene was originally identified in patients with camptomelic dysplasia, a congenital disease of bone and cartilage formation that is often associated with XY sex reversal (Wagner et al, 1994). **The gene is structurally quite similar to the *SRY*, with 71% similarity of the *SOX-9* HMG-box amino acid sequence to that of *SRY*.** Expression of the gene in adults is greatest in the testes. It

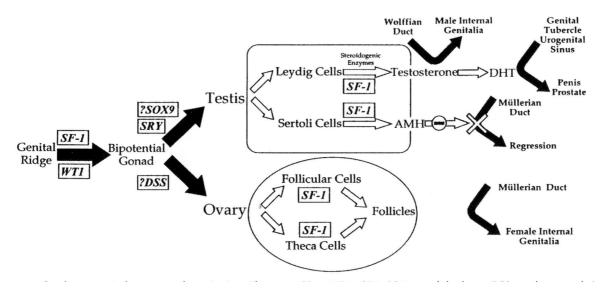

Figure 68–5. Molecular events in human sex determination. The genes *SF-1, WT-1, SRY, SOX-9,* and the locus *DSS* are shown at their position in the sex determination pathway. AMH, anti-müllerian hormone; DHT, dihydrotestosterone. (From Schafer AJ: Sex determination and its pathology in man. Adv Genet 1995;33:294, with permission.)

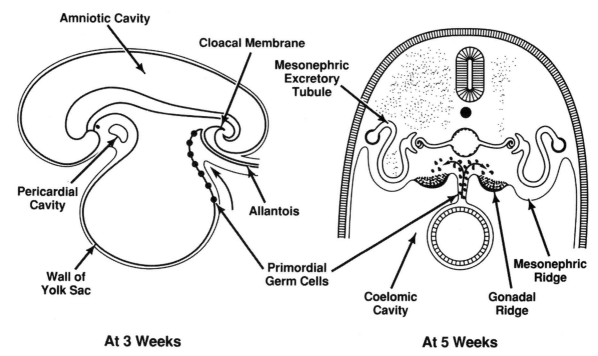

At 3 Weeks   **At 5 Weeks**

Figure 68–6. Migration of primordial germ cells. At 3 weeks, primordial germ cells are being formed and migrate along the wall of the yolk sac to reach the caudal part of the fetus. By 5 weeks, they have reached the level of the gonadal ridge. (From Migeon CJ, Berkovitz GD, Brown TR: Sexual differentiation and ambiguity. In Kappy MS, Blizzard RN, Migeon CJ (eds): Wilkins, The Diagnosis and Treatment of Endocrine Disorders in Childhood and Adolescence. Springfield, Ill, Charles C Thomas, 1994, p 584, with permission.)

is thought likely that the gene is involved in gonadal differentiation (Josso and Rey, 1996).

DSS (DAX-1)

The first indication that an X-specific gene was involved in human sex determination was provided in 1978 with the identification of a family with an X-linked mode of inheritance of 46,Y gonadal dysgenesis. Subsequent studies of a number of sex-reversed subjects confirmed the presence of X-chromosomal genetic duplication and a normal Y chromosome (Ogata et al, 1992). **This finding has suggested that the duplicated X chromosome causes XY sex reversal by expressing a double dose of the gene normally subject to X inactivation. Screening of XY females with a normal *SRY* gene detected such a submicroscopic duplication, a 160-kb region designated *DSS* (dosage-sensitive sex reversal).** Subsequent study of this region revealed a gene, *DAX-1*, that was implicated in adrenal hypoplasia congenita, an inherited disorder of adrenal gland development (Guo et al, 1995). The common origin of adrenals and gonads from primordial mesenchyme and their shared steroidogenic properties support *DAX-1* as the probable gene for both adrenal hypoplasia congenita and *DSS*.

Gonadal Stage of Differentiation

During the first 6 weeks of embryonic development, the gonadal ridge, germ cells, internal ducts, and external genitalia are bipotential in both 46,XY and 46,XX embryos. Under the genetic influences of sex determination, the bipotential gonadal ridges differentiate into either ovaries or testes and germ cells develop into either oocytes or spermatocytes.

Primordial germ cells can be recognized in the 3rd week of gestation on the posterior wall of the secondary yoke sac. **Migration of the germ cells begins in the 5th week of gestation as a result of ameboid movements through the mesentery to the medial ventral aspect of the urogenital ridge** (Jirasek, 1998) (Fig. 68–6). Overall, a population of 1000 to 2000 primordial germ cells reaches the gonadal blastema by the 6th week of gestation.

Transformation of the germ cells into spermatogonia and oogonia results from differentiation of the epithelial gonadal compartments referred to as testicular and ovarian "cords." ***SRY* initiates the switch that induces a cascade of genes directing the indifferent gonad toward testicular organogenesis.** The precise moment at which this occurs remains unknown. Initially, differentiation of Sertoli cells is noted as testicular cords form at 6 to 7 weeks' gestation, creating the basement membrane, or blood-testis barrier, of spermatogonia and Sertoli cells on one side and mesenchymal fibroblasts on the other. **The differentiation of Sertoli cells is associated with the production of MIS, a glycoprotein encoded by a gene on the short arm of chromosome 19** (Haqq et al, 1994).

In males, a second line of primordial cells of steroidogenic mesenchyme remain among the testicular cords and represent future Leydig cells, which differentiate at 8 to 9 weeks.

In the absence of *SRY*, ovarian organogenesis results. Little is known about the genetic control of ovarian development. **It does appear necessary that there be duplicate copies of at least one X chromosomal locus (which presumably explains the dysgenetic ovaries in the 45,XO**

Turner's syndrome patients). A potential candidate is *DSS* on Xp-21, which, when duplicated, promotes male-to-female "sex reversal" (Lopez et al, 1998).

Unlike the testis, which functions primarily as a fetal endocrine organ, the ovary has primarily exocrine activity. **In embryonal ovaries, germ cells undergo intense mitotic proliferation (preceding the onset of meiotic prophase) and in the process exhaust their entire mitotic potential prenatally, reaching a maximum endowment of 20 million cells by 20 weeks' gestation.** The presence of two X chromosomes appears to be responsible for differentiation of the granulosa cells into the protective mantle of the granulosa layer and "rescue" of 30% of germ cells (approximately 2 million) (Byskov and Westergaard, 1998).

Gonadal Function

The initial endocrine function of the fetal testes is the secretion of MIS by the Sertoli cells at 7 to 8 weeks' gestation. MIS, one of the two hormones necessary for male sexual differentiation, acts locally to produce müllerian regression. It is a member of the transforming growth factor–β (TGF-β) family, and the human gene has been cloned and mapped to chromosome 19 (Cate et al, 1986). Little is known about the cellular mechanism of action of MIS. Because the hallmark of MIS-mediated müllerian duct regression is the formation of a ring of connective tissue around the epithelial cells, it is likely that the mesenchyme is the primary target of MIS.

Testosterone secretion by the fetal testes is detectable shortly after the formation of Leydig cells in the interstitium at approximately 9 weeks' gestation (Siiteri and Wilson, 1974). There is a rise in serum and testicular testosterone to a peak concentration at 13 weeks and then a decline. The rate-limiting enzyme for fetal testosterone synthesis is 3-β-hydroxysteroid dehydrogenase, which is approximately 50 times higher in the fetal testes than in the ovary. **Jost and colleagues (1973) clearly demonstrated that androgen is essential for virilization of wolffian duct structures, the urogenital sinus and genital tubercle. Testosterone, the major androgen secreted by the testes, enters target tissues by passive diffusion.** Organs such as the wolffian duct, adjacent to the fetal testis, also take up testosterone by pinocytosis. **The local source of androgen is important for wolffian duct development, which does not occur if testosterone is supplied only via the peripheral circulation. In some cells, such as those in the urogenital sinus, testosterone is converted to dihydrotestosterone (DHT) by intracellular 5α-reductase.** Testosterone or DHT then binds to a high-affinity intracellular receptor protein, and this complex enters the nucleus, where it binds to acceptor sites on DNA, resulting in new messenger RNA and protein synthesis (Fig. 68–7). The androgen receptor has been characterized as a high-affinity receptor that mediates the action of testosterone and DHT in all androgen-dependent tissues. In disorders of the androgen receptor, such as androgen insensitivity syndrome, testosterone production is normal but the hormone is unable to reach the nucleus and interact with DNA. Various defects in the androgen receptor result in a spectrum of phenotypic abnormalities in the genetic male. Because gonadal females have androgen receptor within their tissues, exogenous androgen produces virilization.

DHT binds to the androgen receptor with greater affinity and stability than does testosterone. Therefore, in tissues equipped with 5α-reductase at the time of sexual differentiation (e.g., prostate, urogenital sinus, external genitalia), DHT is the active androgen (George and Peterson, 1988). The 5α-reductase activity has two optimal pH values in cultured genital skin fibroblasts—one at pH 5.5 and a second one near pH 8—which correspond to two distinct enzymes (Jenkins et al, 1992). The alkaline

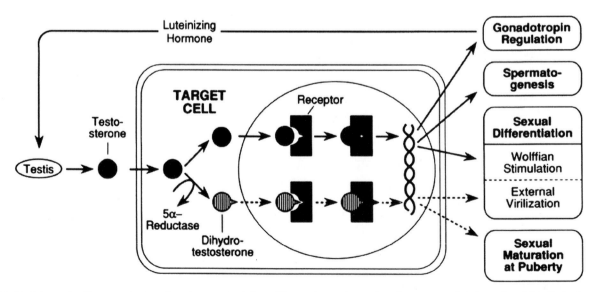

Figure 68–7. Schematic diagram of normal androgen physiology. The major actions of androgens are listed on the right. Testosterone enters androgen target tissues and either binds to the androgen receptor in cell nuclei or is converted by 5α-reductase to dihydrotestosterone (DHT). DHT binds to the same receptor but with greater affinity. Androgen actions mediated by testosterone are indicated by solid arrows, and those mediated by DHT are indicated by the dashed arrows. (From Griffin JE, Wilson JD: Syndromes of androgen resistance. Hosp Pract 1987;22:99–114, with permission.)

enzyme, human steroid 5α-reductase 1, was cloned first; however, the primary enzyme in the prostate is 5α-reductase 2 (Andersson and Russell, 1990). A deletion in the gene coding for this enzyme has been discovered in intersex patients with 5α-reductase deficiency (Andersson et al, 1991).

The gene encoding the androgen receptor has been cloned and mapped to the X chromosome between the centromere and q13 (Lubahn et al, 1988).

Ovary

Estrogen synthesis is detectable in the female embryo just after 8 weeks of gestation. The rate-limiting enzyme is aromatase, which is higher in the fetal ovary than in the fetal testis. Estrogens are not required for normal female differentiation of the reproductive tract, but they can interfere with male differentiation. Estrogen can block the effect of MIS on müllerian ducts, and prenatal estrogen treatment of mothers has been associated with male reproductive tract abnormalities (Gill et al, 1979; Vigier et al, 1989).

Phenotypic Sexual Differentiation

Before the 8th week of gestation, the urogenital tract is identical in the two sexes. Both the wolffian and the müllerian duct systems are present as anlagen of the internal accessory organs of reproduction (Fig. 68–8). In addition, at this stage, the anlagen of the external genitalia of male and female embryos are indistinguishable (Fig. 68–9).

In the male fetus, Sertoli cells produce MIS, which acts locally and unilaterally to suppress the müllerian ducts, and Leydig cells produce testosterone, which permits local development of the wolffian ducts. By 10 weeks of gestation, degeneration of the müllerian ducts is almost complete and the wolffian ducts have become more prominent (see Fig. 68–8). Adjacent to the testes, convolutions of the ducts organize to form the epididymis. The wolffian ducts of the epididymis join with the collecting portion of the testicular tubules (rete testes). Distally, the ducts join the urogenital sinus by about 30 days' gestation, where they develop into the seminal vesicles.

In the female fetus, testosterone is not secreted by the ovaries and therefore the wolffian ducts regress. Because the ovary does not produce MIS, the müllerian ducts are maintained and develop into the female internal reproductive tract. The cephalic ends are anlagen of the fallopian tubes, and the caudal ends fuse to form the uterus (see Fig. 68–8). Contact of the müllerian ducts with the urogenital sinus induces formation of the uterovaginal plate, which ultimately forms the lumen of the vagina. The relative contributions of the müllerian ducts and urogenital sinus to the formation of the vagina remain somewhat controversial; however, there is some agreement that the proximal two thirds of the vagina is contributed by the müllerian ducts and the distal one third by the urogenital sinus.

Masculinization of the male fetus starts between 7 and 8 weeks of gestation (Fig. 68–10). **The first sign of male phenotypic differentiation is degeneration of the müllerian ducts adjacent to the testes as a result of MIS**

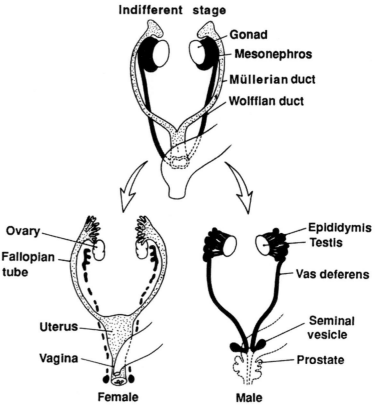

Figure 68–8. Differentiation of the wolffian and müllerian duct and urogenital sinus in the male and female. (From Wilson JD: Embryology of the genital tract. In Harrison HH, Gittes RF, Perlmutter AD, et al (eds): Campbell's Urology, 4th ed. Philadelphia, WB Saunders, 1979, p 1473, with permission.)

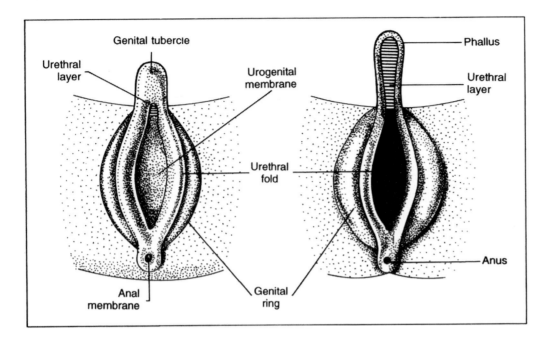

Figure 68–9. Schematic diagram of external genitalia in the undifferentiated period. (From Martinez-Mora J: Development of the genital tract. In Martinez-Mora J: Intersexual States: Disorders of Sex Differentiation. Barcelona, Ediciones Doymer, 1994, p 52, with permission.)

secretion by the Sertoli cells. **Whereas the effects of androgen on the wolffian ducts are related to diffusion of testosterone from the adjacent gonad, masculinization of the external genitalia results from the systemic delivery of testosterone with local conversion to dihydrotestosterone.** By 10 weeks, an increase in distance between genital tubercle and anal folds can be seen. The genital tubercle thickens and elongates to become the penis, and the urethral folds fuse from posterior to anterior over the urethral groove (Fig. 68–11). Near the bladder, the urethra is surrounded by the prostate. The urogenital swellings migrate posteriorly to the genital tubercle and fuse to form the scrotum. **By 12 to 13 weeks' gestation,** the genitalia of the male fetus is completed with closure of the elongated urogenital cleft. Under the influence of androgen secreted by the fetal testes, penile growth and testicular descent occur in the third trimester (see Fig. 68–10).

In the female fetus, the absence of circulating testosterone maintains the appearance of the external genitalia at the 6-week gestational stage. The genital tubercle develops only slightly to form the clitoris. The lateral genital swellings become labia majora, and the adjacent urethral folds become the labia minora (Fig. 68–12). Between the labia minora will develop the vaginal introitus and urethral meatus.

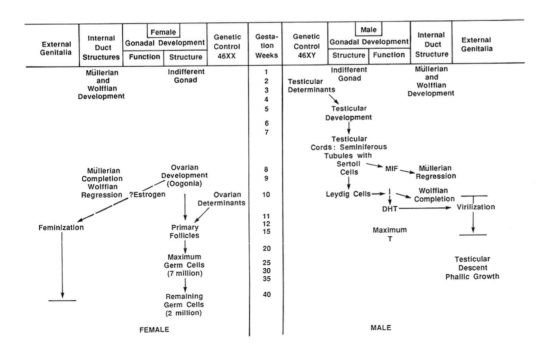

Figure 68–10. Timetable of normal sexual differentiation. (From Diamond D: Intersex disorders: Parts I and II. AUA Update Series, Vol IX, Lessons 9 and 10, Houston, TX, American Urological Association Office of Education, 1990, with permission.)

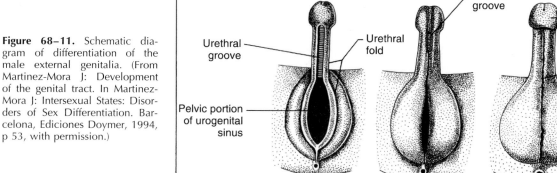

Figure 68–11. Schematic diagram of differentiation of the male external genitalia. (From Martinez-Mora J: Development of the genital tract. In Martinez-Mora J: Intersexual States: Disorders of Sex Differentiation. Barcelona, Ediciones Doymer, 1994, p 53, with permission.)

Psychosexual Differentiation

Humans have been recognized as having sexually dimorphic behavior, which has several aspects: (1) *gender identity,* the identification of self as either male or female; (2) *gender role,* aspects of behavior in which males and females appear to differ; (3) *gender orientation,* or choice of sexual partner (heterosexual, homosexual, or bisexual); and (4) *cognitive differences* (Grumbach and Conte, 1998).

Gender identity is a complex and poorly understood phenomenon in humans, and the mechanisms appear multifactorial. Experience in patients with congenital adrenal hyperplasia (CAH) who were exposed prenatally to androgen and in patients reared in a sex opposite to their chromosomal or gonadal sex have provided evidence to indicate that gender identity is not merely a function of chromosomal complement or prenatal endocrine milieu. Postnatal environmental factors and learning appear to have an important effect. However, strong evidence has accumulated for the impact of prenatal hormonal influences on sexually dimorphic behavior or gender role. Long-term follow-up with CAH patients has supported a greater interest in "tomboyish behavior" than in unaffected girls, although these patterns are not abnormal in relation to female behavior in Western society (Erhardt and Meyer-Bahlberg, 1981).

The previously accepted dogma that children are psychosexually neutral at birth and capable of being environmentally oriented (the blue room/pink room theory) has been seriously challenged by those who support the concept of prenatal psychosexual differentiation (Money and Erhardt, 1972; Diamond and Sigmundson, 1997). Support for either theory in humans is based on the assessment of a limited number of affected patients. In the hope of resolving this dilemma, a national task force has been organized to study larger numbers of affected patients. An improved understanding of the "nature versus nurture" controversy will probably prove important in the optimal management of patients with intersex disorders.

ABNORMAL SEXUAL DIFFERENTIATION

The classification of intersex disorders has undergone evolutionary change as understanding of the etiologic mechanisms of normal and abnormal sexual differentiation has improved. As a result, classification systems vary. We have borrowed from the system utilized by Grumbach and Conte (1998), which incorporates the historical emphasis on classification by gonadal morphology. The first cate-

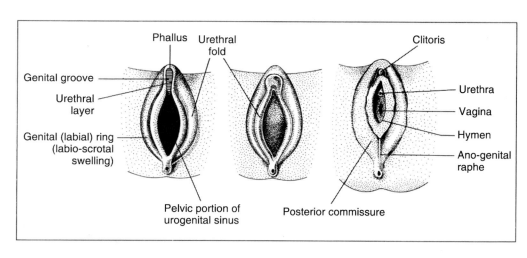

Figure 68–12. Schematic diagram of differentiation of the female external genitalia. (From Martinez-Mora J: Development of the genital tract. In Martinez-Mora J: Intersexual States: Disorders of Sex Differentiation. Barcelona, Ediciones Doymer, 1994, p 52, with permission.)

gory comprises disorders of gonadal differentiation, the second includes female pseudohermaphroditism (i.e., ovaries present, but external genitalia exhibiting evidence of masculinization), the third includes male pseudohermaphroditism (i.e., testes present, but genital ducts and/or external genitalia incompletely masculinized), and the fourth category comprises unclassified forms. Within each category, remarkable advances in chromosomal and biochemical information have allowed subclassification of disorders based on etiologic mechanisms, contributing to a more rational classification system (Table 68–1).

Disorders of Gonadal Differentiation and Development

Seminiferous Tubule Dysgenesis (Klinefelter's Syndrome and Variants)

In 1942, Klinefelter, Reifenstein, and Albright described a syndrome characterized by eunuchoidism, gynecomastia, azoospermia, increased gonadotropin levels, and small, firm testes (Klinefelter et al, 1942). By

Table 68–1. ABNORMAL SEXUAL DIFFERENTIATION

Disorders of gonadal differentiation
  Seminiferous tubule dysgenesis
  Klinefelter's syndrome
  46,XX male
  Syndromes of gonadal dysgenesis
    Turner's syndrome
    Pure gonadal dysgenesis
    Mixed gonadal dysgenesis
    Dysgenetic male pseudohermaphroditism
    Bilateral vanishing testes/testicular regression syndromes
  True hermaphroditism
Female pseudohermaphroditism
  Congenital adrenal hyperplasia (21-hydroxylase, 11β-hydroxylase, 3β-hydroxysteroid dehydrogenase deficiencies)
  Maternal androgens
Male pseudohermaphroditism
  Leydig cell agenesis, unresponsiveness
  Disorders of testosterone biosynthesis
  Variants of congenital adrenal hyperplasia affecting corticosteroid and testosterone synthesis
    Congenital lipoid adrenal hyperplasia
    3β-hydroxysteroid dehydrogenase deficiency
    17α-hydroxylase deficiency
  Disorders of testosterone biosynthesis
    17,20-Lyase deficiency
    17β-hydroxysteroid oxidoreductase deficiency
  Disorders of androgen-dependent target tissue
    Androgen receptor and postreceptor defects
    Syndrome of complete testicular feminization
    Syndrome of partial androgen resistance
    Androgen resistance in infertile men
  Disorders of testosterone metabolism by peripheral tissues
    5α-reductase deficiency
  Disorders of synthesis, secretion, or response to müllerian inhibiting substance
    Persistent müllerian duct syndrome
Unclassified forms
  In males
    Micropenis (covered in Chapter 66)
  In females
    Mayer-Rokitansky-Kuster-Hauser syndrome

1959, these patients were noted to have a 47,XXY karyotype (Jacobs and Strong, 1959).

Klinefelter's syndrome represents the most common major abnormality of sexual differentiation. **By definition, males with at least one Y chromosome and at least two X chromosomes have Klinefelter's syndrome.** The classic 47,XXY complement arises as a result of nondisjunction during meiosis; it occurs in 1 of 1000 liveborn males. But the phenotype is also associated with 48,XXYY and 49,XXXYY, and an exaggerated form of the phenotype is associated with 48,XXXY and 49,XXXXY. The mosaic form 46,XY/47,XXY is associated with a milder version of the phenotypic features of classic 47,XXY Klinefelter's syndrome.

In 47,XXY adults, seminiferous tubules degenerate and are replaced with hyaline. As a result, testes are small and firm, less than 3.5 cm in length. Histologically, Leydig cells appear to be present in large numbers, because they are seen in large clumps in certain areas of the testes, sometimes resembling Leydig cell tumors. However, the absolute volume of Leydig cells is not increased and is probably lower than normal. Serum testosterone is low-normal and gonadotropins are elevated. Plasma estradiol levels tend to be high, with gynecomastia the result of an increased ratio of estradiol to testosterone. The vast majority of patients are azoospermic, and the presence of sperm suggests 46,XY/47,XXY mosaicism. Fertility, with the benefit of intracytoplasmic sperm injection, has been reported in a patient with Klinefelter's syndrome (Kitamura et al, 2000).

The decreased androgen production prevents normal secondary sexual development. Muscle development is poor, and the fat distribution is more female than male. Normal amounts of pubic and axillary hair may be present, but facial hair is sparse. Patients tend to be taller than average, mainly because of the disproportionate length of their legs, which is present even in childhood. Otherwise, few if any distinguishing features are present in the prepubertal child.

Gynecomastia, which can be quite marked, is a common pubertal development in patients with Klinefelter's syndrome. As a result, these patients have 8 times the risk for development of breast carcinoma compared with normal males (Harnden et al, 1971). In addition, they are predisposed to developing malignant neoplasms of extragonadal germ cell origin.

Management of Klinefelter's syndrome entails careful androgen supplementation in selected male patients to improve libido and reduction mammoplasty if necessary. Surveillance for breast carcinoma is also appropriate.

46,XX Males

The condition of 46,XX maleness, which occurs in 1 of every 20,000 males, may be closely related to that of Klinefelter's syndrome. Historically, the genetic analysis of subjects with sex reversal who had a phenotypic sex different from that anticipated based on karyotype was crucial for identification of the SRY gene.

XX maleness, first recognized by de la Chappelle and coworkers in 1964, is characterized by testicular development in subjects who have two X chromosomes and

lack a normal Y chromosome. **Most of these subjects have normal male external genitalia, but 10% have hypospadias and all are infertile.** Among infertile adults, 2% have XX maleness (Van Dyke et al, 1991).

Two categories of patients with XX maleness have been identified—the 80% who are *SRY* positive and those who are *SRY* negative (Weil et al, 1994). The *SRY*-positive group rarely have genital abnormalities, but they have phenotypic features of Klinefelter's syndrome, including hypogonadism, gynecomastia, azoospermia, and hyalinization of seminiferous tubules with altered hormonal levels at puberty (low testosterone, increased follicle-stimulating hormone [FSH] and luteinizing hormone [LH]) (Fechner et al, 1993). Often, the diagnosis is made in a pubertal male who presents for evaluation of gynecomastia. **These patients differ from those with Klinefelter's syndrome in that they are shorter (mean height, 168 cm) and have normal skeletal proportions.**

Three mechanisms have been proposed to explain XX sex reversal. **The most common is translocation of Y chromosomal material, including *SRY*, to the X chromosome.** Clearly, this can be proven in the majority of patients. Alternatively, sex reversal could result either from the mutation of an autosomal or X chromosomal gene, permitting testicular differentiation downstream from *SRY*, or from undetected mosaicism with a Y-bearing cell line. Clinical studies to date have demonstrated XX sex reversal to be a genetically and phenotypically heterogeneous condition (Fechner et al, 1993). However, some series of XX sex reversal include genetically mosaic patients with ovotestes, who are by definition true hermaphrodites.

Treatment of XX maleness is similar to that for Klinefelter's syndrome. Androgen replacement benefits selected patients, and reduction mammoplasty may be beneficial. It is likely that these patients will also be at increased risk for breast carcinoma. Because of their lack of germ cell elements, those classic patients presenting with infertility would not benefit from testicular biopsy for potential intracytoplasmic sperm injection.

Turner's Syndrome

In 1938, Henry Turner described the combination of sexual infantilism, webbed neck, and cubitus valgus (increased carrying angle at the elbows) as a distinct entity. Subsequently, gonadal dysgenesis was recognized as part of this syndrome (Hall and Gilchrist, 1990). It was not until 1959 that Ford recognized that one missing X chromosome was the etiologic basis for the syndrome. Subsequent chromosomal studies showed that **Turner's syndrome is characterized by the presence of only one normally functioning X chromosome.** The other sex chromosome may be absent or abnormal, or mosaicism may be present.

Turner's syndrome, with a 45,X karyotype, is associated with four classic features: female phenotype, short stature, lack of secondary sexual characteristics, and a variety of somatic abnormalities. But the clinical features of Turner's syndrome are quite variable, and almost any combination of physical features may be seen with any X chromosomal abnormality. The severity of phenotypic features does not necessarily correlate with karyotypic findings. The diagnosis of Turner's syndrome should be considered in any infant with lymphedema or any young woman with short stature or primary amenorrhea.

Turner's syndrome has an incidence of 1 in 2500 live births. Half of the patients have a 45,X karyotype in all cells; this is believed to be secondary to loss of an X chromosome through nondisjunction in gametogenesis or an error in mitosis. From 12% to 20% of patients with Turner's syndrome have an isochrome X (duplication of one arm of the X chromosome with loss of the other arm). Mosaicism—the presence of two or more chromosomally different cell lines—occurs in 30% to 40% of these patients, the majority (10% to 15%) being 45,X/46,XX and 2% to 5% being 45,X/46,XY (Zinn et al, 1993). **The presence of Y chromosomal material is of critical importance in patients with Turner's syndrome because it predisposes them to potential masculinization and gonadoblastoma.**

It is postulated that in Turner's syndrome follicular cells that normally surround the germ cells and provide a protective mantle for the oocytes are inadequate (Stanhope et al, 1992). As a result, the rate of attrition of oocytes is so rapid that by birth few or no oocytes remain in the **ovaries, which become streaks** (Epstein, 1990). Typically, these streaks are white, fibrous structures, 2 to 3 cm long and approximately 0.5 cm wide, located in the broad ligament. Histologically, the streak possesses interlacing waves of dense fibrous stroma that is devoid of oocytes but is otherwise indistinguishable from normal ovarian stroma. Both estrogen and androgen are decreased, and FSH and LH are increased. Secondary sexual development does not, as a rule, occur. Pubic and axillary hair fails to develop in normal abundance, and the well-differentiated external genitalia, vagina and müllerian derivatives, and breasts remain small (Saenger, 1996). Turner's syndrome is a common cause of primary amenorrhea, and the diagnosis is frequently made because pubertal development never occurs.

The associated congenital anomalies that are thought typical in Turner's syndrome include short stature, broad chest, widespread nipples, webbing of the neck, peripheral edema at birth, short fourth metacarpal, hypoplastic nails, multiple pigmented nevi, coarctation of the aorta, and renal anomalies (Fig. 68–13). The majority of the associated congenital anomalies can be explained by the presence of lymphedema at critical points in development, leading to an imbalance in growth forces. This may be secondary to failed opening of embryonic lymphatic channels (Zinn et al, 1993).

Of paramount importance in the assessment of the patient with Turner's syndrome is identification of Y chromosomal material or 45,X/46,XY mosaicism, whose detection has been enhanced by use of the polymerase chain reaction (PCR). **In patients with occult Y chromosomal material, the risk of gonadoblastoma, an in situ germ cell cancer, is approximately 30%** (Hall and Gilchrist, 1990). Gonadoblastoma is associated with dysgerminoma or other germ cell neoplasms in 50% to 60% of cases, sometimes associated with virilization. **Because the age of occurrence of gonadoblastoma is variable and has been reported as early as age 6 years, timely prophylactic excision of the streak gonads in the Y mosaic Turner's patient is advised.** This may be well performed laparoscopically. Streak

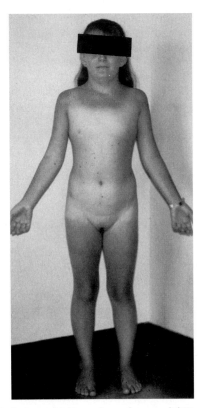

Figure 68–13. Patient with Turner's syndrome exhibiting short stature, low-set ears, webbed neck, shield chest, and widely spaced, hypoplastic nipples. (From Diamond D: Intersex disorders: Parts I and II. AUA Update Series, Vol IX, Lessons 9 and 10, Houston, TX, American Urological Association Office of Education, 1990, with permission.)

gonads confirmed to be in 45,XO patients need not be removed.

Between 33% and 60% of patients with Turner's syndrome have structural or positional abnormalities of the kidney; this occurs most frequently in the classic 45,XO karyotype (Hall and Gilchrist, 1990). **Horseshoe kidney accounts for 10%, duplication or renal agenesis for 20%, and malrotation for 15% of these abnormalities.** Multiple renal arteries have been noted in 90% of patients with Turner's syndrome as a result of their cardiovascular evaluation (Hall and Gilchrist, 1990).

The contemporary treatment of patients with Turner's syndrome has undergone considerable advances. In the neonate, it entails a concerted search for occult Y chromosomal material and subsequently prophylactic gonadectomy if necessary, as well as ultrasound screening for renal and cardiac abnormalities. **In the child, human growth hormone has successfully been employed** to achieve increased adult height (Saenger, 1993). At an appropriate age, typically between 12 and 15 years, exogenous hormonal therapy to induce puberty and then to maintain a normal female endocrine status is begun. An improved understanding of the long-term medical management of these patients, including cardiac surveillance and management of glucose intolerance and osteoporosis, has also resulted in considerable progress. **Finally, with the remarkable advances in assisted reproductive technology, pregnancy is a realistic possibility for patients with**

Turner's syndrome. A spectrum of potential gonadal function has been noted in large series of patients with Turner's syndrome (Kaneko et al, 1990). In one series, nonstreak gonads were reported in one third of such patients and were more commonly noted in girls with loss of only the short arm of the X chromosome. To date, more than 50 pregnancies have been reported among spontaneously menstruating Turner's syndrome patients. For the vast majority with true streak gonads, for whom egg donor implantation is used, 60% pregnancy rates have been reported by centers specializing in in vitro fertilization (Saenger, 1993).

46,XX "Pure" Gonadal Dysgenesis

Patients with 46,XX "pure" gonadal dysgenesis are closely related to those with Turner's syndrome. **They are characterized by normal female external genitalia, normal müllerian ducts with absence of wolffian duct structures, a normal height, bilateral streak gonads, sexual infantilism, and a normal 46,XX karyotype.** The streak gonads result in elevated serum gonadotropins. **Because these subjects exhibit none of the somatic stigmata associated with Turner's syndrome and their condition entails gonadal dysgenesis only, it has been regarded by some authors as "pure."**

A familial incidence of 46,XX gonadal dysgenesis has been reported as an autosomal recessive trait (Espiner et al, 1970). This suggests the possibility that autosomal genes in addition to genes on the X chromosome may be involved in ovarian maintenance.

Management of patients with 46,XX "pure" gonadal dysgenesis entails proper cyclic hormone replacement with estrogen and progesterone. In contrast to Turner's syndrome, growth is not abnormal with this condition, and therefore growth hormone should not be required.

Mixed Gonadal Dysgenesis

The term *mixed gonadal dysgenesis* was coined by Sohval in 1963. In 1975, Zah and associates reported on their series of more than 100 patients with 45,X/46,XY karyotypes, 72 of whom had mixed gonadal dysgenesis with a streak gonad on one side and a testis on the other. This group of patients was categorized by Migeon (1980) as having "partial gonadal dysgenesis" as a result of mosaicism involving the Y chromosome, to distinguish them from patients having complete gonadal dysgenesis with bilateral dysgenetic gonads.

Mixed gonadal dysgenesis is characterized by a unilateral testis, which is often intra-abdominal, a contralateral streak gonad, and persistent müllerian structures associated with varying degrees of inadequate masculinization. Most patients with mixed gonadal dysgenesis have a 45,XO/46,XY karyotype, which is probably the result of anaphase lag during mitosis. The 45,X/46,XY mosaicism is the most common form of mosaicism involving the Y chromosome.

The phenotypic spectrum of patients with XO/XY mosaicism extends from phenotypic females with Turner's syndrome (25%), to those with ambiguous genitalia, to, rarely, those appearing as normal males (Berkovitz et al, 1991). **In** the newborn period, mixed gonadal dysgenesis is the **second most common cause of ambiguous genitalia (after CAH) and must be in the differential diagnosis.** The majority of these patients present with varying degrees of phallic enlargement, a urogenital sinus and labioscrotal fusion, and an undescended testis. In virtually all of these patients, a uterus, vagina, and fallopian tube are present. Short stature and associated somatic stigmata are variable features.

The phenotypic asymmetry of the internal ducts epitomizes the mechanism of local testosterone and MIS production on müllerian and wolffian duct regression and development. In the series of Mendez and colleagues (1993) comprising 16 patients, all had a fallopian tube accompanied by a streak gonad, consistent with absent MIS. **Therefore, although a dysgenetic or streak gonad is associated with ipsilateral müllerian derivatives (uterus, fallopian tube), a well-differentiated testis with functional Sertoli and Leydig cells will have ipsilateral wolffian but no müllerian ducts** (Davidoff and Federman, 1973). In addition, the presence of severe external genital ambiguity in many of these patients suggests that testosterone production in utero was inadequate to promote complete differentiation of the external genitalia. Paradoxically, the dysgenetic testis is capable of responding to gonadotropins and secreting testosterone in normal quantities at puberty. Yet, despite normal postpubertal endocrine function, it is postulated that fetal testicular endocrine function is either delayed or deficient. Histologically, the testes lack germinal elements, so infertility is the rule.

The risk of developing a gonadal tumor (gonadoblastoma, dysgerminoma) is increased in mixed gonadal dysgenesis, with an estimated incidence of 15% to 20% (Robboy et al, 1982; Wallace and Levin, 1990). Gonadoblastoma, a tumor of low malignant potential, is the most common. It was so named because it recapitulates gonadal development more completely than any other tumor (Scully, 1970). **Although germ cell tumors occur both in the dysgenetic testes and in the streak gonads of individuals with 46,X/46,XY mosaicism, the risk of tumor is higher in the former** (Verp and Simpson, 1987).

Patients with mixed gonadal dysgenesis are also at increased risk for Wilms' tumor. Rajfer (1981) reported that 50% of 10 patients with an intersex disorder and Wilms' tumor had mixed gonadal dysgenesis. He postulated that there was a genetic or teratogenetic defect involving the urogenital ridge, the common embryonic anlage of both kidney and gonad. This concept was borne out by improved understanding of the Denys-Drash syndrome. In 1967, Denys and colleagues described a child with XX/XY mosaicism, nephropathy, genital abnormalities, and Wilms' tumor. Drash and coworkers reported two further examples in 1970. **The full triad of the syndrome includes nephropathy, characterized by the early onset of proteinuria and hypertension, and progressive renal failure in most of the patients.** Renal histology demonstrates diffuse focal mesangial sclerosis. **Because incomplete forms of the syndrome may occur, the nephropathy has become regarded as the common denominator of the syndrome** (Habib et al, 1985). Wilms' tumor may be diagnosed before, after, or simultaneously with presentation with nephropathy. The majority of the tumors are of favorable

triphasic histology (Beckwith and Palmer, 1978). However, there is a high incidence of bilateral Wilms' tumor in this syndrome. The genital abnormalities include frank ambiguity, hypospadias, and cryptorchidism. **A large number of patients with Denys-Drash syndrome have been noted to have mixed gonadal dysgenesis.** A relatively new and consistent finding with Denys-Drash syndrome is that of caliceal blunting without obstruction (Jadresic et al, 1990). The high mortality rate associated with this syndrome has prompted an aggressive treatment approach with prophylactic bilateral nephrectomy in an attempt to improve the prognosis for these children (Jadresic et al, 1990).

The management of mixed gonadal dysgenesis entails gender assignment, appropriate gonadectomy, and proper screening for Wilms' tumor. If the diagnosis is made in the neonatal period, the decision regarding sex of rearing should be based on the potential for normal function of the external genitalia and gonads. Historically, two thirds of patients with mixed gonadal dysgenesis have been raised as female. Potential fertility is not a significant issue in this disorder, and therefore the anatomy of the reproductive tract may direct the decision making. The likelihood of significant androgen imprinting is greater in association with a better-masculinized phenotype, and this may serve as the best clinical guide. For patients with Turner's stigmata and growth below the 5th percentile, growth hormone may be appropriate. If the male gender is elected and the testes can be brought to the scrotum, the decision between careful screening for gonadoblastoma (with physical examination and ultrasound) versus prophylactic gonadectomy and androgen replacement must be made.

The expanded use of prenatal diagnosis has changed the understanding of 45,X/46,XY mosaicism. Studies have shown that 90% to 95% of all infants with 45,X/46,XY mosaicism have normal-appearing male genitalia (Hsu, 1989). Approximately 25% have abnormal gonadal histology (Chang et al, 1990). Because only a small proportion of those with dysgenetic gonads actually have ambiguous genitalia, the possibility exists that some males with gonadal dysfunction have 45,X/46,XY mosaicism.

Dysgenetic Male Pseudohermaphroditism

In 1967, Federman coined the term *dysgenetic male pseudohermaphroditism,* which is a **condition closely related to mixed gonadal dysgenesis in that patients with abnormal sex differentiation have two dysgenetic testes rather than one dysgenetic testis and a streak gonad.** As with mixed gonadal dysgenesis, these individuals typically have a 45,X/46,XY or 46,XY karyotype. They may present with a spectrum of external genital abnormalities, depending on the capability of the dysgenetic gonads to produce testosterone. Similarly, persistent müllerian structures are typically present, but to varying degrees depending upon MIS secretion by the dysgenetic gonads.

On histology, the dysgenetic testis is found to be composed of immature hypoplastic seminiferous tubules and persistent stroma resembling that seen in the streak gonad.

Patients with dysgenetic male pseudohermaphroditism are at increased risk for gonadal malignancy. Manuel and colleagues (1976) reported that the incidence of gonado-blastoma or dysgerminoma was 46% by age 40 years. These patients are also at risk for Denys-Drash syndrome (Borer et al, 1995).

The management of dysgenetic male pseudohermaphro-ditism, in terms of gender assignment and surveillance for malignancy, is similar to that for patients with mixed go-nadal dysgenesis.

46,XY Complete Gonadal Dysgenesis

Just as 46,XX males were of great importance in discov-ery of the TDF, so too have been the 46,XY females. **Patients with 46,XY complete gonadal dysgenesis are characterized by normal female genitalia, well-devel-oped müllerian structures, bilateral streak gonads, and a nonmosaic karyotype.** Because there is complete ab-sence of testicular determination in this condition, ambigu-ity of genitalia is not an issue, but **sexual infantilism is the primary clinical problem.**

The etiology of 46,XY complete gonadal dysgenesis may well be an abnormality of the *SRY* gene that elimi-nates SRY function, or loss of another gene downstream from *SRY* that is necessary for SRY protein action. In either case, the absence of testicular determination would permit ovarian differentiation. Work with a group of indi-viduals with 46,XY complete gonadal dysgenesis has helped to narrow the chromosome interval containing the sex reversal gene to 9p24—a very small region (Mc-Donald et al, 1997).

The majority of individuals with 46,XY complete go-nadal dysgenesis present in their teens with delayed puberty. In addition to amenorrhea, breast development is usually absent. The serum concentration of gonadotropins is abnormally elevated, which leads the clinician to the determination of karyotype and the subsequent diagnosis

(Grumbach and Conte, 1998). The high concentration of serum LH in these patients is thought to be responsible for the increased androgen levels that lead to clitoromegaly in some individuals (Fig. 68–14).

The histology of the streak gonad is similar to that of Turner's syndrome, with fibrous connective tissue resem-bling wavy ovarian stroma but without follicles. Some his-tologic variability has been noted, with more proliferative-appearing stroma in some and, rarely, preservation of intact primordial follicles. This variability in ovarian histology is thought to support the hypothesis that these gonads devel-oped as ovaries in utero (German et al, 1978). This would resemble the process that occurs in the streak gonad of Turner's syndrome.

Patients with 46,XY complete gonadal dysgenesis are at significant risk for germ cell tumors. There appears to be a 30% risk of tumor development by age 30 years (Manuel et al, 1976). Gonadoblastoma is most common, and it is frequently bilateral (Fig. 68–15). Other tumors that may arise in this patient population include embryonal carcinoma, endodermal sinus tumor, choriocarcinoma, and immature teratoma. These more highly malignant tumors occur in fewer than 10% of patients with 46,XY complete gonadal dysgenesis (Scully, 1981).

Management of 46,XY complete gonadal dysgenesis entails removal of both streak gonads and proper cyclic hormone replacement with estrogen and progesterone.

Embryonic Testicular Regression and Bilateral Vanishing Testes Syndromes

The syndromes of embryonic testicular regression and bilateral vanishing testes are characterized by **patients with a 46,XY karyotype and absent testes in whom there is clear evidence of testicular function at some point dur-**

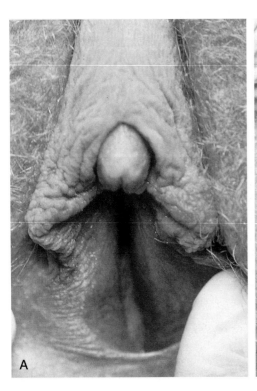

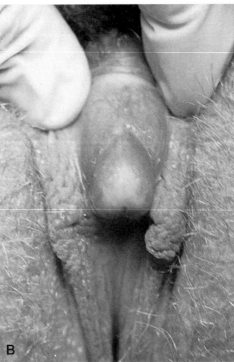

Figure 68–14. *A* and *B*, External genitalia of a 15-year-old female presenting with amenorrhea and hirsutism who was diagnosed with 46,XY gonadal dysgenesis, demonstrating clitoromegaly and urogenital sinus. (Courtesy of S. Bauer, MD.)

A

B

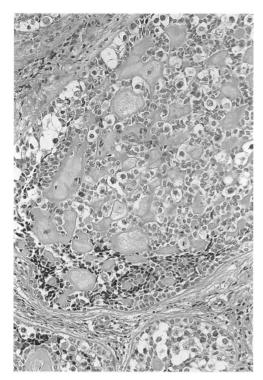

Figure 68–15. Pathology of gonadoblastoma discovered in the patient shown in Figure 68–14 with 46,XY gonadal dysgenesis. (Courtesy of S. Bauer, MD.) Encapsulated nests of gonadoblastoma comprise small sex cord–type cells arranged around rounded spaces of amorphous eosinophilic material and interspersed germ cells.

ing embryogenesis. The syndrome entails the presence of testes that "vanish" during embryogenesis and is distinguished from pure gonadal dysgenesis, in which there is no evidence of testicular function in utero.

These syndromes have been regarded as synonymous by some authors. Other authors, including Migeon and colleagues (1994), have suggested a rational stratification whereby "embryonic testicular regression" refers to loss of testicular tissue within the first trimester and is associated with ambiguity of external genitalia, whereas "bilateral vanishing testes syndrome" refers to individuals in whom male sexual differentiation of ducts and genitalia took place but loss of testicular tissue occurred subsequently in utero.

The etiology of these disorders remains unclear. **It is possible that regression of the testes in utero is caused by a genetic mutation, a teratogen, or bilateral torsion.** A genetic cause is supported by the finding of familial instances of XY agonadism that might be consistent with the rare recessive trait. Marcantonio and associates (1994) suggested the possibility that embryonic testicular regression represents a variant of 46,XY gonadal dysgenesis. They noted a group of patients with absent testes but evidence of incongruity between the extent of Leydig cell and Sertoli cell function, suggesting that gonadal tissue in these subjects was intrinsically abnormal before the testicular regression occurred. The occurrence of embryonic testicular regression in several subjects from one family in their series suggested a genetic basis for the condition, and the pattern of inheritance implicated the involvement of an X chromosome gene. In another group of patients, these au-

thors noted multiple congenital anomalies, suggesting either a mutation in a single gene that functions in several developmental pathways or a defect of multiple genes that might be the result of a large chromosomal deletion.

Clinically, these two syndromes represent a spectrum of phenotypes ranging in severity from complete female, to varying degrees of genital ambiguity in the embryonic testicular regression syndrome, to a normal male phenotype with microphallus and empty scrotum in the bilateral vanishing testes syndrome (Edman et al, 1977). **The diagnosis can be made on the basis of a 46,XY karyotype and castrate levels of testosterone despite persistently elevated serum LH and FSH** (Jarow et al, 1986). In the most severe form of embryonic testicular regression syndrome, agonadism is discovered in a 46,XY phenotypic female with no internal genital structures. This picture is presumed to result when the testis has elaborated MIS but vanishes at approximately day 60 to 70 of gestation, before the elaboration of androgen. In this setting, a belated Jost model is created and the individual goes on to develop a sexually infantile female phenotype but lacks any internal ductal structures. At an intermediate point in the clinical spectrum is the 46,XY patient with absent gonads and internal ductal structures but with ambiguous genitalia owing to incomplete elaboration of androgen by the vanishing testes. Finally, in bilateral vanishing testes syndrome, patients may present as agonadal XY phenotypic males with fully developed wolffian structures, but an empty scrotum, absent prostate, and microphallus. This represents testicular loss after complete anatomic development of the male external genitalia within the first trimester.

On surgical exploration of patients with bilateral vanishing testes syndrome, rudimentary cord structures are usually identified and biopsy of their distal ends demonstrates no recognizable testicular tissue histologically (Bergada et al, 1962). Atrophic epididymal remnants are occasionally seen.

The management of patients with embryonic testicular regression syndrome or bilateral vanishing testes syndrome is dictated by their position in the clinical spectrum of either disorder. Sexually infantile phenotypic females require estrogen supplementation at the time of expected puberty for development of secondary sexual characteristics and may require vaginoplasty. Similarly, phenotypic males require long-term androgen replacement beginning at the time of expected puberty. A study of 21 males so treated demonstrated that replacement therapy started at the correct time caused a normal pubertal growth spurt with normal secondary sex characteristics including penile growth, together with normal bone maturation (Aynsley-Green et al, 1976). In addition, these patients may benefit from placement of testicular prostheses. Patients with embryonic testicular regression syndrome and ambiguous genitalia require individualized assessment to determine the optimal gender assignment.

True Hermaphroditism

True hermaphrodites are individuals who have both testicular tissue with well-developed seminiferous tubules and ovarian tissue with primordial follicles, which

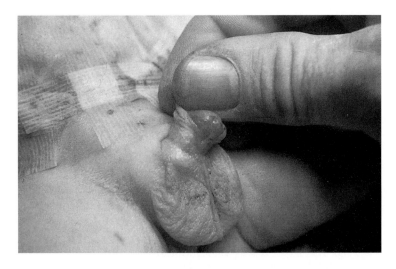

Figure 68–16. Infant with penile hypospadias, chordee, and bilaterally undescended testes who was found to have true hermaphroditism. (From Diamond D: Intersex disorders: Parts I and II. AUA Update Series, Vol IX, Lessons 9 and 10. Houston, TX, American Urological Association Office of Education, 1990, with permission.)

may take the form of one ovary and one testis or, more commonly, one or two ovotestes.

Both the external genitalia and internal duct structures of true hermaphrodites display gradations between male and female. **In most patients, the external genitalia are ambiguous but masculinized to variable degrees, and 75% are raised as male.** Among those raised as male, hypospadias and chordee occur in approximately 80%. Among those patients raised as females, two thirds have clitoromegaly. Virtually all patients have a urogenital sinus, and in most cases a uterus is present (Figs. 68–16 and 68–17). The ovary is found in a normal location, more commonly on the left side. The testis or ovotestis may reside at any point along the path of testicular descent. Testes are more commonly located on the right side (Blyth and Duckett, 1991). Sixty percent of gonads palpable in the inguinal canal or labioscrotal folds are ovotestes, which may be clinically suspected on the basis of a difference in firmness at either end of the gonad, consistent with polar segregation of ovarian and testicular tissue (Grumbach and Conte, 1998).

Approximately two thirds of true hermaphrodites have a 46,XX karyotype; however, 46,XY, and 46,XX/46,XY, 46,XX/47,XXY chimerism occurs less commonly. Chimerism has been thought to result from fertilization infusion of an ovum and its polar body, fusion of two nuclei, or double fertilization. It has also been suggested that true hermaphroditism may result from hidden mosaicism with an XY cell line. Studies have demonstrated heterogeneity of Y-specific DNA regions detected in patients with true hermaphroditism (Hadjiathanasiou et al, 1994). This supports a non–Y-related mechanism responsible for 46,XX true hermaphroditism, such as mutation in an autosomal or X-linked gene involved in sex determination. Berkovitz and colleagues (1991) suggested that 46,XY true hermaphroditism may be a form of partial gonadal dysgenesis. According to this theory, a partial defect in testis determination results in both testicular and ovarian development. This is supported by the finding of ovarian stroma in some dysgenetic testes (Berkovitz et al, 1991).

Just as the differentiation of external genitalia is variable in true hermaphroditism, differentiation of the internal ducts is also quite variable and is related to the function of the ipsilateral gonad. Fallopian tubes are consistently present on the side of the ovary, and a vas deferens is always present adjacent to a testis (Berkovitz et al, 1991). The ovotestis, which comprises two thirds of gonads in true hermaphroditism, is associated with a fallopian tube in two thirds of cases and with either a vas deferens only or both structures in one third of cases.

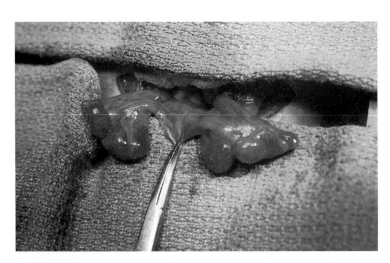

Figure 68–17. Laparotomy findings from true hermaphrodite noted in Figure 68–16; clamp on uterus with bilateral, fimbriated fallopian tubes and bilateral ovotestes. (From Diamond D: Intersex disorders: Parts I and II. AUA Update Series, Vol IX, Lessons 9 and 10. Houston, TX, American Urological Association Office of Education, 1990, with permission.)

The ovarian portion of the ovotestis is frequently normal, whereas the testicular portion is typically dysgenetic. Therefore, although ovulation and pregnancy have been reported for female 46,XX true hermaphrodites, male fertility has not been clearly documented.

The incidence of gonadal tumors is approximately 10% in 46,XY true hermaphroditism and 4% in 46,XX true hermaphroditism. Both gonadoblastoma and dysgerminoma have been described (Verp and Simpson, 1987).

The most important aspect of management in true hermaphroditism is gender assignment. Sex assignment should be based on the functional potential of external genitalia, internal ducts, and gonads, according to the findings at laparoscopy or laparotomy. **Unlike patients with most other forms of gonadal dysgenesis, true hermaphrodites have the potential for fertility if raised as female with the appropriate ductal structures.** Pregnancies have been reported in eight patients with true hermaphroditism, seven with the 46,XX karyotype and one with 46,XX/46,XY (Starceski et al, 1988). If the patient is to be raised as female, all testicular and wolffian tissue should be removed. For those patients with an ovary, this is straightforward; if an ovotestis is present, surgical cleavage of the gonad with excision of the testicular portion has been performed successfully by Nihoul-Fekete and colleagues (1984). They recommend postoperative stimulation with human chorionic gonadotropin (hCG) to confirm that all testicular tissue has been removed. In some settings, the cleavage plane between testicular and ovarian tissues is unclear and gonadectomy is advisable. When ovarian tissue is preserved, normal ovarian function can occur at puberty, although hormonal replacement may be necessary. Careful surveillance for potential gonadal tumors in the patient raised as female is also advisable. If a male gender is assigned, as has been most common historically, all ovarian and müllerian tissue should be removed. Consideration should be given to gonadectomy at puberty with appropriate androgen replacement in this setting, given the high risk of malignancy and unlikelihood of male fertility.

Female Pseudohermaphroditism

Female pseudohermaphroditism is a disorder of phenotypic sexual development in which 46,XX individuals with ovaries have a partially masculinized phenotype and ambiguous genitalia. By far the most common cause of female pseudohermaphroditism is CAH, which is the most common cause of ambiguous genitalia in the newborn. Two very rare causes of female pseudohermaphroditism are maternal ingestion of androgens and virilizing tumors in the mother.

Congenital Adrenal Hyperplasia

The adrenogenital syndrome caused by CAH is a classic example of an inborn error of metabolism—in this case, an error involving cortisol synthesis. A defect in any one of the five enzymes involved in the cortisol biosynthetic pathway (cholesterol side chain cleavage enzyme, 3β-hydroxysteroid dehydrogenase, 17-hydroxylase, 21-hydroxylase, and 11-hydroxylase) may result in CAH. **The most commonly recognized syndromes result from a deficiency of one of the terminal two enzymes of glucocorticoid synthesis (21-hydroxylase or 11-hydroxylase)** (New and Levine, 1984) (Fig. 68–18). As a result of deficiency of either terminal enzyme, formation of hydrocortisone is impaired, causing a compensatory increase in the secretion of adrenocorticotrophic hormone (ACTH). This increase enhances formation of adrenal steroids proximal to the enzymatic defect and a secondary increase in the formation of testosterone, the active androgen in CAH.

A deficiency of steroid 21-hydroxylase is responsible for 95% of cases of CAH; it occurs with an incidence ranging from 1 in 5000 to 1 in 15,000 in the United States and Europe. The highest incidence, 1 in 490, is reported in the Yup'ik Alaskan Eskimo population (New et al, 1994). **Clinically, patients are divided into three categories: (1) salt wasters (patients with virilization and aldosterone**

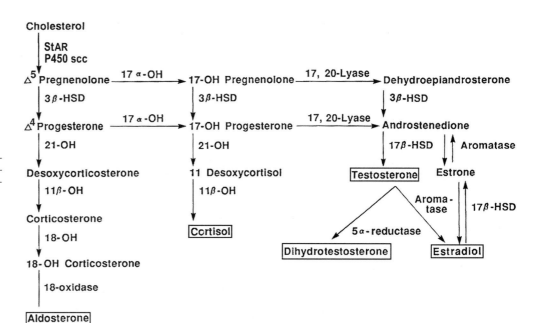

Figure 68–18. Steroid biosynthetic pathway for mineralocorticoid, glucocorticoid, and sex steroid hormone production.

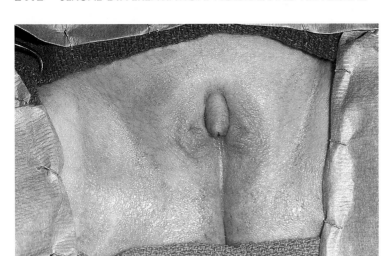

Figure 68–19. External genitalia of a patient with congenital adrenal hyperplasia secondary to 21-hydroxylase deficiency, showing labioscrotal fusion and clitoromegaly.

deficiency), (2) simple virilizers (patients with virilization, but without salt wasting), and (3) nonclassic patients (those without evidence of virilization or salt wasting). Dramatic progress has been made in understanding the molecular basis of CAH, and 95% of the mutations that account for CAH have been identified. An attempt has been made to correlate mutational abnormalities with phenotypic expressions of the disease.

The 21-hydroxylase gene (*CYP-21*) is located on the short arm of chromosome 6, within the large human leukocyte antigen (HLA) locus, and is transmitted in an autosomal recessive pattern (Wilson et al, 1995). Adjacent to the *CYP-21* gene is the CYP-21 pseudogene (*CYP-21P*), so called because it encodes no proteins and is therefore inactive (Tusie-Luna and White, 1995). The inactive *CYP-21P* is 98% homologous to the active gene, *CYP-21*. During meiosis, a gene conversion may occur that transfers deleterious point mutations from the *CYP-21P* gene to the *CYP-21* gene, rendering it inactive. **Mutations leading to conversion of the active *CYP-21* gene into the inactive gene occur in 65% to 90% of cases of classic 21-hydroxylase deficiency (i.e., salt wasting and simple virilizing forms) and in all nonclassic cases** (Kohn et al, 1995; Laue and Rennert, 1995). Gene deletions are responsible for 10% to 35% of the remainder of mutations that produce 21-hy-

droxylase deficiency. About 10 different mutations have been described in the vast majority of patients with classic and nonclassic CAH (Hughes, 1998).

The majority of patients with CAH secondary to 21-hydroxylase deficiency exhibit one of the two classic forms of the disease—**75% present with salt wasting and 25% with simple virilization** (Kohn et al, 1995). The higher proportion of patients with the salt wasting form of the disease recognized in more recent series has been attributed to improved diagnostic capabilities and newborn screening for 21-hydroxylase deficiency as well as to increased survival owing to mineralocorticoid supplementation (Fife and Rappaport, 1983).

In the female with the simple virilizing form of the disorder, female pseudohermaphroditism results. Because impaired steroidogenesis begins early in life—at the time of formation of the external genitalia (beginning at 10 weeks' gestation)—there is virtually always evidence of some degree of masculinization at birth. This is manifested by enlargement of the clitoris and varying degrees of labial fusion (Figs. 68–19 and 68–20). In addition, the vagina and urethra open into a common urogenital sinus. The enlargement of the clitoris may be so dramatic as to make it appear to be a hypospadiac penis with bilateral cryptorchidism, and cases of complete formation of a masculin-

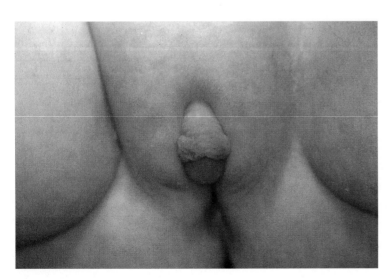

Figure 68–20. Patient with congenital adrenal hyperplasia secondary to 21-hydroxylase deficiency, demonstrating marked virilization of hypospadiac-appearing phallus.

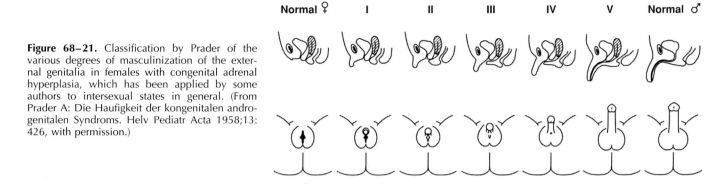

Figure 68–21. Classification by Prader of the various degrees of masculinization of the external genitalia in females with congenital adrenal hyperplasia, which has been applied by some authors to intersexual states in general. (From Prader A: Die Haufigkeit der kongenitalen androgenitalen Syndroms. Helv Pediatr Acta 1958;13: 426, with permission.)

ized urethra to the tip of an enlarged clitoris have been reported. The severity of the virilization is usually greater in infants who experience salt wasting, but not uniformly so. Prader (1958) classified the degrees of virilization of external genitalia in females with CAH (Fig. 68–21). The müllerian structures in these patients are typically normal.

In both males and females with the salt-losing variant of CAH, symptoms begin within the first few weeks after birth, with failure to regain birth weight, progressive weight loss, and dehydration. In severely affected infants, adrenal crises occur within the first 10 to 21 days of life (Grumbach and Conte, 1998). **Vomiting is prominent and can be so extreme that a mistaken diagnosis of pyloric stenosis is made, particularly in the male.** Without therapy, death may rapidly ensue from hyperkalemia, dehydration, and shock. After birth, there is progression of masculinization of the untreated female; pubic and axillary hair develop prematurely, acne appears, and the voice deepens. There is rapid somatic maturation, resulting in premature epiphyseal closure and short adult stature. Although the internal genitalia are female, breast development and menstruation do not occur unless the excessive androgen production is suppressed by adequate steroid therapy.

In the male without salt wasting, the chief clinical manifestations are those of isosexual precocity. The infant appears normal at birth, but signs of sexual and somatic precocity appear within the first 2 to 3 years of life. Although the testes remain normal in size, enlargement of the penis, scrotum, and prostate occur, accompanied by the appearance of pubic hair, acne, and deepening of the voice. The musculature is well developed (prompting the descriptive term "little Hercules"), and bone age is more advanced than appropriate for the chronologic age. The syndrome often goes unrecognized in the non–salt-wasting male until signs of androgen excess, such as accelerated height and precocious sexual hair, appear later in childhood.

In classic 21-hydroxylase deficiency, plasma levels of progesterone and 17-hydroxyprogesterone are markedly elevated. Urinary 17-ketosteroids and pregnanetriol are elevated. **The diagnosis may be made biochemically with the use of radioimmunoassay of plasma 17-hydroxyprogesterone,** which has replaced the more cumbersome 24-hour urine collection of metabolites (e.g., pregnanetriol). **A pelvic ultrasound study demonstrating the presence of müllerian tissues is confirmatory.**

More aggressive screening for 21-hydroxylase deficiency has provided considerable benefits. In one series, despite

sexual ambiguity, one third to one half of the affected female newborns were not diagnosed as having 21-hydroxylase deficiency until they were identified by the screening test (Pang et al, 1985).

Nonclassic 21-hydroxylase deficiency represents an attenuated, late-onset form that is variable in its clinical severity and timing of onset. The presenting symptoms in females are commonly hirsutism and oligomenorrhea, male pattern baldness, and polycystic ovaries. In men with the nonclassic form of 21-hydroxylase deficiency, oligospermia and subfertility have been presenting features, and reversal of infertility with glucocorticoid therapy has been reported. Typically, lower doses of glucocorticoid are required for management of the nonclassic form of CAH.

A deficiency of 11β-hydroxylase accounts for roughly 5% of cases of CAH. Both classic and mild forms have been recognized. Unlike 21-hydroxylase, 11β-hydroxylase is not HLA linked. The defect results from mutations in the *CYP-11B1* gene (Merke et al, 1998). To date, 11 mutations have been described which result in enzyme inactivation. Like 21-hydroxylase deficiency, the nonclassic variant of 11β-hydroxylase deficiency (late onset) is characterized by signs and symptoms of androgen excess in childhood or adolescence. **Hypertension is a common finding in patients with this type of CAH, and it is believed to be secondary to increased serum levels of deoxycorticosterone (DOC).** Although most of the patients are hypertensive, some are normotensive and others experience only intermittent hypertension. Marked virilization occurs in the severe form of the defect and may be as severe as in those patients with a 21-hydroxylase deficiency. In the late-onset form, mild virilization occurs in prepubertal and postpubertal patients.

The diagnosis of 11β-hydroxylase deficiency can be confirmed by finding increased plasma levels of 11-deoxycortisol and 11-DOC. Urinary 17-ketosteroids and 17-hydroxycorticoids are increased. **The treatment with glucocorticoid is identical to that of patients with 21-hydroxylase deficiency.**

The least common enzyme deficiency responsible for a virilizing form of CAH is 3β-hydroxysteroid dehydrogenase. This deficiency affects the early steps in steroid biosynthesis in both adrenals and gonads, resulting in inability to convert 3β-hydroxysteroids to 3-ketosteroids. As a result, the severe form leads to impaired synthesis of aldosterone, cortisol, and sex steroids. Affected females exhibit mild clitoromegaly and labial fusion accompanied by symptoms of aldosterone and cortisol deficiency.

Two homologous genes have been identified for 3β-hydroxysteroid dehydrogenase, both of which contain four exons (Merke et al, 1998). A number of mutations giving rise to the syndrome have been described. This defect has an autosomal recessive inheritance pattern and is heterogeneous in its biochemical and clinical appearance. A non–salt-losing form and mild- and late-onset forms have been described.

The diagnosis of 3β-hydroxysteroid dehydrogenase is based on finding increased serum levels of 17-hydroxypregnenolone and dehydroepiandrosterone (DHEA). The pelvic ultrasound, confirming presence of müllerian tissue, would be supportive. Treatment is similar to that of patients with 21-hydroxylase deficiency.

Currently, one of the most exciting aspects of CAH is the capability of diagnosing and treating the disorder prenatally. **Prenatal diagnosis of CAH in the at-risk fetus is most specifically made by a measurement of amniotic fluid for 17-hydroxyprogesterone** (Laue and Rennert, 1995). The diagnosis may be made during the first trimester by HLA genotyping or by DNA analysis of genes within the HLA complex in cells obtained by chorionic villous sampling. **Treatment of the mother with dexamethasone, which crosses the placenta, suppresses fetal secretion of ACTH, thereby preventing virilization of the genitalia.** There are certain complexities to this form of management, however. The diagnosis of CAH in the fetus can be determined on chorionic villous cells at 8 to 10 weeks or on cells from amniotic fluid at 16 to 17 weeks. However, treatment should be instituted at 5 to 6 weeks of gestation, before initial development of the external genitalia. **Therefore, it is not possible to confirm the diagnosis before therapy is initiated.** Because virilization is not a concern with the male fetus and three of four female fetuses at risk are unaffected, given the autosomal recessive pattern of inheritance, seven of eight fetuses may be treated unnecessarily. Therefore, one goal in therapy is earlier diagnosis to avoid unnecessary treatment.

A number of series have established the effectiveness of prenatal treatment for CAH with dexamethasone (Migeon, 1990; Pang et al, 1990; Speiser et al, 1990). In some neonates, there is no evidence of masculinization, suggesting totally successful therapy. In another group, there is milder masculinization than that noted in an affected sibling. Although compliance and timing of initiation of treatment have been variable from series to series, this heterogeneity of response to therapy raises intriguing questions about the mechanisms involved in virilization of the CAH fetus. In addition, prenatal treatment with dexamethasone has raised ethical concerns. **Although there is no arguing its ability to prevent androgen effects on the genitalia and brain of affected females, the long-term effects of dexamethasone on unaffected fetuses undergoing treatment prenatally remain unknown.** Miller (1999) and others have advocated the use of prenatal treatment for CAH only as an experimental therapy in large centers and under institutional review board scrutiny. The importance of long-term follow-up of these neonates has been emphasized (Speiser, 1999).

The treatment of affected children with hydrocortisone in childhood and adolescence achieves a number of goals, as noted by Bongiovanni and Root (1963): "to supply the deficient hormone; to suppress pituitary ACTH secretion and hence adrenal androgens and clinical virilization; to forestall abnormally rapid somatic growth and osseous advance; to permit normal gonadal development; and to correct salt-water loss or hypertension in the complicated forms." The required dose of glucocorticoid is empirical and should be adjusted for the individual patient based on bone age, linear growth, 24-hour excretion of ketosteroids, and clinical evidence of glucocorticoid deficiency or excess (Grumbach and Conte, 1998). The effectiveness of therapy may be assessed by measuring morning plasma 17-hydroxyprogesterone levels. Those children with the salt-losing form of the disease require increased salt intake and mineralocorticoid treatment in addition to hydrocortisone therapy. After control of electrolytes and blood pressure has been achieved in the acute setting, maintenance therapy with fludrocortisone (0.05 to 2.5 mg daily) should be instituted (Laue and Rennert, 1995; Grumbach and Conte, 1998). The administration of hydrocortisone and, when required, fludrocortisone is continued indefinitely in all patients. Typically, patients are instructed to triple their oral dose of hydrocortisone during stressful events such as surgery or infection.

In the majority of children (who will not have been diagnosed and treated prenatally), it is appropriate to perform feminizing genitoplasty at 3 to 6 months of age, when a well-established course of medical therapy has been instituted, the risks of anesthesia have become minimal, and the child has grown large enough to make the procedure technically feasible (Passerini-Glazel, 1990). **Long-term fertility in males and feminization, menstruation, and fertility in females can be anticipated in the well-treated patient.** Indeed, this potential in even the most masculinized female CAH patient has provided support for feminizing genitoplasty in virtually all 46,XX CAH patients. Proper psychological support should be a component of long-term follow-up.

An intriguing area of surgical innovation in the management of CAH has been the experimental use of "prophylactic" adrenalectomy for selected patients. This approach is based on the premise that in certain patients it is more difficult to maintain adrenal suppression than to prevent adrenal crises. Clinically, these patients are the salt losers and extremely virilized females. For those with this most severe form of 21-hydroxylase deficiency, adequate suppression of adrenal production has required significant degrees of hypercortisolism, associated with poor growth, obesity, and infertility. For the 25% of CAH patients who completely lack 21-hydroxylase enzyme activity and therefore produce neither cortisol nor aldosterone, adrenalectomy may be a practical approach (VanWyk et al, 1996). In general, these patients may be identified genotypically as homozygotes or compound heterozygotes for "null alleles" of the *CYP-21* gene (VanWyk et al, 1996).

Although these patients are rendered Addisonian by this surgery, those with the most severe form of CAH would have a poor intrinsic adrenal response to metabolic stress (Gunther et al, 1997). One theoretical disadvantage of this approach is that if gene therapy were to one day allow functional *CYP-21* genes to be introduced into adrenal cortical tissue, adrenalectomized patients would not be candidates for such therapy (VanWyk et al, 1996).

Female Pseudohermaphroditism Secondary to Maternal Androgens and Progestins and Maternal Tumors

The masculinization of a female fetus as a result of maternal administration of synthetic progestational agents or androgens is a rare occurrence; lessons have been learned from prior unfortunate experience. Historically, progestational agents were used to prevent threatened abortion. In one large series, masculinization occurred in 2% of female infants whose mothers were treated with progestins during pregnancy (Ishizura et al, 1962). In addition, Danazol, a testosterone derivative used to treat endometriosis, has been associated with virilization of the female fetus. **The degree to which any androgen or progestational agent affects female fetal development is a function of the strength of the agent, its maternal dosage, and timing and duration of administration** (Bongiovanni and McFadden, 1960).

Very rarely, a maternal ovarian or adrenal tumor has virilizing effects on a female fetus. More typically, such a tumor has virilizing effects on the mother but no apparent effect on the fetus. Ovarian tumors that have resulted in masculinization of the female fetus include arrhenoblastoma, hilar cell tumor, lipoid cell tumor, ovarian stromal cell tumor, luteoma of pregnancy, and Krukenberg's tumor (Calaf et al, 1994).

Rarer still are maternal adrenal tumors, which have masculinizing effects on the female fetus. Adrenocortical carcinoma and adenoma have been reported.

In any case of exogenous androgen effect on a female fetus, normal endocrine status is recognized postnatally and management is confined to external genital reconstruction, as required.

Male Pseudohermaphroditism

The term *male pseudohermaphroditism* refers to 46,XY individuals with differentiated testes who exhibit varying degrees of feminization phenotypically. Impaired male differentiation in these patients is secondary to inadequate secretion of testosterone by the testes at the necessary period in development, inability of target tissue to respond to androgen appropriately, or impaired production or action of MIS.

Leydig Cell Aplasia (Luteinizing Hormone Receptor Abnormality)

Leydig cell aplasia as a cause of male pseudohermaphroditism was first reported by Berthezene and colleagues in 1976. **In its pure form, this rare disorder is characterized by a normal 46,XY male karyotype associated with a normal-appearing female phenotype. Typically, testes are palpable in the inguinal canals or labia majora.** On investigation, there are no müllerian structures and the vagina is short. A low testosterone level is noted in conjunction with an elevated LH concentration. **The absence of a rise in serum testosterone after human chorionic gonadotropin stimulation is characteristic of this** disorder (Brown et al, 1978). Physiologically, this disorder represents a spectrum between absent Leydig cells and Leydig cells with abnormal LH receptor (David et al, 1984). It is transmitted as an autosomal recessive trait expressed only in males. Incomplete forms of the syndrome occur, with the mildest form being expressed as primary hypogonadism with normal male external genitalia (Lee et al, 1982).

The clinical diagnosis of Leydig cell aplasia, or LH receptor abnormality, is typically made as a result of sexual infantilism and the absence of development of secondary sexual characteristics or the discovery of palpable gonads in the inguinal canal or labia on physical examination (Arnholt et al, 1985). The differential diagnosis includes androgen insensitivity syndrome or a terminal defect in androgen synthesis. The histology of the abnormal testes demonstrates absence of Leydig cells in intratubular spaces with normal Sertoli cells.

Disorders of Testosterone Biosynthesis

A defect in any of the five enzymes required for the conversion of cholesterol to testosterone can cause incomplete (or absent) virilization of the male fetus during embryogenesis. The first three enzymes (cholesterol side chain cleavage, 3β-hydroxysteroid dehydrogenase, and 17α-hydroxylase) are present in both adrenals and testes. **Therefore, their deficiency results in impaired synthesis of glucocorticoids and mineralocorticoids in addition to testosterone.** For all five enzyme deficiencies, the pattern of inheritance is autosomal recessive.

CHOLESTEROL SIDE CHAIN CLEAVAGE DEFICIENCY (StAR DEFICIENCY)

The first step in gonadal and adrenal steroidogenesis is conversion of cholesterol to pregnenolone, which is mediated by a single cholesterol side chain cleavage enzyme known as 450SCC (previously known as 20–22 desmolase). A defect in this enzyme, first described by Prader and Gurtner in 1955, was believed to result in the rare condition congenital lipoid adrenal hyperplasia, so named because the adrenal glands became large and lipid laden. However, more recent **evidence suggests that a defect in cholesterol transport rather than a defective enzyme is etiologically responsible** (Saenger, 1997). The steroidogenic acute regulatory protein (StAR) stimulates cholesterol transport from the outer to the inner mitochondrial membrane (site of the cholesterol side chain cleavage complex). This appears to be the rate-limiting step in acute steroid synthesis.

Affected 46,XY individuals have female or ambiguous external genitalia with a blind-ending vaginal pouch; intraabdominal, inguinal, or labial testes; and absence of müllerian structures, consistent with functioning Sertoli cells (Hauffa et al, 1985). Wolffian ducts are present but rudimentary. Infants often present in the first few weeks of life with severe adrenal insufficiency and salt wasting.

A diagnosis of cholesterol side chain cleavage deficiency should be entertained in any newborn with nonvirilized female external genitalia and evidence of cortisol and aldosterone deficiency with hyponatremia,

hyperkalemia, and metabolic acidosis. Abdominal CT scanning demonstrates large, lipid-laden adrenal glands.

Management is similar to that for 21-hydroxylase deficiency. To date, all surviving 46,XY patients with this disorder have been raised as females and have undergone gonadectomy (Laue and Rennert, 1995). Because testosterone production was never significant, brain imprinting is not a factor in gender assignment.

3β-Hydroxysteroid Dehydrogenase

3β-Hydroxysteroid dehydrogenase catalyzes the 3β-hydroxysteroids (pregnenolone, 17-hydroxypregnenolone, and DHEA) to the three ketosteroids, progesterone, 17-hydroxyprogesterone, and androstenedione. A congenital deficiency of 3β-hydroxysteroid dehydrogenase was first described by Bongiovanni in 1962.

Affected individuals present with various degrees of incomplete masculinization resulting from a block in testosterone biosynthesis and with salt-wasting adrenal insufficiency resulting from impaired synthesis of aldosterone and cortisol. The lack of salt-retaining hormone and cortisol results in a salt-losing crisis soon after birth. However, partial deficiencies associated with severe salt wasting occur, consistent with genetic heterogeneity. The gene has been cloned and localized to chromosome 1 at locus p11–p13 (Chang et al, 1993).

Males with this deficiency usually exhibit incomplete virilization of the external genitalia, with a small phallus, hypospadias with labioscrotal fusion, a urogenital sinus, and a blind-ending vaginal pouch. Testes are often scrotal, and wolffian ducts develop normally. As with other defects in testosterone biosynthesis, in which normal Sertoli cell function is preserved, müllerian structures are absent.

The diagnosis should be considered in 46,XY males with ambiguous genitalia and signs of adrenal insufficiency. Endocrine study demonstrating increased levels of 3β-hydroxysteroids confirms the diagnosis.

Management of 3β-hydroxysteroid dehydrogenase is similar to that for patients with 21-hydroxylase deficiency.

17α-Hydroxylase Deficiency

17α-Hydroxylase catalyzes the conversion of pregnenolone and progesterone to 17-hydroxypregnenolone and 17-hydroxyprogesterone, respectively, in adrenal and gonadal steroidogenesis. The first case of male pseudohermaphroditism due to this enzyme deficiency was reported by New in 1970. The gene for this enzyme has been localized to chromosome 10 (Laue and Rennert, 1995).

Affected 46,XY individuals usually have female external genitalia with absent to slight masculinization. **A deficiency in 17α-hydroxylase activity impairs cortisol production, causing ACTH hypersecretion and resulting in increased levels of DOC, corticosterone, and 18-hydroxycorticosterone in the adrenals. These compounds with mineralocorticoid activity produce excess salt and water retention, hypertension, and hypokalemia.**

The phenotype of affected individuals varies from female external genitalia with a blind-ending vaginal pouch to male with perineal hypospadias and chordee.

The diagnosis should be considered in a male pseudohermaphrodite with hypertension. Endocrine laboratory evaluation demonstrates elevated serum progesterone, DOC, corticosterone, 18-hydroxycorticosterone, and ACTH.

Therapy with glucocorticoid replacement brings blood pressure and hypokalemia back to normal by suppressing ACTH and hence adrenal cortical stimulation. Some patients have been raised as females with gonadectomy and estrogen replacement at puberty. In partial forms, typically with reasonable phallic size, patients may be raised as male with testosterone replacement at puberty. **Fertility has not been reported in patients with testosterone biosynthetic defects, and inadequate testosterone production makes androgen imprinting a less significant issue for these patients.** Therefore, the phenotype may dictate gender assignment.

17,20-Lyase Deficiency

The enzyme 17,20-lyase has been demonstrated to be related to 17α-hydroxylase in that the activities of both are linked to the same gene product on chromosome 10 (Laue and Rennert, 1995). However, in some patients with the genetic defect both biologic activities are absent, but with others only the 17,20-lyase function appears deficient. Zachmann and colleagues first described this clinical entity in 1972.

In cases where the deficiency primarily involves 17,20-lyase, cortisol and ACTH secretion are normal. Aldosterone is secreted normally, and hypertension does not result. **However, impaired biosynthesis of testosterone in the 46,XY individual results typically in ambiguous rather than totally female genitalia at birth.** The deficient masculinization of the external genitalia can range from severe, resulting in a female gender assignment in the neonate, to mild, resulting only in hypospadias. At puberty, the secretion of testicular androgen remains low. Zachmann has postulated that there are two types of 17,20-lyase deficiency—one that is partial and another that is a complete defect (Zachmann et al, 1982).

The diagnosis may be suspected in male pseudohermaphrodites with absent müllerian derivatives and no defect in glucocorticoid or mineralocorticoid synthesis. At the time of expected pubertal development, the patients may present with failure to develop secondary sexual characteristics and elevated gonadotropin levels. The diagnosis may be made prepubertally using hCG and ACTH stimulation.

Management entails plastic reconstruction of the external genitalia and appropriate sex steroid replacement at puberty.

17β-Hydroxysteroid Oxidoreductase Deficiency

This last enzyme in the testosterone biosynthetic pathway catalyzes the conversion of androstenedione to testosterone, DHEA to androstenediol, and estrone to estradiol. Male pseudohermaphroditism resulting from a deficiency in 17β-hydroxysteroid oxidoreductase was first described by Saez and associates in 1971.

Clinically, this is the most interesting enzymatic de-

fect in testosterone biosynthesis in its similarities to 5α-reductase deficiency. **At birth, affected individuals appear to have a normal female phenotype, without significant evidence of virilization.** Therefore, a female gender assignment is usually made. However, these individuals have well-differentiated testes located intra-abdominally, inguinally, or in the labia and no müllerian structures. **At puberty, there is phallic growth and progressive development of male secondary sexual characteristics.** These include increased muscle mass, development of pubic, axillary, and facial and body hair with male distribution. Gynecomastia may occur, and the testes may become palpable (Saez et al, 1972). In some cases, gender reassignment to male has been reported (Imperato-McGinley et al, 1979; Rosler and Kohn, 1983).

The late onset of virilization is related to the pubertal increase in gonadotropin production, which may partially overcome the block in testosterone biosynthesis.

There is a characteristic hormonal profile in this disorder. In the prepubertal patient, plasma androstenedione and estrone levels may not be increased. At puberty, androstenedione, the immediate precursor of testosterone, is increased to 10 to 15 times the normal plasma concentration (Virdis and Saenger, 1984). Earlier precursors are within normal levels. Plasma testosterone is in the low-normal range. Serum LH and FSH are markedly elevated, typically 4 to 6 times normal.

As a result of biochemical characterization and molecular cloning, five different 17β-hydroxysteroid dehydrogenase isozymes have been identified to date. **The type III 17β-hydroxysteroid dehydrogenase isozyme, cloned by Andersson and colleagues (1997), catalyzes the biosynthesis of testosterone from androstenedione. A mutation involving this gene is responsible for male pseudohermaphroditism.** The type III isozyme is apparently expressed early in utero and is responsible for testosterone biosynthesis during the critical period of sexual differentiation, based on the observation that male adults homozygous for 17β-hydroxysteroid dehydrogenase type III gene defects have ambiguous genitalia (Zhu et al, 1998).

The diagnosis is rarely made in the newborn period. It may become apparent on discovery of a testis during a hernia repair in infancy or childhood. An hCG stimulation test would confirm the diagnosis. **The primary management issue for patients with 17β-hydroxysteroid oxidoreductase deficiency has been gender assignment.** At this early stage, maintenance of the female sex of rearing with gonadectomy is usually elected. If the diagnosis is not made until puberty, when dramatic changes in virilization occur, certain families prefer a gender change to male. Traditionally, this decision has been strongly culturally influenced.

If a female sex of rearing is elected, gonadectomy, plastic reconstruction of the genitalia as necessary, and estrogen replacement therapy at puberty are indicated. For the patient maintained in the male gender, orchidopexy and reconstruction of the external genitalia are required. This entails hypospadias repair and chordee correction, which can be quite successful. However, phallic size remains small, and infertility is the rule. Usually endogenous androgen levels are adequate.

Two hypotheses have been proposed to explain the fre-

quency of gender change from female to male with this enzyme deficiency, particularly among the cohort of Arab male pseudohermaphrodites with 17β-hydroxysteroid dehydrogenase type III deficiency. One entails the potential male imprinting of the brain in utero due to the conversion of androstenedione to estrone; this theory is supported by studies in rats and rabbits demonstrating that administration of estrogen or androstenedione is capable of inducing male sexual behavior (Reddy et al, 1974). The second is the possibility that 17β-hydroxysteroid dehydrogenase activity is not deficient in the brain, its effect being mediated by the conversion of androstenedione to testosterone or estrogen (Imperato-McGinley et al, 1979).

Androgen Receptor and Postreceptor Defects

Disorders of androgen receptor function represent the most common definable cause of male pseudohermaphroditism. These patients characteristically have a 46,XY karyotype and testes and present with a spectrum of phenotypic abnormalities that vary from complete external feminization (syndrome of complete androgen insensitivity), to ambiguous genitalia (partial androgen insensitivity, Reifenstein's syndrome), to the phenotypically infertile male. Although the clinical presentations vary according to the severity of the receptor disorder, the pathophysiology is similar (Wiener et al, 1997).

SYNDROME OF COMPLETE ANDROGEN INSENSITIVITY

The syndrome of complete androgen insensitivity (testicular feminization) is characterized clinically by a 46,XY karyotype, bilateral testes, female-appearing external genitalia, and absence of müllerian derivatives. Wilkins first suggested in 1950 (Wilkins, 1950) that the clinical features of this syndrome were the result of androgen resistance. This condition has an incidence of 1 in 20,000 to 1 in 60,000 males, and it is transmitted as an X-linked trait.

The androgen receptor regulates the transcription of other specific genes, once activated by testosterone or DHT. This results in new mRNA synthesis from the downstream genes and protein production. The androgen receptor has been mapped to the X chromosome at Xq11–12 (Brown et al, 1989). Males have only one copy of this gene. Point mutations of the gene account for more than 90% of cases of androgen insensitivity (Quigley et al, 1995). **The identifiable molecular alterations of the androgen receptor gene cannot predict the resulting phenotype of the affected individual unless there is total loss of the receptor, which occurs in only 1% of all patients** (Quigley et al, 1995).

Patients with complete androgen insensitivity have a normal female phenotype with the exception of diminished axillary and pubic hair. Their breast development and body habitus are feminine in character, and their external genitalia are unequivocally female, although the vagina is short and blind-ending. In utero resistance to testosterone action prevents stabilization of the wolffian ducts. However, because the fetal testes secrete MIS, internal genitalia are absent, with the exception of the testes, which may be found in the labia, inguinal canal, or abdomen. These patients are rarely diagnosed in the newborn period, unless a prenatal diagnosis is made on the basis of female phenotype and 46,XY karyotype on amniocentesis. With the increase in prenatal diagnostics, this is becoming a more common occurrence (Hughes and Patterson, 1994). More typically, however, the diagnosis is made as a result of primary amenorrhea or the finding of a testis at inguinal herniorrhaphy. Fifty percent of patients with complete androgen insensitivity syndrome have an inguinal hernia (Conte and Grumbach, 1989). Conversely, 2% of apparently female infants with inguinal hernia are found to have a 46,XY karyotype and complete androgen insensitivity syndrome (Wiener et al, 1997). Therefore, routine vaginoscopy to confirm the presence of a cervix before inguinal herniorrhaphy in female patients is a prudent maneuver. Histologically, the testes exhibit incomplete or absent spermatogenesis, with normal or hyperplastic Leydig cells. They are comparable to immature, cryptorchid testes.

Endocrine evaluation in the newborn period demonstrates normal levels of testosterone, DHT, and gonadotropins. At puberty, gonadotropin levels rise, leading to increased levels of plasma estradiol, which results in feminization, including breast development.

Several types of receptor abnormality that would account for this syndrome have been described, including (1) a decreased amount of apparently normal receptor; (2) absence of receptor binding; (3) a qualitatively abnormal receptor (thermolabile, or unstable in the presence of molybdate); (4) other "receptor-positive" forms, including increased rate of dissociation of steroid receptor complex, defective up-regulation of the androgen receptor, decreased affinity of ligand binding, and impaired nuclear retention of the ligand (Grumbach and Conte, 1998). In general, the severity of the defect in androgen receptor (quantity or quality) correlates with the phenotype.

The diagnosis of complete androgen insensitivity may readily be made in the postpubertal patient on the basis of clinical and hormonal findings of amenorrhea, absence of pubic hair, or inguinal hernias containing testes. It is confirmed by a 46,XY karyotype and a normal male androgen and gonadotropin profile. Pelvic ultrasound examination confirms the absence of müllerian tissue, and a vaginal examination confirms a blind-ending vagina without a cervix.

In the prepubertal child, diagnosis is more difficult and requires an hCG stimulation test and determination of androgen receptor binding activity in cultured genital skin fibroblasts. Because of the time required for receptor binding quantification, it is desirable to use the PCR to characterize the androgen receptor gene in DNA obtained from a venous blood sample, in order to detect a genetic marker for androgen insensitivity syndrome.

Management of complete androgen insensitivity relates primarily to the optimal timing of gonadectomy. Because the testes produce estradiol, which results in the appropriate changes for the female phenotype, it is considered preferable to leave the testes in situ until puberty is complete. Potential exceptions to the policy of delayed gonadectomy are palpable testes or testes associated with an inguinal hernia. One important caveat in deciding to leave the testes in situ is the need to confirm with absolute certainty that complete rather than partial androgen insensitivity exists. If an incomplete form should exist, virilization at puberty could result (Batch et al, 1993).

A competing concern for retention of testicular tissue is the potential for malignant degeneration of the testes. In patients with complete androgen insensitivity who reach adulthood with a retained testis, the risk for development of a testis tumor—usually seminoma or gonadoblastoma—is thought to be 2% to 5%, only slightly higher than for a cryptorchid testis (Manuel et al, 1976; Muller and Skakkebaek, 1984). Before adulthood the risk is extremely low; therefore, delayed gonadectomy after puberty is believed to be safe.

After orchiectomy, cyclic estrogen/progestin therapy is begun. Some patients with a short vagina may benefit from vaginoplasty. **Currently, all studies of patients with complete androgen insensitivity support an unequivocal female gender identity, consistent with androgen resistance of brain tissue as well.** To date, there has been no report of a patient raised as a female who needed gender reassignment to male (Meyer-Bahlberg, 1999).

SYNDROME OF PARTIAL ANDROGEN RESISTANCE (REIFENSTEIN'S SYNDROME)

The syndrome of partial androgen resistance (Reifenstein's syndrome) includes syndromes that were once thought to represent separate entities: Reifenstein's, Gilbert-Dreyfus, Rosewater's, and Lubs' syndromes (Griffin, 1992). **These are X-linked disorders** of incomplete male pseudohermaphroditism that represent a spectrum of phenotypic abnormalities. **The major finding is ambiguity of the external genitalia to varying degrees.** The partial form of androgen insensitivity may be expressed variably even within the same family. **The classic phenotype is that of a male with perineoscrotal hypospadias, cryptorchidism, rudimentary wolffian duct structures, gynecomastia, and infertility. However, the phenotypic spectrum can range from hypospadias and a pseudovagina to gynecomastia and azoospermia** (Wilson et al, 1974). The endocrine profile of partial androgen insensitivity syndrome is similar to that of the complete androgen insensitivity syndrome.

At puberty, gynecomastia may develop. The phallus may enlarge slightly, but it remains small.

Androgen receptor studies in cultured fibroblasts (Wilson et al, 1983) have demonstrated **two forms of receptor defect in the partial androgen insensitivity syndrome: (1) a reduced number of normally functioning androgen receptors, and (2) a normal receptor number but decreased binding affinity** (Griffin and Durrant, 1982).

The diagnosis of partial androgen insensitivity syndrome can be difficult. In the newborn period, it may be made in the setting of a 46,XY karyotype, ambiguous external genitalia, and absent müllerian structures on pelvic ultrasound. Endocrine evaluation confirms normal testosterone and gonadotropin levels and a normal testosterone/DHT ratio. An hCG stimulation test and studies of DHT binding to receptors and cultured genital skin fibroblasts should confirm the diagnosis. A family history consistent with X-linked inheritance of ambiguous genitalia is of great assistance.

Management must be individualized depending on the degree of genital ambiguity. In patients assigned a female gender, gonadectomy and surgical reconstruction of the external genitalia are indicated; at puberty, estrogen/progestin replacement is instituted. Those individuals raised as males would require treatment of their cryptorchidism, reduction of gynecomastia, and genitalia reconstruction. Phallic size remains small, however, and the effects of supraphysiologic doses of testosterone have been disappointing (Migeon et al, 1994). Of importance in considering gender assignment in patients with partial androgen insensitivity is the recognition that the receptor defect affecting the external genitalia appears to affect brain receptors for testosterone similarly.

The most recently discovered and mildest form of androgen receptor abnormality is that of the *infertile male syndrome* (Aiman et al, 1979). Men with this syndrome are normal phenotypically but are azoospermic or severely oligospermic. They have been found to have normal to elevated serum testosterone with normal to elevated LH and decreased androgen receptor binding to DHT in genital skin fibroblasts (Aiman and Griffin, 1982). This suggests that infertility in otherwise normal males may be the clinical manifestation of partial androgen insensitivity—representing the far end of a variable phenotypic spectrum.

5α-Reductase Deficiency

The disorder of 5α-reductase deficiency is one of the most fascinating forms of male pseudohermaphroditism. The clinical presentation of this enzyme disorder was actu-

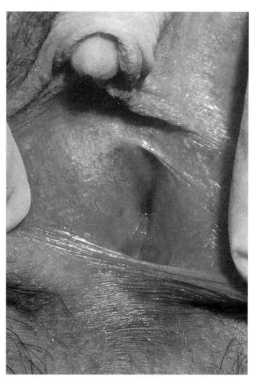

Figure 68–23. Intraoperative view of urogenital sinus in a patient with 5α-reductase deficiency; note enlarged clitoris, urogenital sinus with separate urethral and vaginal openings, and posterior labioscrotal fusion. (From Diamond D: Intersex disorders: Parts I and II. AUA Update Series, Vol IX, Lessons 9 and 10. Houston, TX, American Urological Association Office of Education, 1990, with permission.)

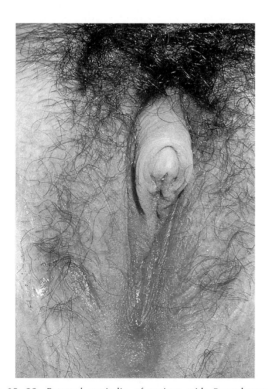

Figure 68–22. External genitalia of patient with 5α-reductase deficiency. Note clitoromegaly with marked labioscrotal fusion and small vaginal introitus. (From Diamond D: Intersex disorders: Parts I and II. AUA Update Series, Vol IX, Lessons 9 and 10. Houston, TX, American Urological Association Office of Education, 1990, with permission.)

ally predicted in 1972, before the description of such patients in 1974 by Walsh and Imperato-McGinley and their colleagues (Wilson, 1972; Walsh et al, 1974; Imperato-McGinley et al, 1974). Extensive characterization of the disease has been achieved since that time.

5α-Reductase is a microsomal enzyme that catalyzes the conversion of testosterone to DHT. The condition is transmitted in an autosomal recessive pattern, and only homozygous males are affected. Two 5α-reductase genes have been cloned; they encode different isoenzymes. The type I isoenzyme, encoded on chromosome 5, is expressed in low levels in the prostate and external genitalia. The type II isoenzyme is encoded on chromosome 2 and is expressed in high levels in the prostate and external genitalia (Thigpen et al, 1992b). **Male pseudohermaphroditism due to 5α-reductase deficiency is secondary to mutations in the type II gene.** At least 20 mutations have been identified (Thigpen et al, 1992a). Identical mutations in individuals with widely different geographic and ethnic backgrounds support the concept of mutational "hot spots" on the gene.

Individuals with this disorder present as newborns with a 46,XY karyotype and a phenotype that may vary from penoscrotal hypospadias to, more commonly, markedly ambiguous genitalia. Typically, the phallus is quite small, appearing as a normal or enlarged clitoris (Fig. 68–22). A urogenital sinus is present, with separate vaginal and urethral openings and labioscrotal fusion (Fig. 68–23). The vaginal pouch is short and blind-ending. Testes and epididymides are located in the labia, inguinal canals, or abdomen, and the vasa terminate in the blind-ending vaginal pouch. At puberty, partial masculinization occurs with an increase in muscle mass, development of male body habitus, increase in phallic size, and onset of erections (Peterson et al, 1977). Sperm production and fertility in affected individuals have been reported (Imperato-McGinley et al, 1982; Zhu et al, 1998). Other secondary sexual characteristics, including enlargement of the prostate and hairline recession do not develop.

On endocrine evaluation, these individuals have elevated mean plasma testosterone, but low DHT levels. After hCG stimulation, the testosterone/DHT ratio increases from the range of 3 to 25 in normal subjects to a range of 75 to 160 (Kupfer et al, 1992). Genital skin fibroblast cultures demonstrate diminished to absent 5α-reductase activity (Migeon et al, 1994). At puberty, virilization is presumed to occur because the androgen receptor binds markedly higher levels of testosterone at low affinity or because the enzyme defect is not a complete one. Indeed, the enzyme abnormalities in this disorder have been shown to be biochemically heterogeneous, ranging from reduced affinity of the enzyme for testosterone and reduced affinity for reduced nicotinamide adenine dinucleotide phosphate (NADPH) to altered pH activity profiles (Kupfer et al, 1992).

The phenotypic characteristics of this disorder have helped to clarify the roles of testosterone and DHT in normal development. **Although DHT appears to be critical for the development of normal external genitalia in utero, testosterone alone appears sufficient for wolffian duct development.**

Individuals in the pedigree studied by Imperato-McGinley in the Dominican Republic underwent gender reversal at puberty and were known within the community as *guavedoces* ("penis at 12") (Imperato-McGinley et al, 1979). This strong tendency toward reversal of gender identity in 5α-reductase deficiency has been one of the most intriguing aspects of the disorder. It has lent support to the concept that testosterone exerts the primary male imprinting effect on the brain. However, the discovery that there are two isoenzymes for 5α-reductase, only type II being deficient in this syndrome, allows for the possibility that 5α-reductase type I has some impact on the brain (Thigpen et al, 1992b). As a result, with early diagnosis of 5α-reductase deficiency, a male gender assignment is generally favored, bearing in mind that the studies strongly supporting male gender identity in this disorder were performed in sociologically unique environments (Zhu et al, 1998). The clinician must be open to familial cultural considerations regarding the value of male gender as well as the significance of penile size. In the setting of male gender assignment, cryptorchidism and hypospadias should be surgically corrected. Fertility is possible. Exogenous DHT could be used at puberty in an attempt to promote phallic growth, but it would be likely to impair spermatogenesis. For some individuals, based primarily on extremely small phallic size, a female gender is assigned. For these patients, gonadectomy should be performed as early as possible and certainly well before puberty to prevent virilization. Estrogen/progestin should be administered at the expected time of puberty. Vaginoplasty and clitoral reduction may be performed within the first year of life in those with a severe defect to provide for normal appearance of the external genitalia and to allay parental anxiety.

Persistent Müllerian Duct Syndrome

Persistent müllerian duct syndrome (PMDS), or *hernia uteri inguinale,* the term originally used by Nilson (1939), characteristically describes a group of **patients with a 46,XY karyotype and normal male external genitalia but internal müllerian duct structures. Typically, these phenotypic males have unilateral or bilateral undescended testes, bilateral fallopian tubes, a uterus, and an upper vagina draining into a prostatic utricle.** The condition is commonly diagnosed after müllerian tissue is encountered during inguinal herniorrhaphy or orchidopexy.

Clarnette and coworkers (1997) suggested three categories for patients with PMDS: (1) The majority (60% to 70%) with bilateral intra-abdominal testes in a position analogous to ovaries; (2) a smaller group (20% to 30%) in which one testis is found in a hernia sac or scrotum in association with a contralateral inguinal hernia (the classic presentation of hernia uteri inguinale); and (3) the smallest group (10%), in which both testes are located in the same hernia sac (as a result of transverse testicular ectopia) along with the fallopian tubes and uterus. Indeed, **PMDS is believed to be etiologically important in transverse testicular ectopia, occurring in 30% to 50% of cases** (Fujita, 1980).

The MIS gene was cloned in 1986 and localized on the short arm of chromosome 19 (Cates et al, 1986). It shows homology with the TGF-β super family of growth and differentiation factors (Imbeaud et al, 1995). **PMDS is thought to be a heterogeneous disorder genetically in which some subjects have decreased secretion of MIS and others have an abnormality of the MIS receptor.** Those patients who are positive for the gene are presumed to have a receptor or postreceptor defect. The condition may occur sporadically or be inherited as an X-linked (or autosomal dominant, sex-limited) trait (Migeon et al, 1994).

The treatment of persistent müllerian duct syndrome is relatively straightforward, in that all patients are phenotypic males who require orchidopexy. The cases of adult patients with associated testis tumor (most commonly seminoma) probably reflect the increased risk of malignancy in intra-abdominal undescended testes. One treatment caveat relates to management of the rudimentary müllerian structures. **The vasa deferentia are in close proximity to the uterus and proximal vagina, and preservation of the necessary müllerian structures to avoid injury to the vasa is recommended to preserve fertility** (Sloan and Walsh, 1976). Although fertility has been reported with this syndrome, malignancy of retained müllerian structures has not (Berkmen, 1997).

Unclassified Forms: Mayer-Rokitansky-Kuster-Hauser Syndrome

The Mayer-Rokitansky-Kuster-Hauser (MRKH) syndrome is a rare disorder entailing congenital absence of

the uterus and vagina. It occurs in approximately 1 of every 4000 to 5000 female births. Patients with MRKH syndrome have a 46,XX karyotype and are normal-appearing females with normal secondary sex characteristics. The external genitalia appear normal, but only a shallow vaginal pouch is present. In the typical form of the syndrome, there is symmetrical anatomy with absence of both vagina and uterus. Normal ovaries and fallopian tubes are present, and ovarian function is normal, but only symmetrical uterine remnants are found (Griffin et al, 1976).

The most common clinical presentation for MRKH syndrome is primary amenorrhea, but patients may present with infertility or dyspareunia. **Upper urinary tract anomalies occur in approximately one third of patients and include renal agenesis, pelvic kidney, and horseshoe kidney.**

Atypical forms of MRKH syndrome have been described in up to 10% of cases, in which asymmetrical uterine remnants and/or aplasia of one or both fallopian tubes is discovered. As a result, endometrial tissue or variable development of the uterus with hematometra may be present, resulting in a clinical presentation with cyclic abdominal pain. **Urinary tract anomalies occur more commonly in patients with the atypical form of MRKH.** In a study of 100 patients with MRKH syndrome, 38 (68%) of 56 patients with the atypical form of the condition had upper urinary tract abnormalities. Not one of 44 patients with the typical form of MRKH syndrome had an upper urinary tract anomaly (Strubbe et al, 1994).

A radiologic evaluation with ultrasound and MRI may define müllerian anatomy accurately in MRKH and distinguish between typical and atypical forms of the disorder (Nussbaum Blask et al, 1991; Reinhold et al, 1997).

Treatment entails surgical creation of a neovagina to allow for sexual function and drainage of menstrual fluid if necessary.

EVALUATION AND MANAGEMENT OF THE NEWBORN WITH AMBIGUOUS GENITALIA

The evaluation and initial management of the newborn with ambiguous genitalia must be regarded as a medical and psychosocial emergency and be handled with great sensitivity toward the family. Ideally, a medical team including a pediatric urologist, an endocrinologist, and a psychologist experienced in managing intersex patients should work closely with the family. **The team's goal should be to make a precise diagnosis of the intersex disorder (which can be achieved in virtually every case) and, with the involvement of the parents, to assign a proper sex of rearing based on the diagnosis, the status of the child's anatomy, and the functional potential of the genitalia and reproductive tract.**

In obtaining the history, certain pieces of information may be particularly valuable. A history of infant death within the family might suggest the possibility of CAH, and infertility, amenorrhea, or hirsutism might also suggest possible familial patterns of intersex states. Certainly, ma-

ternal use of medications, in particular steroids or contraceptives, during the pregnancy is of great importance.

The critical finding on physical examination is the presence of one or two gonads. This finding effectively rules out female pseudohermaphroditism. Because ovaries do not descend, a distinctly palpable gonad along the pathway of descent is highly suggestive of a testis. Rarely, an ovotestis undergoes descent and may be suspected on the basis of asymmetry of tissue texture of the poles of the gonad. This suspicion may be further supported by ultrasound findings. **The patient with bilaterally impalpable testes or a unilaterally impalpable testis and hypospadias should be regarded as having an intersex disorder until proven otherwise, whether or not the genitalia appear ambiguous.** Kaefer and associates (1999) studied the incidence of intersex disorders in patients with cryptorchidism and hypospadias and without ambiguous genitalia. **With a unilateral cryptorchid testis, the incidence of intersex was 30% overall—15% if the undescended testis was palpable and 50% if it was impalpable. In the setting of bilateral undescended testes and hypospadias, the incidence of intersexuality was quite similar—32% overall but only 16% if both gonads were palpable. If one of two undescended testes was impalpable, the incidence of intersex tripled to 47%, comparable to the rate in those with a unilateral, impalpable, cryptorchid testis.** In addition, posterior urethral meatal position was noted to be a strong predictor of intersex in this group of patients—65%, versus 5% to 8% with a midshaft to anteriorly located hypospadiac meatus (Kaefer et al, 1999).

In addition to gonadal examination, penile size should be assessed and an accurate measure of stretched penile length recorded.

An additional important finding on physical examination is the presence of a uterus, which is noted as an anterior midline cord-like structure on rectal examination. **A more precise means of assessing müllerian anatomy is by pelvic ultrasound, which may be performed immediately in the newborn period.** In addition to defining müllerian anatomy and confirming the presence or absence of a uterus, the gonads and adrenals should be studied. Normal anatomy of an undescended gonad should be confirmed, and a cyst within the gonad, consistent with ovotestis, should be ruled out.

Within the immediate newborn period, a karyotype should be obtained. Typically this requires 2 to 3 days to perform. Therefore, an attractive approach to obtain chromosomal data quickly is fluorescent in situ hybridization (FISH), which rapidly identifies X and Y chromosomes. It is typically used to confirm the presence of a second X chromosome. The technique is much more rapid than karyotyping, producing results in a few hours.

Serum studies should be immediately sent to rule out a salt-wasting form of CAH. In addition to serum electrolytes, testosterone and DHT should be measured early. Migeon and colleagues (1994) emphasized that the androgen levels may drop quickly, necessitating early study. In addition, they suggested that serum 17-hydroxyprogesterone should not be measured until day 3 or 4 in order to rule out 21-hydroxylase deficiency, because the stress of delivery may result in physiologic elevation of this steroid precursor in the first day or two of life.

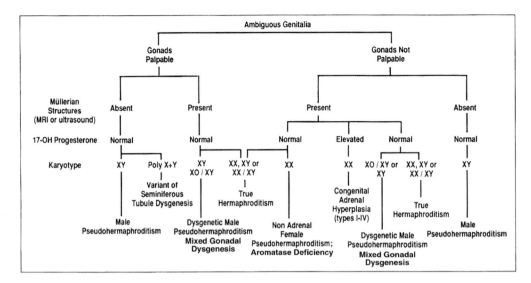

Figure 68–24. Diagnostic algorithm for a newborn with ambiguous genitalia based on gonadal palpability, presence or absence of müllerian structures, 17-hydroxyprogesterone concentration, and karyotype. (After Grumbach MM, Conte FH: Disorders of sex differentiation. In Wilson JD, Foster DW [eds]: Williams Textbook of Endocrinology. Philadelphia, WB Saunders, 1998, p 1401, with permission.)

In the absence of palpable testes, the presence or absence of testicular tissue should be determined by documentation of a markedly elevated LH, consistent with anorchia, or by means of an hCG stimulation test, which can demonstrate normally functioning testicular tissue (Jarow et al, 1986). In addition to ruling out anorchia, the study can enable diagnosis of 5α-reductase deficiency (by virtue of an increased ratio of testosterone to DHT) and can help distinguish between impaired testosterone synthesis (deficient response to hCG) and androgen insensitivity (normal response to hCG).

Based on physical examination (largely, gonadal palpability) the presence or absence of müllerian structures on ultrasound, 17-hydroxyprogesterone concentration, and the karyotype, a reasonable differential diagnosis may be formulated (Fig. 68–24).

Laparotomy and gonadal biopsy is usually the next definitive clinical step required when a firm diagnosis based on the aforementioned data is impossible. The laparoscopic approach can yield comparable information with less morbidity and is being used more widely for this purpose. **Laparotomy or laparoscopy in this setting remains a diagnostic maneuver; removal of gonads or reproductive organs should be deferred until the final pathology report is available and a gender has been assigned.** Biochemical studies on cultured genital skin fibroblasts, obtained at the time of gonadal biopsy, may define the precise cellular abnormality responsible for a given intersex disorder, be it abnormal androgen receptor or an enzyme abnormality. These studies should be performed in specialized laboratories where normal values are well established.

Finally, anatomic definition of the urogenital sinus and ductal structures contributes to the correct diagnosis and is necessary before any surgical intervention. The urogenital sinus is well imaged by retrograde contrast injection, which also opacifies ductal structures, defines the entry of urethra and vagina into the sinus, and outlines the cervical impression within the vagina. Endoscopy can define these relationships further but is usually not necessary until surgical reconstruction becomes imminent.

Gender Assignment

After a definitive diagnosis has been reached, a thorough and candid discussion with the family regarding gender assignment should take place. **Issues related to the diagnosis-specific potential for normal sexual functioning and fertility and the risk of gonadal malignancy should be addressed.** Parents should understand that high-quality data regarding the long-term psychosocial outcomes of gender assignment for the majority of intersex conditions are lacking, although longitudinal studies are being pursued. Parental involvement in the decision-making process is essential.

In the setting of a 46,XX karyotype, gender assignment is usually appropriately female. In CAH, cortisol suppresses the undesired androgen, and if maternal androgen is responsible for virilization, its discontinued stimulation is corrective. In both cases there are normal ovaries and müllerian ducts and a normal reproductive potential exists. **If the karyotype is 46,XY, the issue is a more complex one and includes factors such as penile length and evidence of androgen insensitivity.** For example, 46,XY patients with complete androgen insensitivity are appropriately assigned a female gender, whereas those with 5α-reductase deficiency may be more appropriately assigned a male gender. The most frequent abnormal karyotype is 45,X/46,XY mosaicism, which presents a variable phenotypic spectrum. The degree of masculinization of the external genitalia appears to vary with the amount of testicular tissue present, and gender assignment depends on the functional potential of the gonadal tissue, reproductive tracts, and genitalia.

Overall, it is well to remember in the management of ambiguous genitalia the parameters of optimal gender policy proposed by Meyer-Bahlburg (1998):

1. **Reproductive potential (if attainable at all)**
2. **Good sexual function**
3. **Minimal medical procedures**
4. **An overall gender-appropriate appearance**

5. **A stable gender identity**
6. **Psychosocial well being**

Ultimately, management of patients with intersex disorders remains a challenging and humbling process. On the one hand physicians have at their disposal sophisticated molecular biologic techniques that have enabled them to identify genetic disorders responsible for the majority of intersex conditions. On the other hand, the mysteries of brain dimorphism in the setting of sexual ambiguity remain to be solved in order to optimize the long-term psychosocial outcome of gender assignment for the individual patient.

REFERENCES

Normal Sexual Differentiation

Andersson S, Berman DM, Jenkins EP, et al: Deletion of steroid 5 alpha reductase #2-gene in male pseudohermaphroditism. Nature 1991;354:159–161.

Andersson S, Russell DW: Structural and biochemical properties of cloned and expressed human and rat steroid 5 alpha reductases. Proc Natl Acad Sci U S A 1990;87:3640–3644.

Bogan JS, Page DC: Ovary? Testis?—A mammalian dilemma. Cell, 1994;76:603–607.

Bridges CB: Triploid intersexes in *Drosophila melanogaster.* Science 1921;54:252–254.

Byskov AG, Westergaard LG: Differentiation of the ovary. In Polin RA, Fox WW (eds): Fetal Neonatal Physiology, 2nd ed. Philadelphia, WB Saunders, 1998, pp 2484–2491.

Call KM, Glaser T, Ito CY, et al: Isolation and characterization of zinc finger polypeptide gene at the human chromosome 11 Wilms' tumor locus. Cell 1990;60:509.

Cate RL, Mattaliano RJ, Hession C, et al: Isolation of the bovine and human genes for müllerian inhibiting substance and expression of the human gene in clinical cells. Cell 1986;45:685–698.

Eichwald EJ, Silmser CR: Untitled communication. Transplant Bull 1955;2:148–149.

Ford CE, Jones KW, Polani P, et al: A sex chromosome anomaly in a case of gonadal sex dysgenesis (Turner's syndrome). Lancet 1959;1:711–713.

George FW, Peterson KG: Five alpha dihydrotestosterone formation is necessary for embryogenesis of the rat prostate. Endocrinology 1988;122:1159–1164.

Gill WB, Schumacher GFB, Bibbo M, et al: Association of diethyl stilbestrol exposure in utero with cryptorchidism, testicular hypoplasia, semen abnormalities. J Urol 1979;122:36–39.

Goodfellow PN, Lovell-Badge R: SRY and sex determination in mammals. Ann Rev Genet 1993;27:71–92.

Gubbay J, Vivian N, Economou A, et al: Inverted repeat structure of the Sry locus in mice. Proc Natl Acad Sci U S A 1992;89:7953–7957.

Guo WW, Mason JS, Stone CG, et al: Diagnosis of X-linked adrenal hypoplasia congenita by mutation analysis of the Dax 1 gene. JAMA 1995;274:324–330.

Haqq CM, King C, Ukiyama E, et al: Molecular basis of mammalian sexual determination: Activation of müllerian inhibiting substance gene expression by SRY. Science 1994;266:1494–1500.

Imbeaud S, Faure E, Lamarre I, et al: Insensitivity to anti-Müllerian hormone due to a spontaneous mutation in the human anti-Müllerian hormone receptor. Nat Genet 1995;11:382–388.

Jacobs PA, Strong JA: A case of human intersexuality having a possible XXY sex-determining mechanism. Nature 1959;183:302–303.

Jenkins EP, Andersson S, Imperato-McGinley J, et al: Genetic and pharmacological evidence for more than one human steroid 5 alpha reductase. J Clin Invest 1992;89:293–300.

Jirasek JA: Germ cells and the indifferent gonad. In Polin RA, Fox WW (eds): Fetal and Neonatal Physiology, 2nd ed. Philadelphia, WB Saunders, 1998, pp 2478–2483.

Josso N, Rey R: Genetic mechanisms of sex differentiation. Pediatrics 1996;8:396–400.

Jost A, Vigier B, Prepin J, Perchellet JP: Studies on sex differentiation in mammals: Recent progress in hormone research. Recent Prog Horm Res 1973;29:1–41.

Koopman P, Gubbay J, Vivian M, et al: Male development of chromosomally female mice transgenic for Sry. Nature 1991;351:117–121.

Koopman P, Münsterberg A, Capel B, et al: Expression of a candidate sex determining gene during mouse testis differentiation. Nature 1990;348:450–452.

Kreidberg JA, Sariola H, Loring JM, et al: WT-1 is requirement for early kidney development. Cell 1993;74:679–691.

Lim HN, Hawkins JR: Genetic control of gonadal differentiation. Baillieres Clin Endocrinol Metab 1998;12:2–15.

Lopez ML, Erickson RP, Blecher SR: Sex determination. In Polin RA, Fox WW (eds): Fetal Neonatal Physiology, 2nd ed. Philadelphia, WB Saunders, 1998, pp 2469–2474.

Lubahn DB, Joseph DR, Sullivan PM, et al: Cloning of human androgen receptor complementary DNA and localization to the X chromosome. Science 1988;240:327–330.

Lukusa T, Fryns JP, van Der Berghe H: The role of the Y chromosome in sex determination. Genet Couns 1992;3:1–11.

Magenis RE, Webb MJ, McKean RS, et al: Translocation (X;Y) (p23.33; p11.2) in XX males: Etiology of male phenotype. Hum Genet 1982;62:271–276.

McLaren A, Simpson E, Tomonari K, et al: Male sexual differentiation in mice lacking HY antigen. Nature 1984;312:552–555.

Ogata T, Hawkins JR, Taylor A, et al: Sex reversal in a child with a 46Xyp+ karyotype: Support for the existence of a gene, located in distal Xp, involved in testis formation. J Med Genet 1992;29:226–230.

Page DC, Mosher R, Simpson EM, et al: The sex determining region of the human Y chromosome encodes a finger protein. Cell 1987;51:1091–1104.

Painter TS: The Y chromosome in mammals. Science 1921;53:503–504.

Palmer MS, Sinclair AH, Berta P, et al: Genetic evidence that ZFY is not the testis determining factor. Nature 1989;342:937–939.

Pelletier J, Bruning W, Kashtan CE, et al: Germline mutations in the Wilms' tumor suppressor urogenital development in Denys-Drash syndrome. Cell 1991a;67:437–447.

Pelletier J, Schalling M, Buckler AJ, et al: Expression of the Wilms' tumor gene WT-1 in the murine urogenital system. Development 1991b;5:1345–1356.

Shen WH, Moore CCD, Ikeda Y, et al: Nuclear receptor steroidogenic factor 1 regulates the müllerian inhibiting substance gene: A link to the sex determination cascade. Cell 1994;77:651–661.

Siiteri PK, Wilson JD: Testosterone formation and metabolism during male sexual differentiation in the human embryo. J Clin Endocrinol Metab 1974;38:113.

Sinclair AH, Berta P, Palmer MS, et al: A gene from the human sex determining region encodes a protein with homology to a conserved DHA-binding motif. Nature 1990;346:240–244.

Sinclair AH, Poster JW, Spencer JA, et al: Sequences homologous to ZFY, a candidate human sex determining gene, are autosomal in marsupials. Nature 1988;336:780–783.

Vigier B, Forest MG, Eychenne B, et al: Anti-müllerian hormone produces endocrine sex reversal of fetal ovaries. Proc Natl Acad Sci U S A 1989;86:3684–3688.

Wachtel SS: HY antigen and the genetics of sex determination. Science 1977;198:797–799.

Wagner T, Wirth J, Meyer J, et al: Autosomal sex reversal and camptomelic dysplasia are caused by mutations in and around the SRY-related gene Sox 9. Cell 1994;79:1111–1120.

Psychosexual Differentiation

Diamond M, Sigmundson K: Sex reassignment at birth. Arch Pediatr Adolesc Med 1997;151:248–304.

Erhardt AA, Meyer-Bahlburg HFL: Effects of prenatal sex hormones on gender-related behavior. Science 1981;211:1312–1318.

Grumbach MM, Conte FA: Disorders of sex differentiation. In Wilson JD, Foster DW, Kronenberg HM, Larsen PR (eds): Williams Textbook of Endocrinology, 9th ed. Philadelphia, WB Saunders, 1998, pp 1303–1426.

Money J, Erhardt AA: Man and woman, boy and girl: The differentiation and dimorphism of gender identity from conception to maturity. Baltimore, Johns Hopkins University Press, 1972.

Seminiferous Tubule Dysgenesis

Harnden DG, Maclean N, Langlands AO: Carcinoma of the breast and Klinefelter's syndrome. J Med Genet 1971;8:460–461.

Jacobs PA, Strong JA: A case of human intersexuality having a possible XXY sex-determining mechanism. Nature 1959;183:302.

Kitamura M, Matsumiya K, Koga M, et al: Ejaculated spermatozoa in patients with non-mosaic Klinefelter's syndrome. Int J Urol 2000;7:88–92.

Klinefelter HP Jr, Reifenstein EC Jr, Albright F: Syndrome characterized by gynecomastia, aspermatogenesis, without a-Leydigism and increased excretion of follicle stimulating hormone. J Clin Endocrinol 1942;2:615.

46, XX Male

de la Chappelle A, Hortling H, Niemi M, et al: Sex chromosomes in a human male: First case. Acta Med Scand Suppl 1964;412:25.

de la Chappelle A: Nature and origin of males with XX sex chromosomes. Am J Med Genet 1972;24:71.

Fechner PY, Marcantonio SM, Jaswaney V, et al: The role of the sex determining region Y gene (SRY) in the etiology of 46XX maleness. J Clin Endocrinol Metab 1993;76:690–695.

Van Dyke DC, Hansen JW, Moore JW, et al: Clinical management issues in males with sex chromosomal mosaicism and discordant phenotype/sex chromosomal patterns. Clin Pediatr 1991;30:15–21.

Weil D, Wang I, Deitrich A, et al: Highly homologous loci on the X and Y chromosomes are hot-spots for ectopic recombinations leading to XX maleness. Nat Genet 1994;7:414–419.

Turner's Syndrome

Epstein CJ: Mechanisms leading to the phenotype of Turner syndrome. In Rosenfeld RG, Grumbach MM (eds): Turner syndrome. New York, Marcel Dekker, 1990, pp 13–25.

Ford CE, Jones KW, Polani PE: A sex chromosomal anomaly in a case of gonadal dysgenesis (Turner's syndrome). Lancet 1959;1:711–713.

Hall JG, Gilchrist DM: Turner syndrome and its variants. Pediatr Clin North Am 1990;37:1421–1441.

Kaneko N, Kawagoe S, Hizoi M: Turner's syndrome: Review of the literature with reference to a successful pregnancy outcome. Gynecol Obstet Invest 1990;29:81–87.

Saenger P: Clinical review 48: The current status of diagnosis and therapeutic intervention in Turner's syndrome. J Clin Endocrinol Metab 1993;77:297–301.

Saenger P: Turner's syndrome. N Engl J Med 1996;335:1749–1754.

Stanhope RG, Massarano AA, Brook CGD: The natural history of ovarian demise in the Turner's syndrome (Abstract.). Proceedings of the Third International Symposium on Turner's Syndrome, London, April 9, 1992, p 34.

Turner HH: A syndrome of infantilism, congenital webbed neck and cubitus valgus. Endocrinology 1938;23:566.

Zinn AR, Page DC, Fisher ENC: Turner syndrome: The case of the missing sex chromosome. Trends Genet 1993;9:90–93.

46,XX "Pure" Gonadal Dysgenesis

Espiner A, Veale AMD, Sands VE, et al: Familial syndrome of streak gonads and normal male karyotype in five phenotypic females. N Engl J Med 1970;283:6.

Mixed Gonadal Dysgenesis

Beckwith JB, Palmer NF: Histopathology and prognosis of Wilms' tumor: Results from the first national Wilms tumor study. Cancer 1978;41:1937–1948.

Berkovitz GD, Fechner PY, Zacur HW, et al: Clinical and pathologic spectrum of 46,XY gonadal dysgenesis: Its relevance to the understanding of sex determination. Medicine (Baltimore) 1991;70:375.

Chang HG, Clark RD, Bachman H: The phenotype of 45X/46XY mosaicism: An analysis of 92 prenatally diagnosed cases. Am J Hum Genet 1990;46:156.

Davidoff F, Federman DB: Mixed gonadal dysgenesis. Pediatrics 1973;52:725–742.

Denys P, Malvaux P, van der Berghe H, et al: Association d'un syndrome anatomo-pathologique de pseudohermaphrodisme masculin, d'une tumeur de Wilms'; d'une nephropathie parenchymateuse et d'un mosaisism XX/XY. Arch Fr Pediatr 1967;24:729–739.

Drash A, Sherman F, Hartmann WH, Blizzard RM: A syndrome of pseudo-hermaphrodism, Wilms' tumor, hypertension and degenerative disease. J Pediatr 1970;76:585–593.

Habib R, Loirat C, Gubler MC, et al: The nephropathy associated with male pseudohermaphrodism and Wilms' tumor (Drash syndrome): A distinctive glomerular lesion—report of ten cases. Clin Nephrol 1985;24:269–278.

Hsu LYF: Prenatal diagnosis of 45/46XY mosaicism: A review and update. Prenat Diagn 1989;9:31.

Jadresic L, Leake J, Gordon I, et al: Clinico-pathologic review of 12 children with nephropathy, Wilms' tumor, genital abnormalities (Drash syndrome). J Pediatr 1990;117:717–725.

Mendez JP, Ulloa-Aguirre A, Kofman-Alfaro S, et al: Mixed gonadal dysgenesis: Clinical cytogenetic, endocrinological and histopathological findings in 16 patients. Am J Med Genet 1993;46:263–267.

Migeon CJ: Male pseudohermaphrodism. Ann Endocrinol (Paris) 1980;41:311.

Rajfer J: Association between Wilms' tumor and gonadal dysgenesis. J Urol 1981;125:388–390.

Robboy SJ, Miller T, Donahoe PK, et al: Dysgenesis of testicular and streak gonads in a syndrome of mixed gonadal dysgenesis. Hum Pathol 1982;13:700.

Scully RE: Gonadoblastoma. Cancer 1970;25:1340.

Sohval AR: Mixed gonadal dysgenesis: A variety of hermaphroditism. Am J Hum Genet 1963;15:155.

Verp NS, Simpson JL: Abnormal sexual differentiation and neoplasia. Cancer Genet Cytogenet 1987;25:191.

Wallace T, Levin HS: Mixed gonadal dysgenesis. Arch Pathol Lab Med 1990;114:679.

Zah W, Kalderone HE, Tucci JR: Mixed gonadal dysgenesis. Acta Endocrinol 1975;79:3–39.

Dysgenetic Male Pseudohermaphroditism

Borer JB, Nitti VW, Glassberg KI: Mixed gonadal dysgenesis and dysgenetic male pseudohermaphroditism. J Urol 1995;153:1267–1273.

Federman DD: Disorders of sexual development. N Engl J Med 1967;277:351.

Manuel M, Katayama KP, Jones HW Jr: The age of occurrence of gonadal tumors in intersex patients with a Y chromosome. Am J Obstet Gynecol 1976;124:293.

46,XY Complete Gonadal Dysgenesis

German J, Simpson JL, Chaganti RSK, et al: Genetically determined sex reversal in 46XY humans. Science 1978;202:53.

Grumbach MM, Conte FA: Disorders of sexual differentiation. In Wilson JD, Foster DW, Konenberg HM, Larsen PR (eds): Williams Textbook of Endocrinology. Philadelphia, WB Saunders, 1998, pp 1303–1425.

Manuel M, Katayama KP, Jones HW Jr: The age of occurrence of gonadal tumors in intersex patients with a Y chromosome. Am J Obstet Gynecol 1976;124:293.

McDonald MT, Flejter W, Sheldon S, et al: XY sex reversal and gonadal dysgenesis due to 9p 24 monosomy. Am J Med Genet 1997;73:321–326.

Scully RE: Neoplasia associated with anomalous sexual development and abnormal sex chromosomes. In Josso N (ed): The Intersex Child. Basel, S. Carter, 1981, p 203.

Embryonic Testicular Regression and Bilateral Vanishing Testes Syndromes

Aynsley-Green AA, Zachman NM, Illig R, et al: Congenital bilateral anorchia in childhood: A clinical and endocrine and therapeutic evaluation of 21 cases. Clin Endocrinol 1976;5:381–391.

Bergada C, Cleveland WW, Jones HW Jr, Wilkins L: Variants of embryonic testicular dysgenesis: Bilateral anorchia and the syndrome of rudimentary testes. Acta Endocrinol 1962;40:521–536.

Edman CD, Winters AJ, Porter JC, et al: Embryonic testicular regression:

A clinical spectrum of XY agonadal individuals. Obstet Gynecol 1977;
49:208–217.

Jarow JP, Berkovitz GD, Migeon CJ, et al: Elevation of serum gonadotropins established the diagnosis of anorchism in prepubertal boys with bilateral cryptorchidism. J Urol 1986;136:277.

Marcantonio SM, Fechner PY, Migeon CJ, et al: Embryonic testicular regression sequence: A part of the clinical spectrum of 46XY gonadal dysgenesis. Am J Med Genet 1994;49:1–5.

Migeon CJ, Berkovitz GD, Brown TR: Sexual differentiation and ambiguity. In Kappy MS, Blizzard RN, Migeon CJ (eds): Wilkins, The Diagnosis and Treatment of Endocrine Disorders in Childhood and Adolescence. Springfield, Ill, Charles C Thomas, 1994, pp 573–716.

True Hermaphroditism

Berkovitz GD, Fechner PY, Zacur HW, et al: Clinical and pathologic spectrum of 46XY gonadal dysgenesis: Its relevance to the understanding of sex differentiation. Medicine (Baltimore) 1991;70:375–383.

Blyth B, Duckett JW Jr: Gonadal differentiation: A review of the physiological process and influencing factors based on recent experimental evidence. J Urol 1991;145:689–694.

Grumbach MM, Conte FA: Disorders of sex differentiation. In Wilson JD, Foster DW, Kronenberg HM, Larsen PR (eds): Williams' Textbook of Endocrinology, 9th ed. Philadelphia, WB Saunders, 1998, pp 1303–1426.

Hadjiathanasiou CG, Brauner R, Lortat-Jacob S, et al: True hermaphroditism: Genetic variants and clinical management. J Pediatr 1994;125:738–744.

Nihoul-Fekete C, Lortat-Jacob S, Cachin O, Josso N: Preservation of gonadal function in true hermaphroditism. J Pediatr Surg 1984;19:50–55.

Starceski PJ, Sieber WK, Lee PA: Fertility and true hermaphroditism. Adolesc Pediatr Gynecol 1988;1:55–56.

Verp MS, Simpson JL: Abnormal sexual differentiation and neoplasia. Cancer 1987;25:191–218.

Congenital Adrenal Hyperplasia

Bongiovanni AM, McFadden AJ: Steroids during pregnancy and possible fetal consequences. Fertil Steril 1960;11:181.

Bongiovanni AM, Root AW: The adrenogenital syndrome. N Engl J Med 1963;268:1391–1399.

Calaf J, Prats J, Esteban-Altirriba J: Female pseudohermaphroditism caused by maternal hyperandrogenism. In Martinez-Mora J: Intersexual States: Disorders of Sex Differentiation. Barcelona, Ediciones Doyma, 1994, pp 187–197.

Fife D, Rappaport EB: Prevalence of salt-losing among congenital adrenal hyperplasia patients. Clin Endocrinol 1983;18:259.

Grumbach MM, Conte FA: Disorders of sex differentiation. In Wilson JD, Foster DW, Kronenberg HM, Larsen PR (eds): Williams' Textbook of Endocrinology, 9th ed. Philadelphia, WB Saunders, 1998, pp 1303–1426.

Gunther DF, Bukowski TP, Ritzen EM, et al: Prophylactic adrenalectomy of a three year old girl with congenital adrenal hyperplasia: Pre- and post-operative studies. J Clin Endocrinol Metab 1997;82:3324–3327.

Hughes IA: Congenital adrenal hyperplasia: A continuum of disorders. Lancet 1998;352:752–754.

Ishizura N, Kawashima P, Nakanish T, et al: Statistical observations on genital anomalies of newborns following the administration of progestins to their mothers. J Jpn Obstet Gynecol Soc 1962;9:271.

Kohn B, Day D, Alenzadeh R, et al: Splicing mutation in CYP-21 associated with delayed presentation of salt wasting congenital adrenal hyperplasia. Am J Med Genet 1995;57:450–454.

Laue L, Rennert OM: Congenital adrenal hyperplasia: Molecular genetics and alternative approaches to treatment. Adv Pediatr 1995;42:113–143.

Merke DP, Tajima T, Chhabra A, et al: Novel CYP-11B1 mutations in congenital adrenal hyperplasia due to steroid-11 beta-hydroxylase deficiency. J Clin Endocrinol Metab 1998;83:270–273.

Migeon CJ: Comments about the need for prenatal treatment of congenital adrenal hyperplasia due to 21-hydroxylase deficiency. J Clin Endocrinol Metab 1990;70:836–837.

Miller WL: Dexamethasone treatment of congenital adrenal hyperplasia in utero: An experimental therapy of unproven safety. J Urol 1999;162:537–540.

New MI, Levine LS: Steroid 21-hydroxylase deficiency in adrenal dis-

eases in childhood. In New MI, Levine LS (eds): Pediatric and Adolescent Endocrinology, vol 13: Adrenal Disease in Childhood. Basel, Karger, 1984 pp 1–46.

New MI, White PC, Speiser P: Congenital adrenal hyperplasia. In Martinez-Mora J (ed): Intersexual States: Disorders of Sex Differentiation. Barcelona, Ediciones Doyma, 1994, pp 162–186.

Pang S, Pollack MS, Marshall RN, Immken L: Prenatal treatment of congenital adrenal hyperplasia due to 21-hydroxylase deficiency. N Engl J Med 1990;322:111–115.

Pang S, Spence D, New MI: Newborn screening for congenital adrenal hyperplasia with special reference to screening in Alaska. Ann N Y Acad Sci 1985;458:90–102.

Passerini-Glazel G: Feminizing genitoplasty (Editorial). J Urol 1990;161:1592–1593.

Speiser PW, Laforgia N, Kato K, et al: First trimester prenatal treatment and molecular genetic diagnosis of congenital adrenal hyperplasia. J Clin Endocrinol Metab 1990;70:838–848.

Speiser PW: Prenatal treatment of congenital adrenal hyperplasia. J Urol 1999;162:534–536.

Tusie-Luna M, White PC: Gene conversions and unequal crossovers between CYP-21 (steroid 21-hydroxylase gene) and CYP-21P involve different mechanisms. Proc Natl Acad Sci U S A 1995;92:10796–10800.

VanWyk JJ, Gunther DF, Ritzen EM, et al: The use of adrenalectomy as a treatment for congenital adrenal hyperplasia. J Clin Endocrinol Metab 1996;81:3180–3190.

Wilson RC, Mercado AB, Cheng KC, New MI: Steroid 21-hydroxylase deficiency: Genotype may not predict phenotype. J Clin Endocrinol Metab 1995;80:2322–2329.

Leydig Cell Aplasia/Receptor Abnormality

Arnholt JP, Mendonca BB, Bloise W, Toledo SPA: Male pseudo-hermaphroditism resulting from Leydig cell hyperplasia. J Pediatr 1985;106:1057.

Berthezene F, Forest MG, Grimaud JA, et al: Leydig cell agenesis: A cause of male pseudohermaphroditism. N Engl J Med 1976;295:969–972.

Brown DM, Markland C, Dehner LP: Leydig cell hyperplasia: Cause of male pseudohermaphroditism. J Clin Endocrinol Metab 1978;46:1–7.

David R, Yoon DJ, Landin L, et al: A syndrome of gonadotropin resistance possibly due to a luteinizing hormone receptor defect. J Clin Endocrinol Metab 1984;59:156–160.

Lee PA, Rock JA, Brown TR, et al: Leydig cell hypofunction resulting in male pseudohermaphroditism. Fertil Steril 1982;37:675–679.

Disorders of Testosterone Biosynthesis

Andersson S, Moghrabi N: Physiology and molecular genetics of 17-beta-hydroxysteroid dehydrogenase. Steroids 1997;62:143–147.

Bongiovanni AM: The adrenogenital syndrome with deficiency of 3-beta-hydroxy-steroid dehydrogenase. J Clin Invest 1962;41:2086–2092.

Chang YT, Kappy MS, Iwamoto K, et al: Mutations in type-2 3-beta-hydroxy-steroid dehydrogenase gene in a patient with classic salt wasting 3-beta-hydroxy-steroid dehydrogenase deficiency congenital adrenal hyperplasia. Pediatr Res 1993;34:698–700.

Hauffa BT, Miller WL, Grumbach MM, et al: Congenital adrenal hyperplasia due to deficient cholesterol side chain cleavage activity (20–22 desmolase) in a patient treated for 18 years. Clin Endocrinol 1985;23:481–493.

Imperato-McGinley J, Peterson RE, Stoller R, Goodwin WE: Male pseudohermaphroditism secondary to 17-hydroxysteroid dehydrogenase deficiency: Gender role change with puberty. J Clin Endocrinol Metab 1979;49:391–395.

Laue L, Rennert OM: Congenital adrenal hyperplasia: Molecular genetics and alternative approaches to treatment. Adv Pediatr 1995;42:113–143.

New MI: Male pseudohermaphrodism due to a 17-alpha-hydroxylase deficiency. J Clin Invest 1970;49:1930–1941.

Prader A, Gurtner HP: Das syndrom des pseudohermaphroditismus masculinus bei kongenitaler nebennierenrinden hyperplasie ohne androgenuberproduktion (adrenaler pseudohermaphroditismus masculinus). Helv Pediatra Acta 1955;10:397–412.

Reddy VV, Naftolin F, Ryan KJ: Conversion of androstenedione to estrone by neural tissues from fetal and neonatal rats. Endocrinology 1974;94:117–121.

Rosler A, Kohn G: Male pseudohermaphroditism due to 17 beta-hydroxysteroid dehydrogenase deficiency: Studies on the natural history of the defect and the effect of androgens on gender role. J Steroid Biochem 1983;39:663–674.

Saenger P: New developments in congenital lipoid adrenal hyperplasia and steroidogenic regulatory protein. Pediatr Endocrinol 1997;44:397–421.

Saez JM, DePeretti E, Morera AM, et al: Familial male pseudohermaphroditism with gynecomastia due to a testicular 17-ketosteroid reductase defect. In vivo studies. J Clin Endocrinol Metab 1971;32:604–610.

Saez JM, Morera AM, DePeretti E, Bertrand J: Further in vivo studies in male pseudohermaphroditism with gynecomastia due to a testicular 17-ketosteroid reductase defect (compared to a case of testicular feminization). J Clin Endocrinol Metab 1972;34:598–600.

Virdis R, Saenger P: 17 Beta-hydroxy steroid dehydrogenase deficiency. In New MI, Levine LS (eds): Pediatric and Adolescent Endocrinology, vol 13: Adrenal Disease in Childhood. Basel, Karger, 1984, pp 110–124.

Zachmann M, Vollmin JA, Hamilton W, Prader A: Steroid 17,20-desmolase deficiency: A new cause of male pseudohermaphroditism. Clin Endocrinol 1972;1:369–385.

Zachmann M, Werder EA, Prader A: Two types of male pseudohermaphroditism due to 17,20-desmolase deficiency. J Clin Endocrinol Metab 1982;55:487–490.

Zhu Y, Katz MD, Imperato-McGinley J: Natural potent androgens: Lessons from human genetic models. Baillieres Clin Endocrinol Metab 1998;12:83–113.

Androgen Receptor and Postreceptor Defects

Batch JA, Davies HR, Evans BA, et al: Phenotypic variation and detection of carrier status in the partial androgen insensitivity syndrome. Arch Dis Child 1993;68:453.

Brown CJ, Goss SJ, Lubahn DB, et al: Androgen receptor locus on the human X chromosome: Regional localization to Xq11-12 and description of a DNA polymorphism. Am J Hum Genet 1989;44:264.

Conte FA, Grumbach MM: Pathogenesis, classification, diagnosis and treatment of anomalies of sex. In Besset GM, Cahill GF Jr, Marshall JC, et al (eds): Endocrinology, 2nd ed. Philadelphia, WB Saunders, 1989, pp 1810–1847.

Grumbach MM, Conte FA: Disorders of sex differentiation. In Wilson JD, Foster DW, Kronenberg HM, Larsen PR (eds): Williams' Textbook of Endocrinology, 9th ed. Philadelphia, WB Saunders, 1998, pp 1303–1426.

Hughes IA, Patterson MN: Prenatal diagnosis of androgen insensitivity. Clin Endocrinol 1994;40:295.

Manuel M, Katayama KP, Jones HW Jr: The age of occurrence of gonadal tumors in intersex patients with a Y chromosome. Am J Obstet Gynecol 1976;124:293.

Meyer-Bahlburg HFL: Gender assignment and reassignment in 46XY pseudo-hermaphroditism and related conditions. J Clin Endocrinol Metab 1999;84:3455–3458.

Muller J, Skakkebaek NE: Testicular carcinoma in situ in children with the androgen insensitivity (testicular feminization) syndrome. BMJ 1984;288:1419.

Quigley CA, DeBellis A, Marschke KB, et al: Androgen receptor defects: Historical, clinical, molecular perspectives. Endocr Rev 1995;16:271.

Wiener JS, Teague JL, Roth DR, et al: Molecular biology and function of the androgen receptor in genital development. J Urol 1997;157:1377–1386.

Wilkins L: The Diagnosis and Treatment of Endocrine Disorders in Childhood and Adolescence. Springfield, Ill, Dulcy Thomas, 1950.

Syndrome of Partial Androgen Resistance

Aiman J, Griffin JE, Gazak JM, et al: Androgen insensitivity as a cause of infertility in otherwise normal men. N Engl J Med 1979;300:223.

Aiman J, Griffin JE: The frequency of androgen receptor deficiency in infertile men. J Clin Endocrinol Metab 1982;54:725.

Griffin JE, Durrant JL: Qualitative receptor defects in families with androgen resistance: Failure of stabilization of the fibroblast cytosol androgen receptor. J Clin Endocrinol Metab 1982;55:465–474.

Griffin JE: Androgen resistance: The clinical and molecular spectrum. N Engl J Med 1992;326:611–618.

Migeon CJ, Berkovitz GD, Brown TR: Sexual differentiation and ambigu-

ity. In Kappy MS, Blizzard RN, Migeon CJ (eds): Wilkins, The Diagnosis and Treatment of Endocrine Disorders in Childhood and Adolescence. Springfield, Ill, Charles C Thomas, 1994, pp 573–716.

Wilson JD, Griffin JE, Leshin M, Macdonald PC: The androgen resistant syndromes: Five alpha reductase deficiency, testicular feminization, related disorders. In Stanbury JB, Wyngaarden JB, Frederickson DS, et al (eds): The Metabolic Basis of Inherited Disease. New York, McGraw-Hill, 1983, pp 1001–1026.

Wilson JD, Harrod MJ, Goldstein JL, et al: Familial incomplete male pseudohermaphroditism, type I. N Engl J Med 1974;290:1097–1103.

5α-Reductase Deficiency

Imperato-McGinley JL, Guerrero L, Gautier T, et al: Steroid 5 alpha-reductase deficiency in men: An inherited form of male pseudohermaphroditism. Science 1974;186:1213.

Imperato-McGinley J, Peterson RE, Gautier T, et al: Hormonal evaluation of a large kindred with complete androgen insensitivity: Evidence for secondary 5 alpha-reductase. J Clin Endocrinol Metab 1982;54:931–941.

Imperato-McGinley J, Peterson RE, Gautier T, Sturla E: Androgens and the evolution of male-gender identity among male pseudohermaphrodites with 5 alpha-reductase deficiency. N Engl J Med 1979;300:1233–1237.

Kupfer SR, Quigley CA, French FS: Male pseudohermaphroditism. Semin Perinatol 1992;16:319–331.

Migeon CJ, Berkovitz GD, Brown TR: Sexual differentiation and ambiguity. In Kappy MS, Blizzard RN, Migeon CJ (eds): Wilkins, The Diagnosis and Treatment of Endocrine Disorders in Childhood and Adolescence. Springfield, Ill, Charles C Thomas, 1994, pp 573–716.

Peterson RE, Imperato-McGinley J, Gautier T, Sturla E: Male pseudohermaphroditism due to steroid 5 alpha-reductase deficiency. Am J Med 1977;62:170–191.

Thigpen AE, Davis DL, Gautier T, et al: Brief report: The molecular basis of steroid 5 alpha-reductase deficiency in a large Dominican kindred. N Engl J Med 1992a;327:1216–1219.

Thigpen AE, Davis DL, Milatovich A, et al: Molecular genetics of steroid 5 alpha-reductase 2 deficiency. J Clin Invest 1992b;90:799–809.

Walsh PC, Madden JD, Harrod MJ, et al: Familial incomplete male pseudo-hermaphroditism, type II: Decreased dihydrotestosterone formation in pseudovaginal perineal scrotal hypospadias. N Engl J Med 1974; 291:944.

Wilson JD: Recent studies on the mechanism of action of testosterone. N Engl J Med 1972;287:1284–1291.

Zhu Y, Katz MD, Imperato-McGinley J: Natural potent androgens: Lessons from human genetic models. Baillieres Clin Endocrinol Metab 1998;12:83–113.

Persistent Müllerian Duct Syndrome

Berkmen F: Persistent Müllerian duct syndrome with or without transverse testicular ectopia and testis tumors. Br J Urol 1997;79:122–126.

Cates RL, Mattaliano RJ, Hession C, et al: Isolation of the bovine and human genes from Müllerian inhibiting substance and expression of the human gene in animal cells. Cell 1986;45:685.

Clarnette TD, Sugita Y, Hutson JM: Genital anomalies in human and animal models reveal the mechanisms and hormones governing testicular descent. Br J Urol 1997;79:99–112.

Fujita J: Transverse testicular ectopia. Urology 1980;16:400–402.

Imbeaud S, Faure E, Lamarre I, et al: Insensitivity to anti-Müllerian hormone due to a mutation in the human anti-Müllerian hormone receptor. Res Genet 1995;11:382–388.

Migeon CJ, Berkovitz GD, Brown TR: Sexual differentiation and ambiguity. In Kappy MS, Blizzard RN, Migeon CJ (eds): Wilkins, The Diagnosis and Treatment of Endocrine Disorders in Childhood and Adolescence. Springfield, Ill, Charles C Thomas, 1994, pp 573–716.

Nilson O: Hernia uteri inguinalis beim Manne. Acta Chir Scand 1939;83: 231.

Sloan WR, Walsh PC: Familial persistent Müllerian duct syndrome. J Urol 1976;115:459–461.

Mayer-Rokitansky-Kuster-Hauser Syndrome

Griffin JE, Edwards C, Madden JD, et al: Congenital absence of the vagina: The Mayer-Rokitansky-Kuster-Hauser syndrome. Ann Intern Med 1976;85:224–236.

Nussbaum Blask AR, Sanders RC, Rock JA: Obstructed uterovaginal anomalies: Demonstration with sonography. Radiology 1991;179:84–88.

Reinhold C, Hricak H, Forstner R, et al: Primary amenorrhea: Evaluation with MR imaging. Radiology 1997;203:383–390.

Strubbe EH, Cremers CWRJ, Willemsen WNP, et al: The Mayer-Rokitansky-Kuster-Hauser (MRKH) syndrome without and with associated features: Two separate entities? Clin Dysmorphol 1994;3:192–199.

Evaluation and Management of the Newborn with Ambiguous Genitalia

Jarow JP, Berkovitz GD, Migeon CJ, et al: Elevation of serum gonadotropins established the diagnosis of anorchism in prepubertal boys with bilateral cryptorchidism. J Urol 1986;136:277.

Kaefer M, Diamond D, Hendren WH, et al: The incidence of intersexuality in children with cryptorchidism and hypospadias: Stratification based on gonadal palpability and meatal position. J Urol 1999;162:1003–1007.

Meyer-Bahlburg HFL: Gender assignment in intersexuality. J Psychol Hum Sex 1998;10:1–21.

Migeon CJ, Berkovitz GD, Brown TR: Sexual differentiation and ambiguity. In Kappy MS, Blizzard RN, Migeon CJ (eds): Wilkins, The Diagnosis and Treatment of Endocrine Disorders in Childhood and Adolescence. Springfield, Ill, Charles C Thomas, 1994.

69

SURGICAL MANAGEMENT OF INTERSEXUALITY, CLOACAL MALFORMATION, AND OTHER ABNORMALITIES OF THE GENITALIA IN GIRLS

Richard C. Rink, MD
Martin Kaefer, MD

As with all other organ systems, genital development in the female occurs in an orderly fashion through multiple complex steps that result in an anatomically and functionally normal child in the vast majority of cases. However, errors in development can occur, ranging from minor, clinically insignificant disorders to severe abnormalities that are devastating to the child and parents. The abnormalities may affect the external genitalia alone or in combination with internal genital anomalies, and in some they may involve other organ systems. This chapter briefly describes normal urogenital and anorectal development and then discusses anomalies that arise when abnormal development occurs. Genital ambiguity is often the initial finding in these disorders. This chapter discusses only reconstruction along female lines; male reconstruction (i.e., hypospadias, chordee repair, and orchiopexy) is discussed in Chapters 65 and 67.

Genital reconstruction for intersex conditions at this time is very controversial. Although significant advances in surgical techniques have occurred since Young's early work (1937), well-controlled studies with regard to not just cosmetic results but functional and psychological results are almost nonexistent. Historically, reconstruction in intersex conditions has been surrounded by secrecy, and decisions have been made without scientific studies and often without the patient's knowledge. Questions regarding genital sensitivity, orgasmic potential, gender identity, and psychological aspects in those undergoing early genital surgery currently exist. It is beyond the scope of this chapter to discuss all the pros and cons of this controversy, but it is clear that further studies are warranted.

The recently established multispecialty task force on intersex conditions may answer many of the questions surrounding treatment. It is strongly recommended that these physicians honestly discuss with the parents of these children all aspects of care, including options, risks and benefits, and negative aspects of both observation and surgical therapy. A team of physicians, including a neonatologist, endocrinologist, geneticist, psychiatrist, psychologist, and pediatric urologist, should participate with the parents in decision making. This writing addresses current surgical techniques that are available should surgical therapy be chosen for the intersex child. It also addresses other female genital anomalies not associated with genital ambiguity.

FEMALE REPRODUCTIVE AND CAUDAL EMBRYOLOGY

A comprehensive description of genitourinary embryology can be found elsewhere in these volumes. To foster a deeper understanding of the complex combination of anomalies that can be found in patients with vaginal and cloacal anomalies, a brief review of relevant embryologic events is presented here.

The cloaca is an endoderm-lined primordial organ that is first apparent at the beginning of the 2nd week of gestation (Grosfeld, 1996). This structure, which represents a confluence of the primitive hindgut (dorsally) and the allantois (ventrally) just before the 4th week of gestation, receives the mesonephric ductal system (Stephens, 1983). The urorectal septum, which first appears during the 4th week of development, serves to separate the urogenital sinus (ventrally) from the anal canal (dorsally) (Moore and Persaud, 1995). The urorectal septum actually consists of two components. The first element is Tourneux's fold, which develops along the coronal plane in the angle between the allantois and the hindgut and grows in a caudal fashion toward the cloacal membrane. As this septum nears the cloacal membrane, infoldings of the lateral walls of the cloaca form Rathke's plicae, which coalesce in the coronal midline and form the urorectal septum caudally. By weeks 6 to 7 of development, the urorectal septum has fused with the cloacal membrane, dividing it into a ventral urogenital membrane and a dorsal anal membrane. The fibromuscular node of tissue that results from the contact of the septum with the cloacal membrane serves as a critical insertion site for the perineal muscles and as the dividing point of the primitive cloacal sphincter complex into anterior (urogenital diaphragm) and posterior (external anal sphincter) components. The common ontogeny of these two sphincter complexes explains why the pudendal nerve supplies all of these muscles.

While the urorectal anlage is undergoing division, the developing mesonephric ducts, which have contacted the cloaca, enter the urogenital sinus near the müllerian tubercle (Churchill and Hardy, 1978). An offshoot of the mesonephric duct, the ureteric bud, extends cranially to induce development of the metanephric blastema. The terminal branch point of the ureteral bud from the mesonephric duct is later absorbed into the wall of the urogenital sinus. Proper incorporation of this complex results in the ureters' opening at the lateral aspect of the trigone.

During this critical phase of cloacal development, paired müllerian ducts, which form from the coelomic epithelium, develop lateral to the mesonephric ducts and cross medially to fuse in the midline. **The close proximity of these two ductal systems helps explain the common association of paramesonephric abnormalities and ipsilateral renal anomalies.** The paired müllerian ducts then proceed caudally to join the urogenital sinus, where they produce an elevation called the müllerian tubercle. The caudal fusion of portions of these ducts normally leads to dissolution of the shared midline partition and formation of a common uterovaginal canal, which, as the name implies, gives rise to the uterus as well as the upper vagina.

As first delineated by Koff in 1933, **contact of the uterovaginal primordium with the urogenital sinus forms the müllerian tubercle, which in turn induces the formation of paired caudal endodermal outgrowths called sinovaginal bulbs.** Evidence suggests that these outpouchings may in fact represent the terminal segments of the wolffian ducts (Bok and Drews, 1983). Regardless of origin, **the cells within these sinovaginal bulbs then proliferate to form a cord of tissue which creates a distal vaginal plate that later is canalized in a caudal to cranial direction to form the distal aspect of the vagina** (Fig. 69–1). The portion of the urogenital sinus distal to the müllerian tubercle subsequently exstrophies and everts to become the vestibule. As a result of this process, the urethra and the vagina acquire separate openings in the vulva. The lumen of the vagina is separated from the cavity of the urogenital sinus by the hymen, an invagination of the posterior wall of the urogenital sinus. Rupture of the hymen should occur during the perinatal period.

Various cystic structures may form along the luminal aspect of the vagina. Remnants of the prostatic ductal system and the wolffian duct give rise to the paraurethral glands of Skene and Gardner, respectively. Outgrowths from the urogenital sinus form the greater vestibular glands

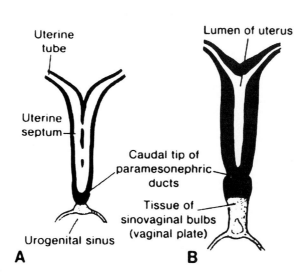

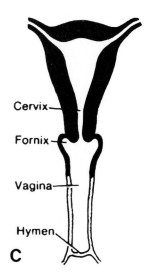

Figure 69–1. Formation of the vagina from the sinovaginal bulbs. (From Saler TW: Langman's Medical Embryology, 6th ed. Baltimore, Williams & Wilkins, 1990, with permission.)

of Bartholin, which are homologues of the bulbourethral glands in the male.

Key events in skeletal formation occur concurrently with cloacal division and proper formation of the mesonephric and paramesonephric ductal systems (Churchill and Hardy, 1978). The vertebrae develop in a craniocaudal direction, with the lower-extremity limb buds developing from condensation of somites 25 through 29. These somites undergo critical differentiation from the 4th through the 8th weeks of development.

From the foregoing brief description of caudal embryology, it should be evident that a disturbance in segmentation at the level of the caudal somites when the fetus is less than 10 mm in size (4th to 5th weeks of human development) can affect many different organ systems. In 1960, Duhamel described the association of the above-described "coincidentally" occurring congenital malformations and introduced the term *caudal regression syndrome* (Duhamel, 1961). Laboratory data with teratogens support the concept that a key event occurs between the 4th and 5th weeks of gestation, which results in an error in the simultaneous development of the terminal bowel, kidney, bladder, paramesonephric ductal system, and lumbosacral spine (Mesrobian et al, 1994). The actual inciting event remains unclear, although disordered mesodermal migration, reduced cellular proliferation, and premature apoptosis have all been proposed as potential mechanisms (Kallen and Winberg, 1974; Alles and Sulik, 1993). Elements of the caudal regression syndrome are seen with increased frequency in infants of diabetic mothers, but the exact mechanism is still in question (Deuchar, 1978; Lynch et al, 1995). Specific gene deletions in the homeobox region of the mammalian genome (the region critical for proper mammalian spatial orientation and segmentation) have been shown to result in a constellation of anatomic findings, as predicted by Duhamel (Warot et al, 1997). Because differentiation of the somites progresses in a cranial-to-caudal direction, it would follow that the most complex anomalies (higher anorectal malformations) would occur as a result of aberrations at an earlier stage of development. This also helps to explain the greater association of severe upper urinary tract malformations, internal genital duct abnormalities, and spinal anomalies in these patients compared with less severe cases of imperforate anus.

Mesodermal disturbances are not limited to the caudal somites. As seen in the VATER and MURCS associations, mesodermally derived organs as cranial as the C1 vertebra and tracheoesophageal anlagen can be affected in association with congenital abnormalities of the mesonephric and paramesonephric ductal systems (Quan and Smith, 1973; Duncan et al, 1979).

STRUCTURAL ANOMALIES OF THE FEMALE INTERNAL GENITALIA

Anomalies of the female reproductive system can be grouped into three main categories: those resulting from either hypoplasia or agenesis, those caused by vertical fusion (canalization abnormalities resulting from abnormal contact of the müllerian structures with the urogenital sinus), and those resulting from lateral fusion (duplication). The mode of presentation, physical findings,

evaluation, and subsequent therapy vary considerably among these groups. Radiographic imaging is of central importance in determining the correct diagnosis. Ultrasound is helpful not only in identifying the genital anatomy but also in screening for associated upper urinary tract abnormalities (Rosenberg et al, 1986; Fernandez et al, 1996). MRI is considered by many to be the "gold standard" for defining internal müllerian anatomy (Fedele et al, 1996; Russ et al, 1997; Lang et al, 1999). It is especially useful in determining the presence or absence of the cervix and the presence of functioning endometrium in complex anomalies. In complicated cases, additional information can be obtained by examination under anesthesia, vaginoscopy, hysteroscopy, and/or laparoscopy (Major et al, 1997). **Obstructive anomalies typically require immediate intervention, but nonobstructive anomalies often do not require surgical intervention unless the patient has reached reproductive age and the condition affects intercourse or adversely affects fertility.** Various systems have been proposed for the classification of these anomalies, with the system proposed by the American Society for Reproductive Medicine being the most inclusive (Anonymous, 1998).

Obstructive Genital Anomalies

Transverse Vaginal Septum

Transverse vaginal septa are believed to arise from a failure in fusion and/or canalization of the urogenital sinus and müllerian ducts. A complete transverse vaginal septum may be located at various levels in the vagina. In one large series the distribution was upper vagina, 46%; middle vagina, 40%; and lower vagina, 14% (Lodi, 1951)

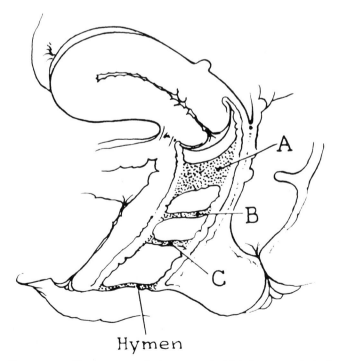

Hymen

Figure 69–2. Transverse vaginal septum. A, high (upper vagina); B, middle; C, low. (From Yerkes EB, Rink RC: What urologists should know about pediatric gynecologic abnormalities. Contemporary Urology 2002;14(1):12.)

(Fig. 69–2). The septa are usually less than 1 cm thick and often have a small central or eccentric perforation (Suidan and Azoury, 1979). Even in cases where a perforation is present, significant obstruction and ascending infection can occur.

Transperineal, transrectal, and abdominal ultrasonography and MRI may be beneficial in establishing the diagnosis and determining the location and thickness of a transverse vaginal septum (Ammann et al, 1983; Doyle, 1992; Meyer et al, 1995; Caloia et al, 1998; Fedele et al, 1999; Lang et al, 1999). MRI can help to determine whether a cervix is present, in order to differentiate between a high septum and congenital absence of the cervix. Failure to differentiate between these diagnoses can result in significant patient morbidity (Casey and Laufer, 1997).

Treatment of the transverse vaginal septum is primarily surgical. The procedure involves resection of the septal tissue and approximation of the vaginal mucosa, which will theoretically **reduce the incidence of subsequent stenosis. Many of the patients present with amenorrhea and a distended upper vagina.**

Vaginal Atresia

Vaginal atresia occurs when the urogenital sinus fails to contribute to the formation of the lower (distal) portion of the vagina. This condition differs from vaginal agenesis and testicular feminization in that the müllerian structures are not affected. As a result, the uterus, cervix, and upper vagina are normal. A very shallow dimple caudal to the urethral opening may be appreciated on physical examination. Palpation of a distended vagina on rectal examination may help to distinguish this condition from testicular feminization or vaginal agenesis. Radio-

graphic evaluation in the form of ultrasound and/or MRI is mandatory to adequately define the müllerian anatomy before intervention.

Surgical correction consists of a transverse incision at the level of the hymenal ring. Dissection is carried out through the fibrous area of the absent lower vagina, until the upper vagina is reached. After the obstruction is drained and the vaginal mucosa is identified, a pull-through procedure can be performed to bring the distended vagina down to the introitus. Ramenofsky and Raffensperger (1971) described a combined abdominoperineal approach that has proved to be very useful for exposing and anastomosing the distal vagina to the perineal skin. As in treatment of transverse vaginal septum, distention of the vagina with retained menstrual blood products can prove extremely beneficial in that it acts as a tissue expander. In vaginal atresia, the distance to bridge between the vagina and perineal surface can almost always be successfully managed with perineal skin flaps and/or simple mobilization of the vagina itself.

Vaginal Agenesis (Müllerian Aplasia)

GENERAL

Vaginal agenesis, which occurs with an incidence of approximately 1 in 5000 live female births, is the congenital absence of the proximal portion of the vagina in an otherwise phenotypically (i.e., normal secondary sexual characteristics), **chromosomally** (i.e., 46,XX), **and hormonally** (i.e., normal levels of luteinizing hormone and follicle-stimulating hormone) **intact female** (Bryan et al, 1949; Griffin et al, 1976). Although Realdus Columbus is credited by some authors as the first to describe a case of

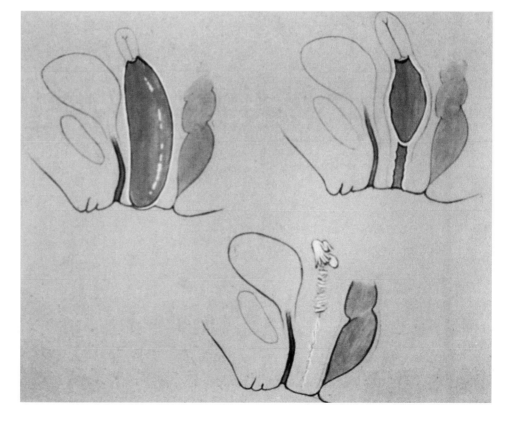

Figure 69–3. Forms of vaginal obstruction. *Upper left,* Imperforate hymen. *Upper right,* Transverse vaginal septum. *Lower,* Vaginal agenesis. (From Yerkes EB, Rink RC: What urologists should know about pediatric gynecologic abnormalities. Contemporary Urology 2002;14(1):12.)

vaginal agenesis, Mayer was one of the first to report vaginal agenesis in stillborn children (Mayer, 1829; Lesavoy, 1985). In 1838, Rokitansky reported 19 adult autopsy cases of uterovaginal agenesis, including 3 with associated unilateral renal agenesis. In 1910, Kuster recognized urologic associations, such as renal ectopy and agenesis, along with skeletal deformities. Hauser brought further attention to the frequent association of renal and skeletal anomalies in these patients and stressed the differences between patients with these findings and those with testicular feminization (Hauser and Schreiner, 1961).

The Mayer-Rokitansky-Kuster-Hauser (MRKH) syndrome, as the entity of müllerian aplasia has come to be known, results from a failure of the sinovaginal bulbs to develop and form the vaginal plate (Fig. 69–3). This may be caused by improper induction of the sinovaginal bulbs from the neighboring uterovaginal primordium. Chronologically, the uterovaginal canal develops at a point in embryogenesis during which other critical mesodermally derived organ systems are also forming. This in part explains the many associated findings. Müllerian aplasia has also been associated with maternal deficiency of galactose 1-phosphate uridyltransferase (Cramer et al, 1996). In contrast to vaginal atresia, the hymenal fringe is usually present along with a small vaginal pouch, because they are both derived embryologically from the urogenital sinus.

Most patients with MRKH present to the physician after the expected age of menarche because of primary amenorrhea. MRKH is in fact second only to gonadal dysgenesis as a cause of primary amenorrhea. A minority of patients present with cyclic abdominal pain caused by the retention of menstrual blood in the uterus. Physical examination reveals absence of the vagina. Inguinal hernia is less common in this disorder than in the testicular feminization syndrome (Schmid-Tannwald and Hauser, 1973). The karyotype is that of a normal 46,XX woman. Radiographic evaluation is indicated to more fully delineate remnant müllerian structures and search for associated anomalies involving the renal and skeletal systems.

ASSOCIATED FINDINGS

MRKH syndrome is associated with the variable absence or hypoplasia of the cervix, uterus, and fallopian tubes. In approximately 10% of patients, a normal but obstructed uterus or a rudimentary uterus with functional endometrium is present (Murray and Gambrell, 1979; Singh and Devi, 1983; Bates and Wiser, 1985). In one of the largest single series to date, Salvatore and Lodovicci (1978) reported that, of 91 patients with vaginal agenesis, almost 25% lacked a uterus, 55% had a solid rudimentary uterus, and the remaining 30% had other abnormalities of this organ. In addition, they demonstrated that, although the fallopian tubes were normal in 32% of cases, they were rudimentary in almost 50% of cases and completely absent in 10%. Although occasionally cystic, the ovaries were almost always present and functional (Salvatore and Lodovicci, 1978). It was subsequently recognized based on the morphology of the retained müllerian structures that the MRKH syndrome could be divided into typical and atypical forms (Schmid-Tannwald and Hauser, 1977).

In the typical form of MRKH (type A), the patient has symmetrical uterine remnants and normal fallopian tubes. The atypical form (type B) comprises patients with asymmetrical uterine buds or abnormally developed fallopian tubes. This is an important distinction, because the overwhelming majority of associated findings in other organ systems have been reported to be present with the atypical form, whereas in the typical form these findings are usually absent (Strubbe et al, 1992, 1993).

The association between vaginal agenesis and developmental abnormalities of the kidney was first recognized by Rokitansky (1838). Approximately one third of patients are found to have abnormal renal findings on intravenous pyelogram and/or ultrasound examination (Strubbe et al, 1993). Renal anomalies are found almost exclusively in the patients with the atypical subtype of vaginal agenesis (type B). In Strubbe's series, 34 of 51 patients with type B anatomy had renal anomalies, but none of the 40 patients with type A (symmetrical) anatomy demonstrated such a deformity (Strubbe et al, 1993). A meta-analysis published by Griffin and associates (1976) demonstrated that the renal anomaly consists of either unilateral renal agenesis or ectopia of one or both kidneys in 74% of those affected. The close proximity of the mesonephric and paramesonephric structures during the early phase of fetal development is thought to be the reason for this frequent association of renal anomalies. Not surprisingly, the converse is also true: The incidence of associated genital abnormalities in female patients with renal anomalies ranges between 25% and 89% (Thompson and Lynn, 1966).

Associated congenital abnormalities of the skeletal system have been described in 10% to 20% of cases (Turunen, 1967; Willemsen, 1982; Strubbe et al, 1987). Congenital fusion (failure of segmentation) of the cervical vertebrae is known as the Klippel-Feil syndrome. The Klippel-Feil syndrome occurs approximately once in 30,000 to 40,000 live births (Gunderson et al, 1967). An association between this abnormality of cervical somite development and vaginal agenesis was first recognized by Duncan (1977). **He proposed the term *MURCS association* to describe the combination of *mü*llerian duct aplasia, *r*enal aplasia, and *c*ervicothoracic *s*omite dysplasia, which many believe is caused by a generalized disordered development of mesodermal differentiation during the 4th week of fetal life** (Duncan et al, 1979). Strubbe demonstrated that the Klippel-Feil abnormality was found only in patients with the atypical form of the MRKH (type B). Additional, albeit less common, skeletal abnormalities include scoliosis and abnormalities of the hands and face (Willemsen, 1982; Fisher et al, 2000). Unlike müllerian anomalies that are associated with abnormal cloacal septation, vaginal agenesis is not associated with an increased incidence of lumbosacral spinal disorders or occult spinal dysraphism (Gunderson et al, 1967).

TREATMENT (VAGINAL REPLACEMENT)

Skin Neovagina

Both nonoperative and operative treatment options exist for this anomaly. Regardless of the method used, it can be very helpful to have the patient speak with a patient who has previously undergone treatment before treatment is initiated (Ingram, 1981). **The nonoperative approach, initially popularized by Frank (1938), involves gentle pressure of graduated hard dilators against the perineal surface in order to create a progressive invagination of the vaginal dimple.** Ingram (1981) modified this technique by using a bicycle seat mounted on a stool. The nonoperative approach has greatest success when a vaginal dimple or pouch is already present (Williams et al, 1984, 1985). With proper patient compliance, this method can achieve a functional vagina in approximately 4 to 6 months.

Modifications of the Frank technique of perineal pressure have been developed that incorporate the surgical placement of tension sutures to aid in directing pressure from a Plexiglas dilator against the vaginal dimple (Vecchietti, 1979). The mold, often referred to as an "olive," has sutures attached to it that are guided in a cranial direction through the vesicorectal space into the perineal cavity and brought out through the abdominal wall (Vecchietti technique). Tension is progressively increased via the abdominal wall sutures until sufficient vaginal length has been achieved (Vecchietti, 1979). In order to avoid a formal laparotomy, laparoscopic techniques have been described to assist in the dissection of the tissue plane for the Vecchietti technique (Borruto, 1992; Gauwerky et al, 1992; Fedele et al, 1994, 1996). In Fedele's more recent series, all patients were found to have healthy vaginal mucosa, with the average vaginal length being almost 8 cm at 3 months. This technique has had limited use by urologists.

If the Frank method has been unsuccessful or is not accepted as a reasonable option by the patient or parents, creation of a functional vagina can be achieved by one of several techniques (Abbé, 1898; McIndoe and Banister, 1938; Hendren and Atala, 1994). **The first landmark advance in vaginal reconstruction is attributed to Abbé in 1898. Abbé described dissecting a canal between the rectum and urethra and lining this area with split-thickness skin grafts. This procedure was later popularized by McIndoe,** and the procedure that bears his name has gained wide acceptance in the United States (McIndoe and Banister, 1938). Preoperative preparation consists of a full mechanical and antibiotic bowel preparation. A split-thickness graft of skin is taken from the buttocks (0.018 to 0.022 inches) and tubularized over a stent (Fig. 69–4). A transverse incision is made at the level of the perineal

dimple, and the potential space between the urethra and the rectum is carefully dissected up to the level of the peritoneal reflection. The graft and mold are then inserted into the potential space, and the labia minora are sutured around the stent to prevent extrusion during the initial healing phase (McIndoe, 1950). Many types of vaginal stents have been used for this purpose, including packed gauze, wood covered with a condom, silicone foam, acrylic, various metals, and an inflatable vaginal stent (Concannon et al, 1993; Chen, 1994; Barutcu and Akguner, 1998). The Foley catheter is replaced by a suprapubic catheter, and postoperatively the patient is kept at strict bed rest for 1 full week. **A high incidence of postoperative vaginal stenosis necessitates postoperative vaginal dilation** (Ingram, 1981). Excellent patient satisfaction has been reported in most large series (Martinez-Mora et al, 1992; Strickland et al, 1993; Alessandrescu et al, 1996).

Other options for creation of a neovagina using local tissues include the use of full-thickness skin grafts from the buttock or full-thickness skin flaps based on the labia majora. Those who champion the use of full-thickness skin grafts report a lower incidence of graft contracture compared with split-thickness graft techniques (Sadove and Horton, 1988). The Williams vaginoplasty involves the creation of a vaginal pouch from the labia majora (Williams, 1964). The combination of this procedure and Frank-type dilation along the vaginal axis can provide a satisfactory result.

Many other surgical procedures have been developed for creation of a functional neovagina using various muscle flaps (e.g., pudendal thigh, rectus abdominis, buttock) (McCraw et al, 1976; Lilford et al, 1989; Dumanian and Donahoe, 1992; Wang and Hadley, 1993; Joseph, 1997). The pelvic peritoneum and human amnion are two other donor sites that have been used to create a neovagina (Davydov, 1977; Ashworth et al, 1986; Morton and Dewhurst, 1986; Tamaya and Imai, 1991).

Intestinal Neovagina

Baldwin first described the use of bowel for the creation of the vagina in 1907. The procedure involved anastomosis of a U-shaped segment of sigmoid to the perineum with subsequent division of the intervening septum (Hensle and

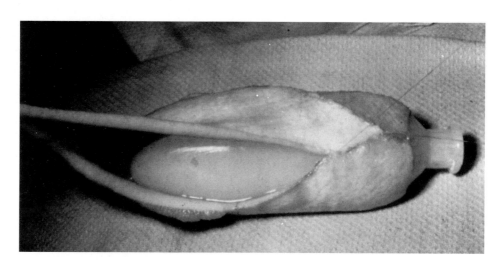

Figure 69–4. McIndoe skin vagina sewn over a vaginal stent.

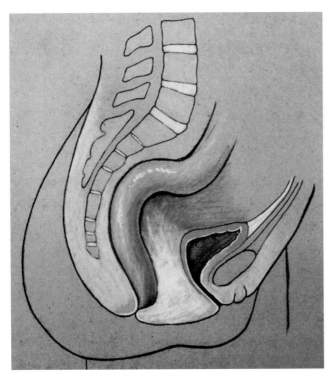

Figure 69–5. Vaginal agenesis.

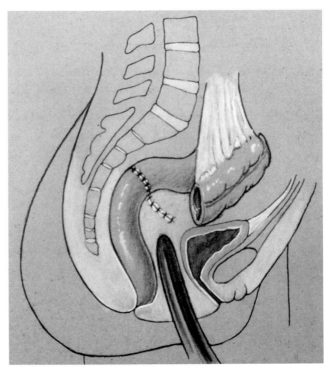

Figure 69–6. Bowel vagina: harvest of colonic segment and creation of vaginal space.

Dean, 1992). Additional experience with this technique was reported by Fall in 1940, but the technique did not gain widespread acceptance until the 1970s due to high patient morbidity and mortality (Fall, 1940; Pratt, 1972). Subsequent improvements in technique and postoperative care resulted in renewed enthusiasm for these techniques (Turner-Warwick and Kirby, 1990; Hensle and Dean, 1992; Hendren and Atala, 1994; Hensle and Reiley, 1998). Sigmoid, cecum, and small intestine have all been used successfully for the creation of a functional neovagina.

The day before surgery, the patient undergoes a full mechanical and antibiotic cleansing of the alimentary tract. The procedure is performed with the patient supine, the legs spread, and the knees bent (frog-leg position). In the case of the older child, Allen stirrups can be used. For the sigmoid vaginoplasty, the intra-abdominal portion of the procedure commences by first identifying an appropriate length of distal sigmoid with a blood supply that will comfortably reach the peritoneum (Figs. 69–5 and 69–6). The distal end of the proposed segment is then divided and anastomosed to the perineum (Fig. 69–7). An intervening segment of sigmoid (approximately 3 cm) is then excised in order to create a space between the oversewn proximal edge of the bowel vagina and the end of the sigmoid, which is anastomosed to the rectum. This maneuver prevents an overlap of suture lines and thereby has the potential advantage of limiting the incidence of fistula formation. The bowel vagina is thereafter fixed to the posterior peritoneum to prevent prolapse.

Although we have had the most success with sigmoid, a small-bowel segment may be chosen with a vascular pedicle that is of adequate length to reach the perineum. After isolating an appropriate length of ileum and reestablishing bowel continuity, the segment is detubularized and recon-

figured in a conical configuration to provide an increased internal diameter (Hendren and Atala, 1994) (Figs. 69–8 and 69–9). The segment is then brought down to the perineum and sewn in place, as in the case of the sigmoid neovagina. In order to avoid a formal laparotomy, laparos-

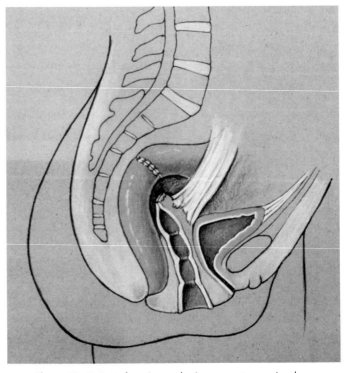

Figure 69–7. Bowel vagina: colonic segment sewn in place.

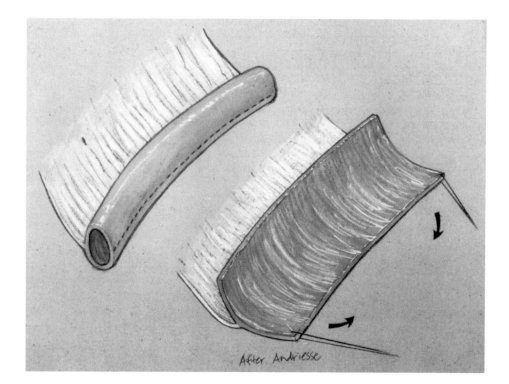

Figure 69–8. Bowel vagina: harvest of ileal segment.

copy-assisted techniques have been described for harvest and delivery of the bowel segment to the perineal location (Ota et al, 2000).

If there is a perineal dimple (i.e., the segment of vagina contributed by the urogenital sinus is present), the bowel segment should be anastomosed directly to it. When a direct perineal anastomosis is required, it is of critical importance to create a large enough space between the rectum and bladder to avoid compromise of the intestinal blood supply. Creation of such a space can be facilitated by the use of progressively larger Hegar dilators.

Gentle passage of the intestinal segment into position is facilitated by placing the segment in a large lubricated Penrose drain before transfer to the perineum.

The functional results of bowel vaginoplasty have been excellent. Of the 65 cases reported by Hendren, 16 experienced mild eversion of the bowel segment, which in every case was amenable to simple trimming. Eight patients ex-

Figure 69–9. Bowel vagina: reconfiguration of ileal segment to create larger luminal diameter.

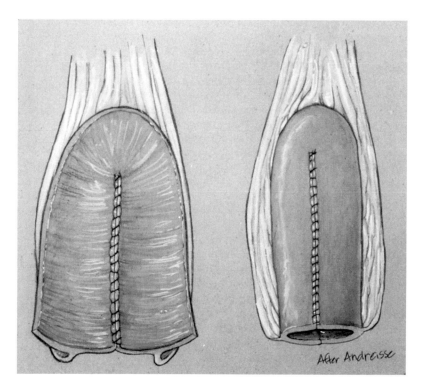

perienced mild stenosis that was later corrected by appropriate Z-plasties to increase the circumference of the mucocutaneous junction (Hendren and Atala, 1994). Patient satisfaction is high, and the majority of patients who are old enough to engage in sexual relations are able to achieve adequate coitus (Hensle and Reiley, 1998).

Stenosis has been reported more frequently after the use of ileum (Hensle and Dean, 1992; Hensle and Reiley, 1998). **As a result, we and others believe that large intestine is the bowel segment of choice.** Two specific indications for use of an ileal segment for bowel vaginoplasty are prior radiation to the deep pelvis and the absence of large intestine (i.e., cloacal exstrophy). When ileum is used, various methods of reconfiguration can be used to increase diameter (Hendren and Atala, 1994). **Advantages of a bowel vagina over the McIndoe procedure include the lubricating properties of mucus** (which may help to facilitate intercourse) **and the reduced incidence of postoperative contracture** (and hence the reduced need for postoperative dilatation). Disadvantages include the frequent need to wear pads because of the chronic vaginal discharge. Daily douching may be necessary to evacuate the mucus (Hendren and Atala, 1994). **Finally, the potential transmission of bloodborne pathogens such as hepatitis and HIV may be increased (in comparison with a squamous epithelium–lined vagina) because of the poor barrier effect of the gastrointestinal tract.**

All patients undergoing creation of a functional vagina with perineal skin require annual examinations, because there have been reports of condylomata acuminata and squamous cell carcinoma involving grafts (Duckler, 1972; Rotmensch et al, 1983; Buscema et al, 1987). Annual examination of the bowel vagina is also indicated because adenocarcinoma has been identified after this procedure (Andryjowicz et al, 1985).

The optimal timing of surgery remains a source of debate. The majority of surgeons who favor the McIndoe procedure for construction of the neovagina believe that it is better to wait until adulthood to perform the procedure, because a degree of maturity is required to perform daily dilatations. Many surgeons who favor the use of bowel for neovaginal reconstruction do not believe that vaginoplasty should be deferred until the patient reaches adulthood. Hendren and associates believe that delaying creation of the neovagina until adulthood may be psychologically traumatic to a young girl (Hendren and Atala, 1994). We have based timing on the underlying diagnosis and need for a neovagina.

Cervical Atresia

Cervical agenesis is an uncommon disorder that manifests with symptoms common to other obstructive entities of the female reproductive tract (i.e., primary amenorrhea, cyclic or chronic abdominal pain). Failure to establish the correct diagnosis and thereby choose the appropriate method of surgical intervention can be fraught with disaster and possible patient mortality. Under many circumstances, the patient is best served by hysterectomy with subsequent vaginal replacement by one of the previously described techniques (Rock et al, 1984; Cukier et al, 1986). Direct anastomosis of the neovagina to the uterine remnant has

been reported, but this procedure carries with it the life-threatening risk of ascending infection in the absence of the normal endocervical barrier (Casey and Laufer, 1997).

Female Circumcision (Infibulation)

Acquired vaginal obstruction may be secondary to a number of ritual female genital mutilation procedures that are widespread in many countries in Africa (stretching in a band from the Horn of Africa through Central Africa to parts of Nigeria), **the Middle East, and Muslim populations of Indonesia and Malaysia** (Toubia, 1994; JAMA, 1995; Dorkenoo, 1996). Although similar procedures were prescribed to U.S. and British women during the 19th century for treatment of ailments ranging from epilepsy to lesbianism, all forms of genital mutilation are now illegal in these Western countries. Often referred to as "female circumcision," the procedure continues to affect an estimated 80 to 110 million women worldwide (Toubia, 1994).

The age at which this procedure is performed ranges from birth to just before marriage. However, it is typically performed on preadolescent children between the ages of 4 and 10 years, most commonly at age 7 (JAMA, 1995). The procedure is typically performed without anesthesia in the context of a ceremony designating the rite of passage into adult society (JAMA, 1995). The extent of the mutilation varies according to ritual, but the practice predates Islam

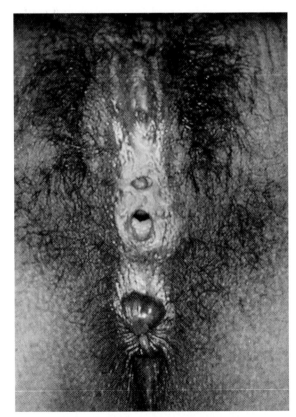

Figure 69–10. Female infibulation. Note the scarred labia majora with only a pinhole opening for passage of menstrual fluid and urine. (From Gonzales ET, Bauer SB [eds]: Pediatric Urology Practice. Philadelphia, Lippincott Williams & Wilkins, 1999, p 599, with permission.)

and therefore is not part of a religion (McCaffrey et al, 1995). In many countries, the women have a deinfibulation procedure performed just before consummating the marriage.

The type of mutilation ranges from simple excision of the prepuce of the clitoris (termed "sunna") to complete excision of all elements of the vulvar region (McCaffrey et al, 1995).

Toubia (1994) classified the more extensive female genital mutilation procedures according to the amount of tissue destruction:

Type I: Complete or partial removal of the clitoris.

Type II: Excision of the clitoris and a portion of the labia minora.

Type III: Excision of the entire clitoris and labia minora with incision of the labia majora along its medial aspect to create raw surfaces. The anterior two thirds of the labia majora are approximated to cover the urethra and introitus, leaving the lower third at the level of the posterior fourchette for the passage of urine and menstrual fluid.

Type IV: Excision of the entire clitoris and labia minora with near-complete approximation of the labia majora, leaving only a pinhole opening near the posterior fourchette for the passage of urine and menstrual fluid (Fig. 69–10).

Closing of the introitus, typically referred to as infibulation or pharaonic circumcision, is performed by a variety of means, including absorbable and nonabsorbable suture materials, thorns, and twigs. The child's legs are then bound for up to 40 days to ensure secondary healing in the ventral midline (McCaffrey et al, 1995).

The physical, psychological, and reproductive repercussions of these forms of genital mutilation are numerous and include immediate destruction and infection of local tissues (e.g., rectum, urethra). Long-term risks include chronic pain, recurrent urinary tract and vaginal infections, dysmenorrhea, dyspareunia, and apareunia. For those individuals with the most narrowing, additional "surgeries" to revise the introital opening may be necessary for both intercourse and vaginal delivery (Aziz, 1980; Toubia, 1994).

Care of the patient who has undergone infibulation must be individualized, not only to provide functionality but also to respect the cultural and ritual desires of the woman. Educating the patient as to the normal appearance of the external female genitalia is critical. Visual aids including photographs and or hand-drawn illustrations of the patient's anatomy and of the planned revision have been used as part of informed consent in order to avoid misunderstanding.

Duplication of the Uterus and Cervix with Unilaterally Imperforate Vagina

Although the majority of obstructive lesions are caused by abnormalities of vertical fusion, occasionally an obstructive process can be encountered in the context of an abnormality of lateral fusion (Figs. 69–11 and 69–12). More than 50 cases of uterus didelphys with unilateral imperforate vagina have been reported in the

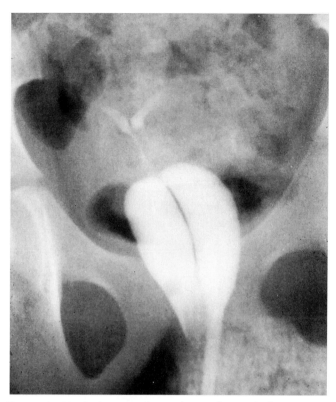

Figure 69–11. Genitogram of complete müllerian duplication (septated vagina and separate uteri).

world's literature (Allan and Cowan, 1963; Burbige and Hensle, 1984). As with other obstructive disorders, the patient may present with cyclic or chronic abdominal pain. However, **unlike other obstructive processes, duplication anomalies with unilateral obstruction do not result in primary amenorrhea.** On physical examination, a unilateral abdominal-pelvic mass that terminates in a bluish bulge in the lateral vaginal wall is often appreciated (Eisenberg et al, 1982). Abdominal ultrasound or MRI or both are excellent at defining the anatomy in a suspected case of unilateral noncommunicating uterine horn. Renal anomalies are frequently encountered on the ipsilateral side to the obstructed system, with renal agenesis being the most common (Eisenberg et al, 1982; Tridenti and Bruni, 1995). A prompt and accurate diagnosis is necessary to prevent injury to the genital organs due to chronic cryptomenorrhea and endometriosis. Treatment consists of wide incision of the vertical vaginal septum to release the entrapped menstrual blood.

Nonobstructive Genital Anomalies

Most abnormalities of lateral fusion have no functional significance. With the exception of those with uterus didelphys and unilateral vaginal obstruction, most patients are asymptomatic. Although an exhaustive description of the defects of lateral fusion is beyond the scope of this chapter, some general comments can be made.

True duplication of the uterus is a rare event. This anomaly results from duplication of the müllerian ducts

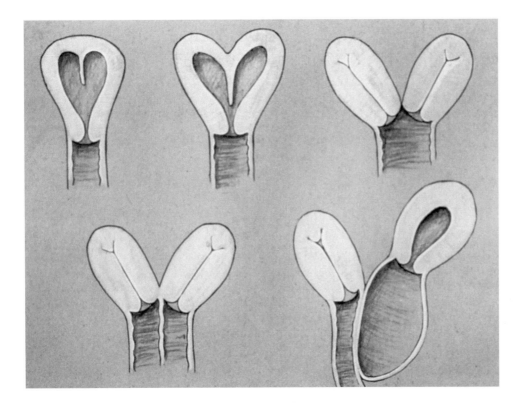

Figure 69–12. Fusion anomalies of the müllerian system. *Upper left to lower right,* Bicornuate uterus (partial); bicornuate uterus; uterine duplication; complete uterine and vaginal duplication; duplication of uterus and cervix with unilateral imperforate vagina. (From Yerkes EB, Rink RC: What urologists should know about pediatric gynecologic abnormalities. Contemporary Urology 2002;14(1): 12.)

and subsequent doubling of the reproductive structures on one or both sides. The much more frequently encountered anomaly of uterine didelphys consists of two separate uterine cavities and cervices as a result of failed resorption of the common medial wall of the paired müllerian duct structures during development. Although up to 75% of patients also have a septate vagina, most have adequate reproductive outcomes and do not require surgical intervention. If later in life the patient experiences difficulty with intercourse, vaginal delivery, or the need to wear two tampons, then surgical excision of the vaginal septum should be undertaken. If only the most cranial portion of the septum remains, a bicornuate uterus will result. The vagina is typically normal, and surgical incision of the uterine septum is rarely indicated except in cases of recurrent pregnancy loss (Decherney and Russel, 1986).

Interlabial Masses

GENERAL

The differential diagnosis of the interlabial mass in the neonate and young child is broad and requires a thorough understanding of the diagnostic possibilities and a systematic evaluation. The age and racial background of the patient can help narrow the differential diagnosis, but physical examination remains the most useful tool for determining the specific pathology.

The physician must be sure to specifically reassure the girl that the examination will not be painful. With the child in the frog-leg position, the physician should note the size of the clitoris, the configuration of the hymen, the location of the urethra, and the character of the interlabial mass (e.g., smooth, lobulated, hemorrhagic). To aid in visualization, the labia majora can be gently grasped and pulled

caudally to enable funneling of the introitus and vagina (the so-called pull-down maneuver). Determining the nature of a specific mass can be facilitated by establishing the location of expected anatomic landmarks. In certain circumstances, the relationship of the mass to the vagina and urethra can be improved by gentle placement of a lubricated cotton applicator posteriorly or placement of a small feeding tube within the suspected urethral orifice, or both. Although an otoscope, nasal speculum, or pediatric vaginal speculum can be useful in evaluating the vagina while the patient is awake, complaints of vaginal origin (i.e., vaginal discharge or bleeding) are often best investigated with a carefully performed examination and vaginoscopy under anesthesia. Renal-pelvic sonography can be a useful adjunct in confirming or establishing the diagnosis in a few of these disorders.

LABIAL ADHESIONS

Labial adhesions are the most common interlabial abnormality identified in a pediatric urologic practice (Fig. 69–13). Fusion of the labia minora originates at the posterior fourchette and progresses for a variable distance toward the clitoris. It is important to differentiate this from the more serious entity of fusion of the labia majora, as is seen in certain intersex disorders. The majority of cases are believed to occur secondary to irritation, infection, or local tissue trauma. Hypoestrogenism is also believed to play a role in this condition. This latter point appears to explain the fact that the overwhelming majority of cases occur in girls between the ages of 3 months and 7 years (Finlay, 1965). Labial adhesions have not been reported in the newborn child, presumably because of the protective effect of maternal estrogen (Leung et al, 1993). These adhesions can

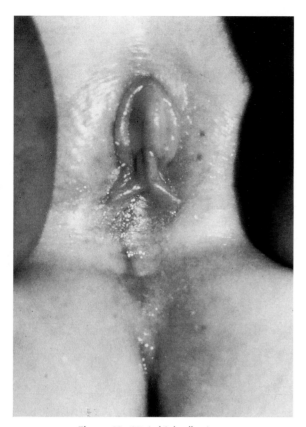

Figure 69–13. Labial adhesions.

rarely be associated with sexual abuse; in such cases, additional physical findings are often noted, such as hematoma and lacerations (McCann et al, 1988). Although labial adhesions are usually asymptomatic, urine pooling within the vagina may lead to postvoid dribbling and perineal irritation and may make it difficult to obtain an accurate urinalysis.

Most children with labial adhesions do not require treatment unless they are symptomatic. When necessary, treatment ranges from the topical application of conjugated estrogens to surgical division. The 90% success rate that has been reported after the topical application of conjugated estrogens supports the concept that this disorder results from a relative hypoestrogenic state (Capraro and Greenberg, 1972). If separation is not noted after 2 weeks of treatment, then manual separation in the outpatient setting may be indicated. After the application of EMLA cream to the introitus, gentle pressure is applied to the thin connecting membrane with the use of a lubricated probe. Rarely, surgical division is required.

INTROITAL CYSTS

Introital cysts in the newborn can represent one of three entities: paraurethral cysts (i.e., Skene's duct cyst), remnants of the mesonephric ductal system (Gartner's duct cyst), and a covered ectopic ureter. When the cyst is large and is clearly emanating from the vaginal introitus, further investigation in the form of a renal-pelvic ultrasound is indicated to look for renal duplication.

Paraurethral cysts **in the newborn represent a dilata-** tion of the periurethral glands, which are located just inside the urethral meatus (Fig. 69–14). **These glands are homologues of the male prostatic glands and number between 6 and 30, with the largest two of these termed the periurethral glands of Skene** (Skene, 1880; Gottesman and Sparkuhl, 1979). In the newborn infant, the periurethral glands occasionally respond to maternal estrogen and secrete mucoid material, which can result in cyst formation. The main distinguishing features of this condition is the displacement of the urethral meatus by the mass, resulting in an eccentric urinary stream. If the urethral meatus can be identified as being completely separate from the mass, then radiographic evaluation is not needed to confirm the diagnosis (Nussbaum and Lebowitz, 1983). These cysts are frequently self-limiting and often rupture spontaneously. If they are persistent, drainage by a small needle is easily achieved at the bedside.

Gartner's duct cysts represent cystic remnants of the wolffian duct system and can be found along the anteromedial wall of the vagina (Pradhan and Tobon, 1986). A cystic structure that is related to the Gartner's duct cyst is the *covered ectopic ureter,* which enters into the vagina (Rosenfeld and Lis, 1993; Holmes et al, 1999). Embryologically, the ureter would not be expected to enter into the vagina. However, an ectopically located ureter may end in a segment of the wolffian duct system, which in the female is represented by a Gartner's duct cyst. In most instances this cystic structure spontaneously ruptures before delivery, resulting in a direct communication between the ectopic ureter and the vagina. However, if the surface epithelium

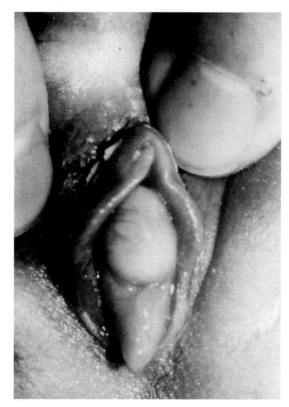

Figure 69–14. Paraurethral cyst. (From Yerkes EB, Rink RC: What urologists should know about pediatric gynecologic abnormalities. Contemporary Urology 2002;14(1):12.)

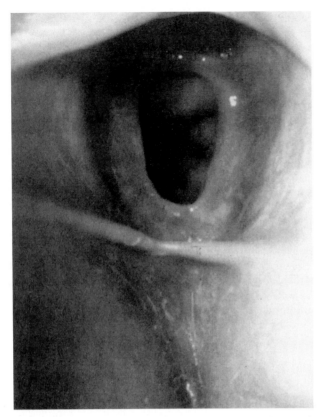

Figure 69–15. Normal hymenal ring. (From Emans SJ: Office evaluation of the child and adolescent. In Emans SJ, Laufer MR, Goldstein DP [eds]: Pediatric and Adolescent Gynecology, 4th ed. Philadelphia, Lippincott Williams & Wilkins, 1998.)

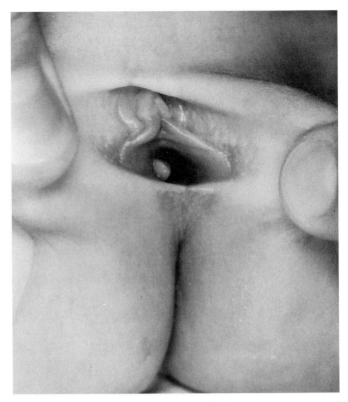

Figure 69–16. Hymenal skin tag.

fails to rupture, a covered, urine-filled cyst will exist within the vagina. Intraoperative injection of the cystic structure with radiographic contrast material may be beneficial in outlining the anatomy. Incision of the cystic structure relieves the obstruction. Subsequent upper pole heminephrectomy may be indicated if negligible function is seen in this moiety after decompression.

Hymenal Disorders

Hymenal skin tags are virtually a normal finding and are rarely symptomatic (Figs. 69–15 and 69–16). When symptomatic (i.e., bleeding), they should be excised to ensure that they do not represent a malignancy and for symptomatic relief. Congenital abnormalities of the hymen are not uncommon and range from imperforate hymen to those with numerous small microperforations.

***Imperforate hymen* is probably the most common congenital obstructive anomaly of the female reproductive tract. The diagnosis is most frequently made at birth by either a bulge along the posterior aspect of the introitus, which represents retained fluid within the vagina, or by a palpable suprapubic mass from a distended vagina** (Fig. 69–17). The buildup of retained vaginal secretions in the newborn period, which results in a whitish appearance to the bulging hymenal membrane, is caused by maternal estradiol stimulation. If the diagnosis is made after the newborn period, then the mucus often will have reabsorbed and a bulge of the hymenal membrane may no

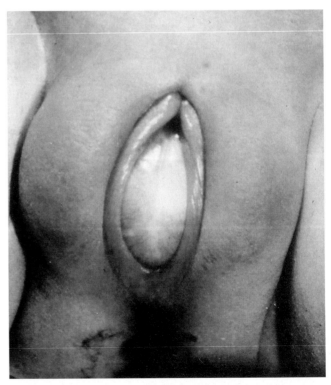

Figure 69–17. Imperforate hymen. Note significant distention from vaginal secretions. (From Yerkes EB, Rink RC: What urologists should know about pediatric gynecologic abnormalities. Contemporary Urology 2002;14(1):12.)

longer be evident. On occasion, the diagnosis is not made until the adolescent period, when the patient presents with amenorrhea and possibly cyclic abdominal pain. Under these circumstances, a bluish bulging hymen may be observed on genital inspection and a mass will be appreciated on rectoabdominal palpation.

In newborns, repair by incision of the hymenal tissue at the bedside is performed in the transverse direction to avoid inadvertent extension of the incision anteriorly or posteriorly (which might injure the urethra or rectal structures). Simple aspiration of the vagina without a definite drainage procedure should be discouraged, because incompletely evacuated material may be prone to ascending bacterial growth. In pubertal girls, general anesthesia with excision of excess hymenal tissues may be indicated (Fig. 69–18).

Acquired abnormalities of the hymenal ring usually result from sexual abuse. The associated finding of a hematoma, abrasion, or laceration in combination with hymenal transection should raise the possibility of this diagnosis. Proper examination under anesthesia and forensic swabbing of affected areas should be undertaken with the use of a standardized protocol.

Prolapsed Urethra

Urethral prolapse usually involves a complete circumferential eversion of the urethral mucosa at the level of the external urethral meatus (Lowe et al, 1986) (Fig. 69–19). **This entity, which was first described by Solinger in 1732, occurs most often in prepubertal black girls and in postmenopausal white women** (Epstein and Strauss, 1937; Richardson et al, 1982). Various etiologies that have been proposed for urethral prolapse include hypoestrogenism (Desai and Cohen, 1997), abnormal connections between the inner longitudinal and outer circular muscle lay-

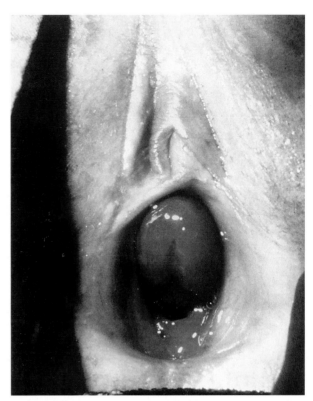

Figure 69–19. Urethral prolapse. (From Yerkes EB, Rink RC: What urologists should know about pediatric gynecologic abnormalities. Contemporary Urology 2002;14(1):12.)

ers of the distal urethra (Lowe et al, 1986), and episodic increases in intra-abdominal pressure (Valerie et al, 1999). The most common presenting complaint is bleeding from the edematous and friable mucosa, which results in blood spotting on the underwear (Richardson et al, 1982; Chaouachi et al, 1989). Urethral prolapse is easily recognized as a doughnut-shaped mass with the urethral meatus at the center. If the diagnosis can be confirmed by passing a urethral catheter, then radiographic evaluation is not indicated (Nussbaum and Lebowitz, 1983). Treatment options include observation, topical steroids, and surgical excision (Redman, 1982; Fernandes et al, 1993). Sitz baths may be helpful. Nonoperative treatment may lead to spontaneous reduction of the prolapse, but a recurrence rate of up to 67% has been noted (Jerkins et al, 1984). Many methods for surgical repair have been described. Circumferential excision of the redundant mucosa with subsequent suturing of the normal urethra to the vestibule is the procedure of choice (Devine and Kessel, 1980). Other methods, including ligation over a transurethral catheter with subsequent sloughing and cryosurgery, should be discouraged (Owens and Morse, 1968; Klaus and Stein, 1973).

Prolapsed Ureterocele

An ectopic ureterocele is a cystic dilatation of the terminal portion of the ureter that occurs predominantly in white females (Mandell et al, 1980). Approximately 90% of ectopic ureteroceles are associated with the upper pole of a duplex collecting system. Although they normally remain positioned proximal to the bladder neck, some may pro-

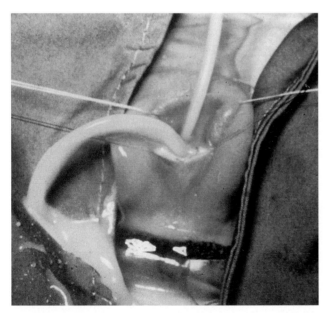

Figure 69–18. Intraoperative photograph: Incisional drainage of imperforate hymen. (From Yerkes EB, Rink RC: What urologists should know about pediatric gynecologic abnormalities. Contemporary Urology 2002;14(1):12.)

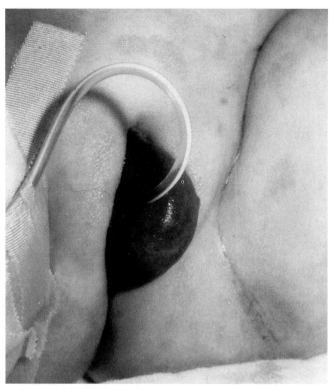

Figure 69–20. Prolapsed ureterocele. Note catheter inserted in urethra.

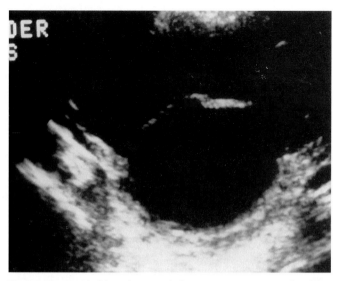

Figure 69–21. Bladder ultrasound demonstrating ureterocele. (From Yerkes EB, Rink RC: What urologists should know about pediatric gynecologic abnormalities. Contemporary Urology 2002;14(1):12.)

lapse through the urethra during micturition, almost always in infancy. This may result in urinary retention and a relative urologic emergency (Gingell et al, 1971). Depending on the length of time the ureterocele has been prolapsed, it may vary in color from pink to dusky purple (Fig. 69–20). **If prolapsed ureterocele is in the differential diagnosis, then a bladder-renal ultrasound should be obtained to look for upper pole hydronephrosis in a duplicated collecting system** (Fig. 69–21).

Treatment of the prolapsed ureterocele consists of needle decompression with reduction and placement of a urethral catheter. Although this can occasionally be achieved in the emergency room setting, abdominal straining by the infant may make this procedure difficult, and treatment under general anesthesia is often preferable.

Injection of radiographic contrast material into the ureterocele can be helpful in identifying the relevant anatomy.

Urethral Polyp

The pediatric equivalent of the urethral caruncle, namely a urethral polyp, is a rare lesion that can manifest as an intralabial mass (Fig. 69–22). The etiology of true lesions has not been completely elucidated, but in the young child they probably represent either hamartomatous growth or a response to inflammation.

We described two young girls who presented with an interlabial mass. Histologic examination of each excised mass revealed a benign urethral polyp covered with transitional and squamous epithelium. Urethral polyps should be included in the differential diagnosis of an interlabial mass in young female patients.

Vaginal Rhabdomyosarcoma

Vaginal rhabdomyosarcoma most often manifests as a grape-like cluster of tissue emanating from the posterior aspect of the vestibule (Fig. 69–23). The mean age of patients with primary vaginal tumors is less than 2 years (Hays et al, 1988). **Of all the female genital tract primary tumors, vaginal primaries appear to have the best prognosis. This excellent prognosis is thought to be a result of the predominance of the embryonal cell type and the relatively early detection due to symptoms of bleeding** (Hays et al, 1988). Once a tissue diagnosis has been made by biopsy, proper staging with abdominal and pelvic CT scanning, chest radiography, and bone marrow biopsy is critical to the optimal stratification of these pa-

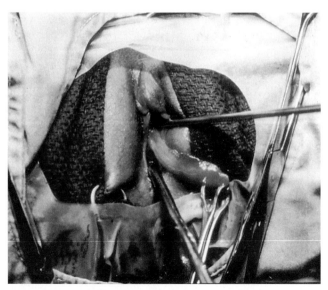

Figure 69–22. Urethral polyp. (From Yerkes EB, Rink RC: What urologists should know about pediatric gynecologic abnormalities. Contemporary Urology 2002;14(1):12.)

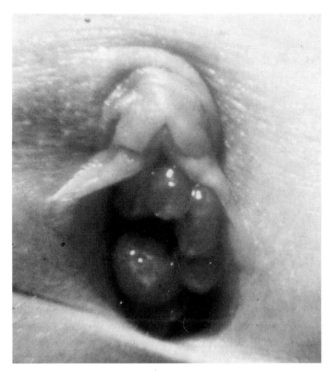

Figure 69–23. Vaginal rhabdomyosarcoma. (From Yerkes EB, Rink RC: What urologists should know about pediatric gynecologic abnormalities. Contemporary Urology 2002;14(1):12.)

some but in others appears more like a normal urethral orifice (Figs. 69–26 and 69–27). **Regardless of how the confluence of the urinary and genital tracts is described, the confluence location is the critical factor in surgical management.** This confluence is known to occur in a spectrum from near-normal anatomy, with the vagina and urethra joining near the perineum, to a communication near the bladder neck, with a long common urogenital sinus channel.

Evaluation

General

Urogenital sinus abnormalities are most often seen in intersex states, most commonly in association with congenital adrenal hyperplasia (CAH), which has been noted to have an incidence as frequent as 1 in 500 in the nonclassic, mild form (Hughes, 1998). The most common enzymatic defect in CAH resulting in genital ambiguity is 21-hydroxylase deficiency, which occurs in approximately 1 in 12,500 persons (Pang, 1997). The initial management of urogenital sinus abnormalities therefore usually focuses on very prompt, careful evaluation of the child with genital ambiguity to identify the genetic gender and endocrinologic abnormalities and to determine the gen-

tients into treatment protocols (Hays et al, 1985, 1988). Advances in chemotherapy have led to a reduction in the role of surgery for this disease with each subsequent Intergroup Rhabdomyosarcoma Study (IRS) trial: IRS-I, 100%; IRS-II, 70%; IRS-III, 30%; and IRS-IV, 13% (Andrassy et al, 1999). After chemotherapy, local resection may be required, but wide excision of the involved organ has no role except in persistent or recurrent disease.

CLASSIFICATION OF UROGENITAL SINUS AND CLOACAL ANOMALIES

Evaluation and medical and surgical management of children with persistent urogenital sinus is one of the most challenging problems a pediatric urologist will face.

In urogenital sinus anomalies, there is a persistent communication of the vagina with the urinary tract. This communication almost always occurs within the urethra, but entry of the vagina into the bladder has been seen. The persistent urogenital sinus is seen most commonly in children with **intersex states** (Fig. 69–24), but it can also occur in two other groups: (a) as an isolated **pure urogenital sinus** (Fig. 69–25) anomaly with no external genital or rectal abnormalities or (b) in patients with associated rectal involvement, in whom all three systems enter a common channel (i.e., **persistent cloaca**).

Early descriptions of this confluence were based on prior medical training. Urologists described the vagina as entering the urethra, whereas gynecologists noted that the urethra entered the vaginal vestibule (Jones and Jones, 1954). Jaramillo and colleagues (1990) noted that on examination the external cloacal orifice appears vaginal in nature in

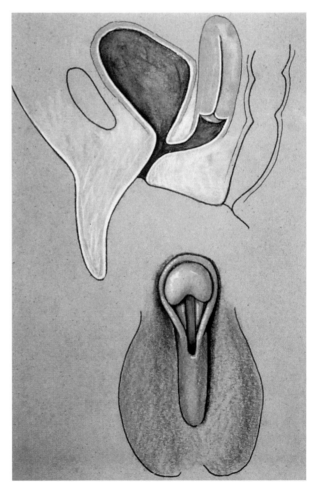

Figure 69–24. Urogenital sinus in a patient with intersex.

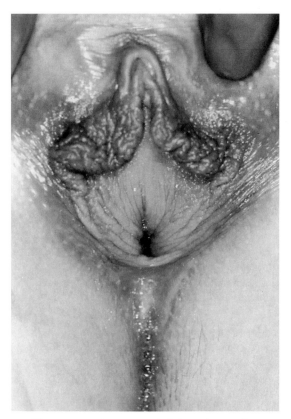

Figure 69–25. Pure urogenital sinus abnormality.

der of rearing. This is done with a team of physicians that includes a neonatologist, endocrinologist, geneticist, psychiatrist, and pediatric urologist in concert with the parents. Every effort is made to complete the evaluation in the first few days of life. The parents need a great deal of emotional support, because this is an extremely stressful time.

The child should not be named until the gender assignment is complete (Rink and Adams, 1999).

Cloacal anomalies are a much more complex problem, but fortunately they occur in only 1 of every 40,000 to 50,000 patients (Karlin et al, 1989). They are the most challenging of the anorectal malformations and make up 13.6% of this group (Fleming et al, 1986). These children present with a very broad spectrum of findings on examination of the external genitalia, but many have a prominent phallic structure and also initially require evaluation for an intersex state.

History and Physical Examination

The history and physical examination are extremely helpful in cases of genital ambiguity and can often lead to the diagnosis itself. It is critical to determine whether the mother ingested any medications, especially androgenic substances, during pregnancy. A family history of early infant death or fluid and electrolyte abnormalities suggests CAH. Have other children had genital ambiguity, or have any changed gender identification at puberty? Notation should be made of any family members with abnormal pubertal development.

The physical examination can at times be very useful in determining the appropriate gender and to help identify other organ system involvement. A general evaluation of the child's overall health should be done before focusing on the genital examination. Abnormal facies suggesting a syndrome should be noted. **Hypertension can occur in children with genital ambiguity secondary to CAH with 11β-hydroxylase deficiency.** Therefore, the blood pressure should be documented. Evidence of dehydration may also lead to a diagnosis of CAH. On abdominal examination a mass, particularly a suprapubic mass, may be present owing to a distended bladder or hydrometrocolpos or both. **Hydrometrocolpos is frequently a presenting sign and is**

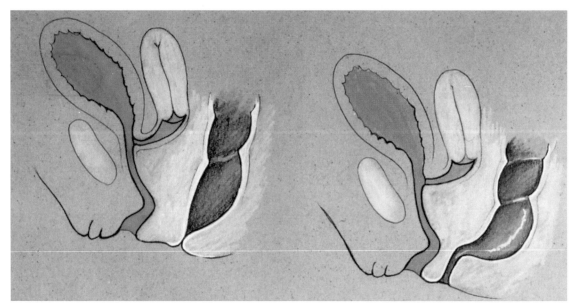

Figure 69–26. *Left,* Urethral-type urogenital sinus. *Right,* Urethral-type urogenital sinus with anteriorly placed rectum.

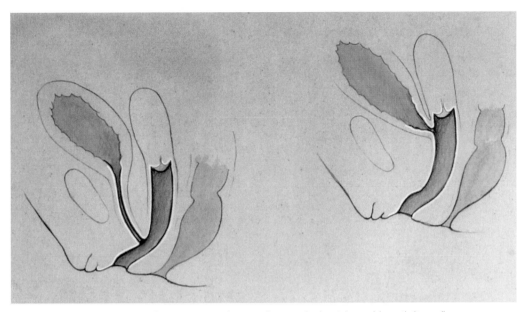

Figure 69–27. Vaginal-type urogenital sinus, showing high *(right)* and low *(left)* confluence.

often the only early finding in pure urogenital sinus abnormalities.

In cloacal anomalies, abdominal distention may be severe, secondary to hydrometrocolpos and bladder and intestinal distention. Hydrometrocolpos was noted commonly in early series (Chappel and Bleloch, 1973; Klugo et al, 1974); its incidence ranged from 29% of Pena's patients (1989) to 63% of those of Bartholomew and Gonzales (1978). It is caused most commonly by preferential flow of urine into the vagina (or vaginas) with voiding and associated poor vaginal drainage. Maternal estrogen stimulation of the cervical glands results in mucus production, adding further to the distention. Urine flow can occur into the rectum also. This distention has resulted in edema-tous, cyanotic legs and respiratory distress (Raffensberger, 1988).

The lower back should be examined to identify any evidence of spinal cord abnormalities, which can be associated with urogenital sinus abnormalities and are very common in cloacal anomalies. These may take the form of a sacral dimple, hair patch, or area of abnormal pigmentation, but more commonly there is evidence of a bone abnormality, such as an abnormal buttocks crease or flattened buttocks due to sacral agenesis.

Genital examination should note the size of the phallus and the consistency of the erectile bodies. Any degree of curvature should be documented. Huffman (1976) multiplied the width of the glans times the length of the phallus

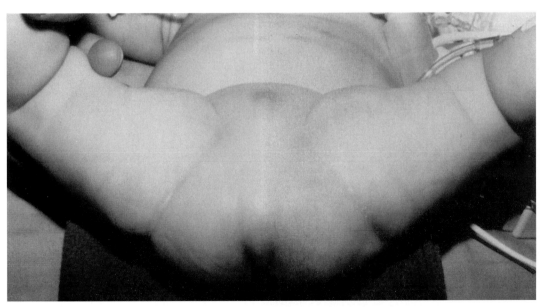

Figure 69–28. Cloaca, showing blank perineal appearance.

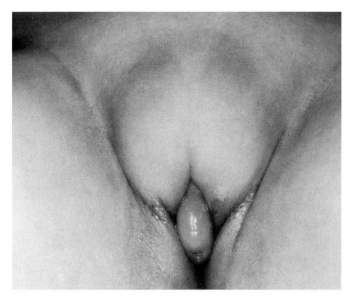

Figure 69-29. Cloaca, showing genital transposition.

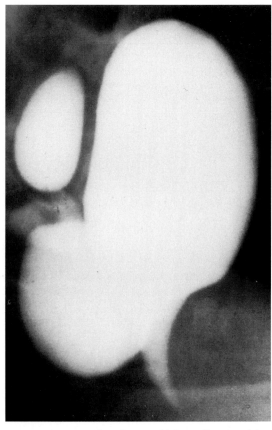

Figure 69-31. Genitography, showing high confluence of the vagina entering near the bladder neck, with flow of contrast material into the uterus.

to determine the "clitoral index," which he noted should be less than 3.5 mm to be normal and was of concern when greater than 10 mm. The gonads should be sought, and, when found, their number, location, and consistency should be noted. If both gonads are descended, it is extremely unlikely to find 46,XX chromosome makeup. The labio-scrotal folds should be examined for their relationship to the phallus and rectum, as well as for the degree of fusion. Increased pigmentation of the labioscrotal folds and areola may be seen in some cases of CAH as a result of increased levels of melanocyte-stimulating hormone.

In urogenital sinus anomalies, the location of the anus should be noted. Although it usually is in the normal location, anterior displacement is not uncommon, and this

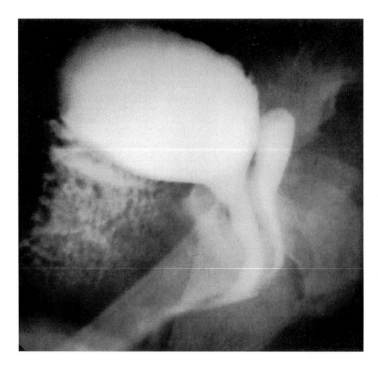

Figure 69-30. Genitography, showing low confluence of urethra and vagina.

bridges the gap to cloacal anomalies (see Fig. 69–26). A gentle rectal examination is helpful to identify a cervix.

Examination of the child with persistent cloaca deserves special mention. There is a single perineal orifice, because the rectum also enters this common channel. The appearance of the external genitalia occurs in a much wider spectrum, from a near-normal female appearance to much more bizarre appearances such as genital transposition or a blank-appearing perineum (Hendren, 1989) (Figs. 69–28 and 69–29). In some instances, there is an enlarged phallic structure, giving the genitalia an ambiguous appearance. The single perineal opening may exit what appears to be a normal vaginal introitus, or it may extend to the tip of a phallic structure. We, as well as others, have encountered children with a secondary accessory channel that exits the tip of the phallus (Hendren, 1989; Karlin et al, 1989).

It is critical to realize that cloacal anomalies are also more often associated with other organ system problems. **Kay and Tank (1977) reported that 13% of patients with cloacal anomalies have cardiovascular abnormalities; central nervous system problems are noted in 10%, and respiratory abnormalities in 5%.** Besides the imperforate anus, other gastrointestinal disorders, such as tracheoesophageal fistula and duodenal atresia, have been seen (Hendren, 1986, 1988). Rectal duplication was found in 2% of Pena's patients (Karlin et al, 1989). **Vertebral, in particular sacral, anomalies are relatively common.**

Laboratory evaluation for genital ambiguity is discussed elsewhere in this volume. It should always be done promptly and include rapid karyotyping of cultured peripheral leukocytes. Results should be available in 48 hours. Biochemical studies to determine the presence of CAH and the specific enzymatic defect are obtained, usually under the direction of the pediatric endocrinologist. Fluid and electrolyte status must be closely monitored in patients with suspected CAH.

Radiographic and Endoscopic Evaluation

UROGENITAL SINUS ABNORMALITIES

Powell and associates (1995) defined four distinct types of urogenital sinus anomalies based on vaginal location: I, labial fusion; II, distal confluence; III, proximal or high confluence; and IV, absent vagina. **Although we agree that Powell's classification can be helpful in teaching and in planning operative procedures, the vaginal confluence with the urogenital sinus is not simply distal or proximal but is a continuum extending from the bladder to a near-normal location in the perineum.** Defining this confluence is critical to operative management in these children, and it is done by a combination of radiographic and endoscopic evaluation.

Radiologic evaluation postnatally begins with ultrasonography of the abdomen and pelvis. The kidneys should be examined, as well as the pelvic anatomy. In intersex individuals, gonads should be identified by location and appearance, and the presence or absence of a uterus should be noted. One should document whether evidence of a distended vagina or bladder is found. Enlarged adrenal glands showing a cerebriform appearance are indicative of CAH (Brock et al, 1998).

Genitography is mandatory and is performed by placing a catheter flush with the urogenital sinus meatus to occlude the opening and then injecting contrast material. This is done in an effort to fill the common sinus, vagina, and bladder with contrast. A catheter is then passed into the bladder to perform a standard voiding cystourethrogram. The location of the vaginal confluence along the common channel, its distance from the bladder neck, and vaginal size are best documented with lateral views (Figs. 69–30 and 69–31). A cervical impression seen at the top of the vagina does document female internal organs. Other radiographic studies for urogenital sinus or intersex abnormalities are generally not done, although in very complex cases and in those where a neurogenic component is suspected MRI may be helpful.

Of even more importance in defining the anatomy and in helping to plan reconstructive surgery is endoscopy, which is usually done at the time of the reconstructive procedure. At times, endoscopy may be necessary to help with gender identity, and in these situations it is done in the first few days of life (Rink and Adams, 1999). As with genitography, the length of the common sinus, the location of the vaginal entry into the sinus, the size of the vagina, and the presence of a cervix should be noted. In a classic article in 1969, and again in several follow-up articles, Hendren noted that in the severely masculinized female an external sphincter may be visualized, and the vagina may be noted to enter proximal to it, having an opening similar to a verumontanum (Hendren and Crawford, 1969; Hendren and Atala, 1995). If noted, this sphincteric mechanism and the vagina's association to it should be defined. **However, although the sphincteric mechanism may masculinize, we have only rarely seen a defined sphincteric mechanism such as Hendren described** (Adams and Rink, 1998).

In the most severely masculinized urogenital sinus patient, the vagina may not be identified by genitography or initially by endoscopy. However, careful examination may reveal single or multiple punctate openings in the area of the proximal urethra (Donahoe and Gustafson, 1994). In these cases, we have found it helpful to pass a ureteral catheter into this opening, place a catheter into the bladder, and then evaluate fluoroscopically to further define the anatomy. The bladder, bladder neck, and ureteral orifices should be identified.

Rarely, even with the evaluation described, some intersex children require gonadal biopsy or evaluation of the internal genitalia. This historically has been done by laparotomy but in most cases can now be easily performed laparoscopically. Regardless of the means, it should be carried out only when the findings would influence the gender of rearing (Rink and Adams, 1999). **If a biopsy is necessary, a deep incision into the gonad should be done, because the ovarian component of an ovatestes may completely surround the testicular component** (Hensle and Kennedy, 1998). Lastly, scrotal skin biopsy may at times be helpful in males with incomplete androgen insensitivity, decreased 5α-reductase activity, or decreased dihydrotestosterone binding (Griffin and Wilson, 1989).

CLOACAL ANOMALIES

Several groups have now reported diagnosis of cloacal anomalies by antenatal ultrasound (Lande and Hamilton, 1986; Petrikovsky et al, 1986; Shalev et al, 1986; Adams et al, 1998; Cacciaguerra et al, 1998; Cilento et al, 1994). **The common findings in all reports have been a cystic pelvic mass between the bladder and rectum, representing a distended vagina.** In some, a distended bladder or rectum has resulted in a bilobed or trilobed cystic structure (Cacciaguerra et al, 1998). Ascites, which develops from voiding into the vagina (or vaginas) with retrograde flow into the uterus and out the fallopian tubes, has been noted (Adams et al, 1998; Cacciaguerra et al, 1998), as has oligohydramnios.

Postnatal radiographic evaluation begins with a plain abdominal film (Jaramillo et al, 1990). A pelvic mass may be obvious. Retrograde flow of urine and meconium, as described earlier, may result in the classic linear calcifications of calcified meconium. More granular calcifications may be noted along the course of the rectum from urine flow into the rectum that yields calcified meconium (Jaramillo et al, 1990).

An abdominal ultrasound is very important not only to visualize the pelvic anatomy but to visualize the kidneys, because hydronephrosis is extremely common (Hendren, 1998) (Fig. 69–32). Hydronephrosis is usually related to hydrocolpos, with the distended vagina compressing the bladder neck and resulting in varying degrees of bladder outlet obstruction (Hendren, 1998).

However, we have seen hydronephrosis caused by primary obstructive megaureters in patients with cloacal anomaly. **Ultrasound may also detect other upper urinary tract anomalies, which were noted in 33% of patients by Kay and Tank (1977).** Renal agenesis, renal dysplasia, and hydronephrosis related to ureteral ectopia or ureterocele have been seen.

As with urogenital sinus abnormalities, genitography and

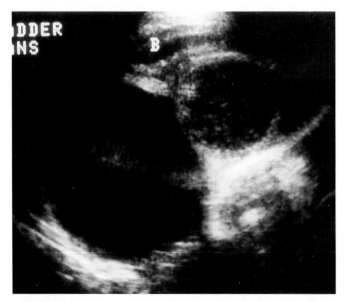

Figure 69–32. Pelvic ultrasound in patient with cloaca. Duplicate fluid-filled vaginas are seen posterior to the decompressed bladder (B).

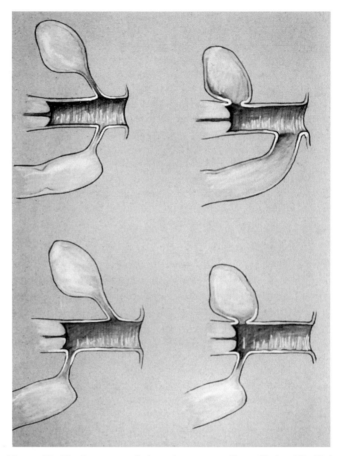

Figure 69–33. Spectrum of cloacal anatomy. (From Yerkes EB, Rink RC: What urologists should know about pediatric gynecologic abnormalities. Contemporary Urology 2002;14(1):12.)

endoscopy are mandatory to define the anatomy, which is even more complex in these cloacal children. The technique and goals of genitography and endoscopy are the same but must now include identification of the rectal as well as the vaginal confluence (Fig. 69–33). The length of the urethra and its communication with the cloaca are important for reconstructive purposes. In Hendren's patients, the urinary communication to the cloaca was urethral in 77%, but in 23% there was virtually no urethra, and the communication was noted at the bladder neck level (Jaramillo et al, 1990). The vaginal anatomy is also much more complex and variable. In Hendren's report of 154 cloaca patients, 66 patients had one vagina, 68 had two vaginas, and the vagina was absent in 20 (Hendren, 1998). The incidence of vaginal duplication has been even higher in our own patient population. The duplication anatomy is also variable. Most authors have observed that the vaginas enter side by side with a single opening into the cloaca, but separate openings have been noted. The vaginas may be of different sizes, and one may enter the sidewall of the other. A cervix is usually seen at the top of each vagina. The entrance into the cloaca again lies along a spectrum from the bladder to near the perineum. Although the uterus usually is similar to the vagina (i.e., two vaginas with two uteri), the vagina may be absent with the uterus still present (Hall et al, 1985).

The rectal confluence is equally as complex, with the

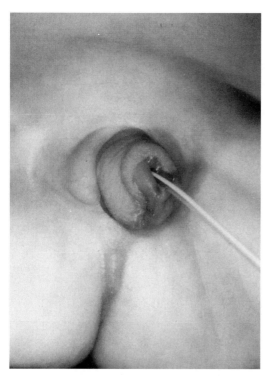

Figure 69–34. Urethral-type external cloacal appearance.

entrance in our experience most commonly just at the level of the vaginal confluence. This rectal opening may be broad, or it may have a long, narrow, fistulous tract. It can even enter into the vagina or bladder with no communication to the cloaca itself. The most common entrance in our experience is within the septum of a duplicated vagina, with all three joining the cloaca together. The various rectal entries are noted in Figure 69–33. **The rectal communication has been noted to be vaginal in 68%, and cloacal in 11%, with the remainder in other locations** (Jaramillo et al, 1990). The length and configuration of the common cloaca should also be noted, because this has important surgical as well as anatomic implications. At times, the common channel is narrow and appears very much like a urethra; in other instances, the channel is much larger and redundant, appearing more like a vagina (Fig. 69–33, *top right*). The urethral appearance was found in 48% of patients, and the vaginal appearance in 52% (Jaramillo et al, 1990). **We have noted that the urethral types result in higher outlet resistance and are more likely to lead to hydrocolpos** (Adams et al, 1998) (Fig. 69–34).

The frequent presence of associated organ system abnormalities necessitates further radiographic evaluation. Echocardiography should always be done. An MRI to evaluate the lumbosacral spine and to assess the pelvic anatomy and musculature is necessary. Historically, it has been well recognized that sacral anomalies are common. Pena (1989) noted a normal sacrum in only 35% of his 54 patients, and Jaramillo and coworkers (1990) reported sacral agenesis in 40% of Hendren's 65 patients. De Filippo and associates (1999) found 10 of 21 patients with imperforate anus or cloaca to have an abnormality of the sacrum and spine. With the use of MRI, spinal cord abnor-

malities have been more commonly detected, with an incidence as high as 43% (Jaramillo et al, 1990). Hendren found that one third of his patients had the spinal cord tethered (Hendren, 1998). MRI has also been very helpful in defining the level of the rectal atresia and in identifying the degree of sphincteric muscle development (Sato et al, 1988).

Because of the complexity of the anatomy and the frequency of hydrometrocolpos, the cloacal child often needs endoscopy early on as a separate procedure to decompress the vagina and bladder and to define the anatomy. As a general rule, visualization of the vagina (or vaginas) is easily done, but entry into the bladder can be very difficult and even impossible at times in the newborn, because it is compressed very anteriorly by the distended vagina. The vagina should always first be emptied. Identification of the rectal fistula can also be difficult at times. Once it is located, the mucus and fecal material should be irrigated from the colon. This can be done by irrigation through the scope in combination with irrigation from the colostomy.

Surgical Reconstruction of Intersex Conditions and Urogenital Sinus

Initial Management, Timing, and Principles

Because the majority of patients with urogenital sinus abnormalities have intersex states, most commonly CAH, the initial medical management involves stabilization of the patient from a metabolic standpoint with replacement cortisol and fludrocortisone (Florinef) if CAH is detected. When the gender of rearing is determined to be female, the timing of feminizing genitoplasty must be discussed. **It must again be stressed that currently there is questioning by both lay and medical personnel as to when and whether to reconstruct.** Current medical practice generally includes early surgical intervention, but some have called for a moratorium on gender-assignment cosmetic surgery when the patient cannot give consent (Diamond, 1999).

The general principles of reconstruction are the same regardless of the age of the patient. **Reconstruction of the masculinized female genitalia involves three steps: clitoral reconstruction, vaginoplasty, and labial reconstruction.** In the mid-1900s, there was not thought to be an optimal timing for reconstruction (Jones and Jones, 1954; Lattimer, 1961), but more recently clitoral reconstruction has been carried out progressively earlier. Gross and colleagues in 1966, and Spence and Allen, in 1973, noted that clitoral surgery could ideally be done when the child was 1 year old. By the 1980s, clitoral surgery was recommended as early as the first few months of life (Snyder et al, 1983). More recently, de Jong and Beomers (1995) reported surgical correction at 1 to 3 weeks of age.

With early diagnosis and safe neonatal anesthesia, most surgeons now agree that clitoral surgery should be carried out in the neonatal period. The optimal timing for vaginoplasty, however, continues to be debated. Simultaneous clitoroplasty, vaginoplasty, and labioplasty has been the standard practice for the child with a low (distal) vaginal confluence. Two separate schools of thought have been put forth for the high vaginal confluence. Many have believed that there is a high rate of vaginal stenosis, warranting delay of vaginal surgery until after puberty, which also avoids any need for vaginal dilation (Sotiropoulos et al, 1976; Snyder et al, 1983; Alizai et al, 1999). **Others, including our group, have believed that vaginoplasty, regardless of the vaginal location, is best combined with clitoroplasty in a single stage. This allows the redundant phallic skin to be used in the reconstruction, adding flexibility for the surgeon, which is compromised when the skin has been previously mobilized** (de Jong and Boemers, 1995; Hendren and Atala, 1995; Rink et al, 1997; Passerini, 1998; Mandell et al, 1988; Gonzales and Fernandez, 1990). **Furthermore, we and others have noted that maternal estrogen stimulation of the child's genitalia results in thicker vaginal tissue that is better vascularized, making vaginal mobilization more easily performed** (Donahoe and Gustafson, 1994; de Jong and Boemers, 1995; Passerini, 1998; Rink and Adams, 1999).

Today, when performing clitoroplasty, every effort is made not only to provide normal cosmesis but to retain normal clitoral innervation for optimal sexual gratification. Clitoral surgery has undergone significant evolution. Initial efforts were primarily done not just to amputate the clitoris but to completely excise all clitoral tissue to avoid any later painful erections (Jones and Jones, 1954; Gross et al, 1966; Hendren and Crawford, 1969). Clitoral amputation was based on reports by both Hampson and Gulliver, noting that the clitoris was not necessary for normal sexual response (Hampson, 1955). As recognition of the importance of the clitoris evolved, several ingenious clitoral recession techniques were reported that preserved the innervation and all clitoral tissue. Lattimer, in 1961, recessed the clitoris in subcutaneous fat and buried it beneath the skin. Kaplan (1967) reported an interesting technique of splitting the two corpora apart and closing in a transverse Henike-Mikulicz fashion. Randolph and Hung (1970) and also Pellerin (1965) buried the corpora beneath the pubis. Efforts to preserve the glans based on a flap were made as early as the 1930s by Young, but the glans sloughed (Young, 1937). In 1961, Schmid was the first to report excising corporal tissue yet preserving the neurovascular bundle with the glans intact. Kumar later noted a similar technique proposed by Keifer the same year (Kumar et al, 1974). Spence and Allen (1973) excised all of the clitoral shaft, leaving the glans intact and attached to the ventral urethral plate. **Virtually all techniques since have been based on Schmid's preservation of the neurovascular bundle** (Shaw, 1977; Barrett and Gonzalez, 1980; Glassberg and Laungani, 1981; Mollard et al, 1981; Rajfer et al, 1982). Although the glans often did well with these techniques, shrinkage and devascularization occurred at times. **Kogan and associates (1983) reported subtunical excision of the erectile tissue done by incising laterally through Buck's fascia to resect the erectile corpus cavernosa tissue.** Clitoroplasty techniques have had only minor technical advances since. The recent demonstration of the neurovascular anatomy of the clitoris by Baskin and coworkers (1999) suggests that a ventromedial incision would preserve not only the main dorsal neurovascular bundle but also the neural branches that fan out laterally.

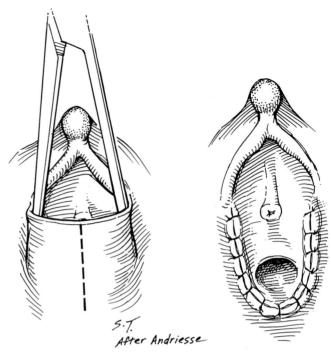

S.T.
After Andriesse

Figure 69–35. Cut-back vaginoplasty. (From Rink RC, Adams MC: Feminizing genitoplasty: State of the art. World J Urol 1998;16:212.)

Vaginoplasty techniques have similarly evolved, with all repairs based on a few landmark reports. **Almost every vaginal repair today uses a posteriorly based perineal flap originally described by Fortunoff and coworkers in 1964. In 1969, Hendren and Crawford reported the "pull-through" vaginoplasty for the high vaginal confluence.** Their efforts to establish the location of the vaginal confluence as the determining factor for the type of vaginoplasty remains the basis for all vaginoplasties today. **Vaginal reconstruction techniques now generally occur in one of four types. (1) The cut-back vaginoplasty is rarely used and is appropriate only for simple labial fusion (Fig. 69–35). (2) The flap vaginoplasty is applicable to the low (distal) vaginal confluence.** In this procedure, the posterior walls of the sinus and vagina are opened but the anterior wall of the vagina is left intact. The posterior perineal flap fits into the opened vagina. **This procedure does not change the level of the confluence; it simply widely opens the urogenital sinus** (Rink and Adams, 1998). Flap vaginoplasty should never be used for those patients with a high vaginal confluence, because it may result in a short hypospadic urethra, vaginal voiding, many infections, and even incontinence (Hendren and Atala, 1995; Rink and Adams, 1999). **(3) The pull-through vaginoplasty is used for the very high vaginal confluence.** In this procedure, the vagina is separated from the urogenital sinus, and the sinus is used to create a urethra. The mobilized vagina may reach the perineum, but in most cases it has required skin flaps to do so. **(4) Complete vaginal replacement can be achieved by several techniques, but it is used only for a rudimentary or absent vagina.**

Labioplasty techniques also continue to evolve. In congenital adrenal hyperplasia and other intersex states, the

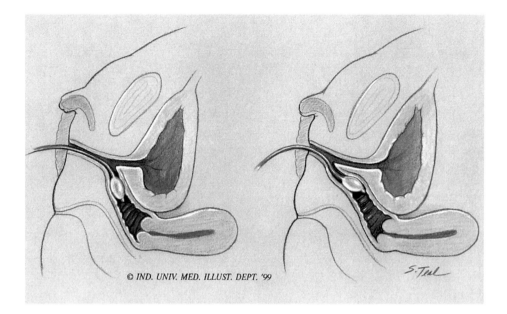

Figure 69–36. Fogarty catheter placed in the vagina in high confluence *(left)* and in low confluence *(right).* (Copyright © 1999 Indiana University Medical Illustration Department.)

© IND. UNIV. MED. ILLUST. DEPT. '99

labia minora are absent and the labia majora are superior to the new vaginal introitus. Labia minora are created by using the phallic skin as described by Marberger (1975). The labioscrotal folds are moved inferiorly by a Y-V-plasty to create normally located labia majora (Hendren and Donahoe, 1980).

Current Operative Techniques for Intersex and Urogenital Sinus Repair

Preoperatively, it is important to ensure that the patient is metabolically stable, particularly the child with CAH. At a minimum, all children undergo an enema, and if there is any indication that a more significant vaginoplasty is required, complete bowel preparation with a polyethylene glycol–electrolyte solution (GoLYTELY) is warranted. All children receive preoperative broad-spectrum antibiotics. After general anesthesia, endoscopy is performed as described previously. **A Fogarty catheter is passed into the vagina, the balloon is inflated to 1 ml, and the catheter is clamped and left indwelling** (Fig. 69–36). **A Foley catheter is then anchored in the bladder.** Both are kept sterile, and the child is prepared with povidone-iodine (Betadine). Many surgeons prefer to place the child in the lithotomy position, but we have found that this position limits vision to only the surgeon, hinders teaching, and does not allow manipulation of child for the unexpected need of a posterior or abdominal approach. All children undergo a complete lower body preparation from nipples to feet. The child's legs are wrapped, and the lower body is passed through the aperture in the drapes; this allows access to the entire perineum and abdomen and further allows the child to be positioned either supine or prone (Fig. 69–37).

LOW VAGINAL CONFLUENCE—CLITORAL HYPERTROPHY

The vast majority of children who undergo surgery for intersex or urogenital sinus conditions have a low vaginal confluence and clitoral hypertrophy. With the child in the supine position, a traction suture is placed through the glans and the proposed incisions are outlined with a skin scribe. Along these lines, 0.5% lidocaine with 1:200,000 epinephrine is injected for hemostasis. Parallel longitudinal lines are drawn on either side of a ventral mucosal strip from around the meatus toward the glans and around the coronal margin (Fig. 69–38A). A perineal inverted U flap is outlined, with the base extending to either ischial tuberosity. A Y incision line is drawn around the inferior aspect of each labia majora (see Fig. 69–38B). The incision begins around the coronal margin, and ultimately the penis is degloved, leaving the ventral strip. Dissection is carried out to the level of the bifurcation of the corporal bodies, with care taken not to injure the neurovascular bundle. A tourniquet is placed at the base of the clitoris. Longitudinal incisions are then made through Buck's fascia on the ventromedial aspect of the corporal bodies, extending from the glans to the bifurcation and exposing the corpora cavernosa tissue, which is dissected from the tunics (Fig. 69–39A). The lateral and dorsal aspects of the tunics are left undisturbed. The proximal ends of the erectile tissue are suture ligated (see Fig. 69–39B). The phallic skin is then split dorsally, similarly to Byar's flaps in hypospadias repair, and secured to the coronal margin. The glans is then secured to the corporal stumps. A better cosmetic result is obtained with this glans location than with approximation to the pubis. If reduction of the glans is indicated, the tissue should be excised from the inferior and medial aspect to avoid injury to the nerves.

With the clitoroplasty completed, the **flap vaginoplasty** is started. The previously outlined U flap is incised, and the underlying fat is mobilized with the flap exposing the urogenital sinus. The flap must be made long enough to provide a tension-free anastomosis to the vagina and wide enough to provide a normal-caliber introitus without compromising the blood supply or the perineal body. The posterior wall of the sinus and vagina is now dissected free from the underlying rectum. With stay sutures in the meatus, the posterior wall of sinus is opened in the midline

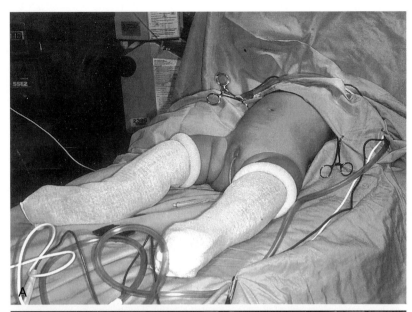

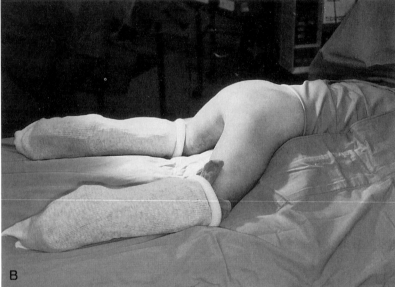

Figure 69–37. Total lower body preparation allows both supine *(A)* and prone *(B)* approaches. (From Rink RC, Adams MC: Feminizing genitoplasty: State of the art. World J Urol 1998;16:212.)

Figure 69–38. Flap vaginoplasty in intersex state. *A,* Proposed incisions. *B,* Clitoroplasty is complete and the flap is developed. The arrow indicates the proposed opening of the sinus. (From Rink RC, Pope JC, Kropp BP, et al: Reconstruction of the high urogenital sinus: Early perineal prone approach without division of the rectum. J Urol 1997;158:1293. Copyright © 1999 Indiana University Medical Illustration Department.)

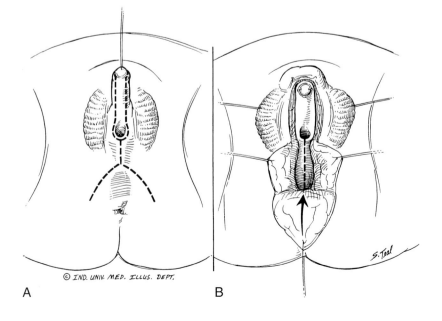

© IND. UNIV. MED. ILLUS. DEPT.

A   B

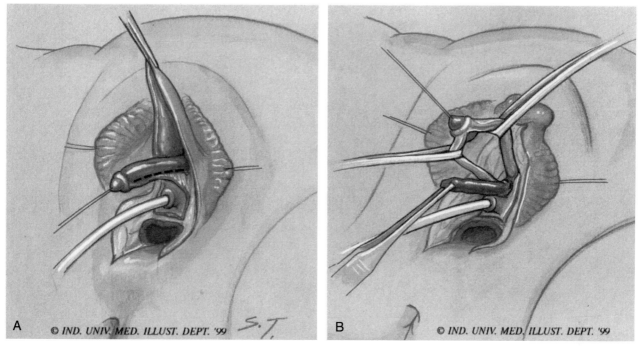

Figure 69-39. Clitoroplasty. *A,* Clitoris degloved; proposed ventromedial incision into Buck's fascia. *B,* Excision of erectile tissue. (Copyright © 1999 Indiana University Medical Illustration Department.)

and is extended proximally into the posterior wall of the vagina (see Fig. 69–38*B*). The distal end of the vagina is usually narrowed; therefore, the posterior wall incision must be carried proximally until the normal-caliber vagina is encountered. Sutures are placed individually through the perineal flap and then through the split posterior wall of the vagina and tied.

Labia minora are now created using the split preputial skin, which is moved inferiorly and anastomosed to the preserved ventral plate and the lateral vaginal wall (Fig. 69–40). The proposed Y incision around the inferior aspect of each labia majora is now made. The labia are mobilized and secured inferiorly alongside the vagina as a Y-V-plasty.

HIGH VAGINAL CONFLUENCE—WITH OR WITHOUT CLITORAL HYPERTROPHY

It is now well established that vaginal separation and a pull-through vaginoplasty, as proposed by Hendren and Crawford (1969), is the best solution to the high vaginal confluence. Fortunately this complex situation is found in only about 5% of patients with CAH (Duman-

Figure 69-40. Labioplasty. *A,* Phallic skin unfurled. *B,* Preputial skin split and used to create labia minora; proposed labia majora Y-V plasty. (From Rink RC, Adams MC: Feminizing genitoplasty: State of the art. World J Urol 1998;16:212. Copyright © 1997 Indiana University Medical Illustration Department.)

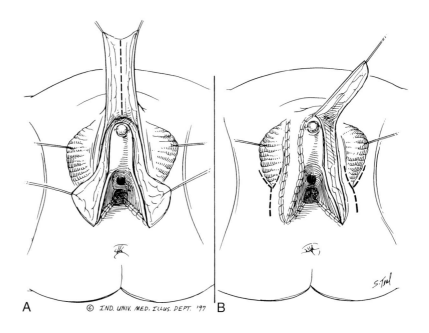

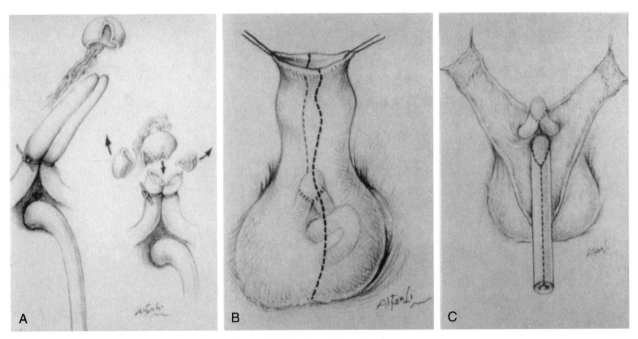

Figure 69–41. Passerini vaginoplasty.

ian and Donahoe, 1992). Although the concept of vaginal separation and pull-through was a major advance, the operation as originally described frequently resulted in an isolated vaginal opening that appeared to be separate from the remainder of the genitalia, and a mucosal lining was lacking (Passerini-Glazel, 1989) (Fig. 69–41). It was also tech-

nically difficult because of poor vision at the critical points (Rink et al, 1997). Several authors addressed these issues. Passerini-Glazel (1989) used the mobilized sinus by dividing it dorsally; when tubularized with the phallic skin and folded back toward the vagina, this created a more normal cosmetic result and provided excellent coverage in the area

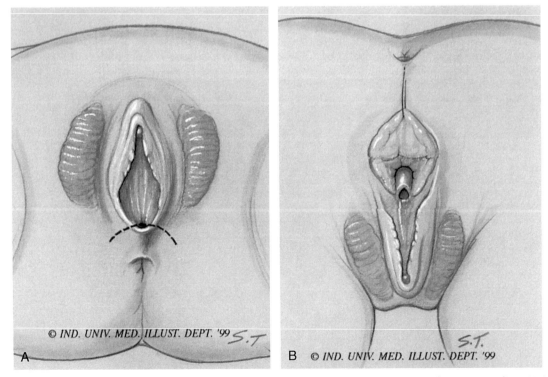

Figure 69–42. Vaginoplasty for patient with pure urogenital sinus begins in the prone position (B). Copyright © 1999 Indiana University Medical Illustration Department.)

of the vaginal separation to prevent urethrovaginal fistula. Gonzalez and Fernandez (1990) used the preputial skin to construct the vaginal vestibule and anterior wall.

The critical and most technically demanding aspect of a pull-through vaginoplasty is separation of the anterior wall of the vagina from the urethra and bladder neck. There is no obvious plane of dissection, and great care must be taken to avoid injury to the urinary tract and its sphincteric mechanism. This area is also the most difficult to visualize, and poor exposure naturally leads to poor results, with the potential for stricture, fistula, diverticulum, or retained distal vagina (Rink and Adams, 1998), Several authors have reported means of improving exposure. Passerini-Glazel mobilized the vagina transtrigonally in difficult cases but has more recently reported that this is seldom necessary (Passerini-Glazel, 1989; Passerini, 1994). Similarly, Di Benedetto and Rossi and their associates proposed an anterior sagittal transanorectal approach with diverting colostomy (Di Benedetto et al, 1997; Rossi et al, 1998). Hendren and Atala reported lateral mobilization of the rectum in 1995 but have since stopped due to the difficulty of this maneuver. Rink and colleagues (1997) reported a midline posterior prone approach with retraction but not division of the rectum that provides excellent exposure for critical aspects of the pull-through vaginoplasty and is described here. Endoscopy with Fogarty and Foley catheter placement and total-body preparation are as described for the flap vaginoplasty. If the child has associated clitoral hypertrophy, the clitoroplasty is performed with the child supine, as described earlier for the low confluence. The child is then rotated to the prone position. In the patient with pure

urogenital sinus, the procedure is started with the patient in the prone position (Fig. 69–42).

The perineal inverted U flap incision is made as previously described, and then the flap is retracted posteriorly, with dissection now carried out in the midline between the posterior wall of the sinus/vagina and rectum. As dissection proceeds proximally, the rectum is easily retracted with a small Deavor retractor (Fig. 69–43A). This exposes the entire urogenital sinus without the need to divide the rectum. The entire length of the sinus is divided in the midline posteriorly to the normal caliber of the vagina. The Deavor retractor is now placed in the vagina and with upward retraction easily exposes the anterior wall of the vagina at its confluence with the sinus (see Fig. 69–43B). This allows dissection of the vagina from the urethra under direct vision (see Fig. 69–43C). The tissues are quite thin in this area, and one should always err on the side of the vagina. More proximally, the dissection becomes easier. Excellent vision is also provided for the tubularization of the sinus to create a urethra. This is closed in two or three layers over a Foley catheter (Fig. 69–44). The anterior wall of the vagina is now mobilized inferiorly, closer to the perineum. If it does not reach the perineum, preputial skin may be sewn to the spatulated anterior vagina, as described by Gonzalez and Fernandez (1990) (Fig. 69–45). When preputial skin is not available, a buttocks flap or a laterally based skin flap can be used (Dumanian and Donahoe, 1992; Parrott and Woodard, 1991) (Fig. 69–46). The child is returned to this supine position, and the posterior perineal flap is anastomosed to the vagina as described for the flap vaginoplasty.

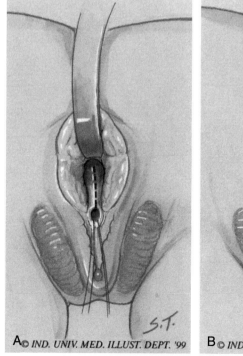
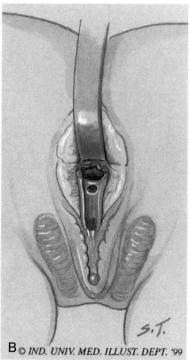
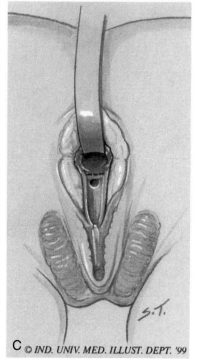

Figure 69–43. A, Posterior flap developed, sinus exposed. B, Sinus opened in posterior midline. C, Retractor in vagina. (Copyright © 1999 Indiana University Medical Illustration Department.)

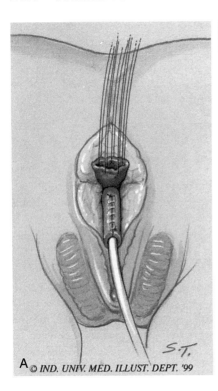

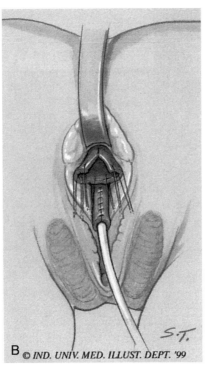

Figure 69–44. *A,* Vagina mobilized, sinus tubularized to create urethra. *B,* Posterior vagina spatulated. (Copyright © 1999 Indiana University Medical Illustration Department.)

Labioplasty is now completed as described earlier. If a laterally based flap is required for the anterior wall, posterior relocation of the labia majora may be done at a later stage.

In those patients with high confluence, particularly if multiple flaps have been used, the legs are bound together loosely postoperatively to prevent tension on the flaps.

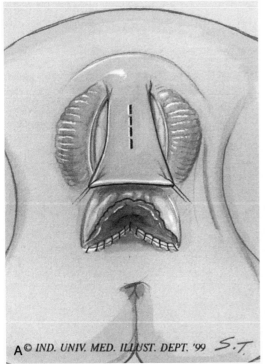

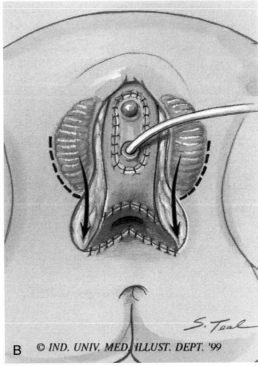

Figure 69–45. Modified Gonzalez preputial flap to create anterior vaginal wall; posterior flap has been anastomosed to spatulated vagina. (Copyright © 1999 Indiana University Medical Illustration Department.)

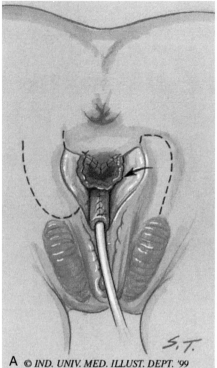
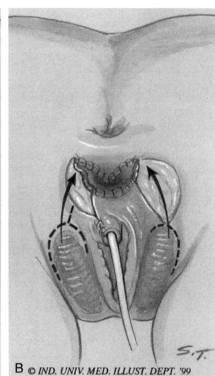

Figure 69–46. A buttock or labial-based flap may be used to create the anterior vaginal wall in a patient with pure urogenital sinus. (Copyright © 1999 Indiana University Medical Illustration Department.)

A © IND. UNIV. MED. ILLUST. DEPT. '99   B © IND. UNIV. MED. ILLUST. DEPT. '99

TOTAL UROGENITAL MOBILIZATION

In 1997, Alberto Pena proposed a maneuver called *total urogenital mobilization* as a means to repair the urogenital sinus component of a cloacal repair. **In this procedure, the entire sinus is dissected circumferentially and mobilized toward the perineum.** Both Ludwikowski and Rink and their colleagues have reported their early experience with urogenital sinus anomalies alone (Ludwikowski et al, 1999; Rink et al, 1999). Pena noted a decrease in operative time by 70%, a superior cosmetic result, and less risk of fistula, vaginal stenosis, or acquired vaginal atresia with total urogenital mobilization. Both Pena (1997) and Ludwikowski's group (1999) reported amputation of the mobilized sinus so that the vagina and urethra are sewn flush to the perineum. **Rink and colleagues (1999) reported use of the mobilized sinus to provide a mucosa-lined vestibule or a Passerini flap to cover the anterior vaginal wall when a pull-through procedure is done.** At the Riley Hospital for Children, we have incorporated this technique into many of the urogenital sinus repairs. It allows the midlevel confluence to reach the perineum without requiring vaginal separation. The highest level confluences may still need a pull-through procedure, but it is much more easily performed after the urogenital sinus has been mobilized (Fig. 69–47).

To begin the total urogenital mobilization procedure, cystoscopy with Fogarty and Foley catheter placement is done as previously described. Clitoroplasty, if necessary, is performed as described earlier. An inverted U-shaped perineal flap is still created as in the standard vaginoplasty, but

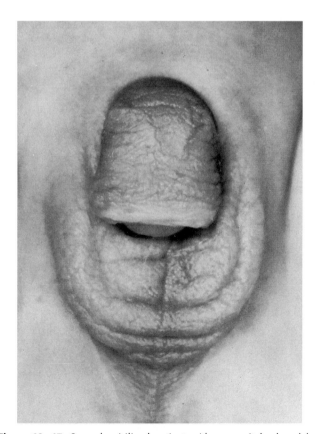

Figure 69–47. Severely virilized patient with congenital adrenal hyperplasia (CAH) before urogenital mobilization.

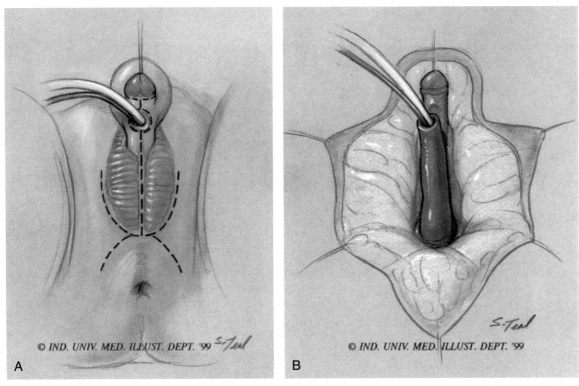

Figure 69–48. Total urogenital mobilization. *A,* Proposed incisions. *B,* Skin mobilized, sinus exposed. (Copyright © 1999 Indiana University Medical Illustration Department.)

the meatus is circumcised and traction sutures are placed (Fig. 69–48A). The initial dissection is carried out in the midline posteriorly until the peritoneal reflection is reached; this allows access to the entire posterior wall of the vagina. The anterior wall is now mobilized from the phallus (see Fig. 69–48B). This circumferential mobilization is done directly on the urogenital sinus and continues proximally beneath the pubis. As the avascular ligaments are divided in this area, the entire urogenital sinus is felt to "give" and move toward the perineum (Fig. 69–49).

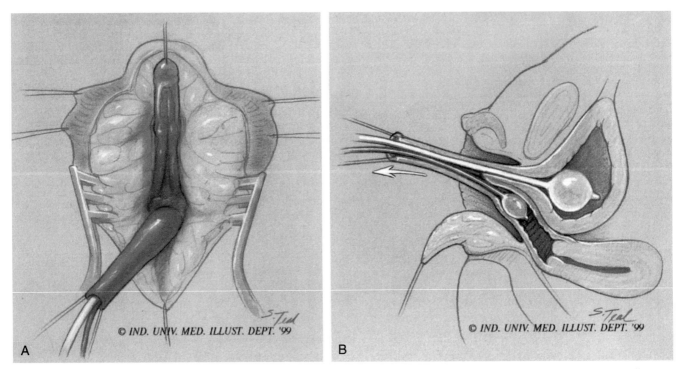

Figure 69–49. Total urogenital mobilization: sinus mobilized to beneath pubis. (Copyright © 1999 Indiana University Medical Illustration Department.)

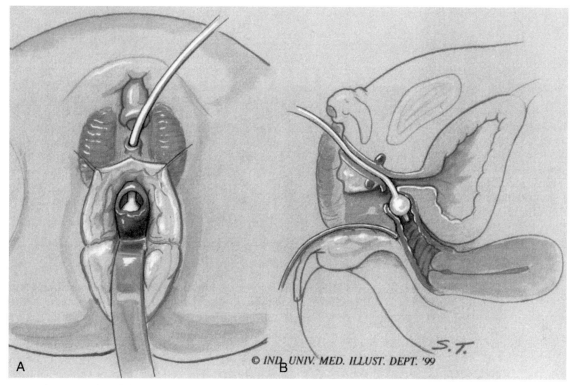

Figure 69–50. Total urogenital mobilization: incision into vagina over palpable Fogarty balloon. *A,* Anteroposterior view. *B,* Lateral view. (Copyright © 1999 Indiana University Medical Illustration Department.)

The Fogarty balloon is now easily palpable in the vagina. The posterior wall of the vagina is opened between stay sutures (Fig. 69–50). If the vagina is now near the perineum, a flap vaginoplasty is easily performed. Rather than discard the mobilized sinus, as previously reported, we have found it helpful to split the sinus ventrally and use it to provide a mucosa-lined vestibule (Fig. 69–51*A*). If the vagina is still quite high, the anterior wall of the vagina should be separated from the urethra and bladder neck, as in the pull-through procedure. We believe that this is most easily performed with the child in the prone position, allowing direct vision. The opening in the urethra is closed in two layers. The mobilized sinus in this situation is split anteriorly and then used as a Passerini flap to create the anterior vaginal wall (see Fig. 69–51*B*). The posterior perineal flap is approximated to the spatulated posterior

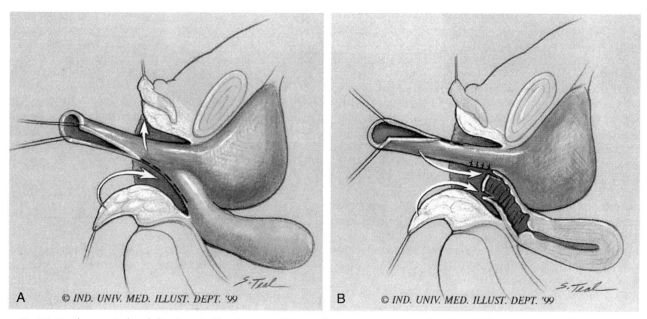

Figure 69–51. Total urogenital mobilization. *A,* The sinus is split ventrally to create a mucosa-lined vestibule in flap vaginoplasty. *B,* The sinus is split dorsally to create an anterior vaginal wall for pull-through vaginoplasty. (From Rink RC: Dial Pediatr Urol [in press].)

vaginal wall. Labioplasty is performed as previously described.

Results of Urogenital Sinus and Intersex Surgery

Well-documented long-term outcomes for clitoroplasty and vaginoplasty are sorely lacking. Most reports have focused on short-term and primarily cosmetic results rather than functional results. **Cosmetic and early functional results have uniformly been reported to be good. Long-term outcomes are more concerning.** Jones and colleagues noted in 1976 that 25 of 84 patients undergoing a vaginoplasty required a secondary procedure to provide a vaginal outlet satisfactory for intercourse; 5 of these 25 also required a third procedure. **The failures were caused by failure to exteriorize the vagina initially or by scar formation.** Sotiropoulos and associates (1976) found that all patients undergoing prepubertal vaginoplasties required revision at puberty. Azziz and coworkers, in 1986, reported results of attempted coitus in 42 women with CAH 23.6 years after vagina repair. Satisfactory coitus was noted in 62% (46% among salt wasters, and 87% among those with the non–salt-losing form). There was a less favorable outcome when the initial procedure was done before 1 year of age. Thirty secondary or tertiary procedures were performed to achieve the final results. In a series from Johns Hopkins, 28 patients had adequate follow-up, of whom 22 (78.5%) needed further vaginal surgery (Bailez et al, 1992). The authors noted that if secondary surgery for vaginal stenosis was needed, success rates were high when the procedure was performed near puberty. This group also noted less favorable results in those younger than 1 year old. Hendren, reporting on 16 patients with high vaginal confluence, noted that 6 of 9 adults had satisfactory coitus and 2 had vaginal stenosis (Hendren and Atala, 1995). More recently, Alizai and colleagues (1999) assessed under anesthesia 14 girls with CAH, aged 11 to 15 years old, who had undergone genitoplasty at a mean age of 2.5 years. Clitoroplasty was thought to be unsatisfactory in 46%, and varying degrees of introital stenosis were noted in 13 of 14 children.

Gearhart and coworkers (1995) looked at pudendal evoked potentials after clitoroplasty and noted that modern clitoroplasties preserve nerve conduction in the dorsal neurovascular bundle. Barrett and Gonzales (1980) noted intact sensation in all of their patients after clitoroplasty. We have not noted vascularization defects after modern clitoroplasty. It is clear that further long-term studies are necessary. Furthermore, sensation alone is a poor indication of clitoral normality after surgery. The potential for orgasm should also be studied.

The results of total urogenital mobilization are very early. It is clear that the procedure is technically easier and the cosmetic results are excellent, but the potential for stress incontinence or denervation of the sphincteric mechanisms is unknown. Until these results are available, this procedure should be used with caution.

Timing of vaginoplasty remains quite controversial. Although the few reported long-term studies suggest that delayed vaginoplasty may be preferable, most surgeons recommend early surgery. They argue that the available long-term studies are based on outdated techniques and that there are tremendous surgical advantages to a single-stage repair. Supporters of early vaginoplasty well recognize that secondary introitoplasty may be necessary, but this usually is easily accomplished. The argument, which will not be settled soon, contrasts two approaches: (1) a simple procedure in an infant (i.e., clitoroplasty) with a postpubertal extensive procedure (i.e., vaginoplasty) or (2) an extensive single-stage clitorovaginoplasty in an infant with a simple introitoplasty in the postpubertal period.

Surgical Reconstruction for Cloacal Malformations

Initial Management, Timing, and Principles

The initial management of cloacal anomaly involves stabilization, because the child is often quite ill with abdominal distention that at times results in respiratory compromise. As with all other anomalies, the management has evolved. Historically, after decompression of the distended organs, it was common practice to perform a rectal pull-through procedure; the genitourinary reconstruction followed at a later date, if at all (Okonkwo and Crocker, 1982). Hall and coauthors (1985) suggested that the vaginal surgery be done after puberty, when estrogen levels are higher. **Although it is tempting to do a pull-through procedure only, it is now clear that this piecemeal repair of the cloaca is a disservice to the child and is contraindicated. It is optimal to repair all abnormalities (i.e., rectal, vaginal, and urethral) in a single stage** (Kay and Tank, 1977; Mollitt et al, 1981). **This allows the best exposure for the difficult rectal and vaginal separation.** Furthermore, the tissues have not been previously violated, and the rectum does not require remobilization. **Hendren pointed out that rectal pull-through should never be done as a separate procedure** (Hendren, 1982, 1986). Of his 154 patients with cloacal anomaly, 60 were secondary cases, many of whom had had a prior pull-through. Definitive repair in this situation often requires repeat rectal mobilization. Raffensberger (1988) proposed neonatal complete repair but later noted that this may not be appropriate.

Surgical management now involves four basic steps: decompression of the gastrointestinal tract, decompression of the genitourinary tract, correction of nephrondestructive or potentially lethal urinary anomalies, and definitive repair of the cloaca.

Decompression of the Gastrointestinal Tract

Decompression of the gastrointestinal tract is done by colostomy. Although all surgeons agree on the need for colostomy initially, the best anatomic location of the colostomy is debated. Hendren initially recommended a low-loop colostomy, but more recently he has performed a right transverse divided colostomy (Hendren, 1982, 1986, 1998). This change was prompted by difficulty with the rectal pull-through and with obtaining a bowel segment for vaginoplasty when a low colostomy has been performed. Divided transverse colostomy preserves intact the left colic blood supply (Hendren, 1992). Pena, as reported by Spitz and Coron (1995), preferred a descending colostomy because there was less surface area for resorption of urine. However, Pena did recommend leaving a long segment of sigmoid to prevent a difficult pull-through requiring abdominal exploration. We have favored a more proximal colostomy but have at times found acidosis, caused by urine absorption through the colonic mucosa, challenging to treat.

At the time of colostomy, endoscopy may be done to more clearly define the anatomy and to aid in decompression of the urinary tract. In our experience, as the cystoscope advances proximally through the cloacal channel, it tends to enter the vagina (or vaginas). In fact, entrance into the urethra/bladder can be extremely difficult in the neonate with a distended vagina, because the vagina compresses the bladder to the anterior abdominal wall, obstructing the bladder neck. Drainage and irrigation of the vagina (or vaginas) not only allow decompression and relief of abdominal distention but may allow visualization of the bladder. Often, the rectal fistula is also difficult to locate; as noted previously, it is most often found within the septum of the duplicated vaginas but can enter in almost any location. With a combination of irrigation through the fistula and through the distal limb of the colostomy, the inspissated mucus and meconium can usually be cleared. It is often helpful to leave small feeding tubes in all channels and then to obtain radiographic studies to further delineate the anatomy. In our experience, this is best done in the radiology suite with fluoroscopy.

Decompression of the Genitourinary Tract

Even after decompression of all structures draining into the cloaca, at times voiding continues into the vagina (or vaginas) and/or the rectum, resulting in rapid redistention of these structures with subsequent poor urinary drainage, persistent hydronephrosis, abdominal distention, urinary infection, and hyperchloremic acidosis. This can usually be managed by intermittent catheterization. The catheter often enters the vagina rather than the bladder, but it still functions to drain and decompress the genitourinary tract (Hendren, 1992). If this does not achieve the desired decompression, then further maneuvers are required. We agree with Hendren that, in the long, urethra-like cloaca, catheterization can at times be difficult and a cut-back procedure (opening the cloaca) may be helpful to aid catheterization. **If this fails, then further decompression can be achieved by either vesicostomy or vaginostomy** (Kay and Tank, 1977) (Fig. 69–52). Some have cautioned against these two procedures, but we have found vesicostomy to be quite helpful at times, and it has not complicated later repair. Vaginostomy, however, should be the last resort because it tethers the vagina to the abdominal wall, making later pull-through difficult. It also necessitates an abdominal procedure.

Repair of Obstructive Urinary Pathology

The third stage of care of the child with a cloacal anomaly is repair of any obstructive urinary tract pathology. At times, these anomalies are ignored early on, awaiting definitive cloacal repair, but this should be avoided. Obstructive lesions should be corrected. However, vesicoureteral reflux, which is quite common, can generally be managed medically if urinary infection is prevented. Other organ system anomalies (e.g., cardiac, spinal cord) may also require repair during this phase.

Definitive Repair of Cloacal Malformations

Definitive repair of the cloaca is usually carried out at 6 to 12 months of age, but obviously the child must be well nourished and thriving in order to proceed with repair. If endoscopy has not been done previously, it may be helpful as a separate procedure before the definitive repair. It can be tedious defining the anatomy, and it is helpful to thoroughly cleanse the distal colonic segment, which usually requires irrigation from the fistula as well as the distal limb of the colostomy. A standard GoLYTELY bowel preparation should also be done.

OPERATIVE TECHNIQUE—CLOACA

The definitive repair begins with endoscopy to reacquaint the surgeon with the anatomy. We have also found

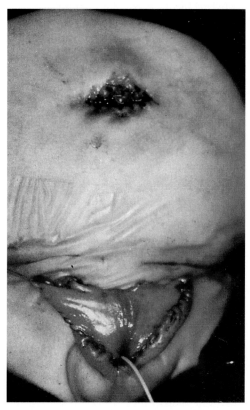

Figure 69–52. Urethra-like cloaca opened, with catheter in place; vesicostomy has also been performed.

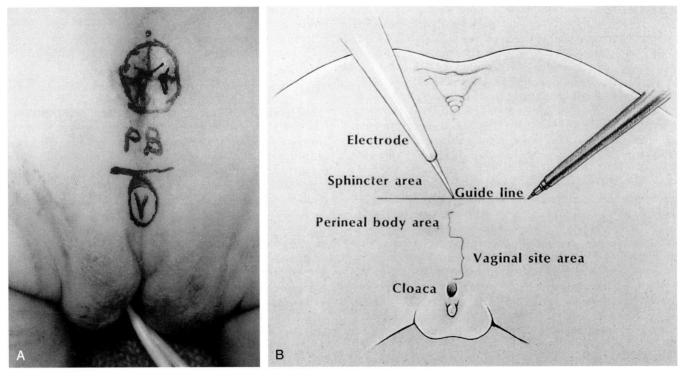

Figure 69–53. Cloaca—proposed location of vagina (V) and perineal body (PB). Rectal location is identified by electrical stimulation.

it helpful to place a Foley catheter in the bladder and different-colored Fogarty catheters in the vagina (or vaginas) and rectum. There, catheters are kept sterile during preparation. As described previously for urogenital sinus repair, a complete lower body Betadine preparation is done circumferentially from the level of the nipples to the toes, and the legs are wrapped. This allows both prone and supine positioning for perineal and abdominal surgery.

The definitive posterior sagittal anorectovaginourethroplasty (PSARVUP) is begun with the child in the prone position and the pelvis elevated on rolls to provide a jackknife position. An electrical simulator is used to determine the area of maximal contraction, which is marked with a skin-scrib and with stay sutures for later rectal placement. The proposed locations of the perineal body and vagina are also marked (Fig. 69–53). We agree with Hendren that it is at times helpful to have a sound in the common cloacal channel, but the Foley and Fogarty catheters usually suffice. The entire dissection is done in the midline until mobilization of the rectum and vagina is begun. The most important advances of Pena's PSARVUP procedure are allowing identification of the external sphincter and muscle complex of the rectum and providing excellent exposure for separation of the rectum and vagina (or vaginas) from the cloaca.

The initial incision extends from the tip of the coccyx in the midline to the posterior aspect of the cloacal orifice. Sutures mark the sphincteric muscular structures on either side as they are encountered. We have found it helpful in the past to open the cloaca in the midline posteriorly to the level of the confluences to allow easy identification of the rectal and vaginal insertions. With total urogenital mobilization, this may be less appropriate. When the rectal fistula is identified, it is opened posteriorly and multiple silk stay sutures are placed. These are helpful in mobilizing the rectum away from the vagina (or vaginas). It is important to remember that the structures share a common wall initially, and it is better to enter the vagina than either the rectum or the urethra. Circumferential dissection of the rectum to well above the sacrum may be necessary. Separation of the peritoneum can be done from this position. Rarely, a child needs to be turned to the supine position for abdominal exploration to free the rectum more proximally. Once adequate rectal mobilization to allow a tension-free anastomosis to the perineal skin has been achieved, the rectal stay sutures are used to retract the rectum away from the genitourinary structures.

Attention is now turned to vaginal separation, which is even more difficult and tedious than the rectal separation. As noted earlier, it is an error to enter the urinary tract during vaginal mobilization. In our experience, side-by-side vaginal duplication is most common, and the midline septum has usually been incised with electrocautery during the initial endoscopy. Hendren (1998) noted that 66 patients had a single vagina, 68 had two, and 20 had none. The Fogarty catheter (or catheters) within the vagina are easily palpable and the posterior aspect of the vagina at the level of the confluence is opened. Again, circumferential stay sutures are very helpful in separating the vagina from the urethra and bladder. A malleable retractor inserted into the opened posterior vaginal wall exposes the anterior wall confluence for separation. Sharp dissection is less apt to injure the urinary tract than is cautery. Making dissection even more difficult is the realization that the vagina often almost encircles the urethra. Failure to recognize this situation can result in injury to these structures. Use of the stay suture for traction aids in further mobilization of the vagina (or vaginas). The outer wall of the vagina appears white, and identification of this color is helpful. Great care should be taken to avoid devascularization of the vagina during its mobilization. Usually, vaginal mobilization allows the vagina to be "pulled through" to near the perineum. If after significant mobilization it still does not reach the perineum, skin flaps can be used to reach the spatulated vagina. With an extremely high vagina or the rare vaginal agenesis, it may be necessary to interpose a bowel segment to reach the perineum, and this obviously requires abdominal surgery. With a very dilated vagina, a vaginal flap can be created to reach the perineum, although care must be taken to avoid devascularization and stenosis (Hendren, 1986; Pena, 1989).

Before the vagina is brought to the perineum, the openings in the common cloacal channel should be closed in two to three layers with absorbable suture to create a urethra. If the cloaca is large and vagina-like, it needs to be opened in its entirety and tailored over the Foley catheter. The vagina is then secured to the perineum. If there is any concern about vaginal injury, the vagina should be rotated to avoid overlapping suture lines (Hendren, 1992). The Foley catheter is left indwelling for 2 weeks.

The perineal body is now reconstructed, and the rectum is pulled through to the perineum. Pena (1989) stressed the importance of tailoring the widened rectum. The amount of tailoring differs in each patient. The muscles must meet posterior to the rectum. The rectum is placed in the center of the sphincteric muscle mass and anastomosed to the skin. Rectal dilation is begun gradually at 2 to 3 weeks after operation, and the colostomy is closed in 3 months if all has healed well.

Once the urethral catheter has been removed, it is imperative to monitor the urinary tract and voiding dynamics closely, because poor emptying secondary to a neuropathic component is seen in almost one third of patients. If any concern arises about the child's ability to empty, clean intermittent catheterization should be started and continued until normal bladder dynamics are ensured. Failure to do this can ultimately result in urinary tract infection, hydronephrosis, and even loss of renal function.

In 1997, Pena described total urogenital mobilization as an easier way to repair cloacal anomalies. The basic technique involves 360-degree mobilization of the entire urogenital sinus after the rectum has been separated. The technique at this point is not different from that described earlier for total urogenital mobilization for urogenital sinus abnormalities. We have found this technique to be extremely helpful. It makes the most difficult part of cloacal surgery (i.e., vaginal separation) much more easily performed, and if the confluence is only 2 to 3 cm from the perineum, separation may not be necessary. In those with high vaginal confluence, separation may still be necessary, but it is much more easily accomplished (Rink et al, 1997). Concerns regarding continence have been raised, but to date the results have not been different than with standard repairs. Long-term results of the total urogenital mobilization are needed.

RESULTS OF CLOACAL SURGERY

Cloacal anomalies are exceedingly challenging to repair. The anatomy is complex and differs from patient to patient. The surgeon must be prepared for a long, tedious

procedure, must be imaginative, and must be willing to handle the tissues with great care. One might assume from this preface that results would be dismal. On the contrary, most patients lead a productive life. It is important to recognize the remarkable efforts of two individuals who have advanced the care of these children: our mentor, Dr. W. Hardy Hendren, and Dr. Alberto Pena. Their tireless efforts and attention to detail have allowed those of us who follow them to achieve excellent results for a most complex problem.

Results have generally been reviewed in terms of urinary continence, fecal continence, and sexual capabilities. Early results from a urinary standpoint were dismal: Chappel and Bleloch (1973) reported that all five of their patients had some degree of incontinence postoperatively, and Bartholomew and Gonzales (1978) had five of seven patients wet after reconstruction. **It is now clear that a high percentage of patients have a neuropathic component to their incontinence.** In 1999, De Filippo and colleagues reported urodynamic data in 26 patients with anorectal malformation (including 6 with cloacal anomalies). Twenty one of the 26 had preoperative leak point pressures greater than 40 cm H_2O, and 15 had normal MRI of the spine. This means that even those not demonstrating a neurologic abnormality may have abnormally high outlet resistance, adding to the risk of incontinence and upper tract changes. Of Hendren's 141 patients, 83 (59%) voided spontaneously with control, 40 (28%) required clean intermittent catheterization, 4 (3%) had undergone urinary diversion, and 1 (0.07%) was continent urinary diversion; only 5 (3.5%) were wet, and in 8 the results were too early to assess. Pena (1989) noted that 6 of 54 patients had a urethrovaginal fistula. Among 26 evaluable patients, Pena (1989) noted urinary continence in 14 of 19 (73%) with a normal sacrum and 2 of 7 (29%) with an abnormal sacrum.

Fecal continence is directly related to neurologic status (Pena, 1989). **Hendren (1992) noted that there are predictors that, when present, bode well for continence: good perineal raphe, well-defined anal dimple, normal spine, normal MRI, and brisk muscle reflex.** In 105 patients, Hendren (1992) noted that 47 had normal bowel function, 27 required enemas, 7 had a colostomy, 7 had fecal soiling, and 4 with anterior anus had normal control. In another series of 19 patients with a normal sacrum, 18 had voluntary bowel movements but 14 had soiling, 3 had diarrhea, and 2 were constipated. Of the 7 patients with an abnormal sacrum, 3 had voluntary bowel movements but 6 had soiling and 2 were constipated (Pena, 1989). Of 24 reported adult patients, 17 had coitus, and 6 had had children (including 5 deliveries by cesarean section and 1 vaginal delivery) (Hendren, 1998).

CONCLUSION

Management of female genital and cloacal anomalies can be exceedingly complex. In those with genital ambiguity, the need for prompt evaluation, family support, and education is mandatory. Differing cultural practices must also be respected and accepted. Surgical reconstruction requires great care of tissues, meticulous attention to detail, and a lifelong commitment by the surgeon. The complex anomalies require an entire team of physicians and nurses dedicated to the care of these problems. This most severe problem should be handled only in centers with great expertise and experience.

REFERENCES

Female Reproductive and Caudal Embryology

Alles AJ, Sulik KK: A review of caudal dysgenesis and its pathogenesis as illustrated in an animal model. Birth Defects 1993;29:83–102.

Bok G, Drews U: The role of the wolffian ducts in the formation of the sinus vagina: An organ culture study. J Embryol Exp Morphol 1983;73: 275–295.

Churchill BM, Hardy BE, et al: Urologic aspects of malformations and common abnormalities of the anus and rectum. Urol Clin North Am 1978;5:141.

Deuchar EM: Culture in vitro as a means of analysing the effect of maternal diabetes on embryonic development in rats. Ciba Found Symp 1978;63:181–197.

Duhamel B: From the mermaid to anal imperforation: The syndrome of caudal regression. Arch Dis Child 1961;36:152.

Duncan PA, Shapiro LR, et al: The MURCS association: Müllerian duct aplasia, renal aplasia, and cervicothoracic somite dysplasia. J Pediatr 1979;95:399–402.

Grosfeld JL: Anorectal anomalies. In Zuidema GD, Condon RE (eds): Shackelford's Surgery of the Alimentary Tract, 4th ed. Philadelphia, WB Saunders, 1996, p 450.

Kallen B, Winberg J: Caudal mesoderm pattern of anomalies: From renal agenesis to sirenomelia. Teratology 1974;9:99–111.

Koff AK: Development of the vagina in the human fetus. Contemp Embryol 1933;24:61.

Lynch SA, Bond PM, et al: A gene for autosomal dominant sacral agenesis maps to the holoprosencephaly region at 7q36. Nat Genet 1995;11: 93–95.

Mesrobian HG, Sessions RP, et al: Cloacal and urogenital abnormalities induced by etretinate in mice. J Urol 1994;152:675–678.

Moore KL, Persaud TVN: The Developing Human, 5th ed. Philadelphia, WB Saunders, 1995, pp 199–200.

Quan L, Smith DW: The VATER association: Vertebral defects, anal atresia, T-E fistula with esophageal atresia, radial and renal dysplasia: A spectrum of associated defects. J Pediatr 1973;82:104–107.

Warot X, Fromental-Ramain C, et al: Gene dosage-dependent effects of the Hoxa-13 and Hoxd-13 mutations on morphogenesis of the terminal parts of the digestive and urogenital tracts. Development 1997;124: 4781–4791.

Young HH: Genital Abnormalities, Hermaphroditism and Related Adrenal Diseases. Baltimore, Williams & Wilkins, 1937.

Structural Anomalies of the Female Internal Genitalia

Anonymous: The American Fertility Society classifications of adnexal adhesions, distal tubal occlusion, tubal occlusion secondary to tubal ligation, tubal pregnancies, mullerian anomalies, and intrauterine adhesions. Fertil Steril 1988;49:944.

Fedele L, Bianchi S, et al: A new laparoscopic procedure for creation of a neovagina in Mayer-Rokitansky-Kuster-Hauser syndrome. Fertil Steril 1996;66:854–857.

Fernandez CO, McFarland RD, et al: MURCS association: Ultrasonographic findings and pathologic correlation. J Ultrasound Med 1996;15: 867–870.

Lang IM, Babyn P, et al: MR imaging of paediatric uterovaginal anomalies. Pediatr Radiol 1999;29:163–170.

Major T, Borsos A, et al: Application of minimally invasive surgery in Mayer-Rokitansky-Kuster-Hauser syndrome. Acta Chir Hung 1997;36: 219–220.

Rosenberg HK, Sherman NH, et al: Mayer-Rokitansky-Kuster-Hauser syndrome: US aid to diagnosis. Radiology 1986;161:815–819.

Russ PD, Allen-Davis JT, et al: Mayer-Rokitansky-Kuster-Hauser syndrome diagnosed by magnetic resonance imaging in a 15-year-old girl. J Pediatr Adolesc Gynecol 1997;10:89–92.

Obstructive Genital Anomalies

Abbé R: New method of creating a vagina in a case of congenital absence. Med Rec 1898;54:836.

Alessandrescu D, Peltecu GC, et al: Neocolpopoiesis with split-thickness skin graft as a surgical treatment of vaginal agenesis: Retrospective review of 201 cases. Am J Obstet Gynecol 1996;175:131–138.

Allan N, Cowan LE: Uterus didelphys with unilateral imperforate vagina: Report of 4 cases. Obstet Gynecol 1963;22:442.

Ammann AM, Brewer WH, et al: A high transverse vaginal septum: Sonographic findings. J Ultrasound Med 1983;2:471–472.

Andryjowicz E, Qizilbash AH, et al: Adenocarcinoma in a cecal neovagina—complication of irradiation: Report of a case and review of literature. Gynecol Oncol 1985;21:235–239.

Ashworth MF, Morton KE, et al: Vaginoplasty using amnion. Obstet Gynecol 1986;67:443–446.

Aziz FA: Gynecologic and obstetric complications of female circumcision. Int J Gynecol Obstet 1980;17:560.

Barutcu A, Akguner M: McIndoe vaginoplasty with the inflatable vaginal stent. (Letter.) Ann Plast Surg 1998;41:568–569.

Bates GW, Wiser WL: A technique for uterine conservation in adolescents with vaginal agenesis and a functional uterus. Obstet Gynecol 1985;66:290–294.

Borruto F: Mayer-Rokitansky-Kuster Syndrome: Vecchietti's personal series. Clin Exp Obstet Gynecol 1992;19:273–274.

Bryan AL, Nigro JA, et al: One hundred cases of congenital absence of the vagina. Surg Gynecol Obstet 1949;88:79.

Burbige KA, Hensle TW: Uterus didelphys and vaginal duplication with unilateral obstruction presenting as a newborn abdominal mass. J Urol 1984;132:1195–1198.

Buscema J, Rosenshein NB, et al: Condylomata acuminata arising in a neovagina. Obstet Gynecol 1987;69:528–530.

Caloia DV, Morris H, et al: Congenital transverse vaginal septum: Vaginal hydrosonographic diagnosis. J Ultrasound Med 1998;17:261–264.

Casey AC, Laufer MR: Cervical agenesis: Septic death after surgery. Obstet Gynecol 1997;90:706.

Chen TH: Refinement of McIndoe's vaginal reconstruction with ORFIT "S" vaginal stent. Plast Reconstr Surg 1994;94:394–396.

Concannon MJ, Croll GH, et al: An intraoperative stent for McIndoe vaginal construction. Plast Reconstr Surg 1993;91:367–368.

Cramer DW, Goldstein DP, et al: Vaginal agenesis (Mayer-Rokitansky-Kuster-Hauser syndrome) associated with the N314D mutation of galactose 1-phosphate uridyltransferase (GALT). Mol Hum Reprod 1996;2: 145–148.

Cukier J, Batzofin JH, et al: Genital tract reconstruction in a patient with congenital absence of the vagina and hypoplasia of the cervix. Obstet Gynecol 1986;68(3 Suppl.):32S–36S.

Davydov SN: Experience in the field of the peritoneal colpopoiesis. In Castelazo-Ayala L, et al (ed): Gynecology and Obstetrics. Amsterdam, Excerpta Medica, 1977, pp 349–353.

Dorkenoo E: Combating female genital mutilation: An agenda for the next decade. World Health Stat Q 1996;49:142–147.

Doyle MB: Magnetic resonance imaging in mullerian fusion defects. J Reprod Med 1992;37:33–38.

Duckler L: Squamous cell carcinoma developing in an artificial vagina. Obstet Gynecol 1972;40:35–38.

Dumanian GA, Donahoe PK: Bilateral rotated buttock flaps for vaginal atresia in severely masculinized females with adrenogenital syndrome. Plast Reconstr Surg 1992;90:487–491.

Duncan PA: Embryologic pathogenesis of renal agenesis associated with cervical vertebral anomalies (Klippel-Feil phenotype). Birth Defects 1977;13:91–101.

Duncan PA, Shapiro LR, et al: The MURCS association: Müllerian duct aplasia, renal aplasia, and cervicothoracic somite dysplasia. J Pediatr 1979;95:399–402.

Eisenberg E, Farber M, et al: Complete duplication of the uterus and cervix with a unilaterally imperforate vagina. Obstet Gynecol 1982;60: 259–262.

Fall FH: A simple method for making an artificial vagina. Am J Obstet Gynecol 1940;40:906.

Fedele L, Bianchi S, et al: A new laparoscopic procedure for creation of a neovagina in Mayer-Rokitansky-Kuster-Hauser syndrome. Fertil Steril 1996;66:854–857.

Fedele L, Busacca M, et al: Laparoscopic creation of a neovagina in Mayer-Rokitansky-Kuster-Hauser syndrome by modification of Vecchietti's operation. Am J Obstet Gynecol 1994;171:268–269.

Fedele L, Portuese A, et al: Transrectal ultrasonography in the assessment of congenital vaginal canalization defects. Hum Reprod 1999;14:359–362.

Fisher K, Esham RH, et al: Scoliosis associated with typical Mayer-Rokitansky-Kuster-Hauser syndrome. South Med J 2000;93:243–246.

Frank RT: The formation of an artificial vagina without operation. Am J Obstet Gynecol 1938;35:1053.

Gauwerky JF, Wallwiener D, et al: An endoscopically assisted technique for construction of a neovagina. Arch Gynecol Obstet 1992;252:59–63.

Griffin JE, Edwards C, et al: Congenital absence of the vagina: The Mayer-Rokitansky-Kuster-Hauser syndrome. Ann Intern Med 1976;85:224–236.

Gunderson CH, Greenspan RH, et al: The Klippel-Feil syndrome: Genetic and clinical reevaluation of cervical fusion. Medicine (Baltimore) 1967;46:491–512.

Hauser GA, Schreiner WE: Mayer-Rokitansky-Kuester syndrome: Rudimentary solid bipartite uterus with solid vagina. Schweiz Med Wschr 1961;91:381.

Hendren WH, Atala A: Use of bowel for vaginal reconstruction. J Urol 1994;152:752–755; discussion, 756–757.

Hensle TW, Dean GE: Vaginal replacement in children. J Urol 1992;148:677–679.

Hensle TW, Reiley EA: Vaginal replacement in children and young adults. J Urol 1998;159:1035–1038.

Ingram JM: The bicycle seat stool in the treatment of vaginal agenesis and stenosis: A preliminary report. Am J Obstet Gynecol 1981;140:867–873.

Joseph VT: Pudendal-thigh flap vaginoplasty in the reconstruction of genital anomalies. J Pediatr Surg 1997;32:62–65.

Kuster H: Uterus bipartitus solidus rudimentarius cum vagina solida. Z Geb Gyn 1910;67:692.

Lang IM, Babyn P, et al: MR imaging of paediatric uterovaginal anomalies. Pediatr Radiol 1999;29:163–170.

Lesavoy MA: Vaginal reconstruction. Urol Clin North Am 1985;12:369–379.

Lilford RJ, Johnson N, et al: A new operation for vaginal agenesis: Construction of a neo-vagina from a rectus abdominis musculocutaneous flap. Br J Obstet Gynaecol 1989;96:1089–1094.

Lodi A: Contributo clinico statistico sulle malformazioni della vagina osservate nella clinica osterica e ginecologica di Milano dal 1906 al 1950. Ann Obstet Ginecol 1951;73:1246.

Martinez-Mora J, Isnard R, et al: Neovagina in vaginal agenesis: Surgical methods and long-term results. J Pediatr Surg 1992;27:10–14.

Mayer CAJ: Uber Verdoppelungen des Uterus und ihre Arten, nebst Bemerkungen uber Hasensharte und Wolfsrachen. J Chir Auger 1829;13:525.

McCaffrey M, Jankowska A, et al: Management of female genital mutilation: The Northwick Park Hospital experience. Br J Obstet Gynaecol 1995;102:787–790.

McCraw JB, Massey FM, et al: Vaginal reconstruction with gracilis myocutaneous flaps. Plast Reconstr Surg 1976;58:176–183.

McIndoe AH: Treatment of congenital absence and obliterative conditions of the vagina. Br J Plast Surg 1950;2:254.

McIndoe AH, Banister JB: An operation for the cure of congenital absence of the vagina. J Obstet Gynaecol Br Commonw 1938;45:490.

Meyer WR, McCoy MC, et al: Combined abdominal-perineal sonography to assist in diagnosis of transverse vaginal septum. Obstet Gynecol 1995;85:882–884.

Morton KE, Dewhurst CJ: Human amnion in the treatment of vaginal malformations. Br J Obstet Gynaecol 1986;93:50–54.

Murray JM, Gambrell RD Jr: Complete and partial vaginal agenesis. J Reprod Med 1979;22:101–105.

Ota H, Tanaka J, et al: Laparoscopy-assisted Ruge procedure for the creation of a neovagina in a patient with Mayer-Rokitansky-Kuster-Hauser syndrome. Fertil Steril 2000;73:641–644.

Pratt JH: Vaginal atresia corrected by use of small and large bowel. Clin Obstet Gynecol 1972;15:639.

Ramenofsky ML, Raffensperger JG: An abdomino-perineal-vaginal pull-through for definitive treatment of hydrometrocolpos. J Pediatr Surg 1971;6:381–387.

Rock JA, Schlaff WD, et al: The clinical management of congenital absence of the uterine cervix. Int J Gynaecol Obstet 1984;22:231–235.

Rokitansky K: Uber die sogenannten Verdoppelungen des Uterus. Med Jahrb Ost Staat 1838;26:39.

Rotmensch J, Rosenshein N, et al: Carcinoma arising in the neovagina:

Case report and review of the literature. Obstet Gynecol 1983;61:534–536.

Sadove RC, Horton CE: Utilizing full-thickness skin grafts for vaginal reconstruction. Clin Plast Surg 1988;15:443–448.

Salvatore CA, Lodovici O: Vaginal agenesis. Acta Obstet Gynecol Scand 1978;57:89–94.

Schmid-Tannwald I, Hauser GA: [Syndrome of testicular feminization and the Mayer-Rokitansky-Kuster-Syndrome: A comparison]. Geburtshilfe Frauenheilkd 1973;33:194–198.

Schmid-Tannwald I, Hauser GA: [Atypical forms of the Mayer-Rokitansky-Kuster-syndrome. (Author's translation.)] Geburtshilfe Frauenheilkd 1977;37:386–392.

Singh J, Devi YL: Pregnancy following surgical correction of nonfused mullerian bulbs and absent vagina. Obstet Gynecol 1983;61:267–269.

Strickland JL, Cameron WJ, et al: Long-term satisfaction of adults undergoing McIndoe vaginoplasty as adolescents. Adolesc Pediatr Gynecol 1993;6:135.

Strubbe EH, Lemmens JA, et al: Spinal abnormalities and the atypical form of the Mayer-Rokitansky-Kuster-Hauser syndrome. (Published erratum appears in Skeletal Radiol 1993;22:120.) Skeletal Radiol 1992;21:459–462.

Strubbe EH, Willemsen WN, et al: Mayer-Rokitansky-Kuster-Hauser syndrome: Distinction between two forms based on excretory urographic, sonographic, and laparoscopic findings. AJR Am J Roentgenol 1993;160:331–334.

Strubbe EH, Thijn CJ, et al: Evaluation of radiographic abnormalities of the hand in patients with the Mayer-Rokitansky-Kuster-Hauser syndrome. Skeletal Radiol 1987;16:227–231.

Suidan FG, Azoury RS: The transverse vaginal septum: A clinicopathologic evaluation. Obstet Gynecol 1979;54:278–283.

Tamaya T, Imai A: The use of peritoneum for vaginoplasty in 24 patients with congenital absence of the vagina. Arch Gynecol Obstet 1991;249:15–17.

Thompson DP, Lynn HB: Genital anomalies associated with solitary kidney. Mayo Clin Proc 1966;41:538–548.

Toubia N: Female circumcision as a public health issue. N Engl J Med 1994;331:712–716.

Tridenti G, Bruni V: Double uterus with a blind hemivagina and ipsilateral renal agenesis: Clinical variants in three adolescent women. Case reports and literature review. Adolesc Pediatr Gynecol 1995;8:201.

Turner-Warwick R, Kirby RS: The construction and reconstruction of the vagina with the colocecum. Surg Gynecol Obstet 1990;170:132.

Turunen A: Spinal changes in patients with congenital aplasia of the vagina. Acta Obstet Gynecol Scand 1967;46:99–106.

Vecchietti G: Le neo-vagin dans le syndrome de Rokitansky-Kuster-Hauser. Rev Med Suisse Romande 1979;99:593.

Wang Y, Hadley HR: The use of rotated vascularized pedicle flaps for complex transvaginal procedures. J Urol 1993;149:590–592.

Williams EA: Congenital absence of the vagina: A simple operation for its relief. J Obstet Gynaecol Br Commonw 1964;71:511.

Williams JK, Ingram JM, et al: Management of noncongenital vaginal stenosis and distortion by the bicycle seat stool pressure technique. Am J Obstet Gynecol 1984;150:166–167.

Williams JK, Lake M, et al: The bicycle seat stool in the treatment of vaginal agenesis and stenosis. J Obstet Gynecol Neonatal Nurs 1985;14:147–150.

Willemsen WN: Combination of the Mayer-Rokitansky-Kuster and Klippel-Feil syndrome: A case report and literature review. Eur J Obstet Gynecol Reprod Biol 1982;13:229–235.

Willemsen WN: Renal-skeletal-ear- and facial-anomalies in combination with the Mayer-Rokitansky-Kuster (MRK) syndrome. Eur J Obstet Gynecol Reprod Biol 1982;14:121–130.

Nonobstructive Genital Anomalies

Andrassy RJ, Wiener ES, et al: Progress in the surgical management of vaginal rhabdomyosarcoma: A 25-year review from the Intergroup Rhabdomyosarcoma Study Group. J Pediatr Surg 1999;34:731–734; discussion, 734–735.

Capraro VJ, Greenberg H: Adhesions of the labia minora. Obstet Gynecol 1972;39:65.

Chaouachi B, Helardot PG, et al: Urethral prolapse in 14 young female patients. Pediatr Surg 1989;4:118.

Decherney AH, Russel JB: Resectoscope management of mullerian fusion defects. Fertil Steril 1986;45:726.

Devine PC, Kessel HC: Surgical correction of urethral prolapse. J Urol 1980;123:856–857.

Desai SR, Cohen RC: Urethral prolapse in a premenarchal girl: Case report and literature review. Aust N Z J Surg 1997;67:660–662.

Epstein A, Strauss B: Prolapse of the female urethra and gangrene. Am J Surg 1937;35:563.

Fernandes ET, Dekermacher S, et al: Urethral prolapse in children. Urology 1993;41:240–242.

Finlay HVL: Adhesions of the labia minora in childhood. Proc R Soc Med 1965;58:929.

Gingell JC, Gordon IR, et al: Acute obstructive uropathy due to prolapsed ectopic ureterocele: Case report. Br J Urol 1971;43:305–308.

Gottesman JE, Sparkuhl A: Bilateral Skene duct cysts. J Pediatr 1979;94:945–946.

Hays DM, Shimada H, et al: Sarcomas of the vagina and uterus: The Intergroup Rhabdomyosarcoma Study. J Pediatr Surg 1985;20:718–724.

Hays DM, Shimada H, et al: Clinical staging and treatment results in rhabdomyosarcoma of the female genital tract among children and adolescents. Cancer 1988;61:1893–1903.

Holmes M, Upadhyay V, et al: Gartner's duct cyst with unilateral renal dysplasia presenting as an introital mass in a newborn. Pediatr Surg Int 1999;15:277–279.

Jerkins GR, Verheeck K, et al: Treatment of girls with urethral prolapse. J Urol 1984;132:732–733.

Klaus H, Stein RT: Urethral prolapse in young girls. Pediatrics 1973;52:645–648.

Leung AK, Robson WL, et al: The incidence of labial fusion in children. J Paediatr Child Health 1993;29:235–236.

Lowe FC, Hill GS, et al: Urethral prolapse in children: Insights into etiology and management. J Urol 1986;135:100–103.

McCann J, Voris J, et al: Labial adhesions and posterior fourchette injuries in childhood sexual abuse. Am J Dis Child 1988;142:659–663.

Mandell J, Colodny AH, et al: Ureteroceles in infants and children. J Urol 1980;123:921–926.

Nussbaum AR, Lebowitz RL: Interlabial masses in little girls: Review and imaging recommendations. AJR Am J Roentgenol 1983;141:65–71.

Owens SB, Morse WH: Prolapse of the female urethra in children. J Urol 1968;100:171–174.

Pradhan S, Tobon H: Vaginal cysts: A clinicopathological study of 41 cases. Int J Gynecol Pathol 1986;5:35–46.

Redman JF: Conservative management of urethral prolapse in female children. Urology 1982;19:505–506.

Richardson DA, Hajj SN, et al: Medical treatment of urethral prolapse in children. Obstet Gynecol 1982;59:69–74.

Rosenfeld DL, Lis E: Gartner's duct cyst with a single vaginal ectopic ureter and associated renal dysplasia or agenesis. J Ultrasound Med 1993;12:775–778.

Skene AJC: The anatomy and pathology of two important glands of the female urethra. Am J Obstet 1880;13:265.

Valerie E, Gilchrist BF, et al: Diagnosis and treatment of urethral prolapse in children. Urology 1999;54:1082–1084.

Classification of Urogenital Sinus and Cloacal Anomalies

Jaramillo D, Lebowitz RL, Hendren WH: The cloacal malformation: Radiologic findings and imaging recommendations. Radiology 1990;177:441–448.

Jones HW, Jones GE: The gynecological aspects of adrenal hyperplasia and allied disorders. Am J Obstet Gynecol: 1954;1330–1361.

Evaluation

Adams MC, Rink RC: Posterior prone approach to the high vagina. Dialogues Pediatr Urol 1998;21:3–4.

Adams MC, Ludlow J, Brock JW III, Rink RC: Prenatal urinary ascites and persistent cloaca: Risk factors for poor drainage of urine or meconium. J Urol 1998;160:2179–2181.

Bartholomew TH, Gonzales ET Jr: Urologic management in cloacal dysgenesis. Urology 1978;11:549–557.

Brock JW III, Hernanz-Schulmann M, Russell WR: Diagnosis of congenital adrenal hyperplasia by ultrasound in the newborn. American Academy of Pediatrics, Urology Section Meeting, San Francisco, 1998.

Cacciaguerra S, Lo Presti L, Di Leo L, et al: Prenatal diagnosis of cloacal anomaly. Scand J Urol Nephrol 1998;32:77–80.

Chappell JS, Bleloch J: Urological aspects of the cloacal type of anorectal anomaly. S Afr Med J 1973;47:817–820.

Cilento BG Jr, Benacerraf BR, Mandell J: Prenatal diagnosis of cloacal malformation. Urology 1994;43:386–388.

De Filippo RE, Shaul DB, Harrison EA, et al: Neurogenic bladder in infants born with anorectal malformations: Comparison with spinal and urologic status. J Pediatr Surg 1999;34:825–827; discussion, 828.

Donahoe PK, Gustafson ML: Early one-stage surgical reconstruction of the extremely high vagina in patients with congenital adrenal hyperplasia. J Pediatr Surg 1994;29:352–358.

Fleming SE, Hall R, Gysler M, et al: Imperforate anus in females: Frequency of genital tract involvement. Incidence of associated anomalies and functional outcome. J Pediatr Surg 1986;21:146–150.

Griffin JE, Wilson JD: The androgen resistance syndromes: 5α-reductase deficiency. Testicular feminization and related syndromes. New York, McGraw-Hill, 1989.

Hall R, Fleming SE, Gysler M, et al: The genital tract in female children with imperforate anus. Surg Gynecol Obstet 1985;151:169–171.

Hendren WH: Repair of cloacal anomalies: Current techniques. J Pediatr Surg 1986;21:1159–1176.

Hendren WH: Urological aspects of cloacal malformations. J Urol 1988;140:1207–1213.

Hendren WH: Cloacal Malformations. Philadelphia, WB Saunders, 1989.

Hendren WH: Cloaca, the most severe degree of imperforate anus: Experience with 195 cases. Ann Surg 1998;228:331–346.

Hendren WH, Atala A: Repair of the high vagina in girls with severely masculinized anatomy from the adrenogenital syndrome. J Pediatr Surg 1995;30:91–94.

Hendren WH, Crawford JD: Adrenogenital syndrome: The anatomy of the anomaly and its repair. J Pediatr Surg 1969;4:49–58.

Hensle TW, Kennedy WA: Surgical management of intersexuality. Philadelphia, WB Saunders, 1998.

Huffman JW: Some facts about the clitoris. Office Gynecology 1976;60:245–247.

Hughes IA: Congenital adrenal hyperplasia: A continuum of disorders. Lancet 1998;352:752–754.

Karlin G, Brock W, Rich M, Pena A: Persistent cloaca and phallic urethra. J Urol 1989;142:1056–1059.

Kay R, Tank ES: Principles of management of the persistent cloaca in the female newborn. J Urol 1977;117:102–104.

Klugo RC, Fisher JH, Retik AB: Management of urogenital anomalies in cloacal dysgenesis. J Urol 1974;112:832–835.

Lande IM, Hamilton EF: The antenatal sonographic visualization of cloacal dysgenesis. J Ultrasound Med 1986;5:275–278.

Pang S: Congenital adrenal hyperplasia. Endocrinol Metab Clin North Am 1997;26:853–891.

Pena A: The surgical management of persistent cloaca: Results in 54 patients treated with a posterior sagittal approach. J Pediatr Surg 1989;24:590–598.

Petikovsky BM, Walzak MP Jr, D'Addario PF: Fetal cloacal anomalies: Prenatal sonographic appearance of persistent cloaca. Acta Obstet Gynecol Scand 1986;65:517–518.

Powell DM, Newman KD, Randolph J: A proposed classification of vaginal anomalies and their surgical correction. J Pediatr Surg 1995;30:271.

Raffensberger JG: The cloaca in the newborn. Birth Defects 1988;24:111–123.

Rink RC, Adams MC: Evaluation and surgical management of the child with intersex. Prog Paediatr Urol 1999;2:67–88.

Sato Y, Pringle KC, Bergman RA, et al: Congenital anorectal anomalies: MR imaging. Radiology 1988;168:157–162.

Shalev E, Feldman E, Weiner E, Zuckerman H: Prenatal sonographic appearance of persistent cloaca. Acta Obstet Gynecol Scand 1986;65:517–518.

Surgical Reconstruction of Urogenital Sinus, Intersex Conditions, and Cloacal Malformations

Alizai NK, Thomas DFM, Lilford RJ, et al: Feminizing genitoplasty for congenital adrenal hyperplasia: What happens at puberty? J Urol 1999;161:1588–1591.

Azziz R, Mulaikal RM, Migeon CJ, et al: Congenital adrenal hyperplasia: Long term results following vaginal reconstruction. Fertil Steril 1986;46:1011–1014.

Bailez MM, Gearhart JP, Migeon CL, Rock J: Vaginal reconstruction after initial construction of the external genitalia in girls with salt-wasting adrenal hyperplasia. J Urol 1992;148:680–682.

Bartholomew TH, Gonzales ET Jr: Urologic management in cloacal dysgenesis. Urology 1978;11:549–557.

Barrett TM, Gonzales ET Jr: Reconstruction of the female external genitalia. Urol Clin North Am 1980;7:455–463.

Baskin LS, Erol A, Wu Y, et al: Anatomical studies of the human clitoris. J Urol 1999;162:1015–1020.

Chappell JS, Bleloch J: Urological aspects of the cloacal type of anorectal anomaly. S Afr Med J 1973;47:817–820.

De Filippo RE, Shaul DB, Harrison EA, et al: Neurogenic bladder in infants born with anorectal malformations: Comparison with spinal and urologic status. J Pediatr Surg 1999;34:825–827; discussion, 828.

de Jong T, Boemers M: Neonatal management of female intersex by clitorovaginoplasty. J Urol 1995;154:830–832.

Diamond M: Pediatric management of ambiguous and traumatized genitalia. J Urol 1999;162:1021–1028.

Di Benedetto V, Gioviale M, Bagnara V, et al: The anterior sagittal transanorectal approach: A modified approach to 1 stage clitoral vaginoplasty in severely masculinized female pseudohermaphrodites. Preliminary results. J Urol 1997;157:330–332.

Donahoe PK, Gustafson ML: Early one-stage surgical reconstruction of the extremely high vagina in patients with congenital adrenal hyperplasia. J Pediatr Surg 1994;29:352–358.

Dumanian GA, Donahoe PK: Bilateral rotated buttock flaps for vaginal atresia in severely masculinized females with adrenogenital syndrome. Plast Reconstr Surg 1992;90:487–491.

Fortunoff S, Lattimer JK, Edson M: Vaginoplasty technique for female pseudohermaphrodites. Surg Gynecol Obstet 1964;118:545–548.

Gearhart JP, Burnett A, Owen JH: Measurement of pudendal evoked potentials during feminizing genitoplasty: Technique and applications. J Urol 1995;153:486.

Glassberg KI, Laungani G: Reduction clitoroplasty. Urology 1981;17:604–605.

Gonzalez R, Fernandes ET: Single stage feminization genitoplasty. J Urol 1990;143:776–778.

Gross RE, Randolph J, Crigler JF, Jr: Clitorectomy for sexual abnormalities: Indications and technique. Surgery: 1966;300–308.

Hall R, Fleming SE, Gysler M, et al: The genital tract in female children with imperforate anus. Surg Gynecol Obstet 1985;151:169–171.

Hampson JG: Hemaphroditic genital appearance, rearing and eroticism in hyperadrenocorticism. Bull J Hopkins Hosp 1955;96:265.

Hendren WH: Further experience in reconstructive surgery for cloacal anomalies. J Pediatr Surg 1982;17:695–717.

Hendren WH: Repair of cloacal anomalies: Current techniques. J Pediatr Surg 1986;21:1159–1176.

Hendren WH: Cloacal malformations: Experience with 105 cases. J Pediatr Surg 1992;27:890–901.

Hendren WH: Construction of a female urethra using the vaginal wall and a buttock flap: Experience with 40 cases. J Pediatr Surg 1998;33:180–187.

Hendren WH, Atala A: Repair of the high vagina in girls with severely masculinized anatomy from the adrenogenital syndrome. J Pediatr Surg 1995;30:91–94.

Hendren WH, Crawford JD: Adrenogenital syndrome: The anatomy of the anomaly and its repair. J Pediatr Surg 1969;4:49–58.

Hendren WH, Donahoe PK: Correction of congenital abnormalities of the vagina and perineum. J Pediatr Surg 1980;15:751–763.

Jones HW, Jones GE: The gynecological aspects of adrenal hyperplasia and allied disorders. Am J Obstet Gynecol 1954;1330–1361.

Jones HW Jr, Garcia SC, Klingensmith G: Secondary surgical treatment of the masculinized external genitalia of patients with virilizing adrenal hyperplasia. Am J Obstet Gynecol 1976;48:73–75.

Kaplan I: A simple technique for shortening of the clitoris without amputation. Obstet Gynecol 1967;29:270–271.

Kay R, Tank ES: Principles of management of the persistent cloaca in the female newborn. J Urol 1977;117:102–104.

Kogan SJ, Smey P, Levitt SB: Subtunical total reduction clitoroplasty: A safe modification of existing techniques. J Urol 1983;130:746–748.

Kumar H, Kiefer JH, Rosenthal IE, Clark SS: Clitoroplasty: Experience during a 19 year period. J Urol 1974;111:81–84.

Lattimer JK: Relocation and recession of the enlarged clitoris with preservation of the glans: An alternative to amputation. J Urol 1961;86:113–116.

Ludwikowski B, Hayward O, Gonzalez R: Total urogenital sinus mobilization: Expanded applications. BJU Int 1999;83:820–822.

Mandell J, Haskins J, Hammond MG: Surgical correction of external genitalia and lower genitourinary tract of markedly virilized child. Urology 1988;31:234–236.

Marberger H: Hunterian Lecture. Royal College of Surgeons, 1975.

Mollard P, Juskiewenski, Sarkissian J: Clitoroplasty in intersex: A new technique. Br J Urol 1981;53:371–373.

Mollitt DL, Schullinger JN, Santulli TV, Hensle TW: Complications at menarche of urogenital sinus with associated anorectal malformations. J Pediatr Surg 1981;16:349–352.

Okonkwo JE, Crocker KM: Cloacal dysgenesis. Obstet Gynecol 1977;50:97–101.

Parrott TS, Woodard JR: Abdominoperitoneal approach to management of the high, short vagina in the adrenogenital syndrome. J Urol 1991;146:647–648.

Passerini G: Vaginoplasty in severely virilized CAH females. Dialogues in Pediatric Urology 1998;21:2–3.

Passerini-Glazel G: A new 1-stage procedure for clitorovaginoplasty in severely masculinized female pseudohermaphrodites. J Urol 1989;142(2 Pt 2):565–568.

Passerini-Glazel G: Vaginoplasty and clitoroplasty for the adrenogenital syndrome. In Hinman F Jr (ed): Atlas of Pediatric Urologic Surgery. Philadelphia, WB Saunders, 1994, p 635.

Pellerin D: La reimplantation du clitoris: Refection plastique du pseudohermaphrodisme feminin. Memoires Acad Chir 1965;91:965–968.

Pena A: The surgical management of persistent cloaca: Results in 54 patients treated with a posterior sagittal approach. J Pediatr Surg 1989;24:590–598.

Pena A: Total urogenital mobilization: An easier way to repair cloacas. J Pediatr Surg 1997;32:267–268.

Raffensberger JG: The cloaca in the newborn. Birth Defects 1988;24:111–123.

Rajfer J, Ehrlich RM, Goodwin WE: Reduction clitoroplasty via ventral approach. J Urol 1982;128:341–343.

Randolph JG, Hung W: Reduction clitoroplasty in females with hypertrophied clitoris. J Pediatr Surg 1970;5:224–231.

Rink RC, Pope JC, Kropp BP, et al: Reconstruction of the high urogenital sinus: Early perineal prone approach without division of the rectum. J Urol 1997;158:1293–1297.

Rink RC, Adams MC: Feminizing genitoplasty: State of the art. World J Urol 1998;16:212–218.

Rink RC, Adams MC: Evaluation and surgical management of the child with intersex. Progr Paediatr Urol 1999;2:67–88.

Rossi F, DeCastro R, Ceccarelli PL, Domini R: Anterior sagittal transanorectal approach to the posterior urethra in the pediatric age group. J Urol 1998;160:1773–1177.

Schmid MA: Plastische korrectur des auBeren Genitale bei einem mannlichen scheinzwitter. Langenbecks Arch Klin Chir 1961;298:977.

Shaw A: Subcutaneous reduction clitoroplasty. J Pediatr Surg 1977;12:331–338.

Snyder H III, Retik AB, Bauer SB, Colodny AH: Feminizing genitoplasty: A synthesis. J Urol 1983;129:1024–1026.

Sotiropoulos A, Morishima A, Homsy Y, Lattimer JK: Long-term assessment of genital reconstruction in female pseudohermaphrodites. J Urol 1976;115:599–601.

Spence HM, Allen TD: Genital reconstruction in the female with the adrenogenital syndrome. Br J Urol 1973;45:126–130.

70
PEDIATRIC UROLOGIC ONCOLOGY

Michael Ritchey, MD

Neuroblastoma
  Epidemiology and Genetics
  Pathology
  Clinical Presentation and Pattern of Spread
  Diagnosis
  Staging
  Treatment

Genitourinary Rhabdomyosarcoma
  Etiology, Epidemiology, and Genetics
  Pathology and Patterns of Spread
  Clinical Grouping and Staging
  Treatment: General Principles
  Specific Sites

Wilms' Tumor
  Epidemiology
  Biology
  Diagnosis and Evaluation
  Staging

  Treatment
Other Renal Tumors
  Clear Cell Sarcoma of the Kidney
  Rhabdoid Tumor of the Kidney
  Congenital Mesoblastic Nephroma
  Solitary Multilocular Cyst and Cystic Partially
    Differentiated Nephroblastoma
  Metanephric Adenofibroma
  Renal Cell Carcinoma
  Angiomyolipoma
  Miscellaneous Tumors
Testicular Tumors
  Etiology and Genetics
  Pathology
  Diagnosis and Staging
  Germ Cell Tumors
  Gonadal Stomal Tumors

NEUROBLASTOMA

Neuroblastoma is known to arise from cells of the neural crest that form the adrenal medulla and sympathetic ganglia. Tumors may occur anywhere along the sympathetic chain within the neck, thorax, retroperitoneum, or pelvis or in the adrenal gland. Seventy-five percent arise in the retroperitoneum, 50% in the adrenal, and 25% in the paravertebral ganglia. The variety of locations in which these tumors can arise and the spectrum of their differentiation result in a wide range of clinical presentations and behaviors (Brodeur, 1991). These tumors can undergo spontaneous regression (Brodeur, 1991), differentiate to benign neoplasms (Everson and Cole, 1966), or exhibit extremely malignant behavior.

Epidemiology and Genetics

Incidence

Neuroblastoma is the most common extracranial solid tumor in children, accounting for 8% to 10% of all childhood cancers. In the United States, the annual incidence is 10 cases per 1 million live births. It is the most common malignant tumor of infancy, with 50% of cases occurring in children younger than 2 years of age and 75% diagnosed by the fourth year of life (Fortner et al, 1968).

Genetics

There have been a number of familial cases reported, which are postulated to represent an autosomal dominant pattern of inheritance (Knudson and Strong, 1972; Robertson et al, 1991). The median age at diagnosis of neuroblastoma is 21 months, but in familial cases it is 9 months (Kushner et al, 1986). At least 20% of patients with familial neuroblastoma have bilateral adrenal or multifocal primary tumors. The risk for development of neuroblastoma in a sibling or offspring of a patient with neuroblastoma is less than 6% (Kushner et al, 1986).

Constitutional Chromosome Abnormalities

Numerous karyotypic abnormalities have been found in neuroblastoma and these are recognized to have prognostic significance. These changes occur in the form of chromosomal deletions, translocations, and cytogenetic evidence of gene amplification. Deletion of the short arm of chromosome 1 is found in 70% to 80% of neuroblastomas and is an adverse prognostic marker (Brodeur et al, 1992; Caron et al, 1996). The deletions are of various lengths, but in a series of eight cases a consensus deletion included the segment 1p36.1–2, suggesting that genetic information related to neuroblastoma tumorigenesis is located in that segment (Weith et al, 1989). There have been two reports of constitutional abnormalities involving the short arm of chromosome 1 (Lampert et al, 1988; Laureys et al, 1990).

Aneuploidy of the tumor DNA occurs in a significant number of cases and is a favorable prognostic indicator, whereas amplification of the N-*myc* oncogene is an adverse prognostic indicator (Look et al, 1991; Muraji et al, 1993). These findings have been so striking that neuroblastoma was the first tumor in which the intensity of chemotherapy was determined not only by the stage and histology of the tumor but by its "biologic markers," which were primarily chromosomal (Matthay et al, 1998).

Embryology and Spontaneous Regression

In 1963, Beckwith and Perrin coined the term *in situ neuroblastoma* for small nodules of neuroblastoma cells, found incidentally within the adrenal gland, that are histologically indistinguishable from neuroblastoma. In situ neuroblastoma was found in 1 of 224 infants younger than 3 months of age during postmortem examination. This represents an incidence approximately 40 to 45 times greater than that of clinical tumors, suggesting that these small tumors regress spontaneously in most cases. Studies have shown that these neuroblastic nodules are found in all fetuses studied and generally regress (Ikeda et al, 1981). Neuroblastoma identified by prenatal ultrasound has also been shown to have a clinically favorable course (Ho et al, 1993).

The concept of in situ neuroblastoma has been used to support the argument that many neuroblastomas arise and regress spontaneously. This concept has been further supported by population-based studies in Quebec province and in Japan, where prospective screening of infants for neuroblastoma has been performed based on urinary catecholamine excretion. An increased number of children were identified with low-stage neuroblastoma, a higher frequency than present clinically, but there was no decrease in the incidence of advanced-stage tumors seen at an older age (Hayashi et al, 1995; Woods et al, 1996). Evaluation of adrenal tumors resected in the neonatal period, whether cystic or solid, showed that in most the "biologic markers" were favorable (Kozakewich et al, 1998). Spontaneous regression of these perinatally identified lesions has also been demonstrated radiographically (Holgerson et al, 1996).

Pathology

Neuroblastoma, ganglioneuroblastoma, and ganglioneuroma display a histologic spectrum of maturation and differentiation. A new grading classification of neuroblastoma introduced in 1984 by Shimada has helped to define subtypes of ganglioneuroblastoma and neuroblastoma (Shimada et al, 1984, 1999a, 1999b). Ganglioneuroma is a histologically benign, fully differentiated counterpart of neuroblastoma. It is unclear whether ganglioneuroma arises de novo or by maturation of a preexisting neuroblastoma or ganglioneuroblastoma. Metastatic lesions have been observed to develop the histology of mature ganglioneuroma, supporting the latter theory (Hayes et al, 1989).

The Shimada classification is an age-linked histopathologic classification. One of its important aspects is determining whether the tumor is stroma poor or stroma rich. Patients with stroma-poor tumors with unfavorable histopathologic features have a very poor prognosis (less than 10% survival) (Shimada et al, 1984). **Stroma-rich tumors can be separated into three subgroups: nodular, intermixed, and well differentiated. Tumors in the latter two categories more closely resemble ganglioneuroblastoma or immature ganglioneuroma and carry a higher rate of survival.** The stroma-poor tumors can be divided into favorable and unfavorable subgroups based on the patient's age at diagnosis, the degree of histologic maturation, and the mitotic rate. When compared with other clinical features, these histologic patterns were independently predictive of outcome (Shimada et al, 1984).

In contrast to neuroblastomas, ganglioneuromas are most often diagnosed in older children and are usually located in the posterior mediastinum and retroperitoneum, with only a small number arising in the adrenal glands (Enzinger and Weiss, 1988). **Ganglioneuromas often grow to a very large size before they cause symptoms as a result of compression of adjacent structures or extension into the spinal canal** (Benjamin et al, 1972).

Clinical Presentation and Pattern of Spread

The clinical manifestations of neuroblastoma vary widely. Although most children present with abdominal pain or a palpable mass, many present with manifestations of their metastatic disease, including bone or joint pain and periorbital ecchymosis. Thoracic lesions may result in respiratory symptoms of cough or dyspnea. Direct extension of the tumor into the spinal canal may produce neurologic deficits as a result cord compression.

Most primary tumors arise within the abdomen (65%); the frequency of adrenal tumors is slightly higher in children than in infants. Physical examination frequently reveals a fixed, hard abdominal mass. Pelvic neuroblastomas arising from the organ of Zuckerkandl account for only 4% of tumors (Haase et al, 1995). Extrinsic compression of the bowel and bladder can produce symptoms of urinary retention and constipation (Fig. 70–1).

Metastases are present in 70% of patients with neuroblastoma at diagnosis and can be responsible for a variety of the clinical signs and symptoms at presentation. A number of unique paraneoplastic syndromes have been associated with both localized and disseminated neuroblastoma. Symptoms produced by catecholamine release may mimic those seen in pheochromocytoma: paroxysmal

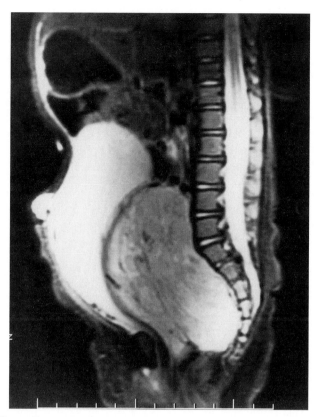

Figure 70–1. MRI demonstrating compression of bowel and bladder by a pelvic neuroblastoma.

hypertension, palpitations, flushing, and headache. Secretion of vasoactive intestinal peptide (VIP) by the tumor can produce severe watery diarrhea and hypokalemia (Cooney et al, 1982). Another unusual presentation of neuroblastoma is acute myoclonic encephalopathy, in which patients develop myoclonus, rapid multidirectional eye movements (opsoclonus), and ataxia. It is thought to result from an interaction between antibodies produced against the neuroblastoma and normal neural tissues (Farrelly et al, 1984; Connolly et al, 1997). Although this syndrome is associated with a favorable outcome from an oncologic perspective (Altman and Baehner, 1976), prolonged neurologic impairment is the rule, and symptomatic therapy is often required (Koh et al, 1994; Russo et al, 1997). Adrenocorticotropic hormone (ACTH) is the most effective therapy, but other treatments include high-dose gammaglobulin and cyclophosphamide.

Diagnosis

Laboratory Evaluation

When sensitive techniques are used, increased levels of urinary metabolites of catecholamines, vanillylmandelic acid (VMA), and homovanillic acid (HVA) are found in 90% to 95% of patients (Williams and Greer, 1963). Therapy with various modalities has been shown to produce a reduction in catecholamine metabolite excretion in most patients (Gerson and Koop, 1974). These metabolites can also be monitored to detect tumor relapse.

Anemia is noted in children with widespread bone marrow involvement. Studies suggest that marrow biopsies add substantially to the detection of marrow involvement by tumor, compared with marrow aspirates alone (Franklin and Pritchard, 1983). It is recommended that two marrow aspirates and two biopsies be performed. In the near future, it is likely that neuroblastoma-specific immunocytology of marrow aspirates will obviate the need for marrow biopsies in most patients (Moss et al, 1985; Hsiao et al, 1990).

Imaging

Imaging studies play an important role in the evaluation of a child with neuroblastoma. Plain radiographs may demonstrate a calcified abdominal or posterior mediastinal mass. Both bone scintigraphy and skeletal survey should be used to detect cortical bone metastases (Heisel et al, 1983). These lesions occur most commonly in the long bones and skull. If the skeletal films are negative, a radionuclide bone scan may detect metastases at an earlier stage. A newer method of imaging both the tumor and metastatic sites is with radiolabeled iodine I 131 metaiodobenzylguanidine (MIBG) (Geatti et al, 1985), which is taken up by the adrenergic secretory vesicles of the tumor cells in both primary and metastatic sites. MIBG scintigraphy can be used to determine the extent of disease and also to detect recurrence of tumor after the completion of therapy (Geatti et al, 1985). Others have reported that the findings of MIBG scans have little impact on patient treatment (Andrich et al, 1996). Ultrasound, CT, and MRI studies provide more information about abdominal disease, including liver metastases. Invasion of the renal parenchyma is not common, but it can be detected radiographically by CT (Albregts et al, 1994). MRI has advantages over CT in the evaluation of intraspinal tumor extension and in demonstrating the relationship between the major vessels and the tumor (Azizhkan and Haase, 1993).

Screening

Mass population screening for neuroblastoma has been widely used in Japan for more than 10 years (Nishi et al, 1987). The goal of screening programs is to detect disease at an earlier stage and to decrease the number of older children with advanced-stage disease, thereby improving survival. An increased number of infants younger than 1 year of age have been diagnosed through the mass screening program (Ishimoto et al, 1990), and most of these patients have lower-stage tumors (Sawada, 1992). Before mass screening started, 20% of neuroblastoma cases were diagnosed before 1 year of age, compared with 55% afterward. However, the number of children older than 1 year of age with advanced-stage disease has not decreased.

There are biologic differences between tumors diagnosed by screening and those detected clinically (Hayashi et al, 1992). In a review of 48 cases discovered by screening, no tumors were observed to have amplified N-*myc* oncogene expression (Ishimoto et al, 1991). Furthermore, 80% had a diploid chromosome pattern, which is associated with a favorable prognosis. On follow-up, all 48 patients were still alive without tumor. In another series of 357 patients whose tumors were diagnosed by mass screening, the over-

Table 70–1. INTERNATIONAL NEUROBLASTOMA STAGING SYSTEM

Stage	Definition
1	Localized tumor with complete gross excision, with or without microscopic residual disease; representative ipsilateral lymph nodes negative for tumor microscopically (nodes attached to and removed with the primary tumor may be positive).
2A	Localized tumor with incomplete gross excision; representative ipsilateral nonadherent lymph nodes negative for tumor microscopically.
2B	Localized tumor with or without complete gross excision, with ipsilateral nonadherent lymph nodes positive for tumor; enlarged contralateral lymph nodes must be negative microscopically.
3	Unresectable unilateral tumor infiltrating across the midline,* with or without regional lymph node involvement; or localized unilateral tumor with contralateral regional lymph node involvement; or midline tumor with bilateral extension by infiltration (unresectable) or by lymph node involvement.
4	Any primary tumor with dissemination to distant lymph nodes, bone, bone marrow, liver, skin, and/or other organs.
4S	Localized primary tumor (as defined for stage 1, 2A, or 2B), with dissemination limited to skin, liver, and/or bone marrow (less than 10% tumor) in infants <1 year of age.

*The midline is defined as the vertebral column. Tumors originating on one side and crossing the midline must infiltrate to or beyond the opposite side of the vertebral column.

all survival rate was 97% (Sawada, 1992). Given the favorable biologic characteristics of tumors discovered by screening, it is possible that they would have the same excellent survival statistics if they were discovered later in life because of clinical symptoms.

Staging

Staging of neuroblastoma is an important aspect of management. The stage of the disease is a significant prognostic variable that determines adjuvant therapy. The International Neuroblastoma Staging System (INSS) is based on clinical, radiographic, and surgical evaluation of children with neuroblastoma (Brodeur et al, 1993) (Table 70–1). Earlier staging systems gave generally comparable results in terms of distinguishing low-stage, good-prognosis disease from high-stage, poor-prognosis disease. The biggest differences arises when the various systems are applied to those with intermediate-stage disease. It is in this cohort of children where use of the Risk Group classification, which combines pathologic findings, stage, and several of the biologic markers, best defines the child's risk for progressive disease (Katzenstein and Cohn, 1998). Although the classification appears complex (Table 70–2), it provides the most accurate assessment of how aggressive chemotherapy and radiotherapy should be to cure the child.

Prognostic Factors

Many variables affect the prognosis of neuroblastoma. In addition to the clinical features, there are now many biologic studies that can be used to stratify patients for treatment.

CLINICAL VARIABLES

Age still remains an important indicator of outcome, as originally reported by Breslow (Breslow and McCann, 1971). **With current treatment, children aged 1 year or younger have an improved survival when compared with older children** (Nitschke et al, 1988). **This may be attributed to more favorable biologic parameters in tumors diagnosed at this age. The** *site of origin* **is of significance: Better survival is noted for nonadrenal primary tumors** (Haase et al, 1995). Most children with thoracic neuroblastoma present at a younger age with localized disease and have improved survival even when corrected for age and stage (Adams et al, 1993). Tumors in this site are less likely to have N-*myc* amplification and more likely to have a DNA index greater than 1.0, both favorable prognostic indicators (Morris et al, 1995).

Stage of the disease is another powerful independent

Table 70–2. RISK GROUP CLASSIFICATION

Risk Group	INSS stage	Age (days)	N-*myc* status	DNA Index	Shimada Histopathology
Low	1	Any	Any	Any	Any
	2A,2B	<365	Any	Any	Any
	2A,2B	≥365	Nonamplified	Any	Any
	2A,2B	≥365	Amplified	Any	Favorable
	4S	<365	Nonamplified	>1.0	Favorable
Intermediate	3	<365	Nonamplified	Any	Any
	3	≥365	Nonamplified	Any	Favorable
	4	<365	Nonamplified	Any	Any
	4S	<365	Nonamplified	1.0	Favorable
	4S	<365	Nonamplified	Any	Unfavorable
High	2A,2B	≥365	Amplified	Any	Unfavorable
	3	<365	Amplified	Any	Any
	3	≥365	Nonamplified	Any	Unfavorable
	3	≥365	Amplified	Any	Any
	4	<365	Amplified	Any	Any
	4	≥365	Any	Any	Any
	4S	<365	Amplified	Any	Any

INSS, International Neuroblastoma Staging System.

prognostic indicator. **Virtually all stage I patients with complete resection of the primary tumor survive. Stage II patients also have a more favorable survival prospect, even though there may be incomplete excision** (Matthay et al, 1989). People with advanced regional disease, stages III and IV, fare less well and require more aggressive treatment. The proportion of patients presenting with localized, regional, or metastatic disease is age dependent (Nitschke et al, 1988). The overall prognosis for stages I, II, or IV-S is between 75% and 90%, whereas those children with stage IV disease have a 2-year disease-free survival range of 19% to 30% despite intensive therapy including bone marrow transplantation. The outcome for infants younger than 1 year of age is substantially better than for older patients with the same stage of disease.

Stage IV-S (S = special) **is a distinct category referring to infants with small primary tumors and liver, skin, and bone marrow metastases without radiographic evidence of bone metastases. It was first proposed by Evans and coworkers in 1980. This group of patients has a good prognosis, ranging from 80% to 87%. Many of these tumors undergo spontaneous regression** (Evans et al, 1987; Haas et al, 1990). The tumors in children with stage IV-S neuroblastoma in general have favorable prognostic findings not typically seen in children with stage IV disease (Hachitanda et al, 1991).

BIOLOGIC VARIABLES

The presence of homogeneously staining regions and double minute chromosomes was noted in approximately one third of neuroblastoma tumors. These abnormalities are cytogenic manifestations of gene amplification, and it was subsequently found that the N-*myc* oncogene was mapped to these regions. The association of N-*myc* amplification with the pathogenesis of neuroblastoma is unclear, but N-*myc* amplification is almost always present at the time of diagnosis (Brodeur, 1991). **Seeger and colleagues (1985, 1988) showed that N-*myc* amplification is associated with rapid tumor progression and a poor prognosis. Amplification is found in 5% to 10% of patients with low-stage or stage IV-S (Hachitanda et al, 1991) but in 30% to 40% of those with advanced-stage disease (Brodeur and Fong, 1989; Brodeur, 1990). The poor prognosis associated with N-*myc* amplification is independent of patient age or stage of disease at presentation.** However, not all patients with a poor outcome have N-*myc* amplification. Many advanced-stage tumors lack N-*myc* at diagnosis, and recurrence or progression of disease develops in most of these patients.

DNA content of tumor cells and ploidy number have been reported to have prognostic value in patients with neuroblastoma (Cohn et al, 1990). Studies of DNA content measured by flow cytometry showed that a "hyperdiploid" karyotype (or increased DNA content) was associated with a favorable outcome (Look et al, 1984: Kusafuka et al, 1994). DNA diploidy and tetraploidy were associated with decreased survival. Deletions of the short arm of chromosome 1 have been found in 70% to 80% of the near-diploid tumors that have been karyotyped (Brodeur and Fong, 1989; Brodeur, 1990). Preliminary studies suggest a correlation between 1p deletion and poor survival (Brodeur

and Fong, 1989; Hayashi et al, 1989). Because there is an association between N-*myc* amplification and 1p deletion, it remains to be determined whether this finding has independent prognostic significance.

Children currently treated on protocols of the Pediatric Oncology Group and the Children's Cancer Group are assigned to a risk group that is determined by age, stage of disease, N-*myc* status, histologic grade, and DNA ploidy (Katzenstein et al, 1998) (see Table 70–2). Other factors that have been demonstrated to have prognostic significance, although they are often associated with these genetic abnormalities, include expression of the gene encoding the high-affinity nerve growth factor receptor (termed *TRKA* proto-oncogene) and the low-affinity nerve growth factor receptor (Tanaka et al, 1995). Both are favorable prognostic predictors and are inversely related to amplification of N-*myc* oncogene (Nakagawara et al, 1993). Lack of expression of CD44 glycoprotein on the tumor cell surface and increased levels of serum ferritin, serum neuron-specific enolase, and serum lactate dehydrogenase are all adverse prognostic factors (Chan et al, 1991; Silber et al, 1991).

Treatment

The treatment modalities primarily used in the management of neuroblastoma are surgery, chemotherapy, and radiation therapy. The role of each in individual patients varies depending on tumor stage, age, and biologic prognostic factors. These can be used to stratify patients into favorable and unfavorable categories by risk group (see Table 70–2).

Surgery

The goals of surgery are to establish the diagnosis, stage the tumor, excise the tumor (if localized), and provide tissue for biologic studies. Resectability of the primary tumor should take into consideration tumor location, mobility, relationship to major vessels, and overall prognosis of the patient. With the efficacy of modern chemotherapy to reduce the size of primary tumors, sacrifice of vital structures to achieve resection at diagnosis should be avoided, particularly in young children in whom prognosis is excellent.

LOW-RISK DISEASE (STAGES I, II, AND IV-S)

Children with stage I neuroblastoma have a disease-free survival rate of greater than 90% with surgical excision alone (O'Neill et al, 1985; Nitschke et al, 1988; DeBernardi et al, 1995). **Chemotherapy is indicated only in the event of recurrence unless the child has N-*myc* amplification and unfavorable histology.** The Pediatric Oncology Group reviewed 101 children with localized neuroblastoma who had complete gross excision of the primary tumor (Nitschke et al, 1988). Nine patients experienced relapse, but six were salvaged with chemotherapy. Radiation therapy has no role in this subset of patients. With current use of the risk factor grading, those children with recurrence in the past may be identified now as the small number with adverse biologic markers.

All patients with INSS stage IIA disease and infants

with INSS stage IIB/III disease should undergo surgical resection followed by postoperative chemotherapy (Green et al, 1981). **Radical resection resulting in removal of normal organs, particularly the kidney, is not justified in this group of patients.** Radiation of the local tumor bed has been advocated for treatment of residual disease in stage II cases. However, a review of 156 patients with stage II neuroblastoma found a 90% 6-year progression-free survival rate regardless of whether radiation therapy was used (Matthay et al, 1989). Therefore, radiation should be reserved for those patients who fail to respond to either primary or secondary chemotherapy. In stage III disease, or in stage II with extensive tumor around the kidney and renal vessels, preoperative treatment with chemotherapy significantly decreases the risk of nephrectomy as a result of resection of the tumor (Shamberger et al, 1998) (Fig. 70–2).

The generally favorable behavior of IV-S disease has been explained with the understanding of biologic markers. The vast majority of these infants have tumors with entirely favorable markers, explaining their favorable behavior. However, a small percentage have adverse markers, and it is these children who have progressive disease that often is fatal. Resection of the primary is not mandatory (Nickerson et al, 1985; Evans et al, 1987). Although excellent survival has been reported after surgery (Martinez et al, 1992), information regarding histologic prognostic factors was not available for all of these patients. In a review of 110 infants with stage IV-S disease, the entire cohort had an estimated 3-year survival rate of 85% ± 4% (Katzenstein et al, 1998). This rate was significantly decreased, to 68% ± 12%, for infants whose tumors were diploid; to 44% ± 33% for those with N-*myc* amplification; and to 33% ± 19% for those with unfavorable histology. Of note, there was no statistical difference in survival rate for infants who underwent complete resection of their primary tumor compared with those who had

partial resection or only biopsy. Patients with extensive metastatic disease and N-*myc* amplification represent a high-risk group (Martinez et al, 1992). These patients should be considered for a more aggressive treatment with multimodal therapy, according to the risk group classification (see Table 70–2).

HIGH-RISK DISEASE (STAGES III AND IV)

There is some debate regarding the extent of surgical resection that is required for stage III lesions. A report from the Children's Cancer Group of 58 patients with stage III disease found that 8 of 12 patients with initial complete excision, and 12 of 14 with subsequent resection of the primary tumor, were long-term survivors (Haase et al, 1989). This contrasts with only 9 of 32 survivors among patients in whom complete tumor excision could not be accomplished. Significant morbidity was reported in association with the surgical procedures, including 21 major complications. The Italian Cooperative Group for Neuroblastoma found that complete resection after chemotherapy of extensive unresectable neuroblastoma was associated with improved survival, compared with partial resection only (Garaventa et al, 1993). Similar results have been noted by others (LeTourneau et al, 1985; O'Neill et al, 1985; Powis et al, 1996). It has been suggested by some that even children with stage III disease do not need cytotoxic therapy if the biologic marker N-*myc* amplification is not present (Kushner et al, 1996). These results are not widely accepted, however, and confirmatory studies are required before this policy can be widely adopted.

The evidence is conflicting in stage IV disease between studies that support (Cecchetto et al, 1983; LeTourneau et al, 1985; Haase et al, 1991; Tsuschida et al, 1992; LaQuaglia et al, 1994; Chamberlain et al, 1995; DeCou et al, 1995) and those that refute (Sitarz et al, 1983; Matsumura et al, 1988; Adams et al, 1993; Kiely, 1994) the role of

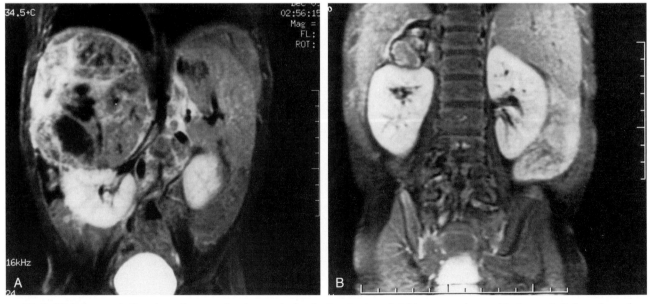

Figure 70–2. CT before and after chemotherapy, showing marked reduction in size of right suprarenal neuroblastoma. *A,* Before chemotherapy. *B,* After chemotherapy.

extensive resection. In a retrospective review, Kiely (1994) compared the results of radical tumor resection with those of more conventional surgery in patients with stage III and IV disease. He found no difference in survival between 46 patients treated with radical surgical procedures and 34 patients treated with more conventional surgery. Shorter and colleagues (1995) also did not find any evidence that the extent of surgical resection had an impact on the survival of stage IV patients.

Usually the safest approach for advanced tumors is to defer tumor resection until after initial chemotherapy (Berthold et al, 1989; Shamberger et al, 1991; Shochat, 1992). **After chemotherapy, the tumors are smaller and firmer, with less risk of rupture and hemorrhage, resulting in a decreased rate of complications, particularly nephrectomy** (Shamberger et al, 1998) (see Fig. 70–2). One specific complication that is encountered after resection of extensive tumor surrounding the celiac axis and the superior mesenteric artery is diarrhea. It is thought to result from resection of the autonomic nerves to the gut that are present anterior to the aorta at the base of the superior mesenteric artery and the celiac axis (Rees et al, 1998).

Surgery usually is performed 13 to 18 weeks after initiation of chemotherapy, allowing three to four courses of treatment (Azizkhan and Haase, 1993). Some tumors remain inoperable even after chemotherapy. Other attempts at local tumor control for unresectable diseases have included the use of intraoperative radiation therapy. This technique has the advantage of delivering a higher dose of radiation to the operative field while sparing normal adjacent tissues (Leavey et al, 1997). As control of distant metastasis in neuroblastoma improves with advances in treatment, surgical resection will become critical.

Chemotherapy

A variety of multiagent treatment regimens have been developed to treat high-risk patients with neuroblastoma. The goal of this treatment intensification is better disease control. Although initial response rates are improving, with a prolonged time to progression of disease, relapse continues to be a major problem, and the 4-year overall survival rate in stage IV disease is 20% (Ikeda et al, 1989; Haase et al, 1991). The dose intensification of chemotherapy needed for local tumor control results in significant myelosuppression, limiting the amount of therapy that can be given. This has prompted the use of autologous bone marrow transplantation after sublethal chemotherapy or total-body irradiation.

The use of marrow-ablative chemoradiotherapy followed by autologous marrow reinfusion has resulted in complete remission in up to 50% of patients with recurrent stage IV disease (Moss et al, 1987; Seeger et al, 1991; Dinndorf et al, 1992; Mugishima et al, 1994; Matthay et al, 1995; Grupp et al, 2000). However, a significant problem is the risk for late relapse. The presence of bulky disease results in increased failure. Tumor debulking with surgery or radiation therapy is warranted before autologous bone marrow transplantation. There are many questions yet to be resolved with this modality of treatment. Toxicity of bone marrow transplantation can be lethal, and the long-term complications that will occur in patients with successful

transplantation are unknown. However, these risks are necessary, given that long-term survival is difficult to achieve in these patients without such aggressive therapy.

Another modality in the treatment of metastatic neuroblastoma is the use of ^{131}I-MIBG (Hutchinson et al, 1992). The finding that both the primary tumor and metastatic areas take up this radiotracer suggested the possibility that therapeutic doses can be delivered to the tumor. Preliminary analysis indicates that objective responses do occur in terms of reduction of tumor volume.

Because increasing the intensity of chemotherapy appears to have reached its limit with the use of double autologous bone marrow transplantation, other routes of treatment must be identified. The use of biologic modifiers is being investigated (Villablanca et al, 1995). The benefit of treatment with 13-*cis*-retinoic acid for a 6-month period after cytotoxic therapy was demonstrated in one population with advanced-stage disease (Matthay et al, 1999). Other avenues of treatment in current phase 1 and phase 2 trials include vaccine therapy and antibody therapy.

GENITOURINARY RHABDOMYOSARCOMA

Rhabdomyosarcoma (RMS) is the most common soft tissue sarcoma in infants and children, accounting for approximately half of all pediatric soft tissue sarcomas and 15% of all pediatric solid tumors. **Fifteen percent to 20% of all cases of RMS arise from the genitourinary system** (Maurer et al, 1988). **The most common genitourinary sites are prostate, bladder, and paratestis; vagina and uterus are relatively unusual sites. Survival rates vary with the site; tumors at certain sites, such as vagina and paratestis, have a better prognosis than bladder or prostate primaries** (Rodary et al, 1988; Crist et al, 1990). There is a bimodal age distribution, with a peak incidence in the first 2 years of life and again at adolescence (La-Quaglia et al, 1994).

Etiology, Epidemiology, and Genetics

Subgroups of children with a genetic predisposition to the development of RMS have been identified. The Li-Fraumeni syndrome associates childhood sarcomas with mothers who have an excess of premenopausal breast cancer and with siblings who have an increased risk of cancer (Li and Fraumeni, 1969). **A mutation of the *p53* tumor suppressor gene was found in the tumors of all patients with this syndrome** (Malkin et al, 1990). An increased incidence of RMS has been found in association with neurofibromatosis (McKeen et al, 1978).

Cytogenetic abnormalities have been noted in RMS. Embryonal RMS demonstrates loss of heterozygosity (LOH) on chromosome 11p15, but at a different location than the *WT2* gene, which has been implicated in the development of some Wilms' tumors (Douglass et al, 1987; Scrable et al, 1990). Alveolar RMS is associated with a translocation between chromosomes 1 or 2 and chromosome 13, resulting in the formation of a chimeric protein (Parham, 1994). PAX3, a DNA-binding protein on chromosome 2, or

PAX7, a DNA-binding protein on chromosome 1, is fused to the *FKHR* gene on chromosome 13. These genes may be involved in the pathogenesis of alveolar RMS. In addition, patients with the t(1;13) translocation are often younger and have a better prognosis than do their counterparts with the t(2;13) abnormality (Barr, 1997; Kelly et al, 1997). Insulin-like growth factor–2 messenger RNA expression has been documented in alveolar and embryonal RMS (Leiroth et al, 1995). Insulin-like growth factors are known to simulate myoblast proliferation and differentiation. Correlation of these molecular abnormalities with clinical behavior has not yet been determined.

Pathology and Patterns of Spread

The histologic variants of RMS were reviewed by the pathology committee of the Intergroup Rhabdomyosarcoma Study Group (IRSG) (Asmar et al, 1994). They developed a new classification, recognizing three major histologic groups that have prognostic significance. **Embryonal RMS is the most common subtype and accounts for most of the genitourinary tumors (Maurer et al, 1977; Newton et al, 1988). It may occur in solid form, arising in muscle groups such as the trunk and extremities, or as the so-called sarcoma botryoides, a polypoid variety that occurs in hollow organs or body cavities such as the bladder or vagina. The botryoid and spindle variants of embryonal RMS are associated with an excellent survival rate.** The second most common form is *alveolar RMS*, which occurs more commonly in the trunk and extremities than in genitourinary sites and has a worse prognosis (Hays et al, 1983; Newton et al, 1988). Alveolar RMS also has a higher rate of local recurrence and spread to regional lymph nodes, bone marrow, and distant sites. The third category consists of *undifferentiated* tumors, which also fare poorly. *Pleomorphic RMS* is now considered to be an anaplastic variant of the more common embryonal or alveolar RMS (Kodet et al, 1993).

The diagnosis of RMS can occasionally be difficult with conventional histologic techniques. In such cases, histology may be complemented by other studies, including electron microscopy, cytogenetics, immunohistochemistry, and DNA

Table 70–3. INTERGROUP RHABDOMYOSARCOMA CLINICAL GROUPING CLASSIFICATION

Group I	Localized disease completely resected
	Confined to organ of origin
	Contiguous involvement
Group II	Total gross resection with evidence of regional spread
	Microscopic residual
	Positive nodes but no microscopic residual
	Positive nodes but microscopic residual in nodes or margins
Group III	Incomplete resection with gross residual disease
	After biopsy only
	After gross or major resection of the primary (>50%)
Group IV	Distant metastasis at diagnosis (lung, liver, bones, bone marrow, brain, nonregional nodes)
	Positive cytology in cerebrospinal, pleural, or peritoneal fluid or implants on pleural or peritoneal surfaces are regarded as stage IV.

Table 70–4. INTERGROUP RHABDOMYOSARCOMA PRETREATMENT TGNM CLINICAL STAGING BASED ON CLINICAL, RADIOGRAPHIC, LABORATORY EXAMINATION AND HISTOLOGY OF BIOPSY

Stage 1 Favorable site, nonmetastatic
Stage 2 Unfavorable, small, negative nodes, nonmetastatic
Stage 3 Unfavorable, big or positive nodes, nonmetastatic
Stage 4 Any site, metastatic
Tumor
  $T_{site\,1}$—Confined to site of origin
  $T_{site\,2}$—Fixation to surrounding tissues
  ≤ 5 cm
  >5 cm
Histology
  G_1—Favorable histology (embryonal, botyroid, spindle-cell)
  G_2—Unfavorable histology (alveolar, undifferentiated)
Regional lymph nodes
  N_0—Regional lymph nodes not clinically involved
  N_1—Regional lymph nodes clinically involved
Metastases
  M_0—No distant metastases
  M_1site—Metastases present

TGNM: T, tumor; G, histology; N, node; M, metastasis.

flow cytometry (Shapiro et al, 1991). Advances in molecular biology have also helped in the identification of difficult cases. Genes of the MyoD family are important in the differentiation of skeletal muscle (Parham, 1994). MyoD gene expression is increased in RMS and is believed to represent failure of differentiation. MyoD expression is not thought to play a role in tumorigenesis but may be a useful marker for identification of these tumors (Dias et al, 1992).

Clinical Grouping and Staging

Tumor stage at diagnosis is most predictive of clinical outcome (Lawrence et al, 1987b). Regional lymph node extension is fairly common and varies with the site of the primary tumor. Metastatic spread of RMS is usually to the lungs. Clinical grouping was employed in the early IRS studies (Table 70–3). One of the difficulties inherent in this system is that the group depends to a large extent on the completeness of surgical excision. As the treatment of RMS has evolved, more patients undergo biopsy only as the initial surgical procedure, leaving gross residual disease. This results in the shifting of more patients from group I to group III. Biologically equivalent tumors could end up in different categories, depending on the aggressiveness of the initial surgical resection. A clinical staging system was devised for IRS-IV (Lawrence et al, 1987a) (Table 70–4). This classification relies on clinical findings from physical examination, laboratory, and imaging studies. Proper assessment for determining the extent of disease includes chest radiography and CT scanning, CT or MRI of the primary site and regional lymph nodes, a bone scan, and bone marrow aspiration and/or biopsy. Sentinel lymph node mapping can be very helpful in distinguishing which patients should receive regional nodal irradiation (Neville et al, 2000a).

In 1997, Lawrence and colleagues applied the staging criteria (see Table 70–4) to patients treated on IRS-III and found that distant metastases at diagnosis, involved regional lymph nodes, and large primary tumors (larger than 5 cm) were relatively unfavorable prognostic signs. This study also showed that patients with small tumors in unfavorable sites (sites other than orbit or head and neck, nonparameningeal or genitourinary sites other than vulvovagina and paratestis) without tumor in the regional lymph nodes (i.e., stage II patients) fare as well as patients with stage I tumors that are located in favorable sites (Lawrence et al, 1997). Data from IRS-IV patients with genitourinary tumors are currently under review. In the meantime, results of treating 139 patients with extremity primary tumors on IRS-IV have recently been published. They show a clear validation of the staging system, with stage II patients faring significantly better than those in stage IV and stage III patients having an intermediate prognosis (Neville et al, 2000b). Options for managing new patients on the IRS-V study are shown in Table 70–5.

Treatment: General Principles

The first effective treatment for RMS was radical surgical excision. The preferred treatment for pelvic genitourinary tumors consisted of total pelvic exenteration. RMS was later found to be radiosensitive, but local tumor control required high doses. In the 1960s, combination therapy was employed (chemotherapy and radiation therapy) after attempts at complete surgical excision (Pinkel and Pickren, 1961). The first large study found that survival was signifi-

cantly enhanced if chemotherapy was routinely administered after surgery (Heyn et al, 1974).

Because of the small numbers of patients encountered at any single institution, a cooperative effort was initiated to study the various therapeutic efforts for RMS (Maurer et al, 1977). During the early years of the IRS (1972 to 1978), radical surgical intervention before chemotherapy with or without radiation was standard. Once it was demonstrated that most patients would survive the disease, investigators explored the use of primary chemotherapy and radiation therapy to avoid exenterative surgery employed for genitourinary RMS (Ortega, 1979; Voute et al, 1981). A major aim of the protocols for patients with primary tumors in these sites in IRS-II (1978 to 1984) was preservation of a functional distal urinary tract while maintaining the high survival rates achieved in IRS-I (Raney et al, 1990). Unfortunately, primary chemotherapy with vincristine, dactinomycin, and cyclophosphamide did not obviate the need for radical surgery or radiation therapy for patients with pelvic RMS. The 3-year survival rate was the same for IRS-II as for IRS-I (Hays, 1993). In IRS-III (1984 to 1991), intensification of therapy using a risk-based study design significantly improved overall treatment outcomes. This required more intensive chemotherapy for stage III tumors, but selected patients were able to receive decreased therapy (Crist et al, 1995).

A number of advances have been made during the IRSG studies, including identification of histology, site, and extent of disease as prognostic factors (Lawrence et al,

Table 70–5. INTERGROUP RHABDOMYOSARCOMA GROUP STUDY V RISK ASSIGNMENTS

Risk (Protocol)	Stage	Group	Site*	Size†	Age (y)	Histology‡	Metastasis§	Nodes‖	Treatment¶
Low, subgroup A (D9602)	1	I	Favorable	a or b	<21	EMB	M0	N0	VA
	1	II	Favorable	a or b	<21	EMB	M0	N0	VA + XRT
	1	III	Orbit only	a or b	<21	EMB	M0	N0	VA + XRT
	2	I	Unfavorable	a	<21	EMB	M0	N0 or NX	VA
Low, subgroup B (D9602)	1	II	Favorable	a or b	<21	EMB	M0	N1	VAC + XRT
	1	III	Orbit only	a or b	<21	EMB	M0	N1	VAC + XRT
	1	III	Favorable (excluding orbit)	a or b	<21	EMB	M0	N0 or N1 or NX	VAC + XRT
	2	II	Unfavorable	a	<21	EMB	M0	N0 or NX	VAC + XRT
	3	I or II	Unfavorable	a	<21	EMB	M0	N1	VAC (+ XRT, Gp II)
	3	I or II	Unfavorable	b	<21	EMB	M0	N0 or N1 or NX	VAC (+ XRT, Gp II)
Intermediate (D9803)	2	III	Unfavorable	a	<21	EMB	M0	N0 or NX	VAC ± Topo + XRT
	3	III	Unfavorable	a	<21	EMB	M0	N1	VAC ± Topo + XRT
	3	III	Unfavorable	a	<21	EMB	M0	N0 or N1 or NX	VAC ± Topo + XRT
	1, 2, or 3	I, II, or III	Favorable or unfavorable	a or b	<21	ALV/UDS	M0	N0 or N1 or NX	VAC ± Topo + XRT
	4	I, II, III, or IV	Favorable or unfavorable	a or b	<10	EMB	M1	N0 or N1	VAC ± Topo + XRT
High (D9802)	4	IV	Favorable or unfavorable	a or b	≥10	EMB	M1	N0 or N1	CPT-11, VAC + XRT
	4	IV	Favorable or unfavorable	a or b	<21	ALV/UDS	M1	N0 or N1	CPT-11, VAC + XRT

*Favorable, orbit/eyelid, head and neck (excluding parameningeal), genitourinary (not bladder or prostate); unfavorable, bladder, prostate, extremity, parameningeal, trunk, retroperitoneal, pelvis, other.
†a, tumor size ≤5 cm in diameter; b, tumor size >5 cm in diameter.
‡ALV, alveolar rhabdomyosarcoma (RMS) or ectomesenchymoma with alveolar RMS; EMB, embryonal, botryoid, or spindle-cell RMS or ectomesenchymoma with embryonal RMS; UDS, undifferentiated sarcoma.
§M0, no metastasis present; M1, metastasis present.
‖N0, regional nodes clinically not involved; N1, regional nodes clinically involved; NX, node status unknown.
¶VAC, vincristine, actinomycin D, cyclophosphamide; XRT, radiotherapy; Topo, topotecan; Gp, group; CPT-11, irinotecan.

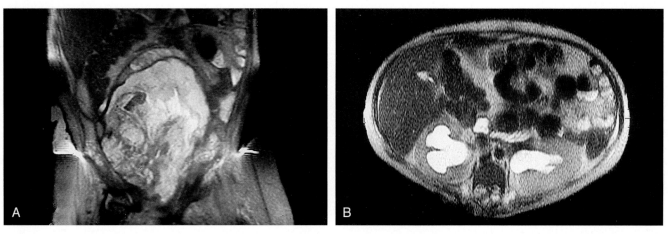

Figure 70–3. CT of a large prostatic RMS extending into the upper abdomen *(A)* with bilateral hydroureteronephrosis *(B)*.

1987a); reduction or elimination of radiation therapy for special groups or sites; reduced need for radical surgery leading to increased bladder salvage from 25% to 60% (Hays et al, 1982; Hays, 1993); and elimination of "routine" lymphadenectomy for some patients with localized paratesticular RMS (Wiener et al, 1994). These advances, as they relate to genitourinary tumors, are addressed in more detail here.

Specific Sites

Bladder and Prostate Tumors

Urinary obstruction is a frequent clinical presentation of RMS of the bladder or prostate (Fig. 70–3). Signs and symptoms include urinary frequency, stranguria, acute urinary retention, and hematuria. On physical examination, an abdominal mass from either tumor or a distended bladder is often present. Tumors of the bladder usually occur as a botryoid form and grow intraluminally, usually at or near the trigone (Hays et al, 1982) (Fig. 70–4). Prostatic RMS tends to manifest as a solid mass rather than the botryoid form seen in the bladder. Determining the actual site of origin can be difficult. Imaging studies show filling defects within the bladder or elevation of the bladder base in prostatic RMS. CT can delineate the extent of tumor and evaluate the pelvic and retroperitoneal nodes. Cystoscopic evaluation establishes the diagnosis, and transurethral biopsy specimens can be obtained.

In recent years, surgical treatment of RMS has become more conservative. Anterior pelvic exenteration is no longer considered to be the initial therapy in pelvic RMS (Raney et al, 1993). Partial bladder resection of the bladder wall for primary tumors affecting the dome or sides of the bladder distant from the trigone is recommended either as initial therapy or as a delayed procedure after chemotherapy. **Although conservative surgical therapy for bladder tumors has not been so successful as for vaginal primaries, the bladder salvage rate has increased** (Hays et al, 1990; Hays, 1993). **With the intensification of treatment for pelvic RMS in IRS-III, 60% of patients retained a functional bladder at 4 years after diagnosis, and the overall survival rate exceeded 85%** (Hays et al, 1995).

There are some concerns about this approach, particularly the number of cases with residual disease after partial cystectomy. Among 22 patients undergoing conservative surgery as primary surgery, there were 5 cases of local

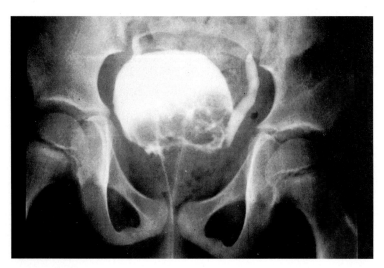

Figure 70–4. Excretory urogram demonstrating filling defects in the bladder caused by rhabdomyosarcoma. (Photograph courtesy of Dr. Stanford Goldman.)

relapse and 1 of distant relapse (Hays et al, 1990). The estimated 3-year survival rate of 79% was similar to that noted for all patients with primary bladder tumors. However, others have noted that a very select group of patients should be expected to have a better prognosis than those with involvement of the bladder base and prostate (Fisch et al, 1995). In the most recent report from the IRS, partial cystectomy had been employed in 40 patients, 33 before any other therapy (Hays, 1993). Seventy-three percent of the long-term survivors in IRS-I and -II had no bladder-related symptoms (Raney et al, 1993). Bladder augmentation or substitution has been used in some of these patients to achieve good functional results (Hicks et al, 1993).

Most of these tumors arise from the trigonal area or prostate and are not amenable to local or partial resection. Prostatic involvement has been reported to be a significant predictor of a poor outcome (Crist et al, 1990). Local recurrence is highly likely if there is incomplete resection or if radiotherapy is omitted. If chemotherapy does not result in adequate shrinkage to allow partial resection, then radical cystectomy may be necessary. Pelvic exenteration is also employed for relapsed tumors (Hays, 1993). **Prostatectomy without cystectomy has been performed in selected patients with persistent disease or local relapse** (McLorie et al, 1989; Hays, 1993; Lobe et al, 1996; Meguerian et al, 1998). **However, local relapses have occurred in 40% of these patients. The completeness of surgical resection may be difficult to determine by frozen section, and there may be an increased likelihood of local recurrence. On the other hand, if the tumor is shrinking during chemotherapy and repeat biopsy after completing radiotherapy shows maturing rhabdomyoblasts without frank tumor cells, total cystectomy may be postponed or avoided altogether** (Ortega et al, 2000). Serial cystoscopic biopsies are especially useful in assessing tumor status in patients with intravesicular RMS (Heyn et al, 1997).

Paratesticular Rhabdomyosarcoma

Among primary genitourinary tumors, 7% to 10% are located in the paratesticular area (Bruce and Gough, 1991). The peak age at presentation is between 1 and 5 years of age (Wiener et al, 1994). Paratesticular RMS arises in the distal portion of the spermatic cord and may invade the testis or surrounding tissues. Paratesticular RMS is usually detected earlier than other genitourinary tumors. Presentation often involves a unilateral, painless scrotal swelling or mass above the testis. On physical examination, a firm mass is present that is usually distinct from the testis. Ultrasound can confirm the solid nature of the lesion. **At diagnosis, 60% of paratesticular tumors are stage I, compared with 13% of RMS overall** (deVries, 1995). **More than 90% of paratesticular RMS are embryonal in histology and have a good prognosis.**

Radical inguinal orchiectomy is recommended for initial treatment. If the tumor has been removed through a prior transcrotal procedure, the risk of local recurrence and nonregional lymph node spread is increased. If cord elements remain after a transcrotal procedure, an inguinal exploration with removal of the remaining spermatic cord and a partial hemiscrotectomy, including the prior scrotal incision, is performed.

Before effective chemotherapy was available, surgery alone produced a 2-year relapse-free survival rate of 50% (Sutow et al, 1970). With current multimodal treatment, survival rates of 90% are expected (Wiener et al, 1994). An imaging evaluation is performed at diagnosis to detect or exclude metastasis. Extension to retroperitoneal lymph nodes occurs in up to 30% of patients. CT is most frequently used to evaluate the retroperitoneum to identify nodal metastases (Lawrence et al, 1987b; Raney et al, 1987), but even with current advances in imaging, there is a significant false-negative rate of CT, which was 14% for IRS-III patients with paratesticular RMS (Wiener et al, 1994).

The role of retroperitoneal lymph node dissection (RPLND) in paratesticular RMS is controversial (Olive et al, 1984; Rodary et al, 1992; Goldfarb et al, 1994; Wiener et al, 1994). The initial use of RPLND was based on the management of non-RMS testicular malignancies. The node dissection itself was not thought to be of therapeutic value but was indicated to stage the disease (Banowsky and Shultz, 1970). Patients found to have positive lymph nodes receive radiation therapy to the involved areas.

Arguments against the routine use of RPLND are that grossly involved retroperitoneal nodes can be detected by preoperative imaging studies, and there is significant morbidity associated with the surgery. Heyn and colleagues (1992) reported a 10% incidence of intestinal obstruction, 8% for ejaculatory dysfunction, and edema of the lower extremities in 5% of patients who had undergone RPLND for paratesticular RMS. However, most of these patients underwent bilateral node dissection. A modified unilateral node dissection is appropriate for staging and, with the addition of nerve-sparing techniques, may avoid some of the reported morbidity of node dissection (LaQuaglia et al, 1989; Donohue et al, 1990). The ability of laparoscopy to identify retroperitoneal nodal disease in this setting remains to be evaluated, but it may offer a less morbid alternative to RPLND.

Another major argument against routine RPLND is that microscopic nodal disease can sometimes be effectively treated by chemotherapy. Olive and coworkers (1984) reported on a group of 19 children with paratesticular RMS who had no clinical evidence of retroperitoneal nodal involvement. Nodal recurrence developed in two patients (10.5%), one of whom did not receive any chemotherapy until relapse occurred. Both parents survived after salvage therapy. A subsequent report of the International Society of Paediatric Oncology (SIOP) experience with 46 children with completely excised tumors and negative CT or lymphangiography results who were treated with intensive chemotherapy alone again found that all children survived (Olive-Sommelet, 1989). However, most of the children did receive doxorubicin or ifosfamide, which has potential for adverse late effects.

During IRS-III, 121 children with paratesticular RMS were reported who underwent RPLND. Fourteen percent of those patients with a negative clinical evaluation were found to have positive lymph nodes on pathologic evaluation (Wiener et al, 1994). Two patients had nodal relapse, one of whom had a prior negative RPLND. This suggests a small risk of nodal relapse in these patients if regional radiation therapy and appropriate chemotherapy are administered. The overall 5-year survival rate for the 98 patients with clinically negative nodes was 96%, and fewer than 10% of patients received doxorubicin or alkylating agents. Although the finding of positive retroperitoneal lymph nodes did identify a group of patients with decreased survival, it is now recommended that patients younger than 10 years of age with clinically negative nodes may undergo treatment with primary chemotherapy alone (Rodary et al, 1992). **Currently, the IRSG recommends that children 10 years of age and older undergo ipsilateral RPLND before chemotherapy. Such patients have an almost 50% chance of having tumor-involved nodes, and radiotherapy is required to prevent recurrence and spread of the disease** (Kattan et al, 1993; Wiener et al, 1994, 2000).

Vaginal and Vulvar Rhabdomyosarcoma

Vaginal and vulvar RMS usually manifests in the first few years of life with vaginal bleeding, discharge, or a vaginal mass. The clinical presentation can be quite striking if there is prolapse of the mass from the vaginal introitus (Fig. 70–5). The diagnosis is made by vaginoscopy and biopsy of the lesion. The vaginal lesions usually arise from the anterior vaginal wall in the area of the embryonic vesicovaginal septum (urogenital sinus). Vaginal tumors may invade the vesicovaginal septum or bladder wall because of their proximity. Cystoscopy is warranted during

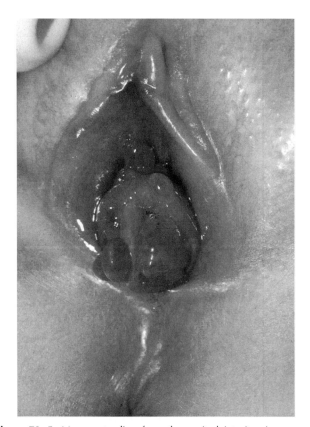

Figure 70–5. Mass protruding from the vaginal introitus in a young girl with vaginal rhabdomyosarcoma.

initial evaluation and at intervals during follow-up (Andrassy et al, 1994).

Vaginal lesions usually have embryonal or botryoid embryonal histology and have an excellent prognosis (Andrassy et al, 1994). Vulvar lesions may have alveolar histology, but because most are localized they also have a good prognosis. In addition to initial biopsy, clinical staging, imaging studies, and bone marrow examination are performed.

Anterior pelvic exenteration was frequently employed to treat these patients in the past. With the development of effective chemotherapy, attempts to preserve the vagina have become a priority. Definitive surgery is delayed until after an initial course of therapy (Hays et al, 1988). Once an adequate response is demonstrated, repeat biopsies are performed. If there is persistence of disease, delayed tumor resection is performed. This may consist of partial vaginectomy or vaginectomy with hysterectomy (Andrassy et al, 1994). In IRS-III, 24 patients with vaginal primaries were treated with a primary chemotherapy protocol. At subsequent surgery, seven patients underwent partial or complete vaginectomy. Six of these seven patients had no viable tumor in the resected specimen, and one had maturing rhabdomyoblasts. The presence of rhabdomyoblasts may not signify persistent active cancer (Andrassy et al, 1999). Heyn and associates (1997) found evidence of cellular maturation in tumors of the bladder on chemotherapy. They hypothesized that, given adequate time, tumor cells with increased maturation after therapy will further mature and ultimately disappear. d'Amore and colleagues (1994) also found maturation in biopsy specimens after just 6 weeks of chemotherapy. They concluded that chemotherapy of RMS tumors causes tumor cell maturation that follows the pathways of normal muscle cell development. Others observed no progression of disease when maturing tumor cells were found (Atra et al, 1994). There was no local recurrence in any of the 24 patients.

During IRS-IV (1988–1996), only 3 (13%) of 21 patients underwent surgical resection after primary chemotherapy. Three patients had rhabdomyoblasts only, whereas one patient who underwent early second-look surgery had rhabdomyoblasts and a small amount of viable tumor. The indications for these surgical procedures are unclear. No patient in IRS-IV had a cystectomy, and all but one patient are alive with no evidence of disease (Andrassy et al, 1999).

Uterine Rhabdomyosarcoma

Uterine RMS may manifest in two ways: as a tumor originating from the cervix, with vaginal bleeding or mass, or as a tumor originating in the uterine body, with an abdominal mass. Diagnosis is made by incisional or excisional biopsy, usually by dilatation and curettage and transvaginal biopsy. More than 90% of uterine tumors are of embryonal histology (Corpron et al, 1995). In addition to biopsy, staging requires a search for metastases, including pelvic examination and CT scans of the pelvis, abdomen, and chest; examination of the bone marrow; cystoscopy; and vaginoscopy.

Older studies reported that uterine RMS occurs in a distinct group of patients who present at an older age and have less response to treatment and therefore poorer prognoses than those with vaginal RMS (Hays et al, 1981, 1985). However, more recent reports suggest that patients with uterine RMS are of the same age group (mean age, 5.5 years) as those with vaginal RMS. Patients treated by primary chemotherapy and delayed resection in IRS-III and the pilot IRS-IV studies responded well to chemotherapy and conservative surgical intervention (Corpron et al, 1995). With this approach, it may be possible to salvage the uterus and vagina as well as the bladder in many of these patients.

WILMS' TUMOR

Wilms' tumor, or nephroblastoma, is the most common primary malignant renal tumor of childhood. This embryonal tumor develops from remnants of immature kidney. The excellent outcome now expected for most children with this tumor is attributed to the combination of effective adjuvant chemotherapy, improved surgical and anesthetic techniques, and the radiosensitivity of the tumor. Treatment of patients with nephroblastoma has been extensively investigated in a number of large, randomized clinical trials. The biology of Wilms' tumor has also been intensively studied by a number of centers. Current management now emphasizes reducing the morbidity of treatment for low-risk patients and reserving more intensive treatment for selected high-risk patients for whom survival remains poor.

Epidemiology

The annual incidence rate of Wilms' tumor in children younger than 15 years of age is about 7 to 10 cases per million. Consequently, approximately 450 new cases are diagnosed each year in North America (Breslow et al, 1993). Wilms' tumor typically affects young children (median age, 3.5 years), with more than 80% of patients identified before 5 years of age. Nevertheless, older children and occasionally even adults can be affected (Arrigo et al, 1990; Kattan et al, 1994). The median age at diagnosis is highest for unilateral unicentric cases and lowest for bilateral cases (Breslow et al, 1993). Wilms' tumor manifests at an earlier age among boys, with the mean age at diagnosis for those with unilateral tumors being 41.5 months, compared with 46.9 months for girls. The mean age at diagnosis for those who present with bilateral tumors is 29.5 months for boys and 32.6 months for girls (Breslow et al, 1993).

Although in North America Wilms' tumor is slightly more frequent in girls than in boys, the worldwide sex ratio is generally believed to be close to 1. With regard to ethnicity, the incidence of Wilms' tumor is lower in East Asian populations and higher in black populations compared with the reported incidence for North American and European Caucasians (Breslow et al, 1994). However, the approximately threefold to fourfold ratio between the maximum and minimum rate worldwide is substantially lower than the 10- to 20-fold ratios typically observed for adult epithelial tumors. The fact that such variations exist and are more closely associated with race than with geography

Table 70–6. INCIDENCE OF CONGENITAL ANOMALIES IN PATIENTS WITH WILMS' TUMOR REPORTED TO THE NATIONAL WILMS' TUMOR STUDY GROUP

Anomaly	Rate (per 1000)
Aniridia	7.6
Beckwith-Wiedemann syndrome	8.4
Hemihypertrophy	33.8
Genitourinary anomalies	
Hypospadias	13.4
Cryptorchidism	37.3
Hypospadias and cryptorchidism	12.0

suggests that environmental risk factors probably play a minor etiologic role, certainly in comparison with adult epithelial cancers (Breslow et al, 1993). Several epidemiologic studies have investigated occupational, environmental, and lifestyle elements as risk factors for Wilms' tumor. Although several studies suggested that a number of parental exposures might be associated with an increased risk of Wilms' tumor, very few have been found conclusively to be associated (Breslow et al, 1993).

A number of recognizable syndromes are associated with an increased incidence of Wilms' tumor (Miller et al, 1964; Clericuzio, 1993) (Table 70–6). **These may be divided into syndromes characterized by overgrowth and those lacking overgrowth. Genitourinary anomalies (renal fusion anomalies, cryptorchidism, hypospadias) are present in 4.5% of patients with Wilms' tumor** (Breslow et al, 1993). **These are common disorders in children, and prospective evaluation for the onset of Wilms' tumor is not necessary in most children with genital anomalies. However, one specific association of male pseudohermaphroditism, renal mesangial sclerosis, and nephroblastoma is known as the Denys-Drash syndrome (DDS)** (Drash et al, 1970). The majority of these patients progress to end-stage renal disease. A specific mutation of the 11p13 Wilms' tumor gene has been identified in these children (Coppes et al, 1993). Although XY individuals have been reported most often, DDS has been reported in genotypic/phenotypic females. One should have a high index of suspicion for the development of renal failure and Wilms' tumor in patients with male pseudohermaphroditism (Tank and Melvin, 1990).

Aniridia is found in 1.1% of patients with Wilms' tumor. Aniridia and Wilms' tumor are most commonly associated in patients with the WAGR (Wilms' tumor, *a*niridia, *g*enital anomalies, mental *r*etardation) syndrome (Clericuzio, 1993). **These patients also have an abnormality of chromosome 11, with a germ line deletion at band p13. Approximately 50% of patients with WAGR syndrome and a constitutional deletion on chromosome 11 develop Wilms' tumor** (Hittner et al, 1980).

An association between Wilms' tumor and horseshoe kidney has been noted. A review of National Wilms' Tumor Study Group (NWTSG) patients found that there was a sevenfold increased risk of Wilms' tumor in patients with a horseshoe kidney (Mesrobian et al, 1985; Neville et al, 1999).

Syndromes with overgrowth features that carry a risk for the development of Wilms' tumor include hemihypertrophy, which may occur alone or as part of the Beckwith-Wiedemann syndrome (BWS) and the Perlman, Soto, and Simpson-Golabi-Behmel syndromes (Perlman et al, 1975; Neri et al, 1998). **BWS is characterized by excess growth at the cellular, organ (macroglossia, nephromegaly, hepatomegaly), or body segment (hemihypertrophy) levels** (Beckwith, 1969; Wiedemann, 1983). **Most cases of BWS are sporadic, but up to 15% exhibit heritable characteristics with apparent autosomal dominant inheritance. The risk of nephroblastoma in children with BWS and hemihypertrophy is estimated to be 4% to 10%** (Tank and Kay, 1980; Beckwith, 1996; Debaun and Tucker, 1998). Adrenocortical neoplasms and hepatoblastoma also occur with increased frequency in BWS. **Children with BWS who are found to have nephromegaly (kidneys greater than or equal to the 95th percentile of age-adjusted renal length) are at the greatest risk for development of Wilms' tumor** (Debaun et al, 1998). The mean age at diagnosis of Wilms' tumor in patients with BWS and hemihypertrophy patients is similar to that in the general Wilms' tumor population (Breslow et al, 1993).

Screening with serial renal ultrasound has been recommended for children with aniridia, hemihypertrophy, and BWS. Review of most studies suggests that 3 to 4 months is the appropriate screening interval. Tumors detected by screening will usually be of a lower stage (Choyke et al, 1999; Green et al, 1993a). Retrospective reviews have been unable to determine whether early detection had an impact on patient survival. Two recent reports called attention to the increased incidence of nonmalignant renal lesions in children with BWS (Borer et al, 1999; Choyke et al, 1999). Recognition of these benign lesions is important to avoid unnecessary nephrectomy when new lesions are identified on screening ultrasound studies (Choyke et al, 1999). Nonmalignant lesions included medullary renal cysts in 13% of patients, hydronephrosis in 12%, and nephrolithiasis in 4%.

Biology

Two classes of genes that lead to cancer have been identified: oncogenes and tumor suppressor genes. Oncogene products activate or repress key regulatory genes whose abnormal expression contributes to the development of cancer. By contrast, the products of tumor suppressor genes provide negative controls of cell proliferation under physiologic conditions and loss of function of a tumor suppressor gene essentially removes the negative control, allowing for uncontrolled growth. Many pediatric tumors result from the loss of function of tumor suppressor genes. The mechanism underlying tumor development as a result of loss of function of a tumor suppressor gene was first proposed by Alfred Knudson in the early 1970s (Knudson and Strong, 1972). Based on the assumption that tumorigenesis is related to discrete changes occurring at random and at a constant average rate, Knudson and Strong suggested a year later that the development of Wilms' tumor also required two rate-limiting genetic events (Knudson and Strong, 1972). The two-event hypothesis, or Knudson model, predicts that two genetic events are *rate-limiting* for tumor formation. Individuals with a genetic predisposition carry an initial lesion in their germ line, either inherited

from a parent or resulting from a de novo germ line mutation. In these individuals, all body cells have already been affected by the first event. Consequently, only one new event in any one cell is required for tumor development. By contrast, individuals who are not genetically predisposed require two relatively rare independent events in the same cell to initiate tumor development (sporadic cases). Subsequent genetic studies in a number of tumors have confirmed the Knudson model, demonstrating that the two postulated "genetic hits" constitute the inactivation of both alleles of a tumor suppressor gene (Comings, 1973). In many cases, the first allele is inactivated by a mutation within the gene itself, and the second allele is inactivated by a gross loss of chromosomal material. The clearest example of tumorigenesis after the inactivation of both copies of a single tumor suppressor gene is the development of retinoblastoma, a rare form of cancer of the retina, after the inactivation of the retinoblastoma gene *RB1*.

The diagnosis of Wilms' tumor usually is made at an earlier age in children with congenital anomalies and also in those with bilateral tumors (Breslow et al, 1993). It was thought that these children had a germ line mutation that predisposed them to both the development of multiple tumors and an earlier age at onset compared with the general population, as had been noted for children with retinoblastoma (Knudson and Strong, 1972). However, the genetic pathways leading to the development of Wilms' tumor are much more complicated than those constituting the genetic basis of retinoblastoma. Several chromosomal regions have been associated with Wilms' tumor, including chromosome 11p13, which harbors the Wilms' tumor suppressor gene *WT1;* chromosome 11p15, which includes the putative Wilms' tumor gene *WT2;* chromosome 16q; chromosome 1p; chromosome 7p; and chromosome 17p (Coppes and Egeler, 1999). The first two loci have been implicated in the actual development of Wilms' tumor; the remaining four do not seem to predispose to Wilms' tumor, but rather seem to be associated with phenotype or outcome.

WT1

The identification and subsequent cloning of *WT1* resulted from cytogenetic observations of gross chromosomal deletions in patients with the WAGR syndrome. These children were shown to have heterozygous germ line deletions at band p13 of chromosome 11 (Riccardi et al, 1978). **Subsequent molecular analysis of the DNA mapping of this specific region led to the identification of the Wilms' tumor suppressor gene *WT1* in 1990** (Bonetta et al, 1990; Call et al, 1990).

Although the exact identity of the genes targeted by the WT1 protein during normal kidney development have not yet been identified, it is now clear that WT1 regulates the transcription of other genes (Rauscher, 1993). The characterization of *WT1* has provided insight into not only the mechanisms underlying the development of Wilms' tumor (Coppes et al, 1993) but also into those involved in genitourinary development (Pritchard-Jones et al, 1990). At first, *WT1* was identified as a classic tumor suppressor gene (i.e., the loss of both copies would be required for tumor development). Although this is indeed the case for several Wilms' tumor types, it has now become clear that specific alterations in only one of the two *WT1* alleles may also contribute to abnormal cell growth. Patients with genitourinary anomalies have an increased risk for carrying a constitutional *WT1* mutation (Diller et al, 1998). No increased risk is observed for patients with nephrogenic rests, bilateral tumors, history of secondary cancers, or family history of Wilms' tumor. This suggests that a constitutional *WT1* mutation encodes truncated WT1 proteins, predisposing to the development of cryptorchidism, hypospadias, and Wilms' tumor.

Germ line mutations in the *WT1* gene are most consistently found in patients with the DDS (Pelletier et al, 1991; Coppes et al, 1992). More than 90% of DDS patients harbor germ line point mutations in only one *WT1* allele. The fact that the phenotype resulting from these heterozygous mutations is far more severe than that resulting from constitutional deletion of one *WT1* allele (i.e., WAGR patients), suggests that the Denys-Drash mutations do not result in inactivation of the WT1 protein but rather in the production of a dysfunctional WT1 protein. It is postulated that this abnormally expressed protein alters regulation of transcription and urogenital development. Of interest, the affected gonads and kidneys in patients with the DDS are heterozygous for germ line mutations, implying that the WT1 mutation acts dominantly with respect to genitourinary abnormalities (Huff et al, 1991).

WT2

Although a large proportion of Wilms' tumors do not harbor alterations at chromosome 11p13, investigators in the field, searching for additional genetic loci, identified chromosome 11p15 as an area harboring a gene, labeled *WT2*, that is important in the development of Wilms' tumor (Koufos et al, 1989; Mannens et al, 1990). Similar to the association between *WT1* and the WAGR syndrome and the DDS, *WT2* has been linked to the BWS (Koufos et al, 1989). Whether the BWS gene and *WT2* are one and the same gene or two distinct but closely linked genes still needs to be elucidated. Many types of tumors show LOH in the 11p15 region (Huff, 1994), and the *WT2* gene may be important in the development of many different tumor types.

Chromosomes 1p and 16q

Loss of the long arm of chromosome 16 has been found in approximately 20% of Wilms' tumors (Maw et al, 1992), **suggesting the presence of a gene at 16q involved in the biology of Wilms' tumor. Similarly, loss of the short arm of chromosome 1p has been found in approximately 10% of cases** (Grundy et al, 1994). **However, because these losses appear to be related to adverse outcome** (Grundy et al, 1994), **both loci are probably involved in tumor progression rather than tumor initiation.** One of the major objectives of the ongoing fifth National Wilms' Tumor Study (NWTS-5) is to confirm the prognostic significance of 1p and 16q loss and to ascertain their potential clinical significance within each tumor stage.

Chromosome 7p

Both cytogenetic analyses of Wilms' tumors and the constitutional karyotypes of patients with Wilms' tumor, have identified recurrent deletions and translocations involving the short arm of chromosome 7 (Rivera, 1995; Miozo et al, 1996). Also, tumor-specific LOH has been noted in approximately 15% of 35 tumors analyzed by NWTSG investigators (Grundy et al, 1996). The combination of constitutional cytogenetic alterations and the observed somatic LOH suggests the presence of yet another putative gene involved in the biology of Wilms' tumor at chromosome 7p. Its exact significance is unknown.

p53 at Chromosome 17p

Alterations of the *p53* tumor suppressor gene and its encoded protein are the most frequently encountered genetic events in human cancer, having been reported in almost every type of sporadic neoplasm (Hollstein et al, 1991). Although the data available at this time indicate that the frequency of *p53* mutations in Wilms' tumor is low, results of one study suggested that *p53* alterations are associated with a specific histopathologic phenotype (Bardeesy et al, 1994). **Because *p53* mutations are seen primarily in anaplastic Wilms' tumors, it has been suggested that the *p53* tumor suppressor gene might underlie the development of a histopathologic variant of Wilms' tumor with poor prognosis. This hypothesis is supported by an observation in tumors in which both anaplastic and nonanaplastic cells could be identified.** In these tumors, *p53* mutations were generally confined to anaplastic cells (Bardeesy et al, 1995). A second study, however, identified a *p53* mutation in a Wilms' tumor with favorable histology (FH), the most common histologic variant, and one that carries an excellent prognosis (Malkin et al, 1994). In this latter study, *p53* mutations were found in tumors from patients with advanced disease (Malkin et al, 1994), suggesting that *p53* mutations are associated with advanced-stage disease in Wilms' tumor, rather than with histologic features.

Familial Wilms' Tumor

In familial Wilms' tumor, cancer susceptibility is transmitted from one generation to the next. Familial Wilms' tumor occurs in 1% to 2% of all cases (Green et al, 1982; Bonaiti-Pellie et al, 1992). Analysis of families with Wilms' tumor has indicated that the predisposition is caused by an autosomal dominant trait with incomplete penetrance (Knudson and Strong, 1972). Attention has been focused on chromosome 19q13.3-q13.4 as an area possibly harboring a gene predisposing to familial Wilms' tumor (McDonald et al, 1998).

Pathology

As a result of many studies by investigators of both the NWTSG and the SIOP, an extensive body of literature on the histopathology of Wilms' tumor is currently available (Beckwith, 1983; Beckwith and Palmer, 1978; Weeks and Beckwith, 1987; Zuppan et al, 1991; Schmidt and Beckwith, 1995). This structural diversity has led to the exploration of correlations between histopathologic features and prognosis. **Markers associated with unfavorable outcome include nuclear atypia (anaplasia, focal or diffuse), and** sarcomatous tumors ("rhabdoid" and "clear cell" types). **The latter two tumor types, however, are tumor categories distinct from Wilms' tumor** (Beckwith and Palmer, 1978; Marsden et al, 1978). **These unfavorable features occurred in approximately 10% of patients but accounted for almost half of the tumor deaths in early NWTSG studies** (Breslow et al, 1985).

The improved histopathologic classification of childhood renal tumors has not only helped to define appropriate treatment strategies for these patients but has also contributed to the understanding of the molecular genetic events underlying the development of Wilms' tumor. For instance, nephrogenic rests, dysplastic lesions of metanephric origin, are now believed to represent precursor lesions (Beckwith, 1993). These lesions are observed in approximately one third of kidneys with Wilms' tumor (Beckwith et al, 1990; Beckwith, 1993). The relationship between the pathology of the nephrogenic rests, the tumor, and congenital disorders predisposing to Wilms' tumor is of particular interest. These associations have been helpful in evaluating a potential correlation between a Wilms' tumor phenotype on the one hand and molecular genetic events leading to the development of that same tumor on the other.

Favorable Histology Wilms' Tumor

Wilms' tumor usually compresses the adjacent normal renal parenchyma, forming a pseudocapsule composed of compressed, atrophic renal tissues. The tumors are usually soft and friable, with necrotic or hemorrhagic areas frequently noted. Most Wilms' tumors are unicentric, but 7% are multicentric unilateral tumors. Derived from primitive metanephric blastema, Wilms' tumor is characterized by tremendous histologic diversity (Beckwith and Palmer, 1978). In addition to expressing a variety of cell types found in a normal developing kidney, Wilms' tumor often contains tissues such as skeletal muscle, cartilage, and squamous epithelium. These heterotopic cell types probably reflect the primitive developmental potential of metanephric blastema that is not expressed in normal nephrogenesis. **The so-called classic Wilms' tumor is characterized by islands of compact, undifferentiated blastema and the presence of variable epithelial differentiation in the form of embryonic tubules, rosettes, and glomeruloid structures separated by a significant stromal component. The proportion of each of these components varies from infrequent to abundant within and among individual tumors. The coexistence of blastemal, epithelial, and stromal cells has led to the term** *triphasic* **to characterize the histologic composition of classic Wilms' tumor.** Some Wilms' tumors, however, are not triphasic but present only biphasic or even monomorphous patterns, so the diagnosis of Wilms' tumor need not be restricted to specimens in which all three cell lines are expressed (Schmidt and Beckwith, 1995). **Wilms' tumors with predominantly epithelial differentiation have a low degree of aggressiveness, and the majority are stage I tumors** (Beckwith et al, 1996). **However, these tumors may be more resistant to therapy if they present as advanced-stage disease. Blastema-predominant tumors are highly aggressive but very responsive to chemotherapy.**

Anaplastic Wilms' Tumor

Anaplasia has been found to be a major indicator of poor outcome. It is characterized by the presence of three abnormalities: nuclear enlargement to three or more times the diameter of the nuclei of the adjacent cells, hyperchromasia of enlarged nuclei, and abnormal mitotic figures. **Anaplasia is rarely seen in tumors of patients younger than 2 years of age at diagnosis (about 2%), but its presence increases to a relatively stable incidence of about 13% in those older than 5 years of age** (Bonadio et al, 1985; Green et al, 1994a). **Anaplasia is associated with resistance to chemotherapy. This is evidenced by the similar incidence of anaplasia (5%) in the NWTSG and SIOP studies** (Vujanic et al, 1999). **Although the presence of anaplasia has clearly been demonstrated to carry a poor prognosis, patients with stage I anaplastic Wilms' tumor and those with higher stages and focal rather than diffuse anaplasia seem to have a more favorable outcome** (Zuppan et al, 1988; Green et al, 1994a). **This confirms the observation that anaplasia is more a marker of chemoresistance than of an inherent aggressiveness of the tumor.** The designation "focal anaplasia" should be based on the distribution of anaplastic cells within the tumor (Schmidt and Beckwith, 1995; Faria et al, 1996), rather than their quantitative density as originally proposed (Beckwith and Palmer, 1978). Diffuse anaplasia is diagnosed when anaplasia is present in more than one portion of the tumor or if it is found in any extrarenal or metastatic site.

Nephrogenic Rests

The presence of Wilms' tumor within a kidney is often associated with additional renal developmental abnormalities. Twenty-five to 40% of children with Wilms' tumor have small foci composed of persistent embryonal cells within otherwise normal kidney tissue (Beckwith et al, 1990; Beckwith, 1993). In the past, several terms were applied to these lesions. In 1990, a new and simplified nomenclature was formulated based on the principle that morphology reflects the developmental history of each lesion (Beckwith et al, 1990). The term *nephrogenic rests* is used for all putative Wilms' tumor precursor lesions, regardless of size, gross feature, or microscopic appearance. The presence of multiple or diffuse nephrogenic rests is referred to as *nephroblastomatosis*. **Nephrogenic rests can be separated into two fundamentally distinct categories:** *perilobar nephrogenic rests* **(PLNRs) and** *intralobar nephrogenic rests* **(ILNRs)** (Beckwith et al, 1990). **These two types are distinguished by their position within the renal lobe (Fig. 70–6). Relative position within the lobe is a direct reflection of the chronology of the embryologic development of the kidney. PLNRs are found only in the lobar periphery, which is elaborated late in embryogenesis, whereas ILNRs are found anywhere within the lobe, or in the renal sinus or the wall of the pelvicaliceal system. Therefore, ILNRs are believed to be the result of earlier gestational aberrations. Of particular interest is the observation that PLNRs are usually found in children with BWS, which is linked to the 11p15 Wilms' locus,**

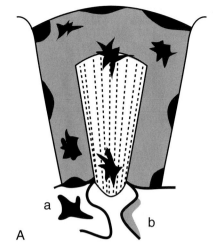

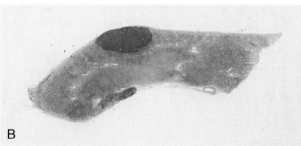

Figure 70–6. *A,* Illustration of renal lobe showing characteristic locations of intralobar nephrogenic rest *(dark gray)* and perilobar nephrogenic rest *(black).* Label *a* indicates intralobar nephrogenic rest in renal sinus; *b* indicates intralobar nephrogenic rest in wall of calyx. (From Beckwith JB: Precursor lesions of Wilms' tumor: Clinical and biological implications. Med Pediatr Oncol 1993;21:158–168, with permission.) *B,* Perilobar nephrogenic rest composed of blastemal cells just beneath the renal capsule (hematoxylin-eosin stain, magnification ×40).

Table 70–7. APPROXIMATE PREVALENCE OF NEPHROGENIC RESTS

Patient Population	PLNR (%)	ILNR (%)
Infant autopsies	1	0.01
Renal dysplasia	3.5	Unknown
Unilateral Wilms' tumor	25	15
Synchronous bilateral Wilms' tumor	74–79	34–41
Metachronous Bilateral Wilms' tumor	42	63–75
Beckwith-Wiedemann, hemihypertrophy	70–77	47–56
Aniridia	12–20	84–100
Drash syndrome	11	78

ILNR, intralobar nephrogenic rests; PLNR, perilobar nephrogenic rests
Adapted from Beckwith JB: Precursor lesions of Wilms' tumor: Clinical and biological implications. Med Pediatr Oncol 1993;21:158–168.

whereas ILNRs are typically seen in children with aniridia, DDS, or other features associated with the 11p13 Wilms' tumor locus (Table 70–7). The age at diagnosis is lower for Wilms' tumor arising in association with ILNR. These observations suggest that the different Wilms' tumor genes may be involved in distinct developmental pathways within the kidney, and that their inactivation may interrupt normal kidney development at different time points. Both types of nephrogenic rests are associated with bilateral Wilms' tumor, where the incidence of nephrogenic rests is much higher than in unilateral Wilms' tumor.

NWTSG investigators have demonstrated the clinical importance of nephrogenic rests. The presence of multiple rests in one kidney usually implies that they are also present in the other kidney. Children younger than 12 months of age who are diagnosed with Wilms' tumor and also have nephrogenic rests, in particular PLNRs, have a markedly increased risk of developing contralateral disease and require frequent and regular

Table 70–8. RECOMMENDED FOLLOW-UP IMAGING STUDIES FOR CHILDREN WITH RENAL NEOPLASMS OF PROVEN HISTOLOGY WHO ARE FREE OF METASTASES AT DIAGNOSIS

Tumor Type	Study	Schedule after Therapy
Favorable histology Wilms' tumor: Stage I anaplastic Wilms' tumor	Chest radiography	6 wk and 3 mo postop; then q 3 mo × 5, q 6 mo × 3, yearly × 2
Irradiated patients only	Irradiated bony structures*	Yearly to full growth, then q 5 yr indefinitely†
Without NRs, stages I and II	Abdominal ultrasound	Yearly × 3
Without NRs, stage III	Abdominal ultrasound	As for chest radiography
With NRs, any stage‡	Abdominal ultrasound	q 3 mo × 10, q 6 mo × 5, yearly × 5
Stage II and III anaplastic	Chest radiography	As for favorable histology
	Abdominal ultrasound	q 3 mo × 4; q 6 mo × 4
Renal cell carcinoma	Chest radiography	As for favorable histology
	Skeletal survey and bone scan	As for CCSK
Clear cell sarcoma (CCSK)	Brain MRI and/or opacified CT	When CCSK is established; then q 6 mo × 10
	Skeletal survey and bone scan	
	Chest radiography	As for favorable histology
Rhabdoid tumor	Brain MRI and/or opacified CT	As for CCSK
	Chest radiography	As for favorable histology
Mesoblastic nephroma (MN)§	Abdominal ultrasound	q 3 mo × 6

*To include any irradiated osseous structures.

†To detect second neoplasms, benign (osteochondromas) or malignant.

‡The panelists at the First International Conference on Molecular and Clinical Genetics of Childhood Renal Tumors, Albuquerque, New Mexico, May 1992 recommended a variation: q 3 mo for 5 yr or until age 7, whichever comes first.

§Data from the files of Dr. J.B. Beckwith reveal that 20 of 293 MN patients (7%) relapsed or had metastases at diagnosis; 4 of the 20 in the lungs, 1 of the 4 at diagnosis. All but 1 of the 19 relapses occurred within 1 year. Chest radiography for MN patients may be elected on a schedule such as q 3 mo × 4, q 6 mo × 2.

Modified, with permission, from D'Angio GJ, Rosenberg H, Sharples K, et al: Position paper. Imaging methods for primary renal tumors of childhood: Cost versus benefits. Med Pediatr Oncol 1993;21:205–212.

surveillance for several years (Table 70–8) (Coppes et al, 1999). Surveillance is also recommended for those diagnosed after 12 months of age who have nephrogenic rests.

Nephrogenic rests display a spectrum of appearances. Hyperplastic rests can produce a renal mass that can be mistaken for a small Wilms' tumor. Incisional biopsy of a hyperplastic rest is of little value in distinguishing this lesion from a Wilms' tumor. The biopsy should include the interface of the rest with the normal renal parenchyma. Wilms' tumor generally compresses the normal kidney with a pseudocapsule at the interface (Beckwith, 1998). Neoplastic induction of cells of a nephrogenic rest can produce Wilms' tumor and possibly other benign or malignant renal neoplasms (Arroyo et al, 2000).

Diagnosis and Evaluation

A palpable, smooth abdominal mass is present on physical examination in more than 90% of children. A family member or primary care provider often discovers the mass incidentally. The tumor is quite large in relation to the size of the child. Other presenting signs and symptoms are gross hematuria, fever, and abdominal pain. Rupture of the tumor with hemorrhage into the free peritoneal cavity can result in the presentation of acute abdomen.

Compression or invasion of adjacent structures may result in an atypical presentation. Extension of Wilms' tumor into the renal vein and inferior vena cava can cause varicocele, hepatomegaly (due to hepatic vein obstruction), ascites, and congestive heart failure. Such symptoms are found in fewer than 10% of patients with intracaval or atrial tumor extension (Ritchey et al, 1988, 1990; Shamberger et al, 2000). Occasionally, children with Wilms' tumor have symptoms resulting from the production of bioactive substances by the tumor (Coppes, 1993). Hypertension is present in 25% of cases and has been attributed to increased plasma renin levels (Voute et al, 1971). During the physical examination, it is important to note signs of associated Wilms' tumor syndromes such as aniridia, hemihypertrophy, and genitourinary anomalies.

Emergent operation is not necessary unless there is evidence of active bleeding or tumor rupture. Laboratory evaluation should include a complete peripheral blood count, platelet count, renal function tests, liver function tests, serum calcium determination, and urinalysis. Acquired von Willebrand's disease has been found in 8% of newly diagnosed Wilms' tumor patients (Coppes, 1993). Elevation of the serum calcium can occur in children with congenital mesoblastic nephroma (CMN) and rhabdoid tumor of the kidney (RTK).

Imaging

A precise diagnosis cannot be obtained on the basis of preoperative imaging studies. All of the solid renal tumors of childhood have some common radiographic features (Broecker, 1991; Glass et al, 1991; White and Grossman, 1991). Other clinical parameters can provide some clues to the diagnosis. The development of a renal tumor in a child known to have aniridia, hemihypertrophy, or other syndromes associated with an increased incidence of nephroblastoma can safely be assumed to be a Wilms'

tumor. Bilateral or multicentric tumors are more typical of Wilms' tumor, but renal lymphoma can also manifest in this fashion. CMN is the most likely diagnosis in a neonate with a renal mass. However, FH Wilms' tumor and RTK of the kidney can also manifest in the first few months of life.

The renal origin of the mass is usually apparent on CT, but it can be mistaken for a neuroblastoma. The preoperative diagnosis was incorrect in 2.5% of the patients in the NWTS-3 (i.e., the child had Wilms' tumor but there was an erroneous diagnosis before surgical exploration) (Ritchey et al, 1992b). Most of these children did not have any preoperative imaging studies performed, and this group of patients had an increased incidence of surgical complications. This emphasizes that defining the exact histology is probably not as important as establishing that a solid renal tumor is present. This information is important for the surgeon to plan for a major cancer operation. Another valuable role of imaging is to confirm that the contralateral kidney is functioning before nephrectomy is performed.

Ultrasound is the first study performed in most children with an abdominal mass. It demonstrates the solid nature of the lesion. **Examination of the inferior vena cava with ultrasound is necessary to exclude intracaval tumor extension, which occurs in 4% of patients with Wilms' tumor** (Ritchey et al, 1988). **MRI is the study of choice if extension of tumor into the inferior vena cava cannot be excluded by ultrasound** (Weese et al, 1991) (Fig. 70–7). CT and MRI studies can further define the extent of the lesion (Broecker, 1991; Glass et al, 1991; White and Grossman, 1991) (Fig. 70–8); however, the role of imaging studies in staging of the renal tumor continues to be defined (Cohen, 1993; D'Angio et al, 1993; Ditchfield et al, 1995). Regional adenopathy and extrarenal tumor extension into the perirenal fat or adjacent structures can be suspected by CT or MRI. However, correlation with pathologic findings to validate the utility of CT staging has not been done. Enlarged retroperitoneal benign lymph nodes are common in children, and correlations between pathologic findings and lymph node evaluation at surgical exploration in patients with Wilms' tumor have resulted in

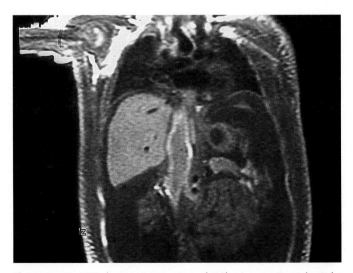

Figure 70–7. MRI depicting extension of Wilms' tumor into the inferior vena cava.

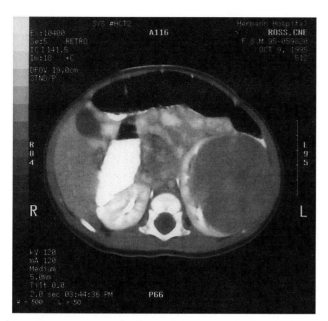

Figure 70-8. CT scan of a left Wilms' tumor with a small rim of functioning renal parenchyma.

significant false-positive and false-negative error rates (Othersen et al, 1990). It should not be expected that CT or MRI would have greater accuracy than visual inspection of these enlarged nodes. Suspected liver invasion on CT is usually found to represent hepatic compression at surgical exploration (Ng et al, 1991).

Positron emission tomography with the glucose analogue 2-deoxy-2-fluoro-D-glucose does show promise in imaging of renal tumors (Shulkin et al, 1997). This technique can provide anatomic imaging of both the primary tumor and metastatic disease, but at present the experience in childhood malignancies is limited.

Bilateral disease occurs in 5% to 7% of patients with Wilms' tumor. Small lesions are often identified in the contralateral kidney on imaging studies. However, a normal CT or MRI should not preclude formal exploration of the contralateral kidney at surgery. Seven percent of children with synchronous bilateral Wilms' tumor enrolled in NWTS-4 had no renal abnormalities identified in the contralateral kidney on preoperative imaging (Ritchey et al, 1995).

The lung is the most common site of distant metastasis in children with Wilms' tumor. Most centers obtain CT of the chest in the initial evaluation of children with Wilms' tumor. Clear cell sarcoma of the kidney (CCSK) and renal cell carcinoma have a propensity to metastasize to the skeleton (D'Angio et al, 1993). Skeletal surveys and bone scans are both recommended after the histologic diagnosis is confirmed. Cranial CT or MRI is performed on all children with CCSK or RTK, because both are associated with intracranial metastases (Weeks et al, 1989).

Staging

The most important determinants of outcome in children with Wilms' tumor are the histopathology and the tumor stage. Accurate staging of Wilms' tumor allows treatment

results to be evaluated and enables universal comparisons of outcomes. The staging system used by the NWTSG (Table 70-9) is based primarily on the surgical and histopathologic findings. Examination for extension through the capsule, residual disease, vascular involvement, and lymph node involvement is essential to properly assess the extent of the tumor.

Stage I tumors are limited to the kidney and are completely resected. However, evidence for tumor extension can be subtle. Tumor invasion of blood and lymphatic vessels in the renal sinus is the first sign of spread outside the kidney in stage II tumors (Weeks and Beckwith, 1987). Penetration through the renal capsule is the next most common site of extrarenal spread. Clear demonstration of tumor cells in the perirenal fat is required to document capsular penetration. For NWTS-4, the distribution by stage for randomly assigned patients was as follows: stage I, 41.8%; stage II, 27.5%; stage III, 21.5%; and stage IV, 9.3% (Green et al, 1998a). Patients with anaplastic tumors are twice as likely to present with stage IV disease than those with FH tumors (Green et al, 1994a).

Prognostic Factors

As the treatment regimens for children with Wilms' tumor have become more effective, the ability of retrospectively determined prognostic factors to predict outcomes is diminished. Traditional staging factors (e.g., tumor size, histology, lymph node metastases), which were relied on in the past to predict risk for tumor progression or relapse, are now less able to stratify patients with FH for treatment. The current NWTS-5 study is evaluating potential biologic factors that may predict tumor behavior. A central tumor bank has been established to maintain biologic specimens from all patients entered on the study.

CHROMOSOMAL ABNORMALITIES

LOH for a portion of chromosome 16q has been noted in 20% of Wilms' tumors (Maw et al, 1992). **A study of 232 patients registered on the NWTSG found LOH for 16q in 17% of the tumors** (Grundy et al, 1994). **Patients with tumor-specific LOH for chromosome 16q**

Table 70-9. STAGING SYSTEM OF THE NATIONAL WILMS' TUMOR STUDY

Stage	Description
I	Tumor limited to the kidney and completely excised. The renal capsule is intact and the tumor was not ruptured before removal. There is no residual tumor.
II	Tumor extends through the perirenal capsule but is completely excised. There may be local spillage of tumor confined to the flank, or the tumor may have been biopsied. Extrarenal vessels may contain tumor thrombus or be infiltrated by tumor.
III	Residual nonhematogenous tumor confined to the abdomen: lymph node involvement, diffuse peritoneal spillage, peritoneal implants, tumor beyond surgical margin either grossly or microscopically, or tumor not completely removed.
IV	Hematogenous metastases to lung, liver, bone, brain, or other organ.
V	Bilateral renal involvement at diagnosis.

had statistically significantly poorer 2-year relapse-free and overall survival rates than did those patients without LOH for chromosome 16q. This difference in outcome persisted after adjustment for histology and stage. This suggests that this chromosomal region may play a role in tumor progression rather than tumor initiation.

Another potential marker is telomerase, a reverse transcriptase that maintains chromosome ends, compensating for the loss of DNA that occurs in replication. High telomerase activity has been found to be an unfavorable prognostic feature for several types of cancers. In a case-cohort study of 78 patients with FH Wilms' tumor, telomerase enzyme activity, expression of hTR (the RNA component of telomerase), and mRNA expression of *hTERT* (the gene that encodes the catalytic component of the enzyme) were measured (Dome et al, 1999). All had detectable expression of hTR, and 97% had detectable *hTERT* transcript. The hTERT mRNA levels correlated with the risk of recurrence even after adjustment for tumor stage. A larger study is underway to determine whether this is an independent prognostic indicator. One of the major objectives of NWTS-5 is to determine whether 16q loss or other molecular markers may serve to further stratify Wilms' tumor patients for treatment. Patients identified with unfavorable molecular findings could be selected for alternate forms of therapy.

DNA CONTENT

The proliferative rate of tumor cells can be estimated by measurement of the DNA content. Flow cytometry has been performed on Wilms' tumor specimens to predict which patients are at risk for metastatic disease (Rainwater et al, 1987). Results from published studies were inconclusive, and DNA content is being examined in the NWTS-5 cohort. Similarly, nuclear morphometric techniques have been evaluated in Wilms' tumor to predict clinical outcome (Partin et al, 1990). A study of 218 patients found that nuclear morphometry was unable to predict disease-free survival (Breslow et al, 1999).

CYTOKINES

The growth of solid tumors is critically dependent on the induction of neovascularity by angiogenic cytokines. Vascular endocrine growth factor (VEGF) is an angiogenic cytokine detected with increased frequency and quantity in experimental and clinical specimens of Wilms' tumor (Kayton et al, 1999; Karth et al, 2000). In experimental animals, lung metastases were far more likely to occur in animals with VEGF-positive tumors. The potential of anti-VEGF therapy to suppress tumor growth has also been assessed (Rowe et al, 2000). Tumors were induced in kidneys of nude mice by the injection of tumor cells. After 1 week, administration of anti-VEGF antibody caused a reduction of more than 95% in tumor weight and abolished lung metastases.

TUMOR MARKERS

Several potential biologic markers for Wilms' tumor have been identified, including hyaluronic acid, hyaluroni-

dase hyaluronic acid–stimulating activity, basic fibroblast growth factor, and serum renin (Coppes, 1993; Lin et al, 1995a, 1995b). Increased urine levels of basic fibroblast growth factor have been found in patients with Wilms' tumor (Lin et al, 1995a). Increased levels of hyaluronic acid and hyaluronic acid–stimulating activity have been reported in both urine and serum of Wilms' tumor patients (Lin et al, 1995b). Patients with persistent disease or relapse had significantly higher levels 1 to 6 months after surgery. Increased plasma renin levels have also been reported in these patients (Voute et al, 1971). There has been no clear correlation with systemic blood pressure, which has been attributed to the elevation of an inactive precursor of renin (prorenin) rather than active renin. Increased plasma renin levels have also been noted with relapse of Wilms' tumor (Coppes, 1993). In all cases, the renin level had decreased after initial tumor excision and then subsequently became elevated. More studies are needed to define the clinical role of these markers in children with Wilms' tumor.

Treatment

SURGICAL CONSIDERATIONS

The initial therapy for most children with Wilms' tumor is radical nephrectomy. Nephrectomy should be done via a transperitoneal approach. The surgeon is responsible for determining tumor extent. Accurate staging is essential for the subsequent determination of the need for radiation therapy and the appropriate chemotherapy regimen. Thorough exploration of the abdominal cavity is necessary to exclude local tumor extension, liver and nodal metastases, and peritoneal seeding. Formal exploration of the contralateral kidney should be performed before nephrectomy. Gerota's fascia is opened, and the kidney is palpated and visually inspected on all surfaces for evidence of a synchronous bilateral tumor or nephrogenic rests. The renal vein and inferior vena cava are palpated to exclude intravascular tumor extension before vessel ligation. Wilms' tumor extends into the inferior vena cava in approximately 6% of cases and may be clinically asymptomatic in more than 50% (Ritchey et al, 1988). Selective sampling of suspicious nodes is an essential component of local tumor staging. Formal retroperitoneal lymph node dissection is not recommended (Othersen et al, 1990; Shamberger et al, 1999).

The other major responsibility when performing a nephrectomy for Wilms' tumor is complete removal of the tumor without contamination of the operative field. Gentle handling of the tumor throughout the procedure is mandatory to avoid tumor spillage, which leads to a sixfold increase in local abdominal relapse (Shamberger et al, 1999). **Shamberger and colleagues (1999) identified risk factors for local tumor recurrence as tumor spillage, unfavorable histology, incomplete tumor removal, and absence of any lymph node sampling. The 2-year survival after abdominal recurrence was 43%, emphasizing the importance of the surgeon's performing a careful and complete tumor resection.**

Removal of a large renal tumor in a small child is associated with some morbidity. NWTS-4 patients undergoing primary nephrectomy had an 11% incidence of surgical complications (Ritchey et al, 1999). The most common complications encountered are hemorrhage and small bowel obstruction (Ritchey et al, 1992, 1993a, 1999). SIOP investigators reported a lower rate of complications when nephrectomy was performed after preoperative chemotherapy (Godzinski et al, 1998). A prospective study comparing the incidence of surgical complications between NWTSG and SIOP is underway.

Cooperative Group Trials

NATIONAL WILMS' TUMOR STUDY GROUP

In North America, pediatric oncologists conduct multi-institutional cooperative trials to study various treatment regimens for pediatric solid tumors. This is the only means to compare outcomes of different treatment modalities in these uncommon neoplasms. The NWTSG was formed in 1969 to study Wilms' tumor. The early NWTSG studies, NWTS-1 (1969–1973) and NWTS-2 (1974–1978), showed that the combination of vincristine (VCR) and dactinomycin (AMD) was more effective than the use of either drug alone. The addition of doxorubicin (DOX) was found to improve survival for stage III and IV patients, and postoperative flank irradiation was unnecessary for group I patients (D'Angio et al, 1976, 1981). **A major accomplishment of the early trials was identification of prognostic factors that allowed stratification of patients into high-risk and low-risk treatment groups. Patients with positive lymph nodes and diffuse tumor spill were found to be at increased risk for abdominal relapse and therefore were considered stage III and given whole abdominal irradiation. One of the most important findings was the identification of unfavorable histologic features that have a very adverse impact on survival.**

The findings of the first two NWTS studies were incorporated into the design of NWTS-3 (1979–1986). Children with stage I FH Wilms' tumor were treated successfully with an 18-week regimen of AMD and VCR without irradiation (D'Angio et al, 1989). The 4-year relapse-free survival rate was 89%, with an overall survival rate of 95.6%. Stage II FH patients treated with the same therapy had a result (4-year overall survival rate, 91.1%) equivalent to that of children who also received DOX with or without radiation therapy. For stage III FH patients, 10.8 Gy of abdominal irradiation was shown to be as effective as 20 Gy in preventing abdominal relapse if DOX was added to the VCR and AMD regimen. The 4-year relapse-free survival rate for stage III patients was 82% in NWTS-3, and the 4-year overall survival rate was 90.9%. Children with stage IV FH tumors received abdominal (local) irradiation based on the local tumor stage and 12 Gy to both lungs, in combination with VCR, AMD, and DOX. The 4-year relapse-free survival rate was 79%, with an overall survival rate of 80.9%. There was no statistically significant improvement in survival when cyclophosphamide was added to the three-drug regimen.

NWTS-4 (1987–1994) compared a pulse-intensive single-dose schedule with divided-dose treatment regimens using AMD and DOX. The pulse-intensive regimens achieved equivalent survival results while decreasing the cost of therapy through modification of the schedule of drug ad-

ministration (Green et al, 1998a). Treatment durations of approximately 6 and 15 months were found to be equally effective in patients with stages II, III, or IV FH tumors (Green et al, 1998b). Overall, the 4-year survival rate for patients with all stages of FH Wilms' tumor now exceeds 90%.

Children with anaplastic Wilms' tumors in NWTS-3 and NWTS-4 were randomly assigned to receive either VCR, AMD, and DOX or those three drugs plus cyclophosphamide. The results were analyzed after the tumors had been reclassified according to the criteria of Faria and Beckwith (Faria et al, 1996). There was no difference in outcome between the regimens for children with focal anaplasia, who had a prognosis similar to that for FH patients (Green et al, 1994a). For stage II to IV diffuse anaplasia, the addition of cyclophosphamide to the three-drug regimen improved the 4-year relapse-free survival rate from 27.2% to 54.8%.

The current NWTS-5 study opened in 1995 as a single-arm therapeutic trial. This study will judge the ability of LOH for chromosomes 16q and 1p to predict the risk for relapse (Grundy et al, 1994). However, many other biologic factors can be studied with the use of banked tumor specimens collected from all enrolled patients (Dome et al, 1999). This tumor bank is available to all investigators and will be useful to evaluate new prognostic factors that may be identified in the future. If molecular genetic markers are predictive of clinical behavior, they may be used in subsequent clinical trials to further stratify patients for therapy.

The treatment regimens used in NWTS-5 are summarized in Table 70–10. Children with stage I or II FH or stage I anaplastic Wilms' tumor receive an 18-week pulse-intensive regimen of VCR and AMD. Patients with stage III FH or stage II or III focal anaplasia are treated with AMD, VCR, and DOX plus 10.8 Gy abdominal irradiation. Patients with stage IV FH tumors receive abdominal irradiation based on the local tumor stage and 12 Gy to both lungs. A new chemotherapeutic regimen combining VCR, DOX, cyclophosphamide, and

Table 70–10. TREATMENT PROTOCOL FOR NATIONAL WILMS' TUMOR STUDY-5

Stage/Histology	Radiotherapy	Chemotherapy
Stage I, II FH	None	EE-4A: pulse-intensive AMD plus VCR (18 wk)
Stage I anaplasia Stage III, IV FH	1080 cGy*	DD-4A: pulse-intensive AMD, VCR, and DOX (24 wk)
Stage II–IV focal anaplasia Stage II–IV diffuse anaplasia Stage I–IV CCSK	Yes†	Regimen I: AMD, VCR, DOX, CPM, and etoposide
Stage I–IV RTK	Yes†	Regimen RTK: carboplatin, etoposide, and CPM

AMD, dactinomycin, CCSK, clear cell sarcoma of the kidney; CPM, cyclophosphamide; DOX, doxorubicin; FH, favorable histology; RTK, rhabdoid tumor of the kidney; VCR, vincristine.
*Stage IV FH patients are given radiation based on the local tumor stage.
†Radiation therapy is given to all patients with CCSK RTK. Consult protocol for specific treatment.

etoposide is being tried in children with stage II or IV diffuse anaplasia.

Accrual of patients for the NWTS-5 study should be completed in late 2001. A portion of the study, examining the role of surgery alone for children younger than 2 years of age with stage I FH tumors weighing less than 550 g, has already been suspended. This part of the study was based on preliminary observation of favorable outcomes in small numbers of such patients when postoperative adjuvant therapy was omitted (Larsen et al, 1990; Green et al, 1994b). It was suspended when the number of tumor relapses exceeded the limit allowed by the design of the study, and the recommendation was made that all children with stage I tumors receive AMD and VCR. The 2-year survival rate of this cohort of patients with small tumors is now 100% with a median follow-up of 1.61 years (Green et al, 2000a), and extended follow-up continues. Observation of untreated children may yield interesting information on the role of chemotherapy in decreasing the incidence of contralateral relapse in patients with neurogenic rests (Green et al, 2000a).

Results from NWTS-3 demonstrated that the risk of tumor relapse at 3 years is 9.6%, 11.8%, 22%, and 22%, respectively, for stages I through IV Wilms' tumor. Relapses occurred in 36% and 45% of those with unfavorable histology stage I through III and stage IV tumors (D'Angio et al, 1989). Children with relapsed Wilms' tumor have a variable prognosis, depending on the initial stage, site of relapse, time from initial diagnosis to relapse, and prior therapy. Adverse prognostic factors include previous treatment that included DOX, relapse less than 12 months after diagnosis, and intra-abdominal relapse in patients previously treated with abdominal irradiation (Grundy et al, 1989). In the past, treatment of these patients has been highly individualized. NWTS-5 is treating children with relapsed Wilms' tumor with a more aggressive approach, particularly for those high-risk patients with adverse prognostic factors at the time of relapse.

INTERNATIONAL SOCIETY OF PAEDIATRIC ONCOLOGY

The other large cooperative group conducting clinical protocols in children with cancer is SIOP. They initiated trials evaluating the role of preoperative therapy for treatment of Wilms' tumor in the early 1970s. It was found that this approach could produce tumor shrinkage (Fig. 70–9), reducing the risk of intraoperative rupture or spill (Lemerle et al, 1976, 1983). SIOP investigators reported a more favorable stage distribution at the time of surgery, with a greater number of patients having "postchemotherapy stage I" tumors. This was thought to be a significant advantage in terms of decreasing morbidity of treatment, particularly the late effects of radiotherapy.

Early SIOP studies evaluated prenephrectomy radiation therapy (Lemerle et al, 1976). **SIOP-5 (1976–1980) showed that 4 weeks of treatment with AMD and VCR was as effective as prenephrectomy radiation therapy in avoiding surgical tumor rupture and increasing the proportion of patients with low-stage disease** (Lemerle et al, 1983). **SIOP-6 (1980–1987) demonstrated that patients with postchemotherapy stage I disease can safely be treated with 18 weeks of AMD and VCR. However, patients' postchemotherapy stage II tumors and negative lymph nodes required more intensive chemotherapy, including the use of an anthracycline, to prevent local relapse** (Tournade et al, 1993). A three-drug chemotherapy regimen after nephrectomy was also needed for postchemotherapy stage II lymph-node positive and stage III disease. SIOP-9 (1987–1993) found no significant additional tumor shrinkage benefit after 4 weeks of preoperative AMD and VCR (Tournade et al, 2001). Patients with stage II or III FH tumors received three drugs (AMD, VCR, and epirubicin). Radiotherapy was limited to patients with stage II N1 or stage III disease; as a result, 18% of patients were irradiated (Graf et al, 2000). Abdominal relapses occurred in 6.6% of stage II N0 patients, and the 2-year relapse-free survival rate was 84%. The rate for stage II N1 and stage III patients was 71%. The latest SIOP study on Wilms' tumor, SIOP 93-01, aims to determine whether postoperative therapy can be omitted in selected patients with stage I disease (Boccon-Gibod et al, 2000) and whether survival can be improved in certain high-risk patients with the use of etoposide, ifosfamide, and carboplatin (Graf et al, 2000).

Both the NWTSG and the SIOP tumor staging system are designed to stratify patients into low-risk and high-risk groups. The goal is to select high-risk patients for more intense therapy while minimizing treatment and thus morbidity for low-risk patients. The NWTSG relies on surgical and pathologic staging, reflecting the extent of disease at diagnosis. Review of the SIOP studies suggests that the "postchemotherapy stage" may inadequately define the risk of intra-abdominal recurrence. An increased frequency of local relapse occurred in unirradiated patients with postchemotherapy stage II tumors without positive lymph nodes (SIOP staging criteria) (Tournade et al, 1993). All patients with postchemotherapy stage II tumors are now given an anthracycline as part of the chemotherapy regimen (Green et al, 1993b). This could increase the incidence of late complications of therapy (see later discussion).

Preoperative Therapy

The current recommendations from the NWTSG are that preoperative chemotherapy is of benefit for patients with bilateral involvement (Blute et al, 1987), **those with inoperable disease at surgical exploration** (Ritchey et al, 1994), **and those with inferior vena cava extension above the hepatic veins** (Ritchey et al, 1993b; Shamberger et al, 2001). All other patients should undergo primary nephrectomy.

INOPERABLE TUMORS

The surgeon determines unresectability of a Wilms' tumor intraoperatively. The surgeon is best able to assess whether primary resection of the tumor will lead to excessive morbidity. Preoperative imaging studies can be misleading. Nephroblastomas are large tumors that often compress and adhere to adjacent structures without frank invasion. Many tumors that appear to invade adjacent organs (e.g., liver) on CT can be easily removed. On the

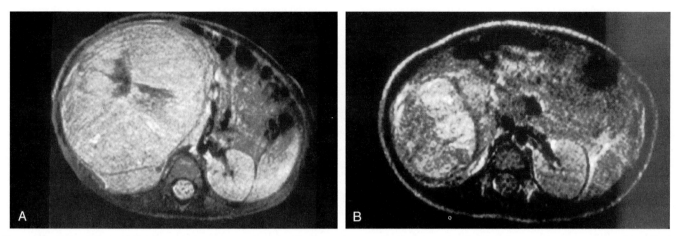

Figure 70–9. *A,* MRI of a Wilms' tumor that was pretreated with chemotherapy. *B,* After 6 weeks of chemotherapy, the tumor is much smaller in size.

other hand, radical en bloc resection of the tumor and surrounding organs is probably not justified in most children, because it is associated with increased surgical morbidity (Ritchey et al, 1992). The gross appearance of the tumor at the time of surgery can be misleading for interpreting tumor extent, and in most cases tumor invasion is not confirmed after the adjacent visceral organs are removed. There may be circumstances when removal of other organs is justified. For example, in a patient with known extracapsular extension, resection of a small portion of liver or of the tail of the pancreas to avoid leaving residual tumor may eliminate the need for radiation therapy and allow a reduction in the amount of chemotherapy. Even if the tumor is confined to the kidney, en bloc resection of nonessential structures may also prevent violation of the tumor capsule and obviate tumor rupture or spill during nephrectomy. The added surgical morbidity of en bloc resection must be weighed against a potential reduction in long-term complications of adjuvant treatment if such treatment can be limited by complete tumor removal.

If the tumor cannot be primarily resected, the patient is treated with a stage III chemotherapy regimen (Ritchey et al, 1994). Definitive resection can usually be

performed within 6 weeks after initiation of therapy. Response of the tumor is assessed with serial imaging studies, but radiographic evidence of persistent disease can occasionally be misleading. Failure of the tumor to shrink could be caused by a predominance of skeletal muscle or benign elements (Zuppan et al, 1991) (Fig. 70–10). Patients with progressive disease have a very poor prognosis (Ritchey et al, 1994).

BILATERAL WILMS' TUMORS

Synchronous bilateral Wilms' tumors occur in about 5% of children (Blute et al, 1987; Coppes et al, 1989; Montgomery et al, 1991). **The preferred approach for patients with bilateral nephroblastoma is initial biopsy followed by preoperative chemotherapy** (Blute et al, 1987; Coppes et al, 1989; Kumar et al, 1998). Radical excision of the tumor should not be done at the initial operation. Partial nephrectomy or wedge excision may be performed at the initial operation only if all tumors can be removed with preservation of two thirds or more of the renal parenchyma on both sides. Bilateral biopsies are obtained to confirm the presence of Wilms' tumor in both

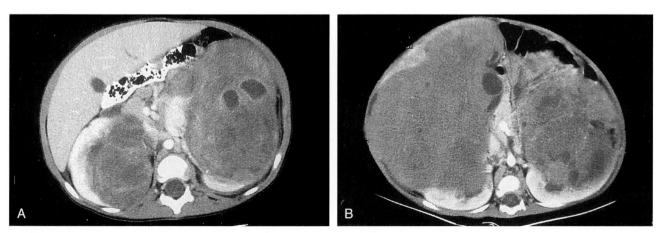

Figure 70–10. Patient with bilateral tumors treated with chemotherapy. *A,* CT before treatment. *B,* CT after 6 months of chemotherapy, showing an increase in the size of the tumors. Bilateral partial nephrectomies were performed, revealing mature tumor elements with rhabdomyoblastic differentiation.

kidneys and to define the histologic type. This is recommended to decrease the incidence of renal failure, which is found in 9.1% and 18.8%, respectively, of patients with synchronous and metachronous bilateral Wilms' tumor (Ritchey et al, 1996). Using this approach, nephrectomy can be avoided entirely in almost 50% of patients (Montgomery et al, 1991; Shaul et al, 1992).

Second-look surgery is performed after completion of the initial course of chemotherapy, usually at 8 to 10 weeks (Ritchey and Coppes, 1995). Preoperative CT or MRI can assess the reduction in tumor volume and the feasibility of partial resection. At the time of the second-look procedure, partial nephrectomies or wedge excisions of the tumors are performed. This should be done only if it will not compromise tumor resection and negative margins can be obtained. One area of controversy is the role of enucleation versus partial nephrectomy when renal salvage procedures are performed in these patients. Enucleation is more likely to result in positive surgical margins (Horwitz et al, 1996). For FH tumors, adjuvant therapy results in a good outcome (Cooper et al, 2000). However, if there is anaplasia in the resected specimen, a positive margin will adversely affect survival.

If there is extensive tumor involvement precluding partial resection, biopsies are obtained. Patients with persistent viable tumor should be changed to a different chemotherapeutic regimen. The patient should be reassessed after an additional 12 weeks to assess the feasibility of resection. If there is a possibility that the remaining kidney can be salvaged, partial nephrectomy or wedge excision of the tumor is performed. If there is extensive tumor involvement precluding partial resection in one kidney, complete excision of tumor from the least involved kidney is performed. If this procedure leaves a viable and functioning kidney, then radical nephrectomy is performed to remove the kidney with extensive tumor involvement. Bilateral nephrectomy and dialysis may be required if the tumors fail to respond to chemotherapy and radiation therapy (Penn, 1979; Rudin et al, 1998). This is the most common cause of renal failure in patients with bilateral Wilms' tumor (Ritchey et al, 1996). The recommended interval before renal transplantation is a minimum of 1 year tumor free after completion of chemotherapy (Penn, 1979; Rudin et al, 1998).

Partial Nephrectomy for Unilateral Tumors

Several centers have explored the role of parenchyma-sparing procedures in children with unilateral Wilms' tumor (McLorie et al, 1991; Cozzi et al, 1995; Moorman-Voestermans et al, 1998). Most tumors are too large at diagnosis to allow partial nephrectomy without pretreatment. After preoperative chemotherapy, partial nephrectomy can be performed in 10% to 15% of patients. Enucleation of the tumor has been used for centrally located tumors in which partial nephrectomy with a rim of renal tissue is not feasible (Cozzi et al, 1995). As noted previously, enucleation increases the risk for positive surgical margins. A review of children with bilateral Wilms' tumor found that the incidence of local recurrence was 7.5% after

partial nephrectomy, compared with 14% after enucleation (NS [not significant]) (Horwitz et al, 1996). Although overall survival was comparable, patients with residual disease and recurrence received added therapy to maintain this survival.

The primary motivation for considering partial nephrectomy is to preserve renal parenchyma and, theoretically, decrease the risk of renal insufficiency. However, **the incidence of renal failure after treatment for unilateral Wilms' tumor is low. Only 0.25% of NWTSG patients developed renal failure after nephrectomy for unilateral tumors** (Ritchey et al, 1996). **Most of those were children with the DDS who had intrinsic renal disease and often progressed to end-stage renal disease. Patients with the WAGR syndrome also have an increased risk of renal failure. One report found a 38% risk of renal failure that occurred at a median of 14 years after diagnosis** (Breslow et al, 2000).

The current recommendation of the NWTSG is to consider partial nephrectomy for patients with bilateral Wilms' tumor, solitary kidney, and renal insufficiency. Also, patients known to have an increased incidence of nephrogenic rests (e.g., BWS, hemihypertrophy, aniridia) are at increased risk for the development of a metachronous tumor and may be considered for parenchyma-sparing procedures (Coppes et al, 1999; Borer et al, 1999). In the latter group, this should be considered only if the tumor can be completely resected with clear margins. The risk of undertreatment and a potentially increased risk of local recurrence must be weighed against the possible benefit of decreasing the incidence of renal failure.

Late Effects of Treatment

Numerous organ systems are subject to the late sequelae of anticancer therapy. Clinicians must be aware of the spectrum of problems that face these children as they grow into adulthood. Musculoskeletal problems (e.g., scoliosis) were significant in children who received irradiation in the early NWTS trials (Evans et al, 1991). Gonadal irradiation can produce hypogonadism and temporary azoospermia in boys (Kinsella et al, 1989). The severity of damage depends on the radiation dose. A 12% incidence of ovarian failure was found in girls who received abdominal radiation therapy (Stillman et al, 1987). Abdominal radiation therapy also increased the risk of adverse pregnancy outcomes (Li et al, 1987). An increased incidence of second malignant neoplasms has been observed in children treated for Wilms' tumor. Two studies in Wilms' tumor survivors noted a 1% cumulative incidence at 10 years after diagnosis and a rising incidence thereafter (Li et al, 1987; Breslow et al, 1988). All but two of these neoplasms occurred in patients who had received radiation therapy, and most often they were located in the radiation field. All of the children who developed hepatocellular carcinoma had received flank irradiation (Kovalic et al, 1991).

In recent years, there has been increasing concern regarding the risk of congestive heart failure in children who receive treatment with anthracyclines such as DOX (Gilladoga et al, 1976). In addition to the acute cardiotoxicity, cardiac failure can develop many years after treatment (Steinherz et al, 1991). In a preliminary review of patients entered on NWTS-1 through -4, the frequency of congestive heart failure was 4.4% among DOX-treated patients who received this drug as part of their initial chemotherapy regimen (Green et al, 2001). The risk was increased if the patient received whole-lung or left-flank irradiation.

It is clear that if radiation therapy and DOX are part of the initial treatment regimen, the risk of late sequelae of therapy is markedly increased. The initial treatment of Wilms' tumor therefore has a significant impact on long-term problems. It is incumbent on the surgeon to completely remove the tumor intact to minimize the therapy needed.

OTHER RENAL TUMORS

Clear Cell Sarcoma of the Kidney

Although it is not currently considered a variant of Wilms' tumor, CCSK accounts for 3% of renal tumors reported to the NWTSG. The age at diagnosis and the location are the same as for nephroblastoma. Although CCSK can pose some serious challenges to the pathologist because it can mimic Wilms' tumor, RTK, and CMN, the classic pattern consists of a cellular lesion of polygonal cells with round oval nuclei having a delicate chromatin pattern and indistinct nucleoli (Schmidt and Beckwith, 1995). Argani and associates recently completed an extensive review of 351 cases of CCSK (Argani et al, 2000). **Important predictors of improved survival were lower stage, younger age at diagnosis, treatment with DOX and absence of tumor necrosis. The addition of DOX improved both overall survival and relapse-free survival** (D'Angio et al, 1989; Argani et al, 2000). **Patients with stage I tumors (using the current criterion of absence of renal sinus invasion) had a 98% survival rate.** Long-term follow-up of patients with CCSK is needed, because 30% of relapses occurred more than 3 years after diagnosis, and some as late as 10 years later. **Unlike Wilms' tumor, CCSK is associated with bone and brain metastases.** Bilateral involvement has thus far not been reported, nor has the presence of congenital anomalies associated with Wilms' tumor (e.g., aniridia, hemihypertrophy).

Rhabdoid Tumor of the Kidney

RTK is the most aggressive and lethal childhood renal tumor; it accounts for 2% of renal tumors registered to the NWTSG. RTK is now considered to be a sarcoma of the kidney and not of metanephric origin (D'Angio et al, 1989). It is characterized by large, uniform cells with abundant acidophilic cytoplasm, frequently containing a discrete zone of pale eosinophilia, made up of fibrillary inclusion bodies, and large nuclei having very prominent nucleoli. RTK and CCSK both occur in renal and extrarenal locations, suggesting an origin from a non–organ-specific mesenchymal cell. Cytogenetic studies have shown that there may be a common genetic basis for renal and extrarenal rhabdoid tumors, deletions and somatic mutations in the *INI1* gene on chromosome 22 in the region of 22q11 (Biegel et al, 1999). Germ line mutations of *INI1* have been identified in renal rhabdoid tumors.

Typical clinical features include early age at diagnosis (median, less than 16 months), resistance to chemotherapy, and high mortality. Unlike Wilms' tumor, which typically metastasizes to the lungs, abdomen or flank, and liver, RTK, which also metastasizes to these sites, is distinguished by its propensity to metastasize to the brain (D'Angio et al, 1993). In addition, RTK is associated with second primary tumors in the brain, including cerebellar medulloblastomas, pineoblastomas, neuroblastomas, and subependymal giant cell astrocytomas (Bonnin et al, 1984).

Congenital Mesoblastic Nephroma

CMN is the most common renal tumor in infants with a mean age at diagnosis of 3.5 months (Howell et al, 1982; Levin et al, 1982). CMN (as well as RTK) should especially be considered in the presence of an intrarenal mass in a young child with hypercalcemia and/or its manifestations, which include nausea, vomiting, anorexia, constipation, and polyuria (Coppes, 1993). Imaging studies cannot reliably distinguish CMN from other renal mass lesions. CMN is a very firm tumor on gross examination, and the cut surface has the yellowish-gray, trabeculated appearance of a leiomyoma. The tumor tends to demonstrate local infiltration into the surrounding perirenal connective tissue and lacks the pseudocapsule typically seen in Wilms' tumor. Unlike Wilms' tumor, CMNs are composed predominantly of bundles of spindle cells resembling fibroblasts or smooth muscle cells. In CMN, tumor induction is postulated to occur at a time when the multipotent blastema is predominately stromagenic (Tomlinson et al, 1992; Snyder et al, 1981). There are no cytogenetic or molecular markers unique to CMN, and *WT1* is not expressed in this tumor (Tomlinson et al, 1992)

The most important aspect of the recognition of these tumors as a separate entity is the usually excellent outcome with radical surgery only (Howell et al, 1982). However, the presence of increased cellularity, either focal or diffuse, and a high mitotic rate are caution signals, because some patients with such lesions have local recurrence and/or distant metastases (Joshi et al, 1986; Beckwith, 1986; Gormley et al, 1989). The risk of recurrence is thought to be less in children who are younger than 3 months of age at diagnosis, but metastases have been reported in a few infants (Heidelberger et al, 1993). Neither chemotherapy nor radiation therapy is routinely recommended (Howell et al, 1982), but consideration for adjuvant treatment should be given to patients with cellular variants that are incompletely resected (Gormley et al, 1989).

Solitary Multilocular Cyst and Cystic Partially Differentiated Nephroblastoma

Solitary multilocular cyst, or multilocular cystic nephroma, is an uncommon, benign renal tumor. Fifty percent of multilocular cysts are found in young children, usually boys. The second peak incidence occurs in young adult women (Johnson et al, 1973; Banner et al, 1981). All cases of multilocular cystic renal disease have been unilateral. The gross appearance of the tumor is its most distinguishing feature. The cut surface reveals a well-encapsulated, multilocular tumor composed of cysts of varying size compressing the surrounding renal parenchyma.

Another entity reported in the literature with similar features is cystic partially differentiated nephroblastoma. Most of these lesions occur during the first year of life (Joshi and Beckwith, 1989). A review of cystic renal tumors in children recommended that multilocular cystic nephroma and cystic partially differentiated nephroblastoma be considered the same entity (Eble and Bonsib, 1998). They are indistinguishable radiographically. Surgery is curative in almost all patients, with recurrence being the result of incomplete resection (Eble and Bonsib, 1998). Histologic examination reveals that blastemal cells or nephrogenic rests may be found in the septa of both tumor types. Some of the smaller lesions can be managed by partial excision, salvaging a portion of the kidney. If partial nephrectomy is considered, frozen section examination is indicated to ensure negative margins (Joshi and Beckwith, 1989).

Metanephric Adenofibroma

Another tumor with prominent stromal features that can resemble CMN is metanephric adenofibroma (Arroyo et al, 2000). The epithelial component of these tumors can range from inactive metanephric adenoma to Wilms' tumor. Other lesions contain areas that are morphologically identical to papillary renal cell carcinoma. This uncommon entity is thought to be derived from ILNR (Arroyo et al, 2000). Metanephric adenofibromas with a composite Wilms' tumor component occur at a young age (mean, 12 months) similar to other ILNR-related Wilms' tumors that develop in patients with DDS and aniridia. None of these tumors has recurred after nephrectomy, but all have been treated with Wilms' tumor chemotherapy.

Renal Cell Carcinoma

Renal cell carcinoma is the most common renal malignancy in the second decade of life. Only 5% of renal cell carcinomas occur in children (Hartman et al, 1982; Broecker, 1991). An abdominal mass is the most common presentation, but hematuria is more common than in Wilms' tumor (Broecker, 1991). Imaging studies cannot differentiate renal cell carcinoma from other solid renal tumors. Reviews of the pathology of renal cell carcinoma have noted a higher incidence of papillary renal cell carcinoma (Carcao et al, 1998; Renshaw et al, 1999). **Complete tumor resection is the most important determinant of outcome.** Raney and colleagues (1983) found that all children with stage I lesions survived, and others have reported 64% to 80% survival for stage I and II tumors (Dehner et al, 1970; Castellanos et al, 1974; Aronson et al, 1996).

Younger age at diagnosis is a favorable prognostic factor (Raney et al, 1983). Like their adult counterpart, renal cell carcinomas are not responsive to chemotherapy or radiation therapy.

Angiomyolipoma

Renal angiomyolipoma is a hamartomatous lesion that is only rarely seen in childhood. There is a clear association with the tuberous sclerosis complex (TSC), and the lesion is more often bilateral in these patients (Blute et al, 1988; Ewalt et al, 1998). **The renal lesions of the TSC include angiomyolipoma, simple cysts, polycystic kidney disease, and renal cell carcinoma. Angiomyolipoma develops in up to 80% of patients with the TSC** (Ewalt et al, 1998). Two genes have been identified in the TSC, on chromosome 9 *(TSC1)* and on chromosome 16 *(TSC2)* (Povey et al, 1994). It has been postulated that these genes act as tumor suppressor genes and that the LOH of *TSC1* or *TSC2* may explain the progressive growth pattern of renal lesions seen in these patients.

The incidence of angiomyolipoma increases with age. Ewalt and coworkers (1998) reported on 60 patients with the TSC who were monitored with periodic ultrasound. The average age at which a normal ultrasound became abnormal was 7.2 years. Angiomyolipomas were found in 45 children. Growth of the lesion was observed in 28 children. Girls were more likely to have an increase in the size of the lesion. All patients with lesions greater than 4 cm in diameter were postpubertal. Annual ultrasound examinations are recommended after puberty. **Children with rowing lesions (Fig. 70–11) can be managed with embolization or partial nephrectomy before they become symptomatic with bleeding** (Lee et al, 1998). **The risk of serious bleeding appears to correlate with a diameter larger than 4 cm** (Blute et al, 1988; Steiner et al, 1993; Dickinson et al, 1998). Nephron-sparing approaches are recommended in children with the TSC because of the presence of multiple, bilateral lesions and the risk of developing of new lesions.

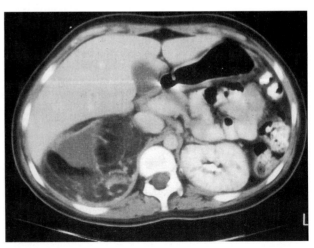

Figure 70–11. Angiomyolipoma of the right kidney in a patient with tuberous sclerosis.

Miscellaneous Tumors

Tumors of the renal collecting system are also very uncommon in childhood. *Transitional cell carcinoma* of the renal pelvis has been reported, and these lesions are managed with nephroureterectomy (Hudson et al, 1981). Fortunately, most filling defects of the upper collecting system represent benign lesions. The most common lesion is a *fibroepithelial polyp* (Gleason and Kramer, 1994). These patients typically present with symptoms secondary to obstruction. Management consists of segmental resection and reconstruction of the urinary tract.

TESTICULAR TUMORS

Testicular tumors are uncommon, accounting for 1% to 2% of all pediatric solid tumors. **Benign lesions represent a greater percentage of cases in children than in adults. Germ cell tumors account for only 65% of prepubertal testicular tumors** (Table 70–11). The incidence of childhood testicular tumors peaks at age 2 years (Li and Fraumeni, 1972; Haas and Schmidt, 1995), tapers after age 4 years, but then begins to rise again at puberty. Testis tumors are rare among black and Asian children.

Etiology and Genetics

A variety of chromosomal abnormalities have been identified in both adolescent and adult germ cell tumors. These include loss of chromosomes 11, 13, and 18, and gain of chromosomes 7 and 8 and the X chromosome (Bussey et al, 1999). The most frequent chromosomal abnormality is the isochromosome of 12p, or i(12p), characteristically composed of two copies of 12p. Testis tumors of infants

Table 70–11. CLASSIFICATION OF PREPUBERTAL TESTICULAR TUMORS

Germ cell tumors
  Yolk sac
  Teratoma
  Mixed germ cell
  Seminoma
Gonadal stromal tumors
  Leydig cell
  Sertoli cell
  Juvenile granulosa cell
  Mixed
Gonadoblastoma
Tumors of supporting tissues
  Fibroma
  Leiomyoma
  Hemangioma
Lymphomas and leukemias
Tumor-like lesions
  Epidermoid cysts
  Hyperplastic nodule secondary to congenital adrenal hyperplasia
Secondary tumors
Tumors of the adnexa

From Kay R: Prepubertal testicular tumor registry. J Urol 1993;150:671–674, with permission.

and young children fail to show the presence of i(12p). Endodermal sinus tumors have been noted to have a deletion of the short arm of chromosome 1, specifically 1p36, in 80% to 100% of cases (Perlman et al, 1996). DNA ploidy analysis reveals that most infantile testicular endodermal sinus tumors are diploid or tetraploid, whereas adult germ cell tumors are typically aneuploid (Silver et al, 1994).

Although the cause of testicular cancer is unknown, a number of etiologic factors have been evaluated. There has been an increasing incidence of testicular cancer in the past few decades (McKiernan et al, 1999). It is suggested that early or prolonged exposure to some carcinogenic stimuli might be implicated. Patients with intersex disorders have an increased incidence of gonadal tumors. **These disorders include androgen insensitivity syndromes (e.g., complete testicular feminization) and gonadal dysgenesis. The risk of tumor formation in gonadal dysgenesis is increased if there is a Y chromosome present; the incidence of tumor development is then approximately 10% by age 20 years. Intratubular germ cell neoplasia has been noted in 6% of children with intersex disorders, with a higher incidence after puberty** (Ramani et al, 1993). The link between cryptorchidism and germ cell tumors of the testis is well known, but these tumors are quite rare in childhood (Kay, 1993).

Pathology

Non–germ cell and germ cell tumors arise from the celomic epithelium and primordial germ cells, respectively. It is postulated that the totipotent germ cells can evolve into seminoma or embryonal carcinoma. Embryonal carcinoma is capable of differentiating into embryonic structures, such as mature or immature teratomas, and extraembryonic structures, such as endodermal sinus tumors and choriocarcinoma. Seminoma or dysgerminoma is a primitive germ cell neoplasm that lacks the capacity for further differentiation. These tumors are unusual in childhood except when related to gonadal dysgenesis.

Yolk sac tumor (YST) is known by a number of other eponyms, including endodermal sinus tumor, embryonal adenocarcinoma, infantile adenocarcinoma of the testis, orchidoblastoma, and Teilum's tumor. Grossly, the tumor is firm and yellow-white on cross section, and hemorrhage is unusual. The microscopic appearance shows a mixture of epithelial and mesenchymal cells in a characteristic organoid pattern. The tumor cells produce the characteristic stages seen in the morphogenesis of extraembryonic membranes (yolk sac and allantoic mesoderm of the placenta). **The characteristic histologic finding in yolk sac tumors is Schiller-Duval bodies** (Wold et al, 1984). The latter are similar to the endodermal sinuses seen in the rat placenta. Eosinophilic cytoplasmic inclusions are common, and specialized staining techniques demonstrate the presence of α-fetoprotein (AFP).

Teratoma is a germ cell tumor with recognizable elements of more than one germ cell layer: endoderm, ectoderm, and mesoderm. Teratomas are classified as mature teratoma, immature teratoma, and malignant teratoma. Mature teratomas generally appear well encapsulated on gross examination. There are multiple cysts, but consistency on cross section varies with the amount of solid tissue present between the cysts. The microscopic appearance varies with the relative amounts of tissue derived from the different germ layers and the degree of maturation (Mostofi and Price, 1973). Cartilage, bone, mucous glands, or muscle may be evident.

Immature teratomas have a gross appearance similar to that of mature teratomas. The pathologic characteristics of immature teratomas in children have been reviewed (Heifetz et al, 1998). It was found that the incidence of foci of YST increased with the grade of the tumor teratoma, and these patients frequently had increased serum AFP preoperatively (Heifetz et al, 1998).

Leydig, Sertoli, and granulosa cells have a common embryologic origin from a mesenchymal stem cell. Pathologic diagnosis can be difficult because of incomplete differentiation (Goswitz et al, 1996). Leydig cell tumors appear well encapsulated with compression of the adjacent testicular tissue. They appear yellow to brown on cross section, reflecting the steroid production by the tumor. Microscopic appearance is similar to that of adrenal rests. The pattern is that of closely packed eosinophilic cells with a granular cytoplasm. **The pathognomonic histologic feature of Leydig cell tumor, Reinke's crystals, is present in only about 40% of tumors** (Mostofi and Price, 1973). **Increased mitotic figures or other features suggestive of malignancy are absent in prepubertal Leydig cell tumors.** A review of 30 cases of Leydig cell tumors identified the following features associated with tumors that metastasized: increased mitotic activity, DNA aneuploidy, infiltrative margins, and angiolymphatic invasion (Cheville et al, 1998). Metastasizing tumors also had higher activity of MIB-1, a cell proliferation marker. None of the prepubertal patients had developed metastatic disease.

Sertoli cell tumors are solid, usually without hemorrhage or necrosis. On cross section they are white to yellow and lobulated in appearance. On microscopic examination, there are large polygonal cells with eosinophilic cytoplasm. Large cell Sertoli cell tumors can be confused with Leydig cell tumors because both are characterized by cells with abundant eosinophilic cytoplasm (Goswitz et al, 1996). The tumors of the adrenogenital syndrome are also another confusing entity in the differential diagnosis (Srikath et al, 1992). Histology does not correlate with outcome, because Sertoli cell tumors often have features of high mitotic rates, nuclear pleomorphism, and increased cellularity.

Gonadoblastomas are small, benign tumors that are bilateral in up to one third of cases. The tumors are composed of large germ cells similar to seminoma, sex cord derivatives resembling immature granulosa and Sertoli cells, and occasionally stromal elements.

Carcinoma In Situ

Carcinoma in situ (CIS) is commonly found in adult patients with testicular cancer and is a precursor to the development of invasive germ cell tumor (Skakkebaek, 1975). CIS has been detected in germ cell tumors in adolescents (Jorgensen et al, 1995), but it has not been identified in children with YST of the testis. The seminiferous tubules adjacent to germ cell tumors in prepubertal children frequently contain cells with enlarged nuclei and clear cytoplasm. However, staining for markers of CIS, placental alkaline phosphatase and c-kit, in seminiferous tubules adjacent to the germ cell tumor was negative in 28 prepubertal testes (Hawkins et al, 1998). CIS is also frequently detected in patients with androgen insensitivity disorders and dysgenetic gonads (Muller et al, 1985; Ramani et al, 1993). These differences suggest that the etiology of germ cell tumor in infants is different than in adults.

There is an association between cryptorchidism and the development of CIS. The incidence of CIS is 1.7% in adults who have previously undergone orchidopexy (Giwercman et al, 1989). **Identification of CIS is more difficult in the prepubertal patient.** Biopsies at the time of orchidopexy in prepubertal children have only rarely demonstrated CIS (Hadziselimovic et al, 1984). Giwercman and colleagues (1988) recommended repeat biopsy after puberty in prepubertal patients with CIS. An exception is the patient with androgen insensitivity or dysgenetic gonads.

Diagnosis and Staging

A painless testicular mass is the most common presentation of a child with a testicular tumor. Disorders that must be excluded are epididymitis, hydrocele, hernia, and spermatic cord torsion. The latter can present as a painless mass in the neonate with little scrotal wall inflammation if the event occurred prenatally. Acute abdominal pain can be the presenting symptom with torsion of an abdominal undescended testicle containing a tumor. Some patients with hormonally active tumors may have small intratesticular lesions that are not palpable on physical examination.

Testicular ultrasound provides important information in the evaluation of testicular masses in children. Color Doppler ultrasound has been reported to be more effective than gray-scale ultrasound in detecting intratesticular neoplasms in the pediatric population (Luker and Siegel, 1994). Ultrasound is particularly useful to identify cystic components of a teratoma of the testis or epidermoid cyst (Fig. 70–12). If these lesions are recognized preoperatively, a testicular sparing procedure can be considered (Rushton et al, 1990; Grunert et al, 1992). MRI has the ability to detect very small functioning Leydig cell tumors that are not evident on ultrasound (Kaufman et al, 1990).

The current staging system used by the Children's Oncology Group is listed in Table 70–12. Staging is based on both tumor markers and pathologic findings. AFP levels are determined at diagnosis and monitored after radical inguinal orchiectomy to determine whether there is an appropriate half-life decline. CT studies of the retroperitoneum and chest are obtained to exclude metastatic lesions. CT imaging of the retroperitoneum can identify most patients with lymph node metastases, but there is a 15% to 20% rate of false-negative findings (Pizzocara et al, 1987).

Tumor Markers

AFP is a single polypeptide chain amino acid produced by the fetal yolk sac, liver, and gastrointestinal tract. YSTs invariably produce AFP, and all AFP-positive tumors are considered to contain yolk sac elements. AFP has a half-life of approximately 5 days, and degradation curves are analyzed after orchiectomy to assess for residual or recurrent disease. **It is important to note that an increased AFP level after orchiectomy for YST in an infant does not always represent persistent disease. Normal adult reference laboratory values for AFP cannot be used in young children because AFP synthesis continues after birth** (Wu et al, 1981; Lahdenne et al, 1991; Brewer and Tank, 1993). **Normal adult levels (less than 10 mg/ml) are not reached until 8 months of age** (Wu et al, 1981). β-Human chorionic gonadotropin (β-hCG) is a glycoprotein produced by embryonal carcinoma and mixed teratomas. The normal value for β-hCG is less than 5 IU/L. The half-life of β-hCG is approximately 24 hours. β-hCG is rarely increased in preadolescent tumors.

Germ Cell Tumors

Mature Teratoma

Teratoma is the second most common testis tumor in children (Brosman, 1979). **Prepubertal mature teratomas have a benign clinical course, in contrast to the clinical behavior of teratomas in adults, which have the propensity to metastasize** (Mostofi and Price, 1973; Haas and Schmidt, 1995; Grady et al, 1997; Gobel et al, 1998). **This benign behavior has led to the consideration of testis-sparing procedures rather than radical orchiectomy** (Marshall et al, 1983; Haas et al, 1986; Altadonna et al, 1988; Rushton et al, 1990; Pearse et al, 1999). All testicular masses in children require ultrasound examination. If this reveals a cystic lesion, the diagnosis of teratoma should be entertained. Other cystic lesions of the testis, such as simple cysts or epidermoid cysts, must be considered in the differential diagnosis. These lesions usually have a hyperechoic center surrounded by an outer hypoechoic rim (Maxwell and Mantora, 1990). Teratoma ap-

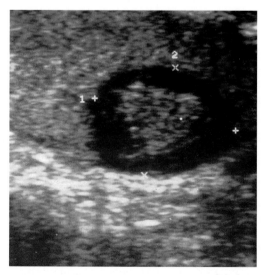

Figure 70–12. Testicular ultrasound demonstrating cystic lesion that proved to be an epidermoid cyst of the testis. The patient underwent a testis-sparing procedure.

Table 70–12. CHILDREN'S ONCOLOGY GROUP STAGING SYSTEM FOR TESTICULAR GERM CELL TUMORS

Stage	Extent of Disease
I	Tumor is limited to the testis. If scrotal orchiectomy has been performed, all margins are negative after resection of proximal cord structures to the level of the internal inguinal ring. Tumor markers are negative after appropriate half-life decline.
II	Microscopic residual disease is present in the scrotum or spermatic cord. Tumor markers remain elevated after appropriate half-life interval. Tumor rupture or scrotal biopsy before complete orchiectomy.
III	Presence of retroperitoneal lymph node involvement.
IV	Distant metastatic deposits.

pears more as a complex hypoechoic area surrounded by highly echogenic signals (Krone and Carroll, 1985). In past years, the majority of these tumors were managed with radical orchiectomy. Although only a limited number of patients have been treated with enucleation of the tumor, there have been no recurrences in those patients reported to date (Rushton et al, 1990). Frozen sections are obtained, and experienced pediatric pathologists can confirm the diagnosis of teratoma from the characteristic histologic features. A detailed review of 21 cases of prepubertal teratoma at the Armed Forces Institute of Pathology did not reveal evidence of multifocal disease or CIS of the adjacent testis (Rushton et al, 1990).

Immature Teratomas

A less common tumor of the testis is immature teratoma. The most common extracranial site is in the ovary; only 10% occur in the testes. Immature teratomas have often been considered to be malignant tumors, but in children they appear to be benign unless they have foci of malignant cells. Because most patients with recurrent tumor can be salvaged with platinum-based chemotherapy, observation alone is recommended for completely resected immature teratoma (Gobel et al, 1998; Marina et al, 1998). Recurrence of immature teratomas after resection occurs almost exclusively in patients with elevated AFP or foci of YST in the initial resection specimens. Recurrent tumors typically are YSTs.

Yolk Sac Tumor

YST is the most common prepubertal testicular tumor of germ cell origin, accounting for 60% of all tumors (Brosman, 1979; Kay, 1993). This tumor occurs primarily in children younger than 2 years of age. The clinical behavior of YST varies considerably from the embryonal carcinoma seen in adults, despite the histologic similarities. Metastasis to the retroperitoneal lymph nodes occurs in 4% to 6% of children with YST (Brosman, 1979; Bracken et al, 1978). **The most common site of distant metastases (20%) is the lung. More than 90% of prepubertal children present with stage I disease** (Haas et al, 1999).

The initial treatment for YST is radical inguinal orchiectomy. This treatment is curative in most children. Routine RPLND and/or adjuvant chemotherapy is not

indicated (Kramer et al, 1984; Mann et al, 1989; Haas and Schmidt, 1995; Haas et al, 1999). Staging of the patient with tumor markers and imaging studies is performed as outlined previously.

Patients with clinical stage I disease do not receive additional adjuvant treatment after radical orchiectomy. Chest radiography, CT, or MRI of the retroperitoneum is recommended monthly for 3 months, again 3 months later, and then every 6 months. This surveillance is continued until 36 months after treatment. Tumor marker studies and physical examinations are performed at more frequent intervals. Approximately 90% of YSTs produce positive serum levels of AFP. Scrotal orchiectomy with negative margins can be treated as stage I, but the proximal cord structures should be resected to the level of the internal ring.

Patients who have undergone prior scrotal biopsy are considered to have stage II disease. A completion orchiectomy with removal of all cord structures is performed. This approach has proved to be of benefit in adult patients with gross contamination during removal of germ cell tumors (Giguere et al, 1988; Capelouto et al, 1995) All patients undergo abdominal CT to examine for retroperitoneal lymphadenopathy. Patients with enlarged lymph nodes should undergo lymph node sampling or biopsy. Patients who have persistent elevation of AFP and retroperitoneal adenopathy are presumed to have metastatic disease. These patients can be treated as stage III.

Combination chemotherapy with platinum-based drugs (cisplatin, etoposide, and bleomycin) is used for pediatric patients with advanced germ cell tumors (Ablin et al, 1991). An intergroup study for the treatment of localized and advanced germ cell tumors in children conducted by the Children's Cancer Group and the Pediatric Oncology Group has been completed (Rescorla, 1998). Persistent retroperitoneal masses after chemotherapy are uncommon (Uehling and Phillips, 1994; Kuo et al, 1999). However, children with clinically evident retroperitoneal disease or elevation of tumor markers after chemotherapy undergo surgery at 12 weeks to establish a histologic diagnosis. Patients with persistent viable tumor are then switched to another treatment regimen. Those patients who develop relapse after initial treatment of a stage I tumor should also undergo biopsy for histologic confirmation.

A similar regimen has been employed by the United Kingdom Children's Cancer Study Group (Mann et al, 1989). Carboplatin has also been used instead of cisplatin in the United Kingdom studies, with equivalent success (Pinkerton et al, 1990). Survival in cases of stage III and IV germ cell tumors (all sites) was 83% and 67%%, respectively. However, overall survival for 68 patients with YSTs of the testis was 99%. Late effects of chemotherapy for childhood germ cell tumors are now being reported (Hale et al, 1999). One frequently noted complication is high-frequency hearing loss in children treated with cisplatin.

Gonadal Stromal Tumors

Gonadal sex-cord stromal tumors are the most common nongerminal testicular tumors in children (Cortez and Kap-

lan, 1993; Goswitz et al, 1996). These benign non–germ cell tumors are more common in children than in adults. They arise from a common mesenchymal stem cell type that can differentiate toward Leydig cells, Sertoli cells, granulosa cells, or a combination of these. An interesting feature of these tumors is their ability to secrete hormones.

Leydig Cell Tumor

Leydig cell tumor is the most common of the sex-cord tumors and has a peak incidence at age 4 to 5 years. Leydig cells produce testosterone, and production of the hormone by the tumor can result in precocious puberty (Urban et al, 1978). This can lead to accelerated skeletal and muscle development and penile growth that does not resolve after treatment (Mengel and Knorr, 1983). Other hormones produced by Leydig cell tumors include corticosteroids, progesterone, and estrogens.

The differential diagnosis of precocious puberty includes pituitary lesions, Leydig cell hyperplasia, large cell Sertoli cell tumors (see earlier discussion), **and hyperplastic testicular nodules that develop in boys with poorly controlled congenital adrenal hyperplasia (CAH)** (Wilson and Netzloff, 1983; Cunnah et al, 1989; Srikath et al, 1992; Walker et al, 1997). Pituitary lesions may be excluded by the finding of an increased serum testosterone concentration with prepubertal levels of luteinizing hormone (LH) and follicle-stimulating hormone (FSH). Children with Leydig cell hyperplasia have normal levels of urinary 17-ketosteroids. Testicular nodules in patients with CAH tend to occur bilaterally, but there have been reports of bilateral Leydig cell tumors (Bokemeyer et al, 1993). A family history of CAH is helpful in making the diagnosis. The hyperplastic nodules that develop in CAH resemble Leydig cells histologically but behave biochemically like adrenal cortical cells. Urinary ketosteroids are increased in patients with 21-hydroxylase deficiency, and serum levels of 17-hydroxyprogesterone are elevated. Regression of the hyperplastic nodules in the testis is usually seen after glucocorticoid replacement (Srikath et al, 1992; Walker et al, 1997). Persistent nodules may result from fibrosis or calcification.

Inguinal orchiectomy is the only treatment required for Leydig cell tumors. Enucleation of the tumor has been reported, with one patient developing local recurrence (Wegner et al, 1997; Konrad and Schoenle, 1999). **Malignancy has not been reported in Leydig cell tumors in children** (Brosman, 1979).

Sertoli Cell Tumor

Sertoli cell tumor is the next most common gonadal stromal tumor in children (Young et al, 1998). This tumor manifests at an earlier age than the Leydig cell tumor, with the usual presentation being a painless testicular mass. These tumors are not as metabolically active as Leydig cell tumors, but gynecomastia has been reported (Gabrilove et al, 1980). There are limited series of children with Sertoli cells tumors (Gabrilove et al, 1980; Goswitz et al, 1996). Most recommend observation in infants, because metastases have not been reported. The treatment is orchiectomy, but examination of the retroperitoneum is warranted to exclude retroperitoneal spread (Rosvoll and Woodward, 1968). Large cell Sertoli cell tumors have been noted with increased frequency in patients with Peutz-Jeghers syndrome and the Carney complex (Chang et al, 1998).

Gonadoblastoma

Gonadoblastomas are the most common tumors found in association with intersex disorders. They occur in dysgenetic gonads and are associated with the presence of a Y chromosome in the karyotype (Manuel et al, 1976). **Children with mixed gonadal dysgenesis have a 25% risk of tumor formation** (Schellas, 1974)**, and the incidence increases with age** (Manuel et al, 1976). **The germ cell component of gonadoblastoma is prone to malignant degeneration into seminoma and nonseminomatous tumors. All streak gonads in patients with gonadal dysgenesis should be removed** (Aarskog, 1970). **Patients with gonadal dysgenesis raised as females should have the gonads removed at diagnosis** (Olsen et al, 1988; Gourlay et al, 1994). Early gonadectomy is advocated, because tumors have been reported in children younger than 5 years of age (Olsen et al, 1988; Gourlay et al, 1994). In mixed gonadal dysgenesis patients reared as males, all streak gonads and undescended testes should be removed. Scrotal testes can be preserved, because they are less prone to tumor development. It has been suggested that gonadal biopsy and histologic examination for CIS in children with gonadal dysgenesis can identify those at risk for development of malignant germ cell tumors (Muller et al, 1985). However, recognition of CIS in prepubertal gonadal biopsies can be difficult, and a negative biopsy does not preclude the later development of a germ cell tumor.

Other Lesions

Leukemia and lymphoma are the most common malignancies to spread to the testicle in children. Children with acute lymphoblastic leukemia who have bulky disease at diagnosis have up to a 20% incidence of testicular relapse (Askin et al, 1981). Routine testicular biopsy after treatment is no longer recommended (Trigg et al, 2000). Positive testis biopsies early in remission identify patients who are at slightly higher risk for adverse events but do not affect survival. Follicular lymphoma can occur as a primary tumor of the testis (Finn et al, 1999). The prognosis is favorable if the tumor is localized. Testicular involvement occurs in 4% of boys with Burkitt's lymphoma and may be the initial clinical presentation (Lamm and Kaplan, 1974).

Testicular cystic dysplasia is a rare benign lesion in boys that has been reported with increasing frequency (Noh et al, 1999; Toffolutti et al, 1999). It is distinguished by the presence of multiple small, irregular cysts localized in the rete testis. Renal agenesis or multicystic renal dysplasia has been noted in more than half of the reported cases. A proposed cause is a defective connection between the efferent ductules originating from the metanephros and the rete testis tubules originating from the gonad. Management options include testis-sparing surgery and nonoperative treat-

ment (Noh et al, 1999). If the latter approach is used, follow-up with serial testicular ultrasound studies is advised.

Testicular microlithiasis has been reported in association with testicular tumors. It has been noted rarely in children. Recommendations have been made for noninvasive ultrasound follow-up until adult age (Furness et al, 1998; Dell'Acqua et al, 1999).

REFERENCES

Neuroblastoma

Adams GA, Shochat SJ, Smith EI, et al: Thoracic neuroblastoma: A Pediatric Oncology Group Study. J Pediatr Surg 1993;28:372–377.

Albregts AE, Cohen MD, Galliani CA: Neuroblastoma invading the kidney. J Pediatr Surg 1994;29:930–933.

Altman AJ, Baehner RL: Favorable prognosis for survival in children with coincident opsomyoclonus and neuroblastoma. Cancer 1976;37:846.

Andrich MP, Shalaby-Rana E, Movassaghi N, et al: The role of iodine-metaiodobenzylguanidine scanning in the correlative imaging of patients with neuroblastoma. Pediatrics 1996;97:246–250.

Azizkhan RG, Haase GM: Current biologic and therapeutic implications in the surgery of neuroblastoma. Semin Surg Oncol 1993;9:493–501.

Beckwith JB, Perrin EV: In situ neuroblastomas: A contribution to the natural history of neural crest tumors. Am J. Pathol 1963;43:1089–1104.

Benjamin SP, McCormack LJ, Effler DB, et al: Primary tumors of the mediastinum. Chest 1972;62:297–303.

Berthold F, Utsch S, Holschneider AM: The impact of preoperative chemotherapy on resectability of primary tumour and complication rate in metastatic neuroblastoma. Z Kinderchir 1989;44:21–24.

Breslow N, McCann B: Statistical estimation of prognosis for children with neuroblastoma. Cancer Res 1971;31:2098–2103.

Brodeur GM: Neuroblastoma: Clinical applications of molecular parameters. Brain Pathol 1990;1:47.

Brodeur GM: Neuroblastoma and other peripheral neuroectodermal tumors. In Fernbach DJ, Vietti TJ (eds): Clinical Pediatric Oncology, 4th ed. St. Louis, Mosby–Year Book, 1991, p 337.

Brodeur GM, Azar C, Brother M, et al: Neuroblastoma: Effect of genetic factors on prognosis and treatment. Cancer Suppl 1992;70:1685–1694.

Brodeur GM, Fong CT: Molecular biology and genetics of human neuroblastoma. Cancer Genet Cytogenet 1989;41:153–174.

Brodeur GM, Pritchard J, Berthold F, et al: Revisions of the international criteria for neuroblastoma diagnosis, staging, and response to treatment. J Clin Oncol 1993;11:1466–1477.

Caron H, VanSluis P, DeKraker J, et al: Allelic loss of chromosome 1p as a predictor of unfavorable outcome in patients with neuroblastoma. N Engl J Med 1996;334:225–230.

Cecchetto G, Luzzatto C, Carli M, et al: The role of surgery in non-localized neuroblastoma: Analysis of 59 cases. Tumori 1983;69:327–329.

Chamberlain RS, Quinones R, Dinndorf P, et al: Complete surgical resection combined with aggressive adjuvant chemotherapy and bone marrow transplantation prolongs survival in children with advanced neuroblastoma. Ann Surg 1995;2:93–100.

Chan HSL, Haddad G, Thorner PS, et al: P-Glycoprotein expression as a predictor of the outcome of therapy for neuroblastoma. N Engl J Med 1991;325:1608–1614.

Cohn SL, Rademaker AW, Salwen HR, et al: Analysis of DNA ploidy and proliferative activity in relation to histology and N-myc amplification in neuroblastoma. Am J Pathol 1990;136:1043–1052.

Connolly A, Pestronk A, Mehta S, et al: Serum autoantibodies in childhood opsoclonus-myoclonus syndrome: An analysis of antigenic targets in neural tissues. J Pediatr 1997;130:878–884.

Cooney DR, Voorhess ML, Fisher JE, et al: Vasoactive intestinal peptide producing neuroblastoma. J Pediatr Surg 1982;17:821–825.

DeBernardi B, Conte M, Mancini A, et al: Localized resectable neuroblastoma: Results of the second study of the Italian Cooperative Group for neuroblastoma. J Clin Oncol 1995;13:884–893.

DeCou JM, Bowman LC, Rao BN, et al: Infants with metastatic neuroblastoma have improved survival with resection of the primary tumor. J Pediatr Surg 1995;30:937–941.

Dinndorf P, Johnson L, Gaynon P, et al: Outcome of autologous (auto) vs. allogeneic (allo) bone marrow transplantation in 25 children with neuroblastoma (nb) and unfavorable features (UPF). (Abstract.) J Cell Biochem 1992;16A(Suppl.):201.

Enzinger FM, Weiss SW: Soft Tissue Tumors. St. Louis, CV Mosby, 1988, pp 828–831.

Evans AE, Chatten J, D'Angio GJ, et al: A review of 17 IV-S neuroblastoma patients at the Children's Hospital of Philadelphia. Cancer 1980; 45:833–839.

Evans AE, D'Angio GJ, Propert K, et al: Prognostic factors in neuroblastoma. Cancer 1987;59:1853–1859.

Everson TC, Cole WH: Spontaneous Regression of Cancer. Philadelphia, WB Saunders, 1966, pp 88–163.

Farrelly C, Daneman A, Chan HSL, et al: Occult neuroblastoma presenting with opsomyoclonus: Utility of computed tomography. AJR Am J Roentgenol 1984;142:807–810.

Fortner J, Nicastri A, Murphy ML: Neuroblastoma: Natural history and results of treating 133 cases. Ann Surg 1968;167:132–142.

Franklin IM, Pritchard J: Detection of bone marrow invasion by neuroblastoma is improved by sampling at two sites with both aspirates and trephine biopsies. J Clin Pathol 1983;36:1215.

Garaventa A, DeBernardi B, Pianca C, et al: Localized but unresectable neuroblastoma: Treatment and outcome of 145 cases. J Clin Oncol 1993;11:1770–1779.

Geatti Ok Shapiro B, Sisson J, et al: Iodine-131 metaiodobenzylguanidine scintigraphy for the location of neuroblastoma: Preliminary experience in ten cases. J Nucl Med 1985;26:736–742.

Gerson JM, Koop CE: Neuroblastoma. Semin Oncol 1974;11:35–46.

Green AA, Hustu HO, Kumar M: Sequential cyclophosphamide and doxorubicin for induction of complete remission in children with disseminated neuroblastoma. Cancer 1981;48:2310.

Grupp SA, Stern JW, Ross AA, et al: Tandem high dose therapy in rapid sequence for children with high-risk neuroblastoma. J Clin Oncol 2000; 35:696–700.

Haas D, Ablin AR, Miller C, et al: Complete pathologic maturation and regression on stage IV-S neuroblastoma without treatment. Cancer 1990;62:2572–2575.

Haase GM, O'Leary MC, Stram DO, et al: Pelvic neuroblastoma: Implications for a new favorable subgroup. A Children's Cancer Group experience. Ann Surg Oncol 1995;2:516–523.

Haase GM, O'Leary MC, Ramsay N, et al: Aggressive surgery combined with intensive chemotherapy improves survival in poor risk neuroblastoma. J Pediatr Surg 1991;26:1119–1123.

Haase GM, Wong KY, DeLorimier AA, et al: Improvement in survival after excision of primary tumor in stage III neuroblastoma. J Pediatr Surg 1989;24:194–200.

Hachitanda Y, Ishimoto K, Shimada H: Stage IVS neuroblastoma: Histopathology of 27 cases compared with conventional neuroblastomas. Lab Invest 1991;64:5P(26).

Hayashi Y, Hanada R, Yamamoto K: Biology of neuroblastomas in Japan found by screening. Am J Pediatr Hematol Oncol 1992;14:342–347.

Hayashi Y, Kanda N, Inaba T, et al: Cytogenetic findings and prognosis in neuroblastoma with emphasis on marker chromosome 1. Cancer 1989;63:126–132.

Hayashi Y, Ohi R, Yaoita S, et al: Problems of neuroblastoma screening for 6 month olds and results of second screening for 18 month olds. J Pediatr Surg 1995;30:467–470.

Hayes FA, Green AA, Rao BN: Clinical manifestations of ganglioneuroma. Cancer 1989;63:1211–1214.

Heisel MA, Miller JH, Reid BS, et al: Radionuclide bone scan in neuroblastoma. Pediatrics 1983;71:206.

Ho PTC, Estroff JA, Kozakewich H, et al: Prenatal detection of neuroblastoma: A ten-year experience from the Dana-Farber Cancer Institute and Children's Hospital. Pediatrics 1993;92:358–364.

Holgerson LO, Subramanian S, Kirpekar M, et al: Spontaneous resolution of antenatally diagnosed adrenal masses. J Pediatr Surg 1996;31:153–155.

Hsiao RJ, Seeger RC, Yu AL, et al: Chromogranin A in children with neuroblastoma. J Clin Invest 1990;85:1555.

Hutchinson RJ, Sisson JC, Shapiro B, et al: I-131-metaiodobenzylguanidine treatment in patients with refractory advanced neuroblastoma. Am J Clin Oncol 1992;15:226–232.

Ikeda Y, Lister J, Bouton JM, et al: Congenital neuroblastoma, neuroblastoma in situ, and the normal fetal development of the adrenal. J Pediatr Surg 1981;16:636.

Ikeda K, Nakagawara A, Yano H, et al: Improved survival rate in children over one year of age with stage III or IV neuroblastoma following an intensive chemotherapeutic regimen. J Pediatr Surg 1989;24:189–193.

Ishimoto K, Kiyokawa N, Fujita H, et al: Problems of mass screening for neuroblastoma: Analysis of false-negative cases. J Pediatr Surg 1990; 25:398–401.

Ishimoto K, Kiyokawa N, Fujita H, et al: Biological analysis of neuroblastoma in mass screened negative cases. In Evans AE, D'Angio G, Brodeur G, et al (eds): Advances in Neuroblastoma Research 3, 1991, pp 602–608.

Katzenstein HM, Bowman LC, Brodeur GM, et al: Prognostic significance of age, MYCN oncogene amplification, tumor cell ploidy, and histology in 110 infants with stage D(S) neuroblastoma: The Pediatric Oncology Group Experience. A Pediatric Oncology Group Study. J Clin Oncol 1998;16:2007–2017.

Katzenstein HM, Cohn SL: Advances in the diagnosis and treatment of neuroblastoma. Curr Opin Oncol 1998;10:43–51.

Kiely EM: The surgical challenge of neuroblastoma. J Pediatr Surg 1994; 29:128–133.

Knudson AG, Jr, Strong LC: Mutation and cancer: Neuroblastoma and pheochromocytoma. Man J Hum Genet 1972;24:514–532.

Koh PS, Raffensperger JG, Berry S, et al: Long-term outcome in children with opsoclonus-myoclonus and ataxia and coincident neuroblastoma. J Pediatr 1994;125:712–716.

Kozakewich HPW, Perez-Atayde AR, Donovan MJ, et al: Cystic neuroblastoma: Emphasis on gene expression, morphology, and pathogenesis. Pediatr Dev Pathol 1998;1:17–28.

Kusafuka T, Fukuzawa M, Oue T, et al: DNA flow cytometric analysis of neuroblastoma: Distinction of tetraploidy subset. J Pediatr Surg 1994; 29:543–547.

Kushner BH, Cheung NKV, LaQuaglia MP, et al: Survival from locally invasive or widespread neuroblastoma without cytotoxic therapy. J Clin Oncol 1996;14:373–381.

Kushner BH, Gilbert F, Helson L: Familial neuroblastoma: Case reports, literature review and etiologic considerations. Cancer 1986;57:1887–1893.

Lampert F, Rudolph B, Christiansen H, et al: Identical chromosome 1p breakpoint abnormality in both the tumor and the constitutional karyotype of a patient with neuroblastoma. Cancer Genet Cytogenet 1988;34:235.

LaQuaglia MP, Kushner BH, Heller G, et al: Stage 4 neuroblastoma diagnosed at more than 1 year of age: Gross total resection and clinical outcome. J Pediatr Surg 1994;29:1162–1166.

Laureys G, Speleman F, Opdenakker G, et al: Constitutional translocation t(1;17)(p36;q12-21) in a patient with neuroblastoma. Genes Chromosomes Cancer 1990;2:252–254.

Leavey PJ, Odom LF, Poole M, et al: Intra-operative radiation therapy in pediatric neuroblastoma. Med Pediatr Oncol 1997;28:424–428.

LeTourneau JN, Bernard JL, Hendren WH, et al: Evaluation of the role of surgery in 130 patients with neuroblastoma. J Pediatr Surg 1985;20:244–249.

Look AT, Hayes FA, Nitschke R, et al: Cellular DNA content as a predictor of response to chemotherapy in infants with unresectable neuroblastoma. N Engl J Med 1984;311:231–235.

Look AT, Hayes FA, Shuster J, et al: Clinical relevance of tumor cell ploidy and N-myc gene amplification in childhood neuroblastoma: A Pediatric Oncology Group Study. J Clin Oncol 1991;9:581–591.

Martinez DA, King DR, Ginn-Pease ME, et al: Resection of the primary tumor is appropriate for children with stage IV-S neuroblastoma: An analysis of 37 patients. J Pediatr Surg 1992;27:1016–1021.

Matsumura M, Atkinson JB, Hays DM, et al: An evaluation of the role of surgery in metastatic neuroblastoma. J Pediatr Surg 1988;23:448–453.

Matthay KK, O'Leary MC, Ramsay NK, et al: Role of myeloablative therapy in improved outcome for high risk neuroblastoma: Review of recent Children's Cancer Group results. Eur J Cancer 1995;31A:572–575.

Matthay KK, Perez C, Seeger RC, et al: Successful treatment of stage III neuroblastoma based on prospective biologic staging: A Children's Cancer Group Study. J Clin Oncol 1998;16:1256–1264.

Matthay KK, Sather HM, Seeger RC, et al: Excellent outcome of stage II neuroblastoma is independent of residual disease and radiation therapy. J Clin Oncol 1989;7:236–244.

Matthay KK, Villablanca JG, Seeger RC, et al: Treatment of high-risk neuroblastoma with intensive chemotherapy, radiotherapy, autologous bone marrow transplantation, and 13-cis-retinoic acid. N Engl J Med 1999;341:1165–1173.

Morris JA, Shochat SJ, Smith EI, et al: Biological variables in thoracic neuroblastoma: A Pediatric Oncology Group Study. J Pediatr Surg 1995;30:296–303.

Moss TJ, Fonkalssrud EW, Feig SA, et al: Delayed surgery and bone marrow transplantation for widespread neuroblastoma. Ann Surg 1987; 206:514–520.

Moss TJ, Seeger RC, Kindler-Rohrborn A, et al: Immunohistologic detection and phenotyping of neuroblastoma cells in bone marrow using cytoplasmic neuron specific enolase and cell surface antigens. Prog Clin Biol Res 1985;175:367.

Mugishima H, Iwata M, Okabe I, et al: Autologous bone marrow transplantation in children with advanced neuroblastoma. Cancer 1994;74: 972–977.

Muraji T, Okamoto E, Fujimoto J, et al: Combined determination of N-myc oncogene amplification and DNA ploidy in neuroblastoma. Cancer 1993;72:2763–2768.

Nakagawara A, Arima-Nakagawara M, Scavarda NJ, et al: Association between high levels of expression of the TRK gene and favorable outcome in human neuroblastoma. N Engl J Med 1993;328:847–854.

Nickerson HJ, Nesbit ME, Grosfeld JL, et al: Comparison of stage IV and IV-S neuroblastoma in the first year of life. Med Pediatr Oncol 1985; 13:261–268.

Nishi M, Miyake H, Takeda T, et al: Effects of the mass screening of neuroblastoma in Sapporo City. Cancer 1987;60:433–436.

Nitschke R, Smith EI, Shochat S, et al: Localized neuroblastoma treated by surgery: A Pediatric Oncology Group Study. J Clin Oncol 1988;6: 1271–1279.

O'Neill JA, Littman P, Blitzer P, et al: The role of surgery in localized neuroblastoma. J Pediatr Surg 1985;20:708–712.

Powis MR, Imeson JD, Holmes SJK: The effect of complete excision on stage III neuroblastoma: A report of the European Neuroblastoma Study Group. J Pediatr Surg 1996;31:516–519.

Rees H, Markley MA, Kiely EM, et al: Diarrhea after resection of advanced abdominal neuroblastoma: A common management problem. Surgery 1998;123:568–572.

Robertson CM, Tyrrell JC, Pritchard J. Familial neural crest tumours. Eur J Pediatr 1991;150:789–792.

Russo C, Cohn SL, Petruzzi, et al: Long-term neurologic outcome in children with opsoclonus-myoclonus associated with neuroblastoma: A report from the Pediatric Oncology Group. Med Pediatr Oncol 1997;29: 284–288.

Sawada T: Past and future of neuroblastoma screening in Japan. Am J Pediatr Hematol Oncol 1992;14:320–326.

Seeger RC, Brodeur GM, Sather H, et al: Association of multiple copies of the N-myc oncogene with rapid progression of neuroblastomas. N Engl J Med 1985;313:1111–1116.

Seeger RC, Villablanca JG, Matthay KK, et al: Intensive chemoradiotherapy and autologous bone marrow transplantation for poor prognosis neuroblastoma. Prog Clin Biol Res 1991;366:527–534.

Seeger RC, Wada R, Brodeur GM, et al: Expression of N-myc by neuroblastomas with one or multiple copies of the oncogene. Prog Clin Biol Res 1988;271:41–49.

Shamberger RC, Allarde-Segundo A, Kozakewich HPW, et al: Surgical management of stage III and IV neuroblastoma: Resection before or after chemotherapy? J Pediatr Surg 1991;26:1113–1118.

Shamberger RC, Smith EI, Joshi VV, et al: The risk of nephrectomy during local control in abdominal neuroblastoma. J Pediatr Surg 1998; 33:161–164.

Shimada H, Ambros IM, Dehner LP, et al: Terminology and morphologic Criteria of neuroblastic tumors: Recommendations by the International Neuroblastoma Pathology Committee. Cancer 1999a;86:349–363.

Shimada H, Ambros IM, Dehner LP, et al: The International Neuroblastoma Pathology Classification (the Shimada system). Cancer 1999b;86: 364–372.

Shimada H, Chatten J, Newton WA, Jr, et al: Histopathologic prognostic factors in neuroblastic tumors: Definition of subtypes of ganglioneuroblastoma and an age-linked classification of neuroblastomas. J Natl Cancer Inst 1984;73:405–416.

Shochat SJ: Update on solid tumor management. Surg Clin North Am 1992;72:1417–1428.

Shorter NA, Davidoff AM, Evans AE, et al: The role of surgery in the management of stage IV neuroblastoma: A single institution study. Med Pediatr Oncol 1995;24:287–291.

Silber JH, Evans AE, Fridman M: Models to predict outcome from childhood neuroblastoma: The role of serum ferritin and tumor histology. Cancer Res 1991;51:1426–1433.

Sitarz A, Finklestein J, Grosfeld J, et al: An evaluation of the role of surgery in disseminated neuroblastoma: A report from the Children's Cancer Study Group. J Pediatr Surg 1983;18:147–151.

Tanaka T, Hiyama E, Sugimoto T, et al: *trk A* gene expression in neuroblastoma: The clinical significance of an immunohistochemical study. Cancer 1995;76:1086–1095.

Tsuchida Y, Yokoyama J, Kaneko M, et al: Therapeutic significance of surgery in advanced neuroblastoma: A report from the Study Group of Japan. J Pediatr Surg 1992;27:616–622.

Villablanca JG, Khan AA, Avramis VI, et al: Phase I trial of 13-cis-retinoic acid in children with neuroblastoma following bone marrow transplantation. J Clin Oncol 1995;13:894–901.

Weith A, Martinsson T, Cziepluch C, et al: Neuroblastoma consensus deletion maps to I p36.1–2. Genes Chromosomes Cancer 1989;1:159–166.

Williams CM, Greer M: Homovanillic acid and vanillylmandelic acid in diagnosis of neuroblastoma. JAMA 1963;183:836–840.

Woods WG, Tuchman M, Robison LL, et al: A population-based study of the usefulness of screening for neuroblastoma. Lancet 1996;348:1682–1687.

Rhabdomyosarcoma

d'Amore ES, Tollot M, Stracca-Pansa V, et al: Therapy-associated differentiation in rhabdomyosarcomas. Mod Pathol 1994;7(1):69–75.

Andrassy RJ, Hays DM, Raney RB, et al: Conservative surgical management of vaginal and vulvar pediatric rhabdomyosarcoma: A report from the Intergroup Rhabdomyosarcoma Study III. J Pediatr Surg 1994;30: 1034–1037.

Andrassy RJ, Wiener ES, Raney RB, et al: Progress in the surgical management of vaginal rhabdomyosarcoma: A 25-year review from the Intergroup Rhabdomyosarcoma Study Group. J Pediatr Surg 1999;34: 731.

Asmar L, Gehan EA, Newton WA, Jr, et al: Agreement among and within groups of pathologists in the classification of rhabdomyosarcoma and related childhood sarcomas: Report of an international study of four pathology classifications. Cancer 1994;74:2579–2588.

Atra A, Ward HC, Aitken K, et al: Conservative surgery in multimodal therapy for pelvic rhabdomyosarcoma in children. Br J Cancer 1994; 70(5):1004–1008.

Banowsky LH, Shultz GN: Sarcoma of the spermatic cord and tunics: Review of the literature, case report and discussion of the role of retroperitoneal lymph node dissection. J Urol 1970;103:628–631.

Barr FG: Molecular genetics and pathogenesis of rhabdomyosarcoma. J Pediatr Hematol Oncol 1997;19:483–491.

Bruce J, Gough DCS: Long-term follow-up of children with testicular tumours: Surgical issues. Br J Urol 1991;67:429–433.

Corpron C, Andrassy RJ, Hays CM, et al: Conservative management of uterine rhabdomyosarcoma: A report from the Intergroup Rhabdomyosarcoma Studies III and IV Pilot. J Pediatr Surg 1995;30:942–944.

Crist WM, Garnsey L, Beltangady MS, et al: Prognostic factors in children with rhabdomyosarcoma: A report of the Intergroup Rhabdomyosarcoma Studies I and II. J Clin Oncol 1990;8:443–452.

Crist W, Gehan EA, Ragab AH, et al: The third intergroup rhabdomyosarcoma study. J Clin Oncol 1995;13:610–630.

deVries JD: Paratesticular rhabdomyosarcoma. World J Urol 1995;13: 213–218.

Dias P, Parham DM, Shapiro DN, et al: Monoclonal antibodies to the myogenic regulatory protein MyoD1: Epitope mapping and diagnostic utility. Cancer Res 1992;52:6431–6439.

Douglass EC, Valentine M, Etucabana E: A specific chromosomal abnormality in rhabdomyosarcoma. Cytogenet Cell Genet 1987;45:148–155.

Donohue JP, Foster RS, Rowland RG, et al: Nerve-sparing retroperitoneal lymphadenectomy with preservation of ejaculation. J Urol 1990;144: 287–292.

Fisch M, Burger R, Barthels U, et al: Surgery in rhabdomyosarcoma of the bladder, prostate and vagina. World J Urol 1995;13:213–218.

Goldfarb B, Khoury A, Greenberg M, et al: The role of retroperitoneal lymphadenectomy in localized paratesticular rhabdomyosarcoma. J Urol 1994;152:785–787.

Hays DM: Bladder/prostate rhabdomyosarcoma: Results of the multi-institutional trials of the Intergroup Rhabdomyosarcoma Study. Semin Surg Oncol 1993;9:520–523.

Hays DM, Lawrence W, Crist W, et al: Partial cystectomy in the management of rhabdomyosarcoma of the bladder: A report from the Intergroup Rhabdomyosarcoma Study (IRS). J Pediatr Surg 1990;25:719–723.

Hays DM, Newton W, Jr, Soule E, et al: Mortality among children with rhabdomyosarcoma of the alveolar histologic subtypes. J Pediatr Surg 1983;18:412–417.

Hays DM, Raney RB, Lawrence W, et al: Rhabdomyosarcoma of the female urogenital tract. J Pediatr Surg 1981;16:828–834.

Hays DM, Raney RB, Lawrence W, et al: Primary chemotherapy in the treatment of children with bladder-prostate tumors in the Intergroup Rhabdomyosarcoma Study (IRS-II). J Pediatr Surg 1982;17:812–820.

Hays DM, Raney RB, Wharam MD, et al: Children with vesical rhabdomyosarcoma (RMS) treated by partial cystectomy with neoadjuvant chemotherapy, with or without radiotherapy: A report from the Intergroup Rhabdomyosarcoma Study (IRS) Committee. J Pediatr Hematol Oncol 1995;17:46–52.

Hays DM, Shimada H, Raney RB, et al: Sarcomas of the vagina and uterus: The Intergroup Rhabdomyosarcoma Study. J Pediatr Surg 1985; 20:718–724.

Hays DM, Shimada H, Raney RB, Jr, et al: Clinical staging and treatment results in rhabdomyosarcoma of the female genital tract among children and adolescents. Cancer 1988;61:1893–1903.

Heyn RM, Holland R, Newton WA, Jr, et al: The role of combined chemotherapy in the treatment of rhabdomyosarcoma in children. Cancer 1974;34:2128–2141.

Heyn R, Raney B, Hays D et al: Late effects of therapy in patients with paratesticular rhabdomyosarcoma. For the Intergroup Rhabdomyosarcoma Study Committee. J Clin Oncol 1992;10:614–623.

Heyn R, Newton WA, Raney RB, et al: Preservation of the bladder in patients with rhabdomyosarcoma. J Clin Oncol 1997;15:69–75.

Hicks BA, Hensle TW, Burbige KA, Altman PR: Bladder management in children with genitourinary sarcoma. J Pediatr Surg 1993;28:1019–1022.

Kattan J, Culine S, Terrier-Lacombe M, et al: Paratesticular rhabdomyosarcoma in adult patients: 16-year experience at Institut Gustav-Roussy. Ann Oncol 1993;4:871–875.

Kelly KM, Womer RB, Sorensen PHB, et al: Common and variant gene fusions predict distinct clinical phenotypes in rhabdomyosarcoma. J Clin Oncol 1997;15:1831–1836.

Kodet R, Newton WA, Jr, Hamoudi AB, et al: Childhood rhabdomyosarcoma with anaplastic (pleomorphic) features. Am J Surg Pathol 1993; 17:443–453.

LaQuaglia M, Ghavimi F, Heller G, et al: Mortality in pediatric paratesticular rhabdomyosarcoma: A multivariate analysis. J Urol 1989; 142:473–478.

LaQuaglia M, Heller G, Ghavami F, et al: The effect of age at diagnosis on outcome in rhabdomyosarcoma. Cancer 1994;73:109–117.

Lawrence W, Jr, Anderson JR, Gehan EA, et al: Pretreatment TNM staging of childhood rhabdomyosarcoma: A report of the Intergroup Rhabdomyosarcoma Study Group. Cancer 1997;80:1165–1170.

Lawrence W, Jr, Hays DM, Heyn R, et al: Lymphatic metastasis with childhood rhabdomyosarcoma. Cancer 1987a;60:910–915.

Lawrence W, Gehan EA, Hays DM, et al: Prognostic significance of staging factors of the UICC staging system in childhood rhabdomyosarcoma: A report from the Intergroup Rhabdomyosarcoma Study (IRS-II). J Clin Oncol 1987b;5:46–54.

Leiroth D, Baserga R, Helman L, Roberts CT, Jr: Insulin-like growth factors and cancer. Ann Intern Med 1995;12:54–59.

Li FP, Fraumeni JF, Jr: Soft-tissue sarcomas, breast cancer, and other neoplasms: A familial syndrome? Ann Intern Med 1969;71:747–752.

Lobe TE, Wiener E, Andrassy RJ, et al: The argument for conservative, delayed surgery in the management of prostatic rhabdomyosarcoma. J Pediatr Surg 1996;31:1084–1087.

Malkin D, Li FP, Strong LC, et al: Germ line p53 mutations in a familial syndrome of breast cancer, sarcomas, and other neoplasms. Science 1990;250:1233–1238.

Maurer HM, Beltangady M, Gehan EA, et al: The Intergroup Rhabdomyosarcoma Study I: A final report. Cancer 1988;61:209–220.

Maurer HM, Moon T, Donaldson M, et al: The Intergroup Rhabdomyosarcoma study: A preliminary report. Cancer 1977;40:2015–2026.

McKeen EA, Bodurtha J, Meadows AT, et al: Rhabdomyosarcoma complicating multiple neurofibromatosis. J Pediatr 1978;93:992–993.

McLorie GA, Abara OE, Churchill BM, et al: Rhabdomyosarcoma of the prostate in childhood: Current challenges. J Pediatr Surg 1989;24:977–981.

Meguerian PA, Agarwal S, Greenberg M, et al: Outcome analysis of rhabdomyosarcoma of the lower urinary tract. J Urol 1998;160:1191–1194.

Neville HL, Andrassy RJ, Lally KP, et al: Lymphatic mapping with sentinel node biopsy in pediatric patients. J Pediatr Surg 2000a;35:961–964.

Neville HL, Andrassy RJ, Lobe TE, et al: Preoperative staging, prognostic factors, and outcome for extremity rhabdomyosarcoma: A preliminary report from the IRS IV (1991–1997). J Pediatr Surg 2000b;35:317–321.

Newton W, Soule EH, Hamoude A, et al: Histopathology of childhood sarcomas, Intergroup Rhabdomyosarcoma Studies I and II: Clinicopathologic classification. J Clin Oncol 1988;6:67–75.

Olive D, Flamant F, Zucker JM, et al: Paraaortic lymphadenectomy is not necessary in the treatment of localized paratesticular rhabdomyosarcoma. Cancer 1984;54:1283–1287.

Olive-Sommelet D: Paratesticular rhabdomyosarcoma. International Society of Pediatric Oncology Protocol. Dial Pediatr Urol 1989;12:4–5.

Ortega JA: A therapeutic approach to childhood pelvic rhabdomyosarcoma without pelvic exenteration. J Pediatr 1979;94:205–209.

Ortega JA, Rowland J, Monforte H, et al: Presence of well-differentiated rhabdomyoblasts at the end of therapy for pelvic rhabdomyosarcoma: Implications for the outcome. J Pediatr Hematol Oncol 2000;22:106–111.

Parham DM: The molecular biology of childhood rhabdomyosarcoma. Semin Diagn Pathol 1994;11:39–46.

Pinkel D, Pickren J: Rhabdomyosarcoma in children. JAMA 1961;175: 293–298.

Raney RB, Gehan EA, Hays DM, et al: Primary chemotherapy with or without radiation therapy and or surgery for children with localized sarcoma of the bladder, prostate, vagina, uterus, and cervix. Cancer 1990;66:2072–2081.

Raney RB, Jr, Heyn D, Hays DM, et al: Sequelae of treatment in 109 patients followed for 5 to 15 years after diagnosis of sarcoma of the bladder and prostate. Cancer 1993;71:2387–2394.

Raney RB, Jr, Tefft M, Lawrence W, Jr, et al: Paratesticular sarcoma in childhood and adolescence: A report from the Intergroup Rhabdomyosarcoma studies I and II, 1973–1983. Cancer 1987;60:2337–2343.

Rodary C, Flamant F, Maurer H, et al: Initial lymphadenectomy is not necessary in localized and completely resected paratesticular rhabdomyosarcoma. (Abstract.) Med Pediatr Oncol 1992;20:430.

Rodary C, Rey A, Olive D, et al: Prognostic factors in 281 children with non-metastatic rhabdomyosarcoma (RMS) at diagnosis. Med Pediatr Oncol 1988;16:71–77.

Scrable HJ, Johnson DK, Rinchik EM, et al: Rhabdomyosarcoma associated locus and MyoD1 are syntenic but separate loci on the short arm of chromosome 11. Proc Natl Acad Sci U S A 1990;87:2182–2186.

Shapiro DM, Parham DM, Douglas EC, et al: Relationship of tumor-cell ploidy to histologic subtype and treatment outcome in children and adolescents with unresectable rhabdomyosarcoma. J Clin Oncol 1991;9: 159–166.

Sutow WW, Sullivan MP, Ried HL, et al: Prognosis in childhood rhabdomyosarcoma. Cancer 1970;25:1385–1390.

Voute PA, Vos A, deKraker J, Behrendt H: Rhabdomyosarcomas: Chemotherapy and limited supplementary treatment to avoid mutilation. Natl Cancer Inst Monogr 1981;56:121–125.

Wiener ES, Anderson JR, Ojimba JI, et al: Controversies in the management of paratesticular rhabdomyosarcoma: Is staging retroperitoneal lymph node dissection necessary for adolescents with resected paratesticular rhabdomyosarcoma? Semin Pediatr Surg 2001;10(3):146–152.

Weiner ES, Lawrence W, Hays D, et al: Retroperitoneal node biopsy in childhood paratesticular rhabdomyosarcoma. J Pediatr Surg 1994;29: 171–178.

Nephroblastoma and Other Renal Tumors

Argani P, Perlman EJ, Breslow NE, et al: Clear cell sarcoma of the kidney: A review of 351 cases from the National Wilms Tumor Study Group Pathology Center. Am J Surg Pathol 2000;24:4–18.

Aronson DC, Medary I, Finlay JL, et al: Renal cell carcinoma in childhood and adolescence: A retrospective survey for prognostic factors in 22 cases. J Pediatr Surg 1996;31:183–186.

Arrigo S, Beckwith JB, Sharples K, et al: Better survival after combined modality care for adults with Wilms' tumor: A report from the National Wilms' Tumor Study. Cancer 1990;66:827–830.

Arroyo M, Green D, Breslow N, et al: Metanephric adenofibroma and related lesions: Clinicopathologic study of 24 cases. Mod Pathol 2000; 13:1P.

Banner MP, Pollack HM, Chatten J, Witzleben C: Multilocular renal cysts: Radiologic-pathologic correlation. AJR Am J Roentgenol 1981; 136:239.

Bardeesy N, Falkoff D, Petruzzi MJ, et al: Anaplastic Wilms' tumour, a subtype displaying poor prognosis, harbours p53 gene mutations. Nat Genet 1994;7:91–97.

Bardeesy N, Beckwith JB, Pelletier J: Clonal expansion and attenuated apoptosis in Wilms' tumors are associated with p53 gene mutations. Cancer Res 1995;55:215–219.

Beckwith JB: Macroglossia, omphalocele, adrenal cytomegaly, gigantism and hyperplastic visceromegaly. Birth Defects 1969;5:188–196.

Beckwith JB: Wilms tumor and other renal tumors of childhood: A selective review from the National Wilms' Tumor Study Pathology Center. Hum Pathol 1983;14:481–492.

Beckwith JB: Congenital mesoblastic nephroma: When should we worry? Arch Pathol Lab Med 1986;110:98–99.

Beckwith JB: Precursor lesions of Wilms tumor: Clinical and biological implications. Med Pediatr Oncol 1993;21:158–168.

Beckwith JB: Certain conditions have an increased incidence of Wilms' tumor. AJR Am J Roentgenol 1996;164:1294–1295.

Beckwith JB: Nephrogenic rests and the pathogenesis of Wilms tumor: Developmental and clinical considerations. Am J Med Genet 1998;79: 268–273.

Beckwith JB, Kiviat NB, Bonadio JF: Nephrogenic rests, nephroblastomatosis, and the pathogenesis of Wilms' tumor. Pediatr Pathol 1990;10:1–36.

Beckwith JB, Palmer NF: Histopathology and prognosis of Wilms tumor: Results from the National Wilms Tumor Study. Cancer 1978;41:1937–1948.

Beckwith JB, Zuppan CE, Browning NG, et al: Histological analysis of aggressiveness and responsiveness in Wilms tumor. Med Pediatr Oncol 1996;27:422–428.

Biegel JA, Zhou JY, Rorke LB, et al: Germ-line and acquired mutations of INI1 in atypical teratoid and rhabdoid tumors. Cancer Res 1999;59:74–79.

Blank E, Neerhout RC, Burry KA: Congenital mesoblastic nephroma and polyhydramnios. JAMA 1978;240:1504–1505.

Blute ML, Kelalis PP, Offord KP, et al: Bilateral Wilms' tumor. J Urol 1987;138:968–973.

Blute ML, Malek RS, Segura JW: Angiomyolipoma: A clinical metamorphosis and concepts for management. J Urol 1988;139:20–24.

Boccon-Gibod L, Rey A, Sandstedt B, et al: Complete necrosis induced by preoperative chemotherapy in Wilms tumor as an indicator of low risk: Report of the International Society of Paediatric Oncology (SIOP) Nephroblastoma Trial and Study 9. Med Pediatr Oncol 2000;34:183–190.

Bonadio JF, Storer B, Norkool P, et al: Anaplastic Wilms' tumor: Clinical and pathological studies. J Clin Oncol 1985;3:513–520.

Bonaiti-Pellie C, Chompret A, Tournade MF, et al: Genetics and epidemiology of Wilms' tumor: The French Wilms' tumor study. Med Pediatr Oncol 1992;20:284–291.

Bonetta L, Kuehn SE, Huang A, et al: Wilms tumor locus on 11p13 defined by multiple CpG island-associated transcripts. Science 1990; 250:994–997.

Bonnin JM, Rubenstein IJ, Palmer NF, Beckwith JB: The association of embryonal tumors originating in the kidney and the brain. Cancer 1984; 54:2137–2146.

Borer JG, Kaefer M, Barnewolt CE, et al: Renal findings on radiological follow-up of patients with Beckwith-Wiedemann syndrome.J Urol 1999; 161:235–239.

Breslow NB, Churchill G, Beckwith JB, et al: Prognosis for Wilms' tumor patients with nonmetatastic disease at diagnosis: Results of the Second National Wilms' Tumor Study. J Clin Oncol 1985;3:521–531.

Breslow NE, Norkool PA, Olshan A, et al: Second malignant neoplasm in survivors of Wilms' tumor: A report from the National Wilms' Tumor Study. J Natl Cancer Inst 1988;80:592–595.

Breslow N, Olshan A, Beckwith JB, Green DM: Epidemiology of Wilms' tumor. Med Pediatr Oncol 1993;21:172–181.

Breslow N, Olshan A, Beckwith JB, et al: Ethnic variation in the incidence, diagnosis, prognosis and follow-up of children with Wilms' tumor. J Natl Cancer Inst 1994;86:49–51.

Breslow NE, Partin AW, Lee BR, et al: Nuclear morphometry and prognosis in favorable histology Wilms tumor: A prospective reevaluation. J Clin Oncol 1999;17:2123–2126.

Breslow NE, Takashima J, Ritchey ML, et al: Renal failure in the Denys-Drash and Wilms tumor aniridia syndromes. Cancer Res 2000;60:4030–4032.

Broecker B: Renal cell carcinoma in children. Urology 1991;38:54–56.

Call KM, Glaser T, Ito CY, et al: Isolation and characterization of a zinc finger polypeptide gene at the human chromosome 11 Wilms' tumor locus. Cell 1990;60:509–520.

Carcao MD, Taylor GP, Greenberg ML, et al: Renal-cell carcinoma in children: A different disorder from its adult counterpart? Med Pediatr Oncol 1998;31:153–158.

Castellanos RD, Aron BS, Evans AT: Renal adenocarcinoma in children: Incidence, therapy and prognosis. J Urol 1974;111:534–537.

Choyke PL, Siegel MJ, Craft AW, et al: Screening for Wilms tumor in children with Beckwith-Wiedemann syndrome or idiopathic hemihypertrophy. Med Pediatr Oncol 1999;32:196–200.

Clericuzio CL: Clinical phenotypes and Wilms tumor. Med Pediatr Oncol 1993;21:182–187.

Cohen MD: Staging of Wilms' tumor. Clin Radiol 1993;47:77–81.

Comings DE: A general theory of carcinogenesis. Proc Natl Acad Sci U S A 1973;70:3324–3328.

Cooper CS, Jaffe WI, Huff DS, et al: The role of renal salvage procedures for bilateral Wilms tumor: A 15-year review. J Urol 2000;163: 265–268.

Coppes MJ: Serum biological markers and paraneoplastic syndromes in Wilms tumor. Med Pediatr Oncol 1993;21:213–221.

Coppes MJ, Arnold M, Beckwith JB, et al: Factors affecting the risk of contralateral Wilms tumor development. Cancer 1999;85:1616–1625.

Coppes MJ, deKraker J, vanKijken PJ, et al: Bilateral Wilms' tumor: Long-term survival and some epidemiological features. J Clin Oncol 1989;7:310–315.

Coppes MJ, Egeler RM: Genetics of Wilms' tumor. Semin Urol Oncol 1999;17:2–10.

Coppes MJ, Huff V, Pelletier J: Denys-Drash syndrome: Relating a clinical disorder to genetic alterations in the tumor suppressor gene WT1. J Pediatr 1993;123:673–678.

Coppes MJ, Liefers GJ, Higuchi M, et al: Inherited WT1 mutations in Denys-Drash syndrome. Cancer Res 1992;52:6125–6128.

Cozzi F, Schiavetti A, Clerico A, et al: Tumor enucleation in unilateral Wilms' tumor: A pilot study. Med Pediatr Oncol 1995;25:313.

D'Angio GJ, Breslow N, Beckwith JB, et al: Treatment of Wilms' tumor: Results of the Third National Wilms' Tumor Study. Cancer 1989;64: 349–360.

D'Angio GJ, Evans AE, Breslow N, et al: The treatment of Wilms' tumor: Results of the National Wilms' Tumor Study. Cancer 1976;38: 633–646.

D'Angio GJ, Evans A, Breslow N, et al: The treatment of Wilms' tumor: Results of the Second National Wilms' Tumor Study. Cancer 1981;47: 2302–2311.

D'Angio GJ, Rosenberg H, Sharples K, et al: Position paper. Imaging methods for primary renal tumors of childhood: Cost versus benefits. Med Pediatr Oncol 1993;21:205–212.

Debaun MR, Siegel MJ, Choyke PL: Nephromegaly in infancy and early childhood: A risk factor for Wilms tumor in Beckwith-Wiedemann syndrome. J Pediatr 1998;132:401–404.

Debaun MR, Tucker MA: Risk of cancer during the first four years of life in children from the Beckwith-Wiedemann syndrome registry. J Pediatr 1998;132:377–379.

Dehner LP, Leestma JE, Price EB, Jr: Renal cell carcinoma in children: A clinicopathologic study of 15 cases and review of the literature. J Pediatr 1970;76:358–368.

Dickinson M, Ruckle H, Beaghler M, Hadley H: Renal angiomyolipoma: Optimal management based on size and symptoms. Clin Nephrol 1998; 49:281–286.

Diller L, Ghhremani M, Morgan J, et al: Constitutional WT1 mutations in Wilms tumor patients. J Clin Oncol 1998;16:3634–3640.

Ditchfield MR, DeCampo JF, Waters KD, Nolan TM: Wilms' tumor: A rational use of preoperative imaging. Med Pediatr Oncol 1995;24:93–96.

Dome JS, Chung S, Bergemann T, et al: High telomerase reverse transcriptase (hTERT) messenger RNA level correlates with tumor recurrence in patients with favorable histology Wilms tumor. Cancer Res 1999;59:4301–4307.

Drash A, Sherman F, Hartmann WH, Blizzard RM: A syndrome of pseudohermaphroditism, Wilms tumor, hypertension and degenerative renal disease. J Pediatr 1970;76:585–593.

Eble JN, Bonsib SM: Extensively cystic renal neoplasms: Cystic nephroma, cystic partially differentiated nephroblastoma, multilocular cystic renal cell carcinoma, and cystic hamartoma of renal pelvis. Semin Diagn Pathol 1998;15:2–20.

Evans AE, Norkool P, Evans I, et al: Late effects of treatment for Wilms' tumor: A report from the National Wilms' Tumor Study Group. Cancer 1991;67:331–336.

Ewalt DH, Sheffield E, Sparagana SP, et al: Renal lesion growth in children with tuberous sclerosis complex. J Urol 1998;160:141–145.

Faria P, Beckwith JB, Mishra K, et al: Focal versus diffuse anaplasia in Wilms tumor. New definitions with prognostic significance. A report from the National Wilms Tumor Study Group. Am J Surg Pathol 1996; 20:909–920.

Gilladoga AC, Manuel C, Tan CT, et al: The cardiotoxicity of Adriamycin and daunomycin in children. Cancer 1976;37:1070–1078.

Glass RBJ, Davidson AJ, Fernbach SK: Clear cell sarcoma of the kidney: CT, sonographic and pathologic correlation. Radiology 1991;180:715–717.

Gleason PE, Kramer SA: Genitourinary polyps in children. Urology 1994; 44:106–109.

Godzinski J, Tournade MF, deKraker J, et al: Rarity of surgical complications after postchemotherapy nephrectomy for nephroblastoma: Experience of the International Society of Paediatric Oncology-Trial and study "SIOP-9." International Society of Paediatric Oncology Nephroblastoma Trial and Study committee. Eur J Pediatr Surg 1998;8:83–86.

Gormley TS, Skoog SJ, Jones RV, Maybee D: Cellular congenital mesoblastic nephroma: What are the options? J Urol 1989;142:479–483.

Graf N, Tournade MF, deKraker J: The role of preoperative chemotherapy in the management of Wilms' tumor. Urol Clin North Am 2000;27: 443–454.

Green DM, Beckwith JB, Breslow NB, et al: The treatment of children with stage II–IV anaplastic Wilms tumor: A report from the National Wilms Tumor Study. J Clin Oncol 1994a;12:2126–2131.

Green DM, Beckwith JB, Weeks DA, et al: The relationship between microsubstaging variables, tumor weight and age at diagnosis of children with stage I/favorable histology Wilms tumor: A report from the National Wilms Tumor Study. Cancer 1994b;74:1817–1820.

Green DM, Breslow NE, Beckwith JB, Norkool P: Screening of children with hemihypertrophy, aniridia, and Beckwith-Wiedemann syndrome in patients with Wilms' tumor: A report from the National Wilms Tumor Study. Med Pediatr Oncol 1993a;21:188–192.

Green DM, Breslow NE, D'Angio GJ: The treatment of children with unilateral Wilms tumor. J Clin Oncol 1993b;11:1009–1010.

Green DM, Breslow NE, Beckwith JB, et al: Comparison between single-dose and divided-dose administration of dactinomycin and doxorubicin for patients with Wilms' tumor: A report from the National Wilms' Tumor Study Group. J Clin Oncol 1998a;16:237–245.

Green DM Breslow NE, Beckwith JBB, et al: Effect of duration of treatment on treatment outcomes and cost of treatment for Wilms' tumor: A report from the National Wilms Tumor Study Group. J Clin Oncol 1998b;16:3744–3751.

Green D, Breslow N, Ritchey M, et al: Treatment with nephrectomy only for small, stage I/favorable histology Wilms tumor: A report from the National Wilms Tumor Study Group. Proc ASCO 2000a;19:582A.

Green DM, Fine NE, nd Li FP: Offspring of patients treated for unilateral Wilms' tumor in childhood. Cancer 1982;49:2285–2288.

Green DM, Nan B, Grigoriev YA, et al: Congestive failure after treatment for Wilms tumor: A report from the National Wilms Tumor Study Group. Med Pediatr Oncol 2001;19:1926–1934.

Grundy P, Breslow N, Green DM, et al: Prognostic factors for children with recurrent Wilms' tumor: Results from the Second and Third National Wilms Tumor Study. J Clin Oncol 1989;7:638–647.

Grundy PE, Telzerow PE, Breslow N, et al: Loss of heterozygosity for chromosomes 16q and 1p in Wilms tumor predicts an adverse outcome. Cancer Res 1994;54:2331–2333.

Grundy PE, Telzerow PE, Moksness J, Breslow NE: Clinicopathologic correlates of loss of heterozygosity in Wilms tumor: A preliminary analysis. Med Pediatr Oncol 1996;27:429–433.

Hartman D, Davis C, Madewell J, Friedman A: Primary malignant tumors in the second decade of life: Wilms tumor versus renal cell carcinoma. J Urol 1982;127:888–891.

Heidelberger KP, Ritchey ML, Dauser RC, et al: Congenital mesoblastic nephroma metastatic to the brain. Cancer 1993;72:2499–502.

Hittner HM, Riccardi VM, Ferrell RE, et al: Genetic heterogeneity of aniridia: Negative linkage data. Metab Pediatr Syst Ophthalmol 1980;4: 179–182.

Hollstein M, Sidransky D, Vogestein B, Harris CC: *p53* mutations in human cancers. Science 1991;253:49–53.

Horwitz J, Ritchey ML, Moksness J, et al: Renal salvage procedures in patients with synchronous bilateral Wilms tumors: A report of the NWTSG. J Pediatr Surg 1996;31:1020–1025.

Howell CJ, Othersen HB, Kiviat NE, et al: Therapy and outcome in 51 children with mesoblastic nephroma: A report of the National Wilms' Tumor Study. J Pediatr Surg 1982;17:826–830.

Hudson HC, Kramer SA, Tatum AH, et al: Transitional cell carcinoma of renal pelvis: Rare occurrence in young male. Urology 1981;18:284–286.

Huff V: Inheritance and functionality of Wilms tumor genes. Cancer Bull 1994;46:255–259.

Huff V, Villalba F, Riccardi VM, et al: Alteration of the WT1 gene in patients with Wilms' tumor and genitourinary anomalies. (Abstract.) Am J Hum Genet 1991;49:44.

Johnson DE, Ayala AG, Medellin H, Wilbur J: Multilocular renal cystic disease in children. J Urol 1973;109:101–103.

Joshi VV, Beckwith JB: Multilocular cyst of the kidney (cystic nephroma) and cystic, partially differentiated nephroblastoma: Terminology and criteria for diagnosis. Cancer 1989;64:466–479.

Joshi VV, Kasznica J, Walters TR: Atypical mesoblastic nephroma: Pathologic characterization of a potentially aggressive variant of conventional congenital mesoblastic nephroma. Arch Pathol Lab Med 1986; 110:100–106.

Karth J, Ferrer F, Hanrahan C, et al: Co-expression of hypoxia inducible factor 1alpha and vascular endothelial growth factor in human Wilms' tumor. J Urol 2000;163:137.

Kattan J, Tournade MF, Culine S, et al: Adult Wilms' tumour: Review of 22 cases. Eur J Cancer 1994;30A:1778–1782.

Kayton ML, Rowe DH, O'Toole KM, et al: Metastasis correlates with production of vascular endothelial growth factor in a murine model of human Wilms tumor. J Pediatr Surg 1999;34:743–748.

Kinsella TJ, Trivette G, Rowland J, et al: Long-term follow-up of testicular function following radiation for early-stage Hodgkin's disease. J Clin Oncol 1989;7:718–724.

Knudson AG, nd Strong LC: Mutation and cancer: A model for Wilms' tumor of the kidney. J Natl Cancer Inst 1972;48:313–324.

Koufos A, Grundy P, Morgan K, et al: Familial Wiedemann-Beckwith syndrome and a second Wilms tumor locus both map to 11p15.5. Am J Hum Genet 1989;44:711–719.

Kovalic JJ, Thomas PRM, Beckwith JB, et al: Hepatocellular carcinoma as second malignant neoplasms in successfully treated Wilms' tumor patients. Cancer 1991;67:342–344.

Kumar R, Fitzgerald R, Breatnach F: Conservative surgical management of bilateral Wilms tumor: Results of the United Kingdom Children's Cancer Study Group. J Urol 1998;160:1450–1453.

Larsen E, Perez-Atayde A, Green DM, et al: Surgery only for the treatment of patients with stage I (Cassady) Wilms' tumor. Cancer 1990;66: 264–266.

Lee W, Kim TS, Chung JW, et al: Renal angiomyolipoma: Embolotherapy with a mixture of alcohol and iodized oil. J Vasc Interv Radiol 1998;9:255–261.

Lemerle J, Voute PA, Tournade MF, et al: Preoperative versus postoperative radiotherapy, single versus multiple courses of actinomycin D, in the treatment of Wilms' tumor: Preliminary results of a controlled clinical trial conducted by the International Society of Paediatric Oncology (SIOP). Cancer 1976;38:647–654.

Lemerle J, Voute PA, Tournade MF, et al: Effectiveness of preoperative chemotherapy in Wilms' tumor: Results of an International Society of Paediatric Oncology (SIOP) clinical trial. J Clin Oncol 1983;1:604–609.

Levin NP, Damjanov I, Depillis VJ: Mesoblastic nephroma in an adult patient: Recurrence 21 years after removal of the primary. Cancer 1982;49:573–577.

Li FP, Yan JC, Sallan S, et al: Second neoplasms after Wilms tumor in childhood. J Natl Cancer Inst 1983;71:1205–1209.

Li FP, Gimbrere K, Gelber RD, et al: Outcome of pregnancy in survivors of Wilms tumor. JAMA 1987;257:216–219.

Lin RY, Argenta PA, Sullivan KM, Adzick NS: Diagnostic and prognostic role of basic fibroblast growth factor in Wilms tumor patients. Clin Cancer Res 1995a;1:327–331.

Lin RY, Argent PA, Sullivan KM, et al: Urinary hyaluronic acid is a Wilms tumor marker. J Pediatr Surg 1995b;30:304–308.

Malkin D, Sexsmith E, Yeger H, et al: Mutations of the p53 tumor suppressor gene occur infrequently in Wilms' tumor. Cancer Res 1994; 54(8):2077–2079.

Mannens M, Devilee P, Bliek J, et al: Loss of heterozygosity in Wilms' tumors, studied for six putative tumor suppressor regions, is limited to chromosome 11. Cancer Res 1990;50:3279–3283.

Marsden HB, Lawler W, Kumar PM: Bone metastasizing renal tumor of childhood: Morphological and clinical features, and differences from Wilms' tumor. Cancer 1978;42:1922–1928.

Maw MA, Grundy PE, Millow LJ, et al: A third Wilms' tumor locus on chromosome 16q. Cancer Res 1992;52:3094–3098.

McDonald JM, Douglass EC, Fisher R, et al: Linkage of familial Wilms' tumor predisposition to chromosome 19 and a two-locus model for the etiology of familial tumors. Cancer Res 1998;58:1387–1390.

McLorie GA, McKenna PH, Greenburg M, et al: Reduction in tumor burden allowing partial nephrectomy following preoperative chemotherapy in biopsy proved Wilms' tumor. J Urol 1991;146:509–513.

Mesrobian H-G, Kelalis PP, Hrabovsky E, et al: Wilms' tumor in horseshoe kidneys. J Urol 1985;133:1002–1003.

Miller RW, Fraumeni JF, Manning MD: Association of Wilms tumor with aniridia, hemihypertrophy and other congenital malformations. N Engl J Med 1964;270:922–927.

Miozo M, Perotti D, Minoletti F, et al: Mapping of a putative tumor suppressor locus to proximal 7p in Wilms tumors. Genomics 1996;37:310–315.

Montgomery BT, Kelalis PP, Blute ML, et al: Extended follow-up of bilateral Wilms' tumor: Results of the National Wilms Tumor Study. J Urol 1991;146:514–518.

Moorman-Voestermans C, Aronson D, Staalman CR, et al: Is partial nephrectomy appropriate treatment for unilateral Wilms' tumor? J Pediatr Surg 1998;33:165–170.

Neri G, Gurrieri F, Zanni G, Lin A: Clinical and molecular aspects of the Simpson-Golabi-Behmel syndrome. Am J Med Genet 1998;79:279–283.

Neville H, Ritchey M, Shamberger R, Haase G, Perlman S: The occurrence of Wilms tumor in horseshoe kidneys: A report from the National Wilms Tumor Study Group (NWTSG). Pediatrics 1999;104:772.

Ng YY, Hall-Craggs MA, Dicks-Mireaux C, Pritchard J: Wilms' tumour: Pre- and post-chemotherapy CT appearances. Clin Radiol 1991;43:255–259.

Othersen HB, Jr, DeLorimier A, Hrabovsky E, et al: Surgical evaluation of lymph node metastases in Wilms' tumor. J Pediatr Surg 1990;25:3:1–2.

Partin AW, Walsh AC, Epstein JI, et al: Nuclear morphometry as a predictor of response to therapy in Wilms' tumor: A preliminary report. J Urol 1990;144:1222–1226.

Pelletier J, Bruening W, Kashtan CE, et al: Germline mutations in the Wilms' tumor suppressor gene are associated with abnormal urogenital development in Denys-Drash syndrome. Cell 1991:67:437–447.

Penn I: Renal transplantation for Wilms' tumor: Report of 20 cases. J Urol 1979;122:793–794.

Perlman M, Levin M, Wittels B: Syndrome of fetal gigantism, renal hamartomas, and nephroblastomatosis with Wilms' tumor. Cancer 1975;35:1212–1217.

Povey S Burley M, Attwood J, et al: Two loci for tuberous sclerosis: One on 9q34 and one on 16p13. Ann Hum Genet 1994;58:107.

Pritchard-Jones K, Fleming S, et al: The candidate Wilms' tumour gene is involved in genitourinary development. Nature 1990;346:194–197.

Rainwater LM, Hosaka Y, Farrow GM, et al: Wilms tumors: Relationship of nuclear deoxyribonucleic acid ploidy to patient survival. J Urol 1987;138:974–977.

Raney RB, Jr, Palmer N, Sutow WW, et al: Renal cell carcinoma in children. Med Pediatr Oncol 1983;11:91–98.

Rauscher III FJ: The WT1 Wilms tumor gene product: A developmentally regulated transcription factor in the kidney that functions as a tumor suppressor. FASEB J 1993;7:896–903.

Renshaw AA, Granter SR, Fletcher JA, et al: Renal cell carcinoma in children and young adults: Increased incidence of papillary architecture and unique subtypes. Am J Surg Pathol 1999;23:795–802.

Riccardi VM, Sujansky E, Smith AC, Francke U: Chromosomal imbalance in the aniridia-Wilms' tumor association: 11p interstitial deletion. Pediatrics 1978;61:604–610.

Ritchey ML, Coppes M: The management of synchronous bilateral Wilms tumor. Hematol Oncol Clin North Am 1995;9:1303–1316.

Ritchey ML, Green DM, Breslow NE, Norkool P: Accuracy of current imaging modalities in the diagnosis of synchronous bilateral Wilms tumor. Cancer 1995;75:600–604.

Ritchey ML, Green DM, Thomas P, et al: Renal failure in Wilms tumor patients: A report of the NWTSG. Med Pediatr Oncol 1996;26:75–80.

Ritchey ML, Kelalis PP, Breslow N, et al: Intracaval and atrial involvement with nephroblastoma: Review of National Wilms' Tumor Study-3. J Urol 1988;140:1113–1118.

Ritchey ML, Kelalis PP, Breslow N, et al: Surgical complications following nephrectomy for Wilms' tumor: A report of National Wilms' Tumor Study-3. Surg Gynecol Obstet 1992;175:507–514.

Ritchey ML, Kelalis P, Breslow N, et al: Small bowel obstruction following nephrectomy for Wilms' tumor. Ann Surg 1993a;218:654–659.

Ritchey ML, Kelalis PP, Haase GM, et al: Preoperative therapy for intracaval and atrial extension of Wilms' tumor. Cancer 1993b;71:414.

Ritchey ML, Othersen HB, Jr, deLorimier AA, et al: Renal vein involvement with nephroblastoma: A report of National Wilms' Tumor Study-3. Eur Urol 1990;17:139–144.

Ritchey ML, Pringle K, Breslow N, et al: Management and outcome of inoperable Wilms' tumor: A report of National Wilms' Tumor Study. Ann Surg 1994;220:683–690.

Ritchey ML, Shamberger RC, Haase G, et al: Surgical complications after nephrectomy for Wilms tumor: Report from the National Wilms Tumor Study Group. Pediatrics 1999;104:816–817.

Rivera H: Constitutional and acquired rearrangements of chromosome 7 in Wilms tumor. Cancer Genet Cytogenet 1995;81(1):97–98.

Rowe DH, Huang J, Kayton ML, et al: Anti-VEGF antibody suppresses primary tumor growth and metastasis in an experimental model of Wilms' tumor. J Pediatr Surg 2000;35:30–33.

Rudin C, Pritchard J, Fernando ON, et al: Renal transplantation in the management of bilateral Wilms' tumour (BWT) and of Denys-Drash syndrome (DDS). Nephrol Dial Transplant 1998;13:1506–1510.

Schmidt D, Beckwith JB: Histopathology of childhood renal tumors. Hematol Oncol Clin North Am 1995;9:1179–1200.

Shamberger RC, Guthrie KA, Ritchey ML, et al: Surgery-related factors and local recurrence of Wilms tumor in National Wilms Tumor Study 4. Ann Surg 1999;229:292–297.

Shamberger RC, Ritchey ML, Haasse GM, et al: Intravascular extension of Wilms tumor. Ann Surg 2001;234:116–121.

Shaul DB, Srikanth MM, Ortega JA, Mahour GH: Treatment of bilateral Wilms' tumor: Comparison of initial biopsy and chemotherapy to initial surgical resection in the preservation of renal mass and function. J Pediatr Surg 1992;27:1009–1015.

Shulkin BL, Chang E, Strouse PJ, et al: PET FDG studies of Wilms tumors. J Pediatr Hematol Oncol 1997;19:334–338.

Snyder HM, III, Lack EE, Chetty-Baktovizian A, et al: Congenital mesoblastic nephroma: Relationship to other renal tumors of infancy. J Urol 1981;126:513–516.

Steiner MS, Goldman SM, Fishman EK, Marshall FF: The natural history of renal angiomyolipoma. J Urol 1993;150:1782–1786.

Steinherz LJ, Steinherz PG, Tan CTC, et al: Cardiac toxicity 4 to 20 years after anthracycline therapy. JAMA 1991;266:1672–1677.

Stillman RJ, Schinfeld JS, Schiff I, et al: Ovarian failure in long term survivors of childhood malignancy. Am J Obstet Gynecol 1987;139:62–66.

Tank ES, Kay R: Neoplasms associated with hemihypertrophy, Beckwith-Wiedemann syndrome and aniridia. J Urol 1980;124:266–268.

Tank ES, Melvin T: The association of Wilms' tumor with nephrologic disease. J Pediatr Surg 1990;25:724–725.

Tomlinson GE, Argyle JC, Velasco S, Nisen PD: Molecular characterization of congenital mesoblastic nephroma and its distinction from Wilms tumor. Cancer 1992;70:2358–2361.

Tournade MF, Com-Nougue C, Voute PA, et al: Results of the sixth International Society of Pediatric Oncology Wilms' tumor trial and study: A risk-adapted therapeutic approach in Wilms' tumor. J Clin Oncol 1993;11:1014–1023.

Tournade MF, Com-Nogoue, deKraker J, et al: Optimal duration of preoperative chemotherapy in unilateral and nonmetastatic Wilms' tumor in children over 6 months of age: Result of the 9th SIOP Wilms' tumor trial and study. J Clin Oncol 2001;19:488–500.

Voute PA, Van Der Meer J, Staugaard-Kloosterziel W: Plasma renin activity in Wilms' tumour. Acta Endocrinologica 1971;67:197–202.

Vujanic GM, Harms D, Sandstedt B, et al: New definitions of focal and diffuse anaplasia in Wilms tumor: The International Society of Paediatric Oncology (SIOP) experience. Med Pediatr Oncol 1999;32:317–323.

Weeks DA, Beckwith JB: Relapse-associated variables in stage I, favorable histology Wilms' tumor. Cancer 1987;60:1204–1212.

Weeks DA, Beckwith JB, Mierau G, Luckey DW: Rhabdoid tumor of kidney: A report of 111 cases from the National Wilms' Tumor Study Pathology Center. Am J Surg Pathol 1989;13:439–458.

Weese DL, Applebaum H, Taber P: Mapping intravascular extension of Wilms' tumor with magnetic resonance imaging. J Pediatr Surg 1991; 26:64–67.

White KS, Grossman H: Wilms' and associated renal tumors of childhood. Pediatr Radiol 1991;21:81–88.

Wiedemann H: Tumors and hemihypertrophy associated with the Wiedemann-Beckwith syndrome. Eur J Pediatr 1983;141:129.

Zuppan CW, Beckwith JB, Luckey DW: Anaplasia in unilateral Wilms' tumor: A report from the National Wilms' Tumor Study Pathology Center. Hum Pathol 1988;19:1199–1209.

Zuppan CW, Beckwith JB, Weeks DA, et al: The effect of preoperative therapy on the histologic features of Wilms' tumor: An analysis of cases from the Third National Wilms' Tumor Study. Cancer 1991;68: 385–394.

Testicular Tumors

Aarskog D: Clinical and cytogenetic studies in hypospadias. Acta Paediatr Scand (Suppl) 1970;203:1–62.

Ablin AK, Krailo M, Ramsey N, et al: Results of treatment of malignant germ cell tumors in 93 children: A report from the Children's Cancer Study Group. J Clin Oncol 1991;9:1782.

Altadonna V, Snyder HM, Rosenberg HK, Duckett JW: Simple cysts of the testis in children: Preoperative diagnosis by ultrasound and excision with testicular preservation. J Urol 1988;140:1505–1507.

Askin FB, Land VJ, Sullivan MP, et al: Occult testicular leukemia: Testicular biopsy at three years continuous complete remission of childhood leukemia. A Southwest Oncology Group Study. Cancer 1981;47: 470–475.

Bokemeyer C, Kuczyk M, Schoffski P, Schmoll H: Familial occurrence of Leydig cell tumors: A report of a case in a father and his adult son. J Urol 1993;150:1509–1510.

Bracken RB, Johnson DE, Cangir A, et al: Regional lymph nodes in infants with embryonal carcinoma of testis. Urology 1978;11:376–379.

Brewer JA, Tank ES: Yolk sac tumors and alpha-fetoprotein in first year of life. Urology 1993;42:79–80.

Brosman SA: Testicular tumors in prepubertal children. Urology 1979;13: 581–588.

Bussey KJ, Lawce HJ, Olson SB, et al: Chromosome abnormalities of eighty-one pediatric germ cell tumors: Sex-, age-, site- and histopathology-related differences. A Children's Cancer Group study. Genes Chromosomes Cancer 1999;25:134–146.

Capelouto CC, Clark PE, Ransil BJ, Loughlin KR: A review of scrotal violation in testicular cancer: Is adjuvant local therapy necessary? J Urol 1995;153:981–985.

Chang B, Borer JG, Tan PE, Diamond D: Large-cell calcifying Sertoli cell tumor of the testis: Case report and review of the literature. Urology 1998;52:520–522.

Cheville JC, Sebo TJ, Lager DJ, et al: Leydig cell tumor of the testis: A clinicopathologic, DNA content, and MIB-1 comparison of nonmetastasizing and metastasizing tumors. Am J Surg Pathol 1998;22:1361–1367.

Cortez JC, Kaplan GW: Gonadal stromal tumors, gonadoblastomas, epidermoid cysts, and secondary tumors of the testis in children. Urol Clin North Am 1993;20:15–26.

Cunnah D, Perry L, Dacie JA, et al: Bilateral testicular tumours in congenital adrenal hyperplasia: A continuing diagnostic and therapeutic dilemma. Clin Encocrinol 1989;30:141–147.

Dell'Acqua A, Toma P, Oddone M, et al: Testicular microlithiasis: US findings in six pediatric cases and literature review. Eur Radiol 1999;9: 940–944.

Finn LS, Viswanatha DS, Belasco JB, et al: Primary follicular lymphoma of the testis in childhood. Cancer 1999;85:1626–1635.

Furness PD, 3rd, Husmann DA, Brock JW, 3rd, et al: Multi-institutional study of testicular microlithiasis in childhood: A benign or premalignant condition? J Urol 1998;160:1151–1154.

Gabrilove JL, Freiberg EK, Leiter E, et al: Feminizing and non-feminizing Sertoli cell tumors. J Urol 1980;124:757–767.

Giguere JK, Stablein DM, Spaulding JT, et al: The clinical significance of unconventional orchiectomy approaches in testicular cancer: A report from the testicular cancer intergroup study. J Urol 1988;139:1225–1228.

Giwercman A, Muller J, Skakkebaek NE: Cryptorchidism and testicular neoplasia. Horm Res 1988;30:157–163.

Giwercman A, Bruun E, Frimont-Moller, C, Skakkebaek NE: Prevalence of carcinoma in situ and other histopathological abnormalities in testes of men with a history of cryptorchidism. J Urol 1989;142:998–1002.

Gobel U, Calaminus G, Engert J, et al: Teratomas in infancy and childhood. Med Pediatr Oncol 1998;31:8–15.

Goswitz, JJ, Pettinato G, Manivel JC: Testicular sex cord-stromal tumors in children: Clinicopathologic study of sixteen children with review of the literature. Ped Pathol Lab Med 1996;16:451–470.

Gourlay WA, Johnson HW, Pantzar JT, et al: Gonadal tumors in disorders of sexual differentiation. Urology 1994;43:537–540.

Grady RW, Ross JH, Kay R: Epidemiological features of testicular teratoma in a prepubertal population. J Urol 1997;158:1191–1192.

Grunert RT, Van Every MJ, Uehling DT: Bilateral epidermoid cysts of the testicle. J Urol 1992;147:1599–1601.

Haas GP, Shumaker BP, Cerny JC: The high incidence of benign testicular tumors. J Urol 1986;136:1219–1220.

Haas RJ, Schmidt P: Testicular germ cell tumors in childhood and adolescence. World J Urol 1995;13:203–208.

Haas RJ, Schmidt P, Gobel U, Harms D: Testicular germ cell tumors, an update: Results of the German cooperative studies 1982–1987. Klin Padiatr 1999;211:300–304.

Hadziselimovic F, Hecker E, Herzog B: The value of testicular biopsy in cryptorchidism. Urol Res 1984;12:171–174.

Hale GA, Marina NM, Jones-Wallace D, et al: Late effects of treatment for germ cell tumors during childhood and adolescence. J Pediatr Hematol Oncol 1999;21:115–122.

Hawkins E, Heifetz SA, Giller R, Cushing B: The prepubertal testis (prenatal and postnatal): Its relationship to intratubular germ cell neoplasia. A combined Pediatric Oncology Group and Children's Cancer Study Group. Human Pathol 1998;28:404–410.

Heifetz SA, Cushing B, Giller R, et al: Immature teratomas in children: Pathologic considerations. A report from the combined Pediatric Oncology Group/Children's Cancer Group. Am J Surg Pathol 1998;22:1115–1124.

Johnstone G: Prepubertal gynecomastia in association with an interstitial cell tumor of the testis. Br J Urol 1967;39:211–220.

Jorgenson N, Muller Giwercman A, et al: DNA content and expression of tumour markers in germ cells adjacent to germ-cell tumours in childhood: Probably a different origin for infantile and adolescent germ cell tumours. J Pathol 1995;176:269.

Kay R: Prepubertal testicular tumor registry. J Urol 1993;150:671–674.

Kaufman E, Akiya F, Foucar E, et al: Virilization due to Leydig cell tumor diagnosis by magnetic resonance imaging. Clin Pediatr 1990;29: 414–417.

Konrad D, Schoenle EJ: Ten-year selective follow-up in a boy with Leydig cell tumor after selective surgery. Horm Res 1999;51:96–100.

Kramer SA, Wold LE, Gilchrist GS, et al: Yolk sac carcinoma: An immunohistochemical and clinicopathological review. J Urol 1984;131: 315–318.

Krone KD, Carroll BA: Scrotal ultrasound. Radiol Clin North Am 1985; 23:121–139.

Kuo JY, Hsieh YL, Chin T, et al: Postchemotherapy retroperitoneal residual mass in infantile yolk sac tumor. Int J Urol 1999;6:116–118.

Lahdenne P, Kuusela P, Siimes MA, et al: Biphasic reduction and concanavalin A binding properties of serum alpha-fetoprotein in preterm and term infants. J Pediatr 1991;118:272–276.

Lamm DL, Kaplan GW: Urologic manifestations of Burkitt's lymphoma. J Urol 1974;112:402–405.

Li FP, Fraumeni JF, Jr: Testicular cancers in children: Epidemiologic characteristics. J Natl Cancer Inst 1972;48:1575–1481.

Luker GD, Siegel MJ: Pediatric testicular tumors: Evaluation with gray-scale and color Doppler US. Radiology 1994;191:561–564.

Mann JR, Pearson D, Barrett A, et al: Results of the United Kingdom Children's Cancer Study Group's malignant germ cell tumor studies. Cancer 1989;63:1657–1667.

Manuel M, Kayatama K, Jones HW, Jr: The age of occurrence of gonadal tumors in intersex patients with a Y-chromosome. Am J Obstet Gynecol 1976;124:293–300.

Marina NM, Cushing B, Giller R, et al: Complete surgical excision is effective treatment for children with immature teratomas with or without malignant elements: A Pediatric Oncology Group/Children's Cancer Group Intergroup Study. Am J Surg Pathol 1998;22:1115–1124.

Marshall S, Lyon RP, Scott MP: A conservative approach to testicular tumors in children: 12 Cases and their management. J Urol 1983;129: 350–351.

Maxwell AJ, Mantora H: Sonographic appearance of epidermoid cyst of the testis. J Clin Ultrasound 1990;18:188–190.

McKiernan JM, Goluboff ET, Liberson GL, et al: Rising risk of testicular cancer by birth cohort in the United States from 1973–1995. J Urol 1999;162:361–363.

Mengel W, Knorr D: Leydig cell tumours in childhood. Prog Pediatr Surg 1983;16:133–138.

Mostofi FK, Price EB: Tumors of the male genital system. In Firminger, HI (ed): Atlas of Tumor Pathology, 2nd series, fascicle 8. Washington, DC, Armed Forces Institute of Pathology, 1973.

Muller J, Skakkebaek NE, Ritzen M, et al: Carcinoma in situ of the testis in children with 45,X/46,XY gonadal dysgenesis. J Pediatr 1985;106: 431–436.

Noh PH, Cooper CS, Snyder HM 3rd: Conservative management of cystic dysplasia of the testis. J Urol 1999;162(6):2145.

Olsen MM, Caldamone AA, Jackson CL, Zinn A: Gonadoblastoma in infancy: Indications for early gonadectomy in 46XY gonadal dysgenesis. J Pediatr Surg 1988;23:270–271.

Pearse I, Glick RD, Abramson SJ, et al: Testicular-sparing surgery for benign testicular tumors. J Pediatr Surg 1999;34:1000–1003.

Perlman EJ, Valentine MB, Griffin CA, Look AT: Deletion of 1p36 in childhood endodermal sinus tumors by two-color fluorescence in situ hybridization: A Pediatric Oncology Group study. Genes Chromosomes Cancer 1996;16:15–20.

Pinkerton CR, Braodbent V, Horwich A, et al: JEB: A carboplatin based regimen for malignant germ cell tumors in children. Br J Cancer 1990; 62:257.

Pizzocara G, Zanoni F, Salvioni R, et al: Difficulties of a surveillance study omitting retroperitoneal lymphadenectomy in clinical stage I non-seminomatous germ cell tumors of the testis. J Urol 1987;138:1393–1396.

Ramani P, Yeung CK, Habeebu S: Testicular intratubular germ-cell neoplasia in children and adolescents with intersex. Am J Surg Pathol 1993;17:1124.

Rescorla FJ: Pediatric germ-cell tumors. In Andrassy RJ (ed): Pediatric Surgical Oncology. Philadelphia, WB Saunders, 1998, pp 239–266.

Rosvoll RV, Woodward JR: Malignant Sertoli cell tumor of the testis. Cancer 1968;22:8–13.

Rushton G, Belman AB, Sesterhenn I, et al: Testicular sparing surgery for prepubertal teratoma of the testis: A clinical and pathological study. J Urol 1990;144:726–730.

Schellas HF: Malignant potential of the dysgenetic gonad, I and II. Obstet Gynecol 1974;44:298–309.

Silver SA, Wiley JM, Perlman EJ: DNA ploidy analysis of pediatric germ cell tumors. Mod Pathol 1994;7:951–956.

Skakkebaek NE: Atypical germ cells in the adjacent "normal" tissue of testicular tumors. Acta Path Microbiol Scand 1975;83:127–130.

Srikath MS, West BR, Ishitani M, et al: Benign testicular tumors in children with congenital adrenal hyperplasia. J Pediatr Surg 1992;27: 639–641.

Toffolutti T, Gamba PG, Cecchetto G, et al: Testicular cystic dysplasia: Evaluation of 3 new cases treated without surgery. J Urol 1999;162: 2146–2148.

Trigg ME, Steinherz PG, Chappell R, et al: Early testicular biopsy in males with acute lymphoblastic leukemia: Lack of impact on subsequent event-free survival. J Pediatr Hematol Oncol 2000;22:27–33.

Uehling DT, Phillips E: Residual retroperitoneal mass following chemotherapy for infantile yolk sac tumor. J Urol 1994;152:185–186.

Urban MD, Lee PA, Plotnick LP, et al: The diagnosis of Leydig cell tumors in childhood. Am J Dis Child 1978;132:494–497.

Walker BR, Skoog SJ, Winslow BH, et al: Testis sparing surgery for steroid unresponsive testicular tumors of the adrenogenital syndrome. J Urol 1997;157:1460–1463.

Wegner HE, Dieckmann KP, Herbst H, et al: Leydig cell tumor: Comparison of results of radical and testis-sparing surgery in a single center. Urol Int 1997;59:170–173.

Wilson BE, Netzloff ML: Primary testicular abnormalities causing precocious puberty Leydig cell tumor, Leydig cell hyperplasia, and adrenal rest tumor. Ann Clin Lab Sci 1983;13:315–320.

Wold LE, Kramer SA, Farrow GM: Testicular yolk sac and embryonal carcinomas in pediatric patients: Comparative immunohistochemical and clinicopathologic study. Am J Clin Pathol 1984;81:427–435.

Wu JT, Book L, Sudar K: Serum alpha-fetoprotein (AFP) levels in normal infants. Pediatr Res 1981;15:50–52.

Young RH, Koeliker DD, Scully RE: Sertoli cell tumors of the testis not otherwise specified: A clinicopathologic analysis of 60 cases. Am J Surg Pathol 1998;22:709–721.

71
URINARY TRACT RECONSTRUCTION IN CHILDREN

Mark C. Adams, MD
David B. Joseph, MD

The goal of this chapter is to review techniques used for lower urinary tract reconstruction in pediatric patients and the principles that guide their use. In general, such intervention is taken in order to reestablish or create anew a system that protects renal function, avoids significant infection, and eventually provides for urinary continence. Those, in simplistic terms, are functions of a "normal" urinary tract.

The scope of the chapter is large. Many specific techniques are presented in detail, particularly those used pri-marily in the pediatric population. For techniques that have been used more extensively in adults, descriptions are brief, with the focus on adaptations for and results of use in children. Urinary diversions, both temporary and permanent with bowel, are discussed elsewhere in the text. Augmentation cystoplasty is reviewed in detail, from preoperative evaluation and surgical techniques to long-term results and newer alternatives. In few areas of urology have intestinal segments been used more extensively than for bladder augmentation in pediatric patients. This experience with augmentation cystoplasty established the basis for later work with continent urinary diversions and orthotopic neobladders.

Patients with complex bladder dysfunction may have bladder neck and external sphincteric problems as well. This chapter covers techniques to increase native outflow resistance in the pediatric population. Certain techniques, such as the Young-Dees-Leadbetter bladder neck repair, are presented in other sections of this text. Others (i.e., sling, collagen injection, and artificial urinary sphincter) have been used more extensively in adults. Again, in that setting, this chapter focuses on adaptations of those procedures for children.

Perhaps the most important contribution affecting lower urinary tract reconstruction was the introduction of clean intermittent catheterization (CIC) by Lapides and colleagues (1972, 1976). Because many pediatric patients with bladder and sphincteric dysfunction do not void adequately after reconstruction, creation of a reliable means to easily catheterize without discomfort is an important part of their care. The work of Mitrofanoff (1980) stimulated interest in continent abdominal wall stomas within pediatric urology, and several effective techniques have since been developed. Review of that experience leads to a discussion of continent urinary diversion in children as construction of an effective efferent limb that provides continence, and a reliable means for catheterization is often the most challenging aspect of such diversion.

"Pure" continent urinary reservoirs, such as the Indiana or Kock pouch, are occasionally performed in children, and that experience is reviewed here. More frequently in children, some of the patient's native urinary tract is used in the reconstruction. This is done to maintain as much urothelial-lined tissue in the urinary tract as possible, to minimize the amount of needed bowel, and, at least potentially, to minimize the morbidity to the patient. The result, then, is a spectrum of repairs between bladder augmentation and continent urinary diversion but rarely a continent reservoir in the classic sense.

Several decades ago, many such reconstructions were undertaken after previous, permanent urinary diversion using bowel (Hendren, 1998). However, today few children are initially treated with permanent diversion. Most reconstructive procedures are now undertaken primarily to correct a problem in the native urinary tract (hydronephrosis, infection, incontinence) that is unresponsive to medical management or after temporary diversion. Children with bladder and sphincteric dysfunction are among the most complex cases seen in pediatric urology; among others, patients with diagnoses such as exstrophy, persistent cloaca and urogenital sinus, posterior urethral valves, bilateral single ectopic ureters, and prune-belly syndrome may be involved. For most pediatric urologists, patients with myelomeningocele make up the great majority of patients requiring this type of surgical intervention. Consequently, many of the results discussed herein focus on the neurogenic population.

Many anomalies affecting the bladder and outlet can be managed so that surgical intervention is not necessary. Once conservative, medical therapy has failed, surgical reconstruction remains an important and effective tool. When reconstruction is considered, it is imperative that the patient be thoroughly evaluated. Each child is unique, and the particular pathophysiology must be understood so that the available surgical techniques may be used thoughtfully to optimize the results while minimizing the morbidity. **The most important factor influencing the outcome of urinary tract reconstruction in children is the commitment of the patient and family to achieving good care.** Evaluating that commitment may at times be difficult, but its importance should not be underestimated.

THE "FUNCTIONAL" URINARY TRACT

The renal pelves and ureters should empty effortlessly into the bladder without any increase in pressure or element of obstruction. The normal ureterovesical junction prevents vesicoureteral reflux. Bladder physiology can be characterized as two different dynamic phases, passive and active. During the passive storage phase, the bladder functions as a reservoir, allowing for an appropriate volume of urine to be stored without leakage while maintaining low pressure to protect the upper tract. In the active voiding phase, the bladder contracts for elimination of urine.

Basic Bladder Function

Passive—Storage

Appropriate urinary storage requires a reservoir that is compliant. By definition this allows for increased urinary capacity without a significant rise in resting pressure. Normally the bladder is considered to be a highly compliant vesicle in that it can accommodate an increasing volume of urine without a corresponding increase in intravesical pressure. Multiple factors contribute to this property. Initially the bladder is in a collapsed state, which allows for the storage of urine at low pressure by simply unfolding. As the bladder expands, detrusor properties of elasticity and viscoelasticity take effect. Elasticity allows the detrusor muscle to stretch without an increase in tension until it reaches a critical volume. This volume should be greater than the expected bladder capacity for age. Viscoelastic bladder properties cause a continual subtle rise in pressure as the bladder fills (Zinner et al, 1976; Wagg and Fry, 1999). When filling is slow (as in a natural state) or stops, there is a rapid decay in this pressure known as stress relaxation (Mundy, 1984; Finkbeiner, 1999). Normally, stress relaxation is in balance with the filling rate and prevents an increase in detrusor pressure. Eventually, with continued filling, the properties of elasticity and viscoelasticity are overcome and pressure rises rapidly. **Favorable dynamics for appropriate urine storage include a thin bladder wall with an appropriate composition of muscle and collagen that allows for expression of normal elastic and viscoelastic properties.** Factors that adversely affect normal compliance include detrusor hypertrophy, fibrosis, outlet obstruction, and recurrent urinary infections (Mundy, 1984; Joseph, 1994).

Continence during urinary storage requires a closed bladder neck at times supported by a contracted external urinary sphincter. Fixed obstruction, neurogenic dysfunction, and chronic inflammation can affect any or all of these passive parameters, resulting in resting bladder hostility and clinical manifestations of poor compliance, upper tract deterioration, and incontinence (Brading, 1997).

Active—Voiding

Under normal conditions, the active phase of voiding requires the bladder to contract after descent of the bladder neck (Morrison, 1997). Reflexive opening of the bladder neck and sequential relaxation of the external urinary sphincter allows for low-pressure, balanced voiding and complete elimination of urine. Again, obstruction, neurogenic dysfunction, and chronic infection can cause physiologic changes that prevent coordinated function of the detrusor, bladder neck, and external sphincter; this is defined as *dyssynergy* (Mundy et al, 1985). A poorly functioning external sphincter caused by denervation fibrosis may also prevent appropriate relaxation, causing elevated voiding pressure against a fixed outlet. Finally, detrusor pathophysiology may prevent a sustained, coordinated bladder contraction and full elimination of all urine.

Dysfunction

Upper Tract

It is critical to understand the dynamics of the entire urinary tract before any major reconstructive procedure is undertaken. Careful evaluation is imperative. In the presence of hydronephrosis, upper tract obstruction must be excluded. With severe and long-standing bladder problems, particularly those involving poor bladder compliance and emptying, upper tract obstruction often occurs secondary to the bladder abnormality. In that setting, secondary obstruction is more common than a second primary problem, namely a separate obstruction at the vesicoureteral junction. Nuclear renography with a catheter in the bladder to keep it empty and at low pressure may be useful to rule out a primary upper tract problem. Antegrade perfusion studies with fluoroscopy and pressure measurement occasionally are necessary. Certainly, if upper tract obstruction is present, it should be corrected at the time of bladder/sphincter reconstruction.

Much like obstruction, vesicoureteral reflux in the presence of a bladder abnormality may be primary or secondary. Differentiation between the two may be difficult. Occasionally, the history is helpful. If reflux was not present initially in a patient with neurogenic dysfunction but developed later, it is typically secondary to bladder hostility. Most reflux in patients with neurogenic dysfunction requiring bladder augmentation is secondary in nature, whereas reflux in patients with other problems (e.g., exstrophy, prune-belly syndrome, posterior urethral valves) may be either primary or a fixed secondary problem if it persists until the time that bladder reconstruction is necessary. Previous work suggested that reflux that is truly secondary to bladder dysfunction may not require surgical correction if the bladder is adequately managed. In those reports, pa-

tients with neurogenic bladder requiring augmentation did not undergo reimplantation for secondary reflux; virtually all of the low-grade reflux resolved with augmentation alone (Nasrallah and Aliabadi, 1991; Morioka et al, 1998).

It is also interesting to speculate whether antireflux surgery is absolutely necessary if a large, compliant bladder is achieved. Bacteria may ascend without reflux after reconstruction (Gonzalez and Reinburg, 1987). Experience with certain forms of continent diversion have not shown an increased risk of pyelonephritis in the absence of any antireflux mechanism if the reservoir is adequate (Helal et al, 1993; Pantuck et al, 2000). Although we would agree that most low-grade, secondary reflux is likely to resolve with adequate treatment of the bladder alone, our preference is to correct reflux that is present at the time of bladder reconstruction, unless low-grade or clearly secondary, because the morbidity is quite low.

After bladder reconstruction, many patients will have chronic bacteriuria, particularly those who catheterize to empty, and the absence of reflux may at least theoretically decrease the likelihood of ascent to the kidney. Caution must be taken when considering the treatment of chronically dilated and scarred ureters. Stopping reflux in that setting is certainly appropriate, but one must be careful not to trade reflux for more problematic obstruction. Overaggressive tapering or tunneling of such ureters may be fraught with complications.

Dysfunction in the upper urinary tract is usually manifested by hydronephrosis, pyelonephritis, or impairment of renal function. When such problems are present in patients with lower tract dysfunction, thoughtful evaluation and treatment are necessary. All problems should be addressed at reconstructive surgery to provide the best result for the patient.

Bladder Dysfunction

Bladder dysfunction is a composite of physiologic abnormalities, and it is helpful to assess each component of passive and active bladder function independently. **Elevated passive filling pressure becomes clinically pathogenic when a pressure greater than 40 cm H$_2$O is chronically reached** (McGuire et al, 1981; Wang et al, 1988; Weston et al, 1989). Pressures at this level sustained over a period of time impair ureteral drainage, which may result in pyelocaliceal changes, hydroureteronephrosis, and decreased glomerular filtration rate. In addition, persistent elevation in filling pressure can result in acquired vesicoureteral reflux (Sidi et al, 1986a; Cohen et al, 1990).

Pharmacologic management can play a role in decreasing the filling pressure, particularly when hyperreflexic detrusor contractions are present. A combination of medications and CIC has a positive impact, particularly in children with neurogenic dysfunction (Rink and Mitchell, 1984). Bladders that are poorly compliant because of neurogenic dysfunction, irradiation, or chronic inflammatory processes are not as likely to respond in a positive fashion to this form of therapy. When compliance is unaffected by medical management, augmentation cystoplasty is required to recreate the filling pressures of a normal bladder. With formal augmentation cystoplasty, the likelihood of detrusor contractions' resulting in effective emptying is significantly diminished. The potential need for CIC is a common theme in any case of urinary reconstruction. **The goals of urinary reconstruction must be clearly stated to the patient, along with the importance of long-term rigid compliance with CIC when clinically indicated.** With rare exceptions, CIC should be taught and accepted by the patient and caretaker before urinary reconstruction is contemplated.

One of the most important contributions in the care of children with bladder dysfunction came with the acceptance of CIC, as described by Lapides and colleagues (1972, 1976), based on the work of Guttmann and Frankel (1966). The effective use of CIC has allowed the application of augmentation and lower tract reconstruction to groups of patients who had not previously been candidates. The principle of CIC allows the reconstructive surgeon to aggressively correct storage problems by providing an adequate reservoir and good outflow resistance. Good spontaneous voiding, although it is a goal, is not imperative because catheterization can be used for emptying. CIC can maintain a physiologic state of complete emptying on a regular basis.

Urinary incontinence is a prominent sign of bladder dysfunction. Continence is based on outflow resistance generated by the bladder neck and external urinary sphincter. Outflow resistance must remain greater than resting bladder pressure throughout normal daily activity and strenuous physical events during storage. When outflow resistance is diminished because of an abnormal bladder neck and external urinary sphincter, incontinence often occurs. Pharmacologic management can enhance outflow resistance when needed, but more commonly operative reconstruction is required in that setting.

When incontinence occurs during the filling phase owing to poor outlet resistance, it is essential to evaluate not only the bladder neck and external urinary sphincter but detrusor characteristics. Clinical experience has shown that once appropriate resistance is achieved at the bladder neck through operative intervention, adverse detrusor characteristics may become unmasked and result in high-pressure urinary storage or uninhibited contractions not previously documented (Bauer et al, 1986; Churchill et al, 1987). For that reason, provocative urodynamic assessment with occlusion of the bladder neck is important before any bladder neck reconstruction in an attempt to identify children who will be at risk.

Normal synergistic voiding occurs when the bladder neck descends, relaxes, and opens, followed by relaxation of the external urinary sphincter and subsequent detrusor contraction. The cascade results in low-pressure, balanced voiding. Dysfunctional voiding during this active bladder phase occurs secondary to discoordinated activity of the bladder neck, external urinary sphincter, and detrusor and can result in urinary incontinence. In addition, when neurogenic dysfunction leads to detrusor sphincter dyssynergy, high-pressure voiding results over a period of time, with negative effects on the upper urinary tract (Mundy et al, 1982; Bauer et al, 1984). A similar clinical situation occurs with a fixed, fibrotic external sphincter. Initial treatment usually centers on pharmacologic management and mechanical elimination of urine from the bladder via CIC in an attempt to bypass the abnormal voiding mechanics.

Other Considerations

Renal function should be assessed in any patient undergoing bladder reconstruction, particularly if hydronephrosis or severe renal scarring is present. **Demos (1962) and Koch and McDougal (1985) demonstrated that urinary solutes, particularly chloride, are absorbed from urine in contact with the mucosa of small and large bowel.** For patients with normal renal function, the kidneys are able to handle the reabsorbed load of chloride and acid without difficulty. However, patients with decreased renal function may develop significant metabolic acidosis secondary to such reabsorption. If acidosis exists preoperatively, it will invariably worsen if urine is stored in small or large intestinal segments (Mitchell and Pizer, 1987). The first component of renal function to deteriorate after obstruction or infection is typically the concentrating ability. Patients with compromised function may generate enormous volumes of urine. **The bladder volume achieved through bladder reconstruction must accommodate the patient's urinary output for an acceptable period, usually about 4 hours.** Patients with renal failure or other medical problems may conversely develop oliguria. Low urinary output may affect an augmented bladder or bowel reservoir, because there is greater potential for collection and inspissation of mucus. There is also less urine for dilution and buffering of gastric secretions if the stomach is used.

Abnormal function of other organ systems also influences the risk of bladder reconstruction with intestinal segments. Reabsorption of ammonia by large or small intestinal segments in contact with urine may be dangerous for patients with hepatic failure (McDougal, 1992a). Some medications excreted in urine may be reabsorbed by bowel mucosa (Savauagen and Dixey, 1969). Therefore, liver function tests and arterial blood gas studies may be appropriate for some patients. Careful history should be taken regarding the patient's preoperative bowel function; this is particularly true for adult patients who may have acquired or secondary gastrointestinal problems. Obviously, short-gut syndrome is a concern in patients with cloacal exstrophy, prior bowel resections, or a history of significant irradiation. A history of chronic diarrhea or fecal incontinence preoperatively should raise concern regarding use of the ileocecal valve in urinary reconstruction.

A critical factor to consider is the commitment of the patient and family. Urinary incontinence at times protects the patient from infection and upper tract deterioration. Effective storage can put the patient at risk for such problems if emptying is not accomplished on a regular basis. Everyone must be aware of the responsibility that goes along with bladder reconstruction and urinary continence.

The timing of appropriate surgical intervention can vary dramatically among patients. It is sometimes necessary to perform early reconstruction when the upper tracts and renal function are threatened. This situation most often occurs in the presence of high-outflow resistance and poor bladder compliance. More commonly, intervention may be undertaken later to achieve urinary continence. The age at which urinary incontinence becomes socially unacceptable varies among patients and families.

When appropriate, it is beneficial for the patient and family to wait for bladder reconstruction until all needs of the patient have been identified. When intervention is contemplated because of infection or hydronephrosis, this is not always possible. When reconstruction is undertaken to achieve continence, it is most efficient to identify all reconstructive issues and address them with one operation. Good urodynamic assessment is usually necessary to determine whether a procedure to increase outflow resistance is necessary in addition to bladder augmentation or replacement. Introducing CIC preoperatively is mandatory in that it allows the patient to demonstrate the ability and desire to use the technique on a regular basis. It is also helpful in determining whether a continent abdominal wall stoma may be helpful to improve the reliability of catheterization and increase the patient's independence. Likewise, particularly in the neurogenic population, it is advantageous to identify those patients who may also benefit from an antegrade colonic enema. In our experience, such enemas are very helpful in treating constipation and fecal incontinence and may dramatically increase the patient's independence of care with what is often a more socially distressing problem than urinary incontinence. It is certainly better for the patient and surgeon to address all of these issues at one operative sitting rather than with sequential procedures.

PATIENT EVALUATION

Each patient should have upper tract imaging before bladder reconstruction is performed. Most patients with significant bladder problems have had routine ultrasonography as part of their surveillance. **If hydronephrosis is present, obstruction and vesicoureteral reflux should be sought with a functional study and voiding cystography.** Nuclear renography with a catheter in the bladder is usually adequate to rule out a primary upper tract obstruction. Reflux should be excluded with a voiding study. That study may be done as part of video urodynamics. In the presence of any hydronephrosis, each patient should have determinations of serum electrolytes, blood urea nitrogen (BUN), and serum creatinine. For patients with elevation of the serum creatinine or significant hydronephrosis, a 24-hour urine collection both for creatinine clearance and urine volume should be obtained.

Urodynamics

Bladder Dynamics—Capacity and Compliance

Urodynamic assessment of the lower urinary tract plays an essential role when bladder reconstruction is considered. It can provide reproducible results in infants and children but requires meticulous attention to detail (Joseph, 1994). With the use of computerized techniques and sophisticated equipment, parameters related to bladder function (i.e., capacity, compliance, contractility, and effective emptying)

and external urinary sphincter activity (synergy/dyssynergy and sphincter length) can be recorded.

Several mechanical factors adversely influence urodynamic data, creating artifacts which, if not recognized, can have a negative impact on the validity of the evaluation. Most often urodynamic testing is undertaken by transurethral catheter placement. A catheter that is too large can lead to the appearance of increased leak or voiding pressure and the inability to empty well, particularly in infants and young boys (Decter and Harpser, 1992). Suprapubic catheter placement circumvents this problem but is not practical in most cases. The testing medium and infusion rate can influence the results. Carbon dioxide is not as reliable as fluid infusion, particularly when evaluating bladder compliance and capacity. The most common fluids used for testing are saline and iodinated contrast agents, both of which provide reproducible results (Joseph, 1993). Use of testing media at body temperature is also appropriate (Joseph, 1996). End filling pressure, and therefore bladder compliance, can be dramatically affected by simply changing the filling rate (Joseph, 1992). That parameter can have a major impact on the clinical decision regarding the need for bladder augmentation. Bauer (1979) suggested that the cystometrogram be performed at a fill rate of no greater than 10% per minute of the predicted bladder capacity for age.

The treatment plans and reconstructive outcome are greatly influenced by passive bladder filling pressure. Based on the work of McGuire et al (1981), a resting pressure exceeding 40 cm H_2O has been considered hostile for upper tract function. Persistently elevated pressure can result in ineffective ureteral peristalsis and relative ureterovesical junction obstruction. Using 40 cm H_2O as a cutoff value helps to identify the "safe period" of bladder filling (Bauer and Joseph, 1990). It should be recognized that this is not an absolute value; in some patients, a lower pressure may be detrimental to the upper tract. **Urinary reconstructive efforts must result in a resting pressure substantially lower than 40 cm H_2O in order to optimize the effect on the upper urinary tract.**

Sphincter Dynamics—Outflow Resistance

The bladder neck and the external urinary sphincter work in synergy, but only one is required to maintain urinary continence. Often neurogenic dysfunction leads to abnormalities of both the structures and may result in diminished outlet resistance during storage, dyssynergic function with voiding, or both. The potential for unmasking bladder hostility by increasing bladder neck or external sphincter resistance must be considered when planning reconstructive procedures (Bauer et al, 1986). Therefore, monitoring of external urinary sphincter electrical activity is required to evaluate coordinated voiding and dyssynergic detrusor sphincter activity. Perineal surface electrodes, abdominal wall sensors, anal plugs, vaginal monitors, electrical wires, and concentric needle electrodes have all been used for electromyography (Joseph, 1996). In children with neurogenic dysfunction, use of a concentric needle electrode or dual-needle electrodes placed through a 25-gauge needle increases accuracy when measuring sphincter activity (Blaivas et al, 1977; Joseph, 1996).

The functional length of the external urinary sphincter also plays a role in outflow resistance, and its measurement can be undertaken with urethral pressure profilometry. Unfortunately, the short length and small diameter of the pediatric urethra makes the mechanics of this study technically more difficult to perform than in the adult. The mechanical pulling device is not practical for pediatric use. To assess the urethral pressure profile, a constant infusion of testing medium at a rate of 2 ml/min using a continuous Harvard pump is required (Joseph, 1996). This eliminates pressure wave artifacts observed with the standard roller ball infusion pumps. Hand withdrawal of the catheter is undertaken, marking every 5 mm on the recording strip. With practice, reliable measurements can be obtained. There is limited value in comparing specific urethral pressure profile results for an individual patient against a standard uroflow nomogram. The preoperative profile for a given patient provides baseline information that can be beneficial when assessing the intraoperative and postoperative functional urethral length.

Some surgeons use leak point pressure (that bladder pressure causing leakage per urethra) to evaluate outflow resistance. It can be determined during passive filling and during Valsalva's maneuver. Fluoroscopy can be informative during those events. It should be recognized that the leak point pressure may be artifactually elevated by the urodynamics catheter in a small male urethra (Decter and Harpser, 1992). Much work remains to determine how well such measurable parameters correlate and how thoroughly each affects emptying.

Bladder Emptying

The patient's ability to empty the bladder before reconstruction should be assessed carefully. Useful parameters related to bladder emptying include synergistic relaxation of the external sphincter on electromyography, urinary flow rates, and measurements of postvoid residual urine. Neurologically normal patients who are able to empty the bladder well preoperatively are much more likely to be able to do so after reconstruction than are patients who have neurogenic dysfunction or are unable to empty well preoperatively. **No test ensures that a patient will be able to void spontaneously and empty well after bladder augmentation or other reconstruction.** Therefore, all patients must be prepared to perform CIC postoperatively. The native urethra should be examined for ease of catheterization. Ideally, the patient should learn CIC and practice it preoperatively until the patient, family, and surgeon are comfortable that catheterization can and will be done reliably. Physical and psychosocial limitations of the patient must be considered in regard to the ability to self-catheterize and perform self-care. **Failure to catheterize and empty reliably after bladder reconstruction may result in upper tract deterioration, urinary tract infection, or bladder perforation despite a technically perfect operation.** Most patients who may catheterize either through the native urethra or through an abdominal wall stoma overwhelmingly prefer the latter (Horowitz et al, 1995).

PATIENT PREPARATION

Bladder and sphincter reconstructive procedures remain some of the most challenging in urology. The patient's general status should be optimized so that he or she has the best chance to achieve a good result with the least risk of morbidity. Each patient's general nutritional and hydrational status should be determined and corrected, if necessary, before surgery. Coexisting medical problems, particularly cardiac and pulmonary problems, should be well managed preoperatively.

Bowel Preparation

Each patient undergoes preoperative bowel preparation to minimize the potential risk of surgery if the use of any bowel is contemplated. Even when ureterocystoplasty or other alternatives are planned, intraoperative findings may dictate the need for use of a bowel segment. Two days of a clear liquid diet before bowel preparation aids in clearing of solid stool. The patient should then undergo full mechanical bowel preparation the day before surgery. Historically, such bowel preparations have been done in the hospital, but recently the trend is toward an outpatient setting. Major reconstructive procedures often require many hours of operative time and large fluid shifts. It is critical that the patient be well hydrated at the time of surgery. There should be a low threshold for the use of intravenous fluids during the preoperative day. The use of oral antibiotics as part of bowel preparation, once dogma, is now a matter of personal preference. Special attention must be paid to the bowel preparation of patients with neurogenic dysfunction. Most of these patients have neuropathic bowel dysfunction as well, usually in association with chronic constipation. Good bowel cleansing is difficult in such patients and should be done aggressively. Several days of oral cathartics and a clear liquid diet at home may be helpful.

Theoretically, the gastric contents are sterile, and use of parenteral antibiotics or routine bowel preparation is not necessary before gastrocystoplasty. Nonetheless, it is safest to follow the guidelines just described for all patients, because intraoperative considerations may preclude the use of stomach or ureter and necessitate ileocystoplasty or colocystoplasty.

Urine Culture

All patients should have a urine culture performed several days before bladder reconstruction. The bladder should not be opened with infected urine, which is likely to spill intraperitoneally. This is particularly true of neurogenic patients with a ventriculoperitoneal shunt. Any patient with a positive preoperative urine culture should undergo treatment and have a second culture documenting sterile urine before the procedure is performed.

Cystoscopy

Preoperative cystoscopy may be the final step in evaluating the native bladder, outflow, or ureteral orifices in pediatric patients. Endoscopy should be performed immediately before bladder reconstruction under the same anesthetic. For adult patients with interstitial cystitis or irritative bladder symptoms requiring augmentation cystoplasty, cystoscopy should be performed well before augmentation to rule out urothelial carcinoma in situ. Bladder biopsy and cytologic examination of the urine may be helpful in excluding tumor. Based on the history, a few patients may warrant endoscopic or radiographic gastrointestinal evaluation.

ANTIREFLUX THERAPY

Ureteral reimplantation into a native bladder, whether the ureter is dilated or not, is a standard procedure familiar to all pediatric urologists and reconstructive surgeons. The long-term success rate is good, and complications are rare. Such reimplantation is certainly preferable and usually possible during lower tract reconstruction.

Transureteroureterostomy and Single Ureteral Reimplantation

Occasionally, the urinary bladder is so small that it is inadequate for bilateral reimplantation, and alternatives must be considered. It is preferable to reimplant both ureters separately, although **if the native urinary bladder is small and adequate for only a single ureteral tunnel, transureteroureterostomy (TUU) and a single reimplantation may be helpful** (Fig. 71–1). Typically, the better

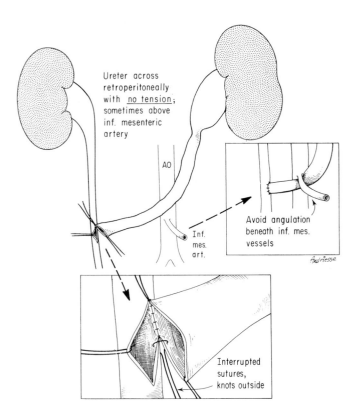

Figure 71–1. Technique for transureteroureterostomy. AO, aorta; Inf. Mes. Art., inferior mesenteric artery. (Illustration courtesy of W. Hardy Hendren, M.D.)

ureter should be implanted into the bladder, draining the other across into it. The crossing ureter should be mobilized to swing gently across the abdomen to the donor side in a smooth course without tension. It should be carefully mobilized with all of its adventitia and as much periureteral tissue as possible to preserve the blood supply. Care must be taken not to angulate the crossing ureter immediately beneath the inferior mesenteric artery. The crossing ureter is widely anastomosed to the posteromedial aspect of the recipient ureter. The recipient is not mobilized or brought medially to meet the end of the other ureter. TUU, when fashioned appropriately, is successful and carries minimal risk of leakage or obstruction (Hodges et al, 1963; Hendren and Hensle, 1980; Noble et al, 1997; Mure et al, 2000). A history of previous calculi remains a relative contraindication to TUU.

The manner in which the bladder is opened may optimize its use for a single reimplantation. Rather than incising the bladder in the anterior midline, a wide, anterior, U-shaped incision based cephalad can be made. This potentially elongates the bladder as a posterior plate which can be brought to one side or the other to meet a single ureter. Incision of the bladder in this way may also be useful in placing a continent catheterizable stoma to the umbilicus when the native bladder otherwise will not reach that far. For ureteral reimplantation after such an incision, a psoas hitch of the bladder fixes it in position for a long, straight ureteral tunnel.

Psoas Hitch

Fixation of the bladder to the psoas muscle allows for precise control of both the length and direction of a ureteral reimplant. Securing the bladder in this manner helps the bladder reach a short ureter or create a long tunnel when necessary. A psoas hitch should prevent any angulation of the ureter with bladder filling. Such angulation may be particularly problematic or obstructive with a dilated and scarred ureter. The bladder should be secured to the psoas muscle and fascia using nonabsorbable sutures. Those sutures must not enter the bladder lumen, or stones will occur. Broad, shallow purchases of the psoas muscle and fascia should be achieved to hold in the long term without approaching the sciatic nerve. The hitching sutures should not be tied too tightly, so as not to cut through either bladder or psoas muscle. The contralateral bladder pedicle may be divided to increase bladder mobility and the length of the hitch on occasion. In general, the ureteral reimplantation should be performed before the bladder psoas hitch (Fig. 71–2).

Antireflux Techniques with Intestinal Segments

The need for ureteral reimplantation into an intestinal segment may occasionally determine the segment to be used for bladder augmentation or replacement. Long experience with ureterosigmoidostomy and colon conduit diversion has established an effective means of keeping reflux out of a colonic segment. A flap valve mechanism can be

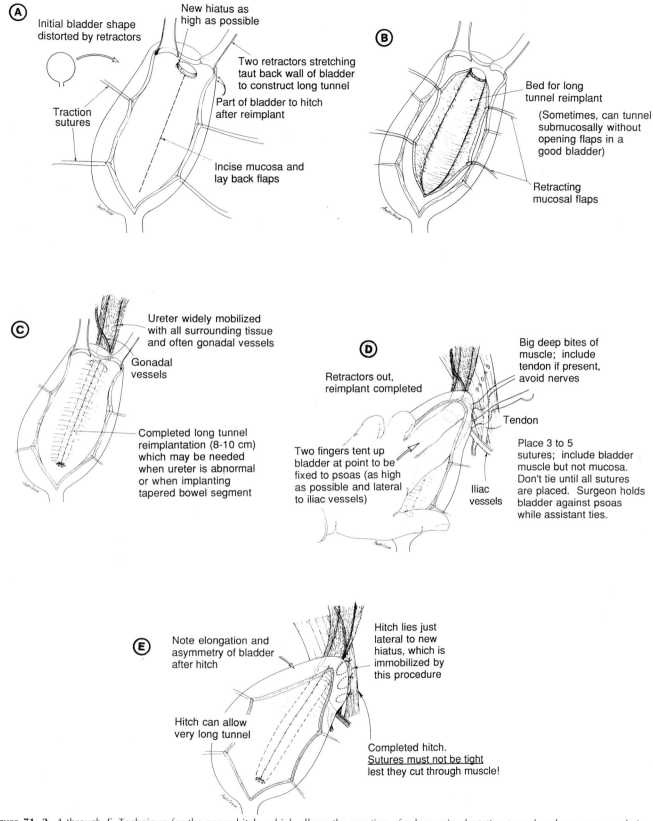

Figure 71–2. *A through E,* Technique for the psoas hitch, which allows the creation of a long reimplantation tunnel and prevents angulation of the ureter or tapered bowel segment when the bladder fills. Monofilament, nonabsorbable suture material is used to fix the bladder to the psoas muscle. Care must be taken to avoid entering the bladder, which might cause stone formation on a suture. (Illustration courtesy of W. Hardy Hendren, M.D.)

created by tunneling the ureter beneath a tenia. Important principles learned from ureterosigmoidostomy include direct mucosa-to-mucosa anastomosis and a submucosal tunnel of adequate length. This technique, familiar to most urologists, has provided favorable long-term results since the 1950s (Nesbit, 1949; Goodwin et al, 1953; Leadbetter and Clarke, 1954) and is based on the initial work of Coffey (1911). Implantation may be done from inside the reservoir with the intestinal segment open or from without after the intestinal segment has been completely reconfigured and closed.

If a gastric segment is used for bladder augmentation or replacement, ureters may be reimplanted into the stomach in a manner remarkably similar to that used in the native bladder. It is easy to create a submucosal tunnel with good muscle backing. The same principles for choosing the length of tunnel in relation to the width of the ureter are used as with bladder. Creating an effective antireflux mechanism into an ileal segment is more difficult. The split/nipple technique described by Griffith may prevent reflux at least at low reservoir pressure (Turner-Warwick and Ashken, 1967; Patil et al, 1976; Stone and MacDermott, 1989; Sagalowsky, 1995). A short longitudinal incision is made in the distal ureter, and the ureteral wall is turned back on itself. The nipple should be at least twice as long as the width of the ureter. The cuff is stabilized by suturing the ureter to itself. The adventitia of the ureter immediately proximal to the cuff is then approximated to the full thickness of the ileal wall at the hiatus so that the cuff protrudes into the lumen. LeDuc and colleagues (1987) described a technique in which the ureter is brought through a hiatus in the ileal wall. From that hiatus, the ileal mucosa is incised and the edges are mobilized so as to create a trough for the ureter. The spatulated ureter is laid into the trough and approximated to the mucosa at the distal end. The ileal mucosa is sutured to the lateral edges of the ureter and should eventually grow over it. Long-term results with these two techniques have been conflicting, but in general they have not proved as reliable as a tunneled ureterocolonic anastomosis in preventing reflux (Patil et al, 1976; LeDuc et al, 1987; Rowland, 1996; Bihrle, 1997), with one exception (Lugagne et al, 1997). It may also be possible to create an antireflux mechanism using a serosa-lined tunnel created between two limbs of ileum, as described by Abol-Enein and Ghoneim (1999).

Reinforced nipple valves of ileum have been used extensively for antireflux with the Kock pouch (Skinner et al, 1989). After several modifications by Skinner, good long-term results have been achieved. His technique requires a relatively long segment of ileum and use of permanent staples. Attempts have been made to secure the nipple for the long term without staples (Gosalbez and Gousse, 1998). Others have tried to avoid using staples and Marlex as well (Hanna and Bloiso, 1987). Maintenance of the intussuscepted cuff is the key to a successful result. The same forces that compress the nipple to achieve continence tend to evert or destabilize it. An ileal nipple valve may be particularly useful with short, dilated ureters; an isoperistaltic segment of ileum may be left with the nipple to replace a short ureter. Likewise, the antireflux mechanism is based on the ileal segment and not on the ureter. Consequently, a very dilated ureter may be anastomosed to the ileum without tapering. In some neobladders, an isoperistaltic limb of ileum is positioned between the reservoir and ureters to discourage reflux, at least at low pressures (Studer and Zingg, 1997).

BLADDER NECK RECONSTRUCTION

One of the greatest technical challenges facing the surgeon in regard to bladder reconstruction is providing adequate outflow resistance. Often the bladder neck is incompetent because of neurogenic dysfunction secondary to spinal dysraphism. Other underlying pathologic conditions, such as exstrophy, bilateral ectopic ureters, or ureteroceles, are unique problems that must be considered when addressing outlet resistance. Many operative techniques have been described for bladder neck reconstruction, indicating that no single option is best for all patients (Kryger et al, 2000). **It cannot be overstated that preoperative evaluation and thorough knowledge of the patient's specific physiologic limitations are required.**

The ability for a sustained bladder contraction to result in complete emptying or the absence of hyperreflexic contractions influences the selection of a technique for gaining outlet resistance. Many operative techniques that create an appropriate increase in outlet resistance do so at the expense of detrusor contractibility. For reasons not clearly defined, increasing outlet resistance can change the behavior of the detrusor, converting a compliant reservoir into a noncompliant, hostile environment (Burbige et al, 1987; Churchill et al, 1987). Provocative cystometry may reveal the patient at risk. This is not always possible, and close postoperative observation is mandatory (Kronner et al, 1998b).

There is a spectrum of techniques in our surgical armamentarium that encompass tightening of the bladder neck, creation of flap valve mechanisms, placement of artificial or autologous bulking agents, and placement of an artificial urinary sphincter (AUS). **The selected option should be individualized to the patient's pathologic process, needs, and personal goals.**

An important consideration is the patient's ability to empty well before reconstruction and its likelihood afterward. Some of these repairs may prohibit spontaneous voiding. In many patients, particularly those with neurogenic dysfunction also requiring bladder augmentation, voiding cannot be expected, and the major concern is providing adequate outflow resistance. For those with other diagnoses, especially if augmentation cystoplasty is not necessary, spontaneous voiding remains a goal.

The following discussion covers a variety of operative techniques used to achieve urinary continence through bladder neck and external urinary sphincter reconstruction. Most of the results are based on experience in individuals with spinal dysraphism, but the techniques may be used with other pathogenic conditions. All techniques have their own learning curve, which necessitates careful analysis of results and forthright reporting. The results of any technique must be kept in perspective, knowing that many studies involve a small patient population with mixed pathologic conditions. Some reports have not examined gender and its effect on choice of procedure or results.

Young-Dees-Leadbetter Repair

The Young-Dees-Leadbetter bladder neck reconstruction is one of the most recognized operative techniques to increase outlet resistance. The original Young procedure has evolved and remains of primary consideration when reconstructing the exstrophic bladder neck. It has been used in patients with many diagnoses.

Technique

Young's initial description (1919) of excising a portion of the bladder neck and significantly tightening the bladder neck over a silver probe was modified by Dees (1949) who extended the length of excised tissue through the trigone. Leadbetter (1964) followed by elevating the ureters off the trigone, placing them in a more cephalic position on the bladder floor. This allowed for tubularization of the trigone and further enhanced lengthening of the urethra. A detailed description and illustrations are found in Chapter 61 in the section on bladder exstrophy.

Results

Reports of success with the Young-Dees-Leadbetter bladder neck reconstruction in children with neurogenic sphincter dysfunction are limited, not only in the number of series but in overall improvement of incontinence. Tanagho (1972) and Leadbetter (1985) independently reviewed their long-term results of this repair showing minimal success in individuals with neurogenic dysfunction. They speculated that the lack of success resulted from a lack of muscle tone and activity in the wrapped muscle related to the neurogenic problem. Many patients in the early series did not undergo bladder augmentation, possibly compromising the continence achieved. Contrary to the results reported in exstrophy patients, the majority of individuals with neurogenic deficiency of the bladder neck require bladder augmentation and CIC. Sidi et al (1987b) documented a 4-hour continence interval in 7 of 11 patients, although 10 required catheterization and 9 augmentation. Five of the seven needed reoperation to achieve continence. This small series represents some of the more recent long-term results of the Young-Dees-Leadbetter reconstruction in children with neurogenic dysfunction, because the technique has largely fallen out of favor.

In an attempt to enhance the Young-Dees-Leadbetter procedure, Mitchell and Rink (1983) described the addition of external support and compression achieved through the placement of a silicone sheath around the reconstructed bladder neck. This was in part done to protect a plane for future placement of an artificial sphincter cuff, if necessary. In place, it seemed to improve the function of the repair by either improving coaptation or maintaining the proximal repair in a better anatomic position. However, most of the thicker Silastic sheaths eventually eroded and disrupted the repairs (Kropp et al, 1993). Quimby and associates (1996) used a thinner Silastic sheath without the same risk of erosion. They also wrapped omentum between the repair and the Silastic wrap. They reported better results of ultimate continence and felt that placement of an artificial sphincter cuff was much easier when needed.

Donnahoo and coworkers (1999) reviewed one of the largest series of this repair used in treating neurogenic incontinence (38 children, 25 of whom were girls). A primary repair was performed in 24 children, a secondary procedure in 6, and a primary repair in conjunction with a Silicone sheath in 8. Partial continence was achieved after the initial repair in 26 children (68%). All children provided with the Silicone sheath were initially continent, but in five sheath erosion occurred. More importantly, 35 (92%) of the children required augmentation cystoplasty to become continent. The authors found that, although continence could be achieved with this technique, it was at the expense of augmentation cystoplasty and multiple procedures.

Fascial Sling

Sling procedures were developed in an attempt to increase resistance at the bladder neck. Both artificial and natural tissues have been used with the same techniques. Resultant coaptation and elevation of the bladder neck should cause approximation of opposing epithelial surfaces and increased outlet resistance that is greater than the resting bladder pressure and greater than the pressure achieved during stressful activity or Valsalva's maneuver. With sling coaptation the bladder neck remains fixed, and, although a strong detrusor contraction can establish a voiding pressure leading to urine flow, it rarely results in adequate bladder emptying in the face of anatomic or neurologic problems. The majority of pediatric patients who undergo a sling procedure must be prepared for CIC. The resistance achieved with bladder neck slings can potentially be overcome by hyperreflexic bladder contractions or elevated pressure due to diminished bladder compliance. Therefore, simultaneous bladder augmentation has been performed in 55% to 100% of patients in order to achieve urinary continence (Bauer et al, 1989; Elder, 1990; Decter, 1993; Kakizaki et al, 1995; Perez et al, 1996a).

Technique

The bladder neck is exposed by clearing fatty tissue overlying the bladder neck and the lateral endopelvic fascia. An incision is made within the endopelvic fascia for approximately 2 cm. The junction between the bladder neck and proximal urethra can be identified by placing a transurethral catheter into the bladder and gently pulling down on the catheter to lodge the balloon at the bladder neck. With the use of blunt dissection, a plane between the posterior bladder neck and vagina in girls or rectal wall in boys is developed. The proper plane may be more easily developed from the cul-de-sac by dissecting behind the bladder and ureters from above (Lottmann et al, 1999; Badiola et al, 2000). If the landmarks are not easily defined, as in a secondary repair, the dissection becomes difficult. It may be appropriate to open the bladder to help prevent inadvertent dissection into the urethra or posterior structures.

When fascial tissue is used, the technique is based on that described by McGuire and Lytton (1978) for stress urinary incontinence. Rectus abdominis fascia 1 cm in width and of an appropriate length is harvested. This fascia can be taken in either vertical or horizontal fashion, depending on the initial skin incision. Fascia from other sites has been used in a similar fashion, but this necessitates a second incision. Cadaveric tissue or biodegradable scaffolds may also be used. All are generally secured to the anterior rectus fascia on either side. Autologous fascial tissue has been used, combining the benefits of a compressive wrap and suspension of the proximal urethra and bladder neck. Several variations of fascial placement and configuration have been described (Woodside and Borden, 1982; McGuire et al, 1986; Elder, 1990; Perez et al, 1996a).

Results

Fascial slings have been used more extensively and with better results in girls with neurogenic sphincter incompetence, although some success has been reported in boys. Overall long-term success with fascial slings in the neurogenic population has varied greatly, from 40% to 100% (Kryger et al, 2000). A variation thought to contribute to a higher rate of success includes a circumferential fascia wrap around the bladder neck. A circumferential wrap equalizes the compressive pressure over a greater surface area of bladder neck and posterior urethra (Walker et al, 1995). In addition to the wrap, simultaneous suspension has been used. Success rates have varied so much that it is difficult to determine whether any modification of the sling technique accounts for an increase in continence. Most patients who have undergone a fascial sling or wrap have also had simultaneous bladder augmentation. **Success of the sling, as with most repairs, appears to be improved with augmentation cystoplasty.** When fascial slings and wraps are used for neurogenic sphincter incontinence, creating a wrap or sling that is too tight is not a concern, because most patients are preferentially managed with CIC.

In contrast to the Silastic sheath, erosion rarely occurs with fascial slings. Gormley et al (1994) reported a revision rate with fascial slings of 15%. Placement of a fascial sling does not eliminate the possibility of later placement of an AUS (Decter, 1993; Barthold et al, 1999). It is not unreasonable to consider placing a fascial sling in a child with a marginally competent bladder neck and posterior urethra if the child is undergoing augmentation cystoplasty and already requires CIC.

Perez et al (1996a) reviewed the outcome of sling cystourethropexy in 39 children, 15 of whom were boys. One of four different techniques was performed. When postoperative continence based on age, sex, underlying diagnosis, preoperative urodynamics, surgical technique, and enterocystoplasty was evaluated, only concomitant enterocystoplasty was predictive of a successful outcome.

Bladder Neck Bulking Agents

Vortsman et al (1985) reported one of the initial descriptions of injection of a bulking agent into the bladder neck in incontinent children. The initial enthusiasm for use of polytetrafluoroethylene was quickly tempered because of concern over migration of particles to regional and distant sites, including pelvic nodes, lungs, brain, kidney, and spleen, found in animal models (Malizia et al, 1984). The technique remains of interest, and several alternatives to polytetrafluoroethylene have been assessed, including glutaraldehyde cross-linked collagen (Leonard et al, 1990a). One concern regarding the use of bovine collagen is the potential for reaction in latex-sensitive children with spina bifida, because the product is not latex-free (Kryger et al, 2000). In an attempt to achieve an ideal substance for injection, investigation is ongoing with the use of autologous cartilage cells harvested from a separate site and then grown in an alginate matrix for endoscopic implantation (Bent et al, 2000). Preliminary results show a positive effect in adult women with stress incontinence. Whether this will be an appropriate alternative for neurogenic sphincter incontinence in children is yet to be seen.

In an attempt to alleviate the risks of injecting a foreign biologic product, alternatives to bovine collagen have been investigated. Polydimethylsiloxane is one such agent. It is composed of sterile, solid, textured Silicone particles, with an average size of 200 μg, which are suspended in a biologic hydrogen carrier. The large size of the particles virtually eliminates the problem of lymphatic and distant migration (Beisang and Ersek, 1992; Guys et al, 1999).

Technique

Endoscopic exposure is used to locate the proximal urethra and bladder neck. Injection can be done directly through the working channel of the endoscope. Ideal placement of the material is in a subepithelial space, mobilizing the epithelium toward the lumen of the bladder neck. When this has been completed in a circumferential fashion, adequate epithelial coaptation occurs, which effectively raises outlet resistance. Alternatively, periurethral injection in women using a long needle placed from the perineum or via a suprapubic approach has been tried. Evidence is lacking whether the exact approach affects success, but accurate placement is important and transurethral injection is generally preferred.

Results

The durability and success of bladder neck and proximal urethral injection remains in doubt for the pediatric population. True continence, as defined by a 4-hour dry period between voidings or catheterizations, has been reported to be at most 64% and has ranged as low as 5% (Leonard et al, 1990a; Capozza et al, 1995; Bomalaski et al, 1996; Perez et al, 1996b; Sundaram et al, 1997; Silveri et al, 1998)). Several factors play a role in the outcome, and in particular any previous operative bladder neck repair. Success is enhanced by elevation of the epithelium of the bladder neck, which may be compromised by scarring from previous operative procedures. **The concept of a minimally invasive operation used to enhance a marginal result gained from a more formal bladder neck repair is enticing, but the data are lacking to show that bladder neck injection is of lasting value.**

Sundaram and colleagues (1997) reported on the efficacy and durability of glutaraldehyde cross-linked bovine collagen in 20 children, 12 of whom had neurogenic sphincter dysfunction. More than half of the children required two or three independent injections. Success was achieved in only 1 patient (5%), who was considered dry; 5 had some improvement, and 10 had either no change or transient improvement of only 2 to 90 days. In their hands, collagen therapy only delayed the ultimate need for bladder neck reconstruction.

Guys and associates (1999) treated 33 children with polydimethylsiloxane, 24 of whom had neurogenic bladder neck and sphincter incontinence. One third of the children achieved continence for longer than 4 hours at a time, and one fourth were continent for approximately 2 hours with minimal pad use. Poor results were reported in approximately 40%. Their results were not affected by previous operative procedures on the bladder neck or by detrusor hyperreflexia. Success was noted to be gender biased, with 47% of girls but only 10% of boys continent.

Submucosal bladder neck injection of bovine dermal collagen was used by Perez and associates (1996b) in 32 patients. Continence was achieved after a single injection in only 20% of those children with neurogenic dysfunction. Complications were limited to febrile urinary infections, one episode of urinary retention, and two instances of worsening incontinence. The authors concluded that, even though their success was limited, the low morbidity and ease of placement justified submucosal injection in selected children.

The cost of the bulking agents can be excessive, and there does not appear to be any financial benefit over a formal repair (Kryger et al, 2000). **At the present time,** **bulking agents play a limited role for increasing outlet resistance and should be reserved for a very select group of patients. The exact criteria that define that group have not been established.** Patients with marginal native outflow resistance are probably better candidates than those with minimal preoperative function.

Artificial Urinary Sphincter

The AUS has been recognized as a device that can result in prompt continence in selected children while preserving their ability to void spontaneously. The AUS was introduced by Scott and colleagues in 1974. The general concept and design of the initial model have been retained, but improvements and enhancements have evolved that have positively affected the long-term success of the AUS. The current AS800 model is the result of multiple refinements, including a seamless, pressurized balloon reservoir, nonkink tubing, and changes in the cuff that facilitate its placement and effectiveness with coaptation of the bladder neck and proximal urethra (Light and Reynolds, 1992; Barrett et al, 1993).

Technique

Placement of the cuff should be at the level of the bladder neck in all girls and prepubertal boys (Fig. 71–3). It is also the most desirable and effective location in pubertal and adult men with neurogenic sphincter incompetence. The bulbar urethra can be used as an alternative site in adult men with a mature spongiosum. Levesque and coworkers (1996) indicated that age is not a factor regarding placement of the cuff around the bladder neck. They found that children do not outgrow the AUS as they progress through puberty, and replacement of the cuff is not routinely necessary. The AUS can be positioned around an intestinal segment used in total urinary reconstruction, but

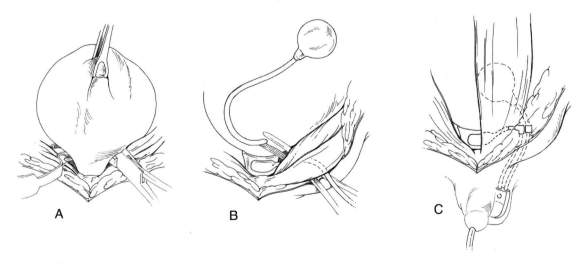

Figure 71–3. Artificial urinary sphincter placement in children. *A,* The cuff is placed around the bladder neck in a prepubertal child. Dissection may be facilitated by palpation of a urethral catheter and balloon or by a posterior approach. If dissection is difficult, the bladder can be opened. *B,* The reservoir is placed beneath the rectus muscle. *C,* A tunnel is then made into the scrotum or labium for positioning of the pump on the same side as the reservoir. Tubing connections are made ventral to the rectus fascia, and the device is initially left deactivated.

it is more prone to erosion there. Several authors have described the successful placement of the cuff around a bowel segment, particularly when omentum is interposed between the cuff and the segment (Burbige et al, 1987; Weston et al, 1991; Light et al, 1995).

Placement of an artificial sphincter in children is the same as for adults. Development of the proper plane for the cuff is similar to that described for a fascial sling. The cuff should be sized snugly, but not tightly, around the bladder neck. Obviously, a sterile environment is critical when considering placement of the AUS to avoid infection. For that reason, preoperative antibiotics are a necessity, and confirmation of sterile urine is required. With those precautions, there is freedom to open the bladder when dissecting around the bladder neck. This often facilitates the dissection and ensures proper placement. Experience has shown that leaving the unit deactivated with the cuff deflated after placement allows formation of a pseudocapsule around the cuff and decreases the risk of erosion (Furlow, 1981; Sidi et al, 1984). The AS800 model has a locking mechanism in the pump which permits the AUS to be deactivated and activated without a second operative procedure.

Results

There are substantial short- and long-term data regarding continence after placement of the AUS. **Continence must be placed in context with the cost experienced by the patient, which is defined by mechanical malformations that result in secondary operative procedures and more catastrophic complications such as device infection or erosion.** Dramatic improvement regarding the need for secondary procedures has occurred with the technical refinements in the device. This is important to consider, because many of the true long-term studies reflect results and revision rates obtained with earlier models. Levesque and coworkers (1996) presented the results of 10 years of follow-up of AUS in children, and Kryger and colleagues (1999) reported data from more than 15 years. Both groups reported an impressive continence rate of 80% and a functioning sphincter in 95% of patients. These reports are consistent with other series in children which have reported continence rates of 75% to 90% and a functioning sphincter in 85% to 97% of patients (Nurse and Mundy, 1988; Gonzalez et al, 1989a; Bosco et al, 1991; O'Flynn and Thomas, 1991; Aprikian et al, 1992; Singh and Thomas, 1996; Simeoni et al, 1996). All of these reports noted a significant reoperative rate, primarily for mechanical problems.

Although the AUS is one of the few surgically created continence mechanisms that does not negatively affect spontaneous voiding, CIC remains an important adjunct in approximately 75% of children with neurogenic sphincter incompetence and can be performed successfully through the cuff (Diokno and Sonda, 1981; Gonzalez et al, 1995; Levesque et al, 1996; Kryger, 1999). As boys approach puberty, spontaneous voiding may become a problem, necessitating CIC for many. It has been speculated that growth of the prostate causes an increase in native outlet resistance. Kaefer and colleagues (1997a) evaluated in-

creases in cuff size as a means to facilitate spontaneous voiding in boys. In their limited series, they did not find that up-sizing restored the ability to void spontaneously. Jumper and associates (1990) reported on prostatic development and sexual function in pubertal boys with spinal dysraphism who had been treated with the AUS. They found that the AUS did not alter sexual development, prostatic growth, or morphology.

Device infection and erosion are the most concerning complications of the AUS. Fastidious attention to detail and sterile technique diminish the risk of infection but do not eliminate it. When infection occurs without erosion, the unit can be removed and later replaced (Nurse and Mundy, 1988). Infections are minimized by sterilization of the urine preoperatively, meticulous cleaning of the wound site, preoperative bowel preparation, perioperative parenteral antibiotics, and copious antibiotic wound irrigation. Newer cuff design and a 6-week delay in activation of the device help formation of a thickened pseudocapsule, which substantially decreases bladder neck and proximal urethral erosion. Kryger and coworkers (1999) indicated that erosion can be virtually eliminated when the cuff has been placed as the primary treatment for bladder neck incompetence. They and others (Aliabadi and Gonzalez, 1990; Gonzalez et al, 1995; Simeoni et al, 1996) have indicated that the risk of erosion substantially increases after previous failed repairs. Identifying the correct plane between the bladder neck and the vagina in girls or rectum in boys preserves the vascularity of the bladder neck and proximal urethra and may decrease the rate of erosion (Aliabadi and Gonzalez, 1990). Initial exposure via a posterior bladder approach, as described by Lottmann and colleagues (1999), may be helpful.

Levesque and associates (1996) evaluated the long-term outcome of the AUS based on date of insertion and location of the placement. Before 1985, the AUS had been inserted in 36 children. Between 1985 and 1990, an additional 18 children underwent placement. In the original group, 24 of the 36 sphincters were in place and 22 were functional. Twelve patients had required at least one revision. The mean survival time of the device was 12.5 years. The success rates at 5 and 10 years were 75% and 72%, respectively. In the group implanted after 1985, 78% retained a functioning sphincter. The overall continence rate in both groups was 59%, and sphincter survival probability at 10 years was approximately 70%. No difference in failure rates was found between boys and girls, with the exception that female patients who had previously undergone bladder neck surgery were more likely to have an erosion. The ability to void independently without the use of CIC was retained in 36 children.

Upper urinary tract changes including hydronephrosis have been reported to occur in up to 15% of children after placement of the AUS (Light and Pietro, 1986; Churchill et al, 1987; Gonzalez et al, 1995; Levesque et al, 1996; Kryger et al, 1999). In extreme cases, renal insufficiency has resulted. **It is now recognized that occlusion of the bladder neck in children with neurogenic sphincter incompetence can result in unmasking or development of detrusor hostility, manifested by a decrease in bladder compliance or an increase in detrusor hyperreflexia**

(Bauer et al, 1986). **Careful preoperative urodynamic assessment identifies only some of the children who are at risk** (Kronner et al, 1998b). When hostile bladder characteristics are found preoperatively, anticholinergic medications can be beneficial for hyperreflexic contractions, but augmentation cystoplasty is usually required for diminished compliance. Churchill and associates (1987) reported on the urodynamic characteristics of capacity and compliance, showing that favorable parameters can be maintained after placement of the AUS. Close observation is still recommended for any child undergoing bladder neck reconstruction to identify early any deterioration in bladder dynamics before upper tract changes occur.

Some children undergoing sphincter placement need bladder augmentation as well, and the timing of the two procedures may be questioned due to the concern for AUS infection. Light and associates (1995) reported a 50% infection rate with simultaneous augmentation, compared with 9.5% when the procedures were staged. On the contrary, a contemporary review by Miller and colleagues (1998) found infection necessitating removal of the device in only 2 (7%) of 29 patients. This low rate is similar to that noted by others (Strawbridge et al, 1989; Gonzalez et al, 1989b). Several reports have evaluated various factors and found that the intestinal segment selected for augmentation appeared to be the only parameter affecting results; gastric augmentation was the least offensive regarding infection (Ganesan et al, 1993; Miller et al, 1998).

The AS800 is the subject of most reviews concerning the AUS, but alternative devices have been reported. Lima and coworkers (1996) reported on the combined use of enterocystoplasty and a "new type" of AUS. The new device was a one-piece adjustable cuff connected to an inflatable port. The injection port was placed subcutaneously and made available for percutaneous access in order to adjust the fluid valve and pressure of the cuff needed to achieve continence. It is too early to determine whether this device will be an acceptable alternative.

The ultimate benefit of the AUS is its ability to achieve a high rate of continence while maintaining the potential for spontaneous voiding. For practical purposes, when CIC is required along with augmentation cystoplasty, use of native tissue for continence eliminates the long-term concern for infection or erosion and the risk of mechanical failure.

Urethral Lengthening

Young's original description of bladder neck reconstruction (1919) consisted of two basic parts—excising a segment of anterior urethral bladder neck tissue and narrowing the remaining posterior portion. This, however, left the tubularized segment in continuity with the bladder, which ultimately led to failure. Refinements by Dees (1949) and Leadbetter (1964) maximized good muscle tone at the bladder neck and extension of the urethral tube through the trigone.

With similar principles, Tanagho (1972) described a cephalad-based anterior detrusor wall tube. Closure of the tubularized bladder neck created circularly oriented muscle fibers, which Tanagho described as a sphincter mechanism. However, he cautioned against using this technique in the neurogenic population. Because of potential breakdown of that tubularized bladder neck and poor results, other techniques have been developed based on the concept of a flap valve to create urinary retention. Kropp and Angwafo (1986) described urethral lengthening and creation of a flap valve for neurogenic bladder neck and sphincter dysfunction. The technique is based on an anterior detrusor wall tube that is kept in continuity with the urethra, tubularized, and implanted into a submucosal tunnel within the trigone. Conceptually this is effective, but difficulty with catheterization is a common problem and a significant concern.

Technique

A Foley catheter is placed intravesically, and the bladder is filled to capacity. The bladder is exposed through a midline or a low transverse abdominal incision. The bladder neck is then identified with application of gentle catheter traction. A 5- $\times$ 1.5-cm rectangular flap based on the bladder neck and urethra is then isolated. Stay sutures are placed, and the flap is mobilized in continuity with the proximal urethra. The detrusor musculature at the bladder neck is then divided, separating the bladder and urethra. The muscle may be left intact at the 5 and 7 o'clock positions. In girls, the anterior vaginal wall is exposed, and in boys the seminal vesicles. The rectangular strip based on the urethra is tubularized posteriorly around the urethral catheter with a continuous absorbable suture. The distal portion of the tubularized strip should be approximated in an interrupted fashion to facilitate excision of excessive tissue without jeopardizing the suture line. A capacious submucosal tunnel through the trigone is then created posteriorly for the proximal neourethra (Fig. 71–4). A wide tunnel is required to prevent kinking at the level of the bladder neck, which would impede catheterization. It is important to eliminate dead space at the entrance of the urethra into the bladder, and this can be accomplished by placing lateral securing sutures in the region of the bladder neck. The detrusor tube must be pulled straight through the tunnel without curves or deviations to facilitate catheterization. Waters and colleagues (1997) and Kropp (1999) have not found it necessary to elevate the native ureters in all cases, reimplanting them in a cephalic location. They now typically reimplant only refluxing ureters (Kropp, 1999). When closing the bladder, the lateral wings in the region of the bladder neck are approximated and incorporate adventitia of the tubularized urethra. This enhances a watertight closure and is continued for 2 or 3 cm anteriorly, often up to the area of augmentation. The tubularized neourethra is long enough to reach the true lumen of the bladder, where it is exposed to pressure as an effective flap valve.

Because of the difficulties with catheterization, modifications of the Kropp bladder neck procedure have been described. Belman and Kaplan suggested a simplified approach (1989). They harvested a rectangular strip from the anterior bladder wall similar to that described by Kropp. However, the lateral and posterior musculature at the bladder wall was not incised, and the proximal urethra and

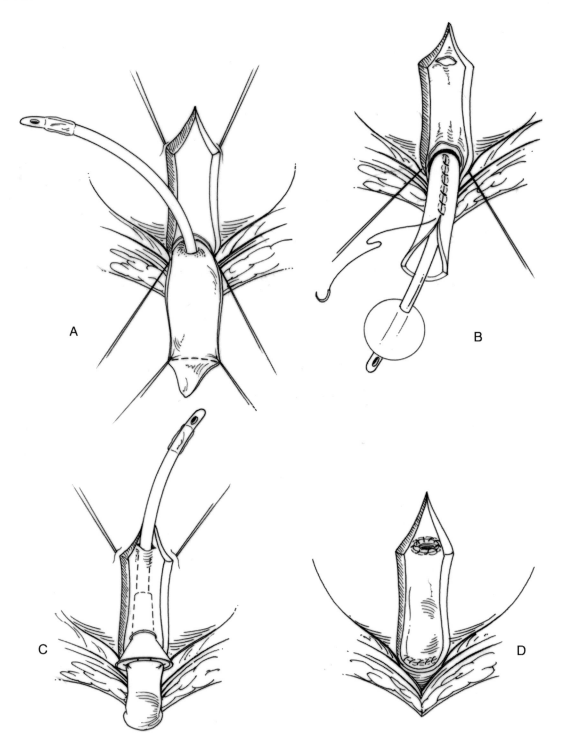

Figure 71–4. Kropp anterior detrusor tube. *A,* An anterior flap of bladder (1.5 cm wide × 4 to 5 cm in length) is created in continuity with the bladder. *B,* The anterior flap is tubularized over a catheter. A tunnel beneath the mucosa of the trigone is created between the ureteral orifices for the length of the tube. *C,* The tubularized flap is brought through the tunnel. *D,* The detrusor tube is secured to the floor of the trigone with interrupted absorbable suture in a straight course.

bladder were not separated. The flap was tubularized over a No. 8 Fr catheter. The epithelium on the floor of the bladder was incised, contrary to the tunnel made by Kropp. The tube was placed within the trough with the proximal meatus secured on the floor of the bladder. The epithelial edges of the trough were then secured to the lateral aspect

of the tube. As with the initial description, the suture line for tubularization of the urethra is posterior, against trigonal muscle. Closure of the bladder begins with reapproximation of the lateral walls of the bladder to the tube until the bladder edges meet. The remaining portion of the bladder is covered by an augmentation.

Results

Snodgrass (1997) examined the results in 23 children, 22 of whom had neurogenic sphincter incompetence, and noted continence in more than 90%. The most common complication was difficult catheterization, particularly in boys. Fewer than half of the boys in Snodgrass' series catheterized through the native urethra; the majority did so via an abdominal wall stoma. Postoperative vesicoureteral reflux was identified in 9 of 18 children; Snodgrass speculated that this was caused by lateral retraction of the ureters resulting from closure of the bladder edges over the detrusor tube. The recommendation was made to leave the posterior bladder wall open and flat when receiving the augmentation in order to prevent this distortion. Kropp (1999) has not had as many problems with catheterization in his patients, and he likewise has achieved a high rate of continence.

Some patients with an effective flap valve mechanism created by urethral lengthening virtually never leak per urethra. This potentially puts them at risk for upper tract deterioration or bladder rupture, particularly if they do not or cannot catheterize reliably. Snodgrass (1997) thought that his modification was beneficial in that it resulted in a shorter intravesical tunnel for the neourethra, allowing for leakage per urethra with overfilling.

Pippi Salle Procedure

In an attempt to maximize the benefits of the Kropp technique and decrease problems with catheterization, Salle and associates (1994) reported use of an anterior bladder onlay flap. With this technique, the posterior wall of the neourethra is intact, theoretically providing less potential hang-up during catheterization. Modifications have been made since the first report to improve flap viability, minimize fistula formation, and extend the indications for the procedure beyond that of the neurogenic bladder (Salle et al, 1997).

Technique

An anterior, full-thickness bladder wall flap measuring 5 × 1 cm is mobilized to the bladder neck with 0.1 cm of its epithelial edges excised in order to avoid overlapping suture lines. Two parallel incisions down to the level of the muscle are made in the mucosa of the trigone from the native bladder neck. The anterior flap is secured to the midline strip of trigone mucosa to create a tube or lengthened urethra, usually in two layers, using absorbable suture. The muscle on either side of the posterior epithelial strip may be incised superficially to provide an edge to which the muscle of the anterior flap may be approximated in an effort to avoid fistula (Fig. 71–5). The more lateral mucosa of the trigone is mobilized and closed over the midline urethra. Distally, the muscle of the bladder neck is wrapped fairly tightly around the urethra with closure. More proximally, the lengthened urethra should extend well into the lumen of the bladder.

Results

Initial complications of this procedure included persistent incontinence, urethrovesical fistula, and partial necrosis of the intravesical neourethra. Widening the base of the urethra at the level of the bladder neck may decrease these problems. Children who have previously undergone bladder surgery can have a secondary Salle repair if the anterior bladder flap is lateralized slightly to avoid any old midline suture line and increased potential for scarring or necrosis.

Salle and associates (1997) found that continence (for longer than 4 hours) was achieved in 12 (70%) of 17 patients. Catheterization difficulties occurred in only 3 of 17 children, 1 of whom subsequently underwent an appendicovesicostomy. Fistula formation at the base of the flap between the proximal, intravesical urethra and the bladder occurred in two children and resulted in recurrent incontinence. This problem appeared to be diminished by creating a wider base to the flap and generously trimming the epithelial edges. This improved the flap width-to-length ratio. Jawaheer and Rangecroft (1999) reported a diurnal continence rate of 61% (for 3 hours or longer) with the Salle procedure. However, only 44% of their patients were dry through the night. Less trouble with catheterization has occurred than with the Kropp technique, but in rare instances it remains a problem. Continence rates have not been quite as high (Rink et al, 1994; Mouriquand et al, 1995).

Bladder Neck Division

The ultimate procedure to increase bladder outlet resistance is to divide the bladder neck so that it is no longer in continuity with the urethra. This must be accompanied by creation of a continent abdominal wall stoma, and it should be performed only in patients who will reliably catheterize. If effective, it prevents any leakage or pop-off per urethra and potentially increases the risk for upper tract deterioration or bladder rupture if emptying is not performed. Division is seldom performed as a primary procedure, but it may be considered if the previously mentioned repairs fail.

Such a procedure effectively moves the reconstructive effort into the realm of continent urinary diversion. The bladder neck is abandoned from a physiologic standpoint, although the bladder may be used as part of the reservoir.

Effective division of the bladder neck is not a simple procedure. The bladder must be aggressively mobilized away from the urethra after complete division of the bladder neck. The bladder should be closed distally in several layers. Omentum has generally been interposed. Without these steps, fistulization and leakage per urethra can occur.

AUGMENTATION CYSTOPLASTY

The initial approach to augmentation cystoplasty is similar regardless of the bowel segment to be used. Cystoscopy should be performed preoperatively to avoid any unsuspected anatomic abnormalities that may affect the surgery or postoperative care. If other bladder procedures (e.g.,

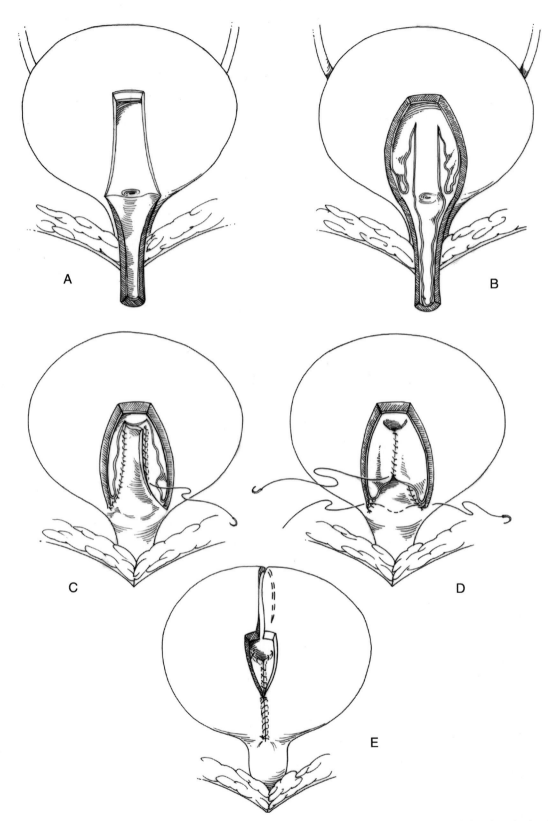

Figure 71–5. Pippi Salle anterior detrusor tube onlay. *A,* An anterior detrusor flap (1 cm × 4 to 5 cm) is mobilized to the level of the bladder neck. *B,* A central strip on the floor of the bladder is created by incising the epithelium on either side. *C,* The anterior detrusor flap is secured to the strip in a two-layer fashion, approximating the epithelium with the first layer and muscle with the second. *D,* The lateral epithelium of the trigone is mobilized and secured over the lengthened urethra. Distally, the bladder is closed to itself and should incorporate a portion of the anterior detrusor flap to ensure a watertight seal. *E,* After distal closure, the remaining portion of the bladder is left open if augmentation cystoplasty is necessary.

ureteral reimplantation) are to be performed, the bladder is left full after cystoscopy. If only augmentation is indicated, the bladder is emptied to allow easy access to the peritoneal cavity.

As a general rule, a midline incision is preferred for intestinal cystoplasty, although these procedures can be performed through a lower transverse incision if there has been no previous abdominal surgery. Laparoscopic assistance with mobilization of the intestine may allow augmentation through a smaller, lower incision (Hedican et al, 1999). Associated bladder procedures should be performed before the peritoneal cavity is opened, to minimize third space fluid loss. For gastrocystoplasty, the incision needs to extend from the pubis to the xiphoid to allow more cephalad exposure.

Management of the Native Bladder

In the past, it was recommended that the majority of the "diseased" bladder be excised in preparation for augmentation. This meant removal of the entire supratrigonal bladder. A cuff of bladder was left surrounding the trigone for anastomosis to the intestinal segment. Despite the cuff, a relatively small area of bladder was left for anastomosis to the bowel segment; most of the bowel was approximated to itself. **More recently, most surgeons have preserved the native bladder as long as it is widely opened to prevent a narrow-mouthed anastomosis, which could result in**

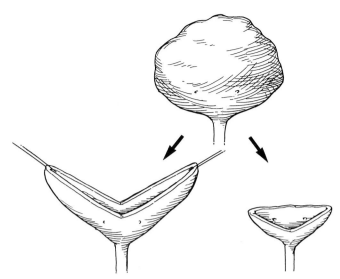

Figure 71–7. The native bladder can be managed by supratrigonal excision of the diseased bladder *(right)*. More typically, the bladder is opened widely in a sagittal plane *(left)*.

the augmentation segment's behaving as a diverticulum (Fig. 71–6). A sagittal incision to bivalve the bladder is generally useful (Fig. 71–7). The incision is carried from a point several centimeters cephalad to the bladder neck anteriorly to a position just above the trigone posteriorly. Such an incision allows a technically easier anastomosis of the bowel segment and leaves the native bladder to add to the overall capacity. A greater circumference for the anastomosis can be provided, if need be, by opening the bladder in a stellate fashion with a second transverse incision into the two bladder halves.

Management of Intestinal Segments

Hinman (1988) and Koff (1988) have well demonstrated the advantages of opening a bowel segment on its antimesenteric border, which allows detubularization and reconfiguration of the segment. **Reconfiguration into a spherical shape provides multiple advantages, including maximization of the volume achieved for any given surface area, blunting of bowel contractions, and improvement of overall capacity and compliance.** All intact, tubular intestinal segments have been noted to generate pressures of 60 to 100 cm H$_2$O with contractions, including ileum (Kock, 1969; Light and Engelmann, 1985; Fowler, 1988; Camey et al, 1991). Detubularization lowered the maximal contractile pressure from 63 to 42 cm H$_2$O in the right colon and from 81 to 28 cm H$_2$O in ileum (Goldwasser et al, 1987). Furthermore, a shorter intestinal segment can be used to achieve the same capacity as when left in tubular form. Detubularization and reconfiguration should always be performed during augmentation cystoplasty. Mathematical models based on the length and width of the bowel segment used may predict the volume needed but are cumbersome (Rink and Mitchell, 1990). Depending on the volume needed, 20 to 40 cm of ileum or approximately 20 cm of colon is usually used for cystoplasty. This somewhat depends on the volume of the native bladder being

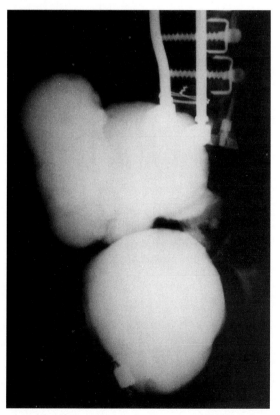

Figure 71–6. Cystogram after augmentation, demonstrating a narrow anastomosis of the bowel segment to bladder. The segment behaves as a diverticulum.

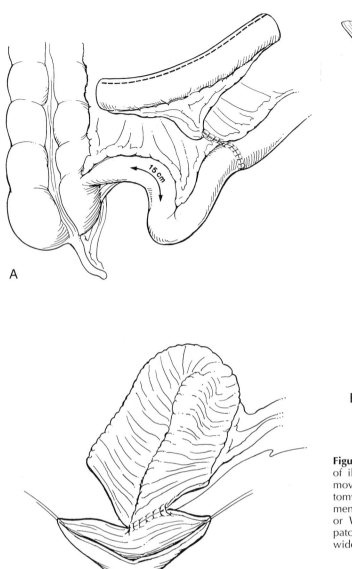

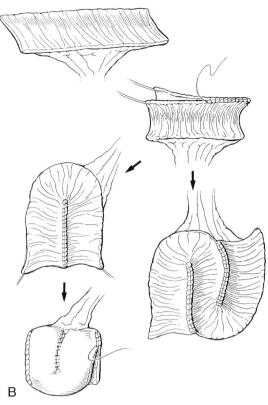

Figure 71–8. *A,* Ileocystoplasty. A 20- to 40-cm segment of ileum at least 15 cm from the ileocecal valve is removed and opened on its antimesenteric border. Ileoileostomy reconstitutes the bowel. *B,* The opened ileal segment should be reconfigured. This can be done in a U, S, or W configuration. It can be further folded as a cup patch. *C,* The reconfigured ileal segment is anastomosed widely to the native bladder.

augmented. If the cystoplasty is being done on a bladder of moderate volume that generates high pressure by uninhibited contractions, less bowel is necessary than for a bladder that is tiny in capacity. Unless otherwise contraindicated, the surgeon should err by making the bladder too large rather than too small. Appreciation of the patient's urinary volumes also should influence the size of the bladder required. Patients with upper tract damage, particularly to concentrating ability, may make huge volumes of urine and require a larger capacity.

Ileocystoplasty

Goodwin and colleagues (1959) were among the first to demonstrate the numerous ways of anastomosing a patch of ileum to the native bladder. Virtually all surgeons recognize that ileum should be detubularized and reconfigured to achieve the most spherical shape possible.

A segment of ileum at least 15 to 20 cm proximal to the ileocecal valve should be selected. The distal portion of terminal ileum is unique from a physiologic standpoint and should be avoided. The isolated segment should be 20 to 40 cm in length, depending on patient size, native bladder capacity, and the desired final capacity. With short ureters, an extra tail of isoperistaltic ileum can be useful to reach the foreshortened ureters. This requires creation of an ileonipple valve to prevent reflux, as in the Kock or hemi-Kock pouch. This type of construction may require up to 60 cm of small intestine. **The segment to be used should have an adequate mesentery to reach the native bladder without tension.** After selecting the appropriate segment, the mesentery is cleared from the bowel at either end for a short distance to create a window. The bowel is divided at these ends, and a handsewn ileoileostomy or stapled anastomosis performed. The harvested ileal segment is irrigated clear with 0.25% neomycin solution and opened on its antimesenteric border (Fig. 71–8*A*). **The ileum is folded**

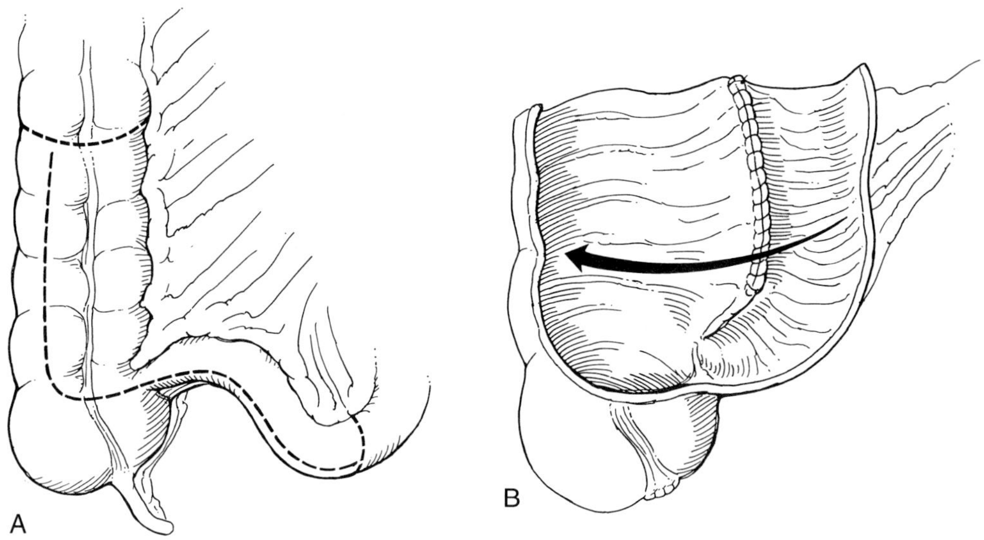

Figure 71–9. Ileocecocystoplasty. *A,* An ileocecal segment is selected. The length of segment chosen depends on the technique employed. After removal, it is opened on the antimesenteric border *(dashed lines). B,* The opened ileal and cecal segments are anastomosed to form a cup in the standard ileocecocystoplasty.

in a **U** shape most commonly, although **longer segments can be folded further into an S or W configuration. The ileum is anastomosed to itself with running absorbable sutures** (see Fig. 71–8B). The suture line should approximate the full thickness of ileum to ileum while inverting the mucosa. If not opened previously, the bladder is incised in a sagittal plane. The anastomosis of the ileum to native bladder is easily done when started posteriorly. The anastomosis may be done in a one- or two-layer fashion, always with absorbable suture (see Fig. 71–8C). Permanent suture should never be used for any cystoplasty because it may serve as a nidus for stone formation. A suprapubic tube is brought out through the native bladder and secured. The anterior aspect of the anastomosis is then completed. The mesenteric window at the bowel anastomosis is closed to prevent an internal hernia. A drain is placed near the bladder and brought out of the pelvis through a separate stab incision. It should be removed promptly if not draining urine, particularly in neurogenic patients with a ventriculoperitoneal shunt. The wound is irrigated, and the abdomen is closed in layers.

Cecocystoplasty and Ileocecocystoplasty

Technique

Couvelair described the use of the cecum for augmentation cystoplasty in 1950. Numerous reports of simple cecocystoplasty have appeared since then. Presently, cecocystoplasty is an uncommon operative procedure; it has largely been replaced by various forms of ileocecocystoplasty and therefore is not discussed further here.

With the ileocecocystoplasty technique, the cecum is opened, reconfigured, and used to augment the bladder alone, leaving a segment of ileum to reach the ureters or to create a continent abdominal wall stoma based on imbrication of the ileocecal valve and proximal ileum. Conversely, the ileal segment can be opened and used as a patch on the cecal segment before augmentation cystoplasty. Many modifications of the technique exist, but all start with mobiliza-

tion of the cecum and right colon by incising the peritoneum along the white line of Toldt up to the hepatic flexure. Approximately 15 to 30 cm of the terminal ileum is used. The length of the ileal segment depends on the technique employed. As with all intestinal cystoplasties, before division of the bowel segment, it should be certain that it will reach the bladder without tension (Fig. 71–9A).

The isolated ileocecal segment is irrigated clear with neomycin solution and opened on its antimesenteric border through the ileocecal valve for its entire length. In the typical ileocecal augmentation, the ileal and cecal segments are of equivalent length such that the borders of the open segment can be anastomosed and then folded on themselves to form a cup cystoplasty (see Fig. 71–9B). The anastomosis of the reconfigured segments is done in a one- or two-layer closure with absorbable suture. The opening should be left large enough to provide a wide anastomosis to the bivalved bladder. **If more volume is necessary, the ileal segment can be significantly longer, allowing it to be folded before anastomosis to the cecum.** The Mainz ileocystoplasty uses an ileal segment twice the length of the cecal segment. The opened edge of the cecal portion is anastomosed to the first portion of the ileal segment. The first and second portions of the ileal segment are next approximated. The compound ileocecal patch is then anastomosed to the bladder (Fig. 71–10). The mesenteric window is closed, and a suprapubic tube is placed through the native bladder and secured through the abdominal wall.

Appendix

One potential advantage of ileocecocystoplasty is the presence of the appendix. Particularly in children, the appendix is useful in the creation of a reliable continent abdominal wall stoma. The appendix may be removed with a small cuff of cecal wall and tunneled into the native bladder or a tenia of the cecal segment to provide a continent mechanism. Likewise, it may be left in situ and the base safely tunneled by creating a window in the mesoappendix. If the appendix is not to be used, an appendectomy is performed with the standard ileocecocystoplasty.

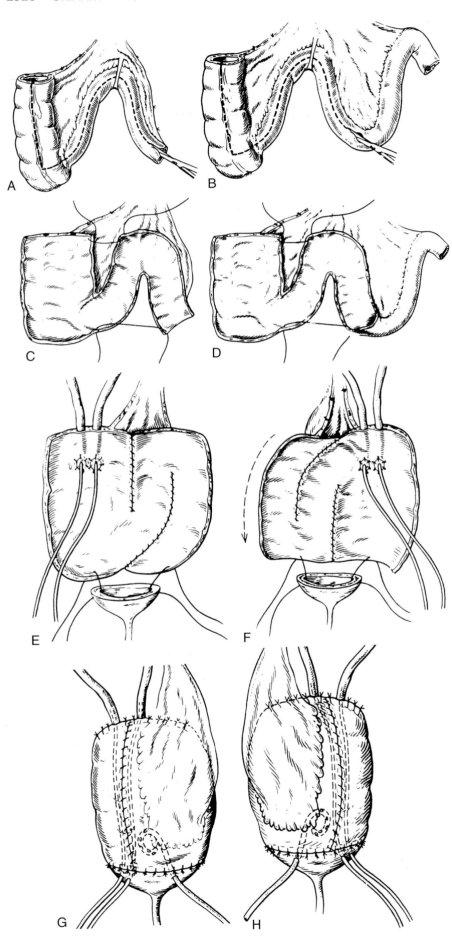

Figure 71–10. The Mainz ileocecocystoplasty. *A* and *B,* The ileal segment is twice the length of the cecal segment. *C* and *D,* It is opened on the antimesenteric border. *E* and *F,* The ureters can be reimplanted into the opened cecal segment if necessary. *G* and *H,* The ileocecal segment is anastomosed to the native bladder. (From Thuroff JW, et al: In King LR, et al [eds]: Bladder Reconstruction and Continent Urinary Diversion. Chicago, Year Book Medical Publishers, 1987.)

Ileocecal Valve

The ileocecal segment has been used extensively for reconstruction and bladder replacement in the adult population. It has been used less frequently in children because most of the patients undergoing augmentation cystoplasty are doing so because of neurovesical dysfunction. Those patients usually have neuropraxic bowel dysfunction as well. Removal of the ileocecal valve in such children can result in intractable diarrhea (Gonzalez and Cabral, 1987; King, 1987). Use of the ileocecal valve in such patients should be avoided unless other advantages of the segment outweigh the risk of diarrhea and fecal incontinence.

There are advantages to the use of the ileocecal segment. Antireflux tunnels can easily be made into the tenia of the cecum when necessary. Again, for the short ureter, a tail of ileum can be left intact to bridge the gap, with the imbricated ileocecal valve used for antireflux. The same imbrication technique can be used to create a continent abdominal wall stoma as with the appendix. Cain and Husmann (1994; Cain et al, 1999) have proposed using the ileocecal segment for augmentation with the plicated ileal segment brought to the abdominal wall as a catheterizable stoma, as in the Indiana pouch.

Sigmoid Cystoplasty

Technique

Use of the sigmoid colon for augmentation cystoplasty was first reported by Lemoine in 1912 (Chargi et al, 1967), and it continues to be used commonly. **Because of the strong unit contractions of the sigmoid, it is imperative to detubularize and reconfigure the segment to provide maximal compliance and disruption of contractions.** Fifteen to 20 cm of sigmoid colon is identified and mobilized. The mesentery is transilluminated to identify the vascular arcade to the segment, after which the surgeon must ensure that the segment can reach the bladder without tension. If so, the bowel segment is divided between clamps and a colocolostomy performed (Fig. 71–11A). The remainder of the abdominal cavity should be carefully packed to prevent contamination from the open sigmoid segment. Detubularization and reconfiguration is done in a fashion determined by the surgeon's preference. The sigmoid patch is anastomosed to the bivalved bladder in a manner similar to that previously described for ileocystoplasty. Again, a large suprapubic tube is brought out through the native bladder and secured to the bladder and skin exit sites. Drains are placed as previously noted.

Reconfiguration of Sigmoid

Sigmoid colon segments are usually reconfigured in one of two ways. Mitchell (1986) suggested closing the two ends and then opening the segment longitudinally opposite its blood supply. The segment easily fits on the bivalved bladder. The bowel segment may fit better in either the sagittal or the coronal plane (see Fig. 71–11B). More radical reconfiguration, and perhaps breakup of unit contractions, may be achieved by folding the sigmoid segment in a U shape, similar to that procedure described for ileocystoplasty (Sidi et al, 1987a) (see Fig. 71–11C). Although the basic procedure is the same, a slightly longer segment of sigmoid may be necessary for effective reconfiguration in this manner.

Gastrocystoplasty

Technique Using Antrum

Two basic techniques exist for use of stomach in bladder augmentation. Leong and Ong (1972) described the use of the entire gastric antrum with a small rim of body for bladder replacement. With their technique, the left gastroepiploic artery is always used as a vascular pedicle. If the right gastroepiploic artery is dominant and the left vessel ends high on the greater curvature, a strip of body along the greater curvature from the left gastroepiploic artery to the antrum is maintained and provides adequate blood supply (Leong, 1988). Continuity of the upper gastrointestinal tract is restored by a Billroth I gastroduodenostomy.

Technique Using Body

In the second type of gastrocystoplasty, a gastric wedge based on the midportion of the greater curvature is used (Adams et al, 1988) (Fig. 71–12A). **The gastric segment used in this technique is made up mainly of body and consequently has a higher concentration of acid-producing cells. The right or left gastroepiploic artery may be used as a vascular pedicle to this segment.** The right artery is commonly dominant and therefore is more frequently used. The wedge-shaped segment of stomach includes both anterior and posterior wall. The segment used may be 10 to 20 cm along the greater curvature, depending on patient age and size as well as the needed volume (see Fig. 71–12B). The incision into the stomach is stopped just short of the lesser curvature to avoid injury to branches of the vagus nerve that control the gastric outlet. Branches of the left gastric artery just cephalad to the apex of this incision are suture ligated in situ before incision to avoid significant bleeding. Parallel atraumatic bowel clamps are placed on either side of the gastric incisions to avoid excessive bleeding or spillage of gastric contents. Alternatively, the stomach may be incised using a gastrointestinal stapling device that places a double row of staples on each side of the incision (Mitchell et al, 1992). The staple lines, however, must be excised. The native stomach is closed in two layers using permanent sutures on the outer seromuscular layer.

Branches of the gastroepiploic artery to the antrum on the right or to the high corpus on the left are divided to provide mobilization of the gastroepiploic pedicle. In order that the eventual pedicle is long enough to reach the bladder, the appropriate segment may be higher on the greater curvature if the right vessel is used as a pedicle, or lower if based on the left. The vascular pedicle, with omentum, should not be free-floating through the abdomen. The segment and pedicle may be passed through windows in the transverse mesocolon and mesentery of the distal ileum and

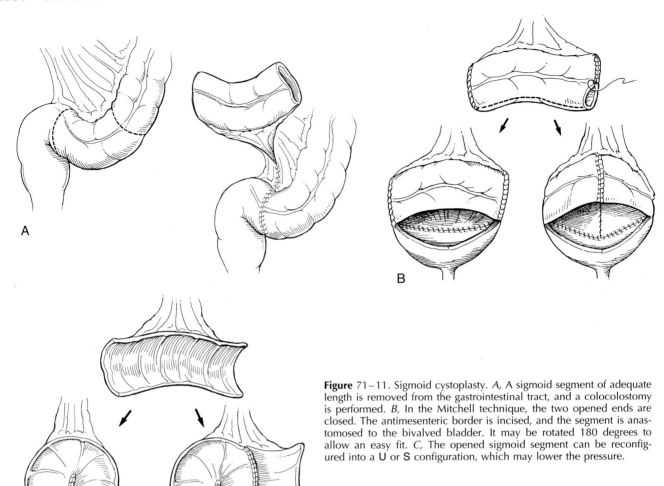

Figure 71–11. Sigmoid cystoplasty. *A,* A sigmoid segment of adequate length is removed from the gastrointestinal tract, and a colocolostomy is performed. *B,* In the Mitchell technique, the two opened ends are closed. The antimesenteric border is incised, and the segment is anastomosed to the bivalved bladder. It may be rotated 180 degrees to allow an easy fit. *C,* The opened sigmoid segment can be reconfigured into a U or S configuration, which may lower the pressure.

carefully secured to the posterior peritoneum. Despite careful consideration for an adequate pedicle length, on occasion the gastric segment initially does not reach the bladder without tension. Either gastroepiploic artery may be mobilized closer to its origin for further length. The first few branches from the gastroepiploic artery to the isolated gastric segment may also be divided. Because of the rich submucosal arterial plexus in the stomach, devascularization of the isolated segment does not result. Rarely, it may be necessary to approximate some of the isolated gastric segment to itself in one corner. The gastric segment should be approximated to the native bladder with one or two layers of absorbable sutures, taking care to invert the mucosa (see Fig. 71–12*C*).

Raz and colleagues (1993) and Lockhart and associates (1993) have described the use of a much longer, more narrow segment of stomach based along the greater curvature. Use of this segment, which includes both body and antrum, somewhat narrows the lumen of the stomach along its entire length except at the fundus and pylorus. Raz and colleagues (1993) isolated this segment with the use of a gastrointestinal stapler so that the native stomach was never open. The segment used in both of these series was

similar to that first described by Sinaiko (1956), the first surgeon to use stomach in bladder replacement. **Postoperative bladder and gastric drainage is no different than that described for intestinal cystoplasty.** Histamine$_2$ (H$_2$)-blockers are often given in the early postoperative period to promote healing (Rink et al, 2000).

Postoperative Management

Early Management

Care of patients after cystoplasty is similar regardless of the gastrointestinal segment used in the procedure. **All patients are maintained on nasogastric decompression until bowel function recovers, including patients who have undergone gastrocystoplasty. Attention to fluid and electrolyte management is important, because third space losses may be significant after extensive reconstructive surgery.** Continuous drainage of the bladder is achieved by suprapubic cystostomy. Mucus production from small or large bowel may be excessive and can potentially occlude the drainage catheter. **The suprapubic tube should be**

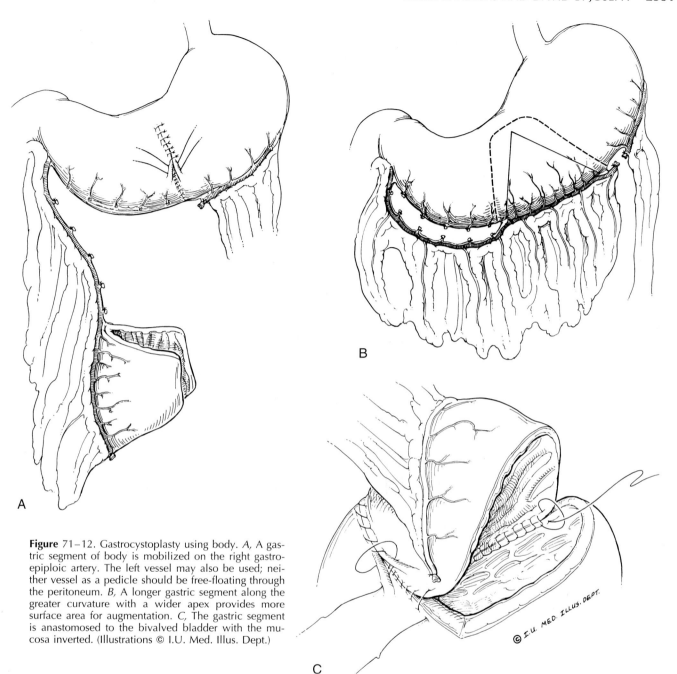

Figure 71–12. Gastrocystoplasty using body. *A,* A gastric segment of body is mobilized on the right gastroepiploic artery. The left vessel may also be used; neither vessel as a pedicle should be free-floating through the peritoneum. *B,* A longer gastric segment along the greater curvature with a wider apex provides more surface area for augmentation. *C,* The gastric segment is anastomosed to the bivalved bladder with the mucosa inverted. (Illustrations © I.U. Med. Illus. Dept.)

irrigated at least three times daily and whenever drainage is slowed by mucus. Suprapubic drainage is continued until approximately 3 weeks after augmentation cystoplasty. Extravesical drains may be removed after several days if drainage of urine is not apparent. The drains are usually removed more promptly in patients with a ventriculoperitoneal shunt to avoid potential infection. Some surgeons prefer that a cystogram be obtained before patient discharge; others wait approximately 3 weeks for the study before clamping the suprapubic tube. All patients begin on CIC every 2 to 3 hours during the day and one or two times at night after bladder healing is documented. The suprapubic tube is removed after catheterization is successfully underway and well tolerated. The duration between catheterizations is gradually increased over several weeks but should not exceed 4 to 5 hours during the day. Patients without neurologic impairment may eventually attempt to void spontaneously. All must check postvoid residual volumes and continue catheterizations if the residuals are significant.

Late Management

Routine radiographic surveillance of the upper urinary tract is indicated at 6 weeks, 6 months, and 1 year after augmentation cystoplasty. Most such surveillance may be done with ultrasonography. Serum electrolytes, BUN and creatinine levels, and urine cultures are performed several times during the first year after surgery. Not all positive urine cultures require treatment in patients using CIC.

Certainly, symptomatic cystitis or an infection involving urea-splitting organisms should be cleared. Evaluation by ultrasonography and serum chemistry analysis is then appropriate once a year. Eventually, yearly endoscopy for tumor surveillance should be performed.

Results and Complications of Augmentation Cystoplasty

The effect of cystoplasty on the patient should be considered in two main categories. First, the effect of removal of a relatively small portion of the gastrointestinal tract for use in urinary reconstruction must be considered. **Any more than rare development of gastrointestinal problems would be prohibitive, even if the results were perfect from the standpoint of the urinary bladder.** Second, the effect of augmentation cystoplasty on the urinary bladder must be reviewed. The primary goal of augmentation is to provide a compliant urinary reservoir. Therefore, **the main consideration after augmentation is the storage pressure and capacity that are achieved. Any other effect on the urinary bladder is a side effect or complication that exists because bowel is not a perfect physiologic substitute for native bladder.**

Gastrointestinal Effects

Postoperative bowel obstruction is uncommon after augmentation cystoplasty, occurring in approximately 3% of patients (Gearhart et al, 1986; King, 1987; Mitchell and Pizer, 1987; Hollensbe et al, 1992; Rink et al, 1995a). **The rate of obstruction is equivalent to that noted after conduit diversion or continent urinary diversion** (Mc-Dougal, 1992b). Delicate handling of tissues, closure of mesenteric windows, and elimination of sites of internal herniation help to avoid obstruction. Some series have suggested differing rates of bowel obstruction depending on the segment used. These differences have not been consistent in most series and therefore probably are not significant; the incidence of bowel obstruction is low regardless of the gastrointestinal segment used and should not influence the choice of a particular segment for enterocystoplasty.

Reports of chronic diarrhea after bladder augmentation alone have been rare. Diarrhea can occur after removal of large segments of ileum from the gastrointestinal tract, although the length of the segments typically used for augmentation rarely are problematic unless other problems coexist. The much longer segments required for continent urinary diversion may increase the risk for chronic diarrhea. The use of a typical colonic segment for augmentation only rarely results in a change in bowel function and is less of a risk than the use of ileum. **Removal of a segment from the gastrointestinal tract that includes the ileocecal valve is the most likely procedure to cause diarrhea.** King (1987) noted that 10% of patients with neurogenic dysfunction have significant diarrhea after such displacement. Other studies have suggested a lower risk, at least among well-selected patients (Husmann and Cain, 1999). Roth et al (1995) reported that 23% of patients in their experience had chronic diarrhea after ileocecal urinary diversion and 11% when ileum alone was used. Some children with neurogenic impairment depend on controlled constipation for fecal continence. Removal of the ileocecal valve from the gastrointestinal tract may significantly decrease bowel transit time. Loss of the valve can also allow bacterial backflow into the ileum, and the organisms may interfere with metabolism of fat and vitamin B_{12}.

Ileum is the sole site of vitamin B_{12} absorption in the bowel. **Removal of the distal ileum from the gastrointestinal tract may result in vitamin B_{12} deficiency and megaloblastic anemia. Certainly the terminal 15 to 20 cm of ileum should not be used for augmentation, although problems may arise even if that segment is preserved** (Steiner and Morton, 1991; Racioppi et al, 1999). Again, the risk is greater if longer segments of ileum are used, as with continent diversion. In one series, 35% of patients monitored for longer than 5 years after construction of a Kock pouch were found to be deficient in vitamin B_{12} (Akerlund et al, 1989). The length of ileum used for augmentation usually is less than half of that used for a Kock pouch, so vitamin B_{12} deficiency seems unlikely after routine bladder augmentation. Canning and associates (1989) evaluated 26 patients after bladder augmentation or replacement and found none with either fat malabsorption or vitamin B_{12} deficiency. Only three patients, however, were observed for longer than 3 years, and longer observation is necessary because existing body vitamin B_{12} stores may last considerably longer (Stein et al, 1997a). Eventually, determination of vitamin B_{12} levels or injections of the vitamin may be appropriate after ileocystoplasty.

Early satiety may occur after gastrocystoplasty, but this usually resolves with time. Disorders of gastric emptying should be extremely rare, particularly when using the gastric body.

Bladder Compliance after Augmentation

An early lesson of past clinical experience with augmentation cystoplasty was the value of detubularization and reconfiguration of the bowel segment (Hinman, 1988; Koff, 1988). **Bowel in its native, tubular form continues to display peristalsis or mass contraction. The tubular form does not maximize the volume achieved for the surface area of bowel used.** Hinman (1988) demonstrated with a mathematical model that the maximum volume achieved for a given surface area occurs when a sphere is created. No finished cystoplasty is a perfect sphere, but it should approach that shape as nearly as possible. Many patients who historically underwent augmentation cystoplasty with a tubular segment of bowel have done well, but there have also been numerous failures caused by continued pressure in the bladder from a segment left in its native form. Some surgeons with extensive experience in augmentation cystoplasty and continent diversion have concluded that ileum is superior to other segments in terms of compliance after augmentation (Goldwasser and Webster, 1986; Rink and McLaughlin, 1994; Studer and Zingg, 1997). Rare reports have suggested superior results with colon compared to ileum (Shekarriz et al, 2000). These

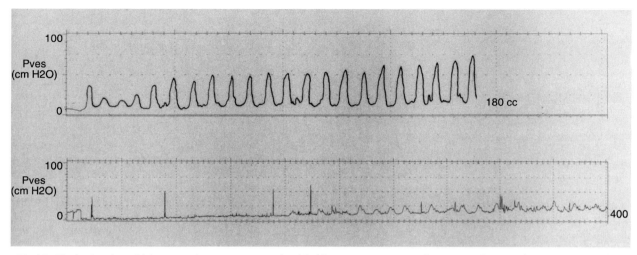

Figure 71–13. Rhythmic, sinusoidal contractions may occur after bladder augmentation, in this case with stomach. Contractions of significant amplitude early in filling occasionally require secondary augmentation.

reports have involved longer colonic segments that were reconfigured in a U shape. Good results have been achieved with all segments in most cases, and it is more important to use a bowel segment well than to choose a particular bowel segment for every patient.

Lytton and Green (1989) demonstrated mass contractions generating pressures of 60 to 110 cm H_2O in right colon reservoirs despite detubularization. Such pressures approach those observed in native cecum (Jakobsen et al, 1987). Hedlund and coworkers (1984) reported pressures of only 25 cm H_2O in detubularized cecal segments 1 year after reconstruction. Placement of an ileal patch on a cecal segment may be a more effective means of decreasing mass contractions than simple reconfiguration (Thuroff et al, 1987). Sidi and associates (1986b) demonstrated early peak bladder pressures of 41 cm H_2O after cup-patch sigmoid cystoplasty that improved with time. Goldwasser's review of enterocystoplasty using detubularized ileum and colon demonstrated contractions greater than 15 cm H_2O in 42% of patients after ileocystoplasty, compared with 60% after colocystoplasty (Goldwasser et al, 1987). Significant contractions, defined as those greater than 40 cm H_2O at a volume of less than 200 ml, were not noted in any of the ileal augmentations but did persist in 10% of cecal cystoplasties. In continent urinary diversion, ileal reservoirs have been noted to have lower basal pressures and less motor activity (Berglund et al, 1987; Studer and Zingg, 1997); cecal reservoirs have been noted to generate more pressure per given volume than ileum despite detubularization and to exhibit more obvious uninhibited contractions (Berglund et al, 1987).

Any problems with pressure after augmentation cystoplasty usually occur because of uninhibited contractions, apparently in the bowel segment. It is extremely rare not to achieve an adequate capacity or flat tonus limb unless a technical error has occurred with use of the bowel segment. Occasionally, a small, scarred pelvis prevents adequate expansion of the augmented bladder. When pressure contractions occur in the bladder after augmentation, they are often noted on a rhythmic or sinusoidal pattern, occasionally with increasing amplitude (Fig. 71–13). For most

patients, the pressure contractions noted urodynamically are of theoretical interest only and have not affected the clinical result. Contractions that begin at low amplitude later in filling and progress only near capacity may be of no clinical significance at all. Early contractions of higher pressure may occasionally result in persistent incontinence, delayed perforation, hydronephrosis, or vesicoureteral reflux. If patients have such clinical problems after augmentation, repeat urodynamic testing is necessary. One cannot assume that the bladder is compliant after augmentation. Rhythmic contractions have been noted postoperatively with all bowel segments, although ileum seems the least likely to demonstrate remarkable urodynamic abnormalities, and stomach the most. Rhythmic contractions after gastrocystoplasty have been noted in up to 62% of patients (Adams et al, 1988; Atala et al, 1993a; Gosalbez et al, 1993a; Roth et al, 2000). The segment of stomach initially described for augmentation using the body was much smaller in size than segments of ileum or colon commonly used for cystoplasty. Use of a slightly larger gastric segment that is longer along the greater curvature results in improved urodynamics after augmentation, with less prominent contractions (Adams et al, 1995; Kurzrock et al, 1998; Koraitim et al, 1999). Leong (1988) suggested that an antral segment of stomach is less likely to demonstrate such contractions.

In perhaps the largest experience with pediatric bladder augmentation, Hollensbe and associates (1992) at Indiana University found that approximately 5% of several hundred patients had significant uninhibited contractions after augmentation cystoplasty causing clinical problems. Pope and Rink (1999) found that 6% of more than 300 patients required secondary augmentation of a previously augmented bladder for similar problems in long-term follow-up. These secondary augmentations represent true failures of the primary cystoplasty, not from any side effect or complication but from failure to achieve the objective—capacity and compliance. In that series, sigmoid colon, followed by stomach and then ileum, was most likely to require reaugmentation. It should be noted that a colonic segment closed at the ends and not generally reconfigured otherwise was typically used in that experience. Other studies have suggested that stomach is more likely than colon to require secondary intervention (El-Ghoneimi et al, 1998).

Metabolic Complications

CHLORIDE ABSORPTION AND ACIDOSIS

The first recognized metabolic complication related to storage of urine within intestinal segments was the occasional development of hyperchloremic metabolic acidosis after ureterosigmoidostomy (Ferris and Odel, 1950). Patients with this metabolic derangement were noted to have fatigue, weakness, anorexia, and polydipsia. **Koch and McDougal (1985) demonstrated the mechanisms by which acid is absorbed from urine in contact with intestinal mucosa.** Resorption in the form of ammonium results in chronic acid loading. Patients with normal renal function usually are able to handle the resorbed load of chloride and acid without frank acidosis. **In 1987, Mitchell and Piser noted that essentially every patient after augmentation with an intestinal segment had an increase in serum chloride and a decrease in serum bicarbonate level, although full acidosis was rare if renal function was normal.** Similar trends of increased serum chloride and decreased bicarbonate have been noted with ileal conduits (Malek et al, 1971) and with continent urinary reservoirs (Allen et al, 1985; McDougal, 1986; Asken, 1987; Thuroff et al, 1987; Boyd et al, 1989). More severe acidosis and electrolyte disturbances requiring treatment have been reported despite normal renal function (Schmidt et al, 1973; Whitmore and Gittes, 1983). Such derangements may be debilitating to the patient if not recognized and treated; patient death has been reported (Heidler et al, 1979). **Hall and colleagues (1991) noted that there is an increase in the urinary acid load with wasting of bony buffers even in the absence of frank acidosis.** Such wasting may result in bone demineralization and can potentially cause retarded growth in children after augmentation cystoplasty. Patients with acidosis should receive bicarbonate therapy. Whether all patients with intestine in the lower urinary tract might benefit from supplemental bicarbonate is controversial. Nurse and Mundy (1989) suggested that arterial blood gas values may be more sensitive than serum bicarbonate or chloride levels for detecting acidosis. Stein and associates (1998) believed that measurements of arterial blood gas for base deficit allowed early treatment of acidosis and avoidance of bone demineralization. In severe cases of acidosis, chloride transport can be blocked with chlorpromazine and nicotinic acid.

Although jejunum is rarely used for bladder reconstruction, storage of urine in this segment results in a unique metabolic pattern of hyponatremic, hypochloremic, and hyperkalemic metabolic acidosis. The problem is often associated with significant hypovolemia.

Gastric mucosa is a barrier to chloride and acid resorption and, in fact, secretes hydrochloric acid (Piser et al, 1987). This difference was the primary factor in the initial consideration of stomach for use in the urinary tract. This secretory nature was shown to be of benefit in azotemic animals during acid loading (Piser et al, 1987; Kennedy et al, 1988). **Serum chloride does decrease and serum bicarbonate increases slightly after gastrocystoplasty whether antrum or body is used in patients with normal or impaired renal function** (Adams et al, 1988; Ganesan et al, 1991; Kurzrock et al, 1998). In 21 patients with renal insufficiency, serum bicarbonate levels improved in all patients but 1 after gastrocystoplasty, and many patients who required oral bicarbonate therapy before cystoplasty did not need it after gastrocystoplasty (Ganesan et al, 1991). A similar benefit was noted in a smaller group of patients with renal failure (Sheldon and Gilbert, 1991).

PATIENT GROWTH

Delayed or slowed growth in children after intestinal cystoplasty has previously been suggested (Wagstaff et al, 1991, 1992; Mundy and Nurse, 1992). A delay in linear growth was noted in 20% of almost 200 pediatric patients without any gross biochemical abnormalities. However, no control patients were included in the series, and body habitus and growth are difficult to measure and predict in children with myelodysplasia. Such patients make up the majority in most series of augmentation cystoplasty cases. More recently, Gros and colleagues (2000) at The Johns Hopkins Hospital evaluated growth in patients with exstrophy. Patients requiring augmentation were matched retrospectively with a similar group not requiring bladder augmentation. Hydronephrosis was not mentioned but was unlikely with a diagnosis of exstrophy. Only one patient was noted to have acidosis in either group. Other factors that might affect growth, such as urinary tract infection, were not controlled. Of 17 patients with adequate measurements before and after augmentation cystoplasty, 14 (82%) had a decline in percentile height postoperatively. The decline corresponded to a 1.5-inch decrease in expected height. No appreciable correlation between the impairment of growth and the segment of bowel used for augmentation was apparent. The pattern of growth was significantly different between patients with and without augmentation in the series. That series was small, and no evaluation of familial growth patterns or ultimate height was possible; however, the findings are worrisome. In the absence of any serum abnormalities, the exact mechanism of delayed growth was not evident, although it seems likely that it was related to chloride absorption and subclinical acidosis (Koch and McDougal, 1988; Bushinsky, 1989; Hochstetler et al, 1997). Better analysis of subtle metabolic alterations after enterocystoplasty may aid in understanding the effect on growth, minimizing changes, or instituting early treatment to avoid the complication.

ALKALOSIS

The secretory nature of gastric mucosa may at times be detrimental to the patient and can result in two unique complications of gastrocystoplasty. Severe episodes of hypokalemic, hypochloremic, metabolic alkalosis after acute gastrointestinal illnesses were observed in 5 of 37 patients who had undergone gastrocystoplasty (Hollensbe et al, 1992). The episodes were significant enough to require hospitalization in all cases and were recurrent in two patients. Three of the five patients with the complication had renal insufficiency and would not have been good candidates for augmentation with other segments due to acidosis. Ganesan and associates (1991) noted similar episodes of alkalosis in 5 of 21 patients with renal insufficiency after gastrocystoplasty. **Those patients with the primary indication for consideration of gastrocystoplasty may be the ones at greatest risk for this unusual complication.** It has been proposed that the alkalosis results from ongoing chloride loss from the gastric segment in the bladder in the face of decreased oral intake. McDougal (1992a) suggested that the decreased ability to excrete bicarbonate from an impaired kidney may compound the problem. Gosalbez and associates (1993b) demonstrated persistently increased fractional excretion of chloride despite profound hypochloremia, suggesting that inappropriate gastric secretion is probably the primary problem. One patient in their series eventually required resection of three quarters of the gastric segment in the bladder because of recurrent problems with alkalosis, and several required therapy with H_2-blockers or H^+-K^+ ion pump inhibitors. All patients and families should be made aware of this potential problem, because it has been reported to occur intermittently in between 3% and 24% of patients. A composite reservoir of stomach and ileum or colon may provide a more metabolically neutral reservoir (McLaughlin et al, 1995; Austin et al, 1997, 1999), although they have typically been constructed only in very complex circumstances. Duel and associates (1996) have used stomach and colon together to advantage in a staged fashion for oncology patients.

HEMATURIA-DYSURIA SYNDROME

Acid secretion by gastric mucosa may result in another unique problem after gastrocystoplasty, the hematuria-dysuria syndrome. Mitchell's group has characterized this syndrome well (Nguyen et al, 1993; Plaire et al, 1999). **Virtually all patients after gastrocystoplasty with normal sensation have occasional hematuria or dysuria with voiding or catheterization beyond that which is expected with other intestinal segments** (Leonard et al, 1999). **All patients should be warned of this potential problem, although in most the symptoms are intermittent and mild and do not require treatment.** The problem has led one group to recommend avoidance of gastrocystoplasty in patients with bladder exstrophy (El-Ghoneimi et al, 1998). The dysuria is certainly not as problematic in patients with neurogenic dysfunction. In the experience of Nguyen and coworkers (1993), 36% of patients developed signs or symptoms of the hematuria-dysuria syndrome after gastrocystoplasty; 14% required treatment with medications, 9% on a regular basis. They believed that patients who are incontinent or have decreased renal function are at increased risk. Others noted a similar requirement for short-term and chronic medical therapy (Hollensbe et al, 1992; Adams et al, 1995). In our experience and that of Nguyen and coworkers, the symptoms of the hematuria-dysuria syndrome respond well to administration of H_2-blockers and hydrogen ion pump blockers. Bladder irrigation with baking soda may also be effective. It has been demonstrated that urinary pH may decrease remarkably after meals in those who have undergone gastrocystoplasty (Bogaert et al, 1995). The signs and symptoms of the hematuria-dysuria syndrome are most

likely secondary to acid irritation. Recent work has suggested that *Helicobacter pylori* may play a role in this complication, as it may in acid complications in the native stomach (Celayir et al, 1999). Such problems can occur but are less frequent after antral cystoplasty, where there is a smaller load of parietal cells (Ngan et al, 1993).

Acid in the urine may also cause external irritation. Leong first noted glanular excoriation after gastrocystoplasty in a patient with voiding symptoms (Ngan et al, 1993). Similar meatal irritation was noted in other patients after gastrocystoplasty; most had significant dysuria. Nguyen and associates (1993) noted skin excoriation in 8 of 57 patients after gastrocystoplasty; all 8 patients had some element of urinary incontinence. **It is imperative to achieve reliable urinary continence in patients undergoing gastrocystoplasty, because urinary leakage may result in exposure of the skin to gastric secretions and in gastric secretions that are poorly diluted and buffered by less urine in the bladder.** Such dilution is important; Reinberg and coworkers (1992) reported perforation of a gastric segment in a defunctionalized bladder after gastrocystoplasty. They then evaluated the influence of urine on gastrocystoplasties in dogs (Castro-Diaz et al, 1992). The animals developed marked inflammation of the gastric segment and native bladder after creation of a dry gastrocystoplasty; three of nine dogs developed ulceration and perforation. Use of H_2-blockers resulted in some protection for the animals; however, such a clinical situation should certainly be avoided. Rare perforations and ulcerations have been noted clinically without defunctionalization (El-Ghoneimi et al, 1998; Mingin et al, 1999b).

Mucus

Intestinal segments continue to produce mucus after placement in the urinary tract. The proteinaceous material can potentially impede bladder drainage during voiding or CIC, particularly in pediatric patients who must use small-caliber catheters. Mucus may serve as a nidus for infection or stone formation when it remains in the bladder for long periods. Mucus production often increases after cystoplasty in the presence of cystitis. Kulb and associates (1986) showed experimentally in dogs that colonic segments produce more mucus than ileum and that gastric segments produce the least amount. This has been noted clinically as well. Most patients do not require any routine bladder irrigations for mucus after gastrocystoplasty. Villous atrophy in the ileum has been documented after long-term placement in the urinary tract. It has been suggested that such atrophy may result in decreased mucus production (Gearhart, 1987), although laboratory demonstration of any decrease in production with time has not been evident (Murry et al, 1987). Hendren and Hendren (1990) noted a decrease in mucus production from colonic segments over years; however, others have not been impressed with such changes (Rink et al, 1995a). Glandular atrophy in colonic mucosa has not been noted histologically (Mansson et al, 1984). **Routine use of daily bladder irrigations to prevent mucus buildup may minimize complications of enterocystoplasty such as urinary tract infection and calculi.**

Urinary Tract Infection

Bacteriuria is very common after intestinal cystoplasty, particularly among patients requiring CIC (Gearhart et al, 1986; Hendren and Hendren, 1990; King, 1991). Recent experience with bowel neobladders has demonstrated that patients who are able to spontaneously void to completion frequently maintain sterile urine. The major difference in the groups of patients with augmentation is the requirement of CIC in most cases because of underlying anatomic or neurologic problems. **It appears that the use of CIC is a prominent factor in the development of bacteriuria after augmentation cystoplasty.** Bacteriuria has been noted even when patients are maintained on daily oral antibiotics or antibiotic irrigation (Gearhart et al, 1986; Casale et al, 1999). In the experience of Hirst (1991), persistent or recurrent bacteriuria occurred in 50% of patients augmented with sigmoid colon, compared with 25% of those undergoing ileocystoplasty. Hollensbe and coworkers (1992) noted bacteriuria much more frequently in patients needing CIC regardless of the segment considered.

The incidence of symptomatic cystitis after cystoplasty probably depends on the length of follow-up and the diligence with which symptoms are sought. All patients and families should be told to expect some signs or symptoms of cystitis. Recurrent episodes of symptomatic cystitis requiring treatment occurred in 23% of patients after ileocystoplasty, 17% after sigmoid cystoplasty, 13% after cecocystoplasty, and 8% after gastrocystoplasty at Indiana University (Hollensbe et al, 1992). Febrile urinary tract infections occurred in 13% of those 231 patients after augmentation. The same trend among different bowel segments was noted for febrile infections, although there was no statistically significant difference among the various segments. **The incidence of pyelonephritis after augmentation cystoplasty, as long as upper tract problems are corrected, is quite similar to that noted for conduit diversion, whether refluxing or not** (McDougal, 1992b). Recurrent infections resulting in deterioration of renal function in the absence of other problems have been quite rare after effective augmentation. Infections may occasionally be more problematic in an immunocompromised patient (Alfrey et al, 1997).

Not every episode of asymptomatic bacteriuria requires treatment in patients performing CIC. Bacteriuria should be treated for significant symptoms such as incontinence or suprapubic pain and perhaps for hematuria, foul-smelling urine, or remarkably increased mucus production. **Bacteriuria should be treated if the urine culture demonstrates growth of a urea-splitting organism that may lead to stone formation.** To minimize infection, patients who need CIC must perform it on a regular basis to avoid increased reservoir pressures and must work to empty the bladder completely. This latter process may require periodic irrigation of mucus as well as patience with the catheter in place. Special care must be taken by patients catheterizing through a continent abdominal wall stoma. Such patients may have more difficulty completely emptying the bladder from a nondependent stoma. Most can do so with effort (Ludlow et al, 1995). Although catheterization is not routinely a sterile technique, proper clean technique should be emphasized.

Calculi

Another long-term complication of augmentation cystoplasty is bladder calculi. In the early 1990s, several series reported calculi in 18% of patients after augmentation cystoplasty (Hendren and Hendren, 1990; Hirst, 1991). Blyth and associates (1992) noted calculus formation in 30% of such patients; they found that patients catheterizing through an abdominal wall stoma had the highest risk, probably because of incomplete emptying. Palmer and associates (1993) noted urolithiasis in 52% of patients after augmentation cystoplasty. Rink and colleagues (1995a) noted only an 8% rate of bladder stone formation in 231 patients with long-term follow-up after enterocystoplasty; the reasons for these remarkable differences are not clear.

The majority of bladder stones in this patient population are struvite in composition, and bacteriuria has been thought to be an important risk factor. Any infection with a urea-splitting organism should therefore be treated aggressively. All patients requiring CIC, particularly those who have already formed stones, should make every effort to empty the bladder completely with each catheterization. If stones are found in patients voiding spontaneously after augmentation, the adequacy of emptying should be reevaluated. The association of urinary stasis with stone formation is well established. Routine bladder irrigations to avoid buildup of inspissated mucus may remove a nidus for stone formation. The group at Indiana University has stressed irrigations and asked patients and families to routinely irrigate the bladder several times a day after augmentation. Compliance with such irrigations may lower the frequency of stone formation. Stones have been noted after the use of all intestinal segments, with no significant difference noted between small and large intestine. Struvite stones are less likely after gastrocystoplasty (Kronner et al, 1998a; Kaefer et al, 1998), probably because of decreased mucus production and acid that minimizes bacteriuria. Uric acid calculi have rarely been noted in the bladder after gastrocystoplasty (Kaefer et al, 1998). Clearly, any foreign body can serve as a nidus for stone formation; for this reason, the use of permanent suture or staples in the urinary tract should be avoided during enterocystoplasty. Khoury and associates (1997) looked for metabolic problems in patients after augmentation and noted low urinary citrate levels in patient with and without stones. They believed that poor emptying and mucus buildup were the most significant factors.

Tumor Formation

A well-recognized complication of ureterosigmoidostomy has been the development of tumors, primarily adenocarcinoma, at the ureterocolonic anastomotic site. In a review by Husmann and Spence (1990) of reported tumors after ureterosigmoidostomy, the latency for development of such tumors averaged 26 years and ranged from 3 to 53 years. Adenocarcinomas were the prominent tumors that developed, but benign polyps and other types of carcinoma were also found. Eraklus and Folkman (1978) estimated that the risk for development of such tumors is increased by 7000-fold over age-matched controls after ureterosigmoidostomy. The exact basis for the increased

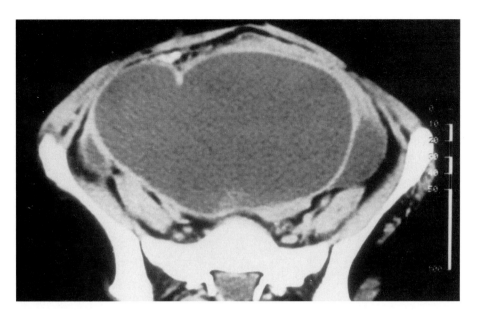

Figure 71–14. Patients with unrecognized spontaneous bladder perforation may occasionally present with an asymptomatic mass (urinoma), here noted on a CT scan.

risk is unknown; however, *N*-nitroso compounds thought to originate from a mixture of urine and feces may be carcinogenic. These compounds have been noted in the urine of patients with conduit diversion and augmentation (Treiger and Marshall, 1991). Husmann and Spence (1990) suggested that those compounds are more likely enhancing agents rather than a lone cause for tumor development. It has been proposed that inflammatory reaction at the anastomotic site may induce growth factor production, which, in turn, increases cellular proliferation. **Filmer and Spencer (1990) identified 14 patients who developed adenocarcinoma in an augmented bladder, and several more have been reported since then.** Nine of those tumors occurred after ileocystoplasty and five after colocystoplasty. **Experimental work in the rat demonstrated hyperplastic growth in the augmented bladder with all intestinal segments, with no segment showing any particularly increased risk** (Klee et al, 1990; Buson et al, 1993; Spencer et al, 1993; Little et al, 1994). The applicability of such findings to humans is uncertain. The long latency period noted for tumor development after ureterosigmoidostomy suggests that short-term follow-up after augmentation cystoplasty is not adequate to evaluate tumor formation. **Patients undergoing augmentation cystoplasty should be made aware of a potentially increased risk for tumor development. Yearly surveillance of the augmented bladder with endoscopy should eventually be performed; the latency period until such procedures are necessary is not well defined. The earliest reported tumor after augmentation was found only 4 years after cystoplasty** (Carr and Herschorn, 1997). Transitional cell carcinoma, hyperplasia, and dysplasia have also been noted near the anastomosis in humans (Gregoire et al, 1993; Barrington et al, 1997). Urine cytology or flow cytometry may ultimately become useful in surveillance.

Delayed Spontaneous Bladder Perforation

Perhaps the most disturbing complication of augmentation cystoplasty is delayed bladder perforation. Patients presenting with spontaneous perforation after augmentation cystoplasty are usually quite ill with abdominal pain, distention, and fever. Sepsis has been common. Nausea, decreased urine output, and shoulder pain from diaphragmatic irritation have also been noted. Perforations have been found in the evaluation of virtually asymptomatic pelvic masses (Pope et al, 1999) (Fig. 71–14). **Patients with neurogenic dysfunction often have impaired lower abdominal sensation and present later in the course of the illness; severe sepsis and death have occurred.** Patients with perforation after gastrocystoplasty often present promptly because of acid irritation. **A high index of suspicion for perforation is necessary. Contrast cystography is diagnostic in most cases** (Braverman and Lebowitz, 1991; Rosen and Light, 1991; Bauer et al, 1992) (Fig. 71–15). Thorough technique is important to identify as many true-positive cases as possible with cystography (Braverman and Lebowitz, 1991). Some reports of perforations have noted a significant false-negative rate on cystography (Rushton et al, 1988; Sheiner and Kaplan, 1988; Pope et al, 1999) and suggested that ultrasonography and CT improve diagnostic accuracy. They recommended that one of those studies be done in any child with suspected perforation if the initial cystogram is negative.

ETIOLOGY

The cause of delayed perforations within a bowel segment is unknown. It has been suggested that perforation might be secondary to traumatic catheterization in some cases (Elder et al, 1988; Rushton et al, 1988). Perforation of a bladder not previously augmented has been recognized after CIC (Reisman and Preminger, 1989). It seems unlikely that catheterization trauma is the lone cause in most patients. The location of the perforations has been variable among patients and even in a single patient with multiple perforations. Perforations have occurred after augmentation in patients who did not catheterize at all. Others have suggested that trauma to the bowel caused by fixed adhesions that result in sheering forces with emptying and fill-

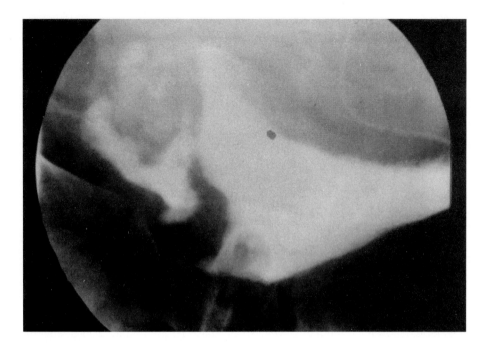

Figure 71–15. After complete filling, a sagittal view on the cystogram demonstrates a spontaneous bladder perforation on the postdrain view.

ing may result in perforation (Elder et al, 1988). Chronic, transmural infection of the bladder wall has also been proposed as a cause. **Histologic examination of bowel segments adjacent to areas of perforation has revealed necrosis, vascular congestion, hemorrhage, and hemosiderin deposition compatible with chronic bowel wall ischemia** (Crane et al, 1991). **Chronic overdistention of the bladder might result in such ischemia.** Decreased perfusion in dog bowel used for augmentation can be induced experimentally with high intravesical pressure (Essig et al, 1991). These changes were noted more prominently at the antimesenteric border of the bowel. Chronic ischemia may thus play a significant role in at least some delayed bladder perforations. Anderson and Rickwood (1991) reported perforations occurring in bladders with significant uninhibited contractions after augmentation as did others (Pope et al, 1998). **High outflow resistance may maintain bladder pressure rather than allowing urinary leakage and venting of the pressure, potentially increasing ischemia.** Hyperreflexia alone is unlikely as a solitary cause of perforation, because the complication was essentially never recognized in the era before bowel detubularization and reconfiguration, when persistent pressure contractions were more common after augmentation cystoplasty. **Once bowel is reconfigured, however, it may be more prone to ischemia if high pressure does persist.**

The majority of patients experiencing perforations after augmentation cystoplasty have had myelodysplasia. The incidence of perforation was lower in series of patients with other diagnoses that required bladder reconstruction (Hendren and Hendren, 1990). The role of neurogenic dysfunction in the origin of these perforations is unclear. No matter what the cause, there is probably some field effect on the entire segment. Once a spontaneous perforation has occurred, the chance of recurrence is significant (Hollensbe et al, 1992). One third of patients with ruptures in one series had a recurrence (Pope et al, 1999). Consideration must eventually be given to removal of the original segment and replacement by another after repeated perforation.

INCIDENCE

This problem has been noted with increasing frequency after augmentation cystoplasty and may involve all segments. Early postoperative leaks from the bowel-to-bowel or bowel-to-bladder anastomoses after augmentation cystoplasty are rare and represent a technical error or problem with early healing. **Delayed perforations more commonly occur within the bowel segment itself and represent a problem with long-term storage of urine within an intestinal segment.** There may be no particular increased risk of one intestinal segment over another. At Indiana University, perforations were noted in 32 of 330 patients undergoing cystoplasty (Pope et al, 1999), at an average of 4.3 years after augmentation. Analysis of this experience suggested that the use of sigmoid colon was the only significant increased risk. However, several other large series of patients with sigmoid cystoplasty have noted a low incidence of delayed perforation (Sidi et al, 1987a; Hendren and Hendren, 1990; Shekarriz et al, 2000). At The Children's Hospital (Boston), the incidence of perforation after augmentation was reported to be highest in ileum (9.3%) and less frequent in ileocecal, sigmoid, and gastric segments (Bauer et al, 1992). **With inconsistent differences across multiple large series, it is unlikely that any given enteric segment is at significantly increased risk for perforation and probable that multiple factors influence the risk for the complication.** Pope, Rink, and the Indiana group (1999) still feel strongly, based on their experience, that sigmoid colon has a greater risk for perforation (a four times higher rate than ileum there). Some other experienced surgeons feel the same (P. Ransley, personal communication, Varese, Italy, 1998).

TREATMENT

The standard treatment for spontaneous perforation of the augmented bladder is surgical repair, as it is for intraperitoneal rupture of the bladder after trauma.

There are reported series of conservative management for suspected perforation (Slaton and Kropp, 1994). Conservative management including catheter drainage, antibiotics, and serial abdominal examinations was successful in 87% of their patients, although only 2 of 13 patients with suspected rupture had x-ray documentation unequivocally identifying a perforation. Even patients who do well with conservative management during the acute episode often require surgical intervention eventually (Pope et al, 1999). Such management may be a consideration in a stable patient with sterile urine. The surgeon should certainly have a low threshold for surgical exploration and repair. The majority of patients with perforations have myelodysplasia and present late in the course of the disease due to impaired sensation. Increasing sepsis and death of the patient may result from a delay in diagnosis or treatment.

Pregnancy

Good success has been reported for women after bladder augmentation, bladder neck repair, or continent urinary diversion in terms of continence and upper tract preservation. Little note has been made of fertility issues. **Limited information exists regarding the outcome of pregnancy in women who have undergone augmentation cystoplasty.** This is partially true because many of the young patients who have undergone these major reconstructive procedures are just reaching the age of potential childbearing. They should become the focus of future evaluations. Older women undergoing bladder replacement for oncologic reasons often are rendered infertile by the nature of the disease and its treatment.

The physiologic and anatomic changes that occur during pregnancy raise a significant set of questions and concerns. **(1) Will the expanding uterus and fetus affect the pedicle to the augmentation, or will the pedicle stretch or deflect out of the way?** Bacteriuria is frequent among patients previously augmented, particularly those requiring CIC to empty. **(2) Is bacteriuria more problematic during pregnancy for women who have undergone previous augmentation or reconstruction?** Little work has been done to establish whether bladder function changes during the course of pregnancy after augmentation or whether upper tract dilatation during pregnancy, common among women without prior reconstruction, is more prevalent or more severe. For that matter, little experience has been reported evaluating the effect of pregnancy on lower urinary tract function after previous reconstruction or vice-versa. At the end of pregnancy, concerns may exist about the method of delivery in terms of safety for the mother and child. **(3) Does prior urinary reconstruction mandate cesarean section? (4) If so, will the augmentation or its pedicle be overlying the uterus and potentially in harm's way? There are no definitive answers to any of these questions.**

Experience during pregnancy related to the pedicle of a prior bladder augmentation is very limited. Hatch and associates (1991) and Schumacher and coworkers (1997) noted that the mesenteric pedicle to bladder augmentations did not appear to be stretched at the time of cesarean section. In those cases, the pedicle was not located near the exposed anterior uterus but was deflected laterally. Schilling et al (1996) recognized a difference between urinary diversion and augmentation. With diversion, the pedicle of the intestinal segment extended cranially and laterally away from the uterus, whereas the pedicle covered the uterus after bladder augmentation. Neither process prevented the rise of the uterus during pregnancy. Those authors speculated that the mesentery underwent changes that enabled deflection or stretch without any adverse effect on circulation.

Although there is a lack of systematic review, most major reconstructive centers have several patients who have completed pregnancies. Loss of the augmentation resulting from a mechanical effect on the pedicle from the enlarging uterus has not been reported. The gradual increase in size may allow the blood supply to deflect or stretch slowly if at all. Pregnancy itself has not had reported detrimental effect on the augmentation.

Successful pregnancy with spontaneous vaginal delivery has been observed after ureterosigmoidostomy and ileal conduit urinary diversion (Pedlow, 1961; Asif and Uehling, 1969). Schumacher et al (1997) reviewed their experience with pregnancy and delivery in patients who had undergone continent catheterizable ileocecal diversion. This represents one of the largest series in the literature, but it included only seven pregnancies among six women. All of the women had a healthy baby by cesarean section. Three pregnancies were completely uneventful. Although these data are specific to the ileocecal pouch, it is not unrealistic to expect a similar outcome with other forms of continent urinary reconstruction. Urgency and late difficulty with catheterization have been noted with Kock continent ileostomies (Ojerskog et al, 1988) and could occur with continent urinary diversion.

Urinary tract infections may be problematic in women who have undergone urinary reconstruction including bladder augmentation. Ureteral dilatation, increased residual urine, and diminished tone to the upper tract may all be important risk factors (Hill et al, 1990; Hatch et al, 1991). Based on those reports, prophylactic antibiotics may be appropriate, particularly once symptomatic infection has occurred. Antibiotics should be chosen that are not teratogenic. Placement of an indwelling stent might benefit some patients. Difficulty with catheterization during the pregnancy or a significant rate of new-onset incontinence has not been reported but also has not been carefully examined. Uterine prolapse has been noted to occur at a higher rate with pregnancy, particularly in patients with exstrophy (Kennedy et al, 1993). Because of such concerns, Stein et al (1994) suggested fixation of the uterus during reconstructive surgery.

It appears unlikely that all women would require cesarean section to deliver after augmentation cystoplasty alone. However, adequate progression of spontaneous vaginal delivery may require flaccid, distensible pelvic tissues. Extensive pelvic surgery to achieve urinary continence may result in scarring and rigid fixation of some of those tissues. Whether this affects or slows the progression of spontaneous vaginal delivery is unknown. Likewise, whether tissues fixed from previous operative repairs can undergo the trauma of delivery and resume the same level of function found before the pregnancy is undetermined. Our bias would be that women who have undergone extensive bladder neck repair would benefit from cesarean delivery, par-

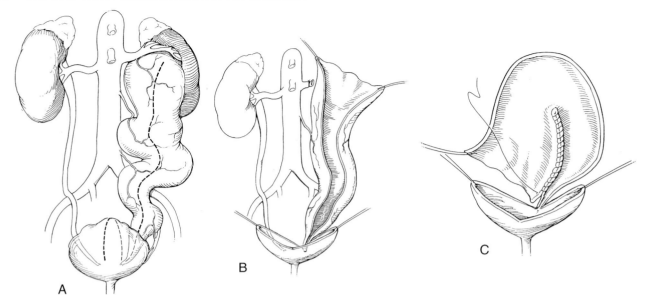

Figure 71–16. Ureterocystoplasty. *A,* After nephrectomy, the bladder is bivalved, with the posterior aspect of the incision carried off the midline to enter the ureteral orifice. The ureter is not detached from the bladder. *B,* The ureter is opened opposite its main blood supply. *C,* The ureter is reconfigured similar to the enterocystoplasty before anastomosis to the bladder.

ticularly if the progression toward spontaneous vaginal delivery is slowed or at all difficult. We well recognize that there is very little scientific information to support or contradict that bias. Although there are reports of spontaneous vaginal delivery in the presence of an AUS (Creagh et al, 1995), the presence of such a prosthetic device raises a concern for erosion with a long, difficult delivery.

If cesarean section is required or selected, it is imperative to protect the augmentation and its pedicle. The anterior uterus can typically be exposed atraumatically, although some time and patience may be required to protect the bladder. Such exposure may be more difficult if multiple abdominal stomas are present. The reconstructive urologist familiar with the patient and her anatomy should be present during cesarean section to maximize safety for the woman.

Choice of Segment

The use of bowel for augmentation of the bladder was first described experimentally by Tizzoni and Foggi in 1888 and was first reported in humans by Mikulicz in 1898 (Orr et al, 1958). Extraordinary advances have been made in the use of the bowel in urinary tract reconstruction since then. Bladder augmentation is used for patients with bladder dysfunction related to a small-capacity, noncompliant reservoir. **Enterocystoplasty improves bladder capacity and compliance in most cases when medical management fails.** It is obvious from the previous discussion that there is no single bowel segment that is perfect for augmentation in all patients. All gastrointestinal segments have been used and continue to be used with good results. Unremitting medical problems or complications requiring surgical intervention are relatively rare after augmentation cystoplasty. No one bowel segment has a clear advantage over others when all such problems are considered. Patient diagnosis, anatomy, and physiology may suggest that one

bowel segment is preferable for a particular patient. Each surgeon interested in augmentation cystoplasty should be familiar with the advantages and disadvantages of each segment in different settings.

In many routine cases, any gastrointestinal segment may be chosen for cystoplasty based purely on the personal preference and familiarity of the surgeon. The surgeon's experience and confidence in using a segment are important. **We believe that no one bowel segment is the best choice in all patients and that optimal results and the most efficient use of bowel are achieved when the bowel segment is chosen based on the needs of the particular patient and then used correctly.** All things being equal, we would prefer to use ileum if there is no clear advantage or reason to use another segment. We would reserve stomach for children with renal insufficiency and acidosis, short gut syndrome, or heavy irradiation. We do continue to use sigmoid cystoplasty in selected patients without reservation; clearly, good results can be expected with any segment if it is used properly.

Alternatives to Gastrointestinal Cystoplasty

Largely because of the complications and side effects just reviewed, alternative methods that can achieve a large-capacity, compliant reservoir remain attractive. Efforts have covered the spectrum from synthetic materials and autologous grafts, to creation of a bladder diverticulum (autoaugmentation), to various forms of neural stimulation. **Some of these alternatives appear to hold promise, but none has stood the test of time for true comparison to intestinal cystoplasty.**

An ideal tissue for increasing capacity and improving compliance would have transitional epithelium so as to be relatively impermeable and avoid metabolic changes. The lining would also prevent mucus production and, probably, the increased potential for tumor development. The ability to augment the bladder without violation of the peritoneal cavity would also decrease morbidity. Two such alternative procedures are ureterocystoplasty and autoaugmentation. With ureterocystoplasty, there is good muscle backing of transitional epithelium, whereas collagen eventually backs the transitional mucosa of an autoaugmentation.

Ureterocystoplasty

TECHNIQUE

It has been noted for years that, in patients with posterior urethral valves, unilateral reflux may behave as a "pop-off" valve to lower intravesical pressures and protect the contralateral upper tract (Hoover and Duckett, 1982; Rittenberg et al, 1988; Kaefer et al, 1995). In many of these patients, the refluxing ureter is massively dilated, draining a poorly functioning or nonfunctioning kidney. **It was a logical extension to use this ureteral tissue to augment the bladder.** Ureterocystoplasty may be performed through a midline, intraperitoneal incision. This incision provides access to the intestine should mobilization of the ureter for augmentation be unsatisfactory. **Bellinger (1993), Dewan and colleagues (1994a), and Reinberg and colleagues (1995) showed that ureterocystoplasty can be done through two incisions, remaining completely extraperitoneal.**

The general technique is the same. A standard nephrectomy is performed with great care to preserve the renal pelvic and upper ureteral blood supply. All adventitia and periureteral tissue is swept from the peritoneum toward the ureter during mobilization to protect the ureteral blood supply. Proximally, this blood supply typically arises medially. As the ureter enters the true pelvis, the blood supply arises posteriorly and laterally. After mobilization of the ureter into the pelvis, the bladder is opened in the sagittal plane. Posteriorly, this incision has typically been carried off-center directly into and through the ureteral orifice of the ureter used for cystoplasty. The ureter is *not* detached from the bladder but is opened longitudinally along its entire length, with care taken to avoid its main blood supply (Fig. 71–16). The incision in the bladder and distal ureter should avoid branches of the superior vesical artery, which serves as an important blood supply to the mobilized ureter. The ureter is folded on itself, and the ureter-to-ureter and ureter-to-bladder anastomoses are performed with running absorbable suture. A suprapubic tube is left indwelling through the native bladder for 3 weeks during healing. After cystography documents the absence of leakage, CIC is started. Patients, particularly those without neurogenic dysfunction, may attempt to void spontaneously. It is our impression that children are more likely to void adequately after ureterocystoplasty than after intestinal cystoplasty, although all must prove that they can empty appropriately by checking postvoid residuals.

Alternatively, the bladder incision can be stopped approximately 2 cm from the orifice, with a similar length of distal ureter left in situ and intact without incision. The resulting small loop of intact ureter does not create clinical problems or adversely affect the end volume in a significant manner (Adams et al, 1998). This modification of technique is easier and may be safer in that it avoids potential injury to the blood supply of the mobilized ureter near the ureterovesical junction.

RESULTS

Early reports suggested that ureterocystoplasty could be technically achieved after nephrectomy by bivalving the bladder through the vesicoureteral junction and laying in the open ureter (Mitchell et al, 1992; Bellinger, 1993). Later reports modified and improved the procedure by noting that, with meticulous care, the vascularity to the entire renal pelvis could be preserved, allowing more tissue for cystoplasty (Churchill et al, 1993; Landau et al, 1994; McKenna and Bauer, 1995; Reinberg et al, 1995). As with intestinal cystoplasty, folding of the ureter into a more spherical configuration, now standard technique, maximizes the volume that can be achieved. In the massively dilated ureter draining a functioning kidney, the distal ureter alone may be used for augmentation, with the proximal ureter either reimplanted into the bladder or anastomosed to the contralateral ureter (Bellinger, 1993).

Numerous series have reported good results after augmentation using ureter, some with follow-up as long as 8 years. The upper tracts have remained stable or improved in virtually all patients. Complications have been uncommon, with only a rare early extravasation of urine reported (Churchill et al, 1993). Landau and colleagues (1994) compared age-matched and diagnosis-matched children who underwent ureterocystoplasty or ileocystoplasty. **The total mean bladder capacity was 470 ml in the ureterocystoplasty group and 381 ml in the ileocystoplasty group. Bladder volumes at 30 cm H_2O were 413 ml and 380 ml after ureterocystoplasty and ileocystoplasty, respectively.** Ureter effectively enhanced both volume and compliance. There was one failure in the group, which occurred in a child in whom the distal ureter did not provide enough volume. Other work has shown that one dilated ureter typically is enough for cystoplasty (Zubieta et al, 1999).

The main disadvantage to ureterocystoplasty is the limited patient population with a nonfunctioning kidney draining into a megaureter. McKenna and Bauer (1995) reported the use of a normal-sized ureter. The ultimate success of ureterocystoplasty using normal ureter requires further follow-up, particularly since Gonzalez (1999) has stated that one quarter of his patients with posterior urethral valves failed ureterocystoplasty with a dilated ureter because of their huge urinary volume. Atala and colleagues (1994) presented an experimental technique to slowly dilate a normal ureter for later use. Work continues to develop such a technique that is clinically applicable for patients (Stifelman et al, 1998).

Autoaugmentation

TECHNIQUES AND RESULTS

Cartwright and Snow (1989a, 1989b) described an ingenious method to improve bladder compliance and capacity using native urothelial tissue. In their procedure, known as autoaugmentation, they excised the detrusor muscle over

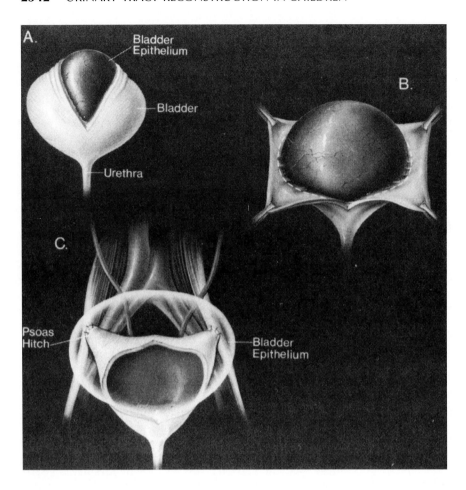

Figure 71–17. Autoaugmentation. *A,* The detrusor is incised. *B,* Detrusor is stripped and excised from mucosa. *C,* The detrusor muscle is anchored bilaterally so that the mucosa bulges with bladder filling. (From Cartwright PC, Snow BW: Bladder autoaugmentation: Early clinical experience. J Urol 1989a;142:505.)

the dome of the bladder, leaving the mucosa intact to protrude as a wide-mouth diverticulum. Initially, they made a midline incision through the bladder muscle (Fig. 71–17*A*). With the bladder distended with saline so that mucosa bulged from the incision, the muscle was mobilized and excised laterally in each direction (see Fig. 71–17*B*). The lateral edges of the detrusor muscle were then secured to the psoas muscle bilaterally to prevent collapse of the diverticulum (see Fig. 71–17*C*). Their early experience with a small group of patients resulted in improved compliance in most, with increasing capacity in some (Cartwright and Snow, 1989a).

This procedure has since been modified by a number of surgeons, particularly in adult patients, each providing a different name for the procedure depending on whether the detrusor muscle was simply incised or excised to create the diverticulum. In an effort to determine whether incision or excision provided superior results, Johnson and colleagues (1994) performed 16 vesicomyotomies and 16 vesicomyectomies in rabbits after previously reducing the bladder capacity. Functional bladder capacity in the animals increased by 43.5%, and there was no statistical difference between the two techniques. They then performed vesicomyotomies (incision) in 12 patients with neurogenic bladder dysfunction and demonstrated a mean increase in capacity of 40% and a mean decrease in leak point pressure of 33% (Stothers et al, 1994). They concluded that detrusor excision offered no advantage over

incision. All patients demonstrated some increase in capacity (15% to 70%), and no patient in early follow-up clinically deteriorated and required enterocystoplasty.

Detrusorectomy, leaving a small cap of muscle at the dome through which a suprapubic tube can be placed, was proposed by Landa and Moorhead (1994). **They have been concerned that, although these procedures usually improve compliance, the increase in volume is "modest at best," a concern shared by others** (Snow and Cartwright, 1996; Snow, personal communication, 1998). In a report of 12 detrusorectomies, five patients were considered to have excellent results, two had acceptable results, and one was lost to follow-up. Failure occurred in four patients (one hydronephrosis, two persistent incontinence, one worsening renal insufficiency), of whom three had undergone gastrocystoplasty or ileocystoplasty (Landa and Moorhead, 1994). In a combined series at the two institutions, only 52% of patients had a good result with autoaugmentation, whereas 20% had a poor outcome (Snow and Cartwright, 1996). Reoperative enterocystoplasty was not hampered by the prior detrusorectomy. The urothelial diverticulum at the time of augmentation cystoplasty was noted to be thick and fibrous, similar to a leather bag.

There are obvious advantages to autoaugmentation and its variants. Native urothelial tissue is used. It is an extraperitoneal procedure, which shortens operative time and avoids the risks of intestinal surgery and adhesions. Autoaugmentation is compatible with CIC and does not seem to complicate subsequent intestinal cystoplasty when necessary.

Complications from the procedures are generally uncommon. Perforation, a major concern after intestinal cystoplasty, has not been reported. Inadvertent opening of the mucosa during the procedure can make subsequent mobilization more difficult and may promote prolonged postoperative extravasation. Such extravasation usually stops with bladder drainage (Landa and Moorhead, 1994; Stothers et al, 1994). Prolonged drainage, however, may lead to compromised results due to collapse of the diverticulum. If concomitant ureteral reimplantation or bladder neck surgery is necessary, various authors have recommended that such procedures should be done first, with the bladder then closed before detrusorectomy (Stothers et al, 1994).

Ehrlich and Gershman (1993) first reported laparoscopic myotomy (incision). A laparoscopic approach uses a smaller incision and perhaps shortens postoperative hospitalization; it may make effective fixation of the detrusor muscle in an open fashion to allow good bulging more difficult. It remains to be seen whether autoaugmentation provides effective long-term results for pediatric patients and whether it can be done as well laparoscopically.

CONCERNS

The main disadvantage of autoaugmentation is a limited increase in bladder capacity; for this reason, adequate preoperative volume may be the most important predictor of success. Landa and Moorhead (1994) noted that if the maximum capacity and the volume of urine held at 40 cm H_2O are similar, the patient may be better served by immediate intestinal cystoplasty. It is of note that many patients have demonstrated clinical improvement after these procedures without a significant change in urodynamics. The exact reasons for the improvement are unknown. In most series of autoaugmentation, no matter what the technique, some patients have been noted or concern has existed at the time of the initial procedure that adequate expansion was not achieved. In most such cases, it was elected to proceed with enterocystoplasty immediately at the time (Landa and Moorhead, 1994). These patients were not included in the failure rate of autoaugmentation. The patient and surgeon must be prepared for such an event on occasion. Stohrer's group (Stohrer et al, 1999), as well as Leng and associates (1999), reported good results with the technique among patients with hyperreflexia.

Even if adequate expansion is achieved initially, there is concern that any improvement may not last in the long term (Dewan et al, 1994b). In animals, the surface area of the autoaugmentation site was observed to decrease by approximately 50% at 12 weeks. Progressive thickening and contracture of the site because of collagenous infiltrate was noted (Johnson et al, 1994). Milam observed that almost one half of his adult patients with hyperreflexia who early on had a good result after autoaugmentation failed with longer follow-up (D.F. Milam, personal communication, 2000). At this point, autoaugmentation probably should be considered only in patients who have reasonable capacity but poor compliance due to uninhibited contractions. If a remarkable increase in capacity is needed, au-

toaugmentation is unlikely to be as definitive as other techniques.

Seromuscular Enterocystoplasty

Based on concerns about collagen deposition and contraction around autoaugmentation, efforts have been made to combine that procedure with demucosalized enteric segments. The use of enteric segments without bowel mucosa within the bladder is not new. As far back as the 1950s, seromuscular augmentation cystoplasty was performed with the serosal side of the bowel turned to the bladder lumen (Shoemaker and Marucci, 1955; Shoemaker et al, 1957). Urothelium soon covered the serosa. Gonzalez's group experienced good results with reversed seromuscular cystoplasty in rats, as did others with rabbits (Celayir et al, 1995), but contracture of the patch occurred in larger animals (De Badiola et al, 1991; Long et al, 1992). Others left the exposed submucosa facing the bladder lumen and noted re-epithelialization with urothelium in animals (Oesch, 1988; Salle et al, 1990). Despite the re-epithelialization, patch contracture occurred (Salle et al, 1990). Several recent series have re-evaluated demucosalized augmentation in humans after taking care to preserve the submucosa. Better results were noted (Lima et al, 1998; De Badiola et al, 1999; Dayanc et al, 1999), although regrowth of metaplastic enteric mucosa was found in the second study.

To avoid contracture, a combination of autoaugmentation after detrusorectomy and coverage with a demucosalized enteric segment has now been used. This has been done to potentially preserve the advantages of both procedures. In a similar fashion, the combination has been undertaken with both colon and stomach. Buson et al (1994) used reconfigured, demucosalized sigmoid colon placed over the urothelium (seromuscular colocystoplasty lined with urothelium, or SCLU). They, and others, noted that the intestinal submucosa should be preserved to avoid contracture (Buson et al, 1994; Vates et al, 1997) (Fig. 71–18). This procedure has been performed clinically, with early reports of good results in most patients (Gonzalez et al, 1994). Postoperative bladder capacity increased an average of 2.4-fold (from 139 to 335 ml) in 14 of their 16 patients, and end filling pressure decreased on average from 51.6 to 27.7 cm H_2O. Two patients failed and required ileocystoplasty; their urodynamic data were excluded. Two other patients developed an hourglass deformity (Gonzalez et al, 1994). Endoscopic biopsy of the segments was interesting: Of 10 biopsies in the series, 1 revealed urothelium with islands of colonic mucosa, and 2 others found only colon mucosa. Removal of all of the enteric mucosa is important when using sigmoid to prevent mucoceles or overgrowth of intestinal mucosa (Gonzalez et al, 1994; Lutz and Frey, 1994). Dewan and associates (1997) believed that preservation of the submucosa eventually promoted regrowth of bowel mucosa. The interaction of the two different tissues will be interesting to follow. The long-term effects on the urothelium by the seromuscular segment and vice versa are unknown. Work has shown that persistent transitional lining will protect from metabolic problems and mucus production (Denes et al, 1997).

Dewan and Byard (1993) alternatively used demucosal-

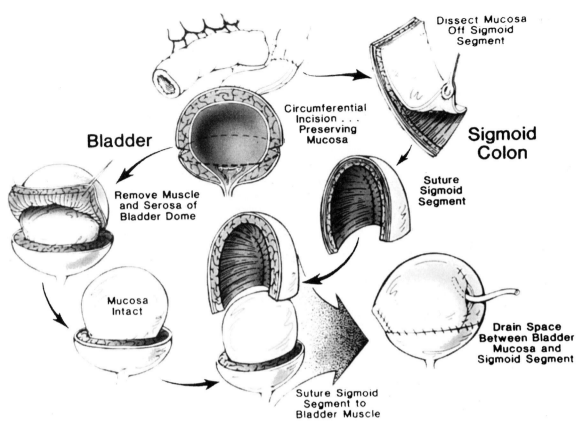

Figure 71–18. Seromuscular enterocystoplasty using sigmoid colon (SCLU). Detrusor incision is performed similar to autoaugmentation; however, the bulging mucosa is covered with a demucosalized segment of sigmoid colon. (From Buson H, Manivel JC, Dayanc M, et al: Seromuscular colocystoplasty lined with urothelium: Experimental study. Urology 1994;44:745, with permission. Copyright © 1994 by Elsevier Science, Inc.)

ized stomach to cover an autoaugmentation, first in sheep and then in patients. Early results showed improved bladder function both clinically and urodynamically (Dewan and Stefanek, 1994; Horowitz and Mitchell, 1993; Horowitz et al, 1994; Robinson et al, 1994) although long-term results have not been as encouraging (Carr et al, 1999). These procedures are technically more demanding than simple augmentation or autoaugmentation and are associated with more blood loss and a longer operative time (Gonzalez et al, 1994; Horowitz et al, 1994). Increased bleeding is particularly likely when using stomach. These urothelium-lined, seromuscular augmentations are theoretically attractive. Thus far, the failure and reoperation rate after such procedures remains higher than that noted for standard enterocystoplasty (Vates et al, 1997; Carr et al, 1999; Shekarriz et al, 2000). The best results have been reported with the use of colon. Those results may be partially attributed to the learning curve with a new, complex procedure. Longer follow-up and more experience are necessary to determine whether the complication rate will decrease with experience or increase because of problems with the combination.

Bladder Regeneration

Other efforts to find alternatives to intestinal cystoplasty in the 1950s included the use of alloplastic materials for bladder substitution (Gleeson and Griffith, 1992). Early research efforts met with very limited success. Further work using biodegradable, collagen-rich tissues to serve as a scaffold for bladder regeneration has also been reported (Kelami, 1971; Fishman et al, 1987; Kambic et al, 1992; Kropp et al, 1995). Atala and coworkers have applied bioengineering techniques to culture and combine various bladder cells in tissue culture for regeneration (Atala et al, 1992, 1993b; Cilento et al, 1994; Oberpenning et al, 1997; Yoo et al, 1998; Fauza et al, 1998). Early efforts are exciting, but preliminary. Clinical applicability in the human with a diseased bladder requires more study. Because enterocystoplasty is not a perfect physiologic substitute for the native bladder, these continued efforts are certainly warranted.

CONTINENT URINARY DIVERSION

The frequency with which continent urinary diversion is performed in children depends on one's definition of continent diversion. In adults, total bladder replacement is not uncommon after cystectomy for transitional cell carcinoma. This has led to extensive experience with continent urinary diversion and orthotopic neobladders that allow spontaneous voiding. Tumors resulting in cystectomy among children are much less common. It is in that setting, and in the occasional child in whom the bladder is congenitally absent or so small as to be virtually useless, that a pure continent urinary diversion in the classic sense of an Indiana or Kock pouch might be performed. Very good results with continent diversion in children have been achieved, equivalent to those reported in adults. Orthotopic neobladders in children are created infrequently. Neurogenic or anatomic problems at the outlet prevent spontaneous voiding in many cases. Even among patients who have undergone cystectomy for tumors, irradiation can interfere with voiding. Occasionally a child with neurogenic dysfunction may be a candidate for orthotopic bladder substitution (Stein et al, 2000). It is not clear how many of those patients with neurogenic dysfunction can be expected to void adequately.

More frequently in children, series of continent diversion have included patients undergoing a mixture of the techniques discussed in this chapter. Some authors have defined combinations of bladder augmentation, continent abdominal wall stoma, and various procedures at the outlet as continent diversions (Kaefer et al, 1997b). Division and closure of the bladder neck to prevent incontinence through the native urethra has typically meant inclusion. Certainly, maximal utilization of the native urinary tract is beneficial to the child. Much as with the discussion of urinary undiversion, these procedures typically have been performed in patients with complex, multiple problems that must be addressed, often after numerous previous surgeries.

Considerations

The amount of bowel used in continent urinary diversion varies depending on the techniques required. Total bladder replacement requires much more intestine than simple augmentation. Typically a 40-cm segment of small bowel is used for an ileal reservoir in a Kock pouch, compared with the 20 cm often used for augmentation. Likewise, the entire right colon with the hepatic flexure may be used in an Indiana pouch with or without a patch of small intestine, whereas only 15 to 20 cm of colon is needed for colocystoplasty. Because of the potential morbidity associated with use of a larger intestinal segment, the native bladder is often incorporated in children if it provides any significant volume. To do so, however, may require repair of the outlet if outflow resistance is low. Otherwise, incontinence per native urethra will result.

Imbrication of the ileocecal valve and terminal ileum has proved to be a simple and reliable means for construction of an effective efferent limb in continent diversion among adults and children. Despite reports to the contrary in selected patients (Husmann and Cain, 1999), concern about fecal incontinence secondary to use of the ileocecal valve remains in patients with neurogenic dysfunction. The flap valve continence mechanism provides numerous alternatives for those surgeons with such concerns in continent diversion. The good results achieved with use of the appendix or tapered intestinal segments have led to their increased use in recent years.

Although maintaining the native urethra for catheterization is ideal, it may not be appropriate or possible in all individuals. As indicated previously, reconstructive bladder neck procedures are often subject to difficulty with catheterization. **Children with neurogenic sphincter incompetence may have associated neurologic limitations that prevent easy access to their native urethra. For children without neurologic deficits, normal sensation of their native urethra can prevent compliance with a routine catheterization schedule because of discomfort. For these reasons, a continent catheterizable stoma provides an adequate, and sometimes a more reliably useful, alternative.**

Continence Mechanisms and Catheterizable Stomas

Ureterosigmoidostomy and Its Variants

Ureterosigmoidostomy can be an effective form of continent urinary diversion in some patients. Its major advantage is the potential for spontaneous emptying by evacuation of urine with stool. The significant complications of hyperchloremic acidosis, infection, hydronephrosis, and the development of colonic malignancies have led to disfavor and disuse, particularly in the United States. **Although good results with standard ureterosigmoidostomy have been reported in some children, the procedure is rarely performed as originally described. The morbidity of acidosis and upper tract changes may increase with time, making those complications particularly worrisome for children with a long life expectancy. The significant risk of adenocarcinoma commits patients to a lifetime of close surveillance for an avoidable tumor.** It is unlikely that ureterosigmoidostomy, as classically described, will regain acceptance for children.

Several modifications of ureterosigmoidostomy have been used in an attempt to decrease its significant complication rate. **The most basic of the modifications is the sigma rectum or the Mainz II pouch.** The colon is incised along the antimesenteric border for 6 cm both proximal and distal to the rectosigmoid junction. The ureters are implanted in an antirefluxing fashion, and that portion of colon is then reconfigured and closed. This is done to create a rectosigmoid reservoir of increased capacity and lower pressure to protect the upper tracts. The Mainz II pouch has been used primarily in children with bladder exstrophy (Stein et al, 1997a). Continence in appropriately selected patients is good, although acidosis is still a significant problem owing to exposure of the entire colon to urine (Fisch et al, 1996; Mingin et al, 1999a; Gerharz et al, 1999). The potential for development of adenocarcinoma still exists with this technique. Long-term follow-up is necessary to determine whether the reconfiguration of the sigmoid in the area of ureteral implantation is truly effective for protection of the upper tracts. Anastomotic stricture at the ureterocolonic anastomosis has been the most common complication in relatively short follow-up (Fisch et al, 1996).

In an effort to control the amount of colon to which urine is exposed, Kock and associates (1988a, 1988b) described creation of a colorectal valve to confine urine to the distal segment. The intussuscepted nipple valve is stabilized with permanent staples. The distal rectal segment is opened and patched with ileum to lower pressure. With short-term follow-up, the valve is effective; no necessity for sodium bicarbonate or potassium citrate therapy was noted (Kock et al, 1988b). Others have demonstrated that the colorectal valve is effective in preventing acidosis by

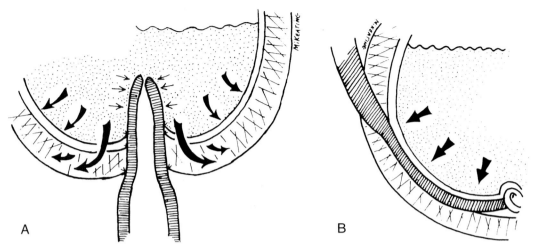

Figure 71–19. Continence mechanisms. *A,* The same pressures that create continence tend to efface nipple valves. *B,* This is not true of flap valves, which have been more reliable in pediatric reconstruction. (Courtesy of Howard M. Snyder III, MD.)

reducing the absorptive surface area exposed to urine (Mahran et al, 1999). Prophylactic alkalinization, necessary for many patients after ureterosigmoidostomy, may be avoided with the creation of such a valve. An increased risk for tumor development still exists with this modification, and long-term follow-up of its use in children is needed to see if it is truly less morbid in terms of infection and upper tract deterioration. Urodynamic evaluation has revealed low pressure in the rectal reservoir (Kock et al, 1988b).

If placement of a colorectal valve avoids most complications of metabolic acidosis from ureterosigmoidostomy and creation of a reservoir with lower pressure better protects the upper tracts, the last remaining major concern about ureterosigmoidostomy is tumor development. The concern is significant: Of 94 children monitored in Boston after ureterosigmoidostomy, 7 developed adenocarcinoma, of whom 4 died from the tumor (Rink and Retik, 1991). Kock and colleagues (1988b), followed by Skinner and associates (1989), used a hemi-Kock pouch to augment the distal rectal segment. A colorectal valve was created to isolate urine to the distal colon. This modification also allowed prevention of reflux to dilated ureters. It may serve to keep the admixture of stool and urine away from the ureteroileal anastomosis, perhaps lowering the risk for tumor development. Simoneau and Skinner (1995) reported their results with the procedure in 15 patients, including 4 children. The complication rate, both early and late, was relatively high. This is not surprising considering the relatively complex nature of the procedure. They did believe that the pediatric patients were better suited for the procedure. Rink and Retik (1991) suggested that the rectum could be augmented with a nonrefluxing ileocecal conduit in a similar fashion.

Before considering any variant of ureterosigmoidostomy, competence of the anal sphincter must be ensured. Tests used to assess sphincter integrity include manometry, electromyography, and practical evaluation of the ability to retain an oatmeal enema in the upright position for a period of time without soilage. Incontinence of a mixture of stool and urine results in foul soilage and must be avoided. Consequently, most patients with neurogenic dysfunction, who are incapable of fecal continence in the presence of diarrhea, are not candidates for these procedures. Proce-

dures that separate the fecal and urinary streams within the rectal sphincter have been described but have not been widely used among children.

Nipple Valves

The greatest experience with nipple valves used to achieve urinary continence has been with the Kock pouch. Skinner and associates (1989) made a series of modifications to aid in maintenance of the efferent nipple. Even with experience and these modifications, a failure rate of 15% or higher can be expected (Benson and Olsson, 1998) (Fig. 71–19). Several authors have reported a reoperation rate of approximately 33% with the Kock pouch, most frequently related to the efferent nipple (DeKernion et al, 1985; Waters et al, 1997). Equivalent results with the nipple valve and a Kock pouch have been achieved in children (Hanna and Bloiso, 1987; Skinner et al, 1988; Kaefer et al, 1997b; Abd-El-Gawad et al, 1999). The last report noted a significant incidence of hyperchloremic acidosis and new hydronephrosis, although those complications were probably a result of the complex nature of the situation rather than the particular continent diversion used.

Intussuscepted nipple valves have also been used with colonic and ileocolonic reservoirs, particularly the Mainz I pouch. Again, evolution of the nipple valve in the Mainz pouch occurred over time (Thuroff et al, 1986, 1988; Hohenfellner et al, 1990; Stein et al, 1995). Most recently, the intussuscepted ileum is fixed with staples, passed through the intact ileocecal valve, and fixed again. Much as with the Kock pouch, the incidence of incontinence has decreased with experience and modifications. The Mainz I pouch has been used in children with good results and low rates of incontinence using the latest modifications (Stein et al, 1995, 1997a; Steiner et al, 1998; Stein et al, 2000). Maintenance of normal upper tracts has been good and metabolic problems rare (Stein et al, 1997b). In fact, improvement of preexisting hydronephrosis has been more common than worsening. For the past several years, the group at Mainz has used a flap valve mechanism and the appendix for a continent catheterizable stoma with less incontinence (Stein et al, 1995; Gerharz et al, 1997).

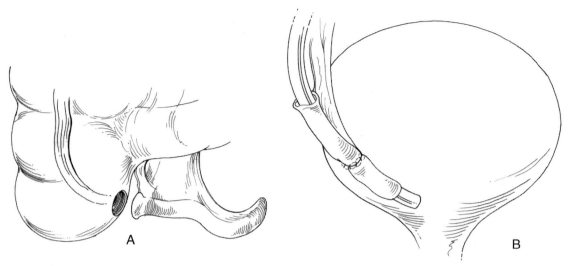

Figure 71–20. Appendicovesicostomy. *A,* The appendix is harvested with a cuff of cecum on a wide pedicle based on the appendiceal artery. A flap of cecum can be harvested in continuity with the appendix and tubularized to increase the length. *B,* The distal appendix is tunneled into the bladder to provide continence after the end is amputated. The proximal end of the appendix, the cecal cuff, is brought to the umbilicus or right lower quadrant as a catheterizable stoma.

Flap Valves and the Mitrofanoff Principle

Mitrofanoff (1980) described a continence mechanism using the appendix or ureter to create a flap valve. He recognized that any tubular structure could be implanted effectively into a low-pressure reservoir. This continence mechanism circumvents many of the secondary potential complications associated with harvesting the ileocecal valve or using other gastrointestinal segments.

The foundation for the success of the Mitrofanoff principle is based on creating a submucosal tunnel for a supple, small-diameter conduit. As the reservoir fills, the rise in intravesical pressure is transmitted through the epithelium and to the implanted conduit, coapting its lumen (see Fig. 71–19). The appendix is an ideal natural tubular structure that can safely be removed from the gastrointestinal tract without significant morbidity. The small caliber of the appendix facilitates creation of a short functional tunnel within the bladder wall. Experience has shown that continence can be achieved with only a 2-cm appendiceal tunnel (Kaefer and Retik, 1997). Whether in a continent urinary reservoir or in native bladder, the appendix has been used as an efferent limb with very good results (Jayanthi et al, 1995; Mollard et al, 1997; Kaefer et al, 1997b; Cain et al, 1999). The appendix has been particularly useful in children because it is relatively longer and the abdominal wall is generally thinner. The flap valve is probably the most reliable of all of the surgically constructed continence mechanisms. This is good in terms of continence when the patient is catheterized reliably. Many patients with good flap valves virtually never leak per stoma. This potentially puts them at greater risk for upper tract deterioration or spontaneous rupture of the bladder or reservoir if catheterization is not performed.

If the appendix is used in situ in a continent urinary reservoir, the reservoir by necessity will include the right colon. Duckett and Snyder (1986, 1987) used the right colon and appendix with good results and called it the Penn pouch. The mesoappendix, in most cases, allows mo-

bilization of the appendix for use in the native bladder or virtually any reservoir.

TECHNIQUE

Appropriate preoperative planning is required to position the skin incision so as to allow for adequate mobilization of the appendix to the bladder. In most children this can be achieved by making a low midline or a transverse incision. On occasion, the cecum may be high in the abdomen. Mobilization of the ascending colon along the line of Toldt may be required to gain mobilization of the appendix and its mesentery. Cadeddu and Docimo (1999) used laparoscopy to aid in the mobilization of the ascending colon and cecum. Once the cecum has been mobilized, the base of the appendix is amputated, leaving a small cuff of cecum with the appendix. This facilitates the stomal anastomosis and decreases the risk of stenosis. The cecum is closed in a fashion similar to an open appendectomy. If the length of the appendix is marginal, a greater portion of the cecum can be harvested, effectively increasing the functional length of the appendix (Cromie et al, 1991). A portion may be tubularized with the appendix (Bruce and McRoberts, 1998).

After harvesting, a location is selected for implantation of the appendix into the bladder. The location is based on the length of the appendix, the mobility of the bladder, and the location for the appendiceal stoma. Typically, the distal end of the appendix is tunneled into a posterolateral position within the bladder (Fig. 71–20).

The base of the appendix is brought to the abdominal wall in a location chosen preoperatively to suit the patient. It should be brought up to reach the skin without tension. Care must be taken not to twist the pedicle or occlude it as it passes through the abdominal wall fascia. The base of the appendix can be hidden within the umbilicus, which allows for easy catheterization and the elimination of a small but obvious abdominal stoma. Because of the small circular diameter of the appendiceal base, stomal stenosis is common, and techniques have been described to prevent this problem. Various flaps have been used as a method for avoiding stomal stenosis (Keating et al, 1993; Kajbafzadeh, et al, 1995; Kaefer and Retik, 1997). **In order to prevent kinking and problems with catheterization, it is advisable to maintain as short a conduit as possible.** Securing the appendix and bladder wall to the peritoneum beneath the fascia helps diminish the problem of conduit kinking with reservoir filling. The importance of meticulous operative detail when securing the Mitrofanoff limb cannot be overemphasized.

When using appendix or any catheterizable stoma, it is advisable to repeatedly catheterize the channel after each step in reconstruction to confirm easy passage. If the catheter does not pass easily into the reservoir, the prior step needs to be revised. Problems with catheterization by the surgeon during the operative procedure usually result in more difficulty for the patient afterward. It is also beneficial to catheterize at variable reservoir volumes to confirm proper fixation of the reservoir and the absence of any kinking. A No. 6 to No. 10 Fr Silastic stent is typically left for 10 to 14 days within the efferent catheterizable channel during the healing process. It is advisable for the surgeon to personally catheterize the efferent limb before allowing the patient or other family members to do so. Catheterization should be repeated at least every 4 hours for reservoir drainage, maintenance of patency, and minimalization of the risk of stomal stenosis.

The appendix may not be available for use in all patients due to previous appendectomy, its location or length, congenital absence, involvement with adhesions, or use for continence enemas. Histologic abnormalities of the appendix have been reported to occur in as many as 30% of patients (Liebovitch et al, 1992) and to increase with age. They rarely are of enough clinical significance to preclude use (Mulvihill et al, 1983).

RESULTS

Several papers have reviewed large series of patients after appendicovesicostomy (Kaefer et al, 1997b; Cain et al, 1999, Harris et al, 2000). The patient populations have been typical of most pediatric groups, the majority having neurogenic dysfunction. Inability to use the appendix, other than for use in situ for antegrade continence enemas, has been rare. The results, in terms of continence, have been superb, usually greater than 95% (Kaefer and Retik, 1997; Suzer et al, 1997; Mor et al, 1997; Gerharz et al, 1997, 1998; Gosalbez et al, 1998; Cain et al, 1999; Castellan et al, 1999). **Incontinence is a rare event with the Mitrofanoff principle; it may result from inadequate length of the flap valve mechanism or persistently elevated reservoir pressure.** Urodynamic assessment is required to evaluate the cause of the incontinence. Although injection of collagen or other biomaterials is a possible treatment for inadequate outflow resistance, a more formal approach with takedown and revision of the leaking Mitrofanoff valve is usually required (Kaefer and Retik, 1997). The most common complication has been stomal stenosis, which has occurred in about 10% to 20% of patients. Such stenosis resulting in difficult catheterization may occur early in the postoperative course and may require formal revision (Harris et al, 2000). Another recognized complication has been

appendiceal perforation. Stricture and necrosis, particularly of cecal extensions of the appendix, have occurred rarely. Abdominal stomas may be associated with a higher risk of reservoir calculi because of the potential for incomplete emptying.

Follow-up in the recent series has averaged approximately 4 years. Patients from Mitrofanoff's early experience (1980) should now have follow-up of more than 20 years, suggesting that the appendix should provide a durable alternative for pediatric patients with a long life expectancy, a finding duplicated by others (Harris et al, 2000).

ALTERNATIVES

When the appendix is unavailable for use, other tubular structures can provide a similar mechanism for catheterization and continence. Mitrofanoff (1980) described a similar technique using ureter (Kaefer et al, 1997b). Care must be taken to preserve the distal blood supply to prevent ischemia. Refluxing ureters have even been used after extravesical reimplantation (Ashcraft and Dennis, 1986; Duel et al, 1996; Kaefer et al, 1997b). Stomal stenosis seems to be more problematic with use of the ureter compared with the appendix, possibly because of a compromised blood supply. In addition, distention of the ureter by catheter passage has caused discomfort in some individuals (Duckett and Lofti, 1993).

Woodhouse and MacNeily (1994), among others, have used the fallopian tube, which can accommodate catheterization. Stenosis appears to be a significant problem with the fallopian tube. In addition, the effect on fertility should be considered when there is a normal ipsilateral gonad. Bihrle and associates (1991) fashioned a gastric tube mobilized on the gastroepiploic artery for implantation in continent reservoirs. Acid irritation of the skin was problematic in some patients. They then used a tapered segment of ileum as well (Adams et al, 1992). By narrowing the segment longitudinally along the mesenteric border using permanent staplers in series, they were able to construct a uniform tube of adequate length that was easy to catheterize and provided good continence rates. Others (Woodhouse and MacNeily, 1994; Hampel et al, 1995) have had similar good results. It is ideal for such tubes to be long enough to bridge the reservoir to skin without tension; however, they should then be kept as short and straight as possible to facilitate easy catheterization. Any long and free catheterizable channel within the abdomen can potentially kink and result in difficult catheterization or perforation.

Monti has been credited with a novel modification of the tapered intestinal segment that can be reimplanted according to the Mitrofanoff principle (Monti et al, 1997). **Recognition should also be directed to another report of this procedure by Yang (1993).** A very short (1 to 2 cm) segment of small bowel is opened longitudinally along the antimesenteric border, the edges spread, and then closed transversely (Fig. 71–21). By this reconfiguration, the initial circumference of the segment is converted to the length and the original length to the circumference. A very uniform tube is created with a small mesentery toward the center. The two ends are devoid of mesentery, making them very easy to tunnel into bladder and bring through

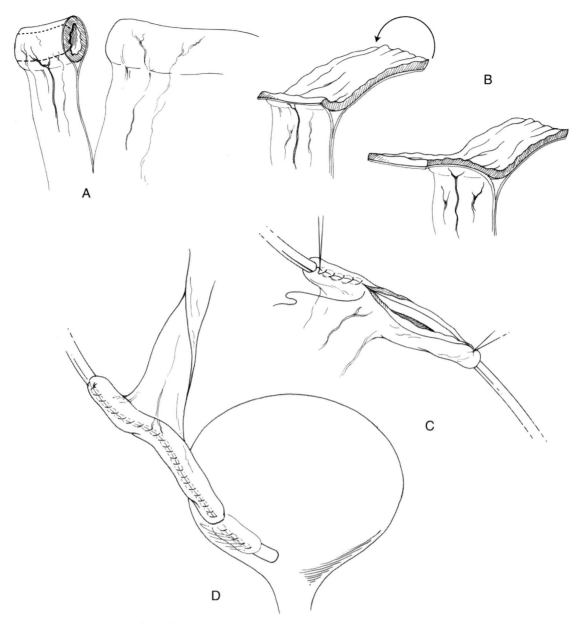

Figure 71–21. Yang-Monti technique for efficient construction of a catheterizable tube. A, A 2-cm length of ileum is harvested either independently or next to a segment isolated for augmentation cystoplasty. The segment is opened horizontally and then tubularized in a longitudinal fashion. B, The initial incision may be made to one side or the other to create a shorter limb for implantation in the bladder and a longer one to be brought through the abdominal wall, or vice-versa. If the segment is opened directly in the midline of the antimesenteric border, two equal-length limbs with a central mesenteric pedicle result. C, The reconfigured ileal segment is tubularized over a No. 12 Fr catheter in a two-layer technique with absorbable sutures. D, A continent catheterizable stoma is created.

the abdominal wall. If the first incision is made directly at the antimesenteric border, both limbs will be of equal length. By making the incision well around one side, one limb may be created much longer than the other. Experience has shown that one need not achieve a long tunnel in the bladder or reservoir to achieve continence with such a small tube, and the longer limb has typically been used to reach the skin through a thick abdominal wall.

Very good results have been achieved with use of the Yang-Monti tube as a catheterizable stoma, and it is certainly an efficient use of bowel. Some surgeons have suggested that it may be easier to catheterize than an ileal segment tapered longitudinally because circular mucosal

folds are redirected longitudinally in the direction of catheter passage. Whether this is truly the case will be determined by longer follow-up data. Flap valves created with ileum may have a lower rate of stomal stenosis than those created with appendix (Kaefer et al, 1999). The one potential disadvantage of the Yang-Monti tube is that it remains relatively short and may not reach the skin without tension in obese patients. Despite extensive use of skin flaps, such tension may lead to stomal stenosis. Two separate reconfigured tubes can be anastomosed together for adequate length (Kaefer and Retik, 1997). Casale (1999) used an initial segment that was twice as long, partially split in the middle, and then opened on opposite sides to create a longer strip, up to 12 cm, that could be tubularized in continuity. One must wonder whether such composite tubes are easier to catheterize than one tapered longitudinally and whether they offer any real advantage.

Ileocecal Valve

Use of the ileocecal valve as a continence mechanism began with Gilchrist and colleagues (1950) and was popularized by the Indiana group (Rowland et al, 1985; Bihrle, 1997). Various modifications exist. In general, a short segment of terminal ileum, whether imbricated or tailored, is used as an efferent limb. This segment should be kept as short and straight as possible to facilitate easy CIC. Continence is based on the imbricated ileocecal valve, not the length of the efferent limb. The imbrication is usually secured with interrupted, permanent sutures, involving the very distal ileum and ileocecal valve. The imbrication is carried well onto the cecum. The reservoir itself is constructed from reconfigured right colon up through the hepatic flexure, with or without a patch of ileum. Standard ureterocolonic anastomoses are done beneath the tenia to prevent reflux. Staplers using absorbable staples have been used for reconfiguration of the reservoir (Kirsch et al, 1996) and may shorten the operative time for reconstruction.

The Indiana pouch has been used in children with excellent results, as it has in adults. Next to the appendix, this continence mechanism is perhaps the simplest and has the shortest learning curve to achieve reliable results. Continence rates are reported to be as high as 95% with preservation of normal upper tracts (Rowland et al, 1985; Rink and Bihrle, 1990; Lockhart et al, 1990; Hensle and Ring, 1991; Rowland, 1995; Kaefer et al, 1997b). Rare reports have noted higher rates of incontinence (Canning et al, 1998). Husmann and Cain (1999) used the cecal segment for bladder augmentation and the efferent limb to construct a continent catheterizable stoma with equally good results. They noted a very low incidence of detrimental effect on gastrointestinal function in a highly selected group of patients with neurogenic dysfunction.

Hydraulic Valves

Benchekroun (1982, 1989) developed an interesting hydraulic valve as a continence mechanism which was modified by Guzman and associates (1989). Urine from the reservoir and any pressure generated there is allowed to enter a sleeve of ileum around the catheterizable channel. Compression of the inner tube theoretically provides continence, and early results were encouraging. Initial continence rates approached 75% and then 90% with a single revision (Benchekroun et al, 1989). Others have not been able to duplicate those results (Sanda et al, 1988; Leonard et al, 1990b), and the valve has largely been abandoned.

Koff and coworkers (1989) added hydraulic compression to the terminal ileum of an Indiana pouch by anastomosing a segment of tubular ileum to the cecum and then wrapping it around the efferent limb. The procedure has not gained popularity, probably because of the excellent success of the standard Indiana pouch.

Continent Vesicostomy

Yachia (1997) described creation of a bladder tube fashioned from a wide-based flap of the anterior bladder wall. No attempt was made to produce continence at the level of the bladder. The continence mechanism was fashioned by weaving the bladder tube through the rectus muscle to produce compression and continence. Continence in their small, short-term series was reported to be 100%, but this has not been duplicated.

Hanna et al (1999) described a continence mechanism based on either a flap of bladder or intestinal tissue fashioned after prior enterocystoplasty. A rectangular flap in continuity with the bladder is tubularized over a No. 14 to 16 Fr catheter. The bladder is plicated around the proximal 3 cm of the tube using nonabsorbable suture to create a type of nipple, similar to gastric fundoplication. No significant morbidity was identified in a limited series of five children, and all five remained dry on CIC. Macedo and Srougi (2000) described a similar continence mechanism created at the time of initial augmentation (Fig. 71–22). They achieved acceptable continence in eight of their first nine patients. The technique is potentially appealing for patients who require augmentation and have no appendix because of its simplicity; however, continence is based on a type of nipple valve that historically has been difficult to keep fixed. The same forces that create continence tend to efface the continence mechanism.

Casale (1991) described a form of continent vesicostomy in which the continence mechanism is based on a flap valve created from an anterior detrusor strip. It is particularly suitable when the bladder is compliant and of large capacity. The anterior detrusor strip is also used to create a catheterizable limb.

TECHNIQUE

Parallel incisions 3 cm apart are made into the anterior bladder and used to create a long rectangular flap. The abdominal wall should be measured to ensure that the strip is long enough to reach the skin without tension. The full-thickness strip is tubularized down to the bladder, typically in two layers. The muscle portion is left broad to come around without tension and provide good blood supply. The mucosa may be trimmed in width before tubularization to avoid redundancy. A strip of mucosa within the bladder, 2 to 3 cm in length and 1.5 cm in width, is incised in a direct line with the mobilized bladder tube. The edges of this strip are mobilized until it can be tubularized along its entire length. It may be beneficial to only mobilize one edge over to the other side, avoiding overlapping suture lines. Casale (1991) originally incised the mucosa transversely at the end of the intravesical strip to be tubularized; Rink and colleagues (1995b) later suggested that it could be left intact (Fig. 71–23). The bladder mucosa from either side of the tube is then mobilized and closed to create a flap valve. More extensive mobilization of the side opposite that mobilized for the inner tube allows closure without overlapping the suture lines, which may help avoid fistula formation and incontinence. A soft stent is usually left through the tube for 3 weeks during healing to prevent

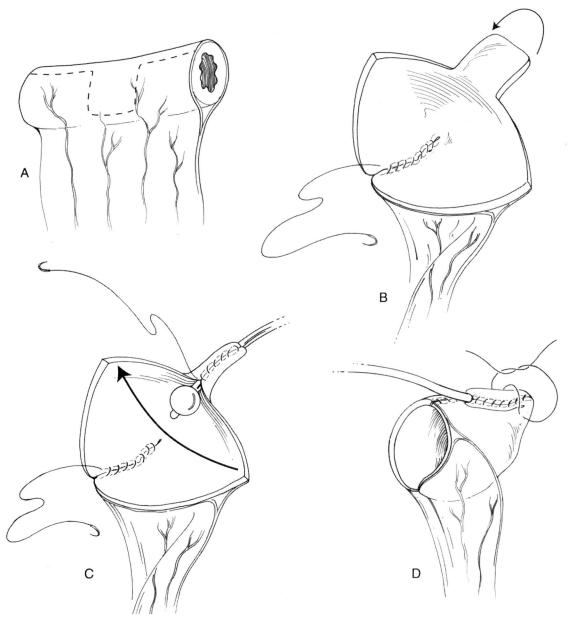

Figure 71–22. The Macedo catheterizable stoma incorporates the creation of a catheterizable intestinal limb in continuity with the augmented segment. *A,* The bowel segment used for augmentation is isolated in a routine fashion. It is opened on its antimesenteric border, creating a central extension with a width of 1.5 to 2 cm. *B,* The intestinal flap is then reconfigured into a U-shaped pouch. *C,* The extension is tubularized over a 12 to 14 Fr catheter, continuing onto the segment for augmentation. *D,* The tubularized segment is then folded onto the pouch and buried with interrupted sutures.

stenosis. It does tend to close if not used and catheterized regularly.

RESULTS

Continence rates have been good as with most flap valve mechanisms (Cain et al, 1999). Stomal stenosis remains a significant problem—29% in the experience at Indiana University. Skin flaps and avoidance of tension to reach the skin may minimize this risk but not remove it. Advantages include avoidance of an intraperitoneal procedure and bowel anastomosis; the appendix can be reserved for use

with enemas. It does use some bladder and decreases capacity, which may not be appropriate for some patients.

Results with Pediatric Continent Diversion

Continent urinary reservoirs have been created in children with very good results, equivalent to those achieved for adults. Creation of an adequate reservoir and an antireflux mechanism has generally been straightforward. For review of issues concerning compliance of the reservoir or

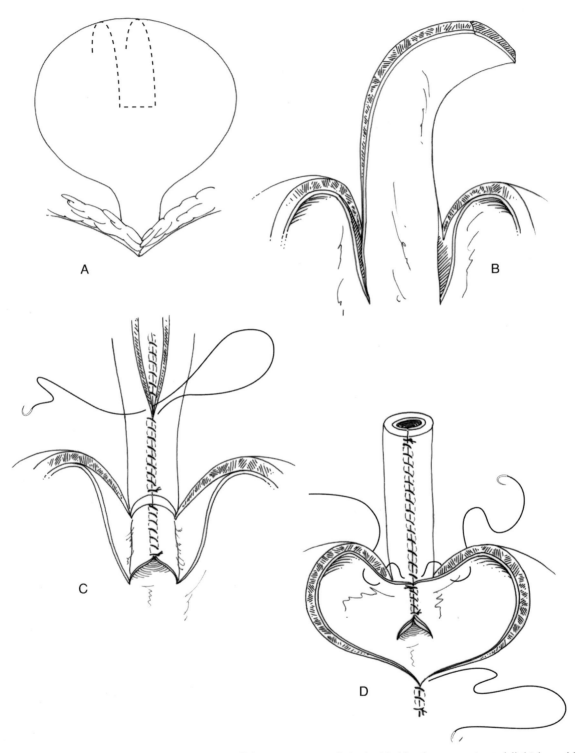

Figure 71–23. Casale continent catheterizable stoma. *A,* Parallel incisions are made in the bladder dome, creating a full-thickness bladder strip. *B,* The epithelium of the bladder is then incised for an additional 2.5 cm. The edges of the epithelium are mobilized, allowing for tubularization. *C,* The epithelium is tubularized from the bladder out to the tip of the strip using an absorbable suture. The muscle of the bladder strip is then tubularized with an absorbable suture. *D,* The lateral edges of the epithelium within the bladder are reapproximated over the tubularized bladder segment with absorbable suture. The bladder is then closed with absorbable suture, incorporating the bladder tube with the initial sutures to prevent kinking.

mechanisms by which reflux can be prevented, the reader may review earlier parts of this chapter or the chapter on continent urinary diversion in adults. The most challenging aspect of continent diversion remains construction of an efferent limb that provides reliable continence and easy catheterization. The continence mechanism most familiar to pediatric urologists is the flap valve. The appendix is simple to use, suitable for most children, and associated with very good continence rates. If the appendix is not present or is to be used for antegrade colonic enemas, tapered intestinal segments provide a nice alternative. Nipple valves are the most complex continence mechanism and therefore have a longer learning curve. Continence rates of approximately 85% can be expected with stapled nipple valves (Kaefer et al, 1997b; Benson and Olsson, 1998), even with extensive experience. With use of the other efferent limbs, continence rates above 90% and approaching 95% have routinely been reported in children (Duckett and Snyder, 1986; Hensle and Ring, 1991; Kaefer et al, 1997b), with preservation of the upper tracts. With proper patient selection and appropriately performed continent diversion, hydronephrosis in children is rare postoperatively. It is more likely to be improved than worsened. New hydronephrosis can occur, particularly if catheterization is not performed reliably (Abd-El-Gawad et al, 1999). There is no evidence that children have more hydronephrosis after continent diversion compared to conduit diversion (Stein et al, 2000).

Children undergoing continent diversion have a long life expectancy. The incidence of complications after continent diversion is likely to increase with longer follow-up. Those patients will be subject to the same complications discussed at length for bladder augmentation. All of those complications, including infection, hydronephrosis, calculi, spontaneous perforation, and tumor, have been reported after continent diversion, in adults if not in children. They are largely a function of the use of intestine as a urinary reservoir. Because more intestine is usually required in continent diversion than in bladder augmentation, the incidence of complications may ultimately be higher than with simple augmentation as follow-up increases. Certainly, serum changes of increased chloride, decreased bicarbonate, and acidosis have been noted in some patients after continent diversion (Allen et al, 1985; McDougal, 1992a; Asken, 1987; Thuroff et al, 1987; Boyd et al, 1989). Spontaneous perforation has occurred in up to 1.5% of patients (Mansson et al, 1997).

The most common complication in pediatric continent diversion thus far has been stomal stenosis. Such stenosis occurs more commonly at the umbilicus and when using appendix rather than tapered ileal segments (Fichtner et al, 1997; Kaefer et al, 1999). Various skin flaps may be placed into the terminal end of the appendix or intestinal segment to lower the rate of stenosis, but they do not eliminate it (Kajbafzadeh et al, 1995).

ANTEGRADE CONTINENCE ENEMAS

Fecal incontinence may be more socially debilitating to patients than urinary incontinence. In a sense, it has been easier to work surgically on urinary incontinence because

urologists and their patients have CIC as a technique for reliable emptying. That has not been the case with constipation and fecal incontinence, particularly among patients with neurogenic dysfunction. **Malone and associates (1990) described use of the appendix for antegrade continence enemas (MACE) to control constipation and achieve fecal continence in patients with complex gastrointestinal disorders refractory to conservative management.** These enemas, usually performed once a day, provide a thorough cleansing in a short period of time. If effective, patients, particularly those with neurogenic dysfunction, often will not stool again until their next enema (Curry et al, 1999). Cecostomy tubes, cecostomy buttons, and tapered intestinal segments tunneled into the cecum have been used for the enemas when the appendix is not suitable or is unavailable. Antegrade continence enemas as originally described by Malone have been used extensively in the neurogenic population (Koyle et al, 1995; Rink et al, 1999; Curry et al, 1999). Enemas are often performed with plain tap water. Metabolic derangements are unusual, although water treated with a softener should be avoided because it can cause hypernatremia (Yerkes et al, 2000). The irrigating volume is increased until a good result is achieved for the patient.

Average volumes in most series have approached 400 ml but occasionally reach 900 ml. The transit time for the enema after insertion varies among patients but averages 25 minutes (range, 15 to 60 minutes) (Rink et al, 1999). Additives to the irrigant may decrease the transit time in some patients (Kajbafzadeh and Chubak, 2000). The enemas are begun daily as soon as bowel function returns after reconstructive surgery. The initial volume used is low and typically is increased every 2 to 3 days until adequate decompression is achieved. Fecal continence until the next enema has been consistent for most patients with neurogenic dysfunction (range, 67% to more than 90%) (Hensle et al, 1998; Rink et al, 1999). Hensle et al (1998) noted occasional soilage requiring a pad in one quarter of their patients who were performing the enemas routinely. Both groups found that the majority of patients could perform the enemas independently. Almost universally, the patients and families have continued to perform the enemas on a regular basis in these series, good evidence that they find the results to be worth any time and effort involved. Rarely, a patient may have severe colonic spasms with flushing that preclude use (Bau et al, 2000). They occasionally respond to multiple flushings with smaller volumes. The most common complication, as with using the appendix as a catheterizable stoma elsewhere, has been stomal stenosis. Stenosis may not occur as commonly as when the appendix is moved to the bladder (Kaefer et al, 2000). Some children require catheterization of the appendix twice a day to avoid contracture or a cicatrix at the skin level. Perforation of the appendix has been noted with catheterization, as has false passage parallel to the appendix. Subsequent intraperitoneal injection of the enema fluid has occurred, resulting in peritonitis. Such patients require antibiotics and close observation. They do not routinely require reoperation (J.W. Brock, III, personal communication, 2000).

The appendix can be used easily in situ (Fig. 71–24). Windows in the mesoappendix may be created and perma-

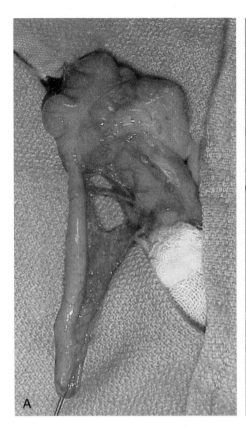
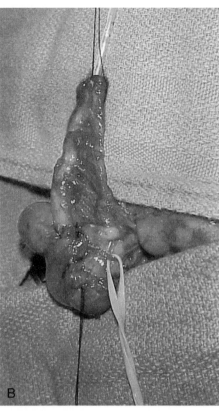

Figure 71–24. The appendix used in situ for antegrade continence enema. *A,* The appendix and its mesentery are mobilized without detachment from the cecum. Windows are carefully made in the mesentery between vessels to the proximal appendix. *B,* The teniae from either side of the cecum are approximated in those windows using permanent sutures to ensure continence of the stoma. The distal end of the appendix is brought to the abdominal wall for catheterization.

nent Lembert sutures used to approximate the cecal wall in each window. This effectively wraps the cecum around the base of the appendix to prevent spillage. Alternatively, one tenia leading to the appendix may be incised longitudinally and reapproximated at the windows of the mesoappendix. Others have made no attempt to create a continence mechanism at the appendicocecal junction, particularly surgeons performing antegrade continence enemas laparoscopically (Cadeddu and Docimo, 1999). Most MACE procedures performed by urologists are done at the time of a major reconstructive procedure involving the bladder. Long experience with construction of continent catheterizable stomas for the urinary bladder has taught them the principles to ensure a good result. Our preference would be to provide some continence mechanism at the base of the appendix in that setting to avoid any spillage.

URINARY UNDIVERSION

The role and frequency of urinary undiversion have changed dramatically over the past several decades. Before the acceptance of CIC (Lapides et al, 1976), many children were not candidates for complex reconstructive procedures because of an inability to empty afterward. Many were initially treated with permanent urinary diversions using an intestinal segment with high expectations. Over time, it became clear that such diversions had significant complications, including infection, stones, and nephropathy (Smith, 1972; Richie et al, 1974; Shapiro et al, 1975; Middleton and Hendren, 1976; Pitts and Muecke, 1979). With the recognition of those complications and the routine use of

CIC, urinary undiversion became a relatively common procedure for the reconstructive surgeon (Hendren, 1974, 1987, 1990; Perlmutter, 1980). With a better understanding of the basic pathophysiology of the urinary tract as well as better options for conservative medical management, fewer patients now require diversion. Better anesthetic and perioperative surgical care has allowed safe definitive repair of primary problems in younger infants. The occasional diversion presently done in extreme cases is usually temporary rather than permanent using bowel. Consequently, undiversion now is quite infrequent and typically involves closure of some portion of the urinary tract rather than takedown of an intestinal segment.

Permanent diversions in children are now typically confined to cancer patients with a poor prognosis and short life expectancy. When their outcome is better than expected, they may still be candidates for undiversion or a change to continent urinary diversion. The Boston group has favored initial temporary diversion with a transverse colon conduit to avoid irradiated bowel. Once the child is cured, the conduit can be converted to a continent reservoir by augmenting the colonic segment with stomach to provide an adequate reservoir and providing a continent catheterizable efferent limb (Duel et al, 1996).

The key to urinary undiversion is understanding the original pathology that led to diversion. This may be relatively easy if the surgeon involved has cared for the patient throughout the course. If the original diversion was done by someone else years previously, such understanding may be difficult and may require very thorough investigation. Accurate understanding of the underlying pathology may be made more difficult because of defunctionalization of the remaining urinary tract. It is important to review the patient's original history and studies to understand the pathophysiology before any intervention is undertaken. For example, failure of the urinary bladder in a patient with neurogenic dysfunction to respond adequately to anticholinergic medication and CIC before vesicostomy diversion might well predict that it will not do so after vesicostomy closure. Special nuances in the current evaluation may also be necessary. Urodynamic evaluation of a bladder diverted for several years with a vesicostomy will virtually always show a small capacity. A repeat study after several days of bladder cycling or occlusion of the vesicostomy may be more predictive of bladder function. The bladder may respond to bladder cycling quickly (Bauer et al, 1986; E.J. McGuire, personal communication, 1996). Temporary occlusion of a vesicostomy with a gastrostomy button may be informative (De Badiola et al, 1995). Occlusion of the vesicostomy during urodynamic studies may be necessary to achieve good bladder filling and pressure so as to accurately define the adequacy of outflow resistance. Such parameters must be evaluated before undiversion and may have changed since the time of diversion, particularly in patients with neurogenic dysfunction. Antegrade perfusion studies may be helpful and necessary when evaluating an upper tract previously diverted by ureterostomy or pyelostomy.

Correcting Original and New Pathology

It is essential that all pathophysiology is appreciated, whether it is original or new. Failure to do so can result in recurrent clinical problems for the patient (i.e., renal insufficiency, hydronephrosis, infection, and incontinence) in the face of a technically perfect operation. Once the reconstructive surgeon well understands those problems, the reconstructive options available at undiversion must be evaluated. Considerations should include the length, dilatation, and scarring of the ureters; the volume, compliance, and fibrosis of the native bladder; and the function of the outlet in terms of resistance for continence and synergistic relaxation for emptying. More global patient problems, such as renal insufficiency and neurogenic dysfunction, may influence the choices of techniques as well. In patients with an existing permanent diversion involving an intestinal segment, the quality, length, and volume of that segment should be considered to determine how it might best be used in reconstruction. An existing ileal conduit might be used as an ileal ureter, as a segment for bladder augmentation, or for tapering as a continent stoma, depending on the needs of the patient.

For examples that illustrate the potentially complex nature of many undiversion cases, the reader is referred to Dr. Hendren's chapter on undiversion in the previous edition of this text (Hendren, 1998). No one has more experience, and his cases demonstrate the total command of all surgical alternatives that is required to manage these patients, as well as the careful preoperative evaluation that allows appropriate choices to be made for each individual patient. They represent the types of patients who typically have undergone undiversion historically.

Results

Hendren (1998) reported a 26-year experience with urinary undiversion in 216 patients. Two thirds of the patients had permanent diversions, many for numerous years. Many of the patients had impaired renal function, either from their underlying problems or as morbidity related to their diversion. More than 10% of the patients required renal transplantation after undiversion, and even more were likely to require transplantation in the future, given the complex nature of their condition. With successful relief of obstruction, prevention of reflux, and provision of a compliant bladder, undiversion prolonged the time to renal failure in some patients and may have avoided it altogether in others. Undiversion may protect renal function rather than contribute to any decline if properly selected and performed.

In Hendren's series, management of the bladder was relatively straightforward and effective, with bladder augmentation as necessary. Inadequate outflow resistance was usually treated with Young-Dees-Leadbetter bladder neck repair. Most complications were related to the ureters: 23 patients required reoperation for persistent reflux and 10 for partial obstruction of the ureter. Those reoperation rates are indicative of the difficulty one faces in dealing with the short, dilated, and scarred ureters which may be present after urinary diversion (Hendren, 1998). Others have had similar good success with undiversion (Gonzalez et al, 1986; Mitchell and Rink, 1987).

The success with many of the techniques necessary for urinary undiversion should be similar to that achieved in primary reconstruction. In other words, the good results of ileocystoplasty or appendicovesicostomy should be equivalent, regardless of whether they are done as part of a urinary undiversion. As noted in Dr. Hendren's cases and series, many problems may be present and multiple techniques may be required for a given patient. **The key to achieving a good result in urinary undiversion is to understand all of the patient's problems and to correct each. The most difficult measure of complex undiversion, and the one most prone to complication, is the short, dilated, and chronically scarred ureter, which may be the residual of the original problem or of previous surgical procedures including diversion.**

In some cases of urinary undiversion, conversion to a continent urinary reservoir is appropriate. This is true of cases in which the native bladder is congenitally absent, removed, or heavily irradiated. In those rare situations, the volume and quality of the patient's native tissue may be so poor that inclusion in the reconstruction is not warranted. **In the majority of cases of urinary undiversion, reconstruction of the native urinary tract is preferable to continent diversion.** Such reconstruction can minimize the morbidity to the patient.

SUMMARY

Before reconstructive surgery for bladder and sphincter dysfunction is done, the patient must be carefully evaluated so that all problems are identified and can be addressed. The surgeon should be flexible and prepared to use the bowel segments and techniques that best fit each patient. **Although a given surgeon's result with any technique may improve with experience and confidence, each patient's unique problems and anatomy may make some choices better than others. Forcing one procedure to fit every patient should be avoided.**

Preoperative evaluation should identify the presence of upper tract obstruction or vesicoureteral reflux. Such problems should be corrected at the time of surgery. It is imperative to provide the patient with an adequate bladder or reservoir, one capable of holding at low pressure the urinary volume that is produced between voidings or catheterizations. This can be accomplished either by augmentation or by construction of a continent reservoir using any gastrointestinal segment. Each has its own set of advantages and disadvantages that should be considered. If adequate outflow resistance is lacking, it should be created at the bladder neck or at the continent catheterizable stoma to prevent incontinence. Any patient undergoing reconstructive surgery for bladder or sphincter dysfunction must be prepared and capable of performing CIC on a reliable basis; many will require it routinely, particularly those patients with neurogenic dysfunction.

As much of the patient's native urinary tract as possible should be preserved in pediatric urologic reconstruction. The urothelial lining avoids much of the morbidity associated with intestinal segments. If necessary, however, virtually any portion of the lower urinary tract may be reconstructed or replaced using intestine. Complications do sometimes occur when intestinal segments are used in this manner; they are not perfect physiologic substitutes. The most important factor in avoiding problems with such complex pediatric cases is the motivation of the patient and family to achieve a successful outcome. Assessment of that commitment is critical.

REFERENCES

Abd-El-Gawad G, Abrahamsson K, Hanson E, et al: Early and late metabolic alterations in children and adolescents with a Kock urinary reservoir. BJU Int 1999;83:285–289.

Abol-Enein H, Ghoneim MA: Serous lined extramural ileal valve: A new continent urinary outlet. J Urol 1999;161:786–791.

Adams MC, Bihrle R, Foster RS, Brito CG: Conversion of an ileal conduit to a continent, catheterizable stoma. J Urol 1992;147:126.

Adams MC, Bihrle R, Rink RC: The use of stomach in urologic reconstruction. AUA Update Series 1995;27:218–223.

Adams MC, Brock JW, 3rd, Pope JC, 4th, Rink RC: Ureterocystoplasty: Is it necessary to detubularize the distal ureter? J Urol 1998;160:851–853.

Adams MC, Mitchell ME, Rink PC: Gastrocystoplasty: An alternative solution to the problem of urological reconstruction in the severely compromised patient. J Urol 1988;140:1152–1156.

Akerlund S, Lelin K, Kock NG, et al: Renal function and upper tract configuration following urinary diversion to a continent ileal reservoir (Kock pouch): A prospective 5 to 11 year follow up after reservoir construction. J Urol 1989;142:964.

Alfrey EJ, Salvatierra O, Jr, Tanney DC, et al: Bladder augmentation can be problematic with renal failure and transplantation. Pediatr Nephrol 1997;11:672–675.

Aliabadi H, Gonzalez R: Success of the artificial urinary sphincter after failed surgery for incontinence. J Urol 1990;143:987.

Allen T, Peters PC, Sagalowaky A: The Camey procedure: Preliminary results in 11 patients. World J Urol 1985;3:167.

Anderson PAM, Rickwood AMK: Detrusor hyperreflexia as a factor in spontaneous perforation of augmentation cystoplasty for neuropathic bladder. Br J Urol 1991;67:210–212.

Aprikian A, Berardinucci G, Pike J, et al: Experience with the AS800 artificial sphincter in myelodysplastic children. Can J Surg 1992;35:396.

Ashcraft KW, Dennis PA: The reimplanted ureter as a catheterizing stoma. J Pediatr Surg 1986;21:1042.

Asif S, Uehling DT: Successful pregnancy following ureteroileostomy. Am J Obstet Gynecol 1969;105:641.

Asken MH: Urinary cecal reservoir. In King LR, Stone AR, Webster GD (eds): Bladder Reconstruction and Continent Urinary Diversion. Chicago, Year Book Medical Publishers, 1987, pp 238–251.

Atala A, Bauer SB, Hendren WH, et al: The effect of gastric augmentation on bladder function. J Urol 1993a;149:1099.

Atala A, Freeman MR, Vacanti JP, et al: Implantation in vivo and retrieval of urothelial structures consisting of rabbit and human bladder muscle. J Urol 1993b;150:608.

Atala A, Lailas NG, Cilento BG, Retik AB: Progressive ureteral dilation for subsequent ureterocystoplasty. Presented at the Section on Urology Meeting, American Academy of Pediatrics, Dallas, TX, 1994.

Atala A, Vacanti JP, Peters CA, et al: Formation of urothelial structures in vivo from disassociated cells attached to biodegradable polymer scaffolds. J Urol 1992;148:658.

Austin PF, DeLeary G, Homsy YL, et al: Long-term metabolic advantages of a gastrointestinal composite urinary reservoir. J Urol 1997;158:1704–1707.

Austin PF, Rink RC, Lockhart JL: The gastrointestinal composite urinary reservoir in patients with myelomeningocele and exstrophy: Long-term metabolic follow-up. J Urol 1999;162:1126–1128.

Badiola F, Gosalbez R, Ruiz E, et al: The posterior approach for bladder neck dissection. Br J Urol 2000;85:59.

Barrett DM, Parulkar BG, Kramer SA: Experience with AS800 artificial sphincter in pediatric and young adult patients. Urology 1993;42:431.

Barrington JW, Fulford S, Griffiths D, Stephenson TP: Tumors in bladder remnant after augmentation enterocystoplasty. J Urol 1997;157:482–486.

Barthold JS, Rodriquez E, Freedman AL, et al: Results of the rectus fascial sling and wrap procedures for the treatment of neurogenic sphincteric incontinence. J Urol 1999;161:272.

Bau MO, Younes S, Aupy A, et al: Continent catheterizable stoma for Mitrofanoff or Malone procedures: Satisfaction index and psychological impact—the patient's perspective. Presented at the Annual Meeting of the European Society of Pediatric Urologists, Tours, France, June 2000.

Bauer SB: Pediatric neurology. In Krane RJ, Sioky MB (eds): Clinical Neurourology. Boston, Little, Brown, 1979, pp 275–294.

Bauer SB, Hallett M, Khoshbin S, et al: Predictive value of urodynamic evaluation in newborns with myelodysplasia. JAMA 1984;252:650.

Bauer SB, Hendren WH, Kozakewich H, et al: Perforation of the augmented bladder. J Urol 1992;148:699.

Bauer SB, Joseph DB: Management of the obstructed urinary tract associated with neurogenic bladder dysfunction. Urol Clin North Am 1990;17:395.

Bauer SB, Peters CA, Colodny AH, et al: The use of rectus fascia to manage urinary incontinence. J Urol 1989;142:516.

Bauer SB, Reda EF, Colodny AH, Retik AB: Detrusor instability: A delayed complication in association with the artificial sphincter. J Urol 1986;135:1212.

Beisang AA, Ersek RA: Mammalian response to subdermal implantation of textured microimplants. Aesthetic Plast Surg 1992;16:83.

Bellinger MF: Ureterocystoplasty: A unique method for vesical augmentation in children. J Urol 1993;149:811–813.

Belman AB, Kaplan GW: Experience with the Kropp anti-continence procedure. J Urol 1989;141:1160.

Benchekroun A: Continent cecal bladder. Br J Urol 1982;54:505–506.

Benchekroun A, Essakalli N, Faik M, et al: Continent urostomy with hydraulic valve in 136 patients: 13 Years of experience. J Urol 1989;142:46.

Benson MC, Olsson CA: Continent urinary diversion. In Walsh PC, Retik AB, Vaughn ED, Jr, Wein AJ (eds): Campbell's Urology, 7th ed. Philadelphia, WB Saunders, 1998, pp 3190–3245.

Bent AE, Tutrone RF, Lloyd K, et al: Treatment of intrinsic sphincter deficiency using autologous ear cartilage as a periurethral bulking agent. J Urol 2000;163:75.

Berglund B, Kock NG, Norlen L, Philipson BM: Volume capacity and pressure characteristics of the continent ileal reservoir used for urinary diversion. J Urol 1987;137:29.

Bihrle R: The Indiana pouch continent urinary reservoir. Urol Clin North Am 1997;24:773.

Bihrle R, Klee LW, Adams MC, Foster RS: The clinical experience with the transverse colon-gastric tube continent urinary reservoir. J Urol 1991;146:751.

Blaivas JG, Labib KB, Bauer SB: A new approach to electromyography of the external urethral sphincter. J Urol 1977;117:773.

Blyth B, Ewalt DH, Duckett JW, Snyder HM: Lithogenic properties of enterocystoplasty. J Urol 1992;148:575.

Bogaert GA, Mevorach RA, Kim J, et al: The physiology of gastrocystoplasty: Once a stomach, always a stomach. J Urol 1995;153:1977.

Bomalaski MD, Bloom DA, McGuire EJ, et al: Glutaraldehyde cross-lined collagen in the treatment of urinary incontinence in children. J Urol 1996;155:699.

Bosco PJ, Bauer SB, Colodny AH, et al: The long-term results of artificial sphincters in children. J Urol 1991;146:396–399.

Boyd SD, Schiff WM, Skinner DG, et al: Prospective study of metabolic abnormalities in patients with continent Kock pouch urinary diversion. Urology 1989;33:85–88.

Brading AF: Alterations in the physiological properties of urinary bladder smooth muscle caused by bladder emptying against an obstruction. Scand J Urol Nephrol Suppl 1997;184:51–58.

Braverman RM, Lebowitz RL: Perforation of the augmented urinary bladder in nine children and adolescents: Importance of cystography. AJR Am J Roentgenol 1991;157:1059.

Bruce RG, McRoberts JW: Cecoappendico-vesicostomy: Conduit-lengthening technique for use in continent urinary reconstruction. Urology 1998;52:702–704.

Burbige KA, Reitelman C, Olsson CA: Complications of artificial urinary sphincter around intestinal segments in reconstructed exstrophy patients. J Urol 1987;138:1123.

Bushinsky DA: Net calcium efflux from live bone during chronic metabolic but not respiratory acidosis. Am J Physiol 1989;256:F836.

Buson H, Castro-Diaz D, Manivel JC, et al: The development of tumors in experimental gastroenterocystoplasty. J Urol 1993;150:730.

Buson H, Manivel JC, Dayanc M, et al: Seromuscular colocystoplasty lined with urothelium: Experimental study. Urology 1994;44:743–748.

Cadeddu JA, Docimo SG: Laparoscopic-assisted continent stomas procedures: Our new standard. Urology 1999;54:909–912.

Cain MP, Casale AJ, King SJ, Rink RC: Appendicovesicostomy and newer alternatives for the Mitrofanoff procedure: Results in the last 100 patients at Riley Children's Hospital. J Urol 1999;162:1749–1752.

Cain MP, Husmann DA: Cecal bladder augmentation with a tapered catheterizable stoma: A modification of the Indiana pouch. Presented at the Urology Section Meeting, American Academy of Pediatrics, Dallas, TX, 1994.

Camey M, Richard F, Botto H: Ileal replacement of bladder. In King LS, Stone AR, Webster GD (eds): Bladder Reconstruction and Continent Urinary Diversion. St. Louis, Mosby–Year Book, 1991, p 389.

Canning DA, Perman JA, Jeffs RD, Gearhart JP: Nutritional consequences of bowel segments in the lower urinary tract. J Urol 1989;142:509.

Canning DC: Continent urinary diversion. In King LR (ed): Urologic Surgery in Infants and Children. Philadelphia, WB Saunders, 1998; 139–161.

Capozza N, Caione P, deGennaro M, et al: Endoscopic treatment of vesico-ureteric reflux and urinary incontinence: Technical problems in the paediatric patient. Br J Urol 1995;75:538.

Carr MC, Docimo SG, Mitchell ME: Bladder augmentation with urothelial preservation. J Urol 1999;162:1133–1137.

Carr LK, Herschorn S: Early development of adenocarcinoma in a young woman following augmentation cystoplasty for undiversion. J Urol 1997;157:2255–2256.

Cartwright PC, Snow BW: Bladder autoaugmentation: Early clinical experience. J Urol 1989a;142:505.

Cartwright PC, Snow BW: Bladder augmentation: Partial detrusor excision to augment the bladder without use of bowel. J Urol 1989b;142:1050.

Casale AJ: A long continent ileovesicostomy using a single piece of bowel. J Urol 1999;162:1743–1745.

Casale AJ: Continent vesicostomy: A new method utilizing only bladder tissue. (Abstract 72.) Presented at the 60th annual meeting of the American Academy of Pediatrics, New Orleans, LA, 1991.

Casale AJ, Such RS, DeMarco RT, et al: The microbiology of bladder augmentation in children. Presented at the Section on Urology Meeting, American Academy of Pediatrics. Washington, DC, 1999.

Castellan MA, Gosalbez R, Labbie A, Monti PR: Clinical applications of the Monti procedure as a continent catheterizable stoma. Urology 1999; 54:152–156.

Castro-Diaz D, Froemming C, Manivel JC, et al: The influence of urinary diversion on experimental gastrocystoplasty. J Urol 1992;148:571–574.

Celayir S, Buyukunal C, Dervisoglu S, Kilic N: Urodynamic investigations in reversed seromuscular enterocystoplasty (RSMEC): An experimental study in a rabbit model. Presented at the Section on Urology Meeting, American Academy of Pediatrics, San Francisco, CA, 1995.

Celayir S, Goksel S, Buyulunal SN: The relationship between *Helicobacter pylori* infection and acid-hematuria syndrome in pediatric patients with gastric augmentation-II. J Pediatr Surg 1999;34:532–535.

Chargi A, Charbonneau J, Gauthier G: Colocystoplasty for bladder enlargement and bladder substitution: A study of late results in 31 cases. J Urol 1967;97:849.

Churchill BN, Aliabadi H, Landau EH, et al: Ureteral bladder augmentation. J Urol 1993;150:716–720.

Churchill BM, Gilmour RF, Khoury AE, McLorie GA: Biological response of bladders rendered continent by insertion of artificial sphincter. J Urol 1987;138:1116.

Cilento BG, Freeman MR, Scheneck FX: Phenotypic and cytogenetic characterization of human bladder urothelia expanded in vitro. J Urol 1994;152:665–670.

Coffey RC: Physiologic implantation of the severed ureter or common bile duct into the intestine. JAMA 1911;56:387.

Cohen RA, Rushton HG, Belman AB, et al: Renal scarring and vesicoureteral reflux in children with myelodysplasia. J Urol 1990;144:541.

Couvelair R: La "Petite Vessle" des tuberculeaux genitourinaires: Essai de classification place et variantes des cysto-intestinoplasties. J Urol 1950; 56:381.

Crane JM, Scherz HS, Billman GF, Kaplan GW: Ischemic necrosis: A hypothesis to explain the pathogenesis of spontaneously ruptured enterocystoplasty. J Urol 1991;146:141–144.

Creagh TA, McInerney PD, Thomas PJ, Mundy AR: Pregnancy after lower urinary tract reconstruction in women. J Urol 1995;154:1323–1324.

Cromie WJ, Barada JH, Weingarten JL: Cecal tubularization: Lengthening technique for creation of catheterizable conduit. Urology 1991;37:41.

Curry JI, Osborne A, Malone PS: The MACE procedure: Experience in the United Kingdom. J Pediatr Surg 1999;34:338–340.

Dayanc M, Kilciler M, Tan O, Gokalp A, et al: A new approach to bladder augmentation in children: Seromuscular enterocystoplasty. BJU Int 1999;84:103–107.

De Badiola F, Manivel JC, Gonzalez R: Seromuscular enterocystoplasty in rats. J Urol 1991;146:559–562.

De Badiola F, Ruiz E, Denes E, et al: New application of the gastrostomy button for clinical and urodynamic evaluation prior to vesicostomy closure. Presented at the Section on Urology Meeting, American Academy of Pediatrics, San Francisco, CA, 1995.

De Badiola F, Ruiz E, Puigdevall J, et al: Seromuscular sigmoidcystoplasty. Presented at the Section on Urology Meeting, American Academy of Pediatrics, Washington, DC, 1999.

Decter RM: Use of the fascial sling for neurogenic incontinence: Lessons learned. J Urol 1993;150:683.

Decter RM, Harpser L: Pitfalls in determination of the leak point pressure. J Urol 1992;148:588–591.

Dees JE: Congenital epispadias with incontinence. J Urol 1949;62:513.

DeKernion JB, Den Besten L, Kaufman J, Ehrlich R: The Kock pouch as a urinary reservoir: Pitfalls and perspectives. Am J Surg 1985;150:83.

Demos MP: Radioactive electrolyte absorption studies of small bowel comparison of different segments for use in urinary diversion. J Urol 1962;88:638.

Denes ED, Vates TS, Freedman AL, Gonzalez R: Seromuscular colocystoplasty lined with urothelium protects dogs from acidosis during ammonium chloride loading. J Urol 1997;158:1075–1080.

Dewan PA, Byard R: Autoaugmentation gastrocystoplasty in a sheep model. Br J Urol 1993;72:56–59.

Dewan PA, Blose CE, Byard RW, et al: Enteric mucosal regrowth after bladder augmentation using demucosalized gut segments. J Urol 1997; 158:1141–1146.

Dewan PA, Nicholls EA, Goh DW: Ureterocystoplasty: An extraperitoneal urothelial bladder augmentation technique. Eur Urol 1994a;26:85–89.

Dewan PA, Stefanek W: Autoaugmentation gastrocystoplasty: Early clinical results. Br J Urol 1994;74:460–464.

Dewan PA, Stefanek W, Lorenz D, Byard RW: Autoaugmentation omentoplasty in a sheep model. Urology 1994b;43:888–891.

Diokno AC, Sonda LP: Compatibility of genitourinary prostheses and intermittent self-catheterization. J Urol 1981;125:659.

Donnahoo KK, Rink RC, Cain MP, Casale AJ: The Young-Dees-Leadbetter bladder neck repair for neurogenic incontinence. J Urol 1999;161: 1946–1949.

Duckett JW, Lofti AH: Appendicovesicostomy (and variations) in bladder reconstruction. J Urol 1993;149:567.

Duckett JW, Snyder HM III: Continent urinary diversion: Variation on the Mitrofanoff principle. J Urol 1986;135:58.

Duckett JW, Snyder HM III: The Mitrofanoff principle in continent urinary reservoirs. Semin Urol 1987;5:55.

Duel BP, Hendren WH, Bauer SB, et al: Reconstructive options in genitourinary rhabdomyosarcoma. J Urol 1996;156:1798.

Ehrlich RM, Gershman A: Laparoscopic seromyotomy (autoaugmentation) for non-neurogenic neurogenic bladder in a child: Initial case report. Urology 1993;42:175–178.

Elder JS: Periurethral and puboprostatic sling repair for incontinence in patients with myelodysplasia. J Urol 1990;144:434.

Elder JS, Snyder HM, Hulbert WC, Duckett JW: Perforation of the augmented bladder in patients undergoing clean intermittent catheterization. J Urol 1988;140:1159–1162.

El-Ghoneimi A, Muller C, Guys JM, et al: Functional outcome and specific complications of gastrocystoplasty for failed bladder exstrophy closure. J Urol 1998;160:1186–1189.

Eraklus AJ, Folkman MJ: Adenocarcinoma at the site of ureterosigmoidostomies for exstrophy of the bladder. J Pediatr Surg 1978;13:730.

Essig KA, Sheldon CA, Brandt MT, et al: Elevated intravesical pressure causes arterial hypoperfusion in canine colocystoplasty: A fluorometric assessment. J Urol 1991;146:551–553.

Fauza DO, Fishman SJ, Mehegan K, Atala A: Videofetoscopically assisted fetal tissue engineering: Bladder augmentation. J Pediatr Surg 1998;33:7–12.

Ferris DO, Odel HM: Electrolyte pattern of the blood after bilateral ureterosigmoidostomy. JAMA 1950;142:634–641.

Fichtner J, Fischer R, Hohenfellner R: Appendiceal continence mechanisms in continent urinary diversion. World J Urol 1997;157:635–637.

Filmer RB, Spencer JR: Malignancies in bladder augmentations and intestinal conduits. J Urol 1990;143:671.

Finkbeiner AE: In vitro responses of detrusor smooth muscle to stretch and relaxation. Scand J Urol Nephrol Suppl 1999;201:5–11.

Fisch M, Wammack R, Hohenfellner R: The sigma rectum pouch (MAINZ pouch II). World J Urol 1996;14:68–72.

Fishman IJ, Flores FN, Scott FB, et al: Use of fresh placental membranes for bladder reconstruction. J Urol 1987;138:1291–1294.

Fowler JE, Jr: Continent urinary reservoirs. Surg Ann 1988;20:201–225.

Furlow WL: Implantation of a new semiautomatic artificial genitourinary sphincter: Experience with primary activation and deactivation in 47 patients. J Urol 1981;126:741.

Ganesan GS, Mitchell ME, Adams MC, et al: Use of stomach for reconstruction of the lower urinary tract in patients with compromised renal function. Presented at the Urology Section Meeting, American Academy of Pediatrics, New Orleans, LA, 1991.

Ganesan G, Nguyen DH, Adams MC, et al: Lower urinary tract reconstruction using stomach and the artificial sphincter. J Urol 1993;149: 1107.

Gearhart JP: Mucus secretions in augmented bladder. Dialog Pediatr Urol 1987;10:6.

Gearhart JP, Albertsen PC, Marchall FF, et al: Pediatric applications of augmentation cystoplasty: The Johns Hopkins experience. J Urol 1986; 136:430.

Gerharz EW, Kohl U, Weingartner K, et al: Complications related to different continence mechanism in ileocecal reservoirs. J Urol 1997; 158:1709–1713.

Gerharz EW, Kohl UN, Weingartner K, et al: Experience with the MAINZ modification of ureterosigmoidostomy. Br J Surg 1999;86:427.

Gerharz EW, Tassadaq T, Pickard RS, et al: Transverse retubularized ileum: Early clinical experience with a new second line Mitrofanoff tube. J Urol 1998;159:525–528.

Gilchrist RK, Merricks JW, Hamlin HH, Rieger IT: Construction of a substitute bladder and urethra. Surg Gynecol Obstet 1950;90:752.

Gleeson MJ, Griffith DP: The use of alloplastic biomaterials in bladder substitution. J Urol 1992;148:1377–1382.

Goldwasser B, Barrett DM, Webster GD, et al: Cystometric properties of ileum and right colon after bladder augmentation, substitution or replacement. J Urol 1987;138:1007.

Goldwasser B, Webster GD: Augmentation and substitution enterocystoplasty. J Urol 1986;135:215–224.

Gonzalez R: Clinical and urodynamic evaluation after ureterocystoplasty. (Discussion.) J Urol 1999;162:1132.

Gonzalez R, Buson H, Reid C, Reinbert Y: Seromuscular colocystoplasty lined with urothelium: Experience with 16 patients. Urology 1994;45: 124–129.

Gonzalez R, Cabral BHP: Rectal continence after enterocystoplasty. Dialog Pediatr Urol 1987;10:3–4.

Gonzalez R, Koleilat N, Austin C, et al: The artificial sphincter AS800 in congenital urinary incontinence. J Urol 1989a;142:512–515.

Gonzalez R, Merino FG, Vaughn M: Long-term results of the artificial urinary sphincter in male patients with neurogenic bladder. J Urol 1995;154:769.

Gonzalez R, Mguyet DH, Koleilat N, et al: Compatibility of enterocystoplasty and the artificial urinary sphincter. J Urol 1989b;142:502.

Gonzalez R, Reinberg Y: Localization of bacteriuria in patients with enterocystoplasty and nonrefluxing conduits. J Urol 1987;138:1104–1105.

Gonzalez R, Sidi A, Zhang G: Urinary undiversion: Indications, technique and results in 50 cases. J Urol 1986;136:13–16.

Goodwin WE, Harris AP, Kaufman JJ, Beal JM: Open, transcolonic ureterointestinal anastomosis. Surg Gynecol Obstet 1953;97:295–330.

Goodwin WE, Winter CC, Barker WF: "Cup-patch" technique of ileocystoplasty for bladder enlargement or partial substitution. Surg Gynecol Obstet 1959;108:240–244.

Gormley EA, Bloom DA, McGuire EJ, et al: Pubovaginal slings for the management of urinary incontinence in female adolescents. J Urol 1994;152:822.

Gosalbez R, Jr, Gousse AE: Reconstruction and undiversion of the short or severely dilated ureter: The antireflux ileal nipple revisited. J Urol 1998;159:530–534.

Gosalbez R, Wei D, Gousse A, et al: Refashioned short bowel segments for the construction of catheterizable channels (the Monti procedure): Early clinical experience. J Urol 1998;160:1099–1102.

Gosalbez R, Jr, Woodard JR, Broecker BH, et al: The use of stomach in pediatric urinary reconstruction. J Urol 1993a;150:438.

Gosalbez R, Jr, Woodard JR, Broecker BH, et al: Metabolic complications of the use of stomach for urinary reconstruction. J Urol 1993b;150: 710–712.

Gregoire M, Kantoff P, DeWolf WC: Synchronous adenocarcinoma and transitional cell carcinoma of the bladder associated with augmentation: Case report and review of the literature. J Urol 1993;149:115.

Gros DA, Dodson JL, Lopatin UA, et al: Decreased linear growth associated with intestinal bladder augmentation in children with bladder exstrophy. J Urol 2000;164:917.

Guttmann L, Frankel H: The value of intermittent self catheterization in the early management of traumatic paraplegia and tetraplegia. Paraplegia 1966;4:63–84.

Guys JM, Simeoni-Alias J, Fakhro A, Delarue A: Use of polydimethylsiloxane for endoscopic treatment of neurogenic urinary incontinence in children. J Urol 1999;162:2133–2135.

Guzman JM, Montes de Oca L, Gonzalez R, et al: Modified Benchekroun technique for continent ileal stoma. J Urol 1989;142:1431.

Hall MC, Koch MO, McDougal WS: Metabolic consequences of urinary diversion through intestinal segments. Urol Clin North Am 1991;18: 725.

Hampel N, Hasan ST, Marshall C, Neal DE: Continent urinary diversion using the Mitrofanoff principle. Br J Urol 1995;74:454–459.

Hanna MK, Bloiso G: Continent diversion in children: Modification of Kock pouch. J Urol 1987;137:1206.

Hanna MK, Richter F, Stock JA: Salvage continent vesicostomy after enterocystoplasty in the absence of the appendix. J Urol 1999;162:826–828.

Harris CF, Cooper CS, Hutcheson JC, Snyder HM: Appendicovesicostomy: The Mitrofanoff procedure—a 15-year perspective. J Urol 2000; 163:1922–1926.

Hatch TR, Steinberg RW, Davis LE: Successful term delivery by cesarean section in a patient with a continent ileocecal urinary reservoir. J Urol 1991;146:1111.

Hedican SP, Schulam PG, Docimo SG: Laparoscopic assisted reconstructive surgery. J Urol 1999;161:267–270.

Hedlund H, Lindstrom K, Mansson W: Dynamics of a continent cecal reservoir for urinary diversion. Br J Urol 1984;56:366–372.

Heidler H, Marberger M, Hohenfellner R: The metabolic situation in ureterosigmoidostomy. Eur Urol 1979;5:39–44.

Helal M, Pow-Sang J, Sanford E, et al: Direct (nontunneled) ureterocolonic reimplantation in association with continent reservoirs. J Urol 1993;150:835–837.

Hendren WH: Urinary tract refunctionalization after prior diversion in children. Ann Surg 1974;180:494–510.

Hendren WH: Techniques for urinary undiversion. In King LR, Stone AR, Webster GD (eds): Reconstruction and Continent Urinary Diversion. Chicago, Year Book Medical Publishers, 1987, p 101.

Hendren WH: Urinary tract refunctionalization after long-term diversion: A 20 year experience with 177 patients. Ann Surg 1990;212:478–495.

Hendren WH: Urinary undiversion: Refunctionalization of the previously diverted urinary tract. In Walsh PC, Retik AB, Vaughan ED, Jr, Wein AJ (eds): Campbell's Urology. Philadelphia, WB Saunders, 1998, p 3247.

Hendren WH, Hendren RB: Bladder augmentation: Experience with 129 cases in children and young adults. J Urol 1990;144:445–453.

Hendren WH, Hensle TW: Transureteroureterostomy: Experience with 75 cases. J Urol 1980;123:826–833.

Hensle TW, Reiley EA, Chang DT: The Malone antegrade continence enema procedure in the management of patients with spina bifida. J Am Coll Surg 1998;186:669–674.

Hensle TW, Ring KS: Urinary tract reconstruction in children. Urol Clin North Am 1991;18:701–715.

Hill DE, Chantigian PM, Kramer SA: Pregnancy after augmentation cystoplasty. Surg Gynecol Obstet 1990;170:485.

Hinman F, Jr: Selection of intestinal segments for bladder substitution: Physical and physiological characteristics. J Urol 1988;139:519.

Hirst G: Ileal and colonic cystoplasties. Prob Urol 1991;5:223.

Hochstetler JA, Flanigan MJ, Kreder KJ: Impaired bone growth after ileal augmentation cystoplasty. J Urol 1997;157:1873–1879.

Hodges CV, Moore RJ, Lehman TH, Behnam AM: Clinical experiences with transureteroureterostomy. J Urol 1963;90:552–562.

Hohenfellner R, Riedmiller H, Thuroff JW: Commentary: The MAINZ pouch. In Whitehead ED (ed): Current Operative Urology. Philadelphia, JB Lippincott, 1990, p 168.

Hollensbe DW, Adams MC, Rink RC, et al: Comparison of different gastrointestinal segments for bladder augmentation. Presented at the American Urological Association Meeting, Washington, DC, 1992.

Hoover DL, Duckett JW: Posterior urethral valves, unilateral reflux and renal dysplasia: A syndrome. J Urol 1982;128:994.

Horowitz M, Kuhr CS, Mitchell ME: The Mitrofanoff catheterizable channel: Patient acceptance. J Urol 1995;153:771.

Horowitz M, Mitchell ME: DAWG procedure (demucosalized augmentation with gastric segment). Presented at the Genitourinary Reconstructive Surgeon's Meeting, San Francisco, CA, 1993.

Horowitz M, Mitchell ME, Nguyen DH: The DAWG procedure: Gastrocystoplasty made better. J Urol 1994;151:503A.

Husmann DA, Cain M: Colocecal bladder augmentation with a tapered continent ileal limb: Use in the neuropathic bladder. Presented at the Section on Urology Meeting, American Academy of Pediatrics, Washington, DC, 1999.

Husmann DA, Spence HM: Current status of tumor of the bowel following ureterosigmoidostomy: A review. J Urol 1990;144:607.

Jakobsen H, Steven K, Stigsby B, et al: Pathogenesis of nocturnal urinary incontinence after ileocecal bladder replacement: Continuous measurement of urethral closure pressure during sleep. Br J Urol 1987;59:148–152.

Jayanthi VR, Churchill BM, McLorie GA, Khoury AE: Concomitant bladder neck closure and Mitrofanoff diversion for the management of intractable urinary incontinence. J Urol 1995;154:886.

Jawaheer G, Rangecroft L: The Pippi Salle procedure for neurogenic urinary incontinence in childhood: A three-year experience. Eur J Pediatr Surg 1999;9:9–11.

Johnson HW, Nigro MK, Stothers L, et al: Laboratory variables of autoaugmentation in an animal model. Urology 1994;44:260–263.

Joseph DB: The effect of medium-fill and slow-fill saline cystometry on compliance and detrusor pressure in infants and children with myelodysplasia. J Urol 1992;143:441–446.

Joseph DB: The use of iothalamate meglumine 17.2% as an effective testing medium in lower urinary tract urodynamic assessment of children. J Urol 1993;149:92.

Joseph DB: Neurogenic bladder dysfunction and myelodysplasia. In Krane RJ, Siroky MB, Fitzpatrick JM (eds): Clinical Urology. Philadelphia, JB Lippincott, 1994, pp 798–813.

Joseph DB: Urodynamics in the pediatric population: Indication and techniques. In Elder JS (ed): Pediatric Urology for the General Urologist. New York, Igaku-Shoin Publishers, 1996, pp 188–201.

Jumper BM, McLorie GA, Churchill BM, et al: Effects of the artificial

urinary sphincter on prostatic development and sexual function in pubertal boys with meningomyelocele. J Urol 1990;144:438.

Kaefer M, Hendren WH, Bauer SB, et al: Reservoir calculi: A comparison of reservoirs constructed from stomach and other enteric segments. J Urol 1998;160:2187–2190.

Kaefer M, Keating MA, Adams MC, Rink RC: Posterior urethral valves, pressure pop-offs and bladder function. J Urol 1995;154:708–711.

Kaefer M, McLaughlin KP, Rink RC, et al: Upsizing of the artificial urinary sphincter cuff to facilitate spontaneous voiding. Urol 1997a;50:106–109.

Kaefer M, Retik AB: The Mitrofanoff principle in continent urinary reconstruction. Urol Clin North Am 1997;24:795–811.

Kaefer M, Rink RC, Cain MP, Casale AJ: Stomal stenosis: Is ileum the ideal substrate for efferent limb construction. Presented at the American Academy of Pediatrics, Washington, DC, October 1999.

Kaefer M, Rink RC, Casale A, Cain M: Stomas stenosis: Appendicovesicostomy vs. appendicocecostomy. Presented at the American Academy of Pediatrics, Urology Section Meeting, Chicago, October 2000.

Kaefer M, Tobin MS, Hendren WH, et al: Continent urinary diversion: The Children's Hospital experience. J Urol 1997b;157:1394–1399.

Kajbafzadeh AM, Chubak N: Simultaneous Malone Antegrade Continent Enema (MACE) and Mitrofanoff principle, using the divided appendix and report of the "V.Q.Q." and "V.Q." technique for prevention of complications at stoma level. Presented at the European Society of Pediatric Urology/American Academy of Pediatrics, Urology Section Meeting, Tours, France, June 2000.

Kajbafzadeh AM, Duffy PG, Carr B, et al: A review of 100 Mitrofanoff stomas and reports of the VQZ technique for prevention of complications at the stomal level. Presented at The European Society of Pediatric Urology Meeting, Toledo, Spain, 1995.

Kakizaki H, Shibata T, Shinno Y, et al: Fascial sling for the management of urinary incontinence due to sphincter incompetence. J Urol 1995;153:644.

Kambic H, Kay R, Chen JF, et al: Biodegradable pericardial implants for bladder augmentation: A 2.5 year study in dogs. J Urol 1992;148:539–543.

Keating MA, Rink RC, Adams MC: Appendicovesicostomy: A useful adjunct to continent reconstruction of the bladder. J Urol 1993;149:1091.

Kelami A: Lyophilized human dura as a bladder wall substitute: Experimental and clinical results. J Urol 1971;105:518–522.

Kennedy HA, Adams MC, Mitchell ME, et al: Chronic renal failure and bladder augmentation: Stomach versus sigmoid colon in the canine model. J Urol 1988;140:1138–1140.

Kennedy WA, Hensle TW, Reiley EA, et al: Pregnancy after orthotopic continent urinary diversion. Gynecol Obstet 1993;177:405.

Khoury AE, Salomon M, Doche R, et al: Stone formation after augmentation cystoplasty: The role of intestinal mucus. J Urol 1997;158:1133–1137.

King LR: Protection of the upper tracts in children. In King LR, Stone AR, Webster GD (eds): Bladder Reconstruction and Continent Urinary Diversion. Chicago, Year Book Medical Publishers, 1987, p 127.

King LR: Cystoplasty in children. In King LR, Stone AR, Webster GD (eds): Bladder Reconstruction and Continent Urinary Diversion, 2nd ed. St. Louis, Mosby–Year Book, 1991, pp 115–125.

Kirsch AJ, Olsson CA, Hensle TW: Pediatric continent reservoirs and colocystoplasty created with absorbable staples. J Urol 1996;156:614–617.

Klee LW, Hooever DM, Mitchell ME, Rink RC: Long-term effects of gastrocystoplasty in rats. J Urol 1990;144:1283.

Koch MO, McDougal WS: The pathophysiology of hyperchloremic metabolic acidosis after urinary diversion through intestinal segments. Surgery 1985;98:561–570.

Koch MO, McDougal WS: Bony demineralization following ureterosigmoid anastomosis: An experimental study in rats. J Urol 1988;140:856.

Kock NG: Internal "reservoir" in patients with permanent ileostomy: Preliminary observations on a procedure resulting in fecal "continence" in five ileostomy patients. Arch Surg 1969;99:223.

Kock NG, Berglund B, Ghoneim MA, et al: Urinary diversion to the augmented and valved rectum: An experimental study in dogs. Scand J Urol Nephrol 1988a;22:227–233.

Kock NG, Ghoneim MA, Lycke KG, Mahran MR: Urinary diversion to the augmented and valved rectum: Preliminary results with a novel surgical procedure. J Urol 1988b;140:1375–1379.

Koff SA: Guidelines to determine the size and shape of intestinal segments used for reconstruction. J Urol 1988;140:1150.

Koff SA, Cirulli C, Wise HA: Clinical and urodynamic features of a new intestinal urinary sphincter for continent urinary diversion. J Urol 1989; 142:293.

Koraitim MM, Khalil MR, Ali GA, Foda MK: Micturition after gastrocystoplasty and gastric bladder replacement. J Urol 1999;161:1480–1484.

Koyle MA, Kaji DM, Duque M, et al: The Malone antegrade continence enema for neurogenic and structural fecal incontinence and constipation. J Urol 1995;154:759–761.

Kronner KM, Casale AJ, Cain MP, et al: Bladder calculi in the pediatric augmented bladder. J Urol 1998a;160:1096–1098.

Kronner KM, Rink RC, Simmons G, et al: Artificial urinary sphincter in the treatment of urinary incontinence: Preoperative urodynamics do not predict the need for future bladder augmentation. J Urol 1998b;160:1093–1095.

Kropp BP, Eppley BL, Prevel CD, et al: Experimental assessment of small intestine submucosa as a bladder wall substitute. Urology 1995;46:396–400.

Kropp BP, Rink RC, Adams MC, et al: Bladder outlet reconstruction: Fate of the silicone sheath. J Urol 1993;150:703.

Kropp KA: Bladder neck reconstruction in children. Urol Clin North Am 1999;26:661–672.

Kropp KA, Angwafo FF: Urethral lengthening and reimplantation for neurogenic incontinence in children. J Urol 1986;135:533.

Kryger JV, Spencer Barthold J, Fleming P: The outcome of artificial urinary sphincter placement after a mean 15 years' follow-up in a paediatric population. Br J Urol 1999;83:1026–1031.

Kryger JV, Gonzalez R, Spencer Barthold J: Surgical management of urinary incontinence in children with neurogenic sphincteric incompetence. J Urol 2000;163:256–263.

Kulb TB, Rink RC, Mitchell ME: Gastrocystoplasty in azotemic canines. Presented at the American Urological Association, North Central Section Meeting, Palm Springs, FL, 1986.

Kurzrock EA, Baskin LS, Kogan BA: Gastrocystoplasty: Long-term follow-up. J Urol 1998;160:2182–2186.

Landa HM, Moorhead JD: Detrusorectomy. Probl Pediatr Urol 1994;8:204–209.

Landau EH, Jayanthi VR, Khoury AE, et al: Bladder augmentation: Ureterocystoplasty versus ileocystoplasty. J Urol 1994;152:716–719.

Lapides J, Diokno AC, Gould FR, Low BS: Further observations on self-catheterization. J Urol 1976;116:169–171.

Lapides J, Diokno AC, Silbert SJ, Lowe BS: Clean intermittent self-catheterization in the treatment of urinary tract disease. J Urol 1972;107:458.

Leadbetter GW: Surgical correction of total urinary incontinence. J Urol 1964;91:261.

Leadbetter GW: Surgical reconstruction for complete urinary incontinence: A 10 to 22 year follow-up. J Urol 1985;133:205.

Leadbetter WF, Clarke BG: Five years' experience with uretero-enterostomy by the "combined" technique. J Urol 1954;73:67–82.

LeDuc A, Camey M, Teillac P: An original antireflux ureteroileal implantation technique: Long-term follow-up. J Urol 1987;137:1156–1158.

Leng WW, Blalock HJ, Fredriksson WH, et al: Enterocystoplasty or detrusor myectomy? Comparison of indications and outcomes for bladder augmentation. J Urol 1999;161:758–763.

Leonard MP, Canning DA, Epstein JI, et al: Local tissue reaction to the suburethral injection of glutaraldehyde cross-linked bovine collagen in humans. J Urol 1990a;143:1209.

Leonard MP, Dharamsi N, Williot PE: Outcome of gastrocystoplasty in tertiary pediatric urology practice. Presented at the Section on Urology Meeting, American Academy of Pediatrics, Washington, DC, 1999.

Leonard MP, Gearhart JP, Jeffs RD: Continent urinary reservoirs in pediatric urological practice. J Urol 1990b;144:330.

Leong CH: The use of gastrocystoplasty. Dialog Pediatr Urol 1988;11:3–5.

Leong CH, Ong GB: Gastrocystoplasty in dogs. Aust N Z J Surg 1972;41:272–279.

Levesque PE, Bauer SB, Atala A, et al: Ten-year experience with the artificial urinary sphincter in children. J Urol 1996;156:625–628.

Liebovitch I, Avigad I, Nativ O, Goldwater B: The frequency of histopathological abnormalities in incidental appendectomy in urological patients: The implications for incorporation of the appendix in urinary tract reconstruction. J Urol 1992;148:41.

Light JK, Engelmann UH: Reconstruction of the lower urinary tract: Observations on bowel dynamics and the artificial urinary sphincter. J Urol 1985;133:594–597.

Light JK, Lapin S, Vohra S: Combined use of bowel and the artificial urinary sphincter in reconstruction of the lower urinary tract: Infectious complications. J Urol 1995;153:331.

Light JK, Reynolds JC: Impact of the new cuff design on reliability of the AS800 artificial urinary sphincter. J Urol 1992;147:609.

Light JK, Pietro T: Alteration in detrusor behavior and the effect on renal function following insertion of the artificial urinary sphincter. J Urol 1986;136:632.

Lima SVC, Araujo LAP, Vilar FO, et al: Combined use of enterocystoplasty and a new type of artificial sphincter in the treatment of urinary incontinence. J Urol 1996;156:622–624.

Lima SVC, Montoro AM, Maciel A, Vilar FO: The use of demucosalized bowel to augment small contracted bladders. Br J Urol 1998;82:436–439.

Little JS, Klee LW, Hoover DM, Rink RC: Long-term histopathologic changes observed in rats subjected to augmentation cystoplasty. J Urol 1994;152:720–724.

Lockhart JL, Lotenfoe RR, Davies R, et al: An alternative continent urinary reservoir for patients with short bowel, acidosis or radiation. Presented at the American Urological Association Meeting, San Antonio, TX, 1993.

Lockhart JL, Pow-Sang JM, Persky L, et al: A continent colonic reservoir: The Florida pouch. J Urol 1990;144:864–867.

Long R, Buson H, Manivel JC, Gonzalez R: Seromuscular enterocystoplasty in dogs. J Urol 1992;147:430A.

Lottmann H, Traxer O, Aigrain X, Melin Y: Posterior approach to the bladder for implantation of the 800 AMS artificial sphincter in children and adolescents: Technique and results in 8 patients. Ann Urol (Paris) 1999;33:357–363.

Ludlow J, McLaughlin KP, Rink RC, et al: Do appendicovesicostomies empty effectively? Presented at the North Central Section—American Urological Association meeting, Minneapolis, MN, 1995.

Lugagne PM, Herve JM, Lebret T, et al: Ureteroileal implantation in orthotopic neobladder with the LeDuc-Camey mucosal-through technique: Risk of stenosis and long-term follow-up. J Urol 1997;158:765–767.

Lutz N, Frey P: Evaluation of modified enterocystoplasties using a pediculated detubularized and demucosed sigmoid patch in the mini-pig. Presented at the Section on Urology Meeting, American Academy of Pediatrics, Dallas, TX, 1994.

Lytton B, Green DF: Urodynamic studies in patients undergoing bladder replacement surgery. J Urol 1989;141:1984.

Macedo A, Jr, Srougi M: A continent catheterizable ileum-based reservoir. BJU Int 2000;85:160–162.

Mahran MR, Dawaba MS, Ghoneim MA: Evaluation of the functional significance of the colorectal valve used in rectal urinary diversion in children: A comparative study between cases with and without the valve. Urology 1999;53:1215–1218.

Malek RS, Burke EC, DeWeerd JH: Ileal conduit urinary diversion in children. J Urol 1971;105:892–900.

Malizia AA, Jr, Reiman HM, Myers RP, et al: Migration and granulomatous reaction after periurethral injection of Polytef (Teflon). JAMA 1984;251:3277.

Malone PS, Ransley PG, Kiely EM: Preliminary report: The antegrade continence enema. Lancet 1990;336:1217.

Mansson W, Bakke A, Bergman B, et al: Perforation of continent urinary reservoirs: Scandinavian experience. Scand J Urol Nephrol 1997;31:529–532.

Mansson W, Colleen S, Sundin R: The continent cecal reservoir for urine. Scand J Urol Nephrol 1984;85(Suppl.):8.

McDougal WS: Bladder reconstruction following cystectomy by uretero-ileo-colourethrostomy. J Urol 1986;135:698–701.

McDougal WS: Metabolic complications of urinary intestinal diversion. J Urol 1992a;147:1199–1208.

McDougal WS: Use of intestinal segments in the urinary tract: Basic principles. In Walsh PC, Retik AB, Stamey TA, Vaughan ED, Jr (eds): Campbell's Urology, 6th ed. Philadelphia, WB Saunders, 1992b, pp 2595–2629.

McGuire EJ, Lytton B: Pubovaginal sling procedure for stress incontinence. J Urol 1978;119:82.

McGuire EJ, Wang CC, Usitalo H, et al: Modified pubovaginal sling in girls with myelodysplasia. J Urol 1986;135:94.

McGuire EJ, Woodside JR, Borden TA, Weiss RM: Prognostic value of urodynamic testing in myelodysplastic patients. J Urol 1981;126:205–209.

McKenna PH, Bauer SB: Bladder augmentation with ureter. Dialog Pediatr Urol 1995;18:4.

McLaughlin KP, Rink RC, Adams MC, Keating MA: Stomach in combination with other intestinal segments in pediatric lower urinary tract reconstruction. J Urol 1995;154:1162–1168.

Middleton AW, Jr, Hendren WH: Ileal conduits in children at the Massachusetts General Hospital from 1955 to 1970. J Urol 1976;115:591–595.

Miller EA, Mayo M, Kwan D, Mitchell M: Simultaneous augmentation cystoplasty and artificial urinary sphincter placement: Infection rates and voiding mechanisms. J Urol 1998;160:750–753.

Mingin GC, Stock JA, Hanna MK: The MAINZ II pouch: Experience in 5 patients with bladder exstrophy. J Urol 1999a;162:846–848.

Mingin GC, Stock JA, Hanna MK: Gastrocystoplasty: Long-term complications in 22 patients. J Urol 1999b;162:1122–1125.

Mitchell ME: Use of bowel in undiversion. Urol Clin North Am 1986;13:349.

Mitchell ME, Piser JA: Intestinocystoplasty and total bladder replacement in children and young adults: Follow-up in 129 cases. J Urol 1987;138:579–584.

Mitchell ME, Rink RC: Experience with the artificial urinary sphincter in children and young adults. J Pediatr Surg 1983;18:700–706.

Mitchell ME, Rink RC: Pediatric urinary diversion and undiversion. Pediatr Clin North Am 1987;34:1319–1332.

Mitchell ME, Rink RC, Adams MC: Augmentation cystoplasty, implantation of artificial urinary sphincter in men and women, and reconstruction of the dysfunction urinary tract. In Walsh PC, Retik AB, Stamey TZ, Vaughn ED, Jr (eds): Campbell's Urology, 6th ed. Philadelphia, WB Saunders, 1992, pp 2630–2653.

Mitrofanoff P: Cystotomie continente trans-appendiculaire dans le traitement des vessies neurologiques. Chir Pediatr 1980;21:297–305.

Mollard P, Gauriau L, Bonnet JP, Mure PY: Continent cystostomy (Mitrofanoff's procedure) for neurogenic bladder in children and adolescent (56 cases: long-term results). Eur J Pediatr Surg 1997;7:34–37.

Monti PR, Lara RC, Dutra MD, et al: New techniques for construction of efferent conduits based on the Mitrofanoff principle. Urology 1997;49:112–115.

Mor Y, Kajbafzadeh AM, German K, et al: The role of ureter in the creation of Mitrofanoff channels in children. J Urol 1997;157:635–637.

Morioka A, Miyano T, Ando K, et al: Management of vesicoureteral reflux secondary to neurogenic bladder. Pediatr Surg Int 1998;13:584–586.

Morrison JFB: The physiological mechanisms involved in bladder emptying. Scand J Urol Nephrol Suppl 1997;184:15–18.

Mouriquand PD, Sheard R, Phillips N, et al: The Kropp-onlay procedure (Pippi Salle procedure): A simplification of the technique of urethral lengthening. Preliminary results in eight patients. Br J Urol 1995;75:656.

Mulvihill S, Goldthorn J, Woolley MM: Incidental appendectomy in infants and children: Risk v. rationale. Arch Surg 1983;118:714.

Mundy AR: Clinical physiology of the bladder, urethra and pelvic floor. In Mundy AR, Stephenson TP, Wein AJ (eds): Urodynamic Principles, Practice and Application. Edinburgh, Churchill Livingstone, 1984.

Mundy AR, Borzskowski M, Saxton HM: Videourodynamic evaluation of neuropathic vesicourethral dysfunction in children. Br J Urol 1982;54:645.

Mundy AR, Nurse DE: Calcium balance, growth and skeletal mineralization in patients with cystoplasties. J Urol 1992;69:257–259.

Mundy AR, Shah PJR, Borzskowski M, Saxton HM: Sphincter behavior in myelomeningocele. Br J Urol 1985;57:647.

Mure PY, Mollard P, Mouriquand P: Transureteroureterostomy in childhood and adolescence: Long-term results in 69 cases. J Urol 2000;163:946–948.

Murry K, Nurse D, Mundy AR: Secreto-motor function of intestinal segments used in lower urinary tract reconstruction. Br J Urol 1987;60:532.

Nasrallah PF, Aliabadi HA: Bladder augmentation in patients with neurogenic bladder and vesicoureteral reflux. J Urol 1991;146:563–566.

Nesbit RM: Ureterosigmoid anastomosis by direct elliptical connection: A preliminary report. J Urol 1949;61:728–734.

Ngan JHK, Lau JLT, Lim STK, et al: Long-term results of antral gastrocystoplasty. J Urol 1993;149:731–734.

Nguyen DH, Bain MA, Salmonson KL, et al: The syndrome of dysuria and hematuria in pediatric urinary reconstruction with stomach. J Urol 1993;150:707–709.

Noble IG, Lee KT, Mundy AR: Transuretero-ureterostomy: A review of 253 cases. Br J Urol 1997;79:20–23.

Nurse DE, Mundy AR: One hundred artificial sphincters. Br J Urol 1988;61:318.

Nurse DE, Mundy AR: Metabolic complications of cystoplasty. Br J Urol 1989;63:165–170.

Oberpenning F, Meng J, Yoo JJ, Atala A: Bladder replacement with tissue-engineered neo-organs. Presented at the Section on Urology Meeting, American Academy of Pediatrics, New Orleans, LA, 1997.

Oesch I: Neourothelium in bladder augmentation: An experimental rat model. Eur Urol 1988;14:328.

O'Flynn KJ, Thomas DG: Artificial urinary sphincter insertion in congenital neuropathic bladder. Br J Urol 1991;67:155.

Ojerskog B, Kock NG, Philipson BM, Philipson M: Pregnancy and delivery in patients with continent ileostomy. Surg Gynecol Obstet 1988;167:61–64.

Orr LM, Thomely MW, Campbell MF: Ileocystoplasty for bladder enlargement. J Urol 1958;79:250.

Palmer LS, Franco I, Koan SJ, et al: Urolithiasis in children following augmentation cystoplasty. J Urol 1993;150:726.

Pantuck AJ, Han KR, Perrotti M, et al: Ureteroenteric anastomosis in continent urinary diversion: Long-term results and complications of direct versus nonrefluxing techniques. J Urol 2000;163:450–455.

Patil U, Glassberg KI, Waterhouse K: Ileal conduit surgery with nippled ureteroileal anastomoses. Urology 1976;7:594–597.

Pedlow PR: Pregnancy associated with uretero-sigmoid anastomosis. J Obstet Gynaecol Br Commonw 1961;68:822.

Perez LM, Smith EA, Broecker BH, et al: Outcome of sling cystourethropexy in the pediatric population: A critical review. J Urol 1996a;156:642–646.

Perez LM, Smith EA, Parrott TS, et al: Submucosal bladder neck injection of bovine dermal collagen for stress urinary incontinence in the pediatric population. J Urol 1996b;156:633–636.

Perlmutter AD: Experiences with urinary undiversion in children with neurogenic bladder. J Urol 1980;123:402–406.

Piser JA, Mitchell ME, Kulb TB, et al: Gastrocystoplasty and colocystoplasty in canines: The metabolic consequences of acute saline and acid loading. J Urol 1987;138:1009–1012.

Pitts WR, Jr, Muecke EC: A 20 year experience with ileal conduits: The fate of the kidneys. J Urol 1979;122:154–157.

Plaire JC, Snodgrass WT, Mitchell ME: Long-term follow-up of the hematuria-dysuria syndrome. Presented at the Section on Urology Meeting, American Academy of Pediatrics. Washington, DC, 1999.

Pope JC, 4th, Albers P, Rink RC, Cain MP, et al: Spontaneous rupture of the augmented bladder from silence to chaos. Presented at the European Society of Pediatric Urologists Meeting, Istanbul, Turkey, 1999.

Pope JC, 4th, Keating MA, Casale AJ, Rink RC: Augmenting the augmented bladder: Treatment of the contractile bowel segment. J Urol 1998;160:854–857.

Pope JC, 4th, Rink RC: Surgical management of the neurogenic bladder. In Gonzalez ET, Bauer SB (eds): Pediatric Urology Practice. Philadelphia, Lippincott-Raven, 1999, pp 401–416.

Quimby GF, Diamond DA, Mor Y, et al: Bladder neck reconstruction: Long-term followup of reconstruction with omentum and silicone sheath. J Urol 1996;156:629–632.

Racioppi MD, Addessi A, Fanasca A, et al: Acid-base and electrolyte balance in urinary intestinal orthotopic reservoir: Ileocecal neobladder compared with ileal neobladder. Urology 1999;54:629–635.

Raz S, Ehrlich RM, Babiarz JW, et al: Gastrocystoplasty without opening the stomach. J Urol 1993;150:713–715.

Reinberg Y, Allen RC, Vaughn M, McKenna PH: Nephrectomy combined with lower abdominal extraperitoneal ureteral bladder augmentation in the treatment of children with the vesicoureteral reflux dysplasia syndrome. J Urol 1995;153:777–779.

Reinberg Y, Manivel JC, Froemming C, et al: Perforation of the gastric segment of an augmented bladder secondary to peptic ulcer disease. J Urol 1992;148:369–371.

Reisman EM, Preminger GM: Bladder perforation secondary to clean intermittent catheterization. J Urol 1989;142:1316–1317.

Richie JP, Skinner DG, Waisman J: The effect of reflux on the development of pyelonephritis in urinary diversion: An experimental study. J Surg Res 1974;16:256–261.

Rink RC, Adams MC, Keating MA: The flip-flap technique to lengthen the urethra (Salle procedure) for treatment of neurogenic urinary incontinence. J Urol 1994;152:799.

Rink RC, Bihrle R: Continent urinary diversion in children and the Indiana pouch. Probl Urol 1990;4:663–675.

Rink RC, Casale AJ, Cain MP, King SJ: In situ imbricated appendix: Experience with a simple MACE technique. Presented at the Annual Meeting of the American Urological Association, Chicago, May 1999.

Rink RC, Hollensbe D, Adams MC: Complications of augmentation in children and comparison of gastrointestinal segments. American Urological Association Update Series 1995a;14:122–128.

Rink RC, McLaughlin KP: Indications for enterocystoplasty and choice of bowel segment. Probl Urol 1994;8:389–403.

Rink RC, McLaughlin KP, Adams MC, Keating MA: Modification of the Casale vesicostomy: Continent diversion without the use of bowel. (Abstract 442.) J Urol 1995b;153:339A.

Rink RC, Mitchell ME: Surgical correction of urinary incontinence. J Pediatr Surg 1984;19:637–641.

Rink RC, Mitchell ME: Role of enterocystoplasty in reconstructing the neurogenic bladder. In Gonzales ET, Roth D (eds): Common Problems in Pediatric Urology. St. Louis, Mosby–Year Book, 1990, pp 192–204.

Rink RC, Renschler T, Adams MC, Mitchell ME: Long term follow-up of the first gastrocystoplasty series. Presented at the European Society of Pediatric Urology/American Academy of Pediatrics, Urology Section Meeting, Tours, France, June 2000.

Rink RC, Retik AB: Ureteroileocecal sigmoidostomy and avoidance of carcinoma of the colon. In King LR, Stone AR, Webster GD (eds): Bladder Reconstruction and Continent Urinary Diversion. St. Louis, Mosby–Year Book, 1991, p 221.

Rittenberg MH, Hulbert WC, Snyder HM, III, Duckett JW: Protective factors in posterior urethral valves. J Urol 1988;140:993.

Robinson RG, Delahunt B, Pringle KC: Autoaugmentation gastrocystoplasty. J Urol 1994;151:500A.

Rosen MA, Light JK: Spontaneous bladder rupture following augmentation enterocystoplasty. J Urol 1991;146:1232–1234.

Roth JA, Borer JG, Hendren WH, et al: Is gastric augmentation a good long-term urodynamic solution to the poorly functioning bladder? Presented at the American Academy of Pediatrics, Urology Section Meeting, Chicago, October 2000.

Roth S, Semjonow A, Waldner M, Hertle L: Risk of bowel dysfunction with diarrhea after continent urinary diversion with ileal and ileocecal segments. J Urol 1995;154:1696–1699.

Rowland RG: Complications of continent cutaneous reservoirs and neobladder-series using contemporary techniques. American Urological Association Update Series 14:lesson 25, 1995;202–207.

Rowland RG: Present experience with the Indiana pouch. World J Urol 1996;14:92–98.

Rowland RG, Mitchell ME, Bihrle R: The cecoileal continent urinary reservoir. World J Urol 1985;3:185.

Rushton HG, Woodard JR, Parrott TS, et al: Delayed bladder rupture after augmentation enterocystoplasty. J Urol 1988;140:344.

Sagalowsky AI: Early results with split-cuff nipple ureteral reimplants in urinary diversion. J Urol 1995;154:2028.

Salle JL, Fraga JC, Amarante A, et al: Urethral lengthening with anterior bladder wall flap for urinary incontinence: A new approach. J Urol 1994;152:803.

Salle JL, Fraga JC, Lucib A, et al: Seromuscular enterocystoplasty in dogs. J Urol 1990;144:454–456.

Salle JL, McLorie GA, Bagli DJ, Khoury AE: Urethral lengthening with anterior bladder wall flap (Pippi Salle procedure): Modifications and extended indications of the technique. J Urol 1997;158:585–590.

Sanda MC, Jeffs RD, Gearhart JP: Evolution of outcomes with the ileal hydraulic continent diversion: Reevaluation of the Benchekroun catheterizable stoma. World J Urol 1988;14:108–111.

Savauagen F, Dixey GM: Syncope following ureterosigmoidostomy. J Urol 1969;101:844.

Schilling A, Krawczak G, Friesen A, Kruse H: Pregnancy in a patient with an ileal substitute bladder followed by severe destabilization of the pelvic support. J Urol 1996;155:1389–1390.

Schmidt JD, Hawtrey CE, Flocks RH, Culp DA: Complications, results, and problems of ileal conduit diversions. J Urol 1973;109:210–216.

Schumacher S, Fichtner J, Stein R, et al: Pregnancy after Mainz pouch urinary diversion. J Urol 1997;158:1362–1364.

Scott FB, Bradley WE, Tumm GW: Treatment of urinary incontinence by an implantable prosthetic urinary sphincter. J Urol 1974;112:75–80.

Shapiro SR, Lebowitz R, Colodny AH: Fate of 90 children with ileal conduit urinary diversion a decade later: Analysis of complications, pyelography, renal function and bacteriology. J Urol 1975;114:89–95.

Sheiner JR, Kaplan GW: Spontaneous bladder rupture following enterocystoplasty. J Urol 1988;140:1157–1158.

Shekarriz B, Upadhyay J, Demirbilek S, et al: Surgical complications of bladder augmentation: Comparison between various enterocystoplasties in 133 patients. Urology 2000;55:123–128.

Sheldon CA, Gilbert A: Gastrocystoplasty allows safe pretransplant urinary reconstruction without acidosis. Presented at the American Urological Association Meeting, Toronto, Canada, 1991.

Shoemaker WC, Bower R, Long DM: A new technique for bladder reconstruction. Surg Gynecol Obstet 1957;105:645–650.

Shoemaker WC, Marucci HD: The experimental use of seromuscular grafts in bladder reconstruction: Preliminary report. J Urol 1955;73:314–321.

Sidi AA, Aliabadi H, Gonzalez R: Enterocystoplasty in the management and reconstruction of the pediatric neurogenic bladder. J Pediatr Surg 1987a;22:153–157.

Sidi AA, Peng W, Gonzalez R: Vesicoureteral reflux in children with myelodysplasia: Natural history results of treatment. J Urol 1986a;136:329.

Sidi AA, Reinberg Y, Gonzalez R: Influence of intestinal segment and configuration on the outcome of augmentation enterocystoplasty. J Urol 1986b;136:1201–1204.

Sidi AA, Reinberg Y, Gonzalez R: Comparison of artificial sphincter implantation and bladder neck reconstruction in patients with neurogenic urinary incontinence. J Urol 1987b;138:1120.

Sidi AA, Sinha B, Gonzalez R: Treatment of urinary incontinence with an artificial sphincter: Further experience with the AS791/792 device. J Urol 1984;131:891.

Silveri M, Capitanucci ML, Mosiello G, et al: Endoscopic treatment for urinary incontinence in children with a congenital neuropathic bladder. Br J Urol 1998;82:694.

Simeoni J, Guys JM, Mollard P, et al: Artificial urinary sphincter implantation for neurogenic bladder: A multi-institutional study in 107 children. Br J Urol 1996;78:287.

Simoneau AR, Skinner DG: Ileo-anal reservoir. J Urol 1995;153:305A.

Sinaiko ES: Artificial bladder from segment of stomach and study effect of urine on gastric secretion. Surg Gynecol Obstet 1956;102:433–438.

Singh G, Thomas DG: Artificial urinary sphincter in patients with neurogenic bladder dysfunction. Br J Urol 1996;77:252.

Skinner DG, Lieskovsky G, Boyd S: Continent urinary diversion: A 51/2 year experience. Ann Surg 1988;208:337–344.

Skinner DG, Lieskovsky G, Boyd S: Continent urinary diversion. J Urol 1989;141:1323–1327.

Slaton JW, Kropp KA: Conservative management of suspected bladder rupture after augmentation enterocystoplasty. J Urol 1994;152:713–715.

Smith ED: Follow-up studies on 150 ileal conduits in children. J Pediatr Surg 1972;7:1–10.

Snodgrass W: A simplified Kropp procedure for incontinence. J Urol 1997;158:1049–1052.

Snow BW, Cartwright PC: Bladder autoaugmentation. Urol Clin North Am 1996;23:323.

Spencer JR, Steckel J, May M, et al: Histological and bacteriological findings in long-term ileocystoplasty and colocystoplasty in the rat. J Urol 1993;150:1321.

Stein R, Fisch M, Andreas J, et al: Whole-body potassium and bone mineral density up to 30 years after urinary diversion. Br J Urol 1998;82:798–803.

Stein R, Fisch M, Beetz R, et al: Urinary diversion in children and young adults using the Mainz Pouch I technique. Br J Urol 1997a;79:354–361.

Stein R, Fisch M, Ermert A, et al: Urinary diversion and orthotopic bladder substitution in children and young adults with neurogenic bladder: A safe option for treatment? J Urol 2000;163:568–573.

Stein R, Fisch M, Schumacher S, et al: Operative Korrektur des äuBeren und inneren weiblichen Genitale bei Blasenekstrophie. Aktuelle Urol 1994;25:1.

Stein R, Fisch M, Stockle M, Hohenfellner R: Urinary diversion in bladder exstrophy and incontinent epispadias: 25 Years of experience. J Urol 1995;154:1177–1181.

Stein R, Lotz J, Fisch M, et al: Vitamin metabolism in patients with a Mainz pouch I: Long-term follow-up. J Urol 1997b;157:44–47.

Steiner G, Muller SC, Bruhl P: Urinary incontinence in neurogenic defects and urogenital anomalies in childhood. Wien Med Wochenschr 1998;148:299–304.

Steiner MS, Morton RA: Nutritional and gastrointestinal complications of the use of bowel segments in the lower urinary tract. Urol Clin North Am 1991;18:743.

Stifelman MD, Ikeguchi FF, Hensle TW: Ureteral tissue expansion for bladder augmentation: A long-term prospective controlled trial in a porcine model. J Urol 1998;160:1826–1829.

Stohrer M, Goepel M, Kramer G, et al: Detrusor myectomy (autoaugmentation) in the treatment of hyper-reflexive low compliance bladder. Urologe A 1999;38:30–37.

Stone AR, MacDermott JA: The split cuff ureteral nipple reimplantation technique: Reliable reflux prevention from bowel segments. J Urol 1989;142:707–709.

Stothers L, Johnson H, Arnold W, et al: Bladder autoaugmentation by vesicomyotomy in pediatric neurogenic bladder. Urology 1994;44:110–113.

Strawbridge LR, Kramer SA, Castillo DA, et al: Augmentation cystoplasty and the artificial genitourinary sphincter. J Urol 1989;142:297.

Studer UE, Zingg EJ: Ileal orthotopic bladder substitutes: What we have learned from 12 years' experience with 200 patients. Urol Clin North Am 1997;24:781–793.

Sundaram CP, Reinberg Y, Aliabadi HA: Failure to obtain durable results with collagen implantation in children with urinary incontinence. J Urol 1997;157:2306–2307.

Suzer O, Vates TS, Freedman AL, et al: Results in the Mitrofanoff procedure in urinary tract reconstruction in children. Br J Urol 1997;79:279–282.

Tanagho EA: Bladder neck reconstruction for total urinary incontinence: 10 Years experience. J Urol 1972;125:321.

Thuroff JW, Alken P, Hohenfellner R: The Mainz pouch (mixed augmentation with ileum 'n' zecum) for bladder augmentation and continent diversion. In King LR, Stone AR, Webster GD (eds): Bladder Reconstruction and Continent Urinary Diversion. Chicago, Year Book Medical Publishers, 1987, p 252.

Thuroff JW, Alken P, Reidmiller H, et al: 100 cases of Mainz pouch: Continuing experience and evolution. J Urol 1988;140:283.

Thuroff JW, Alken P, Reidmiller H, et al: The Mainz pouch (mixed augmentation ileum and cecum) for bladder augmentation and continent diversion. J Urol 1986;136:17.

Tizzoni G, Foggi A: Die Wiederherstellung der Harnblase. Zentralbl Chir 1888;15:921.

Treiger BFG, Marshall FF: Carcinogenesis and the use of intestinal segments in the urinary tract. Urol Clin North Am 1991;18:737.

Turner-Warwick RT, Ashken MH: The functional results of partial, subtotal, and total cystoplasty with special reference to ureterocaecocystoplasty, selective sphincterotomy and cystocystoplasty. Br J Urol 1967;39:3–12.

Vates TS, Denes ED, Rabah R, et al: Methods to enhance in vivo urothelial growth on seromuscular colonic segments in the dog. J Urol 1997;158:1081–1085.

Vortsman B, Lockhart JL, Kaufman M, et al: Polytetrafluoroethylene injection for urinary incontinence in children. J Urol 1985;133:248.

Wagg A, Fry CH: Visco-elastic properties of isolated detrusor smooth muscle. Scand J Urol Nephrol Suppl 1999;201:12–18.

Wagstaff KE, Woodhouse CR, Roose GA, et al: Blood and urine analysis in patients with intestinal bladders. Br J Urol 1991;68:311–316.

Wagstaff KE, Woodhouse CR, Duffy PG, Ransley PG: Delayed linear growth in children with enterocystoplasties. Br J Urol 1992;69:314–317.

Walker RD, Flack CE, Hawkins-Lee B, et al: Rectus fascial wrap: Early results of a modification of the rectus fascial sling. J Urol 1995;154:771.

Wang SC, McGuire EJ, Bloom DA: A bladder pressure management system for myelodysplasia: Clinical outcome. J Urol 1988;140:1499.

Waters PR, Chehade NC, Kropp KA: Urethral lengthening and reimplantation: Incidence and management of catheterization problems. J Urol 1997;158:1053.

Weston PM, Morgan JD, Hussain J, et al: Artificial urinary sphincters around intestinal segments: Are they safe? Br J Urol 1991;67:150.

Weston PM, Robinson LQ, Williams S, et al: Poor compliance early in filling in the neuropathic bladder. Br J Urol 1989;63:28.

Whitmore WF, III, Gittes RF: Reconstruction of the urinary tract by cecal and ileocecal cystoplasty: Review of a 15-year experience. J Urol 1983;129:494–498.

Woodhouse CR, MacNeily AE: The Mitrofanoff principle: Expanding upon a versatile technique. Br J Urol 1994;74:447.

Woodside JR, Borden TA: Pubovaginal sling procedure for the management of urinary incontinence in a myelodysplastic girl. J Urol 1982;127:744.

Yachia D: A new continent vesicostomy technique: Preliminary report. J Urol 1997;157:1633–1637.

Yang W: Yang needle tunneling technique in creating antireflux and continent mechanisms. J Urol 1993;150:830–834.

Yerkes EB, Rink R, King S, et al: Tap water and the MACE: A safe combination? Presented at the American Academy of Pediatrics, Urology Section Meeting, Chicago, October 2000.

Yoo JJ, Meng J, Oberpenning F, Atala A: Bladder augmentation using allogenic bladder submucosa seeded with cells. Urology 1998;51:221–225.

Young HH: An operation for the cure of incontinence of urine. Surg Gynecol Obstet 1919;28:84.

Zinner NR, Ritter RC, Sterling AM: The mechanism of micturition. In Chisholm GD, Williams EI (eds): Scientific Foundation of Urology. London, Heinemann, 1976.

Zubieta R, De Badiola F, Escala JM, et al: Clinical and urodynamic evaluation after ureterocystoplasty with different amounts of tissue. J Urol 1999;162:1129–1132.

72
PEDIATRIC ENDOUROLOGY AND LAPAROSCOPY

Steven G. Docimo, MD
Craig A. Peters, MD

Pediatric Endourology
　Ureteroscopy
　Percutaneous Nephrolithotomy
　Endopyelotomy
　Percutaneous Management of Renal Calyceal
　　Diverticula

Pediatric Laparoscopy
　Diagnostic Laparoscopy
　Operative Laparoscopy

Summary

Pediatric endourology has expanded rapidly from diagnostic cystoscopy and transurethral valve ablation to varied applications comparable to all adult endourologic techniques. This expansion has offered pediatric patients the advantages of less invasive means by which various urologic conditions may be treated, including stones, strictures, and nonfunctioning kidneys, yet it has also posed the challenge of tailoring these techniques to smaller patients with different clinical needs. It is not always self-evident that minimally invasive techniques are better for children. It is not always a matter of downscaling instruments and techniques to apply to small children. This chapter reviews the current applications, techniques, and controversies regarding endourologic practice in children. This topic is divided into a discussion of general endourology, including ureteroscopy and percutaneous renal surgery, and then a review of laparoscopic techniques and their pediatric applications.

PEDIATRIC ENDOUROLOGY

Ureteroscopy

Instruments

Current ureteroscopic instruments permit safe access to the ureter in children as young as 4 months. The importance of appropriate working tools is magnified in the smaller patient. Unfortunately, there is a natural trade-off with smaller instruments in the associated reduction in working channel size that often restricts any manipulation, even when access has been successful. With an appropriate working device, such as a stone basket, there is little room left for irrigation in the working channel and visualization may become limited. These issues must be recognized before a procedure is started, and they must be factored into the clinical balance regarding choice of therapy. Common pediatric ureteroscopic instruments are shown in Table 72–1. Although a range of instruments would be ideal, this is often not practical because of the cost. This is another limitation with pediatric compared with adult endoscopy: one size is largely suitable for adults, whereas the pediatric patient may be a 5-kg infant or a 70-kg adolescent. A practical compromise has been the rigid No. 6.9 Fr cystoureteroscope. This instrument permits safe access to the distal ureter, even in smaller children and without dilation. It has a No. 2 Fr and a No. 3.5 Fr working channel to permit instrumentation with irrigation, thereby making it useful for older children. It can also be used for minipercutaneous access renal procedures. The 15-cm version is probably the most versatile, whereas the longer version is a useful semirigid ureteroscope for the upper tracts in the older child.

Accessory instrumentation is similar to that used in adult ureteroscopic applications, although the need for diagnostic visualization and biopsy in children is rare. Wire sizes need to be smaller to accommodate the generally smaller ureteroscopes, and they must include 0.28-inch and 0.18-inch wires. The rigidity of these wires must be sufficient to permit manipulations of the ureteroscope and passage of stents. Stone baskets and grasping devices are available as small as 1.7 Fr, but they are much less sturdy and may be frustrating to use. Balloon dilation of the ureteral orifice is occasionally needed, but there are few if any dilation bal-

Table 72–1. ENDOSCOPES FOR PEDIATRIC APPLICATIONS

Type	Name	Size	Channel Diameter (Fr)	Length (cm)
Flexible cystoureteroscope	ACMI CAN-1	14.6	6.4	
Flexible ureteropyeloscope	ACMI AUR-7	7.2	3.6	65
Flexible ureteropyeloscope	ACMI AUR-9	9.8	3.6	65
Flexible cystoscope	ACMI AUR-PC	8.5	2.5	20
Semirigid ureteroscope	ACMI MICRO-6	6.9	3.4/2.3	33
Semirigid ureteroscope	ACMI MR-9	9.4	5.4/2.1	33
Semirigid cystoureteroscope	ACMI MRPC	6.9	3.4/2.3	15.5
Semirigid cystoureteroscope	ACMI MR 915	9.4	5.4/2.1	15
Operative ureteroscope	ACMI MRO-6	6.9/8.3	3.4/2.3	33
Rigid ureterorenoscope	Wolf	6/7.5	4.2	43
Rigid ureterorenoscope	Wolf	7.5/9.5	4.2	42
Flexible ureterorenoscope	Wolf	7.5	3.6	70/45/20
Flexible ureterorenoscope	Wolf	9	4.5	70/45
Cystourethroscope	Wolf	11	4	—
Cystourethroscope	Wolf	7.5	—	—
Cystourethroscope	Wolf	8.5	3	—
Cystourethroscope	Wolf	6/7.5	4	14
Cystourethroscope	Wolf	4.5/6	2.4	11
Semirigid ureterorenoscope	Wolf	4.5/6	2.4	31
Cystoureteroscope integrated	Wolf	10.5	5	16
Rigid cystoscope	Storz	7	3	—
Rigid cystoscope	Storz	7.5	3.5	11
Flexible cystoureteroscope	Storz	7.5	3.6	40

loons that are sufficiently small for young children. Use of a smaller ureteroscope is preferable.

Indications

The need for ureteroscopic intervention in children is less than in adults and is largely limited to stone management. There is little need for diagnostic ureteroscopy, nor for tumor resection. Retrograde direct-vision endopyelotomy has not been used in any significant way in children. The choice of ureteroscopic stone removal in a child is a complex one that should balance the relative need for a single-intervention treatment (in contrast to the risk of needing multiple procedures, as with extracorporeal shock wave lithotripsy [ESWL]) with the location and size of the stone. There are few data to indicate the likelihood of stone passage relative to size and location in children. It is clear that children tend to pass stones more readily than adults, and a stone that would appear proportionately to require intervention may actually pass spontaneously in a child. The same indications for urgent intervention are applicable to children, including infection, intractable pain or nausea, and renal impairment. The potential for an associated or causative congenital impairment to urine flow should also be considered in treatment choice. The anatomic conditions may affect the utility of ureteroscopy.

Stone location is not an absolute indicator of the potential use of ureteroscopy in children. Although there are few reports of ureteroscopic management of proximal ureteral or renal pelvic stones, this is possible even in small children (Wollin et al, 1999). It may be necessary to preplace an indwelling stent to facilitate access. Renal pelvic stones are much more difficult to remove ureteroscopically in children because of the progressively limited manipulation ability with smaller, flexible instruments. These are largely technical problems that will become less important with improved instruments. The Holmium laser is one such ad-

vance to facilitate ureteroscopic management of upper tract stones in the small child. The lower pole stone is a well-recognized challenge to ureteroscopic management, particularly in children, where functional access to the lower pole may be limited.

Access

The means of access should be determined by the instruments available for the application and the location of the stone to be removed. Complex procedures that may require several passages of the ureteroscope and prolonged manipulation of the stone and its fragments may benefit from placement of a ureteroscopic sheath to facilitate repeated placements and removals of the ureteroscope. These cannot be placed in small children, and the smallest available size is a No. 10 Fr sheath. This may be passed with care into an 8- to 10-year-old child.

Stone Manipulation and Removal

An appropriate means of stone fragmentation is essential for any pediatric stone manipulation and should be integrated with the ureteroscopic instruments available. The electrohydraulic lithotriptor (EHL) is a useful, all-purpose lithotripter, although it must be used carefully to avoid injury to the ureteral wall. Some surgeons do not use the EHL because of concern about ureteral wall injury; with low power settings and careful application, this is a limited risk. The new holmium:yttrium-aluminum-garnet (YAG) laser system will probably supplant the EHL for most ureteroscopic applications, and it offers the potential for retrograde upper tract stone management in younger children (Reddy et al, 1999; Wollin et al, 1999). The principal benefit with the holmium laser is that stone fragments do not need to be extracted because they are small enough to pass spontaneously. Furthermore, the laser fiber is only 200

Author and Year	No. Patients (age range)	No. Stone Free
Caione et al, 1990	7 (3–8 yr)	7
Scarpa et al, 1995	7 (<10 yr)	7
Shroff and Watson, 1995	13	10 (single procedure)
Smith et al, 1996	11	9 (single procedure)
Fraser et al, 1999	16 (18 mo–15 yr)	14
Jayanthi et al, 1999	12	11
Wollin et al, 1999	15 (4–17 yr)	12 (single procedure)
Van Savage et al, 2000	17 (6 mo to 17 yr)	17
Total	**98**	**87 (89%)**

μm in diameter, which does not restrict irrigant flow or flexibility in smaller endoscopes. An initial concern regarding release of cyanide gas during uric acid stone lithotripsy appears to have been disproven (Teichman et al, 1998).

Postprocedure Management

A temporary indwelling ureteral stent is almost always appropriate after ureteroscopic stone manipulation. The goal is to provide adequate renal drainage until ureteral edema has diminished. This may be as brief as 1 to 2 days or as long as 2 weeks, depending on the degree of stone impaction and the complexity of removal. In children, stent removal usually requires a secondary cystoscopic procedure, except for very short stenting periods, in which a string attached to the stent may be used for withdrawal. After removal, ultrasound is used to monitor upper tract dilation, which may occur with ureteral obstruction. The timing of follow-up should be based on the complexity of the case, but it should not be delayed longer than 4 weeks after the stent is removed. If significant dilation is present, or if the child develops symptoms of obstruction, an intravenous pyelogram (IVP) is used to define the functional anatomy of the ureter. Vesicoureteral reflux is a theoretical complication of ureteral dilation and manipulation, but it has not been reported to be a significant clinical issue (Caione et al, 1990; Scarpa et al, 1995). Routine cystography is not recommended.

Results

There are few reports of ureteroscopic stone manipulation in children (Table 72–2), but all have demonstrated good efficacy and a minimal complication rate. Stone-free rates are about 89%, although this depends on the selection of patients for ureteroscopic intervention. If distal stones alone are approached, a very high stone-free rate may be expected, while proximal and renal stones are more challenging.

Percutaneous Nephrolithotomy

Instruments

A large initial investment in equipment is required for percutaneous renal procedures in children. The proper tools must be available, and assistants in the room must be familiar with both the equipment and the techniques for a successful procedure.

The technology for pediatric-specific applications of percutaneous nephroscopy has improved dramatically over the past decade. Modern sheaths and endoscopes allow adequate access through small tracts, minimizing trauma to the infant kidney. The equipment for obtaining initial percutaneous access will not be discussed here. Many pediatric practitioners have their radiology colleagues obtain initial access to the kidney before the day of the procedure. There is some evidence that this decreases blood loss, and it clearly decreases operating time. Access to the smaller pediatric kidney is facilitated by the ultrasonic and three-dimensional fluoroscopic equipment that usually is not available in the operating room.

Once access has been achieved, equipment can be divided into that needed for dilation and sheath placement, the endoscopes themselves, and equipment for stone manipulation, stone fragmentation or incision, and coagulation.

Traditionally, No. 24- to 30-Fr percutaneous access sheaths and standard adult nephroscopic devices have been used in children with good success. In brief, once the nephrostomy tract has been established, a balloon or set of coaxial dilators is used to create a large enough tract into the kidney for placement of a plastic nephroscopy sheath (LeRoy et al, 1984). The nephroscopes are then introduced through this sheath and can be withdrawn and introduced without losing access to the intrarenal collecting system. The presence of a working sheath dramatically decreases working pressures within the renal pelvis, as measured manometrically, and thereby enhances the safety of percutaneous procedures (Saltzman et al, 1987). Concerns have been raised with the use of these large working sheaths in children, however, including potential damage to the small kidney from tract dilation. Smaller forms of access, including peel-away vascular access introducers, have been used as substitute nephroscopy sheaths (Helal et al, 1997; Jackman et al, 1998b). In one series, a No. 11 Fr Cordis introducer (Cook, Inc., Spencer, IN) was used with good initial success. Although the Cordis set is ideally suited for vascular access, its long trocar increases the potential for renal pelvic or ureteral perforation during sheath introduction. The Cordis sheath was therefore modified to create a purpose-built pediatric renal access sheath (Cook Urological, Spencer, IN) (Jackman et al, 1998b) (Fig. 72–1). In combination with smaller endoscopes, the majority of pediatric percutaneous procedures can be performed through these or similar minipercutaneous sheaths.

Irrigation solutions must be warmed to prevent hypothermia, which can occur quickly in small children. Saline should be used as an irrigant in all cases to avoid dilutional hyponatremia, which can also develop quickly in the small child if extravasation should occur. With smaller endoscopes, irrigant can be introduced under pressure. If this is done, adequate low-pressure efflux via the nephroscopy sheath must be ensured, or significant and life-threatening complications from extravasation may occur (Pugach et al, 1999).

Traditional nephroscopes are available in either rigid or actively deflectable configurations. Rigid nephroscopes have an offset lens system that allows the passage of probes necessary for stone fragmentation and retrieval. The tips of these endoscopes are rounded to decrease the possibility of renal injury. The telescopes come in 0- and 30-

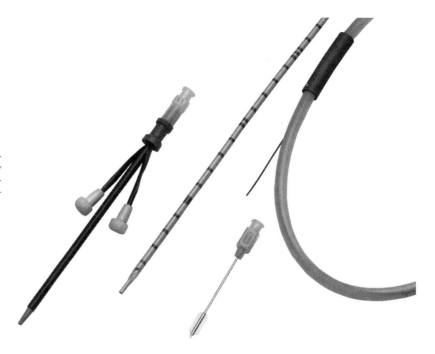

Figure 72–1. A commercially available set for minipercutaneous access to the kidney. The set includes floppy and stiff guide wires, a fascial incising needle, a dual-lumen dilating catheter, and the sheath/trocar combination. (Photograph courtesy of Cook Urological, Inc.)

degree configurations. The outer diameter of the nephroscopes ranges in size from 17 to 24 Fr. Flexible nephroscopes were developed to access all of the calyces of the intrarenal collecting system. These are 15-Fr actively deflectable endoscopes with a 6-Fr working channel. These instruments were specifically manufactured for use in the intrarenal collecting system and have a tip that has a very tight turning radius for working in a small space. In addition to the usual 15-Fr flexible nephroscope, smaller deflectable ureteroscopes can be used to obtain access through narrow infundibula. In addition, if access to a calyx can be obtained by wire, a passive, flexible endoscope with a size as small as 5 Fr can be passed over the wire to visualize the difficult calyx.

Access to these adult nephroscopes is vital for an active percutaneous nephroscopy program, but the majority of pediatric procedures can now be done using one of a number of miniature endoscopes. The No. 7 or No. 8 Fr offset cystoscopes with 5-Fr working ports allow almost any manipulation possible through larger telescopes (Fig. 72–2). The No. 7 and No. 9 Fr flexible ureteroscopes double as nephroscopes, allowing access to all parts of the collecting system. All of these can be used through a No. 11 Fr access sheath with enough clearance to allow low-pressure irrigation.

The ideal instrument for intracorporeal lithotripsy at this time is the holmium laser (Reddy et al, 1999). Proper use of the laser often results in vaporization of the stones, leaving few fragments of significant size. The laser is an expensive instrument and therefore is not universally available for clinical use.

Ultrasonic probes have a long track record for percutaneous lithotripsy, and they have the advantage that the larger probes aspirate stone fragments as they are created. Ultrasonic probes are being developed that will fit through the 5-Fr port of an offset pediatric cystoscope, but their long length at this time limits their utility.

EHL is perhaps the most universally available modality for stone fragmentation. Because EHL probes work equally well in normal saline and water, saline should always be used to decrease the risk of irrigant extravasation in the small child. EHL energy can perforate the renal pelvis or ureter very quickly, so it is imperative that it be used under direct vision at all times. EHL is by far the least expensive form of shock wave lithotripsy, and it is safe and effective under visual control (Denstedt and Clayman, 1990). A newer device, the Swiss lithoclast, consists of a rigid probe that vibrates at a frequency of 12 cycles per second (Denstedt et al, 1992). This instrument acts as a percussive hammer to fragment stones. Probes as small as 3 Fr are available, and it appears that this device may fragment stones more rapidly and efficiently than ultrasonic lithotripsy.

Instruments for incision of ureteropelvic junction (UPJ) or ureteral strictures include cautery probes, laser fibers, small resectoscopes, and visual urethrotomes. A combina-

Figure 72–2. A very useful endoscope for pediatric percutaneous and transurethral procedures is this offset No. 7 Fr cystoscope with a 5-Fr working channel. (Photograph courtesy of Circon, Inc.)

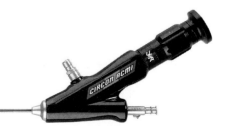

tion dilating balloon and cautery cutting wire (Accucise, Applied Medical, Laguna Hills, CA) has also been used for pediatric endopyelotomy, though its use is somewhat limited by the diameter of the uninflated device (Bolton et al, 1994).

Indications

Percutaneous access in children is used most commonly for stone removal (Docimo, 1996). **Because the ureter in the child is very distensible, allowing passage of relatively large stone fragments, ESWL is the first-line treatment for most renal calculi in children** (Kroovand, 1997). **There is no strict upper limit of stone burden that can be managed with ESWL in children, as there is in adults, although the larger the burden the less likely it is that success will be achieved with one procedure** (Marberger and Hofbauer, 1996). Percutaneous nephrolithotomy is most often used in the case of ESWL failure, or in children whose anatomy would decrease the likelihood of ESWL success. This includes children with neurogenic bladder or bladder exstrophy who have had extensive reconstruction, including ureteral reimplantation or ureteroenterostomy (Cass et al, 1992). In these same children, percutaneous transrenal access may be the preferable route for removal of ureteral stones. Difficult access due to ureteral reimplantation, as well as the risk of causing recurrent vesicoureteral reflux after dilation of the reimplanted ureter (Garvin and Clayman, 1991), are relative contraindications to ureteroscopy, although access is relatively straightforward via a transvesical percutaneous approach (Santarosa et al, 1993).

Percutaneous access to the kidney is also used for ablation of calyceal diverticula, endopyelotomy, or ureterotomy for ureteral stricture. These techniques now can all be performed through miniaturized percutaneous access.

Access

Preoperative imaging of the urinary tract is essential to the planning and performance of endourologic procedures. Bowel preparation and/or simethicone may be used to optimize intraoperative fluoroscopic visualization of the urinary tract, especially in children with neurogenic bowel and bladder who have a tendency toward constipation. Infected urine should be sterilized before endourologic manipulation, and perioperative antibiotics should be used routinely. A ureteral access catheter may be introduced cystoscopically at the beginning of the procedure if it is believed necessary to visualize the collecting system for access. The pediatric ureter is small (Cussen, 1971), and the risk of ureteral injury or stricture, or both, is significant in this population. One should try to limit the number of catheters and wires traversing the ureter at any one time. Ureteral occlusion balloons or ureteral access catheters are not routinely required for percutaneous procedures in children. A Foley catheter is placed in the bladder. Free drainage of urinary stomas, if present, must be ensured when the patient is positioned; augmented bladders or intestinal neobladders should be catheterized with a tube large enough to allow easy passage of mucus to prevent potential rupture due to overdistention.

As mentioned earlier, initial access may be obtained preoperatively by an interventional radiologist. Alternatively, the urologist can obtain access in the operating room at the time of the procedure. Numerous techniques can be used to create a nephrostomy tract. Generally, access is achieved "blind" with the use of a C-arm fluoroscopic unit. The child is placed in the prone position on a fluoroscopic table. Appropriate padding is used for the chest, face, knees, and elbows to prevent injury during potentially prolonged procedures. The flank is prepared and draped with an occlusive drape with a water-collection system. A 22-gauge "finder" needle is introduced from a posterior position, lateral to the quadratus. When urine is aspirated, contrast material can be instilled through this needle to opacify the system. If the contrast agent extravasates, fluoroscopic visualization through the remainder of the case will be compromised; therefore, care should be used, and small amounts should be injected until intrarenal position has been confirmed. Alternatively, the contrast agent can be instilled via a previously placed ureteral catheter. Through either the finder needle or the ureteral catheter, air can be instilled instead of contrast material. The advantage of air is that it outlines first the posterior calyces, which are most advantageous for percutaneous procedures. Air should be instilled in small amounts to prevent the unlikely occurrence of air embolus.

An 18-gauge Chiba or diamond-tip needle is then introduced from a slightly more lateral position. The calyx is chosen for puncture, and the needle is lined up under the fluoroscopic image until it represents just a dot overlying the calyx. Without changing the direction of the needle, the C-arm is tilted to reveal a different view. When the needle tip reaches the calyx in this second dimension, its position is confirmed by aspiration. If urine is obtained, a 0.035- or 0.038-gauge Teflon-coated guide wire is introduced and the needle is withdrawn.

Alternatively, ultrasound guidance may be used to permit needle access to the collecting system. The appropriate calyx is selected and imaged with the use of an ultrasonic probe prepared in a sterile fashion on the operative field. The needle may be advanced under ultrasound guidance or with a biopsy guide placed on the probe to more precisely position the needle. The needle may be observed as it enters the collecting system.

At this point, the procedure is the same whether or not preoperative nephrostomy access has been obtained. Under fluoroscopic guidance, a 0.035-gauge Teflon-coated guide wire is situated in the kidney, and the needle or nephrostomy tube is removed. The guide wire is manipulated down the ureter and into the bladder to obtain nephroureteral access if possible. An angle-tip catheter is sometimes required for this purpose (Kumpe, Cook Urological). For a minipercutaneous procedure, a No. 10 Fr dual-lumen catheter is passed over the wire after the fascia has been incised with a 4.5-mm fascial incising needle. A 0.035-gauge stiff guide wire is then placed alongside the original wire through the second lumen of the catheter, which is then removed. The Teflon-coated wire is sutured to the skin as a safety wire and put aside. Without further dilation, the No. 11 Fr pediatric access sheath is introduced over the guide wire and positioned appropriately in the kidney. The trocar is then removed, and access to the kidney is complete. If larger access is required, an appropriately sized fascial dilating balloon can be inserted over the stiff wire and inflated, with a standard percutaneous access sheath of 24 to 30 Fr introduced over the balloon. Visual confirmation of intrarenal position is always made with the endoscope.

Stone Manipulation

Removal of calculi proceeds as indicated by the size, composition, and location of the stone. Small stones can be withdrawn with the use of baskets or three-prong graspers, or both. Tipless baskets represent a relatively recent innovation that improves access to stones in calyces and tight spaces (Honey, 1998). Lithotripsy may be performed by the techniques described earlier, depending once again on stone composition (which affects the ease of fragmentation) and available equipment. Smaller access sheaths have the disadvantage of requiring smaller stone fragments for removal. This is one of the reasons that the holmium laser, with its ability to vaporize stone, is ideal for use through the minipercutaneous sheath. Despite this, the first reported series of minipercutaneous procedures in children had a high rate of success with EHL (Jackman et al, 1998b).

Postprocedure Management

At the end of the procedure, adequate drainage of the kidney and/or ureter must be achieved in most cases. After minipercutaneous nephrolithotomy, most patients are left with a No. 6 Fr nephroureteral stent with additional side-holes created at the time of surgery to correspond to the location of the renal pelvis (Mitchell stent, Cook Urological) (Jackman et al, 1998b). This allows adequate drainage but can be capped and concealed under a bandage, thus preventing accidental dislodgment by the child. When a small stone has been removed intact, or after a brief procedure when there is no question of residual stone, one may elect to leave no drainage tube. If there is any question, access via a nephrostomy or nephroureteral stent should be maintained until postoperative radiographs confirm the lack of obstruction and extravasation.

After nephrolithotomy with a larger sheath, postoperative drainage may be achieved with a Foley catheter threaded over an angiographic catheter to provide both tamponade of the renal parenchyma and ureteral access (Docimo, 1996). Newer nephroureteral catheters can also provide these functions.

As with any percutaneous nephrolithotomy, postoperative radiologic studies to ensure a stone-free status is imperative. A second-look procedure should be performed in any situation where there is concern about residual stone. The importance of removing all stone fragments may be greater in those children who have abnormal ureteral anatomy and are at higher risk for urinary stasis or poor passage of residual fragments.

Results

Modern series of percutaneous nephrolithotomy in children have demonstrated excellent results (Jackman et al, 1998b; Badawy et al, 1999; Jayanthi et al, 1999). Although any child who is going to undergo percutaneous renal procedures should have at least a type and screen in the blood bank, transfusion rates are quite low. Whether the minipercutaneous techniques will additionally decrease transfusion rates over time remains to be seen.

Endopyelotomy

Indications

Endopyelotomy is an option for the treatment of UPJ obstruction. The principle of the procedure borrows from the Davis intubated ureterotomy (Davis, 1943), in which the strictured ureter is incised longitudinally, stented, and allowed to regenerate over the stenting catheter. The difference in endopyelotomy is that the incision is made from inside the ureter, using endourologic access to achieve the same result.

The indications for endopyelotomy in children are still not clear (Docimo and Kavoussi, 1997). Despite an increasing number of reports, relatively few procedures have been documented in the literature, especially in young children. The success of open pyeloplasty in the infant and toddler (Hendren et al, 1980) far exceeds the expected success rate of endopyelotomy in the adult (Chow et al, 1999) or child (Schenkman and Tarry, 1998), and recommending primary endopyelotomy for this age group is premature.

Endopyelotomy is generally acknowledged to be the procedure of choice after failed pyeloplasty in the adult, and it has a reasonable success rate (Jabbour et al, 1998). **The same may be true in the pediatric population, although fewer cases have been reported** (Capolicchio et al, 1997). **Endopyelotomy should be attempted only when a lumen is recognizable and can be cannulated. Considering the difficulty and morbidity of reoperative pyeloplasty, an attempt at endopyelotomy in most cases is reasonable.**

Although they are not specific contraindications to endopyelotomy, the presence of a large collecting system or poor renal function in the ipsilateral kidney, or both, portends a poorer likelihood of success (Danuser et al, 1998). It is controversial whether high insertion of the UPJ into the pelvis or anomalous crossing renal vessels (or both) is associated with failure (Tawfiek et al, 1998), but evidence suggests that these conditions should not necessarily preclude endopyelotomy (Nakada et al, 1998; Chow et al, 1999).

Access

Access for antegrade endopyelotomy is achieved essentially as described for percutaneous nephrolithotomy. The anatomy of the kidney must be carefully considered, with a posterolateral approach through a middle calyx usually the most effective choice (Bernardo and Smith, 2000). This maximizes the visibility of the UPJ and avoids the potential respiratory complications associated with upper pole access. Endopyelotomy may be effectively performed through a minipercutaneous access, using the holmium laser fiber or a small electrocautery probe to incise the strictured area. As mentioned earlier, access through the UPJ and into the bladder must be obtained before any attempt at incision is made.

Ureteroscopic endopyelotomy has been used with reasonable success in adults and older children (Tawfiek et al, 1998), but its use in younger children is limited by their small ureteral diameter. Very few cases of retrograde endopyelotomy have been reported in children (Gerber et al, 2000), so a recommendation cannot be made as to its use. Endopyelotomy by means of a balloon with an incorporated cutting wire has also been reported in children, but the large size of the catheter and the risk of vascular complications (Schwartz and Stoller, 1999) have dampened enthusiasm for this modality among pediatric urologists. For these reasons, only antegrade endopyelotomy is discussed here.

Incision

The incision of the UPJ must be through the full thickness of the ureteral wall to allow the strictured area to expand and reform around the indwelling ureteral stent. Consequently, renal parenchyma, surrounding structures, and large blood vessels may be encountered. To avoid these structures, a posterolateral incision usually is made in the UPJ. Endoluminal ultrasound has been used to identify vascular structures and modify the angle of incision accordingly, but this modality is not universally available (Tawfiek et al, 1998). The incision can be made with a hook blade, a straight cold knife, nephroscopic scissors, an electrocautery electrode, or a laser fiber (Clayman et al, 1990; Bernardo and Smith, 2000). Incision is made until the outside of the ureter can be seen and the ureteral lumen can be entered with the endoscope (Bernardo and Smith, 2000). Some recommend balloon calibration of the UPJ to ensure complete incision (Kavoussi et al, 1991).

After the incision is made, an appropriate stent is positioned across the UPJ. In adults, an endopyelotomy stent that is 14 Fr in its upper portion and 8.2 Fr in its lower portion is used (Bernardo and Smith, 2000), but this is clearly too large for pediatric use. There is evidence that the size of the stenting catheter may not correlate with success of the procedure (Moon et al, 1995; Anidjar et al, 1997), and in children a size appropriate to age may be used. The stent is conventionally left in situ for 6 weeks, although this might not be necessary, because 2- and 4-week periods have been reported with similar success rates (Kumar et al, 1999).

Postprocedure Management

If percutaneous endopyelotomy is performed, a nephroureteral stent is usually left in place to allow access to the kidney if needed. The stent can be capped and kept under a dressing once it has been demonstrated that there is no extravasation on a nephrostogram (Bernardo and Smith, 2000). It is easily removed after the requisite stenting period, and follow-up studies are obtained at 4 to 6 weeks to demonstrate patency. There is concern for late recurrence of obstruction, especially in the small child, so long-term follow-up with appropriate imaging studies is warranted (Capolicchio et al, 1997).

Results

As mentioned previously, the success rate for endopyelotomy in children is difficult to estimate because of the small numbers reported, but it seems to be approximately 85% at best (Motola et al, 1993; Tan et al, 1993; Bolton et al, 1994; Faerber et al, 1995; Capolicchio et al, 1997; Figenshau and Clayman, 1998; Schenkman and Tarry, 1998; Gerber et al, 2000). The potential for serious complications exists, but they have been reported only rarely. One case of complete ureteral necrosis in an adolescent illustrates the care that must be taken in traversing the ureter, even in older children (Sutherland et al, 1992).

Percutaneous Management of Renal Calyceal Diverticula

Calyceal diverticula in children are uncommon but may manifest with infection, with pain due to stone, or, most often, incidentally on ultrasound examination for nonspecific symptoms (Kottasz and Hamvas, 1977; Siegel and McAlister, 1979). **Their natural history is not well defined, but it is evident that they do persist and many increase in size.** It is not determined that increasing size predicts the development of symptoms. Although the appearance on ultrasound may suggest compression of renal parenchyma, there is no evidence that this is associated with impaired renal function. The strict definition of a calyceal diverticulum includes evidence of accumulation of contrast material into the diverticulum, as seen on IVP or CT imaging (Mosli et al, 1986). Otherwise, the diagnosis of a simple cyst is invoked. We have seen several confirmed calyceal diverticula with contrast accumulation that subsequently lost that property and were then considered to be simple cysts. This evolution raises the possibility that some simple cysts originated as calyceal diverticula. The clinical significance of this is unclear.

The indications for intervention in a calyceal diverticulum include infection, pain, and evidence of stone formation (Gauthier et al, 1983). Occasionally, evidence of stone formation is present as milk of calcium with layering of the echogenic debris (Yeh et al, 1992; Chen et al, 1997). Increasing size is a relative indication for intervention as well, although our practice is to continue to observe these stones, unless otherwise requested by parents.

Percutaneous intervention in children is based on obliteration and scarification of the epithelial lining of the diverticulum, rather than induced drainage through opening of the neck of the diverticulum, as is often performed in adults (Lang, 1991; Baldwin et al, 1998). Any procedure intending to establish free drainage requires temporary indwelling stents and runs the risk of reclosure of the neck. The impact of each of these elements in the child is greater than in the adult. We have therefore used a direct percutaneous access method to ablate the epithelial lining of the diverticulum (Shalhav et al, 1998; Monga et al, 2000).

Access is obtained percutaneously with ultrasound guidance directly into the cavity of the diverticulum, using methods similar to those for renal pelvic access. A flexible wire is coiled in the cavity, but it is unusual that a wire can be passed down the ureter. A working sheath is introduced, as with renal procedures, and the endoscope introduced. The neck of the diverticulum is sought, aided by retrograde instillation of methylene blue dye through a ureteral catheter if desired. The neck is then fulgurated with a Bugbee electrode, followed by cauterization of the epithelial lining. In larger patients, an adult resectoscope can be used to permit use of a roller-ball electrode to hasten the process. After fulguration, a Foley catheter is placed to allow collapse of the diverticulum. This is left in place for 2 to 3 days. The cavity may remain visible on ultrasound after the procedure and may shrink slowly.

Location of the diverticulum can present a technical challenge for access in that anteromedial diverticula require passage of the needle through the renal parenchyma. Laparoscopic resection of these diverticula may be a useful alternative (Gluckman et al, 1993; Ruckle and Segura, 1994; Harewood et al, 1996; Hoznek et al, 1998; Curran et al, 1999). There are few reports of percutaneous management of calyceal diverticula in children. Our experience with six cases suggests adequate outcome with minimal morbidity. In one case the diverticulum did not disappear, although its growth was halted. No significant complications were encountered. One patient required open resection owing to failure of percutaneous access and large size. Retrograde techniques have been described in adults but have not been employed in children. The comparative success rate of direct percutaneous ablation and the need for prolonged intubation and removal of stents in retrograde methods argue in favor of antegrade techniques for pediatric patients.

PEDIATRIC LAPAROSCOPY

Diagnostic Laparoscopy

Indications

Laparoscopic diagnosis has been employed in pediatric urology for more than 25 years, beginning with Cortesi's report of using laparoscopic techniques to identify nonpalpable testes (Cortesi et al, 1976). Further uses in intersex conditions and hernia have been described as well.

Testis

Numerous reports have defined the anticipated outcomes and interpretation of laparoscopic findings associated with cryptorchidism (Garibyan, 1987; Castilho, 1990; Jones and Kern, 1993; Holcomb et al, 1994b; Moore et al, 1994; Tennenbaum et al, 1994; Brock et al, 1996). The true utility of diagnostic laparoscopy has not been completely determined, however, and debate continues (Ferro et al, 1996). **The primary aims of diagnostic laparoscopy are to identify the presence or absence, the location, and the anatomy of the nonpalpable testis.** The use of diagnostic laparoscopy reflects the consistent failure of any imaging modality to accurately identify the location and presence of a nonpalpable testis with certainty. The usual failing is in not being able to definitively prove the absence of a testis; the obvious sequela of missing an intra-abdominal testis would be leaving a testis in the abdomen undetected. For this reason, **any diagnostic technique must have 100% accuracy in determining whether a testis is present in the abdomen or not. Furthermore, when an imaging test identifies a testis, some form of operative intervention is needed to bring the testis into the scrotum or remove it. No imaging test has yet been shown to eliminate the need for surgical intervention.** Several studies have examined this issue but consistently reported a definite incidence of missed intra-abdominal testes and lack of specific identification of absent testes (Kier et al, 1988). Recent reports of complex studies such as MR angiography reveal a greater sensitivity than conventional studies, but their cost and complexity raise a significant question as to their efficacy (Yeung et al, 1999; De Filippo et al, 2000).

Diagnostic laparoscopy has a long record of experience with consistent results (Cisek et al, 1998b). In general there is agreement that laparoscopy should be used only for nonpalpable testes. **It is important to perform a careful examination under anesthesia to detect a small number of testes that were not detected in the office setting. Cisek and associates (1998b) reported an 18% of incidence testes palpable under anesthesia but not palpated in the clinic.** This obviously reduces the number of diagnostic laparoscopies that would reveal a testis that had descended into the inguinal canal.

Reported techniques are similar, with an umbilical port and laparoscopic examination of the area of the internal inguinal ring. Access methods include open and Veress needle techniques. More recently, very small endoscopes (2 mm) have been used (minilap or needlescopic techniques) directly through the Veress needle to eliminate the need for a second, blind trocar insertion after Veress needle insufflation.

Examination of the normal side should be performed first to provide an image of the normal anatomic arrangements in the individual patient. The essential landmarks are illustrated in Fig. 72–3. The triangular arrangement of the medial vas deferens, lateral spermatic vessels, and iliac vessels should provide a basis for comparison to the opposite side. The obliterated umbilical artery is usually the most readily recognized structure in the area of the internal ring. The vas deferens should cross over it from medial to lateral and course toward the internal inguinal ring. It should then be joined by the spermatic vessels, which may be traced cephalad, running parallel to the iliac vessels. The spermatic vessels are usually a very distinct bundle of vessels, but their appearance should be noted because it can indicate the condition of the testis. The internal inguinal ring is usually closed and appears as a flat area of the peritoneum with the vas and vessels passing through it. A patent processus vaginalis may be present, and this is often, but not always, associated with the presence of a testicle. It has been reported that this finding may be used as an indicator that a testis is present in the canal, but this is not always the case and it provides little practical benefit in management beyond what may be learned from the appearance of the vas and vessels (Elder, 1994).

On the affected side, there are three basic patterns

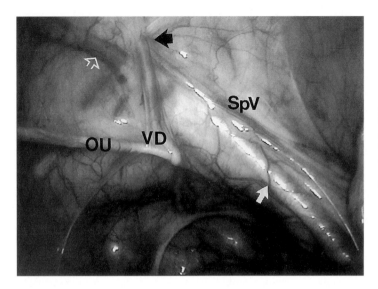

Figure 72–3. Laparoscopic view of normal right inguinal region. The internal inguinal ring *(black arrow)* is marked by the confluence of the vas deferens (VD) and the spermatic vessels (SpV). The vas is readily recognized as it crosses over the obliterated umbilical artery (OU), sometimes incorrectly termed the lateral umbilical ligament. The iliac artery is indicated by the solid white arrow and the inferior epigastric artery by the open white arrow.

that may be seen. **When the vas and the vessels dwindle away before the internal inguinal ring, a vanishing intra-abdominal testis is diagnosed.** This is an important diagnosis that must be made carefully. If both vas and vessels are seen and disappear, there is no reason to explore the inguinal ring, because there will be no structures to identify. Often, however, the vessels are not readily apparent when a vas-like structure is seen. In such cases, it is imperative that a careful examination of the retroperitoneum be performed to identify the vessels, because they may actually be associated with a testicular structure that is completely separate from the vas. **At times, the left colon or the cecum may need to be moved out of the way, or formally mobilized with the use of additional working ports, to confirm the presence of the vessels and the fact that they become atretic** (Fig. 72–4).

The second common appearance is that of vas and vessels that pass through the inguinal ring. This pattern may look very similar to the normal situation, but the important feature to examine is the appearance of the vessels. If they are thick and robust, similar to the normal

opposite side, it is likely that a testis is present. If they are thin and much more delicate than on the contralateral normal side, then it is likely, but not certain, that an atrophic testis will be found in the inguinal canal or scrotum (Plotzker et al, 1992).

The third pattern is that of an intra-abdominal testis, which is usually readily evident. It may be a "peeping" testis that moves between the abdomen and inguinal canal and is always associated with a patent processus vaginalis. Alternatively, the testis may be located in a variety of completely intra-abdominal positions, most commonly along the line of the spermatic vessels, up to the level of the kidney. It may also lie medial to the iliac vessels, even so far inferior as to be adjacent to the bladder or rectum. It may be on a pedicle of the vas and vessels that coils toward the testis (Fig. 72–5). Several very unusual positions have been reported, including adjacent to the liver and passing through the obturator foramen. When the anatomy is not clear, it is best to presume that the testis is in an unusual position and trace the spermatic vessels very carefully. They will usually lead to the testis.

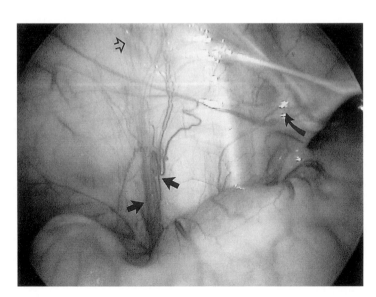

Figure 72–4. Laparoscopic view of a patient with a nonpalpable left testis. The solid straight arrows indicate the spermatic vessels as they disappear approaching the internal ring *(open arrow)*. The vas deferens *(curved arrow)* also vanishes after it crosses over the obliterated umbilical artery. This appearance of vanishing vas and vessels is diagnostic of an intra-abdominal vanishing testis. No further exploration is needed. It is important to note that the sigmoid colon had to be pushed down to confirm the identity of the spermatic vessels.

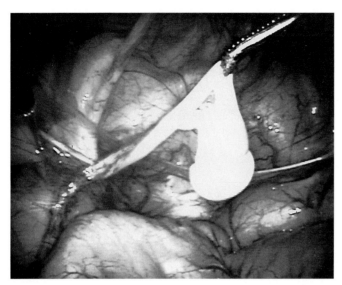

Figure 72–5. Laparoscopic view in a patient with a nonpalpable left testis. This testis was seen deep in the pelvis attached to a long stalk of the spermatic vessels and vas deferens. Laparoscopic orchiopexy was performed.

When an intra-abdominal testis is identified, several aspects should be considered. Beyond the location, the mobility of the testis can be assessed and will affect surgical decision making. If the testis is very atrophic, with minimal structural attachments, removal may be the best option (Thomas et al, 1992). In combination with operative procedures, we measure the position of the testis from the internal inguinal ring to the lower pole of the testis (Fig. 72–6).

A meta-analytic review of published series up to 1996 (1311 patients) was presented by Cisek and associates (1998b), with the results shown in Table 72–3. In general, it may be anticipated that one half of those children with a nonpalpable testis will have a viable testis to salvage; 30% will have a nonviable nubbin of testicular tissue that is usually removed, and the remainder will have evidence of a vanishing testis above the inguinal ring.

Although diagnostic laparoscopy is widely used in the evaluation of the nonpalpable testis, there is lack of universal agreement as to its utility. The principal challenge is that it does not add significant information that alters clinical management for the time and risk involved. This problem was examined in one controlled trial comparing inguinal exploration and diagnostic laparoscopy (Ferro et al, 1999). Operative laparoscopy was not used if an intra-abdominal testis was identified. The authors' conclusions were that laparoscopy did not provide any reduction in time nor improvement in outcomes. The differences between the two arms were relatively slight, and it is important to recognize that the authors did not alter their surgical approach based upon the laparoscopic findings. If the information provided by laparoscopic evaluation is not used in surgical decision making, it will not be of significant benefit. In this study, the authors also recognize differences in practice, in that they used regional anesthesia if laparoscopy is not being performed, whereas this is uncommon in the United States. If operative laparoscopy is integrated with diagnostic laparoscopy, a further benefit will be afforded, because there is a rapid transition to laparoscopic orchiopexy after the diagnosis is made.

The controversy regarding the use of diagnostic laparoscopy also depends on how the surgeon views the impact of various interventions. To some, an unnecessary or unproductive inguinal incision (as in a vanishing abdominal testis) is less morbid than an unnecessary or unproductive diagnostic laparoscopy (Colodny, 1996; Peters, 1996b). It is difficult to directly compare these two, because most young children recover rapidly from both. In a quantitative manner, then, it is difficult to "prove" that laparoscopy is beneficial, and any such "proof" for or against its benefit depends on certain basic assumptions.

The benefit of diagnostic laparoscopy seems to be more intuitive in that it provides specific information regarding the location and character of the testis to permit an informed decision regarding the best surgical approach. Just as preoperative imaging or examination is used in most surgery, laparoscopy provides the surgeon with information regarding the organ that is to be operated

Figure 72–6. Intra-abdominal testis seen laparoscopically in a child with a nonpalpable right testis. The testis is readily seen lying on the iliac vessels. The vas deferens (small solid white arrows) is seen crossing the obliterated umbilical artery, and the epididymis (large white arrow) is seen lateral to the testis (T). To determine whether the testis may be mobilized with the spermatic vessels intact, the distance from the internal inguinal ring (open white arrow) to the distal end of the testis was measured as shown, and was found to be 3.0 cm. This child had a two-stage laparoscopic Fowler-Stephens orchiopexy.

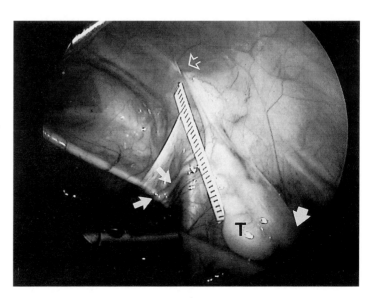

Table 72–3. FINDINGS ON DIAGNOSTIC LAPAROSCOPY FOR NONPALPABLE TESTIS

Finding	No. and Frequency	Management	Comment
Intra-abdominal testis	486 (37%)	Laparoscopic orchiopexy	Excludes transinguinal testes
Transinguinal testes	14 (1%)	Open orchiopexy	Not frequently reported, about 10% when indicated
Vas and vessels through inguinal canal: testicular nubbin	381 (29%)	Limited inguinal exploration to remove nubbin, confirm testicular absence	—
Vas and vessels through inguinal canal: testis present	188 (14%)	Open orchiopexy	More often in heavy children, occasionally with perineal ectopic testis
Intra-abdominal vanishing testis	213 (16%)	No further intervention	Must see vanishing vas and vessels
Nondiagnostic	29 (3%)	—	Various causes

on. In several reports, this has led to a change in surgical therapy for 50% to 60% of patients (Cisek et al, 1998b; Mikaelsson et al, 1999). This seems to be a reasonable goal and benefit.

Our practice is based on this approach, with surgical decision making dependent on laparoscopic findings. If an intra-abdominal testis is identified, operative laparoscopic orchiopexy is performed after placement of two secondary working ports. If an intra-abdominal vanishing testis is evident by vanishing vas and vessels, no further intervention is needed and the procedure is concluded with no incision. **If the vas and vessels pass through the internal inguinal ring and are atretic, it is presumed that a vanishing testis is present and a small, low inguinal exploration is performed at the level of the pubic tubercle.** This permits confirmation of the diagnosis with excision of a nubbin of testis (Rozanski et al, 1996). If the vessels are healthy and similar in size to the contralateral vessels, a formal inguinal incision is used to explore the canal for a testis that could not be palpated under anesthesia. These cases are unusual but may include a perineal ectopic testis. It is also important to recognize the occasional occurrence of the very unusually located testis that is very difficult to detect on conventional inguinal exploration (Moore et al, 1994; Cisek et al, 1998b). We have found testes in locations ranging from near the liver to the

deep pelvis, adjacent to the rectum. Transverse testicular ectopia has also been reported (Fairfax and Skoog, 1995). Given that the principal goal of evaluation of the nonpalpable testis is to prevent misdiagnosis of an intra-abdominal testis, laparoscopy seems to provide the best balance of safety and efficiency (Cortesi et al, 1976; Boddy et al, 1985; Castilho and Ferreira, 1987; Bloom et al, 1988; Guiney et al, 1989; Castilho, 1990; Cortes et al, 1995; Arnbjornsson et al, 1996; Brock et al, 1996). No imaging modality has been shown to be 100% sensitive in the identification of an intra-abdominal testis, and any modality still needs to be paired with surgical manipulation of any testis found. It is unlikely that any imaging study will ever play a significant role in the evaluation of the nonpalpable testis.

Intersex

Diagnostic laparoscopy has been applied to intersex conditions (Yu et al, 1995) and has also been integrated with operative interventions (Martin et al, 1997; Lakshmanan and Peters, 2000). Diagnostic laparoscopy offers direct visualization of the internal genital structures in cases in which the anatomy may not be clear based on imaging studies. It also offers the ability to perform a diagnostic biopsy to establish a histologic diagnosis and the ability to remove aberrant gonadal or ductal structures if necessary.

The principal use of diagnostic laparoscopy for intersex is in conditions where gonadal development may be abnormal or discordant with the sex of rearing (Table 72–4). This includes various forms of gonadal dysgenesis and hermaphroditism. The location and appearance of the gonad may help in making a diagnosis. In true hermaphroditism, the demonstration of testicular and ovarian tissue in one gonad is the diagnostic hallmark and may be established only with biopsy. In such cases, the biopsy should be longitudinal and deep enough to sample the entire gonad. In some situations, the gonad is inappropriate to the sex of rearing and should be removed (Droesch et al, 1990; Shalev et al, 1992; Gililland et al, 1993; Long and Wingfield, 1993; McDougall et al, 1993). Similarly, gonadal removal may be needed in cases of tumor degeneration or risk of degeneration (Wilson et al, 1992). Laparoscopy may also be used when persistent müllerian ductal structures should be removed (McDougall et al, 1994; Ng and Koh, 1997; Wiener et al, 1997).

Occasionally the diagnosis of an unanticipated intersex

Table 72–4. LAPAROSCOPIC EVALUATION OF INTERSEX CONDITIONS

Anatomic Findings	Probable Diagnosis	Laparoscopic Role
Palpable gonads, virilized, possible uterus	Deficiency of müllerian inhibiting substance	Identify and excise müllerian structures
No palpable gonads, virilized	Gonadal dysgenesis, true hermaphroditism	Gonadal biopsy/gonadectomy; define müllerian anatomy
Asymmetry/one palpable gonad, virilized	Gonadal dysgenesis (mixed)	Evaluate opposite gonad; gonadal biopsy/gonadectomy
Female	Male pseudohermaphrodite	
	Testicular feminization	Gonadectomy
	5α-reductase deficiency	Orchiopexy

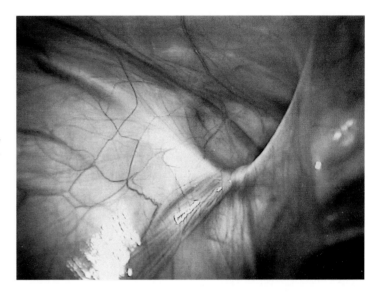

Figure 72–7. Patent processus vaginalis on the left seen laparoscopically during performance of a contralateral hernia repair. There was no clinical evidence of this patent processus.

case occurs intraoperatively, as in the finding of müllerian structures during herniorrhaphy in an apparent male. Laparoscopy permits immediate examination of the internal pelvic structures to facilitate clinical decision making. Similarly, in the female child with a hernia, diagnostic laparoscopy can confirm the presence of normal müllerian structures, obviating the need for vaginoscopy to look for a cervix.

Hernia

Laparoscopic evaluation of the contralateral inguinal ring during hernia repair has emerged as a valuable tool to determine specifically whether contralateral inguinal exploration is needed (Holcomb et al, 1994a, 1996; Wolf and Hopkins, 1994; Fuenfer et al, 1996). Initially this technique was performed with the use of an umbilical laparoscope, but this incurred the small risk of umbilical access. Effective contralateral evaluation is readily accomplished by passing the endoscope through the ipsilateral hernia sac after it has been mobilized from the spermatic cord. A 70- to 90-degree endoscope is ideal and provides a direct view of the contralateral internal ring (Fig. 72–7). A patent processus vaginalis is evident by a gaping passage through the ring. It is usually readily seen, although there are ambiguous cases in which it may be necessary to pull on the contralateral testis to open a patent processus. Scrotal insufflation is an obvious but not universal indicator of a patent processus, as is inguinal crepitus.

Our technique is to isolate the ipsilateral hernia sac, pass the insufflating catheter (No. 8 or No. 10 Fr) into the peritoneum, and instill carbon dioxide (CO_2) to a pressure of 8 to 10 mm Hg. The right-angle endoscope is passed alongside the catheter or through the sac after the catheter is removed. The spermatic vessels and vas permit rapid orientation and examination of the contralateral inguinal ring, and a diagnosis may be made. If there is any uncertainty, the inguinal canal is felt for crepitus and the testis is pulled to determine whether there is a subtle contralateral patent processus vaginalis. If the contralateral processus is patent, a conventional inguinal exploration is performed.

Published reports of diagnostic inguinal laparoscopy demonstrate the utility of laparoscopy in specifically identifying those patients in whom a contralateral inguinal exploration is needed (Kaufman et al, 1996). Although it is uncertain how many of these children would have developed a clinical hernia at some point in the future, it is clear that fewer unnecessary inguinal explorations will be performed with the use of this technique (Rowe et al, 1969). Concurrently, the number of delayed contralateral hernias requiring a subsequent operation will be reduced. Our experience has demonstrated an age-specific incidence of contralateral patent processus vaginalis that is contrary to what might be expected. The incidence of a patent processus in children younger than 2 years of age is less than in children older than 2 years until they reach 4 years. We have also observed three children in whom the processus was unambiguously closed yet developed a clinical hernia from 4 months to 3 years after surgery. All three patients were younger than 2 years of age at the initial surgery. This suggests that caution should be exercised in the interpretation of the endoscopic findings before 24 months, and, perhaps more importantly, that "congenital hernias" in children may actually be "acquired." It is also useful to note that we have identified a widely patent processus vaginalis in older patients (4 [25%] of 16 patients older than 8 years of age) with no clinical signs of a hernia, including a patient as old as 10 years.

Operative Laparoscopy

Indications

Laparoscopy remains a largely diagnostic modality for many pediatric urologists. That is changing, and more extirpative as well as reconstructive procedures are being performed laparoscopically. The era of therapeutic laparoscopy in pediatric urology began with the introduction of spermatic vessel clipping for a first-stage Fowler-Stephens operation (Bloom, 1991), and then laparoscopic orchiopexy (Jordan and Winslow, 1994). Today, laparoscopic orchiopexy is a well-accepted part of the urologist's repertoire for dealing with the high testicle (Jordan, 1997; Lindgren et al, 1998). The techniques of orchiopexy and/or orchiectomy have been expanded to apply to intra-abdominal management of intersex states (Yu et al, 1995).

Experience with laparoscopic techniques in adults led to the now common pediatric laparoscopic nephrectomy (Clayman et al, 1991), as well as laparoscopic partial nephrectomy (Jordan and Winslow, 1993a). Attempts to manage vesicoureteral reflux in a minimally invasive fashion have included laparoscopic extravesical ureteral reimplantation (Atala et al, 1993; Lakshmanan et al, 1998) as well as the development and refinement of endoscopic techniques of ureteral manipulation within the bladder (Cartwright et al, 1996; Okamura et al, 1996; Lakshmanan et al, 1998, 1999).

The reconstructive era of pediatric laparoscopic surgery is just beginning. Upper tract operations, such as pyeloplasty, can be performed in this way but are technically demanding (Peters et al, 1995; Tan, 1999). Although the first laparoscopic bladder augmentation was performed in 1994 (Docimo et al, 1995a), the technique is difficult enough that only a few have been performed since, and most of these in adults (Gill et al, 2000). Autoaugmentation of the bladder has also been applied laparoscopically (McDougall et al, 1995a; Braren and Bishop, 1998). Currently, the most feasible of these techniques is the laparoscopic-assisted bladder reconstruction, which combines the morbidity and cosmetic advantages of laparoscopy with the ability to perform complex tissue assembly through a low abdominal incision (Jordan and Winslow, 1993b; Cadeddu and Docimo, 1999; Hedican et al, 1999).

The field of therapeutic pediatric urologic laparoscopy will expand as technology and experience improve. It is difficult to predict what the indications for minimally invasive abdominal surgery will be in the decades to come, but clearly this is a field that is changing almost daily.

Instruments

Instruments used for therapeutic laparoscopy can be divided into those used for access and those that provide an extension of the surgeon's hands into the peritoneal cavity. Access can be obtained with the use of a Veress needle (Veress, 1938) followed by blind or visually aided trocar introduction, or, alternatively, an open access technique can be used. These techniques include the box stitch technique (Poppas et al, 1999), the Hasson cannula (Hasson, 1998), and the use of a radially dilating trocar system (Schulam et al, 1999; Cuellar et al, 2000). Each of these has its proponents, advantages, and disadvantages. It is important that the surgeon be comfortable with at least one technique of access and preferably have some experience with both open and needle insufflation techniques. A newer option for diagnostic laparoscopy is the introduction of a 2-mm laparoscope through the Veress needle cannula (Molloy, 1995), obviating the need for secondary trocar placement.

Hand instruments for laparoscopy come in three basic sizes. The original laparoscopic hand instruments were almost all 10 mm in diameter. Five-millimeter hand instruments have been the standard for several years. Microlaparoscopic instruments may be either 2 or 3 mm in diameter,

the former more conducive to needle trocar access, the latter somewhat sturdier and more varied in application.

Laparoscopic hand instruments mirror those used for open surgery. The difference, of course, is that the surgeon's actions need to be transmitted from outside the body to the peritoneal cavity. For this reason, most hand instruments consist of a movable handle or grip, a long shaft, and a working end consisting of movable tips. These tips take the shape of scissors, graspers, or forceps of various types; right angle instruments; or clamps. Most of the common hand instruments for open surgery have been duplicated in laparoscopic form. Many of these instruments can be connected to an electrocautery source for hemostatic maneuvers during laparoscopic surgery. For pediatric applications, shorter shaft lengths can be obtained for many of these instruments.

Suturing can be difficult laparoscopically. Laparoscopic needle drivers exist in 10-, 5-, and 3-mm sizes. Because of the limited angle of approach, orienting the needle on the driver and the needle in relation to the tissue can be difficult. Automatic suturing devices have been developed that can increase speed and also make knot tying much easier (Adams et al, 1995). However, automatic suturing instruments remain rather large for pediatric applications. In addition, the most widely available of these incorporates a double-ended needle with a suture coming off at a right angle in the center of the shaft. This of necessity creates a large suture track, which is unacceptable for many pediatric reconstructive applications. For this reason, operations such as laparoscopic pyeloplasty continue to require hand suturing in pediatric patients, even though they are often accomplished with automatic suture devices in the adult (Chen et al, 1996).

Laparoscopic retraction can be difficult and has led to the creation of a number of clever devices, including fan retractors, instruments that form loops or rings after they are inserted into the body, and others. For most pediatric applications, patient positioning is adequate to allow exposure of the area of interest, but with more complex operations on the horizon, laparoscopic retraction may become a necessary part of the pediatric urologist's armamentarium.

Larger operations often require irrigation and/or suction to improve visualization. Suction devices come in 3-, 5- and 10-mm varieties. There are numerous interchangeable tips that allow effective suction under various circumstances. These irrigation-aspiration devices can be connected to reusable suction bottles and pressurized fluid bags, or disposable devices consisting of a battery powered pump directly plugged into a fluid bag can be used. These have the advantage of rapid set-up should the unexpected need for suction and irrigation arise.

Hemostasis can be achieved laparoscopically with the use of electrocautery. Cautery can be delivered via hand instruments, such as scissors, or cautery wands. Both monopolar and bipolar cautery units are available with certain laparoscopic hand tools. Some surgeons prefer bipolar cautery because of theoretically lower risk of inadvertent injury due to accidental touching of vital structures during cauterization. There are also suction devices that have a cautery tip to allow suction and hemostasis to be performed simultaneously. Larger vessels can be controlled using laparoscopic vascular clips (Nelson et al, 1992; Papaioannou et al, 1996). These can be introduced with reusable clip appliers or, more commonly, disposable clip appliers. They come in 5- and 10-mm sizes and should be considered standard equipment if procedures such as nephrectomy or two-stage orchiopexy are likely to be performed. Division of very large vessels, such as a renal vein in an adolescent or adult, might require a vascular gastrointestinal anastomosis stapler (Krasna and Nazem, 1991). These generally require a 12-mm laparoscopic port for introduction. Other methods of hemostasis have been applied, including the laser, the harmonic scalpel, and argon beam coagulation, all of which have been shown to be effective (Jackman et al, 1998a; Spivak et al, 1998; Gill and Mac-Fadyen, 1999; Platt and Heniford, 2000). Specific needs will be dictated by the procedures being performed.

The myriad disposable laparoscopic products for specific indications cannot be covered here. Suffice it to say that the laparoscopic practitioner should remain aware of available devices but at the same time be aware of their potentially high cost.

Anesthetic Issues in Pediatric Laparoscopy

In general, laparoscopy is well tolerated by children, although initial concerns were raised. The principal issues in laparoscopy are the physiologic effects resulting from the creation of a surgical working space using a pneumoperitoneum or retroperitoneum. **Intra-abdominal pressure is increased significantly, and with the common use of CO_2 as the insufflating agent, there is absorption of CO_2 across the peritoneum. There are also risks of CO_2 embolus. In children the key difference from an anesthetic standpoint, compared with adults, is their decreased pulmonary reserve, which results from a relatively low functional reserve capacity and lower oxygen reserve.** Their ability to withstand decreases in oxygen saturation is less that of an adult, reducing the safety margin when any procedure reduces lung volume. Increased intra-abdominal pressure significantly reduces functional reserve capacity (Tobias, 1998). It also increases airway pressures, which may impair ventilation and gas exchange. As a result, children may be more susceptible to oxygen desaturation during a laparoscopic procedure, and this susceptibility may be greater in younger children. Alterations in the mechanical characteristics of ventilation are induced during laparoscopy, reducing airway compliance and increasing resistance (Bergesio et al, 1999). It is important to recognize these issues and adjust intra-abdominal pressures accordingly. **It is helpful that less pressure is required to produce abdominal distention in children because of their greater abdominal compliance.**

Cardiovascular function is altered by pneumoperitoneum in children as a result of increased preload and afterload and filling volumes. Systolic function is not markedly altered. The clinical effect in a child with normal cardiac function is insignificant, but it must be anticipated in the cardiac patient (Gentili et al, 2000).

Hypercarbia caused by CO_2 absorption and decreased ventilatory clearance is well recognized to occur in laparoscopy and is well tolerated in healthy children. The principal effect of hypercarbia is on the myocardium, including inotropic, chronotropic, and arrhythmogenic effects. There is also catecholamine release, which may accentuate these effects and produce vasoconstriction. From a clinical standpoint, these effects are rarely significant in healthy children, but in the susceptible patient potential adverse effects should be anticipated and CO_2 levels adjusted. In general there is no strong indication to alter minute ventilation to control CO_2 levels as measured by the end-tidal CO_2 (ET CO_2), but this requires a clinical judgment by the anesthesiologist. CO_2 embolus may occur when a high volume of CO_2 enters the venous system as a result of vascular injury. Initially heralded by increasing ET CO_2 and decreasing oxygen saturation, cardiovascular collapse may soon follow. At that point, ET CO_2 falls to zero and rapid desaturation occurs. A CO_2 embolus should be suspected and acted on immediately. The classic "mill-wheel" murmur gives evidence to the gas embolus that obstructs right heart outflow and pulmonary circulation. Rapid placement of the patient into the right-side-up position with attempted aspiration of the embolus through a central venous line is appropriate.

Several studies have examined the use of laparoscopy and its impact on anesthetic management in children. In studies of brief laparoscopic procedures used for diagnosis of contralateral hernia, 55 patients were monitored and were without anesthetic complications when endotracheal intubation was used (Tobias et al, 1995). A further study demonstrated that during this brief diagnostic laparoscopy an endotracheal tube was not necessary (Tobias et al, 1994, 1996). Our experience has included only one child who experienced oxygenation problems during laparoscopic orchiopexy. This child had multiple congenital anomalies and a small, kyphotic chest. He desaturated when the intra-abdominal pressure exceeded 10 mm Hg but then did well at 8 mm Hg and the procedure was completed. Neonates may be more prone to such desaturation because they have even less functional pulmonary reserve and higher oxygen consumption, although experimental studies have not shown this to be a major risk (Rubin et al, 1996).

Temperature regulation is another concern in pediatric anesthesia, because children have a greater ratio of surface area to body mass and therefore lose heat more rapidly. Attempts were initially made to warm the insufflating gas to reduce this risk. It has been our experience that heat loss is rare in children undergoing laparoscopic urologic procedures, and indeed it appears as if there are elevations in temperature during renal surgery in infants. The cause of this phenomenon is unknown but has been speculated to be activation of perirenal brown fat with release of catecholamines. We have not seen any adverse effects. For most laparoscopic cases, we do not routinely take extra measures to control temperature.

As with adults, increased intra-abdominal pressure in children reduces urine output, although this effect is transient and has not been observed to cause any permanent renal injury (Razvi et al, 1996). As more procedures are performed in compromised patients, concern has arisen regarding the effect of pneumoperitoneum-induced oliguria on previously compromised renal function. Even in children with chronic renal insufficiency, significant alterations in function have not been observed. In an experimental study using a model of reduced renal function, pneumoperitoneum did not cause further permanent renal dysfunction (Cisek et al, 1998a). That study also examined the physiologic basis for pneumoperitoneum-induced oliguria and suggested that the mechanisms for reduced renal blood flow may not be simple increases in pressure. Distinctly different patterns were seen between the renal circulation and the mesenteric or carotid circulation in response to changes in intra-abdominal pressure. **Renal perfusion returned much more slowly than in the other vascular beds, suggesting regulation by factors other than pressure alone. Whether these are neural or humoral remains to be determined.** It may be possible to pharmacologically control this response to provide the best possible protection to the kidney during laparoscopic surgery.

Complications of Pediatric Laparoscopy

The complications associated with pediatric laparoscopy are no different from those in adults, and similar precautions must be exercised. Several aspects of pediatric laparoscopy, however, increase the risk of certain problems that must be anticipated.

COMPLICATIONS RELATED TO ACCESS

Inadvertent injury to intra-abdominal structures may occur because of the different physical properties of the child's abdomen. The resistance to penetration is much less, and reduced force is needed for access, yet the peritoneum is more likely to separate from the abdominal wall. This may increase the risk of preperitoneal insufflation, and the temptation to push harder may be greater because the tip of the trocar is not yet visible in the field; puncture of abdominal viscera may be more likely. During retroperitoneal procedures, the peritoneum is more easily violated, because of its more posterior reflection and its lesser strength. This can occur even with excessive inflation of a balloon dissector. The relative size of any cannula is greater in a child than in an adult. Where a 5-mm port may not require closure in an adult, it does in a child; otherwise, postoperative hernia may occur. **The lower limit of size requiring suture closure is not firmly established, but a 2-mm port does not require closure, whereas we would suture a 3.5-mm port site.**

Open access technique is not without hazard, including inadvertent injury to a loop of bowel trapped during the opening (Sadeghi-Nejad et al, 1994). As with adult laparoscopy, there is greater risk with the use of Veress needle access (Peters, 1996a), although it should be recognized that this is usually the result of injury from the subsequent blind placement of the first working cannula, rather than the Veress needle itself. With current 2-mm instrumentation, we perform most diagnostic laparoscopies with the combination of a Veress needle and a 2-mm cannula. This requires only one puncture of the needle, whose sheath acts as the cannula for the telescope and insufflation.

OPERATIVE COMPLICATIONS

The principal cause of intraoperative complications in pediatric laparoscopy is likely to be the limited working space in most surgical procedures. Inadvertent injury with cautery or cutting instruments is the consequence of limited space. As a result, extra care is needed when operating in confined spaces. Attention to uninsulated parts of instruments used for cautery is essential. With smaller telescopes, visualization is more easily compromised by smoke, fluid spatter, and the light absorption of blood. All instrument changes must be done with greater care, because the safe range of movement is reduced. Smaller-diameter working instruments also increase the risk for the electrical effects of capacitance coupling, in which induced currents produce thermal injury, usually at port sites (Tucker et al, 1992; Grosskinsky et al, 1993). This is increased with smaller-diameter instruments because the current density is higher, and with thinner abdominal walls because they disperse current less efficiently (Voyles and Tucker, 1992; Willson et al, 1997). Careful attention to the insulation on instruments is important, as is attempting to limit electrocautery use and power.

The effect of pneumoperitoneum on ventriculoperitoneal shunt function has been an issue, yet there does not seem to be a significant risk (Docimo, 1999). One early report suggested that increased intra-abdominal pressure would produce marked increases in intracranial pressure in a noncompliant, chronically drained ventricular system (Uzzo et al, 1997). The authors recommended exteriorization of these shunts during any laparoscopic procedure. However, clinical experience has not confirmed these concerns, and numerous procedures have been performed without ill effect. With a functioning valve in the shunt, there should be no risk of increasing pressure beyond what might be seen with temporarily clamping of the shunt.

As a general practice, we have anticipated major complications by being prepared for emergency open access during laparoscopic procedures, particularly those involving the kidney. This means having blood available in the bank and having an abdominal instrument set with vascular instruments ready in the room. From a practical standpoint, it is essential to have backup laparoscopic instruments during all procedures, as well as two laparoscopic surgical clip appliers in the operating room at all times.

Cryptorchidism

PRIMARY ORCHIOPEXY

Procedure

Examination under anesthesia and diagnostic laparoscopy have been performed as described earlier. If the testis is palpable high in the canal on examination in the operating room, laparoscopy may be used to aid dissection of the intra-abdominal vasculature and vas to prevent the need for an extensive inguinal dissection (Docimo et al, 1995b).

The intra-abdominal testis may be noted anywhere between the internal inguinal ring and the lower edge of the ipsilateral kidney. The testis is evaluated for size and location to determine whether orchiectomy or a two-stage procedure is indicated.

Associated vasal or epididymal anomalies or the appearance of an atrophic testis might suggest orchiectomy as the next logical step. Conversion to a two-stage orchiopexy (see later discussion) is decided by estimating distance of

Prone Retroperitoneal

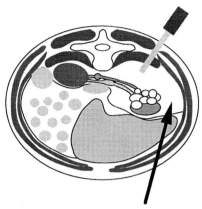

Pneumoretroperitoneum

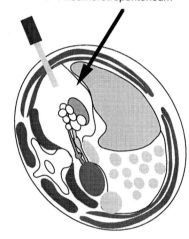

Flank Retroperitoneal

Figure 72–16. Diagram showing the relative positions of the kidney during retroperitoneal nephrectomy using the prone and flank positions. The kidney tends to fall forward and expose the hilum more readily in the prone position. (From Peters, CA: Laparoendoscopic renal surgery in children. J Endourol 2000;14:841–848, with permission.)

ter needs to be removed the lateral approach may be preferable.

Nephrectomy

The surgical technique of laparoendoscopic nephrectomy is similar regardless of the approach used. **In transperitoneal nephrectomy, the colon is first reflected from the kidney by incision of the lateral line of Toldt. In most cases the ureter can be identified and used as a handle to lift the lower pole of the kidney. This facilitates access to the hilar vessels, which are then dissected free and independently ligated.** We have used surgical clips without problems, although some authors suggest using absorbable ties or bipolar cautery for smaller arteries. The security of clips is attractive, and they are efficiently placed. During hilar dissection, there is a tendency in laparoendoscopic procedures to be very close to the kidney; this may lead to ligation of arterial branches, either anterior or posterior. One should always be alert for other branches

still needing ligation before the kidney is removed. With dysplastic kidneys, aberrant arterial supply is common, and these small vessels should be sought. The renal vein can almost always be controlled with a medium or large clip in children and teenagers. It has not been our experience that a gastrointestinal anastomosis stapling device is needed as it can be in adults.

Further dissection of the perinephric tissues may be performed with a combination of rapid blunt and cautery-assisted dissection. **In a cystic kidney, it is best to leave the cysts full until most of the dissection is complete to facilitate blunt dissection. Near completion, it is helpful to drain some of the cysts to permit grasping of the cyst walls for traction on the kidney.**

When the kidney is fully freed, any remaining cysts should be drained to allow removal. In most cases, direct removal is possible through the umbilical port or through the initial port in retroperitoneal access. Larger kidneys may require bag extraction with morcellation.

Instrumentation used for nephrectomy is the same for either approach and includes scissors, delicate dissecting and grasping tools, and a heavy locking grasping device for specimen removal. In most children, 5-mm instruments are easily used and well tolerated. We have used 2-mm working instruments with a 5-mm endoscope, but these instruments are not yet sturdy enough for heavy use (Borer and Peters, 1999). As a compromise, 3.5-mm instrumentation has become available and seems to be effective without creating as large a defect as the 5-mm instruments do. Stapling devices are limited to 5- and 10-mm instruments, so a 5-mm port will always be required. The radially expanding cannula system (Step, InnerDyne, Inc., Salt Lake City, UT) permits moving between 3.5- and 5-mm instruments with the same port, and the claim is made that these ports do not require suture closure. We have not experienced any complications with this system, but the valve mechanisms are fragile and may be damaged with multiple instrument changes.

NEPHROURETERECTOMY

Removal of the ureter along with the kidney is readily accomplished laparoscopically. **In some ways, transperitoneal laparoscopy is ideally suited to nephroureterectomy (see Fig. 72–14), although retroperitoneal approaches usually are adequate.** The extent to which the ureter needs to be removed depends on the pathology. In the setting of obstruction and reflux, the entire ureter must be removed, whereas free reflux with good drainage is unlikely to present any problems with a small, retained stump. In any case of reflux, the stump must be closed with a clip or suture. Reflux of urine into the peritoneum has occurred. The ureter is usually transected just below the lower pole of the kidney and then removed separately, after the kidney has been fully dissected. If a concomitant bladder procedure is to be performed (e.g., contralateral ureteral reimplantation), the distal ureter is dissected from the bladder level, either intravesically or extravesically. Otherwise, the ureter is mobilized using the same three cannulae, with care being taken to pass the ureter under the gonadal vessels. In boys the vas is identified and avoided. The ureter is visualized to its insertion, at which point it is

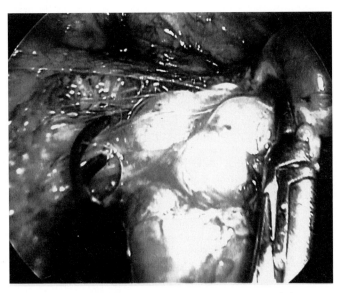

Figure 72–17. Retroperitoneal laparoendoscopic view of the upper pole of a duplex kidney in a child with an ectopic ureter. The upper pole is cystic and is being mobilized on its lateral aspect. The endoscopic grasping instrument is lifting the cystic upper pole upward to facilitate mobilization. The healthy lower pole is visible at the bottom of the image.

closed, with intracorporeal suturing for a large ureter or a ligature for a smaller one. A bladder catheter is left in place overnight.

PARTIAL NEPHRECTOMY

In children, partial nephrectomy is usually performed for a nonfunctioning renal segment of a duplex system. The demarcation between the segments is usually very clear, and the affected unit is often hydronephrotic or cystic, with little blood flow. This facilitates the separation of the two poles for removal. The critical feature in pediatric partial nephrectomy is the delicacy of the renal vasculature of the remnant segment. Open partial nephrectomy is associated with a small but definite incidence of vascular compromise of the remnant pole due to vasospasm of the arterial supply. This may be induced by mobilization of the kidney or during dissection of the vessels to be ligated for removal of the affected pole. Any approach for laparoscopic partial nephrectomy must be done with extra care in protection of the remnant vessels. This is best accomplished by limiting the mobilization of the remnant pole and by isolating the affected vessels close to their renal unit and away from the remnant vessels (Fig. 72–17). A potential advantage with laparoscopic approaches is that wide mobilization of the whole kidney is not necessary in most cases, and therefore the risk to the remnant pole is limited (Janetschek et al, 1997; Yao and Poppas, 2000).

After vascular control has been ensured, the affected pole is separated from the remnant pole with the use of either electrocautery or the harmonic scalpel. This instrument has been very effective in this procedure because it permits efficient cutting and vascular control of the junction between the affected and remnant renal units (Jackman et al, 1998a). The entire collecting system of the affected pole is removed, and this may be aided by development of

the plane between the affected collecting system and the parenchyma of the remnant pole. The only residual tissue attaching the two poles is the thin rim of parenchyma, which may then be incised at its margin with the harmonic scalpel.

Postoperative Management—Renal Laparoscopic Surgery

After a simple nephrectomy, some children may be discharged to home on the same day, depending on age. Younger children often return to their normal diet and exhibit adequate pain control within a few hours after the procedure. Others may need to stay overnight, in part based on parental anxiety. Older children continue to have some element of abdominal discomfort for up to 24 hours, perhaps as a result of the CO_2 distention for transperitoneal procedures. This seems less with retroperitoneal operations. **During the period of hospitalization, children need to be watched for signs of serious complications, which are made more dangerous by their infrequency and possible lack of early recognition.** Hemorrhage is of most concern and is evidenced by alterations in the patient's vital signs. An appropriate level of suspicion is the best means to permit early detection. Similarly, bowel injury may occur without intraoperative recognition during either transperitoneal or retroperitoneal procedures. Bowel injury may not become apparent until after discharge, when fever and evidence of intraperitoneal irritation develop.

Pyeloplasty

Laparoscopic pyeloplasty in children remains a technical challenge, although it has become an established procedure in adults (Chen et al, 1996). The principal difficulty is the need for precise suturing with fine suture material. The automatic suturing devices that are available have not been down-sized adequately to suit the young child. Nevertheless, laparoscopic pyeloplasty is technically feasible and has been reported with adequate early results. There is a clear need for more specific suturing procedures and equipment. With time and experience, laparoscopic pyeloplasty should become a practical, less invasive means of dealing with UPJ obstruction and serve as the foundation of other complex upper tract reconstructive techniques.

Only transperitoneal access techniques have been reported, although retroperitoneal access has been performed (Janetschek et al, 1996). The same methods of access are used as for other renal surgery (Peters et al, 1995; Tan, 1999). Port placement must be specific, to facilitate suturing. We have used three ports for visualization and manipulation, and occasionally a fourth for retraction (Fig. 72–18). The renal pelvis is identified and cleared of surrounding tissues, with attention being paid to a possible crossing lower pole vessel. As with open surgery, minimal handling of the ureter and area of anastomosis reduces postoperative edema. **A hitch stitch is brought through the abdominal wall just below the costal margin, passed through the pelvis, and passed back through the abdominal wall. This lifts and secures the pelvis.** The medial edge of the ureter is cut below the UPJ, and a traction stitch is passed through the distal edge. The rest of the ureter is cut and spatulated laterally. The UPJ segment is

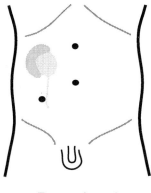

Transperitoneal Pyeloplasty

Figure 72–18. Diagram of port positions for transperitoneal laparoscopic right pyeloplasty. A hitch stitch is placed in the renal pelvis and brought out just below the costal margin in the midclavicular line. (From Peters CA: Laparoendoscopic renal surgery in children. J Endourol 2000;14:841–848, with permission.)

then excised from the pelvis in an oblique angle to create a dependent vertex, to which the vertex of the ureteral spatulation will be sewn. **We do not routinely perform a significant reduction of the pelvis.** We have tried preplacing a ureteral stent to facilitate alignment and suturing but found this to interfere with reconstruction.

The first stitch is passed between the vertex of the ureter and the dependent portion of the pelvis and tied using a preformed slip knot (Tan, 1999). The dependent suture line is sewn first, using this suture. We have used 6-0 braided absorbable suture for small children and 5-0 for older children, as for open surgery. Monocryl is an excellent material, but it is not dyed and is very difficult to see. It also has a significant degree of memory that makes manipulation difficult. A small curved needle (TF) is preferred and can be passed through a 3.5- or 5-mm port. It should be mounted on the needle holder so as to avoid blunting of the point in passage. Depending on the particular anatomy of the pelvis and ureter, it may be preferable to use different ports for suturing. **The aim is to provide an alignment of the needle driver with the line of suturing, and to have the second instrument be about 30 degrees offset from the first.**

Once the back or dependent wall has been sewn, a double-J stent is placed. The stent may be passed through a Veress introducing needle and guided over a wire into the ureter under direct vision. The distal coil needs to be in the bladder based on feel or introduction of blue dye in the bladder and observed reflux into the stent. The proximal coil is positioned into the renal pelvis under direct vision. The anterior wall of the anastomosis is then sewn. With a stent in place, a drain has not been used. Alternatively, a temporary percutaneous nephrostomy may be placed under direct vision. The nephrostomy has the advantage that it permits testing of the anastomosis for patency before access is lost, yet without actually stenting the ureter. A nephroureteral stent may be used, but it must be removed before outcome is assessed. There is insufficient clinical experience to judge which method is most effective.

Double-J stents are removed 2 weeks after the procedure, and ultrasound monitoring in the immediate postoperative period is effective. Functional imaging is used, depending on the clinical scenario and results of ultrasonography.

Miscellaneous Renal Surgery

Laparoscopic renal biopsy for nephrologic disease has been reported, although a comparison with ultrasound-guided needle biopsy has yet to be made. It is performed retroperitoneally, with few reported complications and rapid procedural time (Caione et al, 2000; Takeda et al, 2000). Laparoscopic management of renal malignancy in children has not yet been reported but may ultimately play a role in staging biopsy for Wilms' tumor or perhaps neuroblastoma (Waldhausen et al, 2000).

Laparoscopic adrenal surgery in children has been reported in a few cases, primarily related to cortical adenoma and associated with congenital virilizing adrenal hyperplasia (Schier et al, 1999; Radmayr et al, 2000). The adrenal gland is readily visualized through both retroperitoneal and transperitoneal approaches. There is limited need for adrenalectomy in children, but laparoscopy appears to have a significant potential in this area, as it has in adult surgery.

Results

Overall results of laparoscopic renal surgery in children have been good (Hamilton et al, 2000). There remains uncertainty as to its advantages over conventional open surgery. From one perspective, children, and particularly infants, recover rapidly from most open renal surgery, and they are not saving any lost time at work. Subjectively, however, parents whose children have undergone laparoscopic renal surgery report recoveries that appear to be more rapid than seen in open surgery, and hospital stays are shorter. It is important to recognize that these parameters are subjective and depend on personal and institutional preferences. As laparoscopic renal surgery emerged, several reports of day surgical nephrectomy in infants were published, indicating the rapidity of pediatric recovery, although these procedures were not without risk (Elder et al, 1995).

Operative times for laparoscopic renal surgery have declined with increasing experience and are now reported to be between 60 and 120 minutes in most series for simple nephrectomy. Partial nephrectomy requires somewhat longer but may be performed within 2 hours in many cases. There has been no formal comparison between transperitoneal and retroperitoneal nephrectomy in terms of operative duration, hospital stay, or complications. Laparoscopic nephrectomy in high-risk patients, such as those with renal insufficiency, has been undertaken with good results (El-Ghoneimi et al, 2000).

The incidence of complications has been low in all published series (Ehrlich et al, 1992; Koyle et al, 1993; Diamond et al, 1995; Valla et al, 1996; El-Ghoneimi et al, 1998; Borer and Peters, 1999; Hamilton et al, 2000; Yao and Poppas, 2000; York et al, 2000). **The conversion rate is less than 5%.** No late morbidity has been reported.

Laparoscopic pyeloplasty is too new to adequately assess long-term outcomes, although they should be similar to those for open pyeloplasty (Peters et al, 1995;

Schier, 1998; Tan, 1999). Operative duration is clearly longer but has markedly decreased for the few practitioners using this procedure. Hospital stay is usually overnight, an improvement from most open pyeloplasty reports. Long-term assessment of the role of laparoendoscopic renal surgery will require comparative trials with practitioners who have significant experience. The influences of the learning curve, teaching, and the inherent caution exercised with a new procedure will have to be factored into these results. Subjectively, it is impressive how well the kidney is visualized through endoscopic access and how readily some aspects of the surgery can be performed. It is also apparent how constrained some aspects of the procedure are through endoscopic tools. With improvement in these methods and novel approaches to necessary manipulations, these limitations should vanish.

Bladder Surgery

Laparoscopic surgery involving the bladder can be divided into procedures intended to remove or repair a portion of the bladder or urachus and reconstructive procedures such as bladder augmentation or continent urinary stoma formation. Intravesical surgery is covered in the section dealing with antireflux surgery. Operations to repair the bladder (e.g., diverticulectomy) have been rarely reported in children, so most of the cases in the literature involve adult patients (Das, 1992; Parra et al, 1992; Jarrett et al, 1995; Zanetti et al, 1995; Iselin et al, 1996). This is also true of operations to excise urachal abnormalities (Trondsen et al, 1993; Redmond et al, 1994; Fahlenkamp et al, 1995; Hubens et al, 1995; Linos et al, 1997). The approach to the bladder may be extraperitoneal, working in the space of Retzius, but is more commonly transperitoneal, especially in children. The bladder is relatively easily accessible in children and therefore is well suited for laparoscopic approaches. **For either urachal or bladder procedures, high abdominal access is necessary to allow exposure and room to manipulate instruments.**

Bladder reconstructive procedures have taken three main forms to date: laparoscopic autoaugmentation techniques, laparoscopic enterocystoplasty, and laparoscopic-assisted reconstructive procedures. Augmentation of the bladder with tissue scaffolds (Calvano et al, 2000) or engineered bladder tissue may become important laparoscopic techniques, but they currently are experimental.

LAPAROSCOPIC AUTOAUGMENTATION

Autoaugmentation, or detrusorraphy, is a technique that involves dividing the bladder muscle and dissecting it free of the mucosa (Cartwright and Snow, 1989). This allows the development of a large bladder diverticulum, resulting in improved compliance and low-pressure storage. Because this is a form of bladder augmentation that does not involve the harvesting of gastrointestinal segments and requires very little suturing, it is adaptable to minimally invasive techniques. Laparoscopic autoaugmentation has been performed in animal models (Britanisky et al, 1995) and in children (Ehrlich and Gershman, 1993; Poppas et al, 1996b; Braren and Bishop, 1998), and both transperitoneally and extraperitoneally (McDougall et al, 1995a).

Bladder autoaugmentation requires a large incision of the detrusor with dissection of the underlying mucosa over a large surface area, often followed by fixation of the bladder muscle to the pelvic sidewall to prevent narrowing of the mouth of the newly formed bladder diverticulum. The process of separating bladder muscle from mucosa has been assisted with laser, with the theoretical advantage of a limited depth of tissue destruction (Poppas et al, 1996b). This operation can be done with a very short hospital stay or on an outpatient basis, but it does require postoperative bladder drainage for some period of time because of the possibility of rupture and leakage. Autoaugmentation yields a bladder completely lined with uroepithelium, no mucous formation, no apparent increased risk of stones, and the ability to go on to other forms of augmentation should it become necessary. Autoaugmentation techniques have been combined with extravesical forms of ureteral reimplantation (Carr et al, 1999), and this could theoretically be performed laparoscopically (Atala et al, 1993), although it has not been reported as a combined procedure.

Long-term results of open or laparoscopic autoaugmentation have not been consistent (Gonzalez, 1996), and autoaugmentation has not achieved wide acceptance as a reconstructive technique in children. This is, however, a minimally invasive technique of bladder enlargement, and it may be considered for patients with reasonable capacity but poor compliance and for those who do not require a large increase in bladder capacity. There is little disadvantage to an autoaugmentation if further reconstruction is necessary in the future, especially if it is performed laparoscopically.

LAPAROSCOPIC ENTEROCYSTOPLASTY

The first laparoscopic gastrointestinal bladder augmentation was performed using stomach (Docimo et al, 1995a). The laparoscopic technique involved the use of endoscopic clips to dissect the gastroepiploic pedicle and endoscopic gastrointestinal anastomotic staplers to excise a wedge of stomach. The remaining stomach edge was oversewn with the previously described endoscopic suturing device, and the gastric patch was sewn to the bladder in the same way. **Laparoscopic bladder augmentation has also been performed with the use of small or large intestine, usually with an extracorporeal bowel anastomosis** (Gill et al, 2000)**, and with peritoneum** (L. Kavoussi, personal communication, 1999). These operations require a high degree of laparoscopic skill and involve difficult access for suturing. Development of innovative techniques, including laser welding, tissue adhesives, and newer suturing techniques, may be required to bring laparoscopic bladder augmentation into the mainstream. It is not farfetched to think that most bladder augmentations might be performed laparoscopically in the near future.

LAPAROSCOPIC-ASSISTED RECONSTRUCTIVE SURGERY

At the moment, the state of the art for minimally invasive reconstruction represents a compromise—the laparoscopic-assisted procedure. The concept is based on the premise that bladder reconstructive operations

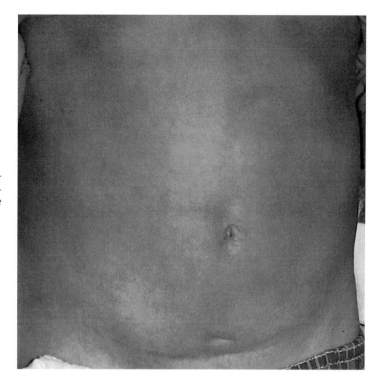

Figure 72–19. This 4-year-old boy with a history of ectopic ureter and poor bladder emptying has undergone laparoscopic nephro-ureterectomy and laparoscopic-assisted appendicovesicostomy. He will have no visible scars as an adult.

can be divided into two stages: in the first, the tissues for the augment and/or the continent stoma are freed and harvested, and in the second, the actual reconstruction is performed. The assembly of parts into a functional bladder unit takes place in the low pelvis and therefore can be accomplished through a small lower abdominal incision (Fig. 72–19). If no continent stoma is to be made and ileum or sigmoid is to be used for the augmentation, the entire operation can be done through this type of incision, and laparoscopic assistance is not employed. If stomach, ureter, or appendix is to be used, an approach to the upper abdomen becomes necessary, and laparoscopy obviates the need for a long midline incision or, in the case of ureter, two incisions. The principle of laparoscopic-assisted reconstructive surgery is simple: use laparoscopy to perform the parts of the operation that require upper abdominal access, and do the technically demanding reconstructive steps through an open lower abdominal incision (Hedican et al, 1999).

Laparoscopic-assisted surgery is widely applicable in patients who require bladder reconstruction and/or antegrade continence enema stoma. The majority of patients reported have had prior abdominal surgery, including ventriculoperitoneal shunt placement and bladder exstrophy closure (Cadeddu and Docimo, 1999; Hedican et al, 1999). The benefit of laparoscopic mobilization is not just cosmetic; in theory, more rapid recovery and decreased intra-abdominal adhesions can be expected. Therefore, even patients with a prior midline incision might benefit. The presence of a ventriculoperitoneal shunt is not a contraindication to laparoscopic surgery (Docimo, 1999; Jackman et al, 2000) and necessitates no special precautions or monitoring.

Laparoscopic-assisted surgery has been applied at only a few centers thus far (Jordan and Winslow, 1993b; Sanchez de Badajoz et al, 1995; Cadeddu and Docimo, 1999; Hedican et al, 1999). The results have generally been as good as those of open operations in terms of surgical outcome, and the cosmetic results are subjectively superior to a standard midline approach (Cadeddu and Docimo, 1999; Hedican et al, 1999). Other advantages of laparoscopic-assisted surgery include the likelihood of fewer intra-abdominal adhesions (Moore et al, 1995b), less postoperative pain, and quicker recovery. The only comparative series of laparoscopic-assisted versus open continent stoma procedures demonstrated a more rapid return to regular diet and a significant decrease in hospital stay with laparoscopy (Cadeddu and Docimo, 1999). Currently, all reconstructive operations that cannot be performed through a small lower abdominal incision can be done in this way, unless there has been extensive prior abdominal surgery.

Ureteral Surgery

ANTIREFLUX SURGERY

Surgery for vesicoureteral reflux has long been a target for those interested in minimally invasive approaches. Most notable among these have been the injection methods (STING procedures) that have been employed for reflux, which are discussed elsewhere. This section deals specifically with the use of laparoscopic techniques in an attempt to correct reflux. These have taken two main forms: transvesical and extravesical techniques.

Strictly speaking, transvesical techniques are not "laparoscopic" or "peritoneoscopic" procedures but rather percutaneous bladder procedures that employ laparoscopic instruments and techniques. Smaller instrumentation has allowed experimentation and clinical experience in intravesical endoscopic surgery. The most common operation through this route has been the percutaneous endoscopic trigonoplasty, a modification of the Gil-Vernet procedure (Okamura et al, 1995; Cartwright et al, 1996). In this operation, a horizontal incision from ureteral orifice to ureteral orifice is closed vertically, incorporating detrusor, pulling the orifices toward the midline, and enhancing the fixation of the ureteral tunnel. Unfortunately, the initial promise of trigonoplasty has not been realized with long term follow-up (Okamura et al, 1996; Gatti et al, 1999). Taking this idea one step further, it has been shown both experimentally (Lakshmanan et al, 1999) and clinically (Gatti et al, 1999) that the ureters can be dissected free of the bladder muscle and reimplanted using endoscopic technique. Once again, the results of the percutaneous reimplantation have not justified its adoption in place of traditional open techniques at this time (Gatti et al, 1999).

The most widely applied laparoscopic approach to vesicoureteral reflux has been the laparoscopic extravesical reimplantation (Atala et al, 1993). This procedure has been used experimentally and clinically at a number of centers (Reddy and Evans, 1994; McDougall et al, 1995b). It is performed in the manner of the Lich-Gregoir operation (Gregoir, 1977). The ureterovesical junction is exposed transperitoneally by incision between the round ligament and the bladder (Lakshmanan et al, 1998). An incision is made in the bladder muscle adjacent to the ureter and is extended cephalad, staying outside of the bladder mucosa. A trough is created with mucosa as its base. The bladder muscle is then closed over the ureter with interrupted laparoscopic suture and tying techniques to effectively create a submucosal tunnel. Results of the largest series to date suggest efficacy similar to that of open surgery (Lakshmanan and Fung, 2000).

It is not clear at this time whether any of these minimally invasive procedures will replace open surgery, which is performed through a small Pfannensteil incision and requires a short hospital stay. The economics of reflux management are such that increased expense for minimally invasive approaches might further tip the balance away from surgical management if cost is the only factor considered (Mathews et al, 2000). Nevertheless, development of these techniques is vital if current reflux management is to be replaced by minimally invasive approaches.

Perivesical Surgery

SEMINAL VESICLE CYST

The potential for perivesical laparoscopic surgery exists, but little has been reported to date. Although surgery for removal of seminal vesicles has been described commonly in adults, mostly related to the management of prostate cancer (Kavoussi et al, 1993), there is one report of excision of a seminal vesicle cyst in a 10-month-old child (Ikari et al, 1999). This was performed transperitoneally. The surgeon incised the retrovesical peritoneum and followed the cystic seminal vesicle, as well as the divided vas deferens on that side, in order to achieve a complete resection. Laparoscopy seems ideally suited to the management of these unusual cases.

VAGINOPLASTY

There are numerous techniques for the creation of a neovagina in children with an absent vagina due to congenital anomalies. Laparoscopic techniques have been used occasionally, mostly in adults. Laparoscopy has been used as an adjunct to the Vecchietti operation for creation of a neovagina in Mayer-Rokitansky-Kuster-Hauser syndrome (Vecchietti, 1965). In this technique, an olive-shaped device is placed at the vaginal dimple, and constant upward traction is applied transabdominally via sutures brought out through the anterior abdominal wall. This creates a neovaginal space in less than 2 weeks. Although this technique would rarely be applicable to pediatric urologic patients, it has been adapted laparoscopically, making it more widely applied for this specific adult population (Fedele et al, 1994; Keckstein et al, 1995; Cooper et al, 1996).

Much more commonly applied in children is the sigmoid (or ileal) vaginoplasty. These operations produce a mucosa-lined neovagina that can be expected to maintain a reasonable lumen without constant dilation. This operation is ideally suited to laparoscopic techniques, avoiding the often large abdominal incision used to harvest the segment of sigmoid. Laparoscopic dissection of the retrovesical space can be combined with perineal dissection to facilitate creation of the neovaginal space (Ota et al, 2000). A similar dissection was used to facilitate skin graft vaginoplasty to an intact uterus in an adolescent girl (Lee et al, 1999).

SUMMARY

The continued expansion of applications of endourologic techniques in pediatric patients holds promise for enhancing care of these patients. Advances in technology will facilitate this expansion, but caution must be exercised so that enthusiasm for the novel does not cloud clinical judgment. It should be clearly evident or at least likely that the "minimally invasive" procedure offers a real advantage to the patient. There is potential for significant harm in misguided applications of these technologies, particularly in inexperienced hands. Properly constructed clinical trials are difficult to accomplish in this setting, but every effort should be made to evaluate in as objective a manner as possible the clinical outcomes of new surgical technologies. If this is not undertaken, new methods with real promise may never fulfill their potential.

REFERENCES

Adams JB, Schulam PG, Moore RG, et al: New laparoscopic suturing device: Initial clinical experience. Urology 1995;46:242–245.

Anidjar M, Meria P, Cochand-Priollet B, et al: Evaluation of optimal stent size after antegrade endopyelotomy: An experimental study in the porcine model. Eur Urol 1997;32:245–252.

Arnbjornsson E, Mikaelsson C, Lindhagen T, Ivarsson SA: Laparoscopy for nonpalpable testis in childhood: Is inguinal exploration necessary when vas and vessels are not seen? Eur J Pediatr Surg 1996;6:7–9.

Atala A, Kavoussi LR, Goldstein DS, et al: Laparoscopic correction of vesicoureteral reflux. J Urol 1993;150:748–751.

Badawy H, Salama A, Eissa M, et al: Percutaneous management of renal calculi: Experience with percutaneous nephrolithotomy in 60 children. J Urol 1999;162:1710–1713.

Baker L, Docimo S, Surer I, et al: A multi-institutional analysis of laparoscopic orchidopexy. BJU Int 2001;87:484–489.

Baldwin DD, Beaghler MA, Ruckle HC, et al: Ureteroscopic treatment of symptomatic caliceal diverticular calculi. Tech Urol 1998;4:92–98.

Bergesio R, Habre W, Lanteri C, Sly P: Changes in respiratory mechanics during abdominal laparoscopic surgery in children. Anaesth Intensive Care 1999;27:245–248.

Bernardo NO, Smith AD: Percutaneous endopyelotomy. Urology 2000;56: 322–327.

Bloom DA: Two-step orchiopexy with pelviscopic clip ligation of the spermatic vessels. J Urol 1991;145:1030–1033.

Bloom DA, Ayers JW, McGuire EJ: The role of laparoscopy in management of nonpalpable testes. J Urol (Paris) 1988;94:465–470.

Boddy SA, Corkery JJ, Gornall P: The place of laparoscopy in the management of the impalpable testis. Br J Surg 1985;72:918–919.

Bolton DM, Bogaert GA, Mevorach RA, et al: Pediatric ureteropelvic junction obstruction treated with retrograde endopyelotomy. Urology 1994;44:609–613.

Borer J, Peters CA: Retroperitoneoscopic nephrectomy in children. J Endourol 2000;14:413–436.

Braren V, Bishop MR: Laparoscopic bladder autoaugmentation in children. Urol Clin North Am 1998;25:533–540.

Britanisky RG, Poppas DP, Shichman SN, et al: Laparoscopic laser-assisted bladder autoaugmentation. Urology 1995;46:31–35.

Brock JW, 3rd, Holcomb GW, 3rd, Morgan WM, 3rd: The use of laparoscopy in the management of the nonpalpable testis. J Laparoendosc Surg 1996;6(Suppl. 1):S35–S39.

Cadeddu JA, Docimo SG: Laparoscopic-assisted continent stoma procedures: Our new standard. Urology 1999;54:909–912.

Caione P, De Gennaro M, Capozza N, et al: Endoscopic manipulation of ureteral calculi in children by rigid operative ureterorenoscopy. J Urol 1990;144:484–485; discussion, 492–493.

Caione P, Micali S, Rinaldi S, et al: Retroperitoneal laparoscopy for renal biopsy in children. J Urol 2000;164:1080–1082; discussion, 1083.

Calvano CJ, Moran ME, Parekh A, et al: Laparoscopic augmentation cystoplasty using the novel biomaterial Surgisis: Small-intestinal submucosa. J Endourol 2000;14:213–217.

Capolicchio G, Homsy YL, Houle AM, et al: Long-term results of percutaneous endopyelotomy in the treatment of children with failed open pyeloplasty [see comments]. J Urol 1997;158:1534–1537.

Carr MC, Docimo SG, Mitchell ME: Bladder augmentation with urothelial preservation. J Urol 1999;162:1133–1136; discussion, 1137.

Cartwright PC, Snow BW: Bladder autoaugmentation: Early clinical experience. J Urol 1989;142:505–508; discussion, 520–521.

Cartwright PC, Snow BW, Mansfield JC, Hamilton BD: Percutaneous endoscopic trigonoplasty: A minimally invasive approach to correct vesicoureteral reflux. J Urol 1996;156:661–664.

Cass AS, Lee JY, Aliabadi H: Extracorporeal shock wave lithotripsy and endoscopic management of renal calculi with urinary diversions. J Urol 1992;148:1123–1125.

Castilho LN: Laparoscopy for the nonpalpable testis: How to interpret the endoscopic findings. J Urol 1990;144:1215–1218.

Castilho LN, Ferreira U: Laparoscopy in adults and children with nonpalpable testes. Andrologia 1987;19:539–543.

Chen RN, Kavoussi LR, Moore RG: Milk of calcium within a calyceal diverticulum. Urology 1997;49:620–621.

Chen RN, Moore RG, Kavoussi LR: Laparoscopic pyeloplasty. J Endourol 1996;10:159–161.

Chiu AW, Chang LS, Birkett DH, Babayan RK: The impact of pneumoperitoneum, pneumoretroperitoneum, and gasless laparoscopy on the systemic and renal hemodynamics. J Am Coll Surg 1995;181:397–406.

Chow GK, Geisinger MA, Streem SB: Endopyelotomy outcome as a function of high versus dependent ureteral insertion. Urology 1999;54: 999–1002.

Cisek LJ, Gobet RM, Peters CA: Pneumoperitoneum produces reversible renal dysfunction in animals with normal and chronically reduced renal function. J Endourol 1998a;12:95–100.

Cisek LJ, Peters CA, Atala A, et al: Current findings in diagnostic laparoscopic evaluation of the nonpalpable testis. J Urol 1998b;160:1145–1149; discussion, 1150.

Clayman RV, Basler JW, Kavoussi L, Picus DD: Ureteronephroscopic endopyelotomy. J Urol 1990;144:246–251; discussion, 251–252.

Clayman RV, Kavoussi LR, Soper NJ, et al: Laparoscopic nephrectomy: Initial case report. J Urol 1991;146:278–282.

Colodny AH: Laparoscopy in pediatric urology: Too much of a good thing? Semin Pediatr Surg 1996;5:23–29.

Cooper MJ, Fleming S, Murray J: Laparoscopic assisted Vecchietti procedure for the creation of a neovagina. J Obstet Gynaecol Res 1996;22: 385–388.

Cortes D, Thorup JM, Lenz K, et al: Laparoscopy in 100 consecutive patients with 128 impalpable testes. Br J Urol 1995;75:281–287.

Cortesi N, Ferrari P, Zambarda E, et al: Diagnosis of bilateral abdominal cryptorchidism by laparoscopy. Endoscopy 1976;8:33.

Cuellar D, Kavoussi P, Baker L, Docimo SG: Open laparoscopic access using a radially dilating trocar: Experience and indications in 50 consecutive cases. J Endourol 2000;14:755–756.

Curran MJ, Little AF, Bouyounes B, et al: Retroperitoneoscopic technique for treating symptomatic caliceal diverticula. J Endourol 1999;13:723–725.

Cussen LJ: The morphology of congenital dilatation of the ureter: Intrinsic ureteral lesions. Aust N Z J Surg 1971;41:185.

Danuser H, Ackermann DK, Bohlen D, Studer UE: Endopyelotomy for primary ureteropelvic junction obstruction: Risk factors determine the success rate [see comments]. J Urol 1998;159:56–61.

Das S: Laparoscopic removal of bladder diverticulum. J Urol 1992;148: 1837–1839.

Davis D: Intubated ureterotomy: A new operation for ureteral and ureteropelvic stricture. Surg Gynecol Obstet 1943;76:513–523.

De Filippo RE, Barthold JS, Gonzalez R: The application of magnetic resonance imaging for the preoperative localization of nonpalpable testis in obese children: An alternative to laparoscopy [comment]. J Urol 2000;164:154–155.

Denstedt JD, Clayman RV: Electrohydraulic lithotripsy of renal and ureteral calculi. J Urol 1990;143:13–17.

Denstedt JD, Eberwein PM, Singh RR: The Swiss Lithoclast: A new device for intracorporeal lithotripsy. J Urol 1992;148:1088.

Diamond DA, Price HM, McDougall EM, Bloom DA: Retroperitoneal laparoscopic nephrectomy in children. J Urol 1995;153:1966–1968.

Docimo SG: The results of surgical therapy for cryptorchidism: A literature review and analysis. J Urol 1995;154:1148–1152.

Docimo SG: Endoscopic surgery in children. In: Marshall FF (ed): Textbook of Operative Urology. Baltimore, WB Saunders, 1996, pp 198–206.

Docimo S: Laparoscopic surgery in children with ventriculoperitoneal shunts is not associated with consequences of increased intracranial pressure. Pediatrics 1999;104:829.

Docimo S, Baker L, Peters C, et al: Multi-institutional analysis of laparoscopic orchidopexy. J Endourol 1999;13:A143.

Docimo SG, Kavoussi LR: The role of endourological techniques in the treatment of the pediatric ureteropelvic junction [editorial; comment]. J Urol 1997;158:1538.

Docimo SG, Moore RG, Adams J, Kavoussi LR: Laparoscopic bladder augmentation using stomach. Urology 1995a;46:565–569.

Docimo SG, Moore RG, Adams J, Kavoussi LR: Laparoscopic orchiopexy for the high palpable undescended testis. J Urol 1995b;154:1513–1515.

Droesch K, Droesch J, Chumas J, Bronson R: Laparoscopic gonadectomy for gonadal dysgenesis. Fertil Steril 1990;53:360–361.

Ehrlich RM, Gershman A: Laparoscopic seromyotomy (auto-augmentation) for non-neurogenic neurogenic bladder in a child: Initial case report. Urology 1993;42:175–178.

Ehrlich RM, Gershman A, Mee S, Fuchs G: Laparoscopic nephrectomy in a child: Expanding horizons for laparoscopy in pediatric urology. J Endourol 1992;6:463–465.

El-Ghoneimi A, Sauty L, Maintenant J, et al: Laparoscopic retroperitoneal nephrectomy in high risk children. J Urol 2000;164:1076–1079.

El-Ghoneimi A, Valla JS, Steyaert H, Aigrain Y: Laparoscopic renal surgery via a retroperitoneal approach in children. J Urol 1998;160: 1138–1141.

Elder JS: Laparoscopy for impalpable testes: Significance of the patent processus vaginalis. J Urol 1994;152:776–778.

Elder JS, Hladky D, Selzman AA: Outpatient nephrectomy for nonfunctioning kidneys. J Urol 1995;154:712–714; discussion, 714–715.

Faerber GJ, Ritchey ML, Bloom DA: Percutaneous endopyelotomy in infants and young children after failed open pyeloplasty. J Urol 1995; 154:1495–1497.

Fahlenkamp D, Schonberger B, Lindeke A, Loening SA: Laparoscopic excision of the sinusoidal remnants of the urachus in a 3-year-old boy. Br J Urol 1995;76:135–137.

Fairfax CA, Skoog SJ: The laparoscopic diagnosis of transverse testicular ectopia. J Urol 1995;153:477–478.

Fedele L, Busacca M, Candiani M, Vignali M: Laparoscopic creation of a neovagina in Mayer-Rokitansky-Kuster-Hauser syndrome by modification of Vecchietti's operation. Am J Obstet Gynecol 1994;171:268–269.

Ferrer FA, Cadeddu JA, Schulam P, et al: Orchiopexy using 2 mm laparoscopic instruments: Two techniques for delivering the testis into the scrotum. J Urol 2000;164:160–161.

Ferro F, Lais A, Gonzalez-Serva L: Benefits and afterthoughts of laparoscopy for the nonpalpable testis. J Urol 1996;156:795–798; discussion, 798.

Ferro F, Spagnoli A, Zaccara A, et al: Is preoperative laparoscopy useful for impalpable testis? J Urol 1999;162:995–996; discussion, 997.

Figenshau RS, Clayman RV: Endourologic options for management of ureteropelvic junction obstruction in the pediatric patient. Urol Clin North Am 1998;25:199–209.

Fowler R, Stephens FD: The role of testicular vascular anatomy in the salvage of high undescended testes. Aust N Z J Surg 1959;29:92.

Fraser M, Joyce AD, Thomas DF, et al: Minimally invasive treatment of urinary tract calculi in children. BJU Int 1999;84:339–342.

Fuenfer MM, Pitts RM, Georgeson KE: Laparoscopic exploration of the contralateral groin in children: an improved technique. J Laparoendosc Surg 1996;6:S1–S4.

Garibyan H: Use of laparoscopy for the localization of impalpable testes. Neth J Surg 1987;39:68–71.

Garvin TJ, Clayman RV: Balloon dilation of the distal ureter to 24F: An effective method for ureteroscopic stone retrieval. J Urol 1991;146:742–745.

Gatti JM, Cartwright PC, Hamilton BD, Snow BW: Percutaneous endoscopic trigonoplasty in children: Long-term outcomes and modifications in technique. J Endourol 1999;13:581–584.

Gauthier F, Montupet P, Valayer J: [Seven cases of calyceal diverticula in children]. Chir Pediatr 1983;24:45–49.

Gentili A, Iannettone CM, Pigna A, et al: Cardiocirculatory changes during videolaparoscopy in children: An echocardiographic study. Paediatr Anaesth 2000;10:399–406.

Gerber GS, Kim J, Nold S, Cromie WJ: Retrograde ureteroscopic endopyelotomy for the treatment of primary and secondary ureteropelvic junction obstruction in children. Tech Urol 2000;6:46–49.

Gililland J, Cummings D, Hibbert ML, et al: Laparoscopic orchiectomy in a patient with complete androgen insensitivity. J Laparoendosc Surg 1993;3:51–54.

Gill BS, MacFadyen BV, Jr: Ultrasonic dissectors and minimally invasive surgery. Semin Laparosc Surg 1999;6:229–234.

Gill IS, Rackley RR, Meraney AM, et al: Laparoscopic enterocystoplasty. Urology 2000;55:178–181.

Gluckman GR, Stoller M, Irby P: Laparoscopic pyelocaliceal diverticula ablation. J Endourol 1993;7:315–317.

Gonzalez R: Re: Laparoscopic laser assisted auto-augmentation of the pediatric neurogenic bladder: Early experience with urodynamic followup [letter; comment]. J Urol 1996;156:1783.

Gregoir W: Lich-Gregoir operation. In: Epstein HB, Hohenfellner R, Williams DI (eds): Surgical Pediatric Urology. Stuttgart, Thieme, 1977, p 265.

Grosskinsky CM, Ryder RM, Pendergrass HM, Hulka JF: Laparoscopic capacitance: A mystery measured. Experiments in pigs with confirmation in the engineering laboratory. Am J Obstet Gynecol 1993;169:1632–1635.

Guiney EJ, Corbally M, Malone PS: Laparoscopy and the management of the impalpable testis. Br J Urol 1989;63:313–316.

Hamilton BD, Gatti JM, Cartwright PC, Snow BW: Comparison of laparoscopic versus open nephrectomy in the pediatric population. J Urol 2000;163:937–939.

Harewood LM, Agarwal D, Lindsay S, et al: Extraperitoneal laparoscopic caliceal diverticulectomy. J Endourol 1996;10:425–430.

Hasson HM: Laparoscopic cannula cone with means for cannula stabilization and wound closure. J Am Assoc Gynecol Laparosc 1998;5:183–185.

Hedican SP, Schulam PG, Docimo SG: Laparoscopic assisted reconstructive surgery. J Urol 1999;161:267–270.

Helal M, Black T, Lockhart J, Figueroa TE: The Hickman peel-away sheath: Alternative for pediatric percutaneous nephrolithotomy. J Endourol 1997;11:171–172.

Hendren WH, Radhakrishnan J, Middleton AW, Jr: Pediatric pyeloplasty. J Pediatr Surg 1980;15:133–144.

Holcomb GW, Brock JW, Morgan WM: Laparoscopic evaluation for a contralateral patent processus vaginalis. J Pediatr Surg 1994a;29:970–973; discussion, 974.

Holcomb GW, Brock JW, Neblett WW, et al: Laparoscopy for the nonpalpable testis. Am Surg 1994b;60:143–147.

Holcomb GW, Morgan WM, Brock JW: Laparoscopic evaluation for contralateral patent processus vaginalis: Part II. J Pediatr Surg 1996;31:1170–1173.

Honey RJ: Assessment of a new tipless nitinol stone basket and comparison with an existing flat-wire basket. J Endourol 1998;12:529–531.

Hoznek A, Herard A, Ogiez N, et al: Symptomatic caliceal diverticula treated with extraperitoneal laparoscopic marsupialization fulguration and gelatin resorcinol formaldehyde glue obliteration. J Urol 1998;160:352–355.

Hubens G, De Vries D, Hauben E, et al: Laparoscopic resection of an adenoma of the urachus in combination with a laparoscopic cholecystectomy. Surg Endosc 1995;9:914–916.

Ikari O, Castilho LN, Lucena R, et al: Laparoscopic excision of seminal vesicle cysts. J Urol 1999;162:498–499.

Iselin CE, Winfield HN, Rohner S, Graber P: Sequential laparoscopic bladder diverticulectomy and transurethral resection of the prostate. J Endourol 1996;10:545–549.

Jabbour ME, Goldfischer ER, Klima WJ, et al: Endopyelotomy after failed pyeloplasty: The long-term results. J Urol 1998;160:690–692; discussion, 692–693.

Jackman SV, Cadeddu JA, Chen RN, et al: Utility of the harmonic scalpel for laparoscopic partial nephrectomy. J Endourol 1998a;12:441–444.

Jackman SV, Hedican SP, Peters CA, Docimo SG: Infant and preschool age percutaneous nephrolithotomy: Experience with a new technique. Urology 1998b;52:697–701.

Jackman SV, Weingart JD, Kinsman SL, Docimo SG: Laparoscopic surgery in patients with ventriculoperitoneal shunts: Safety and monitoring. J Urol 2000;164:1352–1354.

Janetschek G, Peschel R, Bartsch G: [Laparoscopic and retroperitoneoscopic kidney pyeloplasty]. Urologe A 1996;35:202–207.

Janetschek G, Seibold J, Radmayr C, Bartsch G: Laparoscopic heminephroureterectomy in pediatric patients. J Urol 1997;158:1928–1930.

Jarrett TW, Pardalidis NP, Sweetser P, et al: Laparoscopic transperitoneal bladder diverticulectomy: Surgical technique. J Laparoendosc Surg 1995;5:105–111.

Jayanthi VR, Arnold PM, Koff SA: Strategies for managing upper tract calculi in young children. J Urol 1999;162:1234–1237.

Jones C, Kern I: Laparoscopy for the non-palpable testis: A review of twenty-eight patients (1988–1990). Aust N Z J Surg 1993;63:451–453.

Jordan GH: Will laparoscopic orchiopexy replace open surgery for the nonpalpable undescended testis? [editorial; comment]. J Urol 1997;158:1956.

Jordan GH, Winslow BH: Laparoendoscopic upper pole partial nephrectomy with ureterectomy. J Urol 1993a;150:940–943.

Jordan GH, Winslow BH: Laparoscopically assisted continent catheterizable cutaneous appendicovesicostomy. J Endourol 1993b;7:517–520.

Jordan GH, Winslow BH: Laparoscopic single stage and staged orchiopexy. J Urol 1994;152:1249–1252.

Kaufman A, Ritchey ML, Black CT: Cost-effective endoscopic examination of the contralateral inguinal ring. Urology 1996;47:566–568.

Kavoussi LR, Meretyk S, Dierks SM, et al: Endopyelotomy for secondary ureteropelvic junction obstruction in children. J Urol 1991;145:345–349.

Kavoussi LR, Schuessler WW, Vancaillie TG, Clayman RV: Laparoscopic approach to the seminal vesicles. J Urol 1993;150:417–419.

Keckstein J, Buck G, Sasse V, et al: Laparoscopic creation of a neovagina: Modified Vecchietti method. Endosc Surg Allied Technol 1995;3:93–95.

Kier R, McCarthy S, Rosenfield AT, et al: Nonpalpable testes in young boys: Evaluation with MR imaging. Radiology 1988;169:429–433.

Kobashi KC, Chamberlin DA, Rajpoot D, Shanberg AM: Retroperitoneal laparoscopic nephrectomy in children. J Urol 1998;160:1142–1144.

Kottasz S, Hamvas A: Calyceal diverticula: Review of the literature, a hypothesis concerning its aetiology, and report of 17 cases. Acta Chir Acad Sci Hung 1977;18:289–293.

Koyle MA, Woo HH, Kavoussi LR: Laparoscopic nephrectomy in the first year of life. J Pediatr Surg 1993;28:693–695.

Krasna M, Nazem A: Thoracoscopic lung resection: Use of a new endoscopic linear stapler. Surg Laparosc Endosc 1991;1:248–250.

Kroovand RL: Pediatric urolithiasis. Urol Clin North Am 1997;24:173–184.

Kumar R, Kapoor R, Mandhani A, et al: Optimum duration of splinting after endopyelotomy. J Endourol 1999;13:89–92.

Lakshmanan Y, Fung LC: Laparoscopic extravesicular ureteral reimplantation for vesicoureteral reflux: Recent technical advances. J Endourol 2000;14:589–593; discussion, 593–594.

Lakshmanan Y, Mathews RI, Cadeddu JA, et al: Feasibility of total intravesical endoscopic surgery using mini-instruments in a porcine model. J Endourol 1999;13:41–45.

Lakshmanan Y, Peters CA: Laparoscopy in the management of intersex anomalies. Pediatr Endosurg Innov Tech 2000;4:201–206.

Lang EK: Percutaneous infundibuloplasty: Management of calyceal diverticula and infundibular stenosis. Radiology 1991;181:871–877.

Lee CL, Wang CJ, Liu YH, et al: Laparoscopically assisted full thickness skin graft for reconstruction in congenital agenesis of vagina and uterine cervix. Hum Reprod 1999;14:928–930.

LeRoy AJ, May GR, Segura JW, et al: Rapid dilatation of percutaneous nephrostomy tracks. AJR Am J Roentgenol 1984;142:355–357.

Lindgren BW, Darby EC, Faiella L, et al: Laparoscopic orchiopexy: Procedure of choice for the nonpalpable testis? J Urol 1998;159:2132–2135.

Lindgren BW, Franco I, Blick S, et al: Laparoscopic Fowler-Stephens orchiopexy for the high abdominal testis. J Urol 1999;162:990–993; discussion, 994.

Linos D, Mitropoulos F, Patoulis J, et al: Laparoscopic removal of urachal sinus. J Laparoendosc Adv Surg Tech A 1997;7:135–138.

Long MG, Wingfield JG: Laparoscopic gonadectomy in testicular feminization syndrome: A technique for the removal of testes firmly situated within the inguinal canal. Gynecol Endosc 1993;2:43.

Marberger M, Hofbauer J: Ureteroscopy/nephroscopy and percutaneous stone procedures. In: Smith A, ed. Smith's Textbook of Endourology, vol 2. St. Louis, Quality Medical Publishing, 1996, pp 1406–1426.

Martin TV, Anderson KR, Weiss RM: Laparoscopic evaluation and management of a child with ambiguous genitalia, ectopic spleen, and Meckel's diverticulum. Tech Urol 1997;3:49–50.

Mathews R, Naslund M, Docimo S: Cost analysis of the treatment of vesicoureteral reflux: A computer model. J Urol 2000;163:561–566; discussion, 566–567.

McDougall EM, Clayman RV, Anderson K, et al: Laparoscopic gonadectomy in a case of testicular feminization. Urology 1993;42:201–204.

McDougall EM, Clayman RV, Bowles WT: Laparoscopic excision of mullerian duct remnant. J Urol 1994;152:482.

McDougall EM, Clayman RV, Figenshau RS, Pearle MS: Laparoscopic retropubic auto-augmentation of the bladder. J Urol 1995a;153:123–126.

McDougall EM, Urban DA, Kerbl K, et al: Laparoscopic repair of vesicoureteral reflux utilizing the Lich-Gregoir technique in the pig model. J Urol 1995b;153:497–500.

Mikaelsson C, Arnbjornsson E, Lindhagen T, et al: Routine laparoscopy for nonpalpable testes? J Laparoendosc Adv Surg Tech A 1999;9:239–241.

Molloy D: The diagnostic accuracy of a microlaparoscope. J Am Assoc Gynecol Laparosc 1995;2:203–206.

Monga M, Smith R, Ferral H, Thomas R: Percutaneous ablation of caliceal diverticulum: Long-term followup. J Urol 2000;163:28–32.

Moon YT, Kerbl K, Pearle MS, et al: Evaluation of optimal stent size after endourologic incision of ureteral strictures. J Endourol 1995;9:15–22.

Moore RG, Kavoussi LR, Bloom DA, et al: Postoperative adhesion formation after urological. J Urol 1995a;153:792–795.

Moore RG, Kavoussi LR, Bloom DA, et al: Postoperative adhesion formation after urological laparoscopy in the pediatric population. J Urol 1995b;153:792–795.

Moore RG, Peters CA, Bauer SB, et al: Laparoscopic evaluation of the nonpalpable tests: A prospective assessment of accuracy. J Urol 1994;151:728–731.

Mosli H, MacDonald P, Schillinger J: Caliceal diverticula developing into simple renal cyst. J Urol 1986;136:658–661.

Motola JA, Badlani GH, Smith AD: Results of 212 consecutive endopyelotomies: An 8-year followup. J Urol 1993;149:453–456.

Nakada SY, Wolf JS, Jr, Brink JA, et al: Retrospective analysis of the effect of crossing vessels on successful retrograde endopyelotomy outcomes using spiral computerized tomography angiography. J Urol 1998;159:62–65.

Nelson MT, Nakashima M, Mulvihill SJ: How secure are laparoscopically placed clips? An in vitro and in vivo study. Arch Surg 1992;127:718–720.

Ng JW, Koh GH: Laparoscopic orchidopexy for persistent mullerian duct syndrome. Pediatr Surg Int 1997;12:522–525.

Nguyen DH, Mitchell ME: Ureteral obstruction due to compression by the vas deferens following Fowler-Stephens orchiopexy. J Urol 1993;149:94–95.

Okamura K, Ono Y, Yamada Y, et al: Endoscopic trigonoplasty for primary vesico-ureteric. Br J Urol 1995;75:390–394.

Okamura K, Yamada Y, Tsuji Y, et al: Endoscopic trigonoplasty in pediatric patients with primary vesicoureteral reflux: Preliminary report. J Urol 1996;156:198–200.

Ota H, Tanaka J, Murakami M, et al: Laparoscopy-assisted Ruge procedure for the creation of a neovagina in a patient with Mayer-Rokitansky-Kuster-Hauser syndrome. Fertil Steril 2000;73:641–644.

Papaioannou T, Daykhovsky L, Grundfest WS: Safety evaluation of laparoscopically applied clips. J Laparoendosc Surg 1996;6:99–107.

Parra RO, Jones JP, Andrus CH, Hagood PG: Laparoscopic diverticulectomy: Preliminary report of a new approach for the treatment of bladder diverticulum. J Urol 1992;148:869–871.

Peters CA: Complications in pediatric urological laparoscopy: Results of a survey. J Urol 1996a;155:1070–1073.

Peters CA: Laparoscopy in pediatric urology: Challenge and opportunity. Semin Pediatr Surg 1996b;5:16–22.

Peters CA, Kavoussi LR: Pediatric endourology and laparoscopy. In: Walsh PC, Retik AB, Stamey TA, Vaughan ED, Jr (eds): Campbell's Urology, 6th ed. Philadelphia, WB Saunders, 1992:1–18.

Peters CA, Schlussel RN, Retik AB: Pediatric laparoscopic dismembered pyeloplasty. J Urol 1995;153:1962–1965.

Platt RC, Heniford BT: Development and initial trial of the minilaparoscopic argon coagulator. J Laparoendosc Adv Surg Tech A 2000;10:93–99.

Plotzker ED, Rushton HG, Belman AB, Skoog SJ: Laparoscopy for nonpalpable testes in childhood: Is inguinal exploration also necessary when vas and vessels exit the inguinal ring? J Urol 1992;148:635–637.

Poppas DP, Bleustein CB, Peters CA: Box stitch modification of Hasson technique for pediatric laparoscopy. J Endourol 1999;13:447–450.

Poppas DP, Lemack GE, Mininberg DT: Laparoscopic orchiopexy: Clinical experience and description of technique. J Urol 1996a;155:708–711.

Poppas DP, Uzzo RG, Britanisky RG, Mininberg DT: Laparoscopic laser assisted auto-augmentation of the pediatric neurogenic bladder: Early experience with urodynamic followup [see comments]. J Urol 1996b; 155:1057–1060.

Pugach JL, Moore RG, Parra RO, Steinhardt GF: Massive hydrothorax and hydro-abdomen complicating percutaneous nephrolithotomy. J Urol 1999;162:2110; discussion, 2110–2111.

Radmayr C, Neumann H, Bartsch G, et al: Laparoscopic partial adrenalectomy for bilateral pheochromocytomas in a boy with von Hippel-Lindau disease. Eur Urol 2000;38:344–344.

Ransley PC, Vordermark JS, Caldamone AA: Preliminary ligation of the gonadal vessels prior to orchiopexy for the intra-abdominal testicle: A staged Fowler-Stephens procedure. World J Urol 1984;2:266–268.

Razvi HA, Fields D, Vargas JC, et al: Oliguria during laparoscopic surgery: Evidence for direct renal parenchymal compression as an etiologic factor. J Endourol 1996;10:1–4.

Reddy PK, Evans RM: Laparoscopic ureteroneocystostomy [see comments]. J Urol 1994;152:2057–2059.

Reddy PP, Barrieras DJ, Bagli DJ, et al: Initial experience with endoscopic holmium laser lithotripsy for pediatric urolithiasis [see comments]. J Urol 1999;162:1714–1716.

Redmond HP, Ahmed SM, Watson RG, Hegarty J: Laparoscopic excision of a patent urachus. Surg Laparosc Endosc 1994;4:384–385.

Rowe MI, Copelson LW, Clatworthy HW: The patent processus vaginalis and the inguinal hernia. J Pediatr Surg 1969;4:102.

Rozanski TA, Wojno KJ, Bloom DA: The remnant orchiectomy. J Urol 1996;155:712–713.

Rubin SZ, Davis GM, Sehgal Y, Kaminski MJ: Does laparoscopy adversely affect gas exchange and pulmonary mechanics in the newborn? An experimental study. J Laparoendosc Surg 1996;6:S69–S73.

Ruckle HC, Segura JW: Laparoscopic treatment of a stone-filled, caliceal diverticulum: A definitive, minimally invasive therapeutic option. J Urol 1994;151:122–124.

Sadeghi-Nejad H, Kavoussi LR, Peters CA: Bowel injury in open technique laparoscopic cannula placement. Urology 1994;43:559–560.

Saltzman B, Khasidy LR, Smith AD: Measurement of renal pelvis pressures during endourologic procedures. Urology 1987;30:472–474.

Sanchez de Badajoz E, Mate Hurtado A, Jimenez Garrido A, Gutierrez de la Cruz JM: Laparoscopy-assisted cystoplasty. J Endourol 1995;9:269–272.

Santarosa RP, Hensle TW, Shabsigh R: Percutaneous transvesical ureteroscopy for removal of distal ureteral stone in reimplanted ureter. Urology 1993;42:313–316.

Scarpa RM, De Lisa A, Porru D, Canetto A, Usai E: Ureterolithotripsy in children. Urology 1995;46:859–862.

Schenkman EM, Tarry WF: Comparison of percutaneous endopyelotomy with open pyeloplasty for pediatric ureteropelvic junction obstruction. J Urol 1998;159:1013–1015.

Schier F: Laparoscopic Anderson-Hynes pyeloplasty in children [see comments]. Pediatr Surg Int 1998;13:497–500.

Schier F, Mutter D, Bennek J, et al: Laparoscopic bilateral adrenalectomy in a child. Eur J Pediatr Surg 1999;9:420–421.

Schulam PG, Hedican SP, Docimo SG: Radially dilating trocar system for open laparoscopic access. Urology 1999;54:727–729.

Schwartz BF, Stoller ML: Complications of retrograde balloon cautery endopyelotomy. J Urol 1999;162:1594–1598.

Shalev E, Zabari A, Romano S, Luboshitzky R: Laparoscopic gonadectomy in 46XY female patient. Fertil Steril 1992;57:459–460.

Shalhav AL, Soble JJ, Nakada SY, et al: Long-term outcome of caliceal diverticula following percutaneous endosurgical management. J Urol 1998;160:1635–1639.

Shroff S, Watson GM: Experience with ureteroscopy in children. Br J Urol 1995;75:395–400.

Siegel MJ, McAlister WH: Calyceal diverticula in children: Unusual features and complications. Radiology 1979;131:79–82.

Smith DP, Jerkins GR, Noe HN: Urethroscopy in small neonates with posterior urethral valves and ureteroscopy in children with ureteral calculi. Urology 1996;47:908–910.

Spivak H, Richardson WS, Hunter JG: The use of bipolar cautery, laparosonic coagulating shears, and vascular clips for hemostasis of small and medium-sized vessels. Surg Endosc 1998;12:183–185.

Steiger C, Lakshmanan Y, Fung LCT: Laparoscopic extravesical ureteral reimplantation for the correction of vesicoureteral reflux: Recent technical advances. J Urol 1998;159:38.

Sutherland RS, Pfister RR, Koyle MA: Endopyelotomy associated ureteral necrosis: Complete ureteral replacement using the Boari flap. J Urol 1992;148:1490–1492.

Takeda M, Watanabe R, Kurumada S, et al: Endoscopic renal biopsy in pediatric patients: Comparison of retroperitoneoscopy-assisted and retroperitoneoscopic methods [letter]. Nephron 2000;84:199–200.

Tan HL: Laparoscopic Anderson-Hynes dismembered pyeloplasty in children. J Urol 1999;162:1045–1047; discussion, 1048.

Tan HL, Najmaldin A, Webb DR: Endopyelotomy for pelvi-ureteric junction obstruction in children. Eur Urol 1993;24:84–88.

Tawfiek ER, Liu JB, Bagley DH: Ureteroscopic treatment of ureteropelvic junction obstruction. J Urol 1998;160:1643–1646; discussion, 1646–1647.

Teichman JM, Champion PC, Wollin TA, Denstedt JD: Holmium:YAG lithotripsy of uric acid calculi. J Urol 1998;160:2130–2132.

Tennenbaum SY, Lerner SE, McAleer IM, et al: Preoperative laparoscopic localization of the nonpalpable testis: A critical analysis of a 10-year experience. J Urol 1994;151:732–734.

Thomas MD, Mercer LC, Saltzstein EC: Laparoscopic orchiectomy for unilateral intra-abdominal testis. J Urol 1992;148:1251–1253.

Tobias JD: Anesthetic considerations for laparoscopy in children. Semin Laparosc Surg 1998;5:60–66.

Tobias JD, Holcomb GW, Brock JW, et al: Cardiorespiratory changes in children during laparoscopy [see comments]. J Pediatr Surg 1995;30:33–36.

Tobias JD, Holcomb GW, Brock JW, et al: General anesthesia by mask with spontaneous ventilation during brief laparoscopic inspection of the peritoneum in children. J Laparoendosc Surg 1994;4:379–384.

Tobias JD, Holcomb GW, Rasmussen GE, et al: General anesthesia using the laryngeal mask airway during brief, laparoscopic inspection of the peritoneum in children. J Laparoendosc Surg 1996;6:175–180.

Trondsen E, Reiertsen O, Rosseland AR: Laparoscopic excision of urachal sinus. Eur J Surg 1993;159:127–128.

Tucker RD, Voyles CR, Silvis SE: Capacitive coupled stray currents during laparoscopic and endoscopic electrosurgical procedures. Biomed Instrum Technol 1992;26:303–311.

Uzzo RG, Bilsky M, Mininberg DT, Poppas DP: Laparoscopic surgery in children with ventriculoperitoneal shunts: Effect of pneumoperitoneum on intracranial pressure—preliminary experience. Urology 1997;49:753–757.

Valla JS, Guilloneau B, Montupet P, et al: Retroperitoneal laparoscopic nephrectomy in children: Preliminary report of 18 cases. Eur Urol 1996;30:490–493.

Van Savage JG, Palanca LG, Andersen RD, et al: Treatment of distal ureteral stones in children: Similarities to the American Urological Association guidelines in adults. J Urol 2000;164:1089–1093.

Vecchietti G: [Creation of an artificial vagina in Rokitansky-Kuster-Hauser syndrome]. Attual Ostet Ginecol 1965;11:131–147.

Veress J: Neus instrument zur ausfuhrung von brust-oder bachpunktionen und pneumothorax be-handlung. Dtsch Med Wochenschr 1938;64:1480.

Voyles CR, Tucker RD: Education and engineering solutions for potential problems with laparoscopic monopolar electrosurgery [see comments]. Am J Surg 1992;164:57–62.

Waldhausen JH, Tapper D, Sawin RS: Minimally invasive surgery and clinical decision-making for pediatric malignancy. Surg Endosc 2000;14:250–253.

Wiener JS, Jordan GH, Gonzales ET, Jr: Laparoscopic management of persistent mullerian duct remnants associated with an abdominal testis. J Endourol 1997;11:357–359.

Willson PD, van der Walt JD, Moxon D, Rogers J: Port site electrosurgical (diathermy) burns during surgical laparoscopy. Surg Endosc 1997;11:653–654.

Wilson EE, Vuitch F, Carr BR: Laparoscopic removal of dysgenetic gonads containing gonadoblastoma in a patient with Swyer syndrome. Obstet Gynecol 1992;79:842–844.

Wolf SA, Hopkins JW: Laparoscopic incidence of contralateral patent processus vaginalis in boys with clinical unilateral inguinal hernias. J Pediatr Surg 1994;29:1118–1120.

Wollin TA, Teichman JM, Rogenes VJ, et al: Holmium:YAG lithotripsy in children [see comments]. J Urol 1999;162:1717–1720.

Yao D, Poppas DP: A clinical series of laparoscopic nephrectomy, nephroureterectomy and heminephroureterectomy in the pediatric population. J Urol 2000;163:1531–1535.

Yeh HC, Mitty HA, Halton K, et al: Milk of calcium in renal cysts: New sonographic features. J Ultrasound Med 1992;11:195–203.

Yeung CK, Tam YH, Chan YL, et al: A new management algorithm for impalpable undescended testis with gadolinium enhanced magnetic resonance angiography. J Urol 1999;162:998–1002.

York GB, Robertson FM, Cofer BR: Laparoscopic nephrectomy in children. Surg Endosc 2000;14:469–472.

Yu TJ, Shu K, Kung FT, et al: Use of laparoscopy in intersex patients. J Urol 1995;154:1193–1196.

Zanetti G, Trinchieri A, Montanari E, et al: Bladder laparoscopic surgery. Ann Urol (Paris) 1995;29:97–100.

73

TISSUE ENGINEERING PERSPECTIVES FOR RECONSTRUCTIVE SURGERY

Anthony Atala, MD

INTRODUCTION

So the Lord God caused the man to fall into a deep sleep, and while he was asleep, He took part of the man's rib, and closed up the place with flesh. Then the Lord God made a woman from the part He had taken out of the man, and He brought her to the man.

–GENESIS 2:21

Four medical firsts are described in the passage cited above: the use of anesthesia, surgery, cloning, and tissue engineering. Even three decades ago, the performance of two of these, tissue engineering and cloning, was not possible. However, the use of one body part for another or the exchange of parts from one person to another was mentioned in the medical literature even in antiquity. The field of urology was the earliest to gain from the advent of transplantation, with the kidney being the first entire organ to be replaced in a human, in 1955 (Murray et al, 1955).

In the early 1960s, Murray performed a nonrelated kidney transplantation from a nongenetically identical patient into another. This transplant, which overcame the immunologic barrier, marked a new era in medical therapy and opened the door for use of transplantation as a means of therapy for different organ systems. However, lack of good immunosuppression and the ability to monitor and control rejection, as well as a severe organ donor shortage, opened the door for other alternatives.

As times evolved, synthetic materials were introduced to replace or rebuild diseased tissues or parts in the human body. The advent of new manmade materials, such as tetrafluoroethylene (Teflon) and silicone, opened a new field which included a wide array of devices that could be applied for human use. Although these devices could provide for structural replacement, the functional component of the original tissue was not achieved.

Simultaneous with this development was an increased body of knowledge of the biologic sciences that included new techniques for cell harvesting, culture, and expansion. The areas of cell biology, molecular biology, and biochemistry were advancing rapidly. Studies of the extracellular matrix and its interaction with cells, and with growth factors and their ligands, led the way to a further understanding of cell and tissue growth and differentiation.

In the 1960s, a natural evolution occurred wherein researchers started to combine the field of devices and materials sciences with cell biology, in effect starting a new field which is now termed *tissue engineering.* As more scientists from different fields came together with the common goal of tissue replacement, the field of tissue engineering became more formally established. Tissue engineering is now defined as "an interdisciplinary field which applies the principles of engineering and life sciences towards the development of biological substitutes that aim to maintain, restore or improve tissue function" (Atala and Lanza, 2001). The first use of the term "tissue engineering" in the literature can be traced to a reference dealing with corneal tissue in 1985 (Wolter and Meyer, 1985).

In the last two decades, scientists have attempted to engineer virtually every tissue of the human body. This chapter reviews some of the progress that has been achieved in the field of genitourinary tissue engineering.

The genitourinary system is exposed to a variety of possible injuries from the time the fetus develops. Aside from congenital abnormalities, individuals may also suffer from other disorders such as cancer, trauma, infection, inflammation, iatrogenic injuries, or other conditions which may lead to genitourinary organ damage or loss and necessitate eventual reconstruction. **Whenever there is a lack of native urologic tissue, reconstruction may be performed with native nonurologic tissues (skin, gastrointestinal segments, or mucosa from multiple body sites), homologous tissues (cadaver fascia, cadaver or donor kidney), heterologous tissues (bovine collagen), or artificial materials (silicone, polyurethane, Teflon).**

Synthetic materials have been used widely for urologic reconstruction. **The most common type of synthetic prostheses for urologic use are made of silicone.** Silicone prostheses have been used for the treatment of urinary incontinence with the artificial urinary sphincter and detachable balloon system, for treatment of vesicoureteral reflux with silicone microparticles, and for impotence with penile prostheses (Atala et al, 1992a; Riehmann et al, 1993; Levesque et al, 1996; Buckley et al, 1997). There has also been a major effort directed toward the construction of artificial bladders made with silicone. In some disease states, such as urinary incontinence or vesicoureteral reflux, artificial agents (Teflon paste, glass microparticles) have been used as injectable bulking substances; however, these substances are not entirely biocompatible (Atala, 1994; Atala et al, 1994).

Native tissues are usually preferable for reconstruction. The type of tissue chosen for replacement depends on which organ requires reconstruction. Bladder and ureteral reconstruction may be performed with gastrointestinal tissues. Urethral reconstruction is performed with skin or with mucosal grafts from the bladder, rectum, or oral cavity. Vaginas can be reconstructed with skin, small bowel, sigmoid colon, or rectum. **However, a shortage of donor tissue may limit these types of reconstructions, and**

there is a degree of morbidity associated with the harvest. In addition, these approaches rarely replace the entire function of the original organ. The tissues used for reconstruction may lead to complications because of their inherently different functional parameters. In most cases, the replacement of lost or deficient tissues with functionally equivalent tissues would improve the outcome for these patients. This goal may be attainable with the use of tissue engineering techniques.

TISSUE ENGINEERING: STRATEGIES FOR TISSUE RECONSTITUTION

Tissue engineering follows the principles of cell transplantation, materials science, and engineering toward the development of biologic substitutes that can restore and maintain normal function. Tissue engineering may involve matrices alone, wherein the body's natural ability to regenerate is used to orient or direct new tissue growth, or it may use matrices with cells.

When cells are used for tissue engineering, donor tissue is dissociated into individual cells, which are either implanted directly into the host or expanded in culture, attached to a support matrix, and reimplanted after expansion. The implanted tissue can be either heterologous, allogeneic, or autologous. Ideally, this approach allows lost tissue function to be restored or replaced in toto and with limited complications (Atala, 1997). **The use of autologous cells avoids rejection: A biopsy of tissue is obtained from the host, and the cells are dissociated and expanded in vitro, reattached to a matrix, and implanted into the same host** (Atala et al, 1992b, 1993a, 1993b; 1994, 1995, 1999; Cilento et al, 1994; Atala, 1997, 1998; Yoo and Atala, 1997; Fauza et al, 1998a, 1998b; Machluf and Atala, 1998; Yoo et al, 1998a, 1998b; Amiel and Atala, 1999; Kershen and Atala, 1999; Oberpenning et al, 1999; Park et al, 1999).

One of the initial limitations of applying cell-based tissue engineering techniques to urologic organs was the inherent difficulty of growing genitourinary associated cells in large quantities. In the past, it was believed that urothelial cells had a natural senescence that was hard to overcome. Normal urothelial cells could be grown in the laboratory setting, but with limited expansion. Several protocols have been developed over the last two decades that have improved urothelial growth and expansion (Cilento et al, 1994; Scriven et al, 1997; Liebert et al, 1997; Puthenveettil et al, 1999). A system of urothelial cell harvesting was developed that does not use any enzymes or serum and has a large expansion potential. Using these methods of cell culture, it is possible to expand a urothelial strain from a single specimen that initially covers a surface area of 1 cm^2 to one covering a surface area of 4202 m^2 (the equivalent area of one football field) within 8 weeks (Cilento et al, 1994). These studies indicated that it should be possible to collect autologous urothelial cells from human patients, expand them in culture, and return them to the human donor in sufficient quantities for reconstructive purposes. Bladder, ureter, and renal pelvis cells can equally be harvested, cultured, and expanded in a similar fashion (Fig. 73–1). Normal human bladder epithelial and muscle cells

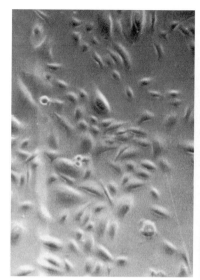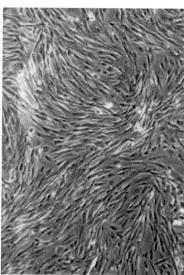

Figure 73–1. Urothelial *(left panel)* and bladder muscle *(right panel)* cells growing in vitro.

can be efficiently harvested from surgical material, extensively expanded in culture, and their differentiation characteristics, growth requirements, and other biologic properties can be studied (Liebert et al, 1991, 1997; Cilento et al, 1994; Tobin et al, 1994; Harriss, 1995; Freeman et al, 1997; Fauza et al, 1998a, 1998b; Solomon et al, 1998; Lobban et al, 1998; Nguyen et al, 1999; Puthenveettil et al, 1999; Rackley et al, 1999).

BIOMATERIALS FOR GENITOURINARY TISSUE ENGINEERING

Biomaterials in genitourinary tissue engineering function as an artificial extracellular matrix (ECM) and elicit biologic and mechanical functions of native ECM found in tissues in the body. Native ECM brings cells together into tissue, controls the tissue structure, and regulates the cell phenotype (Alberts et al, 1994). **Biomaterials facilitate the localization and delivery of cells and/or bioactive factors (e.g., cell adhesion peptides, growth factors) to desired sites in the body; define a three-dimensional space for the formation of new tissues with appropriate structure; and guide the development of new tissues with appropriate function** (Kim and Mooney, 1998a). Direct injection of cell suspensions without biomaterial matrices has been used in some cases (Ponder et al, 1991; Brittberg et al, 1994), but it is difficult to control the localization of transplanted cells. In addition, the majority of mammalian cell types are anchorage dependent and will die if not provided with a cell-adhesion substrate. Biomaterials provide a cell-adhesion substrate and can be used to achieve cell delivery with high loading and efficiency to specific sites in the body. The configuration of the biomaterials can guide the structure of an engineered tissue. The biomaterials provide mechanical support against in vivo forces, thus maintaining a predefined structure during the process of tissue development. The biomaterials can be loaded with bioactive signals, such as cell-adhesion pep-

tides and growth factors, which can regulate cellular function.

Design and Selection of Biomaterials

The design and selection of the biomaterial is critical in the development of engineered genitourinary tissues. The biomaterial must be capable of controlling the structure and function of the engineered tissue in a predesigned manner by interacting with transplanted cells and/or host cells. Generally, the ideal biomaterial should be biocompatible, promote cellular interaction and tissue development, and possess proper mechanical and physical properties.

The selected biomaterial should be biodegradable and bioresorbable to support the reconstruction of a completely normal tissue without inflammation. Such behavior of the biomaterials avoids the risk of inflammatory or foreign-body responses that may be associated with the permanent presence of a foreign material in the body. The degradation products should not provoke inflammation or toxicity and must be removed from the body via metabolic pathways. The degradation rate and the concentration of degradation products in the tissues surrounding the implant must be at a tolerable level (Bergsma et al, 1995).

The biomaterials should provide an appropriate regulation of cell behavior (e.g., adhesion, proliferation, migration, differentiation) in order to promote the development of functional new tissue. Cell behavior in engineered tissues is regulated by multiple interactions with the microenvironment, including interactions with cell-adhesion ligands (Hynes, 1992) and with soluble growth factors (Deuel, 1997). Cell adhesion–promoting factors (e.g., Arg-Gly-Asp [RGD]) can be presented by the biomaterial itself or incorporated into the biomaterial in order to control cell behavior through ligand-induced cell receptor signaling processes (Barrera et al, 1993; Cook et al, 1997). The biomaterial can also serve as a depot for the local release of growth factors and other bioactive agents that induce tissue-specific gene expression of the cells. The biomaterials should possess appropriate mechanical properties to regenerate tissues with predefined sizes and shapes. The biomaterials provide temporary mechanical support sufficient to withstand in vivo forces exerted by the surrounding tissue and maintain a potential space for tissue development. **The mechanical support of the biomaterials should be maintained until the engineered tissue has sufficient mechanical integrity to support itself** (Atala, 1998). This potentially can be achieved by an appropriate choice of mechanical and degradative properties of the biomaterials (Kim and Mooney, 1998a).

The biomaterials need to be processed into specific configurations. A large ratio of surface area to volume is often desirable to allow the delivery of a high density of cells. A high-porosity, interconnected pore structure with specific pore sizes promotes tissue ingrowth from the surrounding host tissue. Several techniques have been developed that readily control porosity, pore size, and pore structure.

Types of Biomaterials

Generally, three classes of biomaterials have been used for engineering of genitourinary tissues: naturally derived materials, such as collagen and alginate; acellular tissue matrices, such as bladder submucosa and small-intestinal submucosa; and synthetic polymers, such as polyglycolic acid (PGA), polylactic acid (PLA), and poly(lactic-co-glycolic acid) (PLGA). These classes of biomaterials have been tested in regard to their biocompatibility with primary human urothelial and bladder muscle cells (Pariente et al, 2001). Naturally derived materials and acellular tissue matrices have the potential advantage of biologic recognition. Synthetic polymers can be produced reproducibly on a large scale with controlled properties of strength, degradation rate, and microstructure.

Collagen is the most abundant and ubiquitous structural protein in the body, and it may be readily purified from both animal and human tissues with an enzyme treatment and salt/acid extraction (Li, 1995). Collagen has long been known to exhibit minimal inflammatory and antigenic responses (Furthmayr and Timpl, 1976), and it has been approved by the U.S. Food and Drug Administration (FDA) for many types of medical applications, including wound dressings and artificial skin (Pachence, 1996). Collagen implants degrade as a result of sequential attacks by lysosomal enzymes. The in vivo resorption rate can be regulated by controlling the density of the implant and the extent of intermolecular cross-linking. The lower the density, the greater the interstitial space, and generally the larger the pores for cell infiltration, leading to a higher rate of implant degradation. Intermolecular cross-linking reduces the degradation rate by making the collagen molecules less susceptible to an enzymatic attack. Intermolecular cross-linking can be accomplished by various physical (e.g., ultraviolet radiation, dehydrothermal treatment) or chemical (e.g., glutaraldehyde, formaldehyde, carbodiimides) techniques (Li, 1995). Collagen contains cell-adhesion domain sequences (e.g., RGD) that exhibit specific cellular interactions. This may help to retain the phenotype and activity of many types of cells, including fibroblasts (Silver and Pins, 1992) and chondrocytes (Sam and Nixon, 1995).

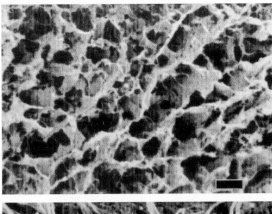
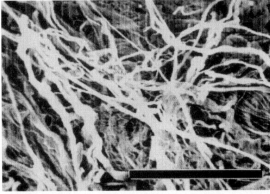
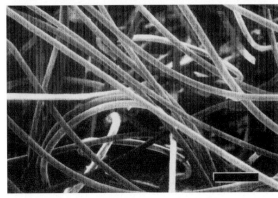

Figure 73–2. Scanning electron micrographs of biomaterials: collagen sponge *(top)*, acellular matrix prepared from pig bladder submucosa *(center)*, and polyglycolic acid fiber-based matrix *(bottom)*. (Size bars = 100 µm.)

Collagen exhibits high tensile strength and flexibility, and these mechanical properties can be further enhanced by intermolecular cross-linking. This material can be processed into a wide variety of structures such as sponges (Fig. 73–2, *top*) fibers, and films (Yannas and Burke, 1980; Li, 1995; Cavallaro et al, 1994).

Alginate, a polysaccharide isolated from seaweed, has been used as an injectable cell delivery vehicle (Smidsrød and Skjåk-Bræk, 1990) and a cell immobilization matrix (Lim and Sun, 1980) owing to its gentle gelling properties in the presence of divalent ions such as calcium. Alginate is relatively biocompatible and is approved by the FDA for human use as wound dressing material. Alginate is a family of copolymers of D-mannuronate and L-guluronate. The physical and mechanical properties of alginate gel are strongly correlated with the proportion and length of polyguluronate block in the alginate chains (Smidsrød and Skjåk-Bræk, 1990).

However, alginate does not possess a biologic recognition domain. In addition, the range of mechanical properties available from alginate hydrogels is quite limited and changes in a noncontrollable manner, presumably because of the loss of ionic cross-linking. Efforts have been made to synthesize biodegradable alginate hydrogels with mechanical properties that are controllable in a wide range by intermolecular covalent cross-linking and with cell-adhesion peptides coupled to their backbones (Rowley et al, 1999).

Acellular tissue matrices are collagen-rich matrices prepared by removing cellular components from tissues (see Fig. 73–2, *center*). The matrices are often prepared by mechanical and chemical manipulation of a segment of bladder tissue (Dahms et al, 1998; Piechota et al, 1998; Yoo et al, 1998b; Chen et al, 1999). The matrices slowly degrade after implantation and are replaced and remodeled by ECM proteins synthesized and secreted by transplanted or ingrowing cells. Acellular tissue matrices have been proved to support cell ingrowth and regeneration of genitourinary tissues, including urethra and bladder, with no evidence of immunogenic rejection (Probst et al, 1997; Chen et al, 1999). Because the structures of the proteins (e.g., collagen, elastin) in acellular matrices are well conserved and normally arranged, the mechanical properties of the acellular matrices are not significantly different from those of native bladder submucosa (Dahms et al, 1998).

Polyesters of naturally occurring α-hydroxy acids, including PGA, PLA, and PLGA, are widely used in tissue engineering. These polymers have gained FDA approval for human use in a variety of applications, including sutures (Gilding, 1981). The ester bonds in these polymers are hydrolytically labile, and these polymers degrade by nonenzymatic hydrolysis. The degradation products of PGA, PLA, and PLGA are nontoxic, natural metabolites that are eventually eliminated from the body in the form of carbon dioxide and water (Gilding, 1981). The degradation rate of these polymers can be tailored from several weeks to several years by altering crystallinity, initial molecular weight, and the copolymer ratio of lactic to glycolic acid. Because these polymers are thermoplastics, they can easily be formed into a three-dimensional scaffold with a desired microstructure, gross shape, and dimension by various techniques, including molding, extrusion (Freed et al, 1994), solvent casting (Mikos et al, 1994), phase separation techniques, and gas foaming techniques (Harris et al, 1998).

Many applications in genitourinary tissue engineering require a scaffold with high porosity and a high ratio of surface area to volume. This need has been addressed by processing biomaterials into configurations of fiber meshes (see Fig. 73–2, *bottom*) and porous sponges using the techniques described previously. The mechanical properties of the scaffold can be controlled by the fabrication process. A drawback of the synthetic polymers is lack of biologic recognition. As an approach toward incorporating cell recognition domains into these materials, copolymers with amino acids have been synthesized (Barrera et al, 1993, 1995; Cook et al, 1997; Intveld et al, 1994). Other biodegradable synthetic polymers, including poly(anhydrides)

and poly(ortho-esters), can also be used to fabricate scaffolds for genitourinary tissue engineering with controlled properties (Peppas and Langer, 1994).

TISSUE ENGINEERING OF UROLOGIC STRUCTURES

Urethra

Various strategies have been proposed over the years for the regeneration of urethral tissue. Woven meshes of PGA (Dexon) were used to reconstruct urethras in dogs. Three to four centimeters of the ventral half of the urethral circumference and its adjacent corpus spongiosum was excised, and the polymer mesh was sutured to the defective area. After 2 weeks, the animals were able to void through the neourethra. At 2 months, the urothelium was completely regenerated. The polymer meshes were completely absorbed after 3 months. No complications occurred. However, the excised corpus spongiosum did not regenerate (Bazeed et al, 1983).

PGA was also used as a cell transplantation vehicle to engineer tubular urothelium in vivo. Cultured urothelial cells were seeded onto tubular PGA scaffolds and implanted into athymic mice. At 20 and 30 days, polymer degradation was evident and tubular urothelium formed in which cells were stained for a urothelium-associated cytokeratin (Atala et al, 1992b).

PGA mesh tubes coated with polyhydroxybutyric acid (PHB) were used to reconstruct urethras in dogs. PHB is a biodegradable thermoplastic polymer produced microbially. PHB degrades by both hydrolysis and enzyme reaction. The hydrolized product, 3-hydroxybutyric acid, is a natural metabolite that is contained in human blood (Holmes, 1985). Eight to 12 months later, complete regeneration of urothelium and adjacent connective tissue occurred. All of the polymers disappeared after 1 year. There were no anastomotic strictures or inflammatory reactions (Olsen et al, 1992).

Small-intestinal submucosa (SIS) was used as an onlay patch graft for urethroplasty in rabbits (Kropp et al, 1998). SIS was compared to full-thickness preputial skin grafts and shams (simple urethrotomy and closure). Animals were sacrificed between 8 and 12 weeks. Histologic evaluation demonstrated that SIS promoted urethral regeneration. Regenerated urethras contained three to four layers of stratified columnar urothelium that was indistinguishable from the normal rabbit urothelium. There was also evidence of circular smooth muscle regeneration underneath the urothelium. This regenerated muscle was contained within an abundant amount of collagen and fibrous connective tissue. Grossly, there was no evidence of diverticulum formation. In contrast, all grafts in the preputial skin group had evidence of diverticulum formation.

A homologous free graft of acellular urethral matrix was used in a rabbit model (Sievert et al, 2000). A 0.8- to 1.1-cm segment of the urethra was resected and replaced with an acellular matrix graft of 1.0 to 1.5 cm. Histologic examination showed complete epithelialization and progressive vessel infiltration. At 3 months, smooth muscle bundles were first observed infiltrating the matrix at the anastomo-

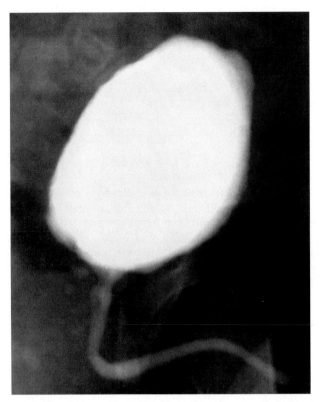

Figure 73–3. Urethrogram 6 months after surgery in a patient who had a portion of his urethra replaced with the use of tissue engineering techniques.

sis; after 6 months, the smooth muscle bundles had grown into one third of the matrix. By 8 months, the host and implant could not be differentiated by urethrography. All tissue components were seen in the grafted matrix after 3 months, with further improvement over time; however, the smooth muscle in the matrix was less than in normal rabbit urethra, and it was not well oriented.

Another acellular collagen matrix has also proved to be a suitable graft for repair of urethral defects both experimentally and clinically. The acellular collagen matrix was obtained from porcine bladder for the animal studies. The neourethras demonstrated a normal urothelial luminal lining and organized muscle bundles, without any signs of strictures or complications. The animals were able to void through the neourethra (Chen et al, 1999). These results were confirmed clinically in a series of patients with a history of failed hypospadias reconstruction wherein the urethral defects were repaired with human bladder acellular collagen matrices (Atala et al, 1999). The neourethras were created by anastomosing the matrix in an onlay fashion to the urethral plate. The size of the created neourethra ranged from 5 to 15 cm. After a 3-year follow-up, three of the four patients had a successful outcome in regard to cosmetic appearance and function (Fig. 73–3). One patient who had a 15-cm neourethra created developed a subglanular fistula. The acellular collagen-based matrix eliminated the necessity of performing additional surgical procedures for graft harvesting, and both operative time and the potential morbidity from the harvest procedure were decreased. Similar results were obtained in pediatric and adult patients with urethral stricture disease (Kassaby et al, 2000).

More than 60 pediatric and adult patients with urethral disease have been successfully treated with the collagen-based matrix. One of its advantages over nongenital tissue grafts used for urethroplasty, such as bladder mucosa (Hendren and Reda, 1986) and buccal mucosa (Kropfl et al, 1998), is that the material is "off the shelf." This eliminates the necessity of additional surgical procedures for graft harvesting, which may decrease operative time, as well as the potential morbidity due to the harvest procedure.

Bladder

Currently, gastrointestinal segments are commonly used as tissues for bladder replacement or repair. However, gastrointestinal tissues are designed to absorb specific solutes, whereas bladder tissue is designed for the excretion of solutes. When gastrointestinal tissue is in contact with the urinary tract, multiple complications may ensue, such as infection, metabolic disturbances, urolithiasis, perforation, increased mucus production, and malignancy (McDougal, 1992; Atala et al, 1993b; Kaefer et al, 1997, 1998). Because of the problems encountered with the use of gastrointestinal segments, numerous investigators have attempted alternative methods, materials, and tissues for bladder replacement or repair. These include autoaugmentation, ureterocystoplasty, methods for tissue expansion, seromuscular grafts, matrices for tissue regeneration, and tissue engineering with cell transplantation.

Autoaugmentation

Recent surgical approaches have relied on native urologic tissue for reconstruction. Autoaugmentation is based on sound surgical principles that allow for the exclusion of nonurologic tissue during augmentation cystoplasty (Cartwright and Snow, 1989a, 1989b; Snow and Cartwright, 1999). The procedure involves extraperitoneal exposure of the bladder and removal of part of the detrusor muscle, which creates a large bladder diverticulum (Fig. 73–4).

In a patient series described by Snow and Cartwright, a total of 30 patients were monitored for longer than 1 year between 1986 and 1997 (Snow and Cartwright, 1999). Fourteen patients (47%) had excellent results, showing a significant improvement in compliance, capacity, and dryness. Seven patients (23%) had fair results, described as stability or improvement of the upper tracts without significant improvement in the urodynamic parameters. Nine patients (30%) had poor results, remaining wet or with worsening hydronephrosis.

Overall, autoaugmentation does not improve bladder capacity consistently, but it is effective in improving hydronephrosis, achieving continence, and diminishing hyperreflexia. In addition, the procedure is associated with a low morbidity rate, in part because of avoidance of the use of bowel and its extraperitoneal surgical approach.

Ureterocystoplasty

Another procedure that relies on native urologic tissue for bladder augmentation is ureterocystoplasty (Bellinger,

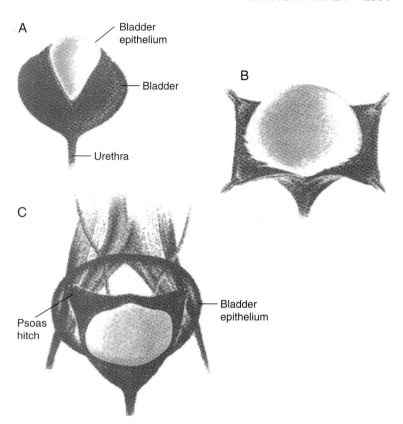

Figure 73–4. Autoaugmentation is performed by incising the detrusor *(A)* and stripping it from intact bladder epithelium *(B)*, which allows the urothelial layer to bulge with bladder filling *(C)*. (From Cartwright PC, Snow BW: Bladder autoaugmentation: Early clinical experience. J Urol 1989;142:505.)

1993; Churchill et al, 1993; Adams et al, 1998). **Uretero-cystoplasty is based on the principle of using a native ureter, which has already been dilated as a result of the patient's inherent pathology. The already dilated ureter is reconfigured and used as a patch for augmentation cystoplasty** (Bellinger, 1993; Churchill et al, 1993). This surgical technique allows for the use of additional urothelium-lined tissue for augmentation.

In a series of 16 patients reported by Churchill (1993), the source of the megaureter for augmentation was a nonfunctioning kidney in 12 patients, a nonfunctioning moiety of a duplex kidney in 2, a horseshoe kidney in 1, and the ipsilateral ureteral segment distal to a transureteroureterostomy in 1. Of the 16 patients, 15 required intermittent catheterization and 1 voided spontaneously at the time of the report. Ten patients were continent day and night, 5 had improved continence, and 1 failed to gain continence. Urodynamic evaluations in 12 of 13 patients showed good capacity with a low-pressure bladder and no instability.

A modification of the procedure involves preservation of the distal ureter during ureterocystoplasty in order to protect the ureteral blood supply. In a series of 13 patients in whom the distal ureter was left intact, mean bladder capacity on cystometrography increased from 103 to 236 ml after reconstruction and reached 137% of expected capacity for age and size (Adams et al, 1998). No uninhibited contractions or problems with compliance were noted. This modified technique appears sound from a physiologic standpoint.

The long-term results of ureterocystoplasty have been satisfactory, with retention of the augmented bladder capacity. However, the procedure is mostly limited to patients

who have a pathologic process, such as reflux or obstruction.

Tissue Expansion for Bladder Augmentation

A system of progressive dilation for ureters and bladders has been proposed but has not yet been attempted clinically (Lailas et al, 1996). **A system wherein progressive dilation could be performed in a normal ureter was designed and could be used for augmentation.**

In an animal experiment, rabbits underwent unilateral ureteral ligation at the ureterovesical junction. A Silastic catheter was threaded into the proximal ipsilateral ureter and connected to an injection port, which was secured subcutaneously. Ten days to 2 weeks after surgery, a saline-antibiotic solution was injected daily subcutaneously into the injection port. After 1 month of daily saline-antibiotic solution injections, the ureteral units were dilated at least 10-fold, as measured by radiography. The dilated ureteral diameter exceeded that of adjacent colon in each instance (Fig. 73–5). Augmentation cystoplasty was performed with the reconfigured dilated ureteral segment. Repeat cystography and cystometrography showed an increased bladder capacity ranging from 190% to 380% (Lailas et al, 1996). In a similar system, a dilating catheter was used to dilate ureteral tissue in pigs (Ikeguch et al, 1998).

A system for the progressive expansion of native bladder tissue has also been used for augmenting bladder volumes (Satar et al, 1999). Beagle dogs underwent urodynamic studies and the bladders were divided horizon-

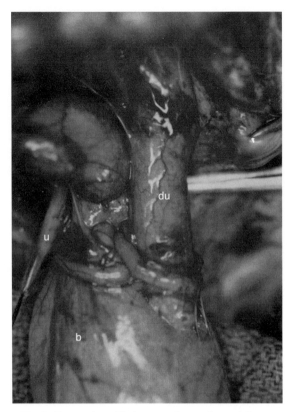

Figure 73–5. Progressive dilation can be performed in a normal-caliber ureter, which can be subsequently used for ureterocystoplasty. After placement of a ureteral dilation device, comparison is made of progressively dilated ureter (du) and native undilated ureter (u) coming off the bladder (b).

tally into two segments: a superior bladder neoreservoir, and an intact smaller bladder inferiorly with both ureters left intact and draining. A Silastic catheter was threaded into the newly formed, superiorly located neoreservoir and connected to an injection port, which was secured subcutaneously. Four weeks after surgery, a saline-antibiotic solution was injected daily into the palpable injection port, dilating the neoreservoir through the Silastic catheter.

Within 30 days after progressive dilation, the neoreservoir volume was expanded at least 10-fold, as measured by radiography and cystometrography (Fig. 73–6). Urodynamic studies of the dilated neoreservoirs showed normal compliance in all animals. Microscopic examination of the expanded neoreservoir tissue showed a normal histology. A series of immunocytochemical studies demonstrated that the dilated bladder tissue maintained normal phenotypic characteristics (Satar et al, 1999).

Ideally, bladder tissue expansion could be performed with an indwelling dilation catheter, similar to a Foley catheter with a large balloon. In the future, one could foresee placing a dilating catheter intravesically in a patient who requires augmentation, either in an intermittent fashion (e.g., four times daily) or left indwelling. An expanding balloon within the catheter could then be filled progressively, with either continuous or intermittent filling until the desired bladder volume is achieved. Studies associated with this concept are currently being conducted in the laboratory.

Seromuscular Grafts and De-epithelialized Bowel Segments

Seromuscular grafts and de-epithelialized bowel segments, either alone or over a native urothelium, have also been attempted (Blandy, 1961, 1964; Harada et al, 1965; Gonzalez et al, 1995; Oesch, 1988; Salle et al, 1990; Cheng et al, 1994; Dewan, 1998). The concept of demucosalizing organs is not new to urologists. More than four decades ago, in 1961, Blandy proposed the removal of submucosa from intestinal segments used for augmentation cystoplasty to ensure that mucosal regrowth would not occur (Fig. 73–7). Hypothetically, this would avoid the complications associated with use of bowel in continuity with the urinary tract (Blandy, 1964; Harada et al, 1965). Since Blandy's initial report, 25 years transpired before there was a renewed interest in demucosalizing intestinal segments for urinary reconstruction (Oesch, 1988).

Since 1988, several other investigators have pursued this line of research (Salle et al, 1990; Cheng et al, 1994;

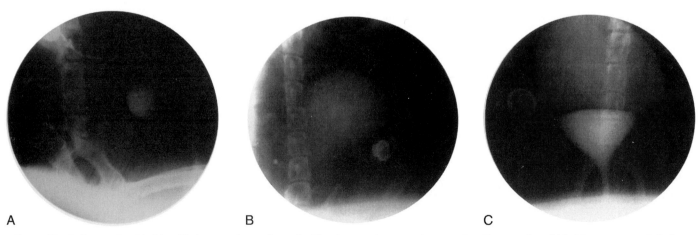

A   B   C

Figure 73–6. Progressive bladder dilation can be performed with adequate increases in capacity. Cystography of bladder neoreservoir before progressive dilation (A) is compared with cystography results after progressive dilation (B) and with cystogram showing dilated neoreservoir and intact bladder segment (C).

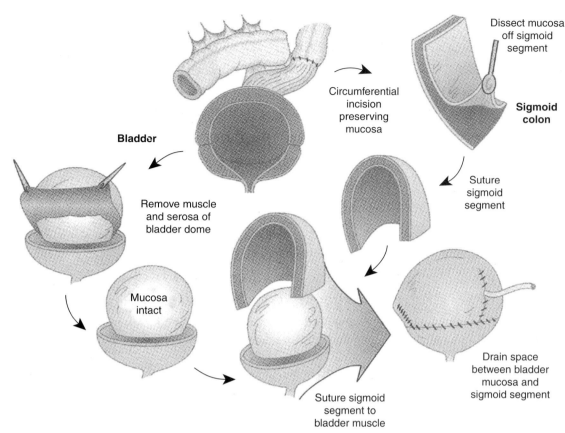

Figure 73–7. Technique for seromuscular enterocystoplasty over bladder diverticulum. (From Buson H, Manivel JC, Dayanc M, et al: Seromuscular colocystoplasty lined with urothelium: Experimental study. Urology 1994;44:745, with permission. Copyright © 1994 by Elsevier Science, Inc.)

Gonzalez et al, 1995; Dewan, 1998). These investigative efforts have emphasized the complexity of both the anatomic and cellular interactions present when tissues with different functional parameters are combined. The complexity of these interactions is emphasized by the observation that the use of demucosalized intestinal segments for augmentation cystoplasty is limited by either mucosal regrowth or contraction of the intestinal patch (Salle et al, 1990; Cheng et al, 1994). **It has been noted that removal of only the mucosa may lead to mucosal regrowth, whereas removal of the mucosa and submucosa may lead to retraction of the intestinal patch** (Atala, 1995, 1998).

Some researchers have combined the techniques of autoaugmentation with those of enterocystoplasty. An autoaugmentation is performed and the diverticulum is covered with a demucosalized gastric or intestinal segment. In a series of autoaugmentation enterocystoplasties (Dewan, 1998), 13 patients with a neurogenic bladder had incorporation of either stomach (7 patients) or colon (6 patients). In both groups, mucosa of the enteric segment was dissected away from the underlying muscle, and the resulting mucosa-free graft was used to cover a newly created bladder diverticulum. A satisfactory increase in bladder capacity and compliance was achieved in most patients.

In another series of patients who underwent seromuscular colocystoplasty, the bladder capacity increased an aver-age of 2.4-fold in 14 patients (Gonzalez et al, 1995). Two patients required reaugmentation. Thirteen patients were dry day and night, 1 was incontinent at night only, and 2 remained wet. Ten patients had a postoperative bladder biopsy. Seven demonstrated urothelium covering the augmented portion of the bladder, 2 had regrowth of colonic mucosa, and 1 showed a mixture of colonic mucosa and urothelium.

Although mucosal regrowth is seen, there is a subset of patients who may benefit from these procedures, in whom mucus secretion may be reduced or eliminated (Gonzalez et al, 1995).

Matrices for Bladder Regeneration

Over the last few decades, several bladder wall substitutes have been attempted with both synthetic and organic materials. The first application of a free tissue graft for bladder replacement was reported by Neuhoff in 1917, when fascia was used to augment bladders in dogs. Since that first report, many other free graft materials have been used experimentally and clinically, including bladder allografts, pericardium, dura, and placenta (Tsuji et al, 1961; Kelami et al, 1970; Fishman et al, 1987; Kambic et al, 1992). Synthetic materials that have been tried in experimental and clinical settings include polyvinyl sponge, Teflon, collagen matrices, Vicryl (PGA) matrices, and silicone (Bona and De Gresti, 1966; Monsour et al, 1987; Gleeson and Griffith, 1992; Rohrmann et al, 1996). Collagen/Vicryl composite membranes were used as a scaffold for tissue ingrowth to repair a full-thickness defect in the bladder of rabbits. The collagen membranes were reinforced with meshes of Vicryl, a biodegradable polymer composed of PLGA, to strengthen the collagen membranes, which are too soft to suture reliably. The results of the initial study were not encouraging because of the occurrence of severe infection (Monsour et al, 1987). However, a later study obtained a high success rate when the experiments were repeated using purification and γ irradiation of collagen and postoperative administration of antibiotics. At 3 weeks, a normal urothelium was noted. At 6 weeks, no implanted biomaterial was identified. At 35 weeks, smooth muscle regeneration was evident. During this period, there was no evidence of urinary leakage, infection, or bladder calculi (Scott et al, 1988).

Most of the these attempts have failed because of mechanical, structural, functional, or biocompatibility problems. **Usually, permanent synthetic materials used for bladder reconstruction succumb to mechanical failure and urinary stone formation, and use of degradable materials leads to fibroblast deposition, scarring, graft contracture, and a reduced reservoir volume over time.**

There has been a resurgence in the use of various collagen-based matrices for tissue regeneration. Fresh placental membranes have been used experimentally in dogs (Fishman et al, 1987). Biodegradable pericardial implants were used for bladder augmentation in dogs (Kambic et al, 1992). Functionally, the implanted bladders showed adequate capacity for up to 36 months, but they were observed grossly to undergo graft shrinkage. Histologically, the epithelial layer was present, but the muscular layer was absent. Bladder grafts, initially used experimentally in 1961, have been used recently by various investigators (Tsuji et al, 1961; Sutherland et al, 1996; Probst et al, 1997; Yoo et al, 1998b).

The allogeneic acellular bladder matrix has served as a scaffold for the ingrowth of host bladder wall components in rats. The matrix was prepared by mechanically and chemically removing all cellular components from bladder tissue (Probst et al, 1997). Partial cystectomy (25% to 50%) was performed, followed by augmentation cystoplasty using acellular bladder matrices. The mucosal lining was complete within 10 days. After 4 weeks, muscular and vascular regeneration was completed. Nerve regeneration continued to improve until week 20 (Probst et al, 1997; Sutherland et al, 1996). The grafted bladders had significantly better capacity and compliance than the autoregenerated bladders after partial cystectomy alone. The bladders regenerated with acellular matrix grafts exhibited contractile activity to electric and carbachol stimulation (Piechota et al, 1998). Clinically relevant antigenicity was not evident (Probst et al, 1997). However, there was a 26% to 63% incidence of bladder stone formation (Probst et al, 1997; Sutherland et al, 1996).

Allogeneic bladder submucosa was used as a biomaterial for bladder augmentation in dogs (Yoo et al, 1998b). The regenerated bladder tissues contained a normal cellular organization consisting of urothelium and smooth muscle and exhibited a normal compliance. **Biomaterials preloaded with cells before their implantation showed better tissue regeneration compared with biomaterials implanted with no cells, in which tissue regeneration depended on ingrowth of the surrounding tissue.** The bladders showed a significant increase (100%) in capacity when augmented with scaffolds seeded with cells, compared to scaffolds without cells (30%).

SIS, a biodegradable, acellular, xenogeneic collagen-based tissue-matrix graft, has been shown to promote regeneration of a variety of host tissues, including blood vessels and ligaments. The matrix is derived from pig small intestine in which the mucosa is mechanically removed from the inner surface and the serosa and muscular layer are removed from the outer surface.

Animal studies have shown that the SIS matrix used for bladder augmentation is able to regenerate in vivo. Augmentation cystoplasty with SIS was performed in eight dogs, with follow-up monitoring lasting 15 months (Kropp et al, 1996a and 1996b). Preoperative mean bladder capacity was 51 ml, compared with a postoperative mean capacity of 55 ml. The mean maximal voiding pressure was 52 cm H_2O preoperatively and 45 cm H_2O postoperatively. Histologically, the transitional layer was the same as that of the native bladder tissue, but, as with other collagen matrices used experimentally, the muscle layer was not fully developed. A large amount of collagen was interspersed among a smaller number of muscle bundles. A computer-assisted image analysis demonstrated a decreased muscle-to-collagen ratio with loss of the normal architecture in the SIS-regenerated bladders.

In vitro contractility studies performed on the SIS-regenerated dog bladders showed a decrease in maximal contractile response by 50% from those of normal bladder tissues. Expression of muscarinic, purinergic, and β-adrenergic receptors and functional cholinergic and purinergic innervation were demonstrated (Kropp et al, 1996b). Cholinergic and purinergic innervation also occurred in rats (Vaught et al, 1996). The regenerated bladders exhibited compliance similar to that of normal bladders (Kropp et al, 1996a).

In multiple studies using various materials as acellular grafts for cystoplasty, the urothelial layer was able to regenerate normally, but the muscle layer, although present, was not fully developed (Kropp et al, 1996b; Sutherland et al, 1996; Probst et al, 1997; Yoo et al, 1998b). Studies involving acellular matrices that may provide the necessary environment to promote cell migration, growth, and differentiation are being conducted. With continued bladder research in this area, these matrices may have a clinical role in bladder replacement in the future.

Tissue Engineering of Bladders with Cell Transplantation

Tissue engineering with selective cell transplantation may provide a means to create functional new bladder segments (Atala, 1997). **The success of cell transplantation strategies for bladder reconstruction depends on the ability to use donor tissue efficiently and to provide the right conditions for long-term survival, differentiation, and growth.**

FORMATION OF BLADDER TISSUE EX SITU

Urothelial and muscle cells can be expanded in vitro, seeded onto the polymer scaffold, and allowed to attach

and form sheets of cells. The cell-polymer scaffold can then be implanted in vivo. A series of in vivo urologic-associated cell-polymer experiments were performed. Histologic analysis of human urothelial, bladder muscle, and composite urothelial and bladder muscle–polymer scaffolds, implanted in athymic mice and retrieved at different time points, indicated that viable cells were evident in all three experimental groups (Atala et al, 1993b). Implanted cells oriented themselves spatially along the polymer surfaces. The cell populations appeared to expand from one layer to several layers of thickness with progressive cell organization over extended implantation times. Cell-polymer composite implants of urothelial and muscle cells, retrieved at extended times (50 days), showed extensive formation of multilayered, sheet-like structures and well-defined muscle layers. Polymers seeded with cells and manipulated into a tubular configuration showed layers of muscle cells lining the multilayered epithelial sheets. Cellular debris appeared reproducibly in the luminal spaces, suggesting that epithelial cells lining the lumens are sloughed into the luminal space. Cell polymers implanted with human bladder muscle cells alone showed almost complete replacement of the polymer with sheets of smooth muscle at 50 days. This experiment demonstrated, for the first time, that composite tissue-engineered structures could be created de novo. Before this study, only single cell–type tissue-engineered structures had been created.

In order to determine the effects of implanting engineered tissues in continuity with the urinary tract, an animal model of bladder augmentation was used (Yoo et al, 1998b). Partial cystectomies, which involved removal of approximately 50% of the native bladder, were performed in 10 beagles. In five, the retrieved bladder tissue was microdissected and the mucosal and muscular layers separated. The bladder urothelial and muscle cells were cultured using the techniques described previously. Urothelial and smooth muscle cells were harvested and expanded separately. A collagen-based matrix, derived from allogeneic bladder submucosa, was used for cell delivery. This material was chosen for these experiments because of its native elasticity. Within 6 weeks, the expanded urothelial cells were collected as a pellet. The cells were seeded on the luminal surface of the allogeneic bladder submucosa and incubated in serum-free keratinocyte growth medium for 5 days. Muscle cells were seeded on the opposite side of the bladder submucosa and subsequently placed in Delbecco's modified Eagle medium (DMEM) supplemented with 10% fetal calf serum for an additional 5 days. The seeding density on the allogeneic bladder submucosa was approximately 1×10^7 cells/cm^2.

Preoperative fluoroscopic cystography and urodynamic studies were performed in all animals. Augmentation cystoplasty was performed with the matrix including cells in one group and the matrix without cells in the second group. The augmented bladders were covered with omentum to facilitate angiogenesis to the implant. Cystostomy catheters were used for urinary diversion for 10 to 14 days. Urodynamic studies and fluoroscopic cystography examinations were performed at 1, 2, and 3 months postoperatively. Augmented bladders were retrieved 2 months (n = 6) and 3 months (n = 4) after surgery and examined grossly, histologically, and immunocytochemically.

Bladders augmented with the matrix seeded with cells showed a 99% increase in capacity compared with bladders augmented with the cell-free matrix, which showed only a 30% increase in capacity (Fig. 73–8). Functionally, all animals showed a normal bladder compliance as evidenced by urodynamic studies; however, the remaining native bladder tissue may have accounted for these results. Histologically, the retrieved engineered bladders contained a cellular organization consisting of a urothelium-lined lumen surrounded by submucosal tissue and smooth muscle. However, the muscular layer was markedly more prominent in the cell-reconstituted scaffold (Yoo et al, 1998b).

Most of the free grafts (without cells) used for bladder replacement in the past were able to show adequate histology in terms of a well-developed urothelial layer, but they were associated with an abnormal muscular layer that varied in terms of its full development (Atala, 1995, 1998). **It has been well established for decades that the bladder is able to regenerate generously over free grafts. Urothelium is associated with a high reparative capacity** (De Boer et al, 1994). **Bladder muscle tissue is less likely to regenerate in a normal fashion. Both urothelial and muscle ingrowth are believed to be initiated from the edges of the normal bladder toward the region of the free graft** (Baker et al, 1955; Gorham et al, 1989). Usually, however, contracture or resorption of the graft has been evident. The inflammatory response toward the matrix may contribute to the resorption of the free graft.

It was hypothesized that building the three-dimensional structure constructs in vitro, before implantation, would facilitate the eventual terminal differentiation of the cells after implantation in vivo and would minimize the inflammatory response toward the matrix, thus avoiding graft contracture and shrinkage. This study demonstrated a major

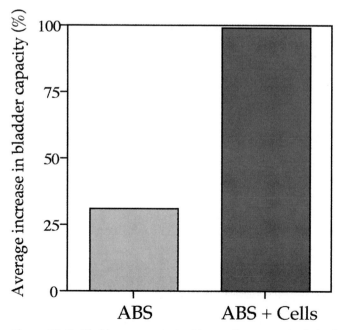

Figure 73–8. Bladders augmented with a collagen matrix derived from bladder submucosa seeded with urothelial and smooth muscle cells (ABS + cells) showed a 100% increase in capacity compared with bladders augmented with the cell-free allogenic bladder submucosa (ABS), which showed only a 30% increase in capacity within 3 months after implantation.

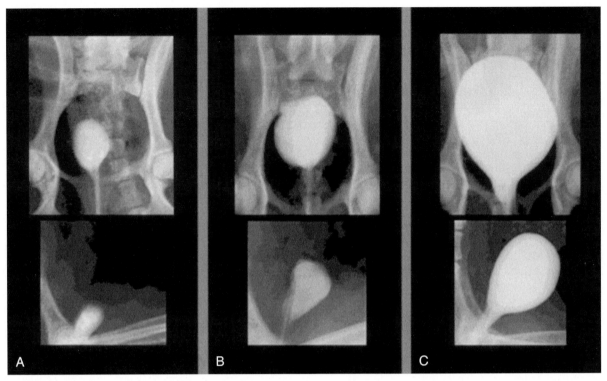

Figure 73–9. Radiographic cystograms in beagles 11 months after subtotal cystectomy without reconstruction *(A)*; with reconstruction using a polymer without cells *(B)*; and with reconstruction with a polymer and cell-seeded tissue-engineered organ *(C)*. Organs after trigone-sparing cystectomy retained a small-sized reservoir. Tissue-engineered neobladders showed a normal configuration and a larger capacity than the trigones grafted with polymer only.

difference between matrices used with autologous cells (tissue-engineered matrices) and those used without cells (Yoo et al, 1998b). Matrices implanted with cells for bladder augmentation retained most of their implanted diameter, as opposed to matrices implanted without cells for bladder augmentation, in which graft contraction and shrinkage occurred. The histomorphology demonstrated a marked paucity of muscle cells and a more aggressive inflammatory reaction in the matrices implanted without cells. Of interest, the urothelial cell layers appeared normal, even though the underlying matrix was significantly inflamed. It was further hypothesized that having an adequate urothelial layer from the outset would limit the amount of urine contact with the matrix and would therefore decrease the inflammatory response, and that the muscle cells were also necessary for bioengineering, because native muscle cells are less likely to regenerate over the free grafts. Further studies confirmed this hypothesis (Oberpenning et al, 1999). It appears that the presence of both urothelial and muscle cells on the matrices used for bladder replacement is important for successful tissue bioengineering.

BLADDER REPLACEMENT USING TISSUE ENGINEERING

The results of initial studies showed that the creation of artificial bladders may be achieved in vivo; however, it could not be determined whether the functional parameters noted were caused by the augmented segment or by the intact native bladder tissue. To better address the functional parameters of tissue-engineered bladders, an animal model was designed that required a subtotal cystectomy with sub-

sequent replacement with a tissue-engineered organ (Oberpenning et al, 1999).

A total of 14 beagle dogs underwent a trigone-sparing cystectomy. The animals were randomly assigned to one of three groups. Group A (n − 2) underwent closure of the trigone without a reconstructive procedure. Group B (n = 6) underwent reconstruction with a cell-free bladder-shaped biodegradable polymer. Group C (n = 6) underwent reconstruction using a bladder-shaped biodegradable polymer that delivered autologous urothelial cells and smooth muscle cells. The cell populations had been separately expanded from a previously harvested autologous bladder biopsy. Preoperative and postoperative urodynamic and radiographic studies were performed serially. Animals were sacrificed at 1, 2, 3, 4, 6, and 11 months postoperatively. Gross, histologic, and immunocytochemical analyses were performed (Oberpenning et al, 1999).

The cystectomy-only controls and polymer-only grafts maintained average capacities of 22% and 46% of preoperative values, respectively. An average bladder capacity of 95% of the original precystectomy volume was achieved in the tissue-engineered bladder replacements. These findings were confirmed radiographically (Fig. 73–9). The subtotal cystectomy reservoirs that were not reconstructed and the polymer-only reconstructed bladders showed a marked decrease in bladder compliance (10% and 42% total compliance). The compliance of the tissue-engineered bladders showed almost no difference from preoperative values that were measured when the native bladder was present (106%). Histologically, the polymer-only bladders presented a pattern of normal urothelial cells with a thickened fibrotic submucosa and a thin layer of muscle fibers. The retrieved tissue-engineered bladders showed a normal cellular organization, consisting of a trilayer of urothelium, submucosa, and muscle (Fig. 73–10). Immunocytochemical analyses for desmin, α-actin, cytokeratin-7, pancytokeratins AE1/AE3, and uroplakin III confirmed the muscle and urothelial phenotype. S-100 staining indicated the presence of neural structures. The results from this study showed that it is possible to tissue-engineer bladders that are anatomically and functionally normal (Oberpenning et al, 1999). Clinical trials for the application of this technology are currently being arranged.

Genital Tissues

Reconstructive surgery is required for a wide variety of pathologic penile conditions, including penile carcinoma, trauma, severe erectile dysfunction, and congenital conditions such as ambiguous genitalia, hypospadias, and epispadias.

One of the major limitations of phallic reconstructive surgery is the availability of sufficient autologous tissue. Nongenital autologous tissue sources have been used for decades. Phallic reconstruction was initially attempted in the late 1930s, with rib cartilage used as a stiffener for patients with traumatic penile loss (Frumpkin, 1944; Goodwin and Scott, 1952). This method, involving multiple staged surgeries, was soon discouraged due to the unsatisfactory functional and cosmetic results. Silicone rigid prostheses were popularized in the 1970s and have been used widely (Bretan, 1989; Small et al, 1975). However, biocompatibility issues have been a problem in selected patients (Thomalla et al, 1987; Nukui et al, 1997). Tissue transfer techniques with flaps from various nongenital sources such as the groin, dorsalis pedis, and forearm, have been used for genital reconstruction (Jordan, 1999). However, operative complications such as infection, graft failure, and donor site morbidity are not negligible. Phallic

reconstruction with autologous tissue, derived from the patient's own cells, may be preferable in selected cases.

Reconstruction of Corporal Tissues

RECONSTRUCTION OF CORPORAL SMOOTH MUSCLE

One of the major components of the phallus is corporal smooth muscle. The creation of autologous functional and structural corporal tissue de novo would be beneficial. Initial experiments were performed to determine the feasibility of creating corporal tissue in vivo using cultured human corporal smooth muscle cells seeded onto biodegradable polymers (Kershen et al, 1998). Primary normal human corpus cavernosal smooth muscle cells were isolated from normal young adult patients after informed consent during routine penile surgery. Muscle cells were maintained in culture, seeded onto biodegradable polymer scaffolds, and implanted subcutaneously in athymic mice. Implants were retrieved at 7, 14, and 24 days after surgery for analyses. Corporal smooth muscle tissue was identified grossly and histologically. Intact smooth muscle cell multilayers were observed growing along the surface of the polymers throughout all time points. Early vascular ingrowth at the periphery of the implants was evident by 7 days. By 24 days, there was evidence of polymer degradation. Smooth muscle phenotype was confirmed immunocytochemically and by Western blot analyses with antibodies to α-smooth muscle actin. This study provided evidence that cultured human corporal smooth muscle cells may be used in conjunction with biodegradable polymers to create corpus cavernosum tissue de novo.

ENDOTHELIAL CELL EXPANSION AND CHARACTERIZATION

In order to engineer functional corpus cavernosum, both smooth muscle and sinusoidal endothelial cells are essen-

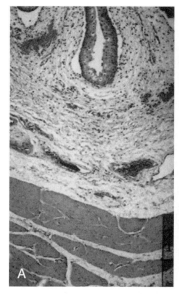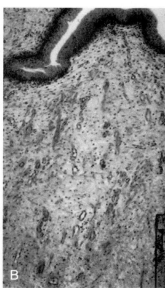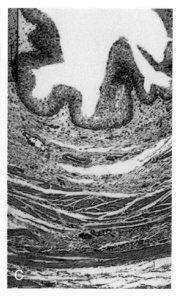

Figure 73–10. Hematoxylin and eosin staining shows histologic results 6 months after surgery (original magnification, ×250). *A,* Normal canine bladder. *B,* The bladder dome of the bladder reconstructed with cell-free polymer consists of normal urothelium over a thickened layer of collagen and fibrotic tissue; only scarce muscle fibers are apparent. *C,* The tissue-engineered neo-organ has a histomorphologically normal appearance. A trilayered architecture consisting of urothelium, submucosa, and smooth muscle is evident.

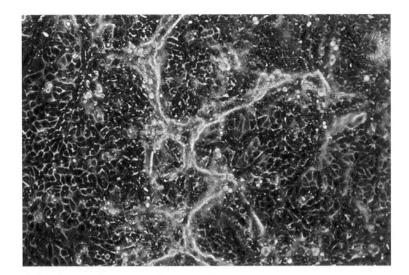

Figure 73–11. Human corporal cavernosal endothelial cells form capillary-like structures in vitro (original magnification, ×100).

tial. However, penile sinusoidal endothelial cells had not been extensively cultured in the past and had not been fully characterized. A method of isolation and expansion of sinusoidal endothelial cells from corpora cavernosa was devised, and cell function and gene expression were characterized.

Corpus cavernosum tissue was digested with collagenase type 2, and the cells were grown in culture. The endothelial cells were isolated from primary culture by magnetic beads coated with anti–bovine E-selectin antibodies. To verify the phenotype, endothelial cells were immunostained with antibodies that recognize endothelial cell–specific markers. To test for the express functional receptors for vascular endothelial growth factor (VEGF), cross-linking of iodine 125–labeled VEGF (^{125}I-VEGF$_{165}$) to the cells was performed, and ^{125}I-VEGF$_{165}$/VEGF-receptor complexes were analyzed by sodium dodecylsulfate–polyacrylamide gel electrophoresis (SDS-PAGE) and autoradiography. The mitogenic responses of the cells to increasing concentrations of VEGF and basic fibroblast growth factor (bFGF) were tested, as well as their ability to form capillaries in three-dimensional collagen gels.

Immunoisolated endothelial cells from corpus cavernosum had a morphology similar to that of endothelial cells and formed a cobblestone-like structure when they reached confluence. The cells were positively stained with anti E-selectin, factor VIII, and Flk-1 antibodies, indicating their endothelial origin. Cross-linking of ^{125}I-VEGF$_{165}$ to VEGF receptors on the cell surface indicated the expression of two VEGF receptors, Flk-1 and neuropilin-1. Increasing concentrations of VEGF and bFGF resulted in 40% and 70% increases in DNA synthesis of corporal cavernosal endothelial cells, respectively. A similar response to VEGF and bFGF was observed with endothelial cells derived from adrenal capillaries. However, endothelial cells did not respond mitogenically to either of the growth factors. **When grown on collagen, corporal cavernosal endothelial cells formed capillary structures that created a complex three-dimensional capillary network** (Fig. 73–11).

These results demonstrate that immunoisolation is a reliable method to obtain endothelial cells from corpus caver-

nosum. Cultured endothelial cells express specific markers, have an endothelial morphology, and express functional VEGF receptors. The cells proliferate in response to endothelial cell growth factors, and they have the capability to form a three-dimensional capillary network. Therefore, corpus cavernosum–derived endothelial cells may be obtained from a biopsy, grown in culture, and expanded while retaining their phenotypic characteristics.

ENGINEERING OF CORPORAL SMOOTH MUSCLE AND ENDOTHELIUM IN VIVO

In a subsequent study, the possibility was investigated of developing human corporal tissue in vivo by combining smooth muscle and endothelial cells (Park et al, 1999). Primary normal human corpus cavernosal smooth muscle cells and ECV 304 human endothelial cells were seeded on biodegradable polymers at concentrations of 20×10^6 and 10×10^6 cells/cm^3, respectively. A total of 80 polymer scaffolds (60 seeded with cells and 20 without cells) were implanted in the subcutaneous space of 20 athymic mice. Each animal had four implantation sites consisting of three polymer scaffolds seeded with muscle and endothelial cells and one control site (polymer alone). Mice were sacrificed at 1, 3, 5, and 7 days, and at 14, 21, 28, and 42 days after implantation. The retrieved structures were analyzed grossly and histologically. Immunocytochemical analyses were performed on cultured cells and retrieved specimens using several specific antibodies. Polyclonal anti-vWF was used to identify infiltrating host vessels. Broadly reacting monoclonal anti-pancytokeratins AE1/AE3 were used to identify ECV 304 human endothelial cells. Corporal smooth muscle fibers were labeled with monoclonal anti–α-smooth muscle actin. The tissue composition of the retrieved specimens was analyzed by computerized morphometry. The percentage and the ratio of muscle and endothelial tissue were calculated with the use of computerized morphometry imaging software.

Human corpus cavernosal smooth muscle cells in culture showed homogeneous populations of spindle-shaped cells under phase contrast microscopy. ECV 304 human endothelial cells were observed as cobblestone monolayers initially, and they progressively aggregated and formed extensive capillary-like networks by 27 days of culture. Immunocytochemical analyses of the cells in vitro were able to identify the ECV 304 human endothelial cells with anti-pancytokeratins and the smooth muscle cells with anti-α-smooth muscle actin. Polyclonal anti-vWF antibodies did not stain the ECV 304 cells.

At retrieval, all polymer scaffolds seeded with cells had formed distinct tissue structures and maintained their preimplantation size. The control scaffolds without cells had decreased in size with time. Histologically, all of the retrieved polymers seeded with corporal smooth muscle and endothelial cells showed survival of the implanted cells. The presence of penetrating native vasculature was observed 5 days after implantation. The formation of multilayered strips of smooth muscle adjacent to endothelium was evident by 7 days after implantation. Increased smooth muscle organization and accumulation of endothelium lining the luminal structures were evident 14 days after implantation. A well-organized construct, consisting of muscle and endothelial cells, was noted at 28 and 42 days after implantation. A marked degradation of the polymer fibers was observed by 28 days. There was no evidence of tissue formation in the controls (polymers without cells).

Immunocytochemical analyses using anti-vWF (identifying native vasculature) and anti-pancytokeratins (identifying ECV 304 endothelial cells) distinguished the origin of the vascular structures in each of the constructs. Anti-vWF antibodies stained the native vessels positively but failed to stain the implanted endothelial cells and reconstituted vascular structures. In contrast, anti-pancytokeratin antibodies identified the implanted endothelial cells and the reconstituted vessels but did not stain the native vascular structures. Anti-α-actin antibodies confirmed the smooth muscle phenotype. Smooth muscle fibers were progressively organized with time.

Computer-assisted quantitative morphometric analysis of the retrieved specimens showed that the tissue was composed of 31.2% $\pm$ 1.6% muscle and 16.4% $\pm$ 1.5% endothelium. These results were consistent throughout the study. The ratio of muscle to endothelial tissue was 1.98 $\pm$ 0.16 to 1, approximately equivalent to the ratio of muscle to endothelial cell seeding before implantation (2:1).

These experiments showed that human corporal smooth muscle cells and endothelial cells seeded on biodegradable polymer scaffolds are able to form vascularized cavernosal muscle when implanted in vivo. Endothelial cells are able to act in concert with the native vasculature. The results of these studies suggested that the creation of well-vascularized, autologous, corporal-like tissue, consisting of smooth muscle and endothelial cells, may be possible.

TISSUE ENGINEERING OF STRUCTURAL CORPORAL TISSUE

The aim of phallic reconstruction is to achieve structurally and functionally normal genitalia. Although it had been shown that human cavernosal smooth muscle and endothelial cells seeded on polymers would form tissue composed of corporal cells when implanted in vivo (see previous discussion), corporal tissue structurally identical to the native corpus cavernosum was not achieved, owing to

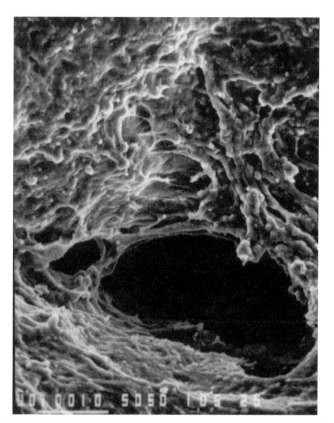

Figure 73–12. Scanning electron microscopy of human cavernosal smooth muscle and endothelial cells seeded on acellular matrices.

the type of polymers used. Therefore, a naturally derived acellular corporal tissue matrix that possesses the same architecture as native corpora was developed (Fig. 73–12). The feasibility of developing corporal tissue consisting of human cavernosal smooth muscle and endothelial cells in vivo, using an acellular corporal tissue matrix as a cell delivery vehicle, was explored (Falke et al, 1999).

Acellular collagen matrices were derived from processed donor rabbit corpora using cell lysis techniques. Human corpus cavernosal muscle and endothelial cells were derived from donor penile tissue, and the cells were expanded in vitro and seeded on the acellular matrices (see Fig. 73–11). A total of 80 matrices, 20 without and 60 with cells, were implanted subcutaneously in 20 athymic mice. Thirty-six matrices with cells were maintained in culture for up to 4 weeks. Hydroxyproline quantification, Western blot analysis, reverse transcriptase–polymerase chain reaction (RT-PCR), and scanning electron microscopy of the matrices, with and without cells, were performed at various time points. Animals were sacrificed at 3 days and at 1, 2, 3, 4, 6, and 8 weeks after implantation. Immunocytochemical and histologic studies were performed to confirm the muscle and endothelial phenotype.

Western blot analysis detected α-actin, myosin, and tropomyosin proteins from human corporal smooth muscle cells. Expression of muscarinic acetylcholine receptor (m-AChR) subtype m4 mRNA was demonstrated by RT-PCR from corporal muscle cells before and 8 weeks after seeding. The implanted matrices showed neovascularity into the sinusoidal spaces by 1 week after implantation. Increasing organization of smooth muscle and endothelial cells lining the sinusoidal walls was observed at 2 weeks and continued with time. The matrices were covered with the appropriate cell architecture 4 weeks after implantation. The matrices showed a stable collagen concentration over 8 weeks, as determined by hydroxyproline quantification. Immunocytochemical studies using α-actin and factor VIII antibodies confirmed the presence of corporal smooth muscle and endothelial cells, both in vitro and in vivo, at all time points. There was no evidence of cellular organization in the control matrices.

This study demonstrated that **human cavernosal smooth muscle and endothelial cells seeded on acellular corporal tissue matrices are able to form vascularized corporal structures in vivo.** The use of these tissue matrices as cell-delivery scaffolds allowed for the development of adequate structural constructs. The formation of corporal tissue, similar to that of the native erectile tissue, may provide an additional armamentarium in the management of complex penile reconstructive challenges.

To apply tissue engineering techniques to reconstruct corporal tissue clinically, further studies must be performed. These include the further development of cell-delivery vehicles identical to native corpus cavernosal architecture and functional and biomechanical studies of the neocorpora. Although smooth muscle and endothelial cells are the major components of erectile tissue, other structures (e.g., connective tissue, nerves) are also needed to achieve normal anatomic and functional corpora.

ENGINEERED CLITORAL TISSUE

The availability of clitoral smooth muscle tissue for use in females with sexual dysfunction may be of clinical utility. Primary cultures of human clitoral smooth muscle cells were derived from operative biopsies obtained during genitoplasty. Cells were maintained in culture for a period of 75 days after the first passage, during which time they multiplied into multilayered tissue-like structures that were readily lifted off the culture plate as a stretchable layer. The layers of clitoral muscle were divided and implanted subcutaneously in athymic mice. Animals were sacrificed at 7, 14, 21, 42, and 84 days after surgery. Implants were examined histologically with hematoxylin and eosin and with Masson's trichrome staining, as well as immunohistochemically with antibodies to the intermediate filaments, α-smooth muscle actin and desmin.

Morphologic analysis of the "neo-tissue" in culture via phase contrast microscopy revealed characteristic spindle-shaped smooth muscle cells growing on top of each other in the typical "hill and valley" appearance. Tissue specimens analyzed before implantation demonstrated the presence of an ECM as well as positive staining for the intermediate filaments α-actin and desmin. Seven days after implantation, intact multilayered smooth muscle strips were identified and there was evidence of early vascular ingrowth at the periphery of the tissue. By 21 days after implantation, there was evidence of more extensive neovascularization, and the smooth muscle maintained its multilayered architecture. The specimens remained immunohis-

tochemically positive for α-actin and desmin after implantation.

This study showed that surgically obtained clitoral smooth muscle may be cultured in vitro, expanded, and developed into multilayered sheets of muscle tissue which can be retransplanted into the in vivo environment. Tissue transplants are neovascularized and can survive in vivo, maintaining smooth muscle phenotype and architecture.

ENGINEERED PENILE PROSTHESES

Although silicone is an accepted biomaterial for penile prostheses, biocompatibility is a concern (Nukui et al, 1997; Thomalla et al, 1987). The use of a natural prosthesis composed of autologous cells may be advantageous. A feasibility study for creating natural penile prostheses made of cartilage was performed initially (Yoo et al, 1998a).

Cartilage, harvested from the articular surface of calf shoulders, was isolated, grown, and expanded in culture. The cells were seeded onto preformed cylindrical polyglycolic acid polymer rods (1 cm in diameter and 3 cm in length). The cell–polymer scaffolds were implanted in the subcutaneous space of 20 athymic mice. Each animal had two implantation sites, consisting of one polymer scaffold seeded with chondrocytes and one control (polymer alone). The rods were retrieved at 1, 2, 4, and 6 months after implantation. Biomechanical properties including compression, tension, and bending were measured on the retrieved structures. Histologic analyses were performed to confirm the cellular composition. At retrieval, all of the polymer scaffolds seeded with cells formed milky-white, rod-shaped, solid cartilaginous structures, maintaining their preimplantation size and shape (Fig. 73–13). The control scaffolds without cells failed to form cartilage. There was no evidence of erosion, inflammation, or infection in any of the implanted cartilage rods.

The compression, tension, and bending studies showed that the cartilage structures were readily elastic and could withstand high degrees of pressure. Biomechanical analyses showed that the engineered cartilage rods possessed the mechanical properties required to maintain penile rigidity. The compression studies showed that the cartilage rods were able to withstand high degrees of pressure. A ramp compression speed of 200 μm/sec, applied to each cartilage rod up to 2000 μm in distance, resulted in 3.8 kg of resistance. The tension-relaxation studies demonstrated that the retrieved cartilage rods were able to withstand stress and were able to return to their initial state while maintaining their biomechanical properties. A ramp tension speed of 200 μm/sec applied to each cartilage rod created a tensile strength of 2.2 kg, which physically lengthened the rods an average of 0.48 cm. Relaxation of tension at the same speed resulted in retraction of the cartilage rods to their initial state. The bending studies performed at two different speeds showed that the engineered cartilage rods were durable, malleable, and able to retain their mechanical properties. Cyclic compression, performed at rates of 500 and 20,000 μm/sec, demonstrated that the cartilage rods could withstand up to 3.5 kg of pressure at a predetermined distance of 5000 μm. The relaxation phase of the cyclic compression studies showed that the engineered rods

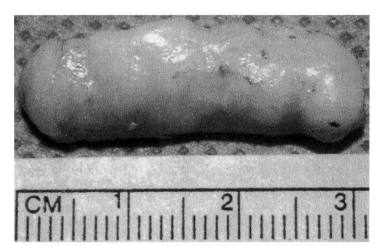

Figure 73–13. Cylindrical polymer scaffolds seeded with chondrocytes and implanted in vivo formed milky-white, rod-shaped, solid cartilaginous structures.

were able to maintain their tensile strength. None of the rods ruptured during the biomechanical stress-relaxation studies.

Histologic examination with hematoxylin and eosin stain showed the presence of mature and well-formed cartilage in all of the chondrocyte-polymer implants. The polymer fibers were progressively replaced by cartilage with time. Undegraded polymer fibers were observed at 1 and 2 months after implantation. However, remnants of polymer scaffolds were not present in the cartilage rods at 6 months. Aldehyde fuchsin-alcian blue and toluidine blue staining demonstrated the presence of highly sulfated mucopolysaccharides, which are differentiated products of chondrocytes. There was no evidence of cartilage formation in the controls.

In a subsequent study using an autologous system, the feasibility of applying the engineered cartilage rods in situ was investigated (Yoo et al, 1999). Autologous chondrocytes harvested from rabbit ear were grown and expanded in culture. The cells were seeded onto biodegradable poly-L-lactic acid coated polyglycolic acid polymer rods at a concentration of 50 μ 10^6 chondrocytes/cm^3. Eighteen chondrocyte-polymer scaffolds were implanted into the corporal spaces of 10 rabbits. As controls, two corpora, one each in two rabbits, were not implanted. The animals were sacrificed at 1, 2, 3, and 6 months after implantation. Histologic analyses were performed with hematoxylin and eosin, aldehyde fuchsin-alcian blue, and toluidine blue staining. All animals tolerated the implants for the duration of the study without any complications. Gross examination at retrieval showed the presence of well-formed, milky-white cartilage structures within the corpora at 1 month. All polymers were fully degraded by 2 months. There was no evidence of erosion or infection in any of the implantation sites. Histologic analyses with alcian blue and toluidine blue staining demonstrated the presence of mature and well-formed chondrocytes in the retrieved implants.

Subsequent studies were performed to assess the long-term functionality of the cartilage penile rods in vivo. To date, the animals have done well and can copulate and impregnate their female partners without problems. Further functional studies need to be completed before this technology can be applied in the clinical setting.

Ureters

Collagen tubular sponges have been used to transplant bladder cells for replacement of ureteral segments in dogs. Five to 12 weeks after implantation, extensive regeneration of uroepithelial cell layers occurred on the luminal side, with no evidence of severe hydronephrosis. However, the study showed severe stricture formation and papillary mucosal thickening at the anastomotic sites. In addition, muscle regeneration into the collagen grafts was not evident. In a urine exposure test, severe salt deposits were noted (Tachibana et al, 1985).

Ureteral acellular matrices were used as a scaffold for the ingrowth of ureteral tissue in rats. The matrices were prepared by removing cell and lipid components from ureters. On implantation, the acellular matrices promoted the regeneration of all ureteral wall components with no evidence of rejection. At 3 weeks, complete epithelialization and progressive vessel infiltration occurred. At 10 weeks, smooth muscle fibers were observed. At 12 weeks, nerve fibers were first detected (Dahms et al, 1997).

Laparoscopic segmental ureteral replacement with free biodegradable grafts was performed in minipigs (Shalhav et al, 1999). A 1.5- to 2.8-cm segment of the upper ureter was excised and laparoscopically replaced by a stinted (No. 6 Fr double-J stent) tube graft made of acellular matrix prepared from minipig ureters, from domestic pig ureters, and from minipig small-intestinal submucosa. In three control animals, the ureteral gap was bridged only by an indwelling stent. The stent was removed at 6 weeks, and retrograde ureteropyelography was performed preoperatively and at 8 and 12 weeks postoperatively. At 12 weeks, all animals had complete obstruction at the level of the replacement, with fibrosis with or without bone formation at the level of the stricture. Regeneration of urothelium occurred in the ureteral segments, but functional replacement was not possible. Ureteral replacement with polytetrafluoroethylene (Teflon) grafts was attempted in dogs, also with poor functional results (Baltaci et al, 1998).

Biodegradable polymer scaffolds have also been used as cell transplantation vehicles to reconstruct ureteral tissues. In one study, urothelial and smooth muscle cells isolated from bladders and expanded in vitro were seeded onto

PGA scaffolds with tubular configurations and implanted subcutaneously into athymic mice. After implantation, the urothelial cells proliferated to form a multilayered luminal lining of tubular structures, while the smooth muscle cells organized into multilayered structures surrounding the urothelial cells. Abundant angiogenesis was evident. The degradation of the polymer scaffolds resulted in the eventual formation of natural urothelial tissues (Atala et al, 1993b). This study suggested that it was possible to engineer urologic tissues containing multiple cell types. This approach was expanded to replacement of ureters in dogs by transplantation of smooth muscle cells and urothelial cells on tubular polymer scaffolds (Yoo et al, 1995).

Formation of Renal Structures

Although the kidney was the first organ to be substituted by an artificial device and the first successfully transplanted organ (Murray et al, 1955), current modalities of treatment are far from satisfactory. Renal transplantation is currently the preferred method of treatment for end-stage renal disease (ESRD). A major problem with transplantation therapy is the shortage of suitable organs. In 1996, 8495 cadaveric kidneys and 3703 kidneys from living donors were transplanted in the United States (Health Care Financing Administration, 1997); in the same year, 34,550 people were on a waiting list for kidney transplants, 1463 were waiting for a combined kidney and pancreas transplant (United Network for Organ Sharing, 1996), and almost 215,000 people (approximately 70% of all ESRD patients in the United States [National Institute of Diabetes and Digestive and Kidney Diseases, 1997]) were treated by various forms of dialysis (Health Care Financing Administration, 1997).

In addition to the inherent shortage of transplant organs, complications associated with renal transplantation are yet to be resolved. Short-term side effects of immunosuppressive therapy, chronic allograft failure due to chronic rejection, increased incidence of cardiovascular disease, infections, increased frequency of cancer, osteoporosis, osteomalacia, and bone disease secondary to hyperparathyroidism are still prevalent (Cohen et al, 1994; Julian et al, 1993; Raine, 1994).

The kidney is probably the most challenging organ in the genitourinary system to reconstruct by tissue engineering techniques, because of its complex structure and function. The formation of a tissue-engineered bioartificial kidney for ESRD or a bioartificial temporary renal assist device for acute renal failure (ARF) may improve many of the current aspects of renal functional replacement. Extracorporeal assist devices may be improved by implanting isolated renal cell lines on bioartificial hemofilters. This may aid in the replacement of specific aspects of renal function, such as improved selected metabolic and endocrinologic parameters. Eventually, reconstruction of a tissue-engineered kidney by renal cell expansion in vitro and subsequent transplantation in vivo may be possible. To achieve this prospect, many technical challenges remain to be solved.

BASIC PRINCIPLES FOR ENGINEERING RENAL STRUCTURES

The challenge in culturing renal cells is the unique structural and cellular heterogeneity present within the kidney. The system of nephrons and collecting ducts is made of up multiple functionally and phenotypically distinct segments. It is believed that identification of growth factors capable of directing tissue development and development of techniques for their delivery would aid in the engineering of human tissue. **Extensive research has been performed on tissue regeneration of the kidney after induced insult and the role of endogenous growth factors in the process. Understanding of these mechanisms may be helpful for the enhancement of engineered renal cell growth.**

It has been well established that during ARF there is significant medullary damage and injury to the vascular endothelium (Brezis and Rosen, 1995). Recovery requires the replacement of damaged tubular cells to restore continuity of the renal epithelium. This process involves a number of growth factors that are originally produced in renal tissue and play a major role in the repair process. These growth factors stimulate cells in the g_0 phase of the cell cycle to initiate DNA synthesis and to undergo mitosis, promoting the cell to the g_1 phase of the cell cycle (Schena, 1998). Epidermal growth factor (EGF), a potent proximal tubule cell mitogen (Milici et al, 1985); transforming growth factor–α (TGF-α), which plays a role in reconstruction of the injured proximal tubule via the EGF receptor (EGFr) (Carley et al, 1988); insulin-like growth factor–1 (IGF-1); and hepatocyte growth factor (HGF) are all endogenous growth factors that play a role during the recovery of the kidney from ATN (Schena, 1998).

To directly assess the role of growth factors in the induction of tubulogenesis in vitro, rabbit proximal tubule cells were treated with TGF-β1, EGF, and *trans*-retinoic acid simultaneously. All three factors were necessary to cause a confluent monolayer of proximal tubular cells to transform within 5 to 6 days to three-dimensional cell aggregates containing lumens and bordered by tubular cells with extensive microvilli formation (Humes and Cieslinski, 1992). It was also shown that deposition of laminin, an ECM molecule for epithelial cell attachment (Hirokoshi et al, 1988), was promoted by *trans*-retinoic acid and that soluble purified laminin could substitute for *trans*-retinoic acid in the promotion of tubulogenesis when combined with TGF-β1 and EGF (Humes and Cieslinski, 1992).

In an attempt to create a functional renal structure in vivo, renal cells were treated with bovine insulin, transferrin, hydrocortisone, and prostaglandin E_2 (PGE$_2$), resulting in tubule- and glomerulus-like structures and angiogenesis (Yoo and Atala, 1997).

Further experiments aimed at the identification of factors capable of increasing tissue proliferation and the development of techniques for the delivery of these factors ex vivo or to transplanted cells may significantly enhance the ability to engineer renal tissue in clinical settings.

The greatest challenge for the evolving discipline of tissue engineering is the generation of whole organs. Emerging concepts for a bioartificial kidney are cur-

rently being explored. Some investigators are pursuing the replacement of isolated kidney function parameters with the use of extracorporeal units, while others are aiming at the replacement of total renal function by tissue-engineered bioartificial structures.

EX VIVO FUNCTIONING RENAL UNITS

Although dialysis is currently the most prevalent form of renal replacement therapy, the relatively high morbidity and mortality have spurred investigators to seek alternative solutions involving ex vivo systems.

Bioartificial Hemofilter

The development of biomaterials with high hydraulic permeability has allowed for the use of continuous hemofiltration as a treatment for acute renal failure. A few considerable limitations have been observed. Thrombotic occlusion and protein deposition result in loss of filtration. The need for anticoagulation in the extracorporeal unit results in frequent bleeding. Another limitation is the need for large amounts of fluids to replace the ultrafiltrate from the filtering unit. Reports on the effects of collagen type I and type IV, laminin, and fibronectin on endothelial cell adherence, growth, and differentiation (Milici et al, 1985; Carley et al, 1988) led to the development of bioartificial hemofilters containing endothelial and other supporting cells. A bioreactor with seeded endothelial cells was created experimentally (Humes et al, 1995). This unit required the use of autologous endothelial cells, since the cells were in continuous contact with blood. Because these hemofilters expose the patient to the risk of thrombosis, transfer of genes that continuously express anticoagulant proteins may be a solution (Wilson et al, 1989; Zweibel et al, 1989). Commercially available bioreactors have been used as a platform for a bioartificial hemofilter. The hollow fibers of the bioreactor were coated with pronectin-F, a nondegradable, stable substrate for cell attachment. Endothelial cells were implanted and grown as a monolayer, and the filtration qualities of the unit were assessed (Woods and Humes, 1997). The filtration rate was 2.2 ml/min, with a filtration fraction of 45%. The leak rate for albumin was found to fall from 83% to 3% compared to the control unit without seeded cells. Although the unit filtered at a low rate, it significantly improved the selectivity to albumin. These promising results warrant future studies.

Bioartificial Renal Tubule

The goal of a bioartificial renal tubule is to reabsorb as much volume of the iso-osmotic ultrafiltrate as possible, aiming at the efficiency of the human kidney. The bioartificial tubule resembles the basic configuration of the bioartificial hemofilter, containing a monolayer of epithelial cells.

In an experimental model of a bioartificial tubule (Woods and Humes, 1997), the cells were grown within the hollow fibers while blood was allowed to flow on the outside of the fibers (i.e., the extracapillary space). Therefore, the cells were immunoisolated by the synthetic membrane. This device managed to transport salt and water along osmotic and oncotic gradients (Nikolovski et al, 1996). A more recent report described a bioartificial renal tubule in which the lumens of single hollow fibers were seeded with Madin-Darby canine kidney cells, a renal epithelial cell line (MacKay et el, 1998). After the introduction of intraluminally perfused (Freed et al, 1994) C-inulin, a recovery rate of 98.9% in the cell-lined units was measured. A control line consisting of hollow fibers without cells obtained less than 7.4% recovery. The baseline transportation rate of the fluid was 1.4 ± 0.4 μl/30 min. Albumin and later ouabain, an inhibitor of Na^+-K^+-ATPase, were introduced to the extracapillary space in order to test the dependency of fluid flux on osmotic and oncotic pressure variance across the tubule. Albumin caused the transport rate to rise to 4.5 ± 0.4 μl/30 min, whereas ouabain caused it to fall to almost the baseline level of 2.1 ± 0.4 μl/30 min. These results demonstrated the functional transport capabilities of an engineered renal epithelial cell confluent monolayer seeded on a support structure.

After the engineering of a single hollow-fiber renal tubule (MacKay et al, 1998), a multifiber renal tubular assist device was constructed that used a confluent monolayer of porcine renal proximal tubular cells grown along the inner surface of polysulphone immunoisolating hollow fibers, allowing for a membrane surface area of 0.7 m²; it contained approximately 2.5×10^9 cells. Active transport properties of sodium, bicarbonate, glucose, and organic anions was demonstrated. Ammoniagenesis, glutathione, metabolism, and synthesis of 1,25-dihydroxyvitamin D_3 by the cell-containing units was also evident.

Combined Extracorporeal Hemofilter and Bioartificial Renal Tubules

In an attempt assess the viability and physiologic functionality of a cell-seeded device to replace the filtration, transport, metabolic, and endocrinologic functions of the kidney in acutely uremic dogs, a combination of a synthetic hemofiltration device and a renal tubular cell therapy device containing porcine renal tubules in an extracorporeal perfusion circuit was introduced (Humes et al, 1999). An attempt was made to duplicate the structural anatomy of the nephron and mimic the functional relationship between the renal glomerulus and tubule. The effects of the assist device on plasma parameters, transport characteristics, and metabolic performance were assessed in a uremic environment. It was shown that levels of potassium and blood urea nitrogen (BUN) were controlled during treatment with the device. The fractional reabsorption of sodium and water reached 40% to 50% of the ultrafiltrate volume. A ratio of tubular fluid to ultrafiltrate concentration of less than 1.0 demonstrated active transport of potassium, bicarbonate, and glucose. A gradual ability to excrete ammonia, up to 100 μmol/hr, was observed over time. Filtered glutathione, an antioxidant that plays an important role in host defense, was recaptured effectively, as was shown by an increase in the level of glutathione in the plasma of the treated uremic dogs. The ability to produce 1,25-vitamin D_3 was demonstrated as well. **These results showed the technologic feasibility of an extracorporeal assist device that is reinforced by the use of proximal tubular cells.**

Creation of Functional Renal Structures In Vivo

Because the kidney is responsible not only for urine excretion but also for several other important metabolic functions, augmentation of either isolated or total renal function with kidney cell expansion in vitro and subsequent autologous transplantation may be a feasible solution.

The simplest devices are targeted at replacing a single aspect of a renal metabolic or endocrinologic function. Metabolic activities include the synthesis of 1,25-vitamin D_3, glutathione, and free radical scavenging enzymes; gluconeogenic and ammoniagenic capabilities; and the production of erythropoietin. An example for this approach could be the implantation of allogeneic or xenogeneic cells for the delivery of a deficient molecule. It has been proposed that erythropoietin-producing cells could be enclosed within a semipermeable membrane, to prevent immunologic attack by host defenses (Humes et al, 1995) after in vivo implantation.

The feasibility of achieving renal cell growth, expansion, and in vivo reconstitution with the use of tissue engineering techniques was explored. In one set of experiments, New Zealand white rabbits underwent nephrectomy and renal artery perfusion with a nonoxide solution that promoted iron particle entrapment in the glomeruli. Homogenization of the renal cortex and fractionation in 83- and 210-μm sieves with subsequent magnetic extraction yielded three separate purified suspensions of distal tubules, glomeruli, and proximal tubules. These cells were plated separately in vitro and seeded onto biodegradable polyglycolic acid polymer scaffolds. Polymer scaffolds were implanted subcutaneously into host athymic mice, including both individual cell types and a mixture of all three cell types. Cell-polymer scaffolds were implanted as sheets in a flat configuration. Cell-free polymer scaffolds served as controls. Animals were sacrificed at 1 week, 2 weeks, and 1 month after implantation, and the retrieved scaffolds were examined histologically. An acute inflammatory phase and a chronic foreign body reaction were seen, accompanied by vascular ingrowth by 7 days after implantation. Histologic examination demonstrated progressive formation and organization of nephron segments within the polymer fibers with time. Renal cell proliferation in the cell-polymer scaffolds was detected by in vivo labeling of replicating cells with the thymidine analog bromodeoxyuridine (BrdU). BrdU incorporation into renal cell DNA was identified immunocytochemically with a monoclonal anti-BrdU antibody (Atala et al, 1995).

These initial results demonstrated that renal-specific cells can be successfully harvested, survive in culture, and attach to artificial biodegradable polymers. The renal cell-polymer scaffolds can be implanted into host animals, where the cells replicate and organize into nephron segments as the polymer, which acts as a cell-delivery vehicle, undergoes biodegradation.

The initial experiments demonstrated that nephron cells or segments seeded onto a biodegradable polymer and reimplanted into a host animal gave rise to renal tubular structures. However, it was unclear whether the tubular structures reconstituted de novo from dispersed renal elements or represented merely fragments of donor tubules that had survived intact.

In order to examine the tubular reconstitution process, nephron elements from animal kidneys were harvested; the cells were expanded in vitro, seeded on biodegradable polymers with a single-cell suspension, and reimplanted into syngeneic hosts. Media conditions commonly used for renal epithelial cell growth proved to be unsuitable for sustaining the cellular developmental potential necessary for this experiment. During the search for an in vitro condition that would optimize cellular developmental potential, it was determined that the cellular expression of the EGFr was inversely proportional to the subsequent ability of the cells to proliferate and to remodel (Fung et al, 1996).

When in vitro conditions that produced minimal EGFr expression were used, renal epithelial cells seeded in a form of a single-cell suspension were found to reconstitute into tubular structures. Sequential retrieval of the seeded polymers over time revealed that the renal epithelial cells first organized into a cord-like structure with a solid center. Subsequent canalization into a hollow tube could be seen by 2 weeks. Histologic examination with nephron segment—specific lactins showed successful reconstitution of proximal tubules, distal tubules, loops of Henle, collecting tubules, and collecting ducts. More importantly, in any given tubular structure either all cells would be positively stained or all cells would be negatively stained. This homogeneous lectin staining pattern suggested that renal epithelial cells from a given nephron segment tended to interact specifically with similarly derived cells, or that each of these tubular structures was clonally derived from a single progenitor cell. The results from the second set of experiments showed that single-cell suspensions of renal epithelial cells characterized by a low level of EGFr expression are capable of reconstituting into tubular structures, with homogeneous cell types within each tubule.

In a third set of experiments, an attempt was made to harness the reconstitution of renal epithelial cells for the generation of functional nephron units. Renal cells were harvested and expanded in culture. The cells were seeded onto a tubular device constructed from a polycarbonate membrane, connected at one end with a Silastic catheter that terminated into a reservoir. The device was implanted in the subcutaneous space of athymic mice. Animals were sacrificed at 1, 2, 3, 4, and 8 weeks after implantation, and the retrieved specimens were examined histologically and immunocytochemically. Yellow fluid was collected from inside the implant, and concentrations of uric acid and creatinine were determined (Yoo et al, 1996).

Histologic examination of the implanted device revealed extensive vascularization with formation of glomeruli and

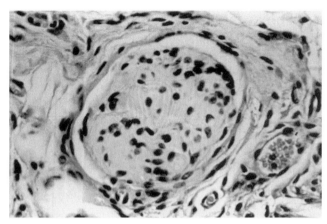

Figure 73–14. Retrieved tissue-engineered renal units demonstrate formation of glomeruli (hematoxylin and eosin stain; original magnification, ×400).

highly organized tubule-like structures. Immunocytochemical staining with anti-osteopontin antibody, which is secreted by proximal and distal tubular cells and the cells of the thin ascending loop of Henle, stained the tubular sections. Immunohistochemical staining for alkaline phosphatase stained proximal tubule-like structures. Uniform staining for fibronectin in the ECM of newly formed tubes was observed. The fluid collected from the reservoir contained 66 mg/dl uric acid (as compared with 2 mg/dl in plasma). The creatinine assay performed on the collected fluid showed an 8.2-fold increase in concentration compared with serum (27.91 ± 7.56 versus 4.49 ± 0.08 mg/dl, respectively). These results suggested that the reconstituted tubules are capable of unidirectional secretion and concentration of solutes. The fluid retrieved was consistent with the makeup of dilute urine in its creatinine and uric acid concentrations.

The results of these studies demonstrate that **renal cells can be successfully harvested, expanded in culture, and implanted in vivo** (Fig. 73–14). **The single cells form multicellular structures and become organized into functional renal units that are able to excrete high levels of solutes through a urine-like fluid.** Further challenges await this technology, including the expansion of this system to larger, three-dimensional structures.

OTHER APPLICATIONS OF GENITOURINARY TISSUE ENGINEERING

Fetal Tissue Engineering

The prenatal diagnosis of fetal abnormalities is now more prevalent. Prenatal ultrasonography allows for a thorough survey of fetal anatomy. For example, the absence of bladder filling, a mass of echogenic tissue on the lower abdominal wall, or a low-set umbilicus on prenatal sonographic examination may suggest the diagnosis of bladder exstrophy. These findings and the presence of intraluminal

intestinal calcifications suggest the presence of a cloacal malformation.

The natural consequence of the evolution in prenatal diagnosis was the use of intervention before birth to reverse potentially life-threatening processes. However, the concept of prenatal intervention itself is not limited to this narrow group of indications. A prenatal rather than a postnatal diagnosis of urologic conditions such as exstrophy may be beneficial under certain circumstances. There is now renewed interest in single-stage reconstruction surgery for some patients with bladder exstrophy. Limiting factors for choosing a single- or multiple-stage approach may include the finding of a small, fibrotic bladder patch without either elasticity or contractility and the finding of a hypoplastic bladder.

There are several strategies that may be pursued, using today's technologic and scientific advances, to facilitate the future prenatal management of patients with urologic disease. Having a ready supply of urologic-associated tissue for surgical reconstruction at birth may be advantageous. Theoretically, once the diagnosis of the pathologic condition is confirmed prenatally, a small tissue biopsy could be obtained under ultrasound guidance. These biopsy materials could then be processed and the various cell types expanded in vitro. Using tissue engineering techniques, reconstituted structures in vitro could then be readily available at the time of birth for reconstruction (Fig. 73–15).

Toward this end, a series of experiments was conducted on fetal lambs (Fauza et al, 1998a, 1998b). Bladder exstrophy was created surgically in 10 fetal lambs at 90 to 95 days' gestation. The lambs were randomly divided into two groups of five. In group I, a small fetal bladder specimen was harvested via fetoscopy. The bladder specimen was separated, and muscle and urothelial cells were harvested and expanded separately under sterile conditions in a humidified 5% CO_2 chamber, as previously described. Seven to 10 days before delivery, the expanded bladder muscle cells were seeded on one side and the urothelial cells on the opposite side of a 20-cm² biodegradable polyglycolic acid polymer scaffold. After delivery, the bladders of all lambs in group I were surgically closed using the tissue-engineered bladder tissue. No fetal bladder harvest was performed in the group II lambs, and bladder exstrophy closure was performed using only the native bladder. Cystograms were performed 3 and 8 weeks after surgery. The engineered bladders were more compliant ($P = .01$) and had a higher capacity ($P = .02$) than the native bladders. Histologic analysis of the engineered tissue showed a normal histologic pattern, indistinguishable from native bladder at 2 months (Fauza et al, 1998b). Similar prenatal studies were performed in lambs with engineering of skin for reconstruction at birth (Fauza et al, 1998a).

With tissue engineering techniques, the bladder exstrophy complex could be managed not only in utero but also after birth in a similar manner, whenever a prenatal diagnosis is not certain. In these instances, bladder tissue biopsies could be obtained at the time of the initial surgery. Various tissues could be harvested and stored for future reconstruction, if necessary. A tissue bank for patients with

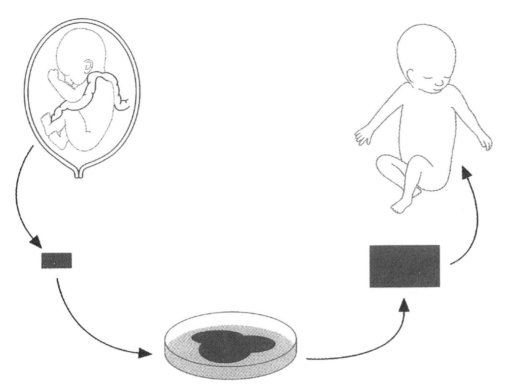

Figure 73-15. In utero tissue engineering strategy. Certain conditions, such as bladder exstrophy, can be diagnosed prenatally. Bladder, cartilage, skin, and other tissues can be retrieved via fetoscopy or percutaneously under ultrasound guidance. Cells can be harvested, expanded in vitro, and reconstituted into tissue structures. Tissue is then readily available at the time of birth for reconstruction.

exstrophy complex could preserve the different cell types indefinitely.

Injectable Therapies

Both urinary incontinence and vesicoureteral reflux are common conditions affecting the genitourinary system for which injectable bulking agents can be used for treatment. There are definite advantages to endoscopic treatment of urinary incontinence and vesicoureteral reflux. The method is simple and can be completed in less than 15 minutes; it has a low morbidity; and it can be performed on an outpatient basis. The goal of several investigators has been to find alternative implant materials that are safe for human use (Kershen and Atala, 1999).

The ideal substance for endoscopic treatment of reflux and incontinence should be injectable, nonantigenic, nonmigratory, volume stable, and safe for human use. Toward this goal, long-term studies were conducted to determine the effect of injectable chondrocytes in vivo (Atala et al, 1993a). It was initially determined that alginate, a liquid solution of glucuronic and mannuronic acid, embedded with chondrocytes, could serve as a synthetic substrate for the injectable delivery and maintenance of cartilage architecture in vivo. Alginate undergoes hydrolytic biodegradation, and its degradation time can be varied depending on the concentration of each of the polysaccharides. The use of autologous cartilage for the treatment of vesicoureteral reflux in humans would satisfy all the requirements for an ideal injectable substance. A biopsy of the ear could be easily and quickly performed, followed by chondrocyte processing and endoscopic injection of the autologous chondrocyte suspension for the treatment of reflux.

Chondrocytes can be readily grown and expanded in culture. Neocartilage formation can be achieved in vitro and in vivo using chondrocytes cultured on synthetic biodegradable polymers (Atala et al, 1993a). In these experiments, the cartilage matrix replaced the alginate as the polysaccharide polymer underwent biodegradation. This system was adapted for the treatment of vesicoureteral reflux in a porcine model (Atala, 1994).

Six miniswine underwent bilateral creation of reflux. All six were found to have bilateral reflux without evidence of obstruction at 3 months after the procedure. Chondrocytes were harvested from the left auricular surface of each miniswine and expanded, with a final concentration of 50×10^6 to 150×10^6 viable cells per animal. The animals underwent endoscopic repair of reflux with the injectable autologous chondrocyte solution on the right side only.

Serial cystograms showed no evidence of reflux on the treated side and persistent reflux in the uncorrected control ureter in all animals. All animals had a successful cure of reflux in the repaired ureter without evidence of hydronephrosis on excretory urography. The harvested ears had evidence of cartilage regrowth within 1 month after chondrocyte retrieval.

At the time of sacrifice, gross examination of the bladder injection site showed a well-defined, rubbery to hard cartilage structure in the subureteral region. Histologic examination of these specimens showed evidence of normal cartilage formation. The polymer gels were progressively replaced by cartilage with increasing time. Aldehyde fuchsin-alcian blue staining suggested the presence of chondroitin sulfate. Microscopic analyses of the tissues surrounding the injection site showed no inflammation. Tissue sections from the bladder, ureters, lymph nodes, kidneys, lungs, liver, and spleen showed no evidence of chondrocyte or alginate migration or granuloma formation. These studies

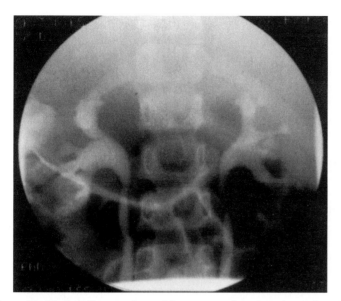
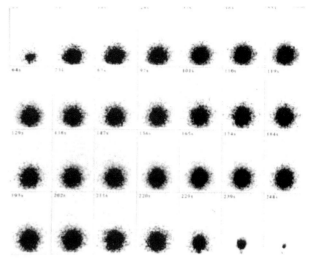

Figure 73–16. *Left,* Preoperative voiding cystourethrogram of a patient showing bilateral reflux. *Right,* Postoperative radionuclide cystography sequence of the same patient 6 months after the injection of autologous chondrocytes.

showed that chondrocytes can be easily harvested and combined with alginate in vitro, the suspension can be easily injected cystoscopically, and the elastic cartilage tissue formed is able to correct vesicoureteral reflux without any evidence of obstruction (Atala, 1994).

Using the same line of reasoning, the possibility of using autologous muscle cells was also investigated (Cilento and Atala, 1995). In vivo experiments were conducted in minipigs, and reflux was successfully corrected. **In addition to its use for the endoscopic treatment of reflux and urinary incontinence, the system of injectable autologous cells may also be applicable for the treatment of other medical conditions, such as rectal incontinence, dysphonia, plastic reconstruction, and wherever an injectable permanent biocompatible material is needed.**

Recently, the first human application of cell-based tissue engineering technology for urologic applications has occurred with the injection of chondrocytes for the correction of vesicoureteral reflux in children (Fig. 73–16) and for urinary incontinence in adults. The clinical trials are currently ongoing (Diamond and Caldamone, 1999; Kershen and Atala, 1999).

The potential use of injectable, cultured myoblasts for the treatment of stress urinary incontinence has been investigated in preliminary experiments (Yokoyama et al, 1999). Primary myoblasts obtained from mouse skeletal muscle were transduced in vitro to carry the β-galactosidase reporter gene and were then incubated with fluorescent microspheres that would serve as markers for the original cell population. Cells were then directly injected into the proximal urethra and lateral bladder walls of nude mice with a microsyringe in an open surgical procedure. Tissue was harvested up to 35 days after injection, analyzed histologically, and assayed for β-galactosidase expression. Myoblasts expressing β-galactosidase and containing fluorescent microspheres were found at each of the retrieved time points. In addition, regenerative myofibers expressing β-galactosidase were identified within the bladder wall. By

35 days after injection, some of the injected cells expressed the contractile filament α-smooth muscle actin, suggesting the possibility of myoblastic differentiation into smooth muscle. The authors reported that a significant portion of the injected myoblast population persisted in vivo. **The fact that myoblasts can be transfected, survive after injection, and begin the process of myogenic differentiation further supports the feasibility of using cultured cells of muscular origin as an injectable bioimplant.**

Testicular Hormone Replacement

Leydig cells are the major source of testosterone production in males. Patients with testicular dysfunction require androgen replacement for somatic development. Conventional treatment for testicular dysfunction consists of periodic intramuscular injections of chemically modified testosterone or, more recently, skin patch applications. However, long-term nonpulsatile testosterone therapy is not optimal and can cause multiple problems, including erythropoiesis and bone density changes.

A system was designed wherein Leydig cells were microencapsulated for controlled testosterone replacement. **Microencapsulated Leydig cells offer several advantages, such as serving as a semipermeable barrier between the transplanted cells and the host's immune system, as well as allowing for the long-term physiologic release of testosterone.**

Purified Leydig cells were isolated, characterized, suspended in an alginate solution, extruded through an air-jet nozzle into a 1.5% $CaCl_2$ solution, where they gelled, and further coated with 0.1% poly-L-lysine (Fig. 73–17). The encapsulated cells were pulsed with human chorionic gonadotropin (hCG) every 24 hours. The medium was sampled at different time points after hCG stimulation and analyzed for testosterone production. Cell viability was confirmed daily. The encapsulated Leydig cells were in-

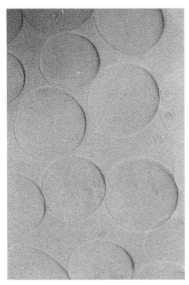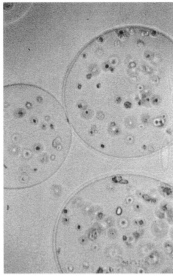

Figure 73-17. *Left,* Hydrogel microcapsules without cells. *Right,* Leydig cells encapsulated in hydrogel microcapsules secrete testosterone in vitro and in vivo.

jected into castrated animals, and serum testosterone was measured serially; the animals were able to maintain testosterone levels in the long term (Machluf et al, 1998). These studies suggest that microencapsulated Leydig cells may be able to replace or supplement testosterone in situations where anorchia or testicular failure is present. A similar system is currently being applied for estrogen.

Gene Therapy and Tissue Engineering

Genetically Engineered Cells

Cells can be engineered to secrete growth factors for various applications, such as promoting angiogenesis for tissue regeneration. Angiogenesis, the process of new blood vessel formation, is regulated by various growth factors (Klagsbrun and D'Amore, 1991; Hanahan and Folkman, 1996; Risau, 1997). These growth factors stimulate endothelial cells that are already present in the patient's body to migrate to the implanted area of need, where they proliferate and differentiate into blood vessels (Polverini, 1996). One of the major molecules that promote and regulate angiogenesis is VEGF (Klagsbrun and D'Amore, 1991; Polverini, 1996). VEGF is the only proangiogenic factor known to act specifically on endothelial cells. Extant amounts of VEGF in patients may induce rapid formation of new blood vessels and capillaries for tissue regeneration. Several methods have been used experimentally to deliver VEGF in vivo. The growth factor protein can be directly injected into tissues (Bauters et al, 1994); however, rapid clearance of VEGF proteins from the vascular system limits its effect to only minutes. The VEGF gene could be delivered to tissues by various techniques; however, the transfection efficiency is low, the onset of action is delayed for up to 48 to 72 hours after the VEGF cDNA is incorporated, and the effect is transient, lasting only several days (Bauters et al, 1994; Takeshita et al, 1996; Taub et al, 1998; Isner and Losordo, 1999). **An approach that has been pursued to increase and stimulate rapid vascularization in vivo is engineering of**

a cell line to secrete high levels of VEGF proteins by transfecting the cells with the VEGF cDNA. The VEGF-secreting cells were encapsulated in polymeric microspheres. The microspheres allowed nutrients to reach the cells while the VEGF proteins secreted from the cells diffused into the surrounding tissues. The microspheres protected the coated cells from the host immune environment. This novel system of neovascularization was tested in vitro and in vivo in an animal model.

CHO cells were chosen for the expression of recombinant VEGF. We had previously cloned the human cDNA encoding $VEGF_{165}$ (Soker et al, 1996) and subcloned it into pRc/CMV expression vector (Invitrogen). In the resulting pCMV-VEGF plasmid, the expression of VEGF is driven by the cytomegalovirus promoter. VEGF expression vector was used to transfect CHO cells, and neomycin-resistant clones were selected. Conditioned medium was collected from individual clones, and proteins were absorbed on heparin Sepharose. Clones that secreted high levels of VEGF as measured by Western blot analysis (CHO/VEGF) were selected for subsequent experiments.

CHO/VEGF cells were encapsulated within microspheres composed of calcium alginate, then coated with the positively charged polyelectrolyte PLL, and recoated with alginate (Machluf et al, 2000). The microcapsules containing the CHO/VEGF cells had a spherical shape with an average diameter of 0.6 ± 0.05 mm. Western blot analyses for human VEGF, performed on the cultured medium of the encapsulated cells, depicted high levels of VEGF at all retrieval time points.

In vivo injected microencapsulated CHO/VEGF cells and the surrounding tissues were harvested from each animal and processed with embedding medium for frozen tissue. Immunostaining with anti–human VEGF showed high levels of VEGF at the inner core of the microcapsules at days 3, 7, and 14 after implantation. Tissues surrounding the microcapsules also stained positively for VEGF. Empty microspheres without CHO/VEGF cells stained negatively for VEGF.

Macroscopic examination of the CHO/VEGF microencapsulated cell implantation sites showed a progressive increase in vascularization. At days 7 and 14, extensive vascularization was evident. Control groups that received empty microcapsules showed only minimal vascularization.

Microscopic examination with CD-31 immunostaining showed positive staining for endothelial cells in the skin harvested from the study groups at all time points. An increase in clusters and sinusoidal structures of newly formed capillaries was seen in the skin over time. A comparison between hematoxylin and eosin staining and CD-31 staining of the skin showed that the newly formed capillaries were scattered around existing blood vessels. Positively stained sinusoidal structures were less numerous in tissues harvested from the control animals.

The microencapsulated engineered cells are a novel system for the delivery of VEGF proteins. The encapsulation of these cells in alginate-PLL capsules protects them from the host immune system while allowing the constant release of VEGF as needed. The release of VEGF over a period of 2 weeks stimulated endothelial cell migration, cluster formation, and formation of new capillaries at the implant sites. The degree of VEGF secretion and the period of delivery can be regulated by modulating the number of engineered cells that are encapsulated per microsphere and the number of microspheres injected. A similar strategy has been pursued for the genetic engineering of anti-angiogenic factor–secreting cells (Joki et al, 2001). These strategies could be useful for antitumor therapy.

Gene Therapy for Tissue-Engineered Constructs

Based on the feasibility of tissue engineering techniques in which cells seeded on biodegradable polymer scaffolds form tissue when implanted in vivo, the possibility was explored of developing a neo-organ system for in vivo gene therapy (Yoo et al, 1997).

In a series of studies conducted in our laboratory, human urothelial cells were harvested, expanded in vitro, and seeded on biodegradable polymer scaffolds. The cell-polymer complex was then transfected with PGL3-luc, pCMV-luc and pCMVβ-gal promoter-reporter gene constructs. The transfected cell-polymer scaffolds were implanted in vivo, and the engineered tissues were retrieved at various time points after implantation. The results indicated that **successful gene transfer may be achieved using biodegradable polymer scaffolds as a urothelial cell-delivery vehicle.** The transfected cell-polymer scaffold formed organ-like structures with functional expression of the transfected genes (Yoo et al, 1997).

This technology is applicable throughout the spectrum of diseases that may be manageable with tissue engineering. For example, one can envision in vivo gene delivery through ex vivo transfection of tissue-engineered cell-polymer scaffolds for the genetic modification of diseased corporal smooth muscle cells harvested from impotent patients. Studies of human corpus cavernosum smooth muscle cells have suggested that cellular overproduction of the cytokine TGF-1 may lead to the synthesis and accumulation of excess collagen in patients with arterial insufficiency resulting in corporal fibrosis. PGE$_1$ was shown to

suppress this effect in vitro. Theoretically, the in vitro genetic modification of corporal smooth muscle cells harvested from an impotent patient, resulting in either a reduction in expression of the TGF-1 gene or overexpression of genes responsible for PGE$_1$ production, could lead to the resumption of erectile functionality once these cells were used to repopulate the diseased corporal bodies.

Stem Cells for Tissue Engineering

Most current strategies for engineering of urologic tissues involve harvesting of autologous cells from the host diseased organ. However, when extensive end-stage organ failure is present, a tissue biopsy may not yield enough normal cells for expansion. Under these circumstances, the availability of pluripotent stem cells may be beneficial. Pluripotent embryonic stem cells are known to form teratomas in vivo, which are composed of a variety of differentiated cells. However, these cells are immunocompetent and would require immunosuppression if used clinically.

The possibility of deriving stem cells from postnatal mesenchymal tissue from the same host and inducing their differentiation in vitro and in vivo was investigated. Stem cells were isolated from human foreskin-derived fibroblasts (Fig. 73–18). Stem cell–derived chondrocytes were obtained through a chondrogenic lineage process. The cells were grown, expanded, seeded onto biodegradable scaffolds, and implanted in vivo, where they formed mature cartilage structures. This was the first demonstration that stem cells can be derived from postnatal connective tissue and can be used for engineering tissues in vivo ex situ (Bartsch et al, 2000).

A second approach that has been pursued for stem lineage isolation involves the isolation of stem cells from individual organs. For example, daily female hormone supplementation is used widely, most commonly in postmenopausal women. A continuous and unlimited hormone supply produced from ovarian granulosa cells would be an attractive alternative. The feasibility of isolating functional human ovarian granulosa stem cells, which, unlike primary cells, may have the ability to proliferate and function indefinitely, was investigated.

Granulosa stem cells were selectively isolated from postmenopausal human ovaries, and their phenotype was confirmed with the stem cell marker antibodies CD34, CD105, and CD90. The granulosa stem cells in culture showed steady-state production of progesterone (5 to 7 ng/ml) and estradiol (2500 to 3000 pg/ml) either with or without hCG stimulation (Raya-Rivera et al, 2000).

Therapeutic Cloning for Tissue Engineering

Recent advances in the cloning of embryos and newborn animals have expanded the possibilities of this technology for tissue engineering and organ transplantation. There are many ethical concerns with cloning in terms of creating humans for the sole purpose of obtaining organs. However, the potential for retrieving cells from

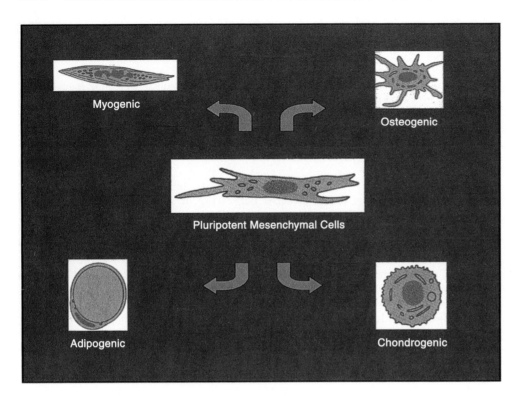

Figure 73–18. Schematic diagram of pluripotential stem cell lineages that can be derived from postnatal tissue.

early-stage cloned embryos for subsequent regeneration is being proposed as an ethically viable benefit of therapeutic cloning (Fig. 73–19). The feasibility of engineering syngeneic tissues in vivo with the use of cloned cells was investigated.

Unfertilized donor bovine eggs were retrieved and the nuclear material was removed. Bovine fibroblasts from the skin of a steer were obtained. The nuclear material was removed from the fibroblast and microinjected into the donor egg shell (nuclear transfer). A short burst of energy was delivered, initiating neoembryogenesis. After 8 days, the embryos were placed in the same steer uterus from which the fibroblasts were obtained. The cloned embryo, with genetic material identical to that of the steer, was retrieved after 40 days for tissue harvest. Various cell types were harvested, expanded in vitro, and seeded on biodegradable scaffolds. The cell-polymer scaffolds were implanted into the back of the same steer from which the cells were cloned. The implants were retrieved at various time points for analyses. Renal tissue; cartilage; and cardiac, skeletal, and smooth muscle were engineered successfully by therapeutic cloning (Fig. 73–20).

These studies demonstrated that cells obtained through nuclear transfer can be successfully harvested, expanded in culture, and transplanted in vivo with the use of biodegradable scaffolds on which the single suspended cells form and organize into tissue structures that are the same genetically as those of the host. These

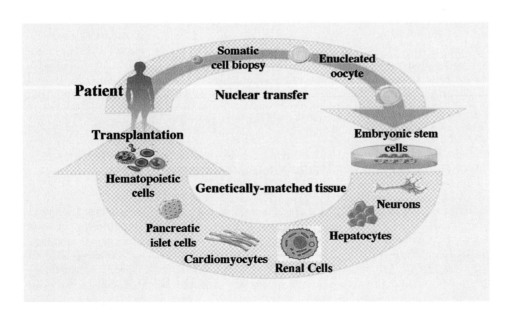

Figure 73–19. Therapeutic cloning strategy and its application to the engineering of tissues and organs.

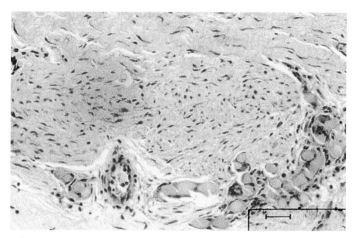

Figure 73–20. Engineered muscle created with the use of therapeutic cloning techniques (bar = 50 μm).

studies were the first demonstration of the use of therapeutic cloning for regeneration of tissues in vivo (Atala et al, 2000).

CONCLUSION

Tissue engineering efforts are currently being undertaken for every type of tissue and organ within the urinary system. Most of the effort expended to engineer genitourinary tissues has occurred within the last decade. **Tissue engineering techniques require a cell culture facility designed for human application. Personnel who have mastered the techniques of cell harvest, culture, and expansion as well as polymer design are essential for the successful application of this technology. Before these engineering techniques can be applied to humans, further studies need to be performed in many of the tissues described.**

The first human use of cell-based tissue engineering technology for urologic applications occurred with the injection of autologous cells for the correction of vesicoureteral reflux in children. These clinical trials are currently ongoing. The same technology has recently been expanded to the treatment of adult patients with urinary incontinence. Furthermore, trials involving urethral tissue replacement using processed collagen matrices are in progress, and those involving bladder replacement using tissue engineering techniques are being arranged. Recent progress suggests that engineered urologic tissues may have clinical applicability in the future.

REFERENCES

Adams MC, Brock JW, Pope JC, Rink RC: Ureterocystoplasty: Is it necessary to detubularize the distal ureter? J Urol 1998;160:851–853.

Alberts B, Bray D, Lewis J, et al: The extracellular matrix of animals. In Alberts B, Bray D, Lewis J, et al (eds): Molecular Biology of the Cell. New York, Garland Publishing, 1994, pp 971–995.

Amiel GE, Atala A: Current and future modalities for functional renal replacement. Urol Clin North Am 1999;26:235–246.

Atala A: Use of non-autologous substances in VUR and incontinence treatment. Dial Pediatr Urol 1994;17:11–12.

Atala A: Commentary on the replacement of urologic associated mucosa. J Urol 1995;156:338.

Atala A: Tissue engineering in the genitourinary system. In Atala A, Mooney D (eds): Tissue Engineering. Boston, Birkhauser Press, 1997, p 149.

Atala A: Autologous cell transplantation for urologic reconstruction. J Urol 1998;159:2.

Atala A: Future perspectives in reconstructive surgery using tissue engineering. Urol Clin North Am 1999;26:157–165, ix–x.

Atala A, Cima LG, Kim W, et al: Injectable alginate seeded with chondrocytes as a potential treatment for vesicoureteral reflux. J Urol 1993a;150:745.

Atala A, Freeman MR, Vacanti JP, et al: Implantation in vivo and retrieval of artificial structures consisting of rabbit and human urothelium and human bladder muscle. J Urol 1993b;150:608–612.

Atala A, Guzman L, Retik A: A novel inert collagen matrix for hypospadias repair. J Urol 1999;162:1148–1151.

Atala A, Kim W, Paige KT, et al: Endoscopic treatment of vesicoureteral reflux with chondrocyte-alginate suspension. J Urol 1994;152:641.

Atala A, Lanza RP: Preface. In Atala A, Lanza RP (eds): Methods of Tissue Engineering. San Diego, Academic Press, 2001.

Atala A, Peters CA, Retik AB, Mandell J: Endoscopic treatment of vesicoureteral reflux with a self-detachable balloon system. J Urol 1992a;148:724–728.

Atala A, Schlussel RN, Retik AB: Renal cell growth in vivo after attachment to biodegradable polymer scaffolds. J Urol 1995;153:4.

Atala A, Vacanti JP, Peters CA, et al: Formation of urothelial structures in vivo from dissociated cells attached to biodegradable polymer scaffolds in vitro. J Urol 1992b;148:658.

Atala A, Yoo J, Cibelli JB, et al: Therapeutic cloning applications for the engineering of kidney tissues. (Abstract.) American Academy of Pediatrics Meeting, Urology Section, Chicago, 2000, p 9.

Baker R, Kelly T, Tehan T, et al: Subtotal cystectomy and total bladder regeneration in treatment of bladder cancer. J Am Med Assoc 1955;168:1178.

Baltaci S, Ozer G, Ozer E, et al: Failure of ureteral replacement with Gore-Tex tube grafts. Urology 1998;51:400–403.

Barrera DA, Zylstra E, Lansbury PT, Langer R: Synthesis and RGD peptide modification of a new biodegradable copolymer poly (lactic acid-co-lysine). J Am Chem Soc 1993;115:11010–11011.

Barrera DA, Zylstra E, Lansbury PT, Langer R: Copolymerization and degradation of poly (lactic acid-co-lysine). Macromolecules 1995;28:425–432.

Bartsch G, Yoo J, Kim B, Atala A: Stem cells in tissue engineering applications for incontinence. J Urol 2000;1009S:227.

Bauters C, Asahara T, Zheng LP, et al: Physiological assessment of augmented vascularity induced by VEGF in ischemic rabbit hindlimb. Am J Physiol 1994;267:263.

Bazeed MA, Thüroff JW, Schmidt RA, Tanagho EA: New treatment for urethral strictures. Urology 1983;21:53–57.

Bellinger MF: Ureterocystoplasty: A unique method for vesical augmentation in children. J Urol 1993;149:811.

Bergsma JE, Rozema FR, Bos RRM, et al: Biocompatibility and degradating mechanism of predegraded and non-degraded poly(lactide) implants: An animal study. J Biomed Mater Res 1995;6:715–724.

Blandy JP: Neal pouch with transitional epithelium and anal sphincter as a continent urinary reservoir. J Urol 1961;86:749.

Blandy JP: The feasibility of preparing an ideal substitute for the urinary bladder. Ann R Coll Surg 1964;35:287.

Bona AV, De Gresti A: Partial substitution of urinary bladder with Teflon prosthesis. Minerva Urol 1966;18:43.

Bretan PN, Jr: History of prosthetic treatment of impotence. In Montague DK (ed): Genitourinary Prostheses. Philadelphia, WB Saunders, 1989, pp 1–5.

Brezis M, Rosen S: Hypoxia of the renal medulla: Its implications for disease. N Engl J Med 1995;332:647–655.

Brittberg M, Lindahl A, Nilsson A, et al: Treatment of deep cartilage defects in the knee with autologous chondrocyte transplantation. N Engl J Med 1994;331:889–895.

Buckley JF, Scott R, Aitchison M, et al: Periurethral microparticulate silicone injection for stress incontinence and vesicoureteric reflux. Minim Invasive Ther 1997;1(Suppl. 1):72.

Carley WW, Milici AJ, Madri JA: Extracellular matrix specificity for the differentiation of capillary endothelial cells. Exp Cell Res 1988;178:426–434.

Cartwright PC, Snow BW: Bladder autoaugmentation: Early clinical experience. J Urol 1989a;142:505–508.

Cartwright PC, Snow BW: Bladder autoaugmentation: Partial detrusor excision to augment the bladder without use of bowel. J Urol 1989b; 142:1050.

Cavallaro JF, Kemp PD, Kraus KH: Collagen fabrics as biomaterials. Biotechnol Bioeng 1994;43:781–791.

Chen F, Yoo JJ, Atala A: Acellular collagen matrix as a possible "off the shelf" biomaterial for urethral repair. Urology 1999;54:407–410.

Cheng E, Rento R, Grayhack TJ, et al: Reversed seromuscular flaps in the urinary tract in dogs. J Urol 1994;152:2252.

Churchill BM, Aliabadi H, London EH, et al: Ureteral bladder augmentation. J Urol 1993;150:716–720.

Cilento BG, Atala A: Treatment of reflux and incontinence with autologous chondrocytes and bladder muscle cells. Dial Pediatr Urol 1995;18: 11.

Cilento BG, Freeman MR, Schneck FX, et al: Phenotypic and cytogenetic characterization of human bladder urothelia expanded in vitro. J Urol 1994;152:655.

Cohen J, Hopkin J, Kurtz J: Infectious complications after renal transplantation. In Morris PJ (ed): Kidney Transplantation: Principles and Practice. Philadelphia, WB Saunders, 1994, pp 364–389.

Cook AD, Hrkach JS, Gao NN, et al: Characterization and development of RGD-peptide-modified poly(lactic acid-co-lysine) as an interactive, resorbable biomaterial. J Biomed Mater Res 1997;35:513–523.

Dahms SE, Piechota HJ, Dahiya R, et al: Composition and biochemical properties of the bladder acellular matrix graft: Comparative analysis in rat, pig and human. Br J Urol 1998;82:411–419.

Dahms SE, Piechota HJ, Nunes L, et al: Free ureteral replacement in rats: Regeneration of ureteral wall components in the acellular matrix graft. Urology 1997;50:818–825.

De Boer WI, Schuller AG, Vermay M, van der Kwast TH: Expression of growth factors and receptors during specific phases in regenerating urothelium after acute injury in vivo. Am J Pathol 1994;145:1199.

Deuel TF: Growth factors. In Lanza RP, Langer R, Chick WL (eds): Principles of Tissue Engineering. New York, Academic Press, 1997, pp 133–149.

Dewan PA: Autoaugmentation demucosalized enterocystoplasty. World J Urol 1998;16:255–261.

Diamond DA, Caldamone AA: Endoscopic correction of vesicoureteral reflux in children using autologous chondrocytes: Preliminary results. J Urol 1999;162:1185.

Falke G, Yoo J, Machado M, et al: Corporal tissue for penile reconstruction. Pediatrics 1999;104s:840.

Fauza DO, Fishman S, Mehegan K, Atala A: Videofetoscopically assisted fetal tissue engineering: Skin replacement. J Pediatr Surg 1998a;33:377.

Fauza DO, Fishman S, Mehegan K, Atala A: Videofetoscopically assisted fetal tissue engineering: Bladder augmentation. J Pediatr Surg 1998b; 33:7.

Fishman IJ, Flores FN, Scott B, et al: Use of fresh placental membranes for bladder reconstruction. J Urol 1987;138:1291.

Freed LE, Vunjak-Novakovic G, Biron RJ, et al: Biodegradable polymer scaffolds for tissue engineering. Bio/Technology 1994;12:689–693.

Freeman MR, Yoo JJ, Raab G, et al: Heparin-binding EGF-like growth factor is an autocrine factor for human urothelial cells and is synthesized by epithelial and smooth muscle cells in the human bladder. J Clin Invest 1997;99:1028.

Frumpkin AP: Reconstruction of male genitalia. Am Rev Sov Med 1944; 2:14.

Fung LCT, Elenius K, Freeman M, et al: Reconstitution of EGFr-poor renal epithelial cells into tubular structures on biodegradable polymer scaffold. Pediatrics 1996;98(Suppl.):S631.

Furthmayr H, Timpl R: Immunochemistry of collagens and procollagens. Int Rev Connect Tiss Res 1976;7:61.

Gilding DK: Biodegradable polymers. In Williams DF (ed): Biocompatibility of Clinical Implant Materials. Boca Raton, FL, CRC Press, 1981, pp 209–232.

Goodwin WE, Scott WW: Phalloplasty. J Urol 1952;68:903.

Gleeson MJ, Griffith DP: The use of alloplastic biomaterials in bladder substitution. J Urol 1992;148:1377.

Gonzalez R, Buson H, Reid C, Reinberg Y: Seromuscular colocystoplasty lined with urothelium (SCLU): Experimental in 16 patients. Urology 1995;45:124.

Gorham SD, French DA, Shivas AA, Scott R: Some observations on the regeneration of smooth muscle in the repaired urinary bladder of the rabbit. Eur Urol 1989;16:440.

Hanahan D, Folkman J: Patterns and emerging mechanisms of the angiogenic switch during a tumorigenesis. Cell 1996;86:353.

Harada N, Yano H, Ohkawa T, et al: New surgical treatment of bladder tumors: Mucosal denudation of the bladder. Br J Urol 1965;37:545.

Harris LD, Kim BS, Mooney DJ: Open pore biodegradable matrices formed with gas foaming. J Biomed Mater Res 1998;42:396–402.

Harriss DR: Smooth muscle cell culture: A new approach to the study of human detrusor physiology and pathophysiology. Br J Urol 1995; 75(Suppl. 1):18–26.

Health Care Financing Administration: End Stage Renal Disease Program Highlights. (Fact sheet.) Washington, DC: U.S. Department of Health and Human Services, 1997.

Hendren WH, Reda EF: Bladder mucosa graft for construction of male urethra. J Pediatr Surg 1986;21:189–192.

Hirokoshi S, Koide H, Shirai T: Monoclonal antibodies against laminin A chain and B chain in the human and mouse kidneys. Lab Invest 1988; 58:532–538.

Holmes P: Applications of PHB-α microbially produced thermoplastic. Phys Technol 1985;16:32–36.

Humes HD, Buffington DA, MacKay SM, et al: Replacement of renal function in uremic animals with a tissue engineered kidney. Nat Biotech 1999;17:451–455.

Humes HD, Cieslinski DA: Interaction between growth factors and retinoic acid in the induction of key tubulogenesis in tissue culture. Exp Cell Res 1992;201:8–15.

Humes HD, Cieslinski DA, Funke AJ: Cell therapy for erythropoietin (EPO) deficient anemias. (Abstract 6.) J Am Soc Nephrol 1995;6:535.

Hynes RO: Integrins: Versatility, modulation and signaling in cell adhesion. Cell 1992;69:11–25.

Ikeguch EF, Stifelman MD, Hensle TW: Ureteral tissue expansion for bladder augmentation. J Urol 1998;159:1665.

Intveld PJA, Shen ZR, Takens GAJ, et al: Glycine glycolic acid based copolymers. J Polym Sci Polym Chem 1994;32:1063–1069.

Isner JM, Losordo DW: Therapeutic angiogenesis for heart failure. Nat Med 1999;5:491.

Joki T, Machluf M, Atala A, et al: Continuous release of endostatin from microencapsulated engineered cells for tumor therapy. Nat Biotechnol 2001;19:35–39.

Jordan GH: Penile reconstruction, phallic construction, and urethral reconstruction. Urol Clin North Am 1999;26:1–13.

Julian BA, Benfield M, Quarles LD: Bone loss after organ transplantation. Transplant Rev 1993;7:82–95.

Kaefer M, Hendren H, Bauer S, et al: Reservoir calculi: A comparison of reservoirs constructed from stomach and other enteric segments. J Urol 1998;160:2187.

Kaefer M, Tobin M, Hendren H, et al: Continent urinary diversion: The Children's Hospital experience. J Urol 1997;157:1394–1399.

Kambic H, Kay R, Chen JF, et al: Biodegradable pericardial implants for bladder augmentation: A 2.5-year study in dogs. J Urol 1992;148:539–543.

Kassaby EA, Yoo J, Retik A, Atala A: A novel inert collagen matrix for urethral stricture repair. J Urol 2000;308S;70.

Kelami A, Ludtke-Handjery A, Korb G, et al: Alloplastic replacement of the urinary bladder wall with lyophilized human dura. Eur Surg 1970; Res. 2:195.

Kershen RT, Atala A: Advances in injectable therapies for the treatment of incontinence and vesicoureteral reflux. Urol Clin North Am 1999;26: 81–94.

Kershen RT, Yoo JJ, Moreland RB, et al: Novel system for the formation of human corpus cavernosum smooth muscle tissue in vivo. J Urol 1998;159(Suppl.):156.

Kim BS, Mooney DJ: Development of biocompatible synthetic extracellular matrices for tissue engineering. Trends Biotechnol 1998a;16:224–230.

Kim BS, Mooney DJ: Engineering smooth muscle tissue with a predefined structure. J Biomed Mater Res 1998b;41:322–332.

Klagsbrun M, D'Amore PA: Regulation of angiogenesis. Annu Rev Physiol 1991;53:217.

Kropfl D, Tucak A, Prlic D, Verweyen A: Using buccal mucosa for urethral reconstruction in primary and re-operative surgery. Eur Urol 1998;34:216–220.

Kropp BP, Ludlow JK, Spicer D, et al: Rabbit urethral regeneration using small intestinal submucosa onlay grafts. Urology 1998;52:138–142.

Kropp BP, Rippy MK, Badylak SF, et al: Small intestinal submucosa: Urodynamic and histopathologic evaluation in long term canine bladder augmentations. J Urol 1996a;155:2098–2104.

Kropp BP, Sawyer BD, Shannon HE, et al: Characterization of using small intestine submucosa regenerated canine detrusor: Assessment of reinnervation, in vitro compliance and contractility. J Urol 1996b;156:599–607.

Lailas NG, Cilento B, Atala A: Progressive ureteral dilation for subsequent ureterocystoplasty. J Urol 1996;156:1151.

Levesque PE, Bauer SB, Atala A, et al: Ten year experience with the artificial urinary sphincter in children. J Urol 1996;156:625.

Liebert M, Hubbel A, Chung M, et al: Expression of mal is associated with urothelial differentiation in vitro: Identification by differential display reverse-transcriptase polymerase chain reaction. Differentiation 1997;61:177–185.

Liebert M, Wedemeyer G, Abruzzo LV, et al: Stimulated urothelial cells produce cytokines and express an activated cell surface antigenic phenotype. Semin Urol 1991;9:124–130.

Lim F, Sun AM: Microencapsulated islets as bioartificial endocrine pancreas. Science 1980;210:908–910.

Li ST: Biologic biomaterials: Tissue-derived biomaterials (collagen). In Brozino JD (ed): The Biomedical Engineering Handbook. Boca Raton, FL, CRC Press, 1995, pp 627–647.

Lobban ED, Smith BA, Hall GD, et al: Uroplakin gene expression by normal and neoplastic human urothelium. Am J Pathol 1998;153:1957–1967.

Machluf M, Atala A: Emerging concepts for tissue and organ transplantation. Graft 1998;1:31.

Machluf M, Amiel G, Soker S, Atala A: A novel system for the enhancement of angiogenesis to free grafts using encapsulated cells engineered to secrete VEGF. J Urol 2000;305S:70.

Machluf M, Boorjian S, Caffaratti J, et al: Microencapsulation of Leydig cells: A new system for the therapeutic delivery of testosterone. Pediatrics 1998;102S:32.

MacKay SM, Funke AJ, Buffington DA, Humes DH: Tissue engineering of a bioartificial tubule. ASAIO J 1998;44:179–183.

McDougal WS: Metabolic complications of urinary intestinal diversion. J Urol 1992;147:1199.

Mikos AG, Thorsen AJ, Czerwonka LA, et al: Preparation and characterization of poly(L-lactic acid) foams. Polymer 1994;35:1068–1077.

Milici AJ, Furie MB, Carley WW: The formation of fenestrations and channels by capillary endothelium in vitro. Proc Natl Acad Sci U S A 1985;82:6181–6185.

Monsour MJ, Mohammed R, Gorham SD, et al: An assessment of a collagen/Vicryl composite membrane to repair defects of the urinary bladder in rabbits. Urology 1987;Res. 15:235.

Murray JE, Merrill JP, Harrison JH: Renal homotransplantation in identical wins. Surg Forum 1955;6:432–436.

National Institute of Diabetes and Digestive and Kidney Diseases: United States Renal Data System: 1997 Annual Data Report. Washington, DC, National Institutes of Health, U.S. Department of Health and Human Services, 1997.

Neuhoff H: Fascial transplantation into visceral defects: An experimental and clinical study. Surg Gynecol Obstet 1917;25:383.

Nikolovski J, Poirier S, Funke AJ, et al: Development of a bioartificial renal tubule for the treatment of acute renal failure. (Abstract 7.) J Am Soc Nephrol 1996;7:1376.

Nguyen HT, Park JM, Peters CA, et al: Cell-specific activation of the HB-EGF and ErbB1 genes by stretch in primary human bladder cells. In Vitro Cell Dev Biol Anim 1999;35:371–375.

Nukui F, Okamoto S, Nagata M, et al: Complications and reimplantation of penile implants. Int J Urol 1997;4:52.

Oberpenning FO, Meng J, Yoo J, Atala A: De novo reconstitution of a functional urinary bladder by tissue engineering. Nat Biotechnol 1999;17:2.

Oesch I: Neourothelium in bladder augmentation: An experimental study in rats. Eur Urol 1988;14:328.

Olsen L, Bowald S, Busch C, et al: Urethral reconstruction with a new synthetic absorbable device. Scan J Urol Nephrol 1992;26:323–326.

Pachence JM: Collagen-based devices for soft tissue repair. J Biomed Mater Res (Appl Biomater) 1996;33:35–40.

Pariente JL, Kim BS, Atala A: In vitro biocompatibility assessment of naturally-derived and synthetic biomaterials using normal human urothelial cells. J Biomed Mater Res 2001;55:33–39.

Park HJ, Kershen R, Yoo J, Atala A: Reconstitution of human corporal smooth muscle and endothelial cells in vivo. J Urol 1999;162:1106–1109.

Peppas NA, Langer R: New challenges in biomaterials. Science 1994;263:1715–1720.

Piechota HJ, Dahms SE, Nunes LS, et al: In vitro functional properties of the rat bladder regenerated by the bladder acellular matrix graft. J Urol 1998;159:1717–1724.

Politano VA: Periurethral polytetrafluoroethylene injection for urinary incontinence. J Urol 1982;127:439–442.

Polverini PJ: The pathophysiology of angiogenesis. Crit Rev Oral Biol Med 1996;6:230.

Ponder KP, Gupta S, Leland F, et al: Mouse hepatocytes migrate to liver parenchyma and function indefinitely after intrasplenic transplantation. Proc Natl Acad Sci U S A 1991;88:1217–1221.

Probst M, Dahiya R, Carrier S, Tanagho EA: Reproduction of functional smooth muscle tissue and partial bladder replacement. Br J Urol 1997;79:505–515.

Puthenveettil JA, Burger MS, Reznikoff CA: Replicative senescence in human uroepithelial cells. Adv Exp Med Biol 1999;462:83–91.

Rackley RR, Bandyopadhyay SK, Fazeli-Matin S, et al: Immunoregulatory potential of urothelium: Characterization of NF-kappaB signal transduction. J Urol 1999;162:1812–1816.

Raine AEG: Cardiovascular complications after renal transplantation. In Morris PJ (eds): Kidney Transplantation: Principles and Practice. Philadelphia, WB Saunders, 1994, pp 339–355.

Raya-Rivera A, Yoo J, Atala A: Hormone producing granulosa stem cells for intersex disorders. (Abstract 29.) American Academy of Pediatrics Meeting, Urology Section, Chicago, 2000.

Riehmann M, Gasser TC, Bruskewitz RC: The hydroflex penile prosthesis: A test case for the introduction of new urological technology. J Urol 1993;149:1304–1307.

Risau W: Mechanisms of angiogenesis. Nature 1997;386:671.

Rohrmann D, Albrecht D, Hannappel J, et al: Alloplastic replacement of the urinary bladder. J Urol 1996;156:2094.

Rowley JA, Madlambayan G, Mooney DJ: Alginate hydrogels as synthetic extracellular matrix materials. Biomaterials 1999;20:45–53.

Salle J, Fraga C, Lucib A, et al: Seromuscular enterocystoplasty in dogs. J Urol 1990;144:454.

Sam AE, Nixon AJ: Chondrocyte-laden collagen scaffolds for resurfacing extensive articular cartilage defects. Osteoarthritis Cartilage 1995;3:47–59.

Satar N, Yoo J, Atala A: Progressive bladder dilation for subsequent augmentation cystoplasty. J Urol 1999;162:829–831.

Schena FP: Role of growth factors in acute renal failure. Kidney Int 1998;53(Suppl. 66):S-11–S-15.

Scott R, Mohammed R, Gorham SD, et al: The evolution of a biodegradable membrane for use in urological surgery. Br J Urol 1988;62:26–31.

Scriven SD, Booth C, Thomas DF, et al: Reconstitution of human urothelium from monolayer cultures. J Urol 1997;158:1147–1152.

Shalhav AL, Elbahnasy AM, Bercowsky E, et al: Laparoscopic replacement of urinary tract segments using biodegradable materials in a large-animal model. J Endourol 1999;13:241–244.

Sievert KD, Bakircioglu ME, Nunes L, et al: Homologous acellular matrix graft for urethral reconstruction in the rabbit: Histological and functional evaluation. J Urol 2000;163:1958–1965.

Silver FH, Pins G: Cell growth on collagen: A review of tissue engineering using scaffolds containing extracellular matrix. J Long-term Effects Med Implants 1992;2:67–80.

Small MP, Carrion HM, Gordon JA: Small-Carrion penile prosthesis: New implant for management of impotence. Urology 1975;5:479.

Smidsrød O, Skjåk-Bræk G: Alginate as an immobilization matrix for cells. Trends Biotechnol 1990;8:71–78.

Snow BW, Cartwright P: Why bladder autoaugmentation is a good choice for detrusor instability or bladder hyperreflexia. Contemp Urol 1999;11:96–100.

Soker S, Fidder H, Neufeld G, Klagsbrun M: Characterization of novel vascular endothelial growth factor (VEGF) receptors on tumor cells that bind VEGF165 via its exon 7-encoded domain. Biol Chem 1996;271:5761.

Solomon LZ, Jennings AM, Sharpe P, et al: Effects of short-chain fatty acids on primary urothelial cells in culture: Implications for intravesical use in enterocystoplasties. J Lab Clin Med 1998;132:279–283.

Sutherland RS, Baskin LS, Hayward SW, Cunha GR: Regeneration of bladder urothelium, smooth muscle, blood vessels, and nerves into an acellular tissue matrix. J Urol 1996;156:571–577.

Tachibana M, Nagamatsu GR, Addonizio JC: Ureteral replacement using collagen sponge tube grafts. J Urol 1985;133:866–869.

Takeshita S, Tsurumi Y, Couffinahl T, et al: Gene transfer of naked DNA encoding for three isoforms of vascular endothelial growth factor stimulates collateral development in vivo. Lab Invest 1996;75:487.

Taub PJ, Marmur JD, Zhang WX, et al: Locally administered vascular endothelial growth factor cDNA increases survival of ischemic experimental skin flaps. Plast Reconstr Surg 1998;102:2033.

Thomalla JV, Thompson ST, Rowland RG, Mulcahy JJ: Infectious complications of penile prosthetic implants. J Urol 1987;138:65–67.

Tobin MS, Freeman MR, Atala A: Maturational response of normal human urothelial cells in culture is dependent on extracellular matrix and serum additives. Surg Forum 1994;45:786.

Tsuji I, Ishida H, Fujieda J: Experimental cystoplasty using preserved bladder graft. J Urol 1961;85:42.

United Network for Organ Sharing. People Awaiting Transplants. Richmond, VA, United Network for Organ Sharing, 1996.

Vaught JD, Kroop BP, Sawyer BD, et al: Detrusor regeneration in the rat using porcine small intestine submucosal grafts: Functional innervation and receptor expression. J Urol 1996;155:374–378.

Wilson JM, Birinyi LK, Salomon RN, et al: Implantation of vascular grafts lined with genetically modified endothelial cells. Science 1989; 244:1344–1346.

Wolter JR, Meyer RF: Sessile macrophages forming clear endothelium-like membrane of successful keratoprosthesis. Trans Am Ophthalmol Soc 1985;82:187–202.

Woods JD, Humes DH: Prospects for a bioartificial kidney. Semin Nephrol 1997;17:381–386.

Yannas IV, Burke JF: Design of an artificial skin: I. Basic design principles. J Biomed Mater Res 1980;14:65–81.

Yokoyama T, Chancellor MB, Watanabe T, et al: Primary myoblasts injection into the urethra and bladder as a potential treatment of stress urinary incontinence and impaired detrusor contractility: Long term survival without significant cytotoxicity. J Urol 1999;161:307.

Yoo JJ, Ashkar, Atala A: Creation of functional kidney structures with excretion of urine-like fluid in vivo. Pediatrics 1996;98(Suppl):605.

Yoo JJ, Atala A: A novel gene delivery system using urothelial tissue engineered neo-organs. J Urol 1997;158:1066–1070.

Yoo JJ, Lee I, Atala A: Cartilage rods as a potential material for penile reconstruction. J Urol 1998a;160:1164.

Yoo J, Park HJ, Lee I, Atala A: Autologous engineered cartilage rods for penile reconstruction. J Urol 1999;162:1119–1121.

Yoo JJ, Meng J, Oberpenning F, Atala A: Bladder augmentation using allogenic bladder submucosa seeded with cells. Urology 1998b;51:221.

Yoo JJ, Satar N, Retik AB, Atala A: Ureteral replacement using biodegradable polymer scaffolds seeded with urothelial and smooth muscle cells. J Urol 1995;153(Suppl.):375A.

Zweibel JA, Freeman SM, Kantoff PW, et al: High-level recombinant gene expression in rabbit endothelial cells transduced by retroviral vectors. Science 1989;243: 220–222.

INDEX

Note: Page numbers followed by the letter f refer to figures; those followed by the letter t refer to tables.

Acetaminophen
  antipyretic therapy with, for children, 1820
  for interstitial cystitis, 654
Acetohydroxamic acid, for struvite calculi, 3263
Acetylcholine (ACh)
  in female sexual function, 1714
  in penile erection, 1599–1600
  in smooth muscle contraction, 838, 838t, 838f
  uropharmacology of, 967–968
N-Acetylglucosamine, in amniotic fluid, prognostic significance of, 1767
N-Acetylglucosaminidase, urinary level of, 2001
Acid(s), renal excretion of. See Acid-base balance.
Acid metabolism, 3241–3242, 3242f
Acid-base balance, 210–220
  adrenergic effects in, 213
  aldosterone in, 213
  ammonium excretion in, 212
  angiotensin II in, 213
  atrial natriuretic peptide in, 213
  bicarbonate buffer system in, 210–211
  cellular buffering in, 211, 211f, 213
  chloride concentration in, 212–213
  disorders of, 214–220, 214t. See also Acidosis; Alkalosis.
    acid-base values in, 48–49, 49f, 214t
  factors affecting, 212–213
  HCO$_3^-$ reabsorption in, 211–212
  in neonates, 1767
  luminal HCO$_3^-$ concentration in, 212
  net acid excretion in, 212
  parathyroid hormone in, 213
  peritubular HCO$_3^-$, PCO$_2$, and pH in, 213
  potassium concentration in, 212–213
  potassium excretion and, 190
  renal acid excretion in, 211–213
  renal base excretion in, 213–214
  respiratory compensation in, 211, 213
  titratable acid excretion in, 212
  with pneumoperitoneum, 3475–3476
Acidosis
  defined, 214
  following augmentation cystoplasty, 2534
  metabolic, 215–218. See also Metabolic acidosis.
  respiratory, 219
    compensatory responses to, 214t
Acoustic-electric conversion, in transrectal ultrasound, 3039
Acquired immunity, 308, 339. See also Immunity.
Acquired immunodeficiency syndrome (AIDS), 693–712. See also Human immunodeficiency virus (HIV).
  acute renal failure in, 276
  aspergillosis in, 706, 806
  blastomycosis in, 811
  candidal infection in, 799
  case definition of, 697, 700, 701t
  cell-mediated immunity in, 697–698
    deficient, 701–702
  coccidioidomycosis in, 812
  cryptococcosis in, 808–809
  cytomegalovirus in, 706, 709–710
  epidemiology of, 703–705
  epididymal infections in, 707
  Fournier's gangrene in, 709
  genitourinary tract involvement in, 706–710
  histoplasmosis in, 814, 815
  invasive cervical carcinoma in, 708
  Kaposi's sarcoma in, 703, 707–708
  lymphadenopathy in, 707

Acquired immunodeficiency syndrome (AIDS) (Continued)
  non-Hodgkin's lymphoma in, 708
  opportunistic infections in, 700–701, 701t
  penile infections in, 706, 706f
  phycomycosis in, 810
  Pneumocystis carinii infection in, 702, 703
  prostatic infections in, 706–707
  renal disease in, 708–709
  schistosomiasis in, 765
  testicular cancer in, 708
  testicular infections in, 707
  toxoplasmosis in, 706
  treatment of
    antiretroviral therapy in, 699–700, 699t
      combination, 700
    currently approved drugs in, 699t
    non-nucleoside reverse transcriptase inhibitors in, 699f, 700
    nucleoside reverse transcriptase inhibitors in, 699–700, 699f
  tuberculosis in, 745
  urethral infections in, 706
  urinalysis in, 710
  urolithiasis in, 709
  urologic malignancies in, 707
  voiding dysfunction in, 709, 943
Acquired renal cystic disease (ARCD), 1976–1982
  and renal cell carcinoma, 1977–1978
  clinical features of, 1978–1979
  computed tomography in, 1976, 1976f, 1978f, 1981
  cysts in, 1937
  differential diagnosis of, 1985, 1985t
  etiology of, 1978
  evaluation of, 1978f, 1980–1981
  histopathology of, 1978f, 1979–1980
  in children, 1977
  incidence of, 1940t, 1976
  magnetic resonance imaging of, 1981
  renal findings in, 1940t
  treatment of, 1979f, 1981–1982
Acrochordons (skin tags), 727
Acrodysostosis, cryptorchidism associated with, 2366t
Acrosome reaction, evaluation of, 1496
ACTH (adrenocorticotropic hormone), secretion of, 1438
Actin, 1243
  of smooth muscle, 378, 382
Actinomycetes
  biology of, 817
  infection with, 817
Action potential, of ureteral smooth muscle, 379–380, 379f
  plateau of, 380, 380f
Activin(s), and FSH secretion, 1438
Activity, restricted, incontinence caused by, in elderly, 1221
Activity product ratio, 3234
Acucise device, for ureteropelvic junction repair, 2003, 2004f
AcuClip, 3468
Acupuncture
  for interstitial cystitis, 657
  for voiding dysfunction, 984
Acute disseminated encephalomyelitis, voiding dysfunction in, 943–944
Acute intermittent porphyria, in children, signs and symptoms of, 1816t
Acute renal failure. See Renal failure, acute.

Acute tubular necrosis (ATN)
  etiology of, 276, 277t, 278t
  in acute renal failure, 276–277
  incidence of, 276
  ischemic-reperfusion injury in, 277–280, 279f–280f
  natural history of, 276–277
  pathophysiology of, 277, 278f
  prevention of, 286
  prognosis of, 286, 286f
Acute tubulointerstitial nephritis, in children
  drug-related, 1843
  immune-mediated, 1843
  infection-related, 1843–1844
Acyclovir, for genital herpes, 682, 682t
  prophylactic, 683
Addison's disease, 3529–3531, 3531f, 3531t, 3532t
  with histoplasmosis, 814
A-delta fibers, in bladder, 847, 847t, 980
Adenine phosphoribosyltransferase deficiency, dihydroxyadenine stones due to, 3265–3266
Adenocarcinoma(s)
  of bladder
    metastatic, 2747
    primary, 2747
  of prostate. See Prostate cancer, adenocarcinoma as.
  of renal pelvis and ureters, 2768
  of rete testis, 2909
  of seminal vesicles, 3877
  with conduit urinary diversion, 3782–3783
Adenofibroma(s), metanephric, 2494
Adenohypophysis, 1438, 1438f
Adenoid cystic carcinoma, of prostate, ultrasound appearance of, 3047–3048
Adenoma(s)
  adrenal
    benign, 3526–3527, 3527f
    Cushing's syndrome due to, 3523
  aldosterone-producing, 3533–3534, 3536
  nephrogenic, in bladder cancer, 2742
  papillary, of seminal vesicles, 3876–3877
  renal
    cortical, 2679–2680, 2679f
    metanephric, 2680, 2680f
Adenomatoid tumor(s), testicular, 2909, 2911–2912
Adenosine A1 agonists, uropharmacology of, 869
Adenosine monophosphate, cyclic (cAMP), in ureteral peristalsis, 384, 384f
Adenosine triphosphatase (ATPase) activity, in ureteral peristalsis, 382, 3834f
Adenosine triphosphate (ATP)
  and purinergic nerves, 858–859
  depletion of, in renal ischemia, 277–278
  in smooth muscle contraction, 838, 838t, 838f
Adenosquamous carcinoma, surface, penile, 2974
Adenoviruses, as gene therapy vectors, 2660
Adhesins
  bacterial, in urinary tract infection, 524, 524f
  E. coli, in preterm births, 581
  X, 525
Adhesion(s)
  homophilic, in T cell-endothelial cell interactions, 331
  in renal cell carcinoma, 2691
  labial, in children, 1825
    management of, 1830
  preputial-glanular, in children, 1823
    management of, 1829–1830

Aminopenicillins, for urinary tract infection, 539t, 540t, 541

Aminophylline, pretreatment with, for shock-wave lithotripsy, 3411

Aminosalicylic acid, in tuberculosis treatment
  adverse effects and side effects of, 757t
  dosage and administration of, 757t

Amitriptyline
  contraindications to, in elderly, 1228–1229
  for interstitial cystitis, 653
  incontinence caused by, in elderly, 1221t
  uropharmacology of, 858t, 866

Ammonia, renal excretion of, 212

Ammonium acid urate calculi, 3266

Amniotic fluid, volume of, 1781, 1784–1785. *See also* Oligohydramnios.

Amoxicillin
  adverse reactions, precautions, and contraindications to, 540t
  for pediatric urinary tract infection
    oral dosage and administration of, 1865t
    prophylactic, 1866t
  for urinary tract infection, 539t, 541
    during pregnancy, 584t

Amoxicillin-clavulanate (Augmentin), for pediatric urinary tract infection, oral dosage and administration of, 1865t

AMPA antagonists, uropharmacology of, 866, 868f, 869

Amphotericin B
  adverse effects and side effects of, 805, 817–818, 820f
  cost of, 818, 818t
  dosage and administration of, 821t
  for aspergillosis, 807, 821t
    in kidney, 806, 821t
    in prostate, 806, 821t
  for blastomycosis, 811–812, 821t
  for candidiasis, 821t
    in children, 802
    in prostate, 800
    in upper urinary tract, 800–801
    intravenous, 804
    irrigant, 803
    liposomal, 804
    with epididymo-orchitis, 799
    with invasive or disseminated infection, 804–805
  for coccidioidomycosis, 812–813, 821t
  for cryptococcosis, 808, 809, 821t
  for histoplasmosis, 814–815, 821t
  for mucormycosis, 810, 821t
  for *Torulopsis glabrata* infection, 805–806
  fungal resistance to, 801, 818
  liposomal, 818
  pharmacology of, 817

Ampicillin
  acute tubulointerstitial nephritis caused by, 1843
  adverse reactions, precautions, and contraindications to, 540t
  effect of, on ureteral function, 403
  for actinomycosis, 817
  for pediatric urinary tract infection
    bacterial resistance to, 1865
    oral dosage and administration of, 1865t
    parenteral dosage and administration of, 1864t
  for urinary tract infection, 539t, 541
    during pregnancy, 584t
  prophylactic, for percutaneous nephrolithotomy, 3416
  serum and urinary levels of, 537t

Amplatz dilator set, metal, 3332–3333, 3332f, 3333f

Amplification, definition of, 2626t

Ampulla(e), 1238
  embryology of, 1238
  of ureteric bud, 1740–1741, 1742, 1742f, 1744f

Amputation, of penis, 3912, 3913f
  during circumcision, 3905

Amyl nitrite, for prevention of erection, in postoperative period after penile surgery, 2303

Amyloid, of seminal vesicles, 3877

Amyloidosis, 944
  nephrogenic diabetes insipidus caused by, 1844

Anaerobes, in urinary tract, 523

Anal folds, 1757

Anal incontinence
  definition of, 1093–1094
  epidemiology of, 1093–1094
  in exstrophy patient, 2142
  with pelvic organ prolapse, 1109

Anal reflex, 904

Anal sphincter, 1099f, 1100f
  components of, 70
  defects of, in exstrophy patient, 2142
  disruption of, obstetric causes of, 1036–1037
  tone, assessment of, 1038, 1111

Anal triangle, 70
  blood supply to, 71, 72f

Anal wink, in elderly, 1225

Analgesia, vanilloid-induced, mechanisms of, 865

Analgesics
  as bladder cancer risk factor, 2739, 2766–2767
  effect of, on ureteral function, 402
  for interstitial cystitis, 654
  nephrogenic diabetes insipidus caused by, 1844

Anaphylactoid reactions, to contrast media, 125

Anaphylotoxin(s), C3 and C5 as, 308

Anastomosis
  bladder neck closure and, in retropubic radical prostatectomy, 3124–3126, 3125f, 3126f
  Bricker, 3765–3766, 3766f
  end-to-end, microsurgical vasoepididymostomy with, 1558t, 1562–1563, 1563f
  hammock, 3768
  ileocolic
    end-to-end, 3754–3755, 3754f
    end-to-side, 3753–3754, 3754f
  intestinal, 3751–3762. *See also* Intestinal anastomosis.
  single-layer suture, enteroenterostomy with, 3753, 3753f
  stricture formation at, following radical prostatectomy, 3088
  two-layer suture, enteroenterostomy with, 3752–3753, 3753f
  ureterocolonic, 3763–3765. *See also* Ureterocolonic anastosmosis.
  ureteroenteric, stricture formation at, 502–505
  ureterointestinal, 3762–3770. *See also* Ureterointestinal anastomosis.
  vascular
    in renal transplantation, 358–359, 360f
    in testis, 77, 77f

Anderson-Hynes pyeloplasty, for ureteropelvic junction repair, 2001, 2002–2003

Androblastoma(s), testicular, 2906–2907

Androgen(s). *See also* Antiandrogen(s); Dihydrotestosterone; Testosterone(s).
  abnormalities of, male infertility with, 1503–1504

Androgen(s) *(Continued)*
  action of, nuclear matrix and, 1261–1262
  adrenal
    effects of, on prostate, 1248
    production of, 1247f, 1248
  age-related changes in, in females, 1715
  and female sexual function, 1714, 1715, 1726–1727
  and hypospadias development, 2287–2288
  and voiding function, 874
  as prostate cancer risk factor, 3007
  central nervous system actions of, 1714–1715
    localization of, 1715
    mechanism of, 1715
  effects of
    in postmenopausal women, 1715
    on epididymis, 1463–1464
    on prostate, 1245, 1245f, 1298–1300, 1299f
      at cellular level, 1250–1252
      estrogen synergism with, 1253–1254, 1367
  excess, in males, 1502
  for micropenis, 2342
  in male gonadal development, 1755–1756, 1757, 2207
  in testicular descent, 2359–2360
  maternal administration of, congenital adrenal hyperplasia due to, 2415
  metabolism of, in prostate, 1252f, 1252–1253
  ovarian, in puberty, 1716
  physiology of, in females, 1714–1715
  preparations of, 1650t
    oral, 1650
    parenteral, 1650
    transdermal, 1650
  prostate cancer resistant to, chemotherapy for. *See* Chemotherapy, for prostate cancer.
  replacement therapy with
    before hypospadias repair, 2294
    for male infertility, 1512
    in erectile dysfunction, 1649–1651
    in women, 1714, 1715
      dosage and administration of, 1727–1728
  sources of, 3183, 3183f
  stimulation with, before hypospadias repair, 2294
  supplementation of, before hypospadias repair, 2294
  testicular, production of, 1246f, 1246–1248, 1247f, 1247t
  therapy with, in hypogonadotropic hypogonadism, 1501
  weak, 1248
  withdrawal of, mechanisms of, 3184

Androgen ablation, neoadjuvant, with radical prostatectomy, 3095–3097, 3098t

Androgen insensitivity, 1503–1504
  complete, 2417–2418

Androgen receptor(s), 1254f, 1254–1255
  abnormalities of, 1439, 1478
    male infertility with, 1503–1504
  activation of, ligand-dependent, 1256f, 1257
  and chromatin remodeling, 1258f, 1259–1261
  and histone acetylation or deacetylation, 1258f, 1260–1261
  and transcriptional regulation, 1258f, 1260–1261
  as prostate cancer risk factor, 3008
  chaparonin binding by, 1255–1256, 1256f
  coactivators of, 1258–1259, 1259f, 1260
  dimerization of, 1256f, 1257
  DNA-binding domain of, 1256–1257

C fibers
  capsaicin and, 978–979
  in bladder instability, after spinal cord injury, 870–871, 871f
  in lower urinary tract, 847t, 847–848, 861–862
C3. *See* Complement component C3 (C3).
C4. *See* Complement component C4 (C4).
C5. *See* Complement component C5 (C5).
Cachexia, erectile dysfunction caused by, 1610
Cactus flower. *See Opuntia*.
Cadaver donor(s), for renal transplantation, 352, 354
  biopsy grading system in, 352, 354t
  goals of resuscitation in, 354
  recipient selection for, 357, 357t
  total midline incision with sternotomy in, 354, 355f–356f
  vs. living donor, 346
Cadherins, 1263, 1264–1265
Cadmium, toxicity of, renal involvement in, 1844
Café-au-lait spots, 1822
Caffeine
  effect of, on spermatogenesis, 1477, 1510
  intake of, and detrusor instability, 1087
CAKUT. *See* Congenital anomalies of the kidney and urinary tract (CAKUT) phenotype.
Calcification(s)
  bladder, in schistosomiasis, 768, 768f, 770, 771f, 772f
  renal, in tuberculosis, 747–748, 748f, 749f
  scrotal, in filariasis, 782–783, 783f
Calcineurin inhibitor toxicity, 365, 368t
  vs. acute kidney graft rejection, 369t
Calcitonin gene-related peptide(s)
  and alprostadil, combined, for erectile dysfunction, 1659
  effect of, on ureteral function, 390
  in lower urinary tract, 861, 862
  in testicular descent, 2361–2362
  intracavernous injection of, 1658
Calcium. *See also* Hypercalcemia; Hypercalciuria.
  dietary
    as prostate cancer risk factor, 3010
    urinary lithiasis related to, 3279, 3279f
  in action potential, 379–380
  in excitation-contraction coupling, 383, 973–974
  in smooth muscle cells, 378, 838, 838t, 838f, 974
  in ureteral peristalsis, 382–383, 382f–383f
  intracellular, activation of, 319
  metabolism of, 3239–3240, 3239f
  renal excretion of, 191–192, 194–195
    in neonate, 1767–1768, 1771
  renal reabsorption of
    calcium-sensing receptors in, 195, 196f
    collecting tubule in, 192
    distal tubule in, 192
    diuretics in, 181, 195
    extracellular fluid volume in, 195
    loop of Henle in, 192
    mechanisms of, 192, 194
    parathyroid hormone in, 194–195, 194f
    proximal tubule in, 192
    vitamin D in, 195
  urinary excretion of, in children, 1837
    normal value for, 1837
    quantitative measurement of, 1837
Calcium antagonists
  effect of, on ureteral function, 403
  for neuromuscular voiding dysfunction, 973–974

Calcium channel(s)
  in male sexual function, 1601, 1602f, 1603f
  in smooth muscle, 837–838, 857–858
Calcium channel blockers
  adverse effects and side effects of, 974
  effect of
    on spermatogenesis, 1477, 1510
    on ureteral function, 403
  for acute renal failure, 284
  for neuromuscular voiding dysfunction, 973–974
  for ureteral obstruction, 433
  for urge incontinence, in elderly, 1229t
  incontinence caused by, in elderly, 1221, 1221t
  uropharmacology of, 858t, 865–866, 974
Calcium hydroxyapatite, as agent for injection therapy, 1183
Calcium load test, in idiopathic hypercalciuria, 3245–3246, 3245t
Calcium oxalate crystals
  in urinary sediment, 109, 109f
  inhibitors of, 3237–3238
Calcium phosphate calculi, renal tubular acidosis and, 3254–3257, 3255f–3257f, 3257t
Calcium transport
  factors regulating, 194–195, 194f, 194t, 196f
  mechanisms of, 192, 194
  sites of, 191–192, 194f
Calcium/creatinine ratio, urinary
  in child, 1771
  in neonate, 1771
Calcium-sensing receptors, in renal reabsorption, 195, 196f
Calculus(i)
  and urethral diverticula, 1208
  bladder, 3384–3386
    after renal transplantation, 369
    following augmentation cystoplasty, 2536
    in children, endemic, 3291–3292
  cultured, in urinary tract infection, 535, 535f
  in children
    computed tomography of, 1820
    with ectopic ureter, 2016
    with ureterocele, 2023, 2034
  prostatic, 605, 607–608
  renal. *See* Urinary lithiasis, renal.
  ureteral. *See* Urinary lithiasis, ureteral.
  video-urodynamics with, 925
Calmodulin, in smooth muscle contraction, 838, 838t, 838f
Calymmatobacterium granulomatis, in granuloma inguinale, 681t, 684
Calyx (calyces). *See* Renal calyx (calyces).
Camera system, for laparoscopy, 3465
Camey II orthotopic substitute, 3851–3852, 3852f
cAMP (cyclic adenosine monophosphate)
  in male sexual function, 1601
  in ureteral peristalsis, 384, 384f
Camper's fascia, 42–43, 43f
Cancer. *See also* at anatomic site, e.g., Prostate cancer; Malignancy; *specific neoplasm, e.g.,* Lymphoma.
  adhesion molecules and, 2650–2651
  after renal transplantation, 372
    risk of recurrence of, 349, 349t
  and female sexual dysfunction, 1718–1719, 1720
  angiogenesis in, 2653–2656
  apoptosis and, 2645
  cell surface and, 2649–2650
  dysregulation and
    hypermethylation and, 2631–2632

Cancer *(Continued)*
    mutation and, 2630–2631
    oncogenes in, 2631
    tumor suppressor genes and, 2631
  gene therapy for, 2660
  growth regulators in, 2646–2649
  hypercalcemia associated with, 3247–3248
  inherited susceptibility to, 2632–2636, 2632t, 2633t
    in genitourinary syndromes, 2633–2635
    polymorphisms and, 2635–2636
    sporadic and hereditary malignancies and, 2632–2633, 2633f, 2634f
  metastatic. *See* Metastasis(es).
  molecular diagnosis of, 2657–2659
    immunohistochemistry in, 2658
    microarray technology in, 2658–2659
    molecular genetics in, 2658
    proteomics in, 2659
  mouse models of, 2656–2657
    genetic engineering and, 2656–2657
    knockout mice as, 2657
    mutagenesis and, 2656
    oncogene-induced tumorigenesis and, 2657
  telomerase and, 2646, 2647f
Cancer therapy. *See also* Brachytherapy; Chemotherapy; Radiation therapy; *specific surgical procedures.*
  target(s) for
    death receptors as, 2644
    ligands as, 2644
Cancer vaccines, 337
Candida
  culture of
    from blood, 802
    from urine, 802
  cystitis caused by, after renal transplantation, 370
  drug resistance in, 801, 819, 821
  identification of, polymerase chain reaction (PCR) for, 802
  in acquired immunodeficiency syndrome, 700
  in blood, 797–798, 801
    bacterial infection and, 801
    in children, 801
    in surgical patients, 801
    laboratory identification of, 802
  in prostatitis, 606–607
  in urine, 797–798, 802, 802f. *See also* Candiduria.
Candida cystitis, after renal transplantation, 370
Candida glabrata. See Torulopsis glabrata.
Candida infection, 797–805
  and obstructive uropathy, 800, 801
    treatment of, 805
  bezoars in
    imaging of, 802–803, 803f
    in bladder, 799, 799f
    in children, 1874
    treatment of, 805
  catheter removal in, 803
  diagnostic studies in, 802–803
  disseminated, treatment of, 804–805
  emphysematous cellulitis in, 799
  emphysematous cystitis in, 799
  epidemiology of, 797–798
  epididymitis caused by, 799
  hematogenous, 801
  historical perspective on, 797
  host factors in, management of, 803
  imaging in, 802–803
  in bladder, 799–800

Candida infection *(Continued)*
  in children, 801–802, 1874
  in collecting system, 800–801
  in kidney, 800–801
    in children, 801–802
  in men, 799
  in prostate, 799–800, 800f
  in renal transplant recipients, 797, 801
  in ureter, 800–801
  invasive, treatment of, 804–805
  local, systemic treatment for, 803–804
  microbiology of, 797–798
  of glans penis, 735f
  perinephric abscess caused by, 800–801
  predisposing factors for, 797–798
  radiographic findings in, 802–803
  renal findings in, 1963f
  serologic studies in, 802
  signs and symptoms of, 798
  sites of involvement in, 798
  superficial, 798, 798f
    diagnosis of, 798
    treatment of, 798
  systemic, 801
    treatment of, 804–805
  treatment of, 803–805, 804f, 821t
    antifungal irrigants for, 803
    endoscopic, 805
    percutaneous, 805
    surgical, 805
  urinalysis in, 802, 802f
  vulvovaginitis caused by, 798–799
Candida intertrigo, of male genitalia, 725–725,
    735f
Candiduria
  epidemiology of, 797–798
  in children, 1874
  in local vs. systemic infection, 802
  laboratory identification of, 802, 802f
  persistent, and disseminated infection, 798
  predisposing factors for, 798
  risk for systemic candidiasis with, 801
  signs and symptoms of, 798
Cantwell-Ransley procedure, modified
  for exstrophy patient, 2160–2162, 2161f–
    2162f, 2169, 2170
  in epispadias patient, 2183–2184
Capacitive coupling, 3484, 3485
Capastat. *See* Capreomycin.
CAPB, prostate cancer and, 3012
Capillary(ies)
  intertubular, 1443
  peritubular, 1443
    in renal hemodynamics, 176–177, 177f
Capillary hemangioma, of male genitalia, 728
Capreomycin
  adverse effects and side effects of, 757t
  dosage and administration of, 757t
  mechanism of action of, 755t
  mutational resistance to, site of, 755t
Capsaicin
  excitation effects of, 865, 979
  for voiding dysfunction, 979
  intravesical therapy with, 979–980
    rationale for, 848, 978–979
  pharmacologic actions of, at receptor level,
    865
  uropharmacology of, 858t, 861, 864–865,
    978–979
Capsaicin lavage, for interstitial cystitis, 656
Capsaicin-sensitive sensory nerves, of ureter,
  390
Capsular artery, 65, 65f

Capsure (urethral meatal device), for stress in-
    continence, 1078
Captopril, incontinence caused by, in elderly,
    1221t
Captopril test, in renovascular hypertension, 243
Captopril-enhanced renography, in renovascular
    hypertension, 244
Carbenicillin, serum and urinary levels of, 537t
Carbon dioxide, for pneumoperitoneum, in lapa-
    roscopic surgery, 3473–3474
  in children, 2577
Carbonic anhydrase-9, in renal cell carcinoma,
    2689
Carboplatin, for prostate cancer, 3214t
Carcinoembryonic antigen (CEA), T cell recog-
    nition of, 334
Carcinoid(s), testicular, 2909
Carcinoma in situ
  of bladder, 2742–2743, 2743f
    chemotherapy for, 2790
  of testis, 2879–2880
    in children, 2496
Carcinosarcoma(s)
  of bladder, 2764
  of renal pelvis and ureters, 2768–2769
Cardiac arrest, anesthesia-related, with laparo-
    scopic surgery, 3490
Cardiac arrhythmia(s). *See* Arrhythmia(s).
Cardiac function, compromised, after renal re-
    vascularization, 250–252
Cardinal ligament(s), 48, 51f, 70, 1101–1102,
    1103f
Cardinal vein(s), 2044–2045, 2045f
Cardiomyopathy, catecholamine-induced, as
    pheochromocytoma mimic, 3541–3542
Cardiopulmonary disease
  erectile dysfunction caused by, 1610
  with radical cystectomy, 2807
Cardiorespiratory function, preoperative evalua-
    tion of, before kidney surgery, 3573
Cardura. *See* Doxazosin.
L-Carnitine, and male fertility, 1512
Carpenter syndrome
  cryptorchidism associated with, 2366t
  multisystem involvement in, 1814t
Cascade phenomenon, in complement, 308
Casodex. *See* Bicalutamide.
Caspases, in regulation of apoptosis, 325–326,
    326f
Castration
  and cell death in prostate, 1274–1276
  chemical, 1245
  medical, for prostate cancer, 3191, 3193–
    3195
  surgical, for prostate cancer, 3190–3191,
    3191t, 3192f
Casts, in urinary sediment, 109, Color Plates I–
    10 to I–12
Catalase, urinary, test for, in pediatric infection,
    1848
Catecholamines
  actions of, 3515, 3516f
  in interstitial cystitis, 642
  metabolism of, 3515, 3516f
  with pheochromocytomas, 3544, 3545t
Catenin(s), 1264
  in renal development, 1928, 1928f, 1929t
Catheter(s)
  condom, for elderly, 1229, 1230
  in cystometrography, 906–907
  in retrograde pyelography, 120, 120f, 128
  inadvertent removal of, during radical prosta-
    tectomy, perineal, 3144

Catheter(s) *(Continued)*
  indwelling, 995–997
    and aspergillosis, 806
    and bladder cancer, 997
    Candida infection with, 798
    complications of, 995–996
    urinary tract infection associated with, 549
      prophylactic antibiotics for, 550
  intraurethral (Nissenkorn), 1382
  prostatic bridge, 1382–1383
  suprapubic, 996
  ureteral
    in localizing site of bacteriuria, 532–533,
      533t
    in urinary tract infection, 548–550
  urethral. *See also* Urethral catheterization.
    and Valsalva leak point pressure measure-
      ment, 912
    for stress incontinence, 1078–1079
    indwelling
      care of, 1231t, 1232
      complications of, 1232
      for underactive detrusor, in elderly,
        1231–1232
      in elderly, 1229–1230, 1231–1232
      precautions with, 1232
      removal of, 1231t
    types of, 112–113, 112f
    urinary tract infection associated with, 548–
      550
      etiology of, 549
      prevention of, 549
      treatment of, 549–550
Catheterization
  after pelvic surgery, 955
  clean intermittent
    candidates for, 995
    complications of, 995
    equipment for, 995
    for urinary tract reconstruction, 2509, 2536
    in children, and risk of urinary tract infec-
      tion, 1863, 1865
    indications for, 995
    patient education about, 995
  continuous, 995–997
    complications of, 995–996
  in detrusor-sphincter dyssynergia, 958
  in sacral spinal cord injury, 948
  in spinal cord injury, 995–997
    and bladder cancer, 997
    in women, 951–952
  in suprasacral spinal cord injury, 947–948
  intermittent, in elderly, with underactive detru-
    sor, 1230–1231
  urethral. *See* Urethral catheterization.
Catheterizing pouches, continent, for continent
    urinary diversion, 3803–3807, 3804f
  care of, 3806–3807
  methodology for, 3805–3806
Cat's eye syndrome, genitourinary anomalies in,
    1815t
Cauda equina, definition of, 953
Cauda equina compression syndrome, priapism
    in, 1611
Cauda equina syndrome, 954
Caudal embryology, 2429–2430, 2429f
Caudal regression syndrome, 2430
  multisystem involvement in, 1814t
Cautery wire, 473f
Cautery wire balloon endopyelotomy, 473–476.
    See also Endopyelotomy.
  complications of, 476
  indications for and contraindications to, 473–
    474, 474f

Cautery wire balloon endopyelotomy
(Continued)
postoperative care in, 475
results of, 475–476
technique of, 474, 475f
wire in, 473f
Cautery wire balloon incision
in endoureterotomy, 493–494
in ureteroenteric stricture repair, 504
Caveolae, in smooth muscle cells, 378
Caveolin, 2651
Caverject. See Alprostadil, intracavernous.
Cavernosal artery, 73, 73f, 74f
of penis, 1593, 1594f
Cavernosal nerves, 56
Cavernosal vein, 74, 74f, 1594, 1594f
Cavernosography, 1646–1647, 1647f
Cavernosometry, 1646
Cavernotome, penile, 1687, 1688f
Cavernous arterial systolic occlusion pressure,
1642, 1647
Cavernous nerves, in exstrophy patient, 2143
Cavernous veno-occlusive dysfunction, 1647
Cavitation, stone comminution by, 3408–3409
CD (cluster of differentiation) markers, 309–
310, 311t
CD4⁺ T cells
activation and expansion of, 321, 322f
antigen-priming of, 322–323, 324f
in HIV infection, 697, 702
in interstitial cystitis, 645
in renal allograft rejection, 363
in tumor immunology, 332
CD4/CD8 T cells, maturation of, 311
CD8⁺ T cells
activation and expansion of, 321, 322f
antigen-priming of, 323
in cytolysis of target cells, 323, 324f, 325
in HIV infection, 702
in interstitial cystitis, 645
in tumor immunology, 332
cDNA. See Deoxyribonucleic acid (DNA), complementary.
CEA (carcinoembryonic antigen), T cell recognition of, 334
Cecocystoplasty, 2527
Cecoureterocele, 2009f
definition of, 2008
Cefaclor, for urinary tract infection
during pregnancy, 584t
in children, 1865t
Cefadroxil, for pediatric urinary tract infection,
1865t
Cefazolin, for pediatric urinary tract infection,
1864t
Cefixime
for classic urethritis, 673t
for pediatric urinary tract infection, 1865t
Cefotaxime, for pediatric urinary tract infection,
1864t
Cefoxitin
for bacteremia, 571t
for pelvic inflammatory disease, 424
Cefpodoxime, for pediatric urinary tract infection, 1865t
Cefprozil, for pediatric urinary tract infection,
1865t
Ceftazidime, for pediatric urinary tract infection,
1864t
Ceftriaxone
for chancroid, 684
for gonococcal urethritis, 673t, 674

Ceftriaxone (Continued)
for pediatric urinary tract infection, 1864t
for syphilis, 683
Celiac plexus, 12
Celiac trunk, 6, 14f
Cell(s). See also named cell, e.g., T cell(s).
aging of, 1274
immortality in, 1274
in urinary sediment, 108–109, Color Plates I–
1 to I–9
proliferation of
in urinary tract obstruction, 441–442
markers of, in bladder cancer, 2753
senescence of, 1274
shape of, and cell function, 1244
smooth muscle. See also Smooth muscle.
anatomy of, 377–378
Cell adhesion molecules, 1250, 1251f, 1263–1265
in bladder cancer, 2751–2752
in prostate, 1244f
Cell cycle, 1267, 1267f, 2636–2640, 2636f
apoptosis and, 2643
G₁S checkpoint in, 2637–2639
cip/kip function and, 2639
cyclin–cyclin-dependent kinases and, 2638
cyclin-dependent kinase inhibitors and,
2638
INK4 function and, 2638–2639
p53 in urologic malignancies and, 2637–2638
p53 regulation of, 2637, 2637f
retinoblastoma protein and, 2639
G₂M checkpoint in, 2640, 2640f
regulation of
in prostate growth, 1272–1273
in renal cell carcinoma, 2690–2691
p53 in, 2637, 2637f
S phase of, 2639
Cell death, 1267, 1267f
programmed. See Apoptosis (programmed cell
death).
Cell population(s), immunoresponsive, 309–313,
311t
antibodies in, 312–313, 313f
antigen-presenting cells in, 312
granulocytes in, 312
homing of, 309
lymphocytes in, 310–312. See also B cell(s);
Natural killer (NK) cells; T cell(s).
macrophages in, 312
monocytes in, 312
vascular endothelial cells in, 312
Cell surface, cancer and, 2649–2650
Cell surface activation, of immune response,
314–318
B cells in, 317–318
major histocompatibility complex in, 314–
315, 314f
presentation of antigen in, 315
recognition of alloantigens in, 316–317, 317t
T cell receptor in, 315, 316f
T cell signals in, 315–316, 317f
Cell transplantation, tissue engineering with, of
bladder, 2602–2605
bladder replacement and, 2604–2605, 2604f,
2605f
ex situ bladder tissue formation and, 2602–
2604, 2603f
Cell-cell interaction, inhibition of, for prostate
cancer, 3222
Cell-mediated immune response, 309
in acquired immunodeficiency syndrome,
697–698
deficient, 701–702

Cellular injury, in kidney transplant preservation,
354–355
Cellulitis
emphysematous, candidal, 799
of male genitalia, 725, 734f. See also Fournier's gangrene.
Centers for Disease Control and Prevention
classification of HIV infection by, 702–703,
702t
Division of Parasitic Diseases, 763
Central nervous system
damage to, and voiding dysfunction in children, 2252–2256
diffuse disease of, voiding dysfunction with,
942–944
female genital innervation by, 1711–1714
in female sexual response, 1713–1714
in schistosomiasis, 780
renin-angiotensin-aldosterone system and, 237
Central perineal tendon, 3898
Central tendon, of perineum, 70
Central venous pressure, readings of, unreliability of, with pneumoperitoneum, 3475
Centrax. See Prazepam.
Cephalexin
for pediatric urinary tract infection
oral dosage and administration of, 1865t
prophylactic, 1866, 1866t
for urinary tract infection, during pregnancy,
584t
prophylactic, for recurrent urinary tract infection, 577, 578t
serum and urinary levels of, 537t
Cephalosporins
acute tubulointerstitial nephritis caused by,
1843
adverse reactions, precautions, and contraindications to, 540t
Fanconi's syndrome caused by, 1844
for pediatric urinary tract infection
oral dosage and administration of, 1865t
parenteral dosage and administration of,
1864t
for urinary tract infection, 539t, 541
during pregnancy, 584t, 585
prophylactic, for percutaneous nephrolithotomy, 3416
c-erb-B2 oncogene, in bladder cancer, 2752
Cerebellar ataxia, voiding dysfunction with, 939
Cerebral palsy
diagnosis of, 2253
etiology of, 2252–2253
findings in, 2253, 2253f, 2253t, 2254t
perinatal risk factors in, 2253, 2254t
treatment recommendations in, 2253–2254
urodynamic evaluation in, 2253, 2253f, 2253t,
2254t
voiding dysfunction with, 933t, 939, 2252–
2254
Cerebro-hepato-renal syndrome, hypospadias
with, 2292t
Cerebro-oculo-facial syndrome, multisystem involvement in, 1814t
Cerebrovascular accident
after renal revascularization, 250
after renal transplantation, 373
and uninhibited neurogenic bladder, 895
brain stem, voiding dysfunction after, 938
erectile dysfunction after, neurophysiology of,
1598
incidence of, 936
incontinence after, 937
postprostatectomy, 1433

Child(ren) *(Continued)*
  voiding dysfunction in
    evaluation of, 1821
    in myelodysplasia, 2234–2245
      with CNS lesions, 2252–2256
      worrisome signs and symptoms in, 2280, 2280t
    voiding pressure in, evaluation of, 2233
  Wilms' tumor in. *See* Wilms' tumor.
  xanthogranulomatous pyelonephritis in, 1857
Child abuse
  evaluation for, 1812, 1817
  genital trauma in, 1824
Childbirth, and pelvic floor dysfunction, 1094
Chills, in patient history, 90
Chinese herb nephropathy, as bladder cancer risk factor, 2767
Chlamydia, in urinary tract infection, 523
Chlamydia infection, vs. cystitis, 574
Chlamydia pneumoniae, in interstitial cystitis, 638
Chlamydia trachomatis
  in lymphogranuloma venereum, 681t, 684
  in nongonococcal urethritis, 673t, 675, 676, 677
  in pelvic inflammatory disease, 424, 675
  in prostatitis, 606
  in urinary schistosomiasis, 769
Chloramphenicol, for bacteremia, 571t
Chlordiazepoxide, 1009
Chloride
  absorption of, following augmentation cystoplasty, 2534
  urinary, in fetus, 1767
m-Chlorophenylpiperazine (mCPP), uropharmacology of, 868
Chlorothiazide, for hyperkalemia, in renal tubular acidosis, in children, 1771
Chlorpromazine, priapism caused by, 1612
Chlorthalidone, for urinary lithiasis, 3281, 3282t
Choledochal cyst, in children, 1816t
Cholelithiasis, in children, 1816t
Cholesterol, in seminal plasma, 1278
Cholesterol embolism, of renal artery, 240
Cholesterol side chain cleavage deficiency, 2415–2416
Cholinergic agonists, effect of, on ureteral function, 388
Cholinergic receptors
  in pontine micturition center, 869
  muscarinic, 857–858
    drug selectivity for, 858, 858t
    in bladder exstrophy, 2143
  supraspinal, and micturition reflex, 869
Cholinomimetic agents
  adverse effects and side effects of, 1001
  contraindications to, 1001
  uropharmacology of, 1000
Chondrocytes, injectable, for vesicoureteral reflux and incontinence, 2614–2615, 2615f
Chondroitin, of prostate, 1244
Chondrosarcoma, of bladder, 2765
Chordee, 1823. *See also* Penile curvature.
  correction of, 3909–3910, 3910f
  definition of, 2284
  etiology of, 2289
  in epispadias patient, 2181
  in prune-belly syndrome, 2120
  release of
    in epispadias patient, 2183
    in exstrophy patient, 2159, 2169, 2170
  without hypospadias, 2289–2290, 3943–3945, 3944f
    class I, 2289–2290

Chordee *(Continued)*
  class II, 2290
  class III, 2290
  etiology of, 2290
Choriocarcinoma, of bladder, 2765
Chromatin, remodeling of, androgen receptor and, 1258f, 1259–1261
Chromosomal abnormality(ies)
  associated with genitourinary anomalies, 1815t
  hypospadias with, 2292t
  in bladder cancer, 2752–2753
  in male infertility, 1497–1500
  in neuroblastoma, 2469–2470
  in Wilms' tumor, 2482–2483, 2487–2488
  with cryptorchidism, 2290
  with hypospadias, 2290
Chromosomal sex, 2395–2399, 2396f
Chromosome(s)
  definition of, 2626t
  translocations of, and male infertility, 1506
Chromosome 1p, in Wilms' tumor, 2483
Chromosome 3q duplication, cryptorchidism associated with, 2366t
Chromosome 4p deletion, cryptorchidism associated with, 2366t
Chromosome 4p duplication, cryptorchidism associated with, 2366t
Chromosome 5p deletion, cryptorchidism associated with, 2366t
Chromosome 7p, in Wilms' tumor, 2483
Chromosome 8p, heterozygosity at, loss of, prostate cancer and, 3013
Chromosome 9p deletion, cryptorchidism associated with, 2366t
Chromosome 9 deletion, in bladder cancer, 2752–2753
Chromosome 10q duplication, cryptorchidism associated with, 2366t
Chromosome 11p deletion, cryptorchidism associated with, 2366t
Chromosome 13p deletion, cryptorchidism associated with, 2366t
Chromosome 13q deletion, in bladder cancer, 2753
Chromosome 15q duplication, cryptorchidism associated with, 2366t
Chromosome 16q, in Wilms' tumor, 2483
Chromosome 18p deletion, cryptorchidism associated with, 2366t
Chromosome 19p deletion, in bladder cancer, 2753
Chronic fatigue syndrome, and interstitial cystitis, 635, 636f
Chronic obstructive pulmonary disease, and incontinence, 1095
Chronic pelvic pain syndrome. *See also* Cystitis, interstitial; Prostatitis.
  classification of, 610
  clinical presentation of, 611, 611f
  cytokines in, 617
  diagnostic algorithm for, 617, 618f
  expressed prostatic secretion in, 615, 615f
  pathogenesis of, 609, 609f
  symptom assessment in, 611–612, 613f
  treatment of
    drug, 618–622
    strategies for, 623, 624f, 624t, 625
Chronic renal failure. *See* Renal failure, chronic.
Chwalle's membrane, 2022
Chylous ascites, following retroperitoneal lymph node dissection, 2938

Chyluria
  in filariasis, 784
  in parasitic disease, 763
Cigarette smoking. *See* Nicotine; Smoking.
Cimetidine
  effect of, on spermatogenesis, 1477
  erectile dysfunction caused by, 1609
  interactions with azoles, 819
cip/kip, G_1S checkpoint and, 2639
Cipro. *See* Ciprofloxacin.
Ciprofloxacin
  adverse effects and side effects of, 757t
  dosage and administration of, 757t
  for actinomycosis, 817
  for chancroid, 684
  for classic urethritis, 673t
  for prostatitis, 619t, 624t
  serum and urinary levels of, 537t
Circinate balanitis (Reiter's disease), 717, 732f
Circle loop nephrostomy, 3337, 3337f
Circulation
  glomerular, 169–170, 170f
    effect of angiotensin II on, 169–170, 214
  pelvic, 49, 51–52, 53f–55f
Circumcaval ureter, 431–432, 431f–432f
Circumcision, 2336–2338, 3905–3906, 3906f
  accidents during, 3905
  and penile prosthesis placement, 1674
  and urinary tract infection, 2054
  clamped, 1823
  complications of, 1818, 1823, 1829, 2336–2337
  controversy regarding, 2336
  female, 2436–2437, 2436f
  in prune-belly syndrome, 2123
  injury in, management of, 1801–1802
  meatal stenosis following, 2337–2338, 2338t
  office procedure for, 1829
  penile squamous cell carcinoma and, 2951, 2952
  techniques for, 1829
  urethral meatal stenosis after, 1818
Circumflex artery, 73f, 74f
Circumflex vein, 74, 74f, 1594, 1594f
Cisapride
  adverse effects and side effects of, 1001
  contraindications to, 1001
  indications for, 1001
  uropharmacology of, 1001
Cisplatin
  discovery of, 2659
  for prostate cancer, 3214t, 3216
Citrate(s)
  for urinary lithiasis, 3283–3284
  metabolism of, 3242–3243
Citric acid, in seminal plasma, 1238, 1276
Clamp(s)
  penile, for incontinence, 991
  vas deferens fixation, ring-tipped, in vasectomy, 1542–1544, 1543f
Classical pathway, of complement activation, 308, 309f
ClC-Kb gene, in Bartter's syndrome, 1844
Clean intermittent catheterization, for urinary tract reconstruction, 2509, 2536
Clean intermittent self-catheterization, in renal transplant recipients, candidates, 351
Clear cell sarcoma, of kidney, 2493
Clenbuterol
  for voiding dysfunction, 975
  indications for, 990–991
  uropharmacology of, 990–991
Climacterium, male, as hormone therapy side effect, 3189

Cystourethrectomy, for interstitial cystitis, 658
Cystourethrocele, repair. *See* Burch culposuspension; Paravaginal fascial repair.
Cystourethrography, 129–131
    complications of, 131
    indications for, 131
    retrograde, 130–131, 131f
    static, 130, 130f
    technique of, 129–131, 130f–131f
    urinary tract anatomy in, 131
    voiding, 130, 130f
        in chronic pyelonephritis, 555
        in prune-belly syndrome, 2124
        in urinary tract infection, 536
        with suprasacral spinal cord injury, 946, 946f
Cystourethropexy. *See* Marshall-Marchetti-Krantz (MMK) procedure; Retropubic suspension surgery.
Cystourethroscope
    flexible, 118, 118f
        advantages of, 117
    rigid, 117–118, 118f
        advantages of, 117
Cystourethroscopy, 117–119
    equipment for, 117–118, 118f–119f
    in postprostatectomy incontinence, 1063
    indications for, 117, 1042
    of ectopic ureter, 2018
    of urethral diverticulum, 1209
    patient preparation for, 117
    technique of, 118–119
    video-, 118, 119f
Cytochrome P450 1A2, in bladder cancer, 2738
Cytokine(s)
    chemoattractant properties of, 25t, 331–332
    during peptide/MHC class II priming, 322–323, 324f
    in growth control, 1250, 1251f
    in nonbacterial prostatitis, 617
    in septic shock, 568f, 569–570, 569f
    in tuberculosis treatment, 756
    in tumor regression, 336–337
    in urinary tract obstruction, 442
    production of, 321–323
    representative, 323t
    type 1, 321–322
    type 2, 322
Cytokine gene expression, Jak/STAT pathway regulating, 320
Cytolytic gene therapy, for prostate cancer, 3166
Cytomatrix, of prostate, 1241t, 1243, 1244f
    intermediate filaments of, 1243
Cytomegalovirus (CMV)
    in acquired immunodeficiency syndrome, 700, 706, 709–710
    infection with, after to renal transplantation, 365
    testing for, prior to renal transplantation, 349
Cytopathology, in bladder cancer, 2772
Cytoplasm, of ureteral smooth muscle cell, 378

Daclizumab, as immunosuppressant, 364t, 365, 365f
Dactinomycin, for Wilms' tumor, 2489
Dandruff (seborrheic dermatitis), genital, 718
Dantrolene
    for malignant hyperthermia, 1010
    for voiding dysfunction, 1010
    uropharmacology of, 1009, 1010
Darifenacin
    for neuromuscular voiding dysfunction, 970
    uropharmacology of, 858, 970

Dartos fascia, 75, 75f
Dartos pouch technique
    for hydrocelectomy, 1580
    for orchiopexy in adults, 1581
Davis intubated ureterotomy, 2002
DAX-1 gene
    in sex determination, 2399
    in sexual differentiation, 1440, 1762f, 1762–1763
Daytime urinary frequency syndrome, in children, 2273
DAZ gene, in spermatogenesis, 1456, 1505
DBY gene, in spermatogenesis, 1505
de Lange syndrome. *See* Brachmann-de Lange syndrome.
Death domains, in apoptosis, 325
Death receptor(s)
    apoptosis and, 2643–2644, 2643f
    as cancer therapy targets, 2644
Death receptor pathway, in apoptosis, 325–326, 326f
Debilitation, erectile dysfunction caused by, 1610
Débridement, for Fournier's gangrene, 591
Decongestants, over-the-counter, incontinence caused by, in elderly, 1221
Deep perineal space, 3897f, 3898, 3899f
Deep plexus, 3888
Deep tendon reflex(es), 903
Deep vein thrombosis
    following laparoscopic surgery, 3489–3490
    postprostatectomy, 1433
    with radical cystectomy, 2824
De-epithelialized bowel segments, 2601
Deflux system, in endoscopic treatment of vesicoureteral reflux, 2093
Degloving injuries, of penis, 3912–3913, 3914f
Dehydration, in early kidney graft dysfunction, 366, 368t
Dehydroepiandrosterone (DHEA), 3511, 3511f
    age-related changes in, 1636
    and erectile dysfunction, 1637
    and female sexual function, 1714
    metabolism of, 3513–3514
    physiologic effects of, 1637
    replacement therapy with, in women, dosage and administration of, 1728
    synthesis of, 1247f, 1248
Dehydroepiandrosterone sulfate (DHEAS)
    age-related changes in, 1636
    synthesis of, 1247f, 1248
Deletion, chromosome. *See also specific chromosomes.*
    definition of, 2626t
Deletion 4p syndrome, hypospadias with, 2292t
Deletion 11q syndrome, hypospadias with, 2292t
Deletion 13q syndrome, hypospadias with, 2292t
Delirium, and incontinence, in elderly, 1220, 1220t
Dementia
    incontinence in, 938, 1223
        in elderly, 938, 1222
        management of, 938, 1228
    voiding dysfunction in, 938
Demyelinating disease. *See also* Acute disseminated encephalomyelitis; Adrenomyeloneuropathy; Guillain-Barré syndrome; Hereditary spastic paraplegia; Multiple sclerosis.
    in males, seminal emission abnormalities in, electroejaculation for, 1565–1566
    reflex neurogenic bladder with, 895
    uninhibited neurogenic bladder with, 895

Dendritic cells
    activation of CD4/CD8 T cells by, 322f
    as target in HIV infection, 696
    in immune response, 320–321
Denervation techniques, for detrusor overactivity, 1044–1045
Denonvillier's fascia, 47, 56, 57, 57f, 1102–1103
Dense bodies, cytoplasmic, 378
Denys-Drash syndrome, 2407, 2481
    Wilms' tumor in, 2635
Deoxyribonucleic acid (DNA), 2626–2627
    complementary, definition of, 2626t
    complementary (cDNA), definition of, 2626t
    content of
        in neuroblastoma, 2473
        in Wilms' tumor, 2488
    hypermethylation of, 2631–2632
    mutation of, carcinogenesis and, 2630–2631
    nuclear, 2629
    repair of, 2640–2643, 2641f, 2642f
        apoptosis and, 2643
        base excision, 2641
        mismatch, 2641–2642
        nucleotide excision, 2641
        of double-stranded breaks, 2642–2643
    transcription of, 2627–2629, 2627f, 2628f
        posttranscriptional modification and, 2629
        regulation of, 2628–2629
    translation of, 2629–2630
    ubiquitinization and, 2630
    viral, transcription of, 696
Deoxyribonucleic acid (DNA) polymerase, HIV-1, 697
Depolarization, of ureteral muscle cells, 379
Depression
    and female sexual dysfunction, 1718–1719, 1720
    cardiovascular morbidity in, 977–978
    incontinence and, 1069
    male sexual dysfunction in, 1649
    with radical cystectomy, 2807–2808
Dercum's disease, 419. *See also* Pelvic lipomatosis.
Dermal nevus, of male genitalia, 729
Dermal skin test, for bovine collagen immunogenicity, 1182
Dermatan sulfate, of prostate, 1244
Dermatitis, of male genitalia
    contact, 719–720
    eczematous or allergic, 719–720, 720t, 733f
    factitial, 721
    seborrheic, 718
Dermatitis artefacta, of male genitalia, 721
Dermatitis herpetiformis, of male genitalia, 721
Dermatofibroma, of male genitalia, 727–728
Dermatomes, 903, 904f
Dermatophyte infection, of male genitalia, 726, 735f
Dermis, papillary, 3887
DES. *See* Diethylstilbestrol (DES).
Descendin, in testicular descent, 2360–2361
Descending perineum syndrome, 1106
Descensus, renal, in ureteral stricture repair, 500
Desipramine, incontinence caused by, in elderly, 1221t
Desmin, 1243
Desmopressin
    contraindications to, 994–995
    for incontinence, in exstrophy patient after reconstruction, 2171
    for nocturnal enuresis, 994, 2277–2278, 2278t
    for nocturnal polyuria, 994

Epispadias (Continued)
  complete, 2182f
  incidence of, 2184
  surgical management of
    continence after, 2185
    objectives for, 2184–2185
    operative techniques for, 2185, 2186f–2187f
    results in, 2185
  glanular, 2181, 2182
  histochemical markers in, 2144
  historical perspective on, 2138
  immunocytochemical markers in, 2144
  male, 2137, 2137f, 2181–2184
    chordee with, 2181
    complete, 2181–2182, 2182f
    embryology of, 2181
    genital reconstruction in, 2183–2184
    incidence of, 2181
    incontinence with, 2182
    surgical management of, 2182–2184
      continence after, 2183t, 2183–2184
      sexual function after, 2184
    types of, 2181–2182
  male-to-female ratio of, 2182
  management of, in neonate, 1802
  penile shaft, 2181, 2182
  penopubic, 2181–2182
    surgical management of, 2182
  repair of
    combined with exstrophy reconstruction, 2147, 2149t, 2150–2151, 2163–2165, 2166f–2168f
      results of, 2171
    in cloacal exstrophy, 2180
    in exstrophy patient, 2159, 2160f
      failed, 2173
      results of, 2169t, 2169–2170
    timing of, 2151
    voiding dysfunction after, artificial sphincter for, 1188. See also Artificial sphincter.
  spectrum of, 2181
  subsymphyseal, 2182
  surgical management of, 2137–2138
Episteride, for benign prostatic hyperplasia, 1364
Epithelial cells
  in urinary sediment, 109, Color Plate I–9
  of prostate, 1240–1241, 1241t
    interactions of, with stromal cells, 1262–1263, 1264f
      in benign prostatic hyperplasia, 1300–1301
    receptivity of, in urinary tract infection, 526–528, 528f
    variation of, 528–529, 528f
Epithelial hyperplasia, in bladder cancer, 2741
Epithelial inclusion cysts, penile, 2338, 2338f
Epithelial tag, 1757, 1760f
Epithelial tumors, testicular, 2910–2911
Epithelioid cells, in chronic inflammation, 339
Epitope, of antigen-binding site, 313
Epoöphoron, 1755f, 1756
  embryology of, 2009, 2014
Epstein-Barr virus (EBV)
  acute tubulointerstitial nephritis caused by, 1843
  cancer related to, 2652
  testing for, prior to renal transplantation, 349
Erectile dysfunction, 1673–1705
  after renal transplantation, 370–371, 372f
    potential causes of, 371t
    treatment options for, 371t

Erectile dysfunction (Continued)
  aging and, 1609–1610
  arteriogenic, 1608
  bicycling and, 1648
  biochemical study in, 1638
  cavernosal (venogenic), 1608–1609
    endothelium in, 1609
    fibroelastic component in, 1608
    gap junctions in, 1609
    smooth muscle in, 1608–1609
  classification of, 1605f, 1605–1610, 1606t
  complex, 1661
    management of, hormones and, 1637
    penile blood flow study in, 1639
  definition of, 1620, 1621, 1623
  dehydroepiandrosterone (DHEA) and, 1637
  diagnosis of, 1620, 1621t
    advances in (future directions for), 1613
    goal-directed approach to, 1621–1627, 1622f
    tests for, 1622f, 1623, 1623t
  drug-induced, 1609
    management of, 1648–1649
  endocrinologic, 1607–1608
  endocrinologic testing in, 1635–1637
  epidemiology of, 1604–1605
  evaluation of patient with, 1620, 1621t
    additional testing in, 1627
    endocrinologic testing in, 1635–1637
    evidence-based assessments in, 1639, 1644
    process of care model for, 1620–1621
    questionnaires for, 1623–1624
    sexual function symptom scores in, 1623
  First International Consultation on, 1621, 1625, 1626
  following cryotherapy, for prostate cancer, 3178
  following radical cystectomy, 2829
  following radical prostatectomy, 3091–3093, 3092f, 3092t, 3093f
    perineal, 3145
    retropubic, 3127–3128
  following urethral injury, 3731, 3732
  historical perspective on, 1591–1592
  history-taking in, 1624t, 1624–1625
  hormonal testing in, 1635–1637
  in estrogen excess, 1503
  in hyperprolactinemia, 1503
  in multiple system atrophy, 941
  in Peyronie's disease, 1698
  in Wernicke's encephalopathy, 962
  incidence of, studies of, 1605
  intraurethral therapy for, 1655–1656
  laboratory testing in, 1626
  naturopathic remedies for, 1620–1621
  neurogenic, 1606–1607
  neurologic testing in, 1633–1635
  nonsurgical treatment of, 1648–1649
  organic, 1624, 1624t
    risk factors for, 1624
  pathophysiology of, 1604–1610
  pharmacotherapy for, 1619–1620
    androgens in, 1649–1651, 1650t
    central conditioners in, 1652
    central initiators in, 1652
    centrally acting drugs for, 1652
    historical perspective on, 1620
    intracavernous injection in, 1656t, 1656–1658
      adverse effects and side effects of, 1660
      contraindications to, 1660
      drug combinations for, 1658–1660

Erectile dysfunction (Continued)
  efficacy of, in different types of erectile dysfunction, 1660
  improvement in spontaneous erection with, 1660
  patient acceptance of, 1660
  patient dropout rate in, 1660
  intraurethral, 1655–1656
  oral preparations for, 1651–1656
  peripheral conditioners in, 1652
  peripheral initiators in, 1652
  peripherally acting drugs for, 1653
  transdermal, 1656
  transglandular, 1656
  physical examination of patient with, 1625–1626
  postprostatectomy, 1433
  prevention of, 1606
  prevalence of, 1604–1605
  priapism-related, 1612
  psychogenic, 1605–1606, 1624, 1624t, 1631–1633
  psychophysiologic testing in, 1631
  referral of patient with, 1627
  surgery for, 1673, 1696
    historical perspective on, 1620
    incision for, 1674
    patient counseling for, 1672t, 1674
    vascular procedures in, 1673. See also Penile revascularization.
  systemic disease and, 1610
  treatment of
    advances in (future directions for), 1613, 1661
    contemporary history of, 1620–1621
    goal-directed approach to, 1620, 1621–1627, 1622f
    historical perspective on, 1673–1674
    hormonal therapy in, 1649–1651
    lifestyle changes in, 1648
    medical. See Erectile dysfunction, pharmacotherapy for.
    nonsurgical, 1648–1649, 1674
    options for, 1621, 1621t
      advantages and disadvantages of, 1627t
      costs of, 1627t
      diagnostic tests for, 1623, 1623t
      discussion of, with patient, 1626–1627
    pelvic floor muscle exercises in, 1649
    placebo effect and, 1673
    process of care model for, 1620–1621
    psychological approach to, 1620
    psychosexual therapy in, 1649
    surgical. See Erectile dysfunction, surgery for.
    vacuum constriction device in, 1660–1661
  vascular evaluation in, 1637–1648
  vascular risk factors for, 1619
  vascular surgery for, 1689–1695
  with tricyclic antidepressants, 977
Erectile dysfunction impact scale, 1625, 1626f
Erectile dysfunction intensity scale, 1625, 1625f
Erectile Dysfunction Inventory for Treatment Satisfaction (EDITS), 1623
Erection. See Penile erection.
Ergot alkaloids, retroperitoneal fibrosis associated with, 505
Erosion(s), skin, 716
Erysipelas, of male genitalia, 725
Erythema, cutaneous, 716
Erythema multiforme, 720
  of penis, 733f
Erythrasma, of male genitalia, 724

Fertility (Continued)
in exstrophy patient, 2143
male
after hypospadias repair, 2324
cryptorchidism and, 2363
in bladder exstrophy, 2174
in prune-belly syndrome, 2121
in testicular germ cell tumors
advanced, 2939–2940
low-stage, 2933
posterior urethral valves and, 2224–2225
normal, 1475–1476
Fertilization rates. See also Pregnancy rates.
with in vitro fertilization (IVF), 1517
Fetal alcohol syndrome, renal findings in, 1963f
Fetal ascites, and prune-belly syndrome, 2118
Fetal diagnosis, 1781–1789. See also Ultrasonography, fetal.
of autosomal recessive polycystic kidney disease, 1788, 1788f, 1943–1944
postnatal evaluation and management with, 1799–1800
of bilateral renal agenesis, 1889
of bladder (classical) exstrophy, 1788, 1788f, 2146, 2148f
of bladder outlet obstruction, 2212–2213, 2213f
of cloacal anomaly, 1789
of cloacal exstrophy, 1788, 2176
of ectopic ureter, 1787, 2016
of genital abnormalities, 1788–1789
of horseshoe kidney, 1905
of imperforate anus, 1789
of megalourethra, 1784, 1784f
of megaureter, 2094–2095
of multicystic dysplastic kidney, 1787f, 1787–1788
of multicystic dysplastic kidney (MCDK), postnatal evaluation and management with, 1799–1800
of neuroblastoma, 1789, 1789f
of patent urachus, 2191
of penile abnormalities, 1788–1789
of posterior urethral valves, 1785–1786, 1786f, 2212–2213, 2213f, 2218, 2220–2223
pitfalls in, 1789
of prune-belly syndrome, 2117, 2122–2123
of renal agenesis, 1788
of ureterocele, 1786f, 1786–1787, 2022–2023
of ureteropelvic junction obstruction, 1785, 1995, 1998
of ureterovesical junction obstruction, 1785
of vesicoureteral reflux, 1785, 2054
pitfalls in, 1789
pitfalls in, 1789
Fetal hydantoin syndrome, hypospadias with, 2292t
Fetal rubella, hypospadias with, 2292t
Fetal trimethadione syndrome, hypospadias with, 2292t
Fetal valproate syndrome, hypospadias with, 2292t
Fetus
kidneys of. See also Kidney(s), fetal.
sexual differentiation in. See Sexual differentiation.
uropathy in
incidence of, 1793
interventions for, 1793–1796
management of, 1793–1796
Fever
effects of, on spermatogenesis, 1477
filarial, 783–784

Fever (Continued)
in Candida infection, 798
in children
management of, 1820
postoperative, evaluation of, 1812
serious illness with
risk of, 1819
types of, 1819, 1819t
with petechiae, 1820, 1820t
in patient history, 90
in urinary tract infection, 532
postoperative, in children, evaluation of, 1812
with bacillus Calmette-Guérin, 2792
with vesicoureteral reflux, 2061–2062
Fexofenadine, for Peyronie's disease, 1700
FG syndrome
cryptorchidism associated with, 2367t
hypospadias with, 2292t
Fiber, dietary, for urinary lithiasis, 3280
Fibroblast(s), interstitial, in urinary tract obstruction, 442
Fibroblast growth factor
in benign prostatic hyperplasia, 1302
in prostate growth, 1268t, 1268–1269, 1301, 1301f
FGF-7. See Keratinocyte growth factor.
FGF-10, 1302
gene disruption, and hypospadias, 2289
in male gonadal development, 1756
in renal development, 1746f, 1747
Fibroblast growth factor-2, as angiogenesis activator, 2653
Fibroepithelial polyp(s), in children, 2495
Fibroid(s), uterine, 426, 426f
Fibroma(s), renal, 2685
Fibromuscular hyperplasia, of renal artery, 231t, 234–235
Fibromyalgia, and interstitial cystitis, 635, 636f
Fibronectin
in bladder cancer, 2751–2752
prostatic, 1243
Fibroplasia
intimal, of renal artery, 231t, 232–233, 233f
medial, of renal artery, 231t, 233, 234f
perimedial, of renal artery, 231t, 233–234, 234f
Fibrosis
in urinary tract obstruction, 440–441, 441f
strategies to affect, 443–444, 443t
pelvic, as laparoscopic surgery contraindication, 3458
retroperitoneal, 505–508. See also Retroperitoneal fibrosis.
Fibrous dysplasia, renovascular hypertension due to, renal arterial reconstruction for, 3615
Filarial fever, 783–784
Filariasis
bancroftian, 780, 781–786
brugian, 780, 781–786
genital, 780–786
incidence of, 763
lymphatic, 780, 781–786
asymptomatic, 783
chronic abnormalities in, 783–784
chyluria in, 784
clinical manifestations of, 783–785
control of, 786
diagnosis of, 785
early established infection, 782
epidemiology of, 781
filarial fever in, 783–784
funiculoepididymitis in, 784
geographic distribution of, 781

Filariasis (Continued)
hydrocele in, 782f, 782–783, 784
late infection, 782f, 782–783, 783f
pathogenesis of, 782–783
pathology of, 782–783
prepatent period of, 782
prevention of, 785–786
prognosis for, 785–786
treatment of, 785
tropical pulmonary eosinophilia in, 785
microbiology of, 780
nonlymphatic, 780
Filiform catheter, 113, 115f
for urethral dilatation, 115–116
Filum terminale, tight, 952
Fimbriae, bacterial, 1850
Finasteride
for benign prostatic hyperplasia, 1360f, 1360–1363, 1361t, 1362f, 1363f, 1364–1365
dosage and administration of, 1359t
mechanism of action of, 1359t, 1360
vs. doxazosin and combination therapy, 1365–1367, 1366t, 1367t
vs. terazosin and combination therapy, 1365f, 1365–1367, 1366t, 1366f, 1367t
for geriatric incontinence, with outlet obstruction, 1230
for lower urinary tract symptoms, with benign prostatic hyperplasia, 1423
for prostate cancer prevention, 3018–3019
for prostatitis, 621, 624t
Fine-needle aspiration. See also Biopsy(ies).
in renal cell carcinoma, 2701
in squamous penile cancer, 2963
of renal masses, 2676
of sperm, 1566t, 1568–1569, 1568f–1569f
First-dose phenomenon, 1007
"Fish-hook" deformity, in circumcaval ureter, 431, 432f
Fistula(s)
arteriovenous, renal, 262, 264, 264f
complex, of posterior urethra, 3941
genitourinary. See also Vesicovaginal fistula(s).
causes of, 1195–1196
historical perspective on, 1195
iatrogenic
clinical features of, 1196
pathogenesis of, 1196
in genitourinary tuberculosis, 750
obstetric, 1195–1196
rectourethral, and vesicoureteral reflux, 2075
rectovesical, and vesicoureteral reflux, 2075
urethral, congenital, 2345–2346, 2345f
urethrocutaneous, 3901–3903, 3902f
after complete primary exstrophy repair, 2205
after exstrophy-epispadias surgery, 2169, 2170, 2171, 2173
prevention of, 2160
after hypospadias repair, 2322
in coccidioidomycosis, 813
urethrovaginal, 1203f, 1203–1207
etiology of, 1196
incontinence with, 1196
urinary, with ureterointestinal anastomoses, 3769–3770
vesicovaginal, 1195–1203. See also Vesicovaginal fistula(s).
in artificial sphincter patient, 1192
video-urodynamics with, 925
with intestinal anastomoses, 3757

Fixed drug eruption, involving male genitalia, 718, 732f

FK-506. *See* Tacrolimus (FK-506).

Flank, anterolateral muscle layers of, 4–5

Flank approach
  to adrenal surgery, 3550–3552, 3552f, 3553f
  to kidney surgery, 3575–3578, 3576f–3579f, 3584–3585, 3587f, 3588f

Flank pain
  in urinary tract infection, 532
  in urinary tract obstruction, 413

Flap(s)
  in reconstructive surgery, 3889–3890, 3889f, 3890f
  tissue
    axial, 2298
    double onlay preputial
      for middle hypospadias repair, 2312
      for posterior hypospadias repair, 2313–2314
    fasciocutaneous, 2298–2299
      in urethroplasty, 2298–2299
    in hypospadias repair, 2308–2311, 2309f–2310f
      Barcat balanic groove technique for, 2311
      Bevan-Mustarde perimeatal-based, ventral skin technique for, 2311
      Mathieu (perimeatal-based) technique for, 2308–2311, 2309f–2310f
    island, 2298
      in urethroplasty
        in epispadias patient, 2183
        in exstrophy patient, 2160
    local, in urethroplasty, 2298–2299, 2303, 2323
    onlay island
      for hypospadias repair, current trends in, 2325
      for middle hypospadias repair, 2311, 2312f–2313f
        split prepuce in situ technique for, 2311–2312, 2314f–2315f
      for posterior hypospadias repair, 2312–2313
    parameatal foreskin, in posterior (proximal) hypospadias repair, 2316–2318
    peninsula, 2298
    random, 2298
    subcutaneous (dartos), for neourethral coverage in hypospadias repair, 2299, 2299f
    transverse preputial island (TPIF), in posterior (proximal) hypospadias repair, 2315–2316, 2316f–2317f

Flap valve(s), for continent urinary diversion, Mitrofanoff principle and, 2547–2550
  alternatives for, 2548–2550, 2549f
  results with, 2548
  technique for, 2547–2548, 2547f

Flap valve mechanism, ureteral, 2013, 2013f

Flavoxate hydrochloride
  for urge incontinence, in elderly, 1228, 1229t
  for voiding dysfunction, 973
  uropharmacology of, 858t, 973, 2235t

Flomax. *See* Tamsulosin.

Flow cytometry, in bladder cancer, 2754, 2770

Floxin. *See* Ofloxacin.

Fluconazole, 819
  adverse effects and side effects of, 820f, 821
  dosage and administration of, 820, 821t
  drug interactions with, 819t
  efficacy of, 820–821

Fluconazole *(Continued)*
  for aspergillosis, 806
  for candidiasis, 804, 821t
    in children, 802
    with epididymo-orchitis, 799
    with invasive or disseminated infection, 805
    with prostatitis, 800
    with vaginitis, 799
  for coccidioidomycosis, 813
  for cryptococcosis, 809, 821t
  for *Torulopsis glabrata* infection, 805–806
  indications for, 820, 821t

Flucytosine
  adverse effects and side effects of, 804, 818–819, 820f
  and amphotericin B, combination therapy with, 804
  dosage and administration of, 821t
  for aspergillosis, 807
  for candidal cystitis, 799
  for candidiasis, 804
  for cryptococcosis, 808, 809, 821t
  for *Torulopsis glabrata* infection, 805
  fungal resistance to, 819
  pharmacology of, 818

Fluid(s)
  body
    composition of, 199–200, 199t
    osmolality of, 199–200, 200f, 200t
  perigraft collection of, after renal transplantation, 368, 369f
  postoperative management of, in renal transplant recipients, 362
  requirements for, in preterm infant, 1772, 1772f

Fluid intake
  deficient, as bladder cancer risk factor, 2741
  excessive, incontinence caused by, in elderly, 1221
  for bladder cancer prevention, 2763
  for urinary lithiasis prevention, 3259–3260
  for urinary lithiasis treatment, 3277–3278
  with cystine stones, 3265

Fluid overload
  in neonates, sequelae of, 1772
  incontinence caused by, in elderly, 1221

Fluid volume, extracellular
  in renal calcium reabsorption, 195
  in renal urate excretion, 197–198

Fluoroquinolones
  adverse reactions, precautions, and contraindications to, 540t
  for acute pyelonephritis, 553, 553f
  for cystitis, 574, 575
  for prostatitis, 619, 619t, 624t
  for urinary tract infection, 539t, 541–542
  prophylactic, for recurrent urinary tract infection, 577, 578t

Fluoroscopy
  for percutaneous puncture
    antegrade approach in, 3323–3325, 3324f–3329f, 3327–3328
    retrograde approach in, 3328–3330
      Hawkins-Hunter system for, 3330
      Lawson system for, 3329–3330, 3329f, 3330f
  for shock-wave lithotripsy, 3403
  of lower urinary tract, 1040, 1041

Fluoroscopy unit, for ureteral access, 3313

Fluorouracil
  for prostate cancer, 3214t, 3216
  for renal cell carcinoma, metastatic, 2717

Fluoxetine
  erectile dysfunction caused by, 1649
  priapism caused by, 1612t

Flurazepam, incontinence caused by, in elderly, 1221t

Flurbiprofen, uropharmacology of, 858t

Flush stoma, 3761

Flutamide
  for benign prostatic hyperplasia, 1364
    dosage and administration of, 1359t
    mechanism of action of, 1359t, 1364
  for prostate cancer, 3196–3197, 3198

Focal glomerulonephritis, in systemic lupus erythematosus, 1840

Foley catheter, 112, 112f
  for nephrostomy drainage, 3335–3336

Foley Y-V-plasty technique
  in pyeloplasty, 481, 482f
  in ureteropelvic junction repair, 2001–2002

Follicle(s), ovarian, origin of, 1755f, 1756

Follicle-stimulating hormone (FSH)
  and Sertoli cell function, 1449
  deficiency of, in males, 1502
  evaluation of, in males, 1484t, 1484–1485
  in male reproductive axis, 1437, 1440–1441
  in spermatogenesis, 1456
  in testicular descent, 2359
  secretion of, 1437–1438
  serum levels of, preoperative analysis of, in vasovasostomy candidate, 1547
  therapy with
    for male infertility, 1511
    in hypogonadotropic hypogonadism, 1501

Folliculitis, of male genitalia, 725

Force-length relations, of smooth muscle, 386–387, 387f

Forceps delivery, stress incontinence after, 1036–1037

Force-velocity relations, of smooth muscle, 387, 387f

Forebrain, in sexual function, 1598t

Foreign body(ies)
  in upper urinary tact, ureteroscopic removal of, 3318
  vesicovaginal fistula caused by, 1196

Foreign body granuloma, with polytetrafluoroethylene (PTFE) injection therapy, 1181–1182

Foreskin. *See also* Circumcision.
  balanoposthitis of, 724
  in neonates, adherent to glans, 1823
  manual retraction of, 2335

Forskolin
  in treatment of erectile dysfunction, 1659
  mechanism of action of, 1659
  source of, 1659

fos oncogene, 320

Fossa navicularis, 3891

Four-corner bladder neck suspension, 1123, 1124, 1125f

Fournier's gangrene, 43, 590–591, 725, 734f
  genital skin loss due to, 3738
  in acquired immunodeficiency syndrome, 709

Fowler syndrome, 960

Fowler-Stephens orchidopexy, 2131

Fowler-Stephens orchiopexy, 2376

Fracture(s)
  compression, stone comminution by, 3406–3407, 3408f
  pelvic
    urethral injuries with, 3725
    voiding dysfunction after, artificial sphincter for, 1188. *See also* Artificial sphincter.

Fracture(s) *(Continued)*
  penile, subclinical, 3946
  risk of, urge incontinence in elderly and, 1069
Frameshift mutations, definition of, 2626t
Fraser syndrome
  cryptorchidism associated with, 2367t
  hypospadias associated with, 2292t
  multisystem involvement in, 1814t
Freeman-Sheldon syndrome, cryptorchidism associated with, 2367t
Frequency
  in acute disseminated encephalomyelitis, 943–944
  in cerebral palsy, 939
  in hereditary spastic paraplegia, 943
  in HIV-infected patients, 943
  in Lyme disease, 942
  in multiple system atrophy, 941
  in Parkinson's disease, 940
  in reflex sympathetic dystrophy, 944
  urinary, 86
    causes of, 661t
    definition of, 901
    in children, with ectopic ureter, 2015–2016
Frequency charts, for incontinent patient, 1039, 1108
Frequency-volume charts, for incontinent patient, 1039, 1108
Frog-leg position, for perineal examination, in female child, 1824, 1824f
Frontometaphyseal dysplasia, cryptorchidism associated with, 2367t
Fructose
  excess, ingestion of, in children, 1816t
  in seminal plasma, 1238, 1277, 1483
Fryns syndrome
  cryptorchidism associated with, 2367t
  hypospadias associated with, 2292t
FSFI (Female Sexual Function Index), 1725
FSH. *See* Follicle-stimulating hormone (FSH).
Functional abdominal pain, 1816t
Fungal balls
  candidal, imaging of, 802–803, 803f
  ureteral obstruction by, 800
Fungal bezoars, percutaneous treatment of, 3351–3352, 3353t
Funguria, in children, 1873–1874
Fungus(i). *See also specific organism.*
  bezoar of
    imaging of, 802–803, 803f
    in bladder, 799, 799f
    in children, 1874
    treatment of, 805
  drug resistance in, 818, 819, 821
  infection with
    epidemiology of, 797–798
    in renal transplant recipients, 797
    predisposing factors for, 798
    primary, 810–815
    sites of involvement in, 798
  opportunistic, 797–810
  rare/unusual, infections with, 815–816
Funiculoepididymitis
  in filariasis, 784
  parasitic, 763
Furosemide
  in neonates, and urinary calcium excretion, 1771
  incontinence caused by, in elderly, 1221t
Furunculosis, of male genitalia, 725
Fusarium infection, 815
Fusiform aneurysm, of renal artery, 262, 263f

G protein, in ureteral peristalsis, 384
G spot, 1711
G syndrome, multisystem involvement in, 1814t
G_1S checkpoint and. *See* Cell cycle, G_1S checkpoint.
G_2M checkpoint, 2640, 2640f
Gadolinium, in magnetic resonance imaging, 146
gag gene, in HIV-1, 694, 695f
Gallium nitrate, for bladder cancer, metastatic, 2813
Gallium-67 citrate radionuclide scan, 161–162
  in children, 1829
Gamma-aminobutyric acid (GABA)
  benzodiazepines and, 1009
  functions of, 1009
  $GABA_A$
    agonists, uropharmacology of, 867, 869
    antagonists, uropharmacology of, 869
    uropharmacology of, 867
  $GABA_B$
    agonists, uropharmacology of, 867, 869
    antagonists, uropharmacology of, 869
    supraspinal, and micturition reflex, 869
Gamma-camera renography, 415f
Gamma-glutamyl-transpeptidase, in testicular germ cell tumors, 2888
Ganglioneuroblastoma(s), in children, 2470
Ganglioneuroma(s), in children, 2470
Gangliosides, in cell-cell interactions, 336
Gangrene
  Fournier's, 43, 590–591, 725, 734f
    in acquired immunodeficiency syndrome, 709
  necrotizing, genital skin loss due to, 3738
GAP (glans approximation procedure), in hypospadias repair, 2305–2306
Gap junctions, in penile function, 1601–1602, 1609
Gardnerella vaginalis, in interstitial cystitis, 638
Gartner's duct
  cysts of, 1755f, 1756, 2439–2440
  embryology of, 2009, 2014
Gas, bowel, plain film radiography of, 123
Gas embolism, with pneumoperitoneum, 3478–3479
Gastric artery, 6
Gastric contents, aspiration of, anesthesia-related, with laparoscopic surgery, 3490–3491
Gastric neobladder, for continent urinary diversion, 3838
Gastric pouches, for continent urinary diversion, 3825–3826, 3826f, 3827f
Gastrocystoplasty, 2529–2530
  antrum technique for, 2529
  body technique for, 2529–2530, 2531f
Gastrointestinal disorders. *See also specific disorders.*
  following radical cystectomy, 2828–2829
  following retroperitoneal lymph node dissection, 2939
  with shock-wave lithotripsy, 3409
Gastrointestinal injury
  during radical nephrectomy, 3601
  in laparoscopy
    electrosurgical, 3483–3485, 3484f
    mechanical, 3485
    with trocar placement, 3483
  with trocar placement, 3480–3481, 3480f
Gastrointestinal surgery, vesicovaginal fistula caused by, 1196
Gastrointestinal tract
  decompression of, for cloacal malformations, 2460–2461

Gastrointestinal tract *(Continued)*
  in prune-belly syndrome, 2121t, 2122
  in schistosomiasis, 779–780
Gastroparesis
  causes of, 962
  definition of, 962
  voiding dysfunction with, 962
Gastroschisis
  in prune-belly syndrome, 2122
  signs and symptoms of, 1822
Gatifloxacin
  adverse effects and side effects of, 757t
  dosage and administration of, 757t
GAX-collagen. *See* Glutaraldehyde cross-linked bovine collagen (GAX-collagen).
GDNF. *See* Glial cell line–derived neurotrophic factor (GDNF).
Gemcitabine (Gemzar), for bladder cancer, metastatic, 2813
Gender assignment, 2422–2423
  in micropenis, 2342
Gender identity, 2403
  hypospadias and, 2324
Gender orientation, 2403
Gender role, 2403
Gene(s). *See also specific gene.*
  cancer. *See* Oncogene(s).
  definition of, 2626t
  disruption of, embryonic lethality in, 1745–1746
  for nitric oxide synthase, 176t
  in disease, 1926
  mutations of, two-hit theory of, 1926–1927
  overexpression of, in bladder cancer, 2737
  products of, 1926
  redundancy of, 1745
  tumor suppressor, 2631
Gene amplification, in bladder cancer, 2737
Gene knock-out studies, of renal development, 1743–1746
Gene therapy, 2660
  for bladder cancer, 2795
  for bladder pain, 876, 876f
  for neurogenic bladder, 876, 876f
  for prostate cancer, 3165, 3166, 3223
  for voiding dysfunction, 876, 876f
  tissue engineering and, 2616–2617
General anesthesia. *See* Anesthesia.
Generators, for shock-wave lithotripsy, 3398–3403
  electrohydraulic (spark gap), 3398, 3399t–3401t, 3401f
  electromagnetic, 3398, 3401–3402, 3401f, 3402f
  microexplosive, 3402–3403
  piezoelectric, 3402, 3402f
Genetic anticipation, 1945
Genetic code, definition of, 2626t
Genetic engineering, mouse models and, 2656–2657
Genetic imprinting, 1945
Genetic regulators, in progressive renal failure, 290
Genetics
  and bacteriuria in children, 1859–1860
  as bladder cancer risk factor, 2741, 2767
  classic, 1926
  of urinary lithiasis, 3231
  polymorphisms and. *See* Polymorphism(s).
Genital mutilation, of females, 2436–2437, 2436f
Genital prolapse. *See* Urogenital prolapse.
  in exstrophy patient, 2175

Hematocolpos, in unilateral renal agenesis, 1890, 1891f

Hematolymphoid malignancies, of prostate, ultrasound appearance of, 3048

Hematoma(s)
  in artificial sphincter implantation, 1192
  in hydrocelectomy, 1580
  in hypospadias repair, 2321
  in testicular biopsy, 1537
  perineal, in children, 1825
  postvasectomy, 1546
  postvasography, 1540
  postvasovasostomy, 1555–1556
  retroperitoneal, percutaneous drainage of, 3347, 3347f

Hematospermia
  in genitourinary tuberculosis, 751
  in patient history, 90

Hematuria, 100–104, 902
  after renal transplantation, 367–368
  anticoagulant-induced, 103
  benign familial, 1841
  benign recurrent, 1841
  conditions mimicking, 1834, 1835t
  definition of, 1834
  differential diagnosis of, 101
  dipstick identification of, 100–101
  evaluation of, 101
  exercise-induced, 103
  following transurethral resection, 2823
  from upper urinary tract, ureteroscopic evaluation of, 3316–3317
  glomerular, 101, 101t, 102f
  gross
    in children, 1826–1827, 1835
      causes of, 1826, 1827f, 1837
    in neonate, evaluation of, 1813
  in Alport's syndrome, 1840
  in benign prostatic hyperplasia, 1325
    medical therapy and, 1346–1347
  in bladder cancer, 2753–2754, 2770
  in children, 1834–1836, 1837–1841
    conditions mimicking, 1834, 1835t
    differential diagnosis of, 1837–1841, 1839f
    etiology of, 1837
    evaluation of, 1812, 1817
      algorithm for, 1826, 1827f, 1837–1841, 1838f
    gross, 1826–1827, 1835
      etiology of, 1826, 1827f, 1837
    in acute tubulointerstitial nephritis, 1843
    laboratory evaluation of, algorithm for, 1827f
    microscopic, 1826–1827
      definition of, 1835, 1837
      etiology of, 1826, 1827f, 1837
      evaluation of, 1818
      prevalence of, 1837
      with proteinuria, 1826–1827
    red blood cell morphology in, 1835f, 1835–1836, 1836f
    with dysmorphic red blood cells, 1835–1836, 1836f, 1838–1841
    with eumorphic red blood cells, 1835f, 1835–1836, 1837–1838
    with glomerular bleeding, 1835–1836, 1836f
    with nonglomerular bleeding, 1835f, 1835–1836
    with ureterocele, 2024
  in genitourinary tuberculosis, 751
  in IgA nephropathy, 101–102

Hematuria *(Continued)*
  in neonates
    evaluation of, 1813
    management of, 1805–1806
    urologic emergency and, 1800t
  in patient history, 85–86
  in schistosomiasis, 768
  in sickle-cell nephropathy, 1841
  in systemic lupus erythematosus, 1840
  in ureteral trauma, 3717
  microscopic
    definition of, 1835
    familial form of, 1841
    in children, 1826–1827
      causes of, 1826, 1827f, 1837
      definition of, 1835, 1837
      evaluation of, 1818
      prevalence of, 1837
      with proteinuria, 1826–1827
    in cystitis, 531
  nonglomerular (essential)
    medical, 102–103, 103f
    surgical, 103–104, 104f
    ureteropelvic junction obstruction and, 1998–2000
  vs. hemoglobinuria and myoglobinuria, 100
  with bacillus Calmette-Guérin, 2792
  with benign prostatic hyperplasia, 1424
  with bladder trauma, 3722
  with renal trauma, 3708
  with shock-wave lithotripsy, 3409
  with ureterocele, 2024

Hematuria-dysuria syndrome, following augmentation cystoplasty, 2535

Hemi-Kock procedures, for continent urinary diversion, with valved rectum, 3800–3802, 3801f

Heminephrectomy
  for ectopic ureter, 2018–2022, 2020f
    flank approach to, 2018, 2020f
    laparoscopic, 2019–2021, 2021f
  in duplicated collecting systems, 3614–3615

Hemizona assay, 1497

Hemizygotes, definition of, 2626t

Hemodiafiltration, in acute and chronic renal failure, 300t

Hemodialysis
  for end-stage renal disease, 346
  in acute renal failure, 285, 300t
  in chronic renal failure, 297, 298–299, 298f, 300t
  renal cystic disease with. See Acquired renal cystic disease (ARCD).

Hemodynamic changes, in unilateral ureteral obstruction, mediator involvement in, 436–439

Hemodynamics
  hypercarbia and, 3476
  patient positioning and, 3476
  renal, 169–186. See also Renal hemodynamics.

Hemofilter, tissue engineering of, 2611–2612

Hemofiltration, in acute and chronic renal failure, 300t

Hemolytic-uremic syndrome
  in children, 1840
  in renal transplant recipient, 348, 1840
  prognosis for, 1840
  treatment of, 1840

Hemolytic-uremic syndrome (HUS), in children, diarrheal vs. nondiarrheal, 1840

Hemophilia, blood-borne transmission of viruses in, 705

Hemorrhage
  adrenal, 3508–3509, 3508f
    in neonate, 1806
  as percutaneous nephrostomy complication, 3337–3339
  at sheath site, in laparoscopy, 3487–3488, 3488f
  following renal revascularization, 3632
  from ileal conduit, in urinary diversion, 3772
  in hypospadias repair, 2321
  in urethral trauma, 3725
  intracranial, in autosomal dominant polycystic kidney disease, 1946–1947
  postoperative, in children, evaluation of, 1812
  renal
    with renal trauma, 3713–3714
    with shock-wave lithotripsy, 3410, 3410f, 3413–3414, 3413f, 3414f
  retroperitoneal, during nephrectomy, management of, 3593–3595, 3595f, 3596f
  with circumcision, 3905
  with intestinal anastomoses, 3759
  with laparoscopic renal surgery, 3680
  with percutaneous nephrolithotomy, 3430
  with radical retropubic prostatectomy, 3126, 3127
  with transrectal ultrasound, 3043

Hemorrhagic cystitis
  acute, in children, 1872
  after renal transplantation, 370

Hemostasis
  in hypospadias repair, 2301–2302
  in laparoscopic surgery, 2576–2577, 3467

Henoch-Schönlein purpura
  in children, 1839–1840
    renal involvement in, 1839–1840
  renal involvement in, 1840–1841
  scrotal swelling due to, 2383
  signs and symptoms of, 1816t

Heparin
  of prostate, 1244
  priapism caused by, 1612t

Heparin lavage, for interstitial cystitis, 656

Heparin-binding EGF, in congenital obstructive uropathy, 1790t

Hepatic artery, 6
  injury of, during renal revascularization, 3635

Hepatic dysfunction, in renal cell carcinoma, 2697

Hepatic vein, 9, 14f

Hepatitis
  sexually-transmitted, 687, 687t
  testing for, prior to renal transplantation, 349

Hepatitis A, 687

Hepatitis B, 687

Hepatitis B surface antigenemia, membranous nephropathy with, in children, 1843

Hepatitis B virus, cancer related to, 2652

Hepatobiliary system, anomalies of, in prune-belly syndrome, 2122

Hepatoblastoma, 1822

Hepatocyte growth factor, in renal cell carcinoma, 2691

Hepatocyte growth factor/scatter factor (HGF/SF), 1271

Hepatorenal bypass, 3622–3623, 3623f, 3624f

Hepatorenal ligament, 22

Hepatorenal syndrome, 274. See also Azotemia, prerenal.

HER-2/neu protein, 333

Herbal remedy(ies), for erectile dysfunction, 1620

Hereditary nonpolyposis colorectal cancer, 2632t, 2635

Hereditary spastic paraplegia, voiding dysfunction in, 942–943

Hermaphroditism, true, 2409–2411, 2410f

Hernia(s)
abdominal wall, in children, 1816t
as laparoscopic surgery contraindication, 3458
cryptorchidism and, 2364–2365
incisional
following laparoscopic surgery, 3489
laparoscopic repair of, 3703
inguinal, 2378–2379
and hypospadias, association of, 2290–2291
in children, 1816t
evaluation of, 1817
in epispadias patient, 2182
in exstrophy patient, 2141
indirect, 1758, 1761
internal, in children, 1816t
laparoscopic evaluation of, 2575, 2575f
parastomal, laparoscopic repair of, 3703
repair, orchialgia after, 1582
sliding, 2047
ultrasound examination of, 1828
umbilical, with bladder exstrophy, 2141

Hernia uteri inguinale, 1754, 2420

Herpes simplex virus (HSV)
infection with. See Herpesvirus infection.
testing for, prior to renal transplantation, 349
types I and II, in genital ulcers, 681t

Herpes zoster, and motor paralytic bladder, 895

Herpes zoster virus, voiding dysfunction caused by, 955

Herpesvirus infection
genital, 680–683, 681t
clinical course of, 681–682
diagnosis of, 682
presentation of, 680
treatment of, 682–683, 682t
of penis, 739f
voiding dysfunction caused by, 955
vs. cystitis, 574

Heterocyclic antidepressants, erectile dysfunction caused by, 1609

Heterozygotes, definition of, 2626t

Hidden penis, 2339–2340, 2339f

Hidradenitis suppurativa, of male genitalia, 724–725

Hinman syndrome, 958
clinical features of, 2263–2264, 2264f–2267f
etiology of, 2265
treatment of, 2265–2267, 2268f
urodynamic diagnosis of, 2264
uropathology of, 2262–2263

Hip dysplasia, with ptosis of eyelids and diastasis recti, cryptorchidism associated with, 2368t

Hirschsprung's disease, in prune-belly syndrome, 2122

Histamine, effect of, on ureteral function, 401–402

Histamine (H_2) antagonists, interactions of, with azoles, 819t

Histiocytes, 312

Histocompatibility antigens, in renal allograft rejection, 363, 363t, 364f

Histones, acetylation or deacetylation of, androgen receptor and, 1258f, 1260–1261

Histoplasmosis
genitourinary manifestations of, 814
predisposing factors for, 813–814
treatment of, 814–815, 821t

History, patient. See Patient history.

HIV. See Human immunodeficiency virus (HIV).

Hives (urticaria), 716

hKLK3 gene, 1280

HLAs (human leukocyte antigens)
classes of, 314–315
in renal allograft rejection, 363, 363t
in urinary tract infection, 526–527

HMG-CoA reductase drugs, for chronic renal failure, 295

Holmium laser, for intracorporeal lithotripsy, 2567

Holmium:yttrium-aluminum-garnet (Ho:YAG) laser, 1395–1396
prostatectomy with, 1398, 1399f
clinical results of, 1402

Holt-Oram syndrome, multisystem involvement in, 1814t

Homatropine, 968

Homeobox genes
in genital development, 1239, 1758
in male gonadal development, 1756

Homing, of immune cells, 309

Homogeneous nucleation, 3235

Homophilic adhesion, in T cell-endothelial cell interactions, 331

Homozygotes, definition of, 2626t

Hormonal therapy
before hypospadias repair, 2294–2295
timing of, 2294–2295
for cryptorchidism, 2369–2370
for endometriosis, 425
for prostate cancer, 3182–3204
5α-reductase inhibition for, 3200
adjuvant, 3202–3203
antiandrogens in, 3195–3199
dosage, side effects, and prospective studies of, 3196–3197
maximal androgen blockade using, 3197–3199
mechanism of action of, 3195, 3195t
pure, as monotherapy, 3196
steroidal, as monotherapy, 3195–3196
end points for, 3184–3187, 3184t
prognostic factors and response criteria and, 3184–3186, 3185t
prostate-specific antigen and, 3186
quality of life and, 3186–3187
endocrine dependence/independence and, 3182–3184, 3183f
androgen sources and withdrawal mechanisms and, 3183–3184, 3183f
growth factors and angiogenesis control and, 3184
intermittent, 3203–3204
method(s) of, 3190–3195
medical castration as, 3191, 3193–3195
surgical castration as, 3190–3191, 3191t, 3192f
node-positive, 3099
patient population and, changes in, 3187–3188
PC-SPES for, 3199–3200
response and progression and, 3188–3189
second-line, 3203
side effects of, 3189–3190
step-up, 3204
survival and, 3188, 3189f
timing of, 3200–3203
ultrasound appearance following, 3047
for prostatitis, 621, 624t
for renal cell carcinoma, metastatic, 2715
for stress incontinence, 1074–1076, 1075f

Hormone(s). See also specific hormone, e.g., Follicle-stimulating hormone (FSH).
in male sexual differentiation, 2354
in renal hemodynamics, 172–175
laparoscopic surgery and, 3476
neural, in male sexual function, 1602–1604
pituitary, in male reproductive axis, 1438–1439
prostate cancer resistant to, chemotherapy for. See Chemotherapy, for prostate cancer.
role of, in interstitial cystitis, 645–646

Hormone response element, and androgen action, 1260–1261

Horseshoe kidney, 1743, 1903–1906, 2046
anomalies associated with, 1905
blood supply to, 1904f, 1904–1905
diagnosis of, 1905f, 1905–1906
embryology of, 1903f, 1903–1904, 1904f
features of, 1904–1905
in exstrophy patient, 2145
incidence of, 1903
isthmusectomy for, 3638–3639
multicystic dysplastic kidney in, 1961, 1962f
percutaneous nephrolithotomy with, 3428–3429
prenatal diagnosis of, 1905
prognosis for, 1906
signs and symptoms of, 1905
tumors in, 1906
ureteropelvic junction obstruction with, 1905, 1998, 1999f
urolithiasis in, 3373

Hospitalization, for chronic renal failure, risk of, 299–300, 299t

Host defense, altered, in bacterial prostatitis, 607

Hot flashes, as side effect of hormone therapy, 3190

Hounsfield units, 141, 141t

HPV. See Human papillomavirus (HPV).

HSV. See Herpes simplex virus (HVS).

HTLV-1 (human T-lymphoproliferative virus type 1), 694

HTLV-2 (human T-lymphoproliferative virus type 2), 694

Human chorionic gonadotropin (hCG)
for cryptorchidism, 2369–2370
for hypospadias repair, 2294
in testicular germ cell tumors, 2887–2888

Human immunodeficiency virus (HIV)
biology of, 693–695
characteristics of, 694–695, 696f
genes of, 694–695, 695f
identification of, 694
infection with. See also Acquired immunodeficiency syndrome (AIDS).
antiretroviral therapy for, 699–700, 699t
combination of agents in, 700
as contraindication in renal transplantation, 349
avoidance of, education in, 699
classification of, 702–703, 702t
clinical spectrum and progression of, 702
deficient cell-mediated immunity in, 701–702
diagnosis of, 701, 701f
epidemiology of, 703–705
hypothetical course of, 698, 698f
natural history of, 701–702
non-nucleoside reverse transcriptase inhibitors for, 699f, 700

Human immunodeficiency virus (HIV)
(*Continued*)
nucleoside reverse transcriptase inhibitors
for, 699–700, 699f
pathogenesis of, 696–698
CD4+ T cell count in, 697
cell-mediated immune response in, 697–
698
lymphoid involvement in, 698
production of virus from infected cells in,
696–697
replication, error rates, and molecular determinants in, 697
role of monocyte-macrophage lineage in,
696
protease inhibitors for, 699f, 700
testing for, 711–712
basic concepts in, 711
wider indications in
arguments against, 712
arguments favoring, 711–712
vaccines against, 699
life cycle of, 694, 695f
origins of, 695
postexposure prophylaxis for, 710–711
removal from semen, 1516
transmission of, 703–705
blood-borne, 704–705
cervical secretions in, 710
heterosexual, 703–704
homosexual, 703
in commercial sex workers, 705
in hemophiliacs, 705
in prison populations, 705
intravenous, 704–705
occupational, 705, 710
perinatal, 705
protection against, 710
semen in, 709–710
sexual, 703–704
risk factors for, 704
unproven modes of, 705
via organ transplantation, 705
via transfusion, 705
type 1 (HIV-1), 694
antiretroviral strategies of, 698–699
genome of, 694–695
isolates of, 697
replication of, 697
type 2 (HIV-2), 694
Human kallikrein 2
activity of, 1279t, 1280
properties of, 1279t, 1280
Human kallikrein-L1
activity of, 1279t
properties of, 1279t, 1280–1281
Human leukocyte antigens (HLAs)
classes of, 314–315
in Reiter's syndrome, 717
in renal allograft rejection, 363, 363t
in urinary tract infection, 526–527
Human papillomavirus (HPV)
as bladder cancer risk factor, 2740
cancer related to, 2652–2653
penile, 2951
in genital warts, 685
penile, 2947–2948
giant condyloma acuminatum due to, 2949–
2950
Human serum albumin, in plasma transport of
testosterone, 1246f, 1249
Human T cell leukemia viruses, cancer related
to, 2652

Human T-lymphoproliferative virus type 1
(HTLV-1), 694
Human T-lymphoproliferative virus type 2
(HTLV-2), 694
Humoral hypercalcemia of malignancy, 3247–
3248
Humoral immune response, 309
Hunner's ulcer, 646f, 648, 649f
transurethral resection of, 657
Hyaluronic acid
in bladder cancer, 2757
of prostate, 1244
Hyaluronic acid and dextranomer microspheres,
for injection therapy, 1183
Hyaluronic acid lavage, for interstitial cystitis,
656
Hyaluronidase, in bladder cancer, 2757
Hybridization, definition of, 2626t
Hydantoin, fetal exposure to, hypospadias with,
2292t
Hydatid cysts, of seminal vesicles, 3877
Hydatid disease, 786–788, 787f, 788f
Hydatid sand, 787f
Hydralazine, priapism caused by, 1612
Hydration, of neonate, 1772, 1772f
Hydraulic valves, for continent urinary diversion, 2550
Hydrocalycosis, 1913–1914, 1914f
Hydrocele, 2377–2379
abdominoscrotal, 2379
after varicocelectomy, 1576–1577
and hypospadias, association of, 2290–2291
asymptomatic, in children, evaluation of, 1818
communicating, 2378–2379
evaluation of, 1817
in filariasis, 782f, 782–783, 784
in infants, 2377–2378
in neonates, 1801
of cord, 2379
parasitic, 763
repair of. *See* Hydrocelectomy.
sclerotherapy for, 1580
simple, 2377–2378
testicular, 96
ultrasound examination of, 1828
with laparoscopy, 3488
Hydrocelectomy, 1579–1581
complications of, 1581
dartos pouch technique for, 1580
excisional techniques for, 1579–1580, 1580f
inguinal approach to, 1579
Jaboulay bottleneck operation for, 1579, 1579f
Lord's plication technique for, 1579, 1580f
methods of, 1579
plication techniques for, 1580, 1580f
scrotal approach to, 1579
window operation for, 1580, 1580f
Hydrocephalus, normal pressure, voiding dysfunction with, 939
Hydrocephaly, 1822
Hydrochlorothiazide
for nephrogenic diabetes insipidus, 1844
for urinary lithiasis, 3281, 3282t
Hydrocolpos
in female neonate, 1802
in unilateral renal agenesis, 1890
Hydrocortisone
for congenital adrenal hyperplasia, 2414
for prostate cancer, 3217t
Hydrogen ion, metabolism of, 3241–3242,
3242f
Hydrolethalus syndrome, hypospadias with,
2292t

Hydrometrocolpos, signs and symptoms of,
1822
Hydronephrosis. *See also* Ureteral obstruction.
after complete primary exstrophy repair, 2205
after renal transplantation, 368–369, 370f
and Down's syndrome, 1789
bilateral
resulting from gravid uterus, 423, 423f
secondary to fibroid uterus, 426f
chronic, nephrogenic diabetes insipidus caused
by, 1844
congenital
diagnosis of, 2000–2001
imaging of, 2000–2001
definition of, 412
detrusor leak point pressure and, 1041
excretory urography of, 421f
experimental, 440
fetal, 1786–1787
and vesicoureteral reflux, 2054–2055
diagnostic workup for, 2062f, 2062–2063
bilateral, postnatal evaluation and management of, 1796–1797
management of, 1793
postnatal evaluation and management of,
1796, 1796t
sex distribution of, 1792
ultrasound appearance of, 1781–1783,
1782t, 1782f, 1783f
unilateral, postnatal evaluation and management of, 1797–1799
following cryotherapy, for prostate cancer,
3180
hypertension and, management of, 433–434
in children, signs and symptoms of, 1816t
in congenital obstructive uropathy, 1789
in endometriosis, 424, 425f
in infants
and growth of contralateral normal kidney,
2000
diagnosis of, 2000
in neonates
clinical features of, 1822
evaluation of patient with, 1812–1813
in nephrogenic diabetes insipidus, 1844
in prune-belly syndrome, 2118, 2123
in schistosomiasis, 777f, 777–779
in spina bifida, 1814
in VATER association, 1998
incidence of, 412
infected, 560
pathophysiology of, 911
physiologic, 1789
prenatal
diagnostic pitfalls in, 1789
evaluation of, 1818–1819, 2000
postnatal evaluation of, 1817
severity of, 1783, 1783f, 1789–1790
ultrasonography of, 134, 413–414
upper pole, with ureterocele, ultrasound of,
2024, 2024f
uterine prolapse associated with, 426
with bilateral single-system ectopic ureters,
2020, 2022f
with cloacal exstrophy, 2177
with ectopic ureter, 2014
with posterior urethral valves, 2215, 2215f,
2216f
with preureteral vena cava, 2044
with ureteral duplication, 2041
with ureterocele, 2023–2024, 2026f
Hydroureter
fetal, ultrasound appearance of, 1783, 1783f

Hydroureter *(Continued)*
  in schistosomiasis, 777f, 777–779
    atonic, 778
    tonic, 778
  with cloacal exstrophy, 2177
  with ectopic ureter, 2014
α-Hydroxy acids, polymers of, for tissue engi-
    neering, 2597
17α-Hydroxycortisone, for benign prostatic hy-
    perplasia
  dosage and administration of, 1359t
  mechanism of action of, 1359t
11β-Hydroxylase deficiency, congenital adrenal
    hyperplasia due to, 2413
17α-Hydroxylase deficiency, 2416
21-Hydroxylase deficiency, congenital adrenal
    hyperplasia due to, 2412, 2412f, 2413
3β-Hydroxysteroid dehydrogenase, deficiency of,
    hypospadias in, 2288
3β-Hydroxysteroid dehydrogenase deficiency,
    2416
  congenital adrenal hyperplasia due to, 2413–
    2414
17β-Hydroxysteroid oxidoreductase deficiency,
    2416–2417
Hydroxyzine
  for interstitial cystitis, 653
  priapism caused by, 1612t
Hylagel Uro, as agent for injection therapy,
    1183
Hymen, 1711
  configurations of, in children and adolescents,
    1825, 1825f
  embryology of, 1756
  imperforate, 1824, 2440–2441, 2440f, 2441f
    evaluation of, 1818
    in female neonate, 1802
  skin tags of, 2440, 2440f
Hyoscyamine
  for urge incontinence, in elderly, 1228
  uropharmacology of, 2235t
L-Hyoscyamine, 969
Hyoscyamine sulfate, 969
Hyperacute rejection, of renal allograft, 363–364
Hyperaldosteronism, primary, 3531–3540
  clinical characteristics of, 3535–3536, 3535t
  diagnostic strategy for, 3538–3539
  diagnostic studies in, 3536–3538, 3536f
    lateralizing, 3537–3538, 3538t
    screening using, 3536–3537
  pathophysiology of, 3532–3535, 3533f, 3534f
  treatment of, 3539
Hypercalcemia
  glucocorticoid-induced, 3248
  granulomatous disease association of, 3248
  hypocalciuric, familial, 3248
  iatrogenic, 3249
  immobilization related to, 3249
  in hyperthyroidism, 3248
  in renal cell carcinoma, 2696
  malignancy-associated, 3247–3248, 3247t
  nephrogenic diabetes insipidus caused by,
    1844
  treatment of, 3249
  with pheochromocytoma, 3248
Hypercalciuria
  absorptive, 3243–3244, 3244f
  calcium oxalate stone formation associated
    with, 3243–3246, 3244f, 3245t
  idiopathic, 3245–3246, 3245t
  in children
    conditions associated with, 1838
    hematuria in, 1838

Hypercalciuria *(Continued)*
  management of, 1838
  nephrolithiasis with, 1838
  screening for, 1837, 1838
  urinary calcium/urinary creatinine (Uca/Ucr)
    ratio in, 1837, 1838
  in neonates, 1771
  renal, 3244–3245, 3244f
  resorptive, 3245
Hypercarbia, laparoscopic surgery and, 3476
Hyperchloremic metabolic acidosis, 216, 216t
  glomerular filtration rate in, 218
  with conduit urinary diversion, 3778–3779
Hypercholesterolemia, erectile dysfunction in,
    1608, 1609
Hyperglycemia
  in diabetes mellitus, and voiding dysfunction,
    956–957
  in early kidney graft dysfunction, 365–366,
    368t
Hyperkalemia
  clinical evaluation of, 193f
  etiology of, 192t
  in renal tubular acidosis, in children, 1771
Hyperlipidemia, erectile dysfunction caused by,
    1610
Hypermethylation, of DNA, 2631–2632
Hypernatremia, 207–210, 208f
  diagnosis and evaluation of, 209, 210f
  electrolyte abnormalities in, 208, 209f
  in diabetes insipidus, 208, 209t
  treatment of, 209–210
Hyperoxaluria, 3249–3252, 3249t
  enteric, 3251
  metabolic, mild, 3251–3252
  overproduction of
    in primary hyperoxaluria, 3249–3250,
      3250f
    increased hepatic conversion causing, 3250
Hyperparathyroidism, primary, renal calculi as-
    sociated with, 3246–3247
Hyperpigmentation, of male genitalia, 728
Hyperplasia, fibromuscular, of renal artery, 231t,
    234–235
Hyperprolactinemia
  causes of, 1637
  erectile dysfunction in, 1503, 1637
    androgen therapy and, 1651
  in males, 1503
    infertility caused by, 1439, 1503
    sexual dysfunction caused by, 1503, 1607
  in females, 1719
Hyperpyrexia, in children, 1820, 1820t
Hypertelorism-hypospadias syndrome, 2292t
Hypertension
  after renal transplantation, 372–373
  and benign prostatic hyperplasia, 1312
  and erectile dysfunction, 1610, 1624
  anesthesia-related, with laparoscopic surgery,
    3490
  definition of, 230–231
  following renal revascularization, 3631–3632
  hydronephrosis and, management of, 433–434
  in autonomic hyperreflexia, 950–951
  in children
    classification of, by age group, 1834,
      1834t
    in renal disease, 1834
  in chronic renal failure, 291
    control of, 294–295
  in neonates, 1806
    urologic emergency and, 1800t
  in renal cell carcinoma, 2696–2697

Hypertension *(Continued)*
  in ureteropelvic junction obstruction, 2000
  multicystic dysplastic kidney and, 1964
  pyelonephritogenic, in children, 1855–1856
  reflux nephropathy and, 2071
  renovascular, 230–261. *See also* Renovascular
    hypertension.
  with benign prostatic hyperplasia, α-adrener-
    gic blockers for, 1357–1358
  with pheochromocytoma, 3540
  with renal trauma, 3714–3715
Hyperthermia
  as angiogenesis inhibitor, 2654
  microwave, for prostatitis, 622–623
Hyperthyroidism
  erectile dysfunction in, 1607
  hypercalcemia in, 3248
  male infertility with, 1503
  voiding dysfunction in, 961
Hypertrophied column of Bertin, 1917, 1917f
Hyperuricemia, in sickle-cell nephropathy, 1841
Hyperuricosuria, 3252
Hypoactive sexual desire disorder
  definition of, 1718
  female, studies of, recommendations of Inter-
    national Consensus Development Panel
    on, 1724
Hypocalciuric hypercalcemia, familial, 3248
Hypocitraturia, 3252–3253, 3253t
Hypogastric nerve, 1711
Hypogastric plexus
  inferior, 56, 56f, 1711
  superior, 55, 56f, 1711
Hypogonadism
  and erectile dysfunction, hormonal therapy
    for, 1649–1651
  hypergonadotropic, 1607
    micropenis in, 2341
  hypogonadotropic, 1607
    anabolic steroid-induced, 1477
    congenital, with anosmia, 1438, 1500–1501
    idiopathic, 1500–1501
    in Kallmann's syndrome, 1477
    isolated, 1500–1501
    testicular biopsy findings in, 1499–1500
Hypohidrotic ectodermal dysplasia, autosomal
    dominant type, hypospadias with, 2292t
Hypokalemia
  clinical evaluation of, 193f
  etiology of, 191t
  in Bartter's syndrome, 1844
  in metabolic acidosis, 217–218
  in primary hyperaldosteronism, 3536
  in renovascular hypertension, 241
  nephrogenic diabetes insipidus caused by,
    1844
  with conduit urinary diversion, 3779
Hypomagnesuria, 3253–3254
Hypomelia-hypotrichosis-facial hemangioma
    syndrome, hypospadias with, 2292t
Hyponatremia, 203–207, 204f
  defined, 203
  diagnosis of, 206
  dilutional, with transurethral resection of pros-
    tate, 1423
  diuretics in, 204–205
  in syndrome of inappropriate antidiuretic hor-
    mone secretion, 206, 206t
  postoperative, 205–206
  treatment of, 206–207, 207f
  with increased plasma osmolality, 204
  with normal body volume, 205
  with normal plasma osmolality, 203–204

Hysterectomy (Continued)
  pseudoincontinence after, 1196
  sexual function after, 1729
  vesicovaginal fistula caused by, 1196
Hysteresis, of smooth muscle, 386f, 387, 394, 394f
Hytrin. See Terazosin.

Iatrogenic calculi, 3266
Ibuprofen
  acute tubulointerstitial nephritis caused by, 1843
  and aplastic anemia, 1820
  antipyretic therapy with, for children, 1820
IC351, 1654
ICDB (Interstitial Cystitis Data Base) study eligibility criteria, 633t
Ice-water test
  bladder, 857
  in spinal cord-injured patient, indications for, 871
  negative, 910
  positive, 910
  technique for, 910
  with lower motor neuron lesion, 910
  with upper motor neuron lesion, 910
Idazoxan, uropharmacology of, 867
Idiopathic hypercalciuria, 3245–3246, 3245t
Idiotope, of antigen-binding site, 313
IDS-89. See Sabal serrulata.
Ifosfamide, for nonseminomatous germ cell tumors, 2904
Ifosfamide toxicity, in children, 1844
IgA (immunoglobulin A)
  in children, and urinary tract infection, 1861
  in prostatitis, 608
  secretion of, 309
IgA nephropathy (Berger's disease)
  hematuria in, 101–102
  in chronic renal failure, 291
IgE (immunoglobulin E), in interstitial cystitis, 639
IgG (immunoglobulin G)
  in prostatitis, 618
  schematic diagram of, 313f
IIEF. See International Index of Erectile Function (IIEF).
IIQ. See Incontinence Impact Questionnaire (IIQ).
IL. See Interleukin (IL) entries.
Ileal antireflux valves, intussuscepted, 3768–3769, 3769f
"Ileal break," with conduit urinary diversion, 3782
Ileal conduit
  Candida infection with, 798
  in conduit urinary diversion, 3771–3772
  complications of, 3772, 3774f, 3774t
  procedure for, 3771–3772, 3772f–3774f
Ileal interposition, for upper ureteral injuries, 3719
Ileal neobladder
  Hautmann, 3852–3853, 3853f
  Studer, 3853, 3854f
  T-pouch, 3854, 3856f–3857f, 3857–3858
Ileal pouch, vesical, 3852
Ileal reservoir
  continent, for continent urinary diversion, 3807, 3808f, 3809f
  Kock, orthotopic, 3853, 3855f

Ileal ureteral substitution, in ureteral stricture repair, 500–501, 502f, 503f
Ileal valve, hydraulic, Benchekroun, for continent urinary diversion, 3824–3825
Ileal vesicotomy, in conduit urinary diversion, 3775
Ileocecal conduit, in conduit urinary diversion, 3775, 3777t, 3778t
Ileocecal valves
  for continent urinary diversion, 2550
  intussuscepted, 3768, 3768f
  in ileocecocystoplasty, 2529
Ileocecocystoplasty, 2527–2529
  appendix in, 2527
  ileocecal valve in, 2529
  technique for, 2527, 2527f, 2528f
Ileocolic anastomosis, sutured
  end-to-end, with discrepant bowel sizes, 3754–3755, 3754f
  end-to-side, 3753–3754, 3754f
Ileocolonic pouch, 3858, 3860f
Ileocystoplasty, 2526–2527, 2526f
Ileostomy, loop end, 3761–3762, 3761f
Ileum, for reconstructive surgery, complications with, 3778–3779
Iliac artery, 7, 14f
  aneurysm of
    as laparoscopic surgery contraindication, 3458
    in urinary tract obstruction, 429, 429f
  common, 49, 53f
  external, 49, 53f, 1593, 1594f
  internal (hypogastric), 49, 51, 53f
  preureteral, 2046, 2047f
Iliac crest, 41, 42f
Iliac lymph nodes, 52
Iliac spine, 41, 42f
Iliac vein, 7, 14f
  external, 1594, 1594f
  internal (hypogastric), 52, 54f, 1594, 1594f
Iliacus muscle, 5, 12f
Iliococcygeus muscle, 46, 49f, 1096, 1096f, 1097, 1097f
Iliococcygeus suspension, for vaginal vault prolapse, 1129
Iliohypogastric nerve, 14, 16f, 54
Ilioinguinal lymphadenectomy
  in penile cancer, 2988–2991, 2990f, 2991f
  in squamous penile cancer, 2964–2965
Ilioinguinal nerve, 14, 16f, 54
Iliopsoas fascia, 45
Iliorenal bypass, 3625–3626, 3625f
Ilium, 42f
Image analysis, in bladder cancer, 2754–2755
Imaging modalities. See specific type, e.g., Magnetic resonance imaging (MRI).
Imbibition
  in tissue transfer, 3888
  of free tissue graft, 2299
Imidazoles, 819–821
  drug interactions with, 819, 819t
  for candidiasis, 799, 803–804
Imipramine
  and MAOIs, interactions of, 978
  cardiotoxicity of, 1077
  effects of
    on lower urinary tract, 1077
    on overactive bladder, 1077
  for detrusor overactivity, 1044, 1088
  for enuresis, in children, 1077
  for geriatric incontinence, 1230
  for nocturnal enuresis, 977, 2277

Imipramine (Continued)
  for postprostatectomy incontinence, 1065
  for stress incontinence, 990
  for urge incontinence, in elderly, 1228, 1229t
  for voiding dysfunction, 976
  incontinence caused by, 1038
  uropharmacology of, 858t, 866, 976–977, 2235t
Immobilization, hypercalcemia due to, 3249
Immotile cilia syndrome, 1477, 1479
Immune function
  laparoscopic surgery and, 3476–3477
  renal cell carcinoma and, 2689–2690
Immune modulators, for prostatitis, 620–621
Immune system
  adhesion molecules and lymphocyte trafficking in, 329–331, 330f, 330t
  apoptosis in, 325–327, 326f
  cell populations in, 309–313, 311t
  cell surface activation of, 314–318, 314f, 316f, 317f, 317t
  chemokines and recruitment of leukocytes in, 331–332, 331t
  complement and, 308–309, 309f
  infections affecting, 338–339, 338f
  lymphocyte tolerance in, 327–329
  lymphoid organs and tissues in, 309, 310f
  phagocytosis in, 308
  relationship between testis and, 339–340
  signal transduction in, 318–320, 318f
  T cell activation and effector function in, 320–325, 322f, 323t, 324f
  tumor immunology and, 332–338, 333t, 335f
Immunity
  acquired, 308, 339
  cell-mediated responses to, 309
    in acquired immunodeficiency syndrome, 697–698
    deficient, 701–702
  humoral responses to, 309
  initiation of, 314
  innate, 308
  passive, 339
  primary, 314
  secondary, 314
  to infection, 338–339, 338f
Immunoglobulin(s), 309. See also Antibody(ies).
  cell surface, on B cells, 310–311
  classes of, 312, 313f
  in seminal plasma, 1238, 1282
Immunoglobulin A (IgA)
  in children, and urinary tract infection, 1861
  in prostatitis, 608
  secretion of, 309
Immunoglobulin A (IgA) nephropathy (Berger's disease), 1841
  hematuria in, 101–102
  in children, 1839
  in chronic renal failure, 291
Immunoglobulin E (IgE), in interstitial cystitis, 639
Immunoglobulin G (IgG)
  in prostatitis, 608
  schematic diagram of, 313f
Immunoglobulin superfamily adhesion molecules, 1263
Immunohistochemistry, in cancer, 2658
Immunologic responses, in urinary tract infection, 533–535
Immunoreceptor tyrosine-based activation motif (ITAM), 315
  phosphorylation of, 318–319

Immunoresponsive cell populations, 309–313, 311t
  antibodies in, 312–313, 313f
  antigen-presenting cells in, 312
  granulocytes in, 312
  homing of, 309
  lymphocytes in, 310–312. *See also* B cell(s); Natural killer (NK) cells; T cell(s).
  macrophages in, 312
  monocytes in, 312
  vascular endothelial cells in, 312
Immunosuppressants
  for interstitial cystitis, 652–653
  in renal transplantation, 364–365
    algorithm for, 365, 366f
    effectiveness, morbidity, and costs of, 365, 367t
    infection and peptic ulcer prophylaxis and, 365, 368t
    mechanism of action of, 364t
    potential drug interactions among, 365, 366t
    sites of action of, 365f
    toxicity of, organ system targets for, 365, 367t
  pregnancy safety information concerning, 372t
Immunosuppression
  aspergillosis in, 806
  coccidioidomycosis in, 812
  histoplasmosis in, 814
  zygomycosis in, 810
Immunosuppressive products, secretion of, as mechanism of tumor escape, 335–336, 335f
Immunotherapy
  for prostate cancer, 3166
  for renal cell carcinoma, 2689–2690
    metastatic, 2715–2718, 2716t, 2717t
  for tumors, 336–337
  for urothelial renal pelvis and ureter tumors, adjuvant, 2869–2870, 2869f
Imperforate anus, 2250–2252
  clinical features of, 1825
  evaluation of, 1812, 2251–2252
  findings associated with, 2251, 2252f
  in neonates, management of, 1804
  in prune-belly syndrome, 2122
  omphalocele with, 1822
  prenatal diagnosis of, 1789
  treatment of, 1813
  urodynamic evaluation with, 2251–2252
Imperforate hymen, 1824, 2440–2441, 2440f, 2441f
  evaluation of, 1818
Impotence. *See also* Detumescence; Erectile dysfunction; *Penile erection*; Priapism.
  in end-stage renal disease, 351
  in patient history, 89
  NIH Consensus Conference on, 1620
  postprostatectomy, and quality of life, 1055
Impress (urethral meatal device), for stress incontinence, 1078
In vitro fertilization (IVF), 1515, 1515t
  efficacy of, 1517
  indications for, 1515, 1516–1517
  methods for, 1516–1517
  sperm retrieval for, 1517–1518
  with intracytoplasmic sperm injection, 1533
    costs of, 1571
    indications for, 1571
    sperm retrieval for, 1566, 1567, 1569
    technique for, 1570, 1570f
Incest, 1824
Incidence, definition of, 1307

"Incidentalomas," 3523–3525, 3524f, 3525t
Incisional hernia(s), following laparoscopic surgery, 3489
Inconspicuous penis, 2338–2340
  concealed (buried; hidden), 2339–2340, 2339f, 3901
  trapped, 2340, 2340f
  webbed, 2339, 2339f
Incontinence, 87–89. *See also* Stress incontinence; Voiding dysfunction.
  after pelvic surgery, 955
  after urethrovaginal fistula repair, 1206–1207
  anal, in exstrophy patient, 2142
  and depression, 1069
  and interstitial cystitis, 635, 636f
  as symptom, sign, and condition, 1027, 1029
  behavioral therapy for, 966–967
  causes of, 832, 832f
    definite, 1027, 1029
    presumed, 1027, 1029
  childhood
    with ectopic ureterocele, 2024
    with recurrent urinary tract infections, 1858–1859
      management of, 1872
  classification of, 1029–1031
  continuous, 87–88, 902
    in females, ectopic ureter and, 2014
  definition of, International Continence Society, 1029
  diagnostic evaluation of, 1037–1043
  drug-induced, 1038
  effect of, on quality of life, assessment of, 1107–1108
  epidemiology of, 1092–1095
  extraurethral, 1029
    signs and symptoms of, 1030t
  geriatric. *See* Geriatric patients, incontinence in.
  giggle, 2272
  grading of, 1179, 1179t
  impact of, 1069–1070
  in benign prostatic hyperplasia, 1325
  in cerebral palsy, 939
  in dementia, 938
  in females
    cure of, definition of, 1148
    ectopic ureter and, 2014
    prevalence of, 1027
    retropubic suspension surgery for, 1140–1149
    risk factors for, 1104, 1104t
    surgery for
      comparison of procedures for, 1148–1149
      follow-up after, duration of, 1148
      intrinsic sphincteric deficiency and, 1148
    with genital prolapse, 1042–1043
    with urethral diverticula, 1208
  in herpes zoster infection, 955
  in HIV-infected patients, 943
  in males
    prevalence of, 1027
    sling procedures for, 1153
  in neurospinal dysraphism, 952
  in patient history, 87–89
  in pregnancy, 1094
  in schistosomiasis, 780, 944
  in schizophrenia, 961–962
  in spinal shock, 945
  in stroke patient, 937
  in tethered cord syndrome, 953
  incidence of, 1093, 1093f

Incontinence (*Continued*)
  male-to-female ratio of, 1070
  mixed
    definition of, 901, 1047
    primary component of, determination of, 1089
    treatment of, 1047
      nonsurgical, 1088–1089
  neuropathic, 891
  nonneurogenic, in males, urodynamic evaluation of, 905
  outlet-related, in males, pathophysiology of, 892
  overflow, 89
    definition of, 901
    in elderly, 1219, 1223, 1226
      treatment of, 1227t
    postprostatectomy, 1057
    signs and symptoms of, 1030
  paradoxical, with urethral diverticula, 1208
  parity and, 1094
  persistent
    after injection therapy, 1181
    with artificial sphincter implantation, 1192
  posthysterectomy, 1094–1095
  postprostatectomy, 1053–1066
    age and, 1059
    ancillary testing in, 1061
    and quality of life, 1053–1055
    bladder dysfunction in, 1056
      and sphincter dysfunction, relative contributions of, 1057–1058, 1058t
      treatment of, 1063
    cystoscopy in, 1063
    evaluation of, 1060–1063
    history-taking in, 1060
    in elderly, 1222–1223
    in myasthenia gravis, 962
    incidence of, 1053–1055
    injection therapy for, 1175, 1178, 1183
      results of, 1179
    pathogenesis of, 1056–1058
    physical examination in, 1060–1061
    preoperative incontinence and, 1059
    prior TURP and, 1059
    radiation therapy and, 1059
    radiologic evaluation in, 1063
    risk factors for, 1058–1059
    severity of, determination of, 1060
    sling procedures for, 1153
    sphincter dysfunction in, 1056–1057
      and bladder dysfunction, relative contributions of, 1057–1058, 1058t
      treatment of, 1063–1065
    treatment of, 1047, 1063–1065. *See also* Artificial sphincter.
    prognostic factors in, 1062–1063
    urodynamic evaluation in, 1061–1063, 1062f, 1063f
  prevalence of, 1027, 1069
    by age group, 1093, 1093f
    in relation to definition of, 1093, 1093f
  recurrent, with artificial sphincter implantation, 1192
  remission rates for, 1093
  severity of, quantitation of, 902–903
  sphincteric, 1034–1036. *See also* Stress incontinence.
    and intrinsic sphincteric deficiency, 1030–1031
    artificial sphincter for, 1188. *See also* Artificial sphincter.
    electrical stimulation for, 988

Interferon-γ (INF-γ)
  antitumor response of, 332–333
  in cell-mediated immune response, 321–322
  in tumor regression, 336
Interlabial mass(es), 2438–2440
  introital cysts as, 2439–2440, 2439f
  labial adhesions as, 2438–2439, 2439f
Interleukin (IL)
  cellular source and activities of, 323t
  in allergic and immune responses, 322–323, 324f
  in Jak signaling pathway, 320
  in tuberculosis treatment, 756
Interleukin-1 (IL-1)
  in nonbacterial prostatitis, 617
  in septic shock, 570
Interleukin-2 (IL-2)
  antitumor response of, 333
  for bladder cancer, superficial, 2795
  for renal cell carcinoma, metastatic, 2716–2717, 2716t
  in renal allograft rejection, 363
  in tumor regression, 336
Interleukin-4 (IL-4), T cell development and, 322
Interleukin-8 (IL-8), in septic shock, 570
Interleukin-10 (IL-10), in septic shock, 570
Interleukin-12 (IL-12)
  antitumor response of, 333
  T cell development and, 322
Interleukin-converting enzyme (ICE), in regulation of cell death, 1276
Intermediate junctions, in cell-to-cell contact, 378
International Classification of Disease (ICD-10)
  classification of sexual dysfunction, 1717
  definition of sexual dysfunction, 1717
International Continence Society
  BPH study of, 915
  classification of voiding dysfunction by, 896t, 896–897
  definition of incontinence by, 1029
  male symptom questionnaire of, 902
  nomenclature of, for pressure-flow micturition studies, 916f, 917–919
  provisional nomogram for analysis of voiding by, 921f, 921–922
  quality of life instrument of, 902
International Index of Erectile Function (IIEF), 1623
International Prostate Symptom Score (I-PSS), 87, 88t, 902, 1309, 1340
International Reflux Study in Children, 2079–2081, 2081t
Intersex condition(s)
  genital reconstruction for, 2428
  laparoscopic evaluation of, 2574–2575, 2574t
  surgical reconstruction of, 2428, 2449–2460
    for high vaginal confluence, 2453–2456, 2454f–2457f
    for low vaginal confluence with clitoral hypertrophy, 2451, 2452f, 2453, 2453f
    initial management, timing, and principles of, 2449–2451, 2450f
    results of, 2460
    total urogenital mobilization as, 2457–2460, 2457f–2459f
  urogenital sinus in, 2443, 2443f
Intersex state, 1478
  clinical features of, 1824
  evaluation for, 2291
  gonadal examination in, 1823
  hypospadias and, 2291

InterStim device, for overactive bladder, 1081–1083
Interstitial cell tumors, testicular, 2905–2906
Interstitial cystitis, 631–660. *See also* Cystitis, interstitial.
Interstitial Cystitis Data Base (ICDB) study eligibility criteria, 633t
Interstitial laser coagulation, 1423
Interstitial nephritis, in acute renal failure, 275–276, 275t
Intervertebral disc(s)
  disease of, voiding dysfunction with, 933t, 953–954
  herniation of, priapism in, 1611
Intestinal anastomosis, 3751–3762
  complications of, 3757–3759, 3758t, 3759f
  stapled, 3755–3757, 3755f, 3756f
    ileal-ileal, end-to-end, 3756, 3756f
    ileocolonic
      end-to-end, 3756, 3756f
      with circular stapling device, 3755–3756, 3755f
  sutured
    ileocolic, end-to-side, 3753–3754, 3754f
    ileocolonic
      end-to-end, with discrepant bowel sizes, 3754–3755, 3754f
      end-to-side, 3753–3754, 3754f
    single-layer, 3753, 3753f
    two-layer, 3752–3753, 3753f
  ureterointestinal, 3762–3770
    complications of, 3769–3770
    intestinal antireflux valves and, 3768–3769, 3768f, 3769f
    small bowel, 3765–3768, 3766f, 3767f
    ureterocolonic, 3763–3765, 3764f, 3764t
  with bifragmentable ring, 3757
Intestinal antireflux valves, 3768–3769
  ileal, intussuscepted, 3768–3769, 3769f
  ileocecal, intussuscepted, 3768, 3768f
  nipple, 3769, 3769f
Intestinal duplication, signs and symptoms of, 1822
Intestinal injury, with laparoscopic renal surgery, 3680–3681
Intestinal malrotation, in prune-belly syndrome, 2122
Intestinal motility
  with conduit urinary diversion, 3782
  with pneumoperitoneum, 3475
Intestinal neobladder, hyperactivity in, drug treatment of, 980
Intestinal obstruction
  following augmentation cystoplasty, 2532
  in children
    pain in, 1821t
    signs and symptoms of, 1822
  with intestinal anastomoses, 3758–3759, 3758t, 3759f
Intestinal perforation, as percutaneous nephrostomy complication, 3339–3340
Intestinal pseudo-obstruction, with intestinal anastomoses, 3759
Intestinal segment(s)
  de-epithelialized, 2601
  elongation of, in isolated intestinal segments, 3759–3760, 3760f
  for augmentation cystoplasty
    choice of, 2540
    management of, 2525–2526
  in reconstructive surgery, 3745–3784
    abdominal stoma(s) in, 3760–3762
      complications of, 3762

Intestinal segment(s) *(Continued)*
    flush, 3761
      loop end ileostomy as, 3761–3762, 3761f
      nipple ("rosebud"), 3760–3761, 3760f, 3761f
    anastomoses in. *See* Intestinal anastomosis.
    bowel preparation for, 3749–3751
      antibiotic, 3750–3751, 3751t
      diarrhea and, 3751
      mechanical, 3749–3750, 3750t
    isolated, complications of, 3759–3760, 3760f
    selection of, 3748–3749
    surgical anatomy for, 3746–3748, 3746f, 3747f
  neuromechanical aspect(s) of, 3783–3784
    motor activity as, 3784, 3784f
    volume-pressure relationships as, 3783–3784, 3783f
  surgical anatomy of, 3746–3748
    of colon, 3747–3748, 3747f
    of small bowel, 3746–3747
    of stomach, 3746, 3746f
Intestinal stenosis, with intestinal anastomoses, 3759
Intestinal stricture, in isolated intestinal segments, 3759
Intestine, ureteral reimplantation into, in antireflux surgery, 2514, 2516
Intimal fibroplasia, of renal artery, 231t, 232–233, 233f
Intra-abdominal pressure
  carbon dioxide to increase, for laparoscopic surgery, in children, 2577
  in testicular descent, 2362
Intracellular mechanisms, in renin-angiotensin-aldosterone system, 236
Intracranial hemorrhage, in autosomal dominant polycystic kidney disease, 1946–1947
Intracrine signals, 1250, 1251f, 1267
Intracytoplasmic sperm injection, 1515, 1515t. *See* In vitro fertilization (IVF), with intracytoplasmic sperm injection.
  sperm retrieval for, 1517–1518
Intraoperative lymphatic mapping, in squamous penile cancer, 2964
Intraprostatic ductal reflux, in prostatitis, 607–608
Intrarenal arterial aneurysm, 262, 263f
Intraurethral catheter (Nissenkorn), 1382
Intrauterine insemination, 1515, 1515t. *See also* Assisted reproductive techniques (ARTs).
Intravenous drug transmission, of human immunodeficiency virus, 704–705
Intravenous pyelography. *See* Pyelography, intravenous.
Intravenous urography. *See* Urography, intravenous.
Intravesical pressure (Pves). *See* Bladder pressure (Pves).
Intravesical therapy, for interstitial cystitis, 655–656
Intrinsic sphincter dysfunction. *See* Intrinsic sphincteric deficiency.
Intrinsic sphincteric deficiency, 892, 901
  and incontinence surgery, 1148
  and urethral hypermobility, 1035–1036, 1140
  injection therapy for, 1173, 1180
  causes of, 1031, 1031t
  definition of, 1031, 1035
  diagnosis of
    in females, 1173
    stress testing for incontinence and, 903

Intrinsic sphincteric deficiency *(Continued)*
  estrogen deficiency-induced, 1036
  in elderly, 1222
  in females, 1030–1031
    age and, 1222
  neurologic lesions causing, 1036
  postoperative, 1036
  pubovaginal sling and, 1145
  radiation-induced, 1036
  risk factors for, 1036
  stress urinary incontinence secondary to, in-
    jection therapy for, 1172–1184
  treatment of, 1043t. *See also* Artificial sphinc-
    ter.
  Valsalva leak point pressure in, 912, 1041
  voiding dysfunction caused by, 1035–1036
Intrinsic sphincteric dysfunction
  definition of, 1152
  maximal urethral closing pressure in, 1152
  treatment of, alternatives for, 1154–1155
Introital cyst(s), 2439–2440, 2439f
Introl bladder neck support prosthesis, for stress
    incontinence, 1079, 1080f
Intron(s), definition of, 2626t
Intubated ureterotomy, for ureteral stricture, 501
Intussusception, in children
  pain in, 1821t
  recurrent, 1816t
Inverted papilloma(s)
  in bladder cancer, 2742, 2742f
  of renal pelvis and ureters, 2768
Ion channels, in male sexual function, 1600–
    1601, 1602f, 1603f
I-PSS (International Prostate Symptom Score),
    87, 88t
Irrigant(s), antifungal, genitourinary, for candidal
    infection, 803
Irrigation
  endoscopic instrumentation for, 3470
  for struvite calculi, 3263–3264
  in laparoscopic surgery, 2576
Irritable bowel syndrome, in children, 1816t
Irritation, as bladder cancer risk factor, 2767
Irritative urinary symptoms, 901, 940
  in acute disseminated encephalomyelitis, 944
  in bladder neck dysfunction, 959
  in patient history, 86
  in tethered cord syndrome, 953
  with pelvic organ prolapse, 1107
  with vesical endometriosis, 964–965
Isaacs' syndrome
  clinical characteristics of, 962
  voiding dysfunction in, 962
Ischemia, renal, 277–280
  cell biology of, 277–279, 279f
  cell injury and repair in, 279, 280f
  hemodynamics of, 280
  intraoperative, 3574–3575
    prevention of, 3574–3575
    renal tolerance to, 3574
  perinatal, functional renal response to, 1776
Ischemic nephropathy, renal arterial reconstruc-
    tion for, 3616
Ischemic-reperfusion injury, in acute tubular ne-
    crosis, 277–280, 279f–280f
Ischial spine, 41, 42f
Ischial tuberosity, 41, 42f
Ischiocavernosus muscles, 71, 71f, 1098, 1099f
  functions of, during penile erection, 1592t
Ischiopubic ramus, 41, 42f
Ischium, 41, 42f
Island flaps, 3890

Isoniazid
  adverse effects and side effects of, 755, 757t
  dosage and administration of, 757t
  for genitourinary tuberculosis, 757–759
  interactions with azoles, 819t
  mechanism of action of, 755, 755t
  mutational resistance to, site of, 755t
  pharmacology of, 755
Isopropamide, 968
Isoproterenol, uropharmacology of, 858t
Isradipine, incontinence caused by, in elderly,
    1221
Isthmusectomy, for horseshoe kidney, 3638–
    3639
ITAM (immunoreceptor tyrosine-based activa-
    tion motif), 315
  phosphorylation of, 318–319
Itraconazole, 819
  adverse effects and side effects of, 820f
  dosage and administration of, 820, 821t
  drug interactions with, 819t
  for aspergillosis, 807, 821t
    in kidney, 806, 821t
    in prostate, 806, 821t
  for blastomycosis, 812
  for coccidioidomycosis, 813
  for histoplasmosis, 814–815, 821t
  indications for, 820
  pharmacology of, 820
Ivemark's syndrome
  clinical features of, 1956t
  genetics of, 1956t
  renal cysts in, 1956t
  renal dysplasia in, 1956t
  renal sequelae of, 1956t
Ivermectin
  for filariasis, 785
    prophylactic, 786
  for onchocerciasis, 786
IVF. *See* In vitro fertilization (IVF).

Jaboulay bottleneck operation, for hydrocelec-
    tomy, 1579, 1579f
Jak kinases, 320
Jak/STAT pathway, in regulation of cytokine
    gene expression, 320
Jejunal conduit, in conduit urinary diversion,
    3772–3773
  complications of, 3773, 3775t
  complications with, 3778
  procedure for, 3772–3773
Jeune's asphyxiating thoracic dystrophy, 1956t
Johanson-Blizzard syndrome
  cryptorchidism associated with, 2367t
  hypospadias with, 2292t
jun oncogene, 320
Junctional nevus, of male genitalia, 728–729
Juvenile nephronopthisis
  associated anomalies in, 1952
  autosomal recessive
    genetics of, 1939t
    incidence of, 1939t
    renal findings in, 1939t
  clinical features of, 1952, 1953t
  evaluation of, 1953–1954
  genetics of, 1952, 1953t
  histopathology of, 1952–1953
  incidence of, 1952, 1953t
  magnetic resonance imaging in, 1953–1954
  renal findings in, 1953t
  tubular basement membrane in, 1953, 1953t

Juvenile nephronopthisis–medullary cystic dis-
    ease complex, 1952–1955
  renal findings in, 1939t
  treatment of, 1954
Juxtaglomerular cells, renin synthesis by, 183
Juxtaglomerular tumors, 2685

K antigens, of *Escherichia coli,* 523, 552
KAL1, in renal development, 1930
KAL1 gene, 1891
Kaliuretic diuretics, 189
Kallikrein(s), and male fertility, 1512
Kallikrein gene family, 1279t, 1280–1281
Kallikrein tumor markers, in prostate cancer,
    3056–3057
Kallmann's syndrome, 1438, 1477, 1500–1501,
    1891
  cryptorchidism associated with, 2367t
Kanamycin
  adverse effects and side effects of, 757t
  dosage and administration of, 757t
  for bowel preparation, 3751t
  serum and urinary levels of, 537t
Kaposi's sarcoma
  in acquired immunodeficiency syndrome, 703,
    707–708
  of male genitalia, 722, 734f
  of penis, 2949
Kartagener's syndrome, 1477, 1479, 1514–1515
Karyotype, definition of, 2626t
Katayama fever. *See* Schistosomiasis, acute.
Kayexalate, for hyperkalemia, in renal tubular
    acidosis, in children, 1771
Kegel exercises. *See also* Pelvic floor exercises.
  for incontinence, 1072
  in behavioral therapy for incontinence, 1070
Keratin, 1243
Keratinocyte growth factor, in prostate, 1275,
    1301–1302
Keratosis, seborrheic, 727
Keratotic balanitis, 2947
  of male genitalia, 723
Ketanserin, uropharmacology of, 864
Ketoconazole, 819
  adverse effects and side effects of, 819, 820f
  dosage and administration of, 819–820, 821t
    in children, 820
  drug interactions with, 819t
  erectile dysfunction caused by, 1609
  for blastomycosis, 811–812, 821t
  for candidiasis, 803–804
    in prostate, 800
    in upper urinary tract, 800
    in vagina, 799
    with cystitis, 799
    with epididymo-orchitis, 799
  for coccidioidomycosis, 812–813
  for cryptococcosis, 809
  for histoplasmosis, 821t
  for mucormycosis, 810
  for prevention of erection, in postoperative
    period after penile surgery, 2303
  for prostate cancer, 3217t
  for *Torulopsis glabrata* infection, 805
  hepatotoxicity of, 2303
  pharmacology of, 819
Ketones, in urine, 106–107
Keyhole sign, 1782t, 1783–1784, 1784f
Keyhole-limpet hemocyanin, for bladder cancer,
    2795

Kidney(s), 19–35. *See also* Neph-; Renal *entries.*
  abdominal, 1894f, 1895
  acid excretion by, 211–213. *See also* Acid-base balance.
    adrenergic receptors in, 213
    aldosterone in, 213
    angiotensin II in, 213
    atrial natriuretic peptide in, 213
    calculation of, 212
    chloride concentration in, 212–213
    extracellular volume in, 212–213
    HCO_3^- in, 213
    net amount of, 212
    neural factors in, 213
    parathyroid hormone in, 213
    PCO_2 in, 213
    pH in, 213
    potassium concentration in, 212–213
    titratable, 212
  after complete primary exstrophy repair, 2205
  agenesis of, 1886–1892
    and ureteropelvic junction obstruction, 1998
    bilateral, 1886–1889, 1930
      associated anomalies in, 1887f, 1887–1888
      diagnosis of, 1888–1889
      embryology of, 1886
      features of, 1886–1887, 1887f
      genetics of, 1886
      in females, 1888
      incidence of, 1886
      prenatal diagnosis of, 1889
      prognosis for, 1889
      sex distribution of, 1886
    genetic defect in, 1747t
    in epispadias patient, 2182
    in neonates, 1805
    prenatal diagnosis of, 1788
    unilateral, 1889–1892, 1930
      and renal function in adulthood, 1777
      associated anomalies in, 1889–1890
      diagnosis of, 1891–1892
      embryology of, 1889
      incidence of, 1889
      left-sided, 1889
      prognosis for, 1892
      sex distribution of, 1889
      syndromes associated with, 1891
    vesicoureteral reflux with, 2074–2075
    with cloacal exstrophy, 2177
  anatomic changes of, after ureteral obstruction, 439–444
    cellular infiltrates and cytokines in, 442
    cellular proliferation and apoptosis in, 441–442
    fibrosis in, 440–441, 441f
      strategies to affect, 443–444, 443t
    gross, 443–441
    microscopic, 441
  anatomic relations of, 21–22, 24, 28f
    anteriorly, 22, 24
    posteriorly, 21–22, 28f, 29f
  anatomy of
    gross, 19–21, 23f–24f
    microscopic, 21, 24f–27f
    surgical, 3571–3573, 3571f, 3572f
  anomaly(ies) of
    classification of, 1885–1886
    in exstrophy patient, 2145
    in females, classification of, 1890f
    in males, 1495

Kidney(s) *(Continued)*
    of ascent, 1885, 1894–1898
    of form and fusion, 1885, 1898–1906
    of number, 1885, 1886–1894
    of rotation, 1885, 1906–1908
    of volume and structure, 1885
    pan-bud, 1936
    vascular, 1885, 1908–1912
    vesicoureteral reflux with, 2074–2075
  aplasia of, 1961
    with ureteral duplication, 2041
  arteries of. *See* Renal artery(ies).
  ascent of
    anomalies of, 1894–1898
    during prenatal development, 1742–1743, 1745f
  Ask-Upmark. *See* Ask-Upmark kidney.
  aspergillosis of, 806, 807f
  base excretion by, 213–214. *See also* Acid-base balance.
  benign multilocular cyst of, 1940t
  bleeding from
    with renal trauma, 3713–3714
    with shock-wave lithotripsy, 3410, 3410f, 3413–3414, 3413f, 3414f
  blood flow in. *See* Renal blood flow (RBF).
  calcification in, in tuberculosis, 747–748, 748f, 749f
  calcium excretion by, 191–192, 194–195. *See also* Calcium, renal reabsorption of.
  cancer of. *See specific type, e.g.,* Renal cell carcinoma.
  candidal infection of, 800–801
  cell differentiation in, congenital obstructive uropathy and, 1790
  clear cell sarcoma of, 2493
  coccidioidomycosis in, 812
  computed tomography of, 139f, 140, 141, 143f
    in children, 1870, 1871f
  congenital disease of
    effect on adult renal function, 1776–1777
    genetic defect in, 1747t
  congenital malformations of, and ureteropelvic junction obstruction, 1997–1998
  cross section through, 24f
  cross-fused ectopy of, 1743
  cryptococcal infection of, 808
  cysts of. *See* Renal cyst(s).
  development of
    apoptosis in, 1747–1748
    cell proliferation in, 1747–1748
    gene expression during, 1743–1747, 1746f, 1747t
    gene knock-out studies of, 1743–1746
    hormonal control of, 1772–1774
    malformation or injury during, functional response to, 1774–1777
    molecular genetics of, 1926–1930
    perinatal ischemia and hypoxia and, 1776
    postnatal, 1767–1768
    prenatal, 1737–1742, 1738f, 1766–1767
      molecular mechanisms of, 1743–1746
    urinary tract obstruction during, functional response to, 1775–1776
  disc, 1899, 1899f, 1901–1902, 1902f
  duplex
    definition of, 2007
    ultrasound of, 2024
    with bifid ureter, embryology of, 2010
    with double ureters, embryology of, 2010, 2012f

Kidney(s) *(Continued)*
  duplication of
    and ureteropelvic junction obstruction, 1998, 1998f
    gradations of, 2038, 2039f
  dwarf, 1935
  dysgenesis of
    definition of, 1930
    genetic defect in, 1747t
  dysplasia of, 1930–1932
    and ureteropelvic junction obstruction, 1998
    congenital obstructive uropathy and, 1790
    cystic, 1930
    definition of, 1930
    etiology of, 1931
    histology of, 1931, 1932f
    in exstrophy patient, 2145
    in prune-belly syndrome, 2118
    multicystic. *See* Multicystic dysplastic kidney (MCDK).
    nephrogenic diabetes insipidus caused by, 1844
    with bilateral single-system ectopic ureters, 2020
    with posterior urethral valves, 2214
    with ureteral duplication, 2041, 2042
  ectopic. *See* Renal ectopia.
  embryology of, 1737–1742, 1738f, 1927–1930, 1928t, 2008–2010
    anatomic stages of, 1737–1742, 1738f, 1765–1766, 1766f
    molecular mechanisms of, 1743–1746
  entrapment of, in laparoscopic nephrectomy, 3653
  familial adysplasia of, 1930, 1931–1932, 1961
  fetal, 1737–1742, 1738f
    and lung development, 1792
    development of
      anatomic stages of, 1737–1742, 1738f, 1765–1766, 1766f
      functional, 1766
    function of, evaluation of, 1766–1767
    hormonal control of, 1772–1774
    inflammatory responses in, in congenital obstructive uropathy, 1791
    injury responses in, in congenital obstructive uropathy, 1791
    lobulations of, 20, 21f
    response to congenital obstructive uropathy, 1790–1791
    ultrasound appearance of, 1781, 1782f, 1782t
  fetal vesicoureteral reflux and, 2055
  functional anatomy of, for percutaneous techniques, 3322–3323, 3323f
  functional development of
    postnatal, 1767–1768
    prenatal, 1766–1767
  Gerota's fascia of, 24–25, 29f
  growth of
    compensatory, in fetus/neonate, with contralateral reduced functioning renal mass, 1774–1775
    nomogram for, 2072, 2072f
    reflux nephropathy and, 2071–2072
  histoplasmosis of, 814
  horseshoe. *See* Horseshoe kidney.
  hypodysplasia of, 1932–1937
    classification of, 1932, 1932t
    definition of, 1930
    in prune-belly syndrome, 1937
    with abnormal ureteral orifice, 1935–1936

Kidney(s) *(Continued)*
  with normal ureteral orifice, 1935
    with obstruction, 1935, 1935f
    without obstruction, 1935
    with urethral obstruction, 1936–1937, 1937f
  hypoplasia of, 1932–1937
    and renal function in adulthood, 1777
    classification of, 1932, 1932t
    definition of, 1930
    in congenital obstruction, 1790
    in exstrophy patient, 2145
    segmental, 1934–1935
    true, 1932–1933
      clinical features of, 1933
      evaluation of, 1933
      histopathology of, 1933
    with ureteral duplication, 2041
  hypoxia in
    interstitial cystitis and, 643
    perinatal, functional response to, 1776
  imaging of, in benign prostatic hyperplasia, 1344
  in amebiasis, 788
  in echinococcosis, 786–788, 788f
  in neonates
    hormonal control of, 1772–1774
    recovery from injury in, relationship to normal development, 1776
  in prune-belly syndrome, 2118, 2123, 2123t, 2124, 2125
  infections of. *See also* Infection(s).
    in children, tests for, 1849
    in prune-belly syndrome, 2118
  inflammation of. *See* Pyelonephritis; Urinary tract infection.
  injury to. *See* Trauma, renal.
  innervation of, 40
  interstitium of, development of, in neonate, 1768
  irrigation of, with antifungal agents, 803
  lobe of, defined, 21
  localization of, in urinary tract infection, 532–535
  L-shaped, 1899, 1899f, 1901, 1901f
  lumbar, 1894f, 1895, 1895f
  lump, 1899, 1899f, 1901, 1901f
  lymphatic drainage of, 29–30, 32f
  magnesium reabsorption by, 195–196, 196t
  magnetic resonance angiography of, 147
  magnetic resonance imaging of, 146–147, 148f, 149
    in children, 1829, 1870, 1871f
  malrotation of, 1906–1908, 1908f
  masses in. *See* Renal tumor(s); *specific mass.*
  medullary sponge. *See* Medullary sponge kidney.
  microscopic changes in, after ureteral obstruction, 440
  multicystic dysplastic. *See* Multicystic dysplastic kidney (MCDK).
  Page's, 266
  pain fibers of, 40, 40f
  pan-bud anomaly of, 1936
  parasitic infections and, 788–789
  pelvic, 1743, 1894f, 1895, 1896f, 3373
    in exstrophy patient, 2145
    with cloacal exstrophy, 2177
  phosphate excretion by, 196–197
  phycomycosis of, 809–810, 810f
  physical examination of, 92–93, 93f
  podocyte processes of, 32, 33f

Kidney(s) *(Continued)*
  polycystic. *See* Autosomal recessive polycystic kidney disease (ARPKD); Multicystic dysplastic kidney (MCDK).
  potassium excretion by, 186–191. *See also* Potassium, renal excretion of.
  pseudotumor of, 1916–1917, 1917f
  pyelonephritic. *See* Pyelonephritis.
  radiologic evaluation of, 904–905
  role of, in volume homeostasis, 184–185, 185f
  scarring of
    in children, 1850–1851, 1851f, 1852, 1853–1855, 1854f, 1870, 1871f
      genetics of, 1860
    in vesicoureteral reflux, 1843, 1855, 1870, 1871f, 2068–2071, 2069f. *See also* Vesicoureteral reflux, renal scarring in.
  shattered, 3709
  sigmoid (S-shaped), 1899, 1899f, 1901
  size of, during pregnancy, 580
  solitary
    glomeruli in, 288
    in exstrophy patient, 2145
  stones in. *See* Urinary lithiasis, renal.
  supernumerary, 1892–1894
  thoracic, 1897–1898
    anomalies associated with, 1898
    diagnosis of, 1898
    embryology of, 1897
    features of, 1897–1898, 1898f
    incidence of, 1897
    prognosis for, 1898
    signs and symptoms of, 1898
  transplantation of. *See* Renal transplantation.
  trauma to. *See* Trauma, renal.
  tuberculosis of, pathology of, 747–748, 748f, 749f
  tubular function in
    in infant/child, evaluation of, 1769–1772
    in neonates, 1767
    prenatal, 1766–1767
    with posterior urethral valves, 2214–2215
  tubulogenesis in, molecular mechanisms of, 1743–1747, 1746f
  ultrasonography of, 134, 135, 135f
    in children, 1827, 1869
  unilateral fused
    with inferior ectopia, 1899, 1899f, 1900, 1901
    with superior ectopia, 1899, 1899f, 1900, 1902
  unipapillary, 1915
  upper pole of, isolation of, in laparoscopic nephrectomy, 3653, 3655f
  urate excretion by, 197–198, 198f
    drugs altering, 198t
    extracellular fluid volume and, 197–198
    pH and, 198
  vascular segments of, 3572, 3572f
  vasculature of, 25–29, 30f–31f. *See also* Renal artery(ies); Renal blood flow (RBF); Renal plasma flow; Renal vein(s).
    anatomic variants in, 27, 31f
    anomalies of, 1885, 1908–1912
    CT angiography of, 140–141
    development of, 1748
    surgical considerations and, 27, 29, 32
  water excretion by, measurement of, 202–203

Kidney Disease Outcome Quality Initiative (K/DOQI), 298

Kidney graft. *See also* Renal transplantation.
  early dysfunction of, 365–366, 368t, 369t
  nephrectomy of, indications for, 366–367
  preparation of
    from cadaveric donor, 358, 358f–359f
    from living donor, 357–358
  preservation of, 354–357
    cellular injury and, 354–355
    clinical, 356–357
    cold storage in, 355–356
  rejection of, 363–365
    cellular interactions in, 363, 364f
    classification of, 363–364
    histocompatibility in, 363, 363t, 364f
    immunosuppression in, 364–365, 364t, 365f, 366f, 366t, 367t
  rupture of, 366
Killian/Teschler-Nicola syndrome, hypospadias with, 2292t
Kinesiologic studies, in voiding dysfunction, 925–928, 926f
Kininase II. *See* Angiotensin-converting enzyme (ACE).
Kinins, effect of, on ureteral function, 402
Kissing balloon technique, of percutaneous transluminal angioplasty, 255
Klinefelter syndrome, 1761
  classic form of, 1504
  diagnosis of, 1504
  genetics of, 1504
  genitourinary anomalies in, 1504, 1815t
  hypospadias with, 2292t
  infertility in, 1504
  mosaic form of, 1504
  nonmosaic, sperm retrieval in, 1569
  phenotype in, 1504
Klinefelter's syndrome, 2404
Klonopin. *See* Clonazepam.
Knee-chest position, for perineal examination, in female child, 1824, 1824f
Knockout mice, 2657
  conditional, 2657
Knot pushers, laparoscopic, 3468
Kocher's maneuver, 16
Kock pouch
  for continent urinary diversion, 3807, 3808f, 3809f
  orthotopic, 3853, 3855f
  urinary stones in, 3386–3387
Kupffer cells, 308, 312

Labia
  adhesions of, 2438–2439, 2439f
  interlabial mass(es) and, 2438–2440
    introital cysts as, 2439–2440, 2439f
    labial adhesions as, 2438–2439, 2439f
Labia majora, 78, 1711, 1712f
  embryology of, 1758, 1759f
  fusion of, in children, 1825
  histoplasmosis of, 814
  masses of
    clinical presentation of, in childhood, 2034
    in children, 1825
Labia minora, 1711, 1712f
  adhesions of, in children, 1825
    management of, 1830
  embryology of, 1758, 1759f
  in exstrophy patient, 2143
Labial fat pads, 78
Labioplasty, for intersex conditions, 2449–2451, 2453, 2453f, 2456

Labioscrotal folds, 1757
Labioscrotal swelling, 1758f, 1759f
Labor and delivery, stress incontinence after, 1036–1037
Laboratory test(s), in neurourologic evaluation, 904
Lacrimo-auriculo-dento-digital syndrome, hypospadias with, 2292t
β-Lactam therapy, for urinary tract infection, during pregnancy, 585
Lactate dehydrogenase
   in prostate, 1282
   in testicular germ cell tumors, 2888
   structure of, 1282
Lactose intolerance, in children, 1816t
Lactotropes, 1438–1439
Lacuna magna, 1757
LADD syndrome, hypospadias with, 2292t
Lamina propria, 3887
Laminin, 1265
   in bladder cancer, 2752
   prostatic, 1243
Langer's lines, 42
Laparoscopes, 3465
Laparoscopic adrenalectomy, 3554–3560
   contraindications to, 3555
   indications for, 3554–3555
   retroperitoneal approach(es) to, 3556–3557, 3556f, 3558–3560
      left, 3556f, 3559–3560
      results with, 3560
      right, 3556f, 3559
   transperitoneal approach(es) to, 3557–3558
      anterior, 3555–3556
      lateral, 3555, 3556f
      left, 3558
      results with, 3558
      right, 3557–3558
Laparoscopic bladder augmentation, 3703
Laparoscopic bladder diverticulectomy, 3702–3703
Laparoscopic cystectomy
   partial, 3702
   radical, 3702
   simple, 3702
Laparoscopic ligation, for varicocele, 2387
Laparoscopic lymphocele ablation, 3701–3702
   anatomic imaging for, 3701
   complications of, 3701
   contraindications to, 3701
   results with, 3702, 3702t
   technique for, 3701
Laparoscopic nephrectomy
   in children, 2583–2584
   in living donors, 3655–3661, 3655f, 3656t
      alternative approaches in, 3661
      left-sided, 3656–3658, 3657f–3659f
      operative preparation for, 3656
      patient positioning for, 3656
      patient selection for, 3655–3656
      procedure for, 3656–3661, 3657f–3659f
      results with, 3659–3661, 3660t
      right-sided, 3658–3659
   partial, 3677–3678, 3678t
   radical, 3671–3677, 3672t
      indications for and contraindications to, 3671
      patient positioning for, 3672
      preoperative evaluation for, 3671–3672
      procedure for, 3672–3674, 3673f–3677f
      results with, 3674–3677
      trocar placement for, 3672
   simple, 3647–3653
      indications and contraindications to, 3647–3648

Laparoscopic nephrectomy (Continued)
      insufflation and trocar placement for, 3648–3649, 3650f, 3651f
      patient positioning for, 3648, 3649f, 3689
      postoperative care for, 3653
      procedure for, 3649, 3651f–3655f, 3653
      results with, 3653
Laparoscopic nephroureterectomy
   radical, 2851, 2853–2855
      results with, 2855
      technique for, 2853–2855, 2853f–2855f
      transperitoneal, in females, 2853–2854, 2853f, 2854f
Laparoscopic pelvic lymph node dissection, 3670–3671, 3687–3691, 3688t
   extended, 3691
   extraperitoneal, 3690
      working space for, 3690, 3690f
   postoperative care for, 3691
   preoperative preparation for, 3688, 3688f
   results with, 3691, 3691t
   transperitoneal, 3688–3690
      steps in, 3689–3690, 3689f, 3690f
      working space for, 3688–3689, 3689f
Laparoscopic radical prostatectomy, 3698–3701
   indications and contraindications to, 3698–3699
   oncologic results with, 3700, 3700t
   surgical morbidity with, 3700–3701
   surgical technique for, 3699–3700, 3699f, 3700f
Laparoscopic retroperitoneal lymph node dissection, 2931
   for testicular cancer, 3691–3695, 3692t
      left-sided, 3694
         operative approach to, 3692
         postchemotherapy or post radiotherapy, 3694
         postoperative care for, 3694
         preoperative preparation for, 3692
         results with, 3694–3695, 3695t
         right-sided, 3693–3694
            interaortocaval dissection in, 3693–3694, 3694f
            para- and precaval dissection in, 3693
            testicular vessel dissection in, 3693
            working space for, 3693
         transperitoneal approach to, 3692–3693, 3693f
Laparoscopic seminal vesicle dissection, 3697–3698
   alternatives to, 3697
   contraindications to, 3697
   indications for, 3697
   results with, 3698
   surgical technique for, 3697–3698, 3697f, 3698f
Laparoscopic surgery, 3455–3504. See also specific procedures.
   complication(s) of, 3477–3491
      anesthesia and, 3490–3491
      exiting abdomen and, 3487–3488, 3488f
      intraoperative, 3483–3487
         bowel injury as, 3483–3485, 3484f
         nerve injury as, 3486–3487
         urinary tract injury as, 3485–3486
         vascular injury as, 3485
      minimizing incidence during learning curve, 3477
      pneumoperitoneum and, 3477–3481, 3480f
      postoperative, 3488–3490
         deep vein thrombosis as, 3489–3490
         incisional hernia as, 3489

Laparoscopic surgery (Continued)
      pain as, 3488–3489
      subcutaneous emphysema as, 3489
      wound infections as, 3490
   trocar placement and, 3481–3483, 3483f
   diagnostic
      in bladder cancer, invasive and metastatic, 2806
      in children, 2571–2575
         in intersex conditions, 2574–2575, 2574t
         indications for, 2571
         of hernia, 2575, 2575f
         of testis, 2571–2574, 2572f, 2573f, 2574t
   exiting abdomen in, 3471–3473
      complications of, 3487–3488, 3488f
      port removal in, 3471–3472, 3473
      port site closure instrumentation for, 3472–3473, 3472f
      postoperative management for, 3473
      skin closure for, 3473
   for cryptorchidism, with intra-abdominal testis, 2374–2376
   for hernia repair, of incisional/parastomal hernias, 3703
   for retropubic suspension surgery, 1146
   for urachal remnant excision, 3702
   for ureteroenteric stricture, 508
   for ureteropelvic junction obstruction, 487–489
      complications of, 488
      indications for and contraindications to, 487
      postoperative care in, 488
      results of, 488–489
      technique of, 487–488, 488f
   for vesicoureteral reflux, 2094
   hand-assisted, 3471, 3471f
   historical background of, 3456–3457
   in children, 2575–2581
      anesthesia for, 2577–2578
      antireflux, 2587–2588
      autoaugmentation as, 2586
      complications of, 2578
      enterocystoplasty as, 2586
      for bladder reconstruction, 2586–2587, 2587f
      for cryptorchidism, 2578–2581, 2579f, 2580f
      for seminal vesicle cysts, 2588
      indications for, 2575–2576
      instruments for, 2576–2577
      renal. See Renal surgery, laparoscopic, in children.
      vaginoplasty as, 2588
   informed consent for, 3458
   instrumentation in, 3465–3471
      for aspiration and irrigation, 3470
      for clipping, 3468–3469
      for grasping and blunt dissection, 3465–3466, 3466f
      for hand-assisted laparoscopy, 3471, 3471f
      for incising and hemostasis, 3466–3467
      for morcellation, 3469–3470
      for port site closure, 3472–3473, 3472f
      for retraction, 3470–3471, 3470f
      for specimen entrapment, 3469, 3469f
      for stapling, 3468, 3468f
      for suturing and tissue anastomosis, 3467–3468
      for visualization, 3465

Ligament(s) *(Continued)*
  Cooper's (pectineal), 42, 47f
  hepatorenal, 22
  inguinal, 44, 46f
  lienorenal, 24
  puboprostatic, 47
  pubourethral, 47, 69, 69f
  round, of uterus, 67, 67f
  sacrospinous, 42
  splenorenal, 24
  suspensory, of clitoris, 69, 69f
  umbilical, median, development of, 1752
  uterosacral, 48, 70
Ligands
  as cancer therapy targets, 2644
  G-protein coupled, cancer and, 2648
Light sources, for laparoscopy, 3465
LIM1 gene, in renal development, 1746
Limb(s), anomalies of
  in prune-belly syndrome, 2122
  with cloacal exstrophy, 2177
Limb contractures, urinary stone treatment with, 3376
Linea alba, 43
Linkage, definition of, 2626t
Linsidomine, intracavernous injection of, 1658
Lioresal. *See* Baclofen.
Lipid(s), in seminal plasma, 1278
Lipid A, endotoxin and, 568–569
Lipoma(s)
  intradural, 952
  renal, 2685
Lipomatosis, pelvic, 419–422, 421f, 421t
  age range for, 420
  cystoscopy in, 422
  imaging appearance of, 420–421, 421f
Lipomeningocele, 952, 2245–2248. *See also* Spinal dysraphism.
  diagnosis of, 2245, 2246f
  with cloacal exstrophy, 2177
Lipomyelomeningocele. *See also* Myelodysplasia.
  definition of, 2234
Liposarcoma(s)
  of bladder, 2765
  paratesticular, 2913
Lipoxins, in renal hemodynamics, 174
Lisinopril, incontinence caused by, in elderly, 1221t
Lithiasis, urinary. *See* Urinary lithiasis.
Lithium
  and female sexual dysfunction, 1720
  priapism caused by, 1612t
Lithium toxicity
  megaureter caused by, 2098
  nephrogenic diabetes insipidus caused by, 1844
Lithotomy, open, for urinary calculi, 3436–3437
  renal, 3436–3437, 3437t
  ureteral, 3437
Lithotripsy
  ballistic, 3395–3396, 3395f
    advantages and disadvantages of, 3395–3396, 3396t
    technique for, 3396
  devices for, comparison of, 3397–3398, 3398t
  electrohydraulic, 3391–3392, 3391f
    for bladder calculi, 3385
  laser, 3392–3393
    for bladder calculi, 3385
  pneumatic, for bladder calculi, 3385
  shock-wave. *See* Shock-wave lithotripsy (SWL).

Lithotripsy *(Continued)*
  ultrasonic, 3396–3397, 3397f
    advantages and disadvantages of, 3397
    for bladder calculi, 3385
    technique for, 3397
  with percutaneous nephrolithotomy, 2567
  with ureteroscopy, 2565
Lithotriptor, electrohydraulic, 2565
Liver
  cirrhosis of
    and benign prostatic hyperplasia, 1312
    erectile dysfunction caused by, 1610
  disease of, blastomycosis with, 811
  in schistosomiasis, 780
Liver injury, as percutaneous nephrostomy complication, 3340
Liverpool nomogram, for uroflowmetry flow rates and bladder volume, 915, 915f
Living donor(s), for renal transplantation, 352
  algorithm for evaluation of, 353f
  laparoscopic nephrectomy in, 3655–3661, 3655f, 3656t
  renal imaging techniques in, 352, 354t
  vs. cadaver donor, 346
LMN lesion. *See* Lower motor neuron (LMN) lesion.
Loa spp. *See* Filariasis.
Lobar nephronia, pediatric, 1852
Local anesthesia. *See also* Anesthesia.
  for hypospadias repair, 2301
  for injection therapy, 1175, 1176
  for vasectomy, 1541f, 1541–1542, 1542f
Locus(i), definition of, 2626t
Lomefloxacin, for prostatitis, 619t, 624t
Loop diuretics
  in acute renal failure, 283
  in renal sodium reabsorption, 180–181
Loop end ileostomy, 3761–3762, 3761f
Loop of Henle, 32. *See also* Nephron(s).
  calcium reabsorption by, 192
  potassium excretion by, 187
  sodium reabsorption by, 180–181, 180f
  urinary concentration and dilution in, 201–202
Loop system (Bradley) classification of voiding dysfunction, 894
Loracarbef, for pediatric urinary tract infection, oral dosage and administration of, 1865t
Lorazepam, 1009
Lord's plication technique, for hydrocelectomy, 1579, 1580f
Losoxantrone, for prostate cancer, 3214t
Lowe syndrome, cryptorchidism associated with, 2367t
Lower motor neuron (LMN) lesion
  ice-water test with, 910
  in spinal dysraphism, 2245–2247, 2247f
  sacral agenesis and, 2249
  voiding dysfunction after
    classification of, 893–894, 895
    treatment of, 1001
Lower urinary tract. *See also* Urinary tract *entries.*
  age-related changes in, 873–874, 1218–1219, 1222–1223
  components of, 1027
  dysfunction of
    incontinence caused by, in elderly, 1222–1223
    neuropathic, in children, 2231–2256
    non-neuropathic, in children, 2261–2280
  endoscopic examination of, 905

Lower urinary tract *(Continued)*
  function of, 1027
    after neurologic injury
      balanced vs. imbalanced, 889t, 893–894
      in children, 2231–2256
    normal, 887–889
    two-phase concept of, 887–889. *See also* Micturition cycle.
    mechanisms underlying, 889–891
  imaging of, 1041
  infection of. *See* Urinary tract infection, lower.
  injury to, in hysterectomy, 1196
  radiologic evaluation of, 905
  symptoms in, 901
    clinical significance of, 919
    patient questionnaire about, 902
    quantification of, 902
    urodynamic evaluation of, 905
Low-protein diets, for chronic renal failure, 295–296
L-selectin, T cell expression of, 329
LU 25-109, for voiding dysfunction, 981t
Lumbar artery, 7, 14f
Lumbar spine
  disc disease in, voiding dysfunction with, 953–954
  stenosis in, 954
    priapism in, 1611
Lumbar vein, 7–8, 14f
Lumbodorsal fascia, 3–4, 11f
Lumbosacral plexus, 14, 16f, 54, 55f
Lumbotomy incision, dorsal, 3578–3579, 3580f
Lung(s). *See also* Pulmonary *entries.*
  abnormalities of, with cloacal exstrophy, 2178
  fetal, development of, 1792
  hypoplasia of, 1785, 1792
    in bilateral renal agenesis, 1888
    in prune-belly syndrome, 2122, 2124
  in prune-belly syndrome, 2121–2122, 2121t, 2123, 2123t, 2124
  injury to, as percutaneous nephrostomy complication, 3339, 3339f
  resection of, postchemotherapy, with testicular tumors, 2938
Lupus erythematosus
  papulosquamous lesions in, 718
  systemic. *See* Systemic lupus erythematosus.
Luteinizing hormone (LH)
  deficiency of, in males, 1499
  effects of, on prostate, 1245, 1245f
  in male reproductive axis, 1437, 1440–1441, 1444, 1446f
  in males, evaluation of, 1484t, 1484–1485
  in spermatogenesis, 1456
  in testicular descent, 2359
  plasma levels of, age-related changes in, 1440
  receptors for, Leydig cell aplasia and, 2415
  secretion of, 1437
  therapy with, for male infertility, 1511
Luteinizing hormone-releasing hormone (LH-RH)
  for cryptorchidism, 2369–2370
  for medical castration, for prostate cancer, 3194–3195
17,20-Lyase deficiency, 2416
Lycopene
  as negative prostate cancer risk factor, 3010
  for prostate cancer prevention, 3018
Lyme disease, voiding dysfunction in, 942
Lymph node(s)
  function of, 309, 310f
  iliac, 52, 55f

Lymph node(s) *(Continued)*
  inguinal, 75–76
Lymph node dissection, pelvic
  in prostate cancer staging, 3072
  laparoscopic. *See* Laparoscopic pelvic lymph node dissection.
Lymph scrotum, in filariasis, 784
Lymphadenectomy
  groin, modified, in penile cancer, 2988, 2988f, 2989f
  ilioinguinal, in penile cancer, 2988–2991, 2990f, 2991f
  in bladder cancer, 2761
  in radical prostatectomy, retropubic, 3112, 3112f
  inguinal. *See* Inguinal lymphadenectomy.
  pelvic
    in prostate cancer staging, 3072
    with radical cystectomy, in females, 2834, 2834f, 2835f
    with radical cystectomy, for invasive bladder cancer, 2807
    with radical nephroureterectomy, technique for, 2850
Lymphadenopathy, in acquired immunodeficiency syndrome, 707
Lymphangiectasia, of male genitalia, 728
Lymphangioma(s), renal, 2685
Lymphangioma circumscriptum, of male genitalia, 728
Lymphangitis, sclerosing, of male genitalia, 727
Lymphatic vessels
  of bladder, 62
  of kidneys, 29–30, 32f
  of pelvis, 52, 55f
  of perineum, 75–76
  of retroperitoneum, 9–10, 15f
  of testes, 10, 15f
  of ureters, 37–38
  testicular, 1444
Lymphedema
  penile, 2343, 2344f
  radiation-induced, 3914
Lymphocele(s)
  after renal transplantation, 368
  after retroperitoneal lymph node dissection, 2938
  laparoscopic ablation of, 3701–3702
    anatomic imaging for, 3701
    complications of, 3701
    contraindications to, 3701
    results with, 3702, 3702t
    technique for, 3701
  percutaneous drainage of, 3346–3347
Lymphocytes, 310–312. *See also* B cell(s); Natural killer (NK) cells; T cell(s).
  circulating pool of, 310
  in immune response, 309
  tolerance of
    central, 327–328
    clonal anergy in, 328
    development of, 327–329
    peripheral, 328
    regulatory T cells in, 329
  trafficking of, adhesion molecules in, 329–331, 330f, 330t
  tumor-infiltrating, 336
Lymphogranuloma venereum, 681t, 684, 740f
Lymphoid tissue, 309, 310f
  in pathogenesis and progression of HIV infection, 698
Lymphoma
  cryptococcosis with, 808
  cutaneous T cell, of male genitalia, 724

Lymphoma *(Continued)*
  non-Hodgkin's, in acquired immunodeficiency syndrome, 708
  of bladder, 2765
  of kidneys, 2720–2721, 2721t
  of testes, 2909–2910
    in children, 2499
  retroviruses in, 694
Lymphoreticular malignancy, penile, 2974
Lynch's syndrome. *See* Hereditary nonpolyposis colorectal cancer.

M line, in magnetic resonance imaging of pelvic floor, 1114, 1115f
M region, 854
Maciol suture needle set, 3472
Macroglossia, in children, 1822
Macrophages, 312
  alveolar, 312
  in prostatitis, 615, 615f
  lipid-laden, associated with xanthogranulomatous pyelonephritis, 565
  role of, in HIV infection, 696
Macroplastique, injection therapy with, 1175
  for female stress incontinence, 1154
  for postprostatectomy incontinence, 1065
Macula densa
  in renin secretion, 183
  in renin-angiotensin-aldosterone system, 235
Macule(s), cutaneous, 716
Magnesium
  deficiency of, potassium excretion and, 190–191
  for urinary lithiasis, 3284–3285
  metabolism of, 3240
  renal reabsorption of, 195–196, 196t
Magnesium oxide, for hypomagnesuria, 3253–3254
Magnetic pressure, 3398
Magnetic resonance angiography (MRA), 146, 150–151
  contrast-enhanced three-dimensional, 151, 153f
  in children, 1829
  in renovascular hypertension, 245–246
  of kidney, 147
  of penis, 1645
  of renal hilum, 149–150, 149f
  of renal masses, 2676, 2677f
Magnetic resonance imaging (MRI), 145–150
  contraindications to, 146
  for percutaneous puncture, 3331
  gadolinium used in, 146
  in children, 1829
  indications for, 146–149
  normal anatomy in, 148f–152f, 149–150
  of acquired renal cystic disease, 1981
  of adrenal gland, 147, 149, 149f
  of autosomal dominant polycystic kidney disease, 1948, 1949f
  of bladder, 147, 150, 151f
  of bladder cancer, 2761, 2771–2772
    invasive, 2804
  of congenital hydronephrosis, 2000–2001
  of ectopic ureter, 2018
  of juvenile nephronopthisis, 1953–1954
  of kidney, 146–147, 148f, 149
    in children, 1870, 1871f
  of pelvic diaphragm, 1097, 1097f
  of pelvic organ prolapse, 1114, 1115f
  of penile cancer, 2954–2955

Magnetic resonance imaging (MRI) *(Continued)*
  of penis, 149, 150, 1645
  of pheochromocytoma, 3545, 3546f, 3547, 3547f
  of preureteral vena cava, 2045
  of prostate, 147, 150, 152f
  of prostate volume, 1310–1311
  of renal cell carcinoma, 2700–2701, 2712, 2713f
  of renal masses, 2675–2676
  of retroperitoneal fibrosis, 419
  of sacral agenesis, 2248–2249, 2250f
  of scrotum, 149, 150
  of seminal vesicles, 149, 3873–3874, 3873f
  of simple renal cysts, 1971, 1973f
  of spinal dysraphism, 2247–2248, 2248f
  of testicular germ cell tumors, 2887
  of testis, 149
  of ureter, 150, 150f
    ectopic, 2018
  of ureteropelvic junction obstruction, 2000–2001
  of urethral diverticulum, 1209, 1211f
  of urinary lithiasis, 3272
  of urinary tract infection, 536
  of urinary tract obstruction, 417
  principles of, 145–146
  pulse sequences in, 146, 147t
  renal function assessment using, 2000–2001
  renal perfusion studies using, 2000–2001
  T_1-weighted, 146, 147t
  T_2-weighted, 146, 147t
Magnetic resonance urography, 146
Magnetic stimulation
  in pelvic floor rehabilitation, for incontinence, 1073–1074
  of sacral nerve root, 983–984
MAINZ pouch
  for continent urinary diversion, 3811–3814
    postoperative care for, 3812, 3814, 3814f–3817f
    procedure for, 3811–3812, 3813f
  orthotopic, 3858, 3859f
MAINZ I pouch, 2546
MAINZ II pouch, 2545
  for continent urinary diversion, 3802–3803, 3802f
Mainz technique, for ureterosigmoidostomy, in exstrophy patient, 2173
Major histocompatibility complex (MHC)
  in allograft rejection, 363, 363t
  in allorecognition, 316–317, 317t
  in immune response, 314–315, 314f
Malabsorption, with conduit urinary diversion, 3782
Malacoplakia
  clinical presentation of, 565
  management of, 566
  pathogenesis and pathology of, 565
  radiologic findings in, 565–566, 566f
Malaria
  nephropathy in, 788
  quartan, 788
Male climacterium, as hormone therapy side effect, 3189
Malecot catheter, 112, 112f
Malignancy. *See also* Cancer; *specific neoplasm, e.g.,* Lymphoma.
  AIDS-associated
    cervical, 708
    urologic, 707
  and metastatic disease. *See* Metastasis(es).
  aspergillosis with, 806

Malignancy *(Continued)*
  blastomycosis with, 811
  Candida infection with, 798
  coccidioidomycosis with, 812
  hemolytic-uremic syndrome caused by, 1840
  involving male genitalia, 722–724, 734f
  priapism caused by, 1612
  vesicovaginal fistula caused by, 1202–1203
  vesicovaginal fistula in, 1196
Malignant hyperthermia, management of, 1010
Malnutrition
  Candida infection with, 798
  in chronic renal failure, 302
Malpighian corpuscle, 32, 33f
Malrotation, of kidney, 1906–1908, 1908f
Mannitol
  before renal arterial occlusion, in partial ne-
    phrectomy, 3604
  in acute renal failure, 283
Mannose-resistant hemagglutination (MRHA),
  524–525
Mannose-sensitive hemagglutination (MSHA),
  524
Mansonella spp. *See* Filariasis.
MAOIs. *See* Monoamine oxidase inhibitors
  (MAOIs).
Marden-Walker syndrome, hypospadias with,
  2292t
Marfan syndrome, multisystem involvement in,
  1814t
Marijuana, effect of, on spermatogenesis, 1477,
  1510
Marimastat, for prostate cancer, 3221–3222
Marlex mesh sling, 1161, 1162
  outcomes with, 1165
Marlex strip sling, outcomes with, 1167
Marshall test, 903, 1110
  in elderly, limited usefulness of, 1226
Marshall-Marchetti-Krantz (MMK) procedure,
  1141
  Burch culposuspension and, comparison of,
    1148–1149
  complications of, 1142, 1146
  for female incontinence, suture material in,
    1141–1142
  in epispadias patient, 2183
  results of, 1142
  technique for, 1142, 1143f
Martius labial interposition graft, for vesicovaginal fistula, 1201, 1201f
Massage
  pelvic floor, 622
  prostatic, 622
Mast cell(s), 312
  involvement of, in interstitial cystitis, 639–
    640, 639f
Mathieu hypospadias repair, 2308–2311, 2309f–
  2310f
Matrix (matrices)
  for bladder regeneration, 2601–2602
  of urinary stones, 3238
Matrix calculi, 3266
Matrix metalloproteinases, 289
  for prostate cancer, 3221–3222
  in prostate cancer, 3016
  inhibitors of, as angiogenesis inhibitors,
    2655–2656
Maximal androgen blockade, for prostate cancer,
  3197–3199
Maximal urethral closing pressure (MUCP)
  age-related changes in, 1218–1219
  and Valsalva leak point pressure, correlation
    between, 912

Maximal urethral closing pressure (MUCP)
  (Continued)
  assessment of, 1156
  clinical significance of, 1156
  definition of, 1152
  drugs affecting, 988–989
  in incontinence, 913
  in intrinsic sphincteric dysfunction, 1152
  in postprostatectomy incontinence, 1061–
    1062
  in spinal shock, 945
  postprostatectomy, 1057
Maximal urethral pressure (MUP), drugs affecting, 988–989
Mayer-Rokitansky syndrome, multisystem involvement in, 1814t
Mayer-Rokitansky-Küster-Hauser syndrome,
  1930, 2420–2421, 2431–2436, 2431f
  findings associated with, 2432
  vaginal replacement for, 2432–2436
    intestinal neovagina in, 2433–2436, 2434f,
      2435f
    skin neovagina in, 2432–2433, 2433f
  with cloacal exstrophy, 2177
McCall culdoplasty, definition of, 1120t
McCall stitch, modified, 1126, 1127f
MCDK. *See* Multicystic dysplastic kidney
  (MCDK).
McDonough syndrome, cryptorchidism associated with, 2367t
Mean arterial pressure, laparoscopic surgery and,
  3476
Meares-Stamey four-hour glass test, for prostatitis, 609, 612–613, 614f
Meatal stenosis, 3904–3905, 3905f
  after hypospadias repair, 2321–2322
  following circumcision, 2337–2338, 2338t
  in balanitis xerotica obliterans, 3900–3901,
    3901f
Meatoplasty. *See also* Meatoplasty and glanuloplasty (MAGPI) technique.
  bulbar elongation anastomotic (BEAM) proce-
    dure for, for hypospadias repair, 2304
  for meatal stenosis, 2338
  in hypospadias repair, 2301
Meatoplasty and glanuloplasty (MAGPI) technique, for hypospadias repair, 2304,
  2306f
Mebendazole, for pelvic enterobiasis, 786
Mechanical properties, of smooth muscle, 386–
  387
Meckel-Gruber syndrome
  cryptorchidism associated with, 2367t
  multisystem involvement in, 1814t
Meckel's diverticulum, in children, 1816t
Meckel's syndrome, 1956
Meconium, passage of, by neonate, 1825
Meconium ileus, 1822
Meconium peritonitis, 2350
Medial fibroplasia
  of renal artery, 231t, 233, 234f
  renovascular hypertension due to, renal arte-
    rial reconstruction for, 3615
Medial preoptic area, in sexual function, 1598,
  1598t
Medial raphe cyst, 726–727, 2350
Median raphe
  development of, 2334
Mediastinal resection, postchemotherapy, with
  testicular tumors, 2938
Mediastinum testis, 76, 76f
Medicated urethral system for erection (MUSE),
  1655–1656

Medullary cystic disease. *See also* Juvenile ne-
  phronopthisis-medullary cystic disease complex.
  clinical features of, 1952, 1953t
  evaluation of, 1953–1954, 1954f
  genetics of, 1952, 1953t
  histopathology of, 1952–1953, 1953f
  in chronic renal failure, 292
  incidence of, 1939t, 1952, 1953t
  renal findings in, 1939t, 1953t
  tubular basement membrane in, 1953, 1953t
  ultrasonography in, 1953, 1954f
Medullary sponge kidney, 1974–1976
  clinical features of, 1974f, 1974–1975
  diagnosis of, 1975
  genetics of, 1940t
  histopathology of, 1975
  incidence of, 1940t, 1974
  prognosis for, 1976
  renal findings in, 1940t
  treatment of, 1975–1976
Megacalycosis, 1914–1915, 1915f, 1916f
  megaureter with, 1915, 1916f
Megacolon, in prune-belly syndrome, 2122
Megacystis
  congenital, 2189
  postnatal evaluation and management of, 1797
Megacystis-megaureter association
  postnatal evaluation and management of,
    1797
  vesicoureteral reflux and, 2075
Megalourethra, 2226f, 2227
  anomalies associated with, 2227
  congenital, in prune-belly syndrome, 2120,
    2120f
  fusiform, 2227
    in prune-belly syndrome, 2120
  in prune-belly syndrome, 1784, 1784f, 2120,
    2120f, 2227
    repair of, 2130f, 2130–2131
  management of, 2227
  prenatal diagnosis, 1784f
  scaphoid, 2227
    in prune-belly syndrome, 2120, 2120f
Megameatus, 1823
  with intact prepuce. *See* Hypospadias, mega-
    meatus/intact prepuce variant of.
Megaprepuce, 2343, 2344f
Megaureter(s), 2094–2108. *See also* Megacystis-
  megaureter association.
  classification of, 2096f, 2096–2097
  congenital, 2189
  definition of, 2095–2096
  discovered in adult, 2098, 2099f
    management of, 2103
  etiology of, 2096f, 2096–2097
  evaluation of, 2100f, 2100–2101, 2101f
  in duplex system, management of, 2107f,
    2107–2108
  in exstrophy patient, 2145
  in neonates, 2096f, 2098
    expectant management of, 2102f, 2103
  in nephrogenic diabetes insipidus, 1844
  nonobstructive nonrefluxing
    clinical correlates of, 2103
  primary
    etiology of, 2096f, 2098
    pathophysiology of, 2098–2100, 2099f,
      2100f
    treatment of, 2103
  secondary
    etiology of, 2096f, 2098
    pathophysiology of, 2098

MRHA (mannose-resistant hemagglutination), 524–525

MRI. *See* Magnetic resonance imaging (MRI).

mRNA (messenger ribonucleic acid), viral, in HIV infection, 696

MSHA (mannose-sensitive hemagglutination), 524

Mucocele, appendiceal, in children, 1816t

Mucormycosis, 809–810, 810f
treatment of, 821t

Mucosa, vaginal, 1710–1711

Mucosal biopsies, in bladder cancer, 2759

Mucosal seal, 890

Mucus, following augmentation cystoplasty, 2535

Müllerian anomalies, with cloacal exstrophy, 2177

Müllerian (paramesonephric) ducts, 1754, 1755f, 1756, 1761, 1766f
differentiation of, 2401, 2401f
formation of, 1753, 1754f
persistent, 2420

Müllerian-inhibiting substance (MIS), 1239, 1268t, 1440, 1754, 1755f
in male sexual differentiation, 2354, 2355
in sexual differentiation, 2401–2402, 2402f

Multicystic, definition of, 1938

Multicystic dysplastic kidney (MCDK), 1960–1965
and ureteropelvic junction obstruction, 1998
and Wilms' tumor, 1963–1964
bilateral, sex distribution of, 1961
bunch of grapes appearance in, 1960, 1960f
clinical features of, 1822, 1961
definition of, 1930
differential diagnosis of, 1787–1788
etiology of, 1961
evaluation of, 1962, 1963f
renal findings in, 1960, 1960f, 1961–1962, 1962f
fetal, ultrasound appearance of, 1783
histopathology of, 1961–1962, 1962f
hydronephrotic form of, 1960, 1960f, 1962
in horseshoe kidney, 1961, 1962f
incidence of, 1940t
outcomes with, 1964t, 1964–1965
prenatal diagnosis of, 1787f, 1787–1788
postnatal evaluation and management with, 1799–1800
prognosis for, 1964–1965
renal findings in, 1940t, 1961
solid cystic form of, 1960, 1960f
treatment of, 1962–1965
unilateral, sex distribution of, 1961
vesicoureteral reflux with, 2074–2075
with cloacal exstrophy, 2177

Multidrug resistance, in renal cell carcinoma, 2690

Multifilamented polyester mesh. *See* Mersilene mesh slings.

Multilocular cyst(s), solitary, in children, 2493–2494

Multimodality therapy
for renal cell carcinoma, metastatic, 2718–2719
for urethral cancer, female, 2998

Multiplane probes, for transrectal ultrasound, 3039

Multiple endocrine neoplasia (MEN), 3543
type I, 2633t
type II, pheochromocytoma associated with, 2632t

Multiple lentigines syndrome
cryptorchidism associated with, 2367t
hypospadias with, 2292t

Multiple sclerosis
and female sexual dysfunction, 1719, 1720, 1722
epidemiology of, 941
erectile dysfunction in, 1477
etiology of, 941
in males, seminal emission abnormalities in, electroejaculation for, 1565–1566
incontinence in, 1034
orgasmic disorder in, 1722
pathophysiology of, 941
urologic sequelae associated with, 90, 941–942
functional classification of, 942
management of, 942
voiding dysfunction in, 933t, 941–942
treatment of, 994

Multiple system atrophy
erectile dysfunction in, 941
parkinsonism in, 940, 941
prostatectomy in, 940, 941
voiding dysfunction in, 941

Mumps orchitis, infertility caused by, 1477, 1508

MUP (maximal urethral pressure), drugs affecting, 988–989

Muscarinic receptor(s)
in bladder, 967–968
locations of, by subtype, 968
nomenclature for, 967

Muscimol, uropharmacology of, 869

Muscle(s). *See also named muscle.*
abdominal wall
anterior, 43–44, 45f
posterior, 3–5, 9f–121f
pelvic, 46, 49f–50f, 70
perineal, 70, 71f
smooth. *See also* Smooth muscle.
of bladder, 59–60, 59f
of ureter, 377–387

Muscle reflex(es), 903

Muscle relaxants, for prostatitis, 621

Muscular dystrophy, pelvic organ prolapse in, 1095

Muscular lesion, and voiding dysfunction, 889t, 894

Musculoskeletal system, in prune-belly syndrome, 2122

MUSE (medicated urethral system for erection), 1655–1656

Mutations
carcinogenesis and, 2630–2631
definition of, 2626t

Myasthenia gravis, voiding dysfunction in, 962

MYC oncogene, in prostate cancer, 3015

Mycobacteria, biology of, 746–747

Mycobacterium africanum, 746

Mycobacterium avium-intracellulare, 747

Mycobacterium bovis, 746

Mycobacterium fortuitum, 747

Mycobacterium kansasii, 747

Mycobacterium microti, 746

Mycobacterium tuberculosis. See also Tuberculosis.
in acquired immunodeficiency syndrome, 700–701, 704
in urinary tract infection, 523

Mycobacterium tuberculosis complex, 746–747

Mycobacterium xenopi, 747

Mycophenolate mofetil
as immunosuppressant, 364, 364t, 365, 365f
toxicity of, organ system target for, 367t

Mycoplasma hominis
in interstitial cystitis, 638
in nongonococcal urethritis, 675

Mycosis fungoides, 724

Myelitis, in schistosomiasis, 780

Myelodysplasia
and age at puberty, 2244
and bowel function, 2244–2245
and continence, 2241–2244, 2242f, 2243f
and sexuality, 2244
detrusor leak point pressure in, 911
epidemiology of, 2234, 2235t
fetal intervention for, 2235
genetics of, 2234, 2235t
in children, and vesicoureteral reflux, 2059
incontinence in, 1034
sling procedures for, 1152–1153, 1153f
neurologic defects caused by, 2235–2236, 2238–2240, 2240f, 2241f
treatment recommendations for, 2239–2240, 2241t
pathogenesis of, 2234–2236
pelvic organ prolapse in, 1095
prevention of, 2234
surveillance of infant with, 2239–2240, 2241t
treatment of, recommendations for, 2238, 2240f
urinary diversion in, 2244
urodynamic evaluation in, 2236–2238, 2237f, 2238f, 2239f
vesicoureteral reflux with, management of, 2240–2241, 2242f
voiding dysfunction with, 933t, 952
in children, 2234–2245

Myelolipoma, 3525–3526, 3526f

Myelomeningocele. *See also* Myelodysplasia.
appearance of, 2236f
definition of, 2234
management of, in neonate, 1805
pathogenesis of, 2234–2236
spinal level of, 2234, 2236t
voiding dysfunction with, 952–953, 954
artificial sphincter for, 1188. *See also* Artificial sphincter.
with cloacal exstrophy, 2177

Myelopathy. *See also* Tropical spastic paraparesis.
cervical, voiding dysfunction in, 952
schistosomal, voiding dysfunction in, 944
syphilitic, voiding dysfunction with, 953

Myeloproliferative disorders, uric acid calculi in, 3259

Myeloschisis, 952

Myoblastoma, granular cell, of bladder, 2765

Myoblasts, injectable, for urinary incontinence, 2615

Myocardial infarction
after renal transplantation, 373
erectile dysfunction caused by, 1610
postprostatectomy, 1433

Myocardial ischemia, in testicular descent, 2360

Myofascial trigger point release, for prostatitis, 622

Myopathy, neurophysiologic recordings in, 926–927

Myoplasty
bladder, to facilitate bladder emptying, 1003
for functional sphincter reconstruction, 993–994

Myosin
  of smooth muscle, 378, 382–383, 382f–383f, 1596
  phosphorylation of, 382
Myosin light-chain kinase, 382, 382f–383f
Myotonic dystrophy
  infertility in, 1508
  voiding dysfunction in, 963–964

N-acetyltransferase, in bladder cancer, 2738
Nafareline acetate, for benign prostatic hyperplasia, 1359t
Naftidine, in antifungal therapy, 821
Nails, examination of, in children, 1822
Nalidixic acid
  for pediatric urinary tract infection
    oral dosage and administration of, 1865t
    prophylactic, 1867
  serum and urinary levels of, 537t
Nalmifene, for interstitial cystitis, 653
Naloxone
  to facilitate bladder emptying, 1002
  uropharmacology of, 870
Nanobacteria, urinary lithiasis related to, 3254
Naproxen, acute tubulointerstitial nephritis caused by, 1843
Narcotic analgesics
  and female sexual dysfunction, 1720
  effect of, on ureteral function, 402
  incontinence caused by, in elderly, 1221t
National Institute of Arthritis, Diabetes, Digestive and Kidney Diseases (NIDDK), 632
  diagnostic criteria of, for interstitial cystitis, 633t
National Institutes of Health Chronic Prostatitis Symptom Index (NIH-CPSI), 613f
National Institutes of Health (NIH) classification, of prostatitis, 610
National Kidney Foundation guidelines, for renal disease education, 303
Natural killer (NK) cells, 311–312
  role of, in tumor immunology, 334
Nausea, in ureteropelvic junction obstruction, 1999
NCCT gene, in Gitelman's syndrome, 1844–1845
Nd:YAG lasers, 1395
  for interstitial cystitis, 657
Neck, webbing of, 1822
Necrospermia, 1481
Necrotizing fasciitis, of male genitalia. See Fournier's gangrene.
Necrotizing gangrene, genital skin loss due to, 3738
Needle holders, laparoscopic, 3467–3468
Needle suspension procedure
  results of, 1152
  retropubic suspension surgery and, comparison of, 1148
nef gene, in HIV-1, 696
Neisseria gonorrhoeae
  in gonococcal urethritis, 673, 673t, 674
  in pelvic inflammatory disease, 424, 685
Nematodes, 788
Neocystostomy, direct
  indications for, 2856–2857
  technique for, 2857, 2858f–2860f
Neodymium:yttrium-aluminum-garnet (Nd:YAG) lasers, 1395
  for interstitial cystitis, 657
Neomycin, for bowel preparation, 3751t

Neonate(s). See also Child(ren); Infant(s).
  abdominal masses in, 1803–1804, 1804t
    distribution of, 1817, 1817t
  absence of voiding in, management of, 1805
  acid-base regulation in, 1767
  adrenal hemorrhage in, 1806
  ascites in, 2211–2212, 2212f
  bladder outlet obstruction in, clinical presentation of, 2211–2212
  cloacal anomaly in, management of, 1804
  collection of urine specimen in, 98, 1847–1848
  febrile, and bacterial infection, 1820, 1820t
  female, perineal mass in, 1802–1803
  fluid and electrolyte management in, 1772, 1772f
  hematuria in
    evaluation of, 1813
    management of, 1805–1806
  hypertension in, 1806
  imperforate anus in, management of, 1804
  kidneys in, functional development of, 1767–1768
  large scrotum in, management of, 1801
  nephrogenic diabetes insipidus in, 1844
  prune-belly syndrome in, 2117
    initial evaluation in, 2124–2125
  renal artery thrombosis in, 1806
  renal vein thrombosis in, 1806
  sepsis in, management of, 1805
  spinal cord injury in, mechanisms of injury in, 2254
  toxic nephropathy in, 1776
  transient nephromegaly in, 1942
  ureteropelvic junction obstruction in, 463–489, 1995. See also Ureteropelvic junction obstruction, congenital.
  urinary ascites in, 1806
  urinary tract infection in, evaluation of, 1813
  urodynamic evaluation in, 2236–2237
  urologic emergencies in, 1800–1806
    clinical presentation of, 1800, 1800t
  voiding cystourethrography in, 1797–1798
  voiding in, 1767
  with ambiguous genitalia. See also Hermaphroditism; Pseudohermaphroditism.
    evaluation and management of, 2421–2423, 2422f
Neostigmine, effect of, on ureteral function, 388
Neourethra
  coverage of. See Urethroplasty.
  formation of. See Urethroplasty.
  in hypospadias repair. See Urethroplasty.
Neovagina, for Mayer-Rokitansky-Küster-Hauser syndrome
  intestines used in, 2433–2436, 2434f, 2435f
  skin used in, 2432–2433, 2433f
Nephrectomy
  allograft, indications for, 366–367
  cadaver donor, surgical approach to, 354, 355f–356f
  for ectopic ureter, laparoscopic, 2019–2021, 2021f
  for perinephric abscess, 562
  for polycystic kidney disease, 3638
  for renal cell carcinoma, metastatic, 2714–2715
  for renal trauma, indications for, 3713
  for ureteral contusion, 3718–3719
  for ureteropelvic junction obstruction, 469
  historical background of, 3571
  in tuberculosis, 759
  laparoscopic. See Laparoscopic nephrectomy.

Nephrectomy (Continued)
  living donor, 352
  partial
    for benign disease, 3613–3615, 3614f
      heminephrectomy as, in duplicated collecting systems, 3614–3615
    for malignancy, 3602–3613, 3603f–3606f
      central tumors and, 3607, 3609–3610, 3610f
      complications of, 3612
      extracorporeal, with autotransplantation, 3610–3612, 3611f
      local recurrence after, 2714, 2714t
      major transverse resection in, 3606–3607, 3609f
      postoperative follow-up for, 3612–3613
      segmental polar nephrectomy as, 3606, 3607f
      simple enucleation in, 3610
      wedge resection in, 3606, 3608f
    for renal pelvis tumors, 2847–2849
    for Wilms' tumor, 2492
    in tuberculosis, 759
    laparoscopic, in children, 2584, 2584f
  polar, segmental, 3606, 3607f
  pretransplantation, indications for, 351, 351t
  radical, 3587–3602
    complications of, 3600–3602
    for renal cell carcinoma
      local recurrence after, 2714
      localized, 2704–2705, 2705t
    indications for, 3587–3588, 3591f
    retroperitoneal hemorrhage during, management of, 3593–3595, 3595f, 3596f
    technique for, 2849–2850, 2851f, 2852f
      standard, 3589–3593, 3591f–3595f
    with vena caval involvement
      infrahepatic, 3595–3596, 3597f–3599f
      intrahepatic or suprahepatic, 3596, 3598–3600, 3600f–3602f
  renal function following, 3573–3574
  simple, 3584–3587
    flank approach to, 3584–3585, 3587f, 3588f
    indications for, 3584
    laparoscopic. See Laparoscopic nephrectomy, simple.
    subcapsular technique for, 3585–3586, 3589f
    transperitoneal approach to, 3586–3587, 3590f
  upper-pole
    for ectopic ureter, 2018–2022, 2020f
    for ureterocele, 2028
Nephritis
  focal bacterial, pediatric, 1852
  in Alport's syndrome, 1840
  in Henoch-Schönlein purpura, 1839–1840
  interstitial, in acute renal failure, 275–276, 275t
Nephroblastoma. See Wilms' tumor.
Nephroblastomatosis, 2484
  computed tomography in, 1829
Nephrocalcin, as calcium oxalate crystal inhibitor, 3237
Nephrocalcinosis, in renal tubular acidosis, in children, 1771
Nephrogenic adenoma, in bladder cancer, 2742
Nephrogenic cords, 1740
Nephrogenic rests, Wilms' tumor and, 2484–2486, 2485f, 2485t
Nephrolithiasis. See Urinary lithiasis, renal.

Perinephric fluid collection, ultrasonography of, 134

Perineum, 70–79
central tendon of, 70
defects of, in exstrophy patient, 2141–2142
fascia of, 48–49, 52f
female, 78–79, 78f–79f, 1710
lymphatic drainage of, 75–76
male, 70–78, 70f, 72f
anatomy of, 3895, 3896f, 3897–3898
muscles and superficial fascia of, 71f
mass in, in female neonate, 1802–1803
muscles of, 1098, 1099f
sensory loss in, in disc disease, 954

Peripheral edema, drug-induced, in elderly, 1221

Peripheral nervous system
and lower urinary tract, 846f, 846–848
female genital innervation by, 1711–1714

Peripheral neuropathy
in diabetes, 956
voiding dysfunction with, 935

Periprostatic plexus, 1594f

Peritoneal dialysis
in acute renal failure, 285–286, 300
in chronic renal failure, 298–299, 300t

Peritoneum
median fold of, 45
umbilical fold of
lateral, 46
medial, 45–46

Peritonitis
in children, signs and symptoms of, 1822
meconium, 2350

Periurethral abscess, 591–592

Periurethral glands, 63

Perivesical fat, 59

Perlman syndrome, cryptorchidism associated with, 2368t

Permethrin cream
for pediculosis pubis infection, 686
for scabies, 685–686

Permixon. See Serenoa repens.

Pernicious anemia
bladder compliance in, 909
sensory neurogenic bladder in, 895
voiding dysfunction with, 933t, 953

Peroneal nerve patch electrode stimulation, 983

Perphenazine, priapism caused by, 1612t

Persistent müllerian duct syndrome, 2420

Pessary(ies), vaginal
and physical examination of patient, 1038
complications of, 1120
for reduction of prolapse, 1042
for stress incontinence, 991–992, 1079–1080, 1080f, 1081f
indications for, 1120
ring, 1120
support, 1120
trial of, before pelvic organ prolapse correction, 1089

PET. See Positron-emission tomography (PET).

Petechiae, in infants, 1822

Peter-plus syndrome
cryptorchidism associated with, 2368t
hypospadias with, 2292t

Peyronie's disease, 94, 1696–1705, 3946
active phase of, 1698
and Dupuytren's contracture, 1696, 1699
and plantar fascial contracture, 1696
and tympanosclerosis, 1696, 1699
areas of induration in, 1699
clinical presentation of, 1699
conditions associated with, 1696

Peyronie's disease (Continued)
dorsal, 1698, 1699, 1700, 1701f
epidemiology of, 1696, 1698
erectile dysfunction in, 1608, 1698
etiology of, 1696
historical perspective on, 1696
history-taking in, 1699
intralesional injections for, 1700
medical management of, 1700
natural history of, 1698
pain in, 1699
patient counseling in, 1698–1699
patients' understanding of, 1699
penile prosthesis for, 1676–1677, 1688–1689
plaque in, 1699
preoperative erectile function in, and postoperative results, 1699
psychological aspects of, 1698–1699
quiescent secondary phase of, 1698
surgical treatment of, 1700–1705, 1701f–1705f
candidates for, 1700
symptomatic incidence of, 1696
vascular testing in, 1699
ventral, 1698, 1699

Pezzer catheter, 112, 112f

Pfannenstiel incisions, for bladder surgery, 2820

pH
blood, calcium excretion and, 191
in acid-base balance, 213
urinary, 99–100
in renal urate excretion, 198

Phaclofen, uropharmacology of, 869

Phaeohyphomycosis, 815

Phagocytosis, 308

Phallic reconstruction. See Penile reconstruction.

Pharmacogenomics, advances in (future directions for), 876

Pharmacology, of bladder, 857–870

Phenacetin, as bladder cancer risk factor, 2739

Phenotype, definition of, 2626t

Phenoxybenzamine
adverse effects and side effects of, 1007
effect of, on ureteral function, 389
erectile dysfunction caused by, 1609
for pheochromocytoma, 3547
for prostatitis, 620, 621, 624t
for voiding dysfunction, 976
incontinence caused by, 1038
indications for, 1007
prophylactic, for postoperative urinary retention, 961
uropharmacology of, 1007, 2235t

Phentolamine
effect of, on ureteral function, 389
erectile dysfunction caused by, 1609
for erectile dysfunction, 1653
intracavernous injection of, 1657
mechanism of action of, 1653

Phenylbutyrate, for prostate cancer, 3222

Phenylephrine
for priapism, 1662, 1662t
uropharmacology of, 867

Phenylpropanolamine
adverse effects and side effects of, 989–990
dosage and administration of, 989
FDA policy on, 989–990
for geriatric incontinence, 1230
for incontinence, 1074
for postprostatectomy incontinence, 1065
for stress incontinence, 989
hemorrhagic stroke caused by, 1074

Phenylpropanolamine (Continued)
uropharmacology of, 858t, 989, 2235t

Phenytoin, interactions with azoles, 819t

Pheochromocytoma, 2632t, 3540–3549
anesthetic management for, 3549, 3549t
during pregnancy, 3541
familial, 3543
hypercalcemia associated with, 3248
imaging of, 3545, 3546f–3548f, 3547
in children, 3544
laboratory diagnosis of, 3544–3545, 3545f, 3545t
of bladder, 2765
preoperative management of, 3547–3549
signs and symptoms of, 3540–3544, 3541t, 3542t, 3543f, 3544f
von Hippel–Lindau disease and, 1959

Phimosis, 94, 2335, 3904

Phocomelia, Roberts-SC, cryptorchidism associated with, 2368t

Phosphatase, in seminal plasma, 1238

Phosphate
dietary, 197
urinary lithiasis related to, 3280
renal excretion of
factors influencing, 197
in neonates, 1767–1768
regulation of, 196–197
serum level of, in Fanconi's syndrome, 1844

Phosphaturia, 99

Phosphodiesterase
in penile detumescence, 1592, 1601, 1602f, 1603f
isoenzymes, 1654
in smooth muscle, 861

Phosphodiesterase activity, in ureteral peristalsis, 384

Phosphodiesterase inhibitors. See also Sildenafil citrate.
for erectile dysfunction, 1653–1655
for voiding dysfunction, 981t
uropharmacology of, 859, 861

Phospholipase C, in ureteral peristalsis, 385, 385f

Phosphorus
fractional tubular reabsorption of, in children, calculation of, 1771
metabolism of, 3240
renal excretion of, in children, evaluation of, 1771

Phosphorylcholine, in prostatic secretions, 1277–1278

Photodynamic therapy, for bladder cancer, 2822–2823
superficial, 2787

Photofrin (porfimer sodium), for bladder cancer, superficial, 2787

Photoplethysmography, vaginal, 1725, 1726f

Phrenic artery, inferior, 6, 14f

Phthiriasis (pediculosis pubis infection), 686

Phycomycosis, 809–810, 810f

Physical examination, 92–98
general observations in, 92
in erectile dysfunction, 1625–1626
in genitourinary fistula patient, 1196–1198
in geriatric incontinence, 1225
in neurourologic evaluation, 903–904
in pelvic organ prolapse, 1109–1112
of bladder, 93–94, 93f–94f
of female pelvis, 97–98
of incontinent patient, 1038
of kidneys, 92–93, 93f
of pediatric patient, 1821–1825

Prostatitis *(Continued)*
  in acquired immunodeficiency syndrome, 707
  in aspergillosis, 806
  in blastomycosis, 811
  interstitial cystitis-like cause of, 608–609
  intraprostatic ductal reflux in, 607–608
  Meares-Stamey four-glass test for, 609, 612–
    613, 614f
  mycotic, 606–607
  neural dysregulation in, 608
  nonbacterial, 625. *See also* Chronic pelvic
    pain syndrome.
    classification of, 610t
    clinical presentation of, 611, 611f
    cytokines in, 617
  nonculturable microorganisms in, 607
  nontuberculous mycobacterial, 747
  pelvic floor musculature abnormalities in, 608
  physical examination of, 612
  prostatic biopsy in, 616–617
  prostatic calculi in, 605, 607–608
  psychologic cause of, 609
  Staphylococcus in, 605
  strategies for, 623, 624f, 624t, 625
  transrectal ultrasonography in, 616
  treatment of, 617–623
    allopurinol in, 621–622
    alpha-blockers in, 620, 624t
    antibiotics in, 617–620, 624t
      clinical trial data for, 619–620, 619t
      pharmacology and pharmacokinetics in,
        617–618
      rationale for, 617
    balloon dilatation in, 622
    biofeedback in, 622
    hormone therapy in, 621, 624t
    immune modulators in, 620–621
    microwave hyperthermia in, 622–623
    minimally invasive surgery in, 622
    muscle relaxants in, 621
    myofascial trigger point release in, 622
    nonsteroidal anti-inflammatory drugs in,
      620–621, 624t
    perineal or pelvic floor massage in, 622
    physical therapy in, 622
    phytotherapeutic agents in, 621, 624t
    prostatic massage in, 622
    strategies for, 623, 624f, 624t, 625
    surgical, 623
    thermotherapy in, 623
  Trichomonas in, 607
  two-glass test for, 614, 615f
  Ureaplasma urealyticum in, 606
  urodynamics for, 616
Prostatodynia, 625. *See also* Chronic pelvic pain
  syndrome; Prostatitis.
  classification of, 610t
  clinical presentation of, 611, 611f
  diagnosis of, 609–610
Prostatron, 1389f, 1389–1390, 1390f
Prostatropin, 1272
Prosthesis, penile. *See* Penile prosthesis.
Prostin VR. *See* Alprostadil, pediatric formula-
  tion of.
Protease(s)
  in renal cell carcinoma, 2691
  in seminal plasma, 1238
Protease inhibitors
  as angiogenesis inhibitors, 2655–2656
  for acquired immunodeficiency syndrome,
    699f, 700
Protective intervention regimens, for chronic renal failure, 294–296

ProteGen, for sling procedures, 1161
Protein(s)
  bcl-2, in regulation of apoptosis, 326
  Bence Jones, 105
  dietary, urinary lithiasis related to, 3278–3279
  HER-2/neu, 333
  in seminal plasma, 1238, 1279t, 1279–1283
  p53, 333
  ras, 319
  responsible for apoptosis, 325–326, 326f
  restriction of, in chronic renal failure, 295–
    296
  smooth muscle, 378, 382–383, 382f–383f
  STAT (signal transducer and activator of tran-
    scription), 320
  Tamm-Horsfall, 105
    in interstitial cystitis, 641
Protein kinase C, activation of, 319
Proteinases, in interstitial cystitis, 639
Proteinuria, 104–106
  detection of, 105
  evaluation of, 105–106, 106f
  glomerular, 105
  in Alport's syndrome, 1840
  in children, 1836–1837, 1841–1844
    in acute tubulointerstitial nephritis, 1843–
      1844
    in glomerular diseases, 1842–1843
    in tubulointerstitial diseases, 1843–1844
    isolated, 1841–1842
    orthostatic, 1841–1842
    persistent asymptomatic, 1842
    qualitative detection of, 1836
    quantitative measurement of, 1836
    transient, 1841
    urinary protein/urinary creatinine (Upr/Ucr)
      ratio in, 1836–1837, 1842
    with hematuria, 1826–1827
  in postinfectious glomerulonephritis, 1839
  in reflux nephropathy, 1843
  in renovascular hypertension, 241
  in systemic lupus erythematosus, 1840
  overflow, 105
  pathophysiology of, 105
  test for, 1841
  tubular, 105
Proteoglycans
  in renal development, 1746f, 1747
  of bladder wall stroma, 840
Proteomics, in cancer, 2659
Proteus mirabilis, in urinary tract infection,
  546–548, 547f
Proto-oncogenes, 2631. *See also* Oncogene(s).
Provirus, 696
Prune-belly syndrome, 2117–2133
  abdominal wall defects in, 2117–2118, 2121,
    2122f
    surgical correction of, 2127f–2128f, 2131–
      2133, 2132f
  and monosomy 16, 2124
  and trisomy 13, 2124
  and trisomy 18, 2124
  and Turner's syndrome, 2124
  bladder diverticulum in, 2189
  bladder in, 2117, 2119, 2119f
    surgical management of, 2127–2129
  cardiac anomalies in, 2121t, 2122, 2124
  category I, 2123, 2123t, 2125
  category II, 2123, 2123t, 2125
    management of, 2125
    prognosis for, 2125
  category III, 2123, 2123t, 2125
    management of, 2125, 2126f

Prune-belly syndrome *(Continued)*
  cause of, 2117–2118
  classification of, 2123, 2123t, 2125
  clinical features of, 1822, 2123
  clinical spectrum of, 2123, 2123t
  cryptorchidism in, 2117–2118, 2120–2121
    management of, 2131
  diagnosis of, 1813
    initial evaluation for, 2124–2125
    prenatal, 2117, 2122–2123
  epidemiology of, 2117
  extragenitourinary abnormalities in, 2121t,
    2121–2122
  fertility in, 2121
  gastrointestinal anomalies in, 2121t, 2122
  genetics of, 2124
  genitourinary abnormalities in, 2118–2121
  in adult, clinical features of, 2123
  in child, clinical features of, 2123
  in female, 2123–2124
  in infant, clinical features of, 2123
  incidence of, 2117
  incomplete, 2124
  infertility in, 1506
  kidneys in, 2118, 2123, 2123t, 2124, 2125
  management of, 1804–1805, 1813, 2124–
    2133
    in utero, 2122–2123
    nonoperative, 2125
    surgical, 2125–2133, 2127f–2132f
    timing of, 2125
  megalourethra in, 1784, 1784f, 2120, 2120f,
    2227
  megaureter in, 2098
  multisystem involvement in, 1814t
  organ involvement in, 2117
  orthopedic deformities in, 2121t, 2122
  pathophysiology of, 2118–2122
  penis in, 2120, 2120f
  posterior urethral valves in, 2211
  prenatal diagnosis of, 2117, 2122–2123
  prognosis for, 2117, 2123, 2133
  prostate gland in, 2118, 2119f, 2120
  pulmonary abnormalities in, 2121t, 2121–
    2122, 2123, 2123t, 2124
  renal hypodysplasia in, 1937
  sex distribution of, 2117
  sexual function in, 2121
  testis in, 2120–2121
  ultrasound in, 2117, 2124, 2124f
  urachal diverticulum in, 2192
  urethra in, 2117–2118, 2119f, 2120, 2123
    surgical management of, 2127–2131,
      2130f
  urinary diversion in, temporary, 2126
  vesicoureteral reflux in, 2119, 2119f
    surgical management of, 2125–2126
  vesicourethral dysfunction in, surgical man-
    agement of, 2127–2131, 2130f
  voiding in, 2119–2120
PSA. *See* Prostate-specific antigen (PSA).
P-selectin glycoprotein ligand, granulocyte and T
  cell expression of, 330
Pseudallescheria boydii infection, 816
Pseudodiverticula, urethral, 1209
Pseudodyssynergia
  causes of, 958
  definition of, 958
  electromyographic characteristics of, 958
  in multiple sclerosis, 942
  with brain tumor, 938
  with cerebrovascular disease, 937

Retrovirus(es). *See also specific virus, e.g.,*
  Human immunodeficiency virus (HIV).
  as gene therapy vectors, 2660
  biology of, 693–695
  cancer and, 694
  flow of genetic information in, 694, 695f
  production of, from infected cells, 696–697
rev gene, in HIV-1, 696
Reverse transcription, of retroviruses, 694, 695f,
  696
Reye's syndrome, aspirin and, 1820
Rhabdoid tumor, renal, 2493
Rhabdomyosarcoma(s), 1789, 2475–2481
  genetics of, 2475–2476
  interlabial, clinical presentation of, 2034
  of bladder, 2478–2479, 2478f, 2765
  paratesticular, 2479–2480, 2912
  pathology of, 2476
  patterns of spread of, 2476
  prostatic, 2478–2479, 2478f
  staging of, 2476–2477, 2476t, 2477t
  treatment of, 2477–2478
    for bladder tumors, 2478–2479, 2478f
    for paratesticular tumors, 2479–2480
    for prostatic tumors, 2478–2479, 2478f
    for uterine tumors, 2480–2481
    for vaginal tumors, 2480, 2480f
    for vulvar tumors, 2480
  uterine, 2480–2481
  vaginal, 2442–2443, 2443f, 2480, 2480f
  vulvar, 2480
Rhabdosphincter, 844, 1028, 1055, 1055f
  age-related changes in, 1219
  development of, 1792
  innervation of, 1056
  postprostatectomy function of, 1059–1060
  skeletal muscle of, 1055
  smooth muscle of, 1055
Rhabdosphincter complex, 3840
Rheumatoid arthritis, and female sexual dysfunction, 1719
Rhinosporidiosis, 816
Rhizomucor spp., 809
Rhizopus spp., 809
rHu-EPO (recombinant human erythropoietin),
  for chronic renal failure, 302
Rib cage, lower, 5, 11f
Ribonucleic acid (RNA)
  messenger (mRNA), in HIV infection, 696
  posttranscriptional modification of, 2629
Rickets, in Fanconi's syndrome, 1844
Rickettsial infection, acute tubulointerstitial nephritis in, 1843
Rieger's syndrome, hypospadias with, 2292t
Rifabutin
  adverse effects and side effects of, 757t
  dosage and administration of, 757t
Rifamate, dosage and administration of, 757t
Rifampin
  acute tubulointerstitial nephritis caused by,
    1843
  adverse effects and side effects of, 756, 757t
  dosage and administration of, 757t
  for genitourinary tuberculosis, 757–759
  interactions with azoles, 819t
  mechanism of action of, 755t, 755–756
  mutational resistance to, site of, 755t
  pharmacology of, 756
Rifapentine
  adverse effects and side effects of, 757t
  dosage and administration of, 757t
Rifater, dosage and administration of, 757t

Right colon pouch(es), 3858
  for continent urinary diversion, surgical tech-
    niques for, 3828–3829, 3829f
  with intussuscepted terminal ileum, for conti-
    nent urinary diversion, 3814–3815,
    3817–3818
    postoperative care for, 3817–3818
    procedures for, 3815, 3817, 3818f–3820f
RigiScan, for nocturnal penile tumescence test-
  ing, 1627, 1628f, 1629, 1630
Rimactane. *See* Rifampin.
River blindness, 780, 786
RNA. *See* Ribonucleic acid (RNA).
RNA viruses, cancer related to, 2652
Roberts syndrome, multisystem involvement in,
  1814t
Roberts-SC phocomelia
  cryptorchidism associated with, 2368t
  hypospadias with, 2292t
Robinow syndrome, multisystem involvement in,
  1814t
Robinson catheter, 112, 112f
Robinul. *See* Glycopyrrolate.
Rofecoxib, for prostatitis, 620, 624t
ROMK gene, in Bartter's syndrome, 1844
Room air, for pneumoperitoneum, in laparo-
  scopic surgery, 3474
Round cells, in semen, 1481, 1491–1492
Round ligament
  embryology of, 1760–1761
  of uterus, 67, 67f
RRT. *See* Renal replacement therapy (RRT).
Rubella, fetal, hypospadias with, 2292t
Rubinstein-Taybi syndrome
  cryptorchidism associated with, 2368t
  multisystem involvement in, 1814t
Rudiger syndrome, multisystem involvement in,
  1814t
Rugae, scrotal, 75
Russell-Silver syndrome
  hypospadias with, 2292t
  multisystem involvement in, 1814t
Rye pollen. *See Secale cereale.*

S phase, of cell cycle, 2639
S phase fraction, as proliferation marker, in
  bladder cancer, 2770
Sabal serrulata, extract of, mechanism of action
  of, 1369
Saccharin, as bladder cancer risk factor, 2739–
  2740
Saccular aneurysm, of renal artery, 262, 263f
Sacher procedure, for priapism, 1695, 1696f
Sacral agenesis, 2248–2250
  definition of, 2248
  diagnosis of, 2248–2249, 2249f, 2250f
  findings in, 2249–2250, 2250f
  incidence of, 2248
  management of, 2250
  risk factors for, 2248
  vesicoureteral reflux in, 2058
  voiding dysfunction with, artificial sphincter
    for, 1188. *See also* Artificial sphincter.
Sacral artery, 7, 14f, 49, 53f
Sacral evoked response-bulbocavernosus reflex
  latency test, in erectile dysfunction, 1633
Sacral micturition center, 1029, 1034
Sacral nerve root electrical stimulation, 1003–
  1004
Sacral nerve root magnetic stimulation, 983–984

Sacral nerve root neuromodulation
  for detrusor overactivity, 1044–1045
  for overactive bladder
    advances in (future directions for), 1083–
      1085
    device for, 1081–1083
    factors affecting, 1083
    overview of, 1081–1082
    percutaneous nerve evaluation in, 1081–
      1082, 1082f, 1088
    rationale for, 1080–1081
    results of, 1082–1083
    stimulator implantation in, 1082
  indications for, 982–983, 1005–1006, 1045
  mechanism of action of, 849, 855–856, 856f
Sacral parasympathetic nucleus, 846
Sacral plexus, 54
Sacral rhizotomy
  for bladder denervation, 985–986
  selective, for bladder denervation, 985–986
Sacral vein, 7, 14f
Sacrospinous ligament, 42, 1095, 1096f
Sacrospinous ligament fixation, for vaginal vault
  prolapse, 1127–1128, 1128f
  and female sexual dysfunction, 1721
Sacrotuberous ligament, 1095, 1096f, 1099f
Sacrum, 41, 42f
Salmonella paratyphi, infection with, in urinary
  schistosomiasis, 769
Salmonella typhi, infection with, in urinary
  schistosomiasis, 769
Salpingitis, coccidioidal, 813
Salvage procedures, for ureteropelvic junction
  obstruction, 484–487
  postoperative care and complication manage-
    ment in, 485, 487
Saphenous vein, 1594, 1594f
Sarcoidosis
  acute tubulointerstitial nephritis in, 1843
  hypercalcemia associated with, 3248
  nephrogenic diabetes insipidus caused by,
    1844
Sarcoma(s), 2633t
  clear cell, of kidney, 2493
  Kaposi's, penile, 2949
  of bladder, 2765
  of prostate, 3033
    ultrasound appearance of, 3048
  of renal pelvis and ureters, 2768–2769
  of seminal vesicles, 3877
  penile, 2973–2974
    Kaposi's, 2949
  renal, 2719–2720, 2720f
    clear cell, 2493
Sarcoplasm, of ureteral smooth muscle cell, 378
Sarcoptes scabiei, in scabies, 685
Saturation, stone formation and, 3234–3235
Saw palmetto berry. *See Serenoa repens.*
S-bladder, 3852
Scabies, 685–686, 726
Scale(s), cutaneous, 716
Scalpels, laparoscopic, 3466
Scardino-prince vertical flap technique, in pyelo-
  plasty, 483, 484f
Scarpa's fascia, 43, 43f
SCH 23390, uropharmacology of, 869
Schafer nomogram, for outflow obstruction, 920,
  920f, 921
Schinzel-Giedion syndrome, hypospadias with,
  2292t
Schistosoma haematobium. See also Schistoso-
  miasis.
  biology of, 764–765
  cercariae of, 764

Sildenafil citrate
  adverse effects and side effects of, 1654
  contraindications to, 1654–1655
  dosage and administration of, 1654
  efficacy of, 1620, 1654
  failure of, androgen therapy in, 1651
  for erectile dysfunction, 1653–1655
  for female sexual arousal disorder, 1728
  for female sexual dysfunction, 1721–1722
  in combination therapy, 1655
  mechanism of action of, 1619, 1653–1654
  prescribing patterns for, 1619–1620
  safety of, 1654
Sildenafil-Trimix, 1655
Silent mutations, definition of, 2626t
Silicate calculi, 3266
Silicon elastomer, for sling procedures, 1161
Silicone
  for reconstructive surgery, 2594
  microimplants, injection therapy with, for female stress incontinence, 1154
Silicone polymers
  injection therapy with, 1046, 1175
    for postprostatectomy incontinence, 1065
    in females, results of, 1180
    in males, results of, 1179
    results of, 1179
  microimplants, in endoscopic treatment of vesicoureteral reflux, 2093
Silk glove sign, 1823
Silver nitrate lavage, for interstitial cystitis, 655
Silver syndrome, hypospadias with, 2292t
Simian immunodeficiency viruses, 695
Simpson-Golabi-Behmel syndrome
  cryptorchidism associated with, 2368t
  hypospadias with, 2292t
Sinequan. *See* Doxepin.
Single-photon emission computed tomography (SPECT), high-resolution, of kidneys, in vesicoureteral reflux, 2065–2066, 2066f
Sinovaginal bulb, 1756, 1757f
Sinus of Guérin, 1757
Sinusal tubercle, 1756
Sinuses, prostatic, 63
Sipple's syndrome, 3543
Sirenomelia, in bilateral renal agenesis, 1888
Sirolimus
  as immunosuppressant, 364, 364t, 365f
  toxicity of, organ system target for, 367t
β-Sitosterol, for benign prostatic hyperplasia, 1371, 1371t
Situs inversus. *See* Kartagener's syndrome.
Six-corner bladder neck suspension, 1122t, 1123–1124, 1124f
Sjögren's syndrome
  acute tubulointerstitial nephritis in, 1843
  and interstitial cystitis, 636
Skeletal muscle, of rhabdosphincter, 1055
Skeleton, anomalies of, with cloacal exstrophy, 2177
Skene's duct cysts, 2439, 2439f
Skene's glands, 68
SKF 38393, uropharmacology of, 869
Skin, examination of, 903
  in children, 1822
Skin coverage, for penile reconstruction, 3911
Skin disorder(s). *See also specific disorder, e.g., Dermatofibroma.*
  of male genitalia
    benign, 727–729
    common, 726–727, 736f, 737f
Skin grafts
  for penile skin loss, 3738–3739
  for scrotal skin loss, 3739

Skin lesions, types of, 716
Skin loss, genital, 3738–3739
  penile, 3738–3739
  scrotal, 3738, 3739
Skin tags, 727
  hymenal, 2440, 2440f
Skin test, for bovine collagen immunogenicity, 1182
Sleep, urine loss in. *See* Enuresis, nocturnal.
Sling procedures
  allograft, 1160–1161
  and cystoceles, 1166
  and destroyed female urethra, 1166
  and urethral diverticula, 1166
  autologous materials for, combined, outcomes with, 1164–1165
  complications of, 1166–1167
  fascia lata for
    allograft
      for sling procedure, 1160
      outcomes with, 1165, 1167
    autologous, 1160
      outcomes with, 1163, 1167
  fascial
    autologous, 1160
      outcomes with, 1163, 1167
    donor, 1160
      outcomes with, 1165, 1167
  for stress incontinence. *See also* Pubovaginal sling.
    historical perspective on, 1151
    indications for, 1153–1154
  for total urethral failure, 1153, 1154f
  in males, 1153
  in myelodysplasia, 1152–1153, 1153f
  in neurogenic conditions, 1152–1153
  indications for, 992
    other than female stress incontinence, 1152–1153
  nonautologous materials for, 1160–1161
  outcomes with
    assessment of, 1162–1163
      characterization of surgical failures for, 1162–1163
      control group for, 1162
      definition of cure and, 1162
      preoperative patient characterization for, 1162
    literature review, 1163–1166, 1164t
    preoperative patient condition and, 1162
  Raz vaginal wall, for stress incontinence, 1116–1118
  sling fixation in, 1158–1159, 1159f
    alternative techniques for, 1161–1162
    to bone, 1161–1162
  surgical failures in, characterization of, 1162–1163
  synthetic materials for, 1161
    complications of, 1167
  technique for, 992–993
  urethral wrap, 1160
  vaginal wall, 1160
    outcomes with, 1163–1164
Sling surgery. *See also* Pubovaginal sling.
  autologous fascial pubovaginal, indications for, 1046, 1047
  efficacy of, 1047
  for geriatric incontinence, 1230
  for postprostatectomy incontinence, 1065
  in females, indications for, 1193
  in males, 1193
    with prostatectomy, 1193
  in prostatectomy patient, 1193

Sling surgery *(Continued)*
  results of, 1179
  safety of, 1047
  suburethral, in females, 1193
Small cell carcinoma, of bladder, 2764
Small intestinal anastomosis, 3765–3768
  Bricker, 3765–3766, 3766f
  hammock, 3768
  LeDuc technique for, 3767–3768, 3767f
  split-nipple, 3767, 3767f
  tunneled, 3766–3767, 3767f
  Wallace technique for, 3766, 3766f
Small intestinal obstruction, following cryotherapy, for prostate cancer, 3180
Small intestine
  anatomy of, 3746–3747
  for reconstructive surgery, 3746–3747
Smith-Lemli-Opitz syndrome
  cryptorchidism associated with, 2368t
  hypospadias with, 2292t
  multisystem involvement in, 1814t
Smoking, 1312–1313
  and erectile dysfunction, 1624, 1648
  and incontinence, 1095
  and spermatogenesis, 1478, 1510
  as bladder cancer risk factor, 2738–2739, 2764, 2766
  as prostate cancer risk factor, 3011
  as risk factor for atherosclerotic disease, 241
  erectile dysfunction caused by, 1608, 1609
  in patient history, 92
  renal cell carcinoma associated with, 2686
Smooth muscle
  actin of, 378, 382
  action potential of, 379–380, 379f–380f
  bladder
    actions of drugs on, 865–866
    contractile properties of, 833
    during bladder filling, 839
    tone of, 839
  calcium channels of, 383
  cavernosal, assessment of, 1647
  cellular anatomy of, 377–378
  cellular mechanics of, 837–839
  characteristics of, 836–839
  clitoral, physiology of, 1717
  contractile activity of, 382–386, 382f
  contractile elements of, 836, 837f
  contraction and relaxation of, molecular mechanisms of, 1600–1601, 1602f, 1603f
  electrical activity of, 378–382
    propagation of, 381–382
  excitation-contraction coupling in, 383, 838, 838t, 838f
  force-length relations of, 386–387, 387f
  force-velocity relations of, 387, 387f
  hysteresis of, 386f, 387
  ion channels in, 837–838
  length-tension relationship in, 839
  mechanical properties of, 386–387
  membrane electrical properties of, 837–838
  morphology of, 836
  myosin of, 378, 382–383, 382f–383f
  of prostate, 1241t, 1243
  of rhabdosphincter, 1055
  pacemaker potential and activity of, 380–381, 381f
  penile
    contraction and relaxation of, molecular mechanisms of, 1600–1601, 1602f, 1603f
    functions of, during penile erection, 1592t
    in erectile dysfunction, 1608–1609

Spermatocyte(s) (Continued)
pachytene, 1452, 1453f
preleptotene, 1452, 1453f
zygotene, 1452, 1453f
secondary, 1452, 1453f
Spermatogenesis, 340
after orchiopexy, 1580
age-related changes in, 1440
blood-testis barrier and, 1450, 1450f, 1451f
cancer treatment and, 1477
chromosomal disorders and, 1504–1506
disorders of, 1504–1512
GnRH therapy for, 1511
in Klinefelter syndrome, 1504
in Noonan's syndrome, 1505
in XX male syndrome, 1504
in XYY syndrome, 1505
in Y chromosome microdeletions, 1505
testicular artery injury and, 1577
testosterone-rebound therapy for, 1511
drugs affecting, 1477, 1510
endocrine control of, 1440–1441, 1456
environmental toxins and, 1510
febrile illness and, 1477
genetic basis of, 1456
heat exposure and, 1509–1510
hormonal regulation of, 1455–1456
in Sertoli cell–only syndrome, 1508
initiation of, in hypogonadotropic hypogonadism, 1501
normal, 1498, 1499f
occupational exposures and, 1510
smoking and, 1478
steps of, 1452–1455, 1453f, 1456
temperature sensitivity of, 1442, 1509–1510, 1580
test for. See also Testis (testes), testicular biopsy findings in atrophy of.
by percutaneous fine-needle aspiration cytology, 1500
varicocele and, 1507–1508
Spermatogonium(a), 1452, 1453f
development of, 1452
proliferation of, 1452–1455
Spermidine, 1277
Spermine, in seminal plasma, 1238, 1277
Spermiogenesis, 1453–1455, 1454f
Sphincter
anal. See Anal sphincter.
artificial. See Artificial sphincter.
bladder. See Urethral sphincter.
smooth. See Urethral sphincter, smooth.
striated. See Urethral sphincter, striated.
urethral. See Urethral sphincter.
Sphincterotomy
in detrusor-sphincter dyssynergia, 958
long-term efficacy of, 1012
outcomes with, 1012
surgical, 1011–1012
12 o'clock, 1011–1012
upper tract complications after, 1012
Spica cast, for postoperative immobilization, with complete primary exstrophy repair, 2200, 2200f
Spina bifida
neonate with
evaluation of, 1812, 1813–1814
management of, 1813–1814
plain film radiography of, 123
presacral dimple in, 1825
vesicoureteral reflux in, 2058
with cloacal exstrophy, 2177
Spina bifida cystica, 952

Spina bifida occulta, 952
plain film radiography of, 123
Spinal cord
abnormalities of, with imperforate anus, 2251, 2252f
anatomy of, 944
disease of, voiding dysfunction with, 941–953, 953–957
in cerebellar ataxia, 939
in cerebral palsy, 939
in multiple system atrophy, 941
in schistosomiasis, 780
sacral, 944, 953
schistosomiasis in, voiding dysfunction with, 944
syringomyelia of, voiding dysfunction in, 944
tethering of, 952
presacral dimple with, 1825
voiding dysfunction with, 953
with imperforate anus, 2251
untethering, in cloacal exstrophy patient, 2181
Spinal cord compression, by prostate cancer, palliative radiation therapy for, 3165
Spinal cord injury
and female sexual dysfunction, 1721, 1722
bladder instability after, mechanisms of, 870–871, 871f
bladder management in, 995–997
catheterization after, 995–997
and bladder cancer, 997
causes of death with, 945
ejaculatory dysfunction in, 1513–1514
epidemiology of, 944–945
general aspects of, 944–945
in children, 2254–2256
age-related incidence of, 2254, 2254f
mechanisms of injury in, 2254
voiding dysfunction in, 2254–2255
management of, 2255–2256
in males, seminal emission abnormalities in, electroejaculation for, 1565–1566
in neonate, mechanisms of injury in, 2254
in women, 951–952
incontinence caused by, 1034
external collecting devices for, 998
infrasacral, and voiding dysfunction, 889t, 894
orgasmic disorder in, 1722
penile erection after, 1597, 1599
priapism in, 1611
sacral
neurologic and urodynamic correlation in, 948–950
urodynamic evaluation in, 948, 949f
voiding dysfunction with, 933t, 935, 948
sexual function in, 945
suprasacral
neurologic and urodynamic correlation in, 948–950
urodynamic evaluation in, 946–947, 947f
voiding dysfunction with, 893t, 894, 894t, 933t, 935, 946f, 946–948, 947f, 1033–1034
traumatic, reflex neurogenic bladder after, 895
urinary tract infection and, 551, 588–590
bacteriology and laboratory findings in, 589–590
clinical presentation of, 589
epidemiology of, 588–589
management of, 590
pathogenesis of, 589
recurrent, 590
urodynamic evaluation in, 906
vesicoureteral reflux and, 951

Spinal cord injury (Continued)
voiding dysfunction after
artificial sphincter for, 1188. See also Artificial sphincter.
classification of (Bors-Comarr), 892–894, 893t, 895
in women, 951–952
vesicoureteral reflux with, 951
voiding dysfunction with, 944–952
Spinal cord tumor, and uninhibited neurogenic bladder, 895
Spinal deformity, urinary stone treatment with, 3376
Spinal dysraphism. See also Lipomeningocele; Neurospinal dysraphism.
clinical findings in, 2245–2247, 2247f
definition of, 952
diagnosis of, 2245, 2246f
magnetic resonance imaging of, 2247–2248, 2248f
occult
types of, 2245, 2245t
voiding dysfunction with, 953, 2245–2248
pathogenesis of, 2247
potential for recoverable function in, 2247, 2247f
ultrasound examination of, 2248, 2248f
urodynamic evaluation in, 906, 2247–2248
voiding dysfunction in, 2245–2248
Spinal shock
bladder compliance in, 909
definition of, 945
reflex neurogenic bladder after, 895
voiding dysfunction in, 893–894, 895, 897, 945
Spinal stenosis
definition of, 954
signs and symptoms of, 954
voiding dysfunction with, 954
Spine
abnormalities of, plain film radiography of, 123
deformities of, in prune-belly syndrome, 2122
lumbosacral, ultrasound examination of, in neonate, 1825
traumatic injury to, in children, 2254–2256
Spiral (helical) computed tomography, 138
for ureterolithiasis, 140, 144
Spironolactone
erectile dysfunction caused by, 1609, 1649
for primary aldosteronism, 3539
Spleen
function of, 309, 310f
injury to, as percutaneous nephrostomy complication, 3340
torsion of, in prune-belly syndrome, 2122
Splenic artery, 6
Splenic vein, 8
Splenorenal bypass, 3621–3622, 3621f, 3622f
Splenorenal ligament, 24
Splicing, definition of, 2626t
Split-nipple small intestinal anastomosis, 3767, 3767f
Sporadic olivopontocerebellar atrophy. See Multiple system atrophy.
Sporotrichosis, 816
Spring-onion deformity, with simple ureterocele, 2034, 2034f
Spurious calculi, 3267
Squamous cell carcinoma
of bladder, 2746–2747
etiology of, 2746

Squamous cell carcinoma *(Continued)*
  histology of, 2746–2747, 2746f
  of penis, 733f. *See* Penile tumor(s), squamous.
  of prostate, ultrasound appearance of, 3047
  of renal pelvis and ureters, 2768
Squamous cell carcinoma in situ, of glans penis, 722, 734f
SRY (sex-determining region of Y chromosome), 1440, 1753, 1755f, 1761f, 1761–1763
SRY gene, in sex determination, 2397, 2398f, 2399
  male, 2354
SSRIs. *See* Selective serotonin reuptake inhibitors (SSRIs).
SST deformity, with penile prosthesis, 1684, 1684f
Staghorn calculi
  renal, 3368–3370
    classification of, 3369, 3369f
    natural history of, 3366
    surgical management of, 3369–3370
  struvite, 3261, 3261f
Stamey needle bladder neck suspension, for stress incontinence, 1116
Stamey percutaneous cystostomy, 114, 116f
Staphylococcus, in prostatitis, 605
Stapled anastomosis, intestinal, 3755–3757
  end-to-end, 3756, 3756f
    with circular stapling device, 3755–3756, 3755f
Stapling devices, for endoscopy, 3468, 3468f
Stapling techniques, absorbable, for continent urinary diversion, 3828
  orthotopic, 3862
StAR. *See* Steroid acute regulatory (StAR) protein.
STAT (signal transducer and activator of transcription) proteins, 320
Static cystography, in bladder trauma, 3723
Stauffer's syndrome, in renal cell carcinoma, 2697
STD. *See* Sexually transmitted disease (STD).
Steinstrasse, with ureteral stones, 3432–3434
Stem cell(s)
  bone marrow, differentiation of, 309. *See also* B cell(s); T cell(s).
  for tissue engineering, 2617, 2618f
  of prostate, 1241–1242
    in benign prostatic hyperplasia, 1298
Stem cell model, of prostate cancer, 3014
Stem cell renewal, testicular, 1453
Stenosis. *See at specific anatomic site, e.g.,* Renal artery(ies), stenosis of.
Stent (stenting)
  Barnes, 1382
  double-J, in ureteroenteric stricture, 504–505
  endopyelotomy, 2003
  in endopyelotomy, 478–479
  intraprostatic, 1380–1385
    biodegradable, 1383
    permanent, 1383–1385
    polyurethane, 1382–1383
    spiral, 1381–1382
      first-generation, 1381
      second-generation, 1381–1382
    temporary, 1381–1383
  renal artery
    complications of, 261, 261t
    indications for, 259
    results of, 259–261, 260f, 260t, 261t
    technique of, 259

Stent (stenting) *(Continued)*
  Trestle, 1382–1383
  ureteral
    after endopyelotomy, 2003
    for ureteral contusion, 3719
    in ureteroscopy, 3308–3309
      coating of, 3308
      design and size of, 3308
      materials for, 3308
      specific, indications for, 3308–3309
    placement of, 3316
  urethral, 1013–1014
    contraindications to, 1089
    for stress incontinence, 1078–1079, 1079f
Sterility, male, 1484
Steroid(s)
  anabolic
    effects of, on males, 1502
    male infertility caused by, 1477
  C18, 1248
  C19, 1248
  C21, adrenal production of, 1248
  in neonates, imprinting of prostate by, 1240
  prepubertal, imprinting of prostate by, 1240
  sex
    plasma levels of, in males, 1247t
    uropharmacology of, 863
  therapy with
    blastomycosis with, 811
    Candida infection with, 798
    coccidioidomycosis with, 812
Steroid acute regulatory (StAR) protein, 1445
  deficiency of, 2415–2416
Steroid receptors, 1254–1255
Steroidogenic factor 1. *See* SF-1 gene.
Stinging nettle. *See Urticaria dioica.*
Stokey nomogram, for uroflowmetry flow rates and bladder volume, 915, 915f
Stoller afferent nerve stimulator (SANS) devices, 984, 1083–1085, 1084f
Stoma(s), abdominal, in intestinal segments, 3760–3762
  complications of, 3762
  flush, 3761
  loop end ileostomy as, 3761–3762, 3761f
  nipple ("rosebud"), 3760–3761, 3760f, 3761f
Stomach. *See also* Gastric *entries.*
  anatomy of, 3746, 3746f
  for reconstructive surgery, 3746
    complications with, 3778
  plain film radiography of, 123
Stone baskets, with ureteroscopy, 3317
Stones. *See* Calculus(i); Urinary lithiasis.
Stool impaction, incontinence caused by, in elderly, 1221
Storage symptoms, 901
Strawberry hemangiomas, of external genitalia, 2349
Streptococcal infection
  group A beta-hemolytic, glomerulonephritis caused by, 1838–1839
  in acute tubulointerstitial nephritis, 1843
Streptococcus pneumoniae, hemolytic-uremic syndrome caused by, 1840
Streptolysin-O, in postinfectious glomerulonephritis, 1838
Streptomycin
  adverse effects and side effects of, 756, 757t
  dosage and administration of, 757t
  for genitourinary tuberculosis, 758
  mechanism of action of, 755t
  mutational resistance to, site of, 755t
  pharmacology of, 756

Streptozyme, in postinfectious glomerulonephritis, 1838
Stress, urinary lithiasis related to, 3234
Stress hyperreflexia
  of detrusor, 1040–1041
  postprostatectomy, evaluation of, 1061
Stress incontinence, 901. *See also* Incontinence; Voiding dysfunction.
  anatomic
    etiology of, 913
    injection therapy for, 1180, 1183
  and urge incontinence, 853
    mixed, in females, 1043
  biofeedback for, 987
  causes of, 832, 901, 1034–1035
  classification of, 892
    anatomic, 1031–1032, 1031f–1033f
  diagnosis of, 1155–1156
  electrical stimulation for, 988
  genuine
    injection therapy for, 1180, 1183
    urethral hypermobility and, 891
  hammock hypothesis for, 892
  in elderly, 1222–1223, 1226–1227
    treatment of, 1227t, 1230
  in females
    age and, 1222
    antihypertensives and, 1221
    causes of, 901
    parity and, 1037
    treatment of, nonsurgical, 1086–1087
  in males, 1226–1227
    age and, 1222–1223
    causes of, 901
  in neurospinal dysraphism, 952
  in patient history, 88–89
  injection therapy for, 1172–1184. *See also* Injection therapy.
  intrinsic sphincteric deficiency and, injection therapy for, 1172–1184
  obstetric risk factors for, 1036–1037
  occult, 1107
  office-based evaluation of, 1113
  paraurethral tissue collagen levels and, 845
  pathophysiology of, 892
  pharmacotherapy for, 988–992, 1074–1076
  postpartum, 1036–1037
  postprostatectomy, 1433
    and sphincter dysfunction, 1060
    evaluation of, 1061
  potential, 1107
  radiographic characterization of, 1151–1152
  retropubic suspension surgery for, 1140–1149
  risk factors for, 1094–1095, 1104, 1104t
  signs and symptoms of, 1029–1030, 1030t
  sling procedures for. *See also* Pubovaginal sling.
    historical perspective on, 1151
  testing for, 1110, 1113–1114, 1114f, 1115f
  treatment of, 988, 1045–1047
    behavioral therapy in, 987, 1087
    devices for, 1077–1079, 1087
      acceptance of, 992, 1078
      arguments for, 1078
      clinical trials of, interpretation of, 1078
      failure of, 992
      occlusive, 991–992, 1078
      patient characteristics and, 992
      societal biases and, 1078
      supportive, 991–992, 1078, 1079–1080, 1080f, 1087, 1089
      urethral meatal, 991, 1078, 1087

Stress incontinence *(Continued)*
  urethral stents and catheters, 1078–1079,
    1087
  vaginal support/pessaries, 991–992,
    1079–1080, 1080f, 1087, 1089
  medical, 988–992, 1074–1076
  nonsurgical, 1045–1046, 1086–1087
  surgical, 1046–1047, 1086, 1104. *See also*
    Stress incontinence, vaginal surgery
    for.
  type 0, 1031
  type I, 1031, 1031f, 1151
  type II, 1151
  type IIA, 1031, 1031f, 1032f
  type IIB, 1031, 1032f
  type III, 892, 1031–1032, 1033f
  urodynamic characterization of, 1151–1152
  vaginal surgery for, 1115–1120
    bone anchoring techniques in, 1119
    complications of, 1119–1120
      intraoperative, 1119
      postoperative, 1119–1120
    Gittes bladder neck suspension in, 1116
    intraoperative management of, 1115
    modified Pereyra approach to, 1115–1116
    outcomes with, 1115
    preoperative preparation for, 1115
    Raz procedures for, 1116–1118, 1117f
    Raz vaginal wall sling procedure in, 1116–
      1118
    Stamey needle bladder neck suspension in,
      1116
    techniques for, 1115–1119
    tension-free vaginal tape procedure in,
      1118f, 1118–1119
  Valsalva leak point pressure in, 912
  with urethral diverticula, 1208
Stress testing, in geriatric incontinence, 1225–
  1226
Striated muscle, urethral, 843–845
  fiber types of, 844–845
Striated sphincter. *See* Urethral sphincter,
  striated.
Striatonigral degeneration. *See* Multiple system
  atrophy.
Stroke. *See* Cerebrovascular accident.
Stromal cells, of prostate, 1241t, 1242–1245
  and epithelial cells, interaction of, 1262–
    1263, 1264f
  in benign prostatic hyperplasia, 1300–1301
Stromal tumors, testicular, 2906–2907
Strongyloides stercoralis, 788
Strontium 90, for prostate cancer, bone
  metastases of, 3165
Struvite calculi, 3260–3264
  bacteriology of, 3260–3261, 3260t
  clinical presentation of, 3261–3262, 3261f
  pathogenesis of, 3260
  staghorn. *See* Staghorn calculi.
  treatment of, 3262–3264, 3262t
Studer ileal bladder substitute, 3853, 3854f
Subarachnoid block, for bladder denervation,
  985
Subcapsular approach, for nephrectomy, 3585–
  3586, 3589f
Subcardinal vein(s), 2044–2045, 2045f
Subcostal nerve, 14, 16f
Subcutaneous hemangioma(s), of external
  genitalia, 2349
Subdermal plexus, 3888
Subfertility, male, 1484
Subinguinal ligation, for varicocele, 2387

Substance P
  in bladder, 861–862, 862t
  in interstitial cystitis, 640
Subtunical venous plexus, 1594f
Sucralfate, interactions with azoles, 819t
Suction, in laparoscopic surgery, 2576
Sulfamethizole, serum and urinary levels of,
  537t
Sulfasalazine, effect of, on spermatogenesis,
  1477, 1510
Sulfisoxazole
  for nongonococcal urethritis, 676
  for pediatric urinary tract infection
    oral dosage and administration of, 1865t
    prophylactic, 1866t
  for urinary tract infection, during pregnancy,
    584t
Sulfonamides
  acute tubulointerstitial nephritis caused by,
    1843
  for pediatric urinary tract infection, oral dos-
    age and administration of, 1865t
  for urinary tract infection, during pregnancy,
    585
Sulfonylureas, interactions with azoles, 819t
Superficial perineal space, 3898
Superficial plexus, 3888
Supernumerary kidneys, 1892–1894
  associated anomalies in, 1893–1894
  diagnosis of, 1894
  embryology of, 1893
  features of, 1893, 1893f
  incidence of, 1892–1893
  signs and symptoms of, 1894
Supersaturation, stone formation and, 3234
Suppressor, definition of, 1266
Suppressor element, definition of, 1266
Supracardinal vein(s), 2044–2045, 2045f
Suprapubic bladder aspiration, 529–530, 530f
Suprapubic cystostomy, for urethral trauma,
  3728
Suprapubic tube tracts, dilation of, 3310–3311
Suprarenal gland(s). *See* Adrenal(s).
Suprasacral spinal lesions, voiding dysfunction
  with, 1033–1034
Supraspinal lesion
  and voiding dysfunction, 889t, 894
  voiding dysfunction with, 1033–1034
Supraspinal neurotransmission, pharmacology of,
  868f, 869–870
Supravesical fissure, 2137, 2137f
Supravesical ureter, dilation of, 3309–3310
Suramin
  for onchocerciasis, 786
  for prostate cancer, 3216, 3217t, 3218
  uropharmacology of, 859
Surgery. *See also specific type, e.g.,* Nephrectomy.
  and pelvic organ prolapse, 1094–1095
  in males, infertility caused by, 1477
Suspensory ligament, of clitoris, 69, 69f
Suture(s)
  absorbable, for continent urinary diversion,
    3791
  for osteotomy, in exstrophy patient, 2153
  in hypospadias repair, 2302
  in laparoscopic surgery, 2576
  in retropubic suspension surgery, 1141–1142
Suture closure techniques, in renal transplantation, 361
Suture introducers, laparoscopic, 3468
Sweating, excess, with tricyclic antidepressants,
  977

Swimmers' itch, 768–769
SWI-SNF complex, 1258f, 1260
SWL. *See* Shock-wave lithotripsy (SWL).
Sympathetic nervous system
  effects of, on epididymis, 1464
  in ureteral function, 389–390
  of lower urinary tract, 846, 846f
Sympatholytic agents
  incontinence caused by, 1038
  uropharmacology of, 2235t
Sympathomimetic agents
  and benign prostatic hyperplasia, 1313
  incontinence caused by, 1038
  uropharmacology of, 2235t
Syndrome of inappropriate antidiuretic hormone
  (SIADH) secretion, in hyponatremia, 206,
  206t
Syneresis
  definition of, 1183
  with polytetrafluoroethylene (PTFE) injection
    therapy, 1178
Syphilis, 681t
  acute tubulointerstitial nephritis in, 1843
  clinical stages and diagnosis of, 683
  etiology of, 683
  secondary, papulosquamous lesions in, 718
  treatment of, 683–684, 683t
Syringomyelia, voiding dysfunction in, 944
Systemic lupus erythematosus
  and interstitial cystitis, 635–636, 636f
  chronic renal failure in, 291–292, 291t
  epidemiology of, 1840
  in children, 1840
  nephropathy in, histologic forms of, 1840
  onset of, clinical features of, 1840
  renal involvement in, 1840–1841
  treatment of, 1840
Systemic sclerosis
  and female sexual dysfunction, 1720, 1722
  erectile dysfunction caused by, 1610
  orgasmic disorder in, 1722
  urodynamic findings in, 963
  voiding dysfunction in, 963

T cell(s), 309, 311. *See also* B cell(s).
  activation of, 315–316, 317f
    NFAT in, 319
    signal 1 step in, 315
    signal 2 step in, 316
    up-regulated adhesion molecule expression
      in, 329–330, 330t
  alloreactive, 316
  antigen-specific, activation of, 320–325
    clonal expansion in, 314, 321, 322f
    cytokine production in, 322–323, 323t,
      324f
    cytolysis of target cells in, 323, 324f, 325
    development of memory cells in, 325
    phenotypic changes in, 325
  CD4⁺. *See* CD4⁺ T cells.
  CD8⁺. *See* CD8⁺ T cells.
  clonal anergy of, 328
  in interstitial cystitis, 645
  interaction of, with endothelial cells, 330–
    331, 330f
  memory, 325
  naïve (antigen-inexperienced), trafficking of,
    329
  peripheral deletion of, 328
  regulatory, 329
  role of, in tumor immunology, 332–333

Testicular tumor(s) *(Continued)*
for seminomas, 2939
lung resection as, 2938
mediastinal resection as, 2938
postchemotherapy retroperitoneal lymph
node dissection as, 2937
preoperative preparation for, 2934
timing of, 2934
histologic classification of, 2876–2878,
2877t
laparoscopic retroperitoneal lymph node
dissection for. *See* Laparoscopic retroperitoneal lymph node dissection, for
testicular cancer.
low-stage
fertility and, 2933
treatment options for, 2931–2933, 2933t
mixed, 2879
natural history of, 2923
nonseminomatous, 2878–2879. *See also*
Nonseminomatous germ cell tumor(s).
pathogenesis and natural history of, 2882–
2883
patterns of spread of, 2882–2883, 2923
retroperitoneal lymph node dissection for.
See Retroperitoneal lymph node dissection.
retroperitoneum and, 2923, 2925, 2925f
seminomatous, 2877–2878. *See also* Semi-
noma(s).
staging of, 2885–2888, 2885t, 2886t
imaging studies in, 2886–2887
orchiectomy findings in, 2886
tumor markers in, 2887–2888
treatment of, 2889–2904
for nonseminomatous tumors, 2894,
2895f, 2896–2904
for seminomas, 2890, 2891f, 2892–2894
monitoring response to, 2888–2889
ultrasonography in, 2884–2885
gonadoblastoma as, 2907–2908
in children. *See* Child(ren), testicular tumors
in.
in neonate, 1801, 1817, 1817t
management of, 2912–2913
mesenchymal, 2908
rhabdomyosarcoma as, 2479–2480
secondary, 2909–2910
leukemic, 2910
lymphoma as, 2909–2910
metastatic, 2910
sex cord–mesenchyma as, 2905–2907
interstitial cell lesions in, 2905–2906
Sertoli cell tumors in, 2906–2907
staging of, 2922–2923, 2924t
surgery of, 2920–2940
orchiectomy as. *See* Orchiectomy.
Testicular vein(s), 77–78, 77f
thrombophlebitis of, 430
Testis (testes), 75–78, 75f–77f
absent, evaluation of, 1818
and vasovasostomy, 1547
androgen production by, 1246f, 1246–1248,
1247f, 1247t
ascending, clinical features of, 1823
atrophy of
in acquired immunodeficiency syndrome,
708
in estrogen excess, 1503
in myotonic dystrophy, 1508
posthypophysectomy, 1455
testicular artery injury and, 1577
testicular biopsy findings in, 1499–1500

Testis (testes) *(Continued)*
testicular germ cell tumors due to, 2882
autotransplantation of, microvascular, 2377
blood supply to, 1442–1444, 1443f, 1534,
1534t. *See also* Testicular artery(ies);
Testicular vein(s).
autoregulation of, 1443–1444
cancer of. *See also* Testicular tumor(s).
in acquired immunodeficiency syndrome,
707, 708
cryptorchid, 1506
cystic dysplasia of, 1961
in children, 2499
cytoarchitecture of, 1444–1451
descent of, during fetal development, 1758–
1760
development of, prenatal, 2354–2355, 2356
dimensions of, by age, 1480, 1480t
dysfunction of, with varicocele, 2385–2386
ectopic, 1506, 2357–2358
embryology of, 1440
endocrinology of, 1440–1441
end-stage, 1499
function of, in exstrophy patient, 2143
hydrocele of, 96
in prune-belly syndrome, 2120–2121
in schistosomiasis, 773
infections of, in acquired immunodeficiency
syndrome, 707
infrapubic, 2357
innervation of, 78, 1441–1442
interstitium of, 1444–1447, 1445f, 1446f
intra-abdominal, 2357
laparoscopic evaluation of, 2572–2573,
2573f
intracanalicular, 2357
laparoscopic examination of, in children,
2571–2574, 2572f, 2573f, 2574t
lymphatic drainage of, 10, 15f
magnetic resonance imaging of, 149
measurement of, 1480
mediastinum of, 76, 76f
microlithiasis of, in children, 2499
microvascular autotransplantation of, in prune-
belly syndrome, 2131
neoplasms of. *See* Testicular tumor(s).
nonandrogenic products of, in benign prostatic
hyperplasia, 1302–1303
nonpalpable, 2358
laparoscopic evaluation of, 2571–2574,
2572f, 2573f, 2574t
pain in. *See also* Orchialgia.
patient history of, 85
postvasectomy, 1546
palpation of, in children, 1823
percutaneous fine-needle aspiration cytology
of, 1500
physical examination of, 96
physiology of, 1441–1456
retractile, 1506, 2358
clinical features of, 1823
in adults, 1581
seminiferous tubules of, 76, 76f. *See also*
Seminiferous tubules.
septa of, 1441
structure of, 1441–1444, 1442f
suprapubic, 2357
surgical anatomy of, 1534, 1534t
temperature of, and fertility, 1440, 1478
tethered, clinical features of, 1823
torsion of. *See* Testicular torsion.
trauma to. *See* Trauma, testicular.
tuberculosis of, 750

Testis (testes) *(Continued)*
tunica albuginea of, 76, 76f
tunica vaginalis of, 76, 76f
ultrasonography of, 135, 137
undescended. *See* Cryptorchidism.
vanishing
bilateral, 2408–2409
laparoscopic evaluation of, 2572, 2572f
varicocele and. *See* Varicocele.
vascularization of, 1441–1444, 1443f
Testis cords, formation of, 1753
Testis-determining factor, 2395–2396
Testolactone, for male infertility, 1511–1512
Testosterone
age-related changes in, in females, 1715
and female sexual function, 1714, 1715,
1726–1727
and male accessory sex gland development,
1238, 1261
and male sexual function, 1607
and Sertoli cell function, 1449
bioavailable, 1636
effects of
on epididymis, 1463–1464
on prostate, at cellular level, 1250–1252,
1251f, 1252f
excess, in males, 1502
free, measurement of, 1636
in males, evaluation of, 1484t, 1484–1485
in spermatogenesis, 1455–1456
metabolism of, 1246f, 1246–1248, 1247f
in prostate, 1250–1252, 1252f
percentage of free, measurement of, 1636
plasma levels of, 1246f, 1246–1248, 1247t,
1447, 1447f
age-related changes in, 1440
plasma protein binding by, 1246f, 1249, 1636
plasma transport of, 1246f, 1249, 1446f
production of, in females, 1714
regulation of pituitary and hypothalamic hormone secretion, 1439
replacement therapy with
adverse effects and side effects of, 1650–
1651
and benign prostatic hyperplasia, 1651
and prostate cancer, 1651
candidates for, 1636
in erectile dysfunction, 1649–1651
in hypogonadotropic hypogonadism, 1501
in women, 1714, 1715, 1727
dosage and administration of, 1727–1728
preparations for, 1650, 1650t
secretion of, fetal, 1440
synthesis of, 1245, 1246f, 1246–1248, 1247f,
1444–1447, 1446f
therapy with
before hypospadias repair, 2294–2295
for exstrophy patient, 2159
total, measurement of, 1636
Testosterone(s). *See also* Dihydrotestosterone
(DHT).
adrenal cortical tumors secreting, 3527
fetal secretion of, 2400, 2400f
in male sexual differentiation, 2354, 2355
in testicular descent, 2359–2360
supplementation of, microencapsulated Leydig
cells for, 2615–2616, 2616f
synthesis of, disorders of, 2415–2417
urinary lithiasis related to, 3254
Testosterone-binding globulin, in plasma transport of testosterone, 1246f, 1249
Testosterone-rebound therapy, for male infertility, 1511

Tethered cord syndrome, voiding dysfunction in, 953

Tetracycline
  Fanconi's syndrome caused by, 1844
  for actinomycosis, 817
  for syphilis, 683
  nephrogenic diabetes insipidus caused by, 1844
  serum and urinary levels of, 537t

Tetralogy of Fallot, in prune-belly syndrome, 2122

Tetrasomy 9-P, genitourinary anomalies in, 1815t

Tetrasomy 12p, hypospadias with, 2292t

Tg737 protein, in renal development, 1926, 1929t

TGF. *See* Transforming growth factor (TGF) *entries*.

α-Thalassemia, X-linked, cryptorchidism associated with, 2369t

Thalidomide, as angiogenesis inhibitor, 2656

Thermal injury, of bowel, electrosurgical, 3483–3485, 3484f

Thermodynamic solubility product, 3234, 3235f

Thermosensor, for cryotherapy, placement of, 3175

Thermotherapy, for prostatitis, 623

Thiamine, deficiency of, 962

Thiazide diuretics
  erectile dysfunction caused by, 1609, 1649
  for hyperoxaluria, 3251
  for urinary lithiasis, 3280–3281, 3282t
  in calcium reabsorption, 181
  in renal calcium reabsorption, 181

Thiersch-Duplay urethroplasty, 2305–2306

Thin glomerular basement membrane disease, in children, 1841

Thioridazine, incontinence caused by, in elderly, 1221t

Thiotepa (triethylenethiophosphoramide), for bladder cancer, superficial, 2793

Thirst, 199

Thoracoabdominal approach
  to adrenal surgery, 3552–3553
  to kidney surgery, 3583–3584, 3585f, 3586f

Threshold potential, of ureteral muscle cells, 379

Thrombophlebitis
  of ovarian vein, 430
  of testicular vein, 430

Thrombosis
  in renal transplant recipients, 350
  of kidney graft, 366
  of renal artery
    following renal revascularization, 3632–3633, 3632f, 3633f
    percutaneous transluminal angioplasty causing, 255
    renal artery, 264–265, 264t

Thromboxane A$_2$, in male sexual function, 1599

Thrush. *See* Candida, infection with.

Thymoxamine. *See* Moxisylyte.

Thymus
  function of, 309, 310f
  maturation of T cells in, 327

Thyroid gland, abnormalities of, male infertility with, 1503

Thyroid-stimulating hormone (TSH), secretion of, 1438

Thyrotoxicosis. *See* Hyperthyroidism.
  hypercalcemia in, 3248

Thyrotropes, 1438

Thyroxine, and male fertility, 1512

Ticarcillin, for pediatric urinary tract infection, parenteral dosage and administration of, 1864t

Ticarcillin plus clavulanate, for bacteremia, 571t

TILs (tumor-infiltrating lymphocytes), 336

Timed voiding, 966
  for detrusor overactivity, 1087
    in elderly, 1228
  in behavioral therapy for incontinence, 1070, 1087
  in diabetes mellitus, 957

Tinea cruris, 726, 735f

Tinea infection, 816

Tinidazole, for amebiasis, 788

Tioconazole, for vaginal candidiasis, 799

Tissue cultures, in urinary tract infection, 535

Tissue engineering, 2593–2619
  advances in (future directions for), 876
  biomaterials for, 2595–2597
    design and selection of, 2595–2596
    types of, 2596–2597, 2596f
  clitoral, 2608
  for genetically engineered cells, 2616–2617
  for in vivo gene therapy, 2617
  for testicular dysfunction, 2615–2616, 2616f
  injectable therapies using, 2614–2615, 2615f
  of bladder, 2598–2605
    autoaugmentation and, 2598, 2599f
    de-epithelialized bowel segments in, 2601
    matrices for, 2601–2602
    seromuscular grafts in, 2600–2601, 2601f
    tissue expansion and, for bladder augmentation, 2599–2600, 2600f
    ureterocystoplasty and, 2598–2599
    with cell transplantation, 2602–2605
      bladder replacement using, 2604–2605, 2604f, 2605f
      bladder tissue formation ex situ and, 2602–2604, 2604f
  of fetal tissue, 2613–2614, 2614f
  of renal structures, 2610–2613
    combined hemofilter and renal tubule as, 2611–2612
    hemofilter as, 2611
    in vivo, 2612–2613, 2613f
    principles for, 2610–2611
    renal tubule as, 2611
  of ureters, 2609–2610
  of urethra, 2597–2598, 2598f
  penile, 2605–2609
    corporal smooth muscle reconstruction using, 2605
    endothelial cell expansion and, 2605–2606, 2606f
    in vivo corporal smooth muscle and endothelium engineering and, 2606–2607
    of structural corporal tissue, 2607–2608, 2607f
    prostheses and, 2608–2609, 2609f
  stem cells for, 2617, 2618f
  strategies for, 2594–2595, 2595f
  therapeutic cloning for, 2617–2619, 2618f, 2619f

Tissue inhibitors of metalloproteinase, as angiogenesis inhibitors, 2655–2656

Tissue inhibitors of metalloproteinases, in urinary tract obstruction, 441

Tissue matrix
  definition of, 1243
  in cancer, 1244
  of prostate, 1241t, 1242–1245, 1244f
  interactions of, 1263–1265

Tissue sloughing, following cryotherapy, for prostate cancer, 3178–3179, 3179f

Tissue transfer, 3887–3890, 3887f–3890f

TKCR syndrome, cryptorchidism associated with, 2368t

TNF. *See* Tumor necrosis factor (TNF) *entries*.

Tobacco use. *See also* Smoking.
  as bladder cancer risk factor, 2738–2739, 2764, 2766
  as prostate cancer risk factor, 3011
  renal cell carcinoma associated with, 2686

Tobramycin
  for bacteremia, 571t
  for pediatric urinary tract infection, parenteral dosage and administration of, 1864t

Toilet dysfunction, in children, 2058–2059

Tolbutamide, interactions with azoles, 819t

Tolterodine
  adverse effects and side effects of, 1076–1077
  and oxybutynin, comparison of, 969
  effects of, on central nervous system, 1077
  for detrusor instability, 1044
  for neuromuscular voiding dysfunction, 969
  for overactive bladder, 969, 1076–1077
    efficacy of, 1076–1077
  for urge incontinence, in elderly, 1228, 1229t
  mechanism of action of, 1076
  pharmacology of, 969
  uropharmacology of, 857–858, 858t, 2235t

Tomoxetine, uropharmacology of, 867

Tonus, of bladder, 909

Topiglan, for erectile dysfunction, 1656

Torsades de pointes, terodiline and, 974

Torsion
  of epididymal appendages, 2381–2382
  of spermatic cord, 2379–2381, 2380f
    perinatal, 2383–2384
  of testicular appendages, 2381–2382
  penile, 2342, 2343f
  testicular, 96
    cryptorchidism and, 2365
    vs. epididymitis, 679–680

Torulopsis glabrata
  in blood, 805
  in urine, 805
  infection with, 805–806
    diagnosis of, 805
    epidemiology of, 805
    genitourinary manifestations of, 805–806
    in children, 1874
    predisposing factors for, 805
    treatment of, 805–806, 821t

Torulosis. *See* Cryptococcosis.

Total parenteral nutrition, priapism caused by, 1612

Total penile disassembly. *See* Penile disassembly technique.

Total prostate volume, in benign prostatic hyperplasia, 1310–1311, 1311f

Townes-Brocks syndrome, hypospadias with, 2292t

Toxicodendron dermatitis (poison ivy), 720

Toxocara canis, 788

Toxoplasmosis
  acute tubulointerstitial nephritis in, 1843
  in acquired immunodeficiency syndrome, 706

T-pouch procedure, 3854, 3856f–3857f, 3857–3858
  for continent urinary diversion, 3807, 3809, 3810f, 3811f
  with valved rectum, 3800–3802, 3801f

Tract dilation, in percutaneous nephrostomy, 3331–3334, 3331f, 3422–3423
  Amplatz dilator set for, 3332–3333, 3332f, 3333f
  balloon catheters for, 3333–3334, 3334f
  fascial dilators for, 3331–3332, 3332f

Transurethral resection of prostate (TURP)
(Continued)
  for chronic prostatitis, 623
  hemostasis in, 1409
  historical perspective on, 1403
  incontinence after
    pathogenesis of, 1056–1057
    prevalence of, 1053, 1054
    radiation and, 1059
    risk factors for, 1059
    sphincter and bladder dysfunction in, 1058,
      1058t
  intraoperative priapism in, 1410
  mortality rate for, 1411–1412
  outcomes with, 1410–1412
  sphincter function after, surgical technique
    and, 1059
  symptom improvement after, 1410
  technique for, 1405–1409, 1406f–1410f
  vs. transurethral incision of prostate, 1415t,
    1415–1416
  vs. transurethral microwave thermotherapy,
    1393–1395
  vs. transurethral vaporization of prostate,
    1413–1414
  vs. watchful waiting, 1348–1349
Transurethral resection syndrome, 1409–1410.
  See also TURP syndrome.
Transurethral ultrasound-guided laser-induced
  prostatectomy (TULIP), 1398–1399
Transurethral vaporization of prostate (TUVP),
  1412–1414
  clinical experience with, 1413
  comparative studies of, 1413–1414
  electrode design for, 1413
  mechanism of action of, 1412–1413
Transurethral vaporization–resection of prostate
  (TUVRP), 1413, 1414
Transvaginal ultrasonography
  guidance, for injection therapy, 1177, 1178f
  of urethral diverticulum, 1209, 1211f
Transvenous occlusion, for varicocele, 2387–
  2388
Transversalis fascia, 5, 45
Transverse myelitis
  in schistosomiasis, 780
  incontinence in, 1034
  reflex neurogenic bladder with, 895
  voiding dysfunction in, 952
Transverse perinei muscle
  deep, 1098
  superficial, 1098, 1099f
Transverse preputial island flap, in posterior
  (proximal) hypospadias repair, 2315–2316,
  2316f–2317f
Transvesical approach, to seminal vesicle surgery, 3879–3880, 3880f
Transversus abdominis muscle, 4, 5, 9f
Tranxene. *See* Clorazepate.
TRAP/DRIP complex, 1258f, 1260
Trapped penis, 2340, 2340f
Trapped prostate, 959
Trauma. *See also under anatomy; specific
  trauma, e.g.,* Fracture(s).
  and motor paralytic bladder, 895
  bladder, 3721–3725
    blunt, 3721, 3722f
    classification and management of, 3723–
      3725
      follow-up cystography in, 3725
      for contusions, 3723
      for extraperitoneal injuries, 3723–3724,
        3724f

Trauma *(Continued)*
      for intraperitoneal injuries, 3724–3725
      prophylactic antimicrobial agents for,
        3725
    delayed perforation as, following augmenta-
      tion cystoplasty, 2537–2539, 2537f,
      2538f
      etiology of, 2537–2538
      incidence of, 2538
      treatment of, 2538–2539
    diagnosis of, 3722–3723
      hematuria in, 3722
      imaging in, 3722–3723, 3722f, 3723f
    etiology of, 3721
      iatrogenic, 3721
      in laparoscopy, 3485–3486
      penetrating, 3721
      perforation as, 2823, 2823f
  brain injury in, voiding dysfunction after, 938
  excretory urography in, 127
  genitourinary, in children, 1824
    evaluation of, 1812
  innocent, to male genitalia, 721
  intestinal, with laparoscopic renal surgery,
    3680–3681
  lower urinary tract, in hysterectomy, 1196
  pelvic, erectile dysfunction caused by, 1608
  penile, 3732–3736
    amputation as, 3732–3733
      cause of, 3732–3733
      during circumcision, 3905
      replantation for, 3733
    and Peyronie's disease, 1696
    buckling, mechanism of injury in, 1697,
      1697f
    fracture as, 3734–3735
    penetrating, 3733–3734
      imaging in, 3733
      management of, 3733–3734
    soft-tissue, 3735–3736
  perineal, erectile dysfunction caused by, 1608
  priapism caused by, 1612
  renal, 3707–3715
    classification of, 3708–3709, 3708t, 3709f
    complications of, 3713–3715
    hematuria with, 3708
    in pediatric urinary tract infection, factors
      affecting, 1859–1863
    nonoperative management of, 3711, 3711f
    operative management of, 3711–3713
      nephrectomy in, 3713
      renal exploration in, 3711–3712, 3712f
      renal reconstruction in, 3712–3713,
        3713f–3715f
    patient factors in, 290–291
    presentation of, 3707–3708
    recovery from, relationship to normal devel-
      opment, 1776
    regulatory substances in, 290
    remodeling events following, 288–289,
      288f
    staging of, 3709–3710
      imaging indications in, 3709–3710,
        3709f
      imaging studies for, 3710, 3710f
    with shock-wave lithotripsy, acute, 3410–
      3411, 3410f, 3411t
  spinal, in children, 2254–2256
  spinal cord. *See* Spinal cord injury.
  testicular, 3736–3738
    blunt, 3736
    clinical findings in, 3736–3737
    imaging in, 3737

Trauma *(Continued)*
    management of, 3737–3738
    outcome with, 3738
    penetrating, 3736
  testicular germ cell tumors due to, 2882
  ureteral, 3715–3721
    diagnosis of, 3717–3718
      hematuria in, 3717
      imaging studies in, 3717–3718, 3717f
      intraoperative recognition in, 3717
    etiology of, 3715–3716
      external, 3715
      laparoscopic, 3716
      open surgical, 3716
      ureteroscopic, 3716
    in laparoscopy, 3486
    in ureteroscopy, perforation as, 3318, 3434
    intraoperative, 426–428, 427f
    management of, 3718–3721, 3718f
      for external trauma, 3718–3720, 3719f
      for surgical injuries, 3720–3721
      for ureteroscopic injuries, 3721
    risk factors for, 427
    sites and number of, 427, 427f
    successful repair of, 427–428
  urethral
    anterior, 3731–3732
    posterior, 3725
      delayed reconstruction for, 3728–3731
        complications of, 3731
        endoscopic, 3729
        preoperative evaluation for, 3728–
          3729, 3729f
        surgical, 3729–3731, 3730f
        timing of, 3728
      diagnosis of, 3725–3727
      initial management for, 3727–3728
        primary realignment in, 3727–3728
        suprapubic cystostomy in, 3728
Trazodone
  and moxisylyte, combined, for erectile dys-
    function, 1652
  and yohimbine, combined, for erectile dys-
    function, 1652
  for erectile dysfunction, 1652
  indications for, 1649
  mechanism of action of, 1652
  priapism caused by, 1612
Trecator-SC. *See* Ethionamide.
Treponema pallidum, 681t, 683. *See also*
  Syphilis.
Trestle stent, 1382–1383
Triad syndrome, 2117
Triamterene calculi, 3266–3267
Triazoles, 819–821
  drug interactions with, 819, 819t
Trichlormethiazide, for urinary lithiasis, 3281,
  3282t
Trichomonas, in prostatitis, 607
Trichomoniasis, vs. cystitis, 574
Trichomycosis, of male genitalia, 724
Trichosporon infection, 816
Tricyclic antidepressants. *See also* Antidepres-
  sants.
  adverse effects and side effects of, 977
    in elderly, 978
  allergic phenomena with, 977
  and MAOIs, interactions of, 978
  and sexual dysfunction, 1721
  cardiotoxicity of, 977–978
  central nervous system side effects of, 977
  effects of, on sexual function, 977
  erectile dysfunction caused by, 1609

Vasoepididymostomy *(Continued)*
  with severely compromised vasal length,
    1562–1564, 1563f
Vasography, 1537–1541, 3874, 3874f
  complications of, 1540
  findings in, interpretation of, 1538–1540,
    1538f–1540f
  fine-needle, 1540
  in infertility work-up, 1492–1493, 1493f
  indications for, 1541
  technique for, 1537–1540, 1537f–1540f
  transrectal, seminal vesiculography combined
    with, 1540–1541
Vasomax. *See* Phentolamine.
Vasopressin
  and renal development, 1774
  in renal hemodynamics, 174
  plasma osmolality and, 199–200, 200f
  precautions with, in elderly, 1229
  secretion of, 1438
    and nocturnal urine production, 2275
Vasovagal reaction, with transrectal ultrasound,
  3043
Vasovasostomy, 1547–1556
  anastomotic techniques in, 1551
    in convoluted vas, 1553–1554, 1555f
  anesthesia for, 1547–1548
  candidate for
    epididymis of, 1547
    laboratory testing in, 1547
    operative scars in, 1547
    sperm granuloma in, 1547
    testis of, 1547
    vasal gap in, 1547
  complications of, postoperative, 1555–1556
  crossed, 1554, 1555f
    testicular transposition used with, 1554–
      1555, 1556f
  incision for
    inguinal, 1548
    scrotal, 1548, 1548f
  indications for, 1550, 1550t
  long-term follow-up evaluation of, 1556
  microsurgical multilayer microdot method for,
    1551–1553, 1552f–1555f
  multiple vasal obstructions and, 1550
  physical examination of candidate for, 1547
  postoperative management of, 1555
  preoperative evaluation for, 1547
  setup for, 1551, 1551f
  surgical approaches for, 1548
  varicocelectomy and, 1550–1551
  vasal fluid in, gross appearance of, and micro-
    scopic findings in, 1550, 1550t
  vasal gap and, 1547, 1548–1549, 1549f
  vasal preparation in, 1548f, 1548–1549, 1549f
  wound closure in, 1555
VATER association, 2250–2251
  and hydronephrosis, 1998
  and ureteropelvic junction obstruction, 1998
  and vesicoureteral reflux, 1998
  multisystem involvement in, 1814t
Vectors, definition of, 2626t
Vein(s)
  adrenal, 8–9, 14f, 18f–21f, 19
  bulbar, 1594, 1594f
  bulbourethral, 1594, 1594f
  cardinal, 2044–2045, 2045f
  cavernosal, 74, 74f, 1594, 1594f
  circumflex, 74, 74f, 1594, 1594f
  cremasteric, 77, 77f
  crural, 1594, 1594f

Vein(s) *(Continued)*
  dorsal, of penis, 49, 51, 53f, 74, 74f, 1594,
    1594f
  emissary, 74, 74f, 1594, 1594f
  gonadal, 8, 14f
  hepatic, 9, 14f
  iliac, 7, 14f
    external, 1594, 1594f
    internal (hypogastric), 52, 54f, 1594, 1594f
  in urinary tract obstruction, 430–432
  lumbar, 7–8, 14f
  mesenteric, 8
  obturator, 52
  penile, 49, 51, 53f, 74, 74f
  portal, 8
  pudendal
    external, 77, 77f, 78f
    internal, 71, 1594, 1594f
  rectal, 71, 72f
  renal. *See* Renal vein(s).
  sacral, 7, 14f
  saphenous, 1594, 1594f
  splenic, 8
  subcardinal, 2044–2045, 2045f
  supracardinal, 2044–2045, 2045f
  testicular, 77–78, 77f, 1443f, 1444
  uterine, 67
  vasal, 77, 77f
  vesical, 52, 54f
Velo-cardio-facial syndrome, hypospadias with,
  2292t
Vena cava
  embryology of, 2044–2045, 2045f
  inferior, 7–9, 14f
    duplication of, with cloacal exstrophy, 2178
    renal cell carcinoma involvement of
      infrahepatic, radical nephrectomy with,
        3595–3596, 3597f–3599f
      suprahepatic, radical nephrectomy with,
        3596, 3598–3600, 3600f–3602f
      treatment of, 2712–2713, 2712f, 2713f
    preureteral, 2044–2045
      anatomy of, 2044, 2045f
      diagnosis of, 2045–2046
      embryology of, 2044–2045, 2045f
      incidence of, 2045
      sex distribution of, 2045
      type I, 2044
      type II, 2044
    right
      bilateral, 2045
      double, 2045, 2046f
      left-sided, 2045
Venography
  intraoperative, for varicocele occlusion, 1571t,
    1576–1577
  of varicocele, 1480, 1494, 1495f
Venous flow, pneumoperitoneum and, 3474
Ventricular septal defect, in prune-belly
  syndrome, 2122
Ventriculoperitoneal shunts, pneumoperitoneum
  effects on, in children, 2578
Verapamil
  effect of, on ureteral function, 403
  for Peyronie's disease, intralesional therapy
    with, 1700
  uropharmacology of, 858t, 865–866
Verrucous carcinoma, of male genitalia, 723,
  734f, 2949–2950
Vertebral anomalies, in cloacal exstrophy patient, 2181
Very-low-birth-weight infants, urolithiasis in,
  3290

Vesical artery, inferior, 65, 65f
Vesical calculi, 3286–3287, 3287f
Vesical ileal pouch, 3852
Vesical pain, in patient history, 85
Vesical vein, 52, 54f
Vesicoamniotic shunting, in utero
  outcomes with, 1795, 1795f
  placement of, 1794, 1795f
Vesicocystourethrography, in urinary schistosomiasis, 770
Vesicostomy
  Blockson technique for, 2220, 2221f–2222f
  continent, 2550–2551, 2551f
    results with, 2551
    technique for, 2550–2551, 2552f
  for posterior urethral valves, 2220, 2221f–
    2222f
  ileal, in conduit urinary diversion, 3775
  in prune-belly syndrome, 2126
Vesicoumbilical fistula, 2190, 2191f
Vesicoureteral reflux
  after antireflux surgery, 2090–2091
  after renal transplantation, 370
  anatomic considerations in, 2056, 2057f
  and megacystis-megaureter association, 2075
  and pregnancy, 2076
  and renal growth, 2071–2072, 2072f
  and risk of urinary tract infection in preg-
    nancy, 1862–1863
  and somatic growth, 2073
  antibiotic therapy for, and reflux nephropathy,
    2070–2071
  associated anomalies and conditions with,
    2073–2076
  bladder diverticula and, 2073–2074, 2075f
  calyceal appearance in, and classification,
    2060–2061
  classification of, 2060f, 2060t, 2060–2061
  clinical correlates of, 2056
  clinical presentation of, 2061–2062
  complete primary exstrophy repair and, 2200,
    2205
  demographics of, 2054–2056
  detrusor leak point pressure and, 1041
  diagnosis of, 2056, 2061–2067
    difficulties in, 2064
  endoscopic treatment of, 2092f, 2092–2094
    anatomic integrity in, 2092
    autologous injectable materials for, 2093–
      2094
    material safety in, 2092
    nonautologous materials for, 2092–2093
    technique for, 2092
  etiology of, 2056–2060
  fetal, 2054–2055
    postnatal evaluation and management of,
      1797–1799
  functional correlates in, 2056–2057
  genetics of, 2055–2056
  grading of, 2060–2061, 2061f, 2077
  historical perspective on, 2054
  imperforate anus and, 2075
  in CHARGE association, 2075
  in children, 2060
    and risk of urinary tract infection, 1862
    associated with dysfunctional elimination
      syndromes and urinary tract infection,
      2271–2272
    clinical correlates of, 2060
    incidence of, 2054–2055, 2055t
    pathogenesis of, 2060
    radiologic examination in, 1828
    voiding cystourethrogram in, 1828

P/N 9997618807

90090

9 789997 618801